19th
EDITION

Handbook of Nonprescription Drugs

An Interactive Approach to Self-Care

19th
EDITION

Handbook of Nonprescription Drugs

An Interactive Approach to Self-Care

EDITOR-IN-CHIEF
Daniel L. Krinsky, MS, RPh
Associate Professor, Department of Pharmacy Practice, Northeast Ohio Medical University, Rootstown, Ohio; Manager, Medication Therapy Management (MTM) Services, Department of Pharmacy, Giant Eagle, Ravenna, Ohio

ASSOCIATE EDITORS
Stefanie P. Ferreri, PharmD, CDE, FAPhA
Clinical Professor, UNC Eshelman School of Pharmacy, The University of North Carolina at Chapel Hill

Brian Hemstreet, PharmD, FCCP, BCPS,
Assistant Dean for Student Affairs and Professor, Regis University School of Pharmacy, Denver, Colorado

Anne L. Hume, PharmD, FCCP, BCPS
Professor of Pharmacy, Department of Pharmacy Practice, University of Rhode Island College of Pharmacy, Kingston; Adjunct Professor of Family Medicine, Brown University/Memorial Hospital of Rhode Island, Providence

Gail D. Newton, PhD, RPh
Associate Professor, Department of Pharmacy Practice, Purdue University College of Pharmacy, West Lafayette, Indiana

Carol J. Rollins, MS, RD, PharmD, BCNSP
Clinical Professor, Department of Pharmacy Practice and Science, The University of Arizona College of Pharmacy, Tucson

Karen J. Tietze, PharmD
Professor of Clinical Pharmacy, Department of Pharmacy Practice and Pharmacy Administration, Philadelphia College of Pharmacy, University of the Sciences, Philadelphia, Pennsylvania

APhA
PUBLICATIONS
Washington, DC

MANAGING EDITOR
Linda L. Young

EDITORIAL SERVICES
Mary Coe, Elizabeth Gailbraith, Terese Platten, Potomac Indexing, Linda L. Young

COMPOSITION SERVICES
Circle Graphics

COVER DESIGNER
Scott Nietzke, APhA Creative Services

ANATOMIC DRAWINGS
Aaron Hilmers, Gray Matter Studio, Walter Hilmers, Jr.

APhA was founded in 1852 as the American Pharmaceutical Association.

Published by the American Pharmacists Association
2215 Constitution Avenue, NW,
Washington, DC 20037-2985
www.pharmacist.com www.pharmacylibrary.com

To comment on this book via e-mail, send your message to the publisher at aphabooks@aphanet.org.

Library of Congress Cataloging-in-Publication Data
Main entry under the title: Handbook of Nonprescription Drugs
ISSN 0889-7816
ISBN-978-1-58212-265-6

CONTENTS

Note: Numbers in parentheses denote each editor's chapter(s) in shared sections.

section III REPRODUCTIVE AND GENITAL DISORDERS
Editor: Anne L. Hume

section IV RESPIRATORY DISORDERS
Editor: Karen J. Tietze

section V GASTROINTESTINAL DISORDERS
Editors: Daniel L. Krinsky (13–17) and Brian Hemstreet (18–22)

section VI NUTRITION AND NUTRITIONAL SUPPLEMENTATION

Editor: Carol J. Rollins

section VII OPHTHALMIC, OTIC, AND ORAL DISORDERS

Editors: Gail D. Newton (28, 29) and Karen J. Tietze (30–32)

section VIII DERMATOLOGIC DISORDERS

Editors: Stefanie P. Ferreri (33–36, 42–45) and Gail D. Newton (37–41)

section IX OTHER MEDICAL DISORDERS

Editors: Anne L. Hume (46) and Daniel L. Krinsky (47)

section X HOME MEDICAL EQUIPMENT

Editor: Gail D. Newton

section XI COMPLEMENTARY THERAPIES

Editor: Anne L. Hume

FOREWORD

Publication of the nineteenth edition of the American Pharmacists Association's (APhA) *Handbook of Nonprescription Drugs: An Interactive Approach to Self-Care* continues a tradition of providing comprehensive content to pharmacists and other health care providers so they can assist patients with the self-care process.

The United States is the world's largest market for nonprescription products, with annual retail sales of approximately $40 billion; these expenditures comprise 60% of the total pharmaceutical units or number of packages sold (source: Consumer Healthcare Products Association's OTC 101 Seminar, October 2015). The anticipated increase in the number of prescription medications that will be reclassified as nonprescription will provide new treatment options but will also further confound the patient's dilemma in selecting appropriate self-treatment.

At state and federal levels, legislation to reduce the environmental impact of nonprescription products banned the use of plastic microbeads in toothpastes and lotions (source: https://www.fda.gov/cosmetics/guidanceregulation/lawsregulations/ucm531849.htm), and approved mandatory drug take-back programs (source: https://www.deadiversion.usdoj.gov/drug_disposal/takeback/). At the state level, the role of pharmacists has been expanded in some states with the creation of a de facto third class of drugs. Specifically, some states grant pharmacists "prescribing" authority for oral contraceptives and naloxone. This intermediate, or third, class of drugs is available without a prescription, but a pharmacist is required to be involved with the sale. In 2012, FDA announced an initiative, *Nonprescription Drug Safe Use Regulatory Expansion* (NSURE), which would expand the conditions under which prescription medicines may be dispensed without a prescription (source: https://www.fda.gov/downloads/ForHealthProfessionals/UCM330650.pdf). As of October 1, 2017, this initiative was still in the discussion phase, and no plans for moving forward had been released. Pharmacists are also charged with overseeing the dispensing of medications classified as "restricted access," namely, pseudoephedrine and dextromethorphan. These two medications have been used to manufacture an illicit drug, methamphetamine, and to elicit a high, respectively.

The 2012 National Health Interview Study reported that Americans are also using natural products (also known as *dietary supplements*), other than vitamins and minerals, for self-treatment: 17.7% of U.S. citizens older than 18 years of age and 4.9% of children between the ages of 4 and 17 years (source: https://www.cdc.gov/nchs/nhis/index.htm). The use of complementary and integrative medicine therapies, dietary supplements, nondrug measures, diagnostic tests, and medical devices is also integral to self-care. However, there is limited clinical evidence as to their safety and effectiveness, and the potential for serious adverse events when these products are combined with prescription or nonprescription medications demands that health care providers be knowledgeable about alternatives to traditional medications and be able to provide therapeutic information and guidance to the consumer. Unlike nonprescription medications, no federal regulatory agency evaluates the safety and effectiveness of CAM therapies.

Numerous other factors have contributed to the growing self-care movement in the United States, including an increase in direct-to-consumer advertising of prescription and nonprescription medications. Information obtained from television commercials, newspaper and magazine advertisements, the Internet, and health-related articles serves to empower consumers to make decisions about their health care. However, individuals who wish to self-treat minor health disorders are faced with a staggering number of single-entity and combination nonprescription products, and they may not have adequate information to determine whether their medical disorder is amenable to self-treatment and whether the self-selected treatment is appropriate for the disorder.

All health care providers should be able to assist individuals in managing their self-care. However, because of their accessibility and expertise with respect to nonprescription and prescription medications, pharmacists are in a unique position to fulfill the self-care needs of most individuals with minor health ailments. Thus, providing a self-care curriculum for pharmacy students with learning outcomes that ensure appropriate knowledge and skills is now more important than ever. The importance of this objective is reflected in the Accreditation Council for Pharmacy Education's (ACPE) Standards 2016 (source: https://www.acpe-accredit.org/pdf/Standards2016FINAL.pdf) and the Competency Statements of the North American Pharmacist Licensure Examination® (NAPLEX®) taken by all United States pharmacy graduates prior to licensure (source: https://nabp.pharmacy/wp-content/uploads/2017/09/NAPLEX-MPJE-Bulletin-August-2017.pdf).

The information in this edition is also available online through the subscription-based PharmacyLibrary portal (www.pharmacylibrary.com). Here you will find the complete *Handbook* content along with many other complementary resources. Through PharmacyLibrary we are also publishing additional case studies to reinforce key concepts discussed in the chapters.

The nineteenth edition of the APhA *Handbook of Nonprescription Drugs: An Interactive Approach to Self-Care* is an excellent and up-to-date resource for all health care educators, students, and providers engaged in self-care.

Thomas E. Menighan, BSPharm, MBA, ScD (Hon)
Executive Vice President & CEO
American Pharmacists Association

PREFACE

The newly revised and updated nineteenth edition of the *Handbook of Nonprescription Drugs: An Interactive Approach to Self-Care* is a comprehensive and authoritative textbook on self-care and nonprescription medications. The major goals for this edition were to

- enhance the content in all chapters from the previous edition with up-to-date information beneficial to all health care providers and students
- update the universal objectives to complement the content in the chapters focused on medical disorders
- add a chapter that focused on pre- and probiotics, because their popularity and science describing their use have grown considerably since the last edition

This edition remains true to the spirit of previous editions, namely to assist health care providers and students in developing knowledge and problem-solving skills needed to

- assess a patient's health status, medical problems, and current practice of self-treatment, including nonprescription and prescription medications, dietary supplements, and other self-care measures
- determine whether self-care and/or self-testing and monitoring are necessary and/or appropriate
- if appropriate, recommend safe and effective self-care measures, taking into account the patient's treatment preferences

Written and reviewed by experts in practice and academia, this edition of the *Handbook* continues to serve as an authoritative source for students and health care providers who guide and care for individuals undertaking self-treatment.

Major Changes in the New Edition

- A rewrite of Chapter 1, "Self-Care and Nonprescription Pharmacotherapy," with a focus on some of the more contemporary issues affecting self-care, the self-care consumer, nonprescription products, the role of health care reform, changes in pharmacy practice as they relate to self-care, and health care in general.
- A rewrite of Chapter 2, "Patient Assessment and Consultation," so that the content is more applicable and practical to the self-care/nonprescription product environment. Case studies that illustrate the use of a more abbreviated problem-solving model were added.
- Addition of a chapter that covers pre- and probiotics.
- Removal of the pregnancy risk categories for all drugs and natural products and, subsequently, the removal of the two appendices that focused on pregnancy risk information.
- Use of standardized, consistent terminology for issues that are discussed in multiple chapters.
- Availability of an online version of the book that will reside on APhA's digital platform PharmacyLibrary (www.pharmacylibrary.com) and allow updating and/or revision of chapters, as needed.
- Incorporation of vaccine information into certain chapters where the content is synergistic.
- For the print and online versions of the book, provision of two new comprehensive patient cases per chapter that are based on the revised eighteenth edition case format.
- For only the online version of the book, provision of additional cases based on the abbreviated case format that was introduced in the seventeenth edition.
- Removal of Chapter 45, "Self-care Components of Selected Chronic Diseases," because a majority of the content was not applicable to self-care.

Removal of Pregnancy Risk Categories

Removal of pregnancy risk categories was based on regulatory action of the Food and Drug Administration (FDA). In 2015 FDA implemented the Pregnancy and Lactation Labeling Rule (PLLR), which replaces the former pregnancy risk letter categories (A, B, C, D, X) for prescription drugs with more descriptive content in the following fields:

- Pregnancy: now includes labor and delivery
- Lactation
- Females and males of reproductive potential

Although this new categorization provides clinicians with more detail for decision making, clinicians still need to apply this information on a case-by-case basis. The PLLR will be implemented in phases, with the final phase to be completed by June 29, 2018.However, this rule is not applicable to self-care and nonprescription products. Readers can find detailed information about the rule at the following websites:

- https://www.fda.gov/drugs/developmentapprovalprocess/developmentresources/labeling/ucm093307.htm

- https://www.federalregister.gov/documents/2014/12/04/2014-28241/content-and-format-of-labeling-for-human-prescription-drug-and-biological-products-requirements-for

Previous editions of the *Handbook* have included pregnancy risk letter designations, where available, and oftentimes this information was based on the designation for the prescription version of the medication. With the changes that have taken place and the lack of support for letter designations to identify pregnancy risk, the editors decided to remove any reference to a pregnancy risk category within the chapters and to remove both appendices. Where this information appeared previously, we now include general language that supports the reader in determining, based on available literature, what is best for their particular patient in each situation. The following is the standard language in all chapters that mention medication or product use in pregnancy:

- See the Preface for a detailed explanation of the pregnancy data.
- Use in pregnancy should be limited to clinical situations in which the potential benefit justifies potential risk to the fetus.

Where a pregnancy issue exists for a nonprescription product, the Drug Facts Label states that the consumer should ask a health care professional before using the product if she is pregnant or breastfeeding. FDA is aware of the limitations of the Drug Facts Label for communicating complex issues such as pregnancy labeling. They attempt to ensure nonprescription labeling is as consistent as possible with the prescription drug labels when a drug is available in both forms. However, the challenge with nonprescription products is to provide information that consumers can understand but is detailed enough to address any concerns. FDA is aware of the inconsistencies this situation has created and, at the time of this writing, was discussing options to enhance information for use of these products during pregnancy.

Use of Consistent Terminology Among Chapters

Another major focus area of the nineteenth edition was ensuring standardized, consistent terminology for issues that are discussed in multiple chapters. Two examples that have significant reach in this edition of the *Handbook* are Reye's syndrome and measurement of liquid medication doses. The manner in which each has been addressed is described here.

Reye's Syndrome Definition

The following information is included in Chapter 5, "Headache" and is the standard; all other chapters that discuss this issue cross-reference Chapter 5.

> Reye's syndrome: Children and teenagers who have or are recovering from chicken pox or flu-like symptoms should not use this product. When using this product, if changes in behavior with nausea and vomiting occur, consult a doctor because these symptoms could be an early sign of Reye's syndrome, a rare but serious illness.

Measurement of Liquid Medications

The following information on measurement of liquid medications is now included in Chapter 11, "Disorders Related to Colds and Allergy," and is the standard; all other chapters that discuss this issue cross-reference Chapter 11.

To address the issue of inaccurate dosing, FDA released guidelines in May 2011 for liquid nonprescription drug products that include any type of dispensing device (dropper, cup, syringe, spoon). (See the full document at http://www.fda.gov/downloads/Drugs/GuidanceComplianceRegulatoryInformation/Guidances/UCM188992.pdf.) Products include liquid analgesics, liquid cough and cold products, and lactase replacement drops. The key points of the guidelines are as follows:

- A dosing device should be included with all oral liquid nonprescription products.
- The device should be calibrated to the dose recommended in the product directions.
- The device should be used only with the product in which it is packaged.
- The markings need to remain visible even when the liquid is in the device.

Objectives of Disorder Chapters

Self-care opportunities exist for many individuals with myriad health disorders. The content presented in this text that focuses on disorders lends itself to the objectives listed below. The editors encourage you to review and utilize these objectives to help you gain the greatest benefit from the information presented in the disorder-related chapters. For each patient complaint

- identify its most likely underlying cause(s)
- identify common signs and symptoms
- determine whether the complaint is amenable to self-care, the patient requires referral, or nothing needs to be done
- identify the FDA-approved monograph active ingredients in a given nonprescription drug category
- determine common side effects for a given category of nonprescription drugs
- determine contraindications to the use of a given category of nonprescription drugs or devices
- distinguish indications and limitations for use of nonprescription drugs or devices in a given category
- explain nondrug measures commonly used in treatment or prevention
- develop an appropriate plan for a given patient who seeks self-care advice
- formulate a list of key counseling points to educate a patient on the appropriate use of nonprescription drugs, nondrug measures, or a device

Highlights of New Features and Revisions

Considerable time and effort have been invested in improving this edition. We are hopeful that the following changes improve the quality and usability of the book, as well as provide increased clarity and convenience.

- Chapter 1, "Self-Care and Nonprescription Pharmacotherapy"
  - New authors, new approach to introducing self-care to the reader
  - Focus on today's health care and self-care consumer
  - Role of health care reform in self-care
  - Role of today's pharmacist and approach to patient care in self-care

  - How self-care fits with the traditional *medication therapy management* model
  - Value of self-care
  - Importance of consumer education
  - Author's vision of the future of self-care
- Chapter 2, "Pharmacists' Patient Care Process in Self-care"
  - Description of the Pharmacists Patient Care Process (PPCP)
  - Description of how more traditional self-care patient assessment processes, such as QuEST/SCHOLAR, relate to PPCP
  - Addition of new case studies to illustrate application of these assessment processes
  - Overview of patient-centered self-care
  - Discussion of special populations and PPCP in self-care
  - A rewrite of Chapter 2 was completed to make the content even more applicable to and practical for the self-care/nonprescription product environment, and to describe the relationship between PPCP and self-care patient assessment processes. As mentioned in the previous edition, part of our responsibility as educators is to expose our students to multiple options for assessing patients in self-care. Although the traditional approach in the *Handbook* was to focus solely on the very complex process, we realized other approaches, such as those that better fit situations when health care providers have more experience and/or limited time to interact with a patient, are important to discuss. One of these abbreviated processes, QuEST/SCHOLAR-MAC, is again used as the basis for the electronic cases written to enhance the application of content in the disorder-related chapters. These supplemental cases are available on APhA's digital subscription product PharmacyLibrary at www.pharmacylibrary.com. In addition, two new comprehensive patient cases are included in each chapter.
- Chapter 3, "Exploring Cultural Aspects of Self-care"
  - Additional emphasis on definitions of key terms
  - Updated demographics to illustrate diversity
  - Discussion of how lack of awareness of culture issues and health disparities among health care providers can contribute to disparities
  - Expanded focus on all minorities who may be affected, including the lesbian, gay, bisexual, and transgender community
  - Detailed information on models for communicating with patients across cultures
  - Comprehensive list of resources for developing a more culturally competent healthcare environment
- Chapter 4, "Legal and Regulatory Issues in Self-care Pharmacy Practice"
  - Description of the history of self-care and list of key FDA guidance documents related to nonprescription products
  - Updated list of Rx-to-OTC switches
  - Factors to address regarding the safe use of nonprescription products
  - Discussion of a third class of drugs and what is happening in the United States versus other countries
  - Cosmetics that could also be considered drugs
  - Point-of-care diagnostic devices and the Clinical Laboratory Improvement Amendments program
  - Liability and nonprescription products
- Chapter 5, "Headache"
  - Updated medication dosing table
  - Detailed information regarding FDA boxed warnings for acetaminophen and hepatotoxicity and severe skin reactions
  - New information about gastrointestinal and cardiovascular risks with nonsteroidal anti-inflammatory drugs
- Chapter 7, "Musculoskeletal Injuries and Disorders"
  - Addition of information regarding the use of topical anesthetics
- Chapter 9, "Disorders Related to Menstruation"
  - Expanded discussion of premenstrual disorders (premenstrual syndrome, premenstrual dysphoric disorder)
- Chapter 10, "Prevention of Pregnancy and Sexually Transmitted Infections"
  - Expanded discussion of human papillomavirus
- Chapter 11, "Disorders Related to Cold and Allergy"
  - Enhanced content in the table Clinically Important Drug–Drug Interactions With Cold and Allergy Products that also includes a management/prevention section
  - Addition of intranasal corticosteroids to the allergic rhinitis section
  - Addition of a new table, Nonprescription Intranasal Corticosteroid Products and Dosage Guidelines
- Chapter 12, "Cough"
  - Addition of a new table, Clinically Important Drug–Drug Interactions With Nonprescription Antitussive Agents
  - Updates regarding the use of codeine in children
- Chapter 13, "Heartburn and Dyspepsia"
  - Addition of a new table, Clinically Important Drug–Drug Interactions With Nonprescription Heartburn and Dyspepsia Agents
- Chapter 16, "Diarrhea"
  - Addition of a new table, Clinically Important Drug–Drug Interactions With Nonprescription Antidiarrheal Agents
- Chapter 19, "Nausea and Vomiting"
  - Addition of a new table, Selected Nonprescription Antiemetic Products and Common Drug Interactions
- Chapter 20, "Prebiotics and Probiotics" (new chapter)
  - Definitions
  - Sources
  - Uses, doses, evidence, and potential risks
- Chapter 23, "Essential and Conditionally Essential Nutrients"
  - Updated information related to calcium and vitamin D
  - Addition of figures for iron, folic acid, and vitamin B_{12}
  - Most nutrients did not have major changes
- Chapter 24, "Functional and Meal Replacement Foods"
  - Removal of "Probiotics" section to new Chapter 20, "Prebiotics and Probiotics"
- Chapter 25, "Sports Nutrition and Performance-Enhancing Nutrients"
  - Discussion of new products and their role, if any, in recreational/nonprofessional sports
  - Addition of two new reviewers who specialize in sports nutrition, including one who works with a national sports team
- Chapter 26, "Infant Nutrition and Special Nutritional Needs of Children"
  - Updated information on available products
  - Updated information on which growth charts to use. Note: Specialized growth charts are no longer recommended by the AAP guidelines for children with Down syndrome.
- Chapter 27, "Overweight and Obesity"
  - Inclusion of most recent revalence data
  - Introduction of the concept of the gut microbiome potentially contributing to obesity
  - Discussion of carbohydrate-restriction versus fat-restriction for weight loss

- Chapter 29, "Otic Disorders"
  - Creation of an enhanced version of the table Selected Products for Use With Gas-Permeable Lenses
- Chapter 31, "Prevention of Hygiene-Related Oral Disorders"
  - Addition of description of ADA Seal of Acceptance
- Chapter 32, "Oral Pain and Discomfort"
  - Information about risks associated with homeopathic teething products
  - Addition of content related to treatment in special populations
- Chapter 33, "Otic Disorders"
  - Addition of content related to treatment in special populations
- Chapter 35, "Contact Dermatitis"
  - Addition of a new table, Usage Guidelines for Products That Remove Urushiol
  - Addition of a new table, Usage Guidelines for Burow's Solution
- Chapter 36, "Diaper Dermatitis and Prickly Heat"
  - Expansion of the table Selected Nonprescription Products for Diaper Dermatitis
- Chapter 37, "Insect Stings and Bites and Pediculosis"
  - Updated information regarding effectiveness of nonprescription pediculicides
- Chapter 38, "Acne"
  - Addition of information on a new antiacne product, adapalene gel 0.1% (Differin Gel)
- Chapter 39, "Prevention of Sun-Induced Skin Disorders"
  - Updated information on use of sunscreens in infants
- Chapter 40, "Skin Hyperpigmentation and Photoaging"
  - Inclusion of a table describing Fitzpatrick skin types as they relate to skin pigmentation
- Chapter 41, "Minor Burns, Sunburn, and Wounds"
  - Inclusion of an update on the role of antibacterial soaps in prevention of infection
- Chapter 43, "Warts"
  - Addition of information on treatment of warts in special populations
- Chapter 44, "Minor Foot Disorders"
  - Discussion of tired aching feet combined with exercise-induced foot injuries
- Chapter 45, "Hair Loss"
  - Addition of information on the management of hair loss in special populations
- Chapter 46, "Insomnia, Drowsiness, and Fatigue"
  - Addition of new drug interaction tables, Clinically Significant Drug Interactions With Diphenhydramine and Clinically Significant Drug Interactions With Caffeine
- Chapter 47, "Tobacco Cessation"
  - Provision of additional information about e-cigarettes
- Chapter 48, "Home Testing and Monitoring Devices"
  - Addition of a case focused on home testing for hepatitis C
- Chapter 51, "Natural Products"
  - Updated list of natural products
  - Revisions focused on enhancing content regarding key uses and issues for each product
  - Addition of a new section, "Weight-Loss Supplements"
  - Updated, detailed information about hepatic risks with kava
  - Information about kratom, an herb to avoid because of significant risks
  - Overview of piperine, an alkaloid found in black pepper that could affect certain medication pharmacodynamics/kinetics
- Chapter 52, "Common Complementary and Integrative Medicine Health Systems"
  - Focus change from complementary and alternative medicine (CAM) to complementary and integrative medicine (CIM)
- For all chapters that discuss disorders, development of new case studies in the comprehensive format

Chapter Features and Content

All chapters that discuss disorders in this edition include the following features and information:

- Up-to-date information on nonprescription medications, including indications, dosages, interactions, supportive evidence for efficacy and safety, medical disorders or symptoms amenable to self-treatment, prescription-to-nonprescription reclassifications, and nonprescription drug withdrawals from the market.
- Treatment algorithms that outline triage and treatment.
- Controversies in self-care therapeutics.
- Self-care treatment or prevention guidelines.
- Product tables with examples of specific nonprescription products.
- New nonprescription medications and dietary supplements, including nutrition-related dietary supplements, such as vitamins and minerals, which are discussed in the nutrition section of the book.

Most chapter features remain unchanged and are intended to promote an interactive approach to self-care. Students and health care providers can use these features to develop or improve problem-solving and critical thinking skills.

- Disorder-related chapters are grouped primarily according to body systems. These chapters begin with a discussion of the epidemiologic, etiologic, and pathophysiologic characteristics and the clinical manifestations of the disorder. These discussions are followed by a comprehensive discussion of self-care options. The inclusion of dietary supplements, as well as nonpharmacologic and preventive measures, completes the discussion of self-care options.
- Case studies, treatment algorithms, comparisons of self-treatments, patient education boxes, and product selection guidelines foster an interactive therapeutic approach to learning.
- Sections on the evaluation of patient outcomes reinforce follow-up of patients who are self-treating. This section defines the parameters for confirming successful self-treatment and those that indicate the need for medical referral.
- Chapters include tables that list interactions (drug–drug, drug–supplement, drug–nutrient), as well as dosage and administration guidelines.
- At the end of each chapter, authors provide a list of key points. These are intended to serve as a summary of critical information in the chapter and can be an excellent resource for educators.
- Authors provide comparisons of agents based on clinical studies of safety and efficacy, as well as product selection guidelines based on patient factors and preferences.
- Authors discuss the role of nonprescription therapies among the available treatment options for a specific disorder and describe other options in the event that nonprescription therapy fails or is not appropriate.

- The book's organization and content allow students and health care providers to quickly identify the information needed to make a treatment recommendation and to counsel patients.

Acknowledgments

We would like to acknowledge the hundreds of individuals who contributed to the new edition of this textbook. We are grateful to each of the authors and reviewers who contributed to this comprehensive and authoritative textbook. These individuals were selected from many practice settings and health professions throughout the country. Their scholarship and clinical experience reflect a broad perspective and interdisciplinary approach to patient care. The dedication of the authors and reviewers in ensuring that chapters were accurate, comprehensive, balanced, and relevant to practice and of the highest quality is deeply appreciated.

The editors of this edition also want to acknowledge the contributions of previous editors, authors, reviewers, and the many health care providers, students, residents, and others who have helped make the *Handbook* the premier resource for self-care content. We also want to thank the staff of the American Pharmacists Association, in particular Julian Graubart, for their ongoing support of our vision for the content and its incorporation into the *Handbook* and PharmacyLibrary.com.

We would like to convey a very special thanks to Linda Young, our managing editor. Ms. Young provided invaluable guidance and support to the editors and authors in all aspects related to the publication of this edition of the textbook. She contributed to the copyediting of chapters, and managed the design, editorial, and composition stages of the book. Without her experience and attention to detail, the improvements in this edition would not have been possible.

We are confident that the combined efforts of these individuals will ensure that the *Handbook of Nonprescription Drugs: An Interactive Approach to Self-care* continues to serve as the worldwide practice and teaching resource on self-care and nonprescription products.

STEFANIE P. FERRERI
BRIAN HEMSTREET
ANNE L. HUME
DANIEL L. KRINSKY
GAIL D. NEWTON
CAROL J. ROLLINS
KAREN J. TIETZE

CONTRIBUTORS

Authors

Note: Numbers in parentheses denote the chapter(s) authored or coauthored.

Donna M. Adkins, BS Pharm, PharmD, BCGP, FASCP (43)
Professor and Chair, Department of Pharmacy Practice and Administration, Wiliam Carey University School of Pharmacy–Tradition Campus, Biloxi, Mississippi

Nicole Paolini Albanese, PharmD, CDE, BCACP (32)
Clinical Associate Professor, Department of Pharmacy Practice, University at Buffalo School of Pharmacy and Pharmaceutical Sciences; PGY2 Ambulatory Care Residency Director, Buffalo Medical Group, P.C., Buffalo, New York

Katelyn Alexander, PharmD (36)
Assistant Professor of Pharmacy Practice, East Tennessee State University Gatton College of Pharmacy, Johnson City

Veronica T. Bandy, MS, PharmD, FCPhA, FCSHP (30)
Clinical Professor, Department of Pharmacy Practice, University of the Pacific Thomas J. Long School of Pharmacy and Health Sciences, Stockton, California

Kimberley W. Benner, PharmD, BCPS, FASHP, FPPAG (33)
Professor of Pharmacy Practice, Samford University McWhorter School of Pharmacy, Birmingham, Alabama; Clinical Pharmacy Specialist, Children's of Alabama, Birmingham

Daphne B. Bernard, PharmD, CACP (41)
Associate Professor, Howard University College of Pharmacy, Washington, DC

Tricia M. Berry, PharmD, BCPS (45)
Professor, Department of Pharmacy Practice, St. Louis College of Pharmacy, St. Louis, Missouri

Elizabeth W. Blake, PharmD, BCPS (37)
Director of Interprofessional Education and Clinical Associate Professor, Department of Clinical Pharmacy and Outcomes Sciences, University of South Carolina College of Pharmacy, Columbia; Clinical Pharmacy Specialist, Primary Care, Palmetto Health Richland, Columbia, South Carolina

Mary M. Bridgeman, PharmD, BCPS, BCGP (23)
Clinical Associate Professor, Rutgers, The State University of New Jersey Ernest Mario School of Pharmacy, Piscataway; Internal Medicine Clinical Pharmacist, Robert Wood Johnson University Hospital, New Brunswick, New Jersey

Geneva Clark Briggs, PharmD, BCPS (48)
President, Briggs and Associates, Richmond, Virginia

Sherrill Brown, DVM, PharmD, BCPS (27)
Associate Professor of Pharmacy Practice and Director of Drug Information Service, College of Health Professions and Biomedical Sciences, The University of Montana Skaggs School of Pharmacy, Missoula

Juliana Chan, PharmD, FCCP, BCACP (17)
Clinical Pharmacist, University of Illinois Medical Center at Chicago; Clinical Associate Professor, Department of Pharmacy Practice, College of Pharmacy, and Department of Medicine, Sections of Digestive Diseases & Nutrition and Section of Hepatology, University of Illinois at Chicago

Aleda M. H. Chen, PharmD, MS, PhD (29)
Assistant Dean and Associate Professor of Pharmacy Practice, Cedarville University School of Pharmacy, Cedarville, Ohio

M. Petrea Cober, PharmD, BCNSP (26)
Pharmacy Clinical Coordinator, Neonatal Intensive Care Unit, Akron Children's Hospital, Akron, Ohio; Associate Professor of Pharmacy Practice, Northeast Ohio Medical University College of Pharmacy, Rootstown, Ohio

Cynthia W. Coffey, PharmD, BCPS (44)
Pharmacist, Riverside Pavilion Pharmacy, Newport News, Virginia

Kimberly M. Crosby, PharmD, BCPS, BCGP, CDE, BC-ADM (39, 40)
Associate Professor, Department of Family Medicine–Tulsa, The University of Oklahoma School of Community Medicine

Barbara Insley Crouch, PharmD, MSPH (21)
Executive Director, Utah Poison Control Center, Salt Lake City; Professor (Clinical), Department of Pharmacotherapy, University of Utah College of Pharmacy, Salt Lake City

Patricia L. Darbishire, PharmD (35)
Director of Introductory Pharmacy Practice Experiences and Clinical Associate Professor, Department of Pharmacy Practice, Purdue University College of Pharmacy, West Lafayette, Indiana

Cathi Dennehy, PharmD (50)
Professor, Department of Clinical Pharmacy, University of California–San Francisco School of Pharmacy

Holly Divine, PharmD, BCACP, BCGP, CDE, FAPhA (2)
Clinical Associate Professor, Pharmacy Practice and Science, University of Kentucky College of Pharmacy, Lexington

Mark Donaldson, BSP, ACPR, PharmD, FASHP, FACHE (32)
Senior Executive Director, Pharmacy Advisory Solutions, Vizient Clinical Pharmacy, Irving, Texas

Shareen Y. El-Ibiary, PharmD, FCCP, BCPS (10)
Professor of Pharmacy Practice, Midwestern University, College of Pharmacy–Glendale, Glendale, Arizona

Patricia H. Fabel, PharmD, BCPS (37)
Assistant Professor, Department of Clinical Pharmacy and Outcomes Sciences, University of South Carolina College of Pharmacy, Columbia

Brett M. Feret, PharmD (6)
Clinical Professor, University of Rhode Island College of Pharmacy, Kingston

Richard G. Fiscella, PharmD, MPH (28)
Clinical Professor Emeritus, Department of Pharmacy Practice, and former Adjunctive Assistant Professor, Department of Ophthalmology, University of Illinois at Chicago College of Pharmacy

Karla T. Foster, PharmD, BCPS (38)
Pharmacist, Walgreens Company, Ridgeland, Mississipi

April Gardner, MSBS, PA-C (42)
Department of Emergency Medicine, The University of Toledo, Toledo, Ohio

Jeffery A. Goad, PharmD, MPH, FAPhA, FISTM (18)
Professor and Chair, Department of Pharmacy Practice, Chapman University School of Pharmacy, Harry and Diane Rinker Health Science Campus, Irvine, California

Jean-Venable "Kelly" R. Goode, PharmD, BCPS (15)
Director of Community Pharmacy Practice and Residency Program, and Professor, Department of Pharmacotherapy and Outcomes Science, Virginia Commonwealth University School of Pharmacy, Richmond

Anita N. Jacobson, PharmD (3)
Clinical Associate Professor of Pharmacy Practice, The University of Rhode Island College of Pharmacy, Kingston; Clinical Pharmacist, Eleanor Slater Hospital, Rhode Island Department of Behavioral Healthcare, Developmental Disabilities and Hospitals, Cranston

Michael K. Jensen, RPh, MS (28)
Clinical Specialist – Ophthalmic Pharmacy and Corporate Compliance Manager – Pharmacy, Intermountain Healthcare, Salt Lake City, Utah

Pramodini Kale-Pradhan, PharmD, FCCP (20)
Professor (Clinical), Department of Pharmacy Practice, Wayne State University Eugene Applebaum College of Pharmacy and Health Sciences, Detroit, Michigan; Clinical Pharmacy Specialist, Infectious Diseases, St. John Hospital and Medical Center, Detroit, Michigan

Cynthia K. Kirkwood, PharmD, BCPP (46)
Professor of Pharmacotherapy and Outcomes Science, and Executive Associate Dean for Academic Affairs, Virginia Commonwealth University School of Pharmacy, Richmond

Wendy Klein-Schwartz, PharmD, MPH (21)
Professor Emeritus, Department of Pharmacy Practice and Science, University of Maryland School of Pharmacy, Baltimore; Associate Professor, Department of Pharmacy Practice and Science, University of Maryland School of Pharmacy, Baltimore

Eunji Michelle Ko, PharmD (52)
Patient Safety Pharmacy Resident, Partners Healthcare, Boston, Massachussets

Barbara A. Kochanowski, PhD (1)
Senior Vice President, Regulatory & Scientific Affairs, Consumer Healthcare Products Association, Washington, DC

Virginia Lemay, PharmD, CDOE, CVDOE (6)
Clinical Associate Professor and PGY1 Community Residency Program Director, University of Rhode Island College of Pharmacy, Kingston; The University of Rhode Island/Rite Aid Community Pharmacist, MTM Specialist, Certified Immunizer, Diabetes Educator, Kingston, Rhode Island

Nicole M. Lodise, PharmD (8)
Professor of Pharmacy Practice–Women's Health/Tobacco Cessation, Albany College of Pharmacy and Health Sciences, Albany, New York; Clinical Pharmacy Specialist, Albany Medical Center, Albany, New York

Rupal Patel Mansukhani, PharmD (34)
Clinical Associate Professor, Department of Pharmacy Practice and Administration, Rutgers, The State University of New Jersey Ernest Mario School of Pharmacy, Piscataway; Clinical Pharmacist, Morristown Medical Center, Morristown, New Jersey

Beth A. Martin, RPh, BSPharm, MS, PhD (47)
Associate Professor (CHS), University of Wisconsin School of Pharmacy, Madison

Tera McIntosh, PharmD, BCACP (2)
Clinical Assistant Professor, Department of Pharmacy Practice and Science, University of Kentucky College of Pharmacy, Lexington

Cydney E. McQueen, PharmD, MSHP (51)
Clinical Associate Professor, Division of Pharmacy Practice and Administration, University of Missouri–Kansas City School of Pharmacy

Karleen Melody, PharmD (31)
Associate Professor of Clinical Pharmacy, University of the Sciences Philadelphia College of Pharmacy, Philadelphia, Pennsylvania

Sarah T. Melton, PharmD, BCPP, BCACP, BCGP, FASCP (46)
Professor of Pharmacy Practice, East Tennessee State University Bill Gatton College of Pharmacy, Johnson City

Sarah J. Miller, PharmD, BCNSP (27)
Professor of Clinical Pharmacy, Department of Pharmacy Practice, University of Montana Skaggs School of Pharmacy, Missoula

Edith Mirzaian, PharmD (18)
Assistant Professor of Clinical Pharmacy, Titus Family Department of Clinical Pharmacy, Pharmaceutical Economics and Policy, University of Southern California School of Pharmacy, Los Angeles

Cortney Mospan, PharmD (36)
Assistant Professor of Pharmacy, Department of Pharmacy Practice, Wingate University School of Pharmacy, Wingate, North Carolina

Mark Newnham, PharmD, BCPS, BCNSP (25)
Clinical Pharmacist, Lawnwood Regional Medical Center and Heart Institute, Fort Pierce, Florida

Julie L. Olenak, PharmD (7)
Assistant Dean of Student Affairs and Associate Professor of Pharmacy Practice, Wilkes University Nesbitt School of Pharmacy, Wilkes-Barre, Pennsylvania

Katherine S. O'Neal, PharmD, MBA, BCACP, CDE, BC-ADM, AE-C (39, 40)
Associate Professor, Department of Pharmacy Practice, The University of Oklahoma College of Pharmacy, Oklahoma City

Christine K. O'Neil, PharmD, BCPS, FCCP, BCGP (49)
Professor of Pharmacy Practice and Director, Curriculum Development, Duquesne University School of Pharmacy, Pittsburgh, Pennsylvania

Katherine Kelly Orr, PharmD (51)
Clinical Professor, Department of Pharmacy Practice, The University of Rhode Island College of Pharmacy, Kingston

Kimberly S. Plake, PhD, FAPhA (35)
Associate Professor, Department of Pharmacy Practice, Purdue University College of Pharmacy, West Lafayette, Indiana

Erin C. Raney, PharmD, BCPS (10)
Professor of Pharmacy Practice, Midwestern University College of Pharmacy–Glendale, Glendale, Arizona

Jennifer Robinson, PharmD (14)
Assistant Dean of Recruitment and Student Success, and Clinical Associate Professor, Washington State University College of Pharmacy, Spokane

Carol J. Rollins, MS, RD, PharmD, BCNSP (23, 24)
Clinical Professor, Department of Pharmacy Practice and Science, The University of Arizona College of Pharmacy, Tucson

Martha M. Rumore, PharmD, JD, MS, LLM, FAPhA (4)
Of Counsel, Sorell, Lenna & Schmidt, LLP, Hauppauge, New York

Kelly L. Scolaro, PharmD (11)
Associate Professor of Pharmacy Practice, Lake Erie College of Osteopathic Medicine (LECOM) School of Pharmacy–Bradenton Campus, Bradenton, Florida

Joan Lerner Selekof, BSN, RN, CWOCN (22)
Manager, WOCN Team, and Certified Wound Ostomy Continence Nurse, University of Maryland Medical Center, Baltimore, Maryland

Leslie A. Shimp, PharmD, MS (9)
Professor Emeritus of Pharmacy, Department of Clinical Pharmacy, The University of Michigan College of Pharmacy, Ann Arbor

Jeri J. Sias, PharmD, MPH (3)
Clinical Professor, Pharmacy Practice & Clinical Sciences, The University of Texas at El Paso School of Pharmacy

Jenelle Sobotka, BS, PharmD, FAPhA (1)
Professor, Department of Pharmacy Practice and Administrative Sciences, and Director of Online Certificate and Master's Programs in Pharmacy Leadership, University of Cincinnati James L. Winkle College of Pharmacy, Cincinnati, Ohio

Sneha Baxi Srivastava, PharmD, BCACP, CDE (44)
Associate Professor, Department of Pharmacy Practice, Rosalind Franklin University of Medicine and Science College of Pharmacy, North Chicago, Illinois

Andrew M. Straw, PharmD (29)
Assistant Professor of Pharmacy Practice, Cedarville University School of Pharmacy, Cedarville, Ohio

Karen J. Tietze, PharmD (12)
Professor of Clinical Pharmacy, Department of Pharmacy Practice and Pharmacy Administration, University of the Sciences Philadelphia College of Pharmacy, Philadelphia, Pennsylvania

Katherine Tromp, PharmD (5)
Associate Professor of Pharmacy Practice, Lake Erie College of Osteopathic Medicine (LECOM) School of Pharmacy–Bradenton Campus, Bradenton, Florida

Candy Tsourounis, PharmD (50)
Professor of Clinical Pharmacy, University of California–San Francisco School of Pharmacy

Catherine Ulbricht, PharmD, MBA [c] (52)
Director of Clinical and Academic Programs, Brigham and Women's Hospital Partners, Boston, Massachusetts; Senior Attending Pharmacist, Massachussetts General Hospital, Boston

Lucio Volino, PharmD (34)
Clinical Associate Professor, Rutgers, The State University of New Jersey Ernest Mario School of Pharmacy, Piscataway; Clinical Pharmacist, RWJBarnabas Health, Livingston, New Jersey

Paul C. Walker, PharmD, FASHP (16)
Director of Experiential Education and Community Engagement, and Clinical Professor, Department of Clinical Sciences, The University of Michigan College of Pharmacy, Ann Arbor; Manager, Pharmacy Patient Outcomes, Department of Pharmacy, The University of Michigan Health System, Ann Arbor

Natalie Walkup, MPAS, PA-C (42)
Assistant Professor, Department of Physician Assistant Studies, University of Toledo College of Medicine Graduate Programs, Toledo, Ohio

Kristin W. Weitzel, PharmD, CDE, FAPhA (15)
Associate Director, University of Florida Health Personalized Medicine Program, and Clinical Associate Professor, Department of Pharmacotherapy and Translational Research, University of Florida College of Pharmacy, Gainesville

Adam C. Welch, PharmD, MBA, BCACP, FAPhA (19)
Associate Dean for Assessment and Academic Affairs, Bill Gatton College of Pharmacy East Tennessee State University, Johnson City

Tara Whetsel, PharmD, BCACP, BC-ADM (13)
Clinical Associate Professor, Department of Clinical Pharmacy, West Virginia University School of Pharmacy, Morgantown

Sheila Wilhelm, PharmD, FCCP, BCPS (20)
Clinical Associate Professor, Department of Pharmacy Practice, Wayne State University Eugene Applebaum College of Pharmacy and Health Sciences, Detroit, Michigan

Julie J. Wilkinson, PharmD, MS, BCPS (5)
Vice Dean for Accreditation, Assessment and Student Success, and Professor of Pharmacy Practice, Lake Erie College of Osteopathic Medicine (LECOM) School of Pharmacy–Bradenton Campus, Bradenton, Florida

Sharon Wilson, PharmD, BCPS (22)
Clinical Specialist–Surgery Critical Care, University of Maryland Medical Center, Baltimore; Assistant Professor, Department of Pharmacy Services, University of Maryland School of Pharmacy, Baltimore

Maria C. Wopat, PharmD (47)
Clinical Pharmacy Specialist and Residency Program Director, William S. Middleton Memorial Veterans Hospital, Madison, Wisconsin

Ann Zweber, BS Pharm (13)
Senior Instructor II, Department of Pharmacy Practice, Oregon State University College of Pharmacy, Corvallis

Reviewers

Note: Numbers in parentheses denote the chapter(s) reviewed.

W. René Acosta, RPh, MS (12)
Associate Dean for Academic Affairs and Clinical Professor, Abbott Endowed Fellow in Pharmacy, Provost's Teaching Fellow, Health Outcomes and Pharmacy Practice Division, The University of Texas at Austin College of Pharmacy

Erin Adams, PharmD, BCACP (42)
Associate Professor of Pharmacy Practice, Shenandoah University Bernard J. Dunn School of Pharmacy—Fairfax Campus, Fairfax, Virginia

Katelyn Alexander, PharmD (39, 41)
Assistant Professor, East Tennessee State University Bill Gatton College of Pharmacy, Johnson City

Karen M.S. Bastianelli, PharmD, BCACP (33)
Director, Pharmaceutical Care Learning Center, and Associate Professor, Department of Pharmacy Practice and Pharmaceutical Sciences, University of Minnesota College of Pharmacy, Duluth

Jessica Bates, PharmD, BCPS (42)
Clinical Coordinator, Pharmacy Skills Lab, The University of Kansas School of Pharmacy, Lawrence, Kansas

Forrest Batz, PharmD (51)
Consultant, Natural Medicines Information & Education, Keaau, Hawaii

Renee Anne Bellanger, PharmD, BCNSP (50)
Professor, Department of Pharmacy Practice, University of the Incarnate Word Joan and Rita Feik School of Pharmacy, San Antonio, Texas; Pharmacy Faculty, Children's Hospital of San Antonio, San Antonio, Texas

Teresa J. Bigler, DHEd, PA-C, DFAAPA (30)
Assistant Professor and Program Director, Physician Assistant Department, School of Allied Health Professions, Louisiana State University Health Sciences Center, Shreveport

Elizabeth W. Blake, PharmD, BCPS (36, 39)
Director, Interprofessional Education, and Clinical Associate Professor, Department of Clinical Pharmacy and Outcomes Sciences, University of South Carolina College of Pharmacy, Columbia; Clinical Pharmacy Specialist, Primary Care, Palmetto Health Richland, Columbia, South Carolina

Sara Elizabeth Bliss, PharmD, BCPS (23, 26)
Surgery/Nutrition Support Pharmacist, Wake Forest University Baptist Medical Center, Winston-Salem, North Carolina

KarenBeth H. Bohan, PharmD, BCPS (44)
Professor, Department of Pharmacy Practice, Binghamton University School of Pharmacy and Pharmaceutical Sciences, Binghamton, New York

Heather S. Boon, BScPhm, PhD (52)
Professor and Dean, Leslie Dan Faculty of Pharmacy, University of Toronto, Toronto, Ontario, Canada

Alaina Borries, PharmD, BCACP, CDE (26)
Ambulatory Care Management Clinical Pharmacist at Carolinas HealthCare System, Monroe, North Carolina

Ashley Branham, PharmD, BCAP (35)
Adjunct Assistant Professor and Preceptor, Community Pharmacy Residency Program, UNC Eshelman School of Pharmacy, The University of North Carolina at Chapel Hill; Director of Clinical Services, Moose Professional Pharmacy, Concord, North Carolina

Mary M. Bridgeman, PharmD, BCPS, BCGP (25)
Clinical Associate Professor, Ernest Mario School of Pharmacy, Rutgers, The State University of New Jersey, Piscataway, New Jersey; Internal Medicine Clinical Pharmacist, Robert Wood Johnson University Hospital, New Brunswick, New Jersey

Kristy L. Brittain, PharmD, BCPS, CDE (4)
Associate Professor, Department of Clinical Pharmacy and Outcomes Sciences, Medical University of South Carolina College of Pharmacy, Charleston

Kimberly Broedel-Zaugg, RPh, MBA, PhD (1)
Professor and Chair, Pharmacy Practice, Administration, and Research, Marshall University School of Pharmacy, Huntington, West Virginia

Wayne Erwin Buff, BS, PharmD (1)
Senior Associate Dean and Clinical Associate Professor, Department of Clinical Pharmacy and Outcomes Sciences, University of South Carolina College of Pharmacy, Columbia

Ann Canales, PharmD, BCPS (6)
Clinical Pharmacist, Allergy Partners of North Texas, Dallas

Kimberly Carter, PharmD (31)
Assistant Professor of Pharmacy Practice, Jefferson College of Pharmacy, Thomas Jefferson University, Philadelphia, Pennsylvania

Mary Chavez, PharmD (52)
Interim Vice Dean, Professor and Chair of Pharmacy Practice, Texas A&M Health Science Center Irma Lerma Rangel College of Pharmacy, Kingsville

Peter A. Chyka, PharmD (21)
Professor, Department of Clinical Pharmacy and Translational Science, and Associate Dean, University of Tennessee Health Science Center College of Pharmacy, Knoxville Campus

Valerie B. Clinard, PharmD (43)
Director for Experiential Education and Associate Professor, Department of Clinical Pharmacy, University of California at San Francisco School of Pharmacy

Mary Petrea Cober, PharmD, BCNSP (6)
Pharmacy Clinical Coordinator, Neonatal Intensive Care Unit, Akron Children's Hospital, Akron, Ohio; Associate Professor of Pharmacy Practice, Northeast Ohio Medical University College of Pharmacy, Rootstown, Ohio

Janice C. Colwell, MS, RN, CWOCN, FAAN (22)
Department of General Surgery, University of Chicago Medical Center, Chicago, Illinois

Steven J. Crosby, BSP, RPh, MA, FASCP (45)
Assistant Dean of Student Engagement and Success, and Associate Professor of Pharmacy Practice, MCPHS University School of Pharmacy, Boston

Erin Dalton, PharmD (35)
Assistant Professor, Department of Pharmacy Practice, and Director, Community-Based Pharmacy Residency Program, South University School of Pharmacy, Savannah, Georgia

Richard H. Dang, PharmD, A Ph, BCACP (16)
Assistant Professor of Clinical Pharmacy, Director of Student Outreach for Community Health, Site Coordinator of PGY-1

Community-Based Pharmacy Residency Program, and Coordinator of APPE Community Pharmacy Professional Experience Programs, University of Southern California College of Pharmacy, Los Angeles, California

Altaf S. Darvesh, M Pharm, PhD (16)
Associate Professor, Pharmaceutical Sciences, College of Pharmacy, and Associate Professor, Psychiatry, College of Medicine, Northeast Ohio Medical University, Rootstown, Ohio

Mark Anthony Della Paolera, BS, RPh, PharmD, BCPS, BCACP (43)
Associate Professor, Pacific University College of Health Professions School of Pharmacy, Hillsboro, Oregon

Erin Dorval, PharmD (34)
Assistant Professor of Pharmacy Practice, Palm Beach Atlantic University, Lloyd L. Gregory School of Pharmacy, West Palm Beach, Florida

Kaelen C. Dunican, PharmD, RPh (43, 45)
Professor of Pharmacy Practice, Massachusetts College of Pharmacy and Health Sciences–Worcester/Manchester

Herbert L. DuPont, MD (16)
Adjunct Professor, Internal Medicine Service, St. Luke's Episcopal Hospital, Houston, Texas; Clinical Professor, Medicine–Infectious Disease, Baylor College of Medicine, Houston, Texas; Professor and Director, Center for Infectious Diseases, University of Texas Houston School of Public Health

Lana Dvorkin Camiel, PharmD (51)
Professor of Pharmacy Practice and Natural Products Division Coordinator, Center for Drug Information and Natural Products, MCPHS University School of Pharmacy, Boston

Margarita Echeverri, PhD (3)
Associate Professor, Division of Clinical and Administrative Sciences, Xavier University of Louisiana College of Pharmacy, New Orleans

Christine Eisenhower, PharmD, BCPS (46)
Clinical Assistant Professor, Department of Pharmacy Practice, University of Rhode Island College of Pharmacy, Kingston

Danielle C. Ezzo, PharmD, BCPS, AE-C (33)
Director, Interprofessional Education, and Clinical Associate Professor, Department of Clinical Health Professions, St. John's University College of Pharmacy and Health Sciences, Queens, New York; Clinical Coordinator of Ambulatory Care & Resident Preceptor of Ambulatory Care Rotation, Northwell Health, New Hyde Park, New York

Patricia H. Fabel, PharmD, BCPS (19)
Assistant Professor, Clinical Pharmacy and Outcomes Sciences Department, University of South Carolina College of Pharmacy, Columbia

Rebecca Falter, PharmD (37)
Associate Professor of Pharmacy Practice, Shenandoah University Bernard J. Dunn School of Pharmacy—Winchester Campus, Winchester, Virginia

Alicia Forinash, PharmD, FCCP, BCPS, BCACP (10)
Professor of Pharmacy Practice and PGY2 Ambulatory Care Residency Program Director, St. Louis College of Pharmacy, St. Louis, Missouri; Clinical Pharmacy Specialist, Maternal & Fetal Care Center, SSM Health at St. Mary's, Clayton/Richmond Heights, Missouri

Karla T. Foster, PharmD, BCPS (19)
Pharmacist, Walgreens Company, Ridgeland, Mississippi

Andrea R. Franks, PharmD, BCPS (17)
Associate Professor, Department of Clinical Pharmacy, University of Tennessee Health Science Center College of Pharmacy, Knoxville; Associate Professor, Department of Family Medicine, University of Tennessee Graduate School of Medicine, Knoxville

Randolph V. Fugit, PharmD, BCPS (13)
Internal Medicine/Infectious Disease Clinical Specialist, and Director, Antimicrobial Stewardship Program, Denver Veterans Affairs Medical Center, Denver, Colorado; Clinical Associate Professor, University of Colorado Skaggs School of Pharmacy and Pharmaceutical Sciences, Anschutz Medical Campus, Aurora

Lauren Garton, PharmD, BCACP (13)
Assistant Professor, Department of Pharmacy Practice, South University School of Pharmacy, Savannah, Georgia

Margaret Goldberg, RN, MSN, CWOCN (22)
Wound Ostomy and Continence Nursing Consultant, Delray Wound Treatment Center, Boca Raton, Florida; President, National Pressure Ulcer Advisory Panel, Washington, DC

Justin Gollon, RN, PharmD, BCPS, BCNSP (25)
Clinical Staff Pharmacist, The University of Arizona Medical Center, Tucson

William C. Gong, PharmD, FASHP, FCSHP (2)
Associate Professor of Clinical Pharmacy and Director, Residency and Fellowship Programs, University of Southern California School of Pharmacy, Los Angeles

Morgan Sayler Herring, PharmD, BCPS (44)
Clinical Assistant Professor, Department of Pharmacy Practice, University of Iowa College of Pharmacy, Des Moines; Clinical Pharmacist, Iowa Lutheran Hospital Family Medicine Residency Program, Family Medicine at East Des Moines–Unity Point Clinic

Karl M. Hess, PharmD, CTH, FCPhA (4, 18)
Vice Chair and Associate Professor of Clinical and Administrative Sciences, Keck Graduate Institute School of Pharmacy, Claremont, California

Michelle L. Hilaire, PharmD, FCCP, CDE, BCPS, BCACP (28)
Clinical Professor, University of Wyoming School of Pharmacy, Laramie; Clinical Pharmacist, Fort Collins Family Medicine Residency Program, Fort Collins, Colorado

Marcella Honkonen, PharmD, BCPS (27)
Assistant Professor, Department of Pharmacy Practice and Science, The University of Arizona College of Pharmacy, Tucson

Amanda Howard-Thompson, PharmD, BCPS (7, 18)
Associate Professor, Department of Clinical Pharmacy, College of Pharmacy, and Associate Professor, Department of Family Medicine, College of Medicine, University of Tennessee Health Science Center-Memphis Campus

Timothy R. Hudd, BS, PharmD, RPh, AE-C (30)
Associate Professor of Pharmacy Practice, MCPHS University School of Pharmacy, Boston; Clinical Pharmacist, Primary Care of the Andovers, North Andover, Massachusetts

Rebekah Jackowski, PharmD (2)
Assistant Professor of Pharmacy Practice, Midwestern University College of Pharmacy–Glendale, Glendale, Arizona

Courtney Izzo Jarvis, PharmD (9)
Associate Professor of Pharmacy Practice, Massachusetts College of Pharmacy and Health Sciences–Worcester/Manchester

Sarah A. Parnapy Jawaid, PharmD (11)
Associate Professor and Vice Chair, Department of Pharmacy Practice, Shenandoah University Bernard J. Dunn School of Pharmacy—Winchester Campus, Winchester, Virginia

Pramodini B. Kale-Pradhan, PharmD, FCCP (12)
Professor (Clinical), Department of Pharmacy Practice, Wayne State University Eugene Applebaum College of Pharmacy and Health Sciences, Detroit, Michigan; Clinical Specialist, Infectious Diseases, Department of Pharmacy Services, St. John Hospital and Medical Center, Detroit, Michigan

Sarah Kelling, PharmD, MPH, BCACP (2)
Clinical Assistant Professor of Pharmacy, Department of Clinical Pharmacy, University of Michigan College of Pharmacy, Ann Arbor, Michigan

Joshua Davis Kinsey, PharmD (45)
Clinical Assistant Professor of Pharmacy Practice and Director of Community Pharmacy Residency Program, Mercer University College of Pharmacy, Atlanta, Georgia

Erika Kleppinger, PharmD, BCPS (29)
Associate Clinical Professor, Department of Pharmacy Practice, Auburn University Harrison School of Pharmacy, Auburn, Alabama

Gregory M. Kwiatkowski, PharmD, BCPS (5)
Clinical Pharmacy Specialist–Emergency Medicine, Department of Pharmacy, Spectrum Health, Grand Rapids, Michigan

Karen W. Lee, PharmD, BCPS (11)
Regional Vice President of Clinical Services, Comprehensive Pharmacy Services, Roxbury, Massachussetts

Thomas L. Lenz, PharmD, MA, PAPHS (25)
Professor of Pharmacy Practice, Director of Pharmacy Distance Pathway, and Clinical Director of Creighton Cardiovascular and Diabetes Risk Reduction Program, Creighton University School of Phamacy and Health Professions, Omaha, Nebraska

Nicholas Leon, PharmD (30)
Associate Professor of Pharmacy Practice, Jefferson College of Pharmacy, Philadelphia, Pennsylvania

Heidi Luder, PharmD, MS, BCACP (33)
Medical Outcomes Specialist, Pfizer Pharmaceuticals, Columbus, Ohio

Janene Marie Madras, BS Pharm, PharmD, BCPS, BCACP (32)
Director of Student Services and Professor of Pharmacy Practice, Lake Erie College of Osteopathic Medicine (LECOM) School of Pharmacy—Erie Campus, Erie, Pennsylvania

Rupal Patel Mansukhani, PharmD (44)
Clinical Associate Professor, Department of Pharmacy Practice and Administration, Rutgers, The State University of New Jersey Ernest Mario School of Pharmacy, Piscataway; Clinical Pharmacist, Morristown Medical Center, Morristown, New Jersey

Michele L. Matthews, PharmD, CPE, BCACP, FASHP (7)
Associate Professor of Pharmacy Practice, MCPHS University School of Pharmacy, Boston; Advanced Practice Pharmacist–Pain Management, Brigham and Women's Hospital, Boston

Melissa Mattison, PharmD (35)
Clinical Assistant Professor of Pharmacy Practice, Community Patient Care Center, Western New England University College of Pharmacy, Springfield, Massachusetts

Jamie Lynn McConaha, PharmD, CTTS, BCACP, CDE (40)
Associate Professor of Pharmacy Practice, Department of Pharmacy Practice, Duquesne University School of Pharmacy, Pittsburgh, Pennsylvania

Marsha McFalls, PharmD, MSEd, RPh (41)
Assistant Professor of Pharmacy Practice and Dir ector of Academic Research Center for Pharmacy Practice, Department of Clinical, Social, and Administrative Sciences, Duquesne University School of Pharmacy, Pittsburgh, Pennsylvania

Bella H. Mehta, PharmD, FAPhA (51)
Professor of Clinical Pharmacy and Family Medicine, Department of Pharmacy Practice and Science, and Director, Continuing Professional Development, The Ohio State University College of Pharmacy, Columbus

Jill E. Michels, PharmD, DABAT (21)
Managing Director, Palmetto Poison Center, and Clinical Assistant Professor, Department of Clinical Pharmacy and Outcomes Sciences, University of South Carolina College of Pharmacy, Columbia

Amee D. Mistry, PharmD (34)
Associate Professor of Pharmacy Practice, MCPHS University School of Pharmacy, Boston

Wendy Mobley-Bukstein, PharmD, BCACP, CDE, CHWC (15)
Assistant Professor of Pharmacy Practice, Drake University College of Pharmacy, Des Moines, Iowa

Anna K. Morin, PharmD, RPh (46)
Dean and Professor, Department of Pharmacy Practice, Massachusetts College of Pharmacy and Health Sciences–Worcester

Cortney Mospan, PharmD, BCACP (13)
Assistant Professor of Pharmacy, Department of Pharmacy Practice, Wingate University School of Pharmacy, Wingate, North Carolina

Leigh Anne Nelson, PharmD, BCPP (46)
Associate Professor, Division of Pharmacy Practice & Administration, University of Missouri–Kansas City School of Pharmacy

Thom Kim Nguyen, PharmD, BCPS, CTTS (44)
Clinical Assistant Professor, Department of Pharmacy Practice and Administration, Rutgers, The State University of New Jersey Ernest Mario School of Pharmacy, Piscataway; Clinical Coordinator, Ambulatory Care, Hunterdon Medical Center, Flemington, NJ

Wesley A. Nuffer, PharmD, BCPS, CDE (27)
Assistant Director of Experiential Programs and Associate Professor, Department of Clinical Pharmacy, University of Colorado Skaggs School of Pharmacy and Pharmaceutical Sciences, Aurora

Monika Majer Nuffer, PharmD (50)
Academic and Experiential Program Coordinator, Distance Degrees and Programs, and Senior Instructor, Department of Clinical Pharmacy and Family Medicine, University of Colorado Skaggs School of Pharmacy and Pharmaceutical Sciences, Aurora; Clinical Pharmacist/Herbal Specialist, The Center for Integrative Medicine at the University of Colorado Hospital, Aurora

Mary Beth O'Connell, PharmD (3)
Professor, Pharmacy Practice Department, Wayne State University Eugene Applebaum College of Pharmacy and Health Sciences, Detroit, Michigan

Rachel R. Ogden, BS Pharm, PharmD, MS, BCGP (12)
Associate Professor of Pharmacy Practice, Associate Dean of Accelerated Pathway, and Director for the PGY2 Pharmacy Geriatric Residency Program, Lake Erie College of Osteopathic Medicine (LECOM) School of Pharmacy—Erie Campus, Erie, Pennsylvania; Clinical Pharmacist, LECOM Institute for Successful Aging, Erie, Pennsylvania

Phung C. On, PharmD, BCPS (7)
Assistant Professor of Pharmacy Practice, MCPHS University School of Pharmacy, Boston, Massachusetts; Clinical Pharmacy Specialist, Transitions of Care, Barbara McInnis House/Boston Medical Center

Katherine Kelly Orr, PharmD (4)
Clinicial Professor, Department of Pharmacy Practice, The University of Rhode Island College of Pharmacy, Kingston, Rhode Island

M. Lisa Pagnucco, BS Pharm, PharmD, BCACP (14)
Associate Professor, Physician Assistant Studies, Grand Valley State University, Cook DeVos Center for Health Sciences, Grand Rapids, Michigan

Krina H. Patel, PharmD, BCPP (42)
Clinical Assistant Professor, Department of Pharmacy Practice and Administration, Rutgers, The State University of New Jersey Ernest Mario School of Pharmacy–Busch Campus, Piscataway

Karen Steinmetz Pater, PharmD, CDE (5)
Associate Professor, Department of Pharmacy and Therapeutics, University of Pittsburgh School of Pharmacy, Pittsburgh, Pennsylvania

Matthew Pitlick, PharmD, BCPS (29)
Associate Professor of Pharmacy Practice, Division of Ambulatory Care Pharmacy, St. Louis College of Pharmacy, St. Louis, Missouri

Kimberly S. Plake, PhD (49)
Associate Professor, Department of Pharmacy Practice, Purdue University College of Pharmacy, West Lafayette, Indiana

Charles D. Ponte, BS, PharmD, FAADE, FAPhA, FASHP, FCCP, FNAP (38)
Professor of Clinical Pharmacy, School of Pharmacy, and Professor of Family Medicine, School of Medicine, West Virginia University Robert C. Byrd Health Sciences Center, Morgantown, West Virginia

Traci M. Poole, PharmD, BCACP, BCGP (15)
Associate Professor of Pharmacy Practice, Belmont University College of Pharmacy, Nashville, Tennessee

Cathy Ramey, PharmD, BCGP (33)
Assistant Professor of Pharmacy Practice, Butler University College of Pharmacy and Health Sciences, Indianapolis, Indiana

Celtina K. Reinert, PharmD (52)
Pharmacy Manager, Queen's Price Chopper Pharmacy, Overland Park, Kansas

Victoria M. Reinhartz, PharmD (17)
Assistant Professor of Pharmacy Practice, Lake Erie College of Osteopathic Medicine (LECOM) School of Pharmacy—Bradenton Campus, Bradenton, Florida

Lorraine M. Reiser, PhD, CRNP, FAANP (26, 27)
Associate Professor of Nursing, Clarion University, Clarion, Pennsylvania

Pamela Ringor, MBA, RPh (37, 39)
Pharmacy Manager, PayLess Pharmacy, Lafayette, Indiana

Ronald J. Ruggiero, PharmD (9)
Clinical Professor, Department of Clinical Pharmacy, School of Pharmacy, and Clinical Professor, Department of Obstetrics, Gynecology, and Reproductive Sciences, School of Medicine, The Medical Center at University of California, San Francisco

Marissa C. Salvo, PharmD, BCACP (8)
Associate Clinical Professor, Department of Pharmacy Practice, University of Connecticut School of Pharmacy, Storrs

G. Blair Sarbacker, PharmD, BCACP (1, 28)
Associate Professor of Pharmacy Practice, Presbyterian College School of Pharmacy, Clinton, South Carolina

Tara Schmitz, PharmD (44)
Owner, Tara's Thrifty White Pharmacy, Oakes, North Dakota

Stacey Schneider, PharmD (32)
Associate Professor of Pharmacy Practice, Northeast Ohio Medical University College of Pharmacy, Rootstown

Emmanuelle Schwartzman, PharmD, BCACP, CDE (38)
Director, Residency and Fellowship Training, and Associate Professor of Pharmacy Practice and Administration, Western University of Health Sciences College of Pharmacy, Pomona, California

Kelly L. Scolaro, PharmD (48)
Associate Professor of Pharmacy Practice, Lake Erie College of Osteopathic Medicine (LECOM) School of Pharmacy–Bradenton Campus, Bradenton, Florida

Leticia A. Shea, PharmD, BCACP (20)
Associate Professor of Pharmacy Practice, Regis University School of Pharmacy, Denver, Colorado

Kayce M. Shealy, PharmD, BCPS, BCACP, CDE (15)
Associate Professor of Pharmacy Practice, Presbyterian College School of Pharmacy, Clinton, South Carolina

Justin J. Sherman, PharmD, MCS (47)
Associate Professor of Pharmacy Practice, School of Pharmacy, and Associate Professor of Family Medicine, School of Medicine, University of Mississippi Medical Center Campus, Jackson

Kelly M. Shields, PharmD (50)
Associate Professor of Pharmacy Practice, Ohio Northern University Raabe College of Pharmacy, Ada

Debra Sibbald, BSc Phm, RPh, ACPR, MA (Adult Education), PhD (Curriculum, Teaching and Learning) (36)
Executive Director of Assessment Programs, Touchstone Institute, Toronto, Ontario, Canada; Senior Lecturer, University of Toronto, Leslie Dan Faculty of Pharmacy

Martha Sikes, MS, RPh, PA-C (31)
Adjunct Clinical Assistant Professor, Mercer University College of Health Professions, Atlanta, Georgia

Dorothy L. Smith, PharmD (2)
Founder and CEO, Consumer Health Information Corporation, McLean, Virginia

Jennifer D. Smith, PharmD (6)
Associate Professor, Department of Pharmacy Practice, Campbell University College of Pharmacy & Health Sciences, Buies Creek, North Carolina

Lisa S. Smith, PharmD, BCPS (20)
Assistant Dean of Faculty and Associate Professor of Pharmacy, Wingate University School of Pharmacy, Wingate, North Carolina

Susan Claire Smolinske, PharmD, DABAT, FAACT (21)
Director, New Mexico Poison and Drug Information Center, and Professor, Pharmacy Practice and Administrative Sciences, University of New Mexico, Albuquerque

Erin L. St. Onge, PharmD (46)
Assistant Dean/Campus Director and Clinical Associate Professor, Deapartment of Pharmacotherapy and Translational Research, University of Florida College of Pharmacy–Orlando Campus

Nora Stelter, PharmD, CHWC (1)
Associate Professor and P3 Introductory Pharmacy Practice Experiences Coordinator, Department of Pharmacy Practice, Drake University College Pharmacy and Health Sciences, Des Moines, Iowa

Rebecca H. Stone, PharmD, BCACP, BCPS (10)
Assistant Professor and Clinical Pharmacist, Department of Clinical and Administrative Pharmacy, University of Georgia, Athens

Sahar Swidan, PharmD (5)
Adjunt Clinical Associate Professor, Department of Clinical Sciences, The University of Michigan College of Pharmacy, Ann Arbor; CEO and President, Pharmacy Solutions, Ann Arbor, Michigan

Jeff G. Taylor, PhD (11)
Professor of Pharmacy, University of Saskatchewan College of Pharmacy and Nutrition, Saskatoon, Saskatchewan, Canada

Renee Ahrens Thomas, PharmD, MBA (17)
Adjunct Associate Professor of Pharmacy Practice, Shenandoah University Bernard J. Dunn School of Pharmacy–Fairfax Campus, Fairfax, Virginia

Dominick P. Trombetta, PharmD, BCPS, BCGP, FASCP (42)
Associate Professor of Pharmacy Practice, Wilkes University Nesbitt School of Pharmacy, Wilkes-Barre, Pennsylvania

Timothy R. Ulbrich, PharmD, RPh (47)
Associate Dean, Workforce Development and Practice Advancement, and Associate Professor of Pharmacy Practice, Northeast Ohio Medical University College of Pharmacy, Rootstown

Tanya Vadala, PharmD (34)
IPRO, Drug Safety Pharmacist, Albany, NY

Amber Verdell, PharmD, BCPS, BCNSP, CNSC (24)
Assistant Professor, Department of Pharmacy Practice, West Coast University School of Pharmacy, Los Angeles, California

Kathleen Vest, PharmD (9)
Professor of Pharmacy, Department of Pharmacy Practice, Midwestern University–Chicago College of Pharmacy, Chicago, Illinois

Kristin R. Villa, PharmD, MS (40, 48)
Graduate Teaching Assistant, Department of Pharmacy Practice, Purdue University College of Pharmacy, West Lafayette, Indiana

Lucio Volino, PharmD (42)
Clinical Associate Professor, Rutgers, The State University of New Jersey Ernest Mario School of Pharmacy, Piscataway; Clinical Pharmacist, RWJBarnabas Health, Livingston, New Jersey

Deepti Vyas, PharmD (3)
Associate Professor of Pharmacy Practice, University of the Pacific Thomas J. Long School of Pharmacy and Health Sciences, Stockton, California

Rashi Chandra Waghel, PharmD, BCACP, CPP (10)
Assistant Professor of Pharmacy, Wingate University School of Pharmacy, Wingate, North Carolina

Paul C. Walker, PharmD, FASHP (36)
Director of Experiential Education and Community Engagement, and Clinical Professor, Department of Clinical Sciences, The University of Michigan College of Pharmacy, Ann Arbor; Manager, Pharmacy Patient Outcomes, Department of Pharmacy, The University of Michigan Health System, Ann Arbor

Kristina E. Ward, BS, PharmD, BCPS (10)
Clinical Professor, Department of Pharmacy Practice, and Director of Drug Information Services, University of Rhode Island College of Pharmacy, Kingston

Miranda Wilhelm, PharmD (35, 36)
Clinical Associate Professor of Pharmacy Practice, Southern Illinois University–Edwardsville School of Pharmacy

Jennifer A. Wilson, PharmD, BCACP (45)
Coordinator of Wellness Clinic and Associate Professor of Pharmacy, Wingate University School of Pharmacy, Wingate, North Carolina

Supakit Wongwiwatthananukit, PharmD, PhD (47)
Professor of Pharmacy Practice, The Daniel K. Inouye College of Pharmacy, University of Hawai'i at Hilo

Tonja M. Woods, PharmD (8)
Associate Dean of Faculty and Clinical Affairs, and Clinical Associate Professor, University of Wyoming School of Pharmacy, Laramie; Clinical Pharmacist, Adult & Geriatric Medical Specialties, Laramie, Wyoming

John R. Yuen, PharmD, BCNP (28, 29)
Board Certified Nuclear Pharmacist, Nuclear Medicine Department, Los Angeles County and USC Medical Center, Los Angeles, California; Adjunct Assistant Professor of Pharmacy Practice, University of Southern California School of Pharmacy, Los Angeles

Kathy Zaiken, PharmD (38)
Professor of Pharmacy Practice, MCPHS University School of Pharmacy, Boston

Deborah Zeitlin, PharmD (31, 32)
Assistant Professor of Pharmacy Practice, Butler University College of Pharmacy and Health Sciences, Indianapolis, Indiana

Ann Zweber, BS Pharm (14)
Senior Instructor II, Department of Pharmacy Practice, Oregon State University College of Pharmacy, Corvallis

section

I

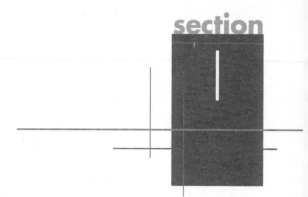

THE PRACTITIONER'S ROLE IN SELF-CARE

CHAPTER 1

SELF-CARE AND NONPRESCRIPTION PHARMACOTHERAPY

JENELLE SOBOTKA AND BARBARA A. KOCHANOWSKI

This chapter introduces the concept of self-care, characteristics of today's self-care consumer, and the growing importance of self-care in our health care system. *Self-care,* as defined by the World Self-Medication Industry, is "The action individuals take for themselves and their families to stay healthy and take care of minor and long term conditions, based on their knowledge and the information available, and working in collaboration with health and social care professionals where necessary."[1] The expanding role of the pharmacist—from medication dispenser to patient care provider—is discussed, with a focus on the pharmacist's role in self-care. An overview of the self-care marketplace, as well as the legislative and regulatory environment, is included, with a brief perspective on future changes expected for expansion of self-care and related health care technology. Because broad public education is a key factor in advancing the consumers' role in prevention of illness and management of their health, several public education programs are described to illustrate pharmacists' role in supporting this effort. The chapter concludes by reviewing the pharmacist's and student pharmacist's role in assisting patients with their self-care needs, while emphasizing the key elements of safety and efficacy in the management of self-care conditions.

The Expanding Definition of Self-Care

A simple definition of *self-care* is the independent act of preventing, diagnosing, and treating one's illnesses without seeking professional advice. However, self-care definitions can vary according to an individual's perspective: health care professionals' definition frequently differs from that of the general public. Health care providers (doctors, pharmacists, nurses, etc.) typically consider self-care to include the management of self-care conditions and the related self-care products available to patients without a prescription. Health care providers who wish to acknowledge the pharmacist's role would add that self-care should include pharmacist assistance in determining whether a patient's condition is appropriate for self-care. Pharmacists are accessible to patients when most self-care decisions are made and are valuable experts in this field. A pharmacist can help a patient improve a condition by recommending the best nonprescription product and/or recommending nonpharmacologic measures (e.g., diet, lifestyle changes). The latter may also be recommended to prevent further occurrences of a condition. In this context, the process becomes "pharmacist-assisted self-care." This textbook primarily covers the pharmacist's role in pharmacist-assisted self-care but also introduces roles that student pharmacists can assume as they develop their patient care skills for self-treatable conditions. Other health care providers (e.g., nurse practitioners, physician assistants) who may also be involved in advising patients on self-care will find significant applications of the concepts, content, and processes provided in this book.

Consumers' perspective and their definitions of self-care can vary from that of health care providers. In a recent survey, consumers were asked to describe what self-care involves.[2] Their responses went far beyond the use of nonprescription medications. The consumers listed healthy habits, such as diet and exercise, but they also noted other important aspects of self-care: screenings and wellness check-ups, preventive care, consults with doctors, and their participation in deciding how to deal with a health problem. All of these factors represent consumers' increasing interest in and expectation to be accountable for their own health and wellness. In the United States, "personal accountability" to manage and improve health is expanding the general public's definition of self-care.

The engagement of a health care provider easily differentiates pharmacist-assisted self-care from self-care. However, when does pharmacist-assisted self-care transition to primary care in a more contemporary health care system? Many people who are not health care professionals would turn to Wikipedia to find common definitions. Wikipedia defines *primary care* as "the day-to-day health care given by a health care provider. Typically, this provider acts as the first contact and principal point of continuing care for patients within a health care system, and coordinates other specialist care that the patient may need."[3] Is the pharmacist considered a health care provider under this definition? Is the pharmacist serving as the first point of contact and principal point of ongoing care for the patient? Many would answer "yes" to these questions, as recognition of pharmacists' evolving role in providing patient care services and medication therapy management (MTM) in their practice settings. In addition, federal legislation to secure pharmacists' recognition as "providers" in the Medicare program (HR592 and S109 introduced in the 2017–18 congressional session) is further advancing this belief.[4] Continued delivery of patient care services, such as immunizations and point-of-care testing, will also advance the public's recognition of pharmacists as primary care providers. In the future, these efforts will contribute to further blurring of the distinguishable differences between pharmacist-assisted self-care and primary care delivery by pharmacists.

Editor's Note: This chapter is based on the 18th edition chapter of the same title, written by Metta Lou Henderson.

The patient-centered care model of health care delivery is gaining popularity as part of ongoing health care reform in the United States. The Institute of Medicine defines *patient-centered care* as "providing care that is respectful of and responsive to individual patient preferences, needs, and values, and ensuring that patient values guide all clinical decisions."[5] This definition implies that patients and their health care providers must have a strong partnership and make decisions together based on the patient's desires and priorities for his or her health goals. As John Gans, former chief executive officer of the American Pharmacists Association (APhA) often said, "All care is self-care!" His message was that the patient is always in charge and will make the final decision on implementing any actions to try to improve his or her health. A key area of emphasis in the patient partnership involves the consideration and integration of cultural beliefs, values, and traditions, because these also play a key role in a patient's personal health care decisions. (See Chapter 3 for further discussion of cultural competency in health care.) Furthering advancements in patient-centered, team-based care, which will involve a multidisciplinary team of providers who honor the health care priorities of the patient, will continue to blur the distinguishable differences between self-care and primary care in our health care delivery system.

It is also important to note that self-care involves the full spectrum of care, including prevention and wellness, diagnosis and screening, and treatment of or relief from symptoms. Preventive self-care involves maintaining well-being and appearance through exercise and a healthy lifestyle. For many individuals, a healthy lifestyle includes controlling their diet; taking vitamins, minerals, and herbal supplements; participating in regular exercise and keeping fit; and maintaining physical appearance by using dental, skin, and hair care products. However, self-care for individuals who are ill involves diagnosing their conditions and then obtaining products for the goal of mitigating illness and relieving symptoms. Examples of self-care in illness include use of dietary options (e.g., warm soup for a cold); use of devices for both disease assessment (e.g., home blood glucose meters, cholesterol tests) and treatment (e.g., ice packs, first-aid bandages, vaporizers, nasal strips); and use of nonprescription medications. In these cases, the use of self-care products typically is limited to mild illness or short-term management of illness, and most products warn users to contact their health care provider if conditions do not improve within a short period of time. However, some self-care involves long-term management of ongoing symptoms or chronic conditions with nonprescription medications, even when the recommendations are made by a physician. For example, ongoing fiber supplementation is used to maintain healthy bowel habits and prevent constipation. Acetaminophen may be used for the ongoing management of arthritis pain. Figure 1–1 provides a depiction of the self-care continuum from "pure self care with individual responsibility" to "pure medical care with professional responsibility," as described by the Self Care Forum.[6]

Globally, the importance of self-care in the overall health care spectrum and the role of the pharmacist are both gaining additional visibility. Most recently the International Pharmaceutical Federation (FIP) released during its 2016 congress a draft of a white paper for public comment.[7] The paper provides a global view of the growing role of pharmacists in self-care and improvement of population health around the world. Once finalized and approved through FIP, the paper will serve as a statement and educational tool for promoting the growing role of pharmacists in self-care to improve global health. The FIP white paper refers to an earlier 2005 report from the London Department of Health that highlighted the large role that self-care plays in the total health care model (Figure 1–2).[8] For professional care, the figure includes primary (1ry) health care as basic medical care, along with secondary (2ry) and tertiary (3ry) health care as more complex medical care services (e.g., specialist physicians, intensive hospitalization care). Compared with self-care, professional care is shown to be a smaller component in a patient's overall health care experience. The FIP white paper also referenced the same London Department of Health report for promoting the importance and value of supporting self-care behaviors for improved population health, as shown in Figure 1–3.[8] Professional care for minor ailments, acute illness,

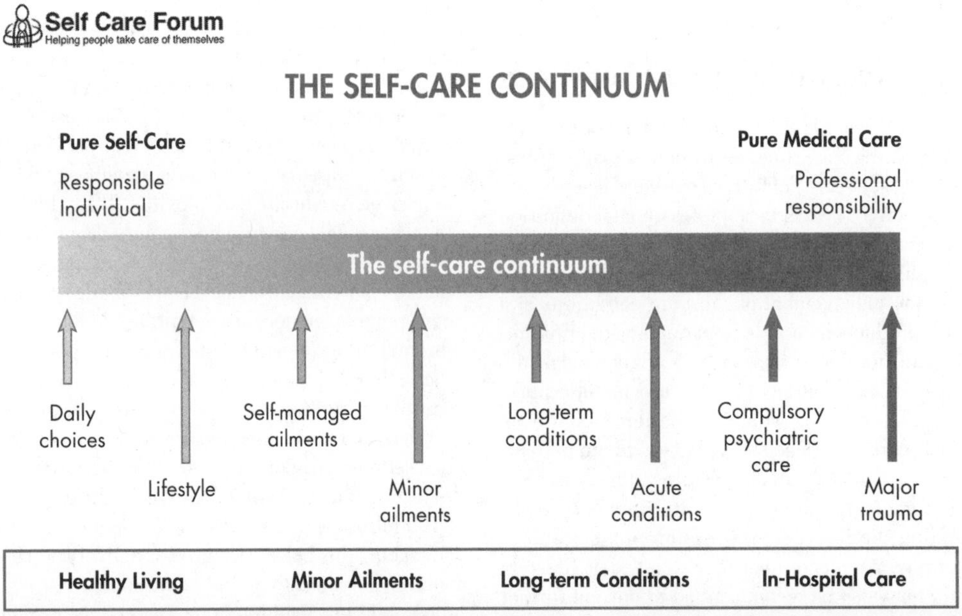

FIGURE 1–1 Self-care continuum developed by the Self Care Forum. (Source: Adapted from reference 6 with the permission of the Self Care Forum. Copyright © 2015.)

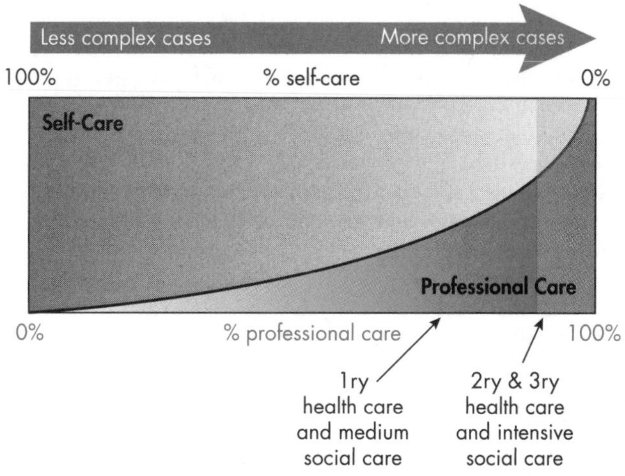

Most care is shared care and can involve a small or large component of self-care.

FIGURE 1-2 Role of self-care in the total health care model. Key: 1ry = Primary; 2ry = secondary; 3ry = tertiary. (Source: Adapted from reference 8 with the permission of the Department of Health, UK.GOV; contains public sector information licensed under the Open Government Licence v1.0.)

and long-term conditions is depicted in the crescent-shaped area of the smaller oval section on the right of the model. Professional care in the patient's self-management of these health issues is depicted as a component of self-care. To the left of the model, self-care measures that are important for maintenance of good health and lifestyle and prevention of illness are depicted as a large component of self-care that does not involve professional care. Again, this model displays visually the important concept of the very large role that self-care plays in the overall health care spectrum. The lower section of the model identifies many important elements for supporting patients' self-care measures. Pharmacists would use most of these elements as tools and processes to assist their patients in implementing self-care approaches.

The International Self-Care Foundation offers additional evidence of the broad scope of self-care, as illustrated by their seven pillars shown in photograph 1 of the Color Plates and outlined in Table 1–1.[9] Clearly, self-care is significant to overall health care, even at the global level, to address patients' active conditions and their preventive health and wellness approaches.

Understanding Today's Self-Care Consumer

Consumers today are motivated and empowered by their ability to use self-care to manage their health. They feel less dependent on physicians and want more control over their health care. Consumers appreciate the convenience of nonprescription medications that enable them to self-treat minor illnesses or injuries, thus avoiding unnecessary treatment from a medical provider.

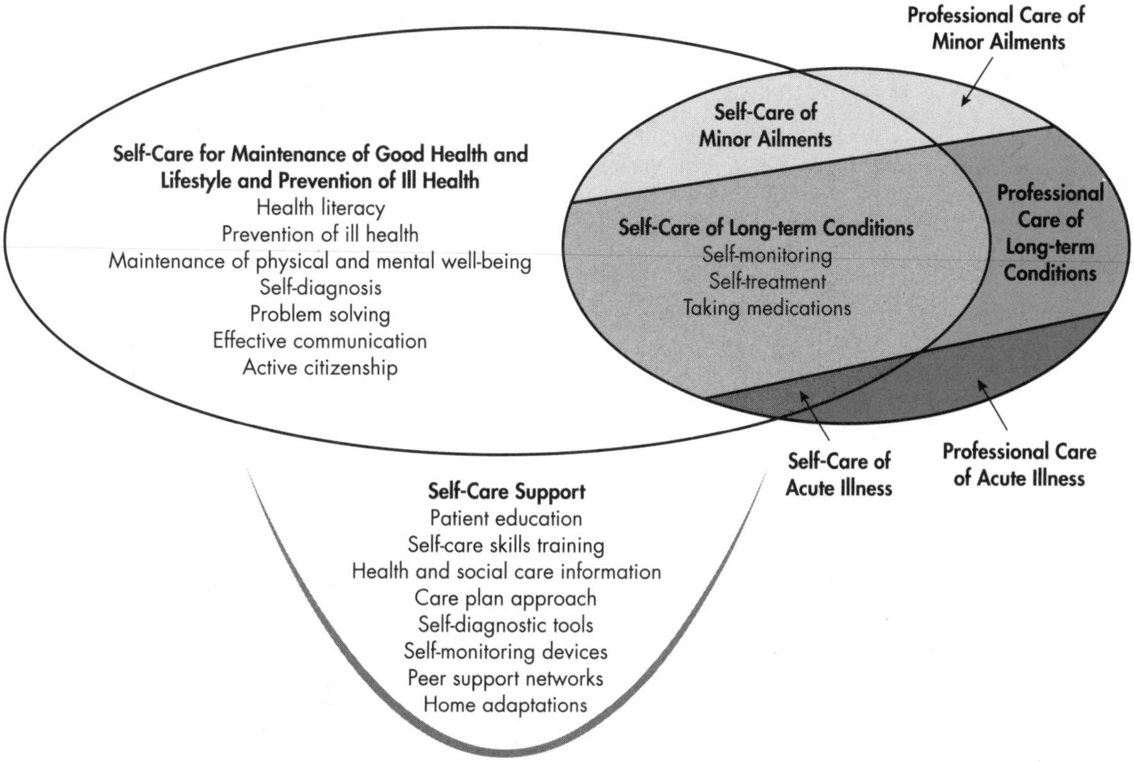

FIGURE 1-3 Self-care and self-care support. (Source: Adapted from reference 8 with the permission of the Department of Health, UK.GOV; contains public sector information licensed under the Open Government Licence v1.0.)

TABLE 1-1 Seven Pillars of Self-Care as Defined by the International Self-Care Foundation

Health literacy	Includes the capacity of individuals to obtain, process, and understand basic health information and services needed to make appropriate health decisions
Self-awareness of physical and mental condition	Includes knowing one's BMI, cholesterol level, and blood pressure; engaging in health screening
Physical activity	Practicing moderate intensity physical activity, such as walking or cycling, or participating in sports at a desirable frequency
Healthy eating	Includes eating a nutritious, balanced diet with appropriate level of caloric intake
Risk avoidance or mitigation	Includes quitting tobacco use, limiting alcohol use, being vaccinated, practicing safe sex, and using sunscreen
Good hygiene	Includes washing hands regularly, brushing teeth, and washing food before consumption
Rational and responsible use of products, services, diagnostics, and medications	Includes being aware of dangers, using responsibly when necessary

Key: BMI = body mass index.
Source: Adapted from reference 9.

A recent survey by the Consumer Healthcare Products Association (CHPA) asked consumers for their perspectives on the role of nonprescription medications in their self-care.[10] A key finding was that consumers trust nonprescription medications, when they are available, for themselves and their children. Key drivers of trust were effectiveness, adverse effects, and doctor recommendation. They also prefer using a nonprescription versus a prescription medication as first-line therapy and for certain ailments such as pain, cough and colds, acid reflux, and upset stomach. Additional data collected in the survey "Your Health at Hand: Perceptions of Over-the-Counter Medicine in the U.S." support the view that both consumers and physicians recognize the role of nonprescription medications in self-care. Key survey results include the following[11]:

- 93% of physicians believe it is important that medications for minor ailments be available over the counter.
- 96% of consumers believe nonprescription medications make it easy to care for minor medical ailments.
- 87% of physicians and 89% of consumers believe nonprescription medications are an important part of overall and family health care.
- 93% of adults prefer to treat minor ailments with nonprescription medications before seeking professional care.
- 88% of physicians recommend patients address minor ailments with self-care, including the use of nonprescription medications, before seeking professional care.

Today's consumer is also much more knowledgeable about health care products and health care in general. In addition, consumers are also more motivated to focus on their health and wellness. For example, consumers are making lifestyle changes, such as drinking more water, taking supplements and vitamins, and eating and exercising more responsibly. Employers, through employee wellness programs, are also offering incentives to improve health. Nearly 90% of employers now offer wellness incentives, such as financial rewards or prizes, to employees who work toward becoming healthier.[12]

The CHPA survey also showed that one in four respondents self-identified as a "family health influencer" based on being knowledgeable about nonprescription medications and playing a role in educating others in the family about their self-care options.[10] These influencers report they are knowledgeable about different nonprescription medications, they avoid going to the doctor unless they absolutely have to, and they choose a medication based on the symptoms it will treat. The family health influencer is more likely to be female, and many are mothers in the family unit. In addition, the survey found that multigenerational households, Hispanic households, and households who care for an adult outside of their home place a high value on a pharmacist's or other in-store health care provider's recommendations. Health care providers must acknowledge and partner with this family health influencer in their caregiver role for the family. Other influencers are also involved in decision making (Figure 1–4).[10]

Internet sources of health information have become increasingly popular across all age groups and demographic populations. Web-based health information is easily and rapidly accessed in the privacy and comfort of one's home. According to a 2013 Pew Internet and American Life Project report, 59% of U.S. adults have searched for online health information in the past year.[13] Most health information seekers, 77%, begin with a major search engine, such as Google, Yahoo, or Bing, whereas another 13% use a more health-specific site such as WebMD. The report has named about a third of adults (35%) as "online diagnosers," because they have gone online to diagnose their or someone else's medical condition.

Individuals who were most likely to search for health information online were white adult women with higher levels of education and income. Dependence on the Internet for self-care information can be problematic. No single organization is accountable for the quality or accuracy of health-related information available on websites. The sheer number and diversity of Internet sources increase the likelihood that patients may unknowingly view biased or outdated information. When asked if the information found online led them to think they needed the attention of a medical professional, 46% of online diagnosers answered "yes," demonstrating the potential role for a pharmacist to provide accurate information and answer questions. Providers should assist their patients in identifying credible resources for health information. A number of valid Internet sources are available to provide information on nonprescription drugs; they include the National Institutes of Health (www.nlm.nih.gov/medlineplus) and sites such as the Cleveland Clinic (www.clevelandclinicmeded.com), WebMD (www.webmd.com), Mayo Clinic (www.mayoclinic.com), and the CHPA Educational Foundation (www.knowyourOTCs.org).

In addition to increased access to health care information, consumers need to be able to understand basic health information to make appropriate health decisions. *Health literacy* is the umbrella term that refers to "the degree to which individuals have the capacity to obtain, process, and understand basic health information and services needed to make appropriate health decisions."[14] Health literacy includes numeracy skills, for example,

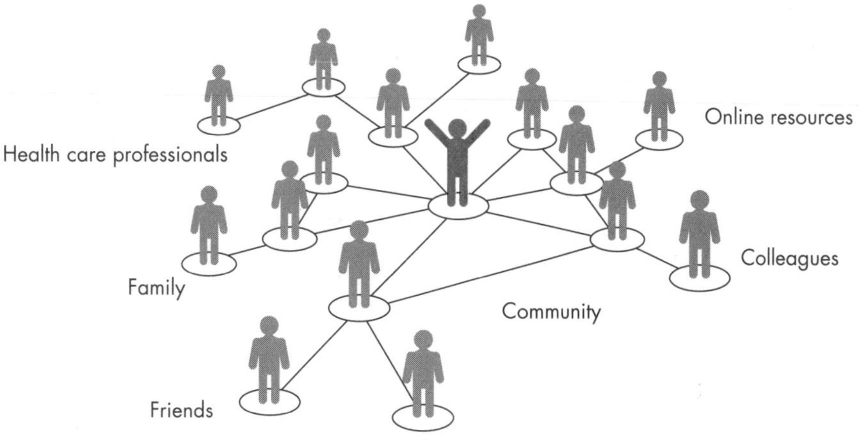

FIGURE 1–4 Influencers of consumers' self-treatment decisions. (Source: Reference 10.)

understanding laboratory values, selecting the proper dose of a medication, and reviewing medical bills. The National Assessment of Adult Literacy showed that only 12% of adults have proficient health literacy and 30% of adults had below basic health literacy.[14] Health literacy affects people's ability to navigate the health care system in a variety of areas: filling out forms, locating physicians and services, discussing their health information, and engaging in self-care. Low literacy has been linked to poor health outcomes, such as higher rates of hospitalization and less frequent use of preventive services.[14]

Health care providers need to be aware that health literacy varies across the population they serve and that they may need to tailor their own language to try to match the patient's skill level. One approach is to use plain language—that is communication that users can understand the first time they read or hear it. Key components of plain language include putting the most important points first, breaking complex concepts into chunks (small bits of information), using simple language, defining technical or medical terms, and using the active voice in which the subject performs the action. Resources for more information include Plain Language.gov (www.plainlanguage.gov) and the Centers for Disease Control and Prevention (CDC) health literacy training module (www.cdc.gov/healthliteracy/training).

The changing demographics of our country's population are also changing the profile of the self-care consumer. The growth of the older population, whose members are known as high users of nonprescription medications, will continue to expand the self-care consumer base. The results of the 2012 National Projections found the number of people ages 65 years or older is expected to more than double from an estimated 43.1 million in 2012 to 83.7 million in 2050.[15] This increase is driven largely by the baby boomers who began turning 65 in 2011. The average life expectancy for Americans has increased, with individuals who reach age 65 years expected to live an additional 16–22 years, depending on gender and race. The fastest growing segment of the elderly is individuals older than 85 years. The racial and ethnic diversity of the older population will also change as the population of Hispanic and non-White groups increases. These individuals will have a significant impact on the future of U.S. health care policy and the health care system as they deal with illness and disability and need long-term care and other resources.

The growth in minority populations in the United States will drive a need for cultural considerations in self-care recommendations. Chapter 3 provides details on cultural considerations in self-care. Chapter 2 provides additional details on self-care for special populations, including geriatric patients, infants and children, and pregnant and breastfeeding patients.

In summary, today's consumer is more empowered and more likely than ever before to take charge of his or her health, often turning to nonprescription medications as first-line therapy for a variety of conditions. In the decades ahead, the older population will be larger and will need information and health care resources, including pharmacists, to manage their health.

Self-Care Changes Driven by Health Care Reform and Changes in Pharmacy Practice

In addition to the consumer factors that affect self-care utilization, notable drivers for self-care utilization are arising from the reform occurring in the U.S. health care system. The passage of the Affordable Care Act (ACA) in 2010 was a key factor in stimulating health care reform. The legislation called for changes to many areas of our health care system, with a focus on increasing access and quality while decreasing costs. The legislation allowed an adoption phase over a series of years for the many new requirements that continue to be implemented. However, even beyond the ACA requirements, the health care market and delivery systems have been actively adopting additional changes that focus on achieving the same goals.

Reform efforts are affecting many areas of the health care system: changes in financial models to drive costs savings, tools and processes to assess and improve quality and patient satisfaction, and new approaches to maximize health care delivery models. Creative financial models are being tested: they feature approaches such as bundled payments and value-based purchasing, as well as new organizational structures, including accountable care organizations, that bring both financial risk and shared savings opportunities to multiple stakeholders in the health care delivery model. In these new models, even care providers are more involved and accountable for the financial impact of health care choices and their patients' outcomes. Patients are also bearing more of the financial burden and accountability for their health care costs through increasing use of high-deductible health care plans and health savings accounts. Quality assessment processes and a focus on indicators of positive outcomes are expanding in all areas of health care. These processes incentivize health care providers to work in closer partnerships with patients to provide health improvement recommendations that patients will adopt to achieve better health outcomes.

Reform is also changing health care delivery to more of an interprofessional team-based model approach in which multidisciplinary health professionals all practice together in a patient-centered focus. This approach should improve the coordination of care for an individual patient across the health care system, while also resulting in improved communications, outcomes, and cost efficiencies in care delivery. Reform, often through legislative changes, is also driving all health care professionals, including pharmacists, to expand their scope of practice and to practice at the top of their capabilities to deliver the most cost-effective care. An overall shortage of primary care providers in the United States has led to an expanding role for nurse practitioners and physician assistants in primary care, while also further increasing demand for the pharmacist's expanding role in self-care and patient care services. Implementation of these reform efforts across the health care continuum is leading toward the common goals of improving health care quality, access, and delivery, while also decreasing costs.

Importantly, many of these health care reform activities can also be linked to influencing changes in the self-care arena. Because health care reform is attempting to improve access, it is driving both patient-initiated self-care and pharmacist-assisted self-care as obvious areas for expansion. The growth of urgent care clinics, some located within pharmacies, is filling a need for better access to primary care. It will be interesting to monitor potential future practice partnerships between pharmacists and other health care providers in these settings and to assess how these partnerships may affect delivery of primary care and pharmacist-assisted self-care.

Insurance plans are also attempting to enhance patients' self-care efforts through programs such as "call a nurse." In this scenario, nurses help patients determine whether medical care is needed or whether other options such as self-care might be appropriate. Some payors have contracted with companies such as OutcomesMTM and Mirixa to compensate pharmacists for providing MTM services, including both self-care interventions with patients and comprehensive medication reviews that include nonprescription medications, vitamins, and supplements. Pharmacists provide MTM services, document the medication-related problems and action steps taken to improve patient outcomes, and then submit a claim and receive payment. Data from OutcomesMTM indicate a return on investment (ROI) of $1.15 for every $1.00 saved in drug product costs.[16] This outcome indicates that the company realizes a positive financial return on payments to pharmacists for MTM interventions that result in drug product cost savings. In other words, for every $1.00 paid to pharmacists, OutcomesMTM can see a $1.15 reduction in their drug product costs. Data from OutcomesMTM also report saving $5.44 for every $1.00 in total estimated cost avoidance for MTM delivery in one health care plan.[16] This outcome indicates that for every $1.00 paid to pharmacists for interventions, OutcomesMTM can see a savings of $5.44 in avoided health care costs. In other words, the insurance plan pays less in health care costs, because pharmacist interventions avoided physician office visits, ER visits, and hospitalizations. It is hoped that the positive ROI, improved access to care, and enhanced access to pharmacist-assisted self-care will encourage insurers to continue to expand these types of new payment models for pharmacists' services.

The incentive for stretching their health care dollars often drives patients to self-care. More individuals and families now have high-deductible insurance plans with potential significant out-of-pocket costs. These patients often may see self-care as a less expensive option to other medical interventions. However, it is best if they consult a pharmacist or other health care provider to ensure that outcome and safety issues are addressed. Many patients have established an employee health savings account that is funded with pretax dollars. Again, self-care can help minimize the spending from this account, so the monies saved can be used for more serious medical issues. For example, a patient with high initial out-of-pocket costs presents to the pharmacy with a sore throat; the cause of the ailment determines its financial consequences. Two possible scenarios, based on the QuEST/SCHOLAR-MAC process[17] (see Chapter 2), include (1) the pharmacist determines that the patient likely has a viral condition and that nonprescription products can be used to help treat the symptoms or (2) the pharmacist determines that the patient likely has strep throat, a bacterial infection that requires antibiotics, and refers the patient to a prescriber. In scenario 1, avoiding an unnecessary physician visit, which can cost a few hundred dollars, is very important to this patient who must pay initial out-of-pocket costs. Such individuals will find the pharmacist to be an accessible, valuable resource to help them sort through their condition to determine whether a medical appointment is truly necessary or whether self-care is appropriate.

In addition to improved access and decreased medical expenses, self-care also offers medications and devices that are typically, but not always, far less expensive than similar prescription products. Occasionally, it may be less expensive for the patient to pay the office visit and prescription copayments, because the cost of an appropriate nonprescription product or device is more expensive. The pharmacist can play an important role in evaluating a patient's overall medication costs by comparing the cost of self-care products with that of similar prescription products, taking into consideration the patient's insurance plan copay and deductible.

In 2012, a survey of more than 3200 individuals provided information regarding the value of nonprescription medications and their contribution to cost savings and quality care in the health care system.[18] Data from the survey showed the following:

- Availability of nonprescription products provides $102 billion in annual savings relative to alternatives, primarily a clinician office visit or phone call. The savings include $77 billion in avoided medical office visits and diagnostic testing and $25 billion in medication cost savings through use of nonprescription treatment options rather than prescription medications (Figure 1–5).
- Each dollar spent on nonprescription medications saves $6–$7 for the health care system.
- In the previous 12 months, 79% of consumers (or approximately 240 million people) reported using a nonprescription product in the categories of allergy, analgesics, antifungals, cough/cold/flu, lower gastrointestinal, upper gastrointestinal, and medicated skin.
- Extrapolating data from the survey nationwide, 180 million individuals would seek treatment from a primary care provider if nonprescription medications were not available. The increased demand for medical care would require an additional 56,000 medical professionals.

The value of self-care is particularly important to the medically underserved and uninsured populations. Without access to self-care, this population often is forced to use the emergency

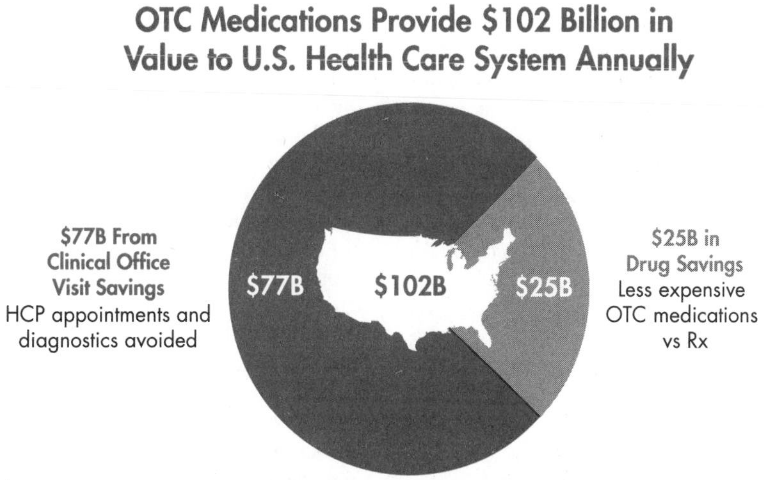

FIGURE 1–5 Annual monetary value of nonprescription medications to U.S. health care system. Key: HCP = Health care provider; OTC = over-the-counter; Rx = prescription. (Source: Adapted from reference 18 with the permission of Booz & Co.)

room for immediate health care needs. The importance of self-care to the patient and payer communities—and providers' recognition of this need—will continue to force reforms in health care delivery that will address the need for increasing access to health care while decreasing costs.

The role of the pharmacist is also changing in how self-care is delivered to patients. As pharmacists' roles evolved over the past few decades, considerable change has occurred in the pharmacy profession: pharmacists have moved from a product-dispensing role to one of a patient care provider who helps patients improve their medication use and advances their health and wellness. This evolution is well stated by the Joint Commission of Pharmacy Practitioners (JCPP) vision for the profession: "Patients will achieve optimal health and medication outcomes when pharmacists are included as essential and accountable members of patient-centered healthcare teams." JCPP represents the combined interests of national organizations of pharmacy practitioners who collectively adopted this new vision for the profession in January 2014.[19] To enable this vision, JCPP approved a standardized Pharmacist Patient Care Process (PPCP) in May 2014. The process is discussed in significant detail in Chapter 2.

At the broader level, the pharmacist's role in MTM is being consistently taught to student pharmacists and pharmacists through the APhA MTM Certificate Training Program.[20] In this program, the five core elements of the MTM service model are defined. The first core element is the medication therapy review (MTR) to gather and evaluate all the patient's medications, including nonprescription medications, nutritional supplements, and herbal products. From this review, the pharmacist prepares the second core element, a personal medication record (PMR) to list all the patient's medications and immunization records identified during the review. The pharmacist also prepares the third core element, a medication action plan (MAP), that identifies medication-related and health-related problems, proposed actions, and results of those actions, when known. The process concludes with the last two core elements: intervention and/or referral followed by documentation of the findings and follow-up plans for the patient's health care needs. It is clear that all five core elements (Table 1–2) include aspects of self-care, nonprescription products, and patient lifestyle and behavior modifications to improve patients' health and quality of life.[20] Most of the following chapters provide comprehensive cases that also demonstrate application of MTM and JCPP elements for patients who are candidates for either self-care or medical referral.

In the past decade, numerous publications have described the value of pharmacists' patient care services in improving health and reducing costs. In 2011, Rear Admiral Scott Giberson was the lead author of the landmark U.S. Public Health Service pharmacy report titled "Improving Patient and Health System Outcomes through Advanced Pharmacy Practice: A Report to the U.S. Surgeon General 2011."[21] This 95-page, evidence-based report included results from federal pharmacists' patient care practices, particularly from the Indian Health Service and Veterans Affairs Hospital System, as well as data referenced from other studies that validated pharmacists' value in the health care system. Additional research projects and publications have also documented the value of pharmacists' patient care services.[22–25] Any of these papers can be used to advocate for pharmacists' expanded patient care roles and for their recognition as health care providers. More

TABLE 1–2 MTM Core Elements

Medication therapy review (MTR)	Collect and evaluate all of the patient's medications.
Personal medication record (PMR)	List all of the patient's medications and immunizations.
Medication action plan (MAP)	Identify medication-related and health-related problems, proposed actions, and results of those actions, when known.
Intervention and/or referral	Take action with patient or health care providers as needed.
Documentation of the findings and follow-up plans	Record notes of the intervention, recommendations, and ongoing care, as needed.

Source: Adapted from reference 20.

recently there has been an emphasis on the pharmacist's role in point-of-care (POC) testing, ranging from blood pressure, cholesterol, blood glucose, and bone density screenings to rapid influenza diagnostic tests and pharmacogenomics. One recent article described the potential benefit of POC testing for patients who visit the pharmacy seeking nonprescription medications for their influenza symptoms.[26] If the pharmacy had the ability to conduct rapid influenza diagnostic testing, the pharmacist could determine who were candidates for self-care and who needed to be referred to their primary care provider, resulting in decreased risk of mortality from influenza. The timeliness of this assessment is critical so that antiviral medication can be prescribed and started within the 48-hour treatment window for a referral patient. If the patient did not test positive for influenza, the pharmacist could assist with cough and cold self-care recommendations, as appropriate.

Legislative and regulatory changes are also allowing the expansion of pharmacists' patient care services. In numerous states, current and new legislation is allowing pharmacists to enter Collaborative Practice Agreements (CPAs) with prescribers.[27] These agreements allow prescribers (primarily physicians) to delegate numerous activities to the pharmacist, including modifying, initiating, or discontinuing patients' drug therapy, and ordering laboratory tests. The National Alliance of State Pharmacists Associations released a report, "Key Elements for CPA Legislative and Regulatory Authority," that offers guidance for further state legislation needed to support this expanding practice area.[28]

Recently, a study to look at the role of pharmacists in expanding access to care was initiated in the state of Washington.[29] Care provided for 20 minor ailments by community pharmacists will be compared with the care received in physician offices, urgent care clinics, and emergency departments. Working under collaborative practice agreements, pharmacists manage patients with conditions that may require prescription therapy and, when appropriate, refer patients for medical care. In other cases, nonprescription therapy and/or nondrug management will be recommended when prescription medication or medical care is not warranted. Comparisons of quality of care, costs per episode, and frequency of follow-up care, along with a review of health outcomes, will be made. Although the study includes the 20 minor ailments listed in Table 1–3, pharmacists in the state of Washington are also comprehensively managing, monitoring, and initiating drug therapy through CPAs for many other conditions.

Changes in pharmacy design and operations are also taking place to improve the accessibility and visibility of pharmacists. For example, Walgreens implemented renovations in numerous pharmacies with store layout designs that allow pharmacists to work at desks in front of the pharmacy.[30] (See the Color Plates, photographs 2A and B, for an illustration of this new model.) Similar attention to changes in pharmacy layout and workflow is occurring in other community pharmacies, with the intent that improved access to the pharmacist will lead to an increase in patient interaction and pharmacist-assisted self-care. In this type of practice model, pharmacy technicians must play an enhanced support role in the prescription preparation and insurance claim management areas to free up the pharmacist's time for patients. Pharmacy technicians have experienced growth in their training and credentialing that better prepares them to assist the pharmacist in a patient care–focused practice: the Pharmacy Technician Certification Board (PTCB) national certification examination is an example. Pharmacy technicians can screen patients to determine who needs to speak with the pharmacist, to assist patients in locating products in the pharmacy aisles, and to help with collecting data from patients, as well as with documentation and billing. Utilizing a new pharmacy layout; enhanced training; and improved teamwork to standardize, validate, promote, and expand the pharmacist's role in patient care will create a strong foundation to drive the pharmacists' availability and capability for a growing role in self-care.

The Current Self-Care Marketplace

Consumers have access to and can purchase many health care products for self-medication. Three general categories of products are available for self-medication: (1) nonprescription medications, (2) dietary supplements, and (3) complementary and integrative health therapies and approaches. Chapter 4 provides details on the regulatory process for nonprescription medications. Chapter 50 covers dietary supplements and natural products, and Chapter 52 covers complementary and integrative medicine.

Nonprescription Medications

The nonprescription drug market represents about $40 billion, or 60%, of the total pharmaceutical volume (units or number of packages) sold in the United States. Figure 1–6 illustrates the details.[31] Five product categories account for more than 70% of sales in the nonprescription medications market: respiratory, oral care,

TABLE 1–3 Minor Ailments Included in the NACDS Institute Study: Expanding Pharmacy Care—Innovative Models from the United States and Abroad

Bronchospasm, wheezing, shortness of breath from asthma or COPD	Acute otitis media	Conjunctivitis	Eye or nasal symptoms from seasonal allergies or other allergic conditions
Nausea and vomiting (not related to motion sickness)	Ear infections caused by bacteria	Migraine headaches	Anaphylactic allergic reactions
Nausea and vomiting caused by motion sickness	Lacerations and abrasions	Contraceptive pregnancy prevention	Allergic reactions from bee stings (not anaphylactic)
Herpesvirus infections (cold sores, genital herpes, shingles)	Wound infections from burns	Vaginal yeast infections	Diarrhea that occurs while traveling
Streptococcal pharyngitis	Animal bite (human, dog, or cat)	Uncomplicated urinary tract infections	Lack of fluoride for oral health

Source: Adapted from reference 29.

Key: COPD = Chronic obstructive pulmonary disease; NACDS = National Association of Chain Drug Stores.

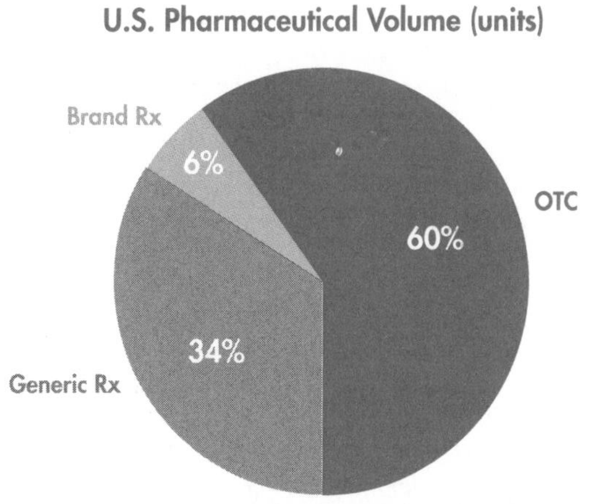

FIGURE 1–6 Breakdown of total U.S. pharmaceutical sales, by market classification. (Source: Reference 31.) Key: OTC = Over-the-counter; Rx = prescription.

gastrointestinal, internal analgesics, and eye care (Figure 1–7). The estimated number of available Food and Drug Administration (FDA)-approved nonprescription drug products is well over 100,000, including more than 400 active ingredients that cover more than 700 therapeutic uses. *Your Health at Hand Book: Guide to OTC Active Ingredients in the United States* provides an extensive list of active ingredients, therapeutic categories, and examples of trade-name products.[32]

Many nonprescription medications were once available only by prescription. A generally favorable environment for reclassification of prescription products to nonprescription status (Rx-to-OTC switch) in the United States has resulted in the availability of more than 700 nonprescription products today that were once available only by prescription. Chapter 4 provides an in-depth discussion of Rx-to-OTC switches.

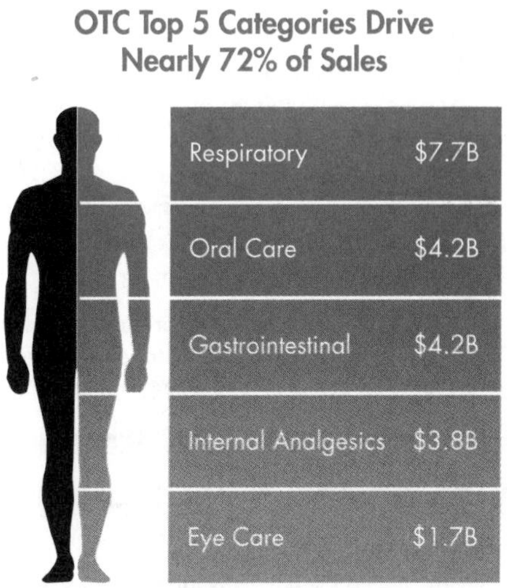

OTC Top 5 Categories Drive
Nearly 72% of Sales
Respiratory $7.7B
Oral Care $4.2B
Gastrointestinal $4.2B
Internal Analgesics $3.8B
Eye Care $1.7B

FIGURE 1–7 Top-selling categories of nonprescription medications. (Source: Reference 31.)

Dietary Supplements

A study by the Council for Responsible Nutrition found that 68% of Americans take dietary supplements, and that this percentage remained stable between 2011 and 2015.[33] Combination vitamin and mineral products remain the most popular dietary supplements, followed by single-ingredient vitamin D, vitamin C, and calcium products. Herbs and botanicals, along with protein and energy supplements, also remained very popular. In the specialty supplements category, fish oil and probiotics continue to see strong sales, with probiotics estimated to reach $2.6 billion in sales by 2020 (see Chapter 20). The overall dietary supplement market sales were $36.7 billion in 2014, an all-time high.[34]

Complementary and Integrative Health Therapies

Factors such as high out-of-pocket health care costs and restricted access to conventional health care providers lead some patients to seek care from complementary and integrative health providers. The National Center for Complementary and Integrative Health (formerly, the National Center for Complementary and Alternative Medicine) reported in the 2012 National Health Interview Survey that 33.2% of U.S. adults and 11.6% of U.S. children used some form of complementary health care in 2012; similar results were reported in 2007.[35] The organization defines *complementary approach* as combining a non-mainstream practice with conventional medicine. Also, as in past surveys, natural products (nonvitamin and nonmineral dietary supplements) were the most commonly used complementary supplements. The mind and body approaches most commonly used by adults include yoga, chiropractic or osteopathic manipulation, meditation, and massage therapy.[35]

Wellness is the primary reason reported by individuals for using natural product supplements or practicing yoga. Data for use of natural product supplements show that more than 85% of U.S. adults report using them for wellness, whereas more than 40% use them for treating a specific condition. More than 90% of U.S. adults who practice yoga do so for wellness, whereas more than 15% practice yoga to treat a health condition. More than two-thirds of U.S. adults report feeling better from using complementary approaches.[35] The pharmacist is ideally situated to advise patients on appropriate choices of complementary and integrative health options. Advising patients on the best approaches requires integrating an understanding of pharmaceutical and natural product ingredients, physiology, pharmacology, potential interactions, and consumer behavior.

Legislative and Regulatory Issues Affecting Self-Care

The self-care environment is shaped by ongoing legislative and regulatory activities. Although a few unique issues are discussed here, details of the regulatory framework for nonprescription medications are provided in Chapter 4.

The basic framework has been in place for decades; however, various state and federal legislative activities impact access and availability of these products. At the federal level, the use of flexible spending accounts that allowed consumers to use pretax dollars to purchase nonprescription medications was disallowed in 2011 as Congress sought ways to pay for the Affordable Care Act.

Legislative efforts to restore this tax-incentivized opportunity are ongoing. At the state level, various legislation has addressed many areas relevant to nonprescription medications, including environmental impact (mandatory drug take-back programs, elimination of plastic microbeads from toothpastes and lotions), which are discussed in this chapter, and pharmacist provider status and pharmacist prescribing authority (e.g., oral contraceptives, naloxone), which are discussed in Chapter 4.

Concerns about pharmaceuticals in the environment, particularly in Washington and California, have led individual counties to pass laws requiring manufacturers to implement take-back programs for drug disposal. Examples include King County, WA, and Alameda County, CA. In Illinois, Indiana, and Wisconsin, the presence of plastic microbeads in lakes led to the passage of laws that ban their use. Subsequently, a federal law that provides a harmonized timeline to ban the use of plastic microbeads in nonprescription medications and personal care products was passed in December 2015.

Educating the Public About Safe Medication Use—Collaborations

It is well known that education is an important component of any program to improve the safe and responsible use of medications. In addition, broad public education can lead to consumer empowerment, resulting in consumers' proactive management of their self-care for health and wellness. Education efforts require people, time, and money. Collaborations between a broad range of stakeholder groups, including health care professionals, government, academia, and industry, can achieve results that are difficult or impossible for one group acting alone. They are an efficient way to utilize unique skill sets to develop and disseminate educational materials and messages to consumers through a variety of media. Impressive examples of public–private partnerships have been formed to educate consumers on the safe use of nonprescription medications. Four such partnerships described in the following sections show that pharmacists are important stakeholders in the development and deployment of educational programming.

NCPIE/BEMedWise and Boy Scouts of America

A partnership between the National Council on Patient Information and Education (NCPIE) and the Boy Scouts of America provides Boy Scouts and Venturers ages 11–17 years the opportunity to earn a patch (see the Color Plates, photograph 3) after completing four lessons on safe and responsible nonprescription medication use. The SCOUTStrong Be MedWise Award program teaches the youths how prescription and nonprescription medications are alike and how they differ, as well as how to use nonprescription medications safely.[36]

Up and Away

The message of the Up and Away campaign is to put medications "up and away," that is, out of sight and reach of young children[37] (see the Color Plates, photograph 4). Led by CDC, this innovative collaboration brings together public health agencies, private sector companies, professional organizations (including the American Pharmacists Association), consumer and patient advocates, and academic experts to develop strategies to keep children safe from unintentional medication overdoses. The developed messages are based on data and consumer research, and campaign partners work to expand the reach of their messages via social media, in-store materials, and in-office materials. Since 2011, emergency department visits for unsupervised pediatric medication exposures have dropped 3.4% each year, suggesting, at least in part, a positive impact of this educational effort.[38] Up and Away provides free educational materials on its website (www.upandaway.org/).[37]

Know Your Dose

The Know Your Dose campaign was developed and launched in 2011 by the Acetaminophen Awareness Coalition (AAC), which consists of leading health, health care provider, and consumer organizations. The coalition's goal is to educate consumers and patients on the importance of knowing the ingredients in their medications and following labeled directions to prevent unintentional acetaminophen overdose. Through outreach to health care providers, patients, and consumers, AAC works to ensure that acetaminophen is used only as directed or labeled. Partner organizations are diverse and include retailers, pharmacists (e.g., American Association of Colleges of Pharmacy, American Pharmacists Association), patient advocacy groups, and other health care practitioner groups. CDC, FDA, and the American Academy of Pediatrics are advisors to the coalition. The Know Your Dose campaign educates consumers and patients on how to use acetaminophen-containing medications safely. Materials are available for distribution to consumers and patients.[39] Although it can be difficult to measure the impact of educational campaigns, data from poison centers show that since 2008, adult exposures to nonprescription acetaminophen combination products have decreased 30.4%[40] (www.knowyourdose.org/).

OTC Medicine Safety Campaign

The APhA Academy of Student Pharmacists (APhA-ASP) partnered with McNeil Consumer Healthcare and Scholastic on the OTC Medicine Safety Campaign to educate 5th- and 6th-grade students and their families about the safe use and storage of nonprescription medications. This campaign is an opportunity for pharmacists and student pharmacists, working through APhA-ASP chapters at colleges of pharmacy, to educate the students and their parents or caregivers about reading medication directions, the importance of following nonprescription label directions, proper measurement of a medication, safe storage and disposal of a medication, and the importance of consulting a parent or guardian before taking medications. Ready-made resources, including E-books, posters, and handouts designed to appeal to 5th and 6th graders, are available through the website (www.pharmacist.com/apha-asp-otc-medicine-safety).[41]

The Future of Self-Care—A Changing Marketplace and Advancements in Technology

Although the self-care market has continued to grow in terms of sales, a trend in the U.S. pharmacy marketplace has been consolidation. Significant changes in the retail environment include acquisition of the Rite Aid Corp. by Walgreens Boots Alliance Inc. and the CVS Health acquisition of Target's pharmacy and clinical businesses. Manufacturers have also driven consolidation through the combination of consumer divisions of Novartis and

GlaxoSmithKline plc, and through Bayer AG's purchase of Merck and Co.'s nonprescription medication and consumer care business.

The self-care marketplace is expected to continue to grow, with more and improved medications and other consumer health care products available to consumers, particularly via community pharmacies. The pharmacist is playing an ever-increasing and influential provider role in assisting patients with self-care. Today, pharmacies offer vaccines and limited diagnostic testing. They also control access to medications such as pseudoephedrine to prevent abuse. In the future, we expect pharmacists to be administering more rapid diagnostic tests and playing a key role in disease identification, tracking, and management. More pharmacists will be prescribing medications such as oral contraceptives and naloxone as additional states pass legislation to make these medications more accessible. The increased utilization of electronic medical record (EMR) systems is allowing more information to be shared by the health professional team, including pharmacists. Eventually, community pharmacists will be able to both review a patient's medical history and enter important information from their self-care interventions into the patient's EMR.

For a pharmacist's self-care activities to expand, their integration in the workflow of pharmacy operations must be addressed. Workflow challenges currently exist with the delivery of patient care services such as immunizations. Any processes established to meet these challenges can be reapplied to self-care and other patient care services. A supportive financial infrastructure that allows compensation for patient care services is also needed to sustain and build patient care practices in pharmacy. Passage of the pharmacist provider status legislation mentioned earlier will help address this need. All of these changes position the pharmacist to play an ever-increasing and influential provider role in aiding self-care.

Technology

For those consumers interested in taking advantage of innovations, technology is enabling and redefining self-care in many ways, but differences among the various demographic groups must be considered. Older, less educated, and poorer Americans are much less likely to be online.[42] For example, a full 80% of people between ages 18 and 29 have broadband in their homes, a number that drops to 43% for those 65 and older. Yet 61% of Americans own a smartphone, and 62% of smartphone owners have used their phone in the past year to look up information about a health condition.[43]

In the past few years, consumer use of health monitoring technology has undergone tremendous growth. Applications available to smartphone users provide health monitoring, exercise tracking, dietary intake analysis, symptom analysis, and many more services. Wearable devices such as Fitbit and Apple Watch can provide feedback on physical fitness, quality of sleep, water intake, and even more health parameters. This collection of consumer health data can be a valuable aid in monitoring outcomes of treatment and lifestyle changes to improve health.

Nonprescription medications and dietary supplement products have also benefited from technology. Product package labels that contain QR codes can provide much more information than usually is printed on a standard Drug Facts label. The consumer simply uses the smartphone app to read the QR code to gain access to the additional content. As one example, these codes can hold multilingual labeling, which allows people in a region where different languages are spoken to use the same product and yet receive labeling information in their preferred language. Technology has also facilitated development of new dosage forms. For example, technology for producing chewable products has produced more pleasing dosage forms, such as chewable tablets and gummies. Rapid-release technology now is used in many nonprescription medications, such as instant-dissolve tablets or melting strips, which can make dosing for children more pleasant. Dosage form features can also offer a safety benefit, such as the flow restrictors in children's liquid acetaminophen products that provide a safeguard against accidental overdose.

The role of technology in health care will continue to expand, particularly in ways to actively engage consumers. Devices to allow POC testing in the pharmacy as well as home-monitoring techniques will continue to expand. For example, the ability to perform DNA testing for pharmacogenomic analysis to address appropriate medication use and the risk of certain diseases is becoming more available to the general public; this technology includes options that involve the pharmacist. For more information about the future vision of diagnostic testing by consumers, view the TED Talk video by Daniel Kraft, MD.[44]

Role of the Pharmacist and Student Pharmacist in Self-Care

As noted earlier, the role of the pharmacist has been slowly evolving from primarily dispensing medications to a health care provider role of improving medication use and health outcomes for patients. A combination of factors, including advanced education, pharmacy layout, and financial models, are supporting this practice change. Student pharmacists can also play increasingly important roles in assisting patients with their self-care needs. During their early professional shadowing experiences or introductory pharmacy practice experiences, student pharmacists can observe the techniques used by the pharmacist to gather information, assess the patient, and provide recommendations. Later, during internships and advanced pharmacy practice experiences, student pharmacists can engage in patient care and apply these same techniques, starting with obtaining initial basic information collection for the pharmacist, helping patients find products in the aisles, and later providing patient assessment and counseling under the supervision of their pharmacist preceptor. Student pharmacists can apply the information that follows in this section to help them develop patient care skills as they progress through pharmacy school.

Although patient counseling commonly occurs in the product aisle or at the pharmacy counter, utilization of private or semi-private counseling areas is increasing, particularly for more extensive conversations. In the practice of pharmacist-assisted self-care, the pharmacist has the expertise to screen patient's health information and apply his or her knowledge and training to select products according to the individual's health care needs (see Chapter 2 for more detail). A 2015 APhA survey of pharmacists reported on the critical role that pharmacists play in supporting patient-initiated self-care.[45] The 394 respondents reported that they provide patient counseling on self-care topics or nonprescription medications an average of 7.2 times each day. They also stated that patients were highly likely to select products consistent with their recommendations. The pharmacists identified the following areas as the most frequent counseling topics:

- Product selection for specific symptoms: 90%
- Potential drug interactions with other medications (prescription and nonprescription): 37%
- Dosing and administration information: 34%

- Signs and/or symptoms that indicate when to seek medical advice: 22%
- Side effects and safety considerations: 14%

The pharmacists reported that patients most frequently requested assistance for the following self-care therapeutic areas:

- Cough and cold: 87%
- Seasonal and environmental allergies: 53%
- Gastrointestinal complaints: 28%
- Dermatologic conditions: 14%
- Dietary supplements: 11%
- Nicotine replacement therapy: 2%

In providing pharmacist-assisted self-care, two key elements are always paramount for the pharmacist to consider. First, the pharmacist must ensure the medication selected for use is the most efficacious, taking into consideration the patient's unique needs and factors such as diseases, current medication use, lifestyle, daily routine, personal priorities and preferences, and desired outcome. The second key area of importance is ensuring the patient's safety by addressing many of the concerns and possible problems that can arise to cause the patient harm. Possible areas of concern and higher risk for safety issues are addressed below.

Specific to product selection, when considering a medication's efficacy, the pharmacist must first help in identifying the best ingredient and device for the patient based on the patient's desired outcome. However, other factors can come into play. The dosage form of the product is an important factor to consider and must meet the needs of the patient. For example, pharmacists can work to enhance adherence and improve outcomes by selecting a coated tablet that is easier for an elderly patient to swallow and recommending an extended-release formulation that requires fewer daily doses for a patient with a busy schedule. Cultural considerations must always be evaluated to ensure patients' needs are met. More information on this topic can be found in Chapter 3.

After helping a patient find the most efficacious medication, the pharmacist must also address other ways to improve the patient's health or condition. Recommendations could include lifestyle, dietary, and behavior changes that will improve the patient's symptoms or condition or help to prevent future illnesses. Sometimes these recommendations become more important in ensuring the patient's wellness than the medication treatment itself. For example, coaching a patient with allergies on prevention and maintenance activities to clear the home of allergens can help prevent the development of allergy-related symptoms in the future.

In addition to efficacy, medication safety is the other paramount concern of the pharmacist. Pharmacists must ensure that their patients understand all aspects of the self-care intervention, including the recommended medication dosage and special administration instructions. This step can be especially important for patients with limited health literacy. A critical counseling point is ensuring that the patient knows the time limit for symptom improvement or, alternatively, if symptoms worsen, at what point to seek medical care. In the previously mentioned survey, pharmacists reported the following three top barriers to patient engagement for self-care[45]:

- Patient is seeking recommendation when medical care is indicated: 66%
- Patients are in a hurry to leave the pharmacy: 65%
- Patients erroneously consider nonprescription products overly safe: 64%

The pharmacist must play a key role in helping the patient understand safety parameters for self-care of his or her condition.

Pharmacists must also consider which patients may fall into the category of special populations, including children and the elderly, patients who are pregnant or breastfeeding, and those with chronic conditions. Patients who are pregnant or breastfeeding are particularly challenging, because it is critical to balance the need for medication with the risk to their unborn child or infant. When possible, nonpharmacologic therapy should be the first option. Pharmacists are trained to assess whether a nonprescription medication is safe for use during pregnancy, yet women often make these decisions independently. The pharmacist can use FDA guidance information, textbooks that provide guidance,[46] and the primary literature to fully assess the potential risks and benefits of a patient's medication choices. Pregnant and breastfeeding patients always should be counseled about potential side effects that could occur in the child.

Elderly patients, with their reduced hepatic and renal function, decreased metabolism and muscle mass, heightened medication sensitivity, multiple disease states, and chronic medication use, are another group for whom special attention must be given to benefits and risks. For example, one study characterized the changes in medication and dietary supplement use from 2005–2006 to 2010–2011 in 2351 participants with mean ages of 70.9 years and 71.4 years, respectively.[47] The prevalence of prescription medication use, polypharmacy (concurrent use of five or more prescription medications), and use of dietary supplements increased, whereas use of nonprescription medications declined during this 5-year period. The use of interacting medications also increased over this time period, reinforcing the need for all health care professionals to reinforce safe use of medications in this population. Use of the Beers Criteria,[48] along with numerous other sources, can be helpful in assessing the risks of nonprescription medication use in the senior population.

Patients with chronic conditions also deserve special attention before a product is recommended. For example, patients with chronic kidney disease can be at risk for further kidney damage with chronic exposure to nonsteroidal anti-inflammatory drugs.[49] Chapters in this book that cover medical conditions will have sections that address management of these special populations.

Key Points

- Self-care involves the full spectrum of care, including prevention and wellness, diagnosis and screening, and treatment or relief of symptoms.
- Self-care is becoming more significant in our overall health care system because of numerous factors. Patients are becoming more accountable and focused on improving their health. Health care reform, combined with cost-reduction pressures, is driving changes in health care delivery and financial models that are all leading to increased use of self-care.
- Both health care professionals and consumers recognize the value and cost savings that self-care and nonprescription products provide to the health care delivery model.
- Consumers are utilizing the Internet and others sources to increase their knowledge about self-care and available nonprescription products. The pharmacist continues to serve as a key resource to aid patients in assessing their condition and selecting appropriate self-care treatments.
- The changing demographics of the U.S. population, including a greater number of older adults and non-Hispanic Whites, and a large population with low health literacy, will require health care professionals to make special considerations for the self-care needs of these patients.

- The pharmacist's role is changing from prescription dispenser to patient care provider, allowing an enhanced role in assisting patients with their self-care needs. The newly established pharmacist patient care process and the core elements of MTM are applicable to the pharmacist's role in assisting with management of prescription and nonprescription medications.
- Although the estimated number of nonprescription drug products is well over 100,000, the self-care marketplace is growing. Fueling this growth is an expanding number of Rx-to-OTC switches and changes in state regulations to allow increased access to prescription products.
- Pharmacists can play a key role in educating consumers on self-care topics through the use of numerous public education programming materials.
- The future of self-care is predicted to continue to expand, with advances in technology, products, devices, and expansion of pharmacists' roles.
- The pharmacist must emphasize efficacy and safety in assisting patients with their self-care needs. Special attention is needed for populations of higher risk, including children, the elderly, pregnant women, and those with chronic conditions.
- Student pharmacists can build their self-care skills as they progress through a pharmacy program—from early shadowing and introductory pharmacy practice experiences to internships and advanced pharmacy practice experiences.

REFERENCES

1. World Self Medication Industry. What is self-care? Available at: http://www.wsmi.org/about-self-care-and-self-medication/what-is-self-care/. Accessed May 5, 2017.
2. Mobihealthnews. Survey: 64 percent of consumers say they can make more health-related decisions themselves [news release]. April 30, 2015. Available at: http://mobihealthnews.com/43085/survey-64-percent-of-consumers-say-they-can-make-more-health-related-decisions-themselves. Accessed May 5, 2017.
3. Primary Care. Available at: https://en.wikipedia.org/wiki/Primary_care. Accessed May 5, 2017.
4. Pharmacistscare.org. Patient Access to Pharmacists Care Coalition. Available at: http://pharmacistscare.org/the-solution/legislative-information/ Accessed May 5, 2017.
5. Institute of Medicine. Crossing the quality chasm: a new healthcare system for the 21st century. March 2001. Available at: http://www.nationalacademies.org/hmd/~/media/Files/Report%20Files/2001/Crossing-the-Quality-Chasm/Quality%20Chasm%202001%20%20report%20brief.pdf. Accessed May 5, 2017.
6. Self Care Forum. What do we mean by self care and why is it good for people? The self-care continuum. Available at: http://www.selfcareforum.org/about-us/what-do-we-mean-by-self-care-and-why-is-good-for-people/. Accessed May 5, 2017.
7. International Pharmaceutical Federation. Pharmacy. Gateway to care—pharmacists supporting self-care. [Draft report for FIP Council review at 2016 FIP Congress]. The Hague, Netherlands: FIP; 2016.
8. Department of Health, GOV.UK. Self care – a real choice: self care support – a practical option. 2005. Available at: http://personcentredcare.health.org.uk/resources/self-care-%E2%80%93-real-choice-self-care-support-%E2%80%93-practical-option. Accessed May 5, 2017.
9. International Self-Care Foundation. The seven pillars of self-care. Available at: http://isfglobal.org/practise-self-care/the-seven-pillars-of-self-care/. Accessed May 5, 2017.
10. Consumer Healthcare Products Association. Understanding trust in OTC medicines: consumer and healthcare provider perspectives. March 6, 2013. Available at: http://www.yourhealthathand.org/images/uploads/Understanding_Trust_in_OTC_Medicines_Research_Findings.pdf. Accessed May 5, 2017.
11. Consumer Healthcare Products Association. Your health at hand: perceptions of over the-counter medicine in the U.S. November 24, 2010. Available at: http://www.yourhealthathand.org/images/uploads/CHPA_YHH_Survey_062011.pdf, Accessed May 5, 2017.
12. Fidelity Investments. Companies expand wellness programs to focus on improving employees' emotional and financial well-being. April 1, 2016. [online survey] Available at: https://www.fidelity.com/about-fidelity/employer-services/companies-expand-wellness-programs. Accessed May 5, 2017.
13. PEW Research Center. Majority of adults look online for health information. February 1, 2013. Available at: http://www.pewresearch.org/daily-number/majority-of-adults-look-online-for-health-information/. Accessed May 5, 2017.
14. U.S. Department of Health and Human Services. Quick guide to health literacy. Available at: http://health.gov/communication/literacy/quickguide/factsbasic.htm. Accessed May 5, 2017.
15. U.S. Census Bureau. 2012 national projections. 2014. Available at: http://www.census.gov/population/projections/data/national/2012.html. Accessed May 5, 2017.
16. OutcomesMTM. MTM Trends Report 2015. Available at: http://outcomesmtm.com/documents/2015MTMTrendsReport.pdf. Accessed May 5, 2017.
17. Burning SM, Kirby J, Conrad W. A structured approach for teaching students to counsel self-care patients. *Am J Pharm Educ.* 2007;71(1):8. PMCID: PMC1847542.
18. Consumer Healthcare Products Association. The value of OTC medicine to the United States. January 2012. Available at: http://www.yourhealthathand.org/images/uploads/The_Value_of_OTC_Medicine_to_the_United_States_BoozCo.pdf. Accessed May 5, 2017.
19. American Pharmacists Association. JCPP approves pharmacists' patient care process[news release], July 2014. Available at: https://www.pharmacist.com/jcpp-approves-pharmacists-patient-care-process. Accessed May 5, 2017.
20. American Pharmacists Association. Delivering medication therapy management services [certificate course]. July 14, 2014. Available at: https://www.pharmacist.com/delivering-medication-therapy-management-services. Accessed May 5, 2017.
21. Giberson S, Yoder S, Lee MP. *Improving Patient and Health System Outcomes through Advanced Pharmacy Practice, A Report to the US Surgeon General.* 2011. Available at: http://www.accp.com/docs/positions/misc/improving_patient_and_health_system_outcomes.pdf. Accessed May 5, 2017.
22. Cranor CW, Bunting BA, Christensen DB. The Asheville Project: long-term clinical and economic outcomes of a community pharmacy diabetes care program. *J Am Pharm Assoc.* 2003;43(2):173–84. PMID: 12688435.
23. Avalere Health. Exploring pharmacists' role in a changing healthcare environment. May 21, 2014. Available at: http://avalere.com/expertise/life-sciences/insights/exploring-pharmacists-role-in-a-changing-health care-environment. Accessed May 5, 2017.
24. Avalere Health. New analysis identifies factors that can facilitate broader reimbursement of pharmacist services. November 6, 2015. Available at: http://avalere.com/expertise/managed-care/insights/new-analysis-identifies-factors-that-can-facilitate-broader-reimbursement-o. Accessed May 5, 2017.
25. American Pharmacists Association. *Pharmacists' Patient Care Services Digest, Building Momentum, Increasing Access.* Washington, DC: American Pharmacists Association. March 2016. Available at: http://media.pharmacist.com/documents/APhA_Digest.pdf. Accessed May 5, 2017.
26. Kuhn C, Klepser D, McCants H. Role of pharmacist-provided point-of-care testing. *JAPhA.* 2015;55(6):572–3. doi: 10.331/JAPhA.2015.15549.
27. American Pharmacists Association. Collaborative practice agreements: NASPA workgroup releases recommendations [news release]. September 1, 2015. Available at: https://www.pharmacist.com/collaborative-practice-agreements-naspa-workgroup-releases-recommendations. Accessed May 5, 2017
28. National Alliance of State Pharmacy Associations. *Key Elements for CPA Legislative and Regulatory Authority: National Alliance of State Pharmacy Associations; Collaborative Practice Workgroup Report.* Richmond, VA: National Alliance of State Pharmacy Associations; July 6, 2015. Available at: http://naspa.us/resource/cpa-report/. Accessed May 5, 2017.
29. National Association of Chain Drug Stores Institute. Expanding pharmacy care – innovative models from the US & abroad [slide presentation]. August 22, 2015. Available at: http://slideplayer.com/slide/7360144/. Accessed May 5, 2017.

30. Drug Store News. With its pharmacists moving out front, Walgreens boosts role of technicians. June 10, 2013. Available at: http://www.drugstorenews.com/article/its-pharmacists-moving-out-front-walgreens-boosts-role-technicians. Accessed May 5, 2017.
31. Consumer Healthcare Products Association. Research by IRI sourced for CHPA's OTC 101 Seminar. October 2015.
32. Consumer Healthcare Products Association. *Your Health at Hand Book: Guide to OTC Active Ingredients in the United States.* April 2011. Available at: http://www.chpa.org/Templates/search.aspx?searchText=your+health+at+hand. Accessed May 5, 2017.
33. Council for Responsible Nutrition. The dietary supplement consumer. 2015 CRN consumer survey on dietary supplements. Available at: http://www.crnusa.org/CRNconsumersurvey/2015/. Accessed May 5, 2017.
34. New Hope Network. 2015 NBJ Supplement Business Report: A Tough Year for Supplements by the Numbers. June 1, 2015. Available at: http://www.newhope.com/managing-your-business/2015-nbj-supplement-business-report-tough-year-supplements-numbers. Accessed May 5, 2017.
35. U.S. Department of Health and Human Services, National Institutes of Health, National Center for Complementary and Integrative Health. Use of complementary health approaches in the U.S.: what complementary and integrative approaches do Americans use? Key findings from the 2012 National Health Interview Survey. Available at: http://nccih.nih.gov/research/statistics/NHIS/2012/key-findings. Accessed May 5, 2017.
36. Boy Scouts of America. What is the SCOUTStrong Be MedWise Award? 2017. Available at: http://www.scouting.org/Home/BSAFit/MedWise_Award.aspx. Accessed May 5, 2017.
37. Up and Away. Put your medicines up and Away and Out of Sight. Available at: http://www.upandaway.org. Accessed May 5, 2017.
38. Lovegrove MC, Weidle NJ, Budnitz DS. Trends in emergency department visits for unsupervised pediatric medication exposures, 2004–2015 *Pediatrics.* 2015 Oct; 136(4):e821–9. doi: 10.1542/peds.2015-2092.
39. Know Your Dose.org, Acetaminophen Awareness Coalition. About acetaminophen. Available at: http://www.knowyourdose.org/. Accessed May 5, 2017.
40. Reynolds KM, Tran AD, Kile DA, et al. *Over-the-Counter (OTC) Acetaminophen Fixed Combination Product Exposures and Case Exposure Rates in Adults Reported to United States Poison Centers (2007–2013).* Alexandria, VA: American Association of Poison Control Centers; 2015.
41. American Pharmacists Association. APhA-ASP OTC Medicine Safety. Available at: http://www.pharmacist.com/apha-asp-otc-medicine-safety. Accessed May 5, 2017.
42. Pew Research Center, Katherine Zickhur, Aaron Smith. Home broadband 2013. Available at: http://www.pewinternet.org/2013/08/26/home-broadband-2013. Accessed May 5, 2017.
43. Pew Research Center, Aaron Smith. Smartphone ownership 2013. Available at: http://www.pewinternet.org/2013/06/05/smartphone-ownership-2013. Accessed May 5, 2017.
44. Daniel Kraft. Medicine's future? There's an app for that. April 2011. Available at: https://www.ted.com/talks/daniel_kraft_medicine_s_future?language=en. Accessed May 5, 2017.
45. American Pharmacists Association. *Practice Insights: Pharmacists as Self-Care Advisors.* Washington, DC: American Pharmacists Association; December 2015. Available at: http://media.pharmacist.com/practice/Practice_Insights_111715.pdf. Accessed May 5, 2017.
46. Briggs G, Freeman R, Yaffee S. *Drugs in Pregnancy and Lactation: A Reference Guide to Fetal and Neonatal Risk.* 9th ed. Philadelphia: Lippincott Williams & Wilkins; 2011.
47. Qato DM, Wilder J, Schumm LP, et al. Changes in prescription and over-the-counter medication and dietary supplement use among older adults in the United States, 2005 vs 2011. *JAMA Intern Med.* 2016;176 (4):473–82. doi: 10.1001/jamainternmed.2015.8581.
48. American Geriatrics Society 2015 Beers Criteria Update Expert Panel. American Geriatrics Society 2015 updated Beers Criteria for potentially inappropriate medication use in older adults. *J Am Geriatr Soc.* 2015;63(11):2227–46. doi: 10.1111/jgs.13702.
49. Gooch K, Culleton B, Manns B, et al. NSAID use and progression of chronic kidney disease. *Am J Med.* 2006;120(3): 280.e1–280.e7. Available at: http://dx.doi.org/10.1016/j.amjmed.2006.02.015. Accessed May 5, 2017.

CHAPTER 2

PHARMACISTS' PATIENT CARE PROCESS IN SELF-CARE

HOLLY DIVINE AND TERA McINTOSH

Pharmacists, and student pharmacists with appropriate supervision and mentoring, can play a valuable role in ensuring medications are used safely and effectively in patients seeking self-care. Although *self-care*, by definition, is treating one's self without accessing professional assistance, inappropriate, ineffective, or unsafe treatment selections can occur when patients are self-medicating, as previously discussed in Chapter 1. The pharmacist can assist patients by identifying their problem, selecting appropriate therapy, and referring them to other health care providers, as needed. The pharmacist's involvement in self-care may also avert medication safety problems, such as drug interactions or adverse drug reactions (see Chapter 1).[1–3] Community pharmacists currently have an active role in counseling patients about nonprescription medications and strongly believe that making nonprescription recommendations is an important part of community practice.[4,5]

The profession of pharmacy continues to evolve from a primary focus on medication distribution to more advanced clinical decision making. As a result, the use of a systematic method or process to arrive at such decisions is desirable.[6,7] The use of a standardized process helps pharmacists provide consistent services to patients, including in self-care encounters.[8]

The pharmaceutical care model originally developed by Hepler and Strand in the 1990s is one of the original systematic blueprints for pharmacists.[9] Other methods and approaches to providing pharmaceutical care, patient assessment, and medication therapy management have been developed, expanded, and used throughout the years; however, the types and levels of pharmacist-provided services vary between these models.[10–14] This variation resulted in the individual pharmacist needing to determine the best model to use in a given situation. In 2014, the Joint Commission of Pharmacy Practitioners (JCPP) released the Pharmacists' Patient Care Process (PPCP), a contemporary, consistent, and comprehensive process. The PPCP is applicable to all areas of pharmacy practice and is built on previous approaches to care.[8] Although this chapter guides the pharmacist on the use of the profession's uniform process to manage a patient's self-care disorders, other health care professionals would use their discipline-specific process to resolve a patient's self-care concern.

Editor's Note: This chapter is based on the 18th edition chapter titled "Patient Assessment and Consultation," written by Gail D. Newton and Holly Divine.

Pharmacists' Patient Care Process

JCPP adopted a vision statement in November 2013 for pharmacists' practice that states "patients achieve optimal health and medication outcomes with pharmacists as essential and accountable providers within patient-centered, team-based healthcare."[15] The need for a uniform patient care process arose as an essential component toward achieving this vision of pharmacists' practice.[8]

The PPCP resulted from a unified pharmacy effort, supported by 13 national pharmacy organizations. It has been incorporated into Key Element 10.8 of the Accreditation Council for Pharmacy Education Standards 2016,[16] thus ensuring that a consistent process is also taught to student pharmacists. Implementation of the process into current practice settings is occurring through strategies that include, but are not limited to, the Pharmacy Health Information Technology Collaborative; the American Society of Health-System Pharmacists Accreditation Standards for Postgraduate Year One residency programs; and other various training programs, projects, and outreach activities.[8]

The PPCP is grounded in a patient-centered care approach that "is applicable to any practice setting where pharmacists provide patient care and for any patient care service provided by pharmacists."[8] For example, this process is just as applicable for the pharmacist working in a community-based or clinic-based ambulatory care setting as it is for someone working in an acute care health system. Similarly, this same process should be used when pharmacists provide patient care in a self-care encounter in a community pharmacy. The differences lie with the level of intensity in each step of the process based on the service provided.[8]

The five core components of the PPCP revolve around patient-centered care and the pharmacists' continual collaboration, documentation, and communication with physicians, other pharmacists, and other health care professionals (see Color Plates, photograph 5).[8] These five components are

1. Collect
2. Assess
3. Plan
4. Implement
5. Follow-up: Monitor and Evaluate

PPCP in Self-Care: The Five Steps

Other available resources provide details about each key component and their implementation in patient care services.[17] The following section provides a brief summary of the five areas and further emphasize how to implement the steps with a focus on self-care encounters. Examples of how to apply PPCP steps in specific self-care encounters are provided. These examples are intended to be snapshots of the entire patient encounter and are not comprehensive. Diverse patient-specific factors may result in an assessment or plan for that patient, disorder, or symptom that differs from what this chapter demonstrates. The specific disorder chapters in this book are referenced with examples for the health care provider to fully research the disorder before engaging in a patient encounter. Where applicable, Cases 2–1 through 2–4 are referenced throughout as examples of how to use the PPCP in self-care encounters; therefore, the cases are grouped at the end of the chapter.

Collect

"The pharmacist assures the collection of the necessary subjective and objective information about the patient in order to understand the relevant medical/medication history and clinical status of the patient."[8]

Self-care encounters in community pharmacies are generally initiated in one of two ways: either the patient or caregiver approaches or contacts the pharmacist, or the pharmacist observes the patient or caregiver in the nonprescription aisle and offers assistance.[18] One survey reported patients initiate the encounter 87% of the time.[19] In either situation, the pharmacist must then engage the patient in this first step of the process by collecting essential information to begin resolving the self-care complaint.

Collection of information from the patient or caregiver can be accomplished through the patient interview (subjective data) and from medical and pharmacy records, direct observation, laboratory test results, and physical assessment (objective data).[20] Subjective data are generally supplied by the patient or caregiver and may not always be accurate or reproducible. Conversely, objective data can be measured or observed and are not influenced by prejudice or emotion.[21]

A comprehensive patient interview would include the following components of the patient's health history[18,20]:

- Chief complaint (CC)
- History of present illness (HPI)
- Past medical history (PMH)
- Health maintenance and immunizations
- Family history (FH)
- Personal and social history (SH)
- Review of systems (ROS) and physical examination (PE)
- Medication history

Although most information in a self-care encounter will be subjective data obtained through the patient interview, objective data may need to be collected. Depending on the presenting situation, physical assessment skills may be employed, such as measuring a blood pressure or taking a temperature. Patients who present with a dermatologic disorder will require PE of the skin. Case 2–1 documents the pharmacist's PE of the affected area under "Characteristics" to assess the medical condition of the reported bee sting. Physical assessment techniques that apply to specific disorders are highlighted in chapter texts and/or tables in subsequent chapters of this book.

The amount and type of information collected for a self-care encounter will be different from other patient care services that involve a greater breadth and depth of care and likely will not require all areas of the health history or full physical assessment.[17] For example, a patient who inquires about nonprescription therapy for sunburn relief may not require that the pharmacist collect the FH, but may need to include the CC, HPI, and PMH, in addition to physically observing the area of concern on the patient's skin (see Chapter 41). Alternatively, identifying an FH of colon cancer would be an important part of the history to collect in a patient who is inquiring about self-care for an anorectal disorder (see Chapter 17). It will be the responsibility of the pharmacist to determine which factors are pertinent to collect in each specific self-care situation. This requires knowledge of various self-care disorders, and subsequent chapters in this book provide a resource for the pharmacist on types of information to collect for specific self-care disorders.[18]

The PPCP explicitly identifies patient-centered factors for which data should be collected. These are patient lifestyle habits, preferences and beliefs, health and functional goals, and socioeconomic factors. Some subsequent chapters in this book have sections titled "Patient Factors" and "Patient Preferences," which focus on the patient-centered areas for which data should be collected and addressed as a part of the developing plan for that specific disorder. Additionally, Chapter 3 goes into further detail about the pharmacist developing cultural competency in self-care and addresses several key areas of the collection step, including but not limited to, cultural beliefs, literacy, and health literacy.

Professionalism, interview proficiency, and interpersonal and communication skills are essential in obtaining effective subjective information.[17] Conducting an efficient patient interview is a skill that develops with practice over time and involves asking appropriate questions and actively listening to the patient.[18] Communication skills are the foundation of many parts of the PPCP and will be discussed in a later section.

Assess

"The pharmacist assesses the information collected and analyzes the clinical effects of the patient's therapy in the context of the patient's overall health goals in order to identify and prioritize problems and achieve optimal care."[8]

The second step involves the assessment and analysis of information collected to identify and prioritize the patient's problem(s).[17] The assess step can be categorized into three areas: (1) medication assessment, (2) patient history and risk assessment, and (3) preventive care assessment.[17] Similar to the collect step, assessing the patient's information may be more focused during a self-care encounter than during a comprehensive medication review. Additionally, it may or may not involve all three of these categories of assessment.

Medication Assessment

Comprehensive medication assessment involves the analysis of each medication for appropriateness, effectiveness, safety, and adherence.[8] Further assessment of medications includes identification and prioritization of drug therapy problems: unnecessary drug therapy, needs additional drug therapy, ineffective drug, dosage too low, adverse drug reaction, dosage too high, and adherence.[22] The term *drug therapy problems* was originally defined in the pharmaceutical care model and has since been rephrased as *medication therapy problems* or *medication-related problems.*[22] In the PPCP, the term *medication-related problems* is used. In a self-care encounter, the most likely medication-related problem is "needs additional drug therapy," as patients are presenting with the intent to purchase a self-care medication to treat a disorder and may require a nonprescription medication for resolution. Other medication-related problems in self-care include but are not limited to "ineffective drug," if a patient is using a self-care medication that is ineffective or is not producing the desired response, or "adverse drug reaction," if the patient is attempting to provide self-care for a disorder or symptom that is the result of another medication. The pharmacist's role in the medication assessment step in self-care is to use the information collected to make appropriate medication recommendations or changes to the medication care plan.[17]

In contrast to a comprehensive medication review during which a pharmacist performs an assessment of all medications the patient is currently taking for appropriateness, effectiveness, safety, and adherence, a self-care encounter is more consistent with a targeted medication review. Generally, self-care encounters require quick assessments because of the nature of their initiation. They may be initiated in an aisle outside the pharmacy, over the telephone by a patient or caregiver, or at the point-of-sale where the pharmacist and the patient have limited time. Time limitations do not excuse the pharmacist from his or her responsibilities in assessing medications, particularly for safety and efficacy. However, in self-care encounters, the assess step in the PPCP can be modified to a more focused approach.

Although the self-care encounter may not include a comprehensive medication review, the pharmacist may have compelling reasons to consider all current medications before making a recommendation. For example, if a patient presents with musculoskeletal pain and the pharmacist is considering a recommendation for a nonsteroidal anti-inflammatory drug (NSAID), the pharmacist should collect information from the patient's profile and interview regarding current NSAID use to assess for duplicate therapy as well as any medications that may potentially cause a drug–drug interaction or drug–disease interaction (see Chapter 7).

Another example of a more focused approach in self-care is assessing the cause of the patient's presenting medical condition or symptom as a potential medication-related problem. If a patient presents with dyspepsia, it would be appropriate to assess the patient's current medication profile to determine whether a current medication is causing an adverse effect, such as the addition of a recent antibiotic to the patient's regimen (see Chapter 13).

Patient History and Risk Assessment

The patient history and risk assessment includes health and functional status, risk factors, health data, cultural factors, health literacy, and access to medications or other aspects of care that would influence decisions on optimal medication regimens for the patient.[8,17] In certain self-care disorders, the collection of key information about the patient's health history, such as health and functional status, could lead the pharmacist to a completely different assessment. The pharmacist should determine whether a patient's disease state could be causing or contributing to the presenting self-care symptom or disorder. For example, if a patient has congestive heart failure (CHF) and is seeking self-care for the relief of a cough, the assessment would be an exclusion for self-care (see Chapter 12). The patient may be experiencing an exacerbation of CHF that requires medical attention beyond that of self-care. Case 2–2 demonstrates how collection of information about the patient's chronic disorder affects the assessment.

Health literacy is an important consideration to ensure patient-centered care is provided (see Chapter 1). Health literacy is defined as "the degree to which individuals have the capacity to obtain, process, and understand basic health information and services needed to make appropriate health decisions."[23] Although validated tools are available to assess health literacy, they may not be feasible to implement in each self-care encounter.[24] An alternative approach is to apply health literacy universal precautions, which assumes that all patients may have difficulty comprehending health information and accessing services.[25] The pharmacist should communicate clearly with everyone involved in the care of the patient and confirm that the patient understands the recommendations.

Cultural factors and health beliefs must be considered in the self-care assessment (see Chapter 3). Health beliefs constitute an array of patient opinions, including ideas about what causes illness and how to treat or prevent it.[26] These beliefs vary in individuals and are greatly influenced by culture. This may influence the kind of treatment a patient prefers, such as conventional nonprescription medications or complementary and alternative products. If a patient preference is identified, the pharmacist can tailor the plan to meet the patient's needs.

Preventive Care Assessment

Preventive care assessment is an important part of the comprehensive assessment of a patient in the PPCP.[8,17] In a self-care encounter, the pharmacist may focus the preventive care assessment on only the presenting disorder or problem. For example, if a patient presents seeking relief from the pain of sunburn, the pharmacist may assess the need for future sunburn prevention and recommend a preventive plan that includes a sunscreen (see Chapter 39). Other opportunities in preventive care assessment should be used, when appropriate. For example, if a patient presents during influenza season, the pharmacist should assess the patient's influenza immunization status.

Exclusions for Self-Treatment

A unique component of PPCP in self-care is the assessment of appropriateness for self-treatment. Within the process, pharmacists should collect the pertinent information for the disorder or problem that would lead to an assessment of "inappropriate for self-treatment." If the pharmacist determines the patient is not a candidate for self-treatment, the medication-related problem may be that the patient "needs additional drug therapy," but the therapy requires an assessment from another health care provider, resulting in treatment with a prescription medication. Another medication-related problem that may result from an exclusion for self-care is "no drug therapy problem exists." If a patient presents with a disorder or injury that requires medical treatment or a procedure from another health care provider as opposed to medication therapy, the patient may not have a medication-related problem to resolve.[22] Exclusions for self-treatment may include but are not limited to the following situations:

- Symptom characteristics or other disorder factors are beyond the scope of self-treatment.
  - Example: Patient presents with symptoms of headache that have persisted for 10 days (see Chapter 5).
- Patient-specific factors preclude treatment with nonprescription medications.
  - Example: For an 8-year-old child with water-clogged ears, nonprescription pharmacologic therapy is not indicated, because he or she is younger than 12 years (see Chapter 30).

- The patient's health status or history precludes self-treatment, even if a nonprescription medication is indicated for the disorder.
  - Example: A pregnant patient presents with heartburn symptoms that have not been previously assessed and diagnosed by another health care provider (see Chapter 13).
- Nonprescription medications are not indicated for the disorder.
  - Example: A patient presents for "bug bites," but lesions have characteristics of scabies, which requires prescription therapy (see Chapter 37).
- Previous treatment with nonprescription medications was ineffective after an adequate trial.
  - Example: Heartburn symptoms persist after 2 weeks of treatment with a nonprescription proton pump inhibitor (see Chapter 13).

The pharmacist is responsible for knowing exclusions for self-treatment for presenting disorders or symptoms and collecting appropriate information that may result in this assessment. In most subsequent chapters, exclusions for self-treatment of one or more disorders are included in text discussion and algorithm(s). Cases 2–2 and 2–3 provide examples of patients who have exclusions for self-treatment.

Plan

"The pharmacist develops an individualized patient-centered care plan, in collaboration with other health care professionals and the patient or caregiver that is evidence-based and cost-effective."[8]

The self-care plan in the patient care process uses the information collected and assessed and will culminate in one of three general recommendations: (1) recommend self-care with pharmacologic, nonpharmacologic, and/or complementary/alternative products; (2) refer the patient to another health care provider for treatment; or (3) recommend self-care until another health care provider can be consulted. The detailed components within the plan should address four key areas: medication-related problems, goals of therapy, patient engagement, and care continuity in collaboration with other health care professionals and the patient or caregiver.[8]

Medication-Related Problems

The plan for the first key area, medication-related problems, generally results in the pharmacist recommending a therapeutic product, such as a nonprescription medication, to resolve the "needs additional drug therapy" problem. Pharmacists should use their knowledge of the medication properties and determine the safest and most cost-effective option while considering all the factors collected from the patient in the first step. These patient-specific and therapy-specific factors include but are not limited to age, gender, medication history, medical conditions, allergies, ingredients, adverse effects, potential drug interactions, and efficacy. The recommendation should also be patient-centered, taking into account, at minimum, patient preferences for dosage forms and dosing regimens, cost, flavors, and previous medication experience. The Drug Facts label on Food and Drug Administration (FDA)-approved nonprescription medications, further described in Chapter 4, includes essential information that should be shared as part of the plan, including uses, warnings, when to use the product, and usage directions, and that should be reviewed with the patient when making the recommendation.

Goals of Therapy

Establishing goals of therapy has been a mainstay of the original pharmaceutical care process and remains central to the plan in PPCP.[8,27] Goals of therapy serve as endpoints to measure outcomes and include both practitioner and patient contributions. They should be realistic, observable, and measurable, and they should contain three components: clinical parameters (signs and symptoms) and/or laboratory values; a desired value or observable change in the parameter; and a specific time frame in which the goal is to be met.[27]

Clinical parameters should include evidence-based guidelines or standards, when available, such as a specific blood pressure measurement for hypertension. In self-care encounters, the clinical parameter is likely to focus on resolution of the presenting sign or symptom, such as "alleviate the discomfort associated with fever" when an antipyretic is recommended (see Chapter 6). Alternatively, the clinical parameter may be a preventive measure. For example, in a patient who presents with vomiting and diarrhea, an oral rehydration solution may not be recommended only to restore hydration status, but also to prevent the progression to severe dehydration (see Chapter 16).

In setting the clinical parameter, the desired value or change in the parameter should also be addressed. The patient should understand if the goal of therapy includes complete resolution of the presenting symptom, a reduction of the symptom, or partial relief. In the fever example, this portion of the goal might be to "*completely* alleviate the symptoms of discomfort associated with fever." The patient-centered perspective may help determine the value of this goal. The patient may be seeking elimination of pain as opposed to pain reduction. Cipolle, Strand, and Morley propose three questions to help establish patient-centered goals[27]:

- What would you like to achieve with your medications?
- What are your goals for this therapy?
- How do you feel about trying to achieve . . . with a new drug therapy?

Finally, the time frame in which the goal is to be met is a critical piece of the self-care plan. Patients should understand how quickly the goal is achieved. Returning to the fever example, the complete goal of therapy including the time frame may be "the patient's discomfort associated with fever will be completely eliminated within 2 hours." The pharmacist should establish the time frame using disorder-specific factors, such as medication onsets and duration of action and appropriate length of time for self-treatment, and patient-specific factors, such as the patient's expectations for symptom relief. Setting a time frame establishes clear expectations. Case 2–4 demonstrates the goal of therapy (see step 8d, "expected time to onset of relief" and step 8e, "degree of relief that can be reasonably expected").

Patient Engagement

Engaging the patient in the plan step involves "education, empowerment, and self-management."[8] Because the patient is presenting with the intent of self-treating the disorder, this portion of the process is essential in the self-care encounter. Every self-care encounter in which the pharmacist provides care should include educating the patient on the presenting disorder, nonpharmacologic measures, nonprescription medications, and when to seek medical attention.

Subsequent chapters that cover disorders include a box that specifically addresses appropriate patient education for the discussed disorder.

The pharmacist needs to identify the medication-specific information that should be communicated to the patient by reviewing and highlighting information on the Drug Facts label in addition to any other medication-related instruction for successful use and therapeutic outcomes. A key part to an effective plan is communicating the goal of therapy and empowering the patient by including him or her in patient-centered goal setting to ensure patient expectations align with the pharmacist's recommendation.

Finally, education on nonpharmacologic recommendations should be identified in the plan. Patients should be educated on nonpharmacologic therapy (which includes nondrug measures, lifestyle recommendations, and preventive measures) for their disorders along with the nonprescription medication education. When a nonpharmacologic therapy is the only recommendation, they should also be counseled on why that was preferable to a nonprescription medication. One example may be a patient who is experiencing insomnia caused by stimulant use, such as caffeine. The most appropriate recommendation may be to discontinue or reduce the stimulant, particularly in late evenings; education on good sleep hygiene should also be provided (see Chapter 46). Furthermore, communicating with the patient regarding the potential risk versus benefit of nonpharmacologic measures for certain disorders may be helpful in acceptance of the nondrug plan.

Care Continuity

Finally, the plan should include care continuity, which involves follow-up, referral, and transitions of care.[8,17] The initial follow-up plan is based on the goal of therapy and advises the patient of what to do once that goal is met, what should occur if the goal is not met, and what steps to take if the patient's condition worsens or the patient experiences an adverse effect. It should include the specific course of action to be taken and when that action is to be taken. The course of action may be a return to the pharmacist for further assessment, selection of a different nonprescription medication therapy, or referral to another health care professional, and should explicitly identify when that action is to be performed. If the patient has multiple goals of therapy, the follow-up plan should address each goal.

To further conceptualize the parts of the follow-up plan that should be addressed by the pharmacist in a self-care encounter, a series of questions is provided for consideration. Using a heartburn encounter as an example, specific follow-up plans addressed to the patient are suggested in response to each question. Note that in the following example, the pharmacist does not have a complete case with all the patient-specific factors, and the example is not intended to serve as a plan for the management of all patients with heartburn. The follow-up plan will not be the same for each patient who presents with heartburn symptoms, and the pharmacist should refer to the disorder-specific chapter for more information. Many factors, which are specific to the presenting disorder, should be considered in developing the follow-up plan. The pharmacist's responsibility is to know the disorder and self-care limitations that would lead to a specific follow-up plan, including but not limited to FDA-approved length of therapy for use of a nonprescription medication for self-care; common adverse effects associated with a nonprescription medication; developing or worsening symptoms that would lead to an exclusion for self-care, necessitating a medical referral; and appropriate stepwise use of an alternative nonprescription medication for efficacy. In case of suspected heartburn (see Chapter 13), the following factors should be considered:

- When should the patient expect results (i.e., clinical outcomes)? This is communicated in the goal of therapy.
  - "Your heartburn symptoms should be completely gone within 10 minutes after taking the antacid."
- What should the patient do if the goal of therapy is not met? For example, complete resolution of symptoms was the goal, but the time frame identified in the goal of therapy has passed and the patient saw no results or only partial results. Options include the following:
  - A return visit to the pharmacist.
    - "If your symptoms aren't completely gone within 10 minutes, contact the pharmacist to help you select a different medication."
  - Selection of a different nonprescription medication.
    - "If your symptoms aren't gone within 10 minutes, discontinue the antacid and begin omeprazole 20 mg once daily."
  - Referral to primary care provider.
    - "If your symptoms aren't gone within 10 minutes, call your primary care provider for an appointment."
- How long should the disorder be treated by self-care before further assessment is warranted by another health care provider (i.e., referral)?
  - "If heartburn symptoms return after taking omeprazole for 14 days, like we discussed, call your primary care provider for an appointment."
- What should the patient do if he or she experiences an adverse drug reaction?
  - "If you develop diarrhea while taking omeprazole, stop taking the drug and call your primary care provider for an appointment."
- What should the patient do if he or she experiences a worsening of his or her condition during the treatment?
  - "If heartburn symptoms get worse or occur more often while taking this medication, call your primary care provider for an appointment."

The pharmacist has the responsibility of identifying exclusions for self-care in the assess step; therefore, the plan may not include any pharmacologic or nonpharmacologic recommendations. The plan may simply be referral to another health care provider. Little is known about how often a pharmacist makes a medical referral in self-care consultations; however, one study identified a medical referral was made in 4.3% of encounters.[1] Cases 2–2 and 2–3 provide examples of medical referrals.

Another unique component of self-care encounters is to recommend self-care until another health care provider can be consulted. The pharmacist may assess the patient and realize referral to another health care provider is warranted. If the situation is not urgent, however, the pharmacist may consider recommending self-care, pharmacologic or nonpharmacologic, while simultaneously referring the patient. For example, a pediatric patient presents with moderate dehydration, but after assessing and taking into consideration patient-specific factors, the pharmacist has concerns that the parent or caregiver may not be successful in preventing further dehydration using an oral rehydration solution. The pharmacist may recommend that the patient see a primary care provider for the disorder while also recommending an oral rehydration solution to attempt to slow the progression to severe dehydration while waiting to see the primary care provider (see Chapter 16). The risk in making a recommendation while waiting for another health care provider consultation is that the patient may ignore the referral and take only the self-care recommendation. The pharmacist must be precise about the referral to ensure the patient understands it (the referral) is the primary recommendation. To avoid patient denial and avoid confusion, the pharmacist should provide explicit instructions, such as, "Contact your primary care provider today and make an appointment. Ask for an appointment today or tomorrow morning, at the latest. In the meantime, use this oral rehydration solution as directed to help alleviate some of your symptoms. This will likely not be enough to prevent serious complications, so do not delay in contacting your primary care provider today."[28] Follow-up with these patients is especially important to ensure that the situation has been properly addressed. Case 2–2 requires a plan for referral because of an exclusion for self-care. Some nonpharmacologic measures, however, are communicated in the case until the patient can see his primary care provider.

Implement

"The pharmacist implements the care plan in collaboration with other health care professionals and the patient or caregiver."[8]

The implement step in PPCP is execution of the developed plan. Of the four main areas in the previous discussion of the plan step, implementation of the first area, "Medication-Related Problems," would include selecting the recommended nonprescription medication from the pharmacy nonprescription section and presenting it to the patient. A full implementation step for self-care would not include sending the patient to the respective aisle number to obtain the product by him- or herself. Implementation also includes communicating the "Goals of Therapy" that were established in the plan.

In the "Patient Engagement" part of the plan, all the pharmacologic and nonpharmacologic educational points were established, and the implementation step is the actual provision of the education to the patient or caregiver. As with the collection step of the process, effective communication skills are required, taking into account health information collected from the initial assessment. In addition to health literacy, patients with low literacy may have difficulties comprehending information on the Drug Facts label and may require additional counseling time to ensure they understand. Using various communication methods, including but not limited to the teach-back method, may confirm that a patient understands the information. The teach-back method involves explaining the information, asking the patient to repeat key points, asking the patient to discuss the information, and actively listening to ensure understanding.[29] Asking patients to repeat back the treatment information provided and giving them easy-to-read patient-centered printed instructions have been shown to improve patient understanding and medication use.[30] Essential communication components are discussed in the "Communicate" section of this chapter.

For "Care Continuity," all the follow-up components to the plan should be communicated to the patient. If one of the follow-up plans includes returning to the pharmacist in a specified time frame, the patient should be provided a specific day or date that the pharmacist will be available for the follow-up visit. Community pharmacists may have various shifts and schedules, so fully implementing the follow-up plan includes information on the pharmacist's availability or the creation of an appointment. Follow-up encounters other than face-to-face meetings may be arranged, when appropriate, using telephone or other communication technologies such as email.

In self-care, implementation may involve a referral to the appropriate health care provider or facility. The pharmacist may contact a patient's primary care provider to communicate patient-specific information obtained during the self-care encounter to facilitate the reason for referral. For patients who do not have a primary care provider, the pharmacist may be integral in connecting the patient to a primary care home or urgent/convenient care facility until a primary care provider can be established. In extreme cases, the pharmacist may call 911 in a medical emergency.

Follow-up: Monitor and Evaluate

"The pharmacist monitors and evaluates the effectiveness of the care plan and modifies the plan in collaboration with other health care professionals and the patient or caregiver as needed."[8]

Follow-up "brings the pharmacist full circle in the ongoing monitoring of the patient."[17] Follow-up may not routinely occur in current self-care encounters, and little is known about the pharmacist's role or outcomes in this area. Some literature suggests that patients may be willing to have a follow-up service for self-care encounters.[2] However, because of the self-limiting nature of most presenting disorders, the pharmacist may not be included in the follow-up plan. For example, if the patient's goal of therapy and follow-up plan included full relief of symptoms within 4 hours and resolution of the disorder within 10 days, and the goal was met, no further follow-up with the pharmacist may be warranted. Similarly, in follow-up plans that include a referral to the primary care provider if the patient's symptoms worsen or do not resolve, the follow-up step may not occur with the pharmacist.

If, however, the follow-up plan includes a return visit to the pharmacist after an identified time frame, the pharmacist should begin the PPCP again by collecting new information and reassessing the patient's condition. The patient's goal of therapy should be reviewed for achievement, as well as an assessment of any new medication-related problems related to the recommended nonprescription medication: appropriateness, efficacy, safety, and adherence. Adherence to recommended therapy should specifically be addressed in the follow-up to determine its contribution to the success of the intended outcome.

The pharmacist's role in a follow-up encounter with the patient after medical referral can be challenging. A patient seeking self-care may not be an established patient at the pharmacy or with the pharmacist. He or she may simply be seeking a consultation for the first time as a walk-in patient. Without a strong pharmacist–patient relationship, the logistics of following up with the patient to determine the outcome of the referral are difficult. The pharmacist may not have the essential demographic information often maintained in pharmacy records for these one-time encounters. For an established patient, following up with the patient to inquire about the outcome of the referral brings closure to the entire PPCP. Future developments in transitions of care for established patients may help close the loop in the process if pharmacists receive discharge information from the health system for patients who have been referred.

PPCP in Self-care: The Core

The PPCP has patient-centered care at its core with continual collaboration, communication, and documentation of care with other health care providers (see Color Plates, photograph 5).[8] Developing the pharmacist–patient relationship helps establish engagement and effective communication with patients and/or caregivers to ensure the process remains patient centered. The following sections further describe each of these core areas with an emphasis on implementing these areas in the self-care encounter.

Patient-Centered Care

Patient-centered care, according to the Institute of Medicine (IOM), is defined as "providing care that is respectful of and responsive to individual patient preferences, needs, and values, and ensuring that patient values guide all clinical decisions."[31] The IOM describes patient-centered care in greater detail in their 2001 report, *Crossing the Quality Chasm: A New Health System for the 21st Century.*" In a self-care encounter, there are many opportunities to center the process around the patient.

The pharmacist must listen to the wants and needs of the patient when collecting information. Careful consideration must be given to ensure relevant patient factors are obtained in order to arrive at an assessment and plan that is truly patient-centered. Lifestyle habits, preferences, and beliefs, as previously described in the five steps, are all important patient-centered collection areas.

Establishing goals of therapy must include the patient's input. Understanding the patient's expectations of the desired outcome and time frame must be carefully considered in developing the plan. Furthermore, patient-centered implementation of the plan involves using collected patient factors regarding literacy, health literacy, and physical functions such as vision or hearing status to tailor the education and counseling to the patient's specific needs.

An additional patient-centered area for consideration is the patient's medication experience. The patient's medication experience is "the sum of all the events a patient has in his [or her] lifetime that involved drug therapy. This is the patient's personal experience with medications. This lived experience shapes his attitudes, beliefs, and preferences about drug therapy."[32] In a brief self-care encounter, the pharmacist may focus on the patient's personal experience with nonprescription medications or specific experiences with a certain self-care disorder. For example, if a patient expresses that he or she is afraid to take a particular nonprescription medication because a family member had a bad experience with that drug, the patient's concerns about drug safety must be recognized and addressed.[32]

Collaborate

Collaboration involves working together to achieve a common goal. In self-care, collaboration occurs most often with patients and/or caregivers to ensure the process is patient-centered and optimal outcomes are achieved. Collaboration with other health care providers is less common in self-care encounters; however, it is essential when referrals are required or more information is needed for safe and effective self-care recommendations.

Communicate

Although communication in the PPCP involves communicating with both providers and patients, most of the communication will be with patients in self-care encounters. Good communication skills are essential in all pharmacist interactions with patients and are not unique to self-care.

Fundamental communication skills, such as active listening and demonstrating empathy, must be mastered in collecting information.[18,33] Active listening requires concentration and a focused effort to minimize external and internal distractions. Empathetic responses are a result of listening, and it is through empathetic response that patients feel understood.[33] Other essential communication skills include asking open-ended questions; avoiding leading questions; being aware of nonverbal communication, such as tone of voice or facial expressions; and using the teach-back method.[18,33]

Pharmacists need to be aware of communication challenges, including but not limited to vision and hearing loss, language barriers, literacy, and health literacy, and to know how to address these challenges. Pharmacists' assumptions in resolving communication challenges are not always appropriate. For example, pharmacists should ask patients who are deaf or hard of hearing about their preferred method of communication, which may be written notes, lip reading, or the use of an interpreter, and should not assume the same communication method applies in every patient.

Maintaining patient privacy in communications for self-care encounters must be carefully regarded, especially considering that the encounter initiation may occur in an open area of the pharmacy where nonprescription medications are located. Additionally, many self-care disorders include sensitive issues or topics that may be difficult or embarrassing for the patient to discuss, including but not limited to anorectal disorders, vaginal and vulvovaginal disorders, and prevention of pregnancy and sexually transmitted infections. Pharmacists must ensure the consultation occurs at the appropriate place. Choosing a private area that minimizes interruption and provides a safe place for the patient to discuss the condition of his or her health is ideal. Being aware of the volume of the conversation to maintain confidentiality is important. Using the foundational skills of active listening and empathy further contribute to developing a trusting relationship that is needed for discussion of sensitive topics.[34]

Document

Documenting pharmacist–patient encounters is an essential part of the PPCP. Documentation demonstrates the pharmacist's contributions to care, ensures continuity of care, provides legal evidence for professional liability, and contributes to billing and reimbursement needs. For these important reasons, pharmacists should document self-care encounters.

Documentation methods in community pharmacy vary. One survey revealed that community pharmacists who currently document patient care services use both paper (54%) and computerized (42%) documentation systems; however, little is known about documentation of self-care encounters.[35] Some sample paper documentation forms have been published and may serve as useful tools.[28,36] Additionally, pharmacy management systems, typically designed for prescription medication use, may have features that provide a venue for self-care documentation. Improved health information technology systems that fully integrate the PPCP steps may improve self-care documentation in community pharmacy.[37] Patient data and health information documented in a self-care encounter would be considered private information and protected under the Health Insurance Portability and Accountability Act (HIPAA).

Efficient Use of PPCP in Self-Care

Efficiency in the PPCP is imperative in a community pharmacy. Self-care encounters are generally not compensated outside the sale of the product; thus, the pharmacist is faced with a time management decision.[38] Pharmacists specifically identify lack of time as a barrier to their involvement in resolving self-care needs in community pharmacies because of their responsibilities in medication distribution.[5] The time pharmacists actually spend with patients or their perception of patients' time expectations for the entire self-care interaction is in the range of 2–6 minutes.[1,19,36,39]

Patients also report an expectation that encounters are brief, indicating a willingness to spend 1–5 minutes for a nonprescription consultation.[40]

Although time constraints are a reality in community practice, professional responsibilities lie with patient care, which includes all steps of the PPCP, from collecting all pertinent information to appropriately assessing the patient and completing, communicating, and implementing the plan.[18] The previous section provides a comprehensive overview of the PPCP, outlining each step within the process and the multiple components of each step. In the overview, it has been noted at each step where modifications may occur for patient care services in self-care encounters.

Tools, mechanisms, and mnemonics have been used in patient assessment in multidisciplinary health care professions for many years.[20,41,42] Some mnemonics developed and used by pharmacists during assessments have been validated and demonstrate improved assessment skills when implemented.[43,44]

TABLE 2–1 QuEST/SCHOLAR-MAC and PPCP

QuEST/SCHOLAR-MAC Components	Pharmacists' Patient Care Process Steps
Quickly and accurately assess the patient SCHOLAR-MAC	Collect Assess
Establish that a patient is an appropriate self-care candidate	Assess
Suggest appropriate self-care strategies	Plan
Talk with the patient	Implement Follow-up

Source: References 8 and 45.

QuEST/SCHOLAR-MAC

One tool designed specifically for self-care encounters, the QuEST/SCHOLAR method, was first presented by Leibowitz and Ginsburg at the inaugural 2002 Self-Care Institute of the American Pharmacists Association.[45] This method employs simple acronyms to prompt health care providers to complete key steps in the self-care problem-solving process. Although no published studies have compared QuEST/SCHOLAR with other tools or mnemonics, the easy-to-remember acronyms may expedite completion of the problem-solving process relative to more structured models that contain no such prompts. One study concluded that its use in teaching student pharmacists improved their ability to provide self-care counseling and elicit important patient information in a consistent manner.[42]

Each letter in the acronym QuEST represents an ordered step in the problem-solving process[45]:

- Quickly and accurately assess the patient (using the SCHOLAR-MAC questioning process described here).
- Establish that a patient is an appropriate self-care candidate.
- Suggest appropriate self-care strategies.
- Talk with the patient.

Similarly, each letter in SCHOLAR represents information that the health care provider should elicit from each patient or caregiver:

- Symptoms: What are the main and associated symptoms?
- Characteristics: What is the situation like? Is it changing?
- History: What has been done so far? Has this ever happened before, and, if so, what was done then? What was successful; what wasn't?
- Onset: When did it start?
- Location: Where is the problem?
- Aggravating factors: What makes it worse?
- Remitting factors: What makes it better?

Because nothing in the SCHOLAR line of questioning is specific to an individual's medical history, the MAC acronym was added to QuEST/SCHOLAR and is intended to prompt users to collect additional key patient information:

- Medications: prescription and nonprescription as well as complementary and alternative products
- Allergies: to medications and other substances
- Conditions: coexisting health conditions

QuEST/SCHOLAR-MAC is not a new problem-solving model or a different process for patient care. It is one option to assist the pharmacist in streamlining the PPCP in self-care encounters by highlighting key areas within the process that are most relevant for self-care. This is important, because tools and mnemonics may be misinterpreted as an entirely new process instead of a tool to assist in learning and in making the existing process efficient. Table 2–1 demonstrates the relationship of the QuEST/SCHOLAR tool to the PPCP steps. Additionally, Cases 2–1 and 2–3 illustrate the application of this tool to the PPCP.

Another tool that may increase efficiency in applying the PPCP in self-care is the use of algorithms or flow charts. Treatment algorithms developed for disorders discussed in this book focus the pharmacist on the most pertinent information to collect and assess within the patient care process for that particular disorder. The algorithms also assist with components of the plan step by identifying appropriate lengths of therapy and follow-up time frames.

Special Populations and PPCP in Self-Care

Providing appropriate recommendations is the goal in every self-care encounter. Special considerations in the PPCP must be given to certain groups of patients known to be at higher risk for medication-related problems. These populations include pediatric, geriatric, pregnant, and lactating patients. Medication-related problems with nonprescription products in these populations can have serious consequences, despite being categorized as self-care. Most disorder-specific chapters in this book include a section titled "Special Populations" under the "Product Selection Guidelines" to address population-specific factors for that disorder. The remainder of this chapter summarizes the characteristics and physiologic and pharmacokinetic considerations of each population and provides general considerations for a self-care encounter using the PPCP in each of these populations.

Pediatric Patients

Pediatric patients present unique challenges in providing self-care recommendations. The pediatric population consists of different sub-populations, broken down into the following subgroups:

neonates (birth to 1 month), infants (1 month to 2 years), children (2–12 years), and adolescents (12–16 years).[46] There are significant differences in the pharmacokinetic and pharmacodynamic profiles between the pediatric subpopulations, as well as differences between each subpopulation and the adult profiles. The pharmacokinetic differences in the pediatric population vary widely, because their body and organ systems are in a continuous state of growth and development.[47] The body is less tolerant of changes, especially at the younger age spectrum, which includes neonates, infants, and children. There are less clinical data for pediatric patients, resulting in insufficient drug labeling and issues with medication dosing and administration.[48] Pharmacists should conservatively evaluate self-care recommendations in the pediatric patient and closely follow approved labeling recommendations when self-treatment is deemed appropriate. Furthermore, the pharmacist will communicate with the parent or caregiver in most encounters, rather than directly with the patient, which must be a consideration in each step of the PPCP for this population.

PPCP Considerations for Pediatric Patients

Specific information to consider during each step of the PPCP for pediatric patients is outlined in this section.

Collect

- Verify patient's age.
  - Several nonprescription medications have exclusions for use based on age. For example, ibuprofen is not indicated in children younger than 6 months (see Chapter 6).
  - Age is an important predictor for general exclusions for self-care regardless of nonprescription product indication and labeling. For example, infants younger than 3 months who present with fever are not candidates for self-care and should receive a medical referral (see Chapter 6).
  - Age can also help guide dosage form selection. In general, younger children (<6–7 years) may have difficulty swallowing solid oral dosage forms. However, this is a patient-specific factor that varies by age and should be reviewed and assessed individually.[49]
- Obtain patient's weight.
  - Nonprescription medications may be dosed according to weight for infants and children. For example, acetaminophen is dosed at 10–15 mg/kg every 4–6 hours (see Chapter 5).
- Consider caregiver factors.
  - Collecting information that leads to an appropriate assessment of the literacy and/or health literacy of the parent or caregiver is important when self-care will be administered to the patient.

Assess

- Determine exclusions for self-treatment.
  - Pediatric patients are more likely to have exclusions for self-treatment for various reasons. Examples include circumstances for which nonprescription medications are not available for the age or the disorder is not self-treatable, given the child's age. For example, girls younger than 12 years who present seeking treatment for vulvovaginal candidiasis should be referred to another health care provider. Referral is required because of the rarity of this disorder in children, which may be indicative of a more serious disorder (see Chapter 8).
- Evaluate for adverse drug effects.
  - Some nonprescription medications have the potential to cause unique adverse effects in children that would not occur in adults. For example, some antihistamines may cause paradoxical effects or excitation in children (see Chapter 11). With this in mind, the pharmacist may recommend dosing the antihistamine earlier in the day to gauge response and account for the potential adverse reaction.

Plan and Implement

- Consider nonpharmacologic therapy.
  - Recommendations for nonpharmacologic measures for self-care may be more common in pediatrics than in the general adult population because of labeling restrictions of nonprescription medications. Recent changes by the FDA to nonprescription medications, particularly for cough and cold products, require nonpharmacologic measures as the primary recommendation for treating colds in younger pediatric patients[50] (see Chapter 11). Pharmacists should assess the need for nonpharmacologic therapy and educate the parent or caregiver when nonpharmacologic recommendations are made. Parents with older children or those who may have used cough and cold products before the FDA changes were made may not be aware of the changes or understand the rationale. Research confirms that parents may be unaware of the FDA changes,[51] may continue to use products despite awareness of the changes,[52] and/or lack confidence in the FDA recommendations.[53] The pharmacist has an important role in educating parents and/or caregivers and may need to spend additional time counseling these individuals.
- Consider specific patient education and counseling.
  - FDA and the Consumer Healthcare Products Association have extensive resources for parents and caregivers on selection, dosing, and administration of nonprescription medications to children.[54,55] The pharmacist's familiarity with these resources may be beneficial in patient-specific communications and also with general educational opportunities within the pharmacy.
- Determine appropriate dosing and administration of medications.
  - Liquid formulations require accurate measuring to ensure appropriate doses are administered and have historically been a source of medication errors and unintentional medication overdoses.[56] FDA released guidelines in May 2011 for liquid nonprescription medication products that include a dispensing device, such as a dropper, cup, syringe, or spoon.[57] There was no standard prior to the guidance, and almost all pediatric nonprescription liquid medications contained highly variable and inconsistent dosing directions and measuring devices.[58] Table 2–2 summarizes the key points of the guidance.
    - Recent recommendations on oral liquid medications by the American Academy of Pediatrics (AAP) have called for exclusive metric-based dosing (i.e., mL) to avoid dosing errors associated with common kitchen spoons (i.e., teaspoons, tablespoons). They include a call for manufacturers to eliminate labeling, instructions, and dosing devices that contain units other than metric units. However, FDA has not made any changes based on these recommendations to date.[56] AAP encourages advanced counseling strategies (e.g., teach-back, drawings/pictures, dose demonstration, show-back) to further reduce dosing

TABLE 2–2 FDA Dosage Delivery Devices for Orally Ingested Nonprescription Liquid Drug Products Key Recommendations

- A dosing device should be included with all oral liquid nonprescription products.
- The device should be calibrated to the dose recommended in the product directions (e.g., teaspoon, tablespoon, milliliter).
- The device should be used only with the product with which it is packaged.
- The markings should remain visible even when the liquid is in the device.

Source: Reference 57.

errors.[56] The pharmacist is uniquely qualified for this role in self-care with oral liquid nonprescription medications for pediatric patients.
  - Age-appropriate tips for oral liquid medication administration are provided in Table 2–3.

Follow-up: Monitor and Evaluate

- Pharmacists should ensure that the parent or caregiver has a clear follow-up plan with a specific time frame and action step. Because of pediatric patients' smaller weight and decreased physiologic tolerance to change, parents and/or caregivers may be directed to follow up with another health care provider sooner rather than later to avoid potential adverse events.

Geriatric Patients

The U.S. geriatric or older adult population, defined as age 65 years and older, is growing rapidly, and they are large consumers of both prescription and nonprescription medications, as previously discussed in Chapter 1.[59,60] Pharmacists can expect a large number of self-care requests and encounters to involve older adults. Understanding the unique characteristics and needs of older adult patients is critical to achieving appropriate patient-centered care.

The aging process includes physiologic changes and decline in the function of many organ systems.[61] A number of these changes and characteristics can affect pharmacokinetic and pharmacodynamic profiles of medications. Absorption, distribution, metabolism, and excretion, the four primary facets of *pharmacokinetics*, or how the body processes a drug, can be altered in older adults. The general age-related pharmacokinetic changes are well described in the literature and are summarized in Table 2–4.[59,62]

The overall effect of changes to absorption, distribution, metabolism, and excretion varies, making it difficult to accurately predict the pharmacokinetic profile of a specific drug in older adults. Older adults experience varying degrees of these changes or may not experience them at all. Without the ability to assess the individual's specific body functionality, the pharmacist must assume that the older adult patient has age-related changes in function and then adjust medication and dosage recommendations

TABLE 2–3 Selected Administration Guidelines for Oral Medications

Infants

- Use a calibrated dropper or oral syringe.
- If a medicine dropper is used, the medication should be squirted into the side of the cheek and not straight back into the throat so that the infant does not choke.
- Do not place the child's medication in the formula, because the baby might not like the taste of the formula and might refuse to take this formula in the future.
- Support the infant's head while holding the infant in the lap.
- Give small amounts of medication at a time to prevent choking.
- If desired, crush non–enteric-coated or non–sustained-release tablets into a powder and sprinkle them on small amounts of food.
- Provide physical comfort while administering medications to help calm the infant.

Toddlers

- Allow the toddler to choose a position in which to take the medication.
- If necessary, disguise the taste of the medication with a small volume of flavored drink or small amounts of food. A rinse with a flavored drink or water will help remove an unpleasant aftertaste.
- If the medication is not palatable, ask the pharmacist whether the pharmacy offers a flavoring service and can add flavoring to the child's medication. Refrigeration also may help.
- Make sure that the medication is not referred to as candy.
- Use simple commands in the toddler's jargon to obtain cooperation.
- Allow the toddler to choose which medication (if multiple) to take first.
- Provide verbal and tactile responses to promote cooperative taking of medication.
- Allow the toddler to become familiar with the oral dosing device.

Preschool Children

- If possible, place a tablet or capsule near the back of the child's tongue, then provide water or a flavored liquid to aid the swallowing of the medication.
- If the child's teeth are loose, do not use chewable tablets.
- Use a follow-up rinse with a flavored drink to help minimize any unpleasant medication aftertaste.
- Allow the child to help make decisions about dosage formulation, place of administration, which medication to take first, and type of flavored drink to use.

TABLE 2-4 General Age-Related Pharmacokinetic Changes in Older Adults

Pharmacokinetics	Physiologic Change
Absorption	Increased GI secretions and motility; decreased surface area and blood flow; increased pH
Distribution	Decreased total body water and muscle mass; increased body fat
Metabolism	Decreased hepatic blood flow and enzyme activity
Elimination	Decreased renal function

Key: GI = Gastrointestinal.
Source: References 59 and 62.

accordingly. For example, if an older adult presents seeking advice for a nonprescription calcium supplement for bone health, the pharmacist may consider a recommendation for a calcium citrate product because of its less reliance on gastric pH for absorption (see Chapter 23). Another example of applying age-related pharmacokinetic changes to nonprescription medications can be illustrated with an older adult who requests assistance in selecting an analgesic. The pharmacist should use more caution in advising older patients regarding use of NSAIDs because of the gastrointestinal changes and renal function concerns associated with aging (see Chapter 5).

In addition to the pharmacokinetic changes of aging for older adults, the following facts and statistics should be considered in the PPCP:

- Polypharmacy (≥5 medications concurrently) and high risk of adverse drug events
  - More than 1 in 3 older adults take 5 or more prescription medications concurrently.[63,64]
  - One in 6 older adults are at risk for major drug–drug interactions.[63]
- Multiple chronic disorders
  - Almost 3 of 4 people ages 65 and older have multiple chronic disorders.[65]
- Alterations in senses[66]
  - One in 6 older adults has impaired vision.
  - One in 4 older adults has impaired hearing.
- Cognition and memory changes
  - Although aging and memory loss are not synonymous, 1 in 9 people ages 65 and older has Alzheimer's disease.[67]
- Misbeliefs that symptoms are part of the aging process instead of a characteristic of a disease or disorder can contribute to underreporting of symptoms.[68]
- *Dysphagia* (difficulty swallowing) affects 15% of the older adult population.[69]
- Sensitivity to anticholinergic medications[70,71]
  - Salivation, lacrimation, urinary output, and gastrointestinal motility are decreased and can cause nutrition problems, blurred vision, urinary retention, and constipation.
  - Cardiovascular system and body temperature regulation are altered.
  - Falls, delirium, and cognitive impairment can occur.
- The role of informal caregivers who provide assistance or participate in making treatment decisions

PPCP Considerations for Geriatric Patients

Specific information to consider during each step of the PPCP for geriatric patients is outlined in this section.

Collect

- Recognize that the collect step may take additional time in older adults because of the amount and complexity of information needed to make an appropriate assessment.
- Perform a more comprehensive review of medical conditions and medication history to avoid potential medication-related problems.
  - Consult the pharmacy's prescription medication profile, when available, to identify potential medication-related problems from multiple medications.
  - Ask about known renal and hepatic disease or impairment.
  - Inquire about chronic health diseases that may affect nonprescription medication recommendations or present exclusions for self-care, such as hypertension, diabetes, lung diseases, or Alzheimer's disease.
- Check for impairments in senses (especially vision and hearing) and memory or signs of cognitive decline.
  - Observe and/or ask about any deficiencies in senses or signs of cognitive dysfunction.
  - Involve family members or caregivers, when available, if memory impairment or cognitive decline is evident.
- Ask more in-depth questions regarding symptoms that could be unrecognized or falsely attributed to age.
- Ask about any swallowing difficulties.
- Inquire about physical limitations that may affect medication use, such as ability to open a medication container or apply topical agents to specific areas.

Assess

- Evaluate for potential duplicate therapy related to polypharmacy.
  - Pharmacists should specifically consider nonprescription medications available with a prescription such as proton pump inhibitors, histamine-2 receptor antagonists, antihistamines, and NSAIDs to avoid duplicate therapy.
- Evaluate for potential adverse drug effects.
  - Polypharmacy increases the likelihood of adverse effects[72]; therefore, current medications should be considered as a cause of any new symptom in the older adults until proven otherwise.
  - Several nonprescription medications are listed in the American Geriatrics Society Updated Beers Criteria of Potentially Inappropriate Medication Use in Older Adults.[73] This resource contains evidence-based information about safe medication use by older patients, including nonprescription medications that have a high likelihood of posing risk in this population. For example, based on these criteria, diphenhydramine may not be an appropriate recommendation in older adults for the treatment of insomnia and would likely pose more risk than benefit[73] (see Chapter 46).
- Evaluate whether the potential dose is too high.
  - Dosage adjustments may be necessary for nonprescription medications in persons who have renal and/or hepatic impairment, just as they are for prescription medications. Because nonprescription medications are labeled for the patient to be able to safely determine the appropriate drug and dosage without the advice of a health care professional, the Drug Facts label may simply state that patients

should avoid taking this medication without medical supervision if they have kidney or liver disease. Labels will not provide the dosage adjustments for specific renal or hepatic dysfunction. The pharmacist's assessment for self-care is to determine the appropriateness of nonprescription therapy for a patient with impaired renal or hepatic function.

Plan and Implement

- Consider concomitant medical conditions and other medications during product selection.
  - Because older adults are more likely to have multiple medical conditions, product selection based on chronic disease status is warranted in this population. In general, consider avoiding elixirs and sugar-sweetened liquids in patients with diabetes and liquids with excessive alcohol for patients on other sedating medications.
- Evaluate for nonadherence to medication regimens.
  - Consider the complexity of the patient's existing medication regimen. Pharmacists should select products that complement or match current regimen timing, when possible.
  - Consider adherence assistive devices, such as medication reminder boxes, or involve caregivers, when appropriate.
- Determine appropriate dosing and administration of medications.
  - Alternative dosage forms or administration methods may be needed for patients with dysphagia. Determining appropriate dosage forms is a complex process and requires that the pharmacist collaborate with the patient or caregiver and the patient's providers. Considerations in making this determination may include, but are not limited to, whether the medication can be crushed, chewed, or thickened, depending on the severity of dysphagia.
- Consider specific patient education and counseling.
  - A patient who is hard of hearing may require the pharmacist to speak slowly in a slightly raised voice, but avoid yelling and consider moving to an area of reduced noise. Other techniques include, but are not limited to, provision of written instructions if the patient prefers this method of communication.
  - A patient with low vision will need clear, audible instructions regarding product use. Other techniques include, but are not limited, to provision of large print instructions.
  - Physical challenges such as decreased dexterity associated with arthritis may require selection of a medication without child-resistant closures and include counseling to keep the product out of the reach of children and pets.
  - Given the high risk of polypharmacy in older adults, explain all active ingredients in the recommended product to avoid duplicate therapy.

Follow-up

- As with pediatric patients, certain characteristics of older adults may cause the pharmacist to refer them to another health care provider sooner rather than later to avoid adverse events. This is particularly true for frail older adults whose nutritional status and lower weight may contribute to higher risk of serious consequences if the disorder suddenly worsens or nonprescription therapy is ineffective. Patients who have limited social support or who may have impairments in cognitive function may also necessitate more intensive follow-up strategies.

Pregnant Patients

Drug therapy may be necessary to treat medical conditions or manage common disorders associated with pregnancy. Many medications cross the placenta to some extent, so there is inherent risk, because a mother who ingests a medication may expose her fetus as well. Consideration to ease the mother's discomfort and the effects of nonprescription medications on the developing fetus is crucial. Patients should never presume that a nonprescription product is safe to use during pregnancy, and pharmacists should be ready to provide guidance to determine when self-care is appropriate and when referral is needed.

PPCP Considerations for Pregnant Patients

Specific information to consider during select steps of the PPCP for the pregnant patient is outlined in this section.

Collect

- The pharmacist should ask all female patients of child-bearing age who present with common symptoms of early pregnancy, such as nausea and vomiting, if they are pregnant or could be pregnant. Visual observation is not reliable, especially at early stages of pregnancy.
- If pregnancy is confirmed, identify the stage of pregnancy. Some medications include specific information regarding safety based on the trimester of pregnancy. For example, the Drug Facts label for ibuprofen specifically warns against use in the last 3 months of pregnancy because of risks to the fetus.[74]

Assess

- Evaluate the safety of medication use during pregnancy.
  - The Drug Facts label for specific nonprescription medications may advise the pregnant patient to consult a health care professional before use. The pharmacist should assess the patient's symptoms and determine whether self-treatment is appropriate with a safe product and/or if referral to another health care professional is needed.
  - FDA recently issued a final rule regarding revised pregnancy and lactation risk categories. Pharmacists should be aware that this new rule applies only to prescription products. The Preface of this book provides a detailed explanation of the pregnancy and lactation data. The new data may include information for some nonprescription medications that are also available as prescriptions. For example, ranitidine is available as both a prescription and nonprescription medication.
- Determine whether the patient's pregnancy status is an exclusion for self-treatment even if a nonprescription product is considered safe for use in pregnancy.
  - For example, calcium carbonate is generally considered the antacid of choice for the pregnant patient; however, heartburn in the absence of an evaluation and diagnosis by a health care provider during pregnancy is an exclusion for self-treatment (see Chapter 13).

Plan and Implement

- Consider nonpharmacologic therapy options in pregnant patients.
  - To minimize medication exposure, the pharmacist might initially recommend nonpharmacologic self-care for pregnant

patients. For example, the pharmacist may provide initial nonpharmacologic recommendations of avoiding triggers, using saline nasal sprays or rinses, or using nasal strips to open passages for the pregnant patient who presents with allergic rhinitis symptoms. Even if a safe nonprescription medication for allergic rhinitis is available, pregnant patients may still be referred to another health care provider to confirm that the nonprescription product is safe for use (see Chapter 11).

- Discourage the use of homeopathic and herbal remedies in pregnancy, because safety and effectiveness are typically not established.
- Evaluate for nonadherence to medication regimens.
  - Because nausea and vomiting are common symptoms in early pregnancy, the pharmacist can provide education to minimize these effects on medication adherence. Advising the patient to eat small meals and frequent snacks and crackers may alleviate or minimize nausea and vomiting. Additionally, the patient can be advised to avoid foods, smells, or situations that cause vomiting (see Chapter 19). When possible, adjust the nonprescription medication schedule to avoid times when nausea and vomiting are typically present or worsened.

Lactating Patients

Similar to considerations in the pregnant patient, the nursing mother's use of medication while breastfeeding has potential for adverse effects on the infant. This potential for infant exposure is affected by the medication-specific properties and concentrations in the mother's blood, the timing of medication administration, and the medication safety profile in the infant.[75] The medication's effect on milk supply, as evidenced by some decongestants, should also be considered.[76] The benefit to the mother must again be weighed against the risks to the infant.

PPCP Considerations for Lactating Patients

Specific information to consider during select steps of the PPCP for the lactating patient is outlined in this section.

Collect

- The pharmacist should ask female patients, particularly those who present with an infant or young child, about breastfeeding status. Assumptions or judgments are not appropriate, and professional communication is essential to collect the appropriate information to make the best assessment.

Assess

- Evaluate the safety of medication use during lactation.
  - The Drug Facts label for specific nonprescription medications may advise the lactating patient to consult a health care professional before use. The pharmacist should assess the patient's symptoms and determine whether self-treatment is appropriate with a safe product and/or if referral to another health care professional is needed.
  - FDA recently issued a final rule regarding revised pregnancy and lactation risk categories. Pharmacists should be aware that this new rule applies only to prescription products. The Preface of this book provides a detailed explanation of the pregnancy and lactation data. The new data may include information for some nonprescription medications that are also available by prescription. For example, ranitidine is available as both a prescription and nonprescription medication.
  - Consult additional, reliable resources.
    - LactMed is a free database, available online and through an application, that is peer reviewed, recommended by AAP, and maintained by the National Library of Medicine.[77] The database contains information on maternal and infant drug levels, effects on lactation and breastfed infants, and alternative drugs to consider.[75,78]

Plan and Implement

- Consider nonpharmacologic therapy options.[79]
- Choose medications with the shortest half-life.[79]
- Discourage the use of homeopathic and herbal remedies during lactation, because safety and effectiveness are typically not established.[75]

CASE 2-1

A 35-year-old female is a regular patient of yours. She was walking into your pharmacy from her car to pick up a prescription and was stung by a bee. She wants to know what she should do to stop the burning.

Information to Obtain from the Patient	What the Patient Told You
Quickly and accurately assess the patient:	
Ask about the current problem (SCHOLAR).	
Symptoms	
What are the main and associated symptoms?	"Pain from a bee sting on my right hand."
Characteristics	
What is the situation like? Is it changing?	"Burning, itching, and redness. Mild, localized erythema with no signs or symptoms of systemic anaphylaxis observed."
History	
What has been done so far? Has this ever happened before, and if so, what was done then? What was successful; what wasn't?	"Nothing."

CASE 2-1 *continued*

Information to Obtain from the Patient	What the Patient Told You
<u>O</u>nset	
When did it start?	"Five minutes ago as I was walking from my car to the pharmacy."
<u>L</u>ocation	
Where is the problem?	"Palm of my right hand."
<u>A</u>ggravating factors	
What makes it worse?	"When I touch the bee sting area."
<u>R</u>emitting factors	
What makes it better?	"Nothing has been tried yet."
Ask about other <u>M</u>edications, <u>A</u>llergies, and <u>C</u>onditions (MAC): Within reason, get as much detail as possible to assist in the decision-making process.	■ "I take levothyroxine 50 mcg every day." ■ "I'm not allergic to any medications." ■ "This is the first time I've ever had a bee sting."
The "E.S.T." pieces of QuEST: Establish, Select, and Talk	**Your Assessment, Recommendation, and Counseling**
<u>E</u>stablish that the patient is an appropriate self-care candidate: ■ Any severe symptoms? ■ Any symptoms that persist or return repeatedly? ■ Is the patient self-treating to avoid medical care?	■ Symptoms are mild and localized to the right hand. Because she is experiencing her first bee sting, the risk of hypersensitivity is low. ■ She is not exhibiting any signs of an anaphylactic reaction, such as hives, swelling, dizziness, weakness, or difficulty breathing.
<u>S</u>uggest appropriate self-care strategies.	■ Nondrug: Remove the stinger by scraping with a credit card immediately; then apply an ice pack or cold compress. ■ Medication: Apply local anesthetic, such as benzocaine 20% aerosol spray, to affected area 3–4 times daily for up to 7 days to reduce itching and burning.
<u>T</u>alk with the patient about ■ Medication action, administration, and adverse effects ■ What to expect from the treatment ■ Appropriate follow-up	**Key Counseling Points:** ■ "I think you can do a few things to help this situation. Benzocaine is a topical anesthetic that will help relieve itching and irritation associated with the bee sting. Spray the affected area 3–4 times daily for up to 7 days. If the site becomes more irritated or redness increases, stop using the spray." ■ "The benzocaine should provide immediate relief. The symptoms should resolve over time and should not last longer than 1 week." ■ "If you experience any hives, excessive swelling, dizziness, vomiting, or difficulty breathing, seek medical attention immediately. If the medical condition worsens or is not resolved by 1 week, seek medical attention." ■ "Keep the area clean by washing regularly with soap and water; do this before each application of benzocaine."

CASE 2-2

Relevant Evaluation Criteria	Scenario/Model Outcome
Collect	
1. Gather essential information about the patient's symptoms and medical history, including	
a. Description of symptom(s) (i.e., nature, onset, duration, severity, associated symptoms)	Patient complains of difficulty sleeping. He describes difficulty falling asleep about 2–3 nights a week and has early awakening with inability to fall back to sleep 5–7 days a week. "I just don't sleep very well anymore, and I wonder if there's something I can take that will help." Symptoms started approximately 1 month ago.
b. Description of any factors that seem to precipitate, exacerbate, and/or relieve the patient's symptom(s)	He sometimes, but not always, has "better sleep" if he sleeps upright in a recliner chair instead of the bed.
c. Description of the patient's efforts to relieve the symptoms	He tried melatonin 3 mg daily before bedtime last week for 3–4 nights with no relief.

CASE 2-2 *continued*

Relevant Evaluation Criteria	Scenario/Model Outcome
d. Patient's identity	James Markum
e. Patient's age, gender, height, and weight	81 years old, male, 5 ft 9 in. tall, 170 lb
f. Patient's occupation	Retired railroad worker
g. Patient's dietary habits	Normal balanced diet; 3 cups of caffeinated coffee daily; no alcohol
h. Patient's sleep habits	Averages 5–6 hours per night. Naps 1–2 times per day in morning and/or afternoon.
i. Concurrent medical conditions, prescription and nonprescription medications, and dietary supplements	Gastroesophageal reflux disease: omeprazole 20 mg daily; hypertension: hydrochlorothiazide 25 mg daily, lisinopril 20 mg daily; depression: sertraline 100 mg daily; Alzheimer's dementia: donepezil 5 mg daily
j. Allergies	NKA
k. History of other adverse reactions to medications	None
l. Other (describe) ______	None
Assess	
2. Differentiate patient's signs/symptoms, and correctly identify the patient's primary problem(s).	Insomnia, possibly secondary to current medical conditions
3. Identify exclusions for self-treatment.	≥65 years, chronic insomnia (>3 weeks), sleep disturbances possibly secondary to medical disorders
4. Formulate a comprehensive list of therapeutic alternatives for the primary problem to determine whether triage to a health care provider is required, and share this information with the patient or caregiver.	Options include (1) Refer patient to his PCP. (2) Recommend self-care with lifestyle modifications for good sleep hygiene and diphenhydramine. (3) Recommend self-care until patient can see his PCP.
Plan	
5. Select an optimal therapeutic alternative to address the patient's problem, taking into account patient preferences.	Patient should consult his PCP.
6. Describe the recommended therapeutic approach to the patient or caregiver.	"I recommend you see your primary care provider for treatment of your sleep problems."
7. Explain to the patient or caregiver the rationale for selecting the recommended therapeutic approach from the considered therapeutic alternatives.	"This is the best option for you since you have had the sleep problems for several weeks and your situation may be related to your current medical conditions. Also, the nonprescription medications we typically use to treat sleep problems are not the best option for you. You may require prescription medications or adjustments of your current medications by your primary care provider."
Implement	
8. When recommending self-care with nonprescription medications and/or nondrug therapy, convey accurate information to the patient or caregiver.	Criterion does not apply in this case.
Solicit follow-up questions from the patient or caregiver.	"Are there any drugs I can take to help until I get an appointment with my physician?"
Answer the patient's or caregiver's questions.	"No, you tried the melatonin and it didn't work. There are no other nonprescription medications that are safe and effective for your sleep problems. I recommend contacting your physician for an appointment. If you are unable to see your physician immediately, you can try to improve sleep by avoiding or reducing caffeine, avoiding daytime naps, and participating in something relaxing prior to bedtime, such as reading."
Follow-up: Monitor and Evaluate	
9. Assess patient outcome.	Contact the patient in 1–2 days to ensure that he sought medical care for insomnia.

Key: NKA = No known allergies; PCP = primary care provider.

CASE 2-3

A mother of a 3-month-old boy calls the pharmacy requesting advice for her son who has had several watery stools since yesterday.

Information to Obtain from the Patient	What the Parent Told You
Quickly and accurately assess the patient:	
Ask about the current problem (SCHOLAR).	
Symptoms	
What are the main and associated symptoms?	"My son has had watery diarrhea since yesterday."
Characteristics What is the situation like? Is it changing?	"The stool is very thin and has no consistency at all. He's breastfed, and he has stopped eating the last few hours. He seems more tired and has not had a wet diaper for several hours."
History	
What has been done so far? Has this ever happened before, and if so, what was done then? What was successful; what wasn't?	"I haven't given him anything to stop the diarrhea."
Onset	
When did it start?	"About 24 hours ago."
Location	
Where is the problem?	"Just diarrhea. No vomiting."
Aggravating factors	
What makes it worse?	"Nothing."
Remitting factors	
What makes it better?	"Nothing."
Ask about other Medications, Allergies, and Conditions (MAC): Within reason, get as much detail as possible to assist in the decision-making process.	■ "My son takes D-Vi-Sol Vitamin D drops daily." ■ "He's not allergic to anything that I know of." ■ "He is otherwise very healthy. This is the first time he has been sick."

The "E.S.T." pieces of QuEST: Establish, Select, and Talk	Your Assessment, Recommendation, and Counseling
Establish that the patient is an appropriate self-care candidate. ■ Any severe symptoms? ■ Any symptoms that persist or return repeatedly? ■ Is the patient self-treating to avoid medical care?	The child's symptoms are severe given that he is younger than 6 months with diarrhea and signs of moderate–severe dehydration. He is not a candidate for self-care.
Suggest appropriate self-care strategies.	"There aren't appropriate nonprescription treatments to help your son, because he is so young. You should call your son's pediatrician immediately. Your son may need fluids that could be given only in an emergency department."
Talk with the patient about ■ Medication action, administration, and adverse effects ■ What to expect from the treatment ■ Appropriate follow-up	**Key Counseling Points:** "Because your child is so young and has diarrhea, you should contact your son's pediatrician immediately to ensure that he gets the fluids and help he needs to prevent becoming dehydrated."

CASE 2-4

Relevant Evaluation Criteria	Scenario/Model Outcome
Collect	
1. Gather essential information about the patient's symptoms and medical history, including	
a. Description of symptom(s) (i.e., nature, onset, duration, severity, associated symptoms)	Patient complains of a burning sensation in her stomach and throat that often is accompanied by feelings of fullness and "acid in my throat." The burning occurs after a heavy meal no more than once weekly. Symptoms last 2–4 hours after a meal and began about 1 month ago.
b. Description of any factors that seem to precipitate, exacerbate, and/or relieve the patient's symptom(s)	Symptoms occur after eating lunch out with coworkers or after potlucks at work and last 2–4 hours after the meal.
c. Description of the patient's efforts to relieve the symptoms	Peppermint candy did not help symptoms. She tried Tums (calcium carbonate 500 mg) once without full symptomatic relief.
d. Patient's identity	Maria Flores
e. Patient's age, gender, height, and weight	43 years old, female, 5 ft 4 in., 175 lb
f. Patient's occupation	Office assistant
g. Patient's dietary habits	Normal balanced diet; 4 or 5 cups of caffeinated coffee daily; 3 or 4 alcoholic beverages once per week
h. Patient's sleep habits	Averages 7–9 hours per night
i. Concurrent medical conditions, prescription and nonprescription medications, and dietary supplements	No concurrent medical conditions; multivitamin daily
j. Allergies	NKA
k. History of other adverse reactions to medications	None
l. Other (describe) _______	Weight gain of 10 lb in the past 3 months
Assess	
2. Differentiate patient's signs/symptoms, and correctly identify the patient's primary problem(s).	Infrequent postprandial burning sensation is consistent with uncomplicated heartburn. Patient denies pregnancy.
3. Identify exclusions for self-treatment.	None
4. Formulate a comprehensive list of therapeutic alternatives for the primary problem to determine whether triage to a health care provider is required, and share this information with the patient or caregiver.	Options include (1) Refer patient to her PCP. (2) Recommend self-care with lifestyle modifications and nonprescription acid-reducing medication. (3) Recommend self-care until patient can see her PCP.
Plan	
5. Select an optimal therapeutic alternative to address the patient's problem, taking into account patient preferences.	A nonprescription acid-reducing medication along with lifestyle modifications should be effective.
6. Describe the recommended therapeutic approach to the patient or caregiver.	"There are a number of things you can do on your own to decrease your symptoms. In addition, I recommend that you use the acid-reducer famotidine 20 mg for additional relief."
7. Explain to the patient or caregiver the rationale for selecting the recommended therapeutic approach from the considered therapeutic alternatives.	"This medication is a reasonable first option in treating your symptoms before consulting your primary care provider. Because the heartburn is predictable with large meals, primarily after lunch, using the famotidine on an as-needed basis should be sufficient."

CASE 2-4 *continued*

Relevant Evaluation Criteria	Scenario/Model Outcome
Implement	
8. When recommending self-care with nonprescription medications and/or nondrug therapy, convey accurate information to the patient or caregiver.	
a. Appropriate dose and frequency of administration	"Swallow one tablet at any time from 10–60 minutes before eating food or drinking beverages that cause heartburn."
b. Maximum number of days the therapy should be employed	"You can use this for up to 14 days in a row, if needed. If you think you need it for a longer period of time, call your primary care provider for an appointment. From what you said, I can't imagine you'll need this more than once a week, if that."
c. Product administration procedures	"Be sure to take this with a full glass of water."
d. Expected time to onset of relief	"You should feel better a few hours after you take this. Often the relief happens sooner."
e. Degree of relief that can be reasonably expected	"You should expect at least some relief; often patients get complete relief with a dose."
f. Most common adverse effects	"Some of the more common adverse effects are headache, diarrhea, dizziness, and constipation, but these don't happen too often and are rarely serious."
g. Adverse effects that warrant medical intervention should they occur	"If you experience any unusual bleeding or bruising, be sure to call your primary care provider and stop using this medicine."
h. Patient options in the event that condition worsens or persists	"If this situation worsens please consult your primary care provider."
i. Product storage requirements	"Store this medicine in a cool dry place out of the reach of children."
j. Specific nondrug measures	"Other things that can help you include eating smaller, more frequent meals and avoiding or eating less of foods and drinks that cause your symptoms."
Solicit follow-up questions from the patient or caregiver.	"May I take the medication after I start the meal if I have forgotten to take it prior?"
Answer the patient's or caregiver's questions.	"Yes, but the medication may not be as effective in preventing heartburn symptoms."
Follow-up: Monitor and Evaluate	
9. Assess patient outcome.	To evaluate efficacy of the treatment, advise the patient to call the pharmacy after using the as-needed medication for heartburn prevention.

Key: NKA = No known allergies; PCP = primary care provider.

Key Points for PPCP in Self-Care

- Pharmacists play an active role in assisting patients with self-care by using the five key PPCP components: collect, assess, plan, implement, and follow-up: monitor and evaluate.
- The PPCP is the same process for self-care encounters as it is with any other pharmacist-provided patient care service and in any practice setting. The process is adaptable depending on the breadth and depth of care needed.
- Collecting essential information for the specific presenting medical condition will lead to an appropriate assessment and may lead to unique considerations in self-care, such as exclusions for self-treatment.
- The plan should include the self-care recommendation, including nonpharmacologic therapies, and the goal of therapy to identify anticipated outcomes of the recommendation and the time frame in which the outcome is expected.
- Follow-up in self-care encounters should include specific guidance on what action to take for efficacy or safety considerations. It may include resolution of the self-care disorder with no further action needed, a return to the pharmacist for additional assessment, selection of an alternative nonprescription medication, or medical referral.
- The PPCP in self-care has patient-centered care at its core with continual collaboration, communication, and documentation of care with other health care providers.
- Efficiency in the PPCP is imperative in a community pharmacy. Tools such as QuEST/SCHOLAR-MAC and the algorithms for specific disorders in this book serve as resources to streamline the process and assist in quickly and accurately using the process in this practice setting.
- Special populations, which include pediatrics, geriatrics, pregnant, and lactating patients, have increased risk of serious adverse events if not appropriately assessed.

- Using PPCP in self-care encounters for special populations may take additional time because of the amount and complexity of information needed for an appropriate assessment.

REFERENCES

1. Sclar DA, Robison LM, Skaer TL. Pharmacy consultation and over-the-counter medication purchasing outcomes. *J Clin Pharm Ther.* 1996;21(3):177–84. doi: 10.1111/j.1365-2710.1996.tb00019.x.
2. Bosse N, Machado M, Mistry A. Efficacy of an over-the-counter intervention follow-up program in community pharmacies. *J Am Pharm Assoc.* 2012;52(4):535–40. doi: 10.1331/JAPhA.2012.10093.
3. Ruiz ME. Risks of self-medication practices. *Curr Drug Saf.* 2010;5(4):315–23. doi: 10.2174/157488610792245966.
4. Pharmacists take center stage in OTC counseling. *US Pharm.* 2007;32(7):4–6. Available at: https://www.uspharmacist.com/article/pharmacists-take-center-stage-in-otc-counseling. Accessed May 23, 2017.
5. Kebodeaux C, Grise WM, Hudspeth B, et al. Chain community pharmacists' willingness, attitudes, and barriers in providing self-care medication and supplement recommendations. *SelfCare.* 2012;3(2):21–32.
6. Harris IM, Phillips B, Boyce E, et al. Clinical pharmacy should adopt a consistent process of direct patient care. American College of Clinical Pharmacy White Paper. *Pharmacotherapy.* 2014;34(8):e133–48. doi: 10.1002/phar.1459.
7. Yee GC, Haas CE. Standards of practice for clinical pharmacists: the time has come. *Pharmacotherapy.* 2014;34(8):769–70. doi: 10.1002/phar.1450.
8. Joint Commission of Pharmacy Practitioners. The pharmacists' patient care process. Available at: http://jcpp.net/patient-care-process. Accessed May 23, 2017.
9. Cipolle RJ, Strand LM, Morley PC. *Pharmaceutical Care Practice: The Patient-Centered Approach to Medication Management.* 3rd ed. New York, NY: McGraw-Hill; 2012:37–72.
10. American Society of Health-System Pharmacists. ASHP guidelines on a standardized method for pharmaceutical care. *Am J Health Syst Pharm.* 1996;53(14):1713–6.
11. American Pharmacists Association; National Association of Chain Drug Stores Foundation. Medication therapy management in pharmacy practice: core elements of an MTM service model (version 2.0). *J Am Pharm Assoc (2003).* 2008;48(3):341–53. doi: 10.1331/JAPhA.2008.08514.
12. Patient-Centered Primary Care Collaborative. *The Patient-Centered Medical Home: Integrating Comprehensive Medication Management to Optimize Patient Outcomes: Resource Guide.* 2nd ed. Washington, DC: Patient-Centered Primary Care Collaborative; June 2012. Available at: https://www.pcpcc.org/sites/default/files/media/medmanagement.pdf. Accessed May 23, 2017.
13. American College of Clinical Pharmacy. Standards of practice for clinical pharmacists. *Pharmacotherapy.* 2014;34(8):794–97. doi: 10.1002/phar.1438.
14. American Pharmacists Association Pharmaceutical Care Guidelines Advisory Committee. Principles of practice for pharmaceutical care. August 1995. Available at: http://www.pharmacist.com/principles-practice-pharmaceutical-care. Accessed May 23, 2017.
15. Joint Commission of Pharmacy Practitioners. Vision for pharmacists' practice. May 29, 2014. Available at: http://jcpp.net/resourcecat/jcpp-vision-for-pharmacists-practice/. Accessed May 23, 2017.
16. Accreditation Council for Pharmacy Education. *Accreditation Standards and Key Elements for the Professional Program in Pharmacy Leading to the Doctor of Pharmacy Degree (Standards 2016).* Chicago, IL: Accreditation Council for Pharmacy Education; February 2, 2015. Available at: https://www.acpe-accredit.org/pdf/Standards2016FINAL.pdf. Accessed May 23, 2017.
17. Bennett MS, Kliethermes MA. *How to Implement the Pharmacists' Patient Care Process.* Washington, DC: American Pharmacists Association; 2015.
18. Lauster CD, Srivastava SB. *Fundamental Skills for Patient Care in Pharmacy Practice.* Burlington, MA: Jones and Bartlett Learning; 2014:1–35.
19. Levy S. Pharmacist knows best: OTC recommendation survey 2007. *Drug Topics.* 2007(May 7). Available at: http://drugtopics.modernmedicine.com/drug-topics/news/modernmedicine/welcome-modernmedicine/pharmacist-knows-best-otc-recommendation-surv?page=full. Accessed May 23, 2017.
20. Herrier R, Apgar D, Boyce R, et al. *Patient Assessment in Pharmacy.* New York, NY: McGraw-Hill; 2015:15–29.
21. Rovers JP, Currie JD. *A Practical Guide to Pharmaceutical Care: A Clinical Skills Primer.* 3rd ed. Washington, DC: American Pharmacists Association; 2007:47–88.
22. Cipolle RJ, Strand LM, Morley PC. *Pharmaceutical Care Practice: The Patient-Centered Approach to Medication Management.* 3rd ed. New York, NY: McGraw-Hill; 2012:141–82.
23. National Network of Libraries of Medicine. Health literacy. Available at: https://nnlm.gov/outreach/consumer/hlthlit.html. Accessed April 5, 2017.
24. Agency for Healthcare Research and Quality. Health literacy measurement tools (revised). Available at: http://www.ahrq.gov/professionals/quality-patient-safety/quality-resources/tools/literacy-toolkit/index.html. Accessed May 23, 2017.
25. Brega AG, Barnard J, Mabachi NM, et al. *Health Literacy Universal Precautions Toolkit.* 2nd ed. Rockville, MD: Agency for Healthcare Research and Quality. Content last reviewed November 2016. Available at: http://www.ahrq.gov/professionals/quality-patient-safety/quality-resources/tools/literacy/index.html. Accessed May 23, 2017.
26. Haubinger C, Ruhl UE, Hach I. Health beliefs and over-the-counter product use. *Ann Pharmacother.* 2009;43:1122–7. doi: 10.1345/aph.1L547.
27. Cipolle RJ, Strand LM, Morley PC. *Pharmaceutical Care Practice: The Patient-Centered Approach to Medication Management.* 3rd ed. New York, NY: McGraw-Hill; 2012:237–64.
28. Rodriguez de Bittner M, Popovich NG. *OTC Advisor: The Pharmacist's Role in Self-Care, Monograph 1.* Washington, DC: American Pharmacists Association; 2009. Available at: http://elearning.pharmacist.com/Portal/Files/LearningProducts/4344c315508d4f889e213ab4bb401e74/assets/09-413_OTC%20Final%20to%20Print.pdf. Accessed May 23, 2017.
29. Lauster CD, Srivastava SB. *Fundamental Skills for Patient Care in Pharmacy Practice.* Burlington, MA: Jones and Bartlett Learning; 2014:125–47.
30. Carlisle A, Jacobson KL, Di Francesco L, et al. Practical strategies to improve communication with patients. *P T.* 2011;36(9):576–80, 89. Available at https://www.ncbi.nlm.nih.gov/pmc/articles/PMC3278143/. Accessed May 23, 2017.
31. Institute of Medicine. *Crossing the Quality Chasm: A New Health System for the 21st Century.* Washington, DC: Institute of Medicine; 2001.
32. Cipolle RJ, Strand LM, Morley PC. *Pharmaceutical Care Practice: The Patient-Centered Approach to Medication Management.* 3rd ed. New York, NY: McGraw-Hill Co; 2012:103–40.
33. Berger BA. *Communication Skills for Pharmacists.* 3rd ed. Washington, DC: American Pharmacists Association; 2009:49–58.
34. Berger BA. *Communication Skills for Pharmacists.* 3rd ed. Washington, DC: American Pharmacists Association; 2009:213–28.
35. Brock KA, Casper KA, Green TR, et al. Documentation of patient care services in a community pharmacy setting. *J Am Pharm Assoc.* 2006;46(3):378–84. doi: 10.1331/154434506777069642.
36. McConaha JL, Finoli LM, Heasley JE. Assessing student pharmacist impact on patient over-the-counter medication selection. *J Pharm Pract.* 2012;26(3):280–7. doi: 10.1177/0897190012465957.
37. Pharmacy Health Information Technology Collaborative. *Workflow of Pharmacist Clinical Documentation Process in Pharmacy Practice Settings.* Alexandria, VA: Pharmacy Health Information Technology Collaborative; July 28, 2014. Available at: http://www.pharmacyhit.org/pdfs/workshop-documents/WG3-Post-2014-03.pdf. Accessed May 23, 2017.
38. Resnik DB, Ranelli PL, Resnik SP. The conflict between ethics and business in community pharmacy: what about patient counseling? *J Bus Ethics.* 2000;28(2):179–86. doi: 10.1023/A:1006280300427.
39. Tsuyuki RT, Landry E, Lalonde L, et al. Results of a national survey on OTC medicines, part 3: perceived time expectations for clinical encounters associated with over-the-counter medicines. *Can Pharm J.* 2012;145(3):116–8. doi: 10.3821/145.3.cpj116.
40. Hong SH, Spadaro D, West D, et al. Patient valuation of pharmacist services for self care with OTC medications. *J Clin Pharm Ther.* 2005;30(3):193–99. doi: 10.1111/j.1365-2710.2005.00625.x.
41. Bates BP, Bates BR, Northway DI. PQRST: a mnemonic to communicate a change in condition. *J Am Med Dir Assoc.* 2002;3(1):23–5. doi: 10.1016/S1525-8610(04)70239-X.
42. Burning SM, Kirby J, Conrad W. A structured approach for teaching students to counsel self-care patients. *Am J Pharm Educ.* 2007;71(1):8. doi: 10.5688/aj710108.

43. Bruno CB, Ip E, Shah B, et al. A mnemonic for pharmacy students to use in pharmacotherapy assessment. *Am J Pharm Educ.* 2012;76(1):16. doi: 10.5688/ajpe76116.
44. Masson SC, Mabasa VH, Malyuk DL, et al. Validity evidence for FASTHUG-MAIDENS, a mnemonic for identifying drug-related problems in the intensive care unit. *Can J Hosp Pharm.* 2013;66(3):157–62. doi: 10.4212/cjhp.v66i3.1252.
45. Leibowitz K, Ginsburg D. Counseling self-treating patients quickly and effectively. Proceedings of the APhA Inaugural Self-Care Institute, May 17–19, 2002, Chantilly, VA.
46. U.S. Food and Drug Administration. *Guidance for Industry: General Clinical Pharmacology Considerations for Pediatric Studies for Drugs and Biological Products.* Silver Spring, MD: FDA Center for Drug Evaluation and Research; 2014. Available at: http://www.fda.gov/downloads/drugs/guidancecomplianceregulatoryinformation/guidances/ucm425885.pdf. Accessed May 23, 2017.
47. Lu H, Rosenbaum S. Developmental pharmacokinetics in pediatric populations. *J Pediatr Pharmacol Ther.* 2014;19(4):262–76. doi: 10.5863/1551-6776-19.4.262.
48. U.S. Food and Drug Administration. Drug research in children. Available at: http://www.fda.gov/Drugs/ResourcesForYou/Consumers/ucm143565.htm. Accessed May 23, 2017.
49. Liu F, Ranmal S, Batchelor HK, et al. Patient-centred pharmaceutical design to improve acceptability of medicines: similarities and differences in paediatric and geriatric populations. *Drugs.* 2014;74(16):1871–89. doi: 10.1007/s40265-014-0297-2.
50. U.S. Food and Drug Administration. Public health advisory: FDA recommends that over-the-counter (OTC) cough and cold products not be used for infants and children under 2 years of age. August 19, 2013. Available at: https://www.fda.gov/NewsEvents/Newsroom/PressAnnouncements/2008/ucm051137.htm. Accessed June 30, 2017.
51. Varney SM, Bebarta VS, Pitotti RL, et al. Survey in the emergency department of parents' understanding of cough and cold medication use in children younger than 2 years. *Pediatr Emerg Care.* 2012;28(9):883–5. doi: 10.1097/PEC.0b013e3182676518.
52. Garbutt JM, Sterkel R, Banister C, et al. Physician and parent response to the FDA advisory about use of over-the-counter cough and cold medications. *Acad Pediatr.* 2010;10(1):64–9. doi: 10.1016/j.acap.2009.07.002.
53. Hanoch Y, Gummerum M, Miron-Shatz T, et al. Parents' decision following the Food and Drug Administration recommendation: the case of over-the-counter cough and cold medication. *Child Care Health Dev.* 2010;36(6):795–804. doi: 10.1111/j.1365-2214.2010.01075.x.
54. U.S. Food and Drug Administration. Tips for parents about the safe use of over-the-counter (OTC) medicine. Available at: http://www.fda.gov/Drugs/ResourcesForYou/Consumers/BuyingUsingMedicineSafely/UnderstandingOver-the-CounterMedicines/TipsForParents/default.htm. Accessed May 23, 2017.
55. Consumer Healthcare Products Association. Pediatric medicines. Available at: http://www.chpa.org/PedMeds.aspx. Accessed May 23, 2017.
56. American Academy of Pediatrics Committee on Drugs. Metric units and the preferred dosing of orally administered liquid medications. *Pediatrics.* 2015;135(4):784–7. doi: 10.1542/peds.2015-0072.
57. U.S. Food and Drug Administration. *Guidance for Industry: Dosage Delivery Devices for Orally Ingested OTC Liquid Drug Products.* Silver Spring, MD: U.S. Department of Health and Human Services, Food and Drug Administration, Center for Drug Evaluation and Research; May 2011. Available at: http://www.fda.gov/downloads/Drugs/GuidanceComplianceRegulatoryInformation/Guidances/UCM188992.pdf. Accessed May 23, 2017.
58. Yin HS, Wolf MS, Dreyer BP, et al. Evaluation of consistency in dosing directions and measuring devices for pediatric nonprescription liquid medications. *JAMA.* 2010;304(23):2595–602. doi: 10.1001/jama.2010.1797.
59. Hajjar ER, Gray SL, Slattum PW, et al. eChapter 8: geriatrics. In: DiPiro JT, Talbert RL, Yee GC, et al., eds. *Pharmacotherapy: A Pathophysiologic Approach.* 9th ed. New York, NY: McGraw-Hill; 2014. Available at: http://accesspharmacy.mhmedical.com/content.aspx?bookid=689&Sectionid=48811433. Accessed May 23, 2017.
60. Centers for Disease Control and Prevention, National Center for Chronic Disease Prevention and Health Promotion. *The State of Aging and Health in America 2013.* Atlanta, GA: Centers for Disease Control and Prevention, U.S. Department of Health and Human Services; 2013. Available at: http://www.cdc.gov/aging/pdf/state-aging-health-in-america-2013.pdf. Accessed May 23, 2017.
61. Olsen C, Tindall W, Clasen M. *Geriatric Pharmacotherapy: A Guide for the Helping Professional.* Washington, DC: American Pharmacists Association; 2007:35–45.
62. Wooten JM. Pharmacotherapy considerations in elderly adults. *South Med J.* 2012;105(8):437–45. doi: 10.1097/SMJ.0b013e31825fed90.
63. Qato DM, Wilder J, Schumm LP, et al. Changes in prescription and over-the-counter medication and dietary supplement use among older adults in the United States, 2005 vs. 2011. *JAMA Intern Med.* 2016;176(4):473–82. doi: 10.1001/jamainternmed.2015.8581.
64. Kantor ED, Rehm CD, Haas JS, et al. Trends in prescription drug use among adults in the United States from 1999–2012. *JAMA.* 2015;314(17):1818–30. doi: 10.1001/jama.2015.13766.
65. Anderson G. *Chronic Care: Making the Case for Ongoing Care.* Princeton, NJ: Robert Wood Johnson Foundation; 2010. Available at: http://www.rwjf.org/content/dam/farm/reports/reports/2010/rwjf54583. Accessed May 23, 2017.
66. Dillon CF, Gu Q, Hoffman HJ, et al. *Vision, Hearing, Balance, and Sensory Impairment in Americans Aged 70 Years And Over: United States, 1999–2006.* Washington, DC: Centers for Disease Control and Prevention; April 2010. NCHS Data Brief No. 31. Available at: http://www.cdc.gov/nchs/data/databriefs/db31.pdf. Accessed May 23, 2017.
67. Alzheimer's Association. 2016 Alzheimer's disease facts and figures. Available at: http://www.alz.org/facts/. Accessed May 23, 2017.
68. Morgan R, Pendleton N, Clague JE, et al. Older people's perceptions about symptoms. *Br J Gen Pract.* 1997;47(420):427–30. Available at: https://www.ncbi.nlm.nih.gov/pmc/articles/PMC1313052/pdf/9281869.pdf. Accessed May 23, 2017.
69. Sura L, Madhavan A, Carnaby G, et al. Dysphagia in the elderly: management and nutritional considerations. *Clin Interv Aging.* 2012;7:287–98. doi: 10.2147/CIA.S23404.
70. Feinberg M. The problems of anticholinergic adverse effects in older patients. *Drugs Aging.* 1993;3(4):335–48. doi: 10.2165/00002512-199303040-00004.
71. Rudolph JL, Salow MJ, Angelini MC, et al. The anticholinergic risk scale and anticholinergic adverse effects in older persons. *Arch Intern Med.* 2008;168(5):508–13. doi: 10.1001/archinternmed.2007.106.
72. Fried TR, O'Leary J, Towle V, et al. Health outcomes associated with polypharmacy in community-dwelling older adults: a systematic review. *J Am Geriatr Soc.* 2014;62(12):2261–72. doi: 10.1111/jgs.13153.
73. American Geriatrics Society 2015 Beers Criteria Update Expert Panel. American Geriatrics Society 2015 updated Beers criteria for potentially inappropriate medication use in older adults. *J Am Geriatr Soc.* 2015 Nov;63(11):2227–46. doi: 10.1111/jgs.13702.
74. U.S. Food and Drug Administration. Ibuprofen drug facts label. Available at: http://www.fda.gov/Drugs/DrugSafety/PostmarketDrugSafetyInformationforPatientsandProviders/ucm125225.htm. Accessed May 23, 2017.
75. Sachs HC; American Academy of Pediatrics Committee on Drugs. The transfer of drugs and therapeutics into human breast milk: an update on selected topics. *Pediatrics.* 2013;132(3):e796–809. doi:10.1542/peds.2013-1985.
76. U.S. National Library of Medicine. LactMed: pseudoephedrine. Record no. 231. Available at: http://toxnet.nlm.nih.gov/newtoxnet/lactmed.htm/. Accessed May 23, 2017.
77. U.S. National Library of Medicine. LactMed: a TOXNET database. Available at: http://toxnet.nlm.nih.gov/newtoxnet/lactmed.htm/. Accessed April 5, 2017.
78. Temming L, Cahill A, Riley L. Clinical management of medications in pregnancy and lactation. *Am J Obstet Gynecol.* 2016;2;1–5. doi: 10.1016/j.ajog.2016.01.187.
79. Spenser J, Gonzalez L, Barnhart D. Medications in the breast-feeding mother. *Am Fam Physician.* 2001;64(1):119–26. Available at: http://www.aafp.org/afp/2001/0701/p119.pdf. Accessed May 23, 2017.

CHAPTER 3

EXPLORING CULTURAL ASPECTS OF SELF-CARE

JERI J. SIAS AND ANITA N. JACOBSON

Patients' cultural and diversity characteristics influence their health care beliefs and behaviors.[1,2] This chapter explores cultural aspects of self-care to guide health care providers (HCPs) to better understand patient health decisions and develop individualized approaches to patient education. HCPs may be able to formulate a more appropriate self-care plan for a given health issue if they understand the patient's point of view and incorporate the patient's health beliefs and behaviors into the plan. If cultural and diversity issues are not considered early in the patient encounter, the HCP may find challenges to assessing and/or educating patients effectively, and patients may have difficulty understanding and following self-care recommendations.[1–3]

In this chapter, demographic shifts in the composition of the U.S. population are outlined to illustrate the relevance of serving diverse populations and socioeconomic considerations in the delivery of self-care health services. Emphasis is placed on defining important cultural and diversity terms and theoretical frameworks for cross-cultural care, so that providers are able to better understand the cultural context in which patients may make self-care decisions related to overall health. Examples of cultural behaviors found in major race and ethnic groups in the United States are discussed, as well as differences in cultural approaches to seeking care, particularly self-care. Attention is given to strategies to assist HCPs in communicating effectively with patients of diverse cultures and backgrounds and in developing more culturally appropriate treatment plans.

Definitions

Culture can be understood as an "integrated pattern of human behavior that includes thoughts, communications, languages, practices, beliefs, values, customs, courtesies, rituals, manners of interacting and roles, relationships and expected behaviors of a race, ethnic, religious or social group."[4] *Cultural identity* is developed on the basis of characteristics such as ethnicity, sex, gender identity and expression, sexual orientation, age, race, country of origin, language, ability level, and religious and spiritual beliefs.[4] Culture can influence all aspects of human behavior. Of particular importance is the role of culture in health-seeking and health maintenance behaviors and how these health beliefs and practices are passed from generation to generation.

Another definition of *culture* is the sum total of socially inherited characteristics of a human group. This definition includes assumptions learned from family and society about the nature of the physical, social, and spiritual world, as well as the goals of life and acceptable ways that one can achieve them.[2] Culture—as a learned set of values, beliefs, and meanings—guides patient decisions, attitudes, and actions.

In this chapter, the term *Western medicine* (also viewed as *allopathic* or *conventional medicine*) represent therapies based on science and regulated by the Food and Drug Administration (FDA), including prescription and nonprescription products. The term *complementary and alternative medicine* (CAM) is used to encompass Eastern and traditional medicine. However, *complementary* often refers to therapy used with Western medicine, and *alternative* often represents therapy used in the place of conventional medicine.[5] Examples include magnet therapy, acupuncture, dietary supplements, mind–body techniques, homeopathy, and massage therapy. The concept of CAM is introduced in this chapter to encourage HCPs to consider the use of these modalities among diverse patient populations. (See Chapters 50 and 51 for an in-depth discussion of CAM.) *Integrative medicine* recognizes evidence-based approaches using the balance of conventional therapies with CAM. (See Chapter 52 for discussion of complementary and integrative medicine [CIM].) These concepts of Western medicine, CAM, and CIM can help to shape how we understand self-care behaviors across cultures and in diverse populations.[5]

Literature suggests that providers who can navigate across diverse cultures and languages are able to demonstrate a combined set of awareness, knowledge, skills, and commitment to develop *cultural respect, sensitivity,* and *competency.*[3,6,7] When providers convey *cultural respect,* they have a "positive effect" on services because they are "respectful of and responsive to the health beliefs, practices and cultural and linguistic needs of diverse patients."[6] As providers portray *cultural sensitivity,* they convey attitudes and behaviors that reflect the patients' views of respect and acceptance of diversity; partner with patients to include their needs, values, and preferences in treatment plans; and empower patients to be in control of their health and health care decisions.[7]

Although several definitions exist, the context of *cultural competency* is described as having the ability to provide "effective, equitable, understandable, and respectful quality care and services" that honor and respond to a diversity of cultural health attitudes, beliefs, practices, and language preferences while accounting for health literacy and other interpersonal communication styles and behaviors.[3,4] When providers are able to communicate information appropriate to populations who have diverse

Editor's Note: This chapter is based on the 18th edition chapter of the same title, written by Magaly Rodriguez de Bittner and Jeri J. Sias.

language, literacy, and abilities in a way that is effective and easy to understand, they are employing *linguistic competency* skills.[8] To support culturally and linguistically competent practices, organizational leadership should be able to plan, implement, and evaluate supportive policies, programs, and interventions to ensure delivery of high-quality services.[4]

Rationale for Exploring Cultural Aspects of Self-Care

Demographic Changes in the U.S. Population

For statistical purposes, the U.S. government classifies five races: (1) Black or African American, (2) Asian, (3) Native Hawaiian or Other Pacific Islanders, (4) American Indian or Alaska Native, and (5) White (Table 3–1).[9–11] In addition to race, individuals may identify themselves in terms of ethnicity as "Hispanic or Latino" or "Not Hispanic or Latino"; race and Hispanic origin are considered two separate categories. For example, individuals may classify themselves as non-Hispanic White, Hispanic White, non-Hispanic Black, or Hispanic Black. The term, *minority* often refers to persons who do not self-identify as non-Hispanic White. To collect data, the U.S. government relies on individuals to self-report or self-identify their race and ethnicity with the opportunity to choose two or more races. The issue of defining race and ethnic background is increasingly complex.

The heterogeneity of the race and ethnicity classification options should be recognized. For example, the groups included under Asian and Pacific Islanders exhibit great variability. This distinction is also true for the Hispanic classification, which includes four diverse groups: Mexican Americans, Puerto Ricans, Cubans, and others (e.g., Central Americans, South Americans, Spaniards). While currently classified as White under the 2010 U.S. Census data, Arab Americans are a growing group, estimated at 0.5% of the population.[12]

The reported number of minorities has resulted in a shift in the composition of the U.S. population (Table 3–2).[13–17] In 2010, the number of foreign-born inhabitants was 40 million, with Mexico as the leading country of origin.[18] In perspective, one of every three U.S. residents identifies as non-White and, by 2044, more than half of the U.S. population is expected to identify with a minority group.[13] Currently, Hispanics comprise the largest minority group followed by African Americans and Asians.

Other changes in the landscape of health care delivery include the increase in adults ages 65 years and older who comprise 14.9% of the population (Table 3–2) and trends in migration patterns that have created unevenly distributed race and ethnic diversity across the United States.[19] Older adults use 30% of nonprescription medications in the United States.[20] Among racial and ethnic minorities, American Indian and Alaska Native populations demonstrate the highest reported CAM use (>50%).[21] These changes have created diversity in ethnic consumer markets that will be more pronounced in certain regions of the United States.

Beyond changes in race, ethnicity, and age characteristics, the U.S. population is becoming more diverse regarding sex, gender identity, gender expression, sexual orientation, socioeconomic status, physical abilities, veteran status, and religious affiliation. An estimated 2.3% of the U.S. population identifies as lesbian, gay, bisexual, and/or transgender (LGBT).[22] In 2010 18.7% of the noninstitutionalized U.S. population reported having a disability, with 12.6% having a severe disability.[23] According to the U.S. Census, 14.8%, or an estimated 1 in 7 Americans, reported living below the poverty level, and more than 21.3 million identify as veterans.[19]

The religious landscape of the United States is changing. Between 2007 and 2014, U.S. population groups who identify themselves as Christian have decreased from 78.4% to 70.6%, and an increasing percentage of the U.S. population does not affiliate with any religion (22.8% in 2014 vs. 16.1% in 2007). Further, nearly 6% of the U.S. population in 2014 is aligned with non-Christian faiths compared with 5% in 2007.[24] These national demographic changes across race, socioeconomic status, religion, and other traits have increased the importance of education and training in diversity, cultural sensitivity, and culturally appropriate services for HCPs. To explore demographic, social, and economic characteristics in any given community in the United States, providers can type in the address or zip code of the population they serve using the U.S. Census resource, American Factfinder (http://factfinder.census.gov).

TABLE 3–1 U.S. Classification of Race and Basis of Origin

Race[a] (self-identified)	Origins
White	Any of the original peoples of Europe, the Middle East, or North Africa
Black or African American	Any of the Black racial groups of Africa
American Indian or Alaska Native	Any of the original peoples of North and South America (including Central America) and who maintains tribal affiliation or community attachment
Asian	Any of the original peoples of the Far East, Southeast Asia, or the Indian subcontinent including, for example, Cambodia, China, India, Japan, Korea, Malaysia, Pakistan, the Philippine Islands, Thailand, and Vietnam
Native Hawaiian or Other Pacific Islander	Any of the original peoples of Hawaii, Guam, Samoa, or other Pacific Islands

[a] In the Census, race represents a "social definition" that is based on "racial and national origin or sociocultural groups." Because race is self-identified in the Census, it does not require a link to a "biologic, anthropologic, or genetic" origin.

Source: References 9–11.

Health Disparities

Although the health of some racial and ethnic groups has improved, health disparities persist among members of diverse cultural groups.[25] In many cases, health disparities cannot be explained solely on the basis of information about the biologic and genetic characteristics of race and ethnic groups. *Health disparities* or inequities occur when differences or gaps exist in health determinants (e.g., clean air, safe communities), health access (e.g., insurance, transportation), and/or health outcomes (e.g., heart disease, diabetes) among particular populations or groups (e.g., based on race, socioeconomic status, disability, or other cultural identities) who have experienced marginalization.[26,27] These

TABLE 3-2 **Population Characteristics in the United States (2000, 2010–2015)**

Characteristics	Total Population[a] 2000 (in percent)	Total Population[a] 2015 (in percent)
Total population[b]	100.0 (281.4 million)	100.0 (321.4 million)
Race (self-identified)		
African American or Black	12.3	13.3
Asian	3.6	5.6
American Indian and Alaska Native	0.9	1.2
Native Hawaiian and Other Pacific Islanders	0.1	0.2
White (non-Hispanic or Latino)	69.1	61.6
Two or more races	2.4	2.6
Ethnicity: Hispanic or Latino	12.5	17.6
Population 65 years and older	12.4	14.9
Education <12th grade[c]	19.6	13.7
Foreign born	11.1	13.1 (2010–2014)
Language other than English spoken at home (≥5 years)	17.9	20.9 (2010–2014)
Persons in poverty	11.3	14.8

[a] Total adds up to greater than 100% because of some cross-classification in Census data.
[b] Based on race alone or in combination with one or more other races.
[c] Less than 9th grade; 9th–12th grade, no diploma (population 25 years and older).
Source: References 15–17.

differences often are connected to socioeconomic and/or environment challenges.

Individuals from some minority groups do not equally experience long life spans, good health, and access to appropriate health care services. For example, low rates of cancer screening and treatment among minority groups are attributed to cultural and linguistic barriers, as well as limited access to health services.[27] Medically diagnosed diabetes prevalence rates are higher among Hispanics and persons with less than a high school education when compared with non-Hispanic Whites and persons with higher education levels. Other health disparities among different races and ethnicities continue to be found (Table 3–3), many of which have a link to self-care.

Among the complex factors explaining health disparities in population groups are race, socioeconomic status, literacy, health practices, psychosocial stressors, lack of resources, environmental exposures, discrimination, policies, and access to health care—often referred to as "determinants of health."[25] These factors influence future patterns of disease, disability, and health care utilization unless they are addressed. For example, when compared with the White population, Hispanics, American Indians, and Alaska Natives experience worse access to care.[28] More than 25% of U.S. adults ages 21–64 years with a disability live below the poverty line.[29]

In an effort to create a healthier society and develop strategies to decrease the gap in health care, the U.S. government has guided public health policy over three decades through the Healthy People initiative.[26] By setting health care priorities and measurable objectives, the Healthy People initiative provides a foundation for the health care agenda for each decade. The Healthy People 2020 overarching goals focus on "(1) attaining high-quality, longer lives free of preventable disease, disability, injury, and premature death; (2) achieving health equity, eliminate disparities, and improve the health of all groups; (3) creating social and physical environments that promote good health for all; and (4) promoting quality of life, healthy development, and healthy behaviors across all life stages."[26]

Several specific objectives within Healthy People 2020 are linked to self-care such as self-monitoring blood glucose in diabetes, taking measures to prevent sunburn, and making attempts to quit smoking. This initiative is a road map to better health and can be used by different populations, communities, professional organizations, and groups to improve overall health.

Culturally Appropriate Health Care and Workforce Diversity

One of the factors identified by government agencies and health care groups contributing to health disparities is the lack of awareness of cultural issues and health disparities among HCPs. This problem may be attributed to inadequate formal education on cultural issues among academic health-related training programs. To ensure effective delivery of culturally and linguistically appropriate health care in cross-cultural and diverse settings, providers should understand basic diversity and cultural issues related to health and illness, health disparities among different groups, and communication strategies for working with culturally diverse patients.[30]

Although cultural competency and diversity education are required as part of accreditation in health professional training, lack of workforce diversity still exists in health care.[31] This reality highlights the need for providers of all races to understand the influences of culture in health care and for health sciences curricula to incorporate content on cultural respect and competency.[32] The

TABLE 3–3 **Examples of Health Disparities Among Race and Ethnic Groups in the United States**

Condition	Rates	Potential Self-Care Link
Obesity prevalence (2007–2010)	Non-Hispanic Black women (53%)[a] Mexican-American women (44%) Non-Hispanic White women (32%)	Approaches to health and wellness, request for diet or weight-loss supplements
HIV/AIDS rate/100,000 among 18 year olds and older (2010)	American Indian/Alaska Native (13.5) Asian (8.4) Black/African American (84.0) Hispanic/Latino (30.9) Native Hawaiian/Other Pacific Islander (27.0) White (9.1)	Acceptance of "safer sex" prevention and practices
Coronary heart disease age-adjusted rate of death/100,000 (2009)	Hispanic (86.5) Non-Hispanic Black (141.3) Non-Hispanic White (117.7) American Indian/Alaska Native (92) Asian/Pacific Islander (67.3)	Willingness to use low-dose aspirin for coronary prevention, use of home blood pressure monitoring

Key: AIDS, Acquired immunodeficiency syndrome; HIV, human immunodeficiency syndrome.
[a] Race and ethnicity are listed as found in Centers for Disease Control and Prevention report.
Source: Reference 27.

current race and ethnic group composition of HCPs in the United States does not reflect the composition of the general population. For example, only 4.4% and 6.8% of first professional degree pharmacy graduates in 2014 were Hispanic and African American, respectively.[33] In 2015, 13.6% of pharmacy students entering professional education were from underrepresented minority groups.[34] The pharmacy student and graduating populations do not proportionately represent the U.S. population that they will serve. Across health professions, there is a need to diversify the health care workforce.[31]

In 2000, the Office of Minority Health developed the National Standards for Culturally and Linguistically Appropriate Services (CLAS) in Health and Health Care.[35] These standards, which were updated in 2013, are based on an in-depth review of the literature, regulations, laws, and standards currently used by federal and state agencies. These enhanced standards provide guidance for individuals and organizations to implement services that are culturally and linguistically appropriate to "advance health equity, improve quality, and eliminate health care disparities." The 15 new standards are divided into four main sections that address (1) the principal standard (used in this chapter's definition for cultural competency); (2) governance, leadership, and workforce; (3) communication and language assistance; and (4) engagement, continuous improvement, and accountability.

Concepts of Working Across Cultures

Stereotyping and Generalization

Unique individuals with slightly different characteristics or beliefs may belong to the same cultural group. However, individual differences within cultural groups must also be considered. There is a great risk in stereotyping and assuming that a person within a group will always behave in the same manner. Stereotyping may be viewed as an assumption (often negative) about behaviors or characteristics exhibited by a group of people.[1] Generalizations may be based on documented or self-described behaviors or characteristics found in groups of people or cultures and may be used as a starting point for understanding cultures. For example, a stereotype would be that all minority groups use CAM. A generalization would be that high CAM use is common in many cultural and ethnic minorities; therefore, it is important to inquire about CAM use. During each consultation, the patient should be treated as an individual with unique beliefs and values. Providers should avoid stereotyping and be cautious of making generalizations about groups of people. Patients should be asked open-ended questions to assess potential mitigating cultural factors including food selection, sexual practices, caregiver responsibilities, living situation, activity level, and alcohol, tobacco, or illicit substance use. However, having a general idea of behaviors and characteristics of groups of people can help providers be aware of potential health beliefs and behaviors. Having some knowledge of typical health-related practices and lifestyles that may influence disease state prevalence or acceptance of self-care treatment for commonly encountered groups is beneficial for shaping patient encounters, treatment plans, and recommendations. Knowing or inquiring about cultural communication preferences, such as salutation, preferred language, eye contact, spatial distance, and physical touch, is also important to facilitating interactions.

Acculturation

Variations in behaviors among members of a group become more important when people belonging to a specific cultural group migrate to and live in places that have a different, but dominant, culture. *Acculturation* is a process by which members of a specific cultural group adopt the beliefs and behaviors of a dominant group, but they may still value and practice their own traditional beliefs and behaviors when in the presence of their own group members.[2] Examples of acculturation can occur when individuals and/or families find themselves adjusting to a different culture, community, regions of a country, as well as to new countries.

One model identifies four levels of acculturation based on the degree that individuals retain a home culture and/or adapt to a new host culture.[36] Individuals who are able to function well in their homes, host culture, and/or language have been able to *integrate* both cultures; these persons are often able to navigate back and forth between cultures. Persons who adopt the new host culture but let go of their original home culture are said to *assimilate*; they function well in the host culture, but may have little knowledge or understanding of the cultural heritage or language of their forebears. Some individuals may live between cultures and feel *separated* because they do not fit into either the new host culture or the home culture. Other individuals who have moved to a new country or region of the United States, but hold onto their home culture and/or language and never fully adopt the new host culture or language may feel *marginalized.* During the acculturation process, people who are influenced by the host culture may behave differently from the norms found in their home culture.

Although acculturation is often directed at an immigrant group adopting habits and language patterns of the dominant host group, the outcomes of acculturation can be reciprocal. The dominant host group may also adopt patterns typical of the immigrant group. The adoption of ethnic or cultural "slang words," the enjoyment of different foods, music, festivities, and dress that represents a particular group are examples of reciprocal acculturation practices. When individuals lose or modify their cultural identity to acquire a new identity that differs from their original cultural group (*assimilation*), these behaviors and adaptations may cause internal conflicts among members of the original group. For example, conflicts can arise when younger members of a cultural group (e.g., second- or third-generation immigrants) do not follow traditions of the older generation and start to exhibit behaviors and beliefs more consistent with the host culture. In some instances, the children of immigrants may not speak their parents' native language.

Culture and acculturation can influence individuals' beliefs and attitudes toward health, illness, and treatment, as well as their decisions regarding health and self-care issues. When providers do not understand a patient's culture, beliefs, and behaviors, the effective delivery of patient-centered care and, consequently, the achievement of optimal health outcomes may be impeded. Incongruent beliefs and expectations between the provider and the patient may lead to misunderstandings, confusion, and, ultimately, refusal of treatment and undesirable therapeutic outcomes.

Cultural Competency Models

Developing cultural competency is a continuous and dynamic process that should be undertaken to ensure that health care is delivered in an effective manner among diverse populations of patients and providers. Several models have been used by providers and educators to better understand stages and processes of cultural competency. Three common models describe cultural competency as a process versus an achievement and can be applied to providers who support patients as they seek self-care therapy options (Table 3–4).[37–39] The Cultural Competence Continuum model developed by Terry Cross explores six stages of cultural competence from cultural destructiveness to cultural proficiency.[37] As providers and educators gain more experience and develop their skills and knowledge they may move toward cultural proficiency.[37]

TABLE 3–4 Cultural Competency Models and Applied Examples for Self-Care

Model	Attributes	Applied Examples in Self-Care
Cultural Competence Continuum (Terry Cross)[37]	**Cultural Destructiveness** (Beginning of the continuum and most negative stage) ■ Attitudes and policies support bigotry, racism, discrimination, and exploitation harmful to cultures and patients. ■ Behavior can be intentional or unintentional. In the Tuskegee study, the U.S. Public Health Service withheld syphilis treatment from African American men.	A health care provider judges a patient who is using CAM and assumes patient is not well educated or informed.
	Cultural Incapacity ■ Organizations or providers do not have any programs or services to respond to needs of patients from other cultures. ■ Ethnocentrism often exists in which a dominant culture makes assumptions about other cultures.	A pharmacy may not carry candles requested by several patients in service area. This common, inexpensive noninvasive adjunct self-care therapy (prayer and candles) is perceived to not be important.
	Cultural Blindness ■ Organizations or individuals try to remain unbiased. ■ Assumption is that culture or race makes no difference; treat everyone "equally." ■ Organizations have programs but do not tailor them to address cultural needs of different groups.	Bandage is "flesh" colored and would be camouflaged on anyone, regardless of skin tone.

(continued)

TABLE 3–4 **Cultural Competency Models and Applied Examples for Self-Care** *(continued)*

Model	Attributes	Applied Examples in Self-Care
	Cultural Precompetence (Skewed toward positive end of continuum) ■ Health care organizations or individuals recognize that cultural differences exist. ■ Organizations may reach out to cultures by hiring diverse workforce, interpreters, or translators for written materials. ■ Organizations limit their efforts to several initiatives and may become frustrated with lack of progress.	Providers might be quick to point to an herbal product line available in their pharmacy targeted for a specific cultural group and assume that this action suffices to care for different cultures.
	Cultural Competence ■ Acceptance and respect for differences among cultural groups is ongoing. ■ Providers and organizations continually increase their cultural competence knowledge and skills. ■ Models are implemented to deliver culturally appropriate care with a true commitment to improve outcomes of patients from diverse cultures. ■ Providers strive to assess personal cultural biases and beliefs. ■ Concerted efforts are made to meet and work with people of diverse backgrounds in the community. ■ Assessments to improve care for different cultures are ongoing.	Organizations may be committed to training their personnel to better understand the self-care needs of patients from different cultural groups.
	Cultural Proficiency (Highest level in the continuum) ■ Organizations and providers have a true commitment to culturally competent practices by engaging in research, evaluating new approaches to care, publishing and disseminating findings, advocating for improvements, and conducting trainings. ■ Work to achieve cultural proficiency is continual, and the positive impact and the transformation of understanding and engaging different cultures are valued.	Providers may work with community members to identify commonly used self-care and herbal products. Ongoing training for staff and students on community health beliefs and values is provided.
Purnell[38]	**Unconsciously Incompetent** Providers do not realize what they do not know about other cultures or the influence of culture across person, family, and community.	A provider encourages influenza vaccine for an individual, not recognizing that the family home is multigenerational and everyone could be vaccinated.
	Consciously Incompetent Providers recognize that they have challenges working with persons from diverse backgrounds.	A provider realizes that there may be different values about contraception in a Nigerian culture and takes time to research information about the beliefs.
	Consciously Competent Providers are aware of their effort to work effectively within or across different cultures.	A provider trains the entire staff on a new refugee population resettled in the community. Key cultural leaders are invited to help role play and address potential cultural beliefs and practices.
	Unconsciously Competent Providers are more easily able to navigate within a different culture or across new cultures; their approach may seem effortless.	Provider has worked with Mexican American patients with diabetes over time and understands different cultural barriers to self-management.
Campinha-Bacote[39]	**Cultural Awareness** Providers explore their own culture and profession through a process of understanding personal biases and assumptions about different cultures.	Providers acknowledge cultural differences in home remedies and self-care treatments used, such as chicken soup and hot tea with lemon to alleviate cold symptoms.

TABLE 3–4 **Cultural Competency Models and Applied Examples for Self-Care** *(continued)*

Model	Attributes	Applied Examples in Self-Care
	Cultural Knowledge	
	Process of gaining more information about diverse cultures, values, beliefs, and practices	Providers learn about common herbs and alternative therapies used in the Vietnamese American Buddhist population living in the neighborhood surrounding the pharmacy or clinic.
	Cultural Skill	
	Providers have the ability to collect, assess, evaluate, and adapt cultural information from diverse patients to improve care.	Providers recognize that when obtaining information about religion and culture in the social history that a woman who identifies as Islamic may prefer to have a female provider to discuss medication for a yeast infection.
	Cultural Encounters	
	Providers actually have the opportunity to interact with one or more patients and families in diverse cultures to enrich their awareness, knowledge, and skills.	Providers are able to see multiple patients who are Hispanic each day and over time understand the importance of family in making decisions about diet and diabetes management.
	Cultural Desire	
	Providers are sincerely motivated to grow in their capacity and skill to navigate across cultures.	In addition to working with patients from the large Catholic parish nearby, the Hindu provider volunteers at the parish community and outreach events.

Key: CAM = Complementary and alternative medicine.
Source: References 37–39.

The Purnell model, which is based in several disciplinary theories (e.g., organizational, family development, religion, political science), describes the interrelationship of several cultural domains such as heritage, family roles, workforce issues, and high-risk behaviors (Figure 3–1).[38] In this model, the providers go through a zigzag process from "unconscious incompetence," where they may not realize that they lack knowledge and skills to work in diverse cultures, toward "unconscious competence," where they have a positive attitude and a more developed foundation of knowledge and skills to adapt care in an efficient manner.

The model developed by Campinha-Bacote has five primary constructs in the cultural competency process: cultural awareness, cultural knowledge, cultural skills, and cultural encounters.[39] Overlapping these constructs is cultural desire—a concept that providers are caring and want to gain knowledge and skills to navigate across cultures. In this model, providers also would accept an attitude of *cultural humility,* recognizing that they will not consider their culture as the right one (ethnocentrism) and will maintain a state of learning about cultures throughout their lives. HCPs can use these models as a framework for working with patients from diverse cultures and backgrounds and developing cultural sensitivity.

Barriers to Self-Care

Differences in patients' language and health literacy (educational), access, capacity, and motivation to take care of themselves (personal), and/or perceived health status and confidence to take care of themselves (sociocultural) pose barriers that can apply to self-care. For example, patients' perceptions of the severity of their health condition may influence whether they pursue care. Providers should be able to recognize the various patient influences that can affect patients' self-care behaviors.

In some cases, providers may miss small differences in the interpretation of language, gesture, or eye contact that can lead to misunderstandings between people of different cultures and their HCPs. The provider's lack of cultural sensitivity and linguistic competency may impede the delivery of appropriate care.

Fear and Mistrust of Health Care Providers

Patients' mistrust of health care systems, providers, and information may create barriers to self-care management, including reduced preventive and follow-up care. Patients may feel that providers do not consider their concerns, and therefore, their expectations were not met. Some health disparities for minority populations, as historically found in African Americans, American Indians, and other groups, have been associated with discriminatory treatment and systemic racism. Many negative institutionalized health care policies and social aspects of provider–patient relationships remain as barriers to effective care. "Racism is insidious, cumulative, and chronic"; its effects can be felt by patients, providers, and all people in health care organizations. Ongoing mistrust and perceptions by patients can adversely affect patient satisfaction and health outcomes.[40]

Persons from diverse races and ethnic minority groups may also differ in their perceptions about research and research participation. For example, in many African American and other communities, mistrust of research exists as a result of the Tuskegee study conducted by the U.S. Public Health Service (USPHS) for 40 years between 1932 and 1972.[41] In the study, African American men with (n = 399) and without (n = 201) syphilis were enrolled without

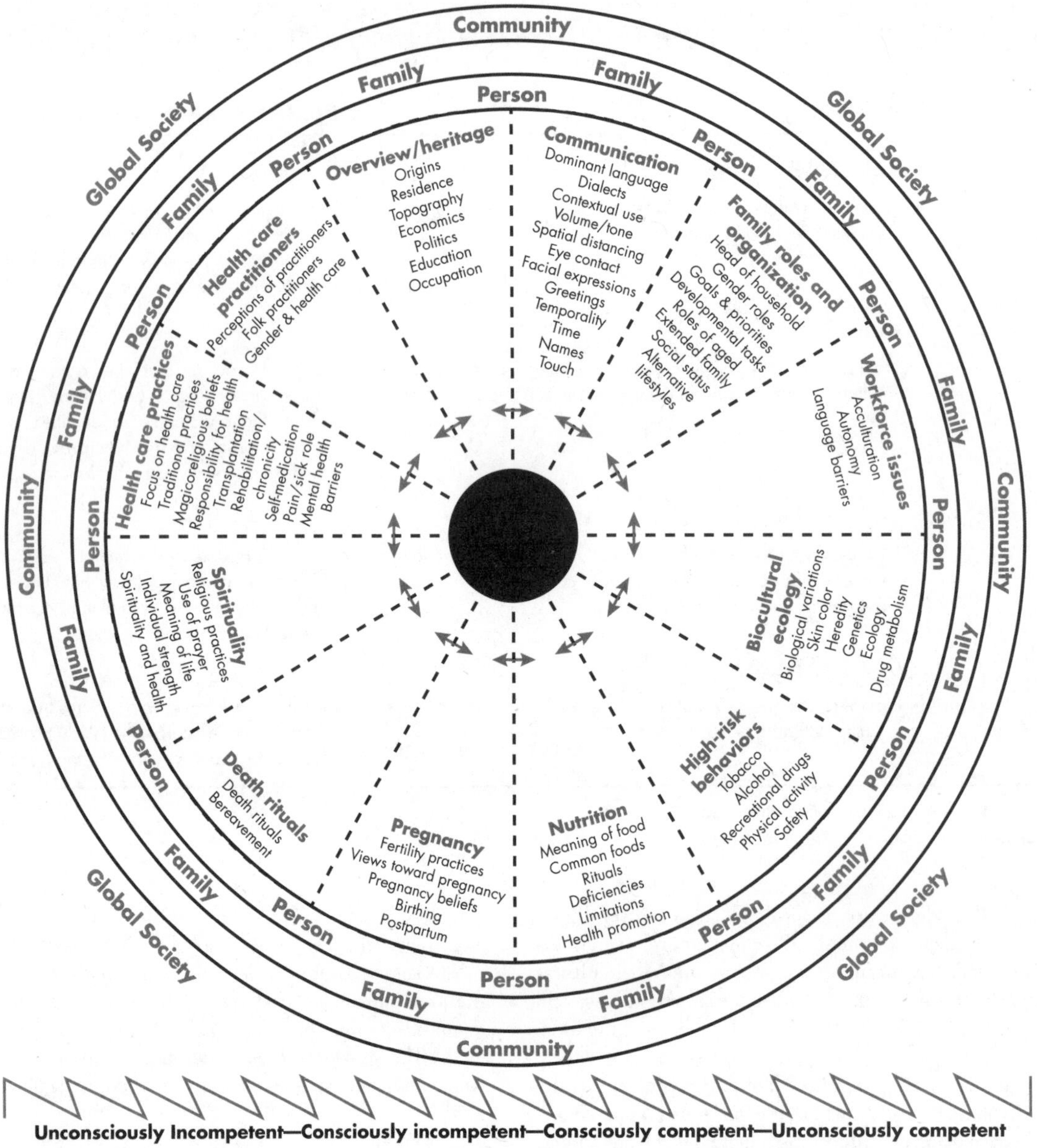

Variant cultural characteristics: age, generation, nationality, race, color, gender, religion, educational status, socioeconomic status, occupation, military status, political beliefs, urban vs. rural residence, enclave identity, marital status, parental status, physical characteristics, sexual orientation, gender issues, and reason for migration (sojourner, immigrant, undocumented status)

Unconsciously incompetent: not being aware that one is lacking knowledge about another culture
Consciously incompetent: being aware that one is lacking knowledge about another culture
Consciously competent: learning about the client's culture, verifying generalizations about the client's culture, and providing culturally specific interventions
Unconsciously competent: automatically providing culturally congruent care to clients of diverse cultures

FIGURE 3-1 The Purnell Model for Cultural Competence. (Source: Reprinted with permission from reference 38.)

informed consent for "free" medical examinations and meals while researchers monitored the effects of the disease. Even when penicillin was discovered as a treatment for syphilis, subjects were not informed of the treatment option nor were they offered the antibiotic. Because of the unethical decisions of that study, many African Americans who are not recent immigrants are unwilling to participate in clinical trials and other aspects of the medical system. Fear persists that unfair treatment and further abuses will occur.[40]

Other minority groups and women have also often been underrepresented in clinical research trials. The National Institutes of Health (NIH) National Institute on Minority Health and Health Disparities has a mission to lead scientific research to improve minority health and eliminate health disparities.[42] NIH and FDA mandates for inclusion of diverse cultures and minorities in research studies have succeeded in encouraging accountability in research design through increased community-based approaches, institutional review board approval, and federal research funding.[40,43]

American Indians have also survived a past that includes government policies and wars that damaged their people and culture. However, since the Indian Health Service was implemented,

American Indian communities are now more protected and have sustained their cultural traditions through family and clan relationships, kinships with homelands, religious ceremonies, and ancient rituals.[40]

The long history of American Indians and African Americans with public health services provided by the USPHS or through the Indian Health Service has led these communities to often mistrust providers and health systems. This mistrust perception may exist based on multiple aspects, such as[44]

- Feelings of prejudice against them
- Fear that their best interests are not considered and that they are treated differently from other patients
- Apprehension that their concerns and problems are not heard
- Concern that their traditional medical practices and/or beliefs will not be affirmed and will be called primitive
- Lack of confidence in HCP skills to diagnose and recommend treatments

Other minorities, such as Hispanics or Asian Americans, may also have perceptions of mistrust derived from sources in their past history outside the United States. Many immigrants may have experienced political oppression or government policies that fostered suspicion or unfair practices. Fears may be centered on deportation if they entered the country undocumented, or skepticism may be present because of prior experiences using different health care systems or experiencing denial to treatment because of language barriers.

Individuals who identify as LGBT also may experience distrust of the health care system and disparities in care. LGBT individuals face potential stigma and lack of understanding of their particular self-care health needs, as well as exclusive health-system practices including barriers to health insurance or visitation restrictions.[45] Providers may be unsure of the appropriate salutations and language to use with transgender patients. Although LGBT individuals experience higher rates of sexually transmitted infections (STIs) and human immunodeficiency virus (HIV) than their heterosexual counterparts, HCP education and medical literature for LGBT communities that focus only on STIs and/or HIV without inclusion of other health care needs promote stereotypes and biases.[46]

Reducing mistrust of the health care system requires repeated positive encounters over time. Some key practices that HCPs can adopt to foster trusting relationships include one-on-one outreach and frequent involvement of the provider with the targeted community. Volunteering and partnering with community leaders, such as clergy, spiritual leaders, or special population advocacy groups, can help to form networks and establish program approval at the earliest stage of the health care–planning process.[44]

Training of community health workers, or other lay community health advocates, can be an effective strategy for garnering trust in the community, especially when time and resources are limited. These community liaisons can help to diffuse health messages, integrate culturally and linguistically diverse prevention programs, provide information about new health technologies, and provide health screenings in the language and the context that the group understands. HCPs should embrace cultural sensitivity training to identify their own potential biases and stereotypes and gain knowledge to better address patients' feelings of mistrust, improve communication, and create trustful relationships.

Language Barriers

The inability to speak or read English makes it difficult for many patients to communicate with their HCPs or to read instructions on prescription and nonprescription labels that are only in English. Limited English proficiency (LEP) creates a significant barrier to seeking self-care or the advice of an HCP when services are only delivered in English. Because of LEP, patients may rely on information from television or magazines that is delivered in their language of origin or on the recommendations of family members, relatives, or community leaders. While many community pharmacies have telephonic interpreter services available, patients who are making self-care decisions in the aisle of the pharmacy may not be aware of this service and may not request assistance from the pharmacist who could subsequently offer information via telephonic interpretation.

According to Title VI of the Civil Rights Act, when organizations receive federal funding, they are responsible for taking measures to provide "meaningful access" for services at no charge to persons with LEP; these measures are based on four primary factors related to frequency of contact and importance of contact (Table 3–5).[47] The federal LEP website includes mapping tools to gather information about English language proficiency demographics reported at a county and state level. Barriers to care occur when organizations and/or providers (1) do not have available interpreter services; (2) do not know how to work with interpreters; (3) are charging patients for interpretation services; (4) request that patients bring family members or friends as interpreters; and (5) signs, forms, and brochures are in English only.

Literacy and Health Literacy

Studies have documented a relationship between poor reading skills and poor health.[48] People who cannot read often hide their limited literacy skills because of shame, embarrassment, low self-esteem, and fear. As a result, many HCPs often overlook this potential source of misinformation concerning self-care products and nonadherence to prescription drugs.

To detect literacy problems, the provider should be sensitive to cues that indicate the patient has difficulty reading. For example, patients may say they "forgot their glasses" when asked to read information. People who read poorly may never join a group education session. Instead, such patients may prefer one-on-one consultations with their HCPs.

Health literacy, or "the degree to which individuals have the capacity to obtain, process, and understand basic health information and services needed to make appropriate health decisions," is also an important skill for self-management and decision making about nonprescription products.[48] A person may have high

TABLE 3–5 Federally Funded Organizational Considerations for Meaningful Access to Persons With Limited English Proficiency

Agencies receiving federal assistance financially must consider the following steps to ensure meaningful access.

1. The number or proportion of LEP persons in the eligible service population
2. The frequency with which LEP individuals come into contact with the program
3. The importance of the service provided by the program
4. The resources available to the recipient

Key: LEP = Limited English proficiency.
Source: Reference 47.

reading literacy but not be able to apply a combination of functional skills, such as reading, calculating basic math, and drawing conclusions, to make an informed decision about his or her health.[48]

In different cultures, styles of communication and belief systems can affect health literacy.[48] Low health literacy is more common in minority groups and may be linked to general literacy levels and/or language. Overall low health literacy makes it difficult for providers to rely on using existing nonprescription labels, drug information pamphlets, or prescription labels produced by the pharmacy computer systems to give to patients. Through verbal communication with the patient, an interpreter, or an adult family member, providers must ensure that the patient understands the instructions and/or prescription label directions. The prerequisite requirements of the Durham–Humphrey (1951) and Kefauver–Harris (1962) amendments to the Federal Food, Drug, and Cosmetic Act, which the FDA uses in evaluating New Drug Applications for proposed nonprescription drugs, demonstrate the need for improved health literacy. The criteria for nonprescription drug approval include evidence that (1) patients can recognize and diagnose themselves for the condition specified in the proposed indication, (2) patients can read the product label and extract the key information necessary to use the drug properly, (3) the drug is effective when used as recommended, and (4) the drug is safe when used as instructed. The consumer must be able to read and understand the information on the label to know the proper dosage, recognize warnings and contraindications, and determine whether contraindications apply.

FDA labeling requirements implemented in 2002 were intended to make it easier for patients to read and understand nonprescription drug labels. The standard product label for nonprescription drugs, titled "Drug Facts," has specific sections for active ingredients, uses, warnings, when to use the product, directions, and inactive ingredients (see Chapters 1 and 4). Manufacturers are required to use large print, simple language, and an easy-to-read format on the labels to help patients with product selection and dosage instruction. In addition to these requirements, pharmacists should be alert to the educational needs of all patients, particularly those with poor reading skills or health literacy levels buying nonprescription products.

Providers can ensure that patients understand aspects of their condition and their responsibility for self-care by integrating the following tips. This approach may also improve adherence to treatment and clinical outcomes. First, the provider should never take for granted that the patient can fully comprehend all instructions, whether written or spoken. Providers should be aware of the potential for shame and treat the patient with respect. Patient education specialists suggest using the teach-back method to ensure the clarity and understanding of the message. This method involves using phrases such as, "Tell me in your own words, how you are going to take this medicine." Gaps in the patient's interpretation will provide additional opportunities to explain the process again or to correct gaps or misunderstandings using different methods to deliver the message. Education should be followed with materials such as pictures or demonstration products, and perhaps with follow-up phone calls.

Sociocultural Framework for Self-Care Practices

Self-care behaviors have not been well described among different population groups. Factors that influence self-care behaviors can include understanding the cultural context of health and attitudes toward taking responsibility for one's own health and illness. Religious beliefs, family and social context, cultural expectations, education and training, and personal experiences affect self-care behaviors. These interpretations are within the foundations of an ethnomedical model of care.[49,50]

According to Kleinman, the patient's understanding of a disease is based on a "consensus of beliefs, information, and expectations pertaining to the illness that are shared with a social network."[49,50] This understanding helps a patient interpret healing and sickness. Normative beliefs are generated by social interaction and personal experiences, which may differ completely from a scientific research approach to evidence-based medicine and the use of technology to diagnose and treat patients, which are within the biomedical model of care.[49,50] For example, some cultures may view hypertension as caused by tension, stress, or worry and may not understand that the disease is the chronic elevation of arterial blood pressure.

Providers who do not consider their patient's beliefs and expectations may encounter resistance to their professional advice. Expecting patients to respond to the provider's advice solely on the basis of biomedical principles may evoke considerable frustration for the patient and the provider. Each patient may have different social support needs and concerns related to making decisions about self-care behaviors and medication use. Providers should remember the significance of extended family and friends often found in minority populations' self-care behaviors. One example involves patients who are neither able nor willing to modify their dietary intake of certain foods (e.g., high fat, salty, and/or low fiber) so as not to impose these restrictions on the whole family. These patients are willing to sacrifice their own health to not inconvenience their family.

Normative beliefs based on the group's experiences also may assist the individual in making decisions whether to seek care from the health system or to use CAM. Self-care practices of many cultural groups involve use of home remedies, herbs, massage therapy, acupuncture, or other treatments that are passed from generation to generation. Communicating within the framework of the patient's culture helps break down barriers while also facilitating trust and understanding between the patient and HCP. Through this knowledge, the HCP can lead a patient away from harmful practices and provide safe, culturally appropriate alternatives. Subsequently, the provider can develop interventions, even biomedical ones, within the context of the patient's belief system. If traditional self-care practices are not harmful or even found to be beneficial to the patient, the provider may be able to accept them as part of a monitored and integrated treatment plan.

For example, a patient who is being monitored and treated through Western medicine might also use a folk or traditional healer. Some common healing methods include prayers, massage, and aromatherapy. Because these practices may be harmless and potentially additive to Western medicine, the provider may accept and even encourage their use as found in CIM. Providers should maintain open and consistent communication with the patient, traditional healer, and other HCPs regarding new information on CAM.

Patients and/or their family members are responsible for the day-to-day management of their illness. Consequently, better methods are needed to determine the patient's health-seeking behaviors, informational needs, preferences, and expectations about treatment management approaches. Providers are encouraged to develop a framework for understanding how patients interpret their experiences. This framework, according to Kleinman[49,50] goes beyond discrete medical episodes of "controlling the biological malfunctioning of disease" to include the psychosocial dynamics of family-based care, healer–patient transactions, spiritualism, shamanic cures, and other important holistic approaches based on the patient's world view. Using this approach reduces the adverse impact of miscommunication, misinformed decisions, and harmful health behaviors.

General Description of Beliefs by Different Population Groups

Some common themes have emerged in the literature related to chronic illness and self-care behaviors in the social context of older adults from African American, American Indian, Asian American, and Latino backgrounds. These self-care behaviors may be found more often among minority groups whose identities are rooted in their home culture and who may have less identity with Western culture and values.[51] The following six concepts highlight how self-care practices may be connected to various cultural ideals or beliefs:

1. *Concepts of independence and interdependence.* In Western medicine, independence, self-determination, and autonomy may be linked to increased self-care. Among African Americans, particularly women, values of self-reliance and independence are consistent with self-care. Among older American Indians and Latinos, family needs may supersede the importance of individual health. Messages of self-care in these populations may need to focus on helping the overall family structure. Among older Asian Americans, a mixed phenomenon may occur because of a higher emphasis on self-discipline consistent with self-care, but family needs may also be valued over those of an individual.
2. *Acceptance of intergenerational households.* European American households are less likely than those of other races and ethnic groups to have older family members living in a household. When households have several generations living together, different dynamics of social and family support for self-care may exist.
3. *Gender roles within the family structure.* Across cultures, women are often given the role of "health manager" in the family, even if the household is patriarchal. When family units are intact, women may have a greater role in influencing self-care practices of the family. When an older married man is widowed, for example, he may have a decreased ability for self-care practices, which may be noted especially among African American and Latino men.
4. *Family traditions related to CAM use.* In general, older adults and immigrants from African, American Indian, Asian, and Latino cultures more often use CAM as part of self-care compared with Whites. However, the level to which these traditions are being passed on to subsequent generations is unclear.
5. *Role of friends.* Friends, godparents, and "fictive kin" (very close friendships that are family-like) can be relied on for support as much as family. For example, in some African American communities, women will rely strongly on each other to help provide childcare. Latinos, American Indians, and Asian Americans also have strong extended friendships that are closely connected to the family.
6. *Religious and spiritual beliefs of different cultures.* The role of God and spiritual healing may influence how persons from a cultural group use and/or accept self-care practices. In some American Indian cultures, physical health is not as important as spiritual or emotional health. In some African American communities, churches have a central role that is sometimes of a familial nature.

Differences in health beliefs and behaviors, as well as the relationship of biological and societal influences, are documented in the literature.[2] Table 3–6 lists some of the characteristics shared

TABLE 3-6 Examples of Cultural Behaviors Among Selected Race and Ethnic Groups[a]

Group (heritage)	General Characteristics
Hispanic	■ Importance of family (family members may be deeply involved in the care of the patient) ■ May use *curanderos* and *curanderas* (traditional healers) ■ May use home remedies, mostly teas or herbal remedies ■ May use religious medals for good luck ■ May believe that health is a matter of "luck" or "fate" ■ May have an attitude toward recovery that is pessimistic ("fatalism") ■ May believe that illnesses are classified as hot and cold with treatment chosen depending on the classification of the disease
Asian	■ Importance of family ■ Balance between forces may define health (*yin* and *yang*) ■ May believe that illnesses may be caused by an imbalance of cold and hot forces ■ May use alternative medicine ■ May use Chinese herbal products or Ayurvedic practices (India) ■ Possible distrust of Western medicine
African American (not recent immigrant)	■ Importance of biological and fictive family ■ May use home remedies and folk medicine ■ May distrust the health care system because of previous experiences with system ■ Importance of religion in achieving cure
American Indian	■ May use sweat lodges as a method of cure ■ May use herbal medicine and natural roots ■ May use prayer for cure of illnesses ■ May believe that health is a harmony with "Mother Earth" ■ May use healers (medicine man or woman)

[a] The described behaviors have been observed in these race and ethnic groups and serve solely as a guide and not as a stereotype.
Source: References 2 and 51.

by people in minority groups in the United States.[2,52] These characterizations are generalizations. Again, not every member of an ethnic or cultural group may conform to these attitudes and beliefs. This chapter uses these examples to help raise provider awareness of aspects of health behavior they may encounter. Awareness of these issues may help providers to deliver more effective care with increased cultural sensitivity.

Religious beliefs are also important in patients' acceptance of the diagnosis and self-care treatment. A set of beliefs, attitudes, and expectations of illness and treatment based on religion may cause friction with the health care system and the health care team. For example, a person whose religious background is Jewish or Islamic may have restrictions on the use of certain nonprescription products (Table 3–7). Consumption of omega-3 fatty acids and other animal-based or gelatin-containing products may or may not comply with strict religious guidelines (kosher or halal) regarding consumption of animal-based products.

Individuals from different cultures may choose to treat illnesses using different rituals and religious items that are outside the realm of Western medicine. For example, patients who identify as Hispanic may use home remedies or other artifacts recommended by spiritual healers, sometimes called *curanderos*. These healers may use a combination of herbal remedies and religious rituals. When providers are nonjudgmental, they can better understand how and when the patient plans to use drug therapy or another alternative treatment. Knowing this information can help providers determine what prior treatments the patient used or is going to use or whether major interactions exist between the nonprescription product and the patient's alternative treatment.

Risks of Self-Medication and Suboptimal Responses to Nonprescription Drug Therapy

Limited data are available specifically on the use of nonprescription products among patients of diverse cultural backgrounds, ability levels, religions, and lifestyles. For many cultural groups, especially those without prescription drug coverage, nonprescription products represent the most frequently used treatments prior to consulting a provider. However, the improper use of nonprescription products places vulnerable populations at an increased risk for adverse drug reactions, drug–drug interactions, and toxicities from long-term exposure. Therefore, the potential for misuse of drugs that are available for self-treatment may outweigh the benefit–risk ratio in some patients. Increased use of nonprescription products by minority groups may create another self-care challenge.

Use of self-care can be important for patients with chronic illnesses. The need for quick relief may prompt more frequent use of nonprescription medicines, thus raising the risk of overmedication and a tendency for people to self-medicate for conditions. Lowered tolerance for discomfort can also lead people to rely on nonprescription drug therapy, especially nonprescription pain relievers, instead of seeking long-term behaviorally oriented prevention strategies. Patients may seek the use of vitamins, laxatives, and antacids to counteract poor eating habits. Checking blood glucose in diabetes is a needed self-care practice. However, poor self-management practices can mask more serious symptoms and complicate the diagnosis of serious diseases.

Low-income patients are often vulnerable to the harmful effects of overuse of nonprescription products for several reasons. First, patients who are chronically ill and have inadequate health insurance may restrict use of prescription drugs when their costs

TABLE 3–7 Resources for Some Religious and Culturally Based Medication Decisions

Provider	Information Provided	Website	Product Symbol
Muslim Consumer Group	List of medication, foods, and other items considered to be halal	www.muslimconsumergroup.com/medicine.html	حلال HALAL
Star-K	Approved Medications 2016 (medications considered kosher)	star-k.org/resources_medicine.php; star-k.org/articles/articles/medicine/452/a-kashrus-guide-to-medications-vitamins-and-nutritional-supplements/	K
OK.org	Kosher Medicine Lists for Pesach and Year Round	ok.org/consumers/passover/kosher-medicine-lists-pesach-year-round/	K
Orthodox Union	Guidelines for Medication—Passover 2016: (Orthodox Union kosher certification)	www.oukosher.org/passover/articles/guidelines-medication-for-passover/	U
Queensland Health	*Healthcare Providers' Handbook on Hindu Patients*	health.qld.gov.au/multicultural/support_tools/hbook-hindu.pdf	n/a
United States Conference of Catholic Bishops	Information on love and sexuality	usccb.org/beliefs-and-teachings/what-we-believe/love-and-sexuality	n/a
Australia Department of Health	Guidance to identify medications and pharmaceuticals of animal origin	https://www.health.qld.gov.au/qhpolicy/docs/gdl/qh-gdl-954.pdf	n/a

Key: n/a = Not applicable.

Note: This table does not provide a comprehensive list of resources used by various religions or cultural groups. Rather it is a guide to explore various beliefs and practices. Individual practices and beliefs may vary.

increase. Many uninsured patients use nonprescription products as alternatives to prescription drugs simply because of cost. These same patients may seek medical care only for the most urgent symptoms, delaying routine visits to their primary care provider's office. HCPs who educate patients on the use of nonprescription products can help prevent delays in seeking medical care. Conditions such as hypertension and hyperlipidemia are often not recognized because of lack of symptoms. Nonprescription products may be used by patients to treat minor symptoms associated with these conditions, such as headache or chest discomfort. The key problem with a suboptimal response to a nonprescription medication is that a more serious condition may not be diagnosed until the patient experiences a complication.

Communication With Culturally Diverse Groups

Gathering and Assessing Patient Information

When interacting with patients from different cultures, providers should use specific communication skills to gather information about the patient's cultural and spiritual health-related beliefs and practices. These communication skills include (1) openness to alternative viewpoints and approaches; (2) routine use of inclusive language (e.g., inquiring about a spouse or partner versus husband or wife, asking sex or gender identity versus assuming male or female) when gathering demographic information; (3) self-awareness of one's own prejudices and biases; (4) engagement to identify the patient's beliefs, expectations, and barriers to treatment; (5) understanding of how patients' beliefs and attitudes may influence the treatment plan; and (6) negotiating treatment that is acceptable to the patient and the provider. Trust is essential to gaining awareness of the issues involved in the interaction, and appropriate language and nonverbal communications and behaviors are crucial to effective communication.[35]

Diverse techniques and models have been suggested to improve communication and care in cross-cultural settings (Table 3–8). One classic model has been described for individual and institutional cross-cultural development.[53] This technique, using the mnemonic LEARN, may be used in clinical encounters. The primary steps (Table 3–9) in LEARN are as follows:

- Listen with sympathy and understanding to the patient's perception of the problem.
- Explain your perceptions of the problem.
- Acknowledge and discuss the differences and similarities.
- Recommend treatment.
- Negotiate a treatment plan that is mutually agreed upon.

TABLE 3-8 Models for Communicating With Patients Across Cultures

Model	Brief Description
CRASH Rust G, Kondwani K, Martinez R, et al. A crash-course in cultural competence. *Ethn Dis.* 2006;16 (2 suppl 3):S3–36.	Consider Culture. Show Respect. Assess and Affirm differences. Show Sensitivity and Self-awareness. Do it all with Humility.
ESTF Betancourt JR, Carrillo JE, Green AR. Hypertension in multicultural and minority populations: linking communication to compliance. *Curr Hypertens Rep.* 1999;1(6):482–8. doi: 10.1007/BF03215777.	Explanatory model of health and illness Social and environmental factors Fears and concerns Therapeutic contracting (treatment)
ETHNICS Levin SJ, Like RC, Gottlieb JE. ETHNIC: a framework for culturally competent clinical practice [special issue]. *Patient Care* 2000;34(9):188.	Explanation Treatment Healers Negotiate Intervention Collaborate Spirituality
RESPECT Bigby JA, ed. *Cross-Cultural Medicine.* Philadelphia, PA: American College of Physicians; 2003:20.	Respect Explanatory model Sociocultural context Power Empathy Concerns and fears Therapeutic alliance and trust

TABLE 3–9 Examples of Ways to Use LEARN

Listen with sympathy to the patient's perception: A woman from the African country of Somali is reluctant to give her mother medication for pain. When asked, she explains that she would prefer to help her mother's pain through massage.[a]

Explain your perceptions of the problem: A pharmacist encounters a patient from Iraq who has received U.S. refugee assistance. The patient has upper respiratory sneezing and coughing and requests an antibiotic because of the wide availability in pharmacies in Iraq without a prescription. The pharmacist tries to explain (1) the differences in pharmacy practice in the two countries and (2) that HCPs are concerned about overprescribing antibiotics, which do not work for viral infections and increase the growth of antibiotic-resistant bacteria. The pharmacist recommends appropriate nonprescription symptomatic therapy, suggests that the patient see a primary care provider, and helps to find a provider.[b]

Acknowledge, Recommend, and Negotiate: A patient from Cambodia complains that her 7-year-old child has had a "fever" for several days. The HCP has read that the word for "fever" in Cambodian may not necessarily mean an elevated temperature. Rather the term may refer to just not feeling well. The HCP clarifies with the mother that the child actually has had a common cold and no elevated temperature.[c] They find an appropriate nonprescription therapy to treat the symptoms. The mother agrees with the plan.

Key: HCP = Health care provider.

[a] Lewis T, Mooney J, Shepodd G. Somali cultural profile. Ethnomed, 2009. Available at: http://ethnomed.org/culture/somali/somali-cultural-profile. Accessed April 5, 2017.

[b] Regester K, Parcells A, Levine Y. Iraqi refugee health cultural profile. Ethnomed, 2012. Available at: http://ethnomed.org/culture/iraqi. Accessed April 5, 2017.

[c] Graham EA. Clinical pearl: "fever" in SE Asians. Does it really mean an elevated body temperature? Ethnomed, 1997. Available at: http://ethnomed.org/clinical/culture-bound-syndromes/pearl_fever. Accessed April 5, 2017.

Within "L" of LEARN, providers can apply the following 4 C's of the patient understanding of illness that have been adapted from Kleinman's Patient Explanatory model.[1] With the 4 C's, providers elicit the following from the patient (and/or family):

1. What do you call the problem? (perception)
2. What do you think caused the problem? (beliefs regarding source of illness)
3. How do you cope with the problem? (use of CAM or other treatments)
4. What concerns do you have about the problem or treatment? (understanding of fears; may also address adherence)

Using Language Assistance and Support

In many instances, the communication barrier may include the patient's inability to speak English. Several websites provide tips for providers to work with health care interpreters and with patients who have limited English proficiency (Table 3–10).

An interpreter provides a means of addressing a language barrier, but this approach has limitations when using untrained interpreters.[1] Problems may arise when family members are used as interpreters because the patient and family members may be put in an uncomfortable position. This situation becomes more critical when a younger family member, sometimes a child, is asked to interpret for older family members, such as parents or grandparents, in a clinical encounter. Putting a child in a position of responsibility is not acceptable and can lead to family conflicts by altering the hierarchy within the family. It also places an undue burden on the child, so this situation should be avoided.

Using family members or untrained personnel to interpret may lead to receiving or transmitting inaccurate information. The HCP may miss relevant and critical information, or information may be misinterpreted by the interpreter and/or patient. These problems can be avoided when the HCP uses personnel who are trained in medical language interpretation and are familiar with the providers. HCPs should be aware that in some cultures, shared health care decision making with other family members, spiritual leaders, and/or cultural leaders is highly valued, and inclusion of these persons may be beneficial to aiding patient comfort with health care recommendations.[1]

Developing a Self-Care Plan

Self-care activities include a range of individual health behaviors such as health maintenance, use of preventive services, symptom evaluation, self-treatment, interaction with HCPs, and seeking advice through lay and alternative care networks. In general, providers should encourage their patients' and their families' participation in self-care behaviors to promote patient empowerment. Unfortunately, some HCPs do not encourage self-care behaviors because they are not aware of appropriately targeted techniques, strategies, and support systems that patients can use.

When assisting patients in their self-care behaviors and self-medication, providers can help to initiate dialogue with the patient for informed decision making. Providers can also participate in health-screening programs to identify health risks in the community and lead health awareness campaigns.

The self-care plan should include the cultural differences and beliefs identified by the patient. These beliefs, as well as the role of the family in the patient's care, will help dictate the most appropriate recommendation. The provider must then use this information to develop self-care recommendations and patient education strategies. Communication with other HCPs about the patient's cultural beliefs and preferences is essential. A collaborative approach helps to ensure that all providers are aware of the patient's preferences. For example, when developing a plan of care for the treatment of a self-limiting illness that requires nonprescription drug therapy, providers can synthesize their knowledge and skills by expanding on "negotiating a treatment plan" from the LEARN model. When negotiating a plan, providers can evaluate

- Communication styles and needs (e.g., interpreter, family support)

TABLE 3-10 Resources for Developing a More Culturally Competent Health Care Environment

Resource	Website
Tips for Using an Interpreter and Linguistic Competency	
Tips for working with an interpreter (American Speech-Language-Hearing Association)	www.asha.org/practice/multicultural/issues/interpret.htm
Best practices for communicating through an interpreter (Refugee Health Technical Assistance Center)	refugeehealthta.org/access-to-care/language-access/best-practices-communicating-through-an-interpreter
National standards for culturally and linguistically appropriate services in health and health care (U.S. Department of Health and Human Services, Office of Minority Health)	thinkculturalhealth.hhs.gov/pdfs/EnhancedNationalCLASStandards.pdf
Limited English proficiency (LEP) resources for effective communication (U.S. Department of Health and Human Services)	hhs.gov/civil-rights/for-individuals/special-topics/hospitals-effective-communication/limited-english-proficiency/index.html
Cultural Competency Assessments	
Health Care Training	
Tool for assessing cultural competence training (Association of American Medical Colleges)	aamc.org/initiatives/tacct
Individual	
Cultural and linguistic competence health practitioner assessment (Georgetown University National Center for Cultural Competence)	clchpa.org
Cultural competence self-test (American Association of Family Physicians)	aafp.org/fpm/2000/1000/p58.html
Individual and Organizational	
Georgetown University National Center for Cultural Competence	nccc.georgetown.edu/resources/assessments.html
Organizational	
Lewin Group. Indicators of cultural competence in health care delivery organizations: an organizational cultural competence assessment profile. Health Resources and Services Administration, U.S. Department of Health and Human Services; 2002	hrsa.gov/culturalcompetence/healthdlvr.pdf
Assessment of organizational cultural competence (Association of University Centers on Disabilities)	aucd.org/docs/councils/mcc/cultural_competency_assmt2004.pdf
Health Literacy Pharmacy Organizational Assessment	
Pharmacy health literacy assessment tool (Agency for Healthcare Research and Quality, 2007)	ahrq.gov/professionals/quality-patient-safety/quality-resources/tools/literacy/index.html
Broad Resources for Cultural Competency and Health Disparities	
Office of Minority Health, U.S. Department of Health and Human Services	minorityhealth.hhs.gov
Culture, language, and health literacy (Health Resources and Services Administration, U.S. Department of Health and Human Services)	hrsa.gov/culturalcompetence
Integrating cultural information into clinical practice (Harborview Medical Center, Ethnomed)	ethnomed.org
Health equity, minority health (Centers for Disease Control and Prevention)	cdc.gov/minorityhealth/

- Patient beliefs, perceptions (4 C's and Patient Explanatory model), and relevant restrictions caused by religion or culture
- Prior treatments (prescription, nonprescription, and CAM) and acceptance of these therapies
- Use of tools to help patient understand and apply recommendation (e.g., medication calendar, pictograms, dosing reminders)
- Appropriate follow-up support (e.g., adverse event, worsening of condition, need to see provider)

Ensuring Cultural Competence in Health Care

Organizational Commitment

Even the most culturally sensitive, respectful, and competent providers will find it difficult to optimize care for patients without having organizational commitment, support, and training to work across diverse cultures. CLAS standards provide guiding principles for organizations.[3] Organizations that support more culturally competent services should have policies and infrastructure (e.g., guiding values and principles, recruitment of diverse providers and staff, policies for using interpreters) to support culturally and linguistically quality health care.[54] Further, these organizations demonstrate a capacity to systematically include feedback from consumers and communities they serve as well as to participate in ongoing self-assessment. Both providers and health system leaders should have a commitment to change, hold a real conviction of the significance of the task, and conduct in-depth self-assessments of the beliefs and attitudes of the personnel and the institution.

Organizational leadership can conduct cultural and linguistic competency self-assessments of their institution and the quality of care being provided (Table 3–10). For example, leaders could form a committee to conduct a baseline self-assessment among department managers, staff members, patients, and community agencies to gain perceptions of the mission, hiring policies, access to interpreters, and community outreach as components of the self-assessment. This process could be evaluated by the committee with recommendations for action. Ongoing organizational support for cultural sensitivity and competency training within the workforce provides a path for continuous improvement. In 2013, five states had legislative requirements to provide cultural sensitivity training to part or all of the health care workforce.[54] Other broad resources in this table may be helpful to learning more about how to improve cultural sensitivity.

Organizations can also evaluate how they serve persons with diverse health literacy skills. The Agency for Healthcare Research and Quality (AHRQ) has a website exploring health literacy issues in a pharmacy setting (Table 3–10).[55] The AHRQ Pharmacy Health Literacy Assessment tool guides an examination of the physical pharmacy layout, assessment of pharmacy staff, and eliciting feedback from patient focus groups. Educational materials should be at a sixth-grade reading level or below and use a variety of media to convey a health message.[56] Creation of a culturally inclusive pharmacy environment can assist with communication and welcome diverse patient groups. Examples include use of diverse individuals in photographs used for advertising or education (e.g., with respect to age, race, ethnicity, ability level, gender expression), bilingual materials and signage, universal symbols, private counseling areas, and communication aids (interpreter services, special phone, and braille). Pharmacy computer databases should record specific cultural needs and behaviors of the patient. These platforms should include information such as religion, language, preferred pronoun and preferred name, gender identity, special needs or accommodations, and health literacy level.

Cases 3–1 and 3–2 illustrate important aspects of culturally sensitive care in the area of self-care. These cases are examples of issues that may commonly be observed in community practice.

Key Points for Multicultural Aspects of Self-Care

- Cultural and diversity issues may affect patients' attitudes and behaviors toward health and illness, as well as their acceptance of and adherence to self-care treatment plans.
- Demographic shifts in the U.S. population from age, race, and language to religion, disability status, and other cultural group changes affect the approach and delivery of care to patients.
- Minority populations (including patients from diverse races and ethnic groups, women, individuals with disabilities,

CASE 3-1

Patient Symptoms and History

Mr. Patel is a 29-year-old man from India who is completing his graduate studies at the state's public university. Mr. Patel, his wife, and 2 children live in graduate housing. Their children attend public elementary schools. He has come into the pharmacy to pick up a prescription for his wife and comments that this summer their family will need to travel to India to take care of family matters. He asks how to ensure that his wife will have 2 months' worth of medication this summer to cover the time they are away.

Clinical and Cultural Considerations

This encounter seems pretty straightforward as the patient is coming in for a prescription. However, opportunities exist with international travel to ensure adequate coverage of travel vaccines. Mr. Patel's children are in public schools and likely will already have had appropriate immunizations prior to being able to enroll. However, if the entire family is traveling to South Asia, there may be opportunities to provide vaccination for hepatitis A.[57,58] Although there may not be any specific cultural beliefs against vaccines in Mr. Patel's culture, an established family-to-provider relationship does exist.

According to the Centers for Disease Control and Prevention, international travelers visiting friends and relatives can benefit from pre-travel counseling regarding vaccine-preventable disease and prophylaxis.[59] When traveling to India, the entire family could benefit from the hepatitis A vaccination series, and typhoid vaccine could be warranted. Depending on the area of travel in India, other prophylaxis could be provided.

Indian Americans represent the third largest group (>18%) among all Asian Americans in the United States.[60] About 70% of Indian Americans (≥25 years of age) have completed a college degree.[60] Although the Patel children are found to be up to date on vaccinations, one large study in more than 100,000 children (ages 12–36 months) found that many children in India remain under-vaccinated or nonvaccinated.[61] Significant differences in immunizations were noted among religious groups (e.g., Muslim Indians increased odds for under-vaccination vs. Hindu, Christian, and Sikh Indians) and location (urban communities with increased odds for under-vaccination compared with rural communities). The government in India is able to use this type of disparity data to target interventions for immunizations. Although this case focused on identifying potential travel vaccine needs for the Patel family, in this global society, there are lessons learned by understanding trends and potential intervention opportunities among culturally diverse groups in other parts of the world.

Source: References 57–61.

CASE 3-2

Patient Symptoms and History

Jorge Ortiz is a 7-month-old Mexican American male baby. His mother comes to the pharmacy requesting information about the best nonprescription medication available to stop the diarrhea that Jorge has been experiencing for 2 days. She has a bottle of bismuth subsalicylate (Pepto-Bismol) in her hand and is requesting information about how quickly it will work as they are planning to leave on a vacation the next day. She expresses concern about the baby having loose stools in the car seat and on the plane. Jorge is experiencing watery, loose stools that differ from his usual bowel movements; they are profuse and occur 8 times or more per day. Mrs. Ortiz reports that he is fussier than usual, seems lethargic, and has not been playing as much as usual with his toys.

Upon further discussion, she reports that he is transitioning from breastfeeding exclusively to using (milk-based) infant formula with some solid foods, including rice cereal and pureed sweet potatoes. She has not taken his temperature but reports that his hands feel warm to the touch. She has offered him white grape juice in a bottle throughout the day since the diarrhea started to avoid his becoming dehydrated.

Clinical and Cultural Considerations

Because of the profuse nature of the diarrhea, symptoms of lethargy, and risk of dehydration, it is important to refer Jorge for medical evaluation. Antidiarrheal agents generally should be avoided in children younger than 2 years of age, and bismuth subsalicylate should be avoided in children younger than 12 years of age. For less severe cases of diarrhea, administration of nonprescription oral rehydration solutions designed for infants and encouragement of maintenance of adequate nutrition through breastfeeding or formula feeding would be appropriate recommendations. Oral rehydration solutions designed for adults or juices and sports drinks should be avoided because of the risk of inducing hypo- or hypernatremia.

Hispanic patients may commonly seek self-treatment, even for serious conditions, because in many Latin countries, pharmaceuticals are available without prescription. Seeking advice and following treatment recommendations from respected family members is a common practice in the Hispanic community, as is using complementary and alternative medicine (CAM) as remedies. Potential barriers to medical care in the Hispanic community include potential lack of health insurance, undocumented status, distrust of health care providers, inability to read, and/or lack of English language fluency.[62] According to the 2014 U.S. Census report, 19.9% of Hispanic Americans are uninsured compared with 7.6% of White non-Hispanic Americans.[63] The pharmacist should offer an open, respectful, personalized discussion with Mrs. Ortiz, acknowledging her desire to stop the diarrhea quickly for the trip, while providing specific information about the risks of dehydration and use of antidiarrheal agents in infants to promote her consideration of the need for evaluation by a medical professional. It is also important to facilitate an accessible and affordable referral for care to Mrs. Ortiz based on her insurance status and/or access to services.

Source: References 62 and 63.

LGBT persons, and older adults) have experienced a range of health disparities. A disproportionately high number of minority patients continue to experience increased burden of disease, lower access to care, and higher rates of complications compared with other populations.

- Mistrust and fear of the U.S. health care system and providers can prevent some minority populations from seeking care. The ability for HCPs to deliver care that is culturally and linguistically sensitive, respectful, and competent can positively affect the quality of care for diverse populations.
- HCPs should assess and evaluate their own values and beliefs about cultures while acquiring knowledge and skills to effectively care for patients from diverse cultures and backgrounds.
- Self-care lends itself very well to the practice of working across diverse cultural groups. Many minority groups seek nonprescription products, as well as CAM therapies, as a main source of care.

REFERENCES

1. Galanti G. *Caring for Patients from Different Cultures.* 5th ed. Philadelphia: University of Pennsylvania Press; 2015.
2. Spector RE. *Cultural Diversity in Health and Illness.* 8th ed. Upper Saddle River, NJ: Pearson; 2013.
3. Office of Minority Health, U.S. Department of Health and Human Services. National CLAS Standards. Available at: https://www.thinkculturalhealth.hhs.gov/clas. Accessed March 12, 2017.
4. Goode TD, Dunne C. Definitions of cultural competence. Curricula enhancement module series. Washington, DC: National Center for Cultural Competence, Georgetown University Center for Child and Human Development. Available at: https://nccc.georgetown.edu/foundations/frameworks.html. Accessed March 12, 2017.
5. National Center for Complementary and Integrative Health. Complementary, alternative, or integrative health: what's in a name? Available at: https://nccih.nih.gov/health/integrative-health. Accessed April 5, 2017.
6. National Institutes of Health. Clear communication: cultural respect. Available at: https://www.nih.gov/institutes-nih/nih-office-director/office-communications-public-liaison/clear-communication/cultural-respect. Accessed April 5, 2017.
7. Tucker CM, Mirsu-Paun A, Van den Berg JJ, et al. Assessments for measuring patient-centered cultural sensitivity in community-based primary care clinics. *J Natl Med Assoc.* 2007;99(6):609–19. PMCID: PMC2574382.
8. Goode TD, Jones W. Linguistic competence. Washington, DC: National Center for Cultural Competence. Available at: http://nccc.georgetown.edu/documents/Definition%20of%20Linguistic%20Competence.pdf. Accessed April 5, 2017.
9. Standards for Maintaining, Collecting, and Presenting Federal Data on Race and Ethnicity. *Fed Regist.* October 30, 1997;62:58782.
10. U.S. Census Bureau. About race. Available at: http://www.census.gov/topics/population/race/about.html. Accessed April 5, 2017.
11. Humes K, Jones N, Ramirez R. Overview of race and Hispanic origin. Washington, DC: U.S. Census Bureau; 2011. 2010 Census Briefs, C2010BR-02. Available at: http://www.census.gov/prod/cen2010/briefs/c2010br-02.pdf. Accessed April 5, 2017.
12. Asi M, Beaulieu D. Arab households in the United States: 2006–2010. Washington, DC: U.S. Census Bureau; 2013. American Community Survey Briefs, ACSBR/10-20. Available at: https://www.census.gov/prod/2013pubs/acsbr10-20.pdf. Accessed April 5, 2017.
13. Colby S, Ortman J. Projections of the size and composition of the U.S. population: 2014 to 2060. Washington, DC: U.S. Census Bureau; 2014. U.S. Census Bureau Current Population Reports, P25-1143. Available at:

https://www.census.gov/content/dam/Census/library/publications/2015/demo/p25-1143.pdf. Accessed April 5, 2017.

14. U.S. Census Bureau. Profiles of general demographic characteristics: 2000 Census of population and housing. Washington, DC: U.S. Census Bureau; 2001. Available at: http://www.census.gov/prod/cen2000/dp1/2khus.pdf. Accessed April 5, 2017.
15. U.S. Census Bureau. Quick facts: United States. Available at: http://www.census.gov/quickfacts/table/PST040215/00. Accessed April 5, 2017.
16. Dalaker J. Poverty in the United States: 2000. Washington, DC: U.S. Government Printing Office; 2001. U.S. Census Bureau Current Population Reports, P60-214. Available at: https://www.census.gov/prod/2001pubs/p60-214.pdf. Accessed April 5, 2017.
17. U.S. Census Bureau. Profile of general demographic characteristics (DP-1), selected social characteristics (DP-2), and selected economic characteristics (DP-3): Census 2000. Available at: https://www.census.gov/census2000/states/us.html. Accessed April 7, 2017.
18. Grieco E, Trevelyan E, Larsen L, et al. The size, place of birth and geographic distribution of the foreign-born population in the United States: 1960 to 2010. Washington, DC: U.S. Census Bureau; 2012. Population Division Working Paper No. 96. Available at: https://www.census.gov/content/dam/Census/library/working-papers/2012/demo/POP-twps0096.pdf. Accessed April 5, 2017.
19. U.S. Census Bureau. QuickFacts: state and county. Available at: http://www.census.gov/quickfacts/table/PST045215/00. Accessed April 5, 2017.
20. Gerontological Society of America. Over-the-counter medication behaviors of older adults: research is needed to better understand and promote safe and effective use. Available at: www.chpa.org/2013medbehaviorolderadults.aspx. Accessed April 5, 2017.
21. National Center for Complementary and Integrative Health. The use of complementary and alternative medicine in the United States. Available at: https://nccih.nih.gov/research/statistics/2007/camsurvey_fs1.htm#most. Accessed April 5, 2017.
22. Ward B, Dahlhamer J, Galinsky A, et al. Sexual orientation and health among U.S. adults: National Health Interview Survey, 2013. *Natl Health Stat Report.* 2014;77:1–10. PMID: 25025690.
23. Brault M. Americans with disabilities: 2010. Washington, DC: U.S. Census Bureau; 2012. U.S. Census Bureau Current Population Reports, P70-131. Available at: https://www.census.gov/content/dam/Census/library/publications/2012/demo/p70-131.pdf. Accessed April 7, 2017.
24. Pew Research Center. America's changing religious landscape. Available at: http://www.pewforum.org/2015/05/12/americas-changing-religious-landscape. Accessed April 5, 2017.
25. U.S. Department of Health and Human Services, Office of Disease Prevention and Health Promotion. Healthy People 2020: disparities. Available at: http://www.healthypeople.gov/2020/about/foundation-health-measures/Disparities. Accessed April 5, 2017.
26. U.S. Department of Health and Human Services. About Healthy People 2020. Available at: http://www.healthypeople.gov/2020/About-Healthy-People. Accessed April 5, 2017.
27. Freiden TR, Meyer PA, Yoon PW et al. Centers for Disease Control and Prevention. CDC Health Disparities and Inequalities Report—United States, 2013. *MMWR Morb Mortal Wkly Rep.* 2013;62(3):1–189. Available at: http://www.cdc.gov/mmwr/pdf/other/su6203.pdf. Accessed April 5, 2017.
28. Agency for Healthcare Research and Quality. 2014 National Healthcare Quality and Disparities Report. Rockville, MD: Agency for Healthcare Research and Quality (AHRQ); 2015. AHRQ Pub. No. 15-0007. Available at: http://www.ahrq.gov/sites/default/files/wysiwyg/research/findings/nhqrdr/nhqdr14/2014nhqdr.pdf. Accessed April 5, 2017.
29. Erickson W, Lee C, von Schrader S. Disability statistics from the 2013 American Community Survey (ACS). Available at: www.disabilitystatistics.org. Accessed June 16, 2016.
30. Betancourt JR, Green AR, Carrillo JE, et al. Cultural competence and health care disparities: key perspectives and trends. *Health Aff (Millwood).* 2005;24(2):499–505. doi: 10.1377/hlthaff.24.2.499.
31. Institute of Medicine of the National Academies. *In the Nation's Compelling Interest: Ensuring Diversity in the Health Care Workforce.* Washington, DC: National Academies Press; 2004.
32. Shaya F, Gbarayor C. The case for cultural competence in health professions education. *Am J Pharm Educ.* 2006;70(6):124. doi: 10.5688/aj7006124.
33. Taylor J, Taylor D, Nguyen N. The pharmacy student population: applications received 2013–14, degrees conferred 2013–14, Fall 2014 enrollments. *Am J Pharm Educ.* 2015;79(5):s3. doi: 10.5688/ajpe795S3.
34. American Association of Colleges of Pharmacy. Academic pharmacy's vital statistics. Available at: http://aacp.org/about/pages/vitalstats.aspx. Accessed April 5, 2017.
35. U.S. Department of Health and Human Services, Office of Minority Health. National standards for culturally and linguistically appropriate services in health and health care. Available at: https://www.thinkculturalhealth.hhs.gov/pdfs/EnhancedNationalCLASStandards.pdf. Accessed April 5, 2017.
36. Sam DL, Berry JW. Acculturation: when individuals and groups of different cultural backgrounds meet. *Perspect Psychol Sci.* 2010; 5(4):472–81. doi:10.1177/1745691610373075.
37. Cross T, Bazron B, Dennis K, et al. *Towards a Culturally Competent System of Care: Volume I.* Washington, DC: CASSP Technical Assistance Center, Georgetown University Child Development Center; 1989.
38. Purnell LD. *Guide to Culturally Competent Health Care.* 3rd ed. Philadelphia, PA: F. A. Davis; 2014.
39. Campinha-Bacote J, Claymore-Cuny D, Cora-Bramble D, et al. Transforming the face of health professions through cultural and linguistic competence education: the role of the HRSA centers of excellence. Available at: http://www.hrsa.gov/CulturalCompetence/cultcompedu.pdf. Accessed April 5, 2017.
40. Benkert R, Peters R, Clark R. Effects of perceived racism, cultural mistrust and trust in providers on satisfaction with care. *J Natl Med Assoc.* 2006;98:1532–40. PMCID: PMC2569718.
41. Tuskegee University. About the USPHS syphilis study. Available at: http://www.tuskegee.edu/about_us/centers_of_excellence/bioethics_center/about_the_usphs_syphilis_study.aspx. Accessed April 5, 2017.
42. National Institutes of Health. Overview: National Institute on Minority Health and Health Disparities. Available at: http://www.nimhd.nih.gov/about/overview. Accessed April 5, 2017.
43. U.S. Food and Drug Administration. FDASIA section 907: inclusion of demographic subgroups in clinical trials. Available at: https://www.fda.gov/regulatoryinformation/lawsenforcedbyfda/significantamendmentstothefdcact/fdasia/ucm389100.htm. Accessed April 7, 2017.
44. Calderon L, Baker R, Fabrega H, et al. An ethno-medical perspective on research participation: a qualitative pilot study. *Med Gen Med.* 2006;8(2):23. PMCID: PMC1785211.
45. The Joint Commission. *Advancing Effective Communication, Cultural Competence, and Patient- and Family-Centered Care: A Roadmap for Hospitals.* Oakbrook Terrace, IL: The Joint Commission; 2010.
46. Snyder JE. Trend analysis of medical publications about LGBT persons: 1950–2007. *J Homosex.* 2011;58(2):164–8. doi: 10.1080/00918369.2011.540171.
47. Limited English proficiency: a federal interagency website. Available at: https://www.lep.gov. Accessed April 5, 2017.
48. National Institutes of Health (NIH), U.S. National Library of Medicine, National Network of Libraries of Medicine. Professional development: health literacy. Available at: http://nnlm.gov/outreach/consumer/hlthlit.html. Accessed April 5, 2017.
49. Kleinman A, Benson P. Anthropology in the clinic: the problem of cultural competency and how to fix it. *PLoS Med.* 2006;3(10):e294–4. doi: 10.1371/journal.pmed.0030294.
50. Kleinman A. *Patients and Healers in the Context of Culture.* Berkeley, CA: University of California Press; 1980.
51. Gallant MP, Spitze G, Grove JG. Chronic illness self-care and the family lives of older adults: a synthetic review across four ethnic groups. *J Cross Cult Gerontol.* 2010;25:21–43. PMCID: PMC2929526.
52. Seidl H, Ball J, Dains J, et al. Cultural awareness. In: *Mosby's Guide to Physical Examination.* 6th ed. St. Louis, MO: Mosby; 2006, pp. 180–6, 347–58, 520–30.
53. Berlin EA, Fowkes WC. A teaching framework for cross-cultural health care. *West J Med.* 1983;139:934–8. PMCID: PMC1011028.

54. U.S. Department of Health and Human Services, Office of Minority Health. CLAS legislation map. Available at: https://www.thinkculturalhealth.hhs.gov/clas/clas-tracking-map. Accessed January 9, 2017.
55. Agency for Healthcare Research and Quality. AHRQ pharmacy health literacy center. Available at: http://www.ahrq.gov/professionals/quality-patient-safety/pharmhealthlit/index.html. Accessed April 5, 2017.
56. DeWalt D, Callahn L, Hawk V, et al. Health literacy universal precautions toolkit. Rockville, MD: Agency for Healthcare Research and Quality; 2010. AHRQ publication 10-0046-EF. Available at: http://www.ahrq.gov/professionals/quality-patient-safety/pharmhealthlit/index.html. Accessed April 5, 2017.
57. Jackson JC. Clinical pearl: pre-travel counseling for persons visiting friends and relatives (VFRs). EthnoMed. Updated March 1, 2013. Available at: http://ethnomed.org/clinical/refugee-health/pre-travel-counseling-for-persons-visiting-friends-and-relatives. Accessed April 5, 2017.
58. Keystone J. Immigrants returning home to visit friends and relatives (VFRs). In: *CDC Health Information for International Travel.* New York: Oxford University Press; 2016. Available at: http://wwwnc.cdc.gov/travel/yellowbook/2016/advising-travelers-with-specific-needs/immigrants-returning-home-to-visit-friends-relatives-vfrs#1966. Accessed April 5, 2017.
59. Centers for Disease Control and Prevention. Health information for travelers to India traveler view. Traveler's Health. Updated July 31, 2015. Available at: http://wwwnc.cdc.gov/travel/destinations/traveler/children.vfr/india?s_cid=ncezid-dgmq-travel-single-001. Accessed April 5, 2017.
60. Social and demographic trends: the rise of Asian Americans. Pew Research Center. Updated April 4, 2013. Available at: http://www.pewsocialtrends.org/2012/06/19/the-rise-of-asian-americans/. Accessed April 5, 2017.
61. Shrivastwa N, Gillespie BW, Kolenic GE, et al. Predictors of vaccination in India for children aged 12–36 months. *Am J Prev Med.* 2015;49 (6 suppl 4):S435–4. doi: 10.1016/j.amepre.2015.05.008.
62. Juckett G. Caring for Latino patients. *Am Fam Physician.* 2013;87(1): 48–4.
63. Smith JC, Medalia C. Health insurance coverage in the United States: 2014. Washington, DC: U.S. Government Printing Office; 2015. U.S. Census Bureau Current Population Reports, P60-253. Available at: https://www.census.gov/content/dam/Census/library/publications/2015/demo/p60-253.pdf. Accessed April 5, 2017.

CHAPTER 4

LEGAL AND REGULATORY ISSUES IN SELF-CARE PHARMACY PRACTICE

MARTHA M. RUMORE

This chapter examines the regulatory and legal aspects of the manufacturing, distribution, labeling, and marketing of nonprescription drug products in the United States. Theories of civil liability, negligence, and breach of warranty are also discussed.

Nonprescription and prescription drugs are regulated differently, but both are held to the same standards for safety and efficacy. Nonprescription medications are actively and stringently regulated by the U.S. Food and Drug Administration (FDA) and the Federal Trade Commission (FTC). It is important that health care providers have an understanding of these regulations so that they can respond to their patients' questions and concerns about the self-care products they use.

Reflecting formal usage in pharmacy practice, the term *nonprescription* replaces *over-the-counter (OTC)* throughout this book. However, historically and in many publications, as well as in common parlance, these designations are used interchangeably.

History of Self-Care

Self-care has evolved over many decades from the era of patent medicine, with often expansive promises of benefit including cure as well as purely fraudulent claims of efficacy, to the current availability of both standard and novel nonprescription therapeutic agents with proven health benefits and cost savings for self-reliant consumers.

In 1906, the Pure Food and Drugs Act[1] prohibited adulteration and misbranding. As a result, many patent medicines were forced off the market. This was followed in 1914 by the Harrison Narcotic Act,[2] which required prescription-only status for opium and other narcotics. In 1938, the Food, Drug & Cosmetic Act (FDCA)[3] mandated safety of foods, drugs, and cosmetics, and in 1951 the Durham-Humphrey Amendment was enacted.[4]

Before the Durham-Humphrey Amendment, the manufacturer determined whether a product would be a prescription or nonprescription drug. Confusion ensued, with some manufacturers of a particular product marketing the drug as a nonprescription medication and other manufacturers of the same drug specifying prescription-only status. There was no FDA listing of prescription medications, and the manufacturer's interpretation of FDA regulations of prescription versus nonprescription status was often arbitrary. If FDA disagreed with a product status determination, its sole recourse for remedy was to sue the manufacturer for misbranding.[5] Many nonprescription drugs were marketed without approved New Drug Applications (NDAs) and were considered "grandfathered" drugs.

In 1937, ingestion of a preparation of sulfanilamide using diethylene glycol as a solvent resulted in the deaths of more than 100 people from kidney failure. At that time, the toxicity of diethylene glycol was unknown. The product was sold over the counter. The event prompted the passage of the 1938 FDCA. However, even the tragedy of the nonprescription sale of sulfanilamide (as Elixir of Sulfanilamide) in 1937 did not clarify when a medication should be available without a prescription, and the confusion continued until 1951 with passage of the Durham-Humphrey Amendment. This amendment provided the statutory basis for two classes of drugs in the United States: prescription and nonprescription. The FDCA required that in the absence of a medical need to restrict distribution, nonprescription availability is the default status for FDA-regulated products.

The next legislation that affected nonprescription drugs was the Kefauver-Harris Drug Amendments of 1962, which required proven efficacy for marketed products, including nonprescription drugs.[6] To address this requirement, the focus was on a review of prescription drugs through a Drug Efficacy Study Implementation (DESI) program. Subsequently, in 1972, FDA instituted the "OTC Review" process, described later in the chapter (see The Nonprescription Drug Review Process).

In 1991, FDA created the Division of Nonprescription Drug Products within the Office of Drug Evaluation in the Center for Drug Evaluation and Research (CDER). FDA has issued more than 25 guidance documents for nonprescription medications. Although not legally enforceable, these directives describe FDA's current opinion on a topic and should be viewed as recommendations. A listing of guidance documents pertaining to nonprescription drugs, with brief content summaries, is presented in Table 4–1.

The Food and Drug Modernization Act of 1997[7] expanded FDA's authority over nonprescription drugs in establishing inactive ingredient labeling requirements. This act preempted states from establishing state-specific labeling requirements when federal requirements exist. In the United States, nonprescription drug manufacturers and distributors are represented by the Consumer Healthcare Products Association (CHPA) (formerly the Proprietary Association and, subsequently, the Nonprescription Drug Manufacturers Association).

Over the past 20 years, legislative and regulatory changes pertaining to nonprescription drugs have been implemented, including standardized labeling called *Drug Facts,* additional final monographs, prescription-to-nonprescription switches for drugs never marketed before, and a mechanism for drugs marketed in foreign countries to be considered for the OTC Review process. In 2014,

TABLE 4-1 **FDA Guidance Documents**

Document (with year of issue)	Summary
Organ-Specific Warnings: Internal Analgesic, Antipyretic, and Antirheumatic (IAAA) Drug Products for Over-the-Counter Human Use—Labeling for Products That Contain Acetaminophen (2015)	Document covers alternative allowable language for acceptable liver warnings for products in view of the fact that some IAAA products have maximum daily doses of acetaminophen that are <4 g.
Over-the-Counter Pediatric Oral Liquid Drug Products Containing Acetaminophen (2015)	Document covers standardization of concentration to 160 mg/5 mL in view of dosing errors from multiple concentrations. The package must include a dosage delivery device. Dosing directions should be provided in milliliter units only.
Nonprescription Sunscreen Products—Content and Format of Data Submissions to Support a GRASE Determination Under the Sunscreen Innovation Act (2015)	Document covers format and content of information needed for 586A requests.
Self-selection Studies for Nonprescription Drug Products (2013)	Document provides recommendations for conducting studies to assess the ability of consumers to apply drug labeling information to their personal health situation to make correct nonprescription purchases.
Labeling and Effectiveness Testing: Sunscreen Products for OTC Human Use (2012)	Document provides information to assist industry to comply with labeling and testing requirements for ultraviolet A and B radiation protection for nonprescription sunscreen products.
Labeling for Bronchodilators: Cough, Cold, Allergy, Bronchodilator, and Asthmatic Drug Products for OTC Human Use (2012)	Document provides information to help industry comply with additional warnings on bronchodilator products (i.e., Asthma Alert and revised indications, warnings, and directions).
Toll-free Number Labeling and Related Requirements for Over-the-Counter and Prescription Drugs Marketed With Approved Applications (2012)	Document provides requirements for toll-free number for ADR reporting (not for medical advice) for products approved pursuant to a monograph and contact for those approved pursuant to an approved application.
Time and Extent Applications for OTC Drug Products (2011)	Document explains what information is required for submission of a TEA to show the product has been used "to a material extent" and "for a material time."
Topical Acne Drug Products for OTC Use—Revision of Labeling and Classification of Benzoyl Peroxide	Document covers addition of benzoyl peroxide as a GRASE active ingredient for nonprescription acne products with new warnings, directions, and labeling requirements.
Label Comprehension Studies for Nonprescription Drug Products (2010)	Document covers recommendations on conducting label comprehension studies.
Organ-Specific Warnings: Internal Analgesic, Antipyretic and Antirheumatic Drug Products (2010)	Document covers labeling requirements for warnings regarding potential liver injury and stomach bleeding.
Postmarketing Adverse Event Reporting for Nonprescription Human Drug Products Marketed Without an Approved Application (2009)	Document covers minimum elements and format for ADR reports and how and where to submit reports.
Labeling of Nonprescription Human Drug Products Marketed Without an Approved Application: Questions and Answers (2009)	Document explains the standardized labeling content and format for products not marketed pursuant to an NDA or ANDA in a Q&A format.
Labeling OTC Human Drug Products—Small Entity Compliance Guide (2009)	Document explains the standardized labeling content and format.
Labeling OTC Human Drug Products—Questions and Answers (2009)	Document clarifies, in Q&A format, the standardized labeling content and format.
Labeling OTC Human Products Updating Labeling in RLDs and ANDAs (2002)	Document assists manufacturers of nonprescription drugs marketed via an ANDA or those holding RLDs to comply with the standardized labeling content and format.
Guidance for Over-the-Counter Human Chorionic Gonadotropin (hCG) 510(k)s (2000)	Document covers pregnancy test kit 510(k) medical device approval and patient labeling requirements.
Labeling of OTC Human Drug Products Using a Column Format (2000)	Document describes how more than one Drug Facts box can be used for each side of a package to allow for the use of columns.
Enforcement Policy on Marketing OTC Combination Products (1984)	Document covers policy regarding marketing of combinations of ingredients.

(continued)

TABLE 4-1 FDA Guidance Documents *(continued)*

Document (with year of issue)	Summary
General Guidelines on OTC Drug Combination Products (1978)	Document describes rules for combinations permitted for marketing. Within each monograph, combinations are detailed: Category I ingredients from *different* therapeutic categories may be combined to treat different symptoms concurrently in certain circumstances. Category I ingredients from the *same* therapeutic category should not be combined if they have the same mechanism of action.
Upgrading Category III Antiperspirants to Category I (1978)	Document details the studies required to bring Category III antiperspirant ingredients into Category I.

Key: ADR = Adverse drug reaction; ANDA = Abbreviated New Drug Application; GRASE = generally recognized as safe and effective; OTC = over-the-counter; Q&A = question-and-answer; RLD = reference-listed drug; TEA = Time and Extent Application.

the Sunscreen Innovation Act (SIA) provided an alternative process for the review of safety and effectiveness of nonprescription sunscreen active ingredients, a category FDA considers as drugs.[8] Most recently, FDA has sought input from stakeholders and the public to improve the regulatory processes for nonprescription drugs.

Nonprescription Drugs: Approval and Regulatory Processes

Definition of Nonprescription Status

Nonprescription medications, by definition, may be used without medical supervision. A drug can be marketed as a nonprescription product if it can be used by a consumer guided by the product label such that the consumer can self-diagnose, self-treat, and self-manage the condition requiring attention and if no health care practitioner is needed for the safe and effective use of the product.[9] The drug must also have a low potential for abuse and misuse, and the benefits of nonprescription availability must outweigh the risks.[9] A state may not allow a prescription drug to be sold as other than prescribed, but a state may restrict a drug with nonprescription status under federal law to prescription status.[10] In *Whitehall Labs v. Wilbar,*[11] the court upheld a Pennsylvania law requiring a prescription for Primatene tablets, which was a nonprescription drug by federal rules, finding the Pennsylvania law to be consistent with tenets of consumer protection. Similarly, in *Northwest Corp. v. Oregon Board of Pharmacy,*[12] the court upheld the states' decision to establish prescription status for ephedrine.

Some nonprescription medications are also available as prescription drugs. In such cases, a determination has been made that the medication is safe for nonprescription use in certain dosages or dosage forms, or for specific indications but not for others. Examples are ibuprofen, for which the 200 mg dose is nonprescription for pain but higher dosages and strengths are prescription-only for such conditions as arthritis; meclizine, which is a prescription drug for vertigo but a nonprescription medication for nausea with motion sickness; and nicotine products, which have nonprescription status in gum, lozenge, and patch formulations but prescription-only status for inhaled and nasal products.

The Nonprescription Drug Review Process

On May 11, 1972, the FDA announced a review of nonprescription products marketed between 1938 and 1962 that were not covered under an NDA. Rather than review the more than 300,000 products,[13] FDA divided the products into categories according to the intended therapeutic effect and active ingredients. It then assigned 17 different panels of experts to review each category (e.g., internal analgesics) and each of the more than 700 listed ingredients for safety and effectiveness. Ingredients were assigned to one of three categories: Category I, generally recognized as safe and effective (GRASE); Category II, not GRASE; Category III, insufficient evidence to prove safety and/or effectiveness (i.e., further information is needed to show safety and efficacy and classify as Category I or II). The panels also considered the first prescription-to-nonprescription (also referred to as "Rx-to-OTC") switches, such as those for diphenhydramine and hydrocortisone. Panel deliberations were published in the *Federal Register,* with a comment period followed by a proposed rule and, finally, formal monographs, also published in the *Federal Register,* detailing the dosages and labeling requirements for each ingredient.

Manufacturers of products containing ingredients in Category II were required to either reformulate or remove products from the market. However, banned products could continue to be sold until the inventory was depleted from the pharmacy or wholesaler stock. In some cases, consumers were actually harmed by banned products (e.g., quinine-induced renal failure) that continued to be sold.[14]

For those ingredients placed in Category III, manufacturers were given more than 15 years to conduct necessary studies or to reformulate their products with Category I ingredients. Other manufacturers simply removed the products from the market promptly, primarily because of the costs of studies in view of the product sale history. Some regulators thought that the 15-year grace period was too long, and in *Cutler v. Kennedy,* several consumers sued to have Category III ingredients removed from the market.[15] To take advantage of Category III classification without fear of regulatory action, a manufacturer must provide timely notification of, and initiate, testing.[16] In *Cutler v. Kennedy,* the court held that the OTC Review required removal of Category III ingredients after the final monograph was published, to prevent exposure to unsafe or ineffective drugs. Consequently, many products were removed from the market, and others were reformulated. Some products were moved from one category to another on the basis of research data regarding safety and efficacy.

After more than 40 years, the OTC Review process continues to be applied for new ingredients, amendments to monographs, unfinished monographs, and switches. This public rule-making process is documented by publication in the *Federal Register,* with a corresponding comment period, for each of the three phases: (1) Advance Notice of Proposed Rulemaking, (2) Tentative Final Monograph, and (3) Final Monograph. These monographs in final form are then codified in the Code of Federal Regulations (CFR), where they can be found in 21 CFR parts 331–358.

Pathways to Nonprescription Status

Two mechanisms exist for marketing nonprescription drug products: NDA and the drug monograph. Today, if a manufacturer follows the monograph, it need not obtain FDA approval for the product. Monographs are tantamount to "recipe books" that specify the active ingredients, dosages, and formulations, as well as the labeling and conditions whereby nonprescription drug ingredients are generally recognized as safe and effective (GRASE), and not misbranded. For products that fall outside the monograph specifications, the manufacturer will need either to pursue an NDA,[17] petition to amend the monograph or to modify the product to comply with the monograph specifications.

New agents that are not included in an OTC Review monograph must be regarded as new drugs. For new sunscreen agents, for example, FDA had taken the position that these are new ingredients requiring an NDA. Under the 2014 SIA, an alternate process known as a 586A request for review of sunscreens was established. In 2015, FDA published four draft guidance documents regarding what scientific testing is required for determination of GRASE status for a sunscreen and the timelines for FDA review.[18–21] Examples of nonprescription medications that have required NDAs for a switch from prescription-to-nonprescription status are oxybutynin, ibuprofen, budesonide, and fluticasone nasal spray.

Various types of NDAs can be submitted for marketing of a nonprescription drug:

- Prescription-to-nonprescription switches effected using an NDA or NDA supplement (e.g., omeprazole, nicotine gum, orlistat)
- "Direct-to-nonprescription" (acetaminophen, nicotine lozenge)
- NDA deviation (for new nonprescription products that differ only slightly from monograph products) (rarely used)[22]
- Abbreviated New Drug Application (ANDA), used for switching a generic drug to nonprescription status (e.g., loratadine).

A product containing an ingredient new to the nonprescription marketplace is regulated under the NDA process under Section 505(b)(1) of the FDCA, such as for a prescription-to-nonprescription switch NDA. An NDA can be used to request approval of a nonprescription drug product that deviates from monograph specifications. The product can be marketed only with the exact formulation and labeling approved by FDA. To make a change, the manufacturer must submit an NDA supplement. Nonprescription products can also be approved by means of a 505(b)(2) application, in which previous safety and efficacy data not conducted by or for the applicant may be used, or using an ANDA under section 505(j) of the FDCA.[23] These applications are confidential, but a fee is required. Nonprescription products approved through the NDA route receive a period of exclusivity whereby no other versions can appear on the market. A comparison of the NDA and monograph routes for nonprescription drug approval is detailed in Table 4–2.

Two mechanisms are available for amending a drug monograph: a Citizen Petition[24] and a Time and Extent Application (TEA).[25] A Citizen Petition can be used to request an amendment or repeal of conditions covered in a monograph at any stage. However, the Citizen Petition is limited to pre-1975 marketing conditions—that is, active ingredient, dosage form, or indication. For petitions, the product cannot be marketed until FDA approves the petition.

A TEA can be used to request that applicable drug products be considered for inclusion in the OTC Review monograph system.[25] A TEA is submitted for drug products that can meet the statutory standard of marketing to a "material extent" and "for a material time." This scenario is defined as follows: Drug products initially marketed under an NDA in the United States after 1972; drug products without any U.S. marketing experience; or those not GRASE (i.e., not meeting monograph specifications) in the original OTC Review but for which additional data are now available. The conditions must have been marketed for nonprescription purchase and for at least 5 continuous years in the same country in sufficient quantity. Several sunscreen ingredients, such as amiloxate and bisoctrizole, have used the TEA process to reach the market.

Consumer behavior studies and label comprehension studies are often used to assess whether consumers can appropriately use the product on a nonprescription basis. Because no learned intermediary (i.e., the prescriber) is involved, as for prescription products, such data are often needed to support a switch from prescription to nonprescription status.

It is also mandatory for nonprescription drug manufacturers to register their establishments and list their drug products with FDA.[26] Additionally, FDA may require in vivo or in vitro finished formulation testing (e.g., dissolution tests for enteric-coated and sustained-release products).

TABLE 4-2 Comparison of New Drug Application (NDA) and Drug Monograph Regulatory Approval Pathways

NDA	Monograph
Premarket approval	No premarket approval
Confidential	Public
Drug product–specific	Applies to all products with the ingredient
Potential for marketing exclusivity	No exclusivity
Application filing fees	No filing fees
GMPs apply	GMPs apply
Clinical development required	No clinical development required

Key: GMPs = Good manufacturing practices.

Prescription-to-Nonprescription Switch

Since the mid-1970s, FDA has switched more than 100 ingredients, dosages, or indications from prescription to nonprescription status (Table 4–3). Switch decisions are made by FDA with the advice of advisory councils. Consumers can benefit from prescription-to-nonprescription switches, because they broaden

TABLE 4-3 **Select Prescription-to-Nonprescription Switches**[a]

Purpose/Class of Drug	Drug Name[b]	Year of Switch
Allergic rhinitis	Xyzal Allergy 24HR Tablets (levocetirizine)	2017
	Children's Xyzal Allergy 24HR Oral Solution (levocetirizine)	
	Rhinocort Allergy Spray (budesonide)	2015
	Flonase Allergy Relief (fluticasone propionate)	2014
	Nasacort Allergy 24 HR (triamcinolone) (nasal spray)	2013
	Nasalcrom (cromolyn sodium)	1996
Analgesic/antipyretic	Motrin Migraine Pain, Advil Migraine Liqui-gels (ibuprofen)	2000
	Excedrin Migraine (aspirin/caffeine/acetaminophen)	1998
	Children's Motrin	1995
	Aleve (naproxen)	1994
	Advil, Nuprin (ibuprofen)	1984
Analgesic/decongestant	Advil Congestion Relief (ibuprofen/phenylephrine)	2010
	Children's Advil Cold (ibuprofen/pseudoephedrine)	2002
	Aleve Cold & Sinus (naproxen/pseudoephedrine)	1999
	Advil Cold & Sinus (ibuprofen/pseudoephedrine)	1989
Anthelminthic	Pyrantel pamoate	1986
Anticandidal	Monistat 3 (miconazole nitrate 4%)	1998
	Vagistat-1 (tioconazole)	1997
	Gyne-Lotrimin 3 (clotrimazole)	1996
	Monistat 3 (miconazole nitrate 2%)	1996
	Femstat 3 (butoconazole nitrate)	1995
	Monistat 7 (miconazole nitrate)	1991
	Gyne-Lotrimin, Mycelex-7 (clotrimazole)	1990
Antidiarrheal	Imodium Advanced	1997
	Imodium A-D (loperamide)	1988
Antihistamine	Allegra (fexofenadine HCl)	2011
	Children's Zyrtec Allergy and Children's Zyrtec Hives Relief (cetirizine), syrup and chewable tablets	2007
	Claritin tablets, reditabs, and syrup (loratadine)	2002
	Tavist-1 (clemastine fumarate)	1992
	Doxylamine	1987
	Diphenhydramine HCl	1985
	Drixoral (dexbrompheniramine maleate)	1982
	Triprolidine	1982
	Chlorpheniramine maleate	1976
Antihistamine eye drop	Zaditor	2006
	Alaway	2006
Antihistamine and decongestant or antitussive	Allegra D (fexofenadine/pseudoephedrine)	2011
	Zyrtec D (cetirizine/pseudoephedrine)	2007
	Claritin-D 24 Hour	2002
	Drixoral Plus (dexbrompheniramine maleate/chlophedianol HCl)	1987
	Actifed (pseudoephedrine/triprolidine)	1985

(continued)

TABLE 4-3 **Select Prescription-to-Nonprescription Switches[a]** *(continued)*

Purpose/Class of Drug	Drug Name[b]	Year of Switch
Acid reducer/PPI	Nexium 24 HR (esomeprazole magnesium)	2014
	Prevacid 24 HR (lansoprazole)	2009
	Prilosec OTC (omeprazole)	2003
	Pepcid Complete (famotidine/calcium carbonate/magnesium hydroxide)	2000
	Zantac 75 (ranitidine)	1995
	Pepcid AC (famotidine)	1995
Anorectal vasoconstrictor	Ephedrine sulfate	1980
	Epinephrine hydrochloride	1980
	Phenylephrine hydrochloride	1980
Antiemetic	Diphenhydramine HCl	1987
Antidandruff	Nizoral (ketoconazole)	1997
Antimicrobial	E-Z Scrub (povidone/iodine sponge)	1987
Antipyretic	Hydrocortisone (>0.5%–1%)	1991
	Hydrocortisone	1979
Cold sores	Abreva (docosanol)	2000
Decongestant	Afrinol Repetabs (pseudoephedrine, timed-release)	1982
	Oxymetazoline	1976
	Pseudoephedrine	1976
	Xylometazoline	1976
Dental rinse	Acidulated phosphate fluoride	1980
	Sodium fluoride; stannous fluoride	1980
Emergency contraception	Plan B One Step (levonorgestrel)	2009
	Plan B (levonorgestrel)	2006
Expectorant/decongestant	Mucinex D ER Tablet	2004
	Mucinex DM ER Tablet	2004
	Mucinex ER Tablet (guaifenesin)	2002
Hair regrowth	Rogaine Extra Strength (minoxidil)	1997
	Rogaine (minoxidil)	1996
Laxative	MiraLax (polyethylene glycol)	2006
Ocular vasoconstrictor/ decongestant	Zaditor (ketoprofen)	2006
	Naphcon A, Opcon A, Ocuhist (pheniramine/naphazoline)	1994
	Vasocon A (antazoline phosphate/naphazoline)	1994
	Ocuclear (oxymetazoline HCl)	1986
Oral anesthetic	Dyclonine HCl (solution, suspension, lozenge)	1982
Overactive bladder	Oxytrol for Women (oxybutynin)	2013
Pediculicide	Nix (permethrin)	1990
Poison ivy protection	Ivy Block (bentoquaram)	1996
Sleep aid	Advil PM (ibuprofen/diphenhydramine)	2005
	Diphenhydramine (HCl and monocitrate)	1982
	Doxylamine succinate	1978
Smoking cessation	Commit (lozenge)	2002
	Nicotrol TD	2002
	Nicorette (gum)	1996
	Nicotrol, Nicoderm CQ (patch)	1996

(continued)

TABLE 4-3 **Select Prescription-to-Nonprescription Switches[a]** *(continued)*

Purpose/Class of Drug	Drug Name[b]	Year of Switch
Sunscreen	Anthelios SX (Ecamsule/avobenzone/octocrylene)	2006
Topical antifungal	Lamisil Derm Gel	2006
	Lotrimin Ultra (butenafine HCl)	2001
	Lamisil AT (terbinafine HCl)	1999
	Lotrimin AF (clotrimazole)	1989
	Miconazole	1982
Weight-loss aid	Alli (orlistat)	2007

Key: PPI = Proton pump inhibitor.

[a] A complete listing can be found at http://www.chpa.org/Switch.aspx.

[b] When a brand name is listed, the switch was affected using the NDA process.

access to important medications. In addition, the nonprescription versions are usually cost-effective for consumers and third-party insurers. A survey found that consumers save up to $750 million a year as a result of using nonprescription cough and cold medications that once were available only by prescription. The same study demonstrated that physician visits for the common cold dropped by 110,000 a year between 1976 and 1989, suggesting that access to OTC products contributed to a reduction in office visits.[27]

Among the first products to be switched to nonprescription status was ibuprofen for the treatment of pain in 1984. In a few cases, a drug that was available as a nonprescription product was returned to prescription status, an example being metaproterenol sulfate. FDA itself switched metaproterenol, a decision that was met with great opposition from physicians and pharmacists.[28] Of note, however, FDA considered that self-diagnosis and self-treatment of asthma with nonprescription metaproterenol may delay physician visits in patients with asthma. Furthermore, a nonprescription product must not require routine medical examinations or laboratory testing, and it was for this reason metaproterenol was returned to prescription status. However, exceptions exist for grandfathered drugs—that is, those available before the FDCA of 1938. This is the reason why Asthmanephrin (racepinephrine) is available over the counter for temporary relief of mild respiratory symptoms of bronchial asthma. An additional requirement for nonprescription status is that the condition must be one that a patient can self-diagnose, thus keeping products like acyclovir for genital herpes or statins for hypercholesterolemia from being switched to nonprescription status.[29] Additional issues for acyclovir pertained to increasing resistance to the drug. Similarly, histamine-2 receptor (H2) blockers cannot be labeled for use in ulcers, because the patient's symptoms may mask the presence of gastric cancer.[30]

Products may be switched from prescription to nonprescription status by any of three routes:

1. Submitting a supplemental NDA (applies to a particular product)
2. Petitioning FDA (may be filed by interested parties such as manufacturers, health insurance companies, associations, or pharmacy benefit managers)
3. Amending the drug monograph (applies to all products with the ingredient)

The supplemental NDA route is the most commonly used for prescription-to-nonprescription switches, because unlike with the other two routes, the proceedings are confidential and allow for 3 years of marketing exclusivity. The exclusivity is an incentive for status switching of medications for which patents are about to expire, with ensuing generic competition. The supplemental NDA route is used if the manufacturer is planning to switch the prescription drug without a change in the previously approved dosage form or route. However, if the manufacturer intends to convert some but not all of the indications to nonprescription status, an NDA must be filed. If the manufacturer intends to market a new product whose active substance, indication, or dosage form has never been nonprescription, either an original NDA (505)(b)(1) or 505(b)(2) is required. After a drug goes off patent, anyone can file a 505(b)(2) NDA to switch the drug to nonprescription status. Additional efficacy studies may be required in these situations or when the nonprescription population differs from the population used to support the original NDA (e.g., ibuprofen, for which the nonprescription indications include pain, fever, and dysmenorrhea, but the prescription indications are osteoarthritis and rheumatoid arthritis). Label comprehension studies may also be required. However, comparative studies with other agents are not required.

The second switch mechanism is to petition FDA. This occurs by a Citizen Petition, which must be accompanied by data demonstrating safety and efficacy. In one instance, a managed care organization petitioned FDA to switch several nonsedating antihistamines to nonprescription status in an effort to save money in plan beneficiary reimbursement. Most insurance plans do not cover nonprescription medications.[31] Additionally, Medicaid and Medicare programs often do not pay for nonprescription products. In the case of the nonsedating antihistamines, the manufacturers objected to any switch to nonprescription status, because they stood to lose revenue if the agents became nonprescription drugs. Profitability of a drug when sold by prescription versus over the counter has a profound effect on whether or not nonprescription status will be sought.

The third switch mechanism is to amend the monograph. A process exists to request amendment or repeal of conditions covered by nonprescription drug monographs. Companies may need to file a complete (not supplemental) NDA to request approval of a nonprescription drug that deviates in any respect from a monograph description. In some cases, FDA itself decided to allow self-use, as with hydrocortisone and diphenhydramine. The respective monographs were then amended to add these drugs.

In some cases (e.g., ibuprofen, naproxen), a partial switch for nonprescription status occurs whereby some doses become nonprescription, whereas others remain prescription. In other instances, two different preparations of a product at the same dose may be marketed as both prescription and nonprescription drugs (e.g., cimetidine 200 mg tablets, loperamide 2 mg capsules). In such cases, the prescription and nonprescription versions may not resemble each other in appearance. Additionally, the indications may differ between the nonprescription and prescription versions (e.g., proton pump inhibitors are nonprescription drugs for heartburn but prescription-only medications for peptic ulcer disease).

Safe Use of Nonprescription Drugs

Adulteration and Misbranding

A nonprescription drug is *adulterated* if it contains a substance that may make the product harmful to consumers under customary conditions for use; if it contains any filthy, putrid, or decomposed substance; if its container is composed of a harmful substance; or if it is manufactured or held under unsanitary conditions. All nonprescription drug manufacturing must adhere to *good manufacturing practices (GMPs)*. Failure to follow GMP requirements may cause adulteration of a nonprescription drug preparation.[32]

A nonprescription medication is considered *misbranded* if its labeling is false or misleading, if it does not bear the required labeling information, or if the container is made or filled in a deceptive manner. *Labeling* refers to all labels and other printed, written, or graphic matter on or accompanying a product.

FDA is authorized to inspect nonprescription drug manufacturing facilities, in a capacity similar to its enforcement powers regarding prescription drugs.[33] It can then use administrative enforcement tools such as issuing warning letters or requesting a product recall, or it may seek judicial enforcement by means of a civil injunction, criminal penalties, or product seizure. FDA can request but not mandate a recall of nonprescription drug products.[34] However, if a manufacturer fails to recall a product pursuant to FDA's request, FDA may apply other enforcement options such as injunction, seizure, or criminal prosecution.[35] Once a manufacturer agrees to recall a product, FDA conducts a health hazard evaluation (HHE), classifies the recall, as described next, and notifies the manufacturer of the classification.[34]

Three recall categories have been defined. For a Class I recall, a reasonable probability exists that the use of, or exposure to, a violative product will cause serious adverse health consequences or death. For a Class II recall, use of, or exposure to, a violative product may cause temporary or medically reversible adverse health consequences or the probability of serious adverse health consequences is remote. For a Class III recall, use of, or exposure to, a violative product is not likely to cause adverse health consequences. Additionally, a recall can extend to the manufacturer, wholesale, or retail or consumer level. Depending on the class or level of recall, the manufacturer's notification can be to direct accounts such as wholesalers or to pharmacies or to the general public by way of the FDA website or media coverage. For recalls at the consumer level, the patient may return the nonprescription product to the place of purchase for a refund. Pharmacists can advise patients about the recall and recommend alternative products to the recalled product. Additionally, in the event of a recall, manufacturers provide a toll-free number for consumers to obtain additional information. FDA has a recall audit program to ensure that the recall has been effective.[34,35] For example, many pediatric (infants and children) acetaminophen products were recalled from stores in 2011 after FDA mandated changes to dosing instructions. Acetaminophen products currently on the shelves immediately became ineligible for sale owing to their nonmonograph status, hence the recall.

Adverse Drug Reaction Reporting

In 2004, a dietary supplement ephedra (i.e., ma huang) was linked to stroke, arrhythmias, and death. The product was banned from the U.S. market. Of importance, the incident prompted the mandatory reporting of serious adverse events for dietary supplements and nonprescription drugs.[36] The Dietary Supplement and Nonprescription Drug Consumer Protection Act of 2006 mandated reporting of serious adverse drug reactions (ADRs) by dietary supplement and nonprescription drug manufacturers.[37] Before this act, ADR reporting was required only for nonprescription drugs marketed pursuant to an NDA or ANDA. Manufacturers should submit all serious ADRs (Table 4–4) to FDA as an Individual Case Safety Report (ICSR) on FDA Form 3500A, together with a copy of the label, via either mail or telephone-transmitted facsimile (fax), within 15 business days of receipt. The ADR may also be reported online using the MedWatch Reporting Form. Consumers may report adverse reactions from nonprescription products using the Medwatch online form or by mail or fax using FDA Form 3500B.

For nonprescription products approved under an NDA or ANDA, the requirements are the same as for prescription products approved under these applications—that is, 15-day, periodic, and annual reports of both serious and nonserious ADRs. All ADR reports must be retained for a 6-year period. For prescription products, labeling warnings are often included in the prescribing information to inform prescribers even when a causal relationship has not been definitely established; however, only clearly documented, clinically significant, and important warnings are required for nonprescription products.[37]

The Dietary Supplement and Nonprescription Drug Consumer Protection Act also requires that a manufacturer of nonprescription products marketed under a monograph must place "responsible person" contact information (i.e., domestic address or phone number) on its labels for consumer reporting of ADRs. The responsible person is defined as the manufacturer, packer, or distributor whose name appears on the label. For nonprescription products marketed pursuant to an NDA or ANDA, a toll-free number is required. If the company does not have a toll-free number, the label may include FDA's toll-free MedWatch telephone

TABLE 4–4 Defining Criteria for Serious Adverse Events

- Death
- Life-threatening
- Hospitalization (initial or prolonged)
- Disability or permanent damage
- Congenital anomaly/birth defect
- Required intervention to prevent permanent impairment or damage (including device placement)
- Other serious important medical events (e.g., allergic bronchospasm requiring treatment in an emergency department; seizure that does not result in hospitalization)

number. However, enforcement of this provision has been problematic. Additionally, consumers may report adverse events to the FDA at www.safetyreporting.hhs.gov.

ADRs have led to various FDA actions including requiring additional warnings, MedWatch Safety Alerts (e.g., methemoglobinemia resulting from benzocaine sprays, gels, or liquids applied topically or to gums), category reclassification (e.g., from I to II), request for a recall, or market removal (e.g., phenylpropanolamine).[38]

Labeling

FDA regulates nonprescription drug labeling. FDA reviews nonprescription drug labels for products marketed under an NDA. Nonprescription products must be labeled with adequate directions for patient use, with accommodation for persons with low-level reading comprehension, without the need for medical consultation. The labeling must be "likely to be read" and "likely to be understood" by the "ordinary individual." All labels must be in English. However, manufacturers may include a toll-free number for Spanish-speaking consumers to call with inquiries.

Since 1999, the content and format requirements for nonprescription drug labeling have been standardized and specific.[39] FDA has even provided guidance on font size for the label, which must be 6-point type or larger.[40] The label must appear on the outside container or wrapper, or the immediate container label if packaging does not include an outside container or wrapper, and begins with a Drug Facts panel. It must further include active ingredient(s), purpose(s), use(s), warning(s), directions, other information, inactive ingredients, and questions (if relevant).[41] Inactive ingredients must be listed in alphabetical order and appear on the outside container. Flavors and fragrances may be listed as "flavors" and "fragrances."[41] Trade secret ingredients may be listed as "and other ingredients." Incidental ingredients present at insignificant levels need not be identified, unless the omission would constitute a failure to reveal a material fact.[41] (See Figures 4–1, 4–2, and 4–3.)

Drug Facts warnings may include but are not limited to the following specific phrases and topics: "for external/rectal/vaginal use only"; Reye's syndrome warning; allergic reaction warning; flammability warning; choking warning; alcohol warning; sore throat warning; dosage warning; "do not use" warning; "ask a doctor if you have"; "ask a doctor or pharmacist before you use"; "stop use and ask a doctor if"; pregnancy/breastfeeding warning; "keep out of reach of children"; and "contains phenylalanine." Drug Facts rules detail how to group warnings and how to bullet-list them. In addition, other rules specify what information should appear on the *principal display panel,* which is defined as "that part of the label that is most likely to be displayed, presented, shown, or examined under normal and customary conditions of display for retail sale."[42]

The labeling permitted for each nonprescription ingredient is detailed in the monograph. Minor changes are permitted, provided that the content is truthful and the language not misleading. Additionally, repackagers of nonprescription products must comply with the same labeling requirements as those for manufacturers. FDA takes action if label claims are false or misleading. Jurisdiction extends to all labels and labeling in any media, including websites and social media.[43] NDA ingredients are not found in the monograph, because only the NDA filer is eligible to market these products. Therefore, no rationale exists for providing information for other manufacturers, because they must still go through the ANDA process once the patents expire.

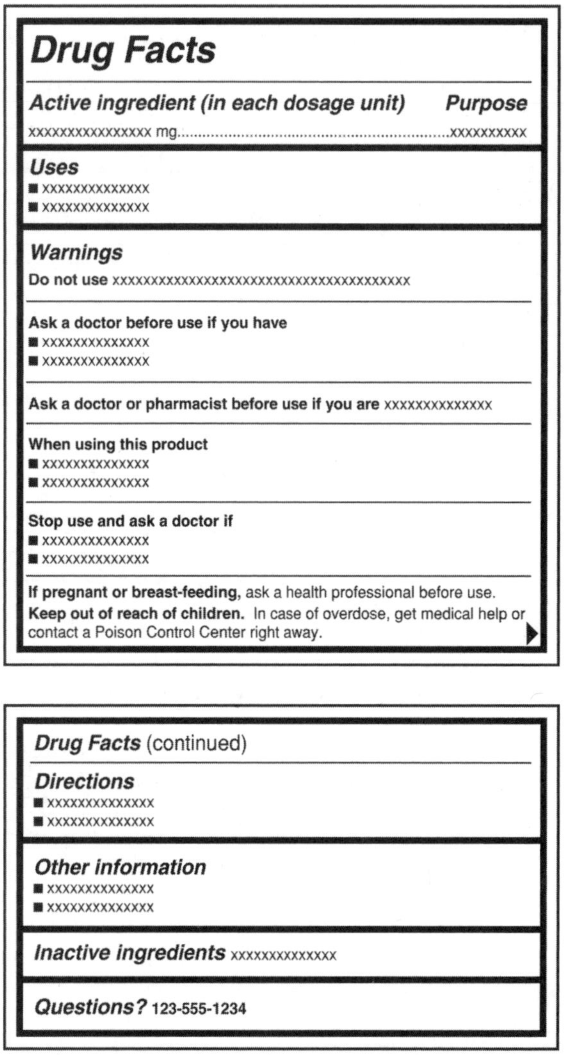

FIGURE **4–1** Drug facts labeling outline. (Source: Reference 40.)

Manufacturers of nonprescription products must warn of foreseeable risks. A voluntary "Flag the Label" program has been adopted by nonprescription drug manufacturers to alert consumers of changes in currently marketed products or labels. *Significant changes* are defined as (1) expansion or limitation of the claims, (2) modification of the dosage level, (3) change in active ingredients or directions for use, (4) new warnings or contraindications, and (5) any other significant new information. The "flag" should be carried on the label for at least 6 months after such a change is made.

An example is product *line extensions,* that is, new products with altered features such as flavors, ingredients, or dosage forms. Line extensions that share the same root name with a suffix or other modifier are prone to patient confusion and errors. FDA reviews and approves proposed trade names for nonprescription products that are approved under the NDA or ANDA process. When products are switched from prescription to nonprescription status, the product may keep its name or use a new name. For partial switches, such as when only one strength formulation is switched to nonprescription status, a new name is usually selected

Drug Facts

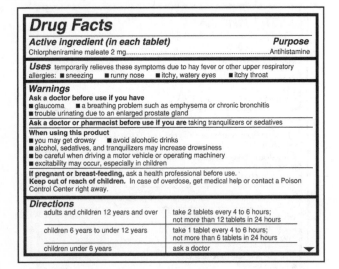

Active ingredient (in each tablet)	*Purpose*
Chlorpheniramine maleate 2 mg	Antihistamine

Uses temporarily relieves these symptoms due to hay fever or other upper respiratory allergies: ■ sneezing ■ runny nose ■ itchy, watery eyes ■ itchy throat

Warnings

Ask a doctor before use if you have
■ glaucoma ■ a breathing problem such as emphysema or chronic bronchitis
■ trouble urinating due to an enlarged prostate gland

Ask a doctor or pharmacist before use if you are taking tranquilizers or sedatives

When using this product
■ you may get drowsy ■ avoid alcoholic drinks
■ alcohol, sedatives, and tranquilizers may increase drowsiness
■ be careful when driving a motor vehicle or operating machinery
■ excitability may occur, especially in children

If pregnant or breast-feeding, ask a health professional before use.
Keep out of reach of children. In case of overdose, get medical help or contact a Poison Control Center right away.

Directions

adults and children 12 years and over	take 2 tablets every 4 to 6 hours; not more than 12 tablets in 24 hours
children 6 years to under 12 years	take 1 tablet every 4 to 6 hours; not more than 6 tablets in 24 hours
children under 6 years	ask a doctor

Drug Facts (continued)

Other information ■ store at 20-25°C (68-77°F) ■ protect from excessive moisture

Inactive ingredients D&C yellow no. 10, lactose, magnesium stearate, microcrystalline cellulose, pregelatinized starch

FIGURE **4-2** Drug facts labeling sample 1. (Source: Reference 40.)

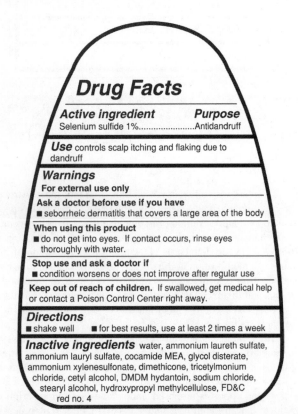

Drug Facts

Active ingredient	*Purpose*
Selenium sulfide 1%	Antidandruff

Use controls scalp itching and flaking due to dandruff

Warnings

For external use only

Ask a doctor before use if you have
■ seborrheic dermatitis that covers a large area of the body

When using this product
■ do not get into eyes. If contact occurs, rinse eyes thoroughly with water.

Stop use and ask a doctor if
■ condition worsens or does not improve after regular use

Keep out of reach of children. If swallowed, get medical help or contact a Poison Control Center right away.

Directions
■ shake well ■ for best results, use at least 2 times a week

Inactive ingredients water, ammonium laureth sulfate, ammonium lauryl sulfate, cocamide MEA, glycol disterate, ammonium xylenesulfonate, dimethicone, tricetylmonium chloride, cetyl alcohol, DMDM hydantoin, sodium chloride, stearyl alcohol, hydroxypropyl methylcellulose, FD&C red no. 4

FIGURE **4-3** Drug facts labeling sample 2. (Source: Reference 40.)

for the nonprescription version. Another example of a change requiring a "Flag the Label" warning is a change in active ingredients. Such was the case when kaolin and pectin were replaced by bismuth subsalicylate in Kaopectate.

Some monographs (e.g., antacid, antiflatulent, topical antifungal, antiemetic, cough and cold) contain professional labeling for health care professionals not included in the nonprescription drug labeling for consumers. The professional labeling is located in the nonprescription monograph. For example, the professional labeling in the monograph for nonprescription antiflatulent products contains additional indications for postoperative gas pain or use in endoscopic examination.[44]

Packaging

Most oral, nasal, otic, ophthalmic, rectal, and vaginal nonprescription medications must be tamper-resistant as required under the Federal Anti-Tampering Act and implementing regulations.[45,46] *Tamper-resistant* refers to a feature of the product packaging that is created to resist access to the product. *Tamper-evident* packaging is characterized by features that make previous unauthorized access to the product easily detectable by the prospective consumer. Exceptions include dermatologics, dentifrices, and insulin. Tamper-resistant packaging is defined as "an indicator or barrier to entry which if breached or missing can reasonably be expected to provide visible evidence to consumers that product tampering has occurred."[45] This requirement was in response to 1982 tampering and adulteration of Extra Strength Tylenol capsules, resulting in several deaths in Chicago. A tamper-resistant statement must be placed on the package and clearly visible to alert consumers about the tamper-evident features. The statement must also advise consumers not to purchase the product if the tamper-evident features are breached or missing.

Nonprescription products must bear an expiration date, which is determined by appropriate stability testing. However, a nonprescription product is exempt from this requirement if its label does not bear any dosage limitations and if the medicine is stable for at least 3 years.

Under the Poison Prevention Packaging Act (PPPA),[47] child-resistant packaging is required for some nonprescription products such as aspirin, acetaminophen, ibuprofen, methyl salicylates, and for any product switched from prescription to nonprescription status.[48] The complete list of products that require child-resistant packaging may be found at 16 CFR. §1700.14. The Consumer Product Safety Commission has authority for enforcement of the PPPA. Manufacturers have the option of choosing one size of their product for a non–child-resistant closure. The label must specify "this package for households without young children." However, if that size is also the most popular size (e.g., bottles of 100 tablets), the manufacturer must also market that size in child-resistant packaging.

Advertising

The Federal Trade Commission (FTC) regulates advertising of nonprescription drugs, devices, and dietary supplements and prohibits false advertisements, which are defined as those that are misleading in a material respect.[49] There is no "fair balance" requirement for benefits versus warnings or contraindications. Advertisements must be supported by the level of data in the manufacturer's files that the ad wording communicates. For example, if the advertisement states "pharmacists and doctors recommend" the product, tests, recommendations, and/or studies must substantiate that statement. A "reasonable basis" standard is applied, meaning that a company must have objective evidence to support a claim before running an advertisement.[50,51] In *Warner Lambert Co v. FTC,* the claims for Listerine in the prevention, cure, and symptomatic alleviation of the common cold were found not to be substantiated, and the company was required not only to stop the advertisement but to run corrective advertisements.[52] In addition to corrective advertising, in other cases FTC has required a manufacturer to conduct at least two clinical trials to substantiate advertising claims.[51]

The National Advertising Division of the Council of the Better Business Bureaus investigates complaints from consumers, competitors, or other parties regarding the truth and accuracy of nonprescription drug advertisements and may escalate the matter to FTC. Additionally, a manufacturer may file private lawsuits against competitors for false claims in advertising, packaging, and labeling through Section 43(a) of the Lanham Act.[53]

FDA has indirect authority over advertising of nonprescription drugs. Advertising claims not included in OTC Review monographs may be subject to agency regulatory action under the misbranding provisions of the FDCA.[54] Additionally, FTC is empowered to issue cease-and-desist orders against false, deceptive, or misleading advertisements of nonprescription drugs. FDA and FTC often act in tandem in reviewing nonprescription drug promotion and have issued joint warning letters to companies that their advertising violates both the FDCA and the FTC Act.

Third Class of Drugs

A little over a decade after passage of the Durham-Humphrey Amendment, various organizations began to advocate for an additional or third class of medications. This intermediate or third class of drugs would be available without a prescription, but a pharmacist would be required to be involved with the sale. Table 4–5 shows drug classification in 10 countries. As can be seen, the two-tier system of prescription and nonprescription in the United States is unique. In fact, the United States and South Africa are the only two countries without such a third class of drugs.

The availability of an intermediate or third class of drugs in the United States, as elsewhere, could be expected to be of considerable benefit in both quality and costs of health care. As a relatively recent example, after the introduction of statins, an important drug class in combating modern diseases, a switch from prescription to nonprescription status would have been not only appropriate but also highly effective in optimizing health care outcomes. With pharmacists involved in the monitoring and education, it is probable that costs, whether economic or health-related (e.g., associated with ADRs), would have been curtailed if these agents had been more readily available as an option for early intervention. An intermediate class of drugs also could be used for those nonprescription products with a potential for abuse or those requiring closer monitoring by a pharmacist.

What is the expected role of pharmacists in this scenario? A tracking system to capture ADRs would be required. Previous concerns have been the time burden such tracking would place on pharmacists and the likelihood of increased costs. The benefits would be obvious when the medication has a potential for abuse or requires closer monitoring or is a first-in-class agent for a new indication.

Pharmacy associations, the National Consumer League, and other consumer groups favor a third or transition class of drugs. CHPA, retail industries, senior citizen groups, and medical groups oppose a third class of drugs. FDA has traditionally opposed a third class of drugs, but in 2012 FDA declared an intent and held a public meeting to clarify parameters for novel switches to nonprescription status. This initiative was termed *Nonprescription Drug Safe Use Regulatory Expansion* (NSURE). Under NSURE, FDA would, for certain common diseases, allow prescription drug products to be available as nonprescription through the use of new technologies (e.g., smartphone applications, point-of-care kiosks) or other conditions for safe use (such as pharmacist interventions).[55] Under NSURE, certain monitoring mechanisms for prescription-to-nonprescription-switch drugs would be allowed, with the proviso of "conditions of safe use." To date, the criteria have not been established, and the conceptional framework

TABLE 4–5 Drug Classification in 10 Countries

Country	Prescription	Pharmacist/Pharmacy Class	Nonprescription
United States	X		X
Australia	X	X	X
Canada	X	X	X
Denmark	X	X	X
France	X	X	
Italy	X	X	
Germany	X	X	X
United Kingdom	X	X	X
Sweden	X	X	X
Switzerland	X	X	X
Netherlands	X	X	

is still in development. However, NSURE has the future potential to increase filings for switches of prescription products that traditionally have been outside the realm of traditional switch candidates, such as first-in-class agents for new indications. Of importance, as a "condition for use," pharmacist interventions under NSURE would undergo definitive expansion with respect to consultation in recommending nonprescription medications.[56]

FDA has emphasized that NSURE was not intended to create a so-called third class of drugs but rather would operate within the existing two classes. Thus, in accordance with the two-tier system in the United States, medications can either be prescription-only or sold in the local convenience store, with no middle ground.[55] Aside from the economic interests of the opposers, FDA has been reluctant to establish a third class, citing reasons that the current two-class system works and that evidence that a third class would improve public health is insufficient for action.[57] These arguments fall short, however, because as discussed further on, strong evidence indicates that the de facto third class of drugs has a tremendous impact on improving public health.

Since 2006, emergency contraception has been nonprescription for women. Additionally, several attempts have been made to allow nonprescription sales of oral contraceptives.

Studies have shown that women in the United States are very interested in access to oral contraceptives without a prescription, that women can accurately identify contraindications to use of oral contraceptives with simple checklists, and that nonprescription contraception would increase use, with consequent reductions in unintended pregnancy rates.[58] Thus far, however, every attempt to change the status of oral contraceptives to nonprescription has been met with strong opposition from "pro-life" groups.[59] Because an OTC Review monograph for oral contraceptives is lacking, a company would have to demonstrate safety and consumers' understanding of the labeling. Health insurers are required under the Affordable Care Act[60] to cover the costs of prescriptions for contraceptives. If contraceptives are moved to nonprescription status, insurers would be less likely to pay for them. Removal of this coverage is a disincentive for nonprescription status. Currently, oral contraceptives are available from pharmacists in several states (e.g., Tennessee, Washington) and Washington, DC, under collaborative practice agreements and in other states (e.g., Oregon, California) through direct pharmacist prescribing.[61,62] However, oral contraceptives remain as prescription products in these scenarios, with pharmacists given additional authority to initiate via protocol or to prescribe them. Although California has no age restrictions, Oregon women under the age of 18 must have a previous prescription from a physician or pharmacist. Several states are considering similar legislation. Alternatively, oral contraceptives could be a candidate for an intermediate or third class of drugs.

In 2007, FDA signaled a possible change in its opposition in calling a meeting to obtain comments about creation of a "behind-the-counter" class of drugs.[63] Unfortunately, the Government Accountability Office (GAO) report issued from that meeting concluded that the experiences in other countries provided little insight into the likely effect of a behind-the-counter class in the United States.[64] As recently as 2012, FDA announced it was considering creation of a class of nonprescription drugs that could be made available to patients "under conditions for safe use," which may potentially include pharmacist intervention.[65] Hearings were held, with the same groups in opposition to the concept. However, no progress has been made moving forward on the concept since then.

De Facto Third Class of Drugs

Some medications are already supplied to patients without a prescription, but consumer access to them is restricted: they are available only "behind the counter"—that is, only by expressly asking a pharmacist for them, thereby creating a de facto third class of medications. This group includes a small number of exempt narcotic combination products placed in Schedule V (e.g., codeine),[66] pseudoephedrine (see Chapter 11), NPH and recombinant (R) U-100 insulin, syringes and needles, and naloxone. Federal requirements for Schedule V medications sold without a prescription are found in Table 4–6.

Another example of voluntary restricted access is dextromethorphan, a cough suppressant. Although dextromethorphan is not a Schedule V medication, drug manufacturers and retailers have imposed state-specific voluntary age restrictions on its purchase,

TABLE 4–6 Federal Requirements for Schedule V Medications

Schedule V definition	■ Codeine preparations: limited to 200 mg/100 mL or 100 g ■ Dihydrocodeine, ethylmorphine, opium preparations: limited to 100 mg/100 mL or 100 g ■ Diphenoxylate: limited to 25 mg/25 mcg atropine sulfate ■ Diphenoxin: limited to 0.5 mg/25 mcg atropine sulfate
Age and personal identification requirement	■ Purchaser must be 18 years of age. ■ Identification is required when pharmacist does not know purchaser.
Seller requirement	■ Dispensed only by pharmacist or intern
Medication limitations	■ Not more than 240 mL (8 ounces) of any such controlled substance containing opium ■ Not more than 120 mL (4 ounces) of any other such controlled substance ■ Not more than 48 dosage units of any such controlled substance containing opium ■ Not more than 24 dosage units of any other such controlled substance may be dispensed at retail to the same purchaser in any 48-hour period.
Documentation requirement	■ Bound record book containing: – Purchaser's name and address – Name and quantity of medication – Date – Name or initials of dispensing pharmacist
Stricter law prevails	■ No state or local law requires a prescription to dispense.

making the drug far less available to teens who might be looking to for a way to get high.[67]

Additionally, in an increasing number of states, pharmacists have been given prescriptive authority to dispense a limited number of prescription medications without a medical prescription. The first state to allow this provider role was Florida, where pharmacists can prescribe medications listed on a formulary that consists of fluoride- or lindane-containing products, some topical anti-infectives, antihistamines and decongestants, and products recommended by an FDA Advisory Panel for transfer to nonprescription status but pending FDA action.[68,69] Currently, six states, Montana, New Mexico, North Carolina, North Dakota, Oregon, and California, give pharmacists midlevel practitioner status, allowing them to initiate and modify drug therapy pursuant to a collaborative practice agreement with a physician.[70] In 2013 and 2016, laws in California and Oregon, respectively, took effect that allow pharmacists to prescribe oral contraceptives to women 18 years and older.[71] In California, the professional scope of practice for pharmacists was expanded to include the following[72]:

- Prescribe nicotine replacement therapy, which normally requires a prescription
- Prescribe medications for travel health purposes (e.g., scopolamine patches)
- Mandate tests to monitor and maintain drug therapy for patients with comorbid conditions such as diabetes, hypertension, and hyperlipidemia

Other states are considering similar legislation.

Pharmacists, who constitute the most accessible interface between the community and the health care system,[73] are ideally positioned to provide overdose education and to expand access to naloxone. As of May 2016, 43 states have laws that permit, under certain circumstances, a person coming off the street to obtain naloxone without a prescription at a pharmacy.[74,75] These laws take many forms: dispensing to any person authorized to receive naloxone by a standing order (e.g., Alabama, Arkansas, New Hampshire, New Jersey, New York); pharmacist prescriptive authority (e.g., Connecticut, Idaho, North Dakota, New Mexico); and collaborative practice agreements (e.g., Idaho, Kentucky, Maryland, Rhode Island, Washington, Tennessee, Wisconsin).[76] The Department of Veterans Affairs and the Indian Health Service have granted independent prescribing authority. Nearly all of these laws grant immunity to pharmacists who prescribe naloxone, provided that the prescriber does not act with gross negligence or reckless indifference to harm. No cases against pharmacists or other prescribers have been reported.[77] The two products currently available are naloxone nasal spray (Narcan) and naloxone autoinjector (Evzio).

Abuse of Nonprescription Medications

A list of nonprescription medications that have been abused, along with legislative and regulatory initiatives to curb such abuse, is presented in Table 4–7. When it comes to protecting the public from abuse of nonprescription medications, pharmacists have made a difference.

TABLE 4-7 Abuse of Various Nonprescription Medications[a]

Medication	Effect(s)/Use	Legislative/Regulatory Action
Dextromethorphan	Dissociative effects; altered mental status; intoxication	Many products reformulated to omit ingredient; in some states, behind-the-counter sale only (e.g., New York, Utah)
Pseudoephedrine (also applied to ephedrine, but sale limits differ)	Precursor used in manufacture of methamphetamine	Combat Methamphetamine Epidemic Act of 2005 (logbook of sales; limits daily purchase amounts to 3.5 g, with 30-day limit of 9 g and mail order 30-day limit 7.5 g) Schedule V in some states (Illinois, Iowa, Kansas), Schedule III (Oregon, Mississippi)[b]
Class V Controlled Substances (e.g., cough syrups)	Opioid abuse	See Table 4–5
Laxatives	Anorexia; electrolyte imbalances; gastrointestinal complications	
Loperamide[c]	Cardiotoxicity; ventricular arrhythmias; QT and QRS prolongation	None
Nonprescription antihistamines; dimenhydrinate	Intoxication; stimulant effects including euphoria and hallucinations	None

[a] See DEA's Office of Diversion Control website for more detailed information regarding sale limits and recordkeeping requirements: https://www.deadiversion.usdoj.gov/pubs/manuals/pharm2/appendix/appdx_g.htm.

[b] U.S. Department of Justice Drug Enforcement Administration. Combat Methamphetamine Epidemic Act 2005. Title VII of USA Patriot Improvement Reauthorization Act of 2005. Pub L No. 109-177. 109th Congress. March 9, 2006. Available at: http://www.deadiversion.usdoj.gov/meth/index.html.

[c] Source: U.S. Food and Drug Administration. Drug Safety Communication: FDA warning about serious heart problems with high doses of the antidiarrheal medicine loperamide (Imodium) including abuse and misuse. Available at: http://www.fda.gov/Drugs/DrugSafety/ucm504617.htm. Accessed April 15, 2017.

From Cosmetic to Drug: Crossing the Line

FDA's authority over cosmetics is less comprehensive than its authority over other FDA-regulated products. Laws that pertain to cosmetics are the FDCA, specifically, the adulteration and misbranding provisions[78]; the Poison Prevention Packaging Act; and the Fair Packaging and Labeling Act.[79] There are no requirements for manufacturer registration, premarket notification, ingredient safety testing, product listing, monographs, GMPs, or ADR reporting.[80] Cosmetic manufacturers may voluntarily decide to register with the FDA and report ingredients in their products. FDA does not have authority to require a manufacturer to recall a cosmetic product from the marketplace.[81] Regulation is under the FDA Center for Food Safety & Applied Nutrition, specifically, the Division of Colors and Cosmetics.

In an early opinion, FDA stated that some cosmetics are also nonprescription drugs. Such products must meet the regulatory requirements (including labeling and packaging) for both cosmetics and drugs. Additionally, many legal precedents are in place for products that have crossed the line from cosmetic to drug—so-called cosmeceuticals.[82] Early cases involved wrinkle removal products for which the product claims included strong therapeutic implications.[83,84] Other cases involve cosmetic product claims that establish the product as intended to treat or prevent disease or otherwise affect the structure or functions of the human body. Often it is not the ingredient used in the product but rather the labeling claims content that determines whether the product is considered a cosmetic or a drug. Some examples are claims that products will restore hair growth, reduce cellulite, treat varicose veins, or regenerate cells. The mere presence of ingredients in low or inactive levels, that is, below those specified in an OTC Review monograph, also does not make a cosmetic a drug. Examples of cosmetic products that may also be drugs are listed in Table 4–8.

If a cosmetic is also a drug, the active ingredients must be listed first, followed by other ingredients, except flavors and fragrances, in descending order of predominance. The "principal display panel" must include the net quantity, name and place of the manufacturer, the declaration of ingredients, and any warning statements. Specific content that determines when a cosmetic should be classified as a drug includes (1) claims to cure, mitigate, treat, or prevent a disease; (2) claims to effect major changes in the structure of the body, or in a major bodily function; and (3) presence of a compendium-listed ingredient intended to serve medicinal purposes.[85]

TABLE 4–8 Cosmetics That May Also Be Drugs

- Topical antimicrobial products (e.g., soaps containing antimicrobials)
- Skin protectants
- Sunscreen products
- Antiperspirant products
- Skin-bleaching products
- Nail hardeners
- Teeth whiteners with bleach
- Indoor and oral tanning preparations
- Hormone creams
- Eye wrinkle creams
- Wrinkle eradicators or antiaging creams

Compounding Nonprescription Drugs

At one time, nonprescription products were routinely compounded as needed. Although explicit guidelines on compounding nonprescription medications are lacking, and the pharmacy compounding provisions of the Food and Drug Modernization Act of 1997 do not directly address nonprescription drugs, pharmacists should rely on guidance established for compounding prescription medications. Pharmacists should not compound any medication for nonprescription use that is intended to be used pursuant to a prescription or one that has not been approved for nonprescription use. Additionally, as with prescription medications, pharmacists should not compound large quantities of nonprescription medications that are essentially copies of commercially available nonprescription drugs.[86] A summary of regulatory requirements for nonprescription drugs is presented in Table 4–9.

Nonprescription Homeopathic Drugs

Homeopathy is a system of alternative medicine based on the practice of treating symptoms of a disease with substances that produce symptoms of the disease in healthy subjects (i.e., "like cures like"). Nonprescription homeopathic preparations are regulated by FDA as drugs[87] and must have a therapeutic indication for a self-limiting, self-diagnosable condition. They are governed by the Homeopathic Pharmacopoeia of the United States (HPCUS) and its supplements, which are produced by the Homeopathic Pharmacopoeia Convention of the United States.[88] The same criteria under the FDCA for a determination of nonprescription or prescription status apply to homeopathic products. The regulatory framework for marketing is found in FDA's Compliance Policy Guide (CPG), specifically, CPG 7132.15.

TABLE 4–9 Summary of Nonprescription Drug Regulations

Labeling	■ Drug Facts format ■ Regulated by FDA ■ Inactive ingredients in alphabetical order
ADR reporting	■ Required for both OTC Review monograph- and NDA-approved nonprescription drugs
Manufacturing	■ GMPs
Advertising	■ Regulated by FTC
Packaging	■ Tamper-resistant ■ Child-resistant
Marketing	■ By NDA ■ By monograph route

Key: ADR = Adverse drug reaction; FDA = U.S. Food and Drug Administration; FTC = Federal Trade Commission; GMPs = good manufacturing practices; NDA = New Drug Application.

Advertising of these products is regulated by FTC. Homeopathic drugs were not included in either the DESI or the Nonprescription Drug Review and have never been required to show safety or efficacy before marketing. These products must comply with display panel requirements but are exempt from expiration dating. However, nonprescription homeopathic drugs cannot be marketed for conditions that require a prescription. Manufacturers must register with FDA, list their products, and adhere to GMPs.[89]

Currently, FDA is taking a closer look at homeopathic products. In 2015, a public hearing was held evaluating FDA's regulatory framework, including labeling, safety and enforcement policies, and mechanisms and means of improving such policies going forward. Homeopathic products and ingredients do not go through any FDA approval process, nor are they subject to any nonprescription monograph. Safety issues have emerged, and many cases of poison exposure related to homeopathic products are reported by the American Association of Poison Control Centers annually.[90]

Dietary Supplements

Although often offered alongside nonprescription drug products on pharmacy shelves, dietary supplements are regulated by FDA's Center for Food Safety and Applied Nutrition as foods, not drugs. Although dietary supplement claims and nonprescription drug claims have different evidence standards, they may be perceived by the consumer as indistinguishable. Dietary supplements belong to a separate category that is not tightly regulated. More than 200 million Americans take dietary supplements, and botanical dietary supplements are used by 17.9% of U.S. adults.[91] Dietary supplements are regulated under the Dietary Supplement Health and Education Act (DSHEA) of 1994.[92] Under the DSHEA, dietary supplements are defined to include "vitamins, minerals, herb or other botanical, amino acid, a substance which increases the dietary intake of it, or a concentrate, metabolite, constituent, extract, or combination of any ingredient described above."[92]

Dietary supplements are not approved by FDA but are subject to the adulteration and misbranding provisions of the FDCA and should be manufactured in accordance with GMPs. However, GMPs are nonbinding on manufacturers, and herbal product manufacturers in particular have largely ignored them because of considerable variation in the ingredients for herbal preparations.[93] A petition must be filed to market new dietary ingredients (i.e., those not already marketed before 1994), thus requiring premarket notification but not an evaluation for efficacy or safety. Enforcement of this provision has been problematic, however, with only approximately 170 notices from 1994 to 2012 despite the introduction of thousands of new supplements to the marketplace.[89] FDA may stop a new dietary ingredient from being marketed if it does not receive enough safety information in advance.

Under the DSHEA, labels must bear the term "dietary supplement," and each ingredient must have the quantity stated. For a proprietary blend, however, the quantities of each ingredient are not stated; only a net contents for the blend is included. Inactive ingredients must be listed in descending order of predominance. The labeling must contain a *Supplement Facts* panel identifying the dietary ingredient(s) contained in the product. When no daily recommended dose has been established, the dietary supplement may be marketed without this information. They may also be marketed in any combination of supplement ingredients (e.g., calcium plus magnesium).[94] Although FDA requires that manufacturers verify that every supplement they produce is safe and accurately labeled, the system essentially operates on the honor code. Under DSHEA, a dietary supplement deemed unsafe may continue to be marketed until the courts rule in FDA's favor.[95]

Advertising claims in all media are regulated by the FTC. However, FDA is responsible for claims on product labeling. Chapter 50 provides information about proper labeling of dietary supplement products.

Dietary supplement manufacturers are subject to GMPs and FDA inspection. Nevertheless, they are often tainted with active pharmaceutical ingredients, are adulterated with other ingredients, fail to contain the purported active ingredient, or may be sold at toxic doses.[96] The DSHEA requires the government to bear the burden of proof to show that a dietary supplement is either adulterated or misbranded, and each case must be tried de novo. Categories of dietary supplements that often have been found to be tainted include male enhancement supplements,[97] herbal products, and weight-loss products. FDA's Medication Health Fraud website (www.fda.gov/Drugs/ucm136245.htm) is a useful resource for information regarding tainted products sold as dietary supplements. Additionally, to improve regulation of dietary supplements, FDA has created an Office of Dietary Supplements Programs. Chapter 50 provides a more in-depth look at dietary supplements.

Point-of-Care Diagnostic Devices

Unlike nonprescription drugs, the point-of-care testing (POCT) devices are reviewed by FDA's Center for Devices and Radiological Health and may be approved via a Premarket Approval (PMA) application or via the 510K route.[98] A company with 510K clearance for a prescription device will need to submit a new 510K to market the product for nonprescription use. Data will be required to show that consumers can use the device and interpret the results without the assistance of a health care professional.[99]

Point-of-care testing can be self-initiated, as when the patient is responding to symptoms, or prescriber-initiated, as when a sample is taken in the home environment and returned to be assayed in a laboratory. Considerable interest in kits for human immunodeficiency virus (HIV) testing, confirmation of streptococcal infection ("Strep"), detection of drugs of abuse, and cholesterol screening and monitoring has been recognized, and much continued discussion in this area is likely.

All point-of-care laboratory testing in pharmacies is subject to regulation by the Centers for Medicare and Medicaid Services as part of the Clinical Laboratory Improvement Amendments (CLIA) program. However, most point-of-care tests conducted in community pharmacies or at health screenings are considered CLIA-waived. To obtain a CLIA waiver, the pharmacy must first obtain a CLIA certificate and then apply for laboratory status at the state level, usually through the state health department.[100] Each state has its own CLIA program and may impose additional requirements or restrictions. Pharmacies with CLIA waivers are still subject to inspection to ensure compliance and must also comply with standards set forth in Occupational Safety and Health Administration (OSHA) universal precautions to reduce risk of exposure to blood-borne pathogens.

Currently, approximately 18% of community pharmacies have a CLIA waiver and can perform CLIA-waived tests such as determination of the international normalized ratio (INR), blood glucose, glycosylated hemoglobin (HgA_1C), and lipid profile.[101] With increased pharmacy-based disease state management programs and health screening-related collaborative practice agreements, the number of pharmacies with CLIA waiver status is likely to increase in the future.

Nonprescription Product Liability

Most cases involving nonprescription drugs are product liability cases, brought against manufacturers, not pharmacies or pharmacists. Although not as common as claims against prescription drugs, nonprescription drugs have been the subject of civil litigation. Claims are brought for breach of the Implied Warranty of Fitness[102] and for breach of the Implied Warranty of Merchantability.[103] Recovery under these legal theories is generally limited to sale of a product, rather than performance of a service in which a defective product may be involved only incidentally. When the service being performed is a professional service, such as with a pharmacist recommendation for a defective nonprescription product, the courts exhibit a reluctance to impose strict liability without fault. However, the pharmacist may still be liable for negligence and/or intentional misconduct as appropriate to the facts of the case.[104] In litigation in which the pharmacist sold the patient camphorated oil instead of castor oil, with subsequent harm to the patient, the court held the pharmacist negligent.[105]

For the nonprescription drug plaintiff, the first evidentiary hurdle is proof of purchase, which can result in a summary judgment on this threshold issue. The injured party will need to furnish a receipt or other evidence of proof of purchase. Causation is another issue, in that a purchased nonprescription product may sit in the medicine cabinet for months before actual use. It is difficult to prove, with mere plaintiff testimony, proximity in time between use of the product and injury. However, unlike the case with prescription drugs, in which the learned intermediary (the prescriber) is a defense for manufacturers, for nonprescription drug products, manufacturer warnings must go directly to the consumer. In *Yugler v. Pharmacia & Upjohn Co.*, the court denied application of the learned intermediary doctrine, even when the provider had initially prescribed prescription Motrin and the patient obtained refills over the counter.[106]

Liability for Advice on Nonprescription Drugs

Pharmacists can be sued for malpractice and negligence for inaccurate advice (with liability requiring affirmative misrepresentations) regarding nonprescription drugs that harm the patient. A recommendation for use of a nonprescription product not in accordance with the labeling may increase the risk for liability if the patient is harmed. Additionally, when a pharmacist recommended a nonprescription product in place of the prescribed one, and the patient was harmed, the court denied the pharmacy's motion for summary judgment that the patient was "contributory negligent" in ignoring the label directions.[107]

One of the most high-profile recent recommendation cases is *Whiting v. Rite Aid Pharmacy*,[108] wherein the patient's estate sued the pharmacist for a recommendation that the patient could safely take phenylpropanolamine and Sudafed. The plaintiff contended that she informed the pharmacist of the patient's prostate problems. The pharmacist denied that the conversation ever occurred. The plaintiff asserted that the use of the drug exacerbated the patient's prostate condition, resulting in the need for several surgeries and, ultimately, his death several years later from an unrelated illness. The pharmacy contended that learned intermediary doctrine protects the pharmacist from such liability and that the pharmacists' duty of care does not require giving adequate advice about nonprescription drugs. Falling under the learned intermediary doctrine is a defense of tort lawsuits stating that the duty to warn of the dangers of a nonprescription product is that of the manufacturer. The court ruled that the learned intermediary doctrine applies only to prescription drugs. Additionally, the court was clear with respect to the duty of care for pharmacists[108]:

> Pharmacists in Utah clearly have duties regarding nonprescription drugs. If a pharmacist answers a customer's question and offers advice about nonprescription drugs, the pharmacist must advise and act in a non-negligent manner consistent with a reasonably prudent pharmacist's response to a customer's question about the safety of a nonprescription drug.

Ingredients in nonprescription drug products change often, and pharmacists should be certain of a product's ingredients and contraindications before recommending it. The Drug Facts labeling of the product should form a basis for any patient consultation and advice on nonprescription drug products. Counseling for patient education should be routinely and briefly documented.[109] As nonprescription marketing of medications becomes more prevalent in the United States, litigation against manufacturers of nonprescription drug products will similarly increase.

Strict Liability Associated With Nonprescription Drugs

Strict liability could apply to pharmacists for failure to effect timely removal of a recalled or expired product from the shelves when a patient is harmed. The courts have generally ruled that no liability accrues to the pharmacist for defective medications sold in prepackaged containers. However, if a pharmacy repackages the drug with its own label, it may be held liable.[110] The label of the repackaged drug should contain the same amount of information as on the original label.[10] In *Patrick v. Carrier Stevens Co.*,[111] the plaintiff prevailed when he purchased a flea repellant warranted by the pharmacist as safe for his pet even if ingested, but which then subsequently harmed his other animals.

Manufacturers are subject to strict liability for harm caused by a "product in a defective condition unreasonably dangerous to the user or consumer."[112] Class action lawsuits for defective nonprescription products continue to be initiated, especially when the company delayed in warning consumers of ADRs. Notable examples of adverse events involving nonprescription drugs leading to class action lawsuits are severe, potentially fatal hypersensitivity allergic reactions from nonprescription acne products; bone fractures and hypomagnesemia from proton pump inhibitors; and Stevens-Johnson syndrome and toxic epidermal necrolysis from ibuprofen.[113–115]

Key Points

- Over the past 100-plus years, regulatory transition of nonprescription medications from patent medicines to scientifically based therapies has occurred.
- Nonprescription medications are vital and one of the least costly components of the U.S. health care system.
- Regulation of nonprescription medications is important to protect the public but should not place limits on achieving an optimal level of personal health.

- Existing overregulation of nonprescription medications prevents patients from gaining control over their health care, increases patient costs, and requires unnecessary use of health care resources to obtain some prescriptions.
- The past few decades have seen a large number of prescription-to-nonprescription switches, and today's consumers are taking greater responsibility for their own health care.
- An essential element of collaborative clinical practice for health care professionals is a full understanding of the regulatory and legal aspects of how nonprescription products are manufactured, labeled, and marketed.

REFERENCES

1. Pure Food and Drugs Act, 34 Stat 768 (1906).
2. Harrison Narcotic Act, Ch. 1, 38 Stat 785 (1914).
3. 21 USC §301, et seq. 52 Stat 1040.
4. Durham Humphrey Amendment, 65 Stat 648 (1951).
5. Abood RR. Federal regulation of medications. In: *Pharmacy Practice and the Law.* 6th ed. Sudbury, MA: Jones & Bartlett; 2011:119.
6. Kefauver Harris Amendment, 76 Stat 780 (1962).
7. Food and Drug Modernization Act of 1997. Pub L No. 105-115, 121 Stat 823.
8. 21 USC Ch. 9 Sub. 5 Part I, enacted November 26, 2014.
9. 21 USC 353(b)(1)(A).
10. Brushwood DB. Nonprescription drugs. In: *Medical Malpractice.* New York, NY: McGraw-Hill; 1996:117–8.
11. 397 Pa 223, 154 A2d 596 (1959).
12. 814 P.2d 191 (Or Ct App 1991).
13. Farley D. Benefit vs. risk. How FDA approves new drugs. *FDA Consum Spec Rep.* 1995;2:23.
14. Podolsky D. Questionable medicine. *US News World Rep.* 1995;118:101.
15. 475 F Supp 838 (DDC 1979).
16. 21 CFR §330.10(a)(13)(iii) and 10(b).
17. Food, Drug & Cosmetic Act, §505(a) and (b) (1938).
18. Guidance for Industry. Nonprescription Sunscreen Drug Products: Safety and Effectiveness Data. U.S. Food and Drug Administration. November 2016. Available at http://www.fda.gov/downloads/drugs/guidancecomplianceregulatoryinformation/guidances/ucm473464.pdf. Accessed April 5, 2017.
19. Guidance for Industry. Sunscreen Innovation Act: Withdrawal of a 586A Request or Pending Request U.S. Food and Drug Administration. October 2016. Available at http://www.fda.gov/downloads/drugs/guidancecomplianceregulatoryinformation/guidances/ucm473467.pdf. Accessed April 5, 2017.
20. Guidance for Industry. U.S. Food and Drug Administration. Sunscreen Innovation Act: Section 586C(c) advisory committee process. October 2016. Available at http://www.fda.gov/downloads/drugs/guidancecomplianceregulatoryinformation/guidances/ucm473770.pdf. Accessed April 5, 2017.
21. Guidance for Industry. Nonprescription Sunscreen Drug Products—Content and Format of Data Submissions. U.S. Food and Drug Administration. November 2016. http://www.fda.gov/downloads/drugs/guidancecomplianceregulatoryinformation/guidances/ucm473772.pdf. Accessed April 5, 2017.
22. Food, Drug & Cosmetic Act, §330.11 (1938).
23. 21 USC 355(b)(2) (2011).
24. 21 CFR 10.30.
25. 21 CFR 330.14.
26. 21 CFR part 207.
27. Temin P. Realized benefits from switching drugs. *J Law Econ.* 1992; 35(2):351–69.
28. FDA's Prescription to Over-the-Counter Drug Switch. Hearing Before the Subcommittee on Oversight and Investigation of the Committee on Energy and Commerce, House of Representatives, Ninety Eighth Congress, Washington, DC, Government Printing Office, 48 *Fed Reg.* 24925 (June 3, 1983).
29. Strom BL. Statins and over-the-counter availability. *N Engl J Med.* 2005;352:1403–5. doi: 10.1056/NEJMp058025.
30. Pray WS. *Nonprescription Product Therapeutics.* 2nd ed. Baltimore, MD: Lippincott Williams & Wilkins; 2006:23–4.
31. Tahmincioclu E. Over-the-counter, yes, but out of the insurance plan. *New York Times.* July 4, 2004.
32. Food, Drug & Cosmetic Act, §505(a)(2)(B) (1938).
33. 21 USC §374(a)(1) (2011).
34. Rumore MM. An analysis of Class I recalls: 1982–1996. *Ther Innov Reg Sci.* 1998;32(1):65–71.
35. U.S. Food and Drug Administration. Recall Procedures Manual. Chapter 7. In: *FDA Enforcement Manual.* Silver Spring, MD: U.S. Food and Drug Administration; Oct 2013.
36. Institute of Medicine. *Use of Dietary Supplements by Military Personnel.* Washington, DC: National Academies Press; 2008. Available at: https://www.nap.edu/catalog/12095/use-of-dietary-supplements-by-military-personnel. Accessed April 5, 2017.
37. Pub L No. 109-462, 120 Stat 4500 (2006).
38. U.S. Food and Drug Administration. Drug Safety Communication: Reports of a rare, but serious and potentially fatal adverse effect with the use of over-the-counter (OTC) benzocaine gels and liquids applied to the gums or mouth. April 7, 2011. Available at: http://www.fda.gov/drugs/drugsafety/ucm250024.htm. Accessed April 5, 2017.
39. 21 CFR 201.66.
40. Guidance for Industry. Labeling for OTC Human Drug Products—Questions and Answers. U.S. Food and Drug Administration. Dec 2008. Available at: http://www.fda.gov/downloads/drugs/guidancecomplianceregulatoryinformation/guidances/ucm078792.pdf. Accessed April 5, 2017.
41. 21 CFR part 201, subparts A and C.
42. 15 USC §1459 (f), Title 15. Commerce and Trade; Chapter 39. Fair Packaging and Labeling Program (2013).
43. FDA Response to Washington Legal Foundation Citizen Petition. Nov. 1, 2001. Available at https://www.regulations.gov/document?D=FDA-2011-P-0497-0003. Accessed April 5, 2017.
44. 21 CFR 332.31.
45. 18 USC 1365.
46. 21 CFR 211.132.
47. Pub L No. 91-601, §7, 84 Stat 1670, 1673 (1970).
48. 21 CFR 1700.14(a)(30).
49. 15 USC §45(a)(1) (2006).
50. Skinner W. Allowable advertising claims for dietary supplements. *J Pharm Law.* 1996;5(2):309–26.
51. Thompson Medical Co, Inc, 104 FTC, 791 F.2d 189 (DC Cir 1986).
52. 562 F2d 749 (DC Cir 1977).
53. 15 USC §1125(a) (1982).
54. 21 CFR 330.1(d).
55. U.S. Food and Drug Administration. Nonprescription Drug Safe Use Regulatory Expansion (NSURE). Oct 4, 2012. Available at: https://www.fda.gov/downloads/ForHealthProfessionals/UCM330650.pdf. Accessed April 5, 2017.
56. Page MR. Rx-to-OTC switches: trends to watch. *Pharm Times.* Feb 9, 2015. Available at: http://www.pharmacytimes.com/publications/issue/2015/february2015/rx-to-otc-switches-trends-to-watch/. Accessed April 5, 2017.
57. APhA policy supports a third class of drugs. *Am Pharm.* 1991;31(2):40.
58. Grossman D. Over-the-counter access to oral contraceptives. *Obstet Clin North Am.* 2015;42:619–29. doi: 10.1016/j.ogc.2015.07.002.
59. FDA's next Rx-to-OTC switch candidate: the pill. *Pharm Times.* 2000;66(7):1.
60. The Patient Protection and Affordable Care Act. Pub L No. 111-148.
61. Mathewson S. Legislators make efforts to give pharmacists prescribing authority for oral contraceptives in multiple states. *Rx Ipsa Loquitur.* 2016;43(5):1, 3.
62. American Pharmacists Association. CEO blog: Oregon continues provider status successes in the West! June 24, 2015. Available at: http://www.pharmacist.com/CEOBlog/oregon-continues-provider-status-successes-west. Accessed April 5, 2017.
63. 72 *Fed Reg.* 56769, Oct. 4, 2007.
64. Nonprescription Drugs: Considerations Regarding a Behind the Counter Drug Class. GAO-09-245. Government Accountability Office. February 20, 2009. Available at: http://www.gao.gov/products/GAO-09-245. Accessed April 5, 2017.

65. Request for Comment. Using Innovative Technologies and Other Conditions of Safe Use to Expand Which Drug Products Can Be Considered Nonprescription. Food and Drug Administration. 77 *Fed Reg.* 12059, Feb. 28, 2012.
66. Controlled Substances Act. Pub L No. 91-513, Title II (1970).
67. Wilson MD, Ferguson RW, Mazer ME, et al. Monitoring trends in dextromethorphan abuse using the National Poison Data System: 2000–2010. *Clin Toxicol* (Phila). 2011 Jun;49(5):409–15. doi: 10.3109/15563650.2011.585429.
68. Florida Pharmacist Self-Care Consultant Law. Oct 1, 1985.
69. Chapter 465, section 186. Florida Stat: Pharmacy. Available at: https://www.flsenate.gov/laws/statutes/2011/465.186. Accessed April 5, 2017.
70. Leheny S. Could prescribing become a daily duty for pharmacists? *Pharm Times.* May 2016. Available at: http://www.pharmacytimes.com/contributor/shelby-leheny-pharmd-candidate-2017/2016/05/could-prescribing-become-a-daily-duty-for-pharmacists/. Accessed April 5, 2017.
71. Yang YT, Kozhimannil KB, Snowden JM. Pharmacist-prescribed birth control in Oregon and other states. *JAMA.* 2016;315(15):1567–8. doi: 10.1001/jama.2016.2327. Available at: http://jamanetwork.com/journals/jama/article-abstract/2506865. Accessed April 5, 2017.
72. Gabay M. A step forward: review of the new California provider status law. *Hosp Pharm.* 2014;49(5):435–6. doi: 10.1310/hpj4905-435.
73. Bratberg J, McLaughlin, Brewster S. Opioid overdose prevention. *J Am Pharm Assoc.* 2015;55:470–6.
74. Davis CS, Carr D. Legal changes to increase access to naloxone for opioid overdose reversal in the United States. *Drug Alcohol Depend.* 2015;157:112–20. doi: 10.1016/j.drugalcdep.2015.10.013.
75. LawAtlas.org. Naloxone overdose prevention laws map. Available at: http://lawatlas.org/datasets/laws-regulating-administration-of-naloxone. Accessed April 5, 2017.
76. Rumore MM. Pharmacy-based naloxone access. *Rx Ipsa Loquitur.* 2016;43(3):1, 3.
77. Wheeler E, Jones TS, Gilbert M, Davidson P. Opioid overdose prevention programs providing naloxone to laypersons. *MMWR Morb Mortal Wkly Rep.* 20;64:631–5.
78. 21 CFR §701.3.
79. Fair Packaging and Labeling Act. 15 USC. 39 Section 1456 et seq. Available at http://uscode.house.gov/view.xhtml?path=/prelim@title15/chapter39&edition=prelim. Accessed April 5, 2017.
80. U.S. Food and Drug Administration. FDA authority over cosmetics: how cosmetics are not FDA-approved, but are FDA-regulated. Available at: https://www.fda.gov/cosmetics/guidanceregulation/lawsregulations/ucm074162.htm. Accessed April 5, 2017.
81. Corby-Edwards AK. FDA regulation of cosmetics and personal care products. Congressional Research Service. CRS Report for Congress No. 7-5700. July 9, 2012. Available at: https://asbcouncil.org/sites/default/files/library/docs/crs_report_fda_regulation_of_cosmetics_and_personal_care_products.pdf. Accessed April 5, 2017.
82. Margolies ME, Rumore MM. From cosmetic to drug: crossing the line. *Drug Info J.* 1993;27:1205–11.
83. *United States v. An Article . . . Line Away,* 415 F2d 369 (3d Cir 1969).
84. *United States v. An Article . . . Helene Curtis Magic Secret,* 331 F Supp 912 (D Md 1971).
85. Preamble to the Tentative Final Monograph for OTC Antimicrobial Products. U.S. Food and Drug Administration. 43 *Fed Reg.* 1209, Jan 6, 1978.
86. Gibbs JN, Mazan KD. Compounding OTC drugs: a legal perspective. *Int J Compounding.* 2000;4(3):180–1.
87. Food, Drug & Cosmetic Act, §201(g)(1) (1938).
88. 21 CFR §210 and §211.
89. 21 CFR §211.137.
90. Krenzelok EP. Rocky Mountain Poison and Drug Center. FDA Public Hearing. Homeopathic Product Exposures National Poison Data System (NPDS) 2006–2013. April 20, 2015. Available at: https://www.fda.gov/downloads/Drugs/newsevents/ucm461658.pdf. Accessed April 5, 2017.
91. Starr RR. Too little, too late: ineffective regulation of dietary supplements. *Am J Public Health.* 2015;105(3):478–85.
92. Pub L No. 103-417, 108 Stat 4325 (1994).
93. Guidance for Industry. Current Good Manufacturing Practice in Manufacturing, Packaging, or Holding Operations for Dietary Supplements. U.S. Food and Drug Administration. 72 *Fed Reg.* 34752, December 2010 (Codified at 21 CFR §-111). Available at: https://www.fda.gov/Food/GuidanceRegulation/GuidanceDocumentsRegulatoryInformation/ucm238182.htm. Accessed April 5, 2017.
94. U.S. Food and Drug Administration. Dietary Supplement Labeling Guide: Chapter IV. Nutrition labeling. Available at: https://www.fda.gov/Food//GuidanceRegulation/GuidanceDocumentsRegulatoryInformation/DietarySupplements/ucm070597.htm. Accessed April 5, 2017.
95. Cohen PA. Assessing supplement safety—the FDA's controversial proposal. *N Engl J Med.* 2012;366(5):389–91. doi: 10.1056/NEJMp1113325.
96. Wheatley VM, Spink J. Defining the public health threat of dietary supplement fraud. *Comp Rev Food Sci Food Safety.* 2013;12(6):599–613.
97. Bonner L. FDA: Sexual enhancement supplements for men often tainted. *Pharm Today.* 2016(Mar):46.
98. Gibbs J. Regulatory pathways for clearance or approval of IVDs. Chapter 3. In: *In Vitro Diagnostics: The Complete Regulatory Guide.* Washington, DC: Food and Drug Law Institute; 2008:43–68.
99. Overview of IVD Regulations. U.S. Food and Drug Administration. Available at: https://www.fda.gov/MedicalDevices/DeviceRegulationandGuidance/IVDRegulatoryAssistance/ucm123682.htm. Accessed April 5, 2017.
100. Centers for Medicare & Medicaid Services. Clinical Laboratory Improvement Amendments (CLIA). CLIA Waiver 42 U.S.C. 26a(d)(3). Available at: http://www.cms.gov/Regulations-and-Guidance/Legislation/CLIA/Index.html?redirect=/CLIA. Accessed April 5, 2017.
101. Gronowski AM, Adams A, Ball C, et al. Pharmacists in laboratory space: friends or foe? *Clin Chem.* 2016;62:679–83.
102. Uniform Commercial Code, Sec 2-315 (1977).
103. Uniform Commercial Code, Sec 2-314 (1977).
104. Carson JJ. The pharmacist: a seller of products vs. a provider of services. *Pharmacy Law Annu.* 1987;3–16.
105. *Moore v. B&C Family Center Inc.,* 85 Mich App 660, 272 NW2d 150 (1978).
106. *Yugler v. Pharmacia & Upjohn Co.,* 2001 NY Misc LEXIS 1356, at 19-20 (NY Sup Ct 2001).
107. *Jacobs Pharmacy v. Gibson,* 116 Ga App 760, 159 SE2d 171 (1967).
108. *Whiting v. Rite Aid Pharmacy,* 2014 US Dist Lexis 87354 (D Utah, June 24, 2014).
109. Brushwood DB. Liability for advice on OTC use. *Pharm Today.* 2014(Aug):48.
110. *Tiege v. Haney,* 184 Minn 569, 239. NW 611 (1931).
111. 358 Mich. 94, 99 NW2d 518 (1959).
112. Restatement (Second) of Torts, American Law Institute, Philadelphia, PA, Section 402A.
113. Stevens-Johnson syndrome class action lawsuit. Available at: http://therappaportlawfirm.com/stevens-johnson-syndrome-class-action-lawsuit/. Accessed April 5, 2017.
114. Schmidt and Clark.com. Acne medication allergic reactions class action lawsuit. Available at: https://www.schmidtandclark.com/acne-medication-allergic-reactions-class-action-lawsuit. Accessed April 5, 2017.
115. Lawyers and Settlements.com. Proton pump inhibitors linked to bone fractures and kidney disease. Available at: https://www.lawyersandsettlements.com/lawsuit/proton-pump-inhibitor-ppi-side-effects-hip-fracture.html. Accessed April 5, 2017.

section

II

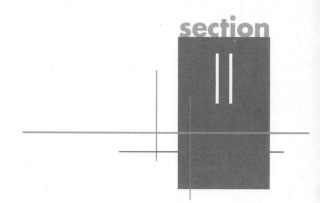

PAIN AND FEVER DISORDERS

CHAPTER 5

HEADACHE

JULIE J. WILKINSON AND KATHERINE TROMP

Worldwide, 47% of the population has suffered from headache within the previous year.[1] Tension-type and migraine headaches are the most common headache types. In some populations, tension-type headache is reported as an episodic event by more than 70% of individuals and as a chronic disorder by 1%–3% of adults. Migraine is more severe, but less common, occurring in 10% of people worldwide.[1] Headaches caused by sinus congestion and those resulting from the overuse of analgesics are also common.

Headaches generally are classified as primary or secondary. *Primary* headaches (approximately 90% of headaches) are not associated with an underlying illness. Examples are episodic and chronic tension-type headaches, migraine headache with and without aura, and cluster headaches. *Secondary* headaches are symptomatic of an underlying condition, such as head trauma, stroke, substance abuse or withdrawal, bacterial and viral diseases, and disorders of craniofacial structures. Medication-overuse headaches are considered primary because they do not have a physiologic origin, even though they are related to a withdrawal effect of medications.

Tension-type headaches, also called stress headaches, can be episodic or chronic. Chronic headaches occur 15 or more days per month for at least 3 months, whereas episodic tension-type headaches occur less than 15 days per month.[1,2] Tension-type headache has the highest prevalence among persons in the age range 40–49 years, occurs in a female-to-male ratio of 5:4, and increases in incidence with higher levels of education.[3]

The prevalence of migraine headache in the United States is approximately 18% for women and 6% for men. Onset usually is in the first three decades of life, with highest occurrence rates of established attacks at around age 40. In children, boys and girls are affected equally, but the frequency of attacks usually greatly decreases in boys after puberty.[4] Migraine without aura (i.e., neurologic symptoms that precede the head pain) occurs almost twice as frequently as migraine with aura, and many affected individuals may have both types of headaches. Up to 70% of patients with migraine have family histories of migraine, suggesting that heredity is a factor in this disorder.

Patients who regularly overuse headache medications for longer than 3 months and experience headache on more than 15 days per month may be suffering from medication-overuse headaches. This correlation is especially likely if the headache frequency or severity has worsened over the period of medication overuse. The prevalence of medication-overuse headache is low in the general population; however, overuse of headache medications has been documented in 18% of patients with chronic tension-type headaches and in 32% of patients with chronic migraine headaches.[5]

Headache is a frequently reported symptom in patients with acute sinusitis. These patients also experience other sinus symptoms such as toothache in the upper jaw, facial pain, nasal stuffiness, and nasal discharge. The prevalence of sinus headache is low, and up to 90% of patients who believe they have sinus headache may actually be experiencing migraine headache.[6]

The economic impact of headache is substantial. Headache is the most common pain condition that results in lost productive time in the U.S. workforce.[7] Most studies looking at the economic burden of headache have focused on migraine headache. Direct costs for medical services for migraine headache have been estimated at $1 billion in the United States. A greater burden comes from lost productivity and wages, with migraine costing $13 billion annually for American employers. Migraine headaches affect health-related quality of life in a manner similar to that for depression.[4]

This chapter focuses on the most common types of headaches that are amenable to self-treatment: tension-type, diagnosed migraine, medication-overuse, and sinus headaches. Nonprescription analgesics are useful for treating headache, either in monotherapy regimens or as adjuncts to nonpharmacologic or prescription therapy. Throughout this chapter, the abbreviation *NSAID* is used to denote the class of nonsteroidal anti-inflammatory drugs (e.g., ibuprofen, naproxen, aspirin). Many headache sufferers self-treat with nonprescription remedies, rather than seeking medical attention. As much as two-thirds of nonprescription analgesic use may be for headache.[8] A recent study found that 24% of patients chronically overused medication and that only 14.5% had ever been advised by a health care provider (HCP) to limit their intake of acute headache remedies.[8] Clearly, an opportunity exists to improve medication use among patients self-treating for various pain syndromes.

Pathophysiology of Headache

Tension-type headaches often manifest in response to stress, anxiety, depression, emotional conflicts, and other stimuli. The episodic tension-type headache subtype is thought to result in pain felt by the peripheral nervous system, whereas the chronic tension-type headache is thought to result from stimuli to the central nervous system.[9] A genetic component appears to influence the presence or absence of tension-type headache. Furthermore, it is likely that tension-type and migraine headaches share pathophysiologic features, making them more similar than distinct.[10]

Migraine headaches probably arise from a complex interaction of neuronal and vascular factors. Stress, fatigue, irregular sleep patterns, fasting or a missed meal, vasoactive substances in food, caffeine, alcohol, changes in female hormones, changes in barometric pressure and altitude, lights, odor, neck pain, exercise, and sexual activity all may trigger migraine.[11] Medications (e.g., reserpine, nitrates, oral contraceptives, postmenopausal hormones) also have been identified as triggers. Menstrual migraines appear at the menstrual stage of the ovarian cycle and occur in less than 10% of women. For some women, these migraine headaches occur at specific times before, after, or during the menstrual cycle.

Most investigation into the pathophysiology of headache has focused on migraine headache. The best evidence suggests that migraine occurs through dysfunction of the trigeminovascular system. Neuronal depolarization that spreads slowly across the cerebral cortex is observed during the aura phase.[12] Magnesium deficiency may contribute to this state.[13] During the headache phase, stimulation (by an axon reflex) of trigeminal sensory fibers in the large cerebral and dural vessels causes neuropeptide release with concomitant neurogenic inflammation, vasodilation, and activation of platelets and mast cells.[12] With menstrual migraine, pathophysiologic changes are mediated by estrogen withdrawal followed by serotonin withdrawal. Decreased serotonin is associated with increased calcitonin gene–related peptide and substance P from trigeminal nerves, leading to vasodilation of vessels and sensitivity of the trigeminal nerves. Estrogen may also influence nitric oxide, magnesium, or prostaglandins, which may contribute to the menstrual migraine.[14,15]

Medication-overuse headache results from excessive use of analgesics, which is thought to cause a change from episodic headaches to chronic headaches. This type of headache differs from headache occurring as an adverse effect of certain medications such as nitrates and phosphodiesterase type-5 inhibitors. Some patients who suffer from migraine or tension-type headaches receive limited relief from analgesics and over time may increase their use of one or more such drugs, which can lead to development of medication-overuse headaches. These headaches are usually associated with frequent medication use (more than twice weekly) for 3 months or longer. Onset of the headache occurs within hours of stopping the agent, and readministration of the agent provides relief.[5] Agents associated with medication-overuse headaches include nonprescription options such as acetaminophen, aspirin, and some other NSAIDs, and caffeine as well as prescription options such as triptans, opioids, butalbital, and ergotamine formulations.[5]

Sinus headache occurs when infection or blockage of the paranasal sinuses causes inflammation or distention of the sensitive sinus walls (see Chapter 11). Sinus congestion may be caused by viral or bacterial infection, or by allergic rhinitis. Pathophysiologic mechanisms at work during migraine headache can result in prominent sinus congestion, leading to confusion about which problem is the cause and which is the effect.

Clinical Presentation of Headache

Headaches can be differentiated by their signs and symptoms; the major defining characteristics are listed in Table 5–1. The severity of pain associated with tension-type headaches is highly variable. Some headaches are so mild they do not require treatment, whereas others are sufficiently severe to be disabling. Episodic tension-type headaches may last a few hours, but duration up to several days has been described. Chronic tension-type headaches are often more severe and frequently last for several days. The pain initially feels like pressure or tightening on both sides of the head and subsequently may spread to feel like a band around the head.[1,3]

Migraine headaches are classified as migraine with or without aura. Aura manifests as a series of neurologic symptoms: ocular perceptions of shimmering or flashing areas or blind spots, visual and auditory hallucinations, muscle weakness that usually is one-sided, and difficulty speaking (rarely). These symptoms may last up to 30 minutes, and the throbbing headache pain that follows may last from several hours to 2 days. Of note, however, aura is not always followed by a migraine headache. Migraines without aura begin immediately with throbbing headache pain. Both forms of migraine often are associated with nausea, vomiting, photophobia, phonophobia, sinus symptoms, tinnitus, light-headedness, vertigo, and irritability and are aggravated by routine physical activity. Premonitory (prodrome) signs and symptoms in migraine can be neuropsychiatric (e.g., anxiety, irritability, yawning, unhappiness, insomnia), sensory (e.g., phonophobia, photophobia, focusing difficulties, speech difficulties), digestive (e.g., food craving, nausea, vomiting, diarrhea, constipation), or general (e.g., asthenia, tiredness, fluid retention, urinary frequency). Premonitory signs and symptoms can be a feature of migraine headaches with and without aura.[16]

Medication-overuse headaches occur as a "rebound phenomenon" after repeated and excessive use of the implicated drug in

TABLE 5-1 Characteristics of Tension-Type, Migraine, and Sinus Headaches

Feature	Tension-Type Headache	Migraine Headache	Sinus Headache
Location	Bilateral Over the top of the head, extending to neck	Usually unilateral	Face, forehead, or periorbital area
Nature	Varies from diffuse ache to tight, pressing, constricting pain	Throbbing; may be preceded by an aura	Pressure behind eyes or face; dull, bilateral pain
Onset	Gradual	Sudden	Simultaneous with sinus symptoms, including purulent nasal discharge
Duration	Hours to days	Hours to 2–3 days	Days (resolves with sinus symptoms)
Non-headache symptoms	Scalp tenderness, neck pain and muscle tension	Nausea, vomiting	Nasal congestion

Source: References 1 and 4.

a patient with an episodic headache disorder. Continued overuse causes headache symptomatology to shift from the baseline headache type to a nearly continuous headache, particularly noticeable on awakening. Additional symptoms may include difficulty concentrating, lethargy, irritability, and nausea.[5]

Sinus headache is usually localized to facial areas over the sinuses and is difficult to differentiate from migraine without aura. The pain of a sinus headache typically is described as dull and pressure-like. Stooping or blowing the nose often intensifies the pain, but the headache is not accompanied by nausea, vomiting, or visual disturbances. Persistent sinus pain and/or discharge suggests possible infection and requires referral for medical evaluation.

Treatment of Headache

Treatment Goals

The goals of treating headache are (1) to reduce the severity and alleviate acute pain, (2) to restore normal functioning, (3) to prevent relapse, and (4) to minimize side effects. For chronic headache, an additional goal is to reduce the frequency of headaches.

General Treatment Approach

Most patients with episodic headaches obtain an adequate response to self-treatment with nonpharmacologic interventions, nonprescription medications, or both. However, some patients with episodic headaches and most with chronic headaches are candidates for prescription treatments.

Episodic tension-type headaches often respond well to nonprescription analgesics, including acetaminophen, NSAIDs, and salicylates, especially when taken at the onset of the headache. If nonprescription analgesics are used to treat chronic headache, frequency of use should be limited to less than 3 days per week, to prevent medication-overuse headache. When medication-overuse headache is suspected, use of the offending agent(s) should be tapered and subsequently eliminated. Most often, tapering of an agent should be done with medical supervision, because use of prescription therapies may be needed to combat the increased headaches that temporarily ensue during the days to weeks of the withdrawal period.[5] With chronic tension-type headaches, in addition to nonprescription or prescription medication, physical therapy and relaxation exercises may be of benefit. Figure 5–1 outlines the self-treatment of headaches and lists exclusions for self-treatment.[17,18]

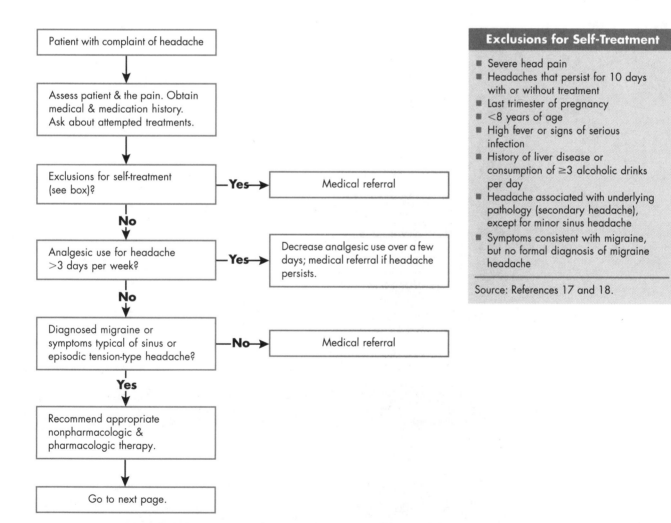

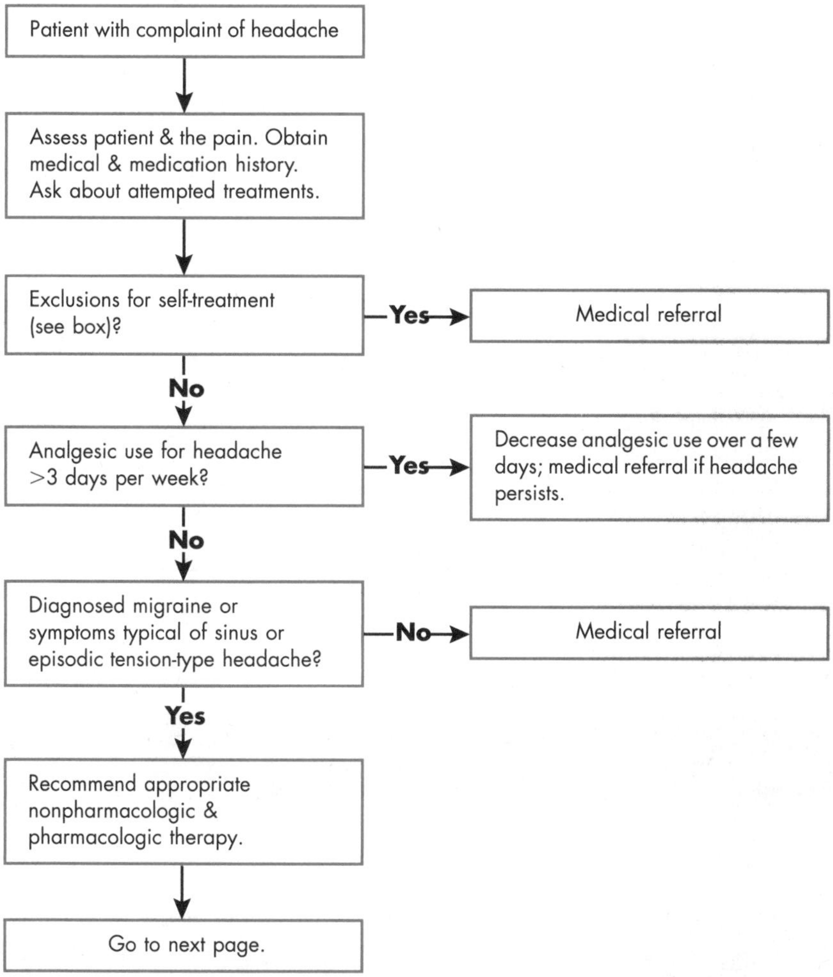
Patient with complaint of headache
Assess patient & the pain. Obtain medical & medication history. Ask about attempted treatments.
Exclusions for self-treatment (see box)?
Yes
Medical referral
No
Analgesic use for headache >3 days per week?
Yes
Decrease analgesic use over a few days; medical referral if headache persists.
No
Diagnosed migraine or symptoms typical of sinus or episodic tension-type headache?
No
Medical referral
Yes
Recommend appropriate nonpharmacologic & pharmacologic therapy.
Go to next page.

Exclusions for Self-Treatment

- Severe head pain
- Headaches that persist for 10 days with or without treatment
- Last trimester of pregnancy
- <8 years of age
- High fever or signs of serious infection
- History of liver disease or consumption of ≥3 alcoholic drinks per day
- Headache associated with underlying pathology (secondary headache), except for minor sinus headache
- Symptoms consistent with migraine, but no formal diagnosis of migraine headache

Source: References 17 and 18.

FIGURE 5–1 Self-care for headache. Key: CABG = Coronary artery bypass graft; CHF = congestive heart failure; GI = gastrointestinal; HBP = high blood pressure; NSAID = nonsteroidal anti-inflammatory drug. (*continued on next page*)

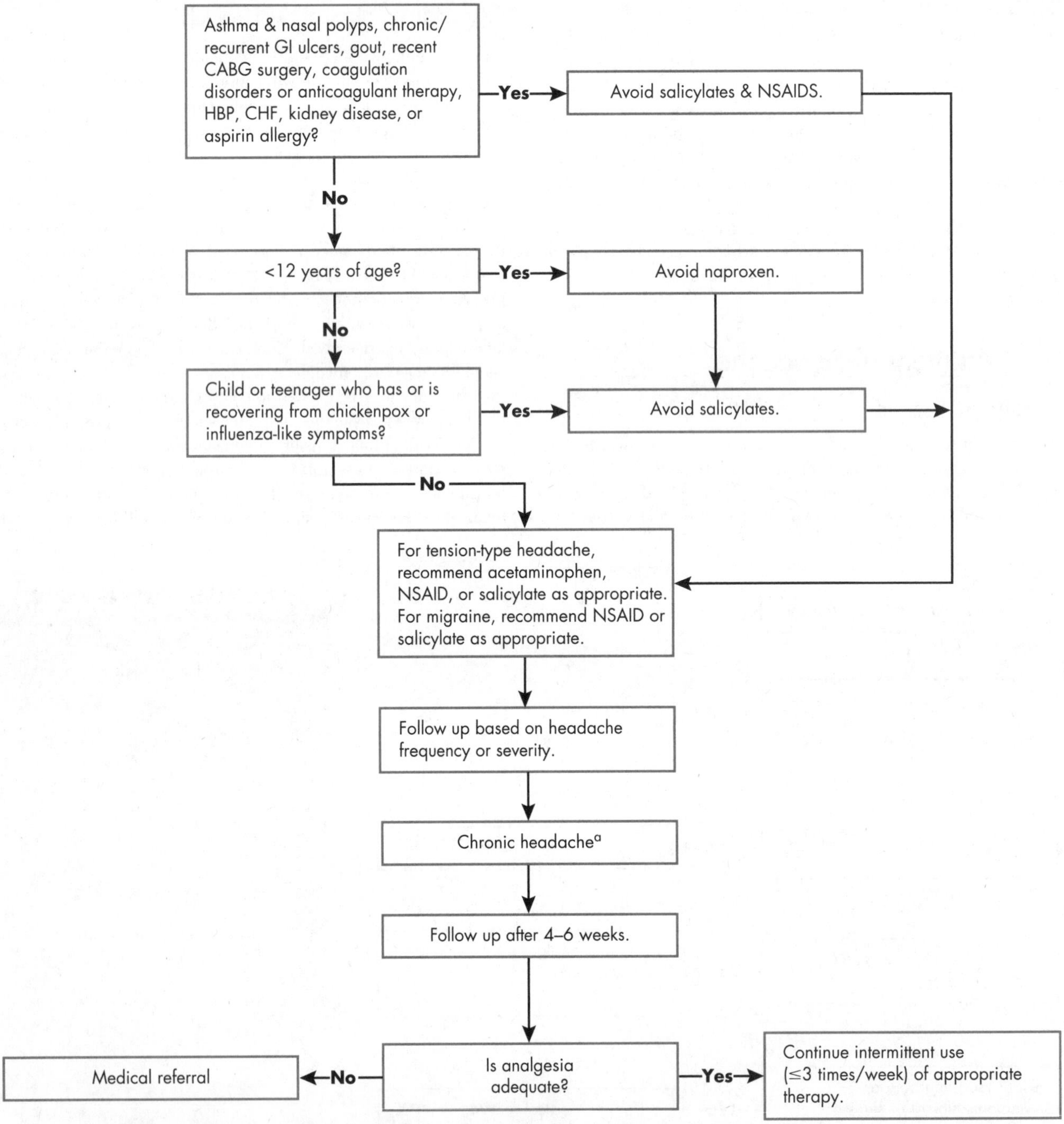

[a] Once a diagnosis of chronic tension-type or migraine headache is established, self-care can resume.

FIGURE 5–1 Self-care for headache. Key: CABG = Coronary artery bypass graft; CHF = congestive heart failure; GI = gastrointestinal; HBP = high blood pressure; NSAID = nonsteroidal anti-inflammatory drug. (*continued*)

A medical diagnosis of migraine headache is required before self-treatment can be recommended. Taking an NSAID or a salicylate at the onset of symptoms can abort mild or moderate migraine headache. Analgesics work best in the early stages of a migraine. Patients with migraines who can predict the occurrence of the headache (e.g., during menstruation) should take an analgesic (usually one of the newer NSAIDs) before occurrence of the event known to trigger the headache, as well as throughout the duration of the event. For patients with coexisting tension and migraine headaches, treatment of the initiating headache type can abort the mixed headache.

Sinus headaches respond well to oral and nasal decongestants (e.g., pseudoephedrine, oxymetazoline), which reduce congestion by causing vasoconstriction in the nasal passages (see Chapter 11). Concomitant use of decongestants and nonprescription analgesics can relieve sinus headache pain. Chronic congestion and sinus infections may be a sign of structural abnormalities and indicate the need for an appropriate medical referral.

Nonpharmacologic Therapy

Chronic tension-type headaches may respond to relaxation exercises and physical therapy that emphasizes stretching and strengthening of head and neck muscles. General treatment measures for migraine include maintaining a regular schedule for sleeping, eating, and exercise; stress management; biofeedback; and cognitive therapy.[11] Some patients obtain relief from the pain of acute migraine attacks by applying ice or cold packs combined with pressure to the forehead or temple areas.

Nutritional strategies are intended to prevent migraine and are based on (1) dietary restriction of foods that contain trigger substances, (2) avoidance of hunger and low blood glucose (a trigger of migraine), and (3) magnesium supplementation.[13,19–20] Advocates of nutritional therapy recommend avoiding known food allergens and foods with vasoactive substances, such as nitrites (found in cured meats), tyramine (found in red wine and aged cheese), phenylalanine (found in the artificial sweetener aspartame), monosodium glutamate (often found in Asian food), caffeine, and theobromines (found in chocolate).[19]

Pharmacologic Therapy

Available nonprescription analgesics for the management of headache include acetaminophen, newer NSAIDs (ibuprofen and naproxen), and salicylates (aspirin and magnesium salicylate). Selection of an analgesic should be based on a careful review of the patient's medical and medication histories. Medical management of nausea accompanying migraine headache may also be indicated to improve symptomatic relief and to facilitate medication delivery by the oral route.

Acetaminophen

Acetaminophen is an effective analgesic and antipyretic. Acetaminophen produces analgesia through central inhibition of prostaglandin synthesis.

Acetaminophen is absorbed rapidly from the gastrointestinal (GI) tract and extensively metabolized in the liver to inactive glucuronic and sulfuric acid conjugates. Acetaminophen is also metabolized by the cytochrome P450 enzyme system to a hepatotoxic intermediate metabolite that is detoxified by glutathione. When given by suppository, acetaminophen has a rectal bioavailability of approximately 50%–60% of that achieved with oral administration. Onset of analgesic activity of acetaminophen occurs approximately 30 minutes after oral administration. Duration of activity is approximately 4 hours and is increased to 6–8 hours with an extended-release formulation.

FDA-approved uses for nonprescription acetaminophen include reducing fever and relieving mild–moderate pain. It is effective in relieving mild–moderate pain of nonvisceral origin (i.e., pain that is not organ-related). Randomized, double-blind studies have documented the effectiveness of acetaminophen 1000 mg over placebo in patients with migraine and tension-type headache.[21]

Recommended child and adult dosages of acetaminophen are provided in Tables 5–2 and 5–3.[22] Table 5–4 lists selected trade name products. Acetaminophen is available for administration in various oral and rectal dosage forms.

Acetaminophen oral capsules contain tasteless granules that can be emptied onto a spoon containing a small amount of cold beverage (hot beverages result in a bitter taste) or soft food. Capsule contents should not be added to a cup of liquid because a large proportion of the granules may adhere to the cup surface.

Acetaminophen is potentially hepatotoxic in doses exceeding 4 g/day, especially with chronic use. Patients should be cautioned

TABLE 5–2 FDA-Approved Dosages for Nonprescription Analgesics in Children Younger Than 12 Years

Dosage Basics	Ibuprofen (mg)	Acetaminophen (mg)
Weight-based dosing	5–10 mg/kg	10–15 mg/kg
Dosing schedule	Every 6–8 hours as needed	Every 4–6 hours as needed
Maximum daily dose	300 mg per dose up to 4 doses, or 1200 mg total daily dose	480 mg per dose up to 5 doses, or 2400 mg total daily dose

Specific Doses by Patient Age/Weight		Ibuprofen	Acetaminophen
Age	**Weight (lb)**		
6–11 months	12–17	50	Ask a doctor.
12–23 months	18–23	75	Ask a doctor.
2–3 years	24–35	100	160
4–5 years	36–47	150	240
6–8 years	48–59	200	320
9–10 years	60–71	250	400
11 years	72–95	300	480

Key: FDA = Food and Drug Administration.
Source: Reference 22.

against exceeding the dose limit. More conservative dosing (i.e., ≤2 g/day) or avoidance may be warranted in patients at increased risk for acetaminophen-induced hepatotoxicity, including those with diagnosed liver disease, concurrent use of other potentially hepatotoxic drugs, poor nutritional intake, or consumption of three or more alcoholic drinks per day.[23] One alcoholic drink is defined as 12 ounces of beer, 5 ounces of wine, or 1.5 ounces of 80-proof liquor.

FDA has required manufacturers to include a boxed warning on acetaminophen products that addresses its potential to cause hepatotoxicity. The basic language of the warning is as follows:

> **Liver warning:** This product contains acetaminophen. Severe liver damage may occur if
>
> - an adult takes more than 4000 mg of acetaminophen in 24 hours
> - a child takes more than 5 doses in 24 hours
> - the product is taken with other drugs containing acetaminophen
> - an adult has 3 or more alcoholic drinks every day while using this product

The warning will vary depending on whether the product is labeled for use in children and/or adults. Also, if it is clearer to communicate the warning in terms of the number of dosage units, rather than the dose in milligrams, the manufacturer may write it in that manner.[24]

FDA has also made recommendations to lower the risk of accidental acetaminophen overdose—for example, reduction of the acetaminophen maximum daily dosage of 3900–4000 mg to 3000–3250 mg. The manufacturer of Tylenol responded to the agency's suggestion and volunteered to reduce its specified maximum daily dosage for Regular Strength Tylenol to 3250 mg (10 tablets) and for Extra Strength Tylenol to 3000 mg (6 tablets). Most generic manufacturers, however, have continued to specify a maximum daily dosage of 4 g/day. Several acetaminophen 650 mg products (tablets and suppositories) are available with labeling that includes a maximum daily dosage of 3900 mg (6 doses).[25] In January 2014, FDA urged health care professionals to no longer prescribe or dispense combination prescription products containing more than 325 mg acetaminophen per dosage unit.[26] Prescription products with more than 325 mg acetaminophen per dosage unit have been voluntarily withdrawn by manufacturers of the drug. The 2011 joint meeting of the Nonprescription Drugs Advisory Committee and the Pediatric Advisory Committee voted in favor of considering a single concentration of pediatric acetaminophen-containing solid oral dosage forms.[27] In accordance with this suggestion, Johnson & Johnson announced in 2017 that the company would no longer manufacture the 80 mg strength of Children's Tylenol tablets and will now manufacture only 160 mg strength tablets for children.[28]

Acetaminophen poisoning is a major reason for contacting poison control centers and constitutes the leading cause of acute liver failure in the United States.[29] Unintended chronic overdose comprises approximately one-half of the cases of acetaminophen-induced acute liver failure. Contributing factors include repeated dosing in excess of package labeling, use of more than one product containing acetaminophen, and alcohol ingestion.[30]

Acetaminophen toxicity evolves in four stages. Stage I includes signs and symptoms of nausea, vomiting, drowsiness, confusion, and abdominal pain, but such early manifestations may be absent or delayed, belying the potential severity of the exposure. Stage II is characterized by emergence of the first symptoms of hepatotoxicity and begins 24–48 hours after acute ingestion of acetaminophen. Stage II signs and symptoms include increased aspartate aminotransferase (AST) and alanine aminotransferase (ALT); increased bilirubin with jaundice; prolonged prothrombin time; and obtundation. Stage III develops after 3–4 days and results in liver failure.

TABLE 5-3 Recommended Dosages of Nonprescription Analgesics for Adults and Children 12 Years and Older

Agent	Dosage Forms	Usual Adult Dosage (maximum daily dosage)
Acetaminophen[a,b]	Immediate-release, extended-release, effervescent, dispersible, and chewable tablets; capsules; liquid; suppositories; powder packet	325–1000 mg every 4–6 hours as needed (4000 mg, suggested 3250 mg[a])
Ibuprofen	Immediate-release and chewable tablets; capsules; suspension	200–400 mg every 4–6 hours as needed (1200 mg)
Naproxen sodium	Immediate-release and delayed release tablets, capsules	220 mg every 8–12 hours as needed For the first dose, you may take 2 tablets within the first hour (660 mg).
Aspirin	Immediate-release, buffered, enteric-coated, film-coated, effervescent, and chewable tablets; suppositories	325–1000 mg every 4–6 hours as needed (4000 mg)
Magnesium salicylate	Tablets	650 mg every 4 hours or 1000 mg every 6 hours as needed (4000 mg)

Key: FDA = Food and Drug Administration.

[a] The manufacturer's voluntary dosing reductions in 2011 resulted in the following dosage for Extra Strength Tylenol: 2 tablets (500 mg each) every 6 hours, with a maximum daily dosage of 3000 mg (6 tablets). The maximum daily dosage for Regular Strength Tylenol was reduced to 3250 mg. However, a maximum daily dosage of 4000 mg is allowed for acetaminophen labeling.[24]

[b] In January 2014, FDA urged health care professionals to no longer prescribe or dispense combination prescription products containing more than 325 mg acetaminophen per dosage unit.[26] Prescription products with more than 325 mg acetaminophen per dosage unit were voluntarily withdrawn.

Source: Reference 22.

TABLE 5-4 **Selected Single-Entity Nonprescription Acetaminophen Products**

Trade Name	Acetaminophen Content
Pediatric Formulations	
FeverAll Infants' Suppository	80 mg
FeverAll Children's Suppository	120 mg
FeverAll Junior Strength Suppository	325 mg
Tylenol Children's Oral Suspension	160 mg/5 mL
Triaminic Fever Reducer Oral Suspension	160 mg/5 mL
Adult Formulations	
Tylenol Tablet/Capsule	325 mg
Tylenol Extra Strength Caplet	500 mg
Tylenol 8 Hour Arthritis Pain Extended Release Caplet	650 mg
Tylenol 8 hour Extended Release Tablet	650 mg
Tylenol Cold + Sore Throat Daytime Liquid	500 mg/15 mL

Source: Reference 22.

Signs and symptoms at this stage may include metabolic acidosis, encephalopathy, cerebral edema, and renal failure. GI symptoms may also be present during this stage. Stage IV begins 4 days after ingestion and can last for several weeks. During this stage, in a majority of cases, hepatic damage is reversible over a period of weeks or months, but more severe cases may require liver transplantation or result in fatal hepatic necrosis.[31]

Because of the potential seriousness of acetaminophen overdose, all cases should be referred to a poison control center or emergency department. Supportive care is provided, along with activated charcoal to reduce acetaminophen absorption in patients who present for treatment within 1 hour after ingestion. When acetaminophen serum levels, with consideration of time since ingestion, exceed those known to cause hepatic injury, prompt administration of acetylcysteine is warranted to supplement glutathione, which is essential for deactivation of a toxic intermediate metabolite of acetaminophen. Acetylcysteine's effectiveness decreases if it is administered more than 8 hours after acute ingestion. Asymptomatic elevations in ALT have been reported in otherwise healthy individuals taking acetaminophen 4 g/day. In a prospective study, 39% of patients experienced ALT elevations to greater than 3 times the upper limit of normal. These elevations generally appeared in the first week of use, with some resolution occurring despite continued dosing. The clinical significance of this observation is uncertain.[32]

Patients with glucose-6-phosphate dehydrogenase deficiency, a hereditary disease that causes premature breakdown of red blood cells, should use caution when taking acetaminophen. It is unclear if regular doses of acetaminophen will cause toxicity in patients with a glucose-6-phosphate dehydrogenase deficiency; however, case reports of hemolysis in patients who took an overdose of acetaminophen and have a glucose-6-phosphate dehydrogenase deficiency have been recorded.[33] In patients with hypersensitivity to acetaminophen, the drug is contraindicated for future use.

Rare but serious cutaneous adverse reactions (SCARs) have been found to be associated with use of acetaminophen as well as other analgesics including NSAIDs. Skin reactions may occur in either new or ongoing users of the drug and have the potential to progress into a life-threatening rash such as Stevens-Johnson syndrome and toxic epidermal necrolysis. Although these events are very rare, it is important to be aware of the possibility and to refer patients for further evaluation.[34] Under a tentative final monograph, FDA is currently recommending that the following language should appear below the liver warning in the Warnings section of the Drug Facts Label for all single ingredient and combination ingredient acetaminophen products:

> **Allergy alert:** Acetaminophen may cause severe skin reactions. Symptoms may include
>
> - skin reddening
> - blisters
> - rash

If a skin rash occurs, stop use and seek medical help right away.[35]

Clinically important drug interactions of acetaminophen are listed in Table 5–5. For patients taking warfarin, acetaminophen is considered the analgesic of choice; however, it has been associated with increases in international normalized ratio (INR). Regular acetaminophen use should be discouraged in patients on warfarin. Patients who require higher scheduled doses (e.g., those with osteoarthritis) should have their INR monitored and warfarin dose adjusted as acetaminophen doses are titrated.

Nonsalicylate Nonsteroidal Anti-inflammatory Drugs

NSAIDs relieve pain through central and peripheral inhibition of cyclooxygenase (COX) with consequent inhibition of prostaglandin synthesis.

All nonprescription NSAIDs are rapidly absorbed from the GI tract, with consistently high bioavailability. They are extensively metabolized, mainly by glucuronidation, to inactive compounds in the liver. Elimination occurs primarily through the kidneys. Time to onset of activity for naproxen sodium and standard ibuprofen is approximately 30 minutes. Duration of activity is up to 12 hours for naproxen sodium and 6–8 hours for ibuprofen. FDA-approved uses for nonprescription NSAIDs include reducing fever and relieving minor pain associated with headache, the common cold, toothache, muscle ache, backache, arthritis, and menstrual cramps. NSAIDs have analgesic, antipyretic, and anti-inflammatory activity, and they are useful in managing mild–moderate pain of nonvisceral origin. Naproxen sodium and ibuprofen became available for nonprescription use in 1994 and 1984, respectively, and both are propionic acid derivatives. Although FDA has approved ketoprofen for nonprescription use, no commercially available nonprescription analgesics currently contain this agent.

Recommended child and adult dosages of nonprescription NSAIDs are provided in Tables 5–2 and 5–3. Table 5–6 lists selected trade name products. Ibuprofen is available as a liquid for pediatric use and comes in two different strengths. This dual option may contribute to the potential for dosing errors. A dose–effect relationship has been demonstrated for ibuprofen analgesia in the range of 100–400 mg.

The most frequent adverse effects of NSAIDs involve the GI tract and include dyspepsia, heartburn, nausea, anorexia, and epigastric pain, even among children using pediatric formulations. NSAIDs may be taken with food, milk, or antacids if upset

TABLE 5-5 **Clinically Important Drug–Drug Interactions with Nonprescription Analgesic Agents**

Analgesic/ Antipyretic	Drug	Potential Interaction	Management/ Preventive Measures
Acetaminophen	Alcohol	Increased risk of hepatotoxicity	Avoid concurrent use if possible; minimize alcohol intake when using acetaminophen.
Acetaminophen	Warfarin	Increased risk of bleeding (elevations in INR)	Limit acetaminophen to occasional use; monitor INR for several weeks when acetaminophen 2–4 grams daily is added or discontinued in patients on warfarin.
Aspirin	Valproic acid	Displacement from protein-binding sites and inhibition of valproic acid metabolism	Avoid concurrent use; use naproxen instead of aspirin (no interaction).
Aspirin	NSAIDs, including COX-2 inhibitors	Increased risk of gastroduodenal ulcers and bleeding	Avoid concurrent use if possible.
Ibuprofen	Aspirin	Decreased antiplatelet effect of aspirin	Aspirin should be taken at least 30 minutes before or 8 hours after ibuprofen. Use acetaminophen (or other analgesic) instead of ibuprofen.
Ibuprofen	Phenytoin	Displacement from protein-binding sites	Monitor free phenytoin levels; adjust dose as indicated.
NSAIDs	Bisphosphonates	Increased risk of GI or esophageal ulceration	Use caution with concomitant use.
NSAIDs	Digoxin	Renal clearance of digoxin inhibited	Monitor digoxin levels; adjust dose as indicated.
Salicylates and NSAIDs	Antihypertensive agents, beta-blockers, ACE inhibitors, vasodilators, diuretics	Antihypertensive effect inhibited; possible hyperkalemia with potassium-sparing diuretics and ACE inhibitors	Monitor blood pressure, cardiac function, and potassium levels.
Salicylates and NSAIDs	Anticoagulants	Increased risk of bleeding, especially GI	Avoid concurrent use, if possible; risk is lowest with salsalate and choline magnesium trisalicylate.
Salicylates and NSAIDs	Alcohol	Increased risk of GI bleeding	Avoid concurrent use, if possible; minimize alcohol intake when using salicylates and NSAIDs.
Salicylates and NSAIDs	Methotrexate	Decreased methotrexate clearance	Avoid salicylates and NSAIDs with high-dose methotrexate therapy; monitor levels with concurrent treatment.
Salicylates (moderate–high doses)	Sulfonylureas	Increased risk of hypoglycemia	Avoid concurrent use, if possible; monitor blood glucose levels when changing salicylate dose.

Key: ACE = Angiotensin-converting enzyme; COX = cyclooxygenase; GI = gastrointestinal; INR = international normalized ratio; NSAID = nonsteroidal anti-inflammatory drug.

Source: Reference 22.

stomach occurs. Tablets should be taken with a full glass of water, suspensions should be shaken thoroughly, and enteric-coated or sustained-release preparations should never be crushed or chewed. Other adverse effects include dizziness, fatigue, headache, and nervousness. Rashes or itching, photosensitivity, and fluid retention or edema may occur in some patients; however, at normal doses, these effects usually are rare.

GI ulceration, perforation, and bleeding are serious potential complications of NSAID use. Risk factors include age older than 60 years, previous ulcer disease in the case of GI bleeding, concurrent use of anticoagulants (including aspirin), higher dose or longer duration of treatment, and consumption of three or more alcoholic drinks per day. Package labeling for NSAIDs includes warnings about stomach bleeding with adult doses (see the box "A Word About NSAIDs and Stomach Bleeding").[36] The prescription products that contain ibuprofen and naproxen include the following warning:

> NSAIDs cause an increased risk of serious gastrointestinal adverse events including bleeding, ulceration, and perforation of the stomach or intestines, which can be fatal. These events can occur at any time during use and without warning symptoms. Elderly patients are at greater risk for serious gastrointestinal events.

TABLE 5–6 Selected Single-Entity Nonprescription Nonsalicylate Nonsteroidal Anti-inflammatory Drugs

Trade Name	Primary Ingredient
Ibuprofen Products (pediatric formulations)	
Children's Advil Suspension	Ibuprofen 100 mg/5 mL
Children's Motrin Suspension	Ibuprofen 100 mg/5 mL
Motrin Infants' Drops Suspension	Ibuprofen 50 mg/1.25 mL
Children's Motrin Chewable Tablet	Ibuprofen 50 mg
Junior Strength Motrin Chewable Tablet	Ibuprofen 100 mg
Ibuprofen Products (adult formulations)	
Advil Tablet/Capsule	Ibuprofen 200 mg
Motrin IB Ibuprofen Tablet	Ibuprofen 200 mg
Advil Migraine Capsule	Ibuprofen 200 mg
Midol Capsule	Ibuprofen 200 mg
Naproxen Products	
Aleve Tablet/Capsule	Naproxen sodium 220 mg
Mediproxen Tablet	Naproxen sodium 220 mg
Pamprin All Day Relief Maximum Strength Tablet	Naproxen sodium 220 mg

NSAID use is associated with increased risk for myocardial infarction, heart failure, hypertension, and stroke. The mechanism by which the risk is conferred is not clear, but it may be related to increased thromboxane A2 activity and suppressed vascular prostacyclin synthesis, resulting in vasoconstriction and platelet aggregation. The cardiovascular risk associated with nonselective NSAIDs appears to depend on dose and duration; people with underlying risk factors such as hypertension, heart failure, and diabetes are at greater risk. Limited data suggest that the risk may not be the same for all nonselective NSAIDs.[37]

The American Heart Association recommends that patients with cardiovascular disease or those at high risk for cardiac events (e.g., hyperlipidemia, hypertension, diabetes, other macrovascular disease) avoid NSAIDs. Patients at low cardiac risk should nevertheless exercise caution with use of NSAIDs by taking the minimum dose for the shortest duration needed to control symptoms. Clinical evidence has shown that the use of NSAIDs in patients with a history of myocardial infarction is associated with an increased risk of future cardiovascular events, extending indefinitely.[38] The prescription products that contain ibuprofen and naproxen include the following warning[22]:

- NSAIDs may cause an increased risk of serious cardiovascular thrombotic events, myocardial infarction, and stroke, which can be fatal. This risk may increase with duration of use. Patients with cardiovascular disease or risk factors for cardiovascular disease may be at greater risk.
- Ibuprofen and naproxen tablets are contraindicated for treatment of perioperative pain in the setting of coronary artery bypass graft (CABG) surgery.

A WORD ABOUT

NSAIDs and Stomach Bleeding

In 2010, FDA approved the following label warning concerning stomach bleeding for nonprescription products that contain NSAIDs in adult doses:

Stomach bleeding warning: This product contains an NSAID, which may cause severe stomach bleeding. The chance is higher if you

- are age 60 or older
- have had stomach ulcers or bleeding problems
- take a blood-thinning (anticoagulant) or steroid drug
- take other drugs containing prescription or nonprescription NSAIDs (aspirin, ibuprofen, naproxen, or others)
- have 3 or more alcoholic drinks every day while using this product
- take more or for a longer time than directed

Ask a doctor before use if the stomach bleeding warning applies to you:

- You have a history of stomach problems, such as heartburn.
- You have high blood pressure, heart disease, liver cirrhosis, or kidney disease.
- You are taking a diuretic.

Stop use and ask a doctor if

- You experience any of the following signs of stomach bleeding:
  - feel faint
  - vomit blood
  - have bloody or black stools
  - have stomach pain that does not get better

Key: FDA = Food and Drug Administration; NSAID = nonsteroidal anti-inflammatory drug.
Source: Reference 36.

Clinically important drug–drug interactions of NSAIDs are listed in Table 5–5. Ibuprofen increases bleeding time by reversibly inhibiting platelet aggregation. Patients on aspirin for cardiovascular prophylaxis should take it at least 1 hour before or 8 hours after ibuprofen to avoid a pharmacodynamic interaction that inhibits the antiplatelet effect of aspirin. In doses of 1200–2400 mg/day, ibuprofen does not appear to affect the INR in patients taking warfarin. However, ibuprofen should not be recommended for self-treatment in patients who concurrently are taking anticoagulants, because its antiplatelet activity could increase GI bleeding. Owing to concerns regarding decreased cardiovascular protection and increased bleeding risk, great caution is warranted in combining aspirin and ibuprofen.

Patients who ingest three or more alcoholic drinks per day should be cautioned about the increased risk of adverse GI events, including stomach bleeding. They also should be referred to their primary care provider (PCP) for monitoring of their NSAID use.

NSAIDs may decrease renal blood flow and glomerular filtration rate through inhibition of renal prostaglandin synthesis. Consequently, blood urea nitrogen and serum creatinine levels can increase, often with concomitant sodium and water retention. Advanced age, hypertension, diabetes, atherosclerotic cardiovascular disease, and use of diuretics appear to increase the risk of renal toxicity with ibuprofen use. Therefore, patients with a history of impaired renal function, congestive heart failure, or diseases that compromise renal hemodynamics should not self-treat with NSAIDs.

NSAID overdoses usually are associated with minimal signs and symptoms of toxicity and are rarely fatal. GI manifestations are common and include nausea, vomiting, abdominal pain, and diarrhea. The most serious effects of large NSAID overdoses include renal failure, neurologic toxicity, and acid–base changes. Examples of specific neurologic symptoms are drowsiness, changes in vision, headache, and confusion. Convulsions have been reported in children who have taken an overdose of ibuprofen. Case reports of GI bleeding also exist.[39]

Salicylates

Salicylates inhibit prostaglandin synthesis from arachidonic acid by inhibiting both isoforms of the COX enzyme (COX-1 and COX-2). The resulting decrease in prostaglandins reduces the sensitivity of pain receptors to the initiation of pain impulses at sites of inflammation and trauma. Although some evidence suggests that aspirin also produces analgesia through a central mechanism, its site of action is primarily peripheral.

Salicylates are absorbed by means of passive diffusion of the nonionized drug in the stomach and small intestine. Factors affecting absorption include dosage form, gastric pH, gastric emptying time, dissolution rate, and the presence of antacids or food. Absorption from immediate-release aspirin products is complete. Rectal absorption of a salicylate suppository is slow and unreliable, as well as proportional to rectal retention time.

Once absorbed, aspirin is hydrolyzed in the plasma to salicylic acid in 1–2 hours. Salicylic acid is widely distributed to all tissues and fluids in the body, including the CNS tissue, breast milk, and fetal tissue. Protein binding is concentration-dependent. At concentrations lower than 100 mg/mL, approximately 90% of salicylic acid is bound to albumin, whereas at concentrations greater than 400 mg/mL, approximately 75% is bound. Salicylic acid is largely eliminated through the kidney. Urine pH determines the amount of unchanged drug that is eliminated, with urinary concentrations increasing substantially in more alkaline urine (pH ~8).

Dosage form alterations include enteric coating, buffering, and sustained release. These formulations were developed to change the rate of absorption and/or to reduce the potential for GI toxicity. Enteric-coated aspirin is absorbed only from the small intestine; its absorption is markedly slowed by food, which is attributed to prolonged gastric emptying time. Hypochlorhydria from acid-suppressing agents (especially proton pump inhibitors) may result in dissolution of enteric-coated products in the stomach, negating any potential benefit in preventing local gastric toxicity. For patients requiring rapid pain relief, enteric-coated aspirin is inappropriate because of the delay in absorption and the time to onset of analgesic effect.

Buffered aspirin products are available in both tablet and effervescent forms. Although buffered products are absorbed more rapidly than nonbuffered products, time to onset of effect is not improved appreciably. Common buffers include aluminum hydroxide; magnesium carbonate, hydroxide, or oxide; calcium carbonate; and sodium bicarbonate (in effervescent formulations). Some effervescent aspirin solutions contain large amounts of sodium and must be avoided by patients who require restricted sodium intake (such as those with hypertension, heart failure, or renal failure). Sustained-release aspirin is formulated to prolong duration of action by slowing dissolution and absorption. Magnesium salicylate is available as a tablet or capsule. Sodium salicylate is approved for nonprescription use, but it is not currently available in a commercial product.

FDA-approved uses for salicylates include treatment of symptoms for osteoarthritis, rheumatoid arthritis, and other rheumatologic diseases, as well as temporary relief of minor aches and pains associated with backache or muscle aches. Salicylates are also effective in treating mild–moderate pain from musculoskeletal conditions and fever. Because of its inhibitory effects on platelet function, aspirin is also indicated for prevention of thromboembolic events (e.g., myocardial infarction, stroke) in high-risk patients. Unlike with the NSAIDs previously discussed, this inhibitory effect is irreversible for aspirin. Thus, the inhibition continues for the duration of the platelet's life. With NSAIDs, the duration of inhibition depends on factors such as dose, serum level, and half-life.

Recommended child and adult dosages of nonprescription salicylates are provided in Tables 5–2 and 5–3. Table 5–7 provides selected salicylate products. Aspirin dosages ranging from 4 to 6 g/day are usually needed to produce anti-inflammatory effects. The maximum analgesic dosage for self-medication with aspirin is 4 g/day; therefore, anti-inflammatory activity often will not occur unless the drug is used at the high end of the acceptable dosage range.

Aspirin is known to commonly cause dyspepsia, which may be minimized by taking it with food. In addition, aspirin is associated with development of gastritis and ulceration of the upper GI tract. It produces GI mucosal damage by compromising the protective mucous and bicarbonate layers of the gastric mucosa, thereby permitting back-diffusion of acid, with consequent cellular and vascular erosion. Two distinct mechanisms are involved: (1) a local irritant effect resulting from contact of the medication with the gastric mucosa and (2) a systemic effect from prostaglandin inhibition. Lack of upper abdominal pain or discomfort is not a reliable indicator for the absence of GI damage associated with use of NSAIDs.[40]

The use of aspirin has been shown to increase the risk for serious upper GI events two- to fourfold.[40] It is recommended that the lowest effective dose be used for cardioprotection (usually 81 mg/day). Patients with risk factors for upper GI bleeding should avoid self-treatment with aspirin. Recognized risk factors are (1) history of uncomplicated or bleeding peptic ulcer; (2) age older than 60 years; (3) concomitant use of NSAIDs, anticoagulants,

TABLE 5–7 Selected Adult Formulations of Nonprescription Single-Entity Salicylate Products

Trade Name	Primary Ingredient
Bayer Low-Dose Aspirin Tablet	Aspirin 81 mg
St. Joseph Chewable Aspirin 81 mg Tablet	Aspirin 81 mg
Ecotrin Enteric-Coated Tablet	Aspirin 325 mg
Bayer Aspirin Delayed Release Tablet	Aspirin 325 mg
Bayer Plus Extra Strength Tablet	Aspirin 500 mg
DeWitts Pain Reliever Tablet	Magnesium salicylate 325 mg
Extra Strength Doan's Tablet	Magnesium salicylate tetrahydrate 580 mg
Percogesic Maximum Strength Backache Relief Coated Caplet/Tablet	Magnesium salicylate tetrahydrate 580 mg

antiplatelet agents, bisphosphonates, selective serotonin reuptake inhibitors, or systemic corticosteroids; (4) infection with *Helicobacter pylori*; (5) rheumatoid arthritis; (6) NSAID-related dyspepsia; and (7) regular use of alcohol.[41]

Various aspirin formulations may have different rates of adverse GI effects. Enteric coating may decrease local gastric irritation. However, with regard to the risk of major GI ulceration and bleeding, no difference has been identified among plain, enteric-coated, and buffered products.[42]

Serious aspirin intolerance is uncommon and consists of two types: *cutaneous* (manifesting as urticaria and angioedema) and *respiratory* (manifesting as bronchospasm, laryngospasm, and rhinorrhea). The mechanism is not immunologically mediated. Risk factors for serious aspirin intolerance include chronic urticaria for the cutaneous type and asthma with nasal polyps for the respiratory type. Ten percent of people diagnosed with asthma have aspirin sensitivity.[43] The degree of intolerance is variable, ranging from minor to severe. Patients with aspirin intolerance generally are advised to avoid NSAIDs. However, the nonacetylated salicylates (magnesium salicylate) and acetaminophen are considered safe.[43]

Nonprescription salicylates interact with several other important drugs and drug classes. Clinically important drug interactions of salicylates are listed in Table 5–5. When monitoring therapy in patients who are taking high-dose salicylates, HCPs should review current drug interaction references for newly identified interactions.

Aspirin ingestion may produce positive results on fecal occult blood testing, so its use should be discontinued at least 3 days before testing. Similarly, aspirin should be discontinued 2–7 days before surgery and should not be used to relieve pain after tonsillectomy, dental extraction, or other surgical procedures, except under the close supervision of an HCP. Aspirin can potentiate bleeding from capillary-rich sites such as the GI tract, tonsillar beds, and tooth sockets.

Because of its effect on hemostasis, aspirin is contraindicated in patients with hypoprothrombinemia, vitamin K deficiency, hemophilia, history of any bleeding disorder, or history of peptic ulcer disease. Patients with compromised renal function have the potential for decreased renal excretion of magnesium, allowing accumulation of toxic levels with regimens including magnesium salicylate. The maximum 24-hour dose of magnesium salicylate contains 264 mg (11 mEq) of magnesium.

All salicylates should be avoided in patients with a history of gout or hyperuricemia because of dose-related effects on renal uric acid handling. In such patients, taking low-dose aspirin for 2 consecutive days is associated with increased risk for onset or reemergence of gout. Serum urate monitoring should be considered in patients with gout who are receiving aspirin therapy.[44]

Reye's syndrome is an acute illness occurring almost exclusively in children and teenagers.[45] The cause is unknown, but the use of salicylates to treat viral illnesses has been associated with the syndrome. Onset usually follows a viral infection with influenza (type A or B) or varicella (chickenpox). Reye's syndrome is characterized by progressive neurologic damage, fatty liver with encephalopathy, and hypoglycemia. Neurologic symptoms may start with lethargy and progress to delirium, confusion, and seizures. The mortality rate may be as high as 50%.

The American Academy of Pediatrics, FDA, the Centers for Disease Control and Prevention, and the Surgeon General have issued warnings that aspirin and other salicylates (including bismuth subsalicylate and nonaspirin salicylates) should be avoided in children and teenagers who have influenza or chickenpox. The following statement is included in the Electronic Code of Federal Regulations[45] and listed on labels of nonprescription aspirin and aspirin-containing products:

> Reye's syndrome: Children and teenagers who have or are recovering from chicken pox or flu-like symptoms should not use this product. When using this product, if changes in behavior with nausea and vomiting occur, consult a doctor because these symptoms could be an early sign of Reye's syndrome, a rare but serious illness.

Although a simple viral upper respiratory infection does not contraindicate aspirin use, it can be difficult to differentiate its symptoms from those of influenza and chickenpox. Many HCPs recommend a conservative approach of avoiding aspirin whenever influenza-like symptoms are present. Use of aspirin as a pediatric antipyretic and reports of Reye's syndrome have all but ceased in the United States.

All nonprescription analgesic and antipyretic products for adult use bear a warning for alcohol use. Use of aspirin with alcohol intake increases the risk of adverse GI events, including stomach bleeding. Patients who consume three or more alcoholic drinks daily should be counseled about the associated risks and referred to their PCP before they use aspirin.

Mild salicylate intoxication (*salicylism*) occurs with chronic toxic blood levels, generally achieved in adults who take 90–100 mg/kg per day of a salicylate for at least 2 days. Symptoms and signs of salicylate toxicity include headache, dizziness, tinnitus, difficulty hearing, dimness of vision, mental confusion, lassitude, drowsiness, sweating, thirst, hyperventilation, nausea, vomiting, and occasional diarrhea. These clinical abnormalities all can be reversed by lowering the plasma concentration to a therapeutic range. Tinnitus, typically an early manifestation, should not be used as a sole indicator of salicylate toxicity.

Acute salicylate intoxication is categorized as mild (ingestion of <150 mg/kg), moderate (ingestion of 150–300 mg/kg), or severe (ingestion of >300 mg/kg). Clinical manifestations depend on the concentration and include lethargy, nausea, vomiting, dehydration, tinnitus, hemorrhage, tachypnea and pulmonary edema, convulsions, and coma. Acid–base disturbances are prominent and range from respiratory alkalosis to metabolic acidosis. Initially, salicylate affects the respiratory center in the medulla, producing hyperventilation and respiratory alkalosis. In severely intoxicated adults and in most salicylate-poisoned children younger than 5 years, respiratory alkalosis progresses rapidly to metabolic acidosis. Children are more likely than adults to exhibit high fever in salicylate poisoning. Hypoglycemia resulting from increased glucose utilization may be especially serious in children. Bleeding may occur from the GI tract or mucosal surfaces, and petechiae are a prominent feature at autopsy in fatal cases.

Emergency management of acute salicylate intoxication is directed at preventing absorption of salicylate from the GI tract and providing supportive care. Activated charcoal should be used at home only if recommended by poison control center or emergency department personnel. In an emergency department setting, GI tract decontamination with gastric lavage or activated charcoal may be undertaken. Enhancing renal elimination can be accomplished through alkalinization of the urine. Dosing recommendations for the use of activated charcoal are included in Chapter 21.

Combination Products

Many nonprescription analgesics are available in combination products (Table 5–8).

Caffeine is used as an adjunct to analgesics for tension-type and migraine headaches. It may also have its own analgesic properties and is known to cause withdrawal headache when taken regularly. Clinical trials have suggested that combining caffeine

TABLE 5-8 Selected Nonprescription Combination Analgesic Products

Trade Name	Primary Ingredients
Acetaminophen-Containing Products	
Excedrin Tension Headache Caplet	Acetaminophen 500 mg; caffeine 65 mg
Excedrin PM Headache Caplet	Acetaminophen 500 mg; aspirin 250 mg; diphenhydramine 38 mg
Goody's Headache Relief Shot Liquid	Acetaminophen 1000 mg; caffeine 65 mg
Percogesic Original Strength Tablet	Acetaminophen 325 mg; diphenhydramine 12.5 mg
Percogesic Extra Strength Tablet	Acetaminophen 500 mg; diphenhydramine 12.5 mg
Sudafed PE Pressure + Pain Caplet	Acetaminophen 325 mg; phenylephrine 5 mg
Tylenol PM Caplet	Acetaminophen 500 mg; diphenhydramine 25 mg
Tylenol Sinus + Headache Caplet	Acetaminophen 325 mg; phenylephrine 5 mg
Tylenol Sinus Severe Caplet	Acetaminophen 325 mg; phenylephrine 5 mg; guaifenesin 200 mg
Nonsalicylate NSAID–Containing Products	
Advil Cold & Sinus Tablet (behind the counter)	Ibuprofen 200 mg; pseudoephedrine 30 mg
Advil Allergy and Congestion Relief	Ibuprofen 200 mg; phenylephrine 10 mg; chlorpheniramine maleate 4 mg
Advil Sinus Congestion and Pain Tablet	Ibuprofen 200 mg; phenylephrine 10 mg
Aleve-D Sinus & Headache Caplet (behind the counter)	Naproxen sodium 220 mg; pseudoephedrine 120 mg
Motrin PM Caplet	Naproxen sodium 200 mg; diphenhydramine 38 mg
Sudafed 12 Hour Pressure + Pain Extended Release Tablet (behind the counter)	Naproxen sodium 220 mg; pseudoephedrine 120 mg
Aspirin-Containing Products	
Anacin Maximum Strength Tablet	Aspirin 500 mg; caffeine 32 mg
Anacin Regular Strength Tablet	Aspirin 400 mg; caffeine 32 mg
Bayer Cafiaspirina Caplet	Aspirin 500 mg; caffeine 40 mg
Excedrin Migraine Caplet	Aspirin 250 mg; acetaminophen 250 mg; caffeine 65 mg
Goody's Cool Orange Powder	Aspirin 500 mg; acetaminophen 325 mg
Goody's Extra Strength Headache Powder	Aspirin 520 mg; acetaminophen 260 mg; caffeine 33.3 mg

Key: NSAID = Nonsteroidal anti-inflammatory drug.

with analgesics may result in better efficacy.[46] Of note, however, caffeine itself may be a trigger for migraines, and withdrawal of caffeine may result in headache. Combination dosage forms containing a decongestant and either acetaminophen or an NSAID are also available. Use of such combinations appears to be logical in sinus headaches or other indications for which both analgesia and decongestion are needed.

Combinations of NSAIDs, aspirin, and/or acetaminophen may achieve goals of pain relief with lower doses of the individual agents; however, insufficient evidence is available to support the safety and effectiveness of this practice. Dosing limits for combination should be closely monitored.

Pharmacotherapeutic Comparison

Aspirin Versus Nonacetylated Salicylates

Although definitive clinical data are lacking, aspirin and nonacetylated salicylates are believed to be of equal anti-inflammatory potency; however, aspirin is thought to be a superior analgesic and antipyretic.

Aspirin Versus Acetaminophen

Numerous controlled studies have demonstrated the equivalent analgesic efficacy of aspirin and acetaminophen on a milligram-for-milligram basis; however, statistical methods used to compare effectiveness among different studies show that acetaminophen may not be quite as effective in some types of pain in which an inflammatory component predominates.[47]

Aspirin Versus Nonsalicylate NSAID

Ibuprofen has been shown to be at least as effective as aspirin in treating various types of pain, including dental extraction pain, dysmenorrhea, and episiotomy pain. Because aspirin must be dosed at levels near the self-care maximum to achieve anti-inflammatory effects, NSAIDs may be preferred for self-treatment of inflammatory disorders such as rheumatoid arthritis or acute muscle injury.[47] NSAIDs have a safety advantage of lower toxicity in overdose.

NSAID Versus Acetaminophen

For episodic tension-type headache, acetaminophen 1000 mg appears to provide relief equivalent to that achieved with naproxen

375 mg.[48] For moderate–severe dental or sore throat pain in children, single doses of acetaminophen 7–15 mg/kg produced pain relief similar to that with ibuprofen 4–10 mg/kg. Ibuprofen was a more effective antipyretic, and both drugs were well tolerated.[49] A review of evidence comparing ibuprofen with acetaminophen for headache treatment in children and adults found that only two trials had shown a modest advantage for ibuprofen, and the researchers concluded that the two agents should be considered equally effective.[50] Acetaminophen does not have anti-inflammatory properties, which may limit its effectiveness in some conditions, including dysmenorrhea and certain types of arthritis.[47]

Naproxen Versus Ibuprofen

Naproxen sodium 220 mg and ibuprofen 200 mg appear to have similar efficacy. Both also have a similar time to onset of activity. The time to onset of activity also is similar for the two NSAIDs. Duration of action of naproxen is longer than that of ibuprofen, with a dosing schedule of every 8–12 hours versus ibuprofen's dosing schedule of every 4–6 hours. Individual patients may report a better response to one NSAID than to another, for reasons that are unclear.

Product Selection Guidelines

Special Population Considerations

Age is an important consideration in the selection of an appropriate nonprescription medication for self-treatment of headache. Parents of children younger than 8 years should consult a pediatrician before giving their children nonprescription medications. Children 2 years and older may use acetaminophen or ibuprofen. Children 12 years and older may use naproxen. To decrease the risk of Reye's syndrome, parents should not use aspirin or aspirin-containing products in children and teenagers who have or are recovering from chickenpox or influenza-like symptoms, unless directed to do so by a PCP.

Older patients are at increased risk for many adverse effects of salicylates and NSAIDs. Comorbid conditions, impaired renal function, and concurrent use of other medications contribute to the increased risk. These patients are more vulnerable to serious GI toxicity and the hypertensive and renal effects of salicylates and NSAIDs.[51] Acetaminophen is generally recognized as the agent of choice to manage mild–moderate pain in the geriatric population.

When aspirin's effect on hemostasis is a concern and peripheral anti-inflammatory activity is not needed, acetaminophen is appropriate for self-medication. If a peripheral anti-inflammatory agent is indicated, prescription salicylate compounds (e.g., salsalate, choline magnesium trisalicylate) are reasonable alternatives.

Many safety considerations have been raised regarding the use of these medications in patients who are pregnant or breastfeeding; however, no such considerations apply for males and females of reproductive potential in general. (See the Preface for a detailed explanation of the pregnancy data.) Acetaminophen crosses the placenta but is considered safe for use during pregnancy. Acetaminophen appears in breast milk, producing a milk-to-maternal plasma ratio of 0.5:1.0. A maternal dose of 1 g correlates with an estimated maximum infant dose that is 1.85% of the maternal dose. The only adverse effect reported in infants exposed to acetaminophen through breast milk is a rarely occurring maculopapular rash, which subsides upon drug discontinuation. Acetaminophen use is considered compatible with breastfeeding.[52]

No evidence exists that NSAIDs are teratogenic in either humans or animals. Use of these agents is contraindicated during the third trimester of pregnancy, however, because all potent prostaglandin synthesis inhibitors can cause delayed parturition, prolonged labor, and increased postpartum bleeding. These agents can also have adverse fetal cardiovascular effects (e.g., premature closure of the ductus arteriosus) when used in pregnancy (particularly in late pregnancy). Reproductive animal studies have not shown evidence of harm to the fetus; however, adequate studies to verify safety have not been conducted in humans. Use in pregnancy should be limited to clinical situations in which the potential benefit justifies potential risk to the fetus.[52,53]

Nursing mothers should not use naproxen. The naproxen anion has been measured in human milk, where it accumulates at a level of 1% of the maximum plasma concentration for naproxen. Prostaglandin-inhibiting drugs have the potential to cause harm in neonates; therefore, this level of exposure in milk has led to the labeling statement to avoid use during lactation.[53] According to the product information for ibuprofen, it is not known whether the drug is excreted in human milk. Given the potential for such excretion and the associated risk of serious adverse reactions in nursing infants, the PCP should carefully assess the need for this medication in breastfeeding patients in light of the potential harm to the infant.[17]

Aspirin should be avoided during pregnancy, especially during the last trimester, and during breastfeeding. Its ingestion during pregnancy may produce maternal adverse effects such as anemia, antepartum or postpartum hemorrhage, and prolonged gestation and labor. Regular aspirin ingestion during pregnancy may increase the risk for complicated deliveries, including unplanned cesarean section, breech delivery, and forceps delivery. Definitive data supporting these concerns, however, are lacking.

Aspirin readily crosses the placenta and can be found in higher serum concentrations in the neonate than in the mother. Salicylate elimination is slow in neonates because of the liver's immaturity and underdeveloped capacity to form glycine and glucuronic acid conjugates and because of reduced urinary excretion resulting from low glomerular filtration rates.

Fetal effects from in utero aspirin exposure include intrauterine growth retardation, congenital salicylate intoxication, decreased albumin-binding capacity, and increased perinatal mortality. In utero death results, in part, from antepartum hemorrhage or premature closure of the ductus arteriosus. In utero aspirin exposure within 1 week of delivery can result in neonatal hemorrhagic episodes and/or pruritic rash. Reported neonatal bleeding complications include petechiae, hematuria, cephalhematoma, subconjunctival hemorrhage, and bleeding after circumcision. An increased incidence of intracranial hemorrhage in premature or low-birth-weight infants associated with maternal aspirin use near the time of birth has also been reported.[52] An association between maternal aspirin ingestion and oral clefting and congenital heart disease has been reported. The relationship between maternal aspirin ingestion and congenital malformation remains unresolved, however, and studies have failed to confirm a relationship between maternal ingestion of aspirin and increased risk of fetal malformation.

Aspirin and other salicylates are excreted into breast milk in low concentrations. After single-dose oral salicylate ingestion, peak milk levels occur at approximately 3 hours, producing a milk–to–maternal plasma ratio of 3:8. Although no adverse effects on platelet function in nursing infants exposed to aspirin via breast milk have been reported, these agents still must be considered to carry a risk for such effects.[52]

Patients with renal impairment should exercise caution when using salicylates and NSAIDs. Clinically important alterations in renal blood flow that result in acute reduction in renal function can result from even short courses of salicylates. Referral for medical evaluation for assistance in selecting an analgesic is appropriate.

Patient Factors

Nonprescription analgesics are available in a number of dosage forms. During patient assessment, the HCP should determine which dosage form will provide an optimal clinical outcome. If rapid response is desired, then immediate-release oral dosage forms are preferred over coated or extended-release forms. For patients experiencing migraine headache with severe nausea, rectal dosage forms may be preferred. Liquid dosage forms often are used in children or adult patients who have difficulty swallowing solid dosage forms. (See Chapter 11, section "Special Populations," for FDA requirements for dispensing devices included in liquid nonprescription products.)

Use of ibuprofen in the pediatric population is complicated by the availability of two liquid formulations of different strengths. Unintended over- or underdosing can occur when parents switch between the concentrated drops (50 mg/1.25 mL) and the suspension (100 mg/5 mL). In addition, rapidly growing infants quickly outgrow previous dose requirements. Therefore, recalculation of the pediatric dose according to present age and body weight is recommended at the time of each treatment course.

Patients with significant alcohol ingestion (three or more drinks per day) should avoid self-treatment with nonprescription analgesics.

Patients with intolerance to aspirin may also experience cross-reactions with other chemicals or drugs. Up to 15% of aspirin-intolerant patients may exhibit signs of cross-reaction when exposed to tartrazine (a dye designated by the FDA-administered Food, Drug, and Cosmetic Act as FD&C Yellow 5), which can be found in many drugs and foods. Among persons with the respiratory type of aspirin sensitivity, rates of cross-reaction between aspirin and acetaminophen, ibuprofen, and naproxen in documented aspirin-intolerant patients are 7%, 98%, and 100%, respectively. High cross-reaction rates are also reported with some prescription NSAIDs. The proposed mechanism of cross-sensitivity between aspirin and NSAIDs involves shunting arachidonic metabolism down the lipoxygenase pathway (consequent to inhibition of the COX-1 enzyme pathway), resulting in accumulation of leukotrienes that can cause bronchospasm and anaphylaxis. Acetaminophen and nonacetylated salicylates are weak inhibitors of COX-1 at moderate doses. Patients with a history of aspirin intolerance should therefore be advised to avoid all aspirin- and NSAID-containing products, and to use acetaminophen or a nonacetylated salicylate, with the caveat that acetaminophen does not offer anti-inflammatory properties.

Patient Preferences

Consideration of dosing frequency in product selection may lead to improved outcomes for individual patients. Naproxen can be taken 2 or 3 times daily, which may improve patient adherence to the medication regimen. By contrast, acetaminophen, ibuprofen, and salicylates may require dosing as frequently as every 4 hours. Because of the delayed absorption of sustained-release aspirin, this dosage form is not appropriate for rapid pain relief but may be useful as a bedtime medication.

Complementary Therapies

Butterbur, feverfew, riboflavin, and coenzyme Q10 commonly are used for the prevention of migraine headaches and are discussed in depth in Chapter 51. These natural products have limited efficacy for the treatment of other types of headaches. Other unproven remedies include peppermint oil applied to the forehead and temples for treatment of tension headache and magnesium for treatment and prevention of migraine headache. Although clinical trials have supported both treatments, sufficient evidence of a clear benefit for use of either peppermint oil or magnesium is lacking, owing to conflicting study outcomes and weaknesses in study methodologies.

Acupuncture has been used to prevent migraine and tension-type headache. Evaluation of acupuncture is complicated by difficulties in blinding and differences in identifying acupuncture points. Overall, results have been variable, but several randomized, placebo-controlled trials found acupuncture to be effective in reducing frequency and severity of headache.[54] Methods focusing on stress relief and relaxation techniques such as massage, yoga, and biofeedback therapy may be useful for the prevention and treatment of headache, but further efficacy studies are needed.

Assessment of Headache: A Case-Based Approach

Before self-treatment of headache can be recommended, the HCP must assess the patient's headaches to determine type, severity, location, frequency, intensity over time, and age at onset. The next step is to obtain a medical and psychosocial history. All current medications should be inventoried, and all past and present headache treatments should be reviewed, with emphasis on determining which treatments, if any, were successful or preferred.

Secondary headaches, other than minor sinus headache, are excluded from self-treatment. Headache associated with seizures, confusion, drowsiness, or cognitive impairment may be a clinical indicator of brain tumor, ischemic stroke, subdural hematoma, or subarachnoid hemorrhage. Headache accompanied by nausea, vomiting, fever, and stiff neck may indicate brain abscess or meningitis. Headache with night sweats, aching joints, fever, weight loss, and visual symptoms (e.g., blurring) in patients with rheumatoid arthritis may indicate cranial arteritis. Headache associated with localized facial pain, muscle tenderness, and limited motion of the jaw may indicate temporomandibular joint disorder.

Cases 5–1 and 5–2 illustrate assessment of two different patients with headache.

Patient Counseling for Headache

To optimize outcomes from therapy, the provider should instruct patients to take an appropriate dose of analgesic early in the course of the headache. The use of nonprescription analgesics to preempt or abort migraine headaches should also be explained to patients with migraines whose headaches are predictable. Patients for whom headache is a relatively common occurrence should be encouraged to keep a log of their headaches to document triggers, frequency, intensity, duration of episodes, and response to treatment. This record may also be helpful in identifying factors that can improve headache prevention and treatment. Patients should be advised that continuing or escalating pain can be a sign of a more serious problem and that such pain warrants prompt medical attention. Appropriate drug and nondrug measures for treating headaches should be explained to the patient. Frequent use of nonprescription analgesics is not appropriate because of the risk for medication-overuse headache. Providers should convey the message that nonprescription analgesics are potent medications with accompanying potential adverse effects, interactions, and precautions and warnings. The box "Patient Education for Headache" lists specific information for patient counseling.

CASE 5-1

Relevant Evaluation Criteria	Scenario/Model Outcome
Collect	
1. Gather essential information about the patient's symptoms and medical history, including	
a. Description of symptom(s) (i.e., nature, onset, duration, severity, associated symptoms)	Patient states that yesterday she had a headache starting in the middle of the day that felt like her head was "about to explode." She stated that the headache did not go away until the next morning. This type of headache happens when her first grade class gets "rowdy," approximately 1 day per week for the last few months.
b. Description of any factors that seem to precipitate, exacerbate, and/or relieve the patient's symptom(s)	The pain feels like constant pain around her head extending to the base of her skull. Acetaminophen has not helped.
c. Description of the patient's efforts to relieve the symptoms	She needs to lie down and go to sleep. Being home where it is quiet helps.
d. Patient's identity	Mary Beth Rodriguez
e. Patient's age, gender, height, and weight	25 years, female, 5 ft 3 in., 150 lb
f. Patient's occupation	First grade teacher
g. Patient's dietary habits	She tries her best to eat a healthy diet, but loves to eat sweets. Her eating schedule is regular most of the time, and she eats lunch in the cafeteria at school. Her husband usually cooks a healthy dinner for her.
h. Patient's sleep habits	She often stays up late grading papers but has to be up early the next morning to start her class.
i. Concurrent medical conditions, prescription and nonprescription medications, and dietary supplements	None
j. Allergies	Peanuts caused a bad rash a few years ago.
k. History of other adverse reactions to medications	None
l. Other (describe) ______	She does not smoke, but she occasionally drinks with friends (1–2 drinks per week).
Assess	
2. Differentiate patient's signs/symptoms, and correctly identify the patient's primary problem(s) (Table 5–1).	Mrs. Rodriguez is having episodic tension-type headache that is most likely due to the stress of her job.
3. Identify exclusions for self-treatment (Figure 5–1).	Mrs. Rodriguez has no exclusions for self-treatment.
4. Formulate a comprehensive list of therapeutic alternatives for the primary problem to determine whether triage to a medical practitioner is required, and share this information with the patient or caregiver.	Options include (1) Refer Mrs. Rodriguez to an appropriate HCP. (2) Recommend self-care with a nonprescription analgesic. (3) Recommend self-care until Mrs. Rodriguez can see an appropriate HCP. (4) Take no action.
Plan	
5. Select an optimal therapeutic alternative to address the patient's problem, taking into account patient preferences.	Mrs. Rodriguez should use a nonprescription analgesic to help relieve her headache pain. Naproxen is an appropriate alternative medication for short-term treatment for her symptoms.
6. Describe the recommended therapeutic approach to the patient or caregiver.	"What you have been experiencing may be tension-type headaches. This is likely a result of the stress you are experiencing from your job. Taking naproxen might help to relieve your symptoms."
7. Explain to the patient or caregiver the rationale for selecting the recommended therapeutic approach from the considered therapeutic alternatives.	"Naproxen may be a good alternative to the acetaminophen you were taking because it is in a different class of medications, so it works in a different way. You will see the most benefit from the medication if you take it at the earliest sign of the headache, rather than waiting for the pain to become worse."

CASE 5-1 *continued*

Relevant Evaluation Criteria	Scenario/Model Outcome
Implement	
8. When recommending self-care with nonprescription medications and/or nondrug therapy, convey accurate information to the patient or caregiver.	
a. Appropriate dose and frequency of administration	"Take naproxen sodium 220 mg, 1 tablet every 8–12 hours as needed. For the first dose, you may take 2 tablets within the first hour. Do not exceed 3 tablets in a 24-hour period."
b. Maximum number of days the therapy should be employed	"Do not use this medication more than 3 days per week."
c. Product administration procedures	"Start naproxen at the first sign of headache."
d. Expected time to onset of relief	"Relief should begin in 30–60 minutes."
e. Degree of relief that can be reasonably expected	"This type of headache may be completely relieved by nonprescription analgesics. However, you may need to decrease your stress level to prevent future headaches."
f. Most common adverse effects	"Upset stomach is a common adverse effect. Taking naproxen with food may help prevent this."
g. Adverse effects that warrant medical intervention, should they occur	"Naproxen should be stopped if you have severe stomach pain, bloody vomit, black stool, abdominal bruising or bleeding, or allergic reaction (swelling of the face or throat, difficulty breathing)."
h. Patient options in the event that condition worsens or persists	"If naproxen does not relieve your headache, you may also try ibuprofen or aspirin. If you continue to have headaches, you may need to see another health care provider for further diagnosis and treatment."
i. Product storage requirements	"Store naproxen in a closed container at room temperature away from moisture and children."
j. Specific nondrug measures	"Managing your stress may help you avoid tension headaches. Relaxation exercises can help with stress management."
Solicit follow-up questions from the patient or caregiver.	"Is it safe to take this medication?"
Answer the patient's or caregiver's questions.	"Naproxen and some other nonsteroidal anti-inflammatory drugs, such as ibuprofen, can cause adverse effects related to irritation of the gastrointestinal tract and increased risk of cardiovascular disease. You do not have risk factors for these problems, but it is best to use the medication sparingly to control the headaches while also making lifestyle changes to decrease the frequency of the headaches."
Follow-up: Monitor and Evaluate	
9. Assess patient outcome.	Call the patient in 6 weeks to determine whether her episodic headaches have been relieved with the recommended therapy.

Key: HCP = Health care provider; NSAID = nonsteroidal anti-inflammatory drug; OTC = over the counter.

CASE 5-2

Relevant Evaluation Criteria	Scenario/Model Outcome
Collect	
1. Gather essential information about the patient's symptoms and medical history, including	
a. Description of symptom(s) (i.e., nature, onset, duration, severity, associated symptoms)	Patient's mother says she had to pick up her son from school today because he was complaining of pain in his head. His teacher reported that he put his head down on his desk during class several times, and he did not eat his usual snack.
b. Description of any factors that seem to precipitate, exacerbate, and/or relieve the patient's symptom(s)	When he is in the sunlight, he squints and complains that the sun is bothering him.

CASE 5-2 *continued*

Relevant Evaluation Criteria	Scenario/Model Outcome
c. Description of the patient's efforts to relieve the symptoms	Sitting quietly in a dark room helped, but the headache continued.
d. Patient's identity	Michael Douglas
e. Patient's age, gender, height, and weight	6 years, male, 3 ft 10 in., 49 lb
f. Patient's occupation	First grader
g. Patient's dietary habits	The patient eats the school lunch and a well-rounded breakfast and dinner at home.
h. Patient's sleep habits	The patient sleeps well at night and generally sleeps from 8 PM until 6:30 AM.
i. Concurrent medical conditions, prescription and nonprescription medications, and dietary supplements	He has mild asthma and has an emergency inhaler that he has used only once in a few months.
j. Allergies	None
k. History of other adverse reactions to medications	None
l. Other (describe) ______	None
Assess	
2. Differentiate patient's signs/symptoms, and correctly identify the patient's primary problem(s) (Table 5–1).	Michael might be having migraine headache as indicated by pain that is exacerbated by light.
3. Identify exclusions for self-treatment (Figure 5–1).	Age <8 years Suspected undiagnosed migraine, based on light sensitivity
4. Formulate a comprehensive list of therapeutic alternatives for the primary problem to determine whether triage to a medical practitioner is required, and share this information with the patient or caregiver.	Options include (1) Refer Michael to an appropriate HCP. (2) Recommend self-care measures until Michael can see an appropriate HCP.
Plan	
5. Select an optimal therapeutic alternative to address the patient's problem, taking into account patient or caregiver preferences.	Referral to an HCP is appropriate for Michael.
6. Describe the recommended therapeutic approach to the patient or caregiver.	"What your son has been experiencing may be a migraine headache. It is recommended that you seek evaluation by your pediatrician to determine appropriate treatment."
7. Explain to the patient or caregiver the rationale for selecting the recommended therapeutic approach from the considered therapeutic alternatives.	"Self-treatment with over-the-counter medications is not recommended until he has been evaluated and diagnosed. His asthma is a complicating factor for the choice of medication."
Implement	
8. When recommending self-care with nonprescription medications and/or nondrug therapy, convey accurate information to the patient or caregiver.	Criterion does not apply in this case.
Solicit follow-up questions from the patient or caregiver.	"Is it unusual for children to have migraine headaches?"
Answer the patient's or caregiver's questions.	"This condition is more common in adults. It is important that you see the pediatrician about this problem."
Follow-up: Monitor and Evaluate	
9. Assess patient outcome.	Contact the mother in 1–2 days to find out if Michael was seen by a pediatrician and what plan was determined.

Key: HCP = Health care provider.

PATIENT EDUCATION FOR

Headache

The objectives of self-treatment are (1) to relieve headache pain, (2) to prevent headaches when possible, and (3) to prevent medication-overuse headaches by avoiding chronic use of nonprescription analgesics. Carefully following product instructions and the self-care measures listed here will help ensure the best results.

Tension-Type Headaches

- Nonprescription pain relievers (analgesics) are usually effective in relieving tension-type headaches. However, consult your primary provider before using them for chronic tension-type headaches that occur more than 15 days per month for 3 months.
- If nonprescription pain relievers are used for chronic headaches, keep records of how often they are used, and share this information with your provider.

Migraine Headache

- Avoid substances (food, caffeine, alcohol, medications) or situations (stress, fatigue, oversleeping, fasting, missing meals) that you know can trigger a migraine.
- Use the following nutritional strategies to prevent migraine:
  - Avoid foods or food additives known to trigger migraines, including red wine, aged cheese, aspartame, monosodium glutamate, coffee, tea, cola beverages, and chocolate.
  - Avoid foods to which you are allergic.
  - Eat regularly to avoid hunger and low blood sugar.
- If onset of migraines is predictable (e.g., headache occurs during menstruation), take aspirin, ibuprofen, or naproxen to prevent the headache. Start taking the analgesic 2 days before you expect the headache and continue regular use during the time the headache might start.
- Try to stop a migraine by taking a nonsteroidal anti-inflammatory agent (NSAID), aspirin, or acetaminophen at the onset of headache pain.
- If desired, use an ice bag or cold pack applied with pressure to the forehead or temples to reduce the pain associated with acute migraine attacks.

Sinus Headache

- Consider using a combination of a decongestant and a nonprescription analgesic to relieve the pain of sinus headache.

Precautions for Nonprescription Analgesics

- If you are pregnant or breastfeeding, consult your primary care provider before taking any nonprescription medications.
- If you have a medical condition or are taking prescription medications, obtain medical advice before taking any of these medications. Nonprescription analgesics are known to interact with several medications.
- Do not take nonprescription analgesics more often than 3 days per week unless a medical provider has recommended prolonged use.
- Do not take these medications if you consume three or more alcoholic beverages daily.
- Do not exceed recommended dosages.
- Products containing aspartame and/or phenylalanine (usually chewable tablets) should not be given to individuals with phenylketonuria.

Salicylates (Aspirin and Magnesium Salicylate) and NSAIDs (Ibuprofen and Naproxen)

- Do not take aspirin during the last 3 months of pregnancy unless a primary care provider is supervising such use. Unsupervised use of this medication could harm the unborn child or cause complications during delivery.
- Do not give aspirin or products that contain aspirin to children and teenagers who have or are recovering from chickenpox or influenza-like symptoms. To avoid the risk of Reye's syndrome, a rare but potentially fatal condition, use acetaminophen for pain relief.
- Do not take aspirin or NSAIDs if you are allergic to aspirin or have asthma and nasal polyps. Take acetaminophen instead.
- Do not take aspirin or NSAIDs if you have stomach problems or ulcers, liver disease, kidney disease, or heart failure.
- Do not take NSAIDs if you have or are at high risk for heart disease or stroke unless the use is supervised by a health care provider.
- Do not take aspirin if you have gout, diabetes mellitus, or arthritis unless the use is supervised by a health care provider.
- Do not take salicylates or NSAIDs if you are taking anticoagulants.
- Do not take magnesium salicylate if you have kidney disease.
- Do not give naproxen to a child younger than 12 years.

When to Seek Medical Attention

- Stop taking salicylates or NSAIDs and seek medical attention if any of the following signs and symptoms are noted:
  - Headache, dizziness, ringing in the ears, difficulty in hearing, dimness of vision, mental confusion, lassitude, drowsiness, sweating, thirst, hyperventilation, nausea, vomiting, or occasional diarrhea. These signs and symptoms indicate mild salicylate toxicity.
  - Dizziness, nausea and mild stomach pain, constipation, ringing in the ears, or swelling in the feet or legs. These signs and symptoms are common adverse effects of salicylates and NSAIDs.
  - Rash or hives, or red, peeling skin; swelling in the face or around the eyes; wheezing or trouble breathing; bloody or cloudy urine; unexplained bruising and bleeding; or signs of stomach bleeding such as bloody or black tarry stools, severe stomach pain, or bloody vomit (see the box "A Word About NSAIDs and Stomach Bleeding"). These signs and symptoms warrant immediate medical attention.

Acetaminophen

- To avoid possible damage to the liver, do not take more than 4 grams of acetaminophen a day (from all nonprescription and prescription single-ingredient or combination products containing acetaminophen).
- Do not drink alcohol while taking this medication.
- Follow dosage instructions for acetaminophen carefully if you have glucose-6-phosphate dehydrogenase deficiency.

When to Seek Medical Attention

- Stop taking acetaminophen and seek medical attention if you develop nausea, vomiting, drowsiness, confusion, or abdominal pain.

Evaluation of Patient Outcomes for Headache

Appropriate follow-up evaluation will depend on headache frequency and severity, as well as patient factors. For patients with episodic headaches, a trial of 6–12 weeks may be needed to assess efficacy of treatment. For chronic headache, follow-up evaluation after 4–6 weeks should be adequate to assess treatment efficacy. In all cases, patients should seek medical attention if headaches persist longer than 3 days or worsen despite self-treatment.

More than one-third of patients with migraine will benefit from preventive therapy, but many do not receive it.[55] Patients with migraine headaches who are not adequately self-treated should be referred for a medical evaluation, because effective prescription therapies are available to substantially limit pain and disability.

Key Points for Headache

- Most tension-type, migraine, and sinus headaches are amenable to treatment with nonprescription medications.
- Patients with symptoms suggestive of secondary headaches (except for minor sinus headache) or of undiagnosed migraine headaches should be referred for medical attention.
- Many patients with frequent headaches may experience improvement after identifying and modifying environmental, behavioral, nutritional, or other triggers for their headaches.
- The choice of nonprescription analgesic depends on patient preferences, presence of precautionary or contraindicating conditions, concomitant medications, cost, and other factors.
- Pharmacists have been identified as key sources of information on nonprescription analgesics to reduce risk for acetaminophen-induced hepatotoxicity and NSAID-induced GI bleeding, cardiovascular events, and nephrotoxicity.
- Use of nonprescription analgesics for headache should be limited to 3 days per week to prevent medication-overuse headache.

REFERENCES

1. World Health Organization. *Headache Disorders.* World Health Organization; 2012. Fact Sheet No. 277. Available at: http://www.who.int/mediacentre/factsheets/fs277/en/. Accessed April 5, 2017.
2. Stovner LJ, Hagen K, Jensen R, et al. The global burden of headache: a documentation of headache prevalence and disability worldwide. *Cephalalgia.* 2007;27(3):193–210. doi: 10.111/j.1468-2982.2007.01288.x.
3. Loder E, Rizzoli P. Tension-type headache. *BMJ.* 2008;336(7635):88–92. doi: 10.1136/bmj.39412.705868.AD.
4. Lipton RB. Migraine: epidemiology, impact, and risk factors for progression. *Headache.* 2005;45(suppl 1):S3–13. doi: 10.1111/j.1526-4610.2005.4501001.x.
5. Dodick D, Freitag F. Evidence-based understanding of medication-overuse headache: clinical implications. *Headache.* 2006;46(suppl 4):S202–11. doi: 10.1111/j.1526-4610.2006.00604.x.
6. Cady RK, Dodick DW, Levine HL, et al. Sinus headache: a neurology, otolaryngology, allergy, and primary care consensus on diagnosis and treatment. *Mayo Clin Proc.* 2005;80(7):908–16. doi: 10.4065/80.7.908.
7. Stewart WF, Ricci JA, Chee E, et al. Lost productive time and cost due to common pain conditions in the US workforce. *JAMA.* 2003;290(18):2443–54. doi: 10.1001/jama.290.18.2443.
8. Mehuys E, Paemeleire K, Van Hees T, et al. Self-medication of regular headache: a community pharmacy-based survey. *Eur J Neurol.* 2012;19(8):1093–9. doi: 10.1001/jama.290.18.2443.
9. The International Classification of Headache Disorders, 3rd Edition. *Cephalalgia.* 2013;33(9):629–808. doi: 10.1177/0333102413485658.
10. Vargas BB. Tension-type headache and migraine: two points on a continuum? *Curr Pain Headache Rep.* 2008;12(6):433–6. PMID: 18973736.
11. Kelman L. The triggers or precipitants of the acute migraine attack. *Cephalalgia.* 2007;27(5):394–404. doi: 10.1111/j.1468-2982.2007.01303.x.
12. Pietrobon D, Moskowitz MA. Pathophysiology of migraine. *Annu Rev Physiol.* 2013;75:365–91. doi: 10.1146/annurev-physiol-030212-183717.
13. Teigen L, Boes CJ. An evidence-based review of oral magnesium supplementation in the preventive treatment of migraine. *Cephalalgia.* 2015;35(10):912–22. doi: 10.1177/0333102414564891.
14. Martin VT, Behbehani M. Ovarian hormones and migraine headache: understanding mechanisms and pathogenesis—part 1. *Headache.* 2006;45(1):3–23. doi: 10.1111/j.1526-4610.2006.00309.x.
15. Martin VT, Behbehani M. Ovarian hormones and migraine headache: understanding mechanisms and pathogenesis—part 2. *Headache.* 2006;46(3):365–86. doi: 10.1111/j.1526-4610.2006.00370.x.
16. Quintela E, Castillo J, Muñoz P, et al. Premonitory and resolution symptoms in migraine: a prospective study in 100 unselected patients. *Cephalalgia.* 2006;26(9):1051–60. doi: 10.1111/j.1468-2982.2006.01157.x.
17. Ibuprofen tablets [product information]. Preferred Pharmaceuticals, Anaheim, CA. January 2015. Available at: https://dailymed.nlm.nih.gov/dailymed/drugInfo.cfm?setid=e31d4be3-e542-43a1-a6e3-4f6937a003ae. Accessed April 5, 2017.
18. Goadsby PJ, Rashkin NH. Headache. In: Kasper D, Fauci A, Hauser S, et al., eds. *Harrison's Principles of Internal Medicine.* 19th ed. New York, NY: McGraw-Hill; 2015. Available at: http://accesspharmacy.mhmedical.com/content.aspx?bookid=1130&Sectionid=79724323. Accessed June 20, 2016.
19. Rockett FC, de Oliveira VR, Castro K, et al. Dietary aspects of migraine trigger factors. *Nutr Rev.* 2012;70(6):337–56. doi: 10.1111/j.1753-4887.2012.00468.x.
20. Dalkara T, Kilic K. How does fasting trigger migraine? A hypothesis. *Curr Pain Headache Rep.* 2013;17(10):368. doi: 10.1007/s11916-013-0368-1.
21. Derry S, Moore RA. Paracetamol (acetaminophen) with or without an antiemetic for acute migraine headache in adults. *Cochrane Database Syst Rev.* 2013;4:CD008040. doi: 10.1002/14651858.CD008040.pub2.
22. Facts and Comparisons E Answers. St. Louis, MO: Wolters Kluwer Health, updated 2016. Available at: http://online.factsandcomparisons.com/login.aspx?url=/index.aspx&qs=. Accessed June 27, 2016.
23. Krahenbuhl S, Brauchli Y, Kummer O, et al. Acute liver failure in two patients with regular alcohol consumption ingesting paracetamol at therapeutic dosage. *Digestion.* 2007;75(4):232–77. doi: 10.1159/000111032.
24. U.S. Food and Drug Administration. Guidance for Industry: Organ-specific warnings: Internal analgesic, antipyretic, and antirheumatic drug products for over-the-counter human use—labeling for products that contain acetaminophen. November 2015. Available at: www.fda.gov/downloads/Drugs/GuidanceComplianceRegulatoryInformation/Guidances/UCM310477.pdf. Accessed April 5, 2017.
25. Krenzelok EP, Royal MA. Confusion: acetaminophen dosing changes based on NO evidence in adults. *Drugs R D.* 2012;12(2):45–8. doi: 10.2165/11633010-000000000-00000.
26. U.S. Food and Drug Administration. FDA recommends health care professionals discontinue prescribing and dispensing prescription combination drug products with more than 325 mg of acetaminophen to protect consumers. Available at: http://www.fda.gov/Drugs/DrugSafety/ucm381644.htm. Accessed April 5, 2017.
27. Food and Drug Administration, Center for Drug Evaluation and Research. Summary Minutes of the Joint Meeting of the Nonprescription Drugs Advisory Committee and the Pediatric Advisory Committee. Available at: https://www.fda.gov/downloads/AdvisoryCommittees/CommitteesMeetingMaterials/Drugs/NonprescriptionDrugsAdvisoryCommittee/UCM264147.pdf. Accessed April 5, 2017.
28. *Tylenol* first to move on single dosage for children's acetaminophen. *Pink Sheet.* March 13, 2017;79(11):24. Available at: https://pink.pharmamedtechbi.com/PS120181/emTylenol-emFirst-To-Move-On-Single-Dosage-For-Childrens-Acetaminophen. Accessed April 5, 2017.
29. Bronstein AC, Spyker DA, Cantilena LR Jr, et al. 2006 annual report of the American Association of Poison Control Centers' National Poison Data System (NPDS). *Clin Toxicol (Phila).* 2007;45(8):815–917.

30. Larson AM, Polson J, Fontana RJ, et al. Acetaminophen-induced acute liver failure: results of a United States multicenter, prospective study. *Hepatology.* 2005;42(6):1364–72. doi: 10.1002/hep.20948.
31. Acetaminophen. Lexicomp Online, Lexi-Tox, Hudson, OH; Lexi-Comp, Inc. Updated 2016. Available at: http://online.lexi.com/action/home. Accessed July 4, 2016.
32. Watkins PB, Kaplowitz N, Slattery JT, et al. Aminotransferase elevations in healthy adults receiving 4 grams of acetaminophen daily. *JAMA.* 2006; 296(1):87–93. doi: 10.1001/jama.296.1.87.
33. Sklar GE. Hemolysis as a potential complication of acetaminophen overdose in a patient with glucose-6-phosphate dehydrogenase deficiency. *Pharmacotherapy.* 2002;22(5):656–8.
34. U.S. Food and Drug Administration. FDA Drug Safety Communication: FDA warns of rare but serious skin reactions with the pain reliever/fever reducer acetaminophen [news release]. August 8, 2013. Available at: http://www.fda.gov/downloads/Drugs/DrugSafety/UCM363052.pdf. Accessed April 5, 2017.
35. U.S. Food and Drug Administration. Recommended warning for over-the-counter acetaminophen-containing drug products and labeling statements regarding serious skin reactions. Guidance for industry. Available at: https://www.fda.gov/downloads/drugs/guidances/ucm424898.pdf. Accessed April 5, 2017.
36. Food and Drug Administration. Over-the-counter drug products containing internal analgesic/antipyretic active ingredients; required warnings and other labeling. CFR: Code of Federal Regulations. Title 21, Part 201, Section 201.326. Updated June 23, 2016. Available at: http://www.ecfr.gov/cgi-bin/text-idx?SID=d896e8f8b1ddcea5d08baa1c5086c5f5&mc=true&node=se21.4.201_1326&rgn=div8. Accessed April 5, 2017.
37. U.S. Food and Drug Administration. FDA Drug Safety Communication: FDA strengthens warning that non-aspirin nonsteroidal anti-inflammatory drugs (NSAIDs) can cause heart attacks or strokes. July 9, 2015. Available at: http://www.fda.gov/Drugs/DrugSafety/ucm451800.htm?source=govdelivery&utm_medium=email&utm_source=govdelivery. Accessed July 31, 2017
38. Olsen AM, Fosbøl EL, Lindhardsen J, et al. Long-term cardiovascular risk of nonsteroidal anti-inflammatory drug use according to time passed after first-time myocardial infarction: a nationwide cohort study. *Circulation.* 2012;126(16):1955–63. doi: 10.1161/CIRCULATIONAHA.112.112607.
39. Hunter LJ, Wood DM, Dargan PI. The patterns of toxicity and management of acute nonsteroidal anti-inflammatory drug (NSAID) overdose. *Open Access Emerg Med.* 2011;39–48. doi: 10.2147/OAEM.S22795. Available at: https://www.dovepress.com/the-patterns-of-toxicity-and-management-of-acute-nonsteroidal-anti-inf-peer-reviewed-article-OAEM. Accessed April 5, 2017.
40. Bhatt DL, Scheiman J, Abraham NS, et al. ACCF/ACG/AHA 2008 expert consensus document on reducing the gastrointestinal risks of antiplatelet therapy and NSAID use: a report of the American College of Cardiology Foundation Task Force on Clinical Expert Consensus Documents. *Circulation.* 2008;118:1894–909. doi: 10.1161/CIRCULATIONAHA.108.191087.
41. Lanas A, Hunt R. Prevention of anti-inflammatory drug-induced gastrointestinal damage: benefits and risks of therapeutic strategies. *Ann Med.* 2006;38(6):415–28. doi: 10.1080/07853890600925843.
42. Kelly JP, Kaufman DW, Jurgelon JM, et al. Risk of aspirin-associated major upper-gastrointestinal bleeding with enteric-coated or buffered product. *Lancet.* 1996;348(9039):1413–6. doi: 10.1016/S0140-6736(96)01254-8.
43. Can individuals with aspirin sensitivity take NSAIDs? *Pharmacist's Letter/Prescriber's Letter.* 2010;26(10). Available at: http://pharmacistsletter.therapeuticresearch.com/pl/ArticleDD.aspx?nidchk=1&cs=FACULTY&s=PL&pt=6&fpt=31&dd=261011&pb=PL&searchid=60315555#dd. Accessed April 5, 2017.
44. Zhang Y, Neogi T, Chen C, et al. Low-dose aspirin use and recurrent gout attacks. *Ann Rheum Dis.* 2014;73(2):385–90. doi: 10.1136/annrheumdis-2012-202589.
45. U.S. Food and Drug Administration. Labeling of drug preparations containing salicylates. *CFR: Code of Federal Regulations.* Title 21, Part 201, Section 201.314. Updated July 27, 2017. Available at: http://www.ecfr.gov/cgi-bin/text-idx?SID=b1b2224711dc88657752be21f12c574a&mc=true&node=se21.4.201_1314&rgn=div8. Accessed July 31, 2017.
46. Diamond S, Freitag FG. The use of ibuprofen plus caffeine to treat tension-type headache. *Curr Pain Headache Rep.* 2001;5:472–8. doi: 10.1067/mcp.2000.109353.
47. Blondell RD, Azadfard M, Wisniewski AM. Pharmacologic therapy for acute pain. *Am Fam Physician.* 2013;87(11):766–72. PMID: 23939498.
48. Prior MJ, Cooper KM, May LG, et al. Efficacy and safety of acetaminophen and naproxen in the treatment of tension-type headache: a randomized, double-blind, placebo-controlled trial. *Cephalalgia.* 2002;22(9):740–8. doi: 10.1046/j.1468-2982.2002.00419.x.
49. Perrott DA, Piira T, Goodenough B, et al. Efficacy and safety of acetaminophen vs ibuprofen for treating children's pain or fever. *Arch Pediatr Adolesc Med.* 2004;158(6):521–6. doi: 10.1001/archpedi.158.6.521.
50. Manzano S, Doyon-Trottier E, Bailey B. Myth: ibuprofen is superior to acetaminophen for the treatment of benign headaches in children and adults. *CJEM.* 2010;12(3):220–2. PMID: 20522287.
51. Tielemans MM, Eikendal T, Jansen JB, van Oijen MG. Identification of NSAID users at risk for gastrointestinal complications: a systematic review of current guidelines and consensus agreements. *Drug Saf.* 2010;33(6): 443–53. doi: 10.2165/11534590-000000000-00000.
52. Briggs G, Freeman R, Yaffe S, eds. *Drugs in Pregnancy and Lactation.* 8th ed. Baltimore, MD: Lippincott Williams & Wilkins; 2008.
53. Naproxen tablets [product information]. Aphena Pharma Solutions, Cookeville, TN. July 2014. Available at: https://dailymed.nlm.nih.gov/dailymed/drugInfo.cfm?setid=502f390d-d69e-4a77-8a59-4eedf91004f3. Accessed April 5, 2017.
54. Linde K, Allais G, Brinkhaus B, et al. Acupuncture for migraine prophylaxis. *Cochrane Database Syst Rev.* 2009;1:CD001218. doi:10.1002/14651858.CD001218.pub2.
55. Holland S, Silberstein SD, Freitag F, et al. Evidence-based guideline update: NSAIDs and other complementary treatments for episodic migraine prevention in adults. *Neurology.* 2012;78:1346–53. doi: 10.1212/WNL.0b013e3182535d0c.

CHAPTER 6

FEVER

VIRGINIA LEMAY AND BRETT M. FERET

Fever is a common reason for visits to pediatricians' offices, with the National Ambulatory Medical Care Survey estimating that 6% of all ambulatory visits to pediatricians are related to fever.[1] Fever is also the leading cause of visits to an emergency department for both male and female children younger than 15 years.[2] In 2012, patients complaining primarily of fever made approximately 10.9 million medical office visits, with a slightly greater number of visits by men.[3] Fever is a more commonly reported symptom in children than in adults: the rate of reported fevers is 10 per 100 children younger than 5 years versus 0.5 per 100 adults. Nonetheless, the rate of fever does not seem to differ significantly with respect to gender, race, or geographic area of residence in the United States.[4]

Most fevers are self-limited and nonthreatening; however, fever can cause a great deal of discomfort and in some cases may indicate a serious underlying pathologic condition (e.g., acute infectious process) for which prompt medical evaluation is indicated. The principal reason for treating fever is to alleviate discomfort, but the underlying cause should be identified and treated appropriately. Fever must be distinguished from hyperthermia and hyperpyrexia. Fever is caused by a regulated rise in body temperature, maintained by the hypothalamus, in response to a pyrogen. *Fever* is defined by a body temperature higher than the normal core (oral) temperature of 100.0°F (37.8°C). It is thus a sign of an increase in the body's thermoregulatory set point.

Hyperthermia, by contrast, represents a malfunctioning of the normal thermoregulatory process at the hypothalamic level caused by excessive heat exposure or production.[5] Because of their different mechanisms, treatment of fever versus hyperthermia also varies.

Hyperpyrexia is defined by a body temperature greater than 106.0°F (41.1°C, oral) that typically is associated with mental and physical signs and symptoms. Hyperpyrexia may develop with either fever or hyperthermia.

Pathophysiology of Fever

Core body temperature is controlled by the hypothalamus and regulated by a feedback system involving information transmitted between the thermoregulatory center in the anterior hypothalamus and the thermosensitive neurons in the skin and central nervous system (CNS). Physiologic (e.g., sweating, vasodilation) and behavioral mechanisms regulate body temperature within the normal range. Although skin temperature may fluctuate greatly in response to environmental conditions, the core temperature is regulated within a narrow range.[6]

Normal thermoregulation prevents wide fluctuations in body temperature, with the average oral temperature usually maintained between 97.5°F and 98.9°F (36.4°C and 37.2°C, respectively). Temperature maintained in this range is considered to be the "set point," or the point at which the physiologic or behavioral mechanisms are not activated. For practical purposes, the commonly accepted core body temperature is usually 98.6°F (37.0°C, oral).

Pyrogens, either exogenous or endogenous, are fever-producing substances that activate the body's host defenses, resulting in an increase in the set point. Exogenous pyrogens (e.g., microbes, toxins) do not independently increase the hypothalamic temperature set point. These substances stimulate the release of endogenous pyrogens (e.g., immune cytokines), thereby increasing the core temperature. Endogenous pyrogens are products released in response to or from damaged tissue such as interleukins, interferons, and tumor necrosis factor.[6–8]

Prostaglandins of the E_2 series (PGE_2) are produced in response to circulating pyrogens and elevate the thermoregulatory set point in the hypothalamus. Within hours, body temperature reaches the new set point, and fever occurs. During the period of upward temperature readjustment, the patient experiences chills, caused by peripheral vasoconstriction and muscle rigidity to maintain homeostasis.[6]

An increase in body temperature may be idiopathic or caused by a variety of mechanisms, including those associated with infectious and other pathologic processes, systemic response to certain drugs, and vigorous activity.

Most febrile episodes are caused by microbial infections (e.g., due to viruses, bacteria, fungi, yeasts, protozoa). No basis has been found for differentiating viral from bacterial infections according to the magnitude of the fever or temperature reduction with antipyretic drug therapy. Fever is often less pronounced in older patients; consequently, infection may not be recognized easily, or early, in this age group if fever is the primary assessment criterion.[9]

Noninfectious pathologic causes of increases in temperature include malignancies, tissue damage (e.g., myocardial infarction, surgery), antigen–antibody reactions, dehydration, heat stroke, CNS inflammation, and metabolic disorders such as hyperthyroidism or gout. Many of these processes may cause hyperthermia, rather than fever, because they interfere with the hypothalamic regulation of temperature.

Drug fever is simply defined as a febrile response to the administration of a medication. Its incidence in ambulatory settings is unknown but among hospitalized patients is approximately 10%[10]

TABLE 6–1 Selected Medications That Induce Hyperthermia

Anti-infectives	Antineoplastics	Cardiovascular	CNS Agents	Other Agents
Aminoglycosides	Bleomycin	Epinephrine	Amphetamines	Allopurinol
Amphotericin B	Chlorambucil	Hydralazine	Barbiturates	Atropine
Cephalosporins	Cytarabine	Methyldopa	Benztropine	Azathioprine
Clindamycin	Daunorubicin	Nifedipine	Carbamazepine	Cimetidine
Chloramphenicol	Hydroxyurea	Procainamide	Haloperidol	Corticosteroids
Imipenem	L-Asparaginase	Quinidine	Lithium	Folate
Isoniazid	6-Mercaptopurine	Streptokinase	MAOIs	Inhaled anesthetics
Linezolid	Procarbazine		Nomifensine	Interferon
Macrolides	Streptozocin		Phenytoin	Iodides
Mebendazole			Phenothiazines	Metoclopramide
Nitrofurantoin			SNRIs	Propylthiouracil
Para-aminosalicylic acid			SSRIs	Prostaglandin E_2
Penicillins			Sumatriptan	Salicylates
Rifampin			Trifluoperazine	Tolmetin
Streptomycin			Thioridazine	
Sulfonamides			TCAs	
Tetracyclines			Topiramate	
Vancomycin			Zonisamide	

Key: CNS = Central nervous system; MAOIs = monoamine oxidase inhibitors; SNRIs = serotonin-norepinephrine reuptake inhibitors; SSRIs = selective serotonin reuptake inhibitors; TCAs = tricyclic antidepressants.

Source: References 5, 10, and 12.

(Table 6–1). With drug-induced fever, temperatures usually range from 98.9°F (37.2°C, oral) to as high as 109.0°F (42.8°C, oral). Drug fever should be suspected in patients without an obvious source of fever; however, this condition often goes unrecognized because of inconsistent signs and symptoms. Failure to discontinue the offending drug may result in substantial morbidity and death.[11,12]

Drug fever may be differentiated from other potentially causative disorders by establishing a temporal relationship between the fever and the administration of a medication, as well as by observing a temperature elevation despite clinical improvement with respect to the underlying disorder.

The management of drug fever involves discontinuing all medications temporarily, if feasible, in addition to the suspected medication whenever possible. If the hyperthermia is drug induced, the patient's temperature generally will decrease within 24–72 hours after the offending agent is withdrawn. After the patient's safety has been considered and the offending medication has been identified and discontinued, each medication may be restarted, one at a time, while monitoring for fever recurrence.[12]

Clinical Presentation of Fever

Because clinical manifestations of fever are nonspecific and do not occur in all patients, the specific cause of a fever may be difficult to determine. The most important indicator of fever is an elevated temperature; therefore, accurate temperature measurement is paramount. Fever is symptomatic of a larger underlying process, whether the process is an infection, due to abnormal metabolism, or drug induced.

Once the presence of fever is established, investigation into the underlying cause is important. Signs and symptoms that typically accompany fever and cause a great deal of discomfort include headache, diaphoresis, generalized malaise, chills, tachycardia, arthralgia, myalgia, irritability, and anorexia. Most children will tolerate a fever well, so if they continue to be alert, play normally, and stay hydrated, the fever is not of great concern. However, high body temperature dulls intellectual function and causes disorientation and delirium, especially in persons with preexisting dementia, cerebral arteriosclerosis, or alcoholism.

Detection of Fever

Subjective assessment of fever typically involves placing a hand on the patient's body, such as on the forehead, to detect warmth. Although this method may identify an increase in skin temperature, it does not accurately detect a rise in core temperature. The most accurate method of assessing for fever is to use a thermometer properly to measure body temperature. The patient's age and level of physical and emotional stress, the environmental temperature, the time of day, and the anatomical site at which the temperature is measured are important considerations in that each factor can affect the results of temperature measurement.

Core temperature is estimated using various types of thermometers at the rectal, axillary, oral, temporal, or tympanic sites. Rectal temperature has long been considered the gold standard measurement; however, its utility has been challenged.[13] Many patients and caregivers prefer other methods of temperature measurement because of comfort and ease of use. Body temperature should be measured with the same thermometer at the same site over the course of an illness, because the readings from different thermometers or sites may vary (Table 6–2). Discrepancy among the various sites of temperature measurement is normal and should not be ascribed to improper measurement technique. On average, a rectal temperature greater than 100.4°F (38.0°C), an oral temperature greater than 99.7°F (37.6°C), an axillary temperature greater than 99.3°F (37.4°C), a tympanic temperature greater than 100.0°F (37.8°C), or a temporal measurement greater than 100.1°F (37.8°C) is considered elevated.[14] The observed variation in temperatures at the different sites is in accord with a simple concept of temperature measurement familiar to the general public: Add 1 degree to an oral temperature to get a rectal or tympanic equivalent, and subtract 1 degree from an oral temperature for an axillary measurement. Normal body temperature may differ by 1.8°F–2.5°F (1.0°C–1.4°C) from these norms. Diurnal rhythms cause body temperature to vary during the day, with higher temperatures typically occurring in the late afternoon to early evening.

Because the U.S. Food and Drug Administration (FDA) regulates thermometers as medical devices, all approved types of thermometers are accurate and reliable, if used appropriately. Today's providers should not recommend mercury-in-glass thermometers for use because of environmental concerns about mercury. Federal and state authorities have lobbied for a ban on mercury thermometers, and 13 states have passed laws that prohibit the manufacture, sale, and distribution of mercury-containing thermometers. In addition, the National Institute of Standards and Technology in conjunction with the Environmental Protection Agency will no longer provide any calibration services for mercury-containing thermometers.[15,16]

TABLE 6–2 Body Temperature Range Based on Site of Measurement

Site of Measurement	Normal Range[a]	Fever[a]
Rectal	97.9°F–100.4°F (36.6°C–38.0°C)	>100.4°F (38.0°C)
Oral	95.9°F–99.5°F (35.5°C–37.5°C)	>99.5°F (37.5°C)
Axillary	94.5°F–99.3°F (34.7°C–37.4°C)	>99.3°F (37.4°C)
Tympanic	96.3°F–100.0°F (35.7°C–37.8°C)	>100.0°F (37.8°C)
Temporal	97.9°F–100.1°F (36.6°C–37.8°C)	*0–2 months of age:* >100.7°F (38.1°C) *3–47 months of age:* >100.3°F (37.9°C) *>4 years of age:* >100.1°F (37.8°C)

[a] Conversion formulas: Celsius = 5/9(°F – 32); Fahrenheit = (9/5 × °C) + 32.

Source: References 14 and 18.

Electronic probe thermometers are available for oral, rectal, and axillary temperature measurements. The probes have an electronic transducer that provides a temperature reading in approximately 10–60 seconds. The oral electronic probes are mostly available as either a pen or a pacifier. The pacifier-shaped electronic thermometer is for oral use only and is useful in infants who are unable to hold a probe under the tongue. The amount of time the pacifier needs to stay in the child's mouth varies depending on the manufacturer, but the time can range from 3 to 8 minutes.[17,18] The pen-shaped probe may be used in the oral, rectal, or axillary area. Because of their electronic digital temperature displays, electronic thermometers provide quick readings, eliminate the possibility of glass breakage, and are easier to read than traditional glass thermometers. The use of disposable probe covers with electronic thermometers also reduces the need for disinfection after their use. Disinfection should still occur if the thermometer is being used for multiple patients. A thermometer that is used rectally should not be used subsequently for oral measurement.

Infrared thermometers are available for tympanic artery and temporal artery temperature measurements. These thermometers use infrared technology to detect heat from the arterial blood supply. They must be placed directly over the line of a blood supply, whether near the temporal artery or the tympanic membrane. Infrared thermometers give a temperature reading in less than 5 seconds and are considered very accurate if used properly. The major problem with infrared thermometers is that the device may not always be placed appropriately, or it may have a dirty lens and consequently may give inaccurate readings. Infrared thermometers are relatively expensive and require batteries, but many families with young children prefer them because of their convenience and noninvasive nature. New technology also includes no-touch infrared thermometers, which offer the advantage of not having to wake a sleeping child to take a temperature.[18,19]

Color-change thermometers are easy to use, but they are not sufficiently accurate or reliable. With these thermometers, an adhesive strip containing heat-sensitive material changes color in response to different temperature gradients. The strip may be placed anywhere on the skin, preferably the forehead, which shows less variation in temperature than other parts of the body. Although this method may detect changes in skin temperature, it does not reliably detect changes in core temperature.

Patient-related factors may preclude the use of a particular type of thermometer. Although a variety of routes for temperature measurement are practicable, rectal temperature measurement historically has been the standard, because the site is not influenced by ambient temperatures, and because this route is appropriate for use in patients of various ages.[14] Oral, tympanic, axillary, and temporal routes are all satisfactory for temperature measurement if the proper procedure is followed.

Table 6–3 describes the proper methods of taking *rectal* temperatures in children and adults. Although the rectal route gives the closest estimate of stable core temperature, its intrusive nature can be very frightening and possibly psychologically harmful to older children. In children younger than 3 months, however, rectal temperature measurement is the preferred method of estimating fever and should be recommended if caregivers are confident they can safely use this route.[18] Risks associated with taking a rectal temperature include retention of the thermometer, rectal or intestinal perforation, and peritonitis. Rectal temperature measurement is also very time consuming, and the patient should never be left unattended while the rectal thermometer remains in place; a positional change may cause the thermometer to be expelled or broken. Rectal temperature measurement is relatively contraindicated in

TABLE 6–3 Guidelines for Rectal Temperature Measurement Using Electronic Thermometers

1. Cover the tip of thermometer with a probe cover.
2. Turn on the thermometer and wait until the device indicates it is ready for use.
3. Apply a water-soluble lubricant to tip of thermometer to allow for easy passage through the anal sphincter and to reduce risk of trauma.
4. For infants or young children, place child face down over your lap, separate the buttocks with the thumb and forefinger of one hand, and insert the thermometer gently in the direction of the child's umbilicus with the other hand. For infants, insert the thermometer to the length of the tip. For young children, insert it about 1 inch into the rectum.
5. For adults, have the patient lie on one side with the legs flexed to approximately a 45-degree angle from the abdomen. Insert the tip 0.5–2 inches into the rectum by holding the thermometer 0.5–2 inches away from the tip and inserting it until the finger touches the anus. Have the patient take a deep breath during this process to facilitate proper positioning of the thermometer.
6. Hold the thermometer in place until it beeps and a temperature is displayed.
7. Remove the thermometer.
8. Dispose of probe cover and clean thermometer with an antiseptic such as alcohol or a povidone/iodine solution by wiping away from the stem toward tip. Rinse with cool water.
9. Wipe away any remaining lubricant from the anus.

patients who are neutropenic, have had recent rectal surgery or injury, or have a pathologic process involving the rectum (e.g., obstructive hemorrhoids, diarrhea). In addition, rectal temperature measurement is slow to detect rapid changes in body temperature because of the large muscle mass and poor blood flow in the area.[14,18,20]

Table 6–4 describes the proper methods of *oral* temperature measurement using electronic thermometers.[18] Oral temperature should not be obtained in a patient who is mouth breathing or hyperventilating; has recently had oral surgery; is not fully alert; or is uncooperative, lethargic, or confused. Oral digital probe thermometers may not be appropriate for use in most children younger than 3 years owing to the difficulty of maintaining a tight seal around the thermometer and keeping the thermometer under the tongue. Accordingly, in these younger children, use of a pacifier thermometer may be recommended. Pacifier thermometers provide reliable temperature readings compared with rectal measurements; however, in children younger than 3 months, pacifier thermometers are less accurate.[21,22]

Table 6–5 describes the proper method of using *tympanic* thermometers, which varies slightly with the age of the patient.[18] Tympanic thermometers have digital readouts, and many can be set to provide either a rectal or an oral temperature equivalent. The tympanic membrane is close to the hypothalamus, and the blood supply to both anatomical areas is at the same temperature, providing an accurate reading of the core body temperature. The thermometer must be positioned in the ear canal properly to ensure the measured infrared radiation is from the tympanic membrane and not from the ear canal or adjacent areas. In clinical trials, accuracy of tympanic thermometers has varied compared with rectal and oral routes.[23,24] Variations in temperature assessment have been attributed to cerumen impaction, inflammation in the ear canal (e.g., otitis media), age of the patient (and corresponding size of the ear canal), and inappropriate technique.[18] Use of tympanic thermometers is not recommended in infants younger than 6 months:

TABLE 6–4 Guidelines for Oral Temperature Measurement Using Electronic Thermometers

Digital Probe

1. Wait 20–30 minutes after drinking or eating.
2. Place a clean disposable probe cover over tip of thermometer.
3. Turn on the thermometer and wait until it is ready for use.
4. Place tip of thermometer under tongue.
5. Close mouth and breathe through nose.
6. Hold thermometer in place until it beeps and temperature has been recorded (usually after 5–30 seconds).
7. Remove the thermometer from mouth and record the displayed temperature.
8. Remove and dispose of probe cover.

Digital Pacifier Thermometer

1. Wait 30 minutes after drinking or eating.
2. Inspect the pacifier for any tears or cracks. Do not use if worn.
3. Press the button to turn on thermometer.
4. Place the pacifier in child's mouth.
5. Have the child hold pacifier in mouth without moving, if possible, for time specified on packaging of thermometer (2–6 minutes).
6. Remove thermometer after the beep and record temperature.

Source: References 17 and 18.

TABLE 6–5 Guidelines for Tympanic Temperature Measurement

1. Place a clean disposable lens cover over ear probe.
2. Turn on thermometer and wait until it is ready for use.
3. For children *younger than 1 year,* pull ear backward to straighten ear canal. Place ear probe into canal, and aim the tip of the probe toward patient's eye.
4. For patients *older than 1 year,* pull ear backward and up to straighten ear canal. Place the ear probe into canal, and aim the tip of probe toward patient's eye.
5. Press the button for temperature measurement, (which usually appears after only 1–5 seconds).
6. Read and record temperature.
7. Discard lens cover.

Source: Reference 18.

their ear canals are not developed fully, leading to inappropriate technique and inaccurate readings. Although not as reliable as the rectal method in children, if used correctly, tympanic thermometry has been found to be more accurate than axillary or oral thermometry in estimating core temperature.[20]

Temporal touch thermometers are placed on the side of the forehead directly over the temporal artery and moved across the forehead (Table 6–6). The temporal artery is directly supplied by the hypothalamus and is near the surface of the skin at the side of the head, permitting surface measurement using infrared technology. The temporal thermometer is capable of providing a reading in a few seconds. The rapid, noninvasive nature of this method makes temporal touch a preferable route of temperature measurement for most patients, and the temporal thermometer is significantly more sensitive than the tympanic thermometer for detecting fever in infants.[25] Of note, however, temporal temperature measurement still has not shown superiority or greater reliability compared with the rectal method.[21] Temporal temperatures may differ from rectal temperatures by ±2.3°F (1.3°C).[22,23] The presence of hair near the temporal area may confound the temperature reading, so hair must be pushed away before a reading is obtained.

No-touch infrared thermometers do not require contact with the body for measurement. Temperature is measured by aiming the thermometer at the center of the patient's forehead. Certain models may also allow use of alternative sites such as the navel and neck, although readings at these sites are less accurate.[18] Although no-touch infrared thermometers are convenient and less invasive, a study of children 1 month to 4 years of age treated in the emergency department found no-touch infrared thermometers to be less accurate and reliable than rectal measurement.[26]

Axillary temperature measurement is frequently used by caregivers and in ambulatory settings, because it is relatively noninvasive. However, axillary measurement performed with digital thermometers (Table 6–7) is not as reliable for detecting fever compared with the oral and rectal methods.[27,28] Reported large variations in temperatures taken by the axillary method are attributable to inappropriate placement of the thermometer, movement of the arm during measurement leading to a poor seal around the thermometer, and insufficient duration of the measurement period. Axillary temperature should not be taken directly after vigorous activity or bathing because both can affect body temperature temporarily without altering the thermoregulatory set point at the hypothalamus. If a fever is detected with the axillary method, a confirmation reading using another method is recommended.

TABLE 6–6 Guidelines for Temporal Artery Temperature Measurement

1. Allow thermometer to acclimatize to the environment for about 30 minutes, if the thermometer was moved from a hot room to a cold room or vice versa.
2. Place probe on one side of forehead (near temporal area).
3. Depress button and hold while scanning for the temporal artery temperature.
4. Sweep thermometer across forehead to the hairline on the opposite side of the head. Ensure that probe remains in contact with skin at all times, and hold button down until finished scanning.
5. If there is sweat on the forehead, sweep the thermometer as normal, but nestle the thermometer on the neck directly behind the ear lobe before releasing the button.
6. Lift thermometer, release the button, and document the recorded temperature.

Source: References 18 and 19.

TABLE 6–7 Guidelines for Axillary Temperature Measurement Using Electronic Thermometer

1. Place a clean disposable probe cover over tip of thermometer.
2. Turn on thermometer and wait until it is ready for use.
3. Place tip of thermometer in armpit. Ensure that armpit is clean and dry. Thermometer must be touching skin, not clothing.
4. If taking a child's temperature, hold child close to secure the thermometer within child's armpit, if necessary.
5. Read and record temperature when thermometer beeps.

Source: Reference 18.

Complications of Fever

The presence of fever is a cause of great concern among caregivers, although in most cases fever may be self-limiting, and serious complications are rare. In one study, 73% of caregivers were "very concerned" about the potential complications of fever, and 88% were "very concerned" when a child's fever was not reduced by antipyretics. There is less concern about complications of fever now than 20 years ago; however, interviewed caregivers still list seizures (32%), brain damage (15%), and death (16%) as the main complications of fever.[29] Overall, the major risks of fever are rare but may include acute complications such as seizures, dehydration, and change in mental status.

Febrile seizure is defined as a seizure accompanied by fever in infants or children who do not have an intracranial infection, a metabolic disturbance, or an otherwise defined cause.[30] Febrile seizures occur in 2%–5% of all children from the ages of 6 months to 5 years, with peak occurrence in those 18–24 months of age. Risk factors for a first febrile seizure include daycare attendance, developmental delay, a family history of febrile seizure, and a neonatal hospital stay longer than 30 days. The severity of the fever and the rate of temperature increase also appear to be critical determinants in the precipitation of a first febrile seizure.[31] The most common seizures associated with fever are simple febrile seizures, which are characterized by nonfocal movements, generally less than 15 minutes in duration, with only one episode in a 24-hour period. Significant neurologic sequelae (e.g., impaired intellectual development, epilepsy) are unlikely after a single pediatric febrile seizure. The risk of recurrence is increased in children who have had multiple febrile seizures, are younger than 1 year at the time of their first seizure, and have a family history of epilepsy. Antipyretics are generally recommended to make the child more comfortable, although they do not reduce the risk of recurrent febrile seizures.[30,32,33] Prophylaxis against simple febrile seizures with antiepileptic or antipyretic drugs is not recommended by the American Academy of Pediatrics.[30]

Serious detrimental effects (e.g., dehydration, delirium, seizures, coma, irreversible neurologic or muscle damage) occur more often in patients with hyperpyrexia (temperatures >106.0°F [41.1°C], oral), which is usually associated with hyperthermia and not fever. Because of the homeostatic mechanisms of the hypothalamus, a core temperature exceeding 106.0°F (41.1°C, oral) in a febrile person is rare. However, even lower body temperature elevations may be life-threatening in patients with heart disease and pulmonary dysfunction. Increased risk of complications is recognized in infants and patients with brain tumors or hemorrhage, CNS infections, preexisting neurologic damage, and a decreased ability to dissipate heat attributed to lower tolerance of elevated body temperature. Older patients are at a higher risk for fever-related complications because of their decreased thirst perception and ability to perspire.[6,34]

Treatment of Fever

Fever is an indicator of an underlying process. Treatment should focus on the primary cause, rather than on the temperature reading. No correlation exists between the magnitude and pattern of temperature elevation (i.e., persistent, intermittent, recurrent, prolonged) and the principal etiologic disorder or severity of the disease. Consequently, determining the cause of the fever on the sole basis of the temperature reading is difficult. The decision to treat fever is based on a patient-specific risk–benefit ratio and the desire to improve comfort.[35] Fever is not associated with many harmful effects unless the temperature exceeds 106.0°F (41.1°C, oral); most fevers are of short duration and may actually have beneficial effects on host defense mechanisms (e.g., antigen recognition, T-helper lymphocyte function, leukocyte motility). Certain microbes are thermolabile, and their growth may be impaired by higher-than-normal temperatures. Accordingly, overtreatment of fever for viral and bacterial infections may be detrimental.[35] Other arguments against treatment include the generally benign and self-limited course of fever, the delayed identification of the diagnosis, and the untoward effects of antipyretic medications.[36]

Treatment Goals

The major goal of self-treatment is to alleviate the discomfort of fever, rather than treating to achieve a specific temperature.[35,37]

General Treatment Approach

Treatment of fever using antipyretics (see Chapter 5, Tables 5–2 and 5–3) is most often indicated for patients with elevated temperatures who also have discomfort. Fever associated with discomfort may be treated with antipyretic agents as well as nonpharmacologic measures.

Self-care measures, including antipyretics, are appropriate initial therapy, unless a patient has exclusions for self-treatment (Figure 6–1). In addition, parents should be urged to call the child's pediatrician immediately or seek urgent medical care if the child has a history of seizure; is unable to stay hydrated; develops a rash; has a rectal temperature of 104.0°F (40.0°C) or higher or its equivalent; or is very sleepy, irritable, or difficult to wake. Children younger than 3 months should be referred for medical evaluation if rectal temperatures reach 100.4°F (38.0°C) or higher, or the equivalent. Children younger than 3 months have immature immune systems and are prone to more serious bacterial infections. In all cases, self-care measures should be started while medical evaluation is being sought.[35,37,38]

Nonpharmacologic Therapy

Nonpharmacologic therapy consists mainly of adequate fluid intake to prevent dehydration. Sponging or baths have limited utility in the management of fever. Body sponging with tepid water may facilitate heat dissipation, in that only a small temperature gradient between the body and the sponging medium is necessary to achieve an effective antipyretic response. However, sponging is not routinely recommended for patients with a temperature less than 104.0°F (40°C, oral); sponging is usually uncomfortable and often induces shivering, which could raise body temperature further. Bathing with ice water or sponging with hydroalcoholic solutions (e.g., isopropyl or ethyl alcohol) is uncomfortable, dangerous, and not recommended. Alcohol poisoning can result from cutaneous absorption or inhalation of topically applied alcohol solutions. Infants and children are at a higher risk of alcohol poisoning because of their smaller body mass. Unlike acetaminophen and nonsteroidal anti-inflammatory drugs (NSAIDs), sponging does not reduce the hypothalamic set point; therefore, implementation of this measure should follow oral antipyretic therapy by 1 hour to permit the appropriate reduction of the hypothalamic set point and a more sustained temperature-lowering response.[39]

Other nonpharmacologic interventions, regardless of the temperature, include wearing lightweight clothing, removing blankets, maintaining a comfortable room temperature of approximately 68.0°F (20.0°C), and drinking sufficient fluid to replenish insensible losses. Because a fever will cause a child to lose fluids more rapidly, sufficient fluid intake is recommended. Fluid intake in fever should be increased by at least 30–60 mL (1–2 ounces) of fluids per hour in children and by at least 60–120 mL (3–4 ounces) of fluids per hour in adults, unless fluids are contraindicated. Sports drinks, fruit juice, water, balanced electrolyte replacement products, or ice pops may be offered. Caution should be exercised in recommending fruit juice and sports drinks to patients with diarrhea; drinks with high sugar loads may worsen concurrent diarrhea.

Pharmacologic Therapy

Antipyretics inhibit PGE_2 synthesis, which decreases the feedback between the thermoregulatory neurons and the hypothalamus, thereby reducing the hypothalamic set point during fever. All antipyretics decrease the production of PGE_2 by inhibiting the cyclooxygenase (COX) enzyme. NSAIDs and aspirin inhibit the COX enzyme in both the peripheral and central nervous systems (CNS) whereas acetaminophen mainly inhibits the COX enzyme in the CNS.[40] Chapter 5 provides an in-depth discussion of the pharmacokinetics, dosing, adverse effect profile, interactions, contraindications, and precautions for nonprescription antipyretic agents.

Acetaminophen typically effects a maximum temperature reduction at 2 hours at usual recommended dosing of 10–15 mg/kg every 4–6 hours, with a maximum of 5 doses/day (see Chapter 5, Tables 5–2 and 5–3). Approximately 80% of children will experience a reduction in their fever with this regimen.[35] Adult dosing ranges from 325 mg to 1000 mg every 4–6 hours, up to a maximum of 4000 mg/day. Some providers have recommended loading doses of acetaminophen for the reduction of fever at 30 mg/kg per dose, after a small study found a faster (one-half hour) and more significant (0.9°F [0.5°C]) decrease than that achieved with a traditional dose.[41] This practice is not recommended, however, because of the lack of any follow-up evidence of benefit, as well as the size and limitations of the study.

Acetaminophen is also available in rectal suppository form. Although a suppository may be an advantage for parents and

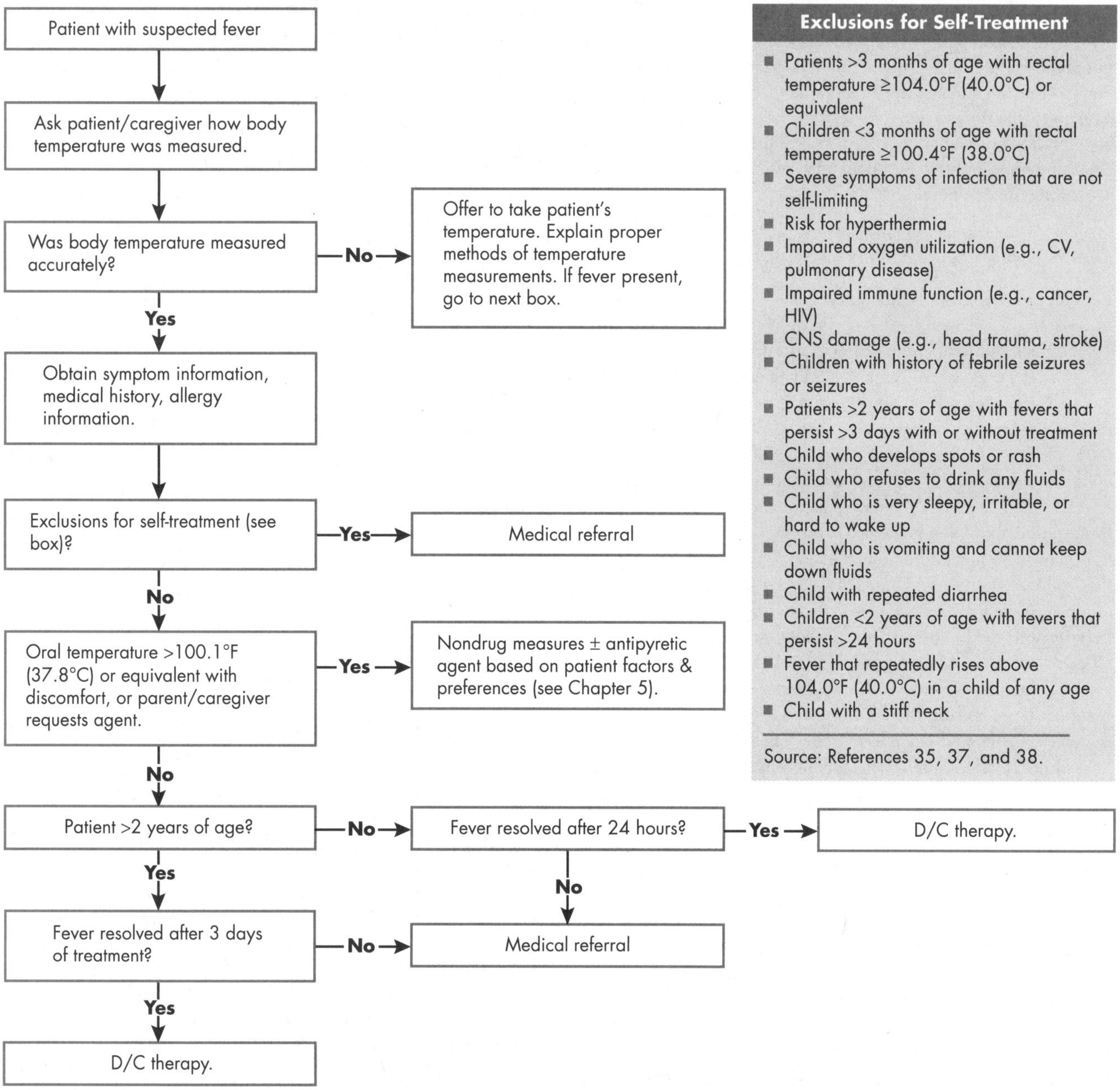

FIGURE **6–1** Self-care for fever. Key: CNS = Central nervous system; CV = cardiovascular; D/C = discontinue; HIV = human immunodeficiency virus.

caregivers who have problems giving their children oral medications, or for children who are vomiting or are having a febrile seizure, absorption with this dosage form is erratic, and studies on its antipyretic activity are conflicting.[42]

Ibuprofen is the most common NSAID used as an antipyretic; maximum temperature reduction typically is achieved at 2 hours at the recommended dosing of 5–10 mg/kg per dose every 6–8 hours, with a maximum of 4 doses per day (see Chapter 5, Tables 5–2 and 5–3). Of note, ibuprofen is approved for the reduction of fever only in patients older than 6 months. Adult dosing ranges from 200 to 400 mg every 4–6 hours, up to a maximum of 1200 mg/day.

Although NSAIDs and acetaminophen are safe and effective when used at low doses for short-duration therapy, they should not be used for more than 3 days to treat fever without medical referral for further evaluation to determine the underlying cause. Common medication errors associated with use of nonprescription antipyretics include overdosing or duplicating therapy, attributed to using multiple products with similar ingredients, and inappropriate dosing for pediatric patients, attributed to mathematical errors in calculating a weight-based dose. A study of dosing by parents demonstrated that 51% of the pediatric patients received an inaccurate dose of medication (62% for acetaminophen and 26% for ibuprofen).[43] Because of these alarming statistics, HCPs should demonstrate to patients and caregivers proper dosing and measurement of the medications with the measuring device provided. In addition, patients should be educated on the appropriate dosing interval and the avoidance of combining antipyretics with cold and cough products containing either acetaminophen or ibuprofen.

Furthermore, owing to safety concerns, FDA issued a guidance statement to companies that manufacture, market, or distribute nonprescription liquid medications regarding the dispensing devices that accompany the drug products. Specifically, FDA recommends that dosage delivery devices such as cups and syringes be included with all nonprescription liquid medications, have clear and appropriate calibrated units, and be used only with the accompanying medication.[44]

Pharmacotherapeutic Comparison

Both ibuprofen and acetaminophen are more effective than placebo in reducing fever, with both showing reductions of approximately 1–2 degrees within 30 minutes to 1 hour. Clinical trials comparing the antipyretic effects of ibuprofen and acetaminophen in recommended dosages have produced variable results, making conclusions on superiority of one or the other agent difficult. A review of the findings in 14 clinical trials comparing ibuprofen and acetaminophen in febrile children found that ibuprofen was slightly more effective than acetaminophen in reducing fever after a single dose; furthermore, ibuprofen was found to be more effective after 6 hours, thus showing a longer duration of action.[45] The same review found that multiple-dose studies failed to show any statistically significant clinical difference. The risk of serious adverse effects did not differ between the medications. The investigators concluded that the efficacy and safety of acetaminophen and of ibuprofen are similar in recommended dosages, with slightly more benefit for ibuprofen in time to onset and duration of action and fever reduction; however, more conclusive findings are needed. A meta-analysis of data for both children and adults also concluded that ibuprofen was more efficacious than acetaminophen in the reduction of fever in both adults and children and both were equally safe.[46] Although ibuprofen has been studied most frequently, other NSAIDs (e.g., naproxen, aspirin) may also be appropriate as antipyretics in adults.

Alternating different antipyretics in the same regimen has become a widespread practice. A survey of 256 caregivers showed that 67% alternated acetaminophen and ibuprofen, and 81% stated their primary care provider or pediatrician advised them to do so. Although alternating the antipyretics was recommended, only 61% of caregivers received any type of written instructions on how to dose the medications, and the dosing intervals varied, ranging from 2 to 6 hours.[47] Despite those practices and clinical trials showing lower temperatures at 4 or more hours with combination therapy, the American Academy of Pediatrics does not recommend alternating antipyretics because of the risk of overdose, medication errors resulting from the complexity of the regimens, and an increased rate of adverse effects.[35,43] In addition, only one study actually showed less stress and time missed from day care with alternating therapy.[48] HCPs should be prepared to provide counseling on the practical application of this mode of treatment if the patient or caregiver has been instructed to use an alternating-drug regimen by a primary care provider. For example, caregivers should be encouraged to write down the generic name, dose, and time of administration for each medication, to minimize the likelihood of duplicate dosing and adverse effects.

The use of antipyretics immediately after vaccine administration is a widespread practice meant to reduce anticipated discomfort and fever. Recently, two open-label randomized trials found the administration of acetaminophen was effective in reducing febrile episodes, but it also significantly reduced the antibody response to several vaccines, although all levels achieved were still considered protective. The clinical significance of these antibody reductions is still unknown; nevertheless, prophylactic antipyretics either before or immediately after vaccine administration should be discouraged. Symptomatic postvaccination reactions may still be treated with antipyretics until additional data indicate otherwise.[49]

Product Selection Guidelines

Age is an important consideration in the selection of an antipyretic, particularly for neonates. Parents and caregivers of children younger than 3 months of age should seek medical evaluation at rectal temperatures or equivalent of 100.4°F (38.0°C) or higher. Children older than 3 months with a rectal temperature or equivalent of 104.0°F (40.0°C) or higher should also be referred. Ibuprofen should be used only in children older than 6 months; because of the risk of Reye's syndrome, children and teenagers who have or are recovering from chickenpox or influenza-like symptoms should not use aspirin or aspirin-containing products.[50] (See Chapter 5 for a complete discussion of these products.) Special populations of patients, such as pregnant women and older adults, may require additional consideration in assessing fever and referring their care. Specifically, as previously stated, fever may be blunted in older patients, thereby predisposing them to a greater risk of complications if a more serious underlying disorder goes unrecognized. Also, pregnant women or patients with uncontrolled high blood pressure, heart failure, renal failure, or an allergy to aspirin should avoid use of the NSAIDs ibuprofen and naproxen sodium or aspirin-containing products. A detailed description of additional criteria for the appropriate use of antipyretic agents is available in Chapter 5, specifically in pediatric and geriatric populations, pregnant and breastfeeding women, and men and women of reproductive capability.

The choice of an antipyretic depends on the patient. Both acetaminophen and ibuprofen are available in a variety of dosage forms and flavors for both children and adults, including tablets, chewable tablets, suspensions, and even suppositories. Selection of a dosage form can be left to patient preference. Consideration of palatability and the taste of the different ibuprofen and acetaminophen suspensions may improve outcomes and adherence to antipyretic regimens in children. (See Chapter 11, section "Special Populations," for FDA requirements for dispensing devices included in liquid nonprescription products.) The dosing frequency of ibuprofen at once every 6–8 hours versus acetaminophen at once every 4–6 hours may also improve adherence and can be considered in product selection, especially in children who have difficulty taking medicine.

Complementary Therapies

Currently, insufficient evidence exists to recommend any dietary supplement or other complementary therapy to treat fever.

Assessment of Fever: A Case-Based Approach

The first step in assessing a patient with symptoms of fever is to obtain an objective temperature measurement to confirm its presence and rule out subjective or inaccurate temperature measurement. If fever is present, assessment of its severity, the seriousness of the underlying cause, and other associated symptoms is indicated. Children who are capable of providing and understanding information should be included in any dialogue concerning their care.

Cases 6–1 and 6–2 are examples of the assessment of two different patients presenting with fever.

CASE 6–1

Relevant Evaluation Criteria	Scenario/Model Outcome
Collect	
1. Gather essential information about the patient's symptoms and medical history, including	
a. Description of symptom(s) (i.e., nature, onset, duration, severity, associated symptoms)	Jessica Smith came home after school and told her mother she was not feeling well. Her mother noticed Jessica was more tired than usual and did not have much of an appetite. Jessica's mother states that before today, Jessica was feeling healthy and well.
b. Description of any factors that seem to precipitate, exacerbate, and/or relieve the patient's symptom(s)	Jessica's mom noticed that Jessica's forehead was warm. When she took Jessica's temperature with an oral thermometer, it was 102.1°F.
c. Description of the patient's/caregiver's efforts to relieve the symptoms	Neither Jessica nor her mother had tried anything to treat her fever up to this point.
d. Patient's identity	Jessica Smith
e. Patient's age, gender, height, and weight	11 years, female, 4 ft 9 in., 82 lb
f. Patient's occupation	Jessica attends fifth grade.
g. Patient's dietary habits	Normal diet
h. Patient's sleep habits	Normal sleep patterns
i. Concurrent medical conditions, prescription and nonprescription medications, and dietary supplements	No medical conditions Flintstones Multivitamin once daily
j. Allergies	NKDA
k. History of other adverse reactions to medications	None
l. Other (describe) ______	Jessica also complains of a dull headache that just started this morning. You retake her temperature in the pharmacy using a temporal thermometer, which reads 102.4°F.
Assess	
2. Differentiate the patient's signs/symptoms, and correctly identify the patient's primary problem(s).	Jessica is experiencing symptoms associated with a fever. When asked, she denies noticing any additional signs or symptoms of a more serious illness that would warrant immediate medical condition.
3. Identify exclusions for self-treatment (Figure 6–1).	None
4. Formulate a comprehensive list of therapeutic alternatives for the primary problem to determine whether triage to a health care provider is required, and share this information with the patient/caregivers.	Options include (1) Refer Jessica for immediate medical attention. (2) Monitor her symptoms and fever, and recommend nondrug measures only. (3) Recommend a medication alone or in combination with nondrug measures. (4) Take no action.
Plan	
5. Select an optimal therapeutic alternative to address the patient's problem, taking into account patient preferences.	Jessica has a fever and is experiencing some discomfort. She has no exclusions for self-care at this time (Figure 6–1), so treatment with either acetaminophen or ibuprofen is appropriate. Drug therapy should be used in conjunction with nondrug measures. She should not receive any aspirin-containing medications.
6. Describe the recommended therapeutic approach to the patient/caregivers.	See Table 5–2 in Chapter 5 for recommended doses of acetaminophen or ibuprofen. "If fever persists >72 hours with or without treatment, Jessica should be seen by a health care provider."
7. Explain to the caregivers the rationale for selecting the recommended therapeutic approach from the considered therapeutic alternatives.	"Jessica has a fever that is causing some discomfort, so minimizing the fever with an antipyretic medication, either acetaminophen or ibuprofen, should help. Her pediatrician should be contacted if her fever gets worse or persists >72 hours or if she complains of other symptoms or signs, such as a stiff neck, severe headache or sore throat, severe ear pain, an unexplained rash, or repeated vomiting or diarrhea."

CASE 6-1 *continued*

Relevant Evaluation Criteria	Scenario/Model Outcome
Implement	
8. When recommending self-care with nonprescription medications and/or nondrug therapy, convey accurate information to the patient/caregivers.	
a. Appropriate dose and frequency of administration	"You can give Jessica acetaminophen chewable tablets (160 mg per tablet) or liquid (160 mg/5 mL). Give 3 chewable tablets or 3 teaspoonsful (15 mL) (480 mg) every 4–6 hours while symptoms last. Do not exceed 5 doses per 24 hours."
b. Maximum number of days the therapy should be employed	"Do not give Jessica the medication for more than 3 days."
c. Product administration procedures	"If taking the chewable tablet, Jessica should chew it completely followed by drinking a full glass of water. If she is taking the liquid, measure the dose using the appropriate dosing syringe or cup provided with the medication, and have Jessica swallow the liquid."
d. Expected time to onset of relief	"A reduction in fever is usually seen within ½–1 hour. Maximum reduction is usually seen within 2 hours."
e. Degree of relief that can be reasonably expected	"A 1- or 2-degree reduction in temperature is expected, but complete resolution of symptoms may vary, depending on the underlying cause of the fever."
f. Most common adverse effects	"Adverse effects are rare, but gastrointestinal effects such as upset stomach or rash are possible. Jessica can take the medication with food if an upset stomach occurs."
g. Adverse effects that warrant medical intervention, should they occur	"Contact a health care provider if signs of an allergic reaction, such as a rash or trouble breathing, occur after a dose is given."
h. Patient's options in the event that condition worsens or persists	"Contact a health care provider in 72 hours if the fever persists or if symptoms worsen."
i. Product storage requirements	"Keep medication in a tightly secured container away from any extreme temperatures and out of reach of children."
j. Specific nondrug measures	"Maintain room temperature at 68°F. Maintain adequate fluid intake and dress her in lightweight clothing."
Solicit follow-up questions from patient/caregivers.	"I read on my 'Mom's Club' Facebook page that I should alternate giving Jessica ibuprofen with acetaminophen. Should I treat Jessica's fever with both drugs?"
Answer patient's/caregivers' questions.	"You should not. Alternating ibuprofen and acetaminophen has not been shown to be more beneficial than using either medication by itself. In fact, there is an increased risk of medication errors and adverse effects if they are used together."
Follow-up: Monitor and Evaluate	
9. Assess patient outcome.	Contact Jessica's mother in 1–2 days to see if Jessica's fever is responding.

Key: NKDA = No known drug allergies.

CASE 6–2

Relevant Evaluation Criteria	Scenario/Model Outcome
Collect	
1. Gather essential information about the patient's symptoms and medical history, including	
a. Description of symptom(s) (i.e., nature, onset, duration, severity, associated symptoms)	Mr. Jones approaches the pharmacy counter looking for a medication to treat his child's fever. He says his son, Jack, has not been sleeping well at night and has not been eating. When taking Jack's temperature rectally for the past 5 days, he had a temperature of 101.4, 101.6, 102.1, 101.7, and 101.5°F.
b. Description of any factors that seem to precipitate, exacerbate, and/or relieve the patient's symptom(s)	Jack's father states lukewarm baths seem to temporarily soothe Jack; however, this has not helped to bring down Jack's temperature.
c. Description of the patient's/caregiver's efforts to relieve the symptoms	Mr. Jones has given Jack 5 mL (1 teaspoonful) of Children's Tylenol liquid (160 mg/5 mL) every 6 hours.
d. Patient's identity	Jack Jones
e. Patient's age, gender, height, and weight	2 years, male, 34 in., 28 lb
f. Patient's occupation	n/a
g. Patient's dietary habits	3 meals a day with 2–3 snacks in between, soy milk
h. Patient's sleep habits	Usually sleeps at least 8–9 hours every night, but during the last few nights, he has been getting only 4–5 hours of sleep and takes 30-minute naps during the day.
i. Concurrent medical conditions, prescription and nonprescription medications, and dietary supplements	Seasonal allergies in the spring
j. Allergies	NKDA
k. History of other adverse reactions to medications	None reported
l. Other (describe) _______	n/a
Assess	
2. Differentiate the patient's signs and symptoms, and correctly identify the patient's primary problem(s).	Jack has a fever that is concerning because of its duration despite treatment.
3. Identify exclusions for self-treatment (Figure 6–1).	Fever lasting for more than 72 hours
4. Formulate a comprehensive list of therapeutic alternatives for the primary problem to determine whether triage to a health care provider is required, and share this information with the patient/caregivers.	Options include (1) Refer Jack to his pediatrician. (2) Refer Jack to a hospital emergency department for immediate medical attention. (3) Monitor his symptoms and fever, and recommend nondrug measures only. (4) Recommend a medication alone or in combination with nondrug measures. (5) Take no action.
Plan	
5. Select an optimal therapeutic alternative to address the patient's problem, taking into account patient preferences.	Jack has an exclusion for self-care in his persistent fever lasting more than 72 hours. Jack's father should contact his pediatrician immediately to rule out any serious conditions.
6. Describe the recommended therapeutic approach to the patient/caregivers.	"No medication recommended at this time. Immediate medical referral is indicated."
7. Explain to the patient/caregivers the rationale for selecting the recommended therapeutic approach from the considered therapeutic alternatives.	"Jack has a fever that has persisted longer than 72 hours even after treatment with appropriate medication."

CASE 6-2 *continued*

Relevant Evaluation Criteria	Scenario/Model Outcome
Implement	
8. When recommending self-care with nonprescription medications and/or nondrug therapy, convey accurate information to the patient/caregivers.	
a. Appropriate dose and frequency of administration	None recommended
b. Patient's options in the event that condition worsens or persists	"If fever worsens or does not improve, you should take Jack to a hospital emergency department after speaking with the pediatrician."
c. Specific nondrug measures	"Maintain room temperature at 68.0°F, and dress him in lightweight clothing."
Solicit follow-up questions from patient/caregivers.	"Can I try giving Jack ibuprofen (Advil) liquid and acetaminophen (Tylenol) liquid at alternating times until I can get him to his pediatrician?"
Answer patient's/caregivers' questions.	"Alternating between acetaminophen and ibuprofen has not been proven to help children feel better faster, and it may increase risk of adverse effects. I am concerned Jack may require additional treatment that is not available over the counter. Please call your pediatrician immediately."
Follow-up: Monitor and Evaluate	
9. Assess patient outcome.	Contact Jack's father in 1–2 days to ensure that he sought medical care for Jack.

Key: n/a = Not applicable; NKDA = no known drug allergies.

Patient Counseling for Fever

Although fever is a common symptom, it often is misunderstood and poorly treated. Studies suggest that fever is incorrectly considered a disease associated with detrimental consequences rather than a symptom, is frequently treated inappropriately, and is evaluated improperly.[51] Many parents and caregivers have "fever phobia" that results in heightened anxiety regarding effects of fever and consequent inappropriate treatment.[29] HCPs can improve patient outcomes by educating patients and caregivers about fever and by teaching self-assessment skills (e.g., the proper methods for measuring body temperature using the variety of thermometers available, as well as proper interpretation of the results). If patients and caregivers are still using mercury-in-glass thermometers, they should be urged to dispose of them according to local environmental standards. HCPs should also explain the appropriate nonpharmacologic and pharmacologic treatments for fever and identify indications for seeking further medical care. Discussions of pharmacologic treatments should highlight methods for safe use of antipyretics and the current evidence available for complementary therapies. The box "Patient Education for Fever" provides specific information to give the patient.

Evaluation of Patient Outcomes for Fever

The primary monitoring parameters for febrile patients are temperature and discomfort. In one study, 32% of caregivers stated they would check a febrile patient's temperature at least every hour.[29] Overaggressive monitoring may result from "fever phobia." Because fever may actually be of physiologic benefit, the ultimate goal of antipyretic therapy is not to normalize temperature but rather to improve overall comfort and well-being.[35] The presence of any associated symptoms (e.g., headache, diaphoresis, generalized malaise, chills, tachycardia, arthralgia, myalgia, irritability, anorexia) should also be monitored daily. Although most patients demonstrate a reduction in temperature after each individual dose of an antipyretic, pharmacologic therapy for fever may take up to 1 day to result in a decrease in temperature. If clinical improvement is not seen or if symptoms are worsening over the course of 3 days of self-treatment, regardless of a drop in temperature, an HCP should be consulted by either phone or appointment for further evaluation.[38] Timeliness of patient follow-up assessment with appropriate medical care is important in identifying a non–self-limiting underlying cause.

Key Points for Fever

- Fever is self-limiting and rarely poses severe consequences unless the core temperature is greater than 106.0°F (41.1°C, oral).
- The main treatment goals for fever are to alleviate the associated discomfort and to eliminate the underlying cause.
- Fever should be confirmed only by means of a thermometer, which is an FDA-regulated medical device.
- Patients should be educated on the proper measurement techniques for the selected thermometry method.
- Patients should be referred for further evaluation if the rectal temperature or its equivalent is greater than 104.0°F (40.0°C), they have a history of febrile seizures, they have comorbid conditions compromising their health, or they are younger than 3 months of age with an oral temperature exceeding 100.4°F (38.0°C) or the equivalent.

PATIENT EDUCATION FOR Fever

The primary objectives of treating fever are (1) to relieve the discomfort of fever and (2) to prevent complications associated with fever. For most patients, carefully following product instructions and the self-care measures listed here will help to ensure optimal therapeutic outcomes.

Temperature Measurement

- Do not rely on feeling the body to detect fever. Take a temperature reading with an appropriate thermometer.
- For children up to 3 months of age, the rectal method of temperature measurement is preferred (Table 6–3). Use of a tympanic thermometer is not recommended in children younger than 6 months because of the size and shape of the infant's ear canal.
- For children ages 6 months to 3 years, the rectal, oral, tympanic, or temporal method may be used if proper technique is followed (Tables 6–3 through 6–6).
- For individuals older than 3 years, the oral, tympanic, or temporal method is appropriate (Tables 6–4 through 6–6).

Nondrug Measures

- Do not use isopropyl or ethyl alcohol for body sponging. Alcohol poisoning can result from skin absorption or inhalation of topically applied alcohol solutions.
- For all levels of fever, wear lightweight clothing, remove blankets, and maintain room temperature at 68°F.
- Unless advised otherwise, drink or provide sufficient fluids to replenish body fluid losses. For children, increase fluids by at least 1–2 ounces per hour; for adults, increase fluids by at least 2–4 ounces per hour. Sports drinks, fruit juice, a balanced electrolyte formulation, and water all are acceptable.

Nonprescription Medications

- Nonprescription analgesics and antipyretics (see Chapter 5, Tables 5–2 and 5–3) help in alleviating discomfort associated with fever and reducing the temperature, respectively.
- Nonprescription analgesics and antipyretics typically take 30 minutes to 1 hour to begin to decrease discomfort and lower body temperature.
- Monitor level of discomfort and body temperature using the same thermometer at the same body site 2 or 3 times per day during a febrile illness.
- Use single-entity nonprescription analgesics and antipyretics at low doses for up to 3 days for treatment of fever (see Chapter 5, Tables 5–2 and 5–3 for dosages), unless you have exclusions for self-care (Figure 6–1).
- Avoid alternating antipyretics because of the complexity of the dosing regimens, increased risk of medication errors, and adverse effects.
- Dosing of either ibuprofen or acetaminophen in children should be based on body weight, not age.
- To avoid incorrect dosing, use the measuring device such as a syringe, dosing spoon, or medicine cup when administering liquid medication that was provided with the medication.
- If you are pregnant or have uncontrolled high blood pressure, congestive heart failure, renal failure, or an allergy to aspirin, avoid use of nonsteroidal anti-inflammatory drugs (ibuprofen and naproxen sodium) or aspirin-containing products.
- To avoid the possible risk of Reye's syndrome, do not use aspirin or aspirin-containing products for fever in children and teenagers who have or are recovering from chickenpox or influenza-like symptoms.

When to Seek Medical Attention

- Seek medical attention if fever or discomfort persists or worsens after 3 days of drug treatment.

- ➤ Sponge baths using topical isopropyl or ethyl alcohol to reduce fever should be discouraged.
- ➤ Referral for further medical evaluation is appropriate to detect an underlying cause if self-treatment for 3 days does not successfully reduce fever in a patient older than 2 years and for at least 24 hours in a child younger than 2 years of age.
- ➤ HCPs should counsel patients on the proper use of nonprescription antipyretic agents (including appropriate use of measuring devices), to limit medication errors and adverse effects. For patients who have been instructed to alternate antipyretic therapies by an HCP, counseling should emphasize the importance of recording the generic name of each drug given, the dose, and the time of administration, to avoid any adverse effects.

REFERENCES

1. Cohee L, Crocetti MT, Serwint JR, et al. Ethnic differences in parental perceptions and management of childhood fever. *Clin Pediatr.* 2010;49(3): 221–7. doi: 10.1177/0009922809336209.
2. Niska R, Bhuiya F, Xu J. *National Hospital Ambulatory Medical Care Survey: 2011 Emergency Department Summary Tables.* Available at: http://www.cdc.gov/nchs/data/ahcd/nhamcs_emergency/2011_ed_web_tables.pdf. Accessed January 19, 2017.
3. Centers for Disease Control and Prevention. *Ambulatory Health Care Data.* Available at: http://www.cdc.gov/nchs/data/ahcd/namcs_summary/2012_namcs_web_tables.pdf. Accessed January 19, 2017.
4. Rehm KP. Fever in infants and children. *Curr Opin Pediatr.* 2001;13(1): 83–8. PMID: 11216593.
5. Halloran LL, Bernard DW. Management of drug-induced hyperthermia. *Curr Opin Pediatr.* 2004;16(2):211–5. PMID: 15021205.
6. Dinarello CA, Porat R. Fever. In: Kasper D, Fauci A, Hauser S, et al., eds. *Harrison's Principles of Internal Medicine,* 19th ed. New York, NY: McGraw-Hill; 2015. Available at: http://accesspharmacy.mhmedical.com/content.aspx?bookid=1130&Sectionid=79724479. Accessed January 19, 2017.
7. Bartfai T, Conti B. Fever [serial online]. *Sci World J.* 2010;10:490–503. doi: 10.1100/tsw.2010.50. Available at http://www.ncbi.nlm.nih.gov/pmc/articles/PMC2850202/pdf/nihms188784.pdf. Accessed January 19, 2017.
8. Barrett KE, Barman SM, Boitano S, Brooks HL. Hypothalamic regulation of hormonal functions. In: Barrett KE, Barman SM, Boitano S, Brooks HL, eds. *Ganong's Review of Medical Physiology.* 24th ed. New York: McGraw-Hill; 2012. Available at: http://accesspharmacy.mhmedical.com/Content.aspx?bookId=393&sectionId=39736759. Accessed January 19, 2017.
9. Norman DC. Fever in the elderly. *Clin Infect Dis.* 2000;31(1):148–51. PMID: 10913413.
10. Musselman ME, Saely S. Diagnosis and treatment of drug-induced hyperthermia. *Am J Health-Syst Pharm.* 2013;70(1):34–42. doi: 10.2146/ajhp110543.
11. DiPiro JT. Allergic and pseudoallergic drug reactions. In: Talbert RL, DiPiro JT, Matzke GR, et al., eds. *Pharmacotherapy: A Pathophysiologic Approach.* 8th ed. New York: McGraw-Hill; 2011. Available at: http://access pharmacy.mhmedical.com/Content.aspx?bookId=462&sectionId=41100876. Accessed January 19, 2017.
12. Cuddy, ML. The effects of drugs on thermoregulation. *ACCN Clin Issues.* 2004;15(2):238–53. PMID: 15461041.
13. Schuh S, Komar L, Stephens D, et al. Comparison of the temporal artery and rectal thermometry in children in the emergency department. *Pediatr Emerg Care.* 2004;20(11):736–41.

14. El-Radhi AS, Barry W. Thermometry in paediatric practice. *Arch Dis Child.* 2006;91(4):351–6. PMCID: PMC2065972.
15. U.S. Environmental Protection Agency. Mercury thermometers. Available at http://www.epa.gov/mercury/mercury-thermometers. Accessed January 19, 2017.
16. Health Care Without Harm. Laws and Resolutions. Available at: https://noharm-uscanada.org/issues/us-canada/laws-and-resolutions. Accessed January 19, 2017.
17. Kaz Inc. Vicks digital pacifier thermometer Model V925P product manual. Available at: http://www.kaz.com/kaz/thermometers/products/vicks-digital-pacifier-thermometer-v925p-a. Accessed January 19, 2017.
18. Thermometer comparison. *Pharm Lett Prescrib Lett.* 2010;26.
19. Exergen Corporation. Exergen temporal artery thermometer instructions for use. Available at: http://www.exergen.com//medical/PDFs/tat2000instrev7.pdf. Accessed January 19, 2017.
20. Robinson JL, Seal RF, Spady DW, et al. Comparison of esophageal, rectal, axillary, bladder, tympanic, and pulmonary artery temperatures in children. *J Pediatr.* 1998;133(4):553–6. PMID: 9787697.
21. Braun CA. Accuracy of a pacifier thermometer in young children. *Pediatr Nurs.* 2006;32(5):413–8. PMID: 17100072.
22. Callanan D. Detecting fever in young infants: reliability of perceived, pacifier, and temporal artery temperatures in infants younger than 3 months of age. *Pediatr Emerg Care.* 2003;19(4):240–3. PMID: 12972820.
23. Paes BF, Vermeulen K, Brohet RM, et al. Accuracy of tympanic and infrared skin thermometers in children [serial online]. *Arch Dis Child.* 2010;95(12):974–8. doi: 10.1136/adc.2010.185801.
24. Craig JV, Lancaster GA, Taylor S, et al. Infrared ear thermometry compared with rectal thermometry in children: a systematic review. *Lancet.* 2002;360(9333):603–9. PMID: 12241932.
25. Greenes DS, Fleisher GR. Accuracy of a noninvasive temporal artery thermometer for use in infants. *Arch Pediatr Adolesc Med.* 2001;155(3):376–81. PMID: 11231805.
26. Fortuna EL, Carney MM, Macy M, et al. Accuracy of non-contact infrared thermometry versus rectal thermometry in young children evaluated in the emergency department for fever. *J Emerg Nurs.* 2010;36(2):101–4. PMID: 20211398.
27. Stine CA, Flook DM, Vincze DL. Rectal versus axillary temperatures: Is there a significant difference in infants less than 1 year of age? *J Pediatr Nurs.* 2012;27(3):265–70. doi: 10.1016/j.pedn.2011.04.004.
28. Klein M, DeWitt TG. Reliability of parent-measured axillary temperatures. *Clin Pediatr.* 2010;49(3):271–3. doi: 10.1177/0009922809350215.
29. Poirier MP, Collins EP, McGuire E. Fever phobia: a survey of caregivers of children seen in a pediatric emergency department. *Clin Pediatr.* 2010;49(6):530–4. doi: 10.1177/0009922809355312.
30. Steering Committee on Quality Improvement and Management, Subcommittee on Febrile Seizures. Febrile seizures: clinical practice guidelines for the long-term management of the child with simple febrile seizures. *Pediatrics.* 2008;121(6):1281–6. PMID: 18519501.
31. Millar JS. Evaluation and treatment of the child with febrile seizure. *Am Fam Physician.* 2006;73(10):1761–4. PMID: 16734052.
32. Strengell T, Uhari M, Tarkka R, et al. Antipyretic agents for preventing recurrences of febrile seizures. *Arch Pediatr Adolesc Med.* 2009;163(9):799–804. doi: 10.1001/archpediatrics.2009.137.
33. Lux AL. Treatment of febrile seizures: historical perspective, current opinions, and potential future directions. *Brain Dev.* 2010;32(1):42–50. PMID: 19854599.
34. High KP, Bradley SF, Gravenstein S, et al. Clinical practice guideline for the evaluation of fever and infection in older adult residents of long-term care facilities: 2008 update by the Infectious Diseases Society of America. *J Am Geriatr Soc.* 2009;57(3):375–94. PMID: 19072244.
35. Section on Clinical Pharmacology and Therapeutics, Committee on Drugs, Sullivan JE, Farra HC. Fever and antipyretic use in children. *Pediatrics.* 2011;127(3):580–7. PMID: 21357332.
36. Mackowiak PA. Concepts of fever. *Arch Intern Med.* 1998;158(17):1870–81. PMID: 9759682.
37. Avner JR. Acute fever. *Pediatr Rev.* 2009;30(1):5–13. PMID: 19118137.
38. American Academy of Pediatrics. When to call the pediatrician: fever. Available at: http://www.healthychildren.org/English/health-issues/conditions/fever/pages/When-to-Call-the-Pediatrician.aspx. Accessed January 19, 2017.
39. Axelrod P. External cooling in the management of fever. *Clin Infect Dis.* 2000;31(Suppl 5):S224–9. PMID: 11113027.
40. Aronoff DM, Neilson EG. Antipyretics: mechanisms of action and clinical use in fever suppression. *Am J Med.* 2001;111(4):304–15. PMID: 11566461.
41. Treluyer JM, Tonnelier S, d'Athis P, et al. Antipyretic efficacy of an initial 30-mg/kg loading dose of acetaminophen versus a 15-mg/kg maintenance dose. *Pediatrics.* 2001 Oct;108(4):E73. PMID: 11581481.
42. Goldstein LE, Berlin M, Berkovitch M, et al. Effectiveness of oral vs. rectal acetaminophen. *Arch Pediatr Adolesc Med.* 2008;162(11):1042–6. doi: 10.1001/archpedi.162.11.1042.
43. Li SF, Lacher B, Crain EF. Acetaminophen and ibuprofen dosing by parents. *Pediatr Emerg Care.* 2000;16(6):394–7. PMID: 11138879.
44. U.S. Department of Health and Human Services, Food and Drug Administration and Center for Drug Evaluation and Research. *Guidance for Industry: Dosage Delivery Devices for Orally Ingested OTC Liquid Drug Products.* May 2011. Available at: http://www.fda.gov/downloads/Drugs/GuidanceComplianceRegulatoryInformation/Guidances/UCM188992.pdf. Accessed January 19, 2017.
45. Goldman RD, Ko K, Linett LJ, et al. Antipyretic efficacy and safety of ibuprofen and acetaminophen in children. *Ann Pharmacother.* 2004;38(1):146–50. PMID: 14742809.
46. Pierce CA, Voss B. Efficacy and safety of ibuprofen and acetaminophen in children and adults: a meta-analysis and qualitative review. *Ann Pharmacother.* 2010;44(3):489–506. doi: 10.1345/aph.1M332.
47. Wright AD, Liebelt EL. Alternating antipyretics for fever reduction in children: an unfounded practice passed down to parents from pediatricians. *Clin Pediatr.* 2007;46(2):146–50. PMID: 17325087.
48. Sarrell EM, Wielunsky E, Cohen HA. Antipyretic treatment in young children with fever. *Arch Pediatr Adolesc Med.* 2006;160(2):197–202. PMID: 16461878.
49. Prymula R, Siegrist CA, Chlibek R, et al. Effect of prophylactic paracetamol administration at time of vaccination on febrile reactions and antibody response in children: two open-label, randomized controlled trials. *Lancet.* 2009;374(9698):1339–50. doi: 10.1016/S0140-6736(09)61208-3.
50. U.S. Food and Drug Administration. Labeling of drug preparations containing salicylates. *CFR: Code of Federal Regulations.* Title 21, Part 201, Section 201.314. Updated July 27, 2017. Available at: http://www.ecfr.gov/cgi-bin/text-idx?SID=b1b2224711dc88657752be21f12c574a&mc=true&node=se21.4.201_1314&rgn=div8. Accessed July 31, 2017.
51. Lagerlov P, Helseth S, Holager T. Childhood illnesses and the use of paracetamol: a qualitative study of parents' management of common childhood illnesses. *Fam Pract.* 2003;20(6):717–23. PMID: 14701898.

CHAPTER 7

MUSCULOSKELETAL INJURIES AND DISORDERS

JULIE L. OLENAK

Pain is one of the most common reasons for visits to health care providers (HCPs). Because pain is a common symptom of disease or injury, patients often seek medical attention, although many seek to relieve the pain by self-treating with nonprescription analgesics. In a large number of cases, the pain that prompts efforts at self-treatment arises from the musculoskeletal system. Musculoskeletal pain may be felt in the affected tissue itself or referred from another anatomic source (e.g., hip pain referred from its primary source in the low back).[1]

Musculoskeletal pain arises from the muscles, bones, joints, and connective tissue. The development of musculoskeletal pain can be acute, such as with sports injuries (e.g., tendonitis, sprains, strains), or it can stem from exacerbation of a pathologic condition (e.g., osteoarthritis). *Acute* pain is typically defined as pain lasting less than 4 weeks. Pain lasting at least 3 months is considered *chronic* pain, which may arise from degenerative joint disease, osteoarthritis, or chronic tendonitis (e.g., carpal tunnel syndrome).[1]

The rate of use of nonprescription systemic and topical analgesics remains high, with more than $4.052 billion and $647 million spent, respectively, per year in the United States on such remedies.[2] Providers need to ask appropriate questions to identify the types of pain for which patients are seeking treatment, to achieve a better understanding of the nature of their pain complaints. Providers must also be ready to offer reasonable recommendations for either treatment or further evaluation.

Musculoskeletal complaints result in a significant amount of lost work days, work limitations, loss of employment, and increased utilization of the health care system. These complaints are believed to be the greatest contributors to the economic burden of chronic pain, costing state and federal agencies $100 billion annually. The total annual cost of persistent chronic pain for adults in the United States is estimated to be between $560 billion and $635 billion. More than 100 million adults in the United States battle chronic pain.[3]

Pathophysiology of Musculoskeletal Injuries and Disorders

The musculoskeletal system includes the muscles, tendons, ligaments, cartilage, and bones. Muscles are attached to bones by tendons, and ligaments connect bone to bone. Tendons and ligaments normally have limited ability to stretch and twist. Because of their high tensile strength, tendons and ligaments rarely rupture unless subjected to intense forces. However, they may become damaged when the articulation (joint) is hyperextended or with overuse.

Synovial bursae are fluid-filled sacs located between joint spaces to provide lubrication and cushioning. Cartilage functions as protective pads between bones in joints and in the vertebral column.[4]

Skeletal, or striated, muscle is composed of cells (myocytes) in which two constituents (actin and myosin) are primarily responsible for contraction. Muscle contraction also involves several electrolytes within the muscle tissue, including calcium and potassium. Pain receptors are located in skeletal muscle and the overlying fascia, and those receptors can be stimulated as a result of overuse or injury to the muscle or surrounding structures.[1,4]

Somatic pain occurs when pain impulses are transmitted from peripheral nociceptors to the central nervous system (CNS) by nerve fibers. Common sites of origin are muscles, fascia, and bones. Somatic pain is most commonly myofascial (e.g., with muscle strain) or musculoskeletal (e.g., with arthritis).[1]

Mechanoreceptors and chemoreceptors mediate muscle pain. These nerve endings are heterogeneous: only a single chemical can stimulate some endings, whereas a variety of chemical, mechanical, and thermal triggers can stimulate others.[1,4]

Erythema (redness), edema, and hyperalgesia (an exaggerated pain response to minor amounts of noxious stimuli[3]) at the affected site characterize the inflammatory response. The inflammatory response develops through participation of multiple mediators, including histamine, bradykinin, serotonin, leukotrienes, and prostaglandin E.[1] Muscle injuries can be categorized as delayed-onset muscle soreness (e.g., overexertion), myalgia, strains, tendonitis, bursitis, and sprains. Low back pain and osteoarthritis are common pathologic conditions associated with musculoskeletal complaints.

Overexertion or *repeated unaccustomed eccentric muscle contraction* is associated with delayed-onset (8 hours or more) muscle soreness, which can last for days, usually peaking at 24–48 hours. This pain reflects muscle damage that presumably was initiated by force generated in the muscle fibers; pathophysiologic components are thought to include inflammation, acidosis, muscle spasms, and/or microlesions. Prolonged tonic contraction produced by exercise, tension, or poor posture and by improper body mechanics can also produce muscle pain. Overexertion injury is common among individuals who do not exercise regularly but then begin an exercise regimen at a level of high intensity.

Myalgia, or *muscle pain,* can result from systemic infections (e.g., influenza), chronic disorders (e.g., fibromyalgia, polymyalgia rheumatica), and medications (e.g., some cholesterol-lowering agents such as hydroxymethylglutaryl–coenzyme A [HMG-CoA] reductase inhibitors). Abuse of alcohol may precipitate acute alcoholic myopathy. Bone and muscle pain may also be related to vitamin D deficiency, as in osteomalacia. In these conditions, the pain typically is widespread or bilateral in distribution and is not specifically associated with a recent injury.[1]

Strains are a result of an injury to a muscle or a tendon. A strain can be caused by an acute injury, or with prolonged overuse, the pathoanatomic changes can result in a chronic condition. The movements that cause a strain involve twisting or pulling. Tendons can become strained when their stretch capacity is exceeded (e.g., hyperextension injury involving an arm or a leg). The strain injury is caused by eccentric contraction of the muscle fibers while the muscle itself is lengthening. A tear of the muscle or tendon can also occur.[5]

Tendonitis is the inflammation of a tendon, which results from acute injury or from chronic repetitive movements of a body part. An example of an overuse injury is carpal tunnel syndrome, a condition characterized by tingling or numbness of the first digits of the hand caused by repetitive use of the hand and wrist. Tendon sheaths become inflamed, with consequent constriction of the median nerve as it passes through a narrow channel between the wrist bones.[4] Tendonitis can also commonly occur in the Achilles tendon, which connects the calf muscle to the heel.

Common terms that describe sports-related tendonitis from overuse include tennis elbow, golfer's elbow, swimmer's shoulder, and jumper's knee. In sports-related overuse injuries, potential contributing factors for tendonitis include older age, poor technique, improper conditioning, exercise of prolonged intensity or duration, and poorly designed equipment for specific activities (e.g., inadequately cushioned athletic shoes).

Finally, certain medications (e.g., fluoroquinolone antimicrobials) are associated with the development of tendonitis or tendon rupture. For these medications, the U.S. Food and Drug Administration (FDA) requires the drug label to carry a boxed warning highlighting the risk of such injury.[6]

Bursitis is a common cause of localized pain, tenderness, and swelling, which is worsened by any movement of the structure adjacent to the bursa, in the joint. Bursitis generally results from an acute injury to the joint or over-repetitive joint action. When pain is accompanied by the presence of a puncture site (possibly from intra-articular injection), an adjacent source of infection, or severe inflammation, an infectious cause should be suspected and ruled out before recommending self-treatment.

Sprains are the most common problem with ligaments. Sprains are graded by their characteristics, with grade I sprains resulting from excessive stretching, grade II sprains resulting from a partial tear, and grade III sprains involving a complete tear of the tissue. Grade II and grade III sprains typically result in moderate–severe pain, loss of function of the affected limb, and an inability to bear weight. Tears and ruptures are more common in ligaments than in tendons. Sprains commonly occur during physical activity. Approximately 628,000 sprains occur annually in the United States.[5]

Low back pain is the fifth most likely reason for a physician visit; the lifetime prevalence of developing low back pain approaches 80%. The National Institute of Arthritis and Musculoskeletal and Skin Disease reports that 25% of people report at least 1 day of back pain in a 3-month period.[4,7]

Main risk factors for the development of low back pain include sedentary lifestyle (particularly one disrupted by bursts of activity), poor posture, improper shoes, excessive body weight, poor mattress and sleeping posture, and improper technique for lifting heavy objects. Most patients recover within a few days to a few weeks, even without treatment; pain that persists for more than 3 months is classified as chronic low back pain.[8] Other causes of low back pain include congenital anomalies, osteoarthritis, vertebral fractures and compressions, spinal tuberculosis, and referred pain from diseased kidneys, pancreas, liver, or prostate.[1]

Osteoarthritis is characterized by a gradual softening and destruction of the cartilage between bones. Over time, cartilage and bone are destroyed in the joint spaces and then regenerate, with consequent rearrangement of the synovial architecture. Often referred to as "degenerative joint disease," osteoarthritis is caused by genetic, metabolic, and environmental factors. Heavy physical activity, repetitive movement, and lifting of heavy weights may aggravate this condition, whereas light–moderate activity does not and is generally helpful.[9] Approximately 52 million people older than 18 years of age in the United States have a diagnosis of osteoarthritis; by 2030, that number is expected to increase to 67 million.[10,11]

Clinical Presentation of Musculoskeletal Injuries and Disorders

Table 7–1 lists many of the presenting signs and symptoms of musculoskeletal disorders and other differentiating factors. Pain is a common symptom among all of these disorders.

In addition to the pain induced by a sprain, impairment of joint function of variable degree will be present. If an apparent sprain is associated with noticeably limited joint function, the injury is most likely to be a grade II or grade III sprain that requires proper workup to rule out a fracture or tear. If the affected joint is visibly deformed, emergency medical assistance is warranted.

Patients with carpal tunnel syndrome often describe a diminished ability to feel heat or cold; a sense that the affected hand is swollen, despite the absence of visible change; a weakness in the hand that may affect performance of fine movements (e.g., buttoning a shirt); and a tendency to drop things. Symptoms persist during sleep and even when the hand is not being used, a characteristic that can be used to distinguish this disorder from others.

The pain of osteoarthritis does not correlate directly with the degree of joint damage. Pain is often referred, and proximal muscles can be involved if a person with osteoarthritis guards the affected joint by changing the gait to reduce discomfort. Low back pain can also be neuropathic in nature, involving the sciatic nerve, with sharp referred pain in one or both legs. Low back pain can often limit the patient's ability to bend, move, sit, or walk.

Complications of untreated pain-inducing injuries include further tissue damage and (in advanced arthritis) bone and cartilage remodeling. Pain is associated with significant limitations, including a reduction in ability to perform activities of daily living (ADLs), disability, loss of work time, and physical impairments (e.g., insomnia).

Treatment of Musculoskeletal Injuries and Disorders

Acute pain is the body's alarm system; it signals injury by trauma, disease, muscle spasms, or inflammation. Chronic pain, conversely, may or may not be indicative of injury and requires a primary care provider's assessment before treatment is initiated.

TABLE 7–1 **Comparison of Musculoskeletal Disorders**

Myalgia	Tendonitis	Bursitis	Sprain	Strain	Osteoarthritis
Location					
Muscles of the body	Tendon locations around joint areas	Inflammation of the bursae within joints; common locations include knee, shoulder, big toe	Stretching or tearing of a ligament within a joint	Hyperextension of a joint that results in overstretching or tearing the muscle or tendon	Weight-bearing joints, knees, hips, low back, hands
Signs					
Possible swelling (rare)	Warmth, swelling, erythema	Warmth, edema, erythema, and possible crepitus	Swelling, bruising	Swelling, bruising	Noninflammatory joints, narrowing of joint space, restructuring of bone and cartilage (resulting in joint deformities), possible joint swelling
Symptoms					
Dull, constant ache (sharp pain relatively rare); weakness and fatigue of muscles also common	Mild-severe pain generally occurring after use; loss of range of motion	Constant pain that worsens with movement or application of external pressure over the joint	Initial severe pain followed by pain, particularly with joint use; tenderness; reduction in joint stability and function	Initial severe pain with continued pain upon movement and at rest; muscle weakness; loss of some function	Dull joint pain relieved by rest; joint stiffness <20–30 minutes; localized symptoms to joint; crepitus
Onset					
Varies depending on cause (i.e., trauma = acute, but drug-induced = insidious)	Often gradual, but can develop suddenly	Acute with injury; recurs with precipitant use of joint	Acute with injury	Acute with injury	Insidious development over years
Modifying Factors					
Elimination of cause; use of stretching, rest, heat, topical analgesics, systemic analgesics	Elimination of cause; use of stretching, rest, ice, topical analgesics, systemic analgesics	Joint rest; immobilization; topical analgesics; systemic analgesics	RICE; stretching; use of protective wraps (e.g., ankle tape, knee brace, cane); topical analgesics; systemic analgesics	RICE; stretching; use of protective wraps; topical analgesics; systemic analgesics	Continuous exercise (light–moderate activity); weight loss, heat, analgesic medication; topical pain relievers

Key: RICE = *Rest, ice, compression, elevation* (Table 7–2).
Source: References 1, 4, 5, and 10.

Treatment Goals

Treatment of the patient with musculoskeletal complaints encompasses many different goals, the most important of which are (1) decreasing the subjective intensity (severity) of pain; (2) decreasing the duration of pain, when possible; (3) restoring function of the affected area; (4) preventing reinjury and disability (i.e., improving capacity for ADLs); and (5) preventing acute pain from becoming chronic persistent pain.

General Treatment Approach

Patients with musculoskeletal injuries present with common symptoms (especially pain and swelling of the affected area) and generally can use similar self-treatment approaches. Nonpharmacologic therapy consisting of rest, ice, compression, and elevation (RICE) along with nonprescription oral analgesics and/or topical analgesics during the first 1–3 days after injury is helpful.[5] Before treatment can be recommended, however, careful screening for warning signs and symptoms that preclude self-treatment is essential to ensure that the patient receives appropriate care. The algorithm in Figure 7–1 presents a stepwise approach to self-management of pain for patients who have none of the exclusions for self-care listed in the algorithm.

Management of acute back pain can include the use of nonprescription analgesics (i.e., NSAIDs) and nonpharmacologic treatments, including the use of heat.[12] Topical analgesics may be considered. Patients with subacute or chronic low back pain require medical evaluation before they initiate self-treatment given the length of time symptoms would be present.

Pain associated with osteoarthritis is approved for self-treatment after an initial medical diagnosis. The general treatment

Exclusions for Self-Treatment

- Severe pain (pain score >6)
- Pain that lasts >10 days
- Pain that continues >7 days after treatment with a topical analgesic
- Increased intensity or change in character of pain
- Pelvic or abdominal pain (other than dysmenorrhea)
- Accompanying nausea, vomiting, fever, or other signs of systemic infection or disorder
- Visually deformed joint, abnormal movement, weakness in any limb, numbness, or suspected fracture
- Pregnancy
- <2 years of age (FDA minimum age)[a]
- Back pain and loss of bowel and/or bladder control

[a] Minimum age for use varies with products. Use with caution and for shortest treatment period possible in children ≤18 years of age.
Source: References 5, 7, 24, and 28.

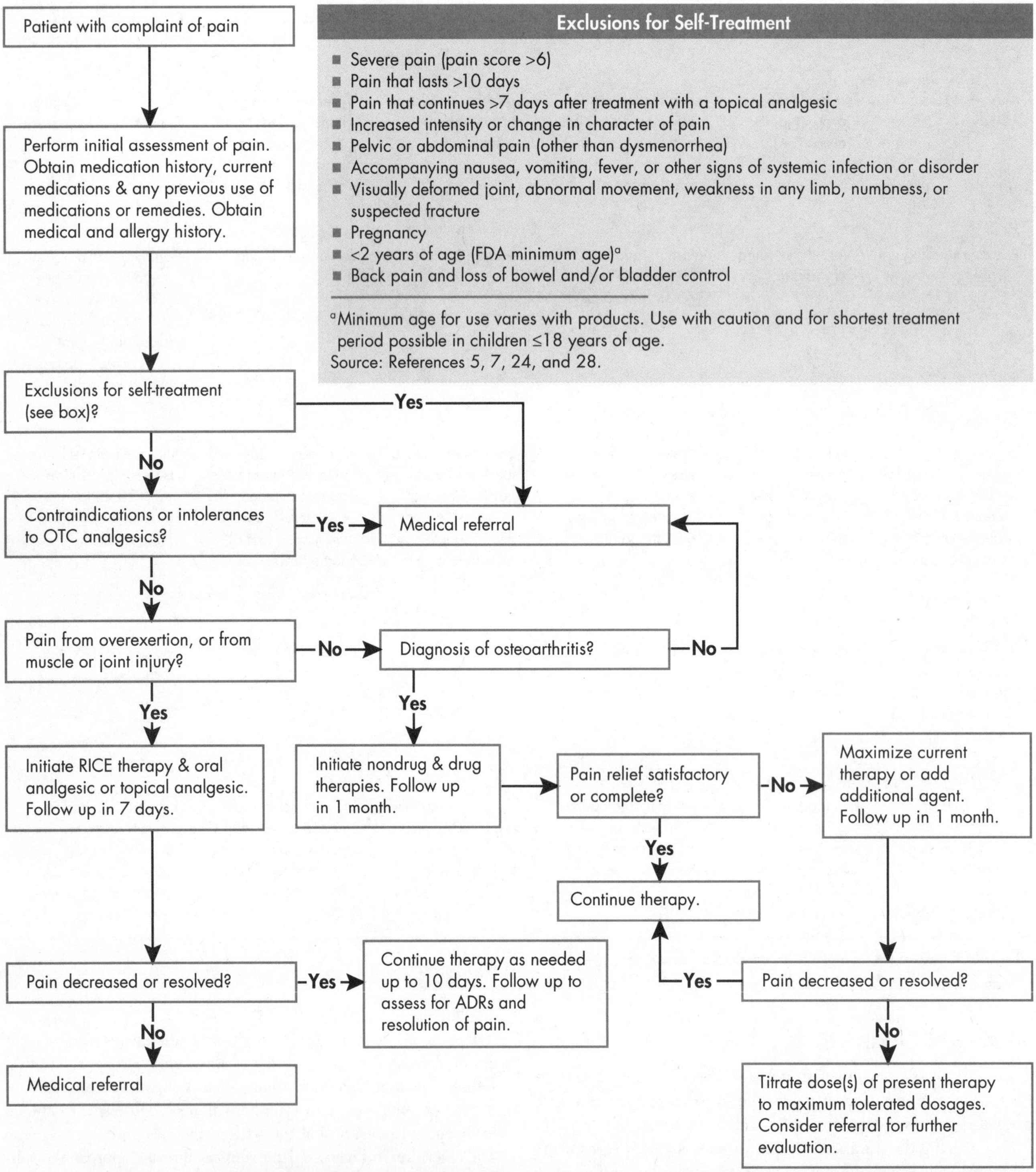

FIGURE 7-1 Self-care for musculoskeletal injuries and disorders. Key: ADR = Adverse drug reaction; FDA = Food and Drug Administration; OTC = over-the-counter; RICE = rest, ice, compression, elevation. (Source: Adapted from Self-care of self-limited pain. In: Albrant DH, ed. *The American Pharmaceutical Association Drug Treatment Protocols.* 2nd ed. Washington, DC: American Pharmaceutical Association; 2001:424–5.)

approach includes appropriate lifestyle changes (incorporating physical activity and weight loss) and use of an analgesic, which may be a nonprescription medication.[9]

Nonpharmacologic Therapy

Injury from playing sports or exercising can be prevented by warming up and stretching muscles before physical activity, ensuring proper hydration, and wearing appropriate footwear. Stretching must be done cautiously—without bouncing—to avoid muscle strain. For muscle cramps, stretching and massaging the affected area followed by immediate rest will loosen the muscle. Appropriate hydration is important, and plain water, sports drinks, or enhanced waters with electrolytes may be used based on patient preference.

RICE therapy promotes healing and helps reduce swelling and inflammation associated with muscle and joint injuries (Table 7–2). Ice should not be applied for more than 15–20 minutes because excessive icing causes considerable vasoconstriction and reduces vascular clearance of inflammatory mediators from the damaged area. Ice therapy can also be recommended for patients with osteoarthritis experiencing pain and/or swelling.[9,13] Both cold and heat, at temperatures outside the skin's threshold for tolerance, can be damaging and can result in blistering or burning; with both types of therapies, therefore, direct application of the medium to the skin is contraindicated.

Heat therapy is an alternative for patients in whom pain of a noninflammatory nature develops and may help with stiffness.

TABLE 7–2 Guidelines for RICE Therapy

- Rest the injured area and continue until pain is reduced (generally 1–2 days). Slings, splints, or crutches can be used if necessary.
- As soon as possible, apply ice to the injured area in 15- to 20-minute increments, at least 3 or 4 times a day. Continue the ice-pack therapy until swelling subsides (usually 1–3 days, depending on the severity of injury).
- Apply compression to the injured area with an elastic support or an elasticized bandage as follows:
  - Choose the appropriate-size bandage for the injured body part. If preferred, a product specifically designed for the injured body part can be purchased.
  - If ice is also being applied to the injured area, soak the bandage in water to aid the transfer of cold.
  - Wrap the injured area by overlapping the previous layer of bandage by approximately one-third to one-half its width.
  - Wrap the point most distal from the injury (e.g., if the ankle is injured, begin wrapping just above the toes).
  - Decrease the tightness of the bandage as you continue to wrap. If the bandage feels tight or uncomfortable, or if circulation is impaired, remove the compression bandage and rewrap it. Cold toes or swollen fingers indicate that the bandage is too tight.
  - After removal, wash the used bandage in lukewarm, soapy water; do not scrub it. Rinse the bandage thoroughly and allow to air dry on a flat surface.
  - Roll up the bandage to prevent wrinkles, and store it in a cool, dry place. Do not iron the bandage to remove wrinkles.
- Elevate the limb or body part with the injured area at or above the level of the heart to decrease swelling and relieve pain.

Key: RICE = *Rest, ice, compression, elevation.*
Source: Reference 5.

It has been studied in the treatment of acute low back pain with favorable effects.[12] In addition, osteoarthritis guidelines recommend heat as adjunct nonpharmacologic therapy.[9,13–16] Although its mechanism of action is not fully understood, heat may alleviate pain by increasing blood flow, reducing muscle spasm, and relieving stiffness. Heat should be applied for 15–20 minutes, 3 or 4 times a day. Heat should not be applied to inflamed areas because it can intensify vasodilation and exacerbate vascular leakage.[17] Furthermore, heat should not be used with topical analgesics or over broken skin.

Heat should be applied to the affected area in the form of a warm wet compress, heating pad, or hot water bottle. Ease of use favors newer, heat-generating adhesive and wrap products (e.g., ThermaCare, Precise, various generic brands), which can be worn on the affected area up to 8 hours (up to 12 hours for some products). The products come in various shapes to accommodate different anatomic areas, including back, hip, neck, knee, wrist and hand, shoulder, elbow, and lower abdomen.

The adhesive products should be applied on dry skin that is free of lotion. In a few exceptions, certain products carry unique directions for use (e.g., ThermaCare menstrual product, BodiHeat), such as placing the adhesive side on the undergarment or clothing.

Heating devices should not be used on areas of skin with decreased sensation, a practice that can lead to a skin burn. Specifically, ThermaCare heat-generating products should not be placed on the back of the knee or inside the bend of the arm.[18]

Although not generally associated with many adverse effects, heat-generating patches can cause skin irritation or even burns. Patients should be advised to remove the patch immediately if they experience any pain or discomfort, itching, or burning. Heat wraps should be worn over a towel or layer of clothing in patients older than 55 years; heat wraps should not be used during sleep.[18]

Limited scientific information is available regarding contrast therapy (alternating heat and ice) to aid in sports injury recovery. Anecdotally, some individuals report relief, but insufficient scientific evidence has accumulated to justify recommendation of this practice.[19,20]

Transcutaneous electrical nerve stimulation (TENS) therapy is used widely by various practitioners (e.g., physicians, physical therapists, chiropractors) in the treatment of pain. FDA has approved TENS therapy for nonprescription use as a class II medical device for the relief of pain associated with sore, aching muscles; joint pain; or chronic intractable pain.[21–23] Pain relief is thought to come from two mechanisms: alteration of pain transmission and an increase in the production of natural endorphins. A TENS device is typically used for an interval of 15–30 minutes up to 3 times daily. The electrode pads can be placed on various areas of the body for pain relief (e.g., back, legs, ankles, arms, shoulders), but placement is product dependent. Because of safety concerns, patients should avoid placing the electrodes on the throat, chest, or head or over the carotid arteries. The electrodes also should not be placed on open wounds, rashes, inflamed skin, cancerous lesions, or areas of skin with altered sensation, or over areas treated with topical analgesics. Patients with internal or attached medical devices (e.g., pacemakers, defibrillators, electrocardiographic monitors, respirators); pregnant patients; and the pediatric population should not use nonprescription TENS devices.[22,23] The directions for proper and safe use of these devices are product specific, so the HCP should review the directions with the patient.

Historically, some patients prefer to use magnesium sulfate (Epsom salt) solution applied to areas of minor sprains and bruises, for a nonpharmacologic treatment for relief of discomfort.

However, scientific evidence to support claims of effectiveness in the general population is lacking. For this self-treatment modality, the magnesium sulfate is dissolved in warm water for soaking the affected part in a bath or for application on wet bandages for an average of 20 minutes.

Heat, massage, acupuncture, and spinal manipulation are nonpharmacologic therapies recommended to treat acute or subacute low back pain. Patients with chronic lower back pain should consider nonpharmacologic recommendations as first-line treatment. Such recommendations include exercise; multidisciplinary rehabilitation; acupuncture; psychological therapies (i.e., mindfulness-based stress reduction, progressive relaxation, cognitive behavioral therapy, electromyography biofeedback, operant therapy); tai chi; yoga; motor control exercise (i.e., focus on strengthening the muscles that support the spine and improving coordination); low-level laser treatments using noninvasive infrared beams as light therapy; or spinal manipulation.[8]

Pharmacologic Therapy

Systemic Analgesics

Acetaminophen, aspirin, and nonaspirin nonsteroidal anti-inflammatory drugs (NSAIDs), such as ibuprofen, naproxen, and magnesium salicylate tetrahydrate, are commonly used nonprescription analgesics; they are often used in the initial treatment of musculoskeletal injuries. Systemic analgesic therapy should be limited to 10 days of self-care use,[24] and patients should seek appropriate medical care if the condition continues beyond this period or worsens during the course of treatment. (See Chapter 5 for dosages, safety, and properties of nonprescription systemic analgesics.)

For the treatment of osteoarthritis of the hip and knee, acetaminophen (rather than NSAIDs) has been recommended historically by some organizations for first-line therapy, despite data suggesting that NSAIDs provide slightly better pain relief.[25] Chronic use of NSAIDs leads to more severe and prevalent adverse effects (e.g., nephropathy, gastrointestinal ulcerations and bleeding, increased risk for cardiac events). The American Association of Orthopedic Surgeons (AAOS) guidelines, alone among similar published directives, state that a recommendation cannot be made specifically for or against acetaminophen, but they include a strong recommendation for oral or topical NSAIDs.[16] Recommendations published by the American College of Rheumatology (ACR), however, include both acetaminophen and NSAIDs among initial therapy options. According to the ACR guidelines, if NSAIDs are used chronically for the management of osteoarthritis, adding a proton pump inhibitor should be considered for gastrointestinal protection. (See Chapter 13 for further information on risks of long-term use of proton pump inhibitors.) The ACR guidelines also express a strong recommendation to consider using topical NSAIDs rather than systemic NSAIDs in patients 75 years of age and older.[9]

The American College of Physicians (ACP) published updated guidelines regarding the management of acute, subacute, and chronic back pain.[8] If a nonprescription medication is recommended by an HCP for the treatment of acute back pain, acetaminophen is no longer considered a first-line therapy. Studies, including a large randomized, placebo-controlled trial, showed no effect on pain and function compared with placebo. If a patient has no contraindication to an NSAID, it should be recommended over acetaminophen. Moderate-quality evidence showed that NSAIDs demonstrated some improvement in pain intensity, and low-quality evidence showed some improvement in function. Additionally, if the patient does not receive adequate relief from NSAIDs or is referred to his or her prescriber, prescription muscle relaxants are also first-line treatment and were shown to be efficacious in acute and subacute lower back pain. A patient with chronic low back pain should consider nonpharmacologic recommendations as first-line treatment. NSAIDs are now considered first-line pharmacologic therapy. Moderate-quality evidence demonstrated some improvement with pain compared with placebo. There was no evidence to evaluate, or recommend, acetaminophen in chronic back pain.[8,12]

Topical Products

Topical analgesics may have local analgesic, anesthetic, antipruritic, and/or counterirritant effects. Nonprescription topical analgesics are approved specifically for the topical treatment of minor–moderate aches and pains of muscles and joints (e.g., simple backache, arthritis pain, strains, bruises, sprains).[26] These agents are recommended as adjuncts to pharmacologic and nonpharmacologic therapy of musculoskeletal injuries and disorders. A topical anesthetic, lidocaine, is now available in a nonprescription cream and patch marketed for nerve pain. Table 7–3 lists examples of commercially available products.

Counterirritants

Topical counterirritants are applied to the skin to relieve pain. Counterirritation is the paradoxical pain-relieving effect achieved by producing a less severe pain to counter a more intense one. The pain relief results more from nerve stimulation than from suppression of the sensation.[26,27] When applied to the skin at pain sites, counterirritants produce a mild, local inflammatory reaction, which provides symptomatic relief at the site underlying the skin surface being treated. These induced sensations distract from the deep-seated pain in muscles, joints, and tendons. Pain is only as intense as it is perceived to be, and the perception of other sensations caused by the counterirritant or its application (e.g., massage, warmth, redness) causes the sufferer to disregard the sensation of pain.[27] On the basis of their topical effects, counterirritants are classified into four groups: rubefacients and those that produce a cooling sensation, cause vasodilation, or incite irritation without rubefaction (Table 7–4).

All regulations and labeling for topical counterirritants are based on the detailed previous proposed rulemaking documents published in the *Federal Register* in 1979 and 1983.[26,28] FDA has recognized the ingredients in Table 7–4 as safe and effective (Category I) counterirritants for use in adults and in children 2 years of age and older.[28] Of note, for many topical nonprescription analgesic products, the lower age limit is older than 2 years.

Labels for most counterirritants indicate that the product is to be used for "the temporary relief of minor–moderate aches and sprains of muscles and joints." In addition, the labeling recommended by most of FDA's review panels includes claims for "simple backache, arthritis pain, strains, bruises, and sprains."[28] In September 2012, FDA issued a Drug Safety Communication about serious burns caused by nonprescription topical counterirritants. Most of the second- and third-degree burn cases were associated with use of topical counterirritant products with higher concentrations of menthol as the single ingredient or with a combination product containing greater than 3% menthol and 10% methyl salicylate. In many of the case reports, the reactions occurred with only one application, and the resulting injury developed within 24 hours. Additionally, some case reports described burns from products containing capsaicin.[29] FDA recommendations for safe use of nonprescription topical analgesic products are presented in

TABLE 7-3 **Selected External Analgesic Products**

Trade Name	Primary Ingredient(s)
Menthol-Containing Products	
Aspercreme Heat Pain Relieving Gel	Menthol 10%
Bengay Ultra Strength Pain Relieving Patch	Menthol 5%
Icy Hot No Mess Applicator	Menthol 16%
Mineral Ice	Menthol 2%
Camphor-Containing Products	
JointFlex Pain Relieving Cream	Camphor 3.1%
Capsaicin-Containing Products	
Capzasin Arthritis Pain Relief No-Mess Applicator	Capsaicin 0.15%
Capzasin-HP Arthritis Pain Relief Cream	Capsaicin 0.1%
Zostrix Hot and Cold Therapy	Capsaicin 0.025%
Zostrix-HP Arthritis Pain Relief Cream	Capsaicin 0.075%
Histamine Dihydrochloride–Containing Products	
Australian Dream Pain Relieving Arthritis Cream	Histamine dihydrochloride 0.025%
Trolamine Salicylate–Containing Products	
Aspercreme Cream/Lotion	Trolamine salicylate 10%
Sportscreme Deep Penetrating Pain Relieving Rub Cream	Trolamine salicylate 10%
Lidocaine-Containing Products	
Aspercreme with Lidocaine Maximum Strength	Lidocaine hydrochloride 4%
Lidocare Patch	Lidocaine 4%
Combination Products	
ActivOn Topical Analgesic Ultra Strength Arthritis	Histamine dihydrochloride 0.025%; menthol 4.127%
Arthritis Hot Cream	Methyl salicylate 15%; menthol 10%
Bengay Ultra Strength Pain Relieving Cream	Methyl salicylate 30%; menthol 10%; camphor 4%
Flexall Ultra Plus Relieving Gel	Menthol 16%; methyl salicylate 10%; camphor 3.1%
Icy Hot Cream Extra Strength/Precise Pain Relieving Cream	Methyl salicylate 30%; menthol 10%
Icy Hot Lidocaine	Lidocaine 4%; menthol 1%
Mentholatum Ointment	Camphor 9%; natural menthol 1.3%
Mentholatum Deep Heating Extra-Strength Pain Relieving Rub Cream	Methyl salicylate 30%; menthol 8%
Salonpas Arthritis Pain Patch	Methyl salicylate 10%; menthol 3%
Salonpas DEEP Relieving Gel	Camphor 3.1%; menthol 10%; methyl salicylate
Salonpas Lidocaine Pain Relieving Gel-Patch	Lidocaine 4%
Sloan's Liniment	Turpentine oil 47%; capsaicin 0.025%
Tiger Balm Arthritis Rub Cream	Camphor 11%; menthol 11%

Table 7–5. A feeling of warmth or coolness is normal with topical counterirritant use, but patients should seek medical attention if burning pain or blistering occurs.[29]

Table 7–4 provides dosing information for the various counterirritants.

Described next are the commonly used counterirritants currently available in the United States.

METHYL SALICYLATE. Methyl salicylate occurs naturally as wintergreen oil or sweet birch oil; gaultheria oil, teaberry oil, and mountain tea are other names for the compound. Methyl salicylate is usually combined with other ingredients (e.g., menthol and/or camphor).

As a rubefacient, methyl salicylate causes vasodilation of cutaneous vasculature, thereby producing reactive hyperemia. This increase in blood pooling and/or flow is hypothesized to be accompanied by an increase in localized skin temperature, which in turn may exert a counterirritant effect. Because of its rubefacient action, methyl salicylate is responsible for the "hot" action in many topical counterirritant products.[27]

TABLE 7–4 Classification and Dosage Guidelines[a] for Nonprescription Counterirritant External Analgesics

Group	Ingredient(s)	Concentration (%)	Mechanism of Action	Frequency and Duration of Use
A	Allyl isothiocyanate Ammonia water Methyl salicylate Turpentine oil	0.5–5.0 1.0–2.5 10–60 6–50	Rubefacients (increase blood flow)	For all counterirritants: Apply no more than 3–4 times/day, as needed, for up to 7 days.
B	Camphor Menthol	3–11 1.25–16.0	Produce cooling sensation	As in group A
C	Histamine dihydrochloride Methyl nicotinate	0.025–0.1 0.25–1.0	Cause vasodilation	As in group A
D	Capsicum Capsicum oleoresin Capsaicin	0.025–0.25 0.025–0.25 0.025–0.25	Incite irritation without rubefaction; are as potent as group A ingredients	*For acute pain:* As in group A *For chronic pain:* Apply 3–4 times/day for duration of pain (often long-term use with medical supervision).

[a] Dosages approved for adults and for children 2 years and older.
Source: Reference 26.

In addition to the mechanisms described previously, topically applied methyl salicylate products inhibit both central and peripheral prostaglandin synthesis. Studies on the rate and extent of percutaneous absorption of various commercially available methyl salicylate preparations show direct tissue penetration rather than redistribution by the systemic blood supply, indicating a localized effect of the topical product.[27]

Localized reactions (e.g., skin irritation, rash) and systemic reactions (e.g., salicylate toxicity) may occur with the use of methyl salicylate. Strong irritation may cause local reactions such as erythema, blistering, neurotoxicity, or thermal hyperalgesia. In addition, heat exposure and exercise after applying methyl salicylate have been associated with a threefold increase in systemic absorption of salicylate, which can lead to increases in adverse systemic reactions.[30] Table 7–5 reviews appropriate precautions to take with use of topical analgesics. Because percutaneous absorption of salicylate can occur, methyl salicylate should be avoided in children and used with caution in individuals who are sensitive to aspirin. Concomitant use of salicylate-containing topical analgesics and maintenance warfarin therapy has been implicated in prolonging prothrombin time.[27] Chapter 5 describes other potential drug interactions related to systemically absorbed salicylates.

The report of the American Association of Poison Control Centers documents 10,000 methyl salicylate exposures in children 6 years of age and younger. In this age group, just a teaspoon of wintergreen oil can cause death.[31] Although an FDA survey found that oral ingestion of methyl salicylate in ointment form caused no deaths and that few cases were associated with severe symptoms, regulations require the use of child-resistant containers for liquid preparations containing concentrations greater than 5%.[26]

CAMPHOR. Although camphor occurs naturally and is obtained from the camphor tree, approximately three-fourths of the camphor used medicinally is prepared synthetically.

In concentrations of 0.1%–3.0%, camphor depresses cutaneous receptors and is used as a topical analgesic, anesthetic, and antipruritic. In concentrations exceeding 3%, particularly when combined with other counterirritant ingredients, camphor stimulates the nerve endings in the skin, thus inducing relief of pain and discomfort by masking moderate–severe deeper visceral pain, with a milder pain arising from the skin at the level of innervation. When applied vigorously, it produces a rubefacient reaction.

Concentrations higher than those recommended are not more effective and can cause more serious adverse reactions if the preparation is accidentally ingested.[28] CNS effects, manifested primarily as tonic–clonic seizures, constitute the major form of toxicity and begin to emerge as early as 10 minutes after ingestion. High doses of camphor can cause nausea, vomiting, colic, headache, dizziness, delirium, convulsion, coma, and death.

Although nonprescription camphor-containing preparations cannot exceed concentrations of 11%, camphor toxicity continues to occur.[32] Parents should be aware of this potential danger, and patient counseling should emphasize use of modalities that do not contain camphor.

MENTHOL. Menthol is either prepared synthetically or extracted from peppermint oil (which contains a 30%–50% concentration of menthol). Menthol may be used safely in small quantities as a flavoring agent and has found wide acceptance in candy,

TABLE 7–5 FDA Recommendations for Application of Nonprescription Topical Analgesic Products

- If pain, swelling, or blistering of the skin occurs after application of a topical analgesic, the patient should immediately discontinue use of the product and seek medical attention.
- Do not bandage the area tightly where the product has been applied.
- Do not use any heat where the product has been applied.
- Do not apply to wounded, damaged, broken, or irritated skin.
- Do not allow these medications to come in contact with the eyes, inside the nose or mouth, or with the genitals.

Key: FDA = U.S. Food and Drug Administration.
Source: Reference 29.

chewing gum, cigarettes, cough drops, toothpaste, nasal sprays, and liqueurs. It is also used as a permeability enhancer to increase absorption of other topically administered medications.[33]

At concentrations less than 1%, menthol depresses cutaneous receptor response (i.e., acts as an anesthetic); at concentrations greater than 1.25%, menthol stimulates cutaneous receptor response (i.e., acts as a counterirritant).

Recent studies have led to the identification of heat- and cold-sensitive receptors within sensory neurons called transient receptor potential (TRP) cation channels. Topically applied menthol activates the TRPM8 menthol receptor, triggering the sensation of cold.[33] The resultant cold sensation travels along pathways similar to the somatic pain sensations from the affected muscle or joint, which distracts from the sensation of pain. The initial feeling of coolness is soon followed by a sensation of warmth.

Menthol is contraindicated in patients with hypersensitivity or sensitization to the agent (e.g., urticaria, erythema, other cutaneous lesions).[33] Treatment should be discontinued if the patient experiences irritation, rash, burning, stinging, swelling, or infection.

METHYL NICOTINATE. Although nicotinic acid is inactive topically, methyl nicotinate readily penetrates the cutaneous barrier. Vasodilation and elevation of skin temperature result from very low concentrations, with higher penetration rates reported for hydrophilic media (i.e., gels). One study showed that indomethacin, ibuprofen, and aspirin significantly depress the skin's vascular response to methyl nicotinate. Because these three drugs suppress prostaglandin biosynthesis, the vasodilator response to methyl nicotinate is thought to be mediated, at least in part, by prostaglandin biosynthesis.[34]

Generalized vascular dilation can occur when methyl nicotinate passes through the skin into the circulatory system. Consequently, persons who apply methyl nicotinate over large areas may experience a drop in blood pressure, a decrease in pulse rate, and syncope caused by the generalized vascular dilation.[34]

CAPSICUM PREPARATIONS. Capsicum preparations—capsaicin, and capsicum oleoresin—are derived from the fruit of various species of pepper plants (in the nightshade family). Capsaicin is the major constituent of hot (chili) peppers. Capsicum oleoresin refers to a concentrated extract, containing capsaicin, which is composed of oil and resin.

When applied to normal skin, capsaicin elicits a transient feeling of warmth through stimulation of the TRPV1 receptor. The mechanism of action is thought to be directly related to capsaicin's effects on the depletion of substance P. This substance is found in slow-conducting, unmyelinated type C neurons that innervate the dermis and epidermis. It is released in the skin in response to endogenous (e.g., stress) and exogenous (e.g., trauma, injury) factors. It appears that pruritic stimuli along with pain impulses are conveyed to central processing centers by type C fibers in the skin, for which capsaicin has selective activity. Local application of capsaicin to the peripheral axon appears to deplete substance P from sensory neurons. The depletion occurs both peripherally and centrally, presumably as the result of impulse initiation. When substance P is released, burning pain occurs, but this effect abates with repeated applications. The diminishing sensation experienced with repeated applications can lead to adherence-related failures; HCPs should inform their patients about such effects and the importance of continuing therapy.[35]

Capsaicin has additional indications beyond those of other counterirritants. Capsaicin is used to reduce the pain—but not the inflammation—of rheumatoid arthritis and osteoarthritis; it is also used in the management of a wide variety of other pain disorders (e.g., postherpetic neuralgia, diabetic neuropathy, back pain).

The optimal dose of capsaicin varies among patients. The efficacy of capsaicin decreases (and local discomfort increases) when capsaicin is applied less often than directed, because the drug's duration of action is 4–6 hours. Pain relief is usually noted within 14 days after therapy has begun, but relief will occasionally be delayed by as much as 4–6 weeks in cases of chronic pain.

Once topical nonprescription capsaicin has begun to relieve pain, its use must continue regularly 3 or 4 times a day, as directed. If capsaicin treatment is stopped and the pain returns, treatment can be resumed. Capsaicin may produce a sensation of burning or stinging pain. As a result of tachyphylaxis, however, this local effect diminishes in intensity with repeated applications, typically within a few days but after as long as 1–2 weeks.[35–37] To reduce the likelihood of capsaicin contact with topically sensitive areas (e.g., mucous membranes), patients should be instructed to use a glove for application and to wash their hands after use.[35] If the hands are the site of application, the patient should wait 30 minutes after application and then wash the hands. During use, capsaicin should not come in contact with the eyes or other sensitive areas of the body, because it will cause a burning sensation.[35] Capsaicin is available in a roll-on applicator or patch formulation, which may be preferred by some patients for its ease of application. Patients using such formulations should still be instructed to wash their hands after handling the product.

Use in patients with hypersensitivity to capsaicin is contraindicated. The agent should be discontinued temporarily if skin breaks down (i.e., the skin is weeping and red, with development of small ulcers), and the agent should not be applied to wounds or damaged skin.

In addition to skin reactions, capsaicin has also been associated with a cough, "runny nose," or sneezing if particles are inhaled.[35] Overdose with use of capsaicin has not been reported, but more serious and intense adverse effects are reported with higher concentrations.[38]

Capsaicin is also available in a prescription patch formulation (Qutenza 8%) approved for the treatment of postherpetic neuralgia.[38]

ADDITIONAL COUNTERIRRITANTS. Allyl isothiocyanate, ammonia water, turpentine oil, and histamine dihydrochloride are also classified as Category I counterirritants by FDA, but few counterirritant preparations contain those ingredients. Most products that contain them also contain other topical analgesics, making any beneficial actions or adverse effects of the products indistinguishable from those of other ingredients. In addition, very little evidence supports the efficacy of such compounds. Allyl isothiocyanate, ammonia water, and turpentine oil are rubefacients, so they should be expected to have effects similar to those of methyl salicylate. However, histamine dihydrochloride causes vasodilation, by mechanisms similar to those for methyl nicotinate.

PHARMACOTHERAPEUTIC EFFICACY AND RECOMMENDATIONS FOR COUNTERIRRITANTS. Literature regarding the efficacy of counterirritants is conflicting, and current studies often are lacking. However, Cochrane reviews evaluating the use of counterirritants in specific conditions and current guidelines for osteoarthritis provide some guidance.

A Cochrane review reports that topical rubefacients (those specifically containing salicylates) are not supported by enough evidence to be recommended for use in acute or chronic pain. The reviewers noted that studies in assessing acute pain were highly variable in design and limited in number, with small trial sizes and very-low-quality evidence; however, the data showed a 50% pain reduction in 64% of the patients treated after 1 week (number needed to treat 3) and a 50% pain reduction in 45% of the patients treated after 2 weeks (number needed to treat 6).[39]

One study evaluated the use of a nonprescription combination methyl salicylate and menthol patch for the treatment of mild–moderate muscle strain; the results showed that pain relief was approximately 40% better in subjects using the 8-hour patch than in the placebo group.[40] These patches (Salonpas Pain Relief Patch and Salonpas Arthritis Pain Patch) are the only nonprescription analgesic patches to undergo FDA approval of a New Drug Application.

Conflicting recommendations have been noted regarding capsaicin. A Cochrane review focused on reevaluating low-concentration (<1%) capsaicin products for the treatment of chronic neuropathic pain. In this report, insufficient evidence was available to allow a conclusion about low-dose capsaicin in treating neuropathic pain, but such preparations were deemed unlikely to have any "meaningful effect."[37] A 2014 Cochrane review concluded that there was moderate evidence for use of capsaicin to reduce low back pain.[41]

The National Institute for Health and Clinical Excellence (NICE) guidelines for osteoarthritis do not support the use of rubefacients, with the exception of capsaicin for the knee and hand.[13] The Osteoarthritis Research Society International (OARSI) guidelines recommend capsaicin as appropriate for managing osteoarthritis of the knee but state that the indications for use on multiple joints remain uncertain.[15] The ACR guidelines for the management of osteoarthritis conditionally recommend topical capsaicin as an initial option for symptom management in the hand. The guidelines also conditionally recommend that capsaicin not be used in the management of osteoarthritis of the knee. No recommendations regarding nonprescription topical analgesics in the management of osteoarthritis of the hip are included.[9]

Other Topical Analgesics

Trolamine Salicylate

Trolamine salicylate is a Category III ingredient (insufficient data are available to establish safety and efficacy). Despite this designation, several nonprescription products contain trolamine salicylate as the primary ingredient (Table 7–3).

Trolamine salicylate, or triethanolamine salicylate, is not a counterirritant analgesic. It has been suggested that trolamine salicylate is absorbed through the skin and results in synovial fluid salicylate concentrations below those of oral aspirin. The recommended topical dosage of trolamine salicylate for adults and for children 2 years of age and older is a 10%–15% concentration applied to the affected area not more than 3 or 4 times a day, as needed. No recent studies have been published regarding the efficacy of topical trolamine salicylate.

Trolamine salicylate is still available as a nonprescription agent and may be most useful to those patients who do not favor the localized irritation or the scent of Category I counterirritants. ACR guidelines conditionally recommend trolamine salicylate as an option for management of osteoarthritis of the hand.[9]

Trolamine salicylate has the same considerations for drug interactions and contraindications as those of other salicylates (see Chapter 5). During use, the agent should not contact the eyes or mucous membranes.

Topical Anesthetics

Lidocaine has widely been available as a nonprescription medication in primarily skin preparations to relieve pain and itching. It is also used for anorectal pain, as a local or injected topical anesthetic, and the prescription patch is approved for postherpetic neuralgia.[42] In the management of injuries, its primary role is in neuropathic pain owing to its mechanism of action. This mechanism of action includes inhibiting the conduction of nerve impulses. As with other topical analgesics, the FDA-approved time frame is 7 days of use. Patients allergic to lidocaine or other amide local anesthetics should avoid this group of agents. Lidocaine is classified by FDA as Category I, as an external analgesic, and is approved in concentrations of 0.5%–4% for nonprescription products. It can be used every 6–8 hours as needed, not to exceed 3 applications in 24 hours. The product should be applied to intact skin.[26,28] If a localized reaction such as a rash, itching, or skin irritation occurs, the product should be removed and the area should be cleansed.

Topical Nonsteroidal Anti-inflammatory Drugs

Traditional topical NSAIDs are not currently available for nonprescription use in the United States, but they are available for prescription use (e.g., diclofenac). Their application for acute soft tissue strains and sprains, where the target tissue is situated closer to the skin surface, is reported to provide the benefits of oral NSAIDs with minimal systemic adverse effects. These agents are recommended in the early management of chronic pain from osteoarthritis.[9,13,25]

Combination Products

Four separate chemical and/or pharmacologic groups of counterirritants provide four qualitatively different types of irritation.[28] Many marketed preparations aim for at least two such effects when greater potency is desired, provided that each active ingredient is from a different group.

Combining counterirritants with skin protectants is not appropriate: the protectants oppose and may nullify counterirritant effects.

Preparation labels must list the active ingredients, including their concentrations, and must identify them by their officially recognized, established names. In addition, manufacturers voluntarily list ingredients on the label. Many manufacturers of combination products list only some of the active ingredients under the "active" heading, and they list many of the other pharmacologically viable products in the inactive ingredients section (e.g., BenGay Vanishing Scent Gel lists camphor and Aspercreme Heat Pain Relieving Gel lists capsaicin under inactive ingredients). Although the concentrations of inactive ingredients are not listed, they are generally below therapeutically determined amounts and are added for reasons other than pain-relieving effects.[26]

Product Selection Guidelines

Special Populations

No significant variability in response has been noted among patients of different ages or racial backgrounds.

The minimum age of patients on product labeling, as specified by the manufacturer, does vary. However, such differences and age limits warrant attention in choosing an appropriate topical preparation. According to the tentative final monograph published in the *Federal Register* in 1983, use of external analgesics, as labeled within the confines of the statement, is to be avoided in children younger than 2 years.[28] However, most available products elect to label the minimum age as older than 12 years, and some products (particularly capsaicin products) specify 18 years and older. Providers should follow labeling instructions for the products used. These products should be used cautiously or avoided entirely in populations in which patients cannot effectively communicate adverse effects they are experiencing after application of a topical analgesic. Of particular concern is use of such products in young children.

Musculoskeletal complaints are common in pregnancy, but complications may occur; therefore, patients should be evaluated by their primary care provider.[43] Limited information is available regarding use of nonprescription topical analgesics in pregnancy. (See the Preface for a detailed explanation of the pregnancy data.) Capsaicin, in the prescription patch formulation, is listed as Pregnancy Category B. The prescription package insert states that no well-controlled human studies have been conducted in pregnant women but that animal studies did not reveal teratogenicity. In addition, although controlled studies in nursing mothers are lacking, capsaicin is known to be excreted in breast milk. According to the prescription insert, the exposure to the child can be reduced by avoiding breastfeeding on the day of treatment.[39] Topical lidocaine, at prescription strength, is listed as Pregnancy Category B. Use of this drug in pregnancy has not been well studied in humans, but animal studies have not shown harm. Lidocaine also has not been studied in nursing mothers.[44] An additional source lists topical lidocaine as compatible in pregnancy and probably compatible with breastfeeding, but human data are limited.[45] Camphor, menthol, methyl salicylate, trolamine salicylate, and methyl nicotinate were not previously categorized. On the basis of limited data suggesting low risk of adverse effects in this setting, topical camphor is suggested to be compatible with use during pregnancy, and although human data are lacking, it is listed as probably compatible with breastfeeding.[46]

Definitive recommendations are not available because of the limited—or in some cases, complete lack of—data that are available on topical analgesic use in pregnancy and lactation. Consideration should be given to the systemic absorption of topical salicylates, particularly in the third trimester. Information regarding use of salicylates in pregnancy can be found in Chapter 5. No information on female and male reproductive potential in general is available for the topical analgesics discussed in this chapter.

Patient Factors

The choice of treatment for acute pain syndromes and chronic conditions such as osteoarthritis is patient dependent. In addition to nonpharmacologic treatment, oral drug therapy is often employed. In such decisions, important considerations include the patient's history (identifying any exclusions for self-treatment), other medications the patient is taking, and any known allergies to medications. Topical analgesics are used as an adjunct or substitute to oral drug therapy. If a counterirritant is selected, an agent with Category I ingredients should be recommended. Product concentrations are variable; in general, the lowest effective dose should be recommended for the shortest duration needed.

Patient Preferences

Factors that affect product selection include dosage form, ease of use, cost, and even odor of the preparation. Dosage forms available include solutions, liniments, gels, lotions, ointments, creams, and patches. Compared with solutions, gels, lotions, and creams, oleaginous preparations (ointments and oil-based liniments) have increased absorption, but owing to their "greasy" feel they generally are less acceptable to patients. The use of patches is becoming more popular because of their simple application and long duration of action. With the exception of patches and solutions, topical products should be rubbed into the skin.

Complementary Therapies

The most common dietary supplement used for osteoarthritis contains glucosamine and chondroitin. Published data regarding these supplements are conflicting because of population size, trial duration, preparations used (e.g., prescription products that are available only in other countries), and outcomes measured (i.e., quality of life, pain indices, and radiologic changes). Initial results from the 6-month Glucosamine/Chondroitin Arthritis Intervention Trial (GAIT) demonstrated no benefit with mild pain but showed a statistically significant reduction with moderate–severe pain. However, only 22% of patients enrolled in the study were categorized as having moderate–severe pain; accordingly, the GAIT investigators concluded that further studies are needed because of the small population size.[47] A 2-year follow-up evaluation in patients from the GAIT study showed no clinical difference in reduction of pain and function and joint space width in comparison with placebo.[48,49] Reflecting the popularity of these supplements, additional studies continue to contribute to the body of literature. An observational study examined the structural effect of glucosamine and chondroitin sulfate on cartilage in patients with moderate osteoarthritis of the knee with meniscal damage at baseline. The study outcome was assessed at 6 years: In this specific population, use of the supplement for 2 or more years reduced the amount of cartilage lost. The protective effect on cartilage was not associated with symptomatic improvement.[50] In the MOVES trial, investigators concluded that a combination of glucosamine hydrochloride and chondroitin sulfate, as a European prescription product, was similar in efficacy to celecoxib in reducing pain over a 6-month period in patients with severe painful knee osteoarthritis.[51] A 2015 Cochrane review of data on chondroitin, while acknowledging that it mostly included low-quality trials, found that this supplement reduced pain by 10% at 6 months in comparison with placebo.[52]

The ACR guidelines conditionally recommend that patients with osteoarthritis of the hip and knee not use glucosamine or chondroitin sulfate.[9] The OARSI guidelines specify that the recommendation for glucosamine for symptom relief remains uncertain but do not recommend it for disease modification.[15] The AAOS guidelines do not recommend the use of glucosamine and chondroitin for patients with symptomatic knee osteoarthritis.[16] The NICE guidelines do not recommend the supplements for treatment.[13] European guidelines support the use of glucosamine and chondroitin but note that this recommendation is based on the availability of a prescription product.[53] These products and other complementary therapies are discussed in greater detail in Chapter 51.

Assessment of Musculoskeletal Injuries and Disorders: A Case-Based Approach

On a routine basis, the HCP should inventory all patient medications, including pain medications, and should note the patient's satisfaction with or preference for past treatments. In addition, the provider should ask about aspects of the patient's medical history that relate directly to the origin or treatment of pain.

Before an attempt is made to treat a pain complaint, the HCP should qualify and quantify the pain. Inquiry about the cause, duration, location, and severity of pain, as well as factors that relieve and exacerbate the pain, will help in completing a thorough assessment of this symptom. Chapter 2 outlines effective strategies for obtaining information from patients about specific complaints. Using a pain scale helps to quantify the intensity of the pain. With the numerical pain scale, the HCP asks the patient to rank the present pain on a scale of 0–10, with 0 being no pain and 10 being the worst pain the patient can imagine. Typically, mild pain is defined as 1–3, moderate pain as 4–6, and severe pain as 7–10 on the numerical pain scale.[1] Initially, pain scores establish a baseline for pain before treatment. In addition, a high pain score can be used to identify patients who would be better served by seeking an appropriate medical evaluation. Pain scores also serve as a metric for assessing therapeutic outcomes. Other scales are available for pain rating in children (e.g., Wong-Baker FACES Pain Scale), adolescents, people who do not speak English, and other special populations.

A chronic painful condition presents a different set of challenges. An observant HCP should intervene with a patient who regularly purchases nonprescription analgesics. If additional interviewing indicates an inadequately treated pain problem, further workup by an appropriate provider is appropriate. Education should be offered regarding the risks of inadequate treatment as well as the overuse of medications.

Cases 7–1 and 7–2 are examples of the assessment of two different patients with a musculoskeletal injury or disorder.

Patient Counseling for Musculoskeletal Injuries and Disorders

Consultation with the patient should include an explanation of the expected benefit of any recommended medication, the appropriate dose and drug administration schedule, application directions, potential adverse reactions, potential drug–drug or drug–disease interactions, and self-monitoring techniques for assessing response to therapy. Printed materials reinforce verbal information. Many such pamphlets or single-page handouts are available from national professional societies (e.g., www.arthritis.org). These materials offer advice on exercise, diet, and sleep habits, as well as outlining the advantages and disadvantages of pharmacologic therapy.

In acute pain management, early administration of nonprescription analgesics is warranted to prevent escalating pain, with downward tapering of the analgesic doses as pain severity allows. Patients should be assessed for the appropriateness of nonprescription oral analgesic regimens (Chapter 5).

Patients should be instructed to notify their primary care provider if the pain worsens in quality or severity, or if new acute pain develops. Other sudden, uncharacteristic pain may be a harbinger of new tissue damage.

The box "Patient Education for Musculoskeletal Injuries and Disorders" lists specific information about topical analgesics, as well as preventive and nondrug measures to provide patients.

CASE 7–1

Relevant Evaluation Criteria	Scenario/Model Outcome
Collect	
1. Gather essential information about the patient's symptoms and medical history, including	
a. Description of symptom(s) (e.g., nature, onset, duration, severity, associated symptoms)	Patient presents with a complaint that his hamstring muscle is sore. He rates his pain right now as 3 on a scale of 0–10.
b. Description of any factors that seem to precipitate, exacerbate, and/or relieve the patient's symptom(s)	He reports that he played 5 soccer games in a tournament over the weekend. The soreness is in his dominant leg that he shoots with.
c. Description of the patient's efforts to relieve the symptom(s)	He increased hydration in case it was a cramp; he did not experience any relief. In addition, he took ibuprofen 400 mg three times yesterday; it provided minimal relief.
d. Patient's identity	Jason Smith
e. Patient's age, gender, height, and weight	15 years old, male, 5 ft 7 in., 140 lb
f. Patient's occupation	High school student
g. Patient's dietary habits	He eats a well-balanced diet. He has noticed an increase in hunger during his last growth spurt.
h. Patient's sleep habits	He is sleeping 6 hours each night.
i. Concurrent medical conditions, prescription and nonprescription medications, and dietary supplements	None
j. Allergies	Cephalosporin antibiotics
k. History of other adverse reactions to medications	None
l. Other patient preferences	n/a
Assess	
2. Differentiate patient's signs/symptoms, and correctly identify the patient's primary problem(s).	Patient is experiencing minor pain in his hamstring, which is most likely from a strain from overuse at his soccer tournament this weekend.

Relevant Evaluation Criteria	Scenario/Model Outcome
3. Identify exclusions for self-treatment (Figure 7–1).	Patient does not have any exclusions for self-care. If his pain were more severe (>6 on pain scale), a medical referral would be recommended.
4. Formulate a comprehensive list of therapeutic alternatives for the primary problem to determine whether triage to a medical provider is required, and share this information with the patient or caregiver.	Options include (1) Refer patient to PCP for further assessment and treatment. (2) Continue NSAID (ibuprofen). (3) Recommend nondrug measures (ice). (4) Recommend a topical analgesic, single or combination product. (5) Take no action.
Plan	
5. Select an optimal therapeutic alternative to address the patient's problem, taking into account patient preferences.	Recommend nondrug measures including rest and ice since this is an acute injury. The patient is a candidate for self-care, and recommended therapy would include a topical analgesic. The patient is not reporting adequate relief from the ibuprofen he tried.
6. Describe the recommended therapeutic approach to the patient or caregiver.	"A topical pain-relieving medicine can be used to help relieve the discomfort, and we can select a cream to be massaged into the muscle."
7. Explain to the patient or caregiver the rationale for selecting the recommended therapeutic approach from the considered therapeutic alternatives.	"Since the ibuprofen is not providing adequate pain relief and the maximum dose is being used, a topical analgesic can be tried as an alternative treatment to relieve the pain."
Implement	
8. When recommending self-care with nonprescription medications and/or nondrug therapy, convey accurate information to the patient or caregiver.	
a. Appropriate dose and frequency of administration	"Apply Bengay Ultra Strength Pain Relieving Cream (methyl salicylate 30%, menthol 10%, camphor 4%) to your hamstring 3 or 4 times a day, as needed."
b. Maximum number of days the therapy should be employed	"This medication can be used for self-treatment for up to 7 days."
c. Product administration procedures	"Rub the cream onto your hamstring where the pain is. It can be used 3 or 4 times a day, as needed. Wash your hands after you apply the cream. It is not recommended to use heat or tightly bandage the area once the medication has been applied."
d. Expected time to onset of relief	"You should expect to get some relief from the pain shortly after application."
e. Degree of relief that can be reasonably expected	"The medicine will help reduce the pain, but it may not completely eliminate it."
f. Most common adverse effects	"It is normal to feel warmth in the area where the medication is applied. Some minor skin irritation may occur."
g. Adverse effects that warrant medical intervention should they occur	"Immediately wash off the product and contact your primary care provider if you notice any skin problems that would indicate a reaction to the product (such as excessive redness, blistering, rash, burning, or stinging)."
h. Patient options in the event that condition worsens or persists	"If the pain worsens or continues beyond 10 days, please contact your primary care provider for further evaluation."
i. Product storage requirements	"Keep the product out of reach of young children."
j. Specific nondrug measures	"Rest for 1 or 2 days so as to not further aggravate the pain. Ice can be used in the first 48 hours, and then heat can be used. Do not apply heat if you have applied the Bengay on your leg."
Solicit follow-up questions from the patient or caregiver.	The parent asks, "How can we prevent this from happening again?"
Answer the patient's or caregiver's questions.	"Proper warm-up and stretching before and after the game will help."
Follow-up: Monitor and Evaluate	
9. Assess patient outcome.	Monitor for a reduction in the patient's reported pain level using a pain scale.

Key: n/a = Not applicable; NSAID = nonsteroidal anti-inflammatory drug; PCP = primary care provider.

CASE 7–2

Relevant Evaluation Criteria	Scenario/Model Outcome
Collect	
1. Gather essential information about the patient's symptoms and medical history, including	
a. Description of symptom(s) (e.g., nature, onset, duration, severity, associated symptoms)	Patient presents with a complaint that she has had a stabbing foot pain that has increased over time. She reports the pain varies throughout the day but rates it as 9 out of 10 at its worst. You observe that she is walking with an altered gait and limp.
b. Description of any factors that seem to precipitate, exacerbate, and/or relieve the patient's symptom(s)	She reports that rest helps but then upon standing the pain is severe. Stretching the foot helps.
c. Description of the patient's efforts to relieve the symptom(s)	She has used ice to try to relieve the pain. A friend told her to roll a frozen water bottle under her foot. She reports this helps a little.
d. Patient's identity	Thelma Jones
e. Patient's age, gender, height, and weight	59 years old, female, 5 ft, 150 lb
f. Patient's occupation	Retired medical biller
g. Patient's dietary habits	She prefers to eat small meals throughout the day.
h. Patient's sleep habits	She has a regular sleeping pattern.
i. Concurrent medical conditions, prescription and nonprescription medications, and dietary supplements	She has a history of asthma and uses an albuterol inhaler as needed. She has not needed to use her inhaler for 3 months. She takes a calcium supplement with vitamin D daily.
j. Allergies	NKA
k. History of other adverse reactions to medications	None
l. Other (describe) _______	n/a
Assess	
2. Differentiate patient's signs/symptoms, and correctly identify the patient's primary problem(s).	The patient appears to have a condition likely affecting the ligament or tendon in the foot.
3. Identify exclusions for self-treatment (Figure 7–1).	The patient is experiencing pain that is severe (9 out of 10 on a pain scale) and is having difficulty walking normally.
4. Formulate a comprehensive list of therapeutic alternatives for the primary problem to determine whether triage to a medical provider is required, and share this information with the patient or caregiver.	Options include (1) Refer patient to PCP for further assessment and treatment. (2) Recommend nondrug measures (ice). (3) Recommend a systemic analgesic. (4) Recommend a topical analgesic. (5) Take no action.
Plan	
5. Select an optimal therapeutic alternative to address the patient's problem, taking into account patient preferences.	Refer the patient to PCP for further evaluation because of the severity of the pain and impaired mobility. The patient can continue to use current therapies (i.e., ice, stretching).
6. Describe the recommended therapeutic approach to the patient or caregiver.	"Based on the severity of your pain, it is recommended you see your primary care provider."
7. Explain to the patient or caregiver the rationale for selecting the recommended therapeutic approach from the considered therapeutic alternatives.	"The severe pain you are experiencing requires further evaluation by your primary care provider."
Implement	
8. When recommending self-care with nonprescription medications and/or nondrug therapy, convey accurate information to the patient or caregiver:	Criterion does not apply in this case.
Solicit follow-up questions from the patient or caregiver.	"My friend told me I can just buy insoles at the pharmacy to relieve the pain." "Is there anything I can do till I see the doctor?"

CASE 7-2 *continued*

Relevant Evaluation Criteria	Scenario/Model Outcome
Answer the patient's or caregiver's questions.	"There are some insoles available, but your foot should be first be evaluated by your primary care provider to determine what is causing the pain and develop a treatment plan. You may continue to use the frozen water bottle if you feel that is providing some pain relief."
Follow-up: Monitor and Evaluate	
9. Assess patient outcome.	Follow up with the patient to determine the outcome of her visit with the PCP.

Key: n/a = Not applicable; NKA = no known allergies; PCP = primary care provider.

PATIENT EDUCATION FOR Musculoskeletal Injuries and Disorders

The objectives of self-treatment are (1) to reduce the severity of pain; (2) to reduce the duration of pain, when possible; (3) to restore function to the affected area; (4) to prevent re-injury and disability; and (5) to prevent acute pain from becoming chronic persistent pain. Certain nondrug measures and nonprescription counterirritants can relieve pain symptoms from a sudden and recent muscle, tendon, or ligament injury; an overuse injury (e.g., tendonitis, bursitis, repetitive stress injury); low back pain; or arthritis. For most patients, carefully following product instructions and the self-care measures listed here will help ensure optimal therapeutic outcomes.

Preventive Measures

- To prevent muscle or joint strains and sprains, do warm-up and stretching exercises before playing sports or exercising, and wrap injured muscle or joint with protective bandage or tape.
- To prevent repetitive strain, exercise the muscles that are vulnerable to the injury, and use ergonomic controls to adjust posture, stresses, motions, and other damaging physical factors.
- To prevent tendonitis and cramps, warm up and stretch muscles before physical activity, drink sufficient fluids, and do not exercise to the point of exhaustion. To help prevent nocturnal leg cramps, raise the foot of the bed. For Achilles tendonitis, wearing better-fitting shoes with heel lifts may help reduce the symptoms.
- To prevent or reduce the occurrence of low back pain, do exercises to strengthen the muscles of the low back and abdomen, and use assistive devices (i.e., cane or walker) if needed.
- To prevent or reduce the occurrence of osteoarthritis, avoid a sedentary lifestyle; keep joints active; lose weight, if overweight; and use assistive devices if needed.

Nondrug Measures

- For pain related to muscle or joint injuries, begin treatment with RICE therapy (Table 7–2).
- For periodic muscle cramps, stretch and massage the affected area immediately; then rest or reduce activity of the muscle to allow it to loosen.
- For stiffness, apply heat to the affected area in the form of a warm wet compress, a heating pad, or a hot water bottle.
- For osteoarthritis, try a combination of nondrug measures, including applying heat or cold to the affected area, supporting the area with splints, and doing range-of-motion and strength maintenance exercises.

Nonprescription Medications

- For mild–moderate muscle pain, take a nonprescription systemic analgesic for no longer than 10 days[24] (see Chapter 5 for a listing of nonprescription analgesics), and/or use a topical analgesic for no longer than 7 days[26] (Table 7–4 provides recommended dosages of counterirritants).
- Do not use topical analgesics if your skin is abraded, sunburned, or otherwise damaged.
- When using counterirritants, especially capsaicin, wash your hands after application and before touching your eyes and mucous membranes, or before handling contact lenses.
- Gently rub a thin layer of counterirritant product into affected muscles or joints until you cannot see the product. Thick application of the product does not make the product work better.
- Do not put a tight bandage or dressing over an area treated with a counterirritant. Do not use heat or warming devices with counterirritants.
- Do not treat a child 2 years of age or younger with counterirritants unless a primary care provider supervises the use. Follow age limits on product labeling.
- If you have asthma and experience worsening of symptoms of wheezing and shortness of breath while you are using a mentholated formulation, stop using it.
- If you are receiving anticoagulation therapy (especially warfarin), do not use products containing salicylates (i.e., methyl salicylate and trolamine salicylate) for prolonged use.
- If a counterirritant causes excessive redness and blistering or hives and vomiting, stop using it.

When to Seek Medical Attention

- A feeling of warmth or coolness is normal; however, if burning pain or blistering occurs, seek medical attention.
- If you experience nausea, vomiting, colic, and other unusual symptoms while using a product containing camphor, seek medical care immediately.
- If the pain has been present for more than 10 days or has worsened, consult a primary care provider.[24]
- If the symptoms persist after more than 7 days of treatment with a topical product, or if the pain is constant and felt in any position, consult a primary care provider.[26]

Key: RICE = *Rest, ice, compression, elevation.*

Evaluation of Patient Outcomes for Musculoskeletal Injuries and Disorders

The primary indicator of treatment effectiveness is the patient's perception of pain relief. If the patient reports that the pain is still present or has worsened after 7 days of using topical nonprescription analgesics,[28] the HCP should refer the patient for further evaluation. In many instances, the lack of a return visit indicates a successful treatment regimen (the provider may call the patient in a few days to determine whether the complaint has resolved). However, a patient who returns with signs of continued swelling, pain, or inflammation should be referred for medical evaluation. The continued pain may indicate an ongoing pathologic process that could lead to long-term disability or decreased mobility.

Key Points for Musculoskeletal Injuries and Disorders

- Self-treatment of patients presenting with pain secondary to an injury or a disorder of the musculoskeletal system should be limited to those with mild–moderate pain who have no exclusions for self-treatment (Figure 7–1).
- Self-treatment of acute musculoskeletal injuries should include nondrug therapy, such as RICE. Heat therapy may also provide benefit after symptoms of inflammation have abated.
- Systemic analgesics are valid first-line agents to treat a majority of musculoskeletal injuries and disorders. Acetaminophen is appropriate in noninflammatory diseases, whereas NSAIDs are preferred if inflammation is present. Adverse effects and drug interactions should be considered before therapy is chosen (see Chapter 5).
- HCPs should counsel patients on the discussion points listed in Table 7–5 to avoid chemical burns with topical nonprescription analgesics.
- HCPs should monitor the outcome of self-treatment regimens and advise patients who self-treat their acute musculoskeletal injury with nonprescription topical analgesics to seek medical attention if they do not obtain symptomatic improvement after 7 days. Patients who experience pain for longer than 10 days, regardless of treatment, should also be referred.

REFERENCES

1. Mense S, Gerwin R. *Muscle Pain: Diagnosis and Treatment.* New York, NY: Springer; 2010:1–84.
2. Consumer Healthcare Products Association. OTC sales by category 2012–2015. March 2016. Available at: http://www.chpa.org/OTCsCategory.aspx. Accessed April 6, 2017.
3. Institute of Medicine. Relieving pain in America: a blueprint for transforming prevention, care, education, and research. June 2011. Available at: https://iprcc.nih.gov/docs/032712_mtg_presentations/IOM_pain_Report_508comp.pdf. Accessed April 6, 2017.
4. Buckwalter J. Musculoskeletal tissues and musculoskeletal system. In: Weinstein S, Buckwalter J, eds. *Tureks Orthopaedics: Principles and Their Application.* 6th ed. Philadelphia, PA: Lippincott Williams & Wilkins; 2005:3–72.
5. National Institute of Arthritis and Musculoskeletal and Skin Disease. Questions and answers about sprains and strains. January 2016. Available at: http://www.niams.nih.gov/Health_Info/Sprains_Strains/default.asp. Accessed April 6, 2017.
6. U.S. Food and Drug Administration. Information for healthcare professionals: fluoroquinolone antimicrobial drugs. April 15, 2013. Available at: http://www.fda.gov/Drugs/DrugSafety/PostmarketDrugSafetyInformationforPatientsandProviders/ucm126085.htm. Accessed April 6, 2016.
7. National Institute of Arthritis and Musculoskeletal and Skin Disease. Handout on health: back pain. March 2015. Available at: http://www.niams.nih.gov/Health_Info/Back_Pain/default.asp. Accessed April 6, 2017.
8. Qaseem A., Wilt T, McLean R., et al. Noninvasive treatments for acute, subacute, and chronic low back pain: a clinical practice guideline from the American College of Physicians. *Ann Intern Med.* 2017;166(7):514–30. doi: 10.7326/M16-2367.
9. Hochberg MC, Altman RD, April KT, et al. American College of Rheumatology 2012 recommendations for the use of nonpharmacologic and pharmacologic therapies in osteoarthritis of the hand, hip, and knee. *Arthritis Care Res.* 2012;64(4):465–74. doi: 10.1002/acr.21596.
10. National Institute of Arthritis and Musculoskeletal and Skin Disease. Handout on health: osteoarthritis. April 2015. Available at: http://www.niams.nih.gov/Health_Info/Osteoarthritis/default.asp. Accessed April 6, 2017.
11. Centers for Disease Control and Prevention. Arthritis: national statistics. January 25, 2016. Available at: http://www.cdc.gov/arthritis/data_statistics/arthritis-related-stats.htm. Accessed April 5, 2016.
12. Chou R, Deyo R, Friedly J, et al. Systemic pharmacologic therapies for low back pain: a systemic review for an American College of Physicians Clinical Practice Guideline. *Ann Intern Med.* 2017;166(7):480–92. doi: 10.7326/M16-2458.
13. National Institute for Health and Clinical Excellence. Osteoarthritis: the care and management of osteoarthritis in adults. Clinical Guideline CG177. February 2014. Available at: https://www.nice.org.uk/guidance/cg177/evidence/full guideline-191761309. Accessed April 5, 2017.
14. Nelson, AE, Allen KD, Golightly YM, et al. A systematic review of recommendations and guidelines for the management of osteoarthritis: the Chronic Osteoarthritis Management Initiative of the U.S. Bone and Joint Initiative. *Semin Arthritis Rheum.* 2014;43:701–12. doi: 10.1016/j.semarthrit.2013.11.012.
15. McAlindon TE, Bannuru RR, Sullivan MC, et al. OARSI guidelines for the non-surgical management of knee osteoarthritis. *Osteoarthr Cartil.* 2014;22:363–88. http://dx.doi.org/10.1016/j.joca.2014.01.003.
16. *Treatment of Osteoarthritis of the Knee: Evidence-Based Guideline.* 2nd ed. Rosemont, IL: American Academy of Orthopaedic Surgeons; 2013. Available at: http://www.aaos.org/uploadedFiles/PreProduction/Quality/Guidelines_and_Reviews/Osteoarthritis%20of%20the%20Knee%20-%20non-arthroplasty.pdf. Accessed April 5, 2017.
17. Brosseau L, Yonge KA, Robinson V, et al. Thermotherapy for treatment of osteoarthritis. *Cochrane Database Syst Rev.* 2011;4:CD004522. doi: 10.1002/14651858.CD004522.
18. ThermaCare.com. ThermaCare frequently asked questions. Available at: http://www.thermacare.com/faqs. Accessed April 6, 2017.
19. Hing WA, White SG, Bouaaphone A, et al. Contrast therapy—a systematic review. *Phys Ther Sport.* 2008;9(3):148–61. doi: 10.1016/j.ptsp.2008.06.001.
20. Bahnert A, Norton K, Lock P. Association between post-game recovery protocols, physical and perceived recovery, and performance in elite Australian football league players. *J Sci Med Sport.* 2013;16(2):151–6. doi: 10.1016/j.jsams.2012.05.008.
21. U.S. Food and Drug Administration. Product classification. August 11, 2014. Available at: http://www.accessdata.fda.gov/scripts/cdrh/cfdocs/cfPCD/classification.cfm?ID=3434. Accessed April 6, 2017.
22. Icy Hot Smart Relief [product information]. Chattam, Inc., Chattanooga, TN. Available at: http://www.smartrelief.com/wp-content/uploads/2014/02/IH_SmartRelief_Inst_Manual.pdf. Accessed April 6, 2017.
23. TENS pain relief systems. AccuRelief web site. Available at: http://www.accurelief.com/products.php. Accessed April 6, 2017.
24. U.S. Food and Drug Administration. Internal analgesic, antipyretic, antirheumatic drug products for over-the-counter human use; tentative final monograph. *Fed Reg.* 1988;53:46204–60. Available at: http://www.fda.gov/downloads/Drugs/DevelopmentApprovalProcess/Development

Resources/Over-the-CounterOTCDrugs/StatusofOTCRulemakings/UCM078460.pdf. Accessed April 6, 2017.
25. American Geriatrics Society panel on the pharmacological management of persistent pain in older persons. *J Am Geriatr Soc.* 2009;57(8):1331–46. doi: 10.1111/j.1532-5415.2009.02376.x.
26. U.S. Food and Drug Administration. External analgesic products for over-the-counter human use; establishment of a monograph and notice of proposed rulemaking. *Fed Reg.* 1979;44(234):69768–874. Available at: http://www.fda.gov/downloads/Drugs/DevelopmentApprovalProcess/DevelopmentResources/Over-the-CounterOTCDrugs/StatusofOTCRulemakings/UCM077916.pdf. Accessed April 6, 2017.
27. Methyl salicylate. In: Brayfield A, ed. *Martindale—The Complete Drug Reference.* 38th ed. London, UK: Pharmaceutical Press; 2014:92.
28. U.S. Food and Drug Administration. External analgesic drug products for over-the-counter human use: tentative final monograph. *Fed Reg.* 1983;48(27):5852–69. Available at: http://www.fda.gov/downloads/Drugs/DevelopmentApprovalProcess/DevelopmentResources/Over-the-CounterOTCDrugs/StatusofOTCRulemakings/UCM077928.pdf. Accessed April 6, 2017.
29. U.S. Food and Drug Administration. FDA Drug Safety Communication: rare cases of serious burns with the use of over-the-counter topical muscle and joint pain relievers. February 11, 2016. Available at: http://www.fda.gov/Drugs/DrugSafety/ucm318858.htm. Accessed April 6, 2017.
30. Danon A, Ben-Shimon S, Ben-Zvi Z. Effect of exercise and heat exposure on percutaneous absorption of methyl salicylate. *Eur J Clin Pharmacol.* 1986;31(1):49–52. doi: 10.1007/bf00870985.
31. Davis JE. Are one or two dangerous? Methyl salicylate exposure in toddlers. *J Emerg Med.* 2007;32(1):63–9. doi: 10.1016/j.jemermed.2006.08.009.
32. Santos C, Cabot J. Persistent effects after camphor ingestions: a case report and literature review. *J Emerg Med.* 2015;48(3):298–304. http://dx.doi.org/10.1016/j.jemermed.2014.05.015.
33. Patel T, Ishiuji Y, Yosipovitch G. Menthol: a refreshing look at this ancient compound. *J Am Acad Dermatol.* 2007;57(5):873–8. doi: 10.1016/j.jaad.2007.04.008.
34. Wilkin JK, Fortner G, Reinhardt LA, et al. Prostaglandins and nicotinate-provoked increase in cutaneous blood flow. *Clin Pharmacol Ther.* 1985;38(3):273–7. doi: 10.1038/clpt.1985.170.
35. Capsaicin. In: Brayfield A, ed. *Martindale—The Complete Drug Reference.* 38th ed. London, UK: Pharmaceutical Press; 2014:35–6.
36. Stanos SP. Topical agents for the management of musculoskeletal pain. *J Pain Symptom Manage.* 2007;33(3):342–55. doi: 10.1016/j.jpainsymman.2006.11.005.
37. Derry S, Moore RA. Topical capsaicin (low concentration) for chronic neuropathic pain in adults. *Cochrane Database Syst Rev.* 2012;9:CD010111. doi: 10.1002/14651858.CD010111.
38. Qutenza [product information]. NeurogesX, Inc., San Mateo, CA. November 2009. Available at: www.qutenza.com. Accessed April 6, 2017.
39. Derry S, Matthews PRL, Moore RA, et al. Salicylate-containing rubefacients for acute and chronic pain in adults. *Cochrane Database Syst Rev.* 2014;11:CD007403. doi: 10.1002/14651858.CD007403.pub3.
40. Higashi Y, Kiuchi T, Furuta K. Efficacy and safety profile of a topical methyl salicylate and menthol patch in adult patients with mild to moderate muscle strain: a randomized, double-blind, parallel-group, placebo-controlled, multicenter study. *Clin Ther.* 2010;32(1):34–43. doi: 10.1016/j.clinthera.2010.01.016.
41. Oltean H, Robbins C, Van Tulder MW, et al. Herbal medicine for low-back pain. Cochrane Database Syst Rev. 2014;12:CD004504. doi: 10.1002/14651858.CD004504.pub4.
42. Lidocaine. Facts and Comparisons eAnswers. St. Louis, MO: Wolters Kluwer Health. Updated April 2015. Available at: http://online.factsandcomparisons.com. Accessed April 6, 2017.
43. Bermas B. Musculoskeletal changes and pain during pregnancy and postpartum. Up to Date. St. Louis, MO: Wolters Kluwer Health. Updated March 3, 2016. Available at: http://www.uptodate.com. Accessed April 6, 2017.
44. Lidocaine patch 5% [product information]. Mylan Pharmaceuticals, Morgantown, WV. January 2015. Available at: http://lidocainepatch.mylan.com/-/media/lidocaine/files/lido-r2%20exhibit%20pdf.pdf. Accessed April 6, 2017.
45. Briggs G, Freeman R. Lidocaine. In: *Drugs in Pregnancy and Lactation.* 10th ed. Philadelphia, PA: Wolters Kluwer Health; 2015:798–99.
46. Briggs G, Freeman R. Camphor. In: *Drugs in Pregnancy and Lactation.* 10th ed. Philadelphia, PA: Wolters Kluwer Health; 2015:188.
47. Clegg DO, Reda DJ, Harris CL, et al. Glucosamine, chondroitin sulfate, and the two in combination for painful knee osteoarthritis. *N Engl J Med.* 2006;354(8):795–808. doi: 10.1056/NEJMoa052771.
48. Sawitzke AD, Shi H, Finco MF, et al. Clinical efficacy and safety of glucosamine, chondroitin sulphate, their combination, celecoxib or placebo taken to treat osteoarthritis of the knee: 2-year results from GAIT. *Ann Rheum Dis.* 2010;69(8):1459–64. doi: 10.1136/ard.2009.120469.
49. Sawitzke AD, Shi H, Finco MF, et al. The effect of glucosamine and/or chondroitin sulfate on the progression of knee osteoarthritis: a report from the glucosamine/chondroitin arthritis intervention trial. *Arthritis Rheum.* 2008;58(10):3183–91. doi: 10.1002/art.23973.
50. Raynauld JP, Pelletier JP, Abraham F, et al. Long-term effects of glucosamine/chondroitin sulfate on the progression of structural changes in knee osteoarthritis: 6-year follow-up data from the osteoarthritis initiative. *Arthritis Care Res (Hoboken).* 2016;68(10):1560–6. doi: 10.1002/acr.22866.
51. Hochberg MC, Martel-Pelletier J, Monfort J, et al. Combined chondroitin sulfate and glucosamine for painful knee osteoarthritis: a multicentre, randomized, double-blind, non-inferiority trial versus celecoxib. *Ann Rheum Dis.* 2016;75:37–44. doi: 10.1136/annrheumdis-2014-206792
52. Singh JA, Noorbaloochi S, MacDonald R, et al. Chondroitin for osteoarthritis. *Cochrane Database Syst Rev.* 2015;9:CD005614. doi: 10.1002/14651858.CD005614.pub2.
53. Bruyere O, Cooper C, Pelleiter JP, et al. A consensus statement on the European Society for Clinical and Economic Aspects of Osteoporosis and Osteoarthritis (ESCEO) algorithm for the management of knee osteoarthritis—from evidence-based medicine to the real-life setting. *Semin Arthritis Rheum.* 2016;45:S3–11. doi: 10.1016/j.semarthrit.2015.11.010.

section

III

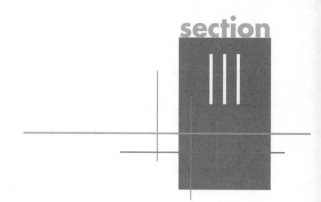

REPRODUCTIVE AND GENITAL DISORDERS

CHAPTER 8

VAGINAL AND VULVOVAGINAL DISORDERS

NICOLE M. LODISE

Vaginal symptoms are among the most common health concerns of both reproductive age and older women. Vaginal symptoms may be experienced by all women whether sexually active or abstinent, homosexual or heterosexual, and premenopausal or postmenopausal.[1] Approximately 65% of women experiencing vaginal symptoms will have one of three common vaginal infections: bacterial vaginosis (BV), vulvovaginal candidiasis (VVC), and trichomoniasis.[1] Infections may also be mixed, with more than one causative organism.

In general, vaginal infections are perceived as minor health problems where patients may consider self-treatment. Women may also self-treat noninfectious vaginal symptoms such as vaginal dryness, atrophic vaginitis, and allergic or chemical dermatologic reactions.[1,2] However, BV and trichomoniasis have been linked to significant health problems, such as pelvic inflammatory disease (PID), preterm birth, and facilitation of the transmission of human immunodeficiency virus (HIV).[2,3] Given the frequency of these vaginal infections and the approval of nonprescription vaginal antifungal products, health care providers (HCPs) need to manage these infections carefully and provide patient education for VVC. HCPs must ensure that patients are making informed self-care decisions by providing them the necessary information and tools to know when and how to self-treat.

The vagina is an elastic fibromuscular tube that extends 8–10 cm from the vulva to the uterus. The upper end of the vagina is closed except for the *cervical os,* the opening to the cervix. Anatomically, the vagina lies between the urinary bladder and the rectum. At the lower (vulvar) end of the vagina are the Bartholin glands, which produce secretions in response to sexual stimulation. At puberty, with the influence of estrogen, the vaginal lining changes to stratified squamous epithelium, which contains glycogen. *Lactobacillus* bacteria convert glycogen to lactic acid, which creates an acidic pH of 4–4.5. This acidic pH and the production of hydrogen peroxide by these bacteria in some patients help protect the vagina from infection with other bacteria. After menopause, thinning of the vaginal lining occurs, concentrations of lactobacilli decline, and pH rises.[4]

The mature vagina is colonized by many organisms. *Lactobacillus* species predominate, accounting for more than 95% of the vaginal flora.[5] Additional species of bacteria, including *Mobiluncus, Gardnerella vaginalis, Prevotella,* and *Bacteroides,* are present in small quantities, with *Candida albicans* isolated in the absence of active infection in approximately 20% of women.[2]

The vaginal ecosystem is affected by the number and types of endogenous organisms, vaginal pH, and glycogen concentration. Hormonal fluctuations during the menstrual cycle, in addition to drug therapy, douching, and number of sex partners, can also influence the vaginal ecosystem.

The healthy vagina is cleansed daily by secretions that lubricate the vaginal tract. Normal vaginal discharge, also known as *leukorrhea,* is odorless, clear or white, and viscous or sticky.[6] This discharge consists of endocervical mucus, endogenous vaginal flora, and epithelial cells.[6] Leukorrhea should not cause irritation, itching, or burning. An increase in vaginal secretions is normal during ovulation, during pregnancy, after menses, and with sexual excitement or emotional flares. An alteration in vaginal secretions may also occur in response to vaginal irritants such as feminine hygiene deodorant products and vaginal douches, as well as contraceptive products or use of tampons.

Differentiation of Common Vaginal Infections

The signs and symptoms for different vaginal infections may be similar, making diagnosis challenging; the characteristic symptoms that often help distinguish infections may also be absent (Table 8–1). Accurately distinguishing VVC from BV and trichomoniasis is important because of the availability of nonprescription vaginal antifungal therapy.

Given the availability of nonprescription vaginal antifungal products and the cost and inconvenience of an office evaluation, many patients prefer to self-treat for presumed VVC, which may result in inappropriate therapy.[7] Women should be encouraged to ask their HCPs, who can educate patients on appropriate self-care treatment.

Many women and HCPs may have trouble identifying VVC on the basis of the symptoms alone.[8,9] Studies have reported that many women who purchased nonprescription antifungal products to treat vaginal symptoms actually did not have VVC infections.[9,10] The symptom most likely to differentiate a *Candida* vaginal infection from that of BV and trichomoniasis is the absence of an offensive odor of the vaginal discharge.[8]

Noninfectious conditions such as irritation or pruritus caused by allergic reactions secondary to douching, feminine hygiene products, latex reactions, spermicides, or soaps may also add to the confusion of diagnosing vaginal infections.[8]

Inappropriate use of vaginal antifungal products has several risks, including unnecessary drug use and a delay in effective

TABLE 8-1 Differentiation of Common Vaginal Infections

Classic Symptoms[1]	Differentiating Signs and Symptoms[1,3,13]	Etiology and Epidemiology[1,3,15]
Bacterial Vaginosis (vaginal pH >4.5)		
Thin (watery), off-white or discolored (green, gray, tan), sometimes foamy discharge; unpleasant "fishy" odor that increases after sexual intercourse or with elevated vaginal pH (e.g., menses)	Vaginal irritation, dysuria, and itching are less frequent with BV than with VVC or trichomoniasis.[15] A foul odor is strongly associated with BV; absence of the odor virtually rules out BV. Increased vaginal discharge ("wetness") is more common with BV than with VVC or trichomoniasis.	Polymicrobial infection resulting from imbalance in normal vaginal flora with increase in *Gardnerella vaginalis* and anaerobes (*Mobiluncus* and *Prevotella*) and decrease in lactobacilli Risk factors: new sexual partner, African American race, use of IUD douching, sexual practices, tobacco use, and prior pregnancy Possible protective factors: use of female hormones, including OC, and condoms Responsible for 30% of vaginal symptoms Predominantly affects young, sexually active women but can arise spontaneously regardless of sexual activity; found in 12% of virginal adolescents; lower prevalence in postmenopausal women, even with use of hormones
Trichomoniasis (vaginal pH >4.5)		
Copious, malodorous, yellow-green (or discolored), frothy discharge; pruritus; vaginal irritation; dysuria No symptoms initially in ~50% of affected women Most men asymptomatic; serve as reservoirs of the infection	Vaginal erythema and possible irritation may occur.[13] Yellow discharge increases likelihood of trichomoniasis.	STI caused by *Trichomonas vaginalis* Risk factors: multiple sex partners, new sexual partner, nonuse of barrier contraceptives, and presence of other STIs Responsible for 15%–20% of vaginal infections
Vulvovaginal Candidiasis (no change in vaginal pH)		
Thick, white ("cottage cheese") discharge with no odor; normal pH (see text for detailed information; also referred to as "yeast infection" or "moniliasis")	Vaginal erythema, irritation, and/or itching, and absence of malodor increase likelihood of VVC; thick, "cheesy" discharge is strongly predictive of VVC.[13,16]	Organisms: *Candida albicans, Candida glabrata, Candida tropicalis,* and *Saccharomyces* Risk factors: medications such as antibiotics and immunosuppressants No identifiable cause for most infections Responsible for 20%–25% of vaginal infections

Key: BV, Bacterial vaginosis; IUD, intrauterine contraception; OC, oral contraceptive; STI, sexually transmitted infection; VVC, vulvovaginal candidiasis.

treatment for the actual condition. The risks of exposure to vaginal antifungal products in the absence of VVC include local irritation and the cost of therapy.[11] Labeling instructions advise patients to seek help for persistent symptoms. If these guidelines are followed, the delay in treatment from misdiagnosis will likely present few serious consequences.

One method to assist patients in appropriate self-care treatment is the use of pH devices to identify whether the vaginal pH is elevated, indicating a need for medical evaluation. One study compared patients' and their HCPs' use of pH devices to ensure ease and accuracy of use by the patient. Nearly 85% of patients obtained pH results similar to their HCPs' results. This outcome demonstrates the benefit and accuracy of patients' using such a tool as an important screening device to assist in self-diagnosis or to encourage further examination by an HCP.[12] The use of vaginal pH self-testing devices may also offer benefit in reducing inappropriate self-treatment with antifungal products.

Table 8–1 describes the classic symptoms of the three most common vaginal infections and the symptoms that women typically experience.[1,3,8,13–19]

VULVOVAGINAL CANDIDIASIS

VVC is also referred to as a *yeast infection* or *moniliasis.* This condition is one of the most common vaginal infections, with nearly 75% of women reporting at least one VVC infection over their lifetimes.[2] Recurrent infections occur in fewer than 5% of women.[3] Approximately 20% of women may be colonized with *C. albicans* but not experience vaginal symptoms.[2,20]

Pathophysiology of Vulvovaginal Candidiasis

Candida fungi are the causative organisms of VVC, with approximately 80%–92% of cases caused by *C. albicans.*[3] The incidence of non–*C. albicans* infections has increased in the past 2 decades.

Candida glabrata, Candida tropicalis, and *Saccharomyces cerevisiae* now account for approximately 10% of *Candida* vaginal infections.[3,6] This increase may be a result of the widespread use of nonprescription antifungals, short courses of topical imidazole therapy, and long-term suppressive therapy with imidazole antifungals.[3]

No single causative factor has been identified for most episodes of VVC. Pregnancy, high-dose combined oral contraceptives, and estrogen therapy may increase vaginal susceptibility to *Candida* vaginal infections by increasing the glycogen content of the vagina, although studies are inconsistent. Vaginal pH increases during menstruation, predisposing women to cyclic fungal vaginal infections. During the reproductive years, the vaginal epithelium cells are thick and contain an abundance of glycogen.[21] These cells exfoliate and continually provide the lactobacilli with the glycogen to produce lactic acid.[21] During and after the menopausal transition, the amount of glycogen declines, leading to decreased lactic acid production and an increased vaginal pH, and predisposes patients to vaginal infections. Women with diabetes are at increased risk for *Candida* vaginal infections, particularly if the glycemic control is poor. Antibiotics may also increase the risk of these infections. Between 25% and 70% of women in studies reported developing *Candida* vaginal infections during or just after treatment with antibiotics such as tetracycline, ampicillin/amoxicillin, and cephalosporins.[22] The proposed mechanism is a decrease in normal vaginal flora, especially lactobacilli, allowing an overgrowth of *Candida* organisms. However, neither an increase in vaginal *Candida* organisms nor a decrease in lactobacilli occurs in all women who take these antibiotics. In addition, patients who have received an organ transplant, have HIV infection, or are taking systemic corticosteroid, antineoplastic, or immunosuppressant drugs may also be at increased risk for developing *Candida* vaginal infections.

An increased frequency of VVC is associated with the onset of regular sexual activity. However, neither the number of sexual partners nor the frequency of sexual intercourse is related to occurrence of VVC episodes.[3] Evidence has suggested an increased risk of VVC associated with receptive oral sex.[1] In addition, use of an intrauterine or vaginal sponge contraceptive has increased the risk for VVC.[3]

A consistent association between tight-fitting, nonabsorbent clothing or pantyhose and the development of VVC has not been demonstrated. However, clothing of this type may increase risk by creating a warm and moist environment. Dietary factors may also be considered: consumption of yogurt has been proposed to provide a potential prophylactic benefit against VVC, but further research is needed.[23]

Treatment of *Candida* vaginal infections does not typically include treatment of the male partner, nor has such treatment been shown to prevent recurrence of *Candida* vaginal infections in women. In women who have recurrent infections or when male partners have balanitis, the men may be treated with a topical imidazole.[13] If treatment is necessary, topical imidazoles may be applied to the infected area twice a day for 2–4 weeks.

Clinical Presentation of Vulvovaginal Candidiasis

The characteristic signs and symptoms of VVC are described in Table 8–1. *Candida* vaginal infections typically do not alter vaginal pH, so a pH greater than 4.5 may indicate a bacterial or trichomonal vaginal infection.[24] Vaginal pH testing devices use pH to assist patients in distinguishing *Candida* vaginal infections that can be self-treated from infections that require medical evaluation and prescription drug therapy. The user-friendly kits use a color test to determine vaginal pH. Limitations with some products include the fact that testing cannot occur until 72 hours after the use of any vaginal preparation, such as a contraceptive spermicide or an antifungal product, and 48 hours after sexual intercourse or douching. In addition, the product cannot be used until 5 days after a menstrual period.

Treatment of Vulvovaginal Candidiasis

The treatment of VVC is determined by the severity of symptoms and the frequency of episodes. VVC can be categorized as uncomplicated or complicated, with recurrent VVC considered a complicated infection.[2] Recurrent or complicated infections are reported in approximately 5% of women; they may be related to host factors such as an inability of normal flora to prevent *Candida* colonization or the presence of potentially resistant organisms.[25]

Treatment Goals

The goals of therapy for vaginal fungal infections are relief of symptoms, eradication of the infection, and reestablishment of normal vaginal flora. A single course of drug therapy is effective in achieving these goals for most women. Some women will experience persistent or recurrent infections and will require prolonged therapy or higher dosages of medication.

General Treatment Approach

Self-treatment of VVC with nonprescription antifungal therapy is appropriate for women with uncomplicated disease, infrequent episodes, and mild–moderate symptoms. Women with more severe symptoms, predisposing illnesses or medications, or recurrent infections should be referred to their HCP for assessment and treatment.

Recurrent VVC occurs when a woman experiences at least four documented infections in a 1-year period.[3] Patients should be evaluated for the possibility of a mixed infection or a strain other than *C. albicans.* In addition, frequent or recurrent episodes of VVC may be an early sign of HIV infection or diabetes. The Food and Drug Administration (FDA) requires labels of nonprescription drug products to include a warning similar to the following[26]:

> Frequent vaginal infections or recurring infections that do not clear up easily with proper treatment require medical evaluation. Possible causes of the infection include pregnancy or a serious underlying medical disorder, such as diabetes or a weakened immune system including exposure to HIV, the virus that causes acquired immunodeficiency syndrome.

Preventive measures are not a standard part of therapy for *Candida* vaginal infections. Women with frequent or unresponsive infections may try dietary changes and other nondrug measures, such as not wearing nonabsorbent clothing. A 3- to 4-month trial of these approaches is sufficient to determine whether they are useful for individual patients.[1] Figure 8–1 outlines the approach to treating a patient with vaginal symptoms.

Exclusions for Self-Treatment

- Pregnancy
- Girls <12 years of age
- Concurrent symptoms: fever or pain in the pelvic area, lower abdomen, back, or shoulder
- Medications that can predispose to VVC: corticosteroids, antineoplastics
- Medical disorders that can predispose to VVC: diabetes, HIV infection
- Recurrent VVC (i.e., >3 vaginal infections per year or vaginal infection in past 2 months)
- First vulvovaginal episode

Source: Reference 13.

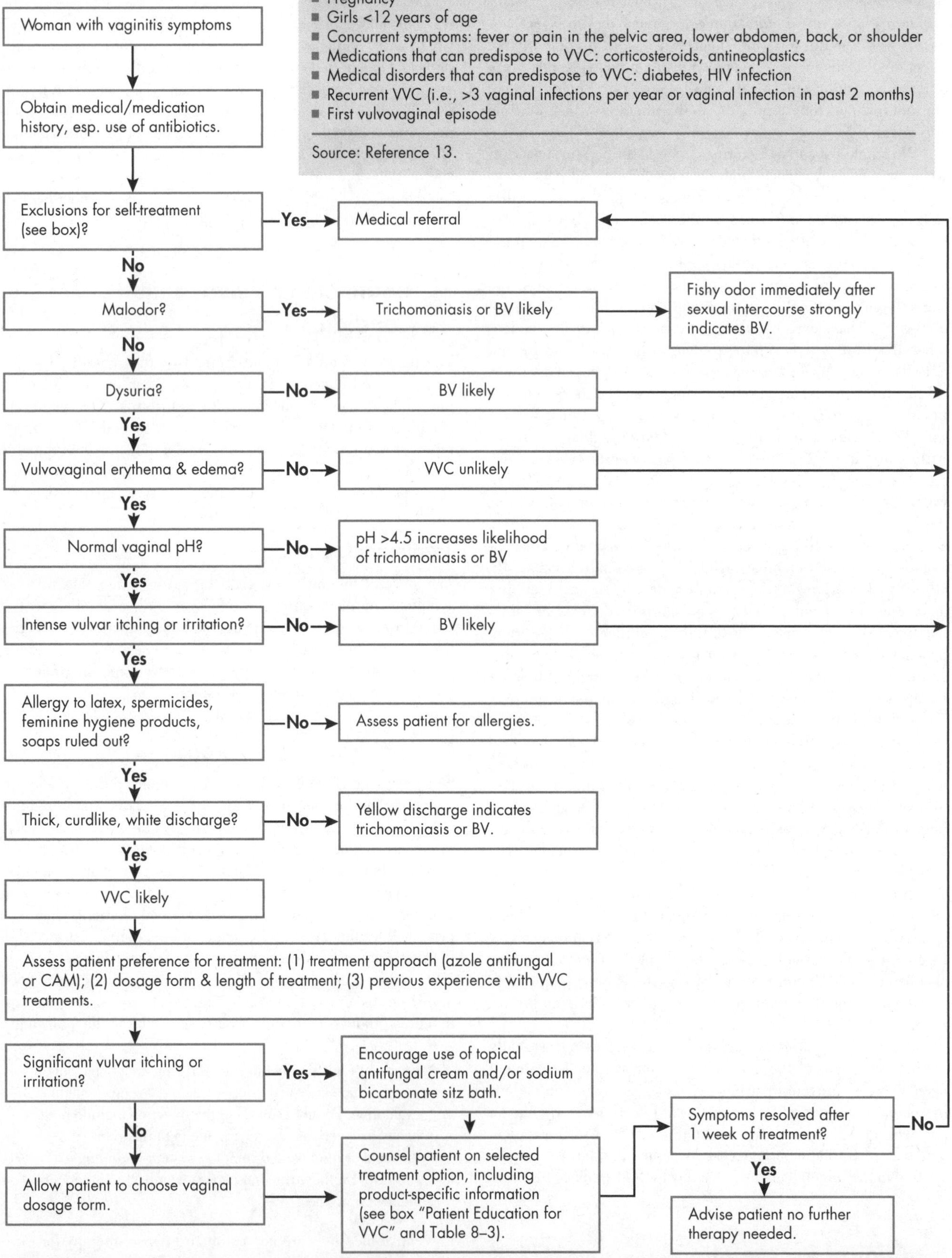

Woman with vaginitis symptoms
Obtain medical/medication history, esp. use of antibiotics.
Exclusions for self-treatment (see box)?
Yes
Medical referral
No
Malodor?
Yes
Trichomoniasis or BV likely
Fishy odor immediately after sexual intercourse strongly indicates BV.
No
Dysuria?
No
BV likely
Yes
Vulvovaginal erythema & edema?
No
VVC unlikely
Yes
Normal vaginal pH?
No
pH >4.5 increases likelihood of trichomoniasis or BV
Yes
Intense vulvar itching or irritation?
No
BV likely
Yes
Allergy to latex, spermicides, feminine hygiene products, soaps ruled out?
No
Assess patient for allergies.
Yes
Thick, curdlike, white discharge?
No
Yellow discharge indicates trichomoniasis or BV.
Yes
VVC likely
Assess patient preference for treatment: (1) treatment approach (azole antifungal or CAM); (2) dosage form & length of treatment; (3) previous experience with VVC treatments.
Significant vulvar itching or irritation?
Yes
Encourage use of topical antifungal cream and/or sodium bicarbonate sitz bath.
No
Allow patient to choose vaginal dosage form.
Counsel patient on selected treatment option, including product-specific information (see box "Patient Education for VVC" and Table 8–3).
Symptoms resolved after 1 week of treatment?
No
Yes
Advise patient no further therapy needed.

FIGURE 8–1 Self-care for vulvovaginal candidiasis. Key: BV = bacterial vaginosis; CAM = Complementary and alternative medicine; HIV = human immunodeficiency virus; VVC = vulvovaginal candidiasis. (Source: References 1, 3, 13, 15, and 16.)

Nonpharmacologic Therapy

Consumption of yogurt-containing live cultures may potentially decrease VVC episodes, particularly for women who experience recurrent infections.[1,23]

Discontinuing a drug known to increase susceptibility to *Candida* vaginal infections might be effective in decreasing the incidence. Low-dose oral contraceptives are unlikely to contribute to the occurrence of VVC, but they might be discontinued to determine whether the frequency of infection is altered. Another form of contraception should be recommended and initiated prior to discontinuing the oral contraceptive. Patients taking antibiotics or immunosuppressant drugs should consult their HCP about these medications.

Pharmacologic Therapy

Vaginal Antifungals

A nonprescription FDA-approved imidazole product is the recommended initial therapy for uncomplicated VVC and relief of external vulvar itching and irritation associated with the infection. Approved nonprescription drugs include clotrimazole, miconazole, and tioconazole, which are available as vaginal creams, suppositories, and tablets. Tables 8–2 and 8–3 provide proper dosing and administration guidelines, respectively.

The major effect of antifungals is altering the fungi's membrane permeability. These drugs inhibit cytochrome P450 (CYP) enzymes in the fungal cell membrane, thereby decreasing synthesis of the fungal sterol ergosterol. The reduced membrane content of ergosterol is accompanied by an increase in lanosterol-like methylated sterols. These sterols cause structural damage to fungal membranes, resulting in the loss of normal membrane function.

Systemic absorption of clotrimazole, miconazole, and tioconazole is about 3%–10%, 1.4%, and a negligible amount of a vaginal dose, respectively.[27] Adverse effects from topical imidazoles include vulvovaginal burning, itching, and irritation in 3%–7% of patients.[28–30] These adverse effects are more likely to occur with the initial application of the vaginal preparation and are similar to symptoms of the vaginal infection. This vaginal irritation may be dose-related; therefore selecting a product formulation with a longer course and lower strength may help. Abdominal cramps (3%), penile irritation, and allergic reactions (3%–7%) are uncommon, and headache may occur in up to 9% of women.[1]

Drug interactions are unlikely because absorption of the antifungals is limited. However, a documented interaction between

TABLE 8–2 Selected Nonprescription Vaginal Antifungal Products and Their Dosages

Trade Name	Primary Ingredient	Dosage
Clotrimazole Products		
Gyne-Lotrimin 7 Cream Mycelex-7 Cream	Clotrimazole 1%	Insert cream into vagina daily for 7 days; apply to vulva twice daily as needed for itching.
Mycelex-7 Combination Pack	Tablet: clotrimazole 100 mg Cream: clotrimazole 1%[b]	Insert tablet into vagina daily for 7 days; apply cream to vulva twice daily as needed for itching up to 7 days.
Gyne-Lotrimin 3 Cream	Clotrimazole 2%	Insert cream into vagina daily for 3 days; apply to vulva twice daily for itching.
Miconazole Nitrate Products		
Monistat 1 Combination Pack Day or Night	Cream: miconazole nitrate 2%[b] Suppository: miconazole nitrate 1200 mg	Apply cream to vulva twice daily as needed for itching up to 7 days; insert suppository into vagina daily (morning or at bedtime) for 1 day.
Monistat 3 Combination Pack[a] Vagistat 3 Combination Pack[a]	Cream: miconazole nitrate 2%[b] Suppository: miconazole nitrate 200 mg	Apply cream to vulva twice daily as needed for itching up to 7 days; insert suppository into vagina daily for 3 days.
Monistat 3 Cream[a]	Miconazole nitrate 4%	Insert cream into vagina daily for 3 days; apply to vulva twice daily as needed for itching.
Monistat 7 Suppository	Miconazole nitrate 100 mg	Insert suppository into vagina daily for 7 days at bedtime.
Monistat 7 Cream	Miconazole nitrate 2%	Insert cream into vagina daily for 7 days; apply to vulva twice daily as needed for itching.
Monistat 7 Combination Pack	Cream: miconazole nitrate 2%[b] Suppository: miconazole nitrate 100 mg	Apply cream to vulva twice daily as needed for itching up to 7 days; insert suppository into vagina daily for 7 days.
Tioconazole Products		
Vagistat-1 Ointment 1-Day Monistat-1 Day	Tioconazole 6.5%	Insert ointment into vagina daily for 1 day.

[a] Prefilled applicators are available for this product.

[b] Use for more than 7 days is not recommended. If no symptom relief occurs, patients should see their HCP.

TABLE 8-3 Guidelines for Applying Vaginal Antifungal Products

1. Start treatment at night before going to bed. Lying down will reduce leakage of the product from the vagina.
2. Wash the entire vaginal area with mild soap and water, and dry completely before applying the product.
3. *Vaginal cream:* (If prefilled applicators are being used, skip to step 4.) Unscrew the cap; place the cap upside down on the end of the tube. Push down firmly until the seal is broken. Attach the applicator to the tube by turning the applicator clockwise. Squeeze the tube from the bottom to force the cream into the applicator. Squeeze until the inside piece of the applicator is pushed out as far as possible and the applicator is completely filled with cream. Remove the applicator from the tube. *Vaginal tablets or suppositories:* Remove the wrapper and place the product into the end of the applicator barrel.
4. While standing with feet slightly apart and knees bent, as shown in drawing A, or while lying on your back with knees bent, as shown in drawing B, gently insert the applicator into the vagina as far as it will go comfortably.
5. Push in the inside piece of the applicator, and place the cream as far back in the vagina as possible. To deposit vaginal tablets or suppositories, insert the applicator into the vagina and press the plunger until it stops.
6. Remove the applicator from the vagina.
7. After use, recap the tube (if using cream). Then clean the reusable applicator by pulling the two pieces apart and washing them with soap and warm water. Throw away disposable applicators after 1 use.
8. If desired, wear a sanitary pad to absorb leakage of the vaginal antifungal. Do not use a tampon to absorb leakage, as this will absorb the medication and reduce its efficacy.
9. Continue using the product for the length of time specified in the product instructions. Use the product every day without skipping any days, even during menstrual flow.

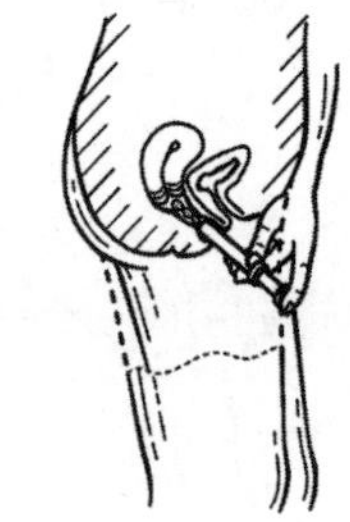

A

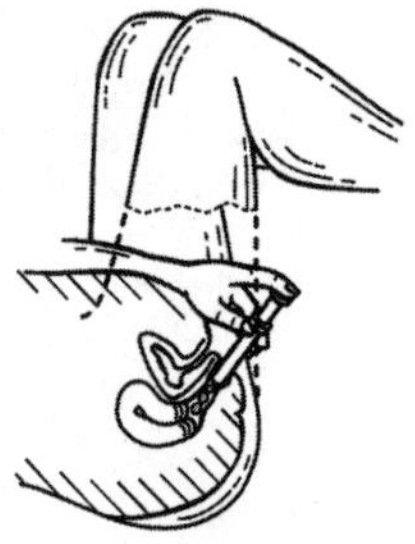

B

miconazole vaginal suppositories and warfarin indicates that their concomitant use might pose an increased bleeding risk, because both medications are metabolized by CYP2C9.[31] Therefore, pharmacists should contact a patient's HCP about reducing the dosage of warfarin during concurrent therapy to avoid an increase in the patient's international normalized ratio (INR). The product information advises women using warfarin in combination with these products that bleeding or bruising might occur. Aside from an allergy to imidazoles, contraindications do not exist with the use of topical imidazoles.

Pharmacotherapeutic Comparison

Studies have shown the imidazoles to be equally effective, with effectiveness rates of about 80%–90%.[3,13] A comparison of miconazole single-dose and 7-day treatments has shown similar overall cure rates, with significantly faster rates of symptom relief by day 3 in the single-dose group compared with the 7-day treatment group.[32] Nonprescription antifungals are available as 7-day regimens of clotrimazole and miconazole; 3-day regimens of clotrimazole and miconazole; and 1-day regimens of clotrimazole, miconazole, and tioconazole. Miconazole nitrate (Monistat 1 Combination pack) has also been approved for insertion in the morning or at bedtime, allowing flexible scheduling for patients. A similar cure rate exists for the daytime and bedtime treatments.[33]

Several other nonprescription vaginal preparations, such as Vagisil cream, containing benzocaine and resorcinol, are also available. These agents may provide relief of itching, but the underlying cause is not addressed. HCPs should counsel patients on the possible risk of methemoglobinemia associated with benzocaine-containing products.[34] Therefore, the use of these agents is rarely, if ever, appropriate given the benefits of the imidazole antifungals, including superior efficacy, improved patient adherence, less frequent local reactions, reduced associated adverse effects, and shorter treatment durations. Rarely, these products and medicated douches may be reserved for vaginal and vulvar irritation and itching; they should be used for a limited time only and on the advice of an HCP (Table 8–4).

TABLE 8-4 Selected Nonprescription Drug Products for Vaginal Itching and Irritation

Trade Name	Primary Ingredients
Benzocaine Products[a]	
Vagisil Anti-Itch Original Formula	Benzocaine 5%; resorcinol 2%
Vagisil Maximum Strength	Benzocaine 20%; resorcinol 3%
Hydrocortisone Products[b]	
Cortizone-10 Feminine Relief	Hydrocortisone 1%
Povidone/Iodine Products	
Summer's Eve Medicated Douche	Povidone/iodine 0.3% (in disposable bottles)
Homeopathic Products	
Yeast-Gard Suppository[c]	*Pulsatilla* (27×); *Candida albicans* (27×) *Candida parapsilosis* (27×)
Yeast-Gard gel treatment[d]	*Pulsatilla* (27×); *Candida albicans* (27×) *Candida parapsilosis* (27×)
Other Products	
Summer's Eve Feminine Powder[e]	
Vagisil Feminine Powder[e]	Cornstarch; aloe; mineral oil (in Summer's Eve)

[a] Apply benzocaine products externally.
[b] Apply hydrocortisone products externally; avoid prolonged use; may use concomitantly with antifungal products.
[c] Use 1 Yeast-Gard suppository daily for 7 days.
[d] Use 1 Yeast-Gard gel treatment daily as needed.
[e] Apply feminine powders externally to absorb moisture.

Product Selection Guidelines

Special Populations

Self-treatment of VVC is not appropriate for girls younger than 12 years. This condition is rare in premenarchal girls. Vaginal symptoms in this age group warrant a medical referral to determine the cause, because infections in prepubertal children may indicate potential sexual abuse.[35]

Self-care in pregnancy is not appropriate. However, when treatment of VVC is indicated, treatment should consist of clotrimazole, miconazole, or tioconazole. When possible, treatment should be withheld during the first trimester.[35] The HCP should evaluate for complications, such as hyperglycemia, and assess for other organisms, because BV and trichomoniasis have the potential for adverse pregnancy outcomes. No special considerations are necessary to treat breastfeeding or older, immunocompetent women presenting with a VVC infection.[13]

Patient Preferences

Selection of cream, tablet, or suppository formulations can be left to the patient, because some women may prefer the convenience of prefilled applicators. Women who have previously experienced VVC may prefer shorter courses of therapy than do those who have not had a prior infection.[1] Once VVC is confirmed, the decision regarding which product to select should be patient specific.[36] If vulvar symptoms are significant, a cream preparation or the combination of a cream with vaginal suppositories or tablets is preferred. Morning or bedtime dosing is available to provide flexibility for patients.

Complementary Therapies

An alternative approach to treating VVC is the use of *Lactobacillus* preparations. The rationale for their use is to reestablish normal vaginal flora and inhibit overgrowth of *Candida* organisms. Data on the effectiveness of this approach are limited and inconsistent. One study of 5 women with positive vaginal cultures for *C. albicans* found 4 women had negative cultures after administration of *Lactobacillus rhamnosus* GG suppositories for 7 days.[23] Another study examining the usefulness of *Lactobacillus* and other probiotic bacteria administered orally, vaginally, and by both routes found that none of the regimens protected against the development of postantibiotic VVC.[37] However, eating 8 ounces of yogurt with live cultures daily may be of some benefit in preventing recurrent VVC.[23] Nonprescription probiotic feminine supplements may be used to reestablish *Lactobacillus*. RepHresh Pro-B probiotic feminine supplement is an easy-to-use, but expensive, product (about $25–$30 for a 30-day supply). Patients take 1 capsule by mouth daily. (See Chapter 20, Table 20–2, for information about probiotics used in vaginosis and vaginitis.)

A sodium bicarbonate sitz bath may provide prompt, temporary relief of vulvar irritation associated with a *Candida* vaginal infection before antifungal agents can provide noticeable benefit.[38]

To manage VVC, some women may prefer natural products such as a vaginal preparation of tea tree oil, which has antibacterial and antifungal properties.[39,40] A 200-mg vaginal suppository containing tea tree oil is available commercially and is used once daily for 6 consecutive nights. Allergic dermatitis may occur. (For information on tea tree oil, see Chapter 51.)

Gentian violet, a dye available in community pharmacies, is an old treatment for VVC. Today, topical gentian violet is used for resistant *Candida* vaginal infections.[41] A tampon may be soaked in gentian violet and inserted into the vagina for several hours or overnight. Often a single application is adequate, but tampons saturated with gentian violet can be used once or twice a day for up to 5 consecutive days.

Another option for the treatment of VVC is boric acid 600 mg in a size 0 gelatin capsule inserted vaginally once daily for 14 days.[3,13,42] Boric acid therapy is useful for non–*C. albicans* infections, which are more likely to be resistant to the imidazole antifungals. Short-term cure rates with boric acid demonstrate efficacy, with approximate cure rates of 70% when used in women whose infection did not respond to vaginal antifungals.[9,13,42,43] For resistant infections, the therapy is used twice weekly for longer durations. Boric acid can be toxic and teratogenic, and human fatalities have been reported from oral ingestion.[44] Boric acid capsules may be compounded in community pharmacies. Patient counseling should stress that the capsule not be ingested. In addition, pregnant women should not use boric acid.

Assessment of Vulvovaginal Candidiasis: A Case-Based Approach

Many episodes of VVC are uncomplicated and can be effectively treated by topical imidazole agents.[3] In particular, the best candidates for self-treatment are otherwise healthy women who experience episodes that are sporadic and uncomplicated and women who predictably experience VVC following a course of antibiotic therapy.[22]

Determining the appropriateness of self-care and the likelihood of a *Candida* vaginal infection are important initial steps in advising a woman about the management of vaginal symptoms with nonprescription drug therapy.

HCPs may advise patients when it is appropriate to self-treat for vaginal symptoms that are consistent with VVC, and when medical evaluation, including pelvic examination and laboratory examination of vaginal secretions, is indicated. Self-treatment is most appropriate when a woman meets the following four criteria[13]:

1. Vaginal symptoms are infrequent (i.e., no more than 3 vaginal infections per year and no vaginal infection within the past 2 months).
2. A medical professional diagnosed at least 1 previous episode of VVC.
3. Symptoms are mild–moderate and consistent with the characteristic signs and symptoms of VVC, particularly in that the discharge does not have a foul odor.
4. If measured, vaginal pH is 4.5 or lower.

Case 8–1 provides an example of the assessment of a patient presenting with a vaginal infection.

Patient Counseling for Vulvovaginal Candidiasis

Counseling of patients who are considering self-treatment with vaginal antifungals should emphasize limiting self-treatment to the presence of mild-moderate classic symptoms, infrequent vaginal symptoms, and predictable antibiotic-associated VVC. Patients with possible recurrent infections or with predisposing illnesses are not candidates for self-care; they should be advised to see their HCP and may require treatment with prescription

CASE 8-1

Relevant Evaluation Criteria	Scenario/Model Outcome
Collect	
1. Gather essential information about the patient's symptoms and medical history, including	
a. Description of symptom(s) (i.e., nature, onset, duration, severity, associated symptoms)	Patient reports experiencing vaginal itching with discharge and redness for the past 2 days but states she has not noticed an odor.
b. Description of any factors that seem to precipitate, exacerbate, and/or relieve the patient's symptom(s)	Patient reports experiencing these symptoms all throughout the day and night.
c. Description of the patient's efforts to relieve the symptoms	Patient reports that she has not tried anything yet.
d. Patient's identity	Emma Givenly
e. Patient's age, weight, gender, and height	29 years old, 5 ft 4 in., female, 130 lb
f. Patient's occupation	Administrative assistant
g. Patient's dietary habits	Reports eating 3 meals/day but states that she does sometimes miss lunch due to work meetings.
h. Patient's sleep habits	Reports sleeping about 6 hours each night usually.
i. Concurrent medical conditions, prescription and nonprescription medications, and dietary supplements	Minastrin 24 Fe 1 daily; ibuprofen 200 mg occasionally for headaches
j. Allergies/other adverse reactions to medications	NKDA
k. History of other adverse reactions to medications	None
l. Other (describe)	Per Emma's medical history, she was diagnosed with a previous VVC infection 3 years ago. Upon further inquiry, she indicates her current discharge is white and states it reminds her of her previous VVC infection.
Assess	
2. Differentiate patient's signs/symptoms, and correctly identify the patient's primary problem(s) (Table 8–1).	Emma has itching, vaginal redness, and white discharge without an odor, symptoms consistent with a *Candida* vaginal infection.
3. Identify exclusions for self-treatment (Figure 8–1).	None
4. Formulate a comprehensive list of therapeutic alternatives for the primary problem to determine whether triage to a medical practitioner is required, and share this information with the patient or caregiver.	Options include (1) Refer Emma for medical evaluation with her HCP. (2) Recommend self-treatment to Emma with an OTC vaginal antifungal product. (3) Take no action.
Plan	
5. Select an optimal therapeutic alternative to address the patient's problem, taking into account patient preferences.	Emma has symptoms associated with an uncomplicated VVC infection. She has had a previous VVC infection and reports no chronic medical problems. She is a candidate for self-treatment. (See Figure 8–1.)
6. Describe the recommended therapeutic approach to the patient or caregiver.	"There are several nonprescription vaginal antifungal products available. Given you have vulvar itching, a combination product with a suppository and a cream may be preferred to assist in relieving your symptoms." (See the box "Patient Education for Vulvovaginal Candidiasis" for instructions on proper use.)
7. Explain to the patient or caregiver the rationale for selecting the recommended therapeutic approach from the considered therapeutic alternatives.	"This treatment is appropriate because you have symptoms common with vulvovaginal candidiasis infections, your symptoms are mild to moderate, and you have no contraindications or exclusions to self-treatment. It is recommended that you see your health care provider if your symptoms do not improve within 3 days or are not gone within 1 week; if the vaginal discharge changes (especially if it becomes malodorous or changes presentation from white to yellow); or if your symptoms return within the next 2 months."

CASE 8-1 *continued*

Relevant Evaluation Criteria	Scenario/Model Outcome
Implement	
8. When recommending self-care with nonprescription medications and/or nondrug therapy, convey accurate information to the patient or caregiver.	
a. Appropriate dose and frequency of administration	"Insert the miconazole cream vaginally once daily for 3 days; apply externally to the vulva as needed for itching up to 7 days."
b. Maximum number of days the therapy should be employed	"Apply the cream for 3 days."
c. Product administration procedures	See Table 8–3.
d. Expected time to onset of relief	"Relief should occur within the first 3 days; often initial relief occurs within hours of the first application."
e. Degree of relief that can be reasonably expected	"All symptoms typically resolve within 1 week after beginning treatment."
f. Most common adverse effects	"Vulvovaginal burning and itching are the most common adverse effects."
g. Adverse effects that warrant medical intervention should they occur	"Significant stinging, burning, or itching that persists beyond the first 48 hours of treatment should be medically evaluated."
h. Patient options in the event that condition worsens or persists	"See your health care provider if symptoms do not improve in 3 days or worsen."
i. Product storage requirements	"The product should be stored in a cool area; storage in the bathroom or bedside is appropriate for ease of use."
j. Specific nondrug measures	None
Solicit follow-up questions from patient or caregiver.	(1) "Are any of the nonprescription vaginal antifungal products more effective than another?" (2) "Should I also use the nonprescription Vagisil Maximum Strength product to help with the itching?"
Answer patient's or caregiver's questions.	(1) "No, all of the products and regimens are equally effective in treating this infection." (2) "These agents may offer relief of itching, but they do not treat the cause. The use of this product is not needed given the benefits of the nonprescription antifungal you are using, which has high efficacy and safety."
Follow-up: Monitor and Evaluate	
9. Assess patient response.	Ask the patient to call you regarding her treatment outcome. Or you could call her in a week to evaluate her response to the treatment. You called the patient 1 week later, and she reported that her symptoms had resolved.

Key: HCP = Health care provider; NKDA = no known drug allergy; OTC = over-the-counter; VVC = vulvovaginal candidiasis.

options. Therefore, a medical evaluation should be obtained if symptoms persist beyond 1 week after treatment or if they recur within 2 months. Also, if vaginal symptoms occur more than 3 times in a 12-month interval, further evaluation is needed. Women taking warfarin should be referred to their primary care provider.

Patients should be informed that a 1- to 7-day course of a nonprescription vaginal antifungal product will kill the "yeast" organisms that caused the infection. Label instructions should be reviewed with the patient. Use of the product only once a day for the specified length of time should be stressed. Patients should be advised that symptomatic relief will likely begin within 2–3 days but that it may take a week for complete resolution of symptoms. The patient should also be advised of signs and symptoms that indicate medical attention is needed. The box Patient Education for Vulvovaginal Candidiasis lists specific information to provide patients.

Evaluation of Patient Outcomes for Vulvovaginal Candidiasis

Symptoms of VVC should improve within 2 or 3 days of initiation of therapy and resolve within 1 week. The length of treatment, particularly for 1- to 3-day treatments, does not directly correspond to the time of resolution of symptoms.

The HCP should advise patients to call if symptoms persist, and women should understand the importance of adherence.

PATIENT EDUCATION FOR Vulvovaginal Candidiasis

The goals of self-treatment are to cure the vaginal fungal infection and reestablish normal vaginal flora. Carefully following the product instructions and the self-care measures will help ensure optimal therapeutic outcomes.

Nondrug Measures

- If significant irritation of the vulva is present, use a sodium bicarbonate sitz bath to provide relief and give the antifungal medication time to become effective.
  - Add 1 teaspoon sodium bicarbonate to 1 pint of water.
  - Add 2–4 tablespoons of the solution to 2 inches of bath water.
  - Sit in the sitz bath or bathtub for 15 minutes as needed for symptom control.
- For recurrent infections, try eating yogurt (1 cup per day of live culture yogurt) and decreasing dietary sugar and refined carbohydrates.

Nonprescription Medications

- Insert the antifungal product into the vagina once a day, preferably at bedtime to minimize leakage from the vagina. Use a sanitary pad or panty liner to avoid staining of underwear.
- Table 8–3 provides instructions on administering vaginal antifungals. Significant relief of symptoms should occur within 24–48 hours, and relief is often apparent within hours after the first dose. However, the length of treatment (particularly for 1- to 3-day treatments) does not directly correspond to the time of resolution of symptoms.
- Continue the therapy for the recommended length of time, even if symptoms are gone. Stopping treatment early is a common reason for recurrence of vaginal symptoms and, possibly, occurrence of difficult-to-treat organisms.
- Vaginal antifungals can be used during a menstrual period. If desired, wait and treat the infection after menses ends. Do not interrupt a course of therapy if menses begins.
- Do not use tampons or douche while using a vaginal antifungal and for 3 days after use.
- Although adverse effects are uncommon, the first dose of the antifungal may cause some vaginal burning and irritation, and a few women (about 1 in 10) experience a headache.
- Refrain from sexual intercourse during treatment with the vaginal antifungal. Vaginal lubricants and vaginal spermicides should not be used at the same time as the vaginal antifungal. Vaginal antifungals can damage latex condoms and diaphragms and may result in unreliable contraceptive effects. Do not use these contraceptives during therapy or for 3 days after therapy, because the antifungal medication remains in the vagina for several days.

When to Seek Medical Attention

- Do not use vaginal antifungals if
  - You have not been medically diagnosed with VVC at least once.
  - You are younger than 12 years old.
  - You are pregnant.
  - You have diabetes; are human immunodeficiency virus (HIV)-positive or have acquired immunodeficiency syndrome (AIDS); or have impaired immune function, including use of medications that may impair function of the immune system.
  - You are using warfarin.
- If you are breastfeeding, consult a health care provider before using a vaginal antifungal.

When to Seek Medical Attention

- Seek medical attention if symptoms do not improve within 3 days or symptoms persist beyond 7 days.
- Seek medical attention if vaginal symptoms worsen or change, especially if the vaginal secretions begin to smell bad, become frothy, or become discolored, or if other symptoms (e.g., abdominal tenderness) occur. These events may indicate that the *Candida* (yeast) organisms are resistant to the nonprescription therapy or that another type of vaginal infection is present.

Persistent or new symptoms that are not consistent with VVC are reasons for advising the patient to seek a medical referral.

ATROPHIC VAGINITIS

Atrophic vaginitis is inflammation of the vagina related to atrophy of the vaginal mucosa secondary to decreased estrogen levels.

Although up to 45% of postmenopausal women may experience symptomatic atrophic vaginitis, only 25% may seek treatment.[45–47] *Dyspareunia,* or painful intercourse, is a symptom sometimes related to inadequate vaginal lubrication or atrophic vaginitis.

Pathophysiology of Atrophic Vaginitis

During menopause, the postpartum period, and breastfeeding, the vaginal epithelium becomes thin, and vaginal lubrication declines secondary to a decrease in estrogen levels. Women may experience atrophic vaginitis and dyspareunia during these intervals.[47] Atrophic vaginitis may also occur among women with decreased ovarian estrogen production, such as that caused by radiation or chemotherapy. Women taking gonadotropin-releasing hormone (GnRH) agonists, antiestrogenic drugs, and aromatase inhibitors may also develop atrophic vaginitis.[47]

Clinical Presentation of Atrophic Vaginitis

Atrophic vaginitis is associated with a decrease in vaginal lubrication.[47] Other symptoms include vaginal irritation, dryness, burning, itching, leukorrhea, and dyspareunia. A thin, watery (occasionally bloody), or yellow malodorous vaginal discharge or "spotting" may also be present.[3,6,47] Sexual activity may result in vaginal bleeding or spotting. A new episode of postmenopausal vaginal bleeding should have a medical referral to rule out endometrial cancer.

Treatment of Atrophic Vaginitis

Self-treatment of atrophic vaginitis is limited to alleviating the primary symptom, vaginal dryness, with lubricant products. To prevent vaginal dryness in women experiencing moderate-severe symptoms, the use of estrogen therapy may be required. Women who are breastfeeding or have recently given birth often have temporary declines in estrogen levels. Vaginal lubricants may be needed only until estrogen levels return to normal.

Treatment Goals

The goals of therapy are to reduce or eliminate the symptoms of vaginal dryness, burning, and itching, and to eliminate dyspareunia if vaginal dryness is the cause of painful sexual intercourse, by providing lubrication to vaginal tissue.

General Treatment Approach

Vaginal dryness may often be treated with a variety of lubricants such as those listed in Table 8–5. Self-treatment is appropriate when the symptoms are mild-moderate and confined to the vaginal area and when no bleeding is present. Women with severe vaginal dryness, dyspareunia, or bleeding should be referred for medical evaluation.

Figure 8–2 outlines the approach to treating vaginal dryness associated with atrophic vaginitis.

TABLE 8-5 Selected Nonprescription Vaginal Lubricants

Trade Names	Primary Ingredients
Astroglide; K-Y Personal Lubricant Liquid[a]	Glycerin; propylene glycol; hydroxyethylcellulose
K-Y Liquibeads	Glycerin; dimethicone; dimethiconol; gelatin
K-Y Warming Liquid Personal Lubricant	Propylene glycol; hydroxypropylcellulose; tocopherol; PEG 8
Replens Gel Silky Smooth Personal Lubricant	Glycerin; mineral oil

Key: PEG = Polyethylene glycol.

[a] Fragrance-free formulation.

Pharmacologic Therapy

Vaginal Lubricants

Multiple water-soluble products, including Astroglide, K-Y Jelly, and Replens, are available for vaginal lubrication. Personal lubricant products temporarily moisten vaginal tissues. These products

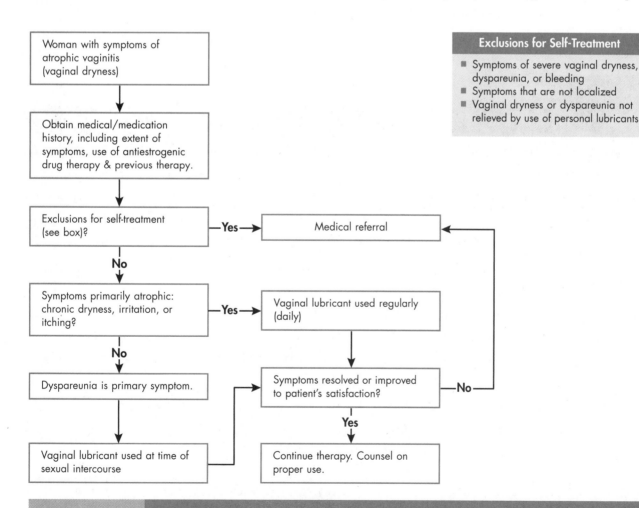

Exclusions for Self-Treatment

- Symptoms of severe vaginal dryness, dyspareunia, or bleeding
- Symptoms that are not localized
- Vaginal dryness or dyspareunia not relieved by use of personal lubricants

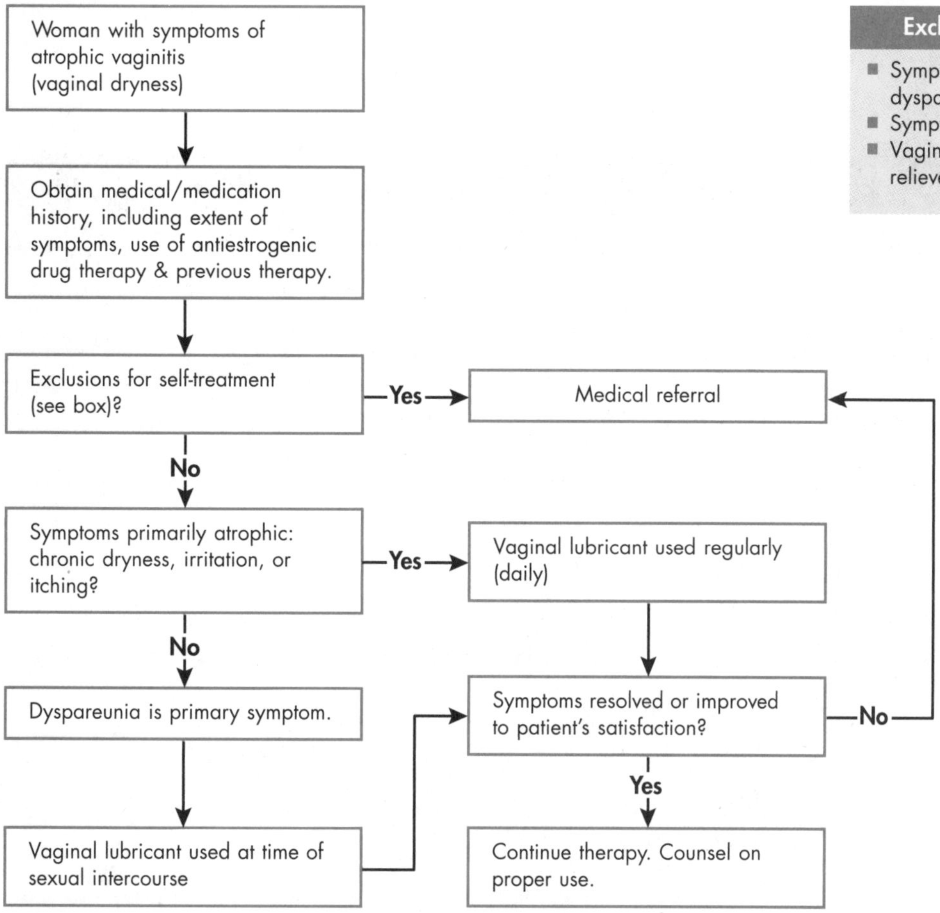

FIGURE 8–2 Self-care for atrophic vaginitis. (Source: Reference 47.)

provide short-term improvement in symptoms such as burning and itching. Personal lubricants can also provide vaginal lubrication to facilitate sexual intercourse.[47]

Petroleum jelly should not be used because it is difficult to remove from the vagina. Only water-soluble lubricants should be used with a latex condom or diaphragm, because other products may damage the latex and impair the efficacy of these contraceptive methods. Water-soluble lubricant gels can be applied both externally and internally. Initially, the patient should be instructed to use a liberal quantity of lubricant (≤2 teaspoons) and then to tailor the quantity and frequency of use to her specific needs. If the patient is treating dyspareunia, the lubricant should be applied to both the vaginal opening and the penis. If the use of lubricants does not produce adequate benefit or is esthetically unappealing to the patient, she should be referred for medical evaluation.

Assessment of Atrophic Vaginitis: A Case-Based Approach

When discussing symptoms of vaginal dryness during the patient assessment, the HCP should obtain a description of symptoms, including their association with sexual intercourse and their severity. The HCP should also ask if the woman has recently given birth, is lactating, or is perimenopausal or postmenopausal. The HCP should also ask patients about the use of any vaginal or feminine hygiene products that may cause or worsen vaginal irritation and dyspareunia.

Case 8–2 provides an example of the assessment of a patient presenting with atrophic vaginitis.

Patient Counseling for Atrophic Vaginitis

The HCP should stress the short-term nature of atrophic vaginitis to women who are breastfeeding or who have recently given birth. Women who are perimenopausal or postmenopausal should know that long-term treatment with vaginal lubricants may be necessary. In either case, the HCP should explain the proper use of the lubricants for treatment of vaginal dryness or dyspareunia. The box "Patient Education for Atrophic Vaginitis" lists specific information.

Evaluation of Patient Outcomes for Atrophic Vaginitis

Symptoms of atrophic vaginitis typically improve within a week. The HCP should advise the patient to call to discuss treatment effectiveness if concerns arise, and to call after 1 week of treatment to report progress in symptom resolution. Symptoms that persist or the presence of bleeding requires medical evaluation.

CASE 8–2

Relevant Evaluation Criteria	Scenario/Model Outcome
Collect	
1. Gather essential information about the patient's symptoms and medical history, including	
a. Description of symptom(s) (i.e., nature, onset, duration, severity, associated symptoms)	Patient is experiencing vaginal dryness and burning with bothersome dyspareunia and reports experiencing these symptoms for several weeks.
b. Description of any factors that seem to precipitate, exacerbate, and/or relieve the patient's symptom(s)	Symptoms are worse during intercourse.
c. Description of the patient's efforts to relieve the symptoms.	Patient reports that she has tried OTC lubricants, but relief has been minimal.
d. Patient's identity	Gia Gardner
e. Patient's age, gender, height, and weight	51 years old, female, 5 ft 5 in., 140 lb
f. Patient's occupation	Elementary school teacher
g. Patient's dietary habits	Reports eating 3 meals per day with 2 snacks as needed and indicates that she focuses on selecting foods low in saturated fat.
h. Patient's sleep habits	Reports sleeping 6–7 hours per night.
i. Concurrent medical conditions, prescription and nonprescription medications, and dietary supplements	Simvastatin 20 mg every night; daily multivitamin
j. Allergies/other adverse reactions to medications	Sulfa: rash
k. History of other adverse reactions to medications	None
l. Other (describe) ______	Gia is postmenopausal and experiencing vaginal dryness, burning, and bothersome dyspareunia not relieved by OTC lubricants. Per her medical history, she has no prior use of estrogen therapy. She also reports a history of a hysterectomy 2 years ago.

CASE 8-2 *continued*

Relevant Evaluation Criteria	Scenario/Model Outcome
Assess	
2. Differentiate patient's signs/symptoms, and correctly identify the patient's primary problem(s).	Gia is postmenopausal. She has vaginal dryness and burning with bothersome dyspareunia but no symptoms indicative of other vaginal infections. These symptoms are consistent with atrophic vaginitis.
3. Identify exclusions for self-treatment (Figure 8–2).	She has vaginal dryness with bothersome dyspareunia as a primary symptom and she has tried OTC lubricants with minimal relief.
4. Formulate a comprehensive list of therapeutic alternatives for the primary problem to determine whether triage to a medical practitioner is required and share this information with the patient or caregiver.	Options include (1) Assess how often Gia is using the OTC lubricants and advise her to use the lubricants daily in addition to using during intercourse until she can see her HCP. (2) Refer Gia to her HCP for possible vaginal estrogen therapy. (3) Take no action.
Plan	
5. Select an optimal therapeutic alternative to address the patient's problem, taking into account patient preferences.	Because Gia has bothersome dyspareunia as a primary symptom and has tried OTC lubricants with minimal relief, she is not a candidate for self-care. The recommended option for this patient would be to see her HCP to further assess her dyspareunia and vaginal dryness and burning in addition to exploring the use of vaginal estrogen therapy to relieve her symptoms.
6. Describe the recommended therapeutic approach to the patient or caregiver.	See the box "Patient Education for Atrophic Vaginitis."
7. Explain to the patient or caregiver the rationale for selecting the recommended therapeutic approach from the considered therapeutic alternatives.	"With your vaginal dryness and dyspareunia symptoms, I recommend that you follow up with your health care provider to consider the use of a vaginal estrogen product, such as tablets. They are generally more effective than lubricants and moisturizers for atrophic vaginitis, such as the product you have been trying. However, you may still use your nonprescription lubricant to assist you with some symptom relief until you see your health care provider."
Implement	
8. When recommending self-care with nonprescription medications and/or nondrug therapy, convey accurate information to the patient or caregiver.	Criterion does not apply to this case.
Solicit follow-up questions from patient or caregiver.	(1) "I was using my lubricant only every few days. How much more often should I try using this nonprescription lubricant?" (2) "Will I have to take oral estrogen or will vaginal estrogen work?"
Answer patient's or caregiver's questions.	(1) "A liberal quantity (2 teaspoons) of nonprescription lubricants may be used. You may use the lubricant daily or as frequently as needed, in addition to using it during intercourse to reduce vaginal dryness." (2) "Oral estrogen therapy is typically not needed for the treatment of atrophic vaginitis, because vaginal estrogen products (creams or tablets) are appropriate options."
Follow-up: Monitor and Evaluate	
9. Assess patient outcome.	Contact the patient in 1–2 days to follow up and confirm she has made an appointment for further evaluation and medical care.

Key: HCP = Health care provider; OTC = over-the-counter.

PATIENT EDUCATION FOR Atrophic Vaginitis

The objective of self-treatment with vaginal lubricants is to relieve vaginal dryness and pain during sexual intercourse related to atrophic vaginitis. Carefully following product instructions and the self-care measures listed here will help to ensure optimal therapeutic outcomes.

- Apply the vaginal lubricant as frequently as needed for relief of vaginal dryness, irritation, burning, itching, or inadequate vaginal lubrication.
- Begin treatment of atrophic symptoms with a liberal quantity of lubricant (2 teaspoons); tailor subsequent doses to the quantity and frequency of use needed to provide relief.
- If using lubricants at the time of sexual intercourse, apply the lubricant to the vagina, particularly at the vaginal opening, and to the penis.
- Some leakage of product will occur. If desired, use a sanitary napkin or panty liner to avoid staining of underwear.
- Relief of symptoms may be apparent within hours after the first dose. Regular application of a lubricant can reverse atrophic symptoms to some extent.
- If no improvement is noticeable within a week, or if symptoms worsen or there is any vaginal bleeding, see your primary care provider.

VAGINAL DOUCHING

Prevalence of Douching

The Centers for Disease Control and Prevention reports that 18.8% of U.S. women practice douching.[48] Douching rates are influenced by race, geographic region, and education.[49] Most women who report douching state they began the practice as adolescents.

The most frequently stated reason for douching is to achieve good vaginal hygiene. Because vaginal douches mechanically irrigate the vagina, clearing away mucus and other accumulated debris, these products may be considered for use as cosmetic cleansing agents.

Potential Adverse Effects of Douching

Douching may lead to adverse health outcomes. Frequent douching has been associated with an increased risk for PID, reduced fertility, ectopic pregnancy, vaginal infections such as BV, sexually transmitted infections, preterm delivery, and cervical cancer.[49] Additional problems include irritation or sensitization from douche ingredients and disruption of normal vaginal flora and vaginal pH. Their effects on vaginal flora vary depending on the ingredients—for example, water/vinegar (acetic acid) douches compared with povidone/iodine douches—and on douching frequency.[50] Local irritation, sensitization, and contact dermatitis are also possible with the antimicrobial agents found in douches. Allergic reactions may occur with intravaginal povidone/iodine, because systemic absorption is possible. This product should not be used by women who are allergic to iodine. Table 8–4 lists examples of douche products that contain povidone/iodine.

Use of Douching Equipment

Two types of syringes are available for douching purposes: douche bags and bulb douche syringes. The douche bag, or fountain syringe or folding feminine syringe, holds 1–2 quarts of fluid and comes with tubing and a shutoff valve. Two types of tips are supplied: one for enema use (the shorter rectal nozzle) and one for douching. The two tips are not interchangeable; vaginal infections may occur if a single tip is used for both douching and enemas.

Bulb douche syringes are available as both disposable and nondisposable products. The nondisposable units hold 8–16 ounces of fluid, whereas the disposable units contain 3–9 ounces. The flow rate is regulated by the amount of hand pressure exerted when the bulb is squeezed. Gentle pressure is recommended, because excess pressure may force fluid through the cervix, causing uterine inflammation. Instructions on proper use of the device are found in Table 8–6.

TABLE 8–6 Administration Guidelines for Douches

Bulb Douche Syringe Method

- Choose a comfortable douching position. Two positions are recommended: (1) sitting on the toilet or (2) standing in the shower. Whichever position is chosen, remember that douching is easier when the user is relaxed.
- Gently insert the nozzle about 3 inches into the vagina. Avoid closing the lips of the vagina.
- Squeeze bottle gently, letting solution cleanse the vagina and then flow freely from the body.
- After douching, throw away bottle and nozzle, if they are disposable.

Douche Bag Method

- Fill the douche bag with the prescribed solution or with a warm water and vinegar solution.
- Lie back in the tub with knees bent. Place the douche bag about 1 foot above the height of hips. Do not place or hang the bag any higher because such height will cause the pressure of fluid entering the vagina to be too high.
- Insert the nozzle several inches into the vagina. Aim the nozzle up and back toward the small of the back. While holding the labia closed around the nozzle, release the clamp slowly to allow fluid to enter the vagina. Rotate the tip and allow fluid to enter the vagina until the vagina feels full. Stop the flow of fluid; then hold the fluid in the vagina for about 30–60 seconds. Release and allow the fluid to flow out; repeat until the douche bag is empty.
- Wash the nozzle with mild soap and water.

PATIENT EDUCATION FOR Douching

Women should be informed that douching is not necessary for cleansing of the vagina. An alternative cleansing method for vaginal and perineal areas should be suggested, such as using the fingers to gently wash the vagina and the vulvar, perineal, and anal regions with lukewarm water and mild soap. Improper methods of douching or too-frequent douching can cause vaginal irritation. Douching can also increase the risk for pelvic inflammatory disease and sterility. Strictly following the product instructions and the self-care measures listed here will help to avoid these problems.

- Keep all douche equipment clean.
- Use lukewarm water to dilute products.
- Follow the appropriate instructions in Table 8–6 for the method of douching being used.
- Never insert a douche with forceful pressure.
- Do not use these products for birth control.
- Do not douche until at least 8 hours after intercourse during which a diaphragm, cervical cap, or contraceptive jelly, cream, or foam was used.
- Do not douche for at least 3 days after the last dose of vaginal antifungal medication.
- Do not douche for 48 hours before any gynecologic examination.
- Do not douche during pregnancy unless under the supervision of a health care provider.
- Use douches only as directed for routine cleansing.
- Do not douche more often than twice a week, except on the advice of a health care provider.
- If vaginal dryness or irritation occurs, discontinue use of the douche.

Patient Counseling for Douching

HCPs should discuss with a woman her reasons for douching. Women should be advised about the possible adverse consequences and that douching is not necessary to cleanse the vagina, because the vagina is a self-cleansing organ. Douching for routine hygienic purposes should be discouraged, and douching is contraindicated during pregnancy. Douching should be delayed at least 6–8 hours after sexual intercourse if a vaginal spermicide was used as a contraceptive agent.

An alternative cleansing method for vaginal and perineal areas should be suggested, such as using the fingers to gently wash the vagina and the vulvar, perineal, and anal regions with lukewarm water and mild soap. If a woman is douching to prevent or treat symptoms of a vaginal infection, such as an abnormal vaginal discharge, she should be counseled about more effective therapy or referred for medical evaluation, as appropriate.

Patients for whom douches have been prescribed or those who insist on douching for other reasons should be instructed on how to use these products safely and effectively. The box "Patient Education for Douching" lists specific information to provide these patients.

Key Points for Vaginal and Vulvovaginal Disorders

- Vaginal symptoms are often nonspecific, and it may be difficult to distinguish symptoms of the three common vaginal infections. The symptom most likely to differentiate a *Candida* vaginal infection from BV and trichomoniasis is the absence of an offensive odor of the vaginal secretions. Measurement of vaginal pH (pH >4.5 rules out a *Candida* infection) may also help to distinguish *Candida* and reduce inappropriate use of nonprescription vaginal antifungals.
- *Candida* vaginal infections are typically caused by *C. albicans*, but non–*C. albicans* vaginal infections have increased. The latter may be more resistant to nonprescription vaginal antifungals.
- Self-treatment for a *Candida* vaginal infection is most appropriate when the patient's symptoms are mild–moderate, when she does not have predisposing illnesses or take predisposing medications, when she has had one previously diagnosed infection, and when her symptoms are not recurrent. Recurrent infections are defined as more than three infections within a 12-month period and symptoms occurring within 2 months of previous vaginal symptoms.
- The nonprescription vaginal antifungals are equally effective. Selection of length of regimen or time of day for administration may be determined by patient preference. A medical referral is advised for women taking warfarin. Patients should be informed that symptoms typically improve within 2–3 days after initiation of the nonprescription vaginal antifungals and resolve within a week. The length of the treatment regimen does not directly correspond to resolution of symptoms.
- Use of a sodium bicarbonate sitz bath may provide relief of itching and irritation prior to the onset of benefit from the antifungal.
- Eating yogurt with live cultures (8 ounces daily) may benefit some patients in preventing recurrent VVC infections.
- Atrophic vaginitis may occur after menopause, after giving birth, during breastfeeding, or as a result of antiestrogenic medications. Vaginal dryness and dyspareunia may be relieved by use of topical personal lubricant products. If symptoms persist, medical evaluation is needed.
- Atrophic vaginitis may cause vaginal bleeding. Any patient who reports postmenopausal bleeding should be referred to an appropriate HCP to rule out endometrial cancer.
- Douching is not recommended for vaginal cleansing, because douching can have adverse consequences. Douching is contraindicated during pregnancy. Douching should be postponed until at least 8 hours after sexual intercourse if a vaginal spermicide was used for contraception.

REFERENCES

1. Reed BD. Vaginitis. In: Sloane PD, Slatt LM, Ebell MH, et al., eds. *Essentials of Family Medicine.* 6th ed. Philadelphia: Lippincott Williams & Wilkins; 2011.
2. Van Schalkwyk J, Yudin MH. Vulvovaginitis: screening for and management of trichomoniasis, vulvovaginal candidiasis, and bacterial vaginosis. *J Obstet Gynaecol Can.* 2015;37(3):266–74. doi: 10.1016/S1701-2163(15)30316-9.
3. Mashburn J. Etiology, diagnosis and management of vaginitis. *J Midwifery Womens Health.* 2006;51(6):423–30. doi: 10.1016/j.jmwh.2006.07.005.
4. Benjamin F. Anatomy, physiology, growth and development. In: Seltzer V, Pearse WH, eds. *Women's Primary Health Care.* 2nd ed. New York: McGraw-Hill; 1999.

5. Bautista CT, Wurapa E, Sateren WB, et al. Bacterial vaginosis: a synthesis of the literature on etiology, prevalence, risk factors, and relationship with chlamydia and gonorrhea infections. *Mil Med Res.* 2016;3(4):1–10. doi: 10.1186/s40779-016-0074-5.
6. Quan M. Vaginitis: diagnosis and management. *Postgrad Med.* 2010; 122(6):117–27. doi: 10.3810/pgm.2010.11.2229.
7. Nyirjesy P, Sobel JD. Advances in diagnosing vaginitis: development of a new algorithm. *Curr Infect Dis Rep.* 2005;7(6):458–62. doi: 10.1007/s11908-005-0048-3.
8. Hainer BL, Gibson MV. Vaginitis: diagnosis and treatment. *Am Fam Physician.* 2011;83(7):807–15. PMID: 21524046.
9. Ferris D, Nyirjesy P, Sobel JD, et al. Over-the-counter antifungal drug misuse associated with patient-diagnosed vulvovaginal candidiasis. *Obstet Gynecol.* 2002;99(3):419–25. doi: 10.1016/S0029-7844(01)01759-8.
10. Schwiertz A, Taras D, Rusch K, Rusch V. Throwing the dice for the diagnosis of vaginal complaints? *Ann Clin Microbiol Antimicrob.* 2006;5:4–10. doi: 10.1186/1476-0711-5-4.
11. Fidler BD. Diagnosis and treatment of vulvovaginal candidiasis. Retail Clinician CE Lesson. 2007:34–42. Available at: at http://www.4healtheducation.com/pdf/retailclinician2007.pdf. Accessed April 6, 2017.
12. Kulp JL, Chaudhry S, Wiita B, Bachmann G. The accuracy of women performing vaginal pH self-testing. *J Womens Health (Larchmt).* 2008; 17(4):523–6. doi: 10.1089/jwh.2007.0446.
13. Centers for Disease Control and Prevention (CDC). Sexually transmitted diseases treatment guidelines, 2015. *MMWR Recomm Rep.* 2015;64(3). Available at: http://www.cdc.gov/std/tg2015. Accessed April 6, 2017.
14. Palmeira-de-Oliveira R, Palmeira-de-Oliveira A, Martinez-de-Oliveira J. New strategies for local treatment of vaginal infections. *Adv Drug Deliv Rev.* 2015;92:105–22. doi: 10.1016/j.addr.2015.06.008.
15. Klebanoff M, Schwebke J, Zhang, J. Vulvovaginal symptoms in women with bacterial vaginosis. *Obstet Gynecol.* 2004;104(2):267–72. doi: 10.1097/01.AOG.0000134783.98382.b0.
16. Owen M, Clenney TL. Management of vaginitis. *Am Fam Physician.* 2004;70(11):2125–32. PMID: 15606061.
17. Soper D. Trichomoniasis: under control or undercontrolled? *Am J Obstet Gynecol.* 2004;190(1):281–90. doi: 10.1016/j.ajog.2003.08.023.
18. Farage MA, Miller KW, Ledger WJ. Determining the cause of vulvovaginal symptoms. *Obstet Gynecol Surv.* 2008;63(7):445–64. doi: 10.1097/OGX.0b013e318172ee25.
19. Biggs WS, Williams RW. Common gynecologic infections. *Prim Care* 2009;36(1):33–51. doi: 10.1016/j.pop.2008.10.002.
20. Pirotta MV, Garland SM. Genital *Candida* species detected in samples from women in Melbourne, Australia, before and after treatment with antibiotics. *J Clin Microbiol.* 2006;44(9):3213–7. doi: 10.1128/JCM.00218-06.
21. Castelo-Branco C, Cancelo MJ, Villero J, et al. Management of postmenopausal vaginal atrophy and atrophic vaginitis. *Maturitas.* 2005; 52(Suppl 1):S46–52. doi: 10.1016/j.maturitas.2005.06.014.
22. Krapf JM, Isaacs C. Vulvovaginitis. Medscape (eMedicine). Updated March 30, 2015. Available at: http://emedicine.medscape.com/article/2188931-overview. Accessed April 6, 2017.
23. Falagas M, Betsi GI, Athanasiou S. Probiotics for prevention of recurrent vulvovaginal candidiasis: a review. *J Antimicrob Chemother.* 2006; 58(2):266–72. doi: 10.1093/jac/dkl246.
24. Roy S, Caillouette JC, Roy T, et al. Vaginal pH is similar to follicle-stimulating hormone for menopause diagnosis. *Am J Obstet Gynecol.* 2004; 190(5):1272–7. doi: 10.1016/j.ajog.2003.12.015.
25. Dovnik A, Golle A, Novak D, Arko D, Takac I. Treatment of vulvovaginal candidiasis: a review of literature. *Acta Dermatovenerologica Alp Pannonica Adriat.* 2015;24(1):5–7. doi: 10.15570/actaapa.2015.2.
26. U.S. Food and Drug Administration. Vaginal candidiasis may sometimes be an early warning of HIV infection [press release]. November 16, 1992. Available at: http://aidsinfo.nih.gov/news/260/vaginal-candidiasis-may-sometimes-be-an-early-warning-of-hiv-infection. Accessed April 6, 2017.
27. Singh S. Treatment of vulvovaginal candidiasis. *CPJ.* 2003;136:26–30.
28. Clotrimazole. Lexi-Drugs Online. Hudson, OH: Lexi-Comp. Available at: http://online.lexi.com/lco/action/search?q=clotrimazole&t=name. Accessed April 6, 2017.
29. Miconazole. Micromedex Online Truven Health Analytics: Micromedex. Available at: http://www.micromedexsolutions.com. Accessed April 6, 2017.
30. Tioconazole. Micromedex Online Truven Health Analytics: Micromedex. Available at: http://www.micromedexsolutions.com. Accessed April 6, 2017.
31. Miconazole. Lexi-Drugs Online Hudson, OH: Lexi-Comp. Available at: http://online.lexi.com/lco/action/search?q=miconazole&t=name. Accessed April 6, 2017.
32. Upmalis D, Cone FL, Lamia CA, et al. Single-dose miconazole nitrate vaginal ovule in the treatment of vulvovaginal candidiasis: two single-blind, controlled studies versus miconazole nitrate 100 mg cream for 7 days. *J Womens Health Gend Based Med.* 2000;9(4):421–9. doi: 10.1089/15246090050020745.
33. Barnhart K. Safety and efficacy of bedtime versus daytime administration of the miconazole nitrate 1200 mg vaginal ovule insert to treat vulvovaginal candidiasis. *Curr Med Res Opin.* 2005;21(1):127–34. doi: 10.1185/030079904X18018.
34. U.S. Food and Drug Administration. Safety: benzocaine topical products: sprays, gels and liquids—risk of methemoglobinemia. Updated April 7, 2011. Available at: https://wayback.archive-it.org/7993/20170112165108/http://www.fda.gov/Safety/MedWatch/SafetyInformation/SafetyAlertsforHumanMedicalProducts/ucm250264.htm. Accessed April 6, 2017.
35. Kohlberger P, Bancher-Todesca D. Bacterial colonization in suspected sexually abused children. *J Pediatr Adolesc Gynecol.* 2007;20(5):289–92. doi: 10.1016/j.jpag.2006.11.004.
36. Sobel JD. Factors involved in patient choice of oral or vaginal treatment for vulvovaginal candidiasis. *Patient Prefer Adherence.* 2013;8:31–4. doi: 10.2147/PPA.S38984.
37. Pirotta M, Gunn J, Chondros P, et al. Effect of lactobacillus in preventing post-antibiotic vulvovaginal candidiasis: a randomized controlled trial. *BMJ.* 2004;329(7465):548–51. doi: 10.1136/bmj.38210.494977.DE.
38. Korenek P, Britt R, Hawkins C. Differentiation of the vaginosis-bacterial vaginosis, lactobacillosis, and cytolytic vaginosis. *Internet J Adv Nurs Pract.* 2002;6(1). Available at: http://ispub.com/IJANP/6/1/12743. Accessed April 6, 2017.
39. Reid G, Bocking A. The potential for probiotics to prevent bacterial vaginosis and preterm labor. *Am J Obstet Gynecol.* 2003;189(4):1202–8. doi: 10.1067/S0002-9378(03)00495-2.
40. Van Kessel K, Assefi N, Marrazzo J, et al. Common complementary and alternative therapies for yeast vaginitis and bacterial vaginosis: a systematic review. *Obstet Gynecol Surv.* 2003;58(5):351–8. doi: 10.1097/01.OGX.0000068791.04785.8D.
41. Watson C, Calabretto H. Comprehensive review of conventional and non-conventional methods of management of recurrent vulvovaginal candidiasis. *Aust N Z J Obstet Gynaecol.* 2007;47(4):262–72. doi: 10.1111/j.1479-828X.2007.00736.x.
42. Sobel JD, Chaim W, Nagappan V, et al. Treatment of vaginitis caused by *Candida glabrata:* use of topical boric acid and flucytosine. *Am J Obstet Gynecol* 2003;189:1297–300. doi: 10.1067/S0002-9378(03)00726-9.
43. Iavazzo C, Gkegkes ID, Zarkado IM, Falagas ME. Boric acid for recurrent vulvovaginal candidiasis: the clinical evidence. *J Womens Health (Larchmt).* 2011;20(8):1245–55. doi: 10.1089/jwh.2010.2708.
44. Allen-Davis J, Beck A, Parker R, et al. Assessment of vulvovaginal complaints: accuracy of telephone triage and in-office diagnosis. *Obstet Gynecol.* 2002;99(1):18–22. doi: 10.1016/S0029-7844(01)01670-2.
45. Santoro N, Komi J. Prevalence and impact of vaginal symptoms among postmenopausal women. *J Sex Med.* 2009;6(8):2133–42. doi: 10.1111/j.1743-6109.2009.01335.x.
46. Nappi R, Kokot-Kierepa M. Women's voices in the menopause: results from an international survey on vaginal atrophy. *Maturitas.* 2010;67(3): 233–8. doi: 10.1016/j.maturitas.2010.08.001.
47. Management of symptomatic vulvovaginal atrophy: 2013 position statement of the North American Menopause Society. *Menopause.* 2013;20(9): 888–902. doi: 10.1097/GME.0b013e3182a122c2.
48. Centers for Disease Control and Prevention (CDC). Key statistics from the National Survey of Family Growth—D listing. Updated April 20, 2015. Available at: http://www.cdc.gov/nchs/nsfg/key_statistics/d.htm#douching. Accessed April 6, 2017.
49. Cottrell BH. An updated review of evidence to discourage douching. *MCM Am J Matern Child Nurs.* 2010;35(2):102–7. doi: 10.1097/NMC.0b013e3181cae9da.
50. Pavlova S, Tao L. In vitro inhibition of commercial douche products against vaginal microflora. *Infect Dis Obstet Gynecol.* 2000;8(2):99–104. doi: 10.1155/S1064744900000090.

CHAPTER 9

DISORDERS RELATED TO MENSTRUATION

LESLIE A. SHIMP

The menstrual cycle is a regular physiologic event for women that begins in adolescence and usually continues through late middle age. Women are able to self-treat for two common menstrual disorders: primary dysmenorrhea and premenstrual syndrome (PMS). Many women use nonprescription products and seek advice from health care providers (HCPs) on how best to manage symptoms of these disorders, including abdominal pain and cramping, irritability, and fluid retention. An understanding of the menstrual cycle will help both patients and HCPs make informed and appropriate decisions about self-care. HCPs should also be familiar with common menstrual symptoms and disorders, as well as the risks for toxic shock syndrome.

Menstruation results from the monthly cycling of female reproductive hormones. A *single menstrual cycle* is the time between the onset of one menstrual flow (menstruation or menses) and the onset of the next. The average age of *menarche* (the initial menstrual cycle) in U.S. women is 12 years, although normal menarche may occur as early as age 11 or as late as age 14.5.[1] The onset of menstruation is influenced by factors such as race, genetics, nutritional status, and body mass. The median menstrual cycle length is 28 days, ranging from 24 to 38 days for adult women; adolescents have a wider cycle length of 20–45 days.[2] Menses lasts 3–7 days, with most blood loss occurring during days 1 and 2.[1,3] The major components of menstrual fluid are blood and endometrial cellular debris; the average blood loss per cycle is 30 mL, with a range of 10–84 mL.[3] A loss of more than 80 mL per cycle or bleeding lasting longer than 7 days is considered abnormal and may be associated with anemia.

The menstrual cycle (Figure 9–1) results from the combined hormonal activity of the hypothalamus, pituitary gland, and ovaries; this is known as the hypothalamic-pituitary-ovarian (HPO) axis. The hypothalamus plays the key role in regulating the menstrual cycle by producing gonadotropin-releasing hormone (GnRH). Low levels of both estradiol and progesterone, present at the end of the previous menstrual cycle, stimulate the hypothalamus to release GnRH, which stimulates pituitary gonadotroph cells to synthesize and secrete luteinizing hormone (LH) and follicle-stimulating hormone (FSH).

Two principal reproductive events occur during each menstrual cycle: the maturation and release of an ovum (egg) from the ovaries and the preparation of the endometrial lining of the uterus for the implantation of a fertilized ovum. The events of the menstrual cycle can be described in phases that reflect changes in either the ovary (follicular/ovulatory and luteal phases) or the uterine endometrium (menstrual/proliferative and secretory phases). The follicular/ovulatory phase correlates with the menstrual/proliferative phase, and the luteal phase correlates with the secretory phase.

Cycle day 1 is the first day of menstrual flow and the beginning of the follicular and menstrual/proliferative phases. The follicular phase can range in length from several days to several weeks, but it lasts an average of 14 days. During the follicular phase, FSH stimulates the maturation of a group of ovarian follicles. These maturing follicles secrete estradiol promoting growth of the uterine endometrium.

By about cycle day 8, a single ovarian follicle usually becomes dominant, which typically results in the release or ovulation of only one mature egg. The ovulatory phase of the cycle is about 3 days in length. During this phase, the pituitary gland secretes high levels of LH for a 48-hour period, which is known as the LH surge. The LH surge catalyzes the final steps in the maturation of the ovum and stimulates production of prostaglandins and proteolytic enzymes necessary for ovulation. Estradiol levels decrease during the LH surge, sometimes resulting in midcycle endometrial bleeding. Ovulation typically occurs 12 hours after the LH surge. Ovulation releases 5–10 mL of follicular fluid, which contains the oocyte mass and prostaglandins; this event may cause abdominal pain (*mittelschmerz,* German for "middle pain") for some women. The HPO axis takes between 6 and 36 months to mature and to establish regular ovulatory cycles. Prior to this, adolescents may experience irregular, unpredictable menses and possibly heavy or prolonged menstrual bleeding associated with anovulatory cycles.[4]

The *luteal phase* is the time between ovulation and the beginning of menstrual blood flow. After the follicle ruptures, it is referred to as the corpus luteum. The luteal phase is typically consistent in length (about 14 ± 2 days) and reflects the 10- to 12-day functional period of the corpus luteum. The corpus luteum secretes progesterone, estradiol, and androgens. The increased levels of estrogen and progesterone alter the uterine endometrial lining. Glands mature, proliferate, and become secretory as the uterus prepares for the implantation of a fertilized egg. Progesterone and estrogen levels increase in the middle of the luteal phase, but LH and FSH levels decline in response to the increased hormone levels. If pregnancy occurs, human chorionic gonadotropin released by the developing placenta supports the function of the corpus luteum until the placenta develops enough to begin secreting estrogen and progesterone. If pregnancy does not occur, the corpus luteum ceases to function. Estrogen and progesterone levels then decline, causing the endometrial lining of the uterus to become edematous and necrotic. The decrease in progesterone also leads to prostaglandin synthesis. Following prostaglandin-initiated vasoconstriction and

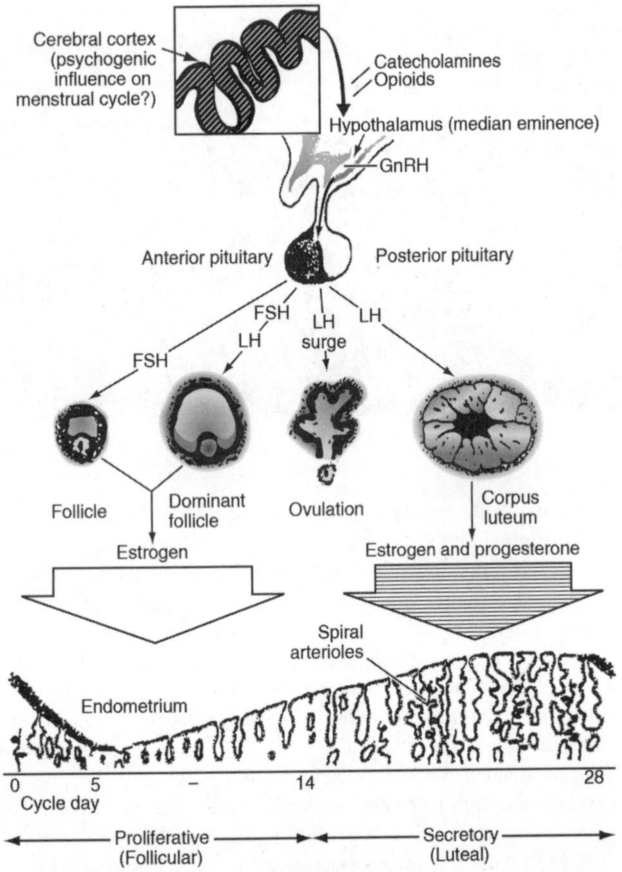

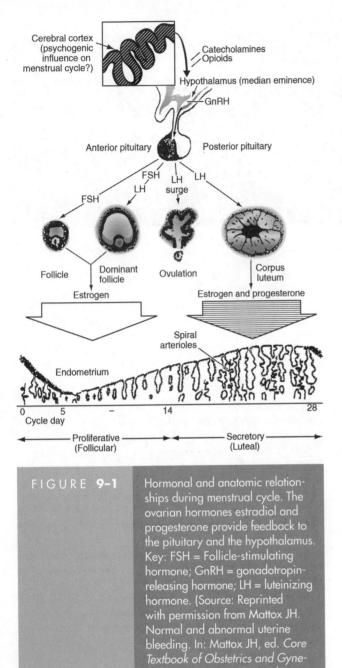

FIGURE 9–1 Hormonal and anatomic relationships during menstrual cycle. The ovarian hormones estradiol and progesterone provide feedback to the pituitary and the hypothalamus. Key: FSH = Follicle-stimulating hormone; GnRH = gonadotropin-releasing hormone; LH = luteinizing hormone. (Source: Reprinted with permission from Mattox JH. Normal and abnormal uterine bleeding. In: Mattox JH, ed. *Core Textbook of Obstetrics and Gynecology*. St. Louis, MO: Mosby-Yearbook; 1998:397.)

uterine contractions, sloughing of the outer two endometrial layers occurs. The decline in estrogen and progesterone results in an increase in GnRH and in the renewed production of LH and FSH, which begins a new menstrual cycle.

DYSMENORRHEA

Dysmenorrhea is the most common gynecologic problem among adolescents and young adult women. The prevalence of dysmenorrhea is highest in adolescence, with up to 93% of young women being affected.[5,6] Dysmenorrhea is divided into primary and secondary disorders by etiology. *Primary dysmenorrhea* is associated with cramp-like lower abdominal pain at the time of menstruation in the absence of pelvic disease. Primary dysmenorrhea usually develops within 6–12 months after menarche, generally affecting women during their teens and early 20s.[7] Primary dysmenorrhea occurs only during ovulatory cycles. Its prevalence increases between early and older adolescence as the regularity of ovulation increases[5] and decreases after age 24.[7,8]

Approximately 10% of women with dysmenorrhea have secondary dysmenorrhea.[9] *Secondary dysmenorrhea* is typically associated with pelvic pathology and is suggested if symptoms initially begin at least 2 years after menarche, if pelvic pain occurs at times other than during menses, if the woman has irregular menstrual cycles or a history of pelvic inflammatory disease (PID), dyspareunia, or infertility.[5,6,10] *Endometriosis,* a growth of cells similar to endometrial cells in locations outside the uterus, is the most common cause of secondary dysmenorrhea. *Adenomyosis,* which is growth of endometrial tissue into the *myometrium*—the muscular wall of the uterus—is another common cause of secondary dysmenorrhea.[11] Adolescents are increasingly being diagnosed with secondary dysmenorrhea, which accounts for symptoms in 47%–73% of teens with severe menstrual pain and no response to nonsteroidal anti-inflammatory drugs (NSAIDs) or oral contraceptives (OCs).[2,10] Secondary dysmenorrhea may also be caused by the presence of an intrauterine contraceptive (IUC).

Severe menstrual pain is reported by 14%–23% of teens.[10] Dysmenorrhea is the leading cause of school absenteeism and lost working hours among adolescent girls and young women. About 26% of adolescent girls report dysmenorrhea-related school absenteeism, which increases to 50% in girls who report severe pain.[10] In addition, adolescents with severe menstrual pain reported that the pain interfered with other life activities, such as social activities, sports, work, and relationships with friends and family.[5,10] Similarly, an estimated 600 million work hours are lost annually because of dysmenorrhea.[8]

The decreased prevalence and severity of dysmenorrhea in women in their mid-20s and older may be partially explained by OC use, which is an effective therapy for primary dysmenorrhea and pregnancy. The use of OCs decreases the amount of endometrium, resulting in lower prostaglandin production. During the last trimester of pregnancy, uterine adrenergic nerves virtually disappear, and only a portion of the nerves regenerate after childbirth. For many women, this phenomenon results in a decreased prevalence of dysmenorrhea following childbirth.[12]

Factors other than young age and nulliparity can increase the risk for or severity of dysmenorrhea. These include early menarche before age 12; heavy menstrual flow; tobacco smoking; low fish consumption; a body mass index of less than 20 kg/m^2 or greater than 30 kg/m^2; premenstrual symptoms; and stress, anxiety, and depression.[6] Obesity is linked to early menarche and can predispose to primary dysmenorrhea.[8] In addition, factors such as attempting to lose weight and stress related to social, emotional, or family issues can all make dysmenorrhea pain more bothersome.[12]

Pathophysiology of Primary Dysmenorrhea

The cause of primary dysmenorrhea is not fully understood. However, prostaglandins and leukotrienes contribute substantially to the occurrence and severity of dysmenorrhea.[5,6,8] Abnormal levels of nitric oxide and vasopressin may also be involved.[6,8] Ovulation increases serum progesterone, which leads to increases in arachidonic acid. During menstruation, arachidonic acid is converted to prostaglandins and leukotrienes, which are then released. Prostaglandin levels are 2–4 times greater in women with dysmenorrhea than in women without dysmenorrhea; the severity of dysmenorrhea is proportional to the endometrial concentration of the prostaglandin $F_2\alpha$ ($PGF_2\alpha$).[7] *Leukotrienes,* inflammatory mediators known to cause vasoconstriction and uterine contractions, are elevated in women with dysmenorrhea; levels are correlated with both occurrence and severity. Leukotrienes may contribute significantly to dysmenorrhea in women who do not respond to NSAIDs.[8] Nitric oxide has also been linked to dysmenorrhea, because transdermal nitroglycerine patches increase nitric oxide and decrease dysmenorrhea-related pain. Nitric oxide is the substance that promotes uterine quiescence during pregnancy, and use of nitric oxide during premature labor can stop uterine contractility.[8] Circulating levels of *vasopressin* (a substance that can produce dysrhythmic uterine contractions) are higher in women with dysmenorrhea than in asymptomatic individuals. However, the role of vasopressin in the etiology of primary dysmenorrhea remains controversial.[5,6]

Prostaglandins stimulate uterine contractions. Normal contractions and vasoconstriction help expel menstrual fluids and control bleeding as the endometrium sloughs. However, the increased levels of prostaglandins and leukotrienes present with dysmenorrhea can lead to strong uterine contractions similar to those experienced during labor and excessive vasoconstriction, resulting in uterine ischemia and pain. In women without dysmenorrhea, uterine contractions are rhythmic, and contraction pressure reaches 120 mm Hg. In contrast, women with dysmenorrhea have more frequent contractions, with pressures up to 180 mm Hg that contribute to ischemia and tissue hypoxia and, thus, pain.

Clinical Presentation of Primary Dysmenorrhea

The pain with primary dysmenorrhea is cyclic in nature and is directly related to the onset of menstruation (Table 9–1). Pain is typically experienced as a continuous dull ache with spasmodic cramping in the lower midabdominal or suprapubic region that may radiate to the lower back and upper thighs. The uterine contractions can force prostaglandins and leukotrienes into the systemic circulation, causing additional symptoms such as nausea, vomiting, fatigue, dizziness, bloating, diarrhea, and headache.[5] A large study of adolescents found that 78% reported fatigue, 71% cramping, 64% headaches, 58% lower back pain, and 37% nausea at the time of menstruation.[10] This clinical presentation can be adequate for the diagnosis of primary dysmenorrhea, if the pain is mild–moderate and the patient responds to NSAID therapy.[5]

Treatment of Primary Dysmenorrhea

Many women self-treat for dysmenorrhea using nonprescription products. In a study of adolescents, 66% self-treated with NSAIDs; fewer used acetaminophen or aspirin.[10] Younger adolescents are less likely than college-aged women to use analgesics.[11] Among those who self-treated, 85% reported moderate–high effectiveness from the analgesic. Other studies have found that self-care may result in use of low or mistimed doses or use of less effective medications, thus increasing the likelihood of school absence and other activity limitations.[5] Inadequate management of dysmenorrhea pain can lead to increased pain sensitivity at times other than during menses and to increased sensitivity to non-uterine pain, thus having important implications for pain perception and quality of life throughout life.[11]

TABLE 9–1 Differentiation of Primary and Secondary Dysmenorrhea

	Primary Dysmenorrhea	Secondary Dysmenorrhea
Age at onset of dysmenorrhea symptoms	As soon as 6–12 months after menarche but typically several years after menarche; age 13–17 years for most girls	At least 2 years after menarche but more typically mid- to late-20s or older or pain begins after years of normal cycles
Menses	More likely to be regular with normal blood loss	More likely to be irregular; menorrhagia and inter-menstrual bleeding more common
Pattern and duration of dysmenorrhea pain	Onset just prior to or coincident with onset of menses; pain with each or most menses, lasting only 2–3 days	Pattern and duration vary with cause; change in pain pattern or intensity may also indicate secondary disease
Pain at other times of menstrual cycle	No	Yes; may occur before, during, or after menses
Response to NSAIDs and/or OCs	Yes	Depends on the cause of secondary dysmenorrhea. Mild–moderate endometriosis may respond to OCs or other hormonal contraceptives, but response to NSAIDs often is absent or inadequate. Adenomyosis is not responsive to NSAIDs or hormonal contraceptives.
Other symptoms	Fatigue, headache, nausea, change in appetite, backache, dizziness, irritability, and depression may occur at same time as dysmenorrhea pain	Vary according to cause of the secondary dysmenorrhea; may include dyspareunia, pelvic tenderness

Key: NSAID = Nonsteroidal anti-inflammatory drug; OC = oral contraceptive.
Source: References 5, 9, 10, and 11.

Treatment Goals

The goals of treating primary dysmenorrhea are to provide relief or a significant improvement in symptoms and minimize the disruption of usual activities.

General Treatment Approach

An important initial step in managing dysmenorrhea is distinguishing between primary and secondary dysmenorrhea. Self-care is appropriate for an otherwise healthy young woman who has a history consistent with primary dysmenorrhea and who is not sexually active or for a woman who has been diagnosed with primary dysmenorrhea.[5] Adolescents with pelvic pain who are sexually active and thus at risk for PID and women with characteristics indicating secondary dysmenorrhea should be referred for medical evaluation. Table 9–1 compares primary and secondary dysmenorrhea. An estimated 80%–90% of women with primary dysmenorrhea can be successfully treated with NSAIDs, OCs, or both.

Other treatment options include use of dietary supplements such as omega-3 fatty acids. These fatty acids are found in fish and fish oil and compete with arachidonic acid in the cyclooxygenase and lipoxygenase pathways, leading to a decrease in the production of the proinflammatory cytokines. Increased consumption of fish rich in omega-3 fatty acids from tuna, salmon, and sardines or use of fish oil supplements may reduce symptoms. Cholecalciferol is known to decrease the production of prostaglandins and increase prostaglandin inactivation.[13] One small study found a reduction in dysmenorrhea pain among women with low serum vitamin D levels who were given a single 300,000 IU dose of cholecalciferol 5 days prior to menses.[14] Women should be counseled to ingest vitamin D_3 600 IU daily. These measures often serve as an adjunct to drug therapy. Figure 9–2 presents an algorithm for managing primary dysmenorrhea.

A patient with more severe dysmenorrhea, a change in the pattern or intensity of pain, or inadequate response or intolerance to NSAIDs should be referred to her primary care provider. An estimated 15% of women do not respond to NSAIDs, cannot tolerate therapy, or prefer not to use medication for dysmenorrhea.[11] Figure 9–2 lists exclusions for self-care.

Nonpharmacologic Therapy

Many women use nonpharmacologic measures to help manage dysmenorrhea and menstrual discomfort. A study of adolescents found that these included sleep, hot baths or a heating pad, and exercise.[5] The use of heat is a commonly recommended nondrug therapy. An abdominal heat patch has been tested for the treatment of dysmenorrhea.[15] The heat patch was significantly better and provided 14% greater pain relief than placebo or acetaminophen. The analgesic effect of the heat patch had a faster onset than drug therapy and was additive to the relief provided by ibuprofen. Evidence regarding the benefit of exercise is conflicting; however, participation in regular exercise may lessen the symptoms of primary dysmenorrhea for some women.[5,6] Nonpharmacologic therapy may be especially useful for women who cannot tolerate or do not respond to nonprescription medications.

Smoking and exposure to secondhand smoke have been associated with more severe and/or chronic dysmenorrhea.[5,16] The severity of dysmenorrhea symptoms reportedly increases with the number of cigarettes smoked per day. The basis for this effect is unknown, but nicotine-induced vasoconstriction may be involved. Discontinuing tobacco smoking or avoiding exposure to tobacco smoke may improve symptoms.

Pharmacologic Therapy

Unfortunately, many women and adolescents with dysmenorrhea remain untreated or are inadequately treated. They continue to experience pain and limitations in their daily activity. The following sections outline the uses and properties of the four nonprescription analgesic medications commonly used by women to treat dysmenorrhea: acetaminophen, aspirin, ibuprofen, and naproxen sodium. Table 9–2 lists their dosages for dysmenorrhea. Chapter 5 provides further discussion of their adverse effects, contraindications, and drug interactions.

Aspirin

Aspirin may be adequate for treating mild symptoms of dysmenorrhea. In typical analgesic dosages, aspirin has only a limited effect on prostaglandin synthesis and is only moderately effective in treating more than minimal symptoms of dysmenorrhea. Aspirin may also increase menstrual flow.

Acetaminophen

Acetaminophen may also be adequate for treating mild symptoms of dysmenorrhea. Acetaminophen is a weak inhibitor of prostaglandin synthesis; however, the reduction of $PGF_2\alpha$ levels is much greater with nonsalicylate NSAIDs than with acetaminophen.[17] Even in dosages of 4 g/day, acetaminophen is less effective than ibuprofen; therefore lower dosages are less likely to be effective.[17]

Nonsalicylate NSAIDs

Nonsalicylate NSAIDs, the first-line treatment for primary dysmenorrhea, include ibuprofen 200 mg and naproxen sodium 220 mg. In clinical trials, NSAIDs were effective in 64%–100% of patients.[11] Relief of dysmenorrhea typically occurs within the first cycle of use. However, dosages used in clinical trials and dosages of prescription drugs for the treatment of dysmenorrhea often are higher than the labeled nonprescription dosages. Therefore, providers may recommend prescription therapy, or they may recommend that a patient who is using nonprescription products use a prescription dosage of an NSAID if the lower dosage does not provide adequate symptom relief.

Therapy with nonsalicylate NSAIDs should begin at the onset of menses or pain. If inadequate pain relief occurs, treatment beginning 1–2 days before expected menses may improve symptomatic relief.[6] If the possibility of pregnancy exists, therapy should be initiated only after menses begins. Patients should be instructed that the NSAID is used to prevent cramps and to relieve pain. Optimal pain relief is achieved when these agents are taken on a schedule, rather than on an as-needed basis. Therefore, ibuprofen should be taken every 4–6 hours and naproxen sodium every 8–12 hours for the first 48–72 hours of menstrual flow, because that time frame correlates with maximum prostaglandin release (Table 9–2). The therapeutic effect usually is apparent within 30–60 minutes, and benefit will be optimal with continued regular use.

A patient with dysmenorrhea may respond better to one NSAID than to another. If the maximum nonprescription dosage of one agent does not provide adequate benefit, switching to another agent is recommended. The analgesic effect for most NSAIDs plateaus, so further dosage increases may increase the risk of adverse effects

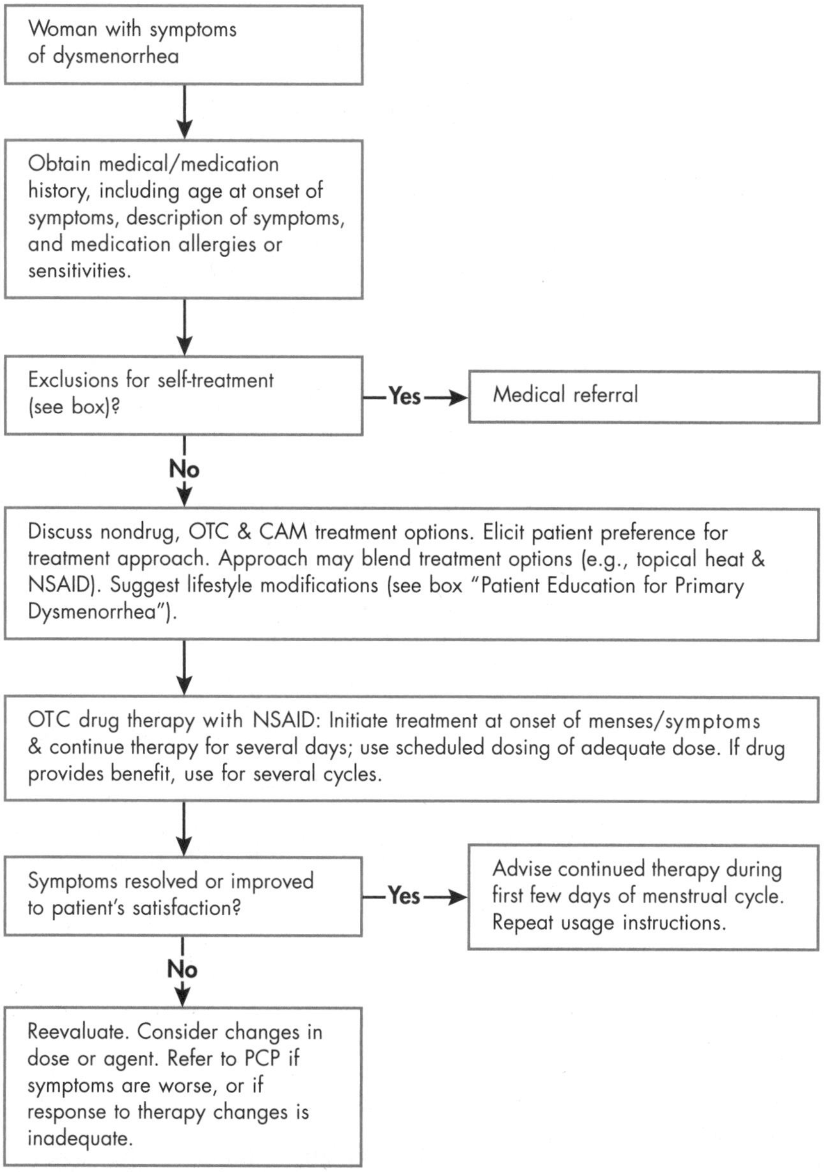

Exclusions for Self-Treatment

- Severe dysmenorrhea and/or menorrhagia
- Dysmenorrhea symptoms inconsistent with primary dysmenorrhea (e.g., age at onset of symptoms, dysmenorrhea pain at times other than onset of menses)
- History of PID, infertility, irregular menstrual cycles, endometriosis, ovarian cysts
- Use of IUC
- Allergy to aspirin or NSAIDs; intolerance for NSAIDs
- Use of warfarin, heparin, or lithium
- Active GI disease (PUD, GERD, ulcerative colitis)
- Bleeding disorder

FIGURE **9–2** Self-care for primary dysmenorrhea. Key: CAM = Complementary and alternative medicine; GERD = gastroesophageal reflux disease; GI = gastrointestinal; IUC = intrauterine contraceptive; NSAID = nonsteroidal anti-inflammatory drug; OTC = over-the-counter; PID = pelvic inflammatory disease; PCP = primary care provider; PUD = peptic ulcer disease.

without providing additional benefit. Therapy with NSAIDs should be undertaken for three to six menstrual cycles, with changes made in the agent, dosage, or both before judging the effectiveness of these agents for a particular patient. If nonprescription NSAID therapy does not provide an adequate therapeutic effect, other therapies that may provide relief from primary dysmenorrhea include prescription NSAIDs; prescription dosages of nonprescription NSAIDs; or use of a combined OC or a progestin implant (Implanon, Nexplanon), estrogen plus progestin vaginal ring (NuvaRing), or the levonorgestrel IUC (Mirena, Skyla).[18]

The usual adverse effects from a few days of intermittent use are gastrointestinal (GI) symptoms such as upset stomach, vomiting, heartburn, abdominal pain, diarrhea, constipation, and anorexia. Adverse effects may also include headache and dizziness. Some GI adverse effects may be decreased by taking the drugs with food.

Pharmacotherapeutic Comparison

A Cochrane review indicated that ibuprofen and naproxen are first-line agents for dysmenorrhea because of their effectiveness and tolerability.[19] Cost and patient preference as to the number of doses and tablets to take should guide agent selection. Because of restrictions on taking medications to school, adolescents may benefit from naproxen's longer duration of action. Women at risk of GI ulceration should consider the use of a gastroprotective agent or another therapeutic option such as an OC. Acetaminophen may provide some relief for patients with hypersensitivity or intolerance to aspirin

TABLE 9-2 **Treatment of Dysmenorrhea With Nonprescription Medications**

Agent	Recommended Nonprescription Dosage (maximum daily dosage)
Acetaminophen	650–1000 mg every 4–6 hours (4000 mg)[a]
Aspirin	650–1000 mg every 4–6 hours (4000 mg)
Ibuprofen	200–400 mg every 4–6 hours[b] (1200 mg)
Naproxen sodium	220–440 mg initially; then 220 mg every 8–12 hours (660 mg)

[a] See Table 5–3 for information on the manufacturer's voluntary reduction of maximum daily dosages of Tylenol (acetaminophen) products sold in the United States.

[b] If 200 mg every 4–6 hours is ineffective, the recommended dosage for dysmenorrhea (400 mg every 6 hours while awake) should be taken.

and for patients with intolerance to the GI and platelet-inhibition adverse effects of aspirin and NSAIDs. Oral contraceptives as well as intravaginal and intrauterine hormonal contraceptives are used for the management of dysmenorrhea. Some trials report benefit in up to 80% of women, but a Cochrane review found limited evidence of effectiveness for the management of dysmenorrhea.[9]

Product Selection Guidelines

Special Populations

The Food and Drug Administration (FDA) recommends that aspirin and aspirin-containing products not be given to children and adolescents who have or are recovering from chickenpox or influenza-like symptoms because of the risk of Reye's syndrome.[20] (See Chapter 5 for further information.) Pregnant or menopausal women will not experience dysmenorrhea. Women attempting to become pregnant should avoid use of NSAIDs in the periconception time, as these agents may impair implantation of the blastocyst. Acetaminophen and ibuprofen can safely be taken by breastfeeding women, as the amounts of both medications are low in breast milk.[21] Women who are breastfeeding should avoid use of aspirin; if a dose of aspirin is taken, a woman should wait 1–2 hours before breastfeeding.[21] Naproxen sodium is a less optimal choice for breastfeeding women; although levels in breast milk are low, this medication has a long half-life, and a report of a serious adverse reaction in a neonate has been published.[21] A nonpharmacologic approach such as using topical heat may also be a good choice for breastfeeding women.

Patient Factors

Given that NSAIDs are used only temporarily and intermittently, the risk for GI toxicity is limited. However, patients who have active peptic ulcer disease, those at risk for GI bleeding, or those with a history of GI ulcers should discuss use of NSAIDs with their primary care provider. Treatment with acetaminophen, nonpharmacologic therapy, or an OC may be more appropriate. NSAIDs can also inhibit platelet activity and increase bleeding time. Women on anticoagulants should avoid NSAID use, and women on other agents that may increase bleeding should use NSAIDs cautiously. Women who consume three or more alcohol-containing beverages daily should discuss use of acetaminophen or aspirin with their primary care provider, because additive liver or GI toxicity, respectively, may occur.

Patient Preferences

Women may prefer to use an NSAID that they are familiar with, or they may prefer to try another agent if adverse effects were experienced previously. Preferences may also be based on tablet/capsule preferences or cost of products.

Complementary Therapies

A 2016 Cochrane review found no high-quality evidence of effectiveness for any dietary supplements in the management of dysmenorrhea.[22] Another Cochrane review found tentative evidence that use of transcutaneous electrical nerve stimulation (TENS) decreases acute pain compared with placebo.[23] Data from several randomized controlled trials have found acupressure to be an easily teachable, effective nonpharmacologic therapy for relieving primary dysmenorrhea.[24] All complementary therapies need further verification.

Assessment of Primary Dysmenorrhea: A Case-Based Approach

Before recommending any product to a patient experiencing symptoms of dysmenorrhea, the HCP should ascertain that the symptoms, particularly the onset and duration of pain in relation to the onset of menses, are consistent with primary dysmenorrhea (Table 9–1).

Case 9–1 illustrates the assessment of a patient with dysmenorrhea.

Patient Counseling for Primary Dysmenorrhea

Adolescents and young women who experience primary dysmenorrhea symptoms should be educated about this condition so they (1) realize primary dysmenorrhea is normal, (2) recognize typical symptoms and symptoms that are inconsistent with primary dysmenorrhea and when to seek medical evaluation, (3) understand that NSAIDs are preferred therapy because of their efficacy, and (4) know how to use these agents for greatest benefit. Patients should also be advised that nonprescription NSAIDs can be appropriate for initial therapy, but that not all women will respond. If response to the first agent is not adequate, another NSAID and/or an OC or a nondrug intervention can be tried. The HCP should explain the proper use of these agents and their potential adverse effects. The box "Patient Education for Primary Dysmenorrhea" lists specific information to provide patients.

Evaluation of Patient Outcomes for Primary Dysmenorrhea

Patient monitoring is accomplished by having the patient report whether her symptoms are improved or resolved. Symptoms should improve within an hour or so of taking an NSAID. The optimal

CASE 9-1

Relevant Evaluation Criteria	Scenario/Model Outcome
Collect	
1. Gather essential information about the patient's symptoms and medical history, including	
a. Description of symptom(s) (i.e., nature, onset, duration, severity, associated symptoms) including age at onset of symptoms	Patient is experiencing painful menstrual cramps. She has had menstrual cramps for most menses over the past 6 months. The cramps occur just during the first 2 days of menses. Prior to that she had cramps only during some menses. Sometimes she also experiences backache and headache during the first couple of days of menses.
b. Description of any factors that seem to precipitate, exacerbate, and/or relieve the patient's symptom(s)	Going to sleep can help sometimes.
c. Description of the patient's efforts to relieve the symptoms	She has tried acetaminophen 325–500 mg, taking it a couple of times a day when the cramps are bad.
d. Patient's identity	Eleanor La Salle; she is accompanied by her mother.
e. Patient's age, gender, height, and weight	14 years old, female, 5 ft 2 in., 100 lb
f. Patient's occupation	High-school student
g. Patient's dietary habits	She reports she eats a good diet overall; she eats meat, likes vegetables and salads; she eats yogurt some days. She does have pizza and fast-food about once weekly. In addition, she consumes chips, candy, and popcorn as snacks.
h. Patient's sleep habits	She sleeps about 8 hours a night; her menstrual cramps usually do not wake her, but occasionally they do.
i. Concurrent medical conditions, prescription and nonprescription medications, and dietary supplements	She has no chronic health conditions but does have occasional headaches or other aches and pains secondary to physical activities. She is on the school cross-country team. Multiple vitamin, 1 daily
j. Allergies	None
k. History of other adverse reactions to medications	None known
l. Other (describe) ______	n/a
Assess	
2. Differentiate patient's signs/symptoms, and correctly identify the patient's primary problem(s).	Ms. La Salle has symptoms that are consistent with mild–moderate primary dysmenorrhea. Her symptoms are cyclic, and the timing follows that of primary dysmenorrhea. She has not described pain at other times during the menstrual cycle. The other symptoms she has experienced (backache, headache) are also consistent with primary dysmenorrhea.
3. Identify exclusions for self-treatment (Figure 9–2).	Ms. La Salle is not experiencing any symptoms that would exclude self-treatment. She is not experiencing pain at times other than at the onset of menses; she does not describe menorrhagia or severe cramps or pain.
4. Formulate a comprehensive list of therapeutic alternatives for the primary problem to determine whether triage to a health care provider is required, and share this information with the patient or caregiver.	Options include (1) Refer patient to an appropriate HCP. (2) Recommend self-care with nonprescription and nondrug measures. (3) Recommend self-care until patient can see an appropriate HCP. (4) Take no action.
Plan	
5. Select an optimal therapeutic alternative to address the patient's problem, taking into account patient preferences.	A trial of nonprescription therapy with an NSAID should be recommended as self-care.
6. Describe the recommended therapeutic approach to the patient or caregiver.	"Your symptoms are consistent with primary dysmenorrhea. This is a condition that can typically be effectively treated with nonprescription NSAID medications. This is the first therapy typically recommended for dysmenorrhea."

Relevant Evaluation Criteria	Scenario/Model Outcome
7. Explain to the patient or caregiver the rationale for selecting the recommended therapeutic approach from the considered therapeutic alternatives.	"You have tried acetaminophen for pain management without much benefit. NSAID medications will provide stronger and more effective pain relief than acetaminophen will, because they target the cause of cramping and pain. Also, the NSAID medication will be more effective if you take it regularly for 2 days beginning as soon as menstrual symptoms or menses begin."
Implement	
8. When recommending self-care with nonprescription medications and/or nondrug therapy, convey accurate information to the patient or caregiver.	Two NSAIDs are available, and they are likely to be equally effective. These agents are ibuprofen and naproxen sodium. Ibuprofen should be taken every 4–6 hours while awake (the maximum daily dose is 1200 mg; suggested initial individual dose is 200–400 mg). For naproxen sodium, the initial dose is 220–440 mg (1–2 tablets) and then doses of 220 mg taken every 8–12 hours with a maximum daily dose of 660 mg. Naproxen sodium has the advantage of one fewer dose per day.
Solicit follow-up questions from the patient or caregiver.	"Why is cramping occurring every month now when it only used to occur some months? Is this a sign that something is wrong?"
Answer the patient's or caregiver's questions.	"Actually, what you are experiencing is completely normal as it takes a young woman's body about a year or so after menses to begin to establish regular ovulatory cycles; dysmenorrhea cramping and pain occur only when ovulation occurs."
Follow-up: Monitor and Evaluate	
9. Assess patient outcome.	"Try the NSAID medication for several months and see if it will help to reduce or alleviate your cramping and pain. You can increase the dose as needed up to the maximum daily dose. These medications are best taken with food to prevent GI upset. If your response to one of these medications is not especially helpful, then try the other NSAID. Sometimes one will work better than the other. Let me know if you have any further questions or if your pain management is not satisfactory. Adding a topical heat patch may help, or you may need stronger doses of these medications than the maximum dose for nonprescription use."

Key: GI = Gastrointestinal; HCP = health care provider; n/a = not applicable; NSAID = nonsteroidal anti-inflammatory drug.

PATIENT EDUCATION FOR Primary Dysmenorrhea

The objective of self-treatment is to relieve or significantly improve symptoms of dysmenorrhea so as to limit discomfort and disruption of usual activities. For most patients, carefully following product instructions and the self-care measures listed here will help ensure optimal therapeutic outcomes.

Nondrug Measures

- If effective, apply topical heat to the abdomen, lower back, or other painful area.
- Stop smoking cigarettes and avoid secondhand smoke.
- Consider eating more fish high in omega-3 fatty acids or taking a fish oil supplement.
- Participate in regular exercise if it lessens the symptoms.
- No dietary supplements have been shown effective for primary dysmenorrhea.

Nonprescription Medications

- Ibuprofen and naproxen sodium are the best type of nonprescription medication for primary dysmenorrhea. The medications stop or prevent strong uterine contractions (cramping).
- Start taking the medication when the menstrual period begins or when menstrual pain or other symptoms begin. Then take the medication at regular intervals following the product instructions, rather than just when the symptoms are present. See Table 9–2 for recommended nonsteroidal anti-inflammatory drug (NSAID) dosages.
- Take the NSAID with food to limit upset stomach and heartburn.
- Do not take NSAIDs if you are allergic to aspirin or any NSAID, or if you have peptic ulcer disease, gastroesophageal reflux disease, colitis, or any bleeding disorder.
- If you have hypertension, asthma, or heart failure, watch for early symptoms that the NSAID is causing fluid retention.
- Do not take a nonsalicylate NSAID if you are also taking anticoagulants or lithium.

When to Seek Medical Attention

- Seek medical attention if the pain intensity increases or if new symptoms occur.
- Seek medical attention if abdominal pain occurs at times other than just before or during the first few days of menses.

effect of drug therapy may not be seen until the woman has used the medication on a scheduled basis. If inadequate pain relief occurs, treatment beginning 1–2 days before expected menses may improve symptomatic relief. The patient with persistent symptoms should be advised to try another nonprescription NSAID, to add adjunct therapy, to consider use of an OC, or to see a primary care provider for evaluation.

PREMENSTRUAL DISORDERS

Almost all women experience some mild physical or mood changes before the onset of menses, and these are normal signs of ovulatory cycles.[25] The changes may include physical symptoms; food cravings; and emotional lability, irritability, or lowered mood. In addition, some women report positive changes, including increased energy, creativity, work productivity, and sexual desire.[26]

Premenstrual disorders are cyclic and composed of a combination of physical, emotional and mood, and behavioral symptoms that occur during the luteal phase of the menstrual cycle. Symptoms improve significantly or disappear by the end of menses and are absent during the first week following menses. The number and severity of symptoms and the extent to which they interfere with functioning distinguish typical premenstrual symptoms, PMS, and premenstrual dysphoric disorder (PMDD)[27] (Table 9–3). PMS is distinguished from normal physiologic premenstrual symptoms by its negative effect on daily functioning and the extent of distress caused by symptoms. PMDD is a severe form of PMS. The diagnosis of PMDD requires a specific constellation of symptoms that occurs on a cyclical basis, the presence of key psychological symptoms, and that symptoms are severe enough to interfere with social and/or occupational functioning.[25]

Of women with premenstrual symptoms, 60%–80% experience only mild, primarily physical symptoms that do not interfere with their lives.[28] An estimated 20%–30% of women experience clinically significant symptoms of PMS, and 3%–8% report symptoms that cause significant impairment that interferes with relationships, lifestyle, or work—PMDD.[25]

Premenstrual disorders can occur any time after menarche. Symptoms usually originate when women are in their teens to early 20s; typically, women wait about a decade to seek care.[5,28] Premenstrual disorder symptoms occur only during ovulatory cycles. Symptoms disappear during events that interrupt ovulation, such as pregnancy and breastfeeding, and at menopause. The use of OCs can cause or exacerbate premenstrual disorder symptoms, and use of hormone therapy in postmenopausal women may result in recurrence of premenstrual disorder symptoms.[29]

Many factors contribute to the development of a premenstrual disorder. Genetic factors likely play a role. Twin studies have shown that premenstrual disorders are inherited, with women whose mothers had a premenstrual disorder being more likely to develop such a disorder.[29,30] In addition, genetic differences exist in the serotonergic 5-HT_{1A} receptor and the estrogen alpha-receptor gene in women with and without premenstrual disorder symptoms.[30] Stress and prior traumatic events, including sexual abuse, are risk factors for premenstrual disorders. Different coping strategies for handling stress, as well as altered psychological and physiologic responses to stress, have been shown in individuals with a history of life stress and abuse.[30] Sociocultural factors can also influence the experience of premenstrual symptoms. Exposure to negative expectations about premenstrual symptoms can lead women to interpret normal symptoms more negatively.[30]

Pathophysiology of Premenstrual Disorders

The etiology of premenstrual disorders is not fully understood. The current consensus is that the fluctuations of estrogen and progesterone caused by normal ovarian function are the cyclic trigger for premenstrual disorder symptoms. Although triggered by hormonal fluctuations, no known hormonal imbalances are present

TABLE 9–3 Differentiation of PMS and PMDD From Other Conditions With Luteal Phase Symptoms

Typical premenstrual symptoms	Mild physical (breast tenderness, bloating, lower backache, food cravings) or mood (irritability, emotional lability, lowered mood, increased energy or creativity) changes before the onset of menses that do not interfere with normal life functions
Premenstrual syndrome	At least one mood (depression, irritability, anger, anxiety) or physical (breast tenderness, abdominal bloating) symptom during the 5 days prior to menses. Symptoms are virtually absent during cycle days 5–10. The symptom or symptoms are severe enough to cause significant distress and/or have a negative effect on normal daily functioning (e.g., interfere with work and school performance) or interpersonal relationships. Symptoms may range from mild–moderate to severe.
Premenstrual dysphoric disorder	Five or more symptoms (mood or physical) are present the last week of the luteal phase of the menstrual cycle, with at least one symptom being significant depression, anxiety, affective lability, or anger. The intensity of the symptoms interferes with work, school, social activities, and social relationships. Symptoms should be absent the week after menses and must not be an exacerbation of the symptoms of another disorder such as depression, panic disorder, or personality disorder.
Premenstrual exacerbation	A worsening of the symptoms of other, typically psychiatric disorders, such as depression and anxiety or panic disorders. Conditions such as asthma, endometriosis, hypothyroidism, irritable bowel syndrome, attention-deficit disorder, diabetes, rheumatoid arthritis, migraine headaches, seizure disorders, and perimenopause can also worsen premenstrually. However, symptoms do not occur only during the luteal phase of the menstrual cycle; there is no symptom-free interval.

Source: Reference 5 and American Psychiatric Association. *Diagnostic and Statistical Manual of Mental Disorders: DSM-5.* 5th ed. Arlington, VA: American Psychiatric Association; 2013.

in women with a premenstrual disorder. Some women are biologically vulnerable or predisposed to experience this type of disorder because of a neurotransmitter sensitivity to physiologic changes in hormone levels.[5,28,30] Serotonin, which is involved in mood and behavior regulation, is affected by estrogen and progesterone levels. Reduced levels of serotonin and serotonin effect in the brain may be linked to certain premenstrual disorder symptoms such as poor impulse control, irritability, carbohydrate craving, and dysphoria.[5,29] Other neurotransmitters and systems that may be important are allopregnanolone and gamma-aminobutyric acid (GABA) receptors. Allopregnanolone is a progesterone metabolite that binds the GABA receptor, leading to an anxiolytic action.[28] Women who have a premenstrual disorder may be less sensitive to the sedating effects of allopregnanolone during the luteal phase and may have different GABA receptor sensitivity.[28,30] These alterations may result in luteal phase symptoms such as anxiety and irritability.[29] In addition, selective serotonin reuptake inhibitors (SSRIs), which are known to relieve premenstrual disorders, affect the synthesis of allopregnanolone. Therefore, for symptoms severe enough to warrant prescription drug therapy, treatment is based on medications that affect the levels of serotonin or suppress ovulation and interrupt hormonal cycling.

The pathophysiology of physical symptoms of premenstrual disorders (e.g., breast tenderness, bloating, and joint/muscle pain) is not as well studied. Studies of fluid retention and breast enlargement have not found tissue changes; abdominal bloating often occurs without weight gain.[27]

Exogenous hormones may influence premenstrual symptoms. Women taking either OCs or postmenopausal hormone therapy may experience adverse effects similar to PMS symptoms as a result of altered hormone levels.[26,29] Conversely, 71% of women reported that the use of their OC had no effect on their PMS symptoms.[5] Certain OCs have been useful in reducing the symptoms of premenstrual disorders, particularly OCs containing drospirenone, those with a lower estrogen dose, those with a shortened hormone-free interval between pill packs, and those with continuous or extended cycles.[18,25]

Clinical Presentation of Premenstrual Disorders

The symptoms of premenstrual disorders are not unique to these conditions; however, the occurrence of specific symptoms and their fluctuation with the phases of the menstrual cycle are diagnostic. Premenstrual symptoms typically begin or intensify about a week prior to the onset of menses, peak near the onset of menses, and resolve within several days after the beginning of menses.[29] Symptoms typically are consistent from month to month. A woman with a premenstrual disorder should experience essentially a symptom-free interval during days 5–10 of her menstrual cycle.

Common symptoms of premenstrual disorders are listed in Table 9–4. Women seeking symptom relief typically report multiple emotional, physical, and behavioral symptoms. Mood and behavioral symptoms are the most upsetting.[29] Most women rate their symptoms as mild–moderate and do not feel that they interfere with their lives. Mood symptoms tend to cause more distress than physical symptoms because of their impact on relationships. A large cross-sectional study conducted in multiple countries found that the most common PMS symptoms reported by women included abdominal bloating, cramps or abdominal pain, irritability, breast tenderness, and joint or back pain.[31] These symptoms may be reported most often to providers and may blur the distinction between dysmenorrhea and PMS. In addition, the presence of dysmenorrhea may be associated with a greater severity of PMS.[32]

TABLE 9-4 Common Premenstrual Syndrome Symptoms

Most Common Negative Symptoms
Fatigue, lack of energy
Irritability, anger
Labile mood with alternating sadness and anger
Depression, decreased interest in usual activities
Anxiety, feeling stressed
Crying spells, oversensitivity
Difficulty concentrating
Abdominal bloating, edema of extremities
Breast tenderness
Appetite changes (overeating and food cravings)
Headache
Hypersomnia/Insomnia
Joint/Muscle pain
Feeling out of control/overwhelmed
Most Common Positive Symptoms
Increased energy, more efficient at work
Increased libido, more affectionate
Increased sense of control, more self-assured

Source: Adapted from reference 25.

Symptoms of PMDD are similar to those of PMS. Compared with women who have PMS, women with PMDD experience more symptoms, symptoms of greater severity, and symptoms that impair personal relationships and the ability to function well at work or school to a greater extent. Among women with PMDD, the most common symptoms are affective in nature. The diagnosis of PMDD requires that a patient experience marked anger or irritability, or depressed mood, anxiety, or emotional lability.[33] Other symptoms of PMDD include difficulty concentrating, lethargy, hypersomnia or insomnia, and physical symptoms such as breast tenderness and bloating. The severity of symptoms must cause significant impairment in the ability to function socially or at work during the week prior to menses.[33] A daily rating of symptoms for several cycles establishes a diagnosis of PMS or PMDD, and these types of symptoms should have occurred during most menstrual cycles over the past year. PMDD symptoms during the last 7 days of the cycle should be at least 30% worse than those experienced during the mid-follicular phase (days 3–9 of the menstrual cycle).

Premenstrual disorders should be distinguished from typical premenstrual symptoms and also from premenstrual exacerbations of other disorders, particularly mood disorders. Some medical conditions can be aggravated during the premenstrual phase.[29,33] In addition, mood disorders not occurring solely during the luteal phase must be distinguished from cyclic mood symptoms (Table 9–3). The lack of a symptom-free interval suggests that the patient has a psychiatric disorder, such as an anxiety or panic disorder, or another health condition, such as the menopausal transition, rather than PMS.

Treatment of PMS

PMS is a multisymptom disorder that involves emotional, behavioral, and physical symptoms. A single therapeutic agent is unlikely to address all symptoms. Thus, treatment should be selected to address the patient's most bothersome symptoms. A symptom log or calendar is a useful tool for documenting the most bothersome symptom(s) and the cyclic nature of this disorder. This information will also be useful in evaluating the efficacy of treatment. Women with severe symptoms are less likely to have symptoms alleviated solely by use of nonprescription therapies. In addition, PMS symptoms are chronic and, in most cases, will continue until menopause. Therefore, the cost of therapy, the possibility that a woman may become pregnant, and the likelihood of adverse effects are important considerations in selecting therapy.

Treatment Goals

The two intended outcomes for women with premenstrual disorders are to better understand premenstrual disorders and to improve or resolve symptoms to reduce the impact on activities and interpersonal relationships. Typically, therapy is considered effective if symptoms are reduced by 50% or more.

General Treatment Approach

Mild–moderate PMS symptoms often are self-treatable and do not require prescription drug therapy. In these cases, initial treatment is generally conservative, and consists of education and nonpharmacologic measures. These include dietary modifications, physical exercise, and stress management. Women should be educated about the syndrome and encouraged to identify techniques for coping with PMS symptoms and stress. Many women are engaged in multiple social roles, which can increase stress. Knowledge of this disorder can allow a woman to exert some control over her symptoms by anticipating and planning. For example, she might schedule more challenging tasks during the first half of the cycle, thus limiting the influence of this condition on her social and work functioning.

In addition to education, treatment options include lifestyle modifications. Nonpharmacologic approaches that can be considered include light therapy, cognitive behavioral therapy, and acupuncture.[29] Supplements with evidence of potential benefit include calcium, pyridoxine, and chasteberry (*Vitex agnus-castus*).[29,30] Preliminary data suggest a potential benefit from ginkgo, magnesium pyrrolidone, St. John's wort, and saffron.[34]

Prescription drug therapy should be considered if the treatments outlined in Figure 9–3 are ineffective or if the patient suffers from moderate–severe PMS or PMDD. SSRIs used daily, only during the luteal phase of the menstrual cycle, or when symptoms occur are the first-line prescription therapy. Agents that suppress ovulation such as OCs and GnRH agonists are also used. Newer OCs containing drospirenone, shortened hormone-free intervals, or extended cycling may also be considered first-line therapy for women who prefer a gynecologic approach rather than a psychological approach.[35] Finally, hysterectomy with bilateral oophorectomy is effective for refractory severe symptoms.[36] Surgery may be appealing for women experiencing significant adverse drug reactions and/or costs.[36]

Nonpharmacologic Therapy

Several nonpharmacologic therapies may improve PMS symptoms. These include aerobic exercise, dietary modifications, and cognitive behavior therapy.[29] Exercise can increase endorphin levels and may help decrease PMS symptoms.[29] Although the benefit of dietary changes is unproven, many HCPs recommend eating a balanced diet while also avoiding salty foods and simple sugars, which may cause fluid retention, and avoiding caffeine and alcohol, which can increase irritability.[29,30] Cravings for foods high in carbohydrates, which contain the serotonin precursor tryptophan, are common in women with PMS. Two studies of a carbohydrate-rich beverage that increased tryptophan levels demonstrated an improvement in emotional symptoms in women with PMS.[30] Consuming foods rich in complex carbohydrates such as whole-grain foods during the premenstrual interval may reduce symptoms.[30]

Stress is reported to increase PMS symptoms. Cognitive behavioral therapy, which emphasizes relaxation techniques and coping skills, may help reduce symptoms.[29,30] These approaches may be helpful used singly or as adjuncts to other therapies. Data that suggest a possible benefit with light therapy, acupuncture, and massage are also available.[29]

Pharmacologic Therapy

A survey of women with PMS found that 80% use some nonprescription therapy including vitamins, minerals, and herbs; a number of products have claims for the management of PMS yet little supporting evidence.[34]

Pyridoxine

Pyridoxine (vitamin B_6) has been suggested as a therapy for PMS. Trials have reported mixed results with no dose–response relationship shown, and no trials were performed in women with PMDD.[30,34] One double-blind, placebo-controlled trial found pyridoxine 80 mg daily improved mood symptoms to a greater extent than placebo.[30] The dosage of pyridoxine should be limited to 100 mg daily because of the risk for peripheral neuropathy with higher dosages.[29]

Calcium and Vitamin D

Data show an inverse relationship between both milk and vitamin D intake, and PMS.[5] An additional study reported that high dietary intake of both calcium and vitamin D may prevent the development of PMS symptoms.[37] Calcium ingestion may reduce fluctuations in calcium levels across the menstrual cycle. Hypocalcemia causes affective symptoms (anxiety, irritability, depression) similar to those of premenstrual disorder.[25] Reduced levels of vitamin D secondary to alterations in calcium and vitamin D metabolism during the luteal phase may trigger PMDD symptoms.

Several randomized trials have evaluated the effect of calcium supplementation on PMS symptoms. The largest trial studied the effect of calcium in a dosage of 600 mg twice daily in 466 women with moderate–severe PMS.[38] Symptoms were significantly reduced by the second month of therapy, and by the third month, calcium had reduced overall symptoms by 48%. Emotional symptoms such as mood swings, depression, and anger, as well as food cravings and physical symptoms, were all reduced. More than 50% of the women taking calcium had a greater than 50% improvement in symptoms; 29% had a greater than 75% improvement in symptoms. Few women experienced adverse effects from calcium; five withdrew from the study because of nausea, and one woman each in the calcium and placebo groups developed kidney stones. The dosage of calcium used in the trial is consistent with the recommended daily calcium intake for women of reproductive age, which is between 1000 and

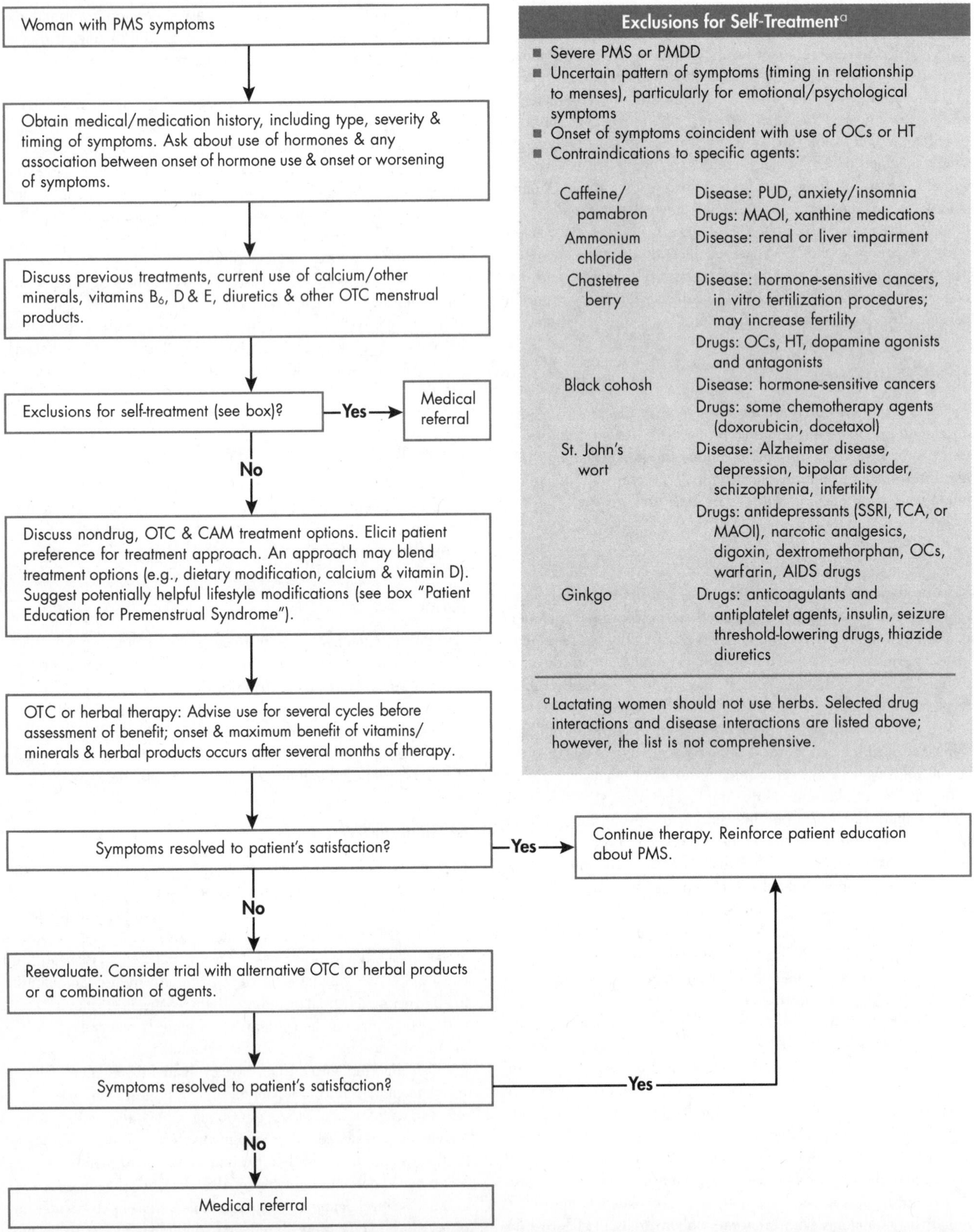

FIGURE 9–3 Self-care for premenstrual syndrome. Key: AIDS = Acquired immunodeficiency syndrome; CAM = complementary and alternative medicine; HT = hormone therapy; MAOI = monoamine oxidase inhibitor; OC = oral contraceptive; OTC = over-the-counter; PMDD = premenstrual dysphoric disorder; PMS = premenstrual syndrome; PUD = peptic ulcer disease; SSRI = selective serotonin reuptake inhibitor; TCA = tricyclic antidepressant.

1300 mg daily. Similar improvements were noted in smaller studies.[27,34,39] Additionally, all HCPs should be reinforcing adequate calcium and vitamin D intake in women to help prevent osteoporosis.

Magnesium

Magnesium deficiency may lead to some PMS-type symptoms (e.g., irritability), and low magnesium levels in red blood cells have been found in women with PMS. Affective symptoms associated with PMS were reduced by magnesium pyrrolidone carboxylic acid in a dosage of 360 mg daily administered during the luteal phase.[33,37] In contrast, two trials of magnesium oxide found no benefit. The dosage of magnesium pyrrolidone carboxylic acid used in the trial was similar to the recommended dietary allowance of magnesium for women (310–360 mg). About 50% of women regularly consume less than that amount, and obtaining adequate magnesium from food sources may be difficult. Food sources of magnesium include spinach, Swiss chard, nuts, legumes (e.g., beans, peas), and whole-grain cereals. Adverse effects other than diarrhea are uncommon.

Nonsteroidal Anti-inflammatory Drugs

NSAIDs reduce some of the physical symptoms such as headache and muscle/joint pains and mood symptoms associated with PMS when taken for several days prior to the onset of and during the first several days of menses.[29] The benefit from these agents may be a result of the coexistence of dysmenorrhea and PMS or PMS manifesting primarily as physical symptoms.

Diuretics

A common premenstrual symptom is the subjective sensation of fluid accumulation, particularly abdominal bloating. However, most women do not experience any true sodium or water retention and do not experience weight gain.[40] Two factors may explain the sense of abdominal bloating. First, a distinction must be made between fluid redistribution (where weight does not change) and fluid retention (which can be detected by weight gain). The abdominal bloating and swelling observed with PMS are primarily caused by a fluid shift to this area. As a result, diuretics that are indicated for relieving fluid retention are unlikely to be helpful for most women with PMS. Second, abdominal distention may occur secondary to relaxation of the gut muscle caused by progesterone.[40] For women who have true water retention and resultant weight gain, a diuretic may be useful.

FDA has approved three nonprescription diuretics as useful for relieving water retention, weight gain, bloating, swelling, and the feeling of fullness. These include ammonium chloride, caffeine, and pamabrom. The latter agent is the most common diuretic in nonprescription menstrual products (Table 9–5).

Ammonium chloride is an acid-forming salt with a short duration of effect. The drug is taken in oral dosages of up to 3 g/day, divided into 3 doses, for no more than 6 consecutive days. Larger dosages of ammonium chloride can produce significant GI and central nervous system adverse effects. Ammonium chloride is contraindicated in patients with renal or liver impairment, because metabolic acidosis may result. Ammonium chloride is no longer available as a nonprescription drug but can be obtained as a dietary supplement.

Caffeine promotes diuresis by inhibiting the renal tubular reabsorption of sodium and water. In doses of 100–200 mg every 3–4 hours, caffeine is safe and effective, although patients may develop tolerance to its diuretic effect. Caffeine may also cause anxiety, restlessness, or insomnia, and it may worsen PMS by causing irritability. Additive adverse effects might occur if other caffeine-containing medications, foods, or beverages especially "energy drinks" are consumed concurrently. Caffeine may also cause GI irritation; thus, it can cause or worsen dyspepsia. Patients taking monoamine oxidase inhibitors (MAOIs) or theophylline should also avoid diuretics that contain caffeine.

Pamabrom, a derivative of theophylline, is used in combination products along with analgesics and antihistamines marketed for the treatment of PMS. Pamabrom may be taken in dosages of up to 50 mg 4 times daily.

TABLE 9–5 Selected Combination Nonprescription Menstrual Products

Trade Name	Diuretic (per tablet/capsule)	Analgesic and/or Antihistamine (per tablet/capsule)
Aqua-Ban Tablets; Diurex Max; Diurex Water Caplets	Pamabrom 50 mg	
Diurex Ultra Water Weight Loss Formula	Caffeine 100 mg	
Pamprin Multi-symptom; Premsyn PMS	Pamabrom 25 mg	Acetaminophen 500 mg; pyrilamine maleate 15 mg
Pamprin Max	Caffeine 65 mg	Acetaminophen 250 mg; aspirin 250 mg
Midol Extended Relief	None	Naproxen sodium 220 mg
Midol Complete	Caffeine 60 mg	Acetaminophen 500 mg; pyrilamine maleate 15 mg
Midol Teen	Pamabrom 25 mg	Acetaminophen 500 mg
Midol PM	None	Acetaminophen 500 mg; diphenhydramine 38 mg

Combination Products

Multi-ingredient nonprescription products are marketed for women with PMS-type symptoms. Two of the most commonly used product brand names are Midol and Pamprin. Some products contain acetaminophen, caffeine/pamabrom, and pyrilamine, whereas others contain only an NSAID or a combination of an analgesic with a diuretic or an antihistamine (Table 9–5). Pain is a less common symptom of PMS, and no evidence exists that the sedative effect of an antihistamine, such as pyrilamine, will provide benefit to women experiencing the emotional symptoms of PMS. Therefore, these types of nonprescription products should not be recommended. More appropriate recommendations are the use of more definitive agents, such as those previously discussed, or referral for prescription drug therapy.

Pharmacotherapeutic Comparison

Calcium can be suggested for the initial treatment of PMS symptoms. If relief is inadequate, another agent or a combination of two or more agents may be tried. Women who experience bloating with documented weight gain might try pamabrom or caffeine. Caffeine and pamabrom may not be an appropriate choice for women who experience irritability as a PMS symptom. Both caffeine and pamabrom should be used cautiously in patients who have a history of peptic ulcer disease or who are taking MAOIs or other xanthine medications such as theophylline. NSAIDs should be reserved for women who experience headache, joint and/or muscle pain, or concomitant dysmenorrhea. Use of combination products containing antihistamines should be discouraged, because drowsiness may impair job performance, schoolwork, and driving.

Product Selection Guidelines

Special Populations

PMS does not occur during pregnancy or after menopause. Adolescents and adult women should initially attempt to manage symptoms with lifestyle changes and therapies such as calcium supplementation. Adolescents should avoid combination products containing aspirin (see "Special Populations" under "Dysmenorrhea"). Women who are breastfeeding should avoid all herbal products, because information about their safety for nursing infants is limited. Vitamins and minerals in the dosages used for PMS are generally compatible with breastfeeding, and magnesium use is unlikely to cause diarrhea in breastfed infants.[20] Diuretics should be avoided during breastfeeding, as caffeine appears in breast milk about 1 hour after maternal ingestion. Caffeine may cause fussiness and poor sleep in infants, especially if consumed in high dosages or if the infant is preterm or younger than 3 weeks of age.[21]

Patient Factors

Patients using proton pump inhibitors and histamine-2 receptor antagonists should use calcium citrate rather than calcium carbonate products, because the latter products are less soluble with a higher gastric pH.

Patient Preferences

Patient preferences for PMS treatment can be accommodated. Women preferring to use dietary supplements should discuss their use with an HCP to ensure that drug–drug or drug–disease interactions do not exist.

Complementary Therapies

Trials have been conducted with botanical therapies, including chasteberry (*Vitex agnus-castus*), St. John's wort (*Hypericum perforatum*), ginkgo (*Ginkgo biloba*), and saffron (*Crocus sativus*).[32] The first three dietary supplements are discussed in depth in Chapter 51.

Chasteberry has shown efficacy in improving mild–moderate PMS symptoms; in four high-quality trials, chasteberry demonstrated a significant improvement compared with placebo.[41] Trials have used different formulations of chasteberry. Two trials using a standardized fruit extract ZE 440 of chasteberry found a significant reduction in PMS symptoms including mood, irritability/anger, pain/headache, breast tenderness, and fluid retention.[42] Two randomized, double-blind, placebo-controlled trials found that chasteberry extract reduced common PMS symptoms and did not cause any serious adverse effects.[42,43] Symptoms were significantly lower by the end of the third cycle of use. In a trial in women diagnosed with PMDD,[44] chasteberry was compared with fluoxetine; a similar percentage of patients improved on both agents. Chasteberry was shown to decrease irritability, breast tenderness, swelling, food cravings, and cramps. In contrast, fluoxetine improved more mood symptoms; symptoms with a 50% reduction included depression, irritability, insomnia, nervous tension, feeling out of control, breast tenderness, and aches. Chasteberry was well tolerated; nausea and headache were the most common adverse effects. Chasteberry may offer more benefit for patients with mild–moderate PMS and for women experiencing breast pain.[44,45] Chasteberry may affect estrogen receptors and inhibit prolactin.[45] Women who are pregnant or lactating should avoid chasteberry, and it should be used cautiously by women taking hormones or who have hormone-sensitive cancers.

One randomized trial of St. John's wort reported a reduction in anxiety-related symptoms in women with PMS, although its effect was not different from placebo.[34] St. John's wort may improve mild–moderate depression. Two high-quality trials did not find a benefit greater than placebo.[41] St. John's wort has many clinically significant drug interactions including reducing the effectiveness of OCs.

A placebo-controlled randomized trial evaluated ginkgo in a dosage of 160–320 mg/day in 165 women with PMS. Symptoms of anxiety, irritability, and depression associated with PMS as well as breast pain were improved with ginkgo.[34,41] Ginkgo has antiplatelet effects and may increase the risk of bleeding.

In one randomized trial comparing saffron extract 30 mg/day with placebo, the saffron extract was found to significantly reduce PMS symptoms and depression symptoms.[34,41]

Assessment of PMS: A Case-Based Approach

The HCP should obtain a complete description of the patient's symptoms and their timing to determine whether the patient has PMS, PMDD, or another disorder with PMS-type symptoms. The severity of premenstrual disorder symptoms is another factor in self-treatment. As with any disorder, the HCP should explore the use of medications that might be causing the symptoms or that might potentially interact with nonprescription agents used to treat PMS. Previous treatments for the symptoms should also be explored.

Case 9–2 illustrates the assessment of a patient with PMS.

Patient Counseling for PMS

Educating women with PMS about the timing of symptoms using a symptom log and calendar and educating women about what might control those symptoms may increase compliance with recommended therapies. HCPs should be prepared to discuss the treatment of behavioral and physical symptoms of mild–moderate PMS. If the patient prefers to use nonprescription medications or vitamins, the proper use and potential adverse effects of these agents should be explained. The patient should also be advised that treatment measures must be implemented during every menstrual cycle, because it may take several cycles for symptomatic relief to occur. The "Patient Education for Premenstrual Syndrome" box lists specific information to provide patients.

CASE 9-2

Relevant Evaluation Criteria	Scenario/Model Outcome
Collect	
1. Gather essential information about the patient's symptoms and medical history, including	
a. Description of symptom(s) (i.e., nature, onset, duration, severity, associated symptoms)	The patient reports that she is experiencing worsening PMS symptoms. She gets symptoms every month about a week prior to menses, and they disappear as soon as menses occur. Most of her symptoms are emotional, such as moodiness (irritability) and being quick to be angry, sometimes out of proportion to the event that triggers her anger. She continues to work full-time, but during the week prior to her period, she often feels overwhelmed and wishes she could just stay at home.
b. Description of any factors that seem to precipitate, exacerbate, and/or relieve the patient's symptom(s)	"It seems worse if I am feeling stressed, like around high-school graduation or the holidays" (when she is in more demand as a photographer).
c. Description of the patient's efforts to relieve the symptoms	"If possible, I try to schedule fewer photo shoots during the weeks before my periods. I took Midol Complete for several days during the week of symptoms a couple of times but found it to be too sedating and otherwise not very helpful. I also tried taking vitamin B_6 at the suggestion of one of my friends, but that did not help me either."
d. Patient's identity	Barbara Kellerman
e. Age, gender, height, and weight	37 years old, female, 5 ft 6 in., 145 lb
f. Patient's occupation	Professional photographer
g. Patient's dietary habits	She typically has 3 meals daily; snacks during the day. Overall she thinks her diet is "OK," although she would like to lose some weight.
h. Patient's sleep habits	She estimates she gets about 7 hours of sleep nightly; she has no problem falling asleep and feels rested when she gets up in the morning.
i. Concurrent medical conditions, prescription and nonprescription medications, and dietary supplements	Hypertension: HCTZ 25 mg daily; seasonal allergies: fluticasone (Flonase) nasal spray once daily April–October Occasional tension headaches: ibuprofen 400 mg Occasional constipation: Metamucil Contraception: her husband had a vasectomy Dietary supplements: MVI, fish oil, vitamin D 2000 IU, probiotic blend (all taken once daily)
j. Allergies	Allergic to pollen, mold
k. History of other adverse reactions to medications	NKDA
l. Other (describe) _______	n/a
Assess	
2. Differentiate patient's signs/symptoms, and correctly identify the patient's primary problem(s).	The symptoms she describes are not consistent with mild–moderate PMS; they are more severe and emotional in nature. The cyclic occurrence of symptoms is consistent with PMS.
3. Identify exclusions for self-treatment (Figure 9–3).	Her symptoms are more severe than what is typical for mild–moderate PMS. She would be better served by referral for more definitive therapy than by an attempt at self-treatment with vitamins, minerals, and herbs.
4. Formulate a comprehensive list of therapeutic alternatives for the primary problem to determine whether triage to a health care provider is required, and share this information with the patient or caregiver.	Options include (1) Refer patient to an appropriate HCP. (2) Recommend self-care with nonprescription and nondrug measures. (3) Recommend self-care until patient can see an appropriate HCP. (4) Take no action.

Relevant Evaluation Criteria	Scenario/Model Outcome
Plan	
5. Select an optimal therapeutic alternative to address the patient's problem, taking into account patient preferences.	Recommend referral to her primary care provider.
6. Describe the recommended therapeutic approach to the patient or caregiver.	"The symptoms you describe are not consistent with mild–moderate PMS, and the emotional symptoms you describe are better managed with prescription medications. You can certainly take calcium 500–600 mg twice daily through diet and/or supplements. And you can consider some stress reduction and relaxation techniques that would help."
7. Explain to the patient or caregiver the rationale for selecting the recommended therapeutic approach from the considered therapeutic alternatives.	"The emotional and mood symptoms you describe are better managed with prescription medications. The nonprescription agents available are not likely to effectively address your symptoms."
Implement	
8. When recommending self-care with nonprescription medications and/or nondrug therapy, convey accurate information to the patient or caregiver.	"If you choose to add calcium to your regimen, it should be taken twice daily, with each dose being not more than 500–600 mg as that is the highest dose the body can absorb at one time. You are not likely to experience adverse effects from calcium, but some women experience gastrointestinal distress or constipation. Let me know if that occurs, and I can suggest how to manage those adverse effects. You are currently taking vitamin D, which will help with the absorption of calcium and may add to the relief of PMS symptoms too."
Solicit follow-up questions from the patient or caregiver.	"What types of prescription medications are used for PMS?"
Answer the patient's or caregiver's questions.	"The most common types of prescription medications used for the management of PMS are in the SSRI family of medications. These medications are regarded as the treatment of choice and have been shown to have good effectiveness for 60%–80% of women with more significant PMS symptoms."
Follow-up: Monitor and Evaluate	
9. Assess patient outcome.	n/a

Key: HCP = Health care provider; HCTZ = hydrochlorothiazide; MVI = multivitamin; n/a = not applicable; NKDA = no known drug allergies; PMS = premenstrual syndrome; SSRI = selective serotonin reuptake inhibitor.

PATIENT EDUCATION FOR Premenstrual Syndrome

The objective of self-treatment is to achieve relief from or significant improvement in premenstrual syndrome (PMS) symptoms to limit discomfort, distress, and the disruption of personal relationships or usual activities. For most patients, carefully following product instructions and the self-care measures listed here will help ensure optimal therapeutic outcomes.

Nondrug Measures

- Try to avoid stress, develop effective coping mechanisms for managing stress, and learn relaxation techniques.
- If possible, participate in regular aerobic exercise.
- During the 7–14 days before your menstrual period, reduce intake of salt, caffeine, chocolate, and alcoholic beverages. Eating foods rich in carbohydrates and low in protein during the premenstrual interval also may reduce symptoms.

Nonprescription Medications

- Nonprescription medications and lifestyle modifications may not improve symptoms for all women, and it may take several months to determine whether these therapies are working.
- Therapy with one nonprescription medication may improve only some of the symptoms; several medications may be needed for optimal symptom control. However, only add one agent at a time so that it is possible to determine which agent causes benefit or adverse effects.
- Follow the guidelines here for the agents that best control your symptoms:
  - Take 1200 mg of elemental calcium daily in divided doses. Calcium can be obtained from food or from supplements. Take no more than 500–600 mg at one time. Calcium may cause stomach upset (if this occurs, take with food) or constipation.
  - Take at least 600 IU of vitamin D daily.
  - Take 300–360 mg of magnesium pyrrolidone daily during the premenstrual interval only. Magnesium may cause diarrhea.
  - Take up to 100 mg of pyridoxine daily. Do not exceed this dosage, or neurologic symptoms caused by vitamin B_6 toxicity may occur.

When to Seek Medical Attention

- If you are taking vitamin B_6 and develop neurologic symptoms (e.g., a sensation of pricking, tingling, or creeping on the skin; bone pain; muscle weakness; or stinging, burning, or itching sensations), stop taking the vitamin and seek medical attention.
- If the PMS symptoms do not improve, or if they worsen, a medical evaluation is suggested.

Evaluation of Patient Outcomes for PMS

Monitoring is accomplished by having the patient report whether the symptoms are resolved. It may take several menstrual cycles to ascertain whether lifestyle changes or nonprescription therapies are reducing the symptoms of PMS. Comparing the occurrence and/or severity of symptoms before and after vitamin or medication use can help determine the value of a therapy. Women should be encouraged to contact their HCP to discuss treatment effectiveness and to clarify information or answer any questions. Reasons for advising the patient to see a provider include persistent symptoms, symptoms that the patient reports are disruptive to personal relationships, or symptoms that affect the patient's ability to engage in usual activities or function productively at work/school.

TOXIC SHOCK SYNDROME

Toxic shock syndrome (TSS) is a severe multisystem illness characterized by high fever, profound hypotension, severe diarrhea, mental confusion, renal failure, erythroderma, and skin desquamation. In 1980, these symptoms were recognized as affecting a relatively large number of young, previously healthy, menstruating women. TSS is commonly divided into menstrual and nonmenstrual cases.

Menstrual TSS affects primarily young women between 13 and 19 years of age.[46] Almost all cases of menstrual TSS have been associated with menstruation and tampon use, especially the use of high-absorbency tampons.[46]

The decrease in cases of menstrual TSS has been attributed to several factors, including removal of superabsorbent tampons from the market; a change in the composition of tampons; an increased awareness of the recommendations to change tampons frequently and to alternate tampon and pad use; and FDA-required standardized labeling of tampons.[46]

The strongest predictor of risk for menstrual TSS is the use of tampons. The greatest risk is associated with the use of higher absorbency tampons; for every 1 g increase in absorbency, the risk for TSS increases 34%–37%. Continuous uninterrupted use of tampons for at least 1 day during menses also has been shown to correlate with an increased risk for menstrual TSS. In addition, using tampons between menstrual periods (to manage vaginal discharge or nonmenstrual bleeding) can increase the likelihood of vaginal ulcers and the risk of TSS.[47] Besides tampons, TSS has been associated with the use of barrier contraceptives, including diaphragms, cervical caps and cervical sponges, and IUCs.

Pathophysiology of Menstrual TSS

Menstrual TSS is caused by the toxin-producing strains of *Staphylococcus aureus*.[48] TSS is an inflammatory immune response to the enterotoxins produced by these bacteria. Toxin-producing strains of *S. aureus* produce the superantigen toxin TSST-1. Most adults have a protective level of antibodies against the TSST-1 toxin. Younger people who lack this antibody protection and who become infected with a toxin-producing strain of *S. aureus* may develop TSS.[48]

Four conditions promote toxin production: elevated protein levels, neutral pH, elevated carbon dioxide levels, and elevated oxygen levels.[46] During menses, menstrual blood provides an increase in protein and also increases vaginal pH to 7, or neutral pH. Tampon use may create the environment for TSS by introducing oxygen into the vagina; oxygen is trapped within the tampon, and higher absorbency tampons carry more oxygen into the vagina.[46,48] Oxygen is a critical factor for the production of TSST-1.[49] After the introduction of a tampon, the vagina takes hours to return to its anaerobic state, with elevated carbon dioxide levels. In addition, tampons, IUCs, and contraceptive sponges create microtrauma, which increases exposure of the toxins to the circulatory and immune systems. Exposure of immune cells to TSST-1 initiates the inflammatory cascade involving interleukin-1 and tumor necrosis factor. This inflammatory response results in the signs and symptoms of TSS.

Clinical Presentation of Menstrual TSS

By definition, menstrual TSS occurs within 2 days of the onset of menses, during menses, or within 2 days after menses. Prodromal symptoms, including malaise, myalgias, and chills, occur for 2–3 days prior to TSS.[48] GI symptoms of vomiting, diarrhea, and abdominal pain typically occur early in the illness and affect almost all patients. After that, TSS evolves rapidly into high fever, myalgias, vomiting and diarrhea, erythroderma, decreased urine output, severe hypotension, and shock. Neurologic manifestations including headache, confusion, agitation, lethargy, and seizures also occur in almost all cases. Acute renal failure, cardiac involvement, and adult respiratory distress syndrome are also common.

Dermatologic manifestations are characteristic of TSS; both early rash and subsequent skin desquamation are required for a definite diagnosis. The early rash often is described as a sunburn-like, diffuse, macular erythroderma that is not pruritic. About 5–12 days after the onset of TSS, desquamation of the skin on the patient's face, trunk, and extremities (including the soles of the feet and the palms of the hands) occurs.

Prevention of Menstrual TSS

Women can almost entirely prevent menstrual TSS by using sanitary pads instead of tampons during their menstrual cycle. Women who use tampons can reduce the risk of developing TSS by following the guidelines in the box Patient Education for Toxic Shock Syndrome.

Women who have had TSS are at risk for recurrence; TSS recurs in about 28%–64% of women with menstrual TSS.[47] Recurrence rates are lower for women who are treated with antibiotics during TSS. Prevention of TSS for these patients includes avoiding tampons, IUCs, diaphragms, cervical caps, and contraceptive sponges.

Assessment of Menstrual TSS: A Case-Based Approach

Obtaining prompt medical attention is an important aspect of care for patients with symptoms consistent with TSS. An HCP can be alert to symptoms of TSS when patients seek nonprescription therapy for a severe "flu" with symptoms such as fever, vomiting, diarrhea, and dizziness, or when patients seek help for an unusual

PATIENT EDUCATION FOR Toxic Shock Syndrome

The objective of self-treatment is to reduce the risk of developing toxic shock syndrome (TSS) associated with the use of tampons or contraceptive devices. For most patients, carefully following product instructions and the self-care measures listed here will help ensure optimal therapeutic outcomes.

- To reduce the risk of TSS to almost zero, use sanitary pads instead of tampons during your period.
- To lower the risk of TSS while using tampons, use the lowest-absorbency tampons compatible with your needs. Also, alternate the use of menstrual pads with the use of tampons (e.g., use pads at night) so that tampons are not used continuously for 24 hours.
- Change tampons four to six times a day and at least every 6 hours; overnight use should be no longer than 8 hours.
- Wash your hands with soap before inserting anything into the vagina (e.g., tampon, diaphragm, contraceptive sponge, or vaginal medication). The bacteria causing TSS usually are found on the skin.
- Do not leave a contraceptive sponge, diaphragm, or cervical cap in place in the vagina longer than recommended; do not use any of them during menstruation.
- Do not use tampons, contraceptive sponges, or a cervical cap during the first 12 weeks after childbirth. It may also be best to avoid using a diaphragm.
- Read the insert on TSS enclosed in the tampon package, and become familiar with the early symptoms of this disorder.

When to Seek Medical Attention

- If you develop symptoms of TSS (high fever, muscle aches, a sunburn-like rash appearing after a day or two, weakness, fatigue, nausea, vomiting, and diarrhea), remove the tampon or contraceptive device immediately, and seek emergency medical treatment. If left untreated, TSS can cause shock and even death.

skin rash that occurs in conjunction with the previously described symptoms. If TSS is suspected, the patient should be advised to seek medical care immediately and to avoid use of NSAIDs for fever and myalgias, because these agents may increase the progression of TSS by increasing the production of tumor necrosis factor.

Patient Counseling for Menstrual TSS

Tampons are used by women of all ages during their reproductive years. HCPs should counsel patients about the prevention of TSS as outlined in the box "Patient Education for Toxic Shock Syndrome." In particular, providers should emphasize the importance of washing the hands before inserting a tampon, which removes organisms causing TSS from the skin. About 18%–36% of women report that they do not always change a tampon at least every 6 hours; providers should counsel patients to change tampons frequently, according to product instructions; to alternate the use of tampons with the use of sanitary pads over a 24-hour period; and to use the lowest absorbency tampons compatible with their needs. The HCP should emphasize, however, that the risk for this condition is quite small. If a patient presents with early symptoms of TSS, she should be advised to remove the tampon or any barrier contraceptive device and to seek emergency medical treatment.

Key Points for Disorders Related to Menstruation

- ➤ Self-care is appropriate for an otherwise healthy young woman whose history is consistent with primary dysmenorrhea and who is not sexually active, or for a woman diagnosed with primary dysmenorrhea. Adolescents with pelvic pain who are sexually active and thus at risk for PID and women with characteristics indicating secondary dysmenorrhea or persistent dysmenorrhea despite treatment with nonprescription agents should be referred for medical evaluation.
- ➤ NSAIDs are the drugs of choice for the management of primary dysmenorrhea. These medications should be taken at the onset of or just prior to menses and should be used in scheduled doses for several days for the optimal reduction in pain and cramping.
- ➤ The use of local topical heat can also provide relief from dysmenorrhea. Its analgesic effect has a faster onset than drug therapy, and it can add to the relief provided by an NSAID. Nonpharmacologic therapy may be especially useful for women who cannot tolerate or who prefer not to use drug therapy or who do not respond to nonprescription NSAIDs.
- ➤ Premenstrual disorders should be distinguished from typical premenstrual symptoms and also from premenstrual exacerbations of other disorders, particularly mood disorders.
- ➤ Premenstrual disorder symptoms typically begin or intensify about a week prior to the onset of menses, peak the 2 days before menses, and resolve within several days to a week after the beginning of menses. A woman with a premenstrual disorder experiences a symptom-free interval during days 5–10 of her menstrual cycle.
- ➤ Premenstrual disorder symptoms are chronic and, in most cases, will continue until menopause. Therefore, the cost of therapy, the possibility that a woman may become pregnant, and the likelihood of adverse effects from therapy are important considerations in selecting therapy.
- ➤ Calcium, pyridoxine, and chasteberry might be suggested to reduce the symptoms of mild–moderate PMS. More severe PMS and PMDD symptoms warrant prescription drug therapy.
- ➤ TSS has been linked to tampon use. To lower the risk for TSS while using tampons, women should use the lowest-absorbency tampons compatible with their needs and should alternate the use of sanitary pads with the use of tampons over a 24-hour period.

REFERENCES

1. Fothergill DJ. Common menstrual problems in adolescence. *Arch Dis Child Educ Pract Ed.* 2010;95(6):199–203. doi: 10.1136/adc.2009.175802.
2. Peacock A, Alvi NS, Mushtaq T. Period problems: disorders of menstruation in adolescents. *Arch Dis Child.* 2012;97(6):554–60. doi: 10.1136/adc.2009.160853.

3. Mihm M, Gangooly S, Muttukrishna S. The normal menstrual cycle in women. *Anim Reprod Sci.* 2011;124(3-4):229–36. doi: 10.1016/j.anireprosci.2010.08.030.
4. Jamison MA. Disorders of menstruation in adolescent girls. *Pediatr Clin North Am.* 2015;62(4):943–61. doi: 10.1016/j.pcl.2015.04.007.
5. Allen LM, Lam ACN. Premenstrual syndrome and dysmenorrhea in adolescents. *Adolesc Med State Art Rev.* 2012;23(1):139–63. PMID: 22764560.
6. Harel Z. Dysmenorrhea in adolescents and young adults: an update on pharmacological treatments and management strategies. *Expert Opin Pharmacother.* 2012;13(15):2157–70. doi: 10.1517/14656566.2012.725045.
7. Mannix LK. Menstrual-related pain conditions: dysmenorrhea and migraine. *J Womens Health (Larchmt).* 2008;17(5):879–91. doi: 10.1089/jwh.2007.0440.
8. Zahradnik HP, Hanjalic-Beck A, Groth K. Nonsteroidal anti-inflammatory drugs and hormonal contraceptives for pain relief from dysmenorrhea: a review. *Contraception.* 2010;81(3):185–96. doi: 10.1016/j.contraception.2009.09.014.
9. Osayande AS, Mehulic S. Diagnosis and initial management of dysmenorrhea. *Am Fam Physician.* 2014;89(5):341–6. PMID: 24695505.
10. Parker A, Sneddon AE, Arbon P. The Menstrual Disorder of Teenagers (MDOT) study: determining typical menstrual patterns and menstrual disturbance in a large population-based study of Australian teenagers. *BJOG.* 2010;117(2):185–92. doi: 10.1111/j.1471-0528.2009.02407.x.
11. Iacovides S, Avidon I, Baker FC. What we know about primary dysmenorrhea today: a critical review. *Hum Reprod Update.* 2015;21(6):762–78. doi: 10.1093/humupd/dmv039.
12. Ju H, Jones M, Mishra G. The prevalence and risk factors for dysmenorrhea. *Epidemiol Rev.* 2014;36:104–13. doi: 10.1093/epirev/mxt009.
13. Bertone-Johnson ER, Manson JE. Vitamin D for menstrual and pain-related disorders in women (comment on "improvement of primary dysmenorrhea caused by single oral dose of vitamin D"). *Arch Intern Med.* 2012;172(4):367–9. doi: 10.1001/archinte.172.4.367.
14. Lasco A, Catalano A, Benvenga S. Improvement of primary dysmenorrhea caused by single oral dose of vitamin D: results of a randomized, double-blind, placebo-controlled study. *Arch Intern Med.* 2012;172(4):366–7. doi: 10.1001/archinternmed.2011.715.
15. Akin M, Price W, Rodriguez G Jr, et al. Continuous, low-level, topical heat wrap therapy as compared to acetaminophen for primary dysmenorrhea. *J Reprod Med.* 2004;49(9):739–45. PMID: 15493566.
16. Ju H, Jones M, Mishra G. Premenstrual syndrome and dysmenorrhea: symptom trajectories over 13 years in young adults. *Maturitas.* 2014; 78(2):99–105. doi: 10.1016/j.maturitas.2014.03.008.
17. Dawood MY, Khan-Dawood FS. Clinical efficacy and differential inhibition of menstrual fluid prostaglandin F2alpha in a randomized, double-blind, crossover treatment with placebo, acetaminophen, and ibuprofen in primary dysmenorrhea. *Am J Obstet Gynecol.* 2007;196(1):35.e1–5. doi: 10.1016/j.ajog.2006.06.091.
18. American College of Obstetricians and Gynecologists. ACOG practice bulletin no. 110: noncontraceptive uses of hormonal contraceptives. *Obstet Gynecol.* 2010;115(1):206–18. doi: 10.1097/AOG.0b013e3181cb50b5.
19. Marjoribanks J, Proctor ML, Farquhar C, et al. Nonsteroidal anti-inflammatory drugs for dysmenorrhea. *Cochrane Database Syst Rev.* 2010; 1:CD001751. doi: 10.1002/14651858.CD001751.
20. U.S. Food and Drug Administration. Labeling of drug preparations containing salicylates. *CFR: Code of Federal Regulations.* Title 21, Part 201, Section 201.314. Updated July 27, 2017. Available at: http://www.ecfr.gov/cgi-bin/text-idx?SID=b1b2224711dc88657752be21f12c574a&mc=true&node=se21.4.201_1314&rgn=div8. Accessed July 31, 2017.
21. U.S. National Library of Medicine. LactMed: drugs and lactation database. Available at: http://toxnet.nlm.nih.gov/cgi-bin/sis/htmlgen?LACT. Accessed May 31, 2013.
22. Pattanittum P, Kunyanone N, Brown J, et al. Dietary supplements for dysmenorrhea. *Cochrane Database Syst Rev.* 2016;3:CD002124. doi: 10.1002/14651858.CD002124.pub2.
23. Johnson MI, Paley CA, Howe TE, et al. Transcutaneous electrical nerve stimulation for acute pain. *Cochrane Database Syst Rev.* 2015;6: CD006142. doi: 10.1002/14651858.CD006142.pub3.
24. Cho SH, Hwang EW. Acupressure for primary dysmenorrhea: a systematic review. *Complement Ther Med.* 2010;18(1):49–56. doi: 10.1016/j.ctim.2009.10.001.
25. Rapkin AJ, Lewis EI. Treatment of premenstrual dysphoric disorder. *Womens Health (Lond).* 2013;9(6):537–56. doi: 10.2217/whe.13.62.
26. Campagne DM, Campagne G. The premenstrual syndrome revisited. *Eur J Obstet Gynecol Reprod Biol.* 2007;130(1):4–17. doi: 10.1016/j.ejogrb.2006.06.020.
27. Freeman EW. Therapeutic management of premenstrual syndrome. *Expert Opin Pharmacother.* 2010;11(17):2879–89. doi: 10.1517/14656566.2010.509344.
28. Jarvis CI, Lynch AM, Morin AK. Management strategies for premenstrual syndrome/premenstrual dysphoric disorder. *Ann Pharmacother.* 2008;42:967–78. doi: 10.1345/aph.1K673.
29. Rapkin A, Mikacich JA. Premenstrual syndrome and premenstrual dysphoric disorder in adolescents. *Curr Opin Obstet Gynecol.* 2008; 20(5):455–63. doi: 10.1097/GCO.0b013e3283094b79.
30. Vigod SN, Ross LE, Steiner M. Understanding and treating premenstrual disorder: an update for the women's health practitioner. *Obstet Gynecol Clin North Am.* 2009;36(4):907–24. doi: 10.1016/j.ogc.2009.10.010.
31. Dennerstein L, Lehert P, Heinemann K. Epidemiology of premenstrual symptoms and disorders. *Menopause Int.* 2012;18(2):48–51. doi: 10.1258/mi.2012.012013.
32. Kitamura M, Takeda T, Koga S, et al. Relationship between premenstrual symptoms and dysmenorrhea in Japanese high school students. *Arch Womens Ment Health.* 2012;15(2):131–3. doi: 10.1007/s00737-012-0266-2.
33. American Psychiatric Association. *Diagnostic and Statistical Manual of Mental Disorders: DSM-5.* 5th ed. Arlington, VA: American Psychiatric Association; 2013.
34. Whelan AM, Jurgens TM, Naylor H. Herbs, vitamins and minerals in the treatment of premenstrual syndrome: a systematic review. *Can J Clin Pharmacol.* 2009;16(3):e407–29. PMID: 19923637.
35. Panay N. Treatment of premenstrual syndrome: a decision-making algorithm. *Menopause Int.* 2012;18(2):90–2. doi: 10.1258/mi.2012.012019.
36. Reid RL. When should surgical treatment be considered for premenstrual dysphoric disorder? *Menopause Int.* 2012;18(2):77–81. doi: 10.1258/mi.2012.012009.
37. Bertone-Johnson ER, Hankinson SE, Bendich A, et al. Calcium and vitamin D intake and risk of incident premenstrual syndrome. *Arch Intern Med.* 2005;165(11):1246–52. doi: 10.1001/archinte.165.11.1246.
38. Thys-Jacobs S, Starkey P, Bernstein D, et al. Calcium carbonate and the premenstrual syndrome: effect on premenstrual and menstrual symptoms. *Am J Obstet Gynecol.* 1998;179(2):444–52. PMID: 9731851.
39. Ghanbari Z, Haghollahi F, Shariat M, et al. Effects of calcium supplement therapy in women with premenstrual syndrome. *Taiwan J Obstet Gynecol.* 2009;48(2):124–9. doi: 10.1016/S1028-4559(09)60271-0.
40. O'Brien PMS, Ismail KMK, Dimmock P. Premenstrual syndrome. In: Shaw RW, Soutter WP, Stanton SL, eds. *Gynecology.* 3rd ed. Edinburgh, UK: Churchill Livingstone; 2003.
41. Dante G, Facchinetti F. Herbal treatments for alleviating premenstrual symptoms: a systematic review. *J Psychosom Obstet Gynaecol.* 2011;32(1): 42–51. doi: 10.3109/0167482X.2010.538102.
42. Ma L, Lin S, Chen R, et al. Treatment of moderate to severe premenstrual syndrome with *Vitex agnus castus* (BNO 1095) in Chinese women. *Gynecol Endocrinol.* 2010;26(8):612–6. PMID: 20334585.
43. He Z, Chen R, Zhou Y, et al. Treatment for premenstrual syndrome with *Vitex agnus castus:* a prospective, randomized, multi-center placebo controlled study in China. *Maturitas.* 2009;63(1):99–103. doi: 10.1016/j.maturitas.2009.01.006.
44. Atmaca M, Kumru S, Tezcan E. Fluoxetine versus *Vitex agnus castus* extract in the treatment of premenstrual dysphoric disorder. *Hum Psychopharmacol.* 2003;18(3):191–5. doi: 10.1002/hup.470.
45. *Vitex agnus-castus.* Monograph. *Altern Med Rev.* 2009;14(1):67–71. PMID: 19364195.
46. McCormick JK, Yarwood JM, Schlievert PM. Toxic shock syndrome and bacterial superantigens: an update. *Annu Rev Microbiol.* 2001;55:77–104. PMID: 11544350.
47. U.S. Food and Drug Administration. Tampons and asbestos, dioxin, & toxic shock syndrome. Available at: https://www.fda.gov/AboutFDA/AboutThisWebsite/ucm450631.htm. [Search on "ucm070003.htm."] April 21, 2017.
48. Reiss MA. Toxic shock syndrome. *Prim Care Update Ob Gyns.* 2000; 7(3):85–90. PMID: 10840210.
49. Strandberg KL, Perterson ML, Schaefers MM, et al. Reduction in *Staphylococcus aureus* growth and exotoxin production and in vaginal interleukin 8 levels due to glycerol monolaurate in tampons. *Clin Infect Dis.* 2009;49(1):1711–7. doi: 10.1086/644614.

CHAPTER 10

PREVENTION OF PREGNANCY AND SEXUALLY TRANSMITTED INFECTIONS

SHAREEN Y. EL-IBIARY AND ERIN C. RANEY

Unprotected sexual activity can result in unintended pregnancy and sexually transmitted infections (STIs), either of which can exact a high physical, psychological, and financial toll on those affected. This chapter discusses how vaccines and properly used nonprescription contraceptive products or methods can reduce the risks of such adverse outcomes.

An estimated 45% of pregnancies in the United States are unintended.[1] Approximately 89% of girls and women at risk for unintended pregnancy use contraception, a rate that is increasing as access to effective contraceptive methods improves.[2] Pharmacists can play an important role in improving these rates further through contraception counseling and provision.

While contraceptive use is increasing, an area of continuing concern is the high risk of pregnancy and STIs in adolescents. The 2011–2013 National Survey of Family Growth (NSFG) found that 40%–50% of teenagers had experienced sexual intercourse.[3] Among sexually active female teenagers, about one-fifth of those at risk for an unintended pregnancy did not use contraception.[3] Low levels of contraceptive use in these teens may be caused by a lack of knowledge and planning, denial, and infrequent or unpredictable intercourse. The teenage pregnancy rate in the United States is one of the highest among developed countries.[3] However, as of 2013, birth rates for U.S. teenagers had reached historic lows for all age and ethnic groups.[3] Adolescents are also particularly vulnerable to STIs, with half of the estimated 20 million people with new STI infections each year occurring in adolescents ages 15–24.[4] Risk factors for these infections include having multiple sexual partners, unprotected intercourse, an inherent biological susceptibility to infection, and barriers to health care utilization.[5]

Women of older reproductive age are also at risk of unintended pregnancies. NSFG found that among women age 35 years or older, 34% of pregnancies were unintended.[1] Postmenopausal women and older men in sexual relationships that are not mutually monogamous are additional groups at risk of STIs.

The availability and relatively low cost of nonprescription contraceptive methods are important, especially for those who are unwilling or unable to access family planning services or use prescription contraceptives. Even if a prescription product is chosen as the primary contraceptive method, low-cost and low-risk nonprescription methods may be appropriate at different times during a person's life. In addition, the widespread accessibility of pharmacist-administered immunizations offers another opportunity for STI prevention.

Overview of Pregnancy and STIs

Pregnancy can result only when a viable egg is available for fertilization by a sperm. (See Chapter 9 for discussion of the reproductive process.) Conception may occur during a 6-day window that begins 5 days before ovulation through the day of ovulation. The estimated risk of pregnancy from unprotected sexual intercourse during this period ranges from 5% to 45%, with peak risk occurring the day before ovulation.[6] Pregnancy can occur despite contraceptive use if the product is used incorrectly or it fails, such as with condom breakage.

STIs are contracted through contact with infected genital tissues, mucous membranes, and/or body fluids. Table 10–1 summarizes the major infections.[5,7,8] Although STIs affect both sexes, women are more likely to develop reproductive consequences, including pelvic inflammatory disease, chronic pelvic pain, pregnancy complications, malignancies, and infertility. This likelihood is possibly related to difficulties in diagnosis, lack of patient recognition of symptoms, and a higher probability of asymptomatic infection.[9]

Prevention of STIs and Pregnancy

Vaccines for STI Prevention

Pharmacist-administered vaccination has become more common. Depending on state laws and regulations, these vaccines may be available for administration in the pharmacy by protocol or without a prescription. States may limit the age range to which a pharmacist may administer vaccines, but if no barriers exist, pharmacists should offer their services to increase the number of vaccinated individuals.

Human Papillomavirus Vaccine

Human papillomavirus (HPV) is a virus that may be transmitted by sexual contact and is a major cause of cervical cancer and genital warts.[5,10] Of the more than 120 different types of HPV identified, HPV types 16 and 18 are responsible for approximately 70% of cervical cancers. HPV types 6 and 11 are responsible for benign cervical cell changes, genital warts, and laryngeal papillomas.[11] HPV is also responsible for a subset of vaginal, vulvar, penile, anal, and some head and neck cancers. HPV infection is the most common STI in the United States, with an estimated 14 million

TABLE 10-1 Sexually Transmitted Infections

Disease [Scientific Name] (Type)	Incubation Period	Symptoms	Diagnosis/ Treatment	Complications	Congenital Transmission/ Neonatal Complications
Noncurable but Vaccine-Preventable STIs					
Genital warts [HPV[a]] (DNA virus)	2–4 months (average)	Asx infections common; warts on external genitalia, rectum, anus, perineum, mouth, larynx, vagina, urethra, cervix	Colposcopy; serology; molecular-based assays/ cryoablation (chemical or physical); antivirals; antimetabolites; immunomodulators	Cervical dysplasia/ neoplasia, anogenital cancers, oropharyngeal cancer	Yes/respiratory papillomatosis
Hepatitis B [hepatitis B virus] (virus)	6 weeks– 6 months	Acute, self-limited, mild	Serology/antivirals	Cirrhosis, hepatocellular cancer	Yes
Curable STIs					
Genital chlamydia [*Chlamydia trachomatis*] (bacterium)	Several weeks	M: range from asx to urethritis, proctitis, urogenital discharge, itching, dysuria F: range from asx to vaginal discharge, postcoital bleeding, cervicitis	NAAT/antibiotics	PID, ectopic pregnancy, infertility	Yes/neonatal conjunctivitis, pneumonia
Gonorrhea [*Neisseria gonorrhoeae*] (bacterium)	Up to 14 days	Urethritis, cervicitis, proctitis, pharyngitis M: mucopurulent urethral discharge F: often asx	Gram stain; culture; NAAT/antibiotics	Septic arthritis, perihepatitis, endocarditis, meningitis, PID, infertility, ectopic pregnancy	Yes/sepsis, meningitis, arthritis, scalp abscess; ophthalmia neonatorum
Nongonococcal urethritis (men) [Various, including *Chlamydia trachomatis, Trichomonas vaginalis, Mycoplasma* sp.] (bacteria)	Varies	M: nonspecific urethritis, discharge, dysuria, pruritus	Gram stain microscopy; NAAT; culture/antibiotics	Epididymitis, proctitis, proctocolitis, Reiter syndrome	—
Syphilis [*Treponema pallidum*] (spirochete)	3 weeks (average)	Primary syphilis: chancre	Darkfield microscopy; treponemal and nontreponemal serologic tests/antibiotics	Secondary syphilis: rash, lymphadenopathy Tertiary syphilis: cardiovascular, gummatous lesions Neurosyphilis: CNS infection	Yes/fetal death, prematurity, congenital syphilis
Trichomoniasis [*Trichomonas vaginalis*] (protozoan)	Unknown (symptoms may appear within 28 days or years later)	M: commonly asx F: ~50% asx, malodorous, frothy green vaginal discharge, itching, dyspareunia, postcoital bleeding	Microscopic exam of vaginal fluids; nucleic acid probe test; PCR/ antibiotics	Pregnancy: preterm labor, low birth weight	Yes

(continued)

TABLE 10-1 **Sexually Transmitted Infections** *(continued)*

Disease [Scientific Name] (Type)	Incubation Period	Symptoms	Diagnosis/ Treatment	Complications	Congenital Transmission/ Neonatal Complications
Noncurable STIs					
AIDS [HIV] (virus)	Up to 10 years	After initial flulike illness, asx until OIs occur	Serologic antibody testing, NAAT/ antivirals; prophylaxis for OIs	OIs, malignancies, death	Yes, also transmitted via breast milk
Genital herpes [HSV-1, HSV-2] (virus)	2–12 days	Asx or vesicular/ ulcerative lesions on mucous membranes	Culture; serology; PCR assay/ antivirals	Disseminated infection, pneumonitis, hepatitis, meningitis/ encephalitis	Yes
Hepatitis C [hepatitis C virus] (virus)[b,c]	8–9 weeks	Asx or mild clinical illness	Serology; immunoassay; EIA; enhanced chemiluminescence immunoassay; NAAT/antivirals	Cirrhosis, hepatocellular cancer	Yes

Key: AIDS = Acquired immunodeficiency syndrome; Asx = asymptomatic; CNS = central nervous system; EIA = enzyme immunoassay; F = female; HIV = human immunodeficiency virus; HPV = human papillomavirus; HSV = herpes simplex virus; M = male; NAAT = nucleic acid amplification test; OI = opportunistic infection; PCR = polymerase chain reaction; PID = pelvic inflammatory disease; STI = sexually transmitted infection.

[a] Self-clearance of HPV virus may occur.

[b] Compared with transmission through blood exposure, sexual transmission of hepatitis C is inefficient but may still occur, especially in those with HIV infection.

[c] Certain hepatitis C genotypes are now considered curable with antiviral treatment.

Source: References 5, 7, and 8.

new cases annually.[11] The highest risk of infection occurs during the first few years after the onset of sexual activity.[11]

Three HPV vaccines have been developed, including Cervarix (bivalent HPV vaccine; HPV subtypes 16, 18), Gardasil (quadrivalent HPV vaccine; HPV subtypes 6, 11, 16, 18), and Gardasil 9 (9-valent HPV vaccine; HPV subtypes 6, 11, 16, 18, 31, 33, 45, 52, 58).[10] Currently, only the 9-valent HPV vaccine is marketed in the United States and is indicated for females and males ages 9–26 years to prevent cervical, vaginal, vulvar, and anal cancers.

The current recommendation of the Advisory Committee on Immunization Practices (ACIP) is for all adolescents 11–12 years of age to receive the applicable HPV vaccine, with vaccination supported as young as age 9 if necessary. Until recently, the vaccine was recommended as a 3-dose series at 0, 1–2 months, and 6 months for all applicable age groups.[10]

The current age range for administration of all three vaccines is wide. ACIP now recommends a 2-dose schedule, given at 0 and 6–12 months, for adolescents up to 15 years of age who are initiating the vaccine. When initiated in this younger cohort, the immune response appears to be similar to that of a 3-dose regimen in older individuals. Those 15 years and older should follow the 3-dose schedule.[10] This wide range accounts for the "catch-up" series that may be used in women up to 26 years of age and in men up to 21 years of age (may be up to 26 years of age in men having sex with men).[10] The vaccines work best prior to HPV exposure from sexual contact, but previous sexual intercourse does not preclude an individual from receiving the vaccine.[11]

ACIP's recommendation for HPV vaccine use has had a profound impact on HPV prevalence in the United States. Comparison of data from a pre-vaccine time period with data collected from 2009 to 2012 showed a decline in HPV subtypes 6, 11, 16, and 18 in girls ages 14–19 years (from 11.5% to 4.3%) and in women ages 20–24 years (from 18.5% to 12.1%).[12] The adverse effects of the three vaccines are similar and may include irritation at the site of administration, malaise, and syncope. Because of the risk of syncope, particularly in younger girls, patients should be monitored for at least 15 minutes after administration of the vaccine.[11]

Hepatitis B Vaccine

Infection with the hepatitis B virus is associated with long-term complications such as hepatitis, cirrhosis, hepatic carcinoma, and death. The virus can be transmitted through contact with blood and other body fluids, and 79% of new infections occur in individuals with high-risk sexual behaviors or injection drug use.[11]

The hepatitis B vaccine is an inactivated injectable formulation with an administration schedule of 0, 1, and 6 months.[11] Recommended as a routine vaccination for all infants starting at birth, the vaccine is also provided to children and adolescents who did not receive the vaccine as an infant or did not complete the series. Adults who meet risk criteria and who were not previously vaccinated should also receive the 3-dose series. Potential candidates for the vaccine include patients with multiple sexual partners; injection drug users; health care and emergency response personnel; patients with diabetes, end-stage renal disease, human immunodeficiency virus (HIV) infection, or liver disease; international travelers; and residents of correctional, drug abuse, or HIV treatment facilities.[11]

TABLE 10-2 **Failure and Use Rates of Various Contraceptive Methods**

Method	Accidental Pregnancy in the First Year of Use (%) Typical Use[a]	Perfect Use[b]	% of Women Using Method[c]
No method at risk for pregnancy	85	85	6.9
Withdrawal	22	4	3.0
Fertility awareness–based methods	24	—	0.8
Calendar method	13	5	—
Cervical mucus method	22	3	—
Symptothermal method	13–20	0.4	—
Lactational amenorrhea method (first 6 months postpartum)	2	0.5	—
Standard days method	12	4	—
TwoDay Method	14	4	—
Spermicides (foam, creams, gels, vaginal suppositories, vaginal film)	28	18	<0.2
Contraceptive sponge	24 (parous women)	20 (parous women)	<0.2
	12 (nulliparous women)	9 (nulliparous women)	
Male condom (without spermicide)	18	2	9.4
Female condom (without spermicide)	21	5	<0.2
Prescription methods	0.05–9	≤0.6	27.6
Sterilization (male/female)	≤0.5	≤0.5	20.6

[a] Among typical couples who initiate use of a method (not necessarily for the first time), the percentage who experience an accidental pregnancy during the first year if they do not stop use for any other reason.

[b] Among typical couples who initiate use of a method (not necessarily for the first time) and who use it consistently and correctly, the percentage who experience an accidental pregnancy during the first year if they do not stop use for any other reason.

[c] Percentage of women ages 15–44 years.

Source: References 13–18.

Contraception for Pregnancy and STI Prevention

The goal of contraceptive use is to prevent unintended pregnancy and STIs with minimal adverse effects. No method of birth control except abstinence is 100% effective, and contraceptive choices may change during a person's life.

The effectiveness of a contraceptive method in preventing pregnancy is reported in two ways: the accidental pregnancy rate in the first year of *perfect* use (method-related failure rate) and the rate in the first year of *typical* use (use-related failure rate; Table 10–2).[13–18] The pregnancy rate with perfect use is difficult to measure and indicates the method's theoretical effectiveness. Perfect use assumes accurate and consistent use of the method every time intercourse occurs. The more realistic rate of typical use includes pregnancies that may have occurred because of inconsistent or incorrect use of the method. Reported use-related failure rates vary, depending on the population studied. Decreased coital frequency and declining fertility in older users may contribute to increased effectiveness rates in this population. Effectiveness also increases the longer an individual uses a particular method.[15]

The most effective way for an individual to avoid contracting an STI is either to abstain from risky sexual activity or to be involved in a long-term mutually monogamous sexual relationship with an uninfected partner.[5] In the absence of those options, preventive strategies (Table 10–3)[5,9] in conjunction with use of

TABLE 10-3 **Prevention Strategies for STIs**

- Abstain from sexual activity.
- Avoid intercourse with a known infected partner.
- Avoid intercourse with an individual having multiple sex partners.
- Use a new condom with each episode of anal, oral, or vaginal intercourse.
- Seek a mutually monogamous relationship with an uninfected partner.
- Discuss partner's past sexual experiences.
- Examine partner for genital lesions.
- Practice genital self-examination.
- Avoid sexual activity involving direct contact with blood, semen, or other body fluids.
- Avoid sharing sexual devices that come in contact with semen or other body fluids.
- Choose safe and effective methods (e.g., mechanical barriers) to reduce the risk of STIs (consider adding more effective methods of pregnancy prevention when necessary).
- Avoid sexual activity if signs/symptoms of an STI are present.
- Consider vaccination if at high risk of a vaccine-preventable STI (e.g., HBV, HPV).

Key: HBV = Hepatitis B virus; HPV = human papillomavirus; STI = sexually transmitted infection.

Source: References 5 and 9.

selected contraceptives may provide the best method for reducing risk of infection (Figure 10–1).[5,9,18–21]

The acceptability of any given contraceptive method is vital for correct and consistent use of the method. Factors that affect acceptability include the user's religious beliefs and future reproductive plans, product effectiveness, partner's preference and support, degree of interruption of spontaneity, ease of use, product accessibility, and cost. To help patients make informed decisions, health care providers should be aware of each method's safety, including potential adverse effects on future fertility and on the fetus, if unintended conception does occur, and the effectiveness, accessibility, and relative cost of different contraceptive methods. The algorithm in Figure 10–1 can assist the provider in making appropriate contraceptive recommendations.

Nonprescription Contraceptive Products

Male Condoms

Condoms, also known as *rubbers, sheaths, prophylactics, safes, skins,* or *pros,* are the most important barrier contraceptive devices that help protect against STIs.[15] Male condoms are available in latex, polyurethane, polyisoprene, and lamb cecum (natural membrane or skin) (Table 10–4).

Latex condoms come in various sizes, colors, styles, shapes, and thicknesses and are degraded by oil-based lubricants. Other features include reservoir tips, ribs, studs, spermicide coating with nonoxynol-9, and lubrication. Latex condoms range in price from $0.18 to $1.08 each.[22] Latex condoms also help protect against STIs.[18]

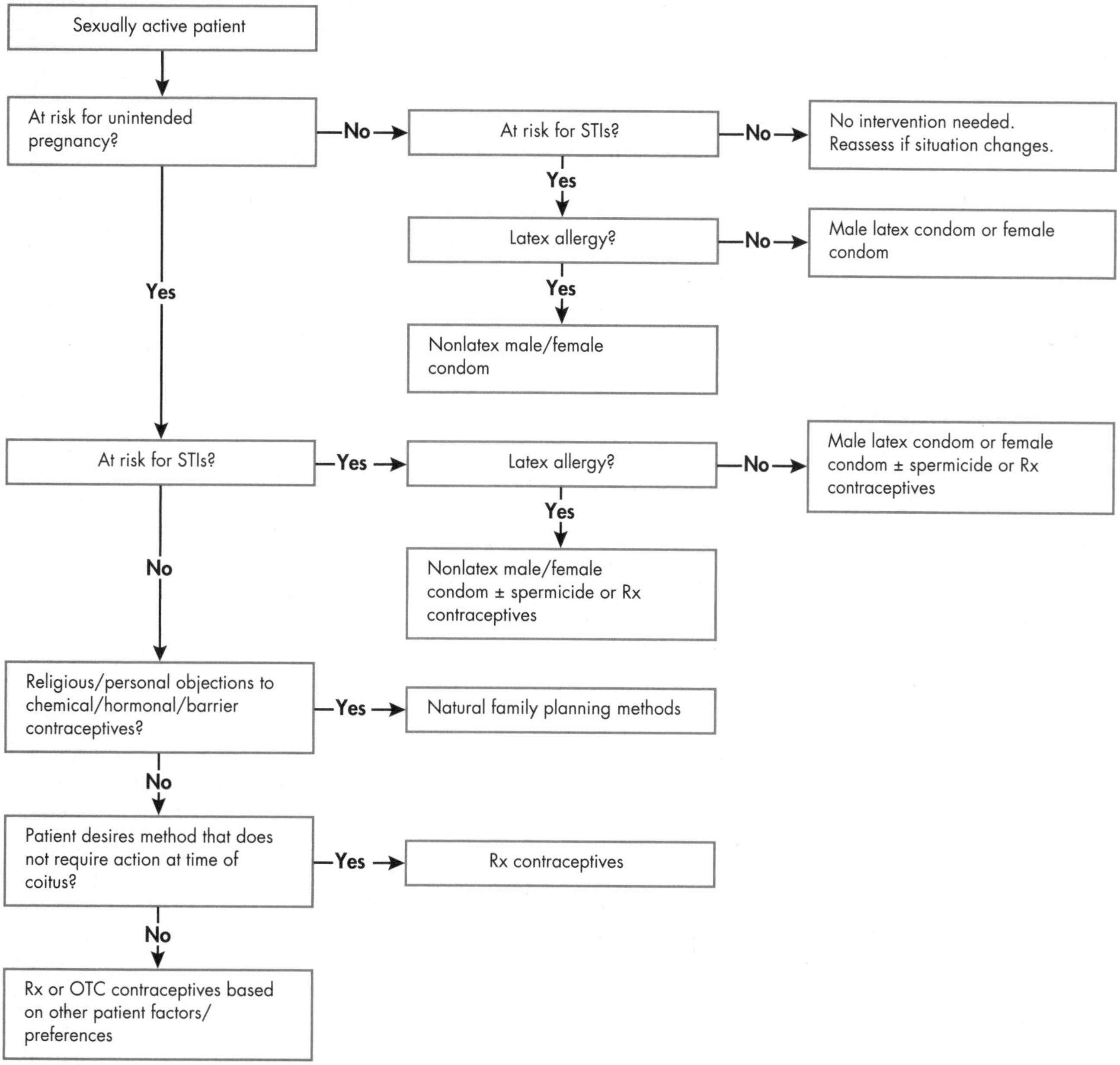

FIGURE 10–1 Prevention of unintended pregnancy and sexually transmitted infections. Key: OTC = Over-the-counter; Rx = prescription; STI = sexually transmitted infection.

TABLE 10–4 Selected Male Condoms

Synthetic, nonlatex condoms	Durex Avanti Bare RealFeel (polyisoprene), Trojan Supra (polyurethane), Lifestyles Skyn (polyisoprene)
Natural membrane condoms	Trojan Naturalamb (lamb cecum)
Latex condoms	Beyond Seven, Billy Boy, Crown, Durex, Kimono, LifeStyles, One, Sir Richard's Condoms, Trojan

Polyurethane condoms conduct heat well, are available prelubricated, are not subject to degradation by oil-based products, but are not as elastic as latex condoms.[23] Another form of condoms include those made of polyisoprene, which are more elastic than those made of polyurethane but can be damaged by oil-based lubricants. Although synthetic and latex condoms are thought to provide similar protection against STIs, prevention of STIs with synthetic condoms has not been well studied. The Food and Drug Administration (FDA) labeling restricts synthetic condom use to latex-sensitive or allergic persons.[18] At a cost of \$0.67–\$1.86 each, polyurethane and polyisoprene condoms are more expensive than latex condoms.[22]

Lamb cecum condoms are labeled only for pregnancy prevention, because the presence of pores in the membrane may allow passage of viral organisms, including HIV and hepatitis B virus.[18] These condoms conduct heat well, are very strong, and are not degraded by oil-based lubricants. With a price of approximately \$2.55 each, these condoms are also more expensive than latex condoms.[22]

FDA regulates condoms as medical devices, and they must meet performance standards for strength and integrity. The true incidence of condom breakage is unknown, and breakage rates from studies vary widely, ranging from 0% to 22%.[24] The overall use-related failure rate for condoms is approximately 18 pregnancies per 100 women during the first year of use (Table 10–2). In some studies, a limited group of patients reported multiple instances of breakage, indicating that breakage may be related as much to the individual user as it is to manufacturing defects. Behaviors that have been associated with an increased risk of condom breakage are (1) incorrect placement of the condom/failure to squeeze air from the receptacle tip; (2) use of an oil-based lubricant with latex condoms; (3) reuse of condoms; (4) increased duration, intensity, or frequency of coitus; (5) prior history of condom breakage or slippage; (6) history of STI; (7) contact with sharp objects; and (8) self-reported problems with fit of a condom.[18,24–26] One study found a decreased incidence of breakage with continued use, indicating that correct use may improve with experience.[24] The benefit of using additional lubrication with lubricated condoms is unclear. One study found that use of additional lubricant increased the risk of condom slippage. However, another study found that use of an additional water-based lubricant was associated with decreased breakage rates but caused no increase in condom slippage rates.[26] A review of comparative studies found that nonlatex synthetic condoms had a significantly higher breakage rate compared with latex condoms.[23,27,28] Two studies also reported a significantly higher pregnancy rate with nonlatex condoms compared with latex condoms.[28,29] Because of these reports, nonlatex condoms should be reserved for use by individuals with intolerance to latex condoms.

Studies support the finding that consistent use of condoms protects against trichomoniasis, bacterial vaginosis, and gonorrhea infections in women, and syphilis, chlamydia, HPV, and herpes simplex virus infections in both men and women.[18] Nonoxynol-9–coated (spermicide-coated) male condoms are no more effective than untreated condoms at preventing STIs and have not been shown to be more effective in pregnancy prevention.[30] Use of nonoxynol-9–treated condoms is discouraged because of the potential risk of irritation from the spermicide in both men and women, resulting in possible increased risk of infection.[18]

Proper use of condoms is essential to their preventing pregnancy and STIs (Table 10–5). For example, a man using a polyurethane condom should be advised that it is not as elastic as the latex condom and will not fit as snugly. In addition, a space must be left at the tip when using condoms without a reservoir.

Prelubricated condoms are a good choice when lubrication is desired. Additional lubrication for use with any latex condom should be selected from products that do not harm or weaken the strength and integrity of the condom (Table 10–6).

Packaged condoms should be kept in their sealed packages until time of use and protected from light and excessive heat, which can rapidly decrease the integrity of the condom material. FDA requires that latex condoms be labeled with an expiration date or date of manufacture. The shelf life of packaged condoms under optimal conditions is 3–5 years. Condoms showing signs of discoloration, brittleness, or stickiness should be discarded, even if they are within their expiration date.

The most frequent complaints about condoms is decreased sensitivity of the glans penis, resulting in decreased sexual pleasure for the man and sensitivity to the condom material. The use of very thin or ridged condoms, nonlatex synthetic condoms, or natural membrane condoms in a monogamous relationship with a partner screened for STI exposure may alleviate decreased sensitivity. Contact dermatitis caused by latex allergy can occur in the male or female partner, and may be characterized by immediate localized itching and swelling (urticarial reaction) or by a delayed eczematous reaction. The sensitizers in latex condoms are usually antioxidants or accelerators used in processing the rubber. In individuals with severe sensitivity, the reaction may include systemic symptoms. Spermicide-treated condoms may enhance latex allergy or cause the sensitivity reactions.[31]

For most people, condoms are an effective, acceptable, inexpensive, safe, and nontoxic method of birth control. Given the range of condoms available, men should be encouraged to try a different style or brand if they are dissatisfied with a condom used previously. Before recommending a latex condom, providers should assess for latex allergy. Ways to assess for possible latex allergy include asking if the patient has any reactions to latex gloves or has any reactions when inflating balloons. If the patient states that he or she has sensitivity to latex products, then an alternate type of condom should be recommended. Some men and women may be sensitized to components of the lubricant or spermicide. Because manufacturers use different processes, changing brands or using a condom without spermicide may resolve the problem.[18] If switching brands does not eliminate the irritation, the man may use nonlatex synthetic condoms. Natural skin condoms may also be used if the individual recognizes the limitations of the product in preventing STIs.

Other uses for barrier methods include prevention of STI transmission via oral sex. A dental dam (square piece of latex or silicone used to cover the vagina or anus during oral sex) or a

TABLE 10–5 Usage Guidelines for Male Condoms

- Use only condoms that are fresh (not previously opened), that are within their expiration date, and that have been stored in a dry, cool place (not a wallet or car glove compartment).
- Do not attempt to test the condom for leaks before using; this step weakens the condom.
- Be aware that long fingernails or jewelry may easily tear condoms.
- As shown in drawing A, unroll the condom onto the erect penis before the penis comes into any contact with the vagina. If you start to put the condom on backward, discard that condom and use a fresh one. (Note: Pre-ejaculate secretions may contain sperm.)
- If you are not using a reservoir-tipped condom, leave one-half inch of space between the end of the condom and the tip of the penis by pinching the top of the condom as you unroll it (drawing B). This method leaves space for the ejaculate (drawing C) and decreases the risk of breakage.
- If your partner has vaginal dryness, use additional lubrication, if desired. This step will help decrease the risk of tears and breakage. Use only water-based lubricants; oil-based lubricants weaken latex condoms and increase the chance of breakage. Spermicidal agents may be used as lubricants with condoms (Table 10–8) and the combination may increase contraceptive effectiveness.
- After ejaculation, withdraw the penis immediately. To prevent the condom from slipping off, hold on to the rim of the condom as you withdraw.
- Check the condom for tears and then discard in a trash can, not a toilet.
- If a tear or break occurs, immediately insert spermicidal foam or jelly containing a high concentration of spermicide into the vagina. Do not use suppositories or a vaginal film in these cases, because the delay time for dissolution may decrease the product's efficacy. Do not douche, because sperm that are present may be forced into the cervical canal. Consider use of emergency contraception as soon as possible and within 72–120 hours after unprotected intercourse if pregnancy is a concern.

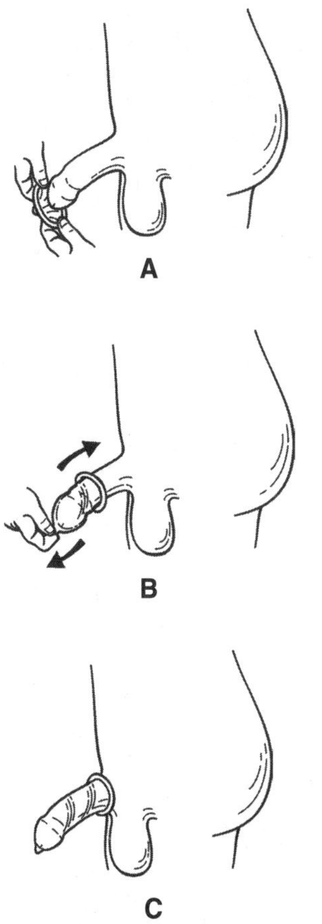

condom cut length-wise may also be used for this purpose.[32] Intact condoms may be used for the penis during oral sex.

Female Condoms

A female condom is another nonprescription contraceptive product. The first female condom, known as the polyurethane F.C. Female Condom (FC1), was approved by FDA in 1993.[33] A second-generation female condom, the FC2, made of nitrile, a synthetic latex, was approved in 2009 and replaced the polyurethane condom as supplies of FC1 were exhausted.[34] The female condom consists of an outer ring, a sheath or pouch that fits over the vaginal mucosa, and an inner ring that secures the sheath by fitting like a diaphragm over the cervix. The female condom is designed for one-time use only and, at a cost of $2.00 each, is more expensive than the latex male condom.[22]

The breakage rate of the female condom has been lower than that of latex male condoms, but slippage rates may be higher, especially with initial use.[25] The 6-month pregnancy failure rate among all users of the FC1 is 12.4%, similar to that for users of diaphragms and cervical caps. Among perfect users, however, 6-month pregnancy failure rates of 0.8%–2.5% have been documented. The extrapolated annual pregnancy failure rate for the FC1 is 21% for all users and 5% for perfect users (Table 10–2).[19,33,34] Although specific data regarding failure rates

TABLE 10–6 Selected Lubricants/Products That Are Safe or Unsafe to Use With Latex Condoms

Safe	Unsafe
Contraceptive foams/gels	Topical oils (e.g., baby oil, mineral oil, massage oil)
Water-based personal lubricants, such as K-Y Jelly	Edible oils/fats (e.g., olive, peanut, corn, canola, and safflower oils; butter; margarine)
Silicone-based lubricants, such as Astroglide	Hemorrhoidal ointments
Glycerin (USP)	Petroleum jelly (e.g., Vaseline)
Replens Inserts	Vaginal creams (e.g., Monistat, Estrace, Vagisil, Premarin)
Saliva	
Water	

Source: Reference 19.

for the FC2 was not available when first released on the market, it was noninferior to the FC1.[34] A more recent study comparing three different female condom brands available outside the United States to the FC2 reported a failure rate of 3.43% for the FC2, confirming its similarity in effectiveness to the FC1.[35] The female condom is an effective barrier to sexually transmitted bacteria and viruses and is similar in efficacy to latex male condoms in decreasing the risk of STIs.[20]

Table 10–7 provides instructions for proper use of the female condom.[36] Skills in correctly using the female condom improve with practice and continued use.[37] The condom may be inserted up to 8 hours before intercourse, but it is effective immediately on insertion. Fresh condoms can be stored at room temperature in their unopened packages. Before inserting the female condom, the woman should ensure that the product is within its expiration date.

The most common complaints about the female condom are vaginal irritation and increased noise ("squeaking"). Additional lubrication may resolve those problems. Some women may have decreased sensation or discomfort, which is caused by the outer ring during intercourse.

The female condom provides a method for women to protect themselves against pregnancy. Compared with vaginal spermicides, the female condom can be inserted much earlier before intercourse and is less messy to use. However, some women may find the female condom cumbersome and unattractive. The female condom should not be used together with the male condom. Use of both products together may cause friction and increase the risk of breakage for either product.[36]

Vaginal Spermicides

Vaginal spermicides use surface-active agents to immobilize and kill sperm. For gels and foams, the spermicide vehicle also acts as a physical barrier against sperm. The effective spermicides include nonoxynol-9, octoxynol-9, and menfegol, but in the United States, all products contain nonoxynol-9 (Table 10–8). Vaginal spermicide products differ in their application method, onset, and duration of action (Table 10–9). The cost of vaginal spermicides ranges from $0.71 to $1.44 per dose.[22]

Vaginal gels (jellies) provide additional lubrication and are safe to use with latex condoms. For convenience, applicators may be prefilled before use. Prefilled unit-dose applicators are also available for some products. Vaginal foams distribute more evenly and adhere better to the cervical area and vaginal walls but provide less lubrication than jellies. A new canister should always be available, because it is difficult to know when the canister is nearly empty.

Vaginal suppositories are solid or semisolid dosage forms that are activated by moisture in the vaginal tract. Incomplete dissolution of the suppository may result in an unpleasant, gritty sensation. Although vaginal suppositories do not require refrigeration, in warmer climates, refrigeration may be desirable to prevent softening.

TABLE 10–7 Usage Guidelines for Female Condoms

- Remove the condom from the package. One end of the condom is closed to form a pouch, as shown in drawing A.
- Gently rub the sides together to evenly distribute the lubricant inside the pouch. If needed, add additional lubrication at this point.
- Add a drop of lubricant on the outside of the pouch to improve the ease of insertion if needed. Oil- or water-based lubricants can be used with this condom.
- To place the pouch properly, grasp the inner ring between the thumb and middle finger of one hand. Place the index finger on the sheath between the other two fingers. (See drawing B.)
- Be careful that sharp fingernails or jewelry does not tear the condom.
- Squeeze the inner ring and with your other hand, spread the lips of the vagina. Then insert the squeezed condom into the vagina as far as possible. (See drawing C.)
- Be sure that the inner ring is placed beyond the pubic (pelvic) bone, that the pouch is not twisted, and that the outer ring is outside the vagina, as shown in drawing D.
- During intercourse, make sure that the penis enters the vagina inside the pouch and that the outer ring remains outside the vagina.
- If desired, add more lubricant during intercourse, without removing the condom.
- Until the couple is comfortable using the female condom, it is recommended that the penis is inserted by hand into the vagina.
- If the female condom is slipping out of the vagina during intercourse or the outer ring is going into the vagina, stop intercourse. Remove the female condom and insert a new condom.
- Remove the pouch before standing by twisting the outer ring and pulling gently. (See drawing E.)
- Discard the used condom in a trash can, not a toilet.
- Insert a new condom for each act of intercourse.
- Do not use a male condom with the female condom. The increased friction could cause displacement of the female condom.

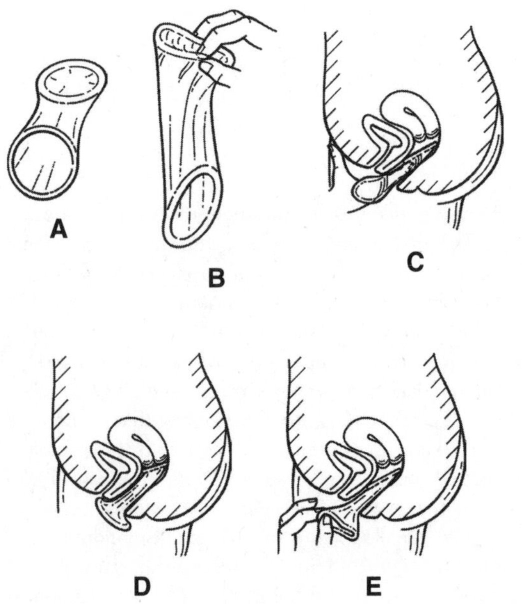

Source: Reference 36.

TABLE 10-8 Selected Nonprescription Vaginal Spermicides Containing Nonoxynol-9

Spermicidal foams	VCF Vaginal Contraceptive Foam 12.5%
Spermicidal gels/jellies	Options Conceptrol Gel 4%, 100 mg
	VCF Vaginal Contraceptive Gel 4%
	Ortho Options Gynol II Extra Strength Vaginal Contraceptive Gel 3%, 150 mg
Spermicidal suppositories	Encare Vaginal Contraceptive Inserts 100 mg
Spermicidal film	VCF Vaginal Contraceptive Film 28%
Spermicidal sponge	Today Contraceptive Sponge 1000 mg

Vaginal contraceptive film contains nonoxynol-9 in paper-thin, 2-inch-square sheets. The film is activated by vaginal secretions. One film is used for each act of intercourse. The practice of inserting the film by placing it over the penis should be avoided, because this method does not ensure proper placement and does not allow adequate time for dissolution. In one comparison of spermicide formulations, the film was rated the most difficult to use but the least messy.[38] Similarly designed vaginal films for cleansing or lubrication do not contain spermicide and should not be used for contraception. Patients should be advised to verify that they are using the correct vaginal film product if they desire contraception.

Spermicides used alone have a relatively high typical rate of usage failure among first-year users (Table 10–2). A review of clinical trials found a similar pregnancy rate between dosage forms containing 100–150 mg nonoxynol-9 per dose.[39] A gel containing 52.5 mg nonoxynol-9 per dose, which is not available in the United States, was significantly less effective at preventing pregnancy than the higher dose formulations.[39] Efficacy improves greatly if spermicides are used with barrier methods, such as diaphragms, cervical caps, or condoms.

Although nonoxynol-9 can inactivate many sexually transmitted pathogens in vitro, clinical studies do not support a protective effect of vaginal spermicides against STI transmission.[19,40] Higher rates of genital lesions, especially in frequent users, have been reported, raising concerns about an increased risk of STI transmission.[19,40] In 2007, FDA ruled that vaginal spermicide products must carry a label stating that the product does not protect against HIV and other STIs.[40] If a risk of STIs exists, spermicides should only be recommended in conjunction with condom use.

Table 10–9 provides guidelines for the proper administration of vaginal spermicides.[19,41,42] When using any vaginal spermicide, a woman should delay douching for at least 6 hours after intercourse. Although allergic reactions are rare, either partner may experience such reactions to spermicides. Couples having oral–genital sex may find the taste of some products unpleasant. Frequent use or use of high-concentration products may irritate or damage vaginal and cervical epithelium,[40] which may be associated with an increased risk for STIs. Despite initial concerns about a possible association between spermicide use and birth defects or miscarriage should an unintended pregnancy occur, current data do not support an increased risk of either attributable to spermicides.[43]

The relatively low effectiveness of spermicides when used alone is their major disadvantage. Studies suggest that simultaneous use of condoms and spermicides, however, provides efficacy rates similar to those of oral contraceptives and intrauterine contraceptives (IUCs).[15] Their availability and ease of use make spermicides a good choice for women who need a backup method. Spermicides are not recommended for women with vaginal anatomic abnormalities that would prevent the proper placement of the spermicide near the cervical opening. Product selection can be based on patient preference and specific product characteristics.

Contraceptive Sponge

The contraceptive sponge marketed as the Today Sponge is a small, circular, disposable sponge made of polyurethane permeated with the spermicide nonoxynol-9. The sponge is believed to act as a contraceptive by serving as a mechanical barrier, providing a spermicide, and absorbing semen. The contraceptive sponge ranges in price from $5 to $8 per sponge.[22]

In two large trials, the failure rate for the contraceptive sponge ranged from 17.4 to 24.5 pregnancies per 100 women in the first year of use.[44] Women who had given birth previously (parous women) had a significantly higher pregnancy rate while using the sponge, compared with women who had never given birth (nulliparous women). That finding may be related to poor fit in women who have delivered vaginally. If the sponge becomes dislodged during intercourse, its efficacy may be decreased.

The contraceptive sponge does not protect against STIs. One study found an increased risk of HIV infection in women with frequent sponge use, possibly because of an increased incidence of vaginal ulceration from the spermicide.[21]

A woman must be able to locate her cervix and must be comfortable in doing so to place the sponge correctly. Table 10–9 provides instructions for proper use. The sponge has a loop attached to the convex side to facilitate removal. Some women have difficulty removing the sponge, and it has been known to fragment on removal. The sponge may be inserted up to 24 hours prior to intercourse but must remain in place for 6 hours after intercourse. The sponge should be stored in its unopened package in a cool place and used before its expiration date.

Some adverse effects, such as vaginal dryness, have been reported with use of the contraceptive sponge. Although the incidence is rare, the contraceptive sponge has been associated with an increased risk of toxic shock syndrome (TSS).[19] Women should take special care to wash their hands before inserting the sponge. The sponge should not be used during menstruation, less than 6 weeks postpartum, or in women with a history of TSS. Use should not exceed the maximum recommended retention time of 30 hours. Women should also be advised to make sure the entire sponge is removed, because fragments left in the vagina may serve as a source for infection.

The contraceptive sponge is convenient, safe, and portable. Contraindications for use include spermicide sensitivity, anatomic abnormalities of the vagina, and a history of TSS. The contraceptive sponge should not be routinely recommended to parous women, because possible problems with adequate cervical coverage may lead to increased risk of pregnancy.

Emergency Contraception

Emergency contraception (EC) involves the use of hormones in the form of oral tablets or a nonhormonal copper IUC to prevent

TABLE 10-9 **Administration Guidelines for Vaginal Spermicides**

Dosage Form	Application Method	Onset/Duration of Action	Application Time Before Intercourse	Reapplication Requirements
Vaginal gel alone	Insert full dose near cervix.	Immediate/1 hour after application	Up to 1 hour	Reapply for each coital act.
Vaginal gel used with diaphragm/cervical cap	Fill barrier device one-third full with gel and place it near cervix. Leave barrier in place for at least 6 hours after intercourse.	Immediate/diaphragm: 6 hours; cervical cap: 48 hours	Up to 1 hour	Diaphragm: for each coital act that occurs within 6 hours of initial insertion of device, reapply spermicide without removing device; for coitus after 6 hours of initial insertion, remove and wash device, fill with new spermicide, and re-insert device. Cervical cap: remove and wash device; then reapply spermicide for each coital act that occurs 48 hours after initial insertion of device.
Vaginal foam	Insert full dose near cervix.	Immediate/1 hour	Up to 1 hour	Reapply for each coital act.
Vaginal suppository	Insert suppository near cervix.	10–15 minutes/1 hour	10–15 minutes	Reapply for each coital act.
Vaginal contraceptive film	Drape film over fingertip; place film near cervix.	15 minutes/3 hours	15 minutes	Reapply for each coital act. Insert at least 15 minutes prior to intercourse and not more than 3 hours prior. If 3 hours have lapsed from the time of insertion before intercourse, insert a new film.
Vaginal contraceptive sponge	Moisten with tap water, insert convex side against cervix.	Immediate/24 hours	Can be inserted up to 24 hours before intercourse.	Leave in for >6 hours after intercourse, but no longer than 30 hours total; polyester loop to facilitate removal.

Source: References 19, 41, and 42.

pregnancy as soon as possible after unprotected intercourse and up to 3–5 days after unprotected sexual intercourse based on product labeling and current practice.[45] Hormones used in EC may include only progestin (synthetic progesterone), estrogen in combination with a progestin, or a selective progesterone receptor modulator. Nonprescription and prescription oral tablet formulations are available. This section focuses on nonprescription progestin-only products.

EC products should be recommended for girls and women of reproductive age who have had recent unprotected intercourse, who experienced method failure such as condom breakage, or who desire advance provision to have the product available in the event of a need for EC.[14,45] Some women may be seeking EC in the case of sexual assault. In addition to providing EC for immediate use, pharmacy staff should refer the individual to health care providers who can evaluate the individual for STIs and report the incident to the authorities as required by state law.

EC products reduce the expected number of pregnancies between 52% and 100% for levonorgestrel users.[45] The efficacy of EC results primarily from the suppression of ovulation. Other possible mechanisms of action include interference with transport of sperm or egg, including thickening of cervical mucus.[14,45] Nonprescription EC products will not affect an implanted embryo or increase the risk of malformations.[45]

Current nonprescription options include levonorgestrel-containing tablets, available as single-tablet formulations in the generic branded products, Aftera, EContra EZ, Fallback Solo, My Way, Next Choice One Dose, Opcicon One-Step, and Take Action, or the branded product Plan B One-Step.[46] Progestin-only products cost between $40 and $50 for single incident use.[22] Nonprescription products each contain 1 tablet of levonorgestrel 1.5 mg labeled to be taken as a single dose within 72 hours after unprotected intercourse or contraceptive failure. Studies have shown effectiveness up to 120 hours after intercourse, although efficacy declines with more time after coitus.[45] Therefore, women presenting within 120 hours of unprotected sex could be offered EC or referred to their provider for ulipristal acetate or the copper IUC. The woman's weight may influence the effectiveness of the levonorgestrel, as it may not be as effective when the body mass index (BMI) is 26 kg/m^2 or greater.[45] Alternative EC products available by prescription may be an option (Table 10–10).[45]

The most common adverse effects reported with oral EC use are nausea and vomiting.[14,45] Nausea occurs in approximately

TABLE 10–10 **Prescription Emergency Contraceptives Available**

Product Name	Dosage	Timing for Use	BMI and Effectiveness
Ulipristal acetate (ella)	30 mg	Within 120 hours post coitus	May start to lose effectiveness at BMI of 30, may become ineffective at BMI of 35; should not be withheld from patient due to BMI
Copper IUC (ParaGard T380A)	n/a	Off-label use, within 120 hours post coitus	No issue with BMI
Estrogen and progestin (combined regimen)	Varies: Ethinyl estradiol 100–120 mcg and levonorgestrel 0.5–0.6 mg (amount per dose, take 2 doses separated by 12 hours)	Off-label use, within 72 hours though studies suggest up to 120 hours post coitus	No information

Key: BMI = Body mass index; IUC = intrauterine contraceptive; n/a = not applicable.
Source: Reference 45.

25% of women using progestin-only products. Vomiting occurs in approximately 5% of progestin-only EC users. An antiemetic is usually not necessary for progestin-only EC but may be recommended 60 minutes before each dose when using combination oral contraceptive regimens.[14,45] If a woman vomits within 1 to 2 hours of taking the dose, she should repeat the dose.[14,45] Headaches, breast tenderness, menstrual changes, and dizziness have also been reported by users.[45]

Patients presenting between 5 and 7 days after unprotected intercourse should be referred to a primary care provider for possible insertion of a copper IUC.[14] Although a copper IUC is usually placed up to 5 days after unprotected intercourse, the IUC can be inserted up to 8 days after intercourse if ovulation is known to have occurred more than 72 hours after intercourse.[14] Therefore, if intercourse occurred 3 days prior to ovulation, the patient could potentially still have an IUC placed up to 5 days after ovulation, though in practice it is usually placed up to 5 days after unprotected intercourse.[14] Table 10–11 provides patient counseling points and information about levonorgestrel EC products.

Fertility Awareness–Based Methods

Examples of contraceptive methods that do not use a chemical or barrier to prevent conception include calendar methods, cervical mucus methods, symptothermal method, and the lactational amenorrhea method (LAM). These fertility awareness–based

TABLE 10–11 **Counseling Points for Emergency Contraception (Levonorgestrel)**

- Identify whether patient has had recent unprotected sex within the past 120 hours or is at risk for unprotected sex and does not want to get pregnant.
- Identify whether patient is appropriate for EC available as nonprescription products.
- Explain how to take EC: Aftera, EContra EZ, Fallback Solo, My Way, Next Choice One Dose, Opcicon One-Step, Take Action, or Plan B One-Step is given as a single dose and should be taken as soon as possible. EC is most effective when taken as soon as possible after unprotected intercourse. The method is effective when taken up to 120 hours after unprotected intercourse though package labeling states within 72 hours.
- Recommend an antiemetic for women using combination oral contraceptives for EC.
- If the woman has a BMI of 26 or greater, explain that the effectiveness of the nonprescription EC products may be reduced, but do not withhold product. Alternative options could include a prescription for ulipristal or see a PCP for the copper IUC.
- Discuss adverse effects of EC, which may include a change in menstrual cycle depending on when emergency contraception is used. Patients may experience their next menstrual cycles early or late or have no change. If a menstrual cycle has not occurred more than 21 days after use of ECPs, the patient should take a pregnancy test.
- Emphasize that EC is not to be used as a regular contraceptive method.
- Recommend that a sexually active woman begin using regular contraception after taking EC. Barrier methods should be used with each subsequent act of intercourse during rest of the current menstrual cycle. Hormonal contraceptive methods may be started with the next menses or may be started the day after taking EC, with 7 days of a backup contraceptive method.
- Explain that EC does not protect against STIs.
- Explain that EC is not 100% effective. Recommend using a pregnancy test if menses is more than 21 days late.
- Recommend a longer term method of contraception if patient is using EC multiple times a month. While it is safe to use EC multiple times a month, it is not intended to be used in this way. A longer-term contraceptive method will provide better protection against pregnancy.
- Provide written instructions.

Key: BMI = Body mass index; EC = emergency contraception; ECP = emergency oral contraceptive; IUC = intrauterine contraceptive; PCP = primary care provider; STI = sexually transmitted infection.
Source: References 14 and 45.

(FAB) methods use various techniques to determine a woman's fertile phase of the menstrual cycle, during which time intercourse should be avoided or another method of contraception used. The techniques are typically chosen, because they pose no health risks to the couple or to the fetus should pregnancy occur or because of decreased cost or religious reasons. In some cases, FAB methods are used because of a lack of access to or knowledge of other methods of contraception. Disadvantages of FAB methods include lack of STI protection, lower efficacy than some other contraceptive methods, and the need for periods of abstinence or the use of another method of contraception, such as condoms, during fertile days.[16]

Calendar Methods

Calendar methods use a woman's monthly menstrual cycle length to calculate the fertile period. These methods factor in the viabilities of ovum (up to 24 hours) and sperm (up to 6 days).[7,17] Menstrual cycles may vary, and therefore, cycle lengths should be recorded for 6–12 cycles to predict the likely range of fertile days. The Calendar Rhythm Method calculates the first fertile day in a woman's menstrual cycle by subtracting 18 from the number of days in her shortest cycle. The last fertile day is calculated by subtracting 11 from the number of days in her longest cycle. Women who have irregular cycles are not optimal candidates for this method as an overestimation of unsafe fertile days could occur.[16] The Standard Days Method is a calendar method recommended only for women with cycles between 26 and 32 days in length. Counting the first day of menstruation as day 1, a woman should avoid intercourse on days 8–19 of her menstrual cycle or use another method of contraception, such as condoms, during this time.[16]

Cervical Mucus Methods

Cervical mucus methods rely on changes in cervical mucus that take place during a normal menstrual cycle.[16] Individuals should be encouraged to work with trained instructors to ensure proper interpretation of mucus as well as to avoid intercourse during the first cycle. Examples of cervical mucus methods include the Billings Ovulation Method, the Creighton Model, and the TwoDay Method.

With the Billings Ovulation Method, the woman observes the cervical mucus on a daily basis and charts its character and quantity. After menstruation, most women notice a sensation of vaginal dryness. Approximately 5–6 days before ovulation, estrogen levels rise, causing the cervical mucus to increase in quantity and elasticity and to become clear, resembling raw egg white. The peak symptom, the last day of the clear, stretchy, estrogenic mucus, has been shown to occur within a day of ovulation for most women. With the postovulatory rise in progesterone, the mucus becomes thick and sticky or is absent. The woman is considered fertile from the first day after menstruation on which mucus is detected until 4 days after appearance of the peak symptom, during which time intercourse should be avoided.[16,47] With experience and assistance, a woman learns to differentiate other vaginal secretions, such as seminal fluid or an infectious discharge, from normal mucus, enabling her to seek early treatment for an infection. Women should be informed that vaginal foams, gels, creams, and douches will interfere with cervical mucus. The Creighton Model involves similar principles, but uses more standardized definitions of cervical secretions, involves the male partner, and requires extensive patient training from certified instructors.[47]

Another method of monitoring cervical secretions is called the TwoDay Method.[16,47] The woman should monitor for secretions on a daily basis, and if she notes any secretions that day or the day before, she is likely to be fertile. If she does not note any secretions, she is unlikely to be fertile. The TwoDay Method is a simple method that does not require keeping records or logs. However, training the woman to identify cervical secretions correctly is still important.[47]

Symptothermal Method

The symptothermal method combines cervical mucus tracking with basal body temperature (BBT) monitoring.[6,16] Observation of the cervical mucus is used to identify the onset of the fertile period, whereas BBT charting is used to identify the end of the fertile period.[16] Monitoring of BBT can also be used to predict ovulation for conception (see Chapter 48).

To monitor BBT, the woman charts her body temperature every morning, preferably with a digital thermometer calibrated in increments of 0.1°F (0.05°C), to detect small changes in body temperature.[16] The temperature must be obtained before getting out of bed at the same time every day and is recorded on a chart (Figure 10–2). At least 3 hours of uninterrupted sleep are required for a reliable reading. The temperature may be taken orally, vaginally, or rectally, but the same site must be used each day.

In some women, the onset of ovulation may be detected by a drop in BBT 12–24 hours before ovulation. At the time of ovulation, BBT rises by at least 0.4°F (0.2°C) above the lowest point (the nadir).[16] The safe (infertile) period begins once there have been 3 consecutive days of rising temperature and lasts until the end of menses. Once menses begins, the unsafe period (fertile) also begins, and the woman repeats the method during her cycle to determine her ovulation time.

Some women do not have a definite or significant temperature dip or rise with ovulation. Stress, inadequate sleep, travel, fever, lactation, or perimenopause may affect BBT.[16] For women who work rotating shifts, an accurate record of BBT may be difficult to maintain. At such times, couples should use an alternative method of contraception.

Home Tests for Ovulation Prediction

Ovulation prediction tests are designed to aid couples in conceiving by detecting the surge in luteinizing hormone that occurs shortly before ovulation (see Chapter 48). These kits detect an increase in urinary excretion of the hormone, which usually occurs 8–40 hours before actual ovulation. These ovulation predictors do not give warning of impending ovulation with enough accuracy to be effective contraceptive agents and are not recommended for use other than as an aid for couples desiring pregnancy.[16]

Lactational Amenorrhea Method

In many developing countries, LAM is used as a contraceptive method for spacing the birth of children. When an infant younger than 6 months of age receives at least 90% of his or her nutrition from breastfeeding, and the mother is amenorrheic, LAM offers

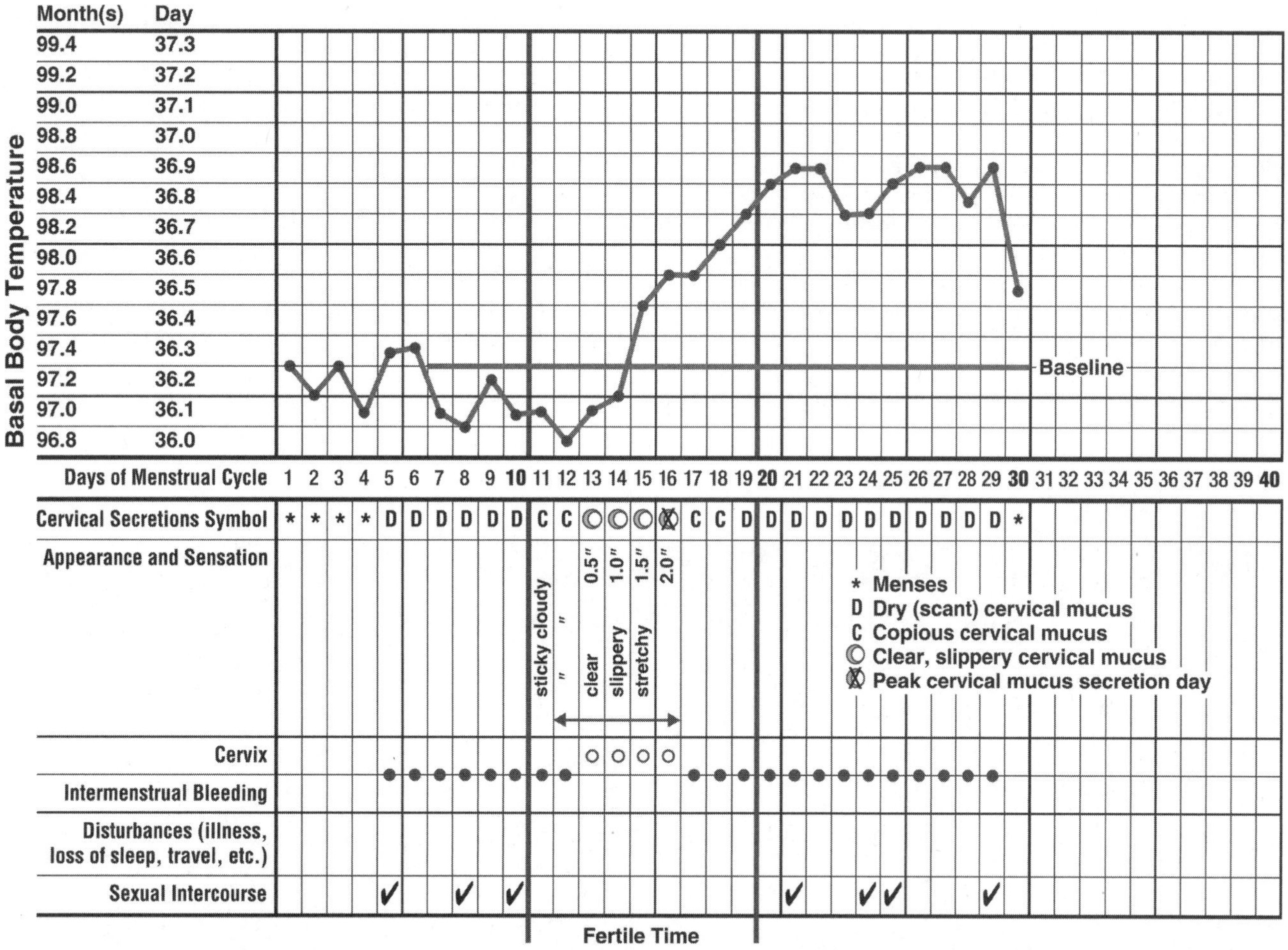

FIGURE 10–2 Symptothermal variations during a model menstrual cycle. (Source: Reprinted with permission from Jennings VH, Arevalo M, Kowal D. Fertility awareness–based methods. In: Hatcher RA, Trussell J, Stewart F, et al., eds. *Contraceptive Technology*. 18th rev ed. New York, NY: Ardent Media; 2004:327.)

more than 98% protection against pregnancy.[14,17] Because the suckling action of the infant on the breast at frequent intervals is necessary for LAM to be effective, milk extraction through a breast pump does not offer the same protection against pregnancy.[17] Although menstrual periods in lactating women may be anovulatory, ovulation may occur before the return of menses. In general, if a breastfeeding woman is having menstrual periods, is supplementing her infant's diet, or is more than 6 months postpartum, she should use an additional method of contraception.[14,17] For a woman who is breastfeeding an infant almost exclusively, studies have reported pregnancy rates of 0.5%–2% for the 6-month period after delivery. Once supplemental feedings begin, the efficacy rate decreases significantly.[17]

Effectiveness of Fertility Awareness–Based Methods

Overall, the pregnancy rate for typical use of FAB methods is approximately 24% (Table 10–2).[15] Compared with condoms, hormonal methods, or the nonhormonal IUC, the risk of pregnancy is higher with any of the FAB methods alone. Consequently, family planners do not recommend using a single method; instead, they suggest using a combination of methods. FAB methods that specifically identify preovulatory and postovulatory changes, such as the symptothermal method, have better outcomes; with perfect use, the annual failure rate is less than 5%.[15] FAB methods also do not provide any protection against STIs and should be recommended solely for couples in mutually monogamous relationships.

Coitus Interruptus

Coitus interruptus (withdrawal) involves coital activity until ejaculation is imminent, followed by withdrawal of the stimulated penis and ejaculation away from the vagina or vulva. Method failures (pregnancy even when the method is used correctly and consistently) occur, in part, because involuntary pre-ejaculation secretions may contain millions of sperm. Disadvantages of this method include the requirement of considerable self-control by the man, the potential for diminished pleasure for the couple because of interrupted lovemaking, and no STI protection. This method has failure rates of 4% with perfect use and 22% with typical use, comparable to those of other barrier methods.[48]

Assessment of Prevention of Pregnancy and STIs: A Case-Based Approach

Before advising a couple on contraception and STI prevention, the health care provider must first identify their level of knowledge about these issues, because they must understand their risk of pregnancy and STIs to select an appropriate product or method. Individuals who prefer FAB methods must understand the reproductive cycle before they can use these methods effectively. Those who prefer nonprescription contraceptive products must know how to use them properly and be prepared to use them with every act of intercourse. The provider should identify individual preferences for products or methods on the basis of the timing of use or religious or cultural practices.

Case 10–1 illustrates the assessment of a woman who is seeking advice on contraception, whereas Case 10–2 deals with the use of EC.

Patient Counseling for Prevention of Pregnancy and STIs

Pharmacists are in a unique position to lower the incidence and consequences of unintended pregnancy and STIs in their communities. The pharmacist should seek opportunities to discuss specific diseases or prevention strategies with individuals who may

CASE 10–1

Relevant Evaluation Criteria	Scenario/Model Outcome
Collect	
1. Gather essential information about the patient's symptoms and medical history, including	
a. Description of symptom(s) (i.e., nature, onset, duration, severity, associated symptoms)	Patient is asking for a recommendation for the best ovulation kit to purchase for use as a contraceptive method. She heard you can identify a "safe time" to have sex where you are not likely to get pregnant. She has not used contraception in the past as she has not been sexually active. However, she plans to begin having intercourse with her current boyfriend. She is not sure of his sexual history but expresses interest in a method that does not require a prescription. She does not have access to a physician at this time because of insurance issues.
b. Patient's identity	Tracy Jones
c. Patient's age, gender, height, and weight	28 years old, female, 5 ft 3 in., 145 lb
d. Concurrent medical conditions, prescription and nonprescription medications, and dietary supplements	None; no history of sexual partners
e. Allergies	NKA
Assess	
2. Differentiate patient's signs/symptoms, and correctly identify the patient's primary problem(s).	Risk of undesired pregnancy and STIs. Patient's choice of avoiding pregnancy through ovulation monitoring with a urine test kit is not appropriate for contraception. In addition, ovulation monitoring does not provide STI protection.
3. Identify exclusions for self-treatment.	None
4. Formulate a comprehensive list of therapeutic alternatives for the primary problem to determine whether triage to a medical provider is required, and share this information with the patient or caregiver.	Options include (1) Recommend use of a male condom (nonspermicidal or spermicidal condom) with or without an additional spermicide to provide STI protection as well as contraception. The use of spermicide (Table 10–8) can enhance the effectiveness of the male condom for pregnancy prevention but has not been shown to improve protection against STIs. (2) Recommend use of a female condom to provide STI protection as well as contraception. (3) Recommend a fertility-awareness–based method such as a calendar method, cervical mucus method, or symptothermal method. When used alone, these methods do not provide STI protection. (4) Refer patient for a prescription hormonal method of contraception to be used in combination with a male or female condom. Self-administered hormonal contraception provided by pharmacists may be available in some states.

CASE 10-1 *continued*

Relevant Evaluation Criteria	Scenario/Model Outcome
Plan	
5. Select an optimal therapeutic alternative to address the patient's problem, taking into account patient preferences.	The patient prefers to use a nonspermicidal male condom with additional spermicide to provide contraception and STI protection. She is interested in learning about options for a fertility-awareness based method. Because she does not have medical insurance, she is not able to pursue a prescription hormonal method at this time.
6. Describe the recommended therapeutic approach to the patient or caregiver.	"Use a nonspermicidal male condom plus additional spermicide with each act of sexual intercourse."
7. Explain to the patient or caregiver the rationale for selecting the recommended therapeutic approach from the considered therapeutic alternatives.	"There are various OTC contraceptive options, including the male and female condom, contraceptive sponge, and various forms of spermicides. Of the OTC methods, only the male or female condom provides protection from STIs, which is important to consider when beginning a sexual relationship. This is important in addition to any other contraception that you use. The use of an ovulation test kit is intended for identifying the fertile period for pregnancy planning and is not intended to identify a time period to avoid before and after ovulation to prevent pregnancy. However, there are methods to monitor cervical mucus and body temperature that can be used to identify fertile phases of the menstrual cycle. These require education from certified trainers or health professionals to be optimally effective and are less effective than condoms when used alone for contraception. This method also would not provide protection from STIs."
Implement	
8. When recommending self-care with nonprescription medications and/or nondrug therapy, convey accurate information to the patient or caregiver.	
a. Appropriate dose and frequency of administration	"Use a fresh male condom and spermicide application with each act of sexual intercourse."
b. Product administration procedures	See Tables 10–5 and 10–9.
c. Expected time to onset of relief	"Once they are correctly placed, male condoms and spermicides are effective immediately."
d. Degree of relief that can be reasonably expected	See Table 10–2 for efficacy rates.
e. Most common adverse effects	"Irritation to the penis or vagina from exposure to latex or spermicide can occur. Some individuals have a sensitivity reaction to nonoxynol-9, the only spermicide currently available. The condom can also break or slip, allowing exposure to sperm and infection. Some men report reduced sensitivity and pleasure when using condoms."
f. Patient options in the event that condition worsens or persists	"Consult your primary care provider."
g. Product storage requirements	See Table 10–5.
Solicit follow-up questions from the patient or caregiver.	"May I use lubricants with the condom?"
Answer the patient's or caregiver's questions.	"Yes. The condom can be used with only certain lubricants that are water-based (Table 10–6). Oil-based lubricants can damage the condom and should be avoided."
Follow-up: Monitor and Evaluate	
9. Assess patient outcome.	Ask the patient to call the pharmacy if she has further questions.

Key: NKA = No known allergies; OTC = over-the-counter; STI = sexually transmitted infection.

CASE 10-2

Relevant Evaluation Criteria	Scenario/Model Outcome
Collect	
1. Gather essential information about the patient's symptoms and medical history, including	
a. Description of symptom(s) (i.e., nature, onset, duration, severity, associated symptoms)	Patient had unprotected intercourse with a partner 3 weeks ago. She is concerned that she may be pregnant and her period is a few days late.
b. Patient's identity	Maggie Jones
c. Patient's age, gender, height, and weight	23 years old, female, 5 ft 4 in., 125 lb
d. Patient's occupation	College student
e. Concurrent medical conditions, prescription and nonprescription medications, and dietary supplements	Occasional tension headaches: ibuprofen 200 mg 2 tablets orally every 8 hours as needed for headache; multivitamin 1 tablet daily; fluticasone (Flonase) nasal spray, 1 spray in each nostril daily as needed for seasonal allergies
f. Allergies	Seasonal, NKDA
g. History of other adverse effects to medications	None
Assess	
2. Differentiate patient's signs/symptoms, and correctly identify the patient's primary problem(s).	Patient has an elevated risk of pregnancy and STI due to unprotected intercourse with partner.
3. Identify exclusions for self-treatment.	Patient has an exclusion for self-treatment with EC due to having unprotected intercourse 3 weeks ago. She is outside the therapeutic window of 120 hours after unprotected intercourse for OTC EC use.
4. Formulate a comprehensive list of therapeutic alternatives for the primary problem to determine whether triage to a medical provider is required, and share this information with the patient or caregiver.	Options include (1) Recommend against use of OTC EC, because it has been longer than 120 hours since the patient had unprotected intercourse. Recommend that she see her health care provider for STI screening and, if applicable, for pregnancy testing and prenatal care. Also, if she is not pregnant, recommend that she seek a longer term prescription contraceptive method, or recommend that she seek a self-administered hormonal contraceptive from a pharmacist if that is allowed in her state. Recommend that she confirm her multivitamin has 400 mcg of folic acid to prevent neural tube defects in case she is pregnant or becomes pregnant in the future. Discuss the need for options such as the male or female condom to reduce risk for STIs in the future. (2) Recommend against use of OTC EC, because it has been longer than 120 hours since she had unprotected intercourse. Recommend that the patient purchase an OTC pregnancy test kit at her local pharmacy. Refer patient to see her PCP if her pregnancy test is positive or period does not begin within 3 weeks. Recommend that she confirm her multivitamin has 400 mcg of folic acid to prevent neural tube defects in case she is pregnant. Discuss the need for options such as the male or female condom to reduce risk for STIs in the future. (3) Take no action.
Plan	
5. Select an optimal therapeutic alternative to address the patient's problem, taking into account patient preferences.	The patient prefers to purchase an OTC pregnancy kit at her local pharmacy. Recommend that she see her PCP to have STI screening and prenatal care, if applicable.

CASE 10-2 *continued*

Relevant Evaluation Criteria	Scenario/Model Outcome
6. Describe the recommended therapeutic approach to the patient or caregiver.	"You should not use the nonprescription emergency contraception products, because you are outside of the window of time that the product is effective in preventing pregnancy. If you are concerned about pregnancy, you should use the pregnancy test at home. Use the test first thing in the morning when you urinate. If the test is positive as indicated in the package information, see your provider promptly. Keep in mind that home pregnancy tests may show false negatives early in the pregnancy, and seeing your primary care provider is the best way to determine whether you are pregnant. Your provider can also screen you for STIs and provide prenatal care or a long-term contraceptive product if needed. Check your multivitamin to make sure it has 400 mcg of folic acid to help prevent neural tube defects in the event you are pregnant or become pregnant in the future."
7. Explain to the patient or caregiver the rationale for selecting the recommended therapeutic approach from the considered therapeutic alternatives.	"Nonprescription emergency contraception is 52% to 100% effective in preventing pregnancy and works better the sooner it is taken. The nonprescription emergency contraception products should be taken as soon as possible within 72 hours of unprotected intercourse, but the product can still be effective up to 120 hours after intercourse. The product will not work 3 weeks after unprotected intercourse. It is not intended to be used during pregnancy. If you are pregnant, it is important to see your provider for prenatal care to ensure the best outcome for you and your child. Continue to take your multivitamin, and check to see that it has 400 mcg of folic acid. In addition, emergency contraception does not protect against sexually transmitted infections. Because you have had unprotected intercourse, you should be screened."
Implement	
8. When recommending self-care with nonprescription medications and/or nondrug therapy, convey accurate information to the patient or caregiver.	(1) "Keep in mind that home pregnancy tests may show false negatives early in the pregnancy. Seeing your primary care provider is the best way to determine whether you are pregnant." (2) "Check your multivitamin to make sure it has 400 mcg of folic acid to help prevent neural tube defects in the event you are pregnant."
Solicit follow-up questions from the patient or caregiver.	(1) "Is there anything I can do to prevent getting an STI?" (2) "Can I use emergency contraception as a regular birth control method?"
Answer the patient's or caregiver's questions.	(1) "Yes, use of a latex male condom or female condom is a good way to prevent STIs (see Tables 10–5 and 10–7 for directions on using these products)." (2) "Emergency contraception is not intended to be a regular form of birth control. For more effective and less expensive ways of contraception, you should see your primary care provider to obtain a prescription for a more regular form of contraception if you are not pregnant. Nonprescription contraceptives such as condoms, spermicides, and the sponge may also be an option."
Follow-up: Monitor and Evaluate	
9. Assess patient outcome.	Contact the patient in a day or two to ensure that she made an appointment and sought the discussed medical care.

Key: EC = Emergency contraception; NKDA = no known drug allergies; OTC = over-the-counter; PCP = primary care provider; STI = sexually transmitted infection.

TABLE 10–12 Provision of Hormonal Contraception by Pharmacists

Provision of hormonal contraception by a pharmacist has been shown to improve access to highly effective methods. Pharmacists in Washington have provided contraception through collaborative practice agreements for several decades. More recently Oregon, California, and Colorado passed legislation allowing pharmacists to provide self-administered hormonal contraception without a prescription. The Oregon and Colorado rulings specify oral and transdermal products, while the California legislation allows oral, transdermal, vaginal, and depot injectable products. The pharmacists are involved in assessing women for potential medical contraindications to hormonal contraception prior to dispensing. Legislation to allow pharmacist contraceptive prescribing is also being pursued in other states such as Tennessee, New Mexico, Alaska, and Hawaii.

Source: References 49 and 50.

be at high risk of unintended pregnancy and STIs. If possible, consultation involving both partners can improve the understanding and acceptance of selected contraceptive methods.

Providers must be familiar with the proper use of available nonprescription contraceptive products and provide easily accessible educational materials and opportunities for consultation by removing barriers that may prevent open conversations. Pharmacists in some states may now provide hormonal contraception without a prescription (Table 10–12).[49,50]

In addition to an educational role, the provider may be able to assist an individual in gaining access to other needed medical and social supportive services. In cases of suspected domestic violence, child abuse, or sexual abuse, pharmacists should act on their role as mandatory reporters as specified by their state laws. A private area for education and counseling is important if adequate discussion is to take place.

Special efforts should be made to offer contraceptive information and services to adolescents. Providers who are uncomfortable discussing reproductive health in a nonjudgmental manner with young people should refer adolescents to a clinic that specializes in services to this age group. Adolescents need clear, accurate information on all aspects of reproductive health. The provider should keep in mind that misconceptions about STI and pregnancy risk as well as proper contraceptive use are common, especially among adolescents; therefore, adequate education is very important. FAB methods are recommended for couples in a stable relationship. These methods, especially the symptothermal and cervical mucus methods, require extensive training and support from health care professionals who have experience with FAB methods. In addition to stocking spermicidal products, BBT thermometers, and monitoring charts, the pharmacist may serve as a referral for individuals who want to use these methods of family planning. A pharmacist with the proper training might consider counseling patients on FAB methods as a unique practice possibility.

Evaluation of Patient Outcomes for Prevention of Pregnancy and STIs

Many sexually active persons are at risk of unintended pregnancy or STIs. The most important factor affecting the ability of a contraceptive to prevent pregnancy and STIs is correct and consistent use with each sexual encounter. Although any of the methods can be used for pregnancy prevention, male condoms (except for lamb cecum) and the female condom are the preferred methods for prevention of STIs. Individuals who experience an adverse effect after use of a nonprescription contraceptive should switch to an alternative brand or agent. If the symptoms do not resolve or if they recur with the use of other agents, the individuals should seek medical attention. A sexually active woman who misses a menstrual period should be encouraged to perform a home pregnancy test or seek medical attention. Symptoms of an STI in a sexually active individual require medical referral (Table 10–1).

Key Points for Prevention of Pregnancy and STIs

- No method of contraception except abstinence is completely effective at preventing unintended pregnancy and STIs.
- The HPV vaccine is an effective method of preventing HPV-related consequences, including genital warts and cervical, vaginal, vulvar, penile, and anal cancers.
- Selection of a contraceptive product or method must be based on individual risk of undesired outcomes (pregnancy and STI) and efficacy, safety, and acceptability.
- Efficacy of nonprescription contraceptives is significantly increased by correct and consistent use of the product or method with each sexual encounter (Tables 10–5 through 10–9).
- Male condoms (latex) and female condoms are the preferred contraceptive products for individuals at risk for STIs. Nonlatex condoms other than lamb cecum may be used in persons with latex hypersensitivity for STI prevention.
- Spermicides decrease risk of unintended pregnancy but may increase risk of STIs.
- Vaginal spermicides are available in different dosage forms to improve patient acceptability.
- EC is an effective method of postcoital contraception that can decrease risk of unintended pregnancy, but the risk of STIs is not decreased. EC should not be used as routine contraception.
- FAB methods are an inexpensive, modestly effective method of contraception that can be used by couples in a mutually monogamous relationship.

REFERENCES

1. Finer LB, Zolna MR. Declines in unintended pregnancy in the United States, 2008–2011. *N Engl J Med* 2016;374;843–52. doi: 10.1056/NEJMsa1506575.
2. Jones J, Mosher WD, Daniels K. Current contraceptive use in the United States, 2006–2010, and changes in patterns of use since 1995. *Natl Health Stat Report.* 2012 Oct 18;(60):1–25. PMID: 24988814.
3. Martinez GM, Abma JC. Sexual activity, contraceptive use, and childbearing of teenagers aged 15–19 in the United States. NCHS data brief, no 209. *NCHS Data Brief.* 2015 Jul;(209):1–8. PMID: 26199985.
4. Centers for Disease Control and Prevention. Reported STDs in the United States: 2014 National Data for Chlamydia, Gonorrhea, and Syphilis. Available at: http://www.cdc.gov/std/stats14/std-trends-508.pdf. Accessed May 1, 2017.
5. Workowski KA, Bolan GA. Centers for Disease Control and Prevention. Sexually transmitted diseases treatment guidelines 2015. *MMWR Recomm Rep.* 2015;64(RR-3):1–135. Available at: https://www.cdc.gov/std/tg2015/tg-2015-print.pdf. Accessed May 1, 2017.
6. Sanford JB, White GL Jr, Hatasaka H. Timing intercourse to achieve pregnancy: current evidence. *Obstet Gynecol.* 2002;100(6):1333–41. PMID: 12468181.

7. Centers for Disease Control and Prevention. Sexually Transmitted Diseases (STDs): CDC Fact Sheets. Available at: www.cdc.gov/std/healthcomm/fact_sheets.htm. Accessed May 1, 2017.
8. Centers for Disease Control and Prevention. HIV Basics. Available at: www.cdc.gov/hiv/basics/index.html. Accessed May 1, 2017.
9. Marrazo JM, Cates W. Reproductive tract infections including HIV and other sexually transmitted infections. In: Hatcher RA, Trussell J, Nelson A, et al., eds. *Contraceptive Technology.* 20th rev ed. New York, NY: Ardent Media; 2011:571–620.
10. Meites E, Kempe A, Markowitz LE. Use of a 2-dose schedule for human papillomavirus vaccination: updated recommendations of the Advisory Committee on Immunization Practices. *MMWR Morb Mortal Wkly Rep.* 2016;65(49):1405–8. doi: 10.15585/mmwr.mm6549a5.
11. Centers for Disease Control and Prevention. *Epidemiology and Prevention of Vaccine-Preventable Diseases: The Pink Book: Course Textbook.* 13th ed. Atlanta, GA: CDC; 2015. Available at: https://www.cdc.gov/vaccines/pubs/pinkbook/index.html. Accessed May 1, 2017.
12. Markowitz LE, Liu G, Hariri S, et al. Prevalence of HPV after introduction of the vaccination program in the United States. *Pediatrics.* 2016;137(3):e20151968. doi: 10.1542/peds.2015-1968.
13. Guttmacher Institute. Contraceptive use in the United States fact sheet. October 2015. Available at: http://www.guttmacher.org/pubs/fb_contr_use.pdf. Accessed May 1, 2017.
14. Zieman M, Hatcher RA. *2012–2014 Managing Contraception.* Tiger, GA: Bridging the Gap Foundation; 2012.
15. Trussell J, Guthrie K. Choosing a contraceptive: efficacy, safety, and personal considerations. In: Hatcher RA, Trussell J, Stewart F, et al., eds. *Contraceptive Technology.* 20th rev ed. New York, NY: Ardent Media; 2011:45–74.
16. Jennings VH, Burke A. Fertility awareness–based methods. In: Hatcher RA, Trussell J, Nelson A, et al., eds. *Contraceptive Technology.* 20th rev ed. New York, NY: Ardent Media; 2011:417–34.
17. Kennedy KI, Trussell J. Postpartum contraception and lactation. In: Hatcher RA, Trussell J, Nelson A, et al., eds. *Contraceptive Technology.* 20th rev ed. New York, NY: Ardent Media; 2011:483–511.
18. Warner DL, Steiner MJ. Male condoms. In: Hatcher RA, Trussell J, Stewart F, et al., eds. *Contraceptive Technology.* 20th rev ed. New York, NY: Ardent Media; 2011:371–86.
19. Cates W Jr, Harwood B. Vaginal barriers and spermicides. In: Hatcher RA, Trussell J, Nelson AL, et al., eds. *Contraceptive Technology.* 20th rev ed. New York, NY: Ardent Media; 2011:392–408.
20. Vijayakumar G, Mabude Z, Smit J, et al. A review of female-condom effectiveness: patterns of use and impact on protected sex acts and STI incidence. *Int J STD AIDS.* 2006;17(10):652–9. doi: 10.1258/095646206780071036.
21. Kreiss J, Ngugi E, Holmes K, et al. Efficacy of nonoxynol 9 contraceptive sponge use in preventing of heterosexual acquisition of HIV in Nairobi prostitutes. *JAMA.* 1992;268(4):477–82. doi:10.1001/jama.1992.03490040053025.
22. Walgreens. Available at: https://www.walgreens.com/. Accessed May 1, 2017.
23. Gallo MF, Grimes DA, Lopez LM, et al. Non-latex versus latex male condoms for contraception (review). *Cochrane Database Syst Rev.* 2006;1:CD003550. doi: 10.1002/14651858.CD0003550.pub2.
24. Crosby RA, Yarber WL, Sanders SA, et al. Men with broken condoms: who and why? *Sex Transm Infect.* 2007;83(1):71–5. doi: 10.1136/sti.2006.021154.
25. Crosby RA, Yarber WL, Graham CS, et al. Does it fit okay? Problems with condom use as a function of self-reported poor fit. *Sex Transm Infect.* 2010;86(1):36–8. doi: 10.1136/sti.2009.036665.
26. Gabbay MB, Thomas J, Gibbs A, et al. A randomized crossover trial of the impact of additional spermicide on condom failure rates. *Sex Transm Dis.* 2008;35(10):862–8. doi: 10.1097/OLQ.0b013e31817fb802.
27. Potter WD, de Villemeur M. Clinical breakage, slippage and acceptability of a new commercial polyurethane condom: a randomized, controlled study. *Contraception.* 2003;68(1):39–45. doi: 10.1016/S0010-7824(03)00075-1.
28. Walsh TL, Frezieres RG, Peacock K, et al. Evaluation of the efficacy of a nonlatex condom: results from a randomized, controlled clinical trial. *Perspect Sex Reprod Health.* 2003;35(2):79–86. doi: 10.1363/3507903.
29. Steiner MJ, Dominik R, Rountree W, et al. Contraceptive effectiveness of a polyurethane condom and a latex condom. *Obstet Gynecol.* 2003;101(3):539–47. PMID: 12636960.
30. World Health Organization. HIV/AIDS: microbicides. Available at: http://www.who.int/hiv/topics/microbicides/microbicides/en/. Accessed May 1, 2017.
31. Liccardi G, Senna G, Rotiroti G, et al. Intimate behavior and allergy: a narrative review. *Ann Allergy Asthma Immunol.* 2007;99(5):394–400. doi:10.1016/S1081-1206(10)60562-5.
32. Centers for Disease Control and Prevention. Oral sex and HIV risk. Available at: https://www.cdc.gov/hiv/risk/oralsex.html. Accessed May 1, 2017.
33. Beksinska M, Smit J, Joanis C, et al. Female condom technology: new products and regulatory issues. *Contraception.* 2011;83(4):316–21. doi: 10.1016/j.contraception.2010.07.022.
34. New female condom clears FDA committee. *AIDS Alert.* 2009;24(4):42–4. PMID: 19382364.
35. Beksinska ME, Piaggio G, Smit JA et al. Performance and safety of the second-generation female condom (FC2) versus the Woman's, the VA worn-of-women and the Cupid female condoms: a randomized controlled non-inferiority crossover trial. *Lancet Glob Health.* 2013;1(3):e146–52. doi: 10.1016/S2214-109X(13)70054-8.
36. Female Health Company. FC2 female condom: how to use. Available at: http://fc2femalecondom.com/how-to-use/fc2-female-condom-step-by-step-instructions-english/. Accessed May 1, 2017.
37. Beksinska M, Smit J, Joanis C, et al. Practice makes perfect: reduction in female condom failures and user problems with short-term experience in a randomized trial. *Contraception.* 2012; 86(2):127–31. doi: 10.1016/j.contraception.2011.11.071.
38. Raymond EG, Chen PL, Condon P, et al. Acceptability of five nonoxynol-9 spermicides. *Contraception.* 2005;71(6):438–42. doi:10.1016/j.contraception.2004.12.023.
39. Grimes DA, Lopez LM, Raymond EG, et al. Spermicide used alone for contraception. *Cochrane Database Syst Rev.* 2013;12:CD005218. doi: 10.1002/14651858.CD005218.pub4.
40. U.S. Food and Drug Administration. Over-the-counter vaginal contraceptive and spermicide drug products containing nonoxynol-9; required labeling. Final rule. *Fed Regist.* 2007;72(243):71769–85.
41. Revive Personal Products. Gynol II Extra Strength Contraceptive Gel: FAQ. Available at: http://www.reviveppc.com/female-sexual-wellness/options/options-faq/. Accessed May 1, 2017.
42. Apothecus Pharmaceutical. Vaginal Contraceptive Film: what is VCF? Available at: http://www.vcfcontraceptive.com/howdoesvcfwork.html. Accessed May 1, 2017.
43. Briggs G, Freeman RK. *Drugs in Pregnancy and Lactation.* 10th ed. Philadelphia, PA: Wolters Kluwer; 2015: 999–1000.
44. Kuyoh MA, Toroitich-Ruto C, Grimes DA, et al. Sponge versus diaphragm for contraception: a Cochrane review. *Contraception.* 2003;67(1):15–8. doi: 10.1002/14651858.CD003172.
45. Trussell J, Raymond EG, Cleland K. *Emergency Contraception: A Last Chance to Prevent Unintended Pregnancy.* Princeton, NJ: Office of Population Research, Princeton University; December 2016. Available at: http://ec.princeton.edu/questions/ec-review.pdf. Accessed May 1, 2017.
46. Clinical Drug Information. Facts & Comparisons eAnswers. Hudson, OH: Wolters Kluwer; 2016. Available at: http://online.factsandcomparisons.com/index.aspx. Accessed February 12, 2016.
47. Pallone SR, Bergus GR. Fertility awareness–based methods: another option for family planning. *J Am Board Fam Med.* 2009;22(2):147–57. doi: 10.3122/jabfm.2009.02.080038.
48. Kowal D. Coitus interruptus (withdrawal). In: Hatcher RA, Trussell J, Nelson A, et al., eds. *Contraceptive Technology.* 20th rev ed. New York, NY: Ardent Media; 2011:409–15.
49. Gardner JS, Miller L, Downing DR, et al. Pharmacist prescribing of hormonal contraceptives: results of the Direct Access study. *J Am Pharm Assoc (2003).* 2008;48(2):212–21. doi: 10.1331/JAPhA.2008.07138.
50. California Board of Pharmacy Proposed Regulation 1746.1 Protocol for Pharmacists Furnishing Self-Administered Hormonal Contraception. Available at: http://www.pharmacy.ca.gov/laws_regs/1746_1_pt.pdf. Accessed May 1, 2017.

section

IV

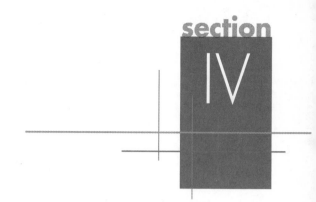

RESPIRATORY DISORDERS

CHAPTER 11

COLDS AND ALLERGY

KELLY L. SCOLARO

Colds and allergic rhinitis are two of the most common conditions for which patients initiate access to the health care system. This chapter reviews the role of the plethora of nonprescription products that patients may use to self-treat symptoms associated with those two disorders.

COLDS

A cold, also known as the common cold, is a viral infection of the upper respiratory tract. According to some estimates, 500 million cases of colds occur annually, making this illness one of the top five diagnosed in the United States.[1] Children usually have 6–10 colds per year.[1] Adults younger than 60 years typically have 2–3 colds per year, whereas adults older than 60 years usually have 1 cold per year.[1] Colds may occur at any time, but in the United States, the cold season extends from late August through early April.[1]

Colds are the leading cause of work and school absenteeism. Colds are usually self-limiting; however, because symptoms are bothersome, patients frequently self-medicate, with an estimated $7 billion spent annually on nonprescription cold and cough products.[2]

Pathophysiology of Colds

Colds are limited to the upper respiratory tract and primarily affect the following respiratory structures: pharynx, nasopharynx, nose, cavernous sinusoids, and paranasal sinuses. The respiratory tract's intricate host defense system usually protects the body from infectious and foreign particles. The respiratory tract, especially the nose, is well perfused and well innervated. The nose contains sensory, cholinergic, and sympathetic nerves. When stimulated by an infectious (e.g., a cold) or allergic (e.g., allergic rhinitis) process, those nerves play a role in the resulting symptoms and are also targets for some nonprescription therapies. Stimulation of sensory fibers by mechanical and thermal stimuli or by mediators such as histamine and bradykinin results in sneezing. Cholinergic and sympathetic nerves are involved in congestion in that they innervate glands and arteries that supply the glands. Cholinergic stimulation dilates arterial blood flow, whereas sympathetic stimulation constricts arterial blood flow. The sensory, cholinergic, and sympathetic nerves also respond to a variety of neuropeptide neurotransmitters.

More than 200 viruses cause colds. A majority of colds in children and adults are caused by rhinoviruses.[1] Other viruses known to cause colds include coronaviruses, parainfluenza, respiratory syncytial virus, adenoviruses, enteroviruses, and human metapneumovirus. Viral and bacterial coinfection (usually with group A beta-hemolytic streptococci) occurs but is rare. Rhinoviruses bind to intercellular adhesion molecule-1 receptors on respiratory epithelial cells in the nose and nasopharynx.[3] Once inside the epithelial cells, the virus replicates, and infection spreads to other cells.[3] Peak viral concentrations are achieved 2–4 days after initial inoculation, and viruses are present in the nasopharynx for 16–18 days.[3] Infected cells release chemokine "distress signals," and cytokines then activate inflammatory mediators and neurogenic reflexes. These activation processes result in recruitment of additional inflammatory mediators, vasodilation, transudation of plasma, glandular secretion, and stimulation of pain nerve fibers and sneeze and cough reflexes. Inflammatory mediators and parasympathetic nervous system reflex mechanisms cause hypersecretion of watery nasal fluid. Viral infection ends once enough neutralizing antibody (secretory immunoglobulin A [IgA] or serum IgG) leaks into the mucosa to end viral replication.

The most efficient mode of viral transmission is self-inoculation of the nasal mucosa or conjunctiva after contact with virus-laden secretions on animate (e.g., hands) or inanimate (e.g., doorknobs, telephones) objects. Transmission by means of inhalation of aerosolized viral particles is also common. Increased susceptibility to colds has been linked to higher exposure rates (e.g., with increased population density in classrooms or day care centers); allergic disorders affecting the nose or pharynx; less diverse social networks; and a weakened immune system due to smoking, a sedentary lifestyle, chronic (i.e., ≥1 month) psychological stress, or sleep deprivation (e.g., poor sleep quality or <7 hours of sleep per night).[1,4,5] Conflicting information has emerged about increased susceptibility due to cold environments, sudden chilling, or exposure to central heating (i.e., low humidity).[6] Walking outside barefoot, teething, and suffering from enlarged tonsils or adenoids have not been shown to increase susceptibility to viral upper respiratory infections.[1]

Clinical Presentation of Colds

A predictable sequence of symptoms begins 1–3 days after infection.[7] Sore throat is the first symptom to emerge, followed by nasal symptoms, which dominate 2–3 days later. Cough develops in 30% of patients by day 4 or 5. Physical assessment may yield the following findings: slightly red pharynx with evidence of postnasal drip, nasal obstruction, and mildly to moderately tender sinuses on palpation.

TABLE 11-1 **Differentiation of Colds and Other Respiratory Disorders**

Illness	Signs and Symptoms
Allergic rhinitis	Watery eyes; itchy nose, eyes, or throat; repetitive sneezing; nasal congestion; watery rhinorrhea; red, irritated eyes with conjunctival injection
Asthma	Cough, dyspnea, wheezing
Bacterial throat infection	Sore throat (moderate–severe pain), fever, exudate, tender anterior cervical adenopathy
Colds	Sore throat (mild–moderate pain), nasal congestion, rhinorrhea, sneezing common; low-grade fever, chills, headache, malaise, myalgia, and cough possible
Croup	Fever, rhinitis, and pharyngitis initially, progressing to cough (may be "barking" cough), stridor, and dyspnea
Influenza	Myalgia, arthralgia, fever with oral T ≥100.4°F–102°F (38°C–38.9°C), sore throat, nonproductive cough, moderate–severe fatigue
Otitis media	Ear popping, ear fullness, otalgia, otorrhea, hearing loss, dizziness
Pneumonia or bronchitis	Chest tightness, wheezing, dyspnea, productive cough, changes in sputum color, persistent fever
Sinusitis	Tenderness over the sinuses, facial pain aggravated by Valsalva maneuver or postural changes, fever with oral T >101.5°F (38.6°C), tooth pain, halitosis, upper respiratory tract symptoms for >7 days with poor response to decongestants
West Nile virus infection	Fever, headache, fatigue, rash, swollen lymph glands, and eye pain initially, possibly progressing to GI distress, CNS changes, seizures, or paralysis
Whooping cough	Initial catarrhal phase (rhinorrhea, mild cough, sneezing) of 1–2 weeks, followed by 1–6 weeks of paroxysmal coughing

Key: CNS = Central nervous system; GI = gastrointestinal; T = temperature.

During the first 2 days of a cold, patients may report clear, thin, and/or watery nasal secretions. As the cold progresses, the secretions become thicker and the color may change to yellow or green. When the cold begins to resolve, the secretions again become clear, thin, and/or watery. Low-grade fever may be present, especially in children, but colds are rarely associated with an oral temperature above 100.4°F (38°C) or rectal or tympanic temperature above 100.9°F (38.3°C). Rhinovirus cold symptoms persist for approximately 7–14 days.[7] Signs and symptoms of a cold may be confused with those of influenza and other respiratory illnesses (Table 11–1).

Most people do not experience complications from colds. However, such complications may be severe and, rarely, life-threatening. Complications include sinusitis, middle ear infections, bronchitis, pneumonia, and exacerbations of asthma or chronic obstructive pulmonary disease.

Treatment of Colds

Treatment Goals

Because there is no known cure for colds, the goal of therapy is to reduce bothersome symptoms and prevent transmission of cold viruses to other persons.

General Treatment Approach

Antibiotics are ineffective against viral infections, and the mainstay of treatment is nonpharmacologic therapy. If a patient desires to self-treat, a stepwise approach using single-entity products targeting specific symptoms is preferred over the use of combination products (Figure 11–1), because symptoms appear, peak, and resolve at different times.[7] Patient education regarding the administration of intranasal drugs (Table 11–2) and ocular drugs (see Chapter 28) is important. Not all patients should self-treat their colds (see the exclusions for self-treatment listed in Figure 11–1).

Nonpharmacologic Therapy

Although evidence of efficacy is lacking, popular therapeutic measures include increased fluid intake, adequate rest, a nutritious diet as tolerated, and increased humidification with steamy showers, vaporizers, or humidifiers. Vaporizers superheat water to produce steam and can accommodate medications such as Vicks Vapo Steam (camphor 6.2%). In contrast, humidifiers use fans or ultrasonic technology to produce a cool mist and cannot accommodate liquid additives. Saline nasal sprays or drops moisten irritated mucosal membranes and loosen encrusted mucus; salt gargles may ease sore throats. Hot tea with lemon and honey, chicken soup, and vegetable and other broths are soothing. Limited evidence suggests that a number of substances in chicken soup could have anti-inflammatory activity.[8] Milk products should not be withheld, in view of the lack of evidence that milk increases cough or congestion. Medical devices, such as Breathe Right nasal strips, are marketed for temporary relief from nasal congestion and stuffiness resulting from colds and allergies. Those devices lift the nares open, thereby enlarging the anterior nasal passages. Aromatic oils (e.g., camphor, menthol, eucalyptus) contained in products such as Vicks VapoRub (for patients 2 years of age and older) ease nasal congestion and improve sleep by producing a soothing sensation.[9] Children should be supervised closely when these products are used because aromatic oils can irritate the eyes and skin and ingestion of large quantities can be toxic.

Nondrug therapy for all patients, especially for infants, includes upright positioning to enhance nasal drainage. Because children typically cannot blow their own noses until the age of approximately 4 years, carefully clearing the nasal passageways with a nasal aspirator may be necessary if accumulation of mucus interferes with sleeping or eating. Nasal aspirators may be

Exclusions for Self-Treatment

- Fever >100.4°F (38.0°C, oral)
- Chest pain
- Shortness of breath
- Worsening of symptoms or development of additional symptoms during self-treatment
- Concurrent underlying chronic cardiopulmonary diseases (e.g., asthma, COPD, CHF)
- AIDS or chronic immunosuppressant therapy
- Frail patients of advanced age
- Infants ≤3 months of age
- Hypersensitivity to recommended OTC medications

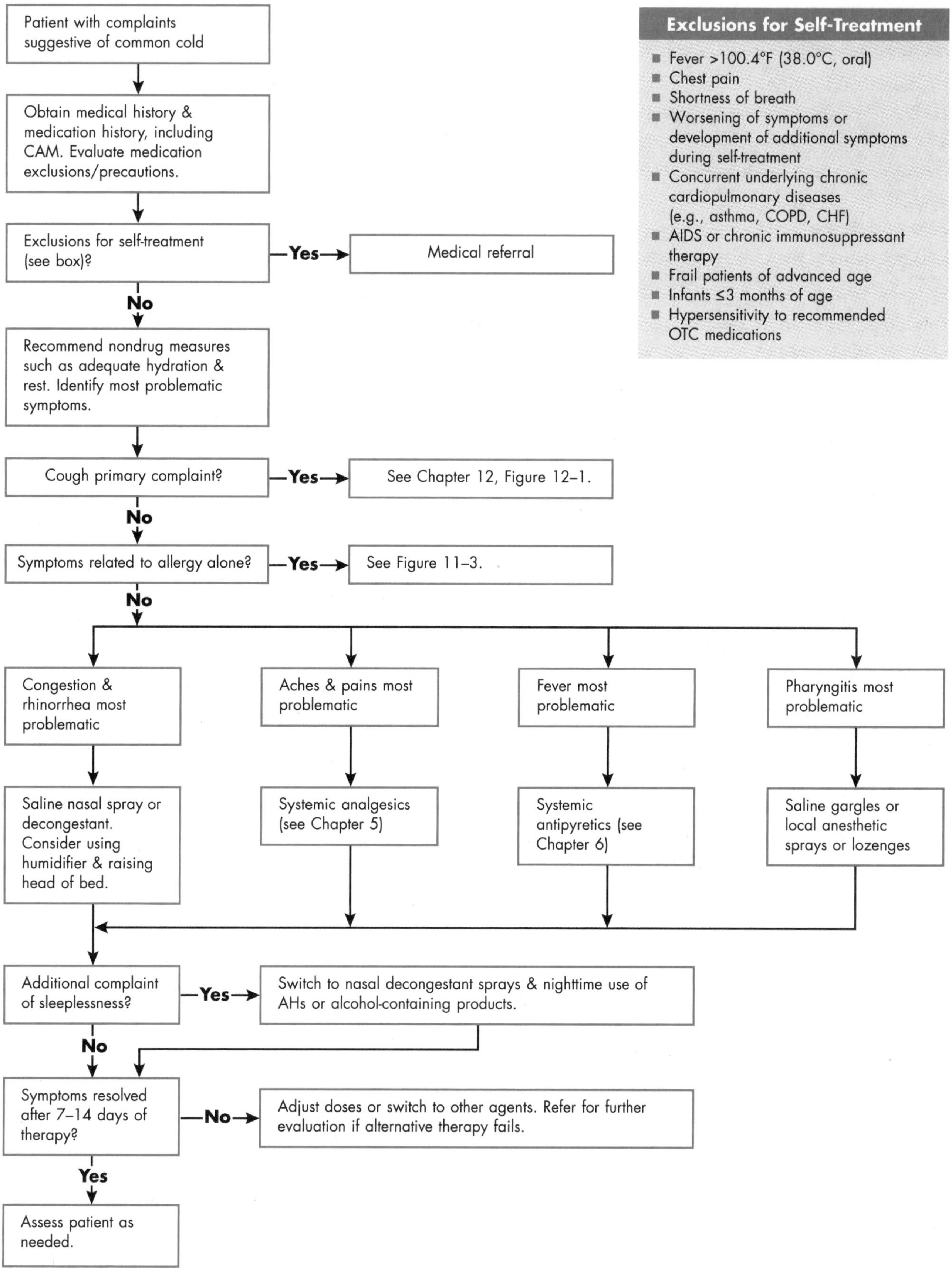
Patient with complaints suggestive of common cold
Obtain medical history & medication history, including CAM. Evaluate medication exclusions/precautions.
Exclusions for self-treatment (see box)?
Yes
Medical referral
No
Recommend nondrug measures such as adequate hydration & rest. Identify most problematic symptoms.
Cough primary complaint?
Yes
See Chapter 12, Figure 12–1.
No
Symptoms related to allergy alone?
Yes
See Figure 11–3.
No
Congestion & rhinorrhea most problematic
Aches & pains most problematic
Fever most problematic
Pharyngitis most problematic
Saline nasal spray or decongestant. Consider using humidifier & raising head of bed.
Systemic analgesics (see Chapter 5)
Systemic antipyretics (see Chapter 6)
Saline gargles or local anesthetic sprays or lozenges
Additional complaint of sleeplessness?
Yes
Switch to nasal decongestant sprays & nighttime use of AHs or alcohol-containing products.
No
Symptoms resolved after 7–14 days of therapy?
No
Adjust doses or switch to other agents. Refer for further evaluation if alternative therapy fails.
Yes
Assess patient as needed.

FIGURE 11–1 Self-care for the common cold. Key: AH = Antihistamine; AIDS = acquired immunodeficiency syndrome; CAM = complementary and alternative medicine; COPD = chronic obstructive pulmonary disease; HF = heart failure; OTC = over-the-counter. (Source: Adapted from references 1 and 7.)

TABLE 11-2 Administration Guidelines for Nasal Dosage Formulations

General Instructions

- Clear nasal passages before administering the product.
- Wash your hands before and after use.
- Gently depress the other side of the nose with finger to close off the nostril not receiving the medication.
- Aim tip of delivery device **away** from nasal septum to avoid accidental damage to the septum.
- Breathe through mouth and wait a few minutes after using the medication before blowing the nose.

Nasal Sprays

- Gently insert the bottle tip into one nostril, as shown in drawing A.
- Keep head upright. Sniff deeply while squeezing the bottle. Repeat with other nostril.

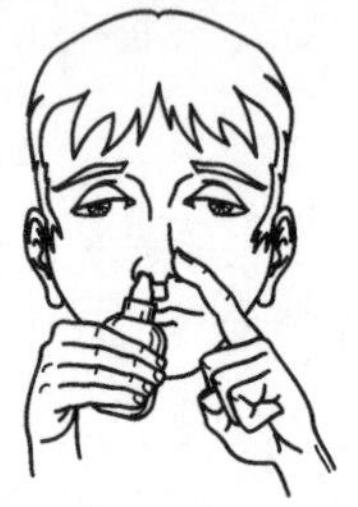

A

Pump Nasal Sprays

- Prime the pump before using it the first time. Hold the bottle with the nozzle placed between the first two fingers and the thumb placed on the bottom of the bottle.
- Tilt the head forward.
- Gently insert the nozzle tip into one nostril, as shown in drawing B. Sniff deeply while depressing the pump once.
- Repeat with other nostril.

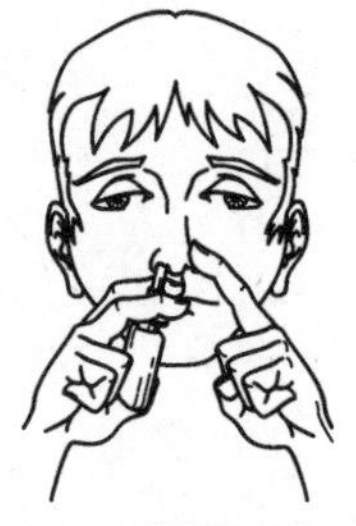

B

Nasal Inhalers

- Warm the inhaler in hand just before use.
- Gently insert the inhaler tip into one nostril, as shown in drawing C. Sniff deeply while inhaling.
- Wipe the inhaler after each use. Discard after 2–3 months even if the inhaler still smells medicinal.

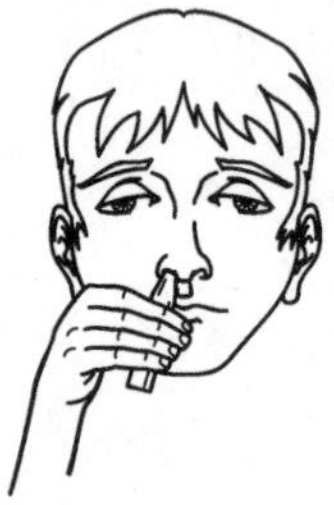

C

Nasal Drops

- Lie on bed with head tilted back and over the side of the bed, as shown in drawing D.
- Squeeze the bulb to withdraw medication from the bottle.
- Place the recommended number of drops into one nostril. Gently tilt head from side to side.
- Repeat with other nostril. Lie on bed for a couple of minutes after placing drops in the nose.
- Do not rinse the dropper.

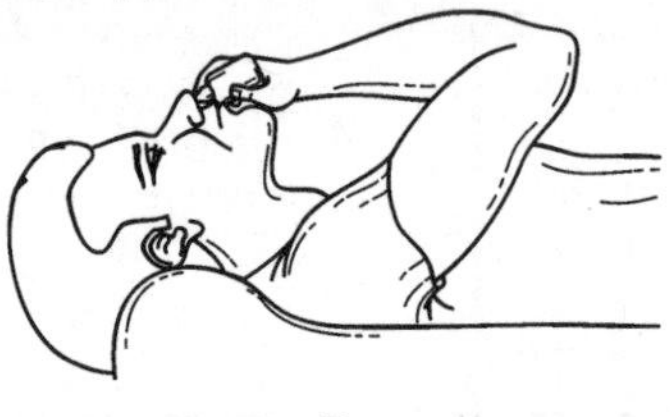

D

Note: Do not share the drug with anyone. Discard solutions if discolored or if contamination is suspected. Remove caps before use and replace tightly after each use. Do not use expired products.

mechanically or manually operated (e.g., bulb syringe). To use a bulb syringe and avoid harm to the child, the caregiver should squeeze the large end of the bulb *before* inserting it, continue to compress the bulb while gently inserting the tip into the infant's nose, and then slowly release the squeezing pressure to draw out fluid. After the pressure is completely released, the syringe is removed from the infant's nose and the fluid expelled from the syringe by again compressing the bulb.

Proper hand hygiene reduces the transmission of cold viruses. The Centers for Disease Control and Prevention (CDC) encourages frequent hand cleansing with soap or soap substitutes such as hand sanitizers.[1] Not all hand sanitizers are effective at eradicating rhinoviruses from hands. Alcohol-based products containing isopropanol or ethanol (60%–80% concentration) are preferred but are short-acting and require frequent reapplication.[10] Chlorhexidine, povidone–iodine, and quaternary ammonium compounds are also effective alone or in combination with alcohol-based products.[10] Alcohol-based nasal sanitizers (e.g., Nozin) are also available, but evidence of their efficacy against cold viruses is lacking. Use of antiviral disinfectants such as Lysol (which kills >99% of rhinoviruses after 1 minute) and antiviral tissues such as Kleenex Anti-Viral (incorporating a tissue layer containing citric acid and sodium lauryl sulfate) may also help prevent transmission to others.

Pharmacologic Therapy

Decongestants

Decongestants specifically treat sinus and nasal congestion. Decongestants are adrenergic agonists (sympathomimetics). Stimulation of alpha-adrenergic receptors constricts blood vessels, thereby decreasing sinusoid vessel engorgement and mucosal edema. Three types of decongestants are available. *Direct-acting* decongestants (e.g., phenylephrine, oxymetazoline, tetrahydrozoline) bind directly to adrenergic receptors. *Indirect-acting* decongestants (e.g., ephedrine) displace norepinephrine from storage vesicles in prejunctional nerve terminals and tachyphylaxis can develop as stored neurotransmitter is depleted. *Mixed* decongestants (e.g., pseudoephedrine) have both direct and indirect activity.

Systemic nonprescription decongestants include pseudoephedrine and phenylephrine. Intranasal nonprescription decongestants include the short-acting decongestants ephedrine, levmetamfetamine (L-desoxyephedrine), naphazoline, phenylephrine, and propylhexedrine, and the long-acting decongestants xylometazoline (8–10 hours) and oxymetazoline (12 hours). Ophthalmic nonprescription decongestants are also available (see Chapter 28).

Systemic decongestants are rapidly metabolized by monoamine oxidase (MAO) and catechol-*O*-methyltransferase in the gastrointestinal (GI) mucosa, liver, and other tissues. Pseudoephedrine is well absorbed after oral administration; phenylephrine has a low oral bioavailability (approximately 38%). Both pseudoephedrine and phenylephrine have short half-lives (pseudoephedrine, 6 hours; phenylephrine, 2.5 hours), and peak concentrations for both drugs are reached at 0.5–2 hours after oral administration.

Decongestants are indicated for temporary relief of nasal and eustachian tube congestion and for cough associated with postnasal drip. Nonprescription decongestants are not approved by the U.S. Food and Drug Administration (FDA) to self-treat nasal congestion associated with sinusitis.

FDA-approved dosages for decongestants are listed in Tables 11–3[11,12] and 11–4.[11] (Note: In 2008, manufacturers voluntarily updated cough and cold products labels to state "do not use" in children under 4 years of age.[13]) Nonprescription decongestants are marketed in a variety of dosage formulations, and many combination products are available (Table 11–5).

Adhering to FDA-approved doses of decongestant products is very important, given that acute overdose can be life-threatening, especially in children. Systemic decongestant overdoses cause excessive central nervous system (CNS) stimulation, paradoxical CNS depression, cardiovascular collapse, shock, and coma. Treatment of decongestant overdoses is supportive.

Adverse effects associated with decongestants include cardiovascular stimulation (leading to elevated blood pressure, tachycardia, palpitations, or arrhythmias) and CNS stimulation (causing restlessness, insomnia, anxiety, tremors, fear, or hallucinations). Children and older adults are more likely than persons in other age groups to experience adverse effects. Adverse effects are more common with systemic decongestants, because topical decongestants are minimally absorbed. However, accidental ingestion of nasal or ocular decongestants can cause adverse effects ranging from nausea, vomiting, and drooling to more serious effects including hypotension, hyperthermia, lethargy, sedation, and coma. Adverse effects specifically related to topical decongestants include propellant- or vehicle-associated effects (e.g., burning, stinging, sneezing, local dryness) and trauma from the tip of the administration device. Rhinitis medicamentosa (RM)—that is, rebound congestion—has been associated with use of topical decongestants. The exact cause is unknown, but short-acting products, preservative agents (e.g., benzalkonium chloride), and long duration of therapy are suspected as contributing factors.[14] Depending on the active ingredient, therapy of 3–7 days is the accepted duration to avoid RM. However, controversy exists, and some studies show that treatment duration of 10 days to 8 weeks appears to be safe and does not cause RM.[15] Further investigation is needed to determine the optimal duration of treatment. Treatment of RM consists of slowly withdrawing the topical decongestant (one nostril at a time); replacing the decongestant with topical normal saline, which soothes the irritated nasal mucosa; and, if needed, using topical corticosteroids and systemic decongestants. A withdrawal period of 2–6 weeks of such measures may be needed before mucous membranes return to normal. A nonprescription kit, RhinoStat, has been advertised to assist health care providers (HCPs) and patients with management of RM. The product creates a patient-specific mixture of the implicated topical decongestant product and a diluent; however, the kit is not FDA approved.

Decongestants interact with numerous drugs, as summarized in Table 11–6. Decongestants are contraindicated in patients receiving concomitant MAO inhibitors (MAOIs).

Decongestants may exacerbate diseases sensitive to adrenergic stimulation, such as hypertension, coronary heart disease, ischemic heart disease, diabetes mellitus, hyperthyroidism, elevated intraocular pressure, and prostatic hypertrophy. Patients with hypertension should use decongestants only with medical advice, and no clear evidence exists that any one agent is safest in this population. Products specifically marketed for patients with hypertension (e.g., Coricidin HBP) do not contain decongestants. Those products usually contain a combination of ingredients that may or may not be appropriate, depending on the patient's symptoms.

TABLE 11-3 Dosage Guidelines for Nonprescription Systemic Nasal Decongestants

	Dosage[a] (maximum daily dosage)		
Drug	**Adults and Children ≥12 Years**	**Children 6 to <12 Years**	**Children 2 to <6 Years[b]**
Phenylephrine HCl	10 mg every 4 hours (60 mg)	5 mg every 4 hours (30 mg)	2.5 mg every 4 hours (15 mg)
Phenylephrine bitartrate	15.6 mg every 4 hours (62.4 mg)	7.8 mg every 4 hours (31.2 mg)	Not recommended for children <6 years except under advice of PCP
Pseudoephedrine	60 mg every 4–6 hours (240 mg)	30 mg every 4–6 hours (120 mg)	15 mg every 4–6 hours (60 mg)

Key: FDA = U.S. Food and Drug Administration; PCP = primary care provider.

[a] Taken as needed.

[b] FDA has advised that cough and cold medications not be used in children younger than 2 years of age.[12] Manufacturers have voluntarily updated cough and cold product labels to state "do not use" in children younger than 4 years of age.[13]

Source: Reference 11.

TABLE 11-4 **Dosage Guidelines for Nonprescription Topical Nasal Decongestants**

Drug	Concentration (%)	Adults and Children ≥12 Years	Children 6 to <12 Years	Children 2 to <6 Years[a]
Sprays/Drops				
Ephedrine[b]	0.5	2–3 drops/sprays in each nostril not more often than every 4 hours	1–2 drops/sprays in each nostril not more often than every 4 hours	Not recommended for children <6 years except under advice of PCP
Levmetamfetamine	0.04–0.15 mg/ 800 mL of air	2 inhalations in each nostril not more often than every 2 hours	1 inhalation in each nostril not more often than every 2 hours	Not recommended for children <6 years except under advice of PCP
Naphazoline	0.05	1–2 drops/sprays in each nostril not more often than every 6 hours	Not recommended for children <12 years except under advice of PCP	Not recommended for children <6 years except under advice of PCP
	0.025	—	1–2 drops/sprays in each nostril not more often than every 6 hours	Not recommended for children <6 years except under advice of PCP
Oxymetazoline	0.05	2–3 drops/sprays in each nostril not more often than every 10–12 hours (maximum: 2 doses/ 24 hours)	2–3 drops/sprays in each nostril not more often than every 10–12 hours (maximum: 2 doses/ 24 hours)	Not recommended for children <6 years except under advice of PCP
	0.025	—	—	2–3 drops/sprays in each nostril not more often than every 10–12 hours (maximum: 2 doses/24 hours)
Phenylephrine	1.0	2–3 drops/sprays in each nostril not more often than every 4 hours	Not recommended for children <12 years except under advice of PCP	Not recommended for children <6 years except under advice of PCP
	0.5	2–3 drops/sprays in each nostril not more often than every 4 hours	Not recommended for children <12 years except under advice of PCP	Not recommended for children <6 years except under advice of PCP
	0.25	2–3 drops/sprays in each nostril not more often than every 4 hours	2–3 drops/sprays in each nostril not more often than every 4 hours	Not recommended for children <6 years except under advice of PCP
	0.125	—	—	2–3 drops/sprays in each nostril not more often than every 4 hours
Propylhexedrine	0.4–0.5 mg/ 800 mL of air	2 inhalations in each nostril not more often than every 2 hours	2 inhalations in each nostril not more often than every 2 hours	Not recommended for children <6 years except under advice of PCP
Xylometazoline[b]	0.1	2–3 drops/sprays in each nostril not more often than every 8–10 hours	Not recommended for children <12 years except under advice of PCP	Not recommended for children <6 years except under advice of PCP
	0.05	—	2–3 drops/sprays in each nostril not more often than every 8–10 hours	2–3 drops/sprays in each nostril not more often than every 8–10 hours (maximum: 3 doses/24 hours)

Key: FDA = U.S. Food and Drug Administration; PCP = primary care provider.

[a] No recommended dosages exist for children younger than 2 years of age, except under the advice and supervision of a PCP.

[b] Products approved by FDA but not currently marketed in the United States.

Source: Reference 11.

TABLE 11-5 **Selected Nonprescription Products for Nasal Decongestion**

Trade Name	Primary Ingredients
Topical Decongestants	
Afrin Original Nasal Spray	Oxymetazoline HCl 0.05%
Vicks Sinex Nasal Spray	Oxymetazoline HCl 0.05%
Zicam Extreme Congestion Relief Nasal Gel	Oxymetazoline HCl 0.05%
4-Way Fast Acting	Phenylephrine HCl 1%
Neo-Synephrine Regular Strength Nasal Spray	Phenylephrine HCl 0.5%
Little Remedies Decongestant Nose Drops	Phenylephrine HCl 0.125%
Otrivin Complete Nasal Care (Canada)	Xylometazoline 0.1%
Nasal Decongestant Inhalers	
Benzedrex Inhaler	Propylhexedrine 250 mg
Vapor Inhaler	Levmetamfetamine (L-desoxyephedrine) 50 mg/inhaler
Systemic Decongestants	
Sudafed PE Congestion	Phenylephrine HCl 10 mg
Sudafed 24 Hour	Pseudoephedrine HCl 240 mg
Sudafed 12 Hour	Pseudoephedrine HCl 120 mg
Nexafed[a]	Pseudoephedrine HCl 30 mg
Zephrex-D[b]	Pseudoephedrine HCl 30 mg
Combination Products	
Sudafed PE Pressure + Pain	Phenylephrine HCl 5 mg; acetaminophen 325 mg
Alka-Seltzer Plus Cold	Phenylephrine bitartrate 7.8 mg; aspirin 325 mg; chlorpheniramine maleate 2 mg
Vicks Dayquil Cold & Flu Relief Liquicaps	Phenylephrine HCl 5 mg; acetaminophen 325 mg; dextromethorphan hydrobromide 10 mg
Tylenol Cold Max Nighttime Cool Burst Liquid	Phenylephrine HCl 5 mg/15 mL; acetaminophen 325 mg/15 mL; dextromethorphan hydrobromide 10 mg/15 mL; doxylamine succinate 6.25 mg/15 mL
Dr. Cocoa Multi-Symptom Mucus Relief	Phenylephrine HCl 2.5 mg/5 mL; guaifenesin 50 mg/5 mL
Aleve-D Sinus & Cold	Pseudoephedrine HCl 120 mg; naproxen sodium 220 mg
Mucinex D	Pseudoephedrine HCl 60 mg; guaifenesin 600 mg
Other Products	
Ocean Premium Saline Nasal Spray	Sodium chloride 0.65%
Simply Saline Nasal Swabs	Glycerin, sodium chloride, methylparaben
Vicks VapoRub	Camphor (4.8%); eucalyptus (1.2%); menthol (2.6%)

[a] Meth-deterring technology (Impede) (i.e., drug is designed to deter the conversion of pseudoephedrine to methamphetamine).
[b] Meth-deterring technology (Tarex).

TABLE 11-6 **Clinically Important Drug–Drug Interactions With Cold and Allergy Products**

Drug/Drug Class	Potential Interaction (drug-specific data)	Management/Prevention
Decongestants		
Ergot derivatives (e.g., dihydroergotamine and ergotamine)	Increased risk of hypertension and vasoconstriction	Avoid combination.
Linezolid	Increased risk of hypertension	Reduce dose of decongestant and monitor closely. Consider therapy modification.
MAOIs (e.g., phenelzine, selegiline)	Increased risk of hypertension	Avoid combination.
Serotonin/norepinephrine reuptake inhibitors	Increased risk of tachycardia	Consider therapy modification
Antihistamines		
Amiodarone	Increased risk of QT interval prolongation (loratadine)	Avoid combination.
Antacids (aluminum and magnesium salts)	Decreased efficacy (fexofenadine)	Separate doses by as much time as possible.
Anticholinergics (e.g., ipratropium, tiotropium, umeclidinium)	Enhanced anticholinergic effects (dry mouth, eyes, urinary retention, sedation)	Avoid combination.
Brexpiprazole	Increased risk of brexpiprazole toxicity (diphenhydramine)	Reduce brexpiprazole dose by 25% or avoid combination.
CNS depressants (alcohol, opiates, sedatives)	Increased sedation (sedating antihistamines; cetirizine, levocetirizine)	Avoid combination.
Erythromycin; ketoconazole	Increased fexofenadine plasma concentration	Monitor therapy closely.
Metoprolol	Increased metoprolol serum concentrations and risk of hypotension (diphenhydramine)	Reduce metoprolol dose or avoid combination.
Phenytoin	Decreased phenytoin elimination (chlorpheniramine)	Monitor therapy or avoid combination.
Potassium chloride (oral)	Increased risk of ulcers	Avoid combination.
Intranasal Corticosteroids		
Protease inhibitors (e.g., ritonavir, tipranavir, telaprevir)	Increased serum concentration of steroids (budesonide, fluticasone)	Avoid combination.

Key: CNS = Central nervous system; MAOI = monoamine oxidase inhibitor.
Source: Lexi-Drugs Online. Hudson, OH: Lexi-Comp. Available at: http://www.crlonline.com. Accessed June 20, 2016.

HCPs should be aware of the possibility that patients may purchase large quantities of pseudoephedrine for illegal use to produce methamphetamine. In 2005, passage of the Combat Methamphetamine Epidemic Act changed the classification of pseudoephedrine to "scheduled listed chemical products."[15] That change in classification allowed limits to be placed on pseudoephedrine sales. All pseudoephedrine products must now be kept in secure areas (e.g., behind a pharmacy counter or in a locked cabinet), and purchases are limited to 3.6 g/day and 9 g per month per patient.[15] The following information from each sale must be entered into a paper or electronic logbook: product name, quantity sold, patient's name and address, and time and date of sale.[15] Patients must show valid identification to purchase pseudoephedrine and then sign the logbook. Some states and corporations have enacted stricter guidelines regarding the sale of pseudoephedrine.

Antihistamines

Monotherapy with nonprescription antihistamines may provide some benefit in adults if started early in the course of a cold (i.e., day 1 or 2 of symptom onset).[16] Also, a combination of first-generation (sedating) antihistamines and decongestants showed some benefit in adults, but the significance of the data is questionable.[17] Apart from questions of efficacy, an important issue is whether potential benefits of sedating antihistamines outweigh known risks associated with these drugs. (See the discussion of antihistamines in the "Allergic Rhinitis" section.)

Local Anesthetics

A variety of products containing local anesthetics (e.g., benzocaine, dyclonine hydrochloride) are available for the temporary relief of sore throats (Table 11–7). Local anesthetic products may be used every 2–4 hours. HCPs should counsel patients with a history of allergic reactions to anesthetics to avoid products containing benzocaine. Benzocaine has also been associated with methemoglobinemia, especially in children younger than 2 years, and should be avoided in this age group. Some products contain local antiseptics (e.g., cetylpyridinium chloride, hexylresorcinol) and/or menthol or camphor. Local antiseptics are not effective

TABLE 11-7 **Selected Nonprescription Products for Sore Throat**

Trade Name	Primary Ingredients
Lozenges	
Cepacol Sore Throat Sugar Free Extra Strength	Benzocaine 15 mg; menthol 3.6 mg
Chloraseptic Sore Throat	Benzocaine 6 mg; menthol 10 mg
Halls Fruit Breezers	Pectin 7 mg
Sucrets Classic	Dyclonine HCl 2 mg
Vicks VapoDrops	Menthol 1.7 mg (cherry)
	Menthol 3.3 mg (menthol)
Throat Sprays	
Cepacol Ultra Sore Throat Spray	Benzocaine 5%; glycerin 33%
Chloraseptic Sore Throat	Phenol 1.4%

for viral infections. Emerging evidence suggests that menthol and camphor may provide pain relief by stimulation of the TRPM8 or "menthol" receptor.[18]

Systemic Analgesics

Systemic analgesics (e.g., aspirin, acetaminophen, ibuprofen, naproxen) are effective for aches or fever sometimes associated with colds. Concerns that use of aspirin and acetaminophen may increase viral shedding and prolong illness have not been validated.[19] Because of the risk of Reye's syndrome, aspirin and aspirin-containing products should not be used in children or teenagers who have or are recovering from chickenpox or influenza-like symptoms. (See Chapter 5 for a complete discussion of those products, including the manufacturer's voluntary reduction of maximum daily dosages of Tylenol products sold in the United States [see the "Acetaminophen" section and Table 5–3], and developments in liquid infant acetaminophen products [see the "Patient Factors" section].)

Antitussives and Protussives (Expectorants)

When present, cough associated with colds is usually nonproductive. Antitussive agents (codeine and dextromethorphan) are of questionable efficacy in colds, and their use in this setting is not recommended.[20] Guaifenesin, an expectorant, has not been proved effective in natural colds.[20] (See Chapter 12 for a complete discussion of these products.)

Combination Products

Decongestants and antihistamines are marketed in many combinations, including combinations with analgesics, expectorants, and antitussives. Products are also marketed for daytime or nighttime use. Products for nighttime use usually contain a sedating antihistamine, whereas daytime products do not. Combination products are convenient, but this benefit must be weighed against the risks associated with taking unnecessary drugs.

Pharmacotherapeutic Comparison

As stated earlier, evidence does not support the use of antitussives and expectorants and is limited for the use of antihistamines to treat symptoms related to colds. The use of local anesthetics and systemic analgesics for treatment of pain related to sore throat or of fever related to colds, however, is supported by good evidence.

Topical decongestants are convenient dosage forms and are effective in relieving nasal congestion; however, duration of their use is limited to 3–7 days owing to concerns about development of RM. The major differences between topical decongestants are in duration of action, dosage formulation (e.g., mist vs. spray vs. drops), moisture content, and preservative content.

Although many manufacturers have reformulated products with phenylephrine as a response to pseudoephedrine regulations, controversy remains with regard to the relative safety and efficacy of the systemic decongestants. Clear evidence that oral phenylephrine is safer than pseudoephedrine has yet to be presented.[21,22] Strong evidence supports the efficacy of oral dosage forms of pseudoephedrine, whereas efficacy of the current FDA-approved dose of phenylephrine has been extensively debated, and a citizen's petition was filed in 2015 to remove it from the nonprescription drug market.[21,22]

Product Selection Guidelines

Special Populations

Drug use during pregnancy and lactation requires a balance between risk and benefit. (See the Preface for a detailed explanation of the pregnancy data.) Because most colds are self-limiting, with bothersome rather than life-threatening symptoms, many HCPs recommend nondrug therapy. When drugs are considered, those with a long record of safety in animals and humans are preferred. To minimize possible adverse effects on the fetus or newborn, pharmacists should advise pregnant or lactating women to avoid products labeled as "extra strength," "maximum strength," or "long-acting," as well as combination products. Systemic decongestants should also be avoided, because human data suggest increased risk of adverse effects based on theoretically decreased fetal blood flow.[23] Oral use of phenylephrine during the first trimester has been associated with minor malformations (e.g., inguinal hernia, hip dislocation).[23] Pseudoephedrine has been linked to abdominal wall defects (gastroschisis) in newborns.[23] No clear association has been found between birth defects and the use of intranasal decongestants during pregnancy.[23] Oxymetazoline is poorly absorbed after intranasal administration and is the preferred topical decongestant during pregnancy. Nonprescription cold products do not appear to affect male reproduction.

The American Academy of Pediatrics has found pseudoephedrine to be compatible with breastfeeding.[23] No human data are available for intranasal phenylephrine and oxymetazoline, so they are considered "probably compatible" in lactating mothers.[23] Because decongestants may decrease milk production, lactating mothers should monitor their milk production and drink extra fluids as needed. Dextromethorphan, guaifenesin, benzocaine, camphor (topical), and menthol (topical) each carry a low risk of birth defects and have been found to be compatible with breastfeeding.[23]

As stated earlier, older patients should use decongestants with caution, because they may be more sensitive to adverse effects and may have a higher prevalence of concomitant disease states (e.g., cardiovascular disease) in which nonprescription cold products may potentially have a negative impact. (See the section "Special

Populations" under "Allergic Rhinitis" later in the chapter for a discussion of antihistamine use in the geriatric population.)

Using nonprescription cold products in children is controversial owing to the lack of clinical evidence of safety and efficacy in this age group. Currently, FDA does not recommend nonprescription cold medications for children younger than 2 years because of the lack of efficacy and risk of misuse or overuse leading to adverse events and death.[12] Manufacturers have voluntarily updated product labeling to include the statement "Do not use in children under four years of age" and added warnings to antihistamine-containing products against their use for sedation purposes.[13] FDA continues to monitor and review the use of nonprescription cold medications in children between the ages of 2 and 11 years.[12] HCPs should emphasize nondrug measures in children, and if pharmacotherapy is deemed necessary, parents should follow dosing instructions carefully and avoid combination products to avoid overdosage. To address the issue of inaccurate dosing, FDA released guidelines in May 2011 for liquid nonprescription drug products that include any type of dispensing device (dropper, cup, syringe, or spoon).[24] Products include liquid analgesics, liquid cough and cold products, and lactase replacement drops. The key points of the guidelines are as follows:

- A dosing device should be included with all oral liquid nonprescription products.
- The device should be calibrated to the dose recommended in the product directions.
- The device should be used only with the product in which it is packaged.
- The markings need to remain visible even when the liquid is in the device.

Patient Factors

As discussed earlier, it may be difficult to differentiate cold symptoms from those of some acute and chronic disorders (Table 11–1). If duration of symptoms is longer than 7–14 days or a chronic condition is suspected, self-treatment is contraindicated. Patients with chronic conditions exacerbated by adrenergic stimulation, or those overly sensitive to such stimulation, should avoid decongestants. HCPs should educate patients who participate in organized sports that oral decongestants are considered "doping" products and should be used only in accordance with sport regulations.

Patient Preferences

Lozenges, soft chews, and nasal drug delivery forms may be preferred by patients who have difficulty swallowing or when access to water is not convenient. Nasal delivery forms, however, may be difficult to use for patients with severe arthritis or coordination problems.

For patients who prefer a nasal delivery form, each dosage form has distinct advantages and disadvantages. Nasal sprays are simple to use, cover a large surface area, are relatively inexpensive, and have a fast onset of action. The disadvantages include imprecise dosage, a tendency for the tip to become clogged with repeated use, and a high risk of contamination from aspiration of nasal mucus into the bottle. Metered pump sprays deliver a more precise dose. Nasal drops are preferred for small children but can be difficult to use, cover a limited surface area, and pass easily into the larynx. A high risk of contamination stemming from the tendency to touch the dropper to the nasal mucosa during administration is also recognized. Nasal inhalers are small, but their use requires an unobstructed airway and sufficient air flow to distribute the drug to the nasal mucosa. Nasal inhalers lose efficacy after 2–3 months, even when tightly capped, because of dissipation of the active ingredient. Nasal polyps, enlarged turbinates, and abnormalities such as septal deviation may reduce the efficacy of topical dosage forms.

Complementary Therapies

Numerous complementary therapies are marketed for the treatment of colds (Table 11–8[25–28]; see also Chapter 51). Zinc and high-dose vitamin C are popular therapies.

High local concentrations of zinc ions purportedly block the adhesion of human rhinovirus to the nasal epithelium and are also thought to inhibit viral replication by disrupting viral capsid formation. However, in vitro studies have shown only a modest antiviral effect. Formulations include tablets, capsules, chews, lozenges, syrups, and oral sprays. Nasal formulations were removed from the market because of associated anosmia (loss of smell).[29] Oral formulations may be associated with GI adverse effects (e.g., nausea, upset stomach, bitter taste). Since the 1980s, the effectiveness of zinc has been highly debated. A meta-analysis of 17 trials concluded that oral zinc (as lozenges or syrup) was effective in reducing cold symptoms or duration of the cold if started within 24 hours of symptom onset and administered every 2 hours while the patient was awake. The study also reported that prophylaxis with zinc for at least 5 months reduced the incidence of colds in healthy patients.[30]

TABLE 11-8 Selected Complementary Therapies for Colds and Allergies

Botanical Natural Product [Scientific Name]	Risks	Effectiveness
African geranium [umckaloabo, active ingredient in Umcka ColdCare products] (*Pelargonium sidoides*)	Allergic reactions or GI disturbances	Some evidence for alleviating symptoms of acute rhinosinusitis associated with colds in adults
Ephedra [ma huang] (*Ephedra sinica*)	Tachycardia, hypertension, heart attack, stroke, seizure	Effective decongestant
Goldenseal (*Hydrastis canadensis*)	Potentially toxic, especially in patients with glucose-6-dehydrogenase deficiency	Some evidence of anti-inflammatory effects of active ingredient berberine for treatment of pulmonary inflammation

Key: GI = Gastrointestinal.

Source: References 25–28.

The efficacy and safety of high-dose (e.g., ≥2 g/day) vitamin C (ascorbic acid) supplementation for prophylaxis and treatment of colds have been debated for more than 70 years. An analysis of 29 trials showed that although routine use of high-dose vitamin C does not appear to prevent colds in the general population, it did reduce the duration by approximately 8% in adults and 14% in children.[31] In contrast, high-dose vitamin C prophylaxis was effective in preventing colds in a subgroup of patients under severe physical stress (e.g., marathon runners).[31] Such use of vitamin C after the onset of a cold, however, was not effective at reducing severity or duration of symptoms.[31] Regular use of high doses may increase the risk of development of kidney stones in men.[32] Doses of 4 g/day or greater are associated with diarrhea and other GI symptoms and therefore should not be recommended.

Products that claim to strengthen the immune system such as Airborne, Emergen-C Immune+, and others have not been proved to be effective in preventing or treating colds. Vitamin D supplementation to prevent colds is controversial, but a recent meta-analysis showed benefit, especially daily use in patients with low vitamin D levels.[33] Docosahexaenoic acid (DHA) supplementation during pregnancy may help to reduce the incidence and duration of colds in infants, but more studies are needed.[34] Homeopathic products containing Galphimia glauca, Sabadilla, and Luffa operculata (e.g., on Zicam nasal swabs) are marketed to reduce severity if taken at the onset of symptoms, but evidence of efficacy and safety is lacking. Various probiotic products are available, and emerging research suggests that they may help support the immune system and prevent colds.[35] (See Chapter 20 for a complete discussion of those products.)

TABLE 11-9 Physical Assessment of Patient Presenting With Cold Symptoms

1. Observe patient (look and listen for signs of chronic conditions, such as red, watery eyes; wheezing; productive cough; barrel chest; poorly perfused areas; enlarged lymph nodes; rash).

If equipment and privacy allow, conduct the following:

2. Obtain vital signs (temperature, respiratory rate, pulse, and blood pressure).
3. Palpate sinuses and neck, and observe for any pain/tenderness.
4. Visually examine throat for redness or exudates. If bacterial pharyngitis is suspected, run rapid strep test.
5. Auscultate chest to detect wheezing, crackles, and rapid or irregular heartbeat.

Assessment of Colds: A Case-Based Approach

After asking questions about the patient's symptoms, medical history, medication use (current and past), and the efficacy of past self-treatment of colds, the HCP should conduct a brief physical assessment (Table 11–9). If the assessment and the patient's answers do not reveal exclusions for self-treatment, the provider should recommend medications that target the patient's most troublesome symptoms.

Case 11–1 is an example of assessment of a patient with a possible cold.

CASE 11-1

Relevant Evaluation Criteria	Scenario/Model Outcome
Collect	
1. Gather essential information about the patient's symptoms and medical history, including	
a. Description of symptom(s) (i.e., nature, onset, duration, severity, associated symptoms)	Patient complains of muscle pain, fatigue, and a sore throat that all began yesterday. In addition, he woke up this morning with a high fever.
b. Description of any factors that seem to precipitate, exacerbate, and/or relieve the patient's symptom(s)	His sore throat has progressively worsened since it began, and nothing seems to relieve the pain.
c. Description of the patient's efforts to relieve the symptoms	Patient ate chicken soup and took Tylenol 500 mg, 2 tablets last night.
d. Patient's identity	William Green
e. Patient's age, gender, height, and weight	55 years, male, 6 ft, 207 lb
f. Patient's occupation	Businessman
g. Patient's dietary habits	Patient eats a healthy, low-carbohydrate, low-fat diet. Patient consumes junk food and alcohol several times during a month because of business trips.
h. Patient's sleep habits	Erratic because of frequent business travel
i. Concurrent medical conditions, prescription and nonprescription medications, and dietary supplements	One A Day Men's Health Formula multivitamin once a day; saw palmetto 450 mg once a day
j. Allergies	Sulfa (he experienced a rash)
k. History of other adverse reactions to medications	None
l. Other (describe) ______	Patient's oral temperature currently is 103°F (39.4°C), and blood pressure is 112/77 mm Hg.

CASE 11-1 *continued*

Relevant Evaluation Criteria	Scenario/Model Outcome
Assess	
2. Differentiate patient's signs/symptoms, and correctly identify the patient's primary problem(s).	Cold signs/symptoms tend to include nasal congestion, sneezing, and low-grade fever. Patient has muscle pain, fatigue, and high fever (T >102°F [38.9°C]), so his symptoms are more indicative of flu.
3. Identify exclusions for self-treatment (Figure 11–1).	His symptoms (such as high fever with T >102°F [38.9°C]) indicate that patient has the flu.
4. Formulate a comprehensive list of therapeutic alternatives for the primary problem to determine whether triage to a medical provider is required, and share this information with the patient or caregiver.	Options include (1) Recommend a combination product because the patient has multiple symptoms that are all severe. (2) Refer patient to his PCP for evaluation and treatment. (3) Recommend self-care until patient can consult his PCP. (4) Take no action.
Plan	
5. Select an optimal therapeutic alternative to address the patient's problem, taking into account patient preferences.	Recommend self-care until patient can consult his PCP.
6. Describe the recommended therapeutic approach to the patient or caregiver.	Patient should consult his PCP for evaluation and treatment. Patient may continue to use acetaminophen (Tylenol) to manage fever and muscle aches while waiting.
7. Explain to the patient or caregiver the rationale for selecting the recommended therapeutic approach from the considered therapeutic alternatives.	Because patient's symptoms seem to be related to the flu and not a cold, he needs to consult his PCP.
Implement	
8. When recommending self-care with nonprescription medications and/or nondrug therapy, convey accurate information to the patient or caregiver.	Criterion does not apply in this case.
Solicit follow-up questions from the patient or caregiver.	"Can I use Chloraseptic Sore Throat lozenges to help with the sore throat?"
Answer the patient's or caregiver's questions.	"Yes. Chloraseptic Sore Throat lozenges can temporarily relieve sore throat." "Take 2 lozenges every 4 hours, but do not exceed 12 lozenges every 24 hours."
Follow-up: Monitor and Evaluate	
9. Assess patient outcome.	Contact patient in 1 week by telephone to ensure that he made an appointment and sought medical care.

Key: PCP = Primary care provider; T = temperature.

Patient Counseling for Colds

Nondrug measures may be effective in relieving the discomfort of cold symptoms. The provider should explain the appropriate nondrug measures for the patient's particular symptoms. With use of nonprescription medications, the purpose of each medication should be described, and the patient should be counseled to use only medications that target his or her specific symptoms. Also needed is a clear explanation of possible adverse effects, drug interactions, and precautions or warnings. Finally, the provider should explain the signs and symptoms that indicate the disorder is worsening and that medical care should be sought. (See the box "Patient Education for Colds.")

Evaluation of Patient Outcomes for Colds

Most colds are self-limiting, so symptoms usually resolve on their own in 7–14 days. For a majority of patients, targeted nonprescription therapy will relieve their cold symptoms. Patients should be monitored for worsening symptoms and progression to complications by measuring their temperature, assessing nasal secretions, assessing respirations for wheezing or shortness of breath, identifying productive cough, and asking about facial or neck pain. If complications are suspected, medical referral is necessary. Referral to a primary care provider (PCP) is also required for patients

PATIENT EDUCATION FOR

Colds

The objectives of self-treatment are (1) to reduce symptoms, (2) to improve functioning and sense of well-being, and (3) to prevent spread of the disease. For most patients, carefully following product instructions and the self-care measures listed here will help ensure optimal therapeutic outcomes.

Nondrug Measures

- To prevent spreading a cold to others, follow these steps:
  - Frequently wash your hands with soap for at least 20 seconds.
  - Use facial tissues to cover your mouth and nose when coughing or sneezing, and then promptly throw the tissues away.
  - Use antiviral products such as Lysol to clean surfaces (e.g., doorknobs, telephones) that you may have touched.
- The following measures may provide relief or speed up recovery from a cold:
  - Getting adequate rest may help you recover more quickly.
  - Drinking fluids and using a humidifier or vaporizer may loosen mucus and promote sinus drainage.
  - Sucking on hard candy, gargling with salt water (½–1 teaspoon of salt per 8 ounces of warm water), or drinking fruit juices or hot tea with lemon may soothe a sore throat.

Nonprescription Medications

- Ask a health care provider to help you select medications that target the most bothersome symptoms.

Sore Throat and Cough

- Sore throat may be treated with anesthetic products and/or systemic pain relievers:
  - Allow lozenges, troches, and orally disintegrating strips to dissolve slowly in the mouth; do not chew or bite these products.
  - Benzocaine and dyclonine may numb the mouth and tongue. If these effects occur, do not eat or drink until they go away.
  - Seek medical attention if any of the following occur after using benzocaine products: pale, gray- or blue-colored skin, lips, and nail beds; headache; lightheadedness; shortness of breath; fatigue; and rapid heart rate.
- Cough related to a runny nose (postnasal drip) may be treated with a sedating antihistamine and decongestant combination.

Rhinorrhea (Runny Nose) and Sneezing

- See the box "Patient Education for Allergic Rhinitis" for treatment of rhinorrhea (runny nose) and sneezing.

Nasal Congestion

- Nasal congestion may be treated with topical or systemic decongestants, which constrict blood vessels in the nose to reduce congestion.
  - Systemic decongestants include pseudoephedrine and phenylephrine. Dosages are listed in Table 11–3.
  - Topical decongestants include ephedrine, naphazoline, oxymetazoline, phenylephrine, and xylometazoline. Dosages are listed in Table 11–4.
- Decongestants have the following adverse effects:
  - The most common adverse effects caused by systemic decongestants are cardiovascular stimulation (leading to elevated blood pressure, rapid heart rate, palpitations, or arrhythmias) and central nervous system stimulation (causing restlessness, insomnia, anxiety, tremors, fear, or hallucinations).
  - Topical decongestants may cause any of the adverse effects listed for systemic decongestants. However, less of the topical medication gets into the body, so these adverse effects are less common.
  - Topical decongestants may irritate the nose or the bottle tip can injure the nose if used forcefully.
  - Topical decongestants may cause rebound congestion if used longer than 3–7 days.
- Note the following precautions for use of decongestants in persons with other medical conditions:
  - Persons with high blood pressure should use decongestants only with medical advice.
  - Persons with thyroid disorders, heart disease, glaucoma, or an enlarged prostate may experience worsening symptoms of their underlying disease if they take decongestants.
  - Persons with diabetes need to closely monitor their blood glucose concentrations and may need to adjust their dose of insulin if they take decongestants.
- Note the following drug interactions for decongestants:
  - Persons taking MAOI antidepressants, ergot derivatives for headaches, and certain antibiotics (linezolid) should not take decongestants.
  - Persons taking SSRI or SNRI antidepressants should use decongestants with caution as these medications may increase heart rate.
- Store all medications according to the manufacturer's recommendations. Do not use expired medications.

When to Seek Medical Attention

- Seek medical attention for the following situations:
  - Sore throat persists more than several days, is severe, or is associated with persistent fever, headache, or nausea or vomiting.
  - Symptoms worsen while nonprescription medications are being taken.
  - Signs and symptoms of bacterial infections develop (e.g., thick nasal or respiratory secretions that are not clear; temperature higher than 101.5°F [38.6°C] [oral]; shortness of breath; chest congestion; wheezing, rash, or significant ear pain).

Note About Pediatric Dosing

- Manufacturers of cough and cold medications have revised the labeling to state that these products should not be used in children younger than 4 years, and FDA has mandated that dosing devices be included with products for children older than 4 years. The dosing device should be used only with the product in which it is packaged. Health care providers should emphasize this information to caregivers of infants and young children.

Key: FDA = U.S. Food and Drug Administration; MAOI = monoamine oxidase inhibitor; SNRI = serotonin-norepinephrine reuptake inhibitor; SSRI = selective serotonin reuptake inhibitor.

who meet the exclusions for self-treatment in Figure 11–1 or the warnings listed in the box "Patient Education for Colds." Follow-up assessment usually is not necessary for patients with uncomplicated colds, but a subsequent telephone call from the provider's office in 7–14 days may be deemed appropriate.

ALLERGIC RHINITIS

Allergic rhinitis, a systemic disease with prominent nasal symptoms, is a worldwide problem that affects both adults and children. An estimated 8% of adults and 10% of children in the United States are newly diagnosed with allergic rhinitis annually.[36] Annual direct costs (e.g., medications, office visits) are estimated to be $3.4 billion.[37] Addition of indirect costs (e.g., related to work and school absenteeism) increases this estimate to $11 billion.[37] Impaired quality of life creates additional significant, but yet to be quantified, intangible costs.

Symptoms of allergic rhinitis generally begin after the second year of life, and the disease is prevalent in children and in adults 18–64 years of age.[38] After the age of 65 years, the number of cases decreases. The prevalence of allergic rhinitis is higher in the southern United States.[38]

Pathophysiology of Allergic Rhinitis

Allergic rhinitis affects the upper respiratory system. (The previous section "Colds" provides a detailed discussion of the respiratory anatomy and physiology.) Risk factors for developing allergic rhinitis include family history of atopy (allergic disorders) in one or both parents; filaggrin (skin barrier protein) gene mutation; elevated serum IgE greater than 100 IU/mL before the age of 6 years; higher socioeconomic level; eczema; and positive reaction to allergy skin tests.[39,40] Emerging evidence also suggests that diet may be a risk factor in children and adolescents. Children who consume three or more fast-food meals per week showed an increased incidence of allergic disorders.[41] The exact mechanism for that increase is not known but is thought to be related to higher dietary content of fatty acids, especially trans fatty acids, which trigger an immune response.[41]

Allergic rhinitis is triggered by indoor and outdoor environmental allergens. Common outdoor aeroallergens (airborne environmental allergens) include pollen and mold spores. Other nonairborne pollens have also been implicated. Pollutants (e.g., ozone, tobacco smoke, diesel exhaust particles) are considered environmental triggers and are becoming more of a concern in highly populated areas. Common indoor aeroallergens include those from house-dust mites and cockroaches, mold spores, and pet dander. Occupational aeroallergens include wool dust, latex, resins, biologic enzymes, organic dusts (e.g., flour), and various chemicals (e.g., isocyanate, glutaraldehyde).

The pathogenesis of allergic rhinitis is complex, involving numerous cells and mediators, and consists of four phases.[42] First is the sensitization phase, which occurs on initial allergen exposure. The allergen stimulates beta-lymphocyte–mediated IgE production. Second is the early phase, occurring within minutes of subsequent allergen exposure. The early phase consists of rapid release of preformed mast cell mediators (e.g., histamine, proteases), as well as the production of additional mediators (e.g., prostaglandins, kinins, leukotrienes, neuropeptides). Figure 11–2 shows mediator-specific symptoms. The third phase is cellular recruitment. Circulating leukocytes, especially eosinophils, are attracted to the nasal mucosa and release more inflammatory mediators. Fourth and last is the late phase, which begins 2–4 hours after allergen

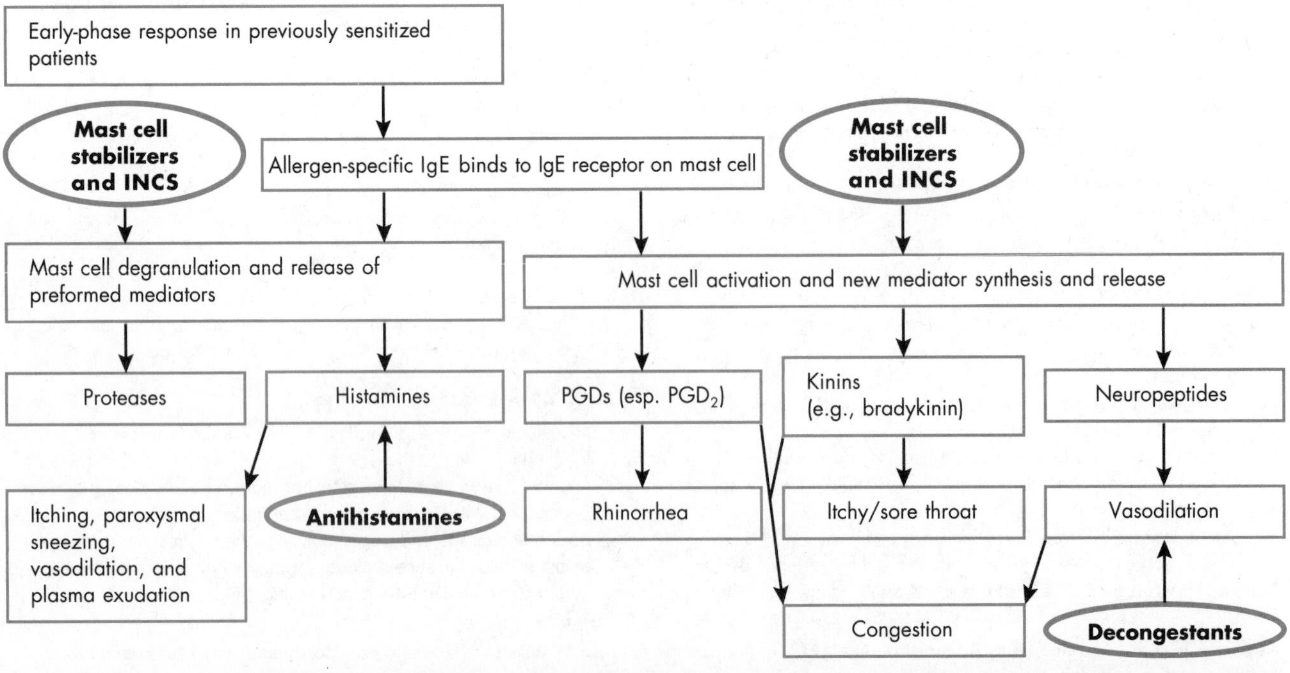

FIGURE 11-2 Mediator-specific symptoms and targeted drug therapy. Key: Ig = Immunoglobulin; INCS = Intranasal corticosteroids; PGD = prostaglandin. (Source: Reference 42.)

exposure; signs and symptoms include mucus hypersecretion secondary to submucosal gland hypertrophy and congestion. Continued persistent inflammation "primes" the tissue, resulting in a lower threshold for allergic- and nonallergic-mediated triggers (e.g., cold air, strong odors).

Clinical Presentation of Allergic Rhinitis

Allergic rhinitis has been classified as seasonal allergic rhinitis ("hay fever") and perennial allergic rhinitis. A newer classification with the categories *intermittent* allergic rhinitis (IAR) and *persistent* allergic rhinitis (PER) was proposed in the late 1990s; this is now the more accepted terminology.[39,40] A third category, *episodic*, has since been added.[39] Classification depends on the timing and duration of symptoms. Symptoms can be further classified as mild or moderate–severe (Table 11–10).[39,40] Symptoms of allergic rhinitis and common physical findings in these patients are summarized in Table 11–11[39,40,42] and can be used to differentiate allergic from nonallergic rhinitis. Table11–12 lists causes of nonallergic rhinitis.[39,40,42] Systemic symptoms include fatigue, irritability, malaise, and cognitive impairment.

TABLE 11-10 Classification of Allergic Rhinitis

Duration	Severity
Intermittent	**Mild**
Symptoms occur ≤4 days per week OR ≤4 weeks.	Symptoms do not impair sleep or daily activities[a]; no troublesome symptoms.
	Moderate–Severe
	One or more of the following occurs: impairment of sleep; impairment of daily activities[a]; troublesome symptoms.
Persistent	**Mild**
Symptoms occur >4 days per week AND >4 weeks.	Symptoms do not impair sleep or daily activities[a]; no troublesome symptoms.
	Moderate–Severe
	One or more of the following occurs: impairment of sleep; impairment of daily activities[a]; troublesome symptoms.
Episodic	
Symptoms occur if an individual is in contact with an exposure that is not normally a part of the individual's environment. (i.e., a cat at a friend's house).	Can be mild, moderate, or severe—based on symptoms

[a] Daily activities include work, school, sports, and leisure.

Source: References 39 and 40.

Acute complications of allergic rhinitis include sinusitis and otitis media with effusion. Complications of a chronic nature include nasal polyps, sleep apnea, sinusitis, and hyposmia (diminished sense of smell).[37,39,40] Allergic rhinitis and asthma share a common pathology, and allergic rhinitis has been implicated in the development of asthma and in exacerbations of preexisting asthma in children and adults. Depression, anxiety, delayed speech development, and facial or dental abnormalities have also been linked to allergic rhinitis.[37,39,40]

Treatment of Allergic Rhinitis

Treatment Goals

Allergic rhinitis cannot be cured. The goals of therapy are to reduce symptoms and to improve the patient's functional status and sense of well-being. Treatment is individualized to provide optimal symptomatic relief and/or control.

General Treatment Approach

Allergic rhinitis is treated in three steps: allergen avoidance, pharmacotherapy, and immunotherapy.[39,40,42] Patient education is an important part of all three steps, especially regarding continuous allergen avoidance and the administration of nonprescription medications (for instructions, see Table 11–2 for intranasal preparations and Chapter 28, "Ophthalmic Disorders," for ocular drugs). The algorithm in Figure 11–3 outlines the self-treatment of episodic allergic rhinitis, IAR, and PER and lists exclusions for self-treatment.[39,40] Because allergen avoidance alone typically is not sufficient to provide complete relief of allergic rhinitis, targeted therapy with single-entity drugs is usually initiated. Nonprescription therapy with intranasal corticosteroids (INCS), antihistamines, or decongestants usually can control most symptoms. Agents with different mechanisms of action or delivery systems may be added if single-drug therapy does not provide adequate relief, or if symptoms are already moderately severe, particularly intense, or long-lasting.

Nonpharmacologic Therapy

Allergen avoidance is the primary nonpharmacologic measure for allergic rhinitis. Avoidance strategies depend on the specific allergen. House-dust mites (*Dermatophagoides* spp.), found in all but the driest regions of the United States, thrive in warm, humid environments. The main allergen is a fecal glycoprotein, but other mite proteins and proteases are also allergenic. Avoidance strategies, targeted at reducing the mite population, include lowering the household humidity to less than 40%, applying acaricides, and reducing mite-harboring dust by removing carpets, upholstered furniture, stuffed animals, and bookshelves from the patient's bedroom and other rooms if possible. Mite populations in bedding are reduced by encasing the mattress, box springs, and pillows with mite-impermeable materials. Bedding that cannot be encased should be washed at least weekly in hot (131°F [55°C]) water. Bedding that cannot be encased or laundered should be discarded.

Outdoor mold spores are prevalent in late summer and fall, especially on calm, clear, dry days. *Alternaria* and *Cladosporium* are common outdoor allergenic molds; *Penicillium* and *Aspergillus* are common indoor molds. Avoiding activities that disturb decaying plant material (e.g., raking leaves) lessens exposure to outdoor mold. Indoor mold exposure is minimized by lowering household

TABLE 11-11 Differentiation of Allergic Rhinitis From Nonallergic Rhinitis

Symptoms/Findings	Allergic Rhinitis	Nonallergic Rhinitis[a]
Symptom presentation	Bilateral symptoms that are worst upon awakening, subside during the day, then may worsen at night	Unilateral symptoms common but can be bilateral; constant day and night
Sneezing	Frequent, paroxysmal	Little or none
Rhinorrhea	Anterior, watery	Posterior, watery or thick and/or mucopurulent (associated with an infection)
Pruritus (itching) of eyes, nose, and/or palate	Frequent	Not present
Nasal obstruction	Variable	Usually present and often severe
Conjunctivitis (red, irritated eyes with prominent conjunctival blood vessels)	Frequent	Not present
Pain	Sinus pain due to congestion may be present; throat pain due to postnasal drip irritation may be present.	Variable depending on cause
Anosmia	Rare	Frequent
Epistaxis	Rare	Recurrent
Facial, nasal, or throat features	"Allergic shiners" (periorbital darkening secondary to venous congestion) "Dennie's lines" (wrinkles beneath the lower eyelids) "Allergic crease" (horizontal crease just above bulbar portion of the nose secondary to the "allergic salute") "Allergic salute" (patient will rub the tip of the nose upward with the palm of the hand) "Allergic gape" (open-mouth breathing secondary to nasal obstruction) Nonexudative cobblestone appearance of posterior oropharynx	Nasal polyps Nasal septal deviation Enlarged tonsils and/or adenoids

[a] Depending on the cause of the nonallergic rhinitis, not all symptoms may be exhibited.
Source: References 39 and 42.

humidity, removing houseplants, venting food preparation areas and bathrooms, repairing damp basements or crawl spaces, and frequently applying fungicide to obviously moldy areas.

Cat-derived allergens (the Fel d1 family of proteins, secreted through sebaceous glands in the skin) are small and light, and they stay airborne for several hours. Cat allergens can be found in the home months after the cat is removed. Although unproven, weekly cat baths may reduce the allergen load.

Cockroaches are a major source of urban allergens; their saliva, feces, and body parts all have been implicated. To eliminate cockroaches, patients should be encouraged to keep kitchen areas clean, to keep stored food tightly sealed, and to treat infested areas with baits or pesticides.

Pollutants (e.g., ozone, diesel fumes) are an additional concern in urban environments. Pollutants such as diesel exhaust particles are especially irritating to the respiratory tract and have been shown to increase the severity of allergic rhinitis.[39,40] Patients whose allergies are triggered by air pollutants should be aware of the air quality index (AQI), (a measure of five major air pollutants per 24 hours) and should plan outdoor activities when the AQI is low.

In general, trees produce pollen in spring, grasses in early summer, and ragweed from mid-August to the first fall frost. Knowledge of pollen counts (the number of pollen grains per cubic meter per 24 hours) helps patients plan outdoor activities. Most patients are symptomatic when pollen counts are very high, and only very sensitive patients have symptoms when pollen counts are low. Pollen counts are highest early in the morning and lowest after rainstorms clear the air. Avoiding outdoor activities when pollen counts are high and closing house and car windows reduce pollen exposure.

Ventilation systems with high-efficiency particulate air (HEPA) filters remove pollen, mold spores, and cat allergens from household air but not fecal particles from house-dust mites, which settle to the floor too quickly to be filtered. Filters need to be changed regularly to maintain effectiveness. The systems are expensive and not effective for all patients. HEPA filters are also found in some vacuum cleaners. Weekly vacuuming of carpets, drapes, and upholstery with a HEPA filter–equipped vacuum cleaner may help reduce household allergens, including those from house-dust mites.[42]

Nasal wetting agents (e.g., saline, propylene, polyethylene glycol sprays, gels) or nasal irrigation with warm saline (isotonic or hypertonic) delivered using a syringe or Neti pot may relieve nasal mucosal irritation and dryness, thus decreasing nasal stuffiness, rhinorrhea, and sneezing. That process also aids in the removal of dried, encrusted, or thick mucus from the nose. No significant adverse effects have been noted with use of nasal wetting agents. Mild stinging or burning has been noted with saline irrigation. Only distilled, sterile, or boiled tap water should be used to prepare nasal irrigation solutions because of the risk of rare but serious infections.

TABLE 11-12 Causes of Nonallergic Rhinitis

Hormonal

Pregnancy, puberty, thyroid disorders

Structural

Septal deviation, adenoid hypertrophy

Drug-Induced

Cocaine, beta blockers, ACEIs, chlorpromazine, clonidine, reserpine, hydralazine, oral contraceptives, aspirin or other NSAIDs, overuse of topical decongestants

Systemic Inflammatory

Eosinophilic nonallergic rhinitis (NARES)

Lesions

Nasal polyps, neoplasms

Traumatic

Recent facial or head trauma

Autonomic (Vasomotor)

Age-related; physical or chemical agent causing parasympathetic hyperactivity

Key: ACEI = Angiotensin-converting enzyme inhibitor; NARES = nonallergic rhinitis with eosinophilia syndrome; NSAID = nonsteroidal anti-inflammatory drug.
Source: Reference 42.

Pharmacologic Therapy

INCS has been shown to be the most effective treatment for most symptoms of allergic rhinitis.[40,42] Until 2013, INCS were available only by prescription, but four nonprescription intranasal preparations are now offered. Other nonprescription options include ocular and oral antihistamines, topical and oral decongestants, and mast cell stabilizers. INCS, antihistamines, and mast cell stabilizers should be used regularly rather than episodically. With these products, patients should start taking the medication at least 1 week before symptoms typically appear or as soon as possible before expected allergen exposures. Length of therapy with those medications should be individualized according to duration and severity of symptoms, pattern of allergen exposure (episodic or continuous), and geographic location.

Intranasal Corticosteroids

INCS, also known as glucocorticoids, are very effective agents for treatment of nasal symptoms such as itching, rhinitis, sneezing, and congestion, because they inhibit multiple cell types and mediators, including histamine, and effectively stop the "allergic cascade."[39,40] Budesonide, fluticasone furoate, fluticasone propionate, and triamcinolone acetonide are FDA approved for nonprescription use for nasal symptoms.[43] Fluticasone furoate and propionate have additional FDA approval for nonprescription use to treat ophthalmic symptoms such as itchy or watery eyes.[43] FDA-approved dosages for INCS are listed in Table 11–13.[43]

INCS usually are well tolerated. Adverse effects typically are minor and include nasal discomfort or bleeding, sneezing, cough, and pharyngitis. INCS have low systemic absorption, however; patients who are sensitive to INCS or use higher-than-recommended doses may experience systemic effects such as headache, dizziness, nausea, and vomiting. Additionally, long-term use has been linked to changes in vision, glaucoma, cataracts, increased risk of infection (e.g., *Candida*), and growth inhibition in children. INCS have few drug interactions, as listed in Table 11–6.

Antihistamines

Since the 1940s, antihistamines have been used to treat allergies.[39] These drugs are classified as sedating (first-generation, nonselective) or nonsedating (second-generation, peripherally selective). The role of sedating antihistamines in treating allergic rhinitis is controversial. Sedating antihistamines are effective, readily available without a prescription, and relatively inexpensive. However, these antihistamines expose patients to risks of anticholinergic effects and should be used with caution.

Antihistamines compete with histamine at central and peripheral histamine-1 (H1) receptor sites, preventing the histamine receptor interaction and subsequent mediator release. In addition, second-generation antihistamines inhibit the release of mast cell mediators and may decrease cellular recruitment.

Differences among antihistamines relate to the rapidity and degree to which they penetrate the blood–brain barrier as well as to their receptor specificity. Sedating antihistamines are highly lipophilic molecules that readily cross the blood–brain barrier. Nonsedating antihistamines, large protein-bound lipophobic molecules with charged side chains, do not readily cross the blood–brain barrier. Both types of antihistamines are highly selective for H1 receptors but have little effect on H2, H3, or H4 receptors. The sedating antihistamines have anticholinergic, antiserotonin, and anti–alpha-adrenergic effects.

Each antihistamine chemical class (Table 11–14) differs slightly in terms of its activity and adverse effect profile.[44,45] Most sedating antihistamines are well absorbed after oral administration, with time to peak plasma concentrations in the range of 1.5–3 hours. Protein binding is in the range of 78%–99%, and sedating antihistamines undergo significant first-pass metabolism through the cytochrome P450 system. Half-lives vary widely—for example, 2–10 hours for diphenhydramine versus 20–24 hours for chlorpheniramine.

The nonsedating antihistamines are also rapidly absorbed after oral administration, with time to peak plasma concentrations in the range of 1–3 hours. Loratadine has the highest protein binding at 97% and is extensively metabolized by the liver to an active metabolite (desloratadine), whereas cetirizine, fexofenadine, and levocetirizine are minimally metabolized. Half-lives range from 8 hours (for cetirizine, levocetirizine, loratadine) to 14 hours (for fexofenadine).

Antihistamines are indicated for relief of symptoms of allergic rhinitis (e.g., itching, sneezing, rhinorrhea) and other types of immediate hypersensitivity reactions. FDA-approved dosages for systemic antihistamines are listed in Table 11–15.[11] Nonprescription antihistamines are marketed as immediate-release and sustained-release tablets and capsules, chewable tablets, oral disintegrating tablets, solutions, and syrups. Alcohol-free, sucrose-free, and dye-free formulations are available. (See Chapter 28 for a discussion of ocular antihistamines.)

Sedating antihistamine overdoses are characterized by excessive H1-, cholinergic-, alpha-adrenergic-, and serotonergic-receptor

Exclusions for Self-Treatment

- Children <12 years[a]
- Pregnant or lactating women[a]
- Symptoms of nonallergic rhinitis (Table 11–11)
- Symptoms of otitis media, sinusitis, bronchitis, or other infection
- Symptoms of undiagnosed or uncontrolled asthma (e.g., wheezing, shortness of breath); COPD; or other lower respiratory disorder
- Severe or unacceptable side effects of treatment

[a] Excluded from self-treatment unless already diagnosed with allergic rhinitis and nonprescription therapy approved by a PCP.

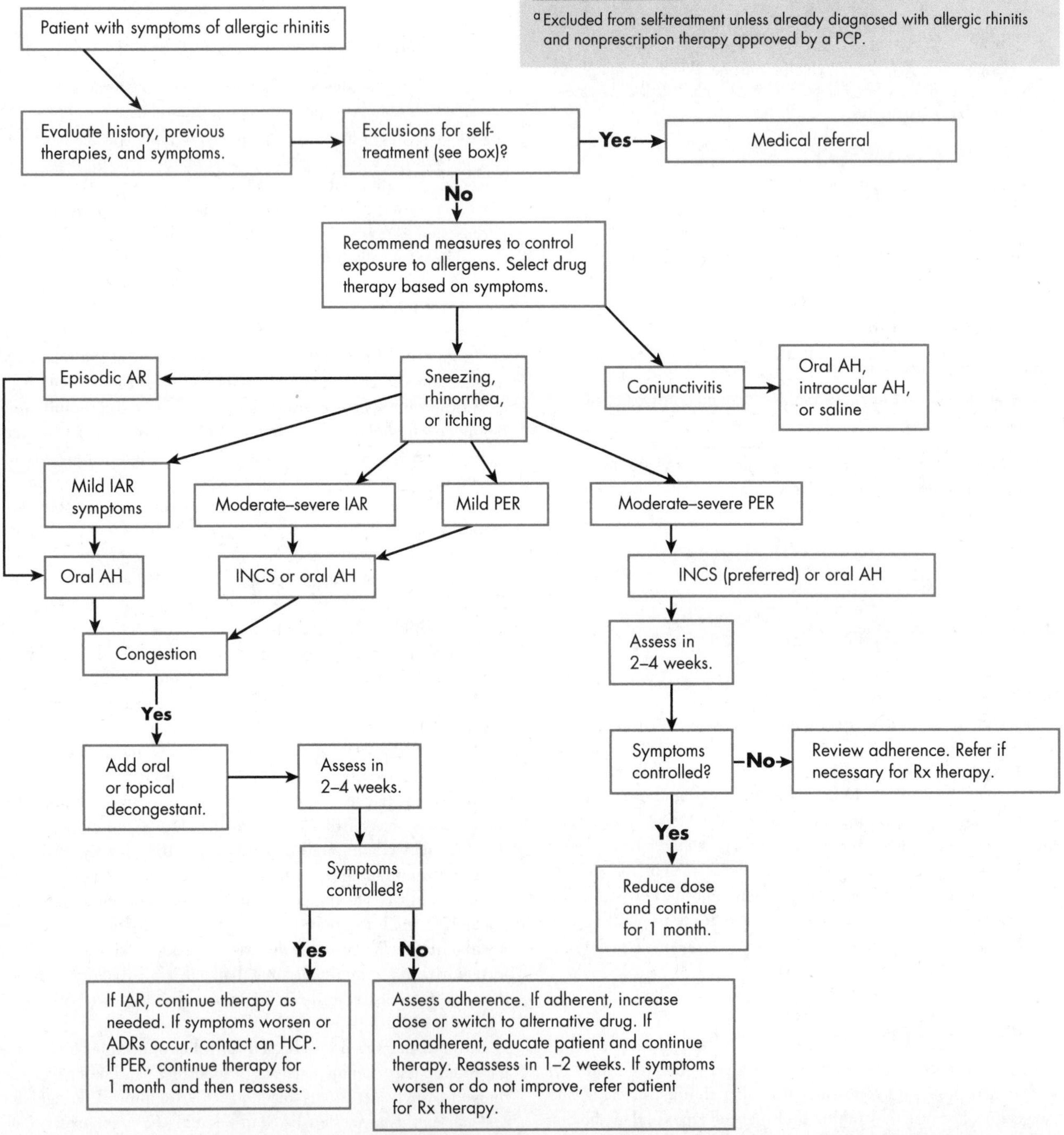

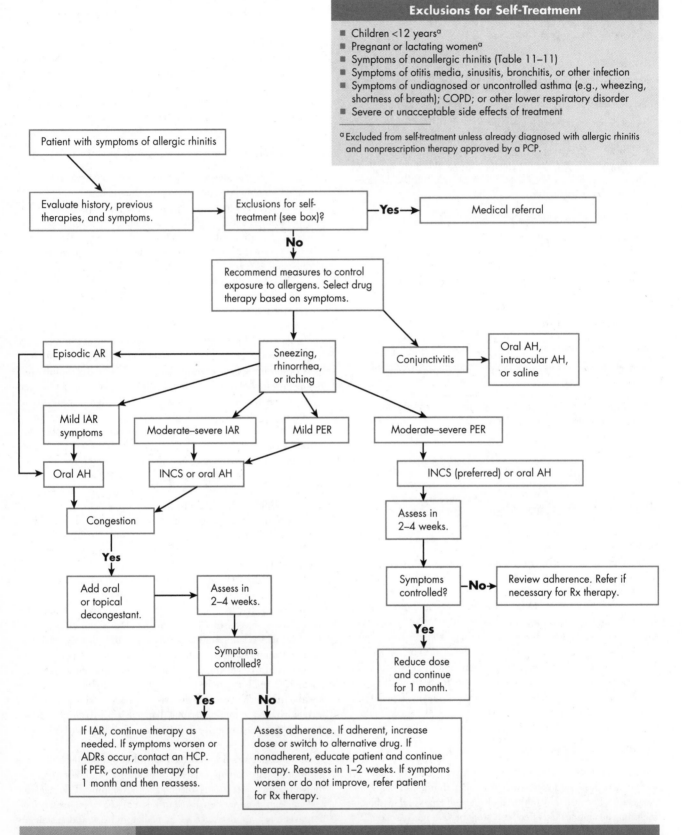

FIGURE 11–3 Self-care for allergic rhinitis. Key: ADR = Adverse drug reaction; AH = antihistamine; AR = allergic rhinitis; COPD = chronic obstructive pulmonary disease; HCP = health care provider; IAR = intermittent allergic rhinitis; INCS = intranasal corticosteroids; PCP = primary care provider; PER = persistent allergic rhinitis; Rx = prescription. (Source: References 42, 43, and 45.)

TABLE 11-13 Nonprescription Intranasal Corticosteroid Products and Dosage Guidelines

Drug	Brand Name	Strength	Dosage[a]
Budesonide	Rhinocort Allergy Spray	32 mcg/spray	*Adults and children ≥12 years:* Use 2 sprays in each nostril once daily; once allergy symptoms improve, reduce to 1 spray in each nostril per day. *Children 6–11 years:* Use 1 spray in each nostril once daily; if allergy symptoms do not improve, may increase to 2 sprays in each nostril per day. Once allergy symptoms improve, reduce to 1 spray in each nostril per day. *Children <6 years*: Do not use.
Fluticasone furoate	Flonase Sensimist	27.5 mcg/spray	*Adults and children ≥12 years:* Week 1: Use 2 sprays in each nostril once daily. Weeks 2–26: Use 1 or 2 sprays in each nostril once daily. After 26 weeks of daily use without improvement, consult an HCP.
	Children's Flonase Sensimist		*Children 2–11 years:* Use 1 spray in each nostril once daily. After 8 weeks of daily use without improvement, consult an HCP. *Child <2 years:* Do not use.
Fluticasone propionate	Flonase Allergy Relief	50 mcg/spray	*Adults and children ≥12 years:* Week 1: Use 2 sprays in each nostril once daily. Weeks 2–26: Use 1 or 2 sprays in each nostril once daily. After 26 weeks of daily use without improvement, consult an HCP.
	Children's Flonase Allergy Relief		*Children 4–11 years:* Use 1 spray in each nostril once daily. After 8 weeks of daily use, consult a health care provider. *Child <4 years:* Do not use.
Triamcinolone acetonide	Nasacort Allergy 24HR	55 mcg/spray	*Adults and children ≥12 years:* Use 2 sprays in each nostril once daily; once allergy symptoms decrease, reduce to 1 spray in each nostril per day.
	Children's Nasacort Allergy 24HR		*Children 6–11 years:* Use 1 spray in each nostril once daily; if allergy symptoms do not subside, may increase to 2 sprays in each nostril per day. Once allergy symptoms decrease, reduce to 1 spray in each nostril per day. *Children 25 years:* Use 1 spray in each nostril once daily. *Children <2 years:* Do not use.

Key: HCP = Health care provider.

[a] Patients should be instructed to shake bottle before use to ensure suspension is mixed and uniform.

Source: Reference 43.

TABLE 11-14 Antihistamine Classes

Class (Specific Drug Entities)	Properties
Alkylamines (brompheniramine, chlorpheniramine, dexbrompheniramine, dexchlorpheniramine, pheniramine, triprolidine)	Moderately sedating; strong anticholinergic effects; higher risk of paradoxical CNS stimulation than with other classes
Ethanolamines (diphenhydramine, doxylamine)	Highly sedating; strong anticholinergic effects; large doses cause seizures and arrhythmias
Ethylenediamines (pyrilamine, thonzylamine)	Weak CNS effects; increased GI effects
Phenothiazines (promethazine)	Highly sedating; strong anticholinergic effects; block alpha-adrenergic receptors; more likely to cause hypotension; akathisia and dystonic reactions may occur
Piperidines (fexofenadine, loratadine)	Nonsedating
Piperazines (cetirizine, chlorcyclizine, hydroxyzine, levocetirizine, meclizine)	Minimally to moderately sedating

Key: CNS = Central nervous system; GI = gastrointestinal.

Source: References 44 and 45.

TABLE 11-15 **Dosage Guidelines for Systemic Nonprescription Antihistamines**

Drug	Dosage[a] (maximum daily dosage)		
	Adults/Children ≥12 Years	Children 6 to <12 Years	Children 2 to <6 Years[b]
Brompheniramine maleate	4 mg every 4–6 hours (24 mg)	2 mg every 4–6 hours (12 mg)	1 mg every 4–6 hours (6 mg)
Cetirizine HCl[c]	10 mg every 24 hours (10 mg)	5–10 mg every 24 hours (10 mg)	2.5 mg every 12 hours or 2.5–5.0 mg every 24 hours (5 mg)
Chlorcyclizine HCl[d]	25 mg every 6–8 hours (75 mg)	Not recommended for children <12 years except under advice of PCP	—
Chlorpheniramine maleate	4 mg every 4–6 hours (24 mg)	2 mg every 4–6 hours (12 mg)	1 mg every 4–6 hours (6 mg)
Dexbrompheniramine maleate	2 mg every 4–6 hours (12 mg)	1 mg every 4–6 hours (6 mg)	0.5 mg every 4–6 hours (3 mg)
Dexchlorpheniramine maleate	2 mg every 4–6 hours (12 mg)	1 mg every 4–6 hours (6 mg)	0.5 mg every 4–6 hours (3 mg)
Diphenhydramine citrate	38–76 mg every 4–6 hours (456 mg)	19–38 mg every 4–6 hours (228 mg)	9.5 mg every 4–6 hours (57 mg)
Diphenhydramine HCl	25–50 mg every 4–6 hours (300 mg)	12.5–25 mg every 4–6 hours (150 mg)	6.25 mg every 4–6 hours (37.5 mg)
Doxylamine succinate	7.5–12.5 mg every 4–6 hours (75 mg)	3.75–6.25 mg every 4–6 hours (37.5 mg)	1.9–3.125 mg every 4–6 hours (18.75 mg)
Fexofenadine[e]	60 mg every 12 hours or 180 mg every 24 hours (180 mg)	30 mg every 12 hours (60 mg)	30 mg every 12 hours (60 mg)
Levocetirizine[e]	5 mg every 24 hours (5 mg)	2.5 mg every 24 hours (2.5 mg)	1.25 mg every 24 hours (1.25 mg)
Loratadine	10 mg every 24 hours (10 mg)	10 mg every 24 hours (10 mg)	5 mg every 24 hours (5 mg)
Phenindamine tartrate[d]	25 mg every 4–6 hours (150 mg)	12.5 mg every 4–6 hours (75 mg)	6.25 mg every 4–6 hours (37.5 mg)
Pheniramine maleate	12.5–25 mg every 4–6 hours (150 mg)	6.25–12.5 mg every 4–6 hours (75 mg)	3.125–6.25 mg every 4–6 hours (37.5 mg)
Pyrilamine maleate	25–50 mg every 6–8 hours (200 mg)	12.5–25 mg every 6–8 hours (100 mg)	6.25–12.5 mg every 6–8 hours (50 mg)
Thonzylamine HCl[d]	50–100 mg every 4–6 hours (600 mg)	25–50 mg every 4–6 hours (300 mg)	12.5–25.0 mg every 4–6 hours (150 mg)
Triprolidine HCl[d]	2.5 mg every 4–6 hours (10 mg)	1.25 mg every 4–6 hours (5 mg)	*Age 4–6 years:* 0.938 mg every 4–6 hours (3.744 mg) *Age 2 to <4 years:* 0.625 mg every 4–6 hours (2.5 mg) *Age 4 months to <2 years:* 0.313 mg every 4–6 hours (1.25 mg)

Key: FDA = U.S. Food and Drug Administration; PCP = primary care provider.

[a] Taken as needed.

[b] With the exception of cetirizine, fexofenadine, levocetirizine and loratadine, these products are not recommended for children younger than 6 years, except with the advice and supervision of a PCP. FDA recommends that the labels on nonprescription products not provide dosing information for children younger than 6 years.

[c] For adults older than 65 years, 10 mg cetirizine is not recommended, except with the advice and supervision of a PCP.

[d] Drug is FDA approved but not currently marketed in the United States.

[e] For adults older than 65 years, fexofenadine and levocetirizine is not recommended, except with the advice and supervision of a PCP.

Source: Reference 11.

blockade.[45] Overdoses also cause excessive blockade of fast sodium channels and potassium channels, thus leading to cardiac symptoms (tachycardia and conduction abnormalities, including torsades de pointes).[45] CNS signs and symptoms include toxic psychosis, hallucinations, agitation, lethargy, tremor, insomnia, and tonic-clonic seizures. Children tend to be more sensitive to CNS excitatory effects, and adults are more likely to experience CNS depression.[45] Peripheral signs and symptoms include hyperpyrexia, mydriasis, vasodilation, decreased exocrine secretion, urinary retention, decreased GI motility, dystonic reactions, and rhabdomyolysis. Overdoses of nonsedating antihistamines are characterized by drowsiness, restlessness/hyperactivity, and tachycardia. Treatment of antihistamine overdoses is supportive.

The adverse effect profile of systemic antihistamines varies widely and depends on the receptor activity, chemical structure, and lipophilicity of the drug. The primary adverse effects, CNS effects (depression and stimulation) and anticholinergic effects, are common with first-generation antihistamines but are rarely seen with second-generation agents. CNS-depressive effects include sedation and impaired performance (e.g., impaired driving performance, poor work performance, incoordination, reduced motor skills, and impaired information processing).[45] CNS-stimulatory effects include anxiety, hallucinations, appetite stimulation, muscle dyskinesias, and activation of epileptogenic foci. Adverse effects associated with cholinergic blockage include dryness of the eyes and mucous membranes (mouth, nose, vagina); blurred vision; urinary hesitancy and retention; constipation; and reflex tachycardia.

Antihistamines interact with numerous drugs (Table 11–6).[44] All antihistamines decrease or prevent immediate dermal reactivity and should be discontinued at least 4 days before scheduled allergy skin testing. Fexofenadine should not be taken with any fruit juices (e.g., grapefruit, apple, or orange). Fruit juice is thought to reduce absorption of fexofenadine by directly inhibiting intestinal organic anion–transporting polypeptides (OATPs), specifically OATP1A2.[46] Separating fexofenadine dose and fruit juice consumption by at least 2 hours will avoid this interaction.[46]

Sedating antihistamines are contraindicated in newborns or premature infants, lactating women, and patients with narrow-angle glaucoma. Additional contraindications include acute asthma exacerbation, stenosing peptic ulcer, symptomatic prostatic hypertrophy, bladder neck and pyloroduodenal obstruction, and concomitant use of MAOIs. Formulations of 12- and 24-hour sustained-release loratadine/pseudoephedrine combination products are contraindicated in patients with esophageal narrowing, abnormal esophageal peristalsis, or a history of difficulty swallowing tablets.

Patients with lower respiratory tract diseases (e.g., emphysema, chronic bronchitis) should use sedating antihistamines with caution. People whose activities require mental alertness should not use sedating antihistamines and should use levocetirizine and cetirizine with caution. Function may be impaired even if the patient does not feel drowsy or took the dose the previous evening. The sedating antihistamines are photosensitizing drugs. Patients should be advised to use sunscreen and to wear protective clothing.

Combination Products

Antihistamines are marketed in combination with decongestants and analgesics. Those combinations are also available in sustained-release formulations, allowing convenient dosage regimens. These combination products should be used with caution, however, because of the increased risk of adverse effects, especially insomnia, which compounds the daytime fatigue already associated with this disease.

Decongestants

Congestion is a common allergic rhinitis symptom controllable with systemic decongestants or with short-term (~5 days) use of topical nasal decongestants. (See earlier discussion of decongestants in the section "Colds.")

Cromolyn Sodium

Cromolyn is a mast cell stabilizer indicated for preventing and treating the symptoms of allergic rhinitis. Cromolyn is thought to work by blocking the influx of calcium into mast cells, thereby preventing mediator release. Less than 7% of an intranasal cromolyn dose is absorbed systemically, and what little is absorbed has no systemic activity. The absorbed drug is rapidly excreted unchanged in the feces and urine, with a half-life of 1–2 hours.

Cromolyn is approved for use in patients 2 years of age or older; the recommended dosage is 1 spray in each nostril 3–6 times daily at regular intervals.[11] Treatment is more effective if started before symptoms begin. It may take 3–7 days for initial clinical improvement to become apparent and 2–4 weeks of continued therapy to achieve maximal therapeutic benefit. Sneezing is the most common adverse effect reported for intranasal cromolyn. Other adverse effects include nasal stinging and burning. No drug interactions have been reported with intranasal cromolyn.

Pharmacotherapeutic Comparison

INCS have been shown to be the most effective agents for treatment of moderate–severe IAR and both types of PER. Monotherapy with INCS is considered first-line.[39,40,42] If additional symptom control is needed, combination therapy with antihistamines, decongestants, or mast cell stabilizers can be initiated. Owing to their quick onset of action, oral antihistamines are first-choice agents for symptom control in episodic allergic rhinitis. Both sedating and nonsedating antihistamines are effective. Some evidence suggests greater efficacy for the sedating type in treating symptoms of allergic rhinitis.[47] However, this evidence is based on trials using the maximum daily dosage (50 mg) of diphenhydramine.[47] Sedating antihistamines have a quick onset of action, but the duration of action is also shorter, and multiple daily doses are required. The risks of cognition impairment and sedation have been well established with this class of drugs.[45] The World Health Organization strongly recommends nonsedating antihistamines on the basis of their efficacy and safety profile, quick onset of action, and longer duration, which allows once-daily dosing.[39,46]

Cetirizine has been shown to be a more potent antihistamine than either loratadine or fexofenadine.[46] However, unlike loratadine and fexofenadine, cetirizine causes sedation (in approximately 10% of patients).

Product Selection Guidelines

Special Populations

Because pregnancy is a common cause of nonallergic rhinitis, pregnant women should be referred for differential diagnosis. If allergic rhinitis is confirmed and nonprescription therapy is approved by a PCP, several treatment choices are available.[23] (Please refer to the Preface for a detailed explanation of the pregnancy data.) Intranasal cromolyn is considered compatible with pregnancy and is a first-line option.[23] Diphenhydramine and chlorpheniramine are considered compatible with pregnancy.[23] Levocetirizine, loratadine and cetirizine are considered to carry a low risk of adverse fetal effects, whereas fexofenadine is associated with moderate risk.[23] Because of minimal systemic absorption, INCS are considered compatible with pregnancy. However, systemic use of budesonide and triamcinolone has been linked to cleft lip and palate and low birth weight.[23] Nonprescription allergy products do not appear to affect male reproduction.

Lactating women diagnosed with allergic rhinitis and approved for self-treatment by a PCP have fewer options. Because of its limited systemic absorption, intranasal cromolyn is a good choice, and adverse effects in nursing infants have not been reported.[23] INCS have low molecular weights and are thought to be excreted in breast milk. Reports of INCS causing harm in nursing infants are lacking, however, and they are considered "probably compatible."[23] Antihistamines are contraindicated during lactation because of their ability to pass into breast milk. Short-acting chlorpheniramine, fexofenadine, or loratadine seems to be the best option if an oral antihistamine is needed, but the antihistamine should be used with caution and under the supervision of a PCP. If an oral antihistamine is used during lactation, the mother should avoid long-acting and high-dose antihistamines and should take the dose at bedtime after the last feeding of the day.[23]

Because of concerns regarding undiagnosed asthma, children younger than 12 years should be referred to a PCP for differential diagnosis.[39,40] If nonprescription therapy is approved by a PCP, several treatment choices are available for children.[39,40,46] Intranasal cromolyn, fluticasone furoate, and triamcinolone acetonide are safe for children 2 years of age and older, intranasal fluticasone propionate is safe for children 4 years and older, and intranasal budesonide is safe for children 6 years and older. However, these products may be difficult for children to self-administer. In addition, all three INCS have been linked to growth inhibition in children; FDA-mandated labeling for the nonprescription products encourages parents to speak to an HCP if they plan to use these products in children for longer than 2 months per year.[43] Loratadine is the nonprescription antihistamine of choice, followed by fexofenadine, levocetirizine, and cetirizine. Sedating antihistamines should be avoided in children because of paradoxical excitation and risk for serious adverse events with misuse.[46]

Sedating antihistamines should be avoided in older patients because they are more likely than younger adults to be taking concomitant medications with anticholinergic properties and are at increased risk of CNS-depressive adverse effects, including confusion as well as hypotension.[48] Those adverse effects contribute to a higher risk of falling in this population.[48] Loratadine and intranasal cromolyn are drugs of choice in older patients. Dosage of fexofenadine and levocetirizine should be adjusted in patients with renal impairment. Loratadine and cetirizine dosage should be adjusted in patients with renal and/or hepatic impairment.

Patient Factors and Preferences

The duration of treatment and the presence of concomitant symptoms will determine which antihistamine product is selected (Table 11–16). Product selection may also be based on adverse effect profiles and cost. For example, all first-generation antihistamines are sedating, but the degree of sedation depends on chemical class (Table 11–14). Nonsedating antihistamines are more expensive but carry less risk of sedation and impairment, which may justify the additional cost. Some patients report that antihistamines are less effective after prolonged use. This decline is most likely not indicative of true tolerance but rather stems from several factors, including patient nonadherence to dosing regimens, an increase in antigen exposure, worsening of disease, limited effectiveness of antihistamines in severe disease, or the development of similar symptoms from unrelated diseases. Chemical class differences make it reasonable to suggest switching to a different class of antihistamine if a patient has a less-than-optimal response to one class of antihistamine. Patient sensory perception of INCS may also influence therapy. Alcohol-free formulations may be preferred by patients who are sensitive to smell, taste, or aftertaste of nasal preparations.

Complementary Therapies

Ephedra (ma huang) and feverfew are commonly suggested herbal remedies for allergic rhinitis. Ephedra-containing products are banned by FDA owing to their serious adverse effects (e.g., stroke). Parthenolide, feverfew's biologically active component, may have anti-inflammatory properties, but its safety and efficacy in allergic rhinitis are unproved. (For further discussion of these types of products, see Chapter 51.) Capsaicin-based nasal sprays (e.g., Sinus Buster) have shown promise in treating nonallergic rhinitis but not allergic rhinitis. Using local honey or homeopathic products containing known allergens (e.g., bioAllers Animal Hair and Dander Allergy Relief Liquid contains cat, cattle, dog, horse, and sheep wool extracts) to induce long-term resistance by repeated exposure to controlled amounts of allergen has not been proved to be safe or effective. Safety and efficacy data are also lacking for symptom-specific homeopathic remedies such as Sabadilla for nasal and ocular symptoms (red, watery eyes) and Wyethia for itching. The role of vitamin D in the treatment of allergic disorders is an emerging area of research.[49] Two small studies showed that patients with low plasma vitamin D levels were more likely to have allergic rhinitis.[49] However, two other studies showed no relationship.[49] More research is needed on the role of vitamin D in the pathophysiology of allergies.

Assessment of Allergic Rhinitis: A Case-Based Approach

Asking the patient for a detailed description of symptoms and obtaining the patient's medical and medication use (previous and current) history are essential to determining whether the patient has allergic rhinitis or rhinitis related to other causes and is eligible for self-care (Tables 11–11 and 11–12).

The medical history may uncover other respiratory illnesses that complicate treatment of allergic rhinitis. The patient's current medication use will also alert the HCP to possible interactions with nonprescription allergy medications. The provider should also ask the patient whether nonprescription products used to treat episodic allergic rhinitis, IAR, or PER were effective and without adverse effects.

TABLE 11-16 Selected Nonprescription Products for Allergic Rhinitis

Trade Name	Primary Ingredients
Systemic First-Generation Antihistamine Products	
Chlor-Trimeton Allergy (4, 8, or 12 Hour) Tablets	Chlorpheniramine 4, 8, or 12 mg, respectively
Benadryl Allergy Tablets	Diphenhydramine HCl 25 mg
Children's Benadryl Allergy Relief Syrup	Diphenhydramine HCl 12.5 mg/5 mL
Systemic Second-Generation Antihistamine Products	
Zyrtec Tablets	Cetirizine 10 mg
Children's Zyrtec Syrup	Cetirizine 5 mg/5 mL
Allegra Allergy 24 hour Tablets	Fexofenadine 180 mg
Children's Allegra Orally Disintegrating Tablets[a]	Fexofenadine 30 mg
Xyzal Allergy 24HR Tablets	Levocetirizine 5 mg
Children's Xyzal Allergy 24HR Oral Solution	Levocetirizine 2.5 mg/5 mL
Claritin Non-Drowsy Tablets	Loratadine 10 mg
Alavert Orally Disintegrating Tablets	Loratadine 10 mg
Combination Systemic Products	
Dimetapp Cold and Allergy Syrup	Brompheniramine 1 mg/5 mL; phenylephrine 2.5 mg/5 mL
Zyrtec D Tablets	Cetirizine 5 mg; pseudoephedrine HCl 120 mg
Actifed Cold and Allergy Tablets	Chlorpheniramine 4 mg; phenylephrine 10 mg
Advil Allergy Sinus Caplets	Chlorpheniramine 2 mg; pseudoephedrine HCl 30 mg; ibuprofen 200 mg
Allegra D 12-Hour Tablets	Fexofenadine 60 mg; pseudoephedrine HCl 120 mg
Claritin-D 24 Hour Tablets	Loratadine 10 mg; pseudoephedrine sulfate 240 mg
Nasal Products	
Ayr Saline Nasal Gel	Sodium chloride; aloe; propylene glycol; glycerin
NasalCrom Spray	Cromolyn sodium 5.2 mg/spray
Ocean Spray	Sodium chloride 0.65%

[a] Contains phenylalanine.

Case 11–2 presents an example of the assessment of a patient with allergic rhinitis.

Patient Counseling for Allergic Rhinitis

The provider should emphasize that the best method of treating allergic rhinitis is to avoid allergens. Many patients, however, have no control over their work environment or are unable to implement all of the preventive measures at home. These patients usually rely on allergy medications for symptom control. Patient counseling should include information about proper use of recommended medication(s) and about possible adverse effects, drug–drug and drug–disease interactions, and other precautions and warnings. The provider should also be aware of duplication of therapy with prescription INCS. Patient counseling should also emphasize signs and symptoms indicating that the disorder has progressed to the point at which medical care is needed. The box "Patient Education for Allergic Rhinitis" presents specific information to provide patients.

Evaluation of Patient Outcomes for Allergic Rhinitis

Many patients achieve symptomatic relief with initial nonprescription drug therapy in 3–4 days, but complete relief of symptoms may take 2–4 weeks. After this time frame, a follow-up telephone call from the provider or a scheduled office appointment is recommended to determine whether symptom control has been achieved or if the patient is encountering any adverse effects or problems. A validated instrument such as the Rhinitis Control Assessment Test may be used to monitor response to therapy.[50] Patients who respond poorly to treatment should be assessed to determine whether they are practicing recommended allergen avoidance strategies and are adhering to medication regimens. Options for patients who do not achieve relief include increasing current medications to maximally effective dosages and changing to a different medication or dosage formulation. Patients who do not respond to nonprescription therapy should be referred back to their PCPs for prescription medications such as intranasal antihistamines, systemic corticosteroids, leukotriene inhibitors, anticholinergics, or immunotherapy. In addition,

CASE 11-2

Relevant Evaluation Criteria	Scenario/Model Outcome
Collect	
1. Gather essential information about the patient's symptoms, including	
a. Description of symptom(s) (i.e., nature, onset, duration, severity, associated symptoms)	Patient has had a runny nose along with itchy eyes and sneezing for approximately 1 week.
b. Description of any factors that seem to precipitate, exacerbate, and/or relieve the patient's symptom(s)	Symptoms are usually worse in the morning, lessen in severity during the day, and then get worse again at night.
c. Description of the patient's efforts to relieve the symptoms	Patient has not taken anything before this visit.
d. Patient's identity	Grady Allen Barr
e. Patient's age, gender, height, and weight	26 years, male, 6 ft 3 in., 210 lb
f. Patient's occupation	College student
g. Patient's dietary habits	Well-balanced diet
h. Patient's sleep habits	Patient usually sleeps around 7–8 hours, but his recent symptoms have been causing him to lose sleep.
i. Concurrent medical conditions, prescription and nonprescription medications, and dietary supplements	Multivitamin 1 tablet every morning
j. Allergies	No known allergies
k. History of other adverse reactions to medications	None
Assess	
2. Differentiate patient's signs/symptoms, and correctly identify the patient's primary problem(s).	Allergic rhinitis commonly manifests as sneezing, itchy nose or eyes, and a runny nose. Symptoms are usually worse in the morning and at night, with some relief during the day. Nonallergic rhinitis symptoms typically are present the entire day and do not include sneezing or itchy eyes and nose.
3. Identify exclusions for self-treatment (Figure 11–3).	None
4. Formulate a comprehensive list of therapeutic alternatives for the primary problem to determine whether triage to a medical provider is required, and share this information with the patient or caregiver.	Options include (1) Recommend an appropriate nonprescription product for symptoms: an oral antihistamine or an intranasal corticosteroid for runny nose, itchy eyes, and sneezing. (2) Refer patient to his PCP for evaluation and treatment. (3) Recommend self-care until patient can consult his PCP. (4) Take no action.
Plan	
5. Select an optimal therapeutic alternative to address the patient's problem, taking into account patient preferences.	Recommend that the patient try a nonsedating oral antihistamine to relieve his allergic rhinitis. Recommend that the patient take loratadine 10 mg by mouth every morning.
6. Describe the recommended therapeutic approach to the patient or caregiver.	At this time, there are no exclusions for self-care. Because allergic rhinitis accounts for all of the present symptoms, monotherapy with an oral antihistamine is appropriate.
7. Explain to the patient or caregiver the rationale for selecting the recommended therapeutic approach from the considered therapeutic alternatives.	This case of allergic rhinitis seems to be mild and intermittent based on the timing and severity of the symptoms. An oral antihistamine is a reasonable option for treatment, because it should relieve these issues within a few days.

CASE 11-2 *continued*

Relevant Evaluation Criteria	Scenario/Model Outcome
Implement	
8. When recommending self-care with nonprescription medications and/or nondrug therapy, convey accurate information to the patient or caregiver.	"Take 1 tablet of loratadine every morning. Allergy symptoms should begin to decrease after approximately 3–4 days of treatment, but full effects may not be seen for 2–4 weeks. Overall, this drug is well tolerated. Adverse effects are minimal but may include drowsiness, headache, somnolence, and anticholinergic effects. Contact your PCP if your symptoms worsen or if you experience any adverse drug reactions."
Solicit follow-up questions from the patient or caregiver.	"Is there anything I can do to keep this from happening again?"
Answer the patient's or caregiver's questions.	"The best nonpharmacologic measure you can take is allergen avoidance. If you know what causes your allergies, you can eliminate that problem or do your best to limit exposure to that allergen. You can also start taking loratadine before symptoms start."
Follow-up: Monitor and Evaluate	
9. Assess patient outcome.	Contact patient in 2–4 weeks to see if symptoms have been relieved.

Key: PCP = Primary care provider.

PATIENT EDUCATION FOR Allergic Rhinitis

The primary objective of self-treatment is to prevent or reduce symptoms, which in turn will improve functioning and enhance a sense of well-being. For some patients, prescription therapy such as a short course of oral corticosteroids may help control symptoms, whereas other therapy is initiated when symptoms are especially severe. For most patients, carefully following instructions for nonprescription allergy medications and the self-care measures listed here will help ensure optimal therapeutic outcomes.

Nondrug Measures

- Avoidance of allergens is important regardless of whether allergy medications are being taken.
- For symptoms that develop mainly when outdoors:
  - Frequently check local pollen counts and air quality index.
  - Keep house and car windows shut; avoid yard work and outdoor sports on days with high levels of pollen (spring/summer), mold (late summer/fall), or pollution.
- For symptoms that occur mainly when indoors:
  - Try to remove the symptom trigger(s) (e.g., cats, house-dust mites, tobacco smoke, and molds) from rooms.
  - Lower the humidity in the home to reduce molds. Use lower settings on humidifiers, repair damp basements and crawl spaces, vent kitchens and bathrooms, and remove houseplants.
  - Wash bedding in hot water (131°F [55°C]) every week, and encase mattresses and pillows in coverings resistant to house-dust mites.
- Nasal saline solutions may relieve nasal irritation and dryness, and aid in the removal of dried, encrusted, or thick mucus from the nose.

Nonprescription Medications

- Ask a health care provider for help in selecting an allergy medication that treats the most bothersome symptoms. If needed, additional medications can be added for other symptoms:
  - Intranasal steroids are effective for itchy eyes and noses, sneezing, runny nose, and congestion.
  - Antihistamines are effective for itching, sneezing, and runny nose but have little effect on nasal congestion.
  - Decongestants are effective for nasal congestion but have little effect on other symptoms.
  - Combination therapy with intranasal steroids, antihistamines, and decongestants is common.
  - Intranasal and ocular preparations are available to reduce nasal and eye symptoms, respectively.
  - Intranasal cromolyn is the preferred initial drug of choice during pregnancy and lactation. This medication is not absorbed into the body.
  - For intranasal products, follow the dosing and administration directions carefully. (See Table 11–2.)
  - The most common adverse effects of nasal preparations include nasal stinging and burning.
- Allergy medications are more effective if they are used regularly rather than episodically:
  - If you have episodic or intermittent allergies, start allergy medications as soon as possible, before exposure to allergen.
  - If you have persistent allergies, take allergy medications on a regular basis.

Nasal Congestion

- See the box "Patient Education for Colds" for information about relieving nasal congestion.

Rhinorrhea (Runny Nose) and Sneezing

- Many factors cause a runny nose, and depending on the factors, nonprescription steroids or antihistamines may only partially treat this symptom. Because some nonprescription antihistamines may make you very drowsy, the potential benefits of the medication must be weighed against the potential risks.
- Sneezing is a common and sometimes bothersome symptom. Sneezing may be reduced with nonprescription intranasal steroids or antihistamines. The potential benefits of using antihistamines must be weighed against the potential risks.

PATIENT EDUCATION FOR Allergic Rhinitis *(continued)*

- Intranasal steroids and oral antihistamines are the preferred initial treatment for runny nose and sneezing in persons who are eligible for self-care (see exclusions in Figure 11–3).
- Note the following precautions for use of nonprescription intranasal corticosteroids:
  - Intranasal corticosteroids may irritate the nose or the bottle tip can injure the nose if used forcefully.
  - Follow the package labeling carefully and use the lowest dose for the shortest amount of time, especially in children.
  - If you have HIV/AIDS and are being treated with protease inhibitors, check with your health care provider before using intranasal corticosteroids.

Antihistamines

- There are two types of antihistamines, sedating and nonsedating. Cetirizine, fexofenadine, levocetirizine, and loratadine are nonsedating antihistamines and usually do not cause significant drowsiness.
- Note the following adverse effects for antihistamines:
  - The sedating antihistamines cause drowsiness and impair mental alertness. Mental alertness is impaired even if you do not feel drowsy or if you took the dose the previous evening. While taking these medications, do not drive a vehicle, operate machinery, or engage in other activities that require alertness.
  - Sedating antihistamines may cause sensitivity to sunlight. Use sunscreens and wear protective clothing when outdoors.
  - Use of sedating antihistamines may cause dryness in your mouth, nose, and other areas of your body.
  - Children and older persons may experience unexpected and paradoxical excitement with sedating antihistamines.
  - Older patients should avoid sedating antihistamines and may need lower doses of nonsedating antihistamines because they are more sensitive to the effects of these medications and more often take other medications that interact with these drugs.
- Do not use antihistamines:
  - If you are allergic to antihistamines or similar medications.
  - If you are breastfeeding.
- Do not give antihistamines to newborns or premature infants unless directed to do so by a primary care provider.
- Note the following precautions for use of nonprescription antihistamines:
  - Persons with glaucoma, stenosing peptic ulcer, symptomatic enlarged prostate, bladder neck obstruction, or stomach or intestinal blockage should not use sedating (first-generation) antihistamines.
  - Persons with lower respiratory tract disease (e.g., emphysema or chronic bronchitis) should use sedating antihistamines with caution.
  - Persons with esophageal narrowing, abnormal esophageal peristalsis, or problems swallowing tablets should not take the 12- or 24-hour sustained-release dosage forms of loratadine combined with pseudoephedrine. There have been reports of esophageal obstruction and perforation with use of these sustained-release dosage forms.
- All antihistamines interact with the following drugs:
  - Alcohol, sedatives, opioid analgesics, and other central nervous system depressants may cause additive depressive effects when taken with antihistamines.
  - Anticholinergic drugs (e.g., ipratropium)
  - Potassium chloride may cause increase in ulcers when taken with antihistamines.
- Specific sedating antihistamines interact with the following drugs:
  - Chlorpheniramine may increase the adverse effects of phenytoin.
  - Diphenhydramine may increase the adverse effects of metoprolol and brexpiprazole.
- Nonsedating antihistamines interact with the following drugs:
  - Fexofenadine interacts with ketoconazole, erythromycin, and antacids. Also avoid taking with fruit juice.
  - Loratadine interacts with amiodarone.
- Store all medications according to the manufacturer's instructions.

When to Seek Medical Attention

- Seek medical attention in the following situations:
  - Your allergy symptoms worsen while you are taking nonprescription medications or do not decrease after 2–4 weeks of treatment.
  - You develop signs or symptoms of secondary bacterial infections (e.g., thick nasal or respiratory secretions that are not clear, oral temperature higher than 101.5°F [38.6°C], shortness of breath, chest congestion, wheezing, significant ear pain, rash).

clinical reassessment is appropriate, and the diagnosis of allergic rhinitis may need to be reconsidered. Patients who demonstrate any of the warning signs or symptoms listed in the box "Patient Education for Allergic Rhinitis" should be referred to a PCP.

Key Points for Disorders Related to Colds and Allergic Rhinitis

- Colds are self-limiting viral infections characterized by initial sore throat followed by nasal symptoms and nonproductive cough.
- Medical referral is appropriate for patients with suspected colds who are immunocompromised, have underlying cardiopulmonary diseases, or have alarm symptoms (high fever, chest pain, shortness of breath, or wheezing).
- Treatment for colds is symptomatic and targeted at the most bothersome symptoms.
- Decongestants are the most common nonprescription agents for treatment for congestion related to colds and allergic rhinitis, but they should be used cautiously in patients with hypertension, diabetes, and other chronic diseases.
- Therapy for allergic rhinitis is sequential and consists of allergen avoidance, pharmacotherapy, and allergen immunotherapy.
- Medical referral is appropriate for patients with symptoms suggestive of nonallergic rhinitis, otitis media, sinusitis, or lower respiratory tract problems such as pneumonia, asthma,

or bronchitis, and for those patients who fail to respond to nonprescription medications.

➤ Antihistamines are commonly used to control allergic rhinitis symptoms. Nonsedating (second-generation) antihistamines are preferred over sedating (first-generation) antihistamines on the basis of safety and efficacy data.

REFERENCES

1. Centers for Disease Control and Prevention. Common colds: protect yourself and others. February 2016. Available at: http://www.cdc.gov/features/rhinoviruses/. Accessed April 5, 2017.
2. Consumer Healthcare Products Association. OTC sales by category 2011–2014. Available at: http://www.chpa.org/OTCsCategory.aspx. Accessed April 5, 2017.
3. Patrick A. Rhinovirus chemotherapy. *Antiviral Res.* 2006;71(2–3):391–6. doi: 10.1016/j.antiviral.2006.03.011.
4. Cohen S, Janicki-Deverts D, Doyle WJ. Self-rated health in healthy adults and susceptibility to the common cold. *Psychosom Med.* 2015;77(9): 959–68. doi: 10.1097/PSY.0000000000000232.
5. Prather AA, Janicki-Deverts D, Hall MH, et al. Behaviorally assessed sleep and susceptibility to the common cold. *Sleep.* 2015;38(9):1353–9. doi: 10.5665/sleep.4968.
6. Eccles R, Wilkinson JE. Exposure to cold and acute upper respiratory tract infection. *Rhinology.* 2015;53(2):99–106. doi: 10.4193/Rhin14.239.
7. Rajnik M. Rhinovirus infection clinical presentation. 2014. Available at: http://emedicine.medscape.com/article/227820-clinical. Accessed April 5, 2017.
8. Rennard BO, Ertl RF, Gossman GL, et al. Chicken soup inhibits neutrophil chemotaxis in vitro. *Chest.* 2000;118(4):1150–7. PMID: 11035691.
9. Paul IM, Beiler J, King TS, et al. Vapor rub, petrolatum, and no treatment for children with nocturnal cough and cold symptoms. *Pediatrics.* 2010;126(6):1092–9. doi: 10.1542/peds.2010-1601.
10. World Health Organization. Guidelines on hand hygiene in health care. 2009. Available at: http://whqlibdoc.who.int/publications/2009/9789241597906_eng.pdf. Accessed April 5, 2017.
11. U.S. Food and Drug Administration. Cold, cough, allergy, bronchodilator, and antiasthmatic drug products for over-the counter human use. *CFR: Code of Federal Regulations.* Title 21, Part 341. Updated March 7, 2016. Available at: http://www.ecfr.gov/cgi-bin/text-idx?SID=694f58669bc9c39632fe5305dd2358e6&mc=true&node=pt21.5.341&rgn=div5#se21.5.341_172. Accessed April 5, 2017.
12. U.S. Food and Drug Administration. Public Health Advisory: FDA recommends that over-the-counter (OTC) cough and cold products not be used for infants and children under 2 years of age. Updated August 20, 2013. Available at: http://www.fda.gov/ForConsumers/ConsumerUpdates/ucm051137.htm. Accessed April 5, 2017.
13. Consumer Healthcare Products Association. CHPA announces voluntary labeling updates for oral OTC children's cough and cold medications. *CHPA Executive Newsletter.* 2008; Issue No. 21-8. Available at: http://www.chpa.org/workarea/downloadasset.aspx?id=911. Accessed April 5, 2017.
14. Mortuaire G, de Gabory L, Francois M, et al. Rebound congestion and rhinitis medicamentosa: nasal decongestants in clinic practice. Critical review of the literature by a medical panel. *Eur Ann Otorhinolaryngol Head Neck Dis.* 2013;130(3):137–44. doi: 10.1016/j.anorl.2012.09.005.
15. U.S. Department of Justice Drug Enforcement Administration. Combat Methamphetamine Epidemic Act 2005. Title VII of USA Patriot Improvement Reauthorization Act of 2005. Pub L No. 109-177. 109th Congress. March 9, 2006. Available at: http://www.deadiversion.usdoj.gov/meth/index.html. Accessed April 5, 2017.
16. De Sutter AI, Saraswat A, van Driel ML. Antihistamines for the common cold. *Cochrane Database Syst Rev.* 2015;11:CD009345. doi: 10.1002/14651858.CD009345.pub2.
17. De Sutter AI, van Driel ML, Kumar AA, et al. Oral antihistamine-decongestant-analgesic combinations for the common cold. *Cochrane Database Syst Rev.* 2012;2:CD004976. doi: 10.1002/14651858.CD004976.pub3.
18. Knowlton WM, McKemy DD. TRPM8: from cold to cancer, peppermint to pain. *Curr Pharm Biotechnol.* 2011;12(1):68–77. PMID: 20932257.
19. Eccles R. Efficacy and safety of over-the-counter analgesics in the treatment of common cold and flu. *J Clin Pharm Ther.* 2006;31(4):309–19. doi: 10.1111/j.1365-2710.2006.00754.x.
20. Bosler DC. Cough suppressant and pharmacologic protussive therapy: ACCP evidence-based clinical practice guidelines. *Chest.* 2006;129(1 Suppl 1): 238–49S. doi: 10.1378/chest.129.1_suppl.238S.
21. Horak F, Zieglmayer P, Zieglmayer R, et al. A placebo-controlled study of the nasal decongestant effect of phenylephrine and pseudoephedrine in the Vienna challenge chamber. *Ann Allergy Asthma Immunol.* 2009;102(2): 116–20. doi: 10.1016/S1081-1206(10)60240-2.
22. Tanzi MG. Lack of efficacy prompts citizen petition to remove phenylephrine from OTC market. *Pharm Today.* 2016;22(1):26.
23. Briggs GG, Freeman RK. *Drugs in Pregnancy and Lactation: A Reference Guide to Fetal and Neonatal Risk.* 10th ed. Philadelphia, PA: Wolters Kluwer Health; 2015:132–3, 162–4, 188, 238–9, 252, 385–7, 414–6, 543–4, 576–7, 643, 818–9, 1041–2, 1110, 1168–70, 1398–1400.
24. U.S. Food and Drug Administration. Guidance for Industry: dosage delivery devices for orally ingested OTC liquid drug products. May 2011. Available at: http://www.fda.gov/downloads/Drugs/GuidanceComplianceRegulatoryInformation/Guidances/UCM188992.pdf. Accessed March 25 2016.
25. Roxas M, Jurenka J. Colds and influenza: a review of diagnosis and conventional, botanical and nutritional considerations. *Altern Med Rev.* 2007;12(1):25–48. PMID: 17397266.
26. National Center for Complementary and Alternative Medicine. Herbs at a glance. Available at: http://nccam.nih.gov/health/herbsataglance.htm. Accessed April 5, 2017.
27. Guo R, Pittler MH, Ernst E. Herbal medicines for the treatment of allergic rhinitis: a systematic review. *Ann Allergy Asthma Immunol.* 2007;99(6): 483–95. doi: 10.1016/S1081-1206(10)60375-4.
28. Timmer A, Gunther J, Rucker G, et al. Pelargonium sidoides extract for acute respiratory tract infections. *Cochrane Database Syst Rev.* 2008;3: CD006323. doi: 10.1002/14651858.CD006323.pub3.
29. U.S. Food and Drug Administration. Public Health Advisory: loss of sense of smell with intranasal cold remedies containing zinc. June 16, 2009. Available at: http://www.fda.gov/drugs/drugsafety/postmarketdrugsafetyinformationforpatientsandproviders/ucm166834.htm. Accessed April 5, 2017.
30. Singh M, Das RR. Zinc for the common cold. *Cochrane Database Syst Rev.* 2011;3:CD001364. doi: 10.1002/14651858.CD001364.pub3.
31. Hemila H, Chalker E. Vitamin C for preventing and treating the common cold. *Cochrane Database Syst Rev.* 2013;1:CD000980. doi: 10.1002/14651858.CD000980.pub4.
32. Ferraro PM, Curhan GC, Gambaro G, et al. Total, dietary, and supplemental vitamin C intake and risk of incident kidney stones. *Am J Kidney Dis.* 2016;67(3):400–7. doi: 10.1053/j.ajkd.2015.09.005.
33. Bergman P, Lindh AU, Björkhem-Bergman L, et al. Vitamin D and respiratory tract infections: a systematic review and meta-analysis of randomized controlled trials. *PLoS One.* 2013;8(6):e65835. doi: 10.1371/journal.pone.0065835.
34. Imhoff-Kunsch B, Stein AD, Martorell R, et al. Prenatal docosahexaenoic acid supplementation and infant morbidity: randomized controlled trial. *Pediatrics.* 2011;128(3):e505–12. doi: 10.1542/peds.2010-1386.
35. Hao Q, Dong BR, Wu T. Probiotics for preventing acute upper respiratory tract infections. *Cochrane Database Syst Rev.* 2015;2:CD006895. doi: 10.1002/14651858.CD006895.pub3.
36. National Center for Health Statistics. Fastats—allergies and hay fever. February 2016. Available at: http://www.cdc.gov/nchs/fastats/allergies.htm. Accessed April 5, 2017.
37. Meltzer EO, Bukstein DA. The economic impact of allergic rhinitis and current guidelines for treatment. *Ann Allergy Asthma Immunol.* 2011; 106(2 Suppl):S12–6. doi: 10.1016/j.anai.2010.10.014.
38. Blackwell DL, Lucas JW. Tables of summary health statistics for U.S. adults: 2014 National Health interview survey. Table A-2a. Available

at: http://www.cdc.gov/nchs/nhis/SHS/tables.htm. Accessed April 5, 2017.

39. Seidman MD, Gurgel RK, Lin SY, et al. Clinical practice guideline: allergic rhinitis. *Otolaryngol Head Neck Surg.* 2015;152(1 Suppl):S1–43. doi: 10.1177/0194599814561600.
40. Bousquet J, Schunemann HJ, Samolinski B, et al. Allergic rhinitis and its impact on asthma (ARIA): achievements in 10 years and future needs. *J Allergy Clin Immunol.* 2012;130:1049–62. doi: 10.1016/j.jaci.2012.07.053.
41. Ellwood P, Asher MI, Garcia-Marcos L, et al. Do fast foods cause asthma, rhinoconjunctivitis and eczema? Global findings from the International Study of Asthma and Allergies in Childhood (ISAAC) phase three. *Thorax.* 2013;68(4):351–60. doi: 10.1136/thoraxjnl-2012-202285.
42. Tran NP, Vickery J, Blaiss MS. Management of rhinitis: allergic and non-allergic. *Allergy Asthma Immunol Res.* 2011;3(3):148–56. doi: 10.4168/aair.2011.3.3.148.
43. U.S. Food and Drug Administration. Drugs@FDA [database]. Available at: http://www.accessdata.fda.gov/scripts/cder/drugsatfda. Accessed April 5, 2017.
44. Lexi-Drugs Online. Hudson, OH: Lexi-Comp. Available at: http://www.crlonline.com. Accessed June 20, 2016.
45. Gharahbaghian L. Cough, cold, and allergy preparation toxicity clinical presentation. December 29, 2015. Available at: http://emedicine.medscape.com/article/1010513-clinical. Accessed April 5, 2017.
46. Golightly LK, Greos LS. Second-generation antihistamines: actions and efficacy in the management of allergic disorders. *Drugs.* 2005;65(3): 341–84. PMID: 15669879.
47. Raphael GD, Angello JT, Wu MM, et al. Efficacy of diphenhydramine vs desloratadine and placebo in patients with moderate-to-severe seasonal allergic rhinitis. *Ann Allergy Asthma Immunol.* 2006;96(4):606–14. doi: 10.1016/S1081-1206(10)63557-0.
48. American Geriatrics Society 2015 Beers Criteria Update Expert Panel. American Geriatrics Society 2015 updated Beers criteria for potentially inappropriate medication use in older adults. *J Am Geriatr Soc.* 2015;63(11):2227–46. doi: 10.1111/jgs.13702.
49. Krinsky DL. Patient self-care and allergic rhinitis: new and emerging issues. *Pharm Today.* 2016;22(2):14.
50. Schatz M, Meltzer EO, Nathan R, et al. Psychometric validation of the Rhinitis Control Assessment Test: a brief patient-completed instrument for evaluating rhinitis symptom control. *Ann Allergy Asthma Immunol.* 2010;104:118–24. doi: 10.1016/j.anai.2009.11.063.

CHAPTER 12

COUGH

KAREN J. TIETZE

Cough is an important defensive respiratory reflex with potentially significant adverse physical and psychological consequences and economic impact. Cough is the most common symptom for which patients seek medical care.[1] Cough is also a common reason for emergency department visits. In 2011, cough was the second most common reason for children younger than 15 years to visit emergency departments and the fifth most common reason for adults.[2] Americans spend more than $8.1 billion annually on nonprescription cough and cold and related medications, more than on any other nonprescription sales category.[3]

Pathophysiology of Cough

Cough is initiated by stimulation of chemically and mechanically sensitive, vagally mediated sensory pathways in pharyngeal, laryngeal, esophageal, and tracheobronchial airway epithelium.[4] The number of afferent nerves activated and the intensity of activation may influence the cough threshold.[5] Receptors in the larynx, trachea, and proximal large airways are more sensitive to mechanical stimulation, whereas distal airways receptors are more sensitive to chemical stimulation.[6] A complex medullary brainstem network ("cough control center") processes the sensory input and stimulates the motor efferents. Voluntary cough is controlled by the cerebral cortex.[7] Viruses promote cough by a different, though not well understood, mechanism.[8]

A cough starts with a deep inspiration, followed by closure of the glottis and forceful contraction of the chest wall, abdominal wall, and diaphragmatic muscles against the closed glottis; pressure within the thoracic cavity may reach 300 mm Hg.[4] When the glottis opens, air is expelled with a velocity of approximately 11–15 m/second, propelling mucus, cellular debris, and foreign material out of the respiratory system.[9] Cough may occur in epochs ("coughing fits").

Cough, classified as *acute* (duration of less than 3 weeks), *subacute* (duration of 3–8 weeks), or *chronic* (duration of more than 8 weeks), is a symptom of diverse infectious and noninfectious disorders (Table 12–1).[10,11] In children, cough may also be a symptom of aspiration caused by poor coordination of sucking and swallowing or esophageal motility disorders. Angiotensin-converting enzyme inhibitors cause dry cough in approximately 20% of patients taking these medications.[12] Systemic and ophthalmic beta-adrenergic blockers may cause cough in patients with obstructive airway diseases (e.g., asthma, chronic obstructive pulmonary disease [COPD]).

Clinical Presentation of Cough

Coughs are described as productive or nonproductive. A *productive* cough (a wet or "chesty" cough) serves a useful physiologic purpose. Productive coughs expel secretions from the lower respiratory tract that, if retained, could impair ventilation and the lungs' ability to resist infection. Productive coughs may be effective (secretions easily expelled) or ineffective (secretions present but difficult to expel). The appearance of the secretions is not always a reliable diagnostic indicator, but secretions typically are clear with bronchitis and purulent with bacterial infection. Anaerobic bacterial infections are associated with a distinct malodor. *Nonproductive* coughs (dry or "hacking" coughs), which are associated with viral and atypical bacterial infections, gastroesophageal reflux disease (GERD), cardiac disease, and some medications, serve no useful physiologic purpose.

Common complications of cough include exhaustion, sleep deprivation, musculoskeletal pain, hoarseness, excessive perspiration, social embarrassment, and urinary incontinence. Less common complications include cardiac dysrhythmias, syncope, stroke, pneumothorax, and rib fractures. Mechanical irritation from coughing may cause sore throat. Cough may cause prolonged absence from work or school, withdrawal from social activities, and anxiety from fear that the cough is a symptom of a serious illness, such as cancer or tuberculosis.

Treatment of Cough

Treatment Goals

The primary goal of self-treatment of cough is to reduce the number and severity of cough episodes. The second goal is to prevent complications. Cough treatment is symptomatic; the underlying disorder must be treated to stop the cough.

General Treatment Approach

Selection of a medication for self-care for cough depends on the nature and underlying cause of the cough. Figure 12–1 lists exclusions for self-care.[13–17] These exclusions are based on the presence of signs and symptoms of potentially serious medical conditions associated with cough that require further evaluation. *Antitussives* (cough suppressants) control or eliminate cough and are the drugs of choice for nonproductive coughs. Antitussives should not be used to treat productive cough unless the potential

TABLE 12-1 **Etiology of Cough**

Classification	Etiology
Acute	Viral URTI, acute bronchitis, pertussis, allergic rhinitis, aspiration syndromes, asthma exacerbations, COPD exacerbations, pneumonia, pulmonary embolism, acute left ventricular failure
Subacute	Postinfectious cough, bacterial sinusitis
Chronic	UACS, asthma, GERD, COPD, chronic bronchitis, ACEIs, bronchogenic carcinoma, carcinomatosis, sarcoidosis, chronic left ventricular failure, aspiration secondary to pharyngeal dysfunction

Key: ACEIs = Angiotensin-converting enzyme inhibitors; COPD = chronic obstructive pulmonary disease; GERD = gastroesophageal reflux disease; UACS = upper airway cough syndrome; URTI = upper respiratory tract infection.

Source: References 10–11.

benefit outweighs the risk (e.g., significant nocturnal cough). Suppression of productive coughs may lead to retention of lower respiratory tract secretions, increasing the risk of airway obstruction and secondary bacterial infection. *Protussives* (expectorants) change the consistency of mucus and increase the volume of expectorated sputum and may provide some relief for patients in whom coughing expels thick, tenacious secretions from the lungs with difficulty.

Cough medications are marketed in a variety of dosage forms—syrups, liquids, solutions, suspensions, tablets, capsules, liquid gels, lozenges, oral granules, oral strips, topical ointments and creams, topical patches, and vaporizer solutions. Generic formulations are widely available. The U.S. Food and Drug Administration (FDA) permits various combinations of antitussives, protussives, analgesics, decongestants, and antihistamines. However, combinations of antitussives and protussives are potentially counterproductive.

Nonpharmacologic Therapy

Nonpharmacologic therapy includes use of nonmedicated lozenges and hard candies, humidification, interventions to promote nasal drainage, and hydration. Nonmedicated lozenges and hard candies may reduce cough by stimulating saliva, thereby decreasing throat irritation. Humidifiers (ultrasonic, impeller, and evaporative) increase the amount of moisture in inspired air, which may soothe irritated airways. However, high humidity may increase environmental mold, dust mites, white dust from minerals released into the air, and microorganisms. Vaporizers (humidifiers with a medication well or cup for volatile inhalants) produce a medicated vapor. Cool-mist humidifiers and vaporizers are preferred because fewer bacteria grow at the cooler temperatures and there is less risk of scalding if they are tipped over. Humidifiers and vaporizers must be cleaned daily and disinfected weekly.

Babies and young children up to approximately 2 years of age cannot blow their noses; a rubber bulb nasal syringe may be used to clear the nasal passages and reduce cough if postnasal drip causes cough. Propping infants upright when they sleep and raising the head of the bed at night promote drainage of nasal secretions. Less viscous and thus easier-to-expel secretions are formed when the patient is well hydrated. Cautious hydration is recommended for patients with lower respiratory tract infections, heart failure, renal failure, or other medical conditions potentially exacerbated by overhydration.

Pharmacologic Therapy

Table 12–2 lists examples of antitussive and expectorant products.

Oral Antitussives

FDA-approved nonprescription oral antitussives include codeine (codeine, codeine phosphate, codeine sulfate), dextromethorphan (dextromethorphan, dextromethorphan hydrobromide), diphenhydramine (diphenhydramine citrate, diphenhydramine hydrochloride), and chlophedianol hydrochloride.[18] Nonprescription oral antitussives are typically used "as needed" (PRN)—within the limits of the maximum recommended daily dose. Nonprescription topical antitussives are also typically used on a PRN basis within the limits of the maximum recommended daily dose.

Codeine

At antitussive dosages, codeine is a Schedule V narcotic available without a prescription in 29 states and Washington, DC (8 of the 29 states limit sales to products sold by a pharmacist in a pharmacy).[19] Codeine-containing Schedule C–V products must contain no more than 200 mg of codeine per 100 milliliters.[20]

Codeine acts centrally on the medulla to increase the cough threshold. Codeine is methylmorphine; metabolites (morphine, norcodone, and others) may be the active antitussive. Codeine is well absorbed orally, with a 15- to 30-minute onset of action and a 4- to 6-hour duration of effect. The elimination half-life is 2.5–3 hours. Ten percent of a codeine dose is demethylated in the liver to form morphine; approximately 3%–16% of codeine is eliminated unchanged in the urine. The complicated metabolic pathway includes cytochrome P450 (CYP) 2D6, CYP3A4, and uridine 5′-diphospho-glucuronosyltransferase (UGT) 2B7.

Codeine is indicated for the suppression of nonproductive cough caused by chemical or mechanical respiratory tract irritation. Codeine's efficacy and safety as an antitussive drug in children are not established; pediatric dosage guidelines are extrapolated from the adult literature. Table 12–3 lists FDA-approved dosages for codeine and other nonprescription cough products. The table also notes manufacturers' voluntary decision in 2008 to update age limits on cough and cold product labels.[21,22] Reduced doses are appropriate for patients of advanced age and the debilitated. Codeine is available as oral solutions, liquids, suspensions, and syrups in combination with other active ingredients, including guaifenesin, antihistamines, and decongestants. Alcohol-, dye-, gluten-, and sucrose-free formulations are available.

Usual antitussive codeine dosages have low toxicity and little risk of addiction. Of note, however, codeine syrup containing the antihistamine promethazine hydrochloride, when mixed with soft drinks and/or alcohol and sometimes candy (common street names include "purple drank," "sizzurp," "syrup," and "lean"), is abused for the sedative effect. The most common adverse effects associated with antitussive codeine dosages are nausea, vomiting, sedation, dizziness, and constipation. The lethal dose of codeine in adults is 0.5–1 g, with death from marked respiratory depression and cardiopulmonary collapse. Concomitant use

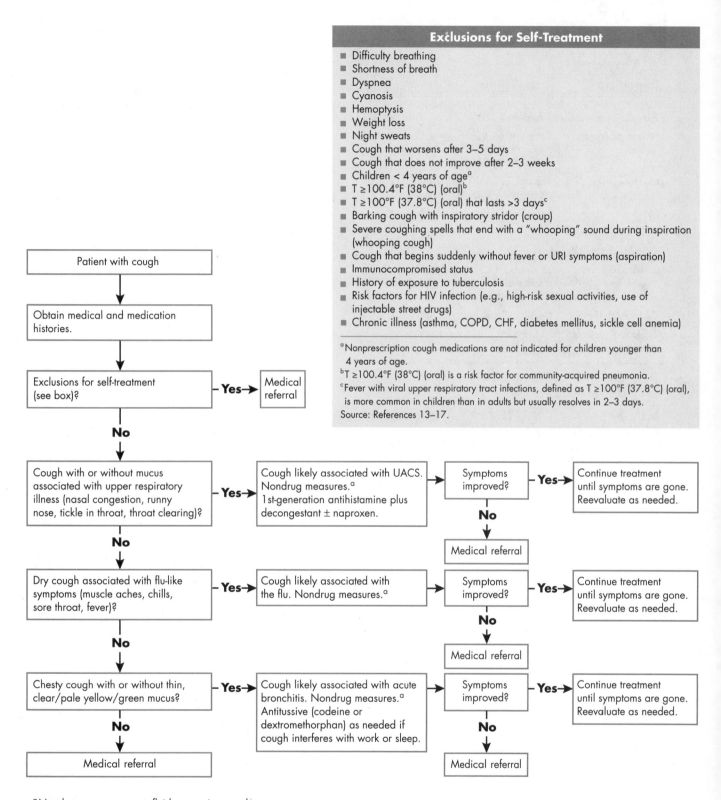

Exclusions for Self-Treatment

- Difficulty breathing
- Shortness of breath
- Dyspnea
- Cyanosis
- Hemoptysis
- Weight loss
- Night sweats
- Cough that worsens after 3–5 days
- Cough that does not improve after 2–3 weeks
- Children < 4 years of age[a]
- T ≥100.4°F (38°C) (oral)[b]
- T ≥100°F (37.8°C) (oral) that lasts >3 days[c]
- Barking cough with inspiratory stridor (croup)
- Severe coughing spells that end with a "whooping" sound during inspiration (whooping cough)
- Cough that begins suddenly without fever or URI symptoms (aspiration)
- Immunocompromised status
- History of exposure to tuberculosis
- Risk factors for HIV infection (e.g., high-risk sexual activities, use of injectable street drugs)
- Chronic illness (asthma, COPD, CHF, diabetes mellitus, sickle cell anemia)

[a] Nonprescription cough medications are not indicated for children younger than 4 years of age.
[b] T ≥100.4°F (38°C) (oral) is a risk factor for community-acquired pneumonia.
[c] Fever with viral upper respiratory tract infections, defined as T ≥100°F (37.8°C) (oral), is more common in children than in adults but usually resolves in 2–3 days.
Source: References 13–17.

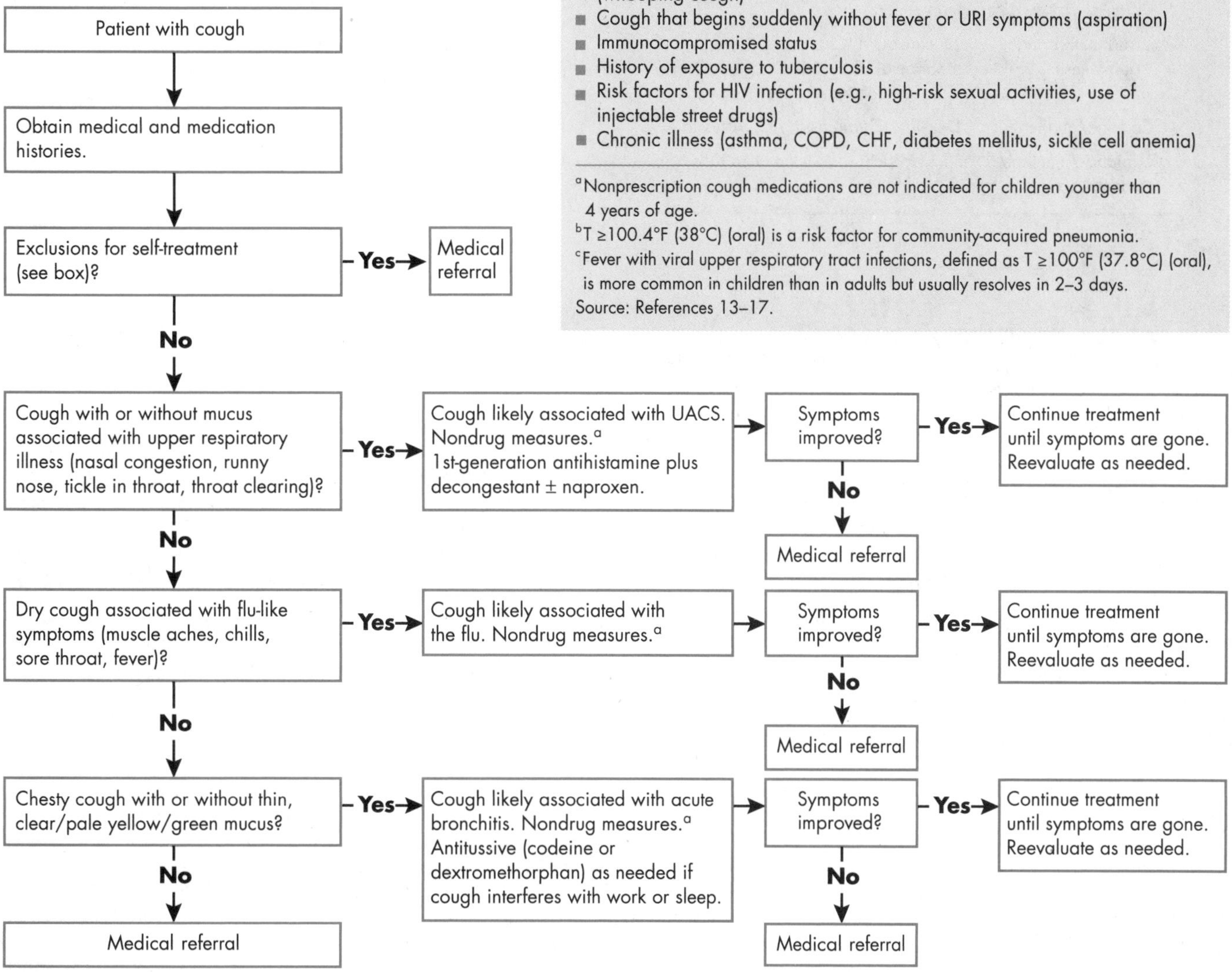
Patient with cough
Obtain medical and medication histories.
Exclusions for self-treatment (see box)?
Yes
Medical referral
No
Cough with or without mucus associated with upper respiratory illness (nasal congestion, runny nose, tickle in throat, throat clearing)?
Yes
Cough likely associated with UACS. Nondrug measures.a 1st-generation antihistamine plus decongestant ± naproxen.
Symptoms improved?
Yes
Continue treatment until symptoms are gone. Reevaluate as needed.
No
Medical referral
No
Dry cough associated with flu-like symptoms (muscle aches, chills, sore throat, fever)?
Yes
Cough likely associated with the flu. Nondrug measures.a
Symptoms improved?
Yes
Continue treatment until symptoms are gone. Reevaluate as needed.
No
Medical referral
No
Chesty cough with or without thin, clear/pale yellow/green mucus?
Yes
Cough likely associated with acute bronchitis. Nondrug measures.a Antitussive (codeine or dextromethorphan) as needed if cough interferes with work or sleep.
Symptoms improved?
Yes
Continue treatment until symptoms are gone. Reevaluate as needed.
No
Medical referral
No
Medical referral

[a] Nondrug measures: rest, fluids, vaporizer, and reassurance.

FIGURE 12–1 Self-care for cough. Key: CHF = Congestive heart failure; COPD = chronic obstructive pulmonary disease; HIV = human immunodeficiency virus; T = temperature; UACS = upper airway cough syndrome; URI = upper respiratory infection.

TABLE 12-2 Selected Nonprescription Products for Cough

Primary Ingredients	Trade Name
Single-Ingredient Products	
Dextromethorphan	Delsym, Robitussin Nighttime Cough DM Max, Hold DM, Children's Triaminic Long-Acting Cough
Guaifenesin	Robafen, Children's Mucinex Chest Congestion, Antitussin
Menthol	Vicks VapoDrops, Halls Mentho-Lyptus Drops
Combination Products	
Dextromethorphan/guaifenesin	Mucinex-DM, Cheracol D Cough Formula, Vicks 44E Cough & Chest Congestion Relief
Codeine/guaifenesin	Dex-Tuss, Guaiatussin AC, Virtussin A/C
Camphor/menthol/eucalyptus oil	Vicks VapoRub, Mentholatum Kids

of codeine and central nervous system (CNS) depressants causes additive CNS depression. Strong CYP2D6 inhibitors may block the conversion of codeine to the active metabolites. Table 12–4 lists clinically important codeine–drug interactions.[23] Codeine is contraindicated in patients with known codeine hypersensitivity and during labor when a premature birth is anticipated. Patients with impaired respiratory reserve (e.g., asthma, COPD) or preexisting respiratory depression, drug addicts, and individuals who take other respiratory depressants or sedatives, including alcohol, should use codeine with caution.

Dextromethorphan

Dextromethorphan is a nonopioid with no analgesic, sedative, respiratory depressant, or addictive properties at usual antitussive doses. Dextromethorphan, the methylated dextrorotatory analogue of levorphanol (itself a codeine analogue), acts centrally in the medulla to increase the cough threshold. It is well absorbed orally, with a 15- to 30-minute onset of action and a 3- to 6-hour duration of effect. Dextromethorphan undergoes polymorphic metabolism, with a usual elimination half-life of 1.2–2.2 hours. However, the half-life may be as long as 45 hours in people with a poor metabolism phenotype.

Dextromethorphan is indicated for the suppression of nonproductive cough caused by chemical or mechanical respiratory

TABLE 12-3 Dosage Guidelines for Nonprescription Oral Antitussives and Expectorants

	Dosage (maximum daily dosage)		
Drug	**Adults/Children ≥12 Years**	**Children 6 to <12 Years**	**Children 2 to <6 Years[a]**
Chlophedianol[b,c]	25 mg every 6–8 hours PRN (100 mg)	12.5 mg every 6–8 hours PRN (50 mg)	12.5 mg every 6–8 hours PRN (50 mg)
Codeine[b–d]	10–20 mg every 4–6 hours PRN (120 mg)	5–10 mg every 4–6 hours PRN (60 mg)	1 mg/kg/day PRN in 4 equal divided dosages or by average body weight
Dextromethorphan hydrobromide[b]	10–20 mg every 4 hours or 30 mg every 6–8 hours PRN (120 mg)	5–10 mg every 4 hours or 15 mg every 6–8 hours PRN (60 mg)	2.5–5 mg every 4 hours or 7.5 mg every 6–8 hours PRN (30 mg)
Diphenhydramine citrate[b,c]	38 mg every 4 hours PRN (228 mg)	19 mg every 4 hours PRN (114 mg)	9.5 mg every 4 hours PRN (57 mg)
Diphenhydramine HCl[b,c]	25 mg every 4 hours PRN (150 mg)	12.5 mg every 4 hours PRN (75 mg)	6.25 mg every 4 hours PRN (37.5 mg)
Guaifenesin[b]	200–400 mg every 4 hours PRN (2.4 g)	100–200 mg every 4 hours PRN (1.2 g)	50–100 mg every 4 hours PRN (600 mg)

[a] The Consumer Health Care Products Association announced in October 2008 that manufacturers were voluntarily updating cough and cold product labels to state "do not use" in children younger than 4 years.[21] In response, FDA announced that it would not object to the more restrictive labeling.[22] These actions have not changed the official monograph for cold, cough, allergy, bronchodilator, and antiasthmatic drug products.[18]

[b] Not recommended for use in children younger than 2 years; no FDA-approved dosing recommendations.

[c] FDA recommends that the labels on nonprescription products not provide dosage information for children younger than 6 years.

[d] Codeine may be dosed by age correlated with average body weight: *2 years of age* (average body weight of 12 kg) = 3 mg every 4–6 hours (maximum in 24 hours: 12 mg); *3 years of age* (average body weight of 14 kg) = 3.5 mg every 4–6 hours (maximum in 24 hours: 14 mg); *4 years of age* (average body weight of 16 kg) = 4 mg every 4–6 hours (maximum in 24 hours: 16 mg); *5 years of age* (average body weight of 18 kg) = 4.5 mg every 4–6 hours (maximum in 24 hours: 18 mg). A dispensing device such as a dropper calibrated for age or weight should be provided along with the product when it is intended for use in children 2 to <6 years of age, to prevent possible overdose from improper measurement of the medication.

Key: FDA = U.S. Food and Drug Administration; PRN = as needed.

Source: Reference 18.

TABLE 12–4 **Clinically Important Drug–Drug Interactions With Nonprescription Antitussive Agents**[a]

Antitussive	Drug/Drug Class	Potential Interaction	Management/ Preventive Measures
Codeine	Alvimopan	Opioid use increases the risk of alvimopan adverse reactions.	Discontinue opioids at least 7 days before initiating alvimopan.
Codeine	CNS depressants, including alcohol, azelastine, doxylamine, droperidol, hydrocodone, orphenadrine, perampanel, sodium oxybate, suvorexant, tapentadol, thalidomide, zolpidem	CNS depressants enhance the CNS depressant effect of codeine.	Avoid concurrent use if possible.
Codeine	Strong CYP2D6 inhibitors, including abiraterone, fluoxetine, paroxetine, quinidine, and panobinostat	Strong CYP2D6 inhibitors may block the metabolism of codeine to the active metabolites.	Avoid concurrent use if possible.
Codeine	Eluxadoline	Codeine may enhance eluxadoline-associated constipation.	Avoid concurrent use if possible.
Codeine	Mixed agonist/antagonist opioids, including buprenorphine	Mixed agonist/antagonists may reduce the therapeutic effect of codeine.	Avoid concurrent use if possible.
Codeine	Naltrexone	Naltrexone may reduce the therapeutic effect of codeine.	Avoid concurrent use if possible.
Dextromethorphan	Strong CYP2D6 inhibitors, including abiraterone, fluoxetine, paroxetine, quinidine, and panobinostat	Strong CYP2D6 inhibitors may decrease dextromethorphan metabolism, increasing the psychoactive effects of dextromethorphan.	Avoid concurrent use if possible.
Dextromethorphan	Serotonin modulators, including fluoxetine and paroxetine	Serotonin modulators may increase the risk of psychoactive effects of dextromethorphan.	Avoid concurrent use if possible.
Dextromethorphan	MAO inhibitors, including rasagiline, selegiline, isocarboxazid, phenelzine, and tranylcypromine	MAO inhibitors may increase dextromethorphan-associated serotonergic adverse effects.	Avoid concurrent use if possible.

[a] See Chapter 11 (Table 11–6) for diphenhydramine–drug interactions.

Key: CNS = Central nervous system; CYP = cytochrome P450; MAO = monoamine oxidase.

Source: Reference 23.

tract irritation. The efficacy and safety of dextromethorphan as an antitussive drug in children have not been established.[24] Table 12–3 lists FDA-approved dextromethorphan dosages. Dextromethorphan, as a single ingredient and in combination with active ingredients such as guaifenesin, acetaminophen, antihistamines, and decongestants, is marketed in the form of syrups, liquids, solutions, extended-release oral suspensions, elixirs, drops, gels, liquid-filled gel caps, tablets, capsules, powders, granules, strips, and lozenges. Alcohol-, sucrose-, gluten-, and dye-free formulations are available.

Dextromethorphan has a wide margin of safety. Adverse effects with usual doses are uncommon but may include drowsiness, nausea or vomiting, stomach discomfort, or constipation. Dextromethorphan overdoses cause confusion, excitation, nervousness, irritability, restlessness, and drowsiness, as well as severe nausea and vomiting; respiratory depression may occur with very high doses. Additive CNS depression occurs with alcohol, antihistamines, and psychotropic medications. The combination of monoamine oxidase inhibitors (MAOIs) and dextromethorphan may cause *serotonergic syndrome* (e.g., increased blood pressure, hyperpyrexia, arrhythmias, myoclonus). Dextromethorphan should not be taken for at least 14 days after the MAOI is discontinued. Table 12–4 lists clinically important dextromethorphan–drug interactions. Patients who have known hypersensitivity to dextromethorphan or who have a previous history of dextromethorphan dependence should not take it.

Dextromethorphan is abused for its phencyclidine-like euphoric effect ("robo-tripping").[25] Euphoric manifestations range from mild stimulation and alcohol-like intoxication to dissociative hallucinations; abuse may be associated with psychosis and mania. Dextromethorphan abuse is especially common among male adolescents.[26]

Diphenhydramine

Diphenhydramine, a nonselective (first-generation) antihistamine with significant sedating and anticholinergic properties, acts centrally in the medulla to raise the cough threshold. Second-generation antihistamines (e.g., loratadine, fexofenadine) lack antitussive activity. Diphenhydramine is well absorbed after oral administration, with a bioavailability of 40%–70%, a time to onset of action of approximately 15 minutes, and a duration of action of approximately

4–6 hours. The volume of distribution is 3.3–4.5 L/kg. Diphenhydramine is hepatically metabolized to *N*-demethyl, urine, and acidic metabolites, with a clearance of 0.4–0.7 L/kg per hour. Less than 4% is excreted unchanged in the urine.

Diphenhydramine is indicated for the suppression of nonproductive cough caused by chemical or mechanical respiratory tract irritation. Table 12–3 lists FDA-approved diphenhydramine dosages. A common ingredient in cold and allergy products, diphenhydramine is available in multiple dosage formulations, including an alcohol-free syrup specifically indicated for cough. Symptoms of diphenhydramine overdose include mild to severe CNS depression (e.g., mental confusion, sedation, respiratory depression), hypotension, and CNS stimulation (e.g., hallucinations, convulsions).

Adverse effects of diphenhydramine include drowsiness, disturbed coordination, respiratory depression, blurred vision, urinary retention, dry mouth, and dry respiratory secretions. Uncommon adverse effects reported with diphenhydramine include acute dystonic reactions such as oculogyric crisis (rotation of the eyeballs), torticollis (contraction of neck muscles), and catatonia-like states, as well as allergic and photoallergic reactions. Diphenhydramine may cause excitability, especially in children. Diphenhydramine potentiates the depressant effects of narcotics, nonnarcotic analgesics, benzodiazepines, tranquilizers, and alcohol on the CNS, and it intensifies the anticholinergic effect of MAOIs and other anticholinergics. (See Table 11–6 in Chapter 11 for clinically important diphenhydramine–drug interactions.) Diphenhydramine is contraindicated in patients with known hypersensitivity to diphenhydramine or structurally similar antihistamines. Diphenhydramine should be used with caution in patients with diseases potentially exacerbated by drugs with anticholinergic activity, including narrow-angle glaucoma, stenosing peptic ulcer, pyloroduodenal obstruction, symptomatic prostatic hypertrophy, bladder neck obstruction, asthma and other lower respiratory tract disease, elevated intraocular pressure, hyperthyroidism, cardiovascular disease, and hypertension. Because of the increased risk of toxicity, diphenhydramine-containing antitussives should not be used with any other diphenhydramine-containing product, including topical products.

Chlophedianol

Chlophedianol is a centrally acting oral antitussive originally marketed in 1960 as a prescription antitussive. Reintroduced as a nonprescription product in late 2009, chlophedianol is an alkylamine antihistamine derivative with antitussive, moderate local anesthetic, and mild anticholinergic effects. Chlophedianol is indicated for the suppression of nonproductive cough caused by chemical or mechanical respiratory tract irritation. Table 12–3 lists the FDA-approved chlophedianol dosage. Chlophedianol is marketed in combination with guaifenesin, antihistamines, and/or decongestants in the form of oral liquids, syrups, and tablets. Sugar-, alcohol-, dye-, and gluten-free products are available.

Published data for chlophedianol are limited. It has a slower time to onset of maximal effect than that for codeine (4 hours versus 30 minutes), in addition to a longer duration of action.[27] Chlophedianol is metabolized hepatically and eliminated renally. Adverse effects include excitation, hyperirritability, nightmares, hallucinations, hypersensitivity, and urticaria. Dry mouth, vertigo, visual disturbances, nausea, vomiting, and drowsiness have been associated with large doses. Chlophedianol–drug interactions have not been evaluated. Chlophedianol is contraindicated in patients with known chlophedianol hypersensitivity.

Protussives (Expectorants)

Guaifenesin (glyceryl guaiacolate), the only FDA-approved expectorant, is indicated for the symptomatic relief of acute, ineffective productive cough.[18] Guaifenesin is not indicated for chronic cough associated with chronic lower respiratory tract diseases such as asthma, COPD, or emphysema, or for smoker's cough. Guaifenesin loosens and thins lower respiratory tract secretions, making minimally productive coughs more productive. However, data supporting its efficacy, especially at nonprescription dosages, are limited.[28] Although the pharmacokinetic properties of guaifenesin are not well described, guaifenesin appears to be well absorbed after oral administration, with a half-life of approximately 1 hour.

Table 12–3 lists FDA-approved dosages of guaifenesin. Guaifenesin is marketed as oral liquids, syrups, solutions, granules, and immediate-release and extended-release tablets. Alcohol-, sucrose-, and dye-free formulations are also available. Most reports of guaifenesin overdose involve combinations of drugs and therefore are difficult to assess. However, signs and symptoms of overdose appear to be extensions of the adverse effects.

Guaifenesin generally is well tolerated. Adverse effects include nausea, vomiting, dizziness, headache, rash, diarrhea, drowsiness, and stomach pain. Large doses of this agent, either as a single agent or in combination with ephedrine or pseudoephedrine, have been associated with renal calculi.[29] No guaifenesin–drug interactions have been reported. Guaifenesin is contraindicated in patients with a known hypersensitivity to guaifenesin.

Topical Antitussives

Camphor and menthol are the only FDA-approved topical antitussives.[18] Other volatile oils (e.g., eucalyptus), common in many cough and cold preparations, impart a strong medicinal odor to products but are not FDA-approved antitussives. At subtherapeutic doses, menthol is a common flavoring agent. Although the mechanism of action is not well described, inhaled camphor and menthol vapors stimulate sensory nerve endings within the nose and mucosa, creating a local anesthetic sensation and a sense of improved airflow; cough reflex sensitivity may be suppressed with these agents.[30] However, objective evidence of antitussive efficacy is very limited. Skin, nose, or eye burning and/or irritation may occur with topical application. A possible drug interaction with menthol cough drops and warfarin resulting in reduced warfarin response has been reported.[31] Table 12–5 provides administration guidelines for these agents.

Camphor- and menthol-containing ointments, creams, and solutions may splatter and cause serious burns if used near an open flame or placed in hot water or in a microwave oven. Camphor and menthol vapors may be ciliotoxic and proinflammatory, especially in young children.[32] These products are also toxic if ingested. Toxic effects include burning sensations in the mouth, nausea and vomiting, epigastric distress, restlessness, excitation, delirium, seizures, and death. Ingestion of as little as 4 teaspoons of products containing 5% camphor may be lethal for children.[33]

Product Selection Guidelines

Efficacy

Although antitussives and expectorants have been marketed for decades, efficacy has been difficult to prove and may depend on the underlying cause of the cough. There is no good evidence that dextromethorphan, codeine, diphenhydramine, and guaifenesin are effective treatment of acute cough in adults or children[34,35];

TABLE 12-5 **Administration Guidelines for Nonprescription Topical Antitussives (Adults and Children ≥2 Years[a])**

Formulation	Administration
Ointments[b]	Rub on the throat and chest in a thick layer; application may be repeated PRN up to 3 times daily or as directed by primary care provider; loosen clothing around throat and chest so vapors reach the nose and mouth; cover with a warm, dry cloth (optional). Do not use in the nostrils, under the nose, by the mouth, on damaged skin, or with tight bandages.
Lozenges[c]	Allow lozenge to dissolve slowly in mouth; repeat hourly or as needed or as directed by a primary care provider.
Inhalation[d]	For products intended to be added directly to cold water for use in a steam vaporizer: add measured solution to cold water; place the mixture in the vaporizer; breathe in the medicated vapors up to 3 times daily PRN. For products to be placed in the medication chamber of a hot steam vaporizer: place water in vaporizer; place solution in medication chamber; breathe in the medicated vapors up to 3 times daily PRN.

Key: PRN = As needed.
[a] For children <2 years of age, consult a primary care provider.
[b] Camphor 4.7%–5.3%; menthol 2.6%–2.8%.
[c] Menthol lozenges, 5–10 mg lozenge; repeat hourly as needed.
[d] Camphor 6.2%; menthol 3.2%.
Source: Reference 18.

there is even less evidence for the efficacy of menthol, camphor, and chlophedianol.[36] Also lacking is evidence for or against the efficacy of nonprescription antitussives as adjuncts to antibiotics for the treatment of acute pneumonia.[37] Factors such as taste, smell, color, viscosity, sugar content, and personal expectation may contribute to a large placebo response (up to 85%).[38] Proof of efficacy will require data from well-designed trials in subjects with natural disease who are assessed with standardized objective outcome parameters.

- The American College of Chest Physicians (ACCP) published updated evidence-based diagnosis and management of cough guidelines in 2006[39]; similar international guidelines are available.[40] The ACCP guidelines state that central cough suppressants are ineffective in cough associated with the common cold, and they recommend a combination of a first-generation antihistamine with a decongestant to treat the viral infection–induced postnasal drip that is most likely the cause of the cough (see Chapter 11).[41] Also, because viral infection increases upper airway afferent nerve sensitivity, the guidelines suggest that the anti-inflammatory naproxen may reduce viral-associated cough.[41] The guidelines also recommend empirical treatment of cough associated with chronic upper airway cough syndrome, for which the etiology is unclear, with a first-generation antihistamine/decongestant combination (see Chapter 11).[42] The guidelines recommend codeine or dextromethorphan for the short-term symptomatic relief of cough associated with acute and chronic bronchitis and postinfectious subacute cough. Guaifenesin is not recommended for any indication. The guidelines do not address chlophedianol.

Dosage Formulations

Cough products are marketed in a variety of dosage formulations. Efficacy appears to be the same for all dosage formulations; patients may select a specific product on the basis of preference and convenience. Most products are formulated for dosage intervals of 4–6 hours, but some liquid and tablet dosage forms are specifically formulated for an extended dosage interval. For example, some dextromethorphan products are formulated with polymer complexes (e.g., sulfonated styrene–divinylbenzene copolymer), conferring an extended dosage interval (8–12 hours). Patients self-treating nocturnal cough may prefer a product with this advantage.

Special Populations

In January 2008, FDA issued a public health advisory recommending that nonprescription cough and cold medicines ". . . not be used to treat infants and children younger than 2 years because several serious and potentially life-threatening side effects can occur."[43] In October 2008, the Consumer Healthcare Products Association (CHPA) announced that manufacturers were voluntarily updating cough and cold product labels to state "do not use" in children younger than 4 years.[21] FDA announced that it would not object to the more restrictive labeling.[22] To address the issue of inaccurate dosing, FDA released guidelines in May 2011 for liquid nonprescription drug products that include any type of dispensing device (dropper, cup, syringe, or spoon).[44] These products include liquid analgesics, liquid cough and cold products, and lactase replacement drops. The key points of the guidance are recommendations that

- A dosing device be included with all oral liquid nonprescription products.
- The device be calibrated to the dose recommended in the product directions.
- The device be used only with the product in which it is packaged.
- The markings remain visible even when the liquid is in the device.

The European Medicines Agency (EMA) announced in 2015 that codeine is not to be used to treat cough and colds in children younger than 12 years and is not recommended for children and adolescents between 12 and 18 years of age who have breathing problems.[45] In 2017, FDA revised the codeine label requirements. The revised label includes a new contraindication against the use of codeine to treat cough or pain in children younger than 12 years of age and a new warning against the use of codeine in adolescents between 12 and 18 years of age who are obese, have obstructive sleep apnea, or have severe lung disease.[46]

An increased risk of congenital birth defects has been recognized if codeine is taken during the first trimester of pregnancy. Codeine should be used during pregnancy only if the potential benefits outweigh the risks. Nonteratogenic concerns include the risk of neonatal respiratory depression if codeine is taken close to the time of delivery and neonatal withdrawal if codeine is used regularly during the pregnancy. Codeine is excreted in breast milk and is associated with drowsiness in nursing infants.[47] (See the Preface for a detailed explanation of the pregnancy data.)

Because older adults may be more susceptible to the sedating effects of codeine, the dose should be started at the lower end of the recommended range and titrated as tolerated, with careful monitoring.

Dextromethorphan is viewed as probably safe for use during pregnancy.[48] It is not known whether dextromethorphan is excreted in breast milk. (See the Preface for a detailed explanation of the pregnancy data.) Because older adults may be more susceptible to the sedating effects of dextromethorphan, the dose should be started at the lower end of the recommended range and titrated as tolerated, with careful monitoring.

Diphenhydramine is commonly used during pregnancy, although no controlled studies have been conducted in pregnant women. Diphenhydramine is excreted in breast milk and may cause unusual excitation and irritability in the infant; it may also decrease the flow of milk. (See the Preface for a detailed explanation of the pregnancy data.) Compared with the general population, the elderly are more likely to experience dizziness, excessive sedation, syncope, confusion, and hypotension with diphenhydramine. The 2015 American Geriatrics Society Beers Criteria identify diphenhydramine, along with other nonprescription and prescription first-generation histamine-1 receptor (H1) antihistamines, as potentially inappropriate medications in older adults.[49] Children and the elderly may experience paradoxical excitation, restlessness, and irritability with diphenhydramine. Dosing for the latter group should be started at the lower end of the dosage range and titrated as tolerated, with careful monitoring.

Controlled studies on the use of guaifenesin or chlophedianol during pregnancy or breastfeeding are lacking. (See the Preface for a detailed explanation of the pregnancy data.) No special considerations have emerged regarding use of guaifenesin by older adults. Chlophedianol should be used with caution in sedated or debilitated patients.

Some cough formulations contain alcohol. Alcohol is a known teratogen and should be avoided during pregnancy.

TABLE 12–6 Signs and Symptoms of Disorders Associated With Cough

Disorder	Signs and Symptoms
Acute bronchitis	Purulent sputum; cough that lasts 1–3 weeks; mild dyspnea, mild bronchospasm and wheezing; usually afebrile, although a low-grade fever may be present
Asthma	Wheezing or chest tightness; shortness of breath, coughing predominantly at night; cough in response to specific irritants, such as dust, smoke, or pollen
Chronic bronchitis	Productive cough most days of the month at least 3 months of the year for at least 2 consecutive years
COPD	Persistent, progressive dyspnea; chronic cough (may be intermittent or unproductive), chronic sputum production
GERD	Heartburn; sour taste in mouth; worsening of symptoms in supine position; improvement with acid-lowering drugs
HF	Fatigue; dependent edema; breathlessness
Lower respiratory tract infection	Fever (mild to high); thick, purulent, discolored phlegm; tachypnea, tachycardia
UACS	Mucus drainage from nose; frequent throat clearing
Viral URTI	Sneezing; sore throat; rhinorrhea; low-grade fever

Key: COPD = Chronic obstructive pulmonary disease; GERD = gastroesophageal reflux disease; HF = heart failure; UACS = upper airway cough syndrome; URTI = upper respiratory tract infection.

Patient Factors

Cough is a symptom of many acute and chronic diseases (Table 12–6). Patients with identified exclusions for self-care (Figure 12–1) should be referred for further evaluation. Patients with known chronic diseases associated with cough, or with signs and symptoms suggestive of such diseases, should not attempt to self-treat cough, even cough caused by an acute viral upper respiratory tract infection (URTI), because the acute infection may exacerbate the underlying disease. Patients with smoker's cough should be counseled regarding smoking cessation options; antitussives and expectorants are not indicated (see Chapter 47).

Dextromethorphan and diphenhydramine should not be taken concurrently with MAOIs. Diphenhydramine is highly sedating and should be avoided by patients for whom the anticholinergic properties of the drug present a risk of adverse effects or complications. First-generation antihistamines and decongestants should be used only if the potential benefit outweighs the risk (see Chapter 11).

Complementary Therapies

Hundreds of herbal and other complementary therapies are marketed for cough. However, available evidence does not support the use of complementary therapies for treating cough, and some products have potential safety issues. (See Chapters 51 and 52, respectively, for information on such therapies.) For example, honey, a common but unproven home remedy, should not be given to children younger than 1 year because of the risk of botulism from ingestion of honey contaminated with *Clostridium botulinum*.[50]

Assessment of Cough: A Case-Based Approach

Before recommending any treatment, the health care provider needs to determine the duration of the cough (acute, subacute, chronic), the nature of the cough (productive or nonproductive), and presence of any associated symptoms suggesting that the patient has an acute or chronic medical condition requiring referral (Figure 12–1). The provider's assessment should also review the patient's current prescription and nonprescription medications, medication allergies, and history of adverse drug reactions. In addition, the provider should inquire how the patient has treated the current cough, as well as previous coughs, and whether these treatments were satisfactory or effective.

Cases 12–1 and 12–2 provide examples of the assessment of two different patients with cough.

CASE 12-1

Relevant Evaluation Criteria	Scenario/Model Outcome
Collect	
1. Gather essential information about the patient's symptoms and medical history, including	
a. Description of symptom(s) (i.e., nature, onset, duration, severity, associated symptoms)	The patient has been coughing for 3 weeks. She presented to her provider 2 weeks ago with fever, dyspnea, and cough productive of copious amounts of yellow-green mucus. She was treated with a 10-day course of antibiotics for a presumed bacterial pneumonia. The fever and dyspnea resolved; the cough is now nonproductive.
b. Description of any factors that seem to precipitate, exacerbate, and/or relieve the patient's symptom(s)	Talking and breathing cold air trigger "coughing spells."
c. Description of the patient's efforts to relieve the symptoms	The patient tried Luden's Wild Cherry cough drops, Ricola Lemon Mint cough drops, and Vicks Menthol cough drops without relief. She prefers to use cough drops or lozenges (she doesn't like the taste of cough syrups).
d. Patient's identity	Betty Wilson
e. Patient's age, gender, height, and weight	61 years, female, 5 ft 4 in., 118 lb
f. Patient's occupation	Administrative assistant
g. Patient's dietary habits	Lacto-ovo-vegetarian
h. Patient's sleep habits	Sleeps 9–10 hours a night
i. Concurrent medical conditions, prescription and nonprescription medications, and dietary supplements	No concurrent medical conditions. No routine nonprescription medications or complementary and alternative medicines.
j. Allergies	NKDA
k. History of other adverse reactions to medications	None
l. Other (describe) ______	None
Assess	
2. Differentiate patient's signs/symptoms, and correctly identify the patient's primary problem(s).	Betty is likely experiencing postinfectious subacute cough.
3. Identify exclusions for self-treatment (Figure 12–1).	None
4. Formulate a comprehensive list of therapeutic alternatives for the primary problem to determine whether triage to a health care provider is required, and share this information with the patient or caregiver.	Options include (1) Take no action. (2) Recommend that the patient see her PCP for further evaluation and treatment. (3) Recommend nondrug treatments (e.g., inhale warm steamy vapors). (4) Recommend self-care with a cough medication containing codeine or dextromethorphan.
Plan	
5. Select an optimal therapeutic alternative to address the patient's problem, taking into account patient preferences.	Betty may treat her cough as needed with a cough drop or lozenge containing dextromethorphan (e.g., Hold DM, Robitussin DM Medi-Soothers, Sucrets DM). The recommended dose for adults is dextromethorphan 10–20 mg every 4 hours as needed.
6. Describe the recommended therapeutic approach to the patient or caregiver.	"Postinfectious cough may be treated with a centrally active cough medication such as codeine or dextromethorphan. In our state, codeine-containing cough medications require a prescription; dextromethorphan medications are available without a prescription. Several companies make cough drops or lozenges containing dextromethorphan. Let the cough drop or lozenge dissolve slowly in your mouth. Do not take more than recommended for the specific product. Some medications may interact with dextromethorphan and some other nonprescription medications may contain dextromethorphan, so ask your provider or pharmacist before starting any new medication."
7. Explain to the patient or caregiver the rationale for selecting the recommended therapeutic approach from the considered therapeutic alternatives.	"Centrally active cough medications such as dextromethorphan and codeine may reduce postinfectious cough."

CASE 12-1 *continued*

Relevant Evaluation Criteria	Scenario/Model Outcome
Implement	
8. When recommending self-care with nonprescription medications and/or nondrug therapy, convey accurate information to the patient or caregiver.	See the box "Patient Education for Cough."
Solicit follow-up questions from the patient or caregiver.	"Is it OK to drive while taking dextromethorphan?"
Answer the patient's or caregiver's questions.	"Dextromethorphan may cause slight drowsiness or dizziness. Use caution when driving or performing tasks that require you to be awake and alert."
Follow-up: Monitor and Evaluate	
9. Assess patient outcome.	Ask Betty to call to update you on her response to treatment.

Key: NKDA = No known drug allergies; PCP = primary care provider.

CASE 12-2

Relevant Evaluation Criteria	Scenario/Model Outcome
Collect	
1. Gather essential information about the patient's symptoms and medical history, including	
a. Description of symptom(s) (i.e., nature, onset, duration, severity, associated symptoms)	The patient has a productive cough that started about 2 weeks ago. Initially the patient had a cold with symptoms of sore throat, nasal congestion, rhinorrhea, and dry hacking cough. Over the next 1–2 weeks, the sore throat and nasal symptoms resolved, but the cough persisted and became productive of large amounts of cream-colored opaque mucus. The patient has felt feverish with intermittent chills for the last 2–3 days but has not taken his temperature.
b. Description of any factors that seem to precipitate, exacerbate, and/or relieve the patient's symptom(s)	The cough has gotten worse over the last 2–3 days. The cough is worse at night and when he lies down.
c. Description of the patient's efforts to relieve the symptoms	The patient took Mucinex DM (600 mg guaifenesin and 30 mg dextromethorphan) for the dry hacking cough. He took Sudafed (pseudoephedrine) 30 mg 3–4 times a day for 4–5 days for the rhinorrhea.
d. Patient's identity	Maxwell Webster
e. Patient's age, gender, height, and weight	45 years, male, 5 ft 9 in., 158 lb
f. Patient's occupation	Architect
g. Patient's dietary habits	Maxwell changed his diet to lean meats (chicken, fish, turkey) and fresh fruits and vegetables 1 year ago after being diagnosed with high cholesterol.
h. Patient's sleep habits	He sleeps 8 hours a night.
i. Concurrent medical conditions, prescription and nonprescription medications, and dietary supplements	Dyslipidemia diagnosed 1 year ago. The patient takes Zetia (ezetimibe) 10 mg daily. He has no other known medical condition and is not taking any routine nonprescription or complementary and alternative medicine.
j. Allergies	None
k. History of other adverse reactions to medications	None
l. Other (describe) ______	The patient started smoking at age 18 years. He currently smokes 1 ppd.

CASE 12-2 *continued*

Relevant Evaluation Criteria	Scenario/Model Outcome
Assess	
2. Differentiate patient's signs/symptoms, and correctly identify the patient's primary problem(s).	The productive cough with fevers and chills may be symptoms of a secondary lower respiratory tract infection such as acute bronchitis or pneumonia.
3. Identify exclusions for self-treatment (Table 12–1).	Exclusions for self-care include cough that does not improve after 2–3 weeks and cough that worsens after 3–5 days.
4. Formulate a comprehensive list of therapeutic alternatives for the primary problem to determine whether triage to a health care provider is required, and share this information with the patient or caregiver.	Options include (1) Take no action. (2) Recommend that the patient see his PCP for further evaluation and treatment. (3) Recommend nondrug treatment (e.g., use nonmedicated lozenges, inhale warm steamy vapors). (4) Recommend self-care with a nonprescription centrally acting antitussive or expectorant. (5) Recommend that the patient stop smoking.
Plan	
5. Select an optimal therapeutic alternative to address the patient's problem, taking into account patient preferences.	Maxwell should be referred to his PCP for further evaluation and treatment of his productive cough, fever and chills. Central cough suppressants are not recommended for productive coughs and may impair clearance of the lower respiratory tract secretions. Expectorants are not recommended for productive coughs. Nonmedicated lozenges may reduce cough from throat irritation. The patient may treat his fever with an antipyretic (see Chapter 6). Recommend smoking cessation.
6. Describe the recommended therapeutic approach to the patient or caregiver.	"You should consult with your primary care provider about your productive cough, fever, and chills."
7. Explain to the patient or caregiver the rationale for selecting the recommended therapeutic approach from the considered therapeutic alternatives.	"Productive cough, fever, and chills after a viral upper respiratory tract infection may be symptoms of a new lower respiratory tract viral or bacterial infection."
Implement	
8. When recommending self-care with nonprescription medications and/or nondrug therapy, convey accurate information to the patient or caregiver.	Criterion does not apply in this case.
Solicit follow-up questions from the patient or caregiver.	"What are my choices if I decide to stop smoking?"
Answer the patient's or caregiver's questions.	"Nonprescription nicotine replacement choices include nicotine-containing patches, gums, and lozenges. Prescription medications include nicotine-containing nasal sprays and inhalers and medications that reduce nicotine cravings such as bupropion and varenicline. Individual or group counseling are also available to help you quit smoking." (See Chapter 47 for information on self-care assessment of and medications for smoking cessation.)
Follow-up: Monitor and Evaluate	
9. Assess patient outcome.	Ask Maxwell to call you after he is evaluated by his PCP to update you on his medical condition and decision regarding smoking cessation.

Key: PCP = Primary care provider; ppd = packs of cigarettes smoked per day.

Patient Counseling for Cough

The provider should identify appropriate drugs and describe nondrug measures for treating the patient's type of cough. After a product is recommended, the dosage guidelines, drug administration techniques (for topical drugs), and possible adverse effects, drug–drug interactions, and precautions or warnings should be fully explained. The provider should ensure that the patient understands when self-care for the cough is no longer adequate and that medical care must be sought. For patients with underlying medical disorders, the provider should identify which nonprescription medications are contraindicated, with specific reasons as appropriate, and what symptoms indicate the need to seek medical care. The box "Patient Education for Cough" lists specific information for patients.

Evaluation of Patient Outcomes for Cough

For most patients with cough who are candidates for self-management, 7 days of nonprescription drug therapy should relieve cough. If, after 7 days of self-management, the cough persists but has lessened in severity, the patient may continue the self-management regimen until the cough resolves. Cough associated with viral URTIs usually resolves within 2 weeks; postviral coughs may persist for 3 weeks or longer. Coughs associated with other respiratory infections typically resolve in 3–4 weeks. In all cases, the patient should be referred for further medical evaluation if the cough worsens or if the patient develops other exclusions for self-treatment (Figure 12–1).

PATIENT EDUCATION FOR Cough

The goals of self-treatment are (1) to reduce the number and severity of cough episodes and (2) to prevent complications. For most patients, carefully following product instructions and the self-care measures listed here will help ensure optimal therapeutic outcomes.

Nondrug Measures

- Stay well hydrated.
- Reduce throat irritation by slowly dissolving nonmedicated lozenges and candies in the mouth.
- Use humidifiers and vaporizers to increase the moisture in the air and possibly soothe irritated airways.
- Treat the underlying cause of cough (e.g., nasal congestion).

Nonprescription Medications

- Cough is a symptom of an underlying disorder. Contact your primary care provider if you have any of the exclusions for self-care listed in Figure 12–1.
- Select a product on the basis of the active ingredients and dosage formulation. Brand names frequently change and may not clearly represent the active ingredients.
- Slowly dissolve medicated lozenges in your mouth; do not chew.
- Swallow tablets and capsules whole; do not crush or chew.
- Follow the recommended dosing guidelines for each medication.
- Store all of these medications according to the manufacturer's recommendations. Do not use any expired drug.

Cough Suppressants (Antitussives)

- Cough suppressants control or eliminate cough and are the drugs of choice for nonproductive coughs.
- Oral nonprescription cough suppressants include codeine (available without a prescription in some states), dextromethorphan, diphenhydramine, and chlophedianol.
- Topical nonprescription antitussives include camphor and menthol.
- Do not heat or microwave topical antitussives or add these preparations to hot water. Do not use topical antitussives near an open flame. Topical antitussive ointments and liquids are toxic if ingested.
- The most common adverse effects of codeine include nausea, vomiting, sedation, dizziness, and constipation.
- Dextromethorphan's adverse effects are uncommon but may include drowsiness, nausea, vomiting, stomach discomfort, and constipation.
- The most common diphenhydramine adverse effects include drowsiness, disturbed coordination, decreased respiration, blurred vision, difficult urination, and dry mouth.
- The most common chlophedianol adverse effects include nausea, dizziness, and drowsiness.
- Codeine, dextromethorphan, diphenhydramine, and chlophedianol interact with drugs that cause drowsiness (e.g., narcotics, sedatives, some antihistamines, alcohol).
- Dextromethorphan interacts with monoamine oxidase inhibitors (e.g., phenelzine, tranylcypromine, isocarboxazid). Do not take dextromethorphan within 14 days of taking one of these medications.
- Diphenhydramine and chlophedianol also interact with drugs that have anticholinergic activity.
- Patients with impaired respiratory reserve (e.g., asthma, chronic obstructive pulmonary disease) should use codeine and diphenhydramine with caution.
- Patients with narrow-angle glaucoma, stenosing peptic ulcer, pyloroduodenal obstruction, symptomatic prostatic hypertrophy, bladder neck obstruction, elevated intraocular pressure, hyperthyroidism, heart disease, or hypertension should use diphenhydramine with caution.
- Talk with your doctor before using any medication while pregnant.
- Codeine and diphenhydramine are excreted in breast milk and may cause adverse effects in the child.
- Older adults and children may exhibit paradoxical excitation, restlessness, and irritability with diphenhydramine or chlophedianol. Older adults are more likely than the general population to experience adverse effects from diphenhydramine.

Expectorants (Protussives)

- Guaifenesin is the only available nonprescription protussive.
- Guaifenesin is generally well tolerated, but adverse effects may include nausea, vomiting, dizziness, headache, rash, diarrhea, drowsiness, and stomach pain.
- There are no reported drug interactions with guaifenesin.
- Guaifenesin is contraindicated in patients with a known hypersensitivity to the medication.
- Guaifenesin is not indicated for chronic cough associated with chronic lower respiratory tract diseases such as asthma, chronic obstructive pulmonary disease, emphysema, or smoker's cough.

Note About Pediatric Dosing

- Manufacturers of cough and cold medications have revised product labeling to state that these products should not be used in children younger than 4 years. Health care providers should stress this information to caregivers of infants and young children.

Key Points for Cough

- Cough is an important respiratory defensive reflex.
- Antitussives (cough suppressants) are the drugs of choice for nonproductive coughs.
- Protussives (expectorants) are the drugs of choice for coughs that expel thick, tenacious secretions from the lungs with difficulty.
- Neither codeine nor dextromethorphan has been shown to be effective for acute coughs associated with viral URTIs in either adults or children.
- In 2008, manufacturers voluntarily updated labels for cough and cold products to state "do not use" in children younger than 4 years.
- Combination products are convenient but are generally more expensive per dose and are associated with increased risk of adverse effects and drug interactions.
- Referral to a primary care provider is warranted if the cough worsens or if the patient develops signs or symptoms of a medical condition requiring further evaluation.
- Referral to a primary care provider is also warranted for patients with cough and a history or symptoms of chronic underlying disease associated with cough (e.g., asthma, COPD, chronic bronchitis, heart failure).

REFERENCES

1. Ambulatory and Hospital Care Statistics Branch. *National Ambulatory Medical Care Survey: 2012 State and National Summary Tables.* Hyattsville, MD: National Center for Health Statistics; 2012. Available at: https://www.cdc.gov/nchs/data/ahcd/namcs_summary/2012_namcs_web_tables.pdf. Accessed April 21, 2017.
2. Ambulatory and Hospital Care Statistics Branch. *National Hospital Ambulatory Medical Care Survey: 2011 Emergency Department Summary Tables.* Hyattsville, MD: National Center for Health Statistics; 2012. Available at: https://www.cdc.gov/nchs/data/ahcd/nhamcs_emergency/2011_ed_web_tables. Accessed April 21, 2017.
3. Consumer Healthcare Products Association. OTC Sales by Category 2013–2016. Available at: http://www.chpa.org/OTCsCategory.aspx. Accessed April 21, 2017.
4. Polverino M, Polverino F, Fasolino M, et al. Anatomy and neuropathophysiology of the cough reflex arc. *Multidiscip Respir Med.* 2012; 7(1):5–12. doi: 10.1186/2049-6958-7-5.
5. Canning BJ. Encoding of the cough reflex. *Pulm Pharmacol Ther.* 2007; 20(4):396–401. doi: 10.1016/jpupt.2006.12.003.
6. Canning BJ, Chang AB, Bolser DC, et al. Anatomy and neurophysiology of cough. *Chest.* 2014;146(6):1633–48. doi: 10.1378/chest.14-1481.
7. Chung KF, Bolser D, Davenport P, et al. Semantics and types of cough. *Pulm Pharmacol Ther.* 2009;22(2):139–42. doi: 10.1016/j.pupt.2008.12.008.
8. Footitt J, Johnston SL. Cough and viruses in airways disease: mechanisms. *Pulm Pharmacol Ther.* 2009;22(2):108–13. PMID:19480062.
9. Kwon SB, Park J, Jang J, et al. Study on the initial velocity distribution of exhaled air from coughing and speaking. *Chemosphere.* 2012;87(11): 1260–4. doi: 10.1016/j.chemosphere.2012.01.032.
10. Dicpinigaitis PV, Colice GL, Goolsby MJ, et al. Acute cough: a diagnostic and therapeutic challenge. *Cough.* 2009;5:11. doi: 10.1186/1745-9974-5-11.
11. De Blasio F, Virchow JC, Polverino M, et al. Cough management: a practical approach. *Cough.* 2011;7(7):1–12. doi:10.1186/1745-9974-7-7.
12. Tumanan-Mendoza BA, Dans AL, Villein LL, et al. Dechallenge and rechallenge method showed different incidences of cough among four ACE-Is. *J Clin Epidemiol.* 2007;60(6):547–53. PMID: 17493508.
13. Lechtzin W. Cough in adults. In: Kaplan JL, Porter RS, eds. *Merck Manual Professional Version.* Kenilworth, NJ: Merck & Co. Available at: http://www.merckmanuals.com/professional/pulmonary-disorders/symptoms-of-pulmonary-disorders/cough-in-adults. Accessed April 21, 2017.
14. Consolini DM. Cough in children. In: Kaplan JL, Porter RS, eds. *Merck Manual Professional Version.* Kenilworth, NJ: Merck & Co. Available at: http://www.merckmanuals.com/professional/pediatrics/symptoms-in-infants-and-children/cough-in-children. Accessed April 21, 2017.
15. Tackett KL, Atkins A. Evidence-based acute bronchitis therapy. *J Pharm Pract.* 2012;25(6):586–90. doi: 10.1177/0897190012460826.
16. Nolt BR, Gonzales R, Maselli J, et al. Vital-sign abnormalities as predictors of pneumonia in adults with acute cough illness. *Am J Emerg Med.* 2007;25(6):631–6. PMID: 17606087.
17. Snellman L, Adams W, Anderson G, et al. *Diagnosis and Treatment of Respiratory Illness in Children and Adults.* Bloomington, MN: Institute for Clinical Systems Improvement. Updated January 2013. Available at: https://www.icsi.org/_asset/1wp8x2/RespIllness.pdf. Accessed April 21, 2017.
18. U.S. Food and Drug Administration. Cold, cough, allergy, bronchodilator, and antiasthmatic drug products for over-the-counter human use. *CFR: Code of Federal Regulations.* Title 21, Part 341. Updated April 1, 2012. Available at: http://www.accessdata.fda.gov/scripts/cdrh/cfdocs/cfcfr/CFRSearch.cfm?CFRPart=341&showFR=1. Accessed April 21, 2017.
19. National Association of Boards of Pharmacy. *2016 Survey of Pharmacy Law.* Mount Prospect, IL: National Association of Boards of Pharmacy; 2016:76–9.
20. U.S. Food and Drug Administration. Controlled Substances Act. Title 21–Food and Drugs, Chapter 13–Drug Abuse Prevention and Control, Subchapter 1–Control and Enforcement, Part B–Authority to Control; Standards and Schedules. Available at: http://www.fda.gov/regulatoryinformation/lawsenforcedbyfda/ucm148726.htm. Accessed April 21, 2017.
21. Consumer Healthcare Products Association. CHPA announces voluntary labeling updates for oral OTC children's cough and cold medications. *CHPA Executive Newsletter.* 2008;21-08. Available at: http://www.chpa.org/workarea/downloadasset.aspx?id=911. Accessed April 21, 2017.
22. U.S. Food and Drug Administration. FDA statement following CHPA's announcement on nonprescription over-the-counter cough and cold medicines in children [news release]. October 8, 2008. Available at: https://www.fda.gov/ForConsumers/ConsumerUpdates/ucm048515.htm. Accessed April 21, 2017.
23. LexiDrugs Online. Hudson, OH: Lexi-Comp. Available at: https://online.lexi.com/lco/action/index/type/dryg. Accessed April 21, 2017.
24. Sharfstein JM, North M, Serwint JR. Over the counter but no longer under the radar—pediatric cough and cold medications. *N Engl J Med.* 2007;357(23):2321–4. doi: 10.1056/NEJMp0707400.
25. Reissig CJ, Carter LP, Johnson MW, et al. High doses of dextromethorphan, an NMDA antagonist, produce effects similar to hallucinogens. *Psychopharmacology.* 2012;223(1):1–15. doi: 10.1007/s00213-012-2680-6.
26. Wilson MD, Ferguson RW, Mazer ME, et al. Monitoring trends in dextromethorphan abuse using the National Poison Data System: 2000–2010. *Clin Toxicol.* 2011;49(5):409–15. doi: 10.3109/15563650.2011.585429.
27. Chen JYP, Biller HF, Montgomery EG Jr. Pharmacologic studies of a new antitussive, *alpha* (dimethylaminoethyl)-*ortho*-chlorobenzhydrol hydrochloride (SL-501, Bayer B-186). *J Pharmacol Exp Ther.* 1960;128(4): 384–91. PMID: 13809592.
28. Hoffer-Schaefer A, Rozycki HJ, Yopp MA, et al. Guaifenesin has no effect on sputum volume or sputum properties in adolescents and adults with acute respiratory tract infections. *Respir Care.* 2014;59(5):631–6. doi: 10.4187/respcare.02640.
29. Song GY, Lockhart ME, Smith JK, et al. Pseudoephedrine and guaifenesin urolithiasis: widening the differential diagnosis of radiolucent calculi on abdominal radiograph. *Abdom Imaging.* 2005;30(5):644–6.
30. Wise PM, Breslin PAS, Dalton P. Sweet taste and menthol increase cough reflex thresholds. *Pulm Pharmacol Ther.* 2012;25(3):236–41. doi: 10.1016/j.pupt.2012.03.005.
31. Coderre K, Faria C, Dyer E. Probable warfarin interaction with menthol cough drops. *Pharmacotherapy.* 2010;30(1):110. doi: 10.1592/phco.30.1.110.
32. Abanses JC, Arima S, Rubin BK. Vicks VapoRub induces mucin secretion, decreases ciliary beat frequency, and increases tracheal mucus transport in the ferret trachea. *Chest.* 2009;135(1):143–8.

33. American Academy of Pediatrics. Committee on Drugs. Camphor revisited: focus on toxicity. *Pediatrics.* 1994;94(1):127–8. PMID: 8008522.
34. Smith SM, Schroeder K, Fahey T. Over-the-counter (OTC) medications for acute cough in children and adults in community settings. *Cochrane Database Syst Rev.* 2014;11:CD001831. doi:10.1002/14651858.CD001831.pub5.
35. Chang AB, Peake J, McElrea MS. Anti-histamines for prolonged non-specific cough in children. *Cochrane Database Syst Rev.* 2010;2:CD005604. doi:10.1002/14651858.CD005604.
36. Paul IM. Therapeutic options for acute cough due to upper respiratory infections in children. *Lung.* 2012;190(1):41–4. doi: 10.1007/s00408-011-9319-y.
37. Chang CC, Cheng AC, Chang AB. Over-the-counter (OTC) medications to reduce cough as an adjunct to antibiotics for acute pneumonia in children and adults. *Cochrane Database Syst Rev.* 2014;3:CD006088. doi:10.1002/14651858.CD006088.pub4.
38. Eccles R. Mechanisms of the placebo effect of sweet cough syrups. *Respir Physiol Neurobiol.* 2006;152(3):340–8. doi: 10.1016/j.resp.2005.10.004.
39. Irwin RS, Baumann MH, Bolser DC, et al. Diagnosis and management of cough executive summary. *Chest.* 2006;129(1 Suppl):1S–23S. doi: 10.1378/chest.129.1.suppl.1S.
40. Gibson PG, Chang AB, Glasgow NJ, et al. CICADA: Cough in children and adults: diagnosis and assessment. *Med J Aust.* 2010;192(5):265–71. PMID: 20201760.
41. Pratter MR. Cough and the common cold: ACCP evidence-based clinical practice guidelines. *Chest.* 2006;129(1 Suppl):72S–74S. PMID: 16428695.
42. Pratter MR. Chronic upper airway cough syndrome secondary to rhinosinus diseases (previously referred to as postnasal drip syndrome): ACCP evidence-based clinical practice guidelines. *Chest.* 2006;129(1 Suppl): 63S–71S. PMID: 16428698.
43. U.S. Food and Drug Administration. Public Health Advisory: FDA recommends that over-the-counter (OTC) cough and cold products not be used for infants and children under 2 years of age. Updated August 20, 2013. Available at: http://www.fda.gov/NewsEvents/Newsroom/PressAnnouncements/2008/ucm051137.htm. Accessed April 21, 2017.
44. U.S. Food and Drug Administration. *Guidance for Industry: Dosage Delivery Devices for Orally Ingested OTC Liquid Drug Products.* Rockville, MD: U.S. Department of Health and Human Services, Food and Drug Administration; May 2011. Available at: https://www.fda.gov/downloads/Drugs/Guidances/UCM188992.pdf. Accessed April 21, 2017.
45. European Medicines Agency. Codeine-containing medicinal products for the treatment of cough or cold in paediatric patients. April 24, 2015. Available at: http://www.ema.europa.eu/ema/index.jsp?curl=pages/medicines/human/referrals/Codeine_containing_medicinal_products_for_the_treatment_of_cough_and_cold_in_paediatric_patients/human_referral_prac_000039.jsp&mid=WC0b01ac05805c516f. Accessed April 21, 2017.
46. U.S. Food and Drug Administration. FDA Drug Safety Communication: FDA restricts use of prescription codeine pain and cough medicines and tramadol pain medicines in children; recommends against use in breastfeeding women. April 20, 2017. Available at: https://www.fda.gov/Drugs/DrugSafety/ucm549679.htm. Accessed August 1, 2017.
47. Sachs HC. The transfer of drugs and therapeutics into human breast milk: an update on selected topics. *Pediatrics.* 2013;132(3):e796-809. doi: 10.1542/peds.2013-1985.
48. Einarson A, Lyszkiewicz D, Koren G. The safety of dextromethorphan in pregnancy: results of a controlled study. *Chest.* 2001;119(2):466–9. PMID: 11171724.
49. American Geriatrics Society 2015 Beers Criteria Update Expert Panel. Updated Beers criteria for potentially inappropriate medication use in older adults. *J Am Geriatr Soc.* 2015;63(11):2227-46. doi: 10.1111/jgs.13702.
50. Oduwole O, Meremikwu MM, Oyo-Ita A, et al. Honey for acute cough in children. *Cochrane Database Syst Rev.* 2014;12:CD007094. doi:10.1002/14651858.CD007094.pub4.

section

V

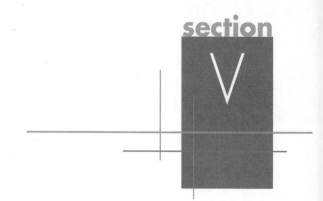

GASTROINTESTINAL DISORDERS

CHAPTER 13

HEARTBURN AND DYSPEPSIA

TARA WHETSEL AND ANN ZWEBER

Heartburn (*pyrosis*), one of the most common gastrointestinal (GI) complaints, is often described as a burning sensation in the stomach or lower chest that rises up toward the neck and occasionally to the back.[1] Patients may also describe it as indigestion, acid regurgitation, sour stomach, or bitter belching. Heartburn is a common symptom of gastroesophageal reflux disease (GERD), but similar symptoms may also occur in patients with peptic ulcer disease (PUD), delayed gastric emptying, gallbladder disease, and numerous other GI disorders. *Dyspepsia,* defined as symptoms originating from the gastroduodenal region, includes bothersome postprandial fullness, early satiation, epigastric pain, and epigastric burning.[2] Patients with dyspepsia may report many of these symptoms, as well as anorexia, belching, nausea and vomiting, and upper abdominal bloating. Heartburn can also occur with dyspepsia. Dyspepsia can be organic (i.e., has an identifiable cause) or functional (i.e., has no identifiable organic, systemic, or metabolic disease that is likely to explain the dyspeptic symptoms).

Although rarely a cause of mortality, dyspepsia, heartburn, and GERD are associated with considerable morbidity and cost. Patients with heartburn may limit their activities and restrict their food choices to reduce symptom frequency and severity. Compared with the general population, patients with heartburn have an impaired quality of life, with symptoms affecting activity and work.[3] Nocturnal symptoms of heartburn were reported in 24.9% of the general population and in up to 79% of patients with heartburn that occurs at least once a week.[4] Nocturnal symptoms are associated with interrupted sleep, decreased health-related quality of life, decreased work productivity, increased daytime sleepiness, and increased complications, such as erosive *esophagitis* (inflammation of the esophagus) and stricture.[4] Patients with dyspepsia report a diminished quality of life similar to that of patients with mild heart failure or menopause.[5] A retrospective analysis of health insurance claims showed that patients with functional dyspepsia incurred $5138 more in annual costs than did people without dyspepsia.[5] The total direct and indirect costs for GERD were over $12.6 billion per year; a large percentage of the costs were for prescription medications.[1]

The prevalence of heartburn and acid regurgitation (as reported over a 1-year period) in a healthy, predominantly white population was 42% and 45%, respectively.[1] Weekly symptoms were reported by 20% of the population, with an equal gender distribution.[1] Most subjects reported their heartburn to be moderately severe. In a cross-sectional study, the prevalence of heartburn was similar among African Americans, Hispanics, Asians, and Whites (23%–27%).[1] However, Whites had significantly more esophagitis. Although men and women are affected almost equally by GERD, males have a higher rate of esophagitis and Barrett's esophagus (a precancerous condition). Older patients have a higher prevalence of GERD complications, but they may experience fewer symptoms because of decreased sensitivity to refluxed acid. The prevalence of GERD has been increasing in Western countries over the past 30 years, while remaining relatively low among residents of Africa and Asia. The rise in Western countries is speculated to be a result of increasing obesity and decreasing prevalence of *Helicobacter pylori* (*H. pylori*) infection.[1] Heartburn is common during pregnancy, with 30%–80% of women complaining of heartburn.[1]

The prevalence of dyspepsia has been estimated to range between 10% and 45%.[2] Much of this variation is influenced by criteria used to define dyspepsia. When heartburn is excluded, the prevalence of uninvestigated dyspepsia is 5%–15%. Compared with men, women have a slightly higher prevalence. The incidence of dyspepsia has been estimated to be 2.8% per year.[5] Among patients with dyspepsia, 5%–10% have a peptic ulcer and approximately 20% have erosive esophagitis.

Pathophysiology of Heartburn and Dyspepsia

Esophageal defense mechanisms (antireflux barriers, esophageal acid clearance, tissue resistance) help protect the esophageal mucosa from acid damage.[1] Antireflux barriers include the intrinsic lower esophageal sphincter (LES), the diaphragmatic crura, the intra-abdominal location of the LES, the phrenoesophageal ligaments, and the acute angle of His (Figure 13–1). These anatomic structures work together to provide a physical barrier against reflux of gastric contents into the esophagus. The major component, the LES, is contracted at rest but relaxes on swallowing to permit the flow of food, liquids, and saliva into the stomach. Transient relaxations occur when there is no swallowing or esophageal peristalsis, allowing retrograde movement of stomach contents into the esophagus. The crural diaphragm provides an extrinsic squeeze to the LES, contributing to resting pressure and augmenting LES pressure during periods of increased abdominal pressure, such as with coughing, sneezing, or bending over. The angle of His creates a flap valve effect that contributes to the antireflux barrier.

When reflux of acidic gastric material does occur, physiologic mechanisms help protect the esophageal mucosa from damage.[1] Esophageal acid clearance occurs when peristalsis moves refluxed material into the stomach, and saliva and esophageal gland secretions neutralize residual acid. Gravity also helps clear the esophagus. Tight junctions in esophageal mucosa and

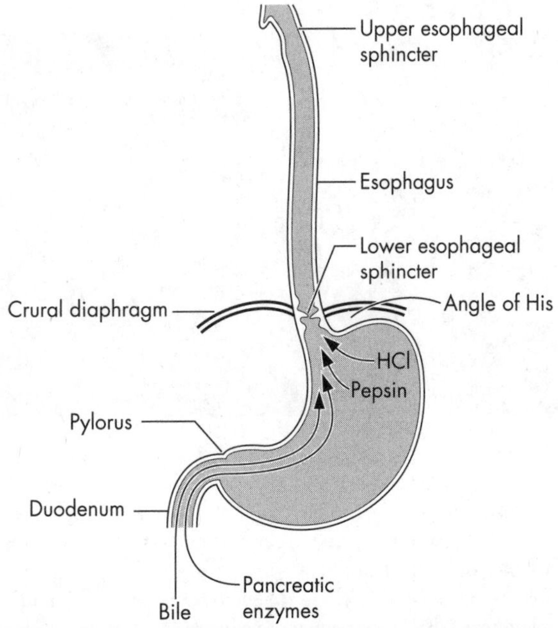

FIGURE 13–1 Esophageal defense mechanisms and offensive factors associated with heartburn.

the intercellular space matrix further reduce epithelial damage from hydrogen ions. Epithelial cells are also capable of buffering and extruding hydrogen ions that do penetrate the cell membrane. Tissue resistance is further aided by the esophageal blood supply, which delivers oxygen, nutrients, and bicarbonate, and removes hydrogen and carbon dioxide, thereby maintaining normal tissue acid–base balance. Even though gastroesophageal reflux is common, particularly postprandially, symptoms and esophageal damage are uncommon because of these esophageal defense mechanisms.

Heartburn is likely related to stimulation of esophageal mucosal chemoreceptors.[6] Acid reflux, weakly acidic reflux, bile reflux, and mechanical stimulation of the esophagus can cause heartburn symptoms.[1,6] It is unclear why some reflux episodes produce symptoms but most do not. Possible contributing factors include mucosal disruption, decreased acid clearance, inflammation, reduced salivary bicarbonate concentration, volume of refluxate, frequency of heartburn, and interaction of pepsin with acid.[1,6] One theory is that the esophagus becomes hypersensitive from repeated acid exposure, causing symptoms to occur from smaller boluses of acid.[6] Any disruption in the esophageal defense mechanisms can lead to increased acid exposure. Distention of the proximal stomach by either food or gas is a major stimulus for transient LES relaxations. Some patients may have decreased LES pressure that can be overcome by an abrupt increase in intra-abdominal pressure from coughing, straining, or bending over. A hiatal hernia impairs LES function and esophageal acid clearance. A hiatal hernia displaces the LES from the crural diaphragm, reduces LES pressure, and results in more frequent transient relaxations of the LES, all of which contribute to increased reflux. Prolonged exposure of the esophagus to the refluxed material can occur in a lying or sleeping position, with decreased salivation or with peristaltic dysfunction. Large volumes of refluxate from overeating or delayed gastric emptying can also increase esophageal acid exposure. As a result, damage to the tight intercellular junctions of the esophageal mucosa can lead to increased cellular permeability to hydrogen ions, with subsequent cellular injury. This increased permeability partly explains the development of heartburn in the absence of overt esophagitis.[1] The composition of the refluxate is an important contributor to the degree of esophageal damage. Pepsin and/or bile salts combined with acid produce greater injury than seen with acid alone. *H. pylori* infection lowers gastric acidity, thereby possibly protecting against heartburn, GERD, and related complications.[1]

A number of risk factors are associated weakly with the development of heartburn (Table 13–1).[1,6–8] Foods (e.g., fat, chocolate, peppermint) and drugs (e.g., theophylline, morphine, calcium channel blockers, diazepam) can decrease LES pressure, leading to increased reflux. Citrus, tomato-based, and spicy foods

TABLE 13–1 Risk Factors That May Contribute to Heartburn and GERD

Dietary	**Medications**
Alcohol (ethanol)	Alpha-adrenergic antagonists
Caffeinated beverages	Anticholinergic agents
Carbonated beverages	Aspirin/NSAIDs
Chocolate	Barbiturates
Citrus fruit or juices	Benzodiazepines
Coffee	Beta$_2$-adrenergic agonists
Fatty foods	Bisphosphonates
Garlic or onions	Calcium channel blockers
Mint (e.g., spearmint, peppermint)	Chemotherapy
	Clindamycin
Salt and salt substitutes	Dopamine
Spicy foods	Doxycycline
Tomatoes/tomato juice	Estrogen
Lifestyle	Iron
Exercise (isometric, running)	Narcotic analgesics
Obesity	Nitrates
Smoking (tobacco)	Potassium
Stress	Progesterone
Supine body position	Prostaglandins
Tight-fitting clothing	Quinidine
Diseases	TCAs
Motility disorders (e.g., gastroparesis)	Tetracycline
	Theophylline
PUD	Zidovudine
Scleroderma	**Other**
Zollinger–Ellison syndrome	Genetics
	Pregnancy

Key: GERD = Gastroesophageal reflux disease; NSAID = nonsteroidal anti-inflammatory drug; PUD = peptic ulcer disease; TCA = tricyclic antidepressant.

Source: References 1 and 6–8.

irritate inflamed esophageal mucosa. Smoking contributes by relaxing LES pressure and decreasing salivation. Anxiety, fear, and worry may lower visceral sensitivity thresholds, leading to increased pain perception. Bending over, straining to defecate, lifting heavy objects, and performing isometric exercises may increase intra-abdominal pressure above the LES pressure, leading to reflux. Obesity increases intra-abdominal pressure, and epidemiologic studies suggest that the prevalence of GERD is considerably higher in obese patients.[1]

Dyspepsia may be caused by PUD, GERD, celiac disease, gastric or esophageal malignancy (rarely), or other GI disorders. Specific foods (e.g., spicy food, coffee, alcohol) and excessive food intake have not been established as causing dyspepsia. Medications (including iron, antibiotics, narcotics, digoxin, estrogens, theophylline, and nonsteroidal anti-inflammatory drugs [NSAIDs]) commonly cause dyspepsia through direct gastric mucosal injury, changes in GI function, exacerbation of reflux, or some other mechanism.[2] The pathophysiology of functional dyspepsia is unclear but may include delayed gastric emptying, impaired gastric accommodation to a meal, hypersensitivity to gastric distention, altered duodenal sensitivity, abnormal intestinal motility, and central nervous system dysfunction.[2] One or more of these disturbances can occur in individual patients. The cause of symptoms in patients with functional dyspepsia has not been established. Population studies have suggested a genetic predisposition. *H. pylori* may play a role in functional dyspepsia, as evidenced by the small improvement in symptoms following eradication of the infection. Patients who have recovered from gastroenteritis may suffer from postinfection functional dyspepsia. Psychosocial factors are an important contributor to symptom severity. Patients with functional dyspepsia may also have anxiety disorders, depression, somatoform disorders, and a recent or remote history of physical or sexual abuse. The exact mechanism is unknown, but some studies have suggested a relationship between psychosocial factors and visceral hypersensitivity.[2]

Clinical Presentation of Heartburn and Dyspepsia

Heartburn may occur alone or as a symptom of other GI disorders, such as GERD and PUD (Table 13–2). Heartburn is noted most frequently within 1 hour after eating, especially after a large meal or ingestion of offending foods and/or beverages. Lying down or bending over may exacerbate heartburn. Regurgitation and, less commonly, water brash may occur. *Regurgitation* is characterized by a bitter acidic fluid in the back of the throat and occurs more commonly at night or upon bending over. It differs from vomiting: nausea, retching, or abdominal contractions do not occur. *Water brash* is the sudden filling of the mouth with clear, slightly salty fluid secreted from the salivary glands. Severity of any of these symptoms is subjective, and no standard definitions exist for classifying symptoms as "mild," "moderate," or "severe." Symptoms may be considered mild if they bother the patient a little but do not interfere with normal activities. Symptoms that are somewhat bothersome or annoying and/or interfere with normal activities may be considered moderate. GERD is suggested by heartburn that occurs 2 or more times a week.[1] GERD can be complicated by erosive esophagitis, hemorrhage, esophageal ulcers, strictures, Barrett's esophagus, and esophageal adenocarcinoma. Heartburn severity is poorly correlated with esophageal damage, especially in older patients who on presentation may have no or mild symptoms despite severe erosive esophagitis or other complications.[1] Upper endoscopy is the standard for determining the presence and extent of esophageal damage.

Alarm symptoms include dysphagia, odynophagia, upper GI bleeding, and unexplained weight loss. These symptoms can indicate more severe disease and/or complications. *Dysphagia* (difficulty swallowing) is slowly progressive for solid food and usually is associated with long-standing heartburn. The most common causes are peptic stricture or Schatzki's ring, but severe esophagitis, peristaltic dysfunction, and esophageal cancer are other potential etiologies.[1] *Odynophagia* (painful swallowing) is less common and may indicate severe ulcerative esophagitis, pill-induced injury (e.g., from tetracycline, potassium chloride, vitamin C, NSAIDs, aspirin, bisphosphonates), or infection. Signs of upper GI bleeding include hematemesis, melena, occult bleeding, and anemia. Patients may also present with atypical or extraesophageal symptoms related to gastroesophageal reflux. These include noncardiac chest pain, asthma, laryngitis, hoarseness, *globus sensation* (sensation of a lump in the throat), chronic cough, recurrent pneumonitis, and dental erosion.[1,9] Alarm symptoms or atypical symptoms should be evaluated by a primary care provider (PCP).

TABLE 13–2 Differentiation of Simple Heartburn From Other Acid-Related Disorders

	Simple Heartburn	GERD	Dyspepsia	PUD
Etiology	See Table 13–1.	See Table 13–1.	Possible contributing factors: food, alcohol, caffeine, stress, and medications Chronic dyspepsia: associated with PUD, GERD, celiac disease, and gastric cancer; or may lack an identifiable cause (functional dyspepsia)	Gastric or duodenal ulcer caused most commonly by *Helicobacter pylori* infection and/or NSAIDs
Typical symptoms	Burning sensation behind the breastbone that may radiate toward the neck, throat, and, occasionally, the back	Heartburn, acid regurgitation	Primary: postprandial fullness, early satiation, epigastric pain, epigastric burning Other: belching, bloating, nausea, vomiting	Gnawing or burning epigastric pain, occurring during day and frequently at night; may be accompanied by heartburn and dyspepsia

Key: GERD = Gastroesophageal reflux disease; NSAID = nonsteroidal anti-inflammatory drug; PUD = peptic ulcer disease.

Dyspepsia can present with one or more of four main symptoms. *Postprandial fullness* is an unpleasant sensation perceived as the prolonged persistence of food in the stomach. *Early satiation* is the feeling of fullness that occurs soon after eating begins and that is out of proportion to the amount of food ingested. (*Early satiety* was the term previously used, but *early satiation* is the correct term according to the most recent diagnostic criteria.[2]) *Epigastric pain* is an unpleasant sensation between the umbilicus and lower end of the sternum. *Epigastric burning* refers to an unpleasant subjective sensation of heat. Less specific symptoms may include bloating, nausea, vomiting, and belching. Symptoms are mostly intermittent and may or may not be related to meals. Weight loss is considered an alarm symptom that should prompt referral for further investigation. Other alarm symptoms include anemia, blood loss, and dysphagia.[2]

Treatment of Heartburn and Dyspepsia

Treatment Goals

The goals of self-treatment of heartburn and dyspepsia are (1) to provide complete relief of symptoms, (2) to reduce recurrence of symptoms, and (3) to prevent and manage unwanted effects of medications.

General Treatment Approach

The approach to self-treatment of heartburn and dyspepsia requires an initial assessment to determine whether the patient is a candidate for self-care (Figure 13–2). Patients with exclusions for self-treatment should be referred for further medical evaluation. If the individual is a candidate for self-treatment, specific nondrug measures discussed in the section "Nonpharmacologic Therapy" should be recommended and continued throughout treatment. If appropriate, a recommendation should also be made for a nonprescription medication. The selection of the medication should be based on the frequency, duration, and severity of symptoms; the cost of the medication; potential drug–drug interactions and adverse effects; and the patient's preference. Antacids and nonprescription histamine-2 receptor antagonists (H2RAs) should be recommended for patients with mild, infrequent heartburn and dyspepsia. Antacids are advantageous because they provide rapid relief of symptoms, but relief is brief when antacids are taken on an empty stomach (Table 13–3). When used in recommended dosages, the different types of antacids are interchangeable despite differences in antacid salts and potency. Antacid/alginic acid combinations have an onset of action that is comparable to that of antacids alone and may also provide better relief and a slightly longer duration of action.[10,11]

A nonprescription H2RA is preferable to an antacid when patients with mild–moderate episodic heartburn require more prolonged relief of symptoms. H2RAs do not relieve heartburn or dyspepsia as rapidly as an antacid does (Table 13–3), but they may be used with an antacid if both quick relief and longer duration of action are desired. H2RAs may also be used to prevent heartburn and acid indigestion if they are given 30 minutes to 1 hour prior to situations in which heartburn is anticipated. Lower dose nonprescription H2RA products (e.g., famotidine 10 mg up to twice daily) should be recommended for patients with mild, infrequent heartburn. Higher dose nonprescription products (e.g., famotidine 20 mg up to twice daily) should be reserved for moderate symptoms. Patients should not exceed 14 days of self-treatment with an H2RA without consulting their PCP.

Nonprescription proton pump inhibitors (PPIs) can be used for treating frequent heartburn (occurring ≥2 days per week) or when patients do not respond to nonprescription H2RAs.[12] The onset of symptomatic relief following a PPI dose is slower than that with an H2RA dose (Table 13–3), and complete relief of symptoms may take several days after initiation of therapy. However, compared with the H2RAs, PPIs provide better symptomatic relief and a prolonged duration of action. Self-treatment with a PPI should be limited to a duration of 14 days and retreatment to every 4 months.[13]

Nonpharmacologic Therapy

Nonpharmacologic measures may benefit some patients, but these changes alone are unlikely to completely relieve symptoms in the majority of patients. Dietary and lifestyle modifications recommended for heartburn are aimed at avoiding foods and beverages that precipitate heartburn and adopting behaviors that reduce esophageal acid exposure. Nonpharmacologic measures should be recommended for all patients with heartburn and dyspepsia despite the fact that evidence supporting their effectiveness is either lacking or equivocal.[5,7,8] A complete and accurate history will assist in identifying contributing factors (Table 13–1). Patients should be asked to keep a diary to track dietary, lifestyle, and medication "triggers." Recommendations should be tailored to the patient's specific history. Weight loss should be advised for overweight patients with heartburn. Elevating the head of the bed by placing 6- to 8-inch blocks underneath the legs at the head of the bed or placing a foam wedge (e.g., GERD pillow) beneath the patient's upper torso and head should be recommended for patients who have heartburn when recumbent. Use of traditional pillows may worsen symptoms, because they cause the patient to bend at the waist, which contributes to an increase in intragastric pressure.

Patients should be educated about factors that contribute to heartburn and be advised how to manage them (see the box "Patient Education for Heartburn and Dyspepsia"). Most importantly, heartburn sufferers should be counseled to eat smaller meals, to reduce intake of dietary fat, and to refrain from eating within 3 hours of going to bed or lying down. Prescription and nonprescription medications should be evaluated for their potential to cause or exacerbate heartburn and dyspepsia (Table 13–1). When possible, patients should be advised to switch to less troublesome nonprescription medications or to consult their prescriber about prescription drugs that may be exacerbating their symptoms. Use of tobacco products should be discouraged. Patients should be advised to limit or discontinue alcohol or caffeine consumption, if either worsens symptoms.

Pharmacologic Therapy

Antacids

Antacids relieve heartburn and dyspepsia by neutralizing gastric acid. Nonprescription antacid products contain at least one of the following salts: magnesium (hydroxide, carbonate, trisilicate); aluminum (hydroxide or phosphate); calcium carbonate; or sodium bicarbonate (Table 13–4). Most antacids are relatively inexpensive, making them affordable products for the temporary relief of mild and infrequent heartburn and dyspepsia.

Exclusions for Self-Treatment

- Frequent heartburn for more than 3 months
- Heartburn while taking recommended dosages of nonprescription H2RA or PPI
- Heartburn that continues after 2 weeks of treatment with a nonprescription H2RA or PPI
- Heartburn and dyspepsia that occur when taking a prescription H2RA or PPI
- Severe heartburn and dyspepsia
- Nocturnal heartburn
- Difficulty or pain on swallowing solid foods
- Vomiting up blood or black material or passing black tarry stools
- Chronic hoarseness, wheezing, coughing, or choking
- Unexplained weight loss
- Continuous nausea, vomiting, or diarrhea
- Chest pain accompanied by sweating, pain radiating to shoulder, arm, neck, or jaw, and shortness of breath
- Children <2 years (for antacids), 12 years (for H2RAs), or 18 years (for PPIs)
- Adults >45 years with new-onset dyspepsia

Source: References 1, 2, and 8.

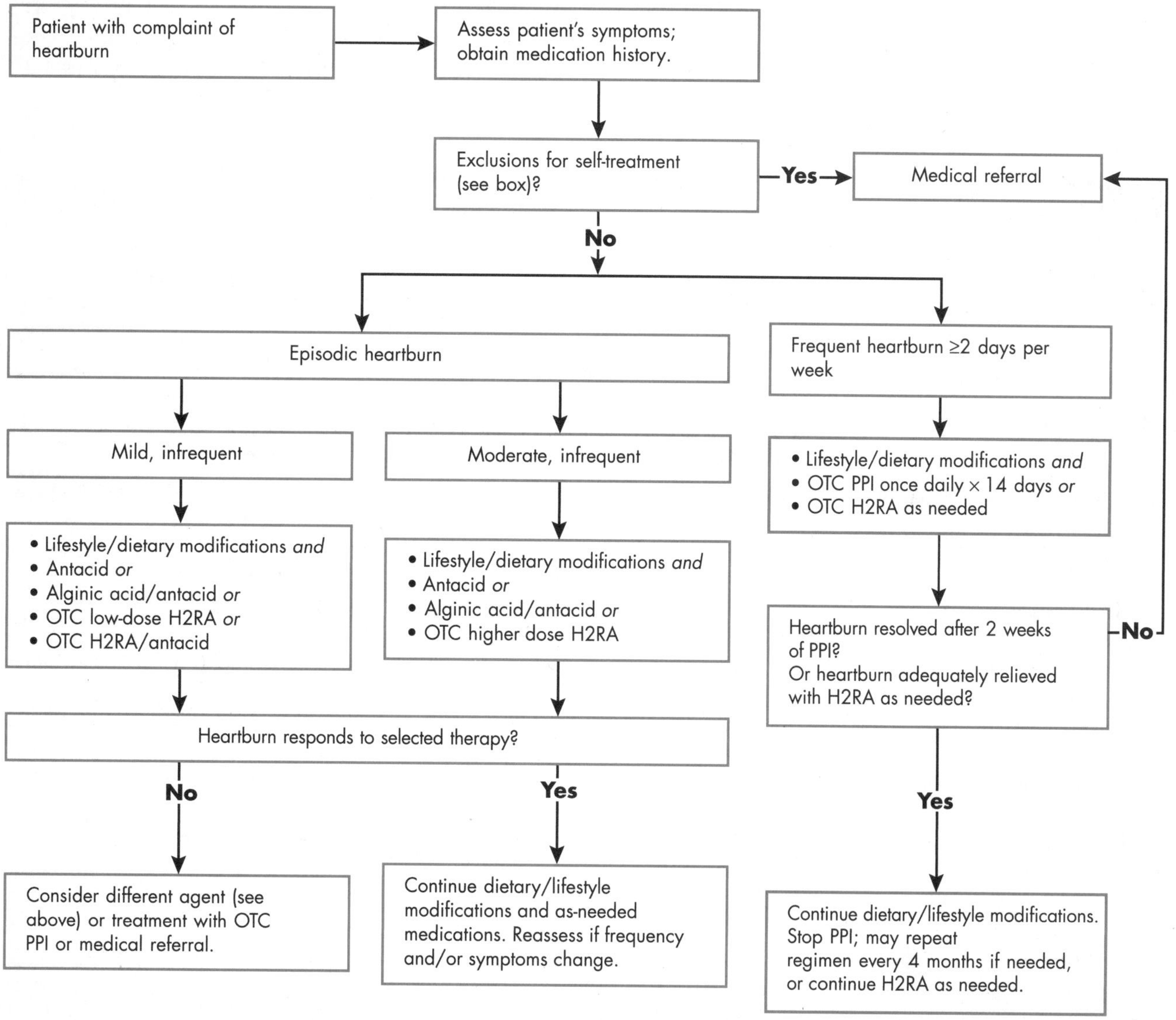

FIGURE 13-2 Self-care for heartburn. Key: H2RA = Histamine-2 receptor antagonist; OTC = over-the-counter; PPI = proton pump inhibitor.

TABLE 13-3 Onset and Duration of Symptomatic Relief With Nonprescription Medications in Relieving Heartburn

Medication	Onset of Relief	Duration of Relief
Antacids	<5 minutes	20–30 minutes[a]
H2RAs	30–45 minutes	4–10 hours
H2RA + antacid	<5 minutes	8–10 hours
PPIs	2–3 hours	12–24 hours

Key: H2RA = Histamine-2 receptor antagonist; PPI = proton pump inhibitor.

[a] Food prolongs duration of relief.

Antacids act as buffering agents in the lower esophagus, gastric lumen, and duodenal bulb. The cations react with chloride, but the anionic portion of the molecule reacts with hydrogen ions to form water and other compounds. Sodium bicarbonate reacts rapidly with gastric acid to form sodium chloride, carbon dioxide, and water. This agent's duration of action is shortened by its quick elimination from the stomach.[14] Of the magnesium salts, magnesium hydroxide is used most often. Magnesium hydroxide reacts rapidly with gastric acid to form magnesium chloride and water. This agent has a shorter duration of action than that of calcium carbonate and aluminum hydroxide. Calcium carbonate is a potent antacid that dissolves slowly in gastric acid to form calcium chloride, carbon dioxide, and water. This agent's onset of action is slower, but its duration of effect is longer than that of magnesium hydroxide or sodium bicarbonate. Aluminum hydroxide reacts with hydrochloric acid to form aluminum chloride and water. This agent has a slower onset and a longer duration than those of magnesium hydroxide. As a result of these reactions, a small but noticeable increase in intragastric pH occurs. Increasing the intragastric pH above 5 blocks the conversion of pepsin to pepsinogen.[14] Antacids also increase LES pressure.[1]

TABLE 13-4 Selected Nonprescription Antacid and Bismuth Products and Their Dosage Regimens

Trade Name	Primary Ingredients	Dosage (maximum daily dosage)
Adults/Children ≥12 Years		
Alka-Seltzer Heartburn	Sodium bicarbonate 1940 mg; anhydrous citric acid 1000 mg	Dissolve 2 tablets in 4 ounces of water every 4 hours as needed (8 tablets)
Alka-Seltzer Original	Sodium bicarbonate 1916 mg; anhydrous citric acid 1000 mg; aspirin 325 mg	Dissolve 2 tablets in 4 ounces of water every 4 hours as needed (8 tablets)
Gaviscon Regular Strength Liquid	Each 15 mL contains[a] aluminum hydroxide 95 mg; magnesium carbonate 358 mg	15–30 mL 4 times a day, after meals and at bedtime (120 mL)
Gelusil Tablets	Aluminum hydroxide 200 mg; magnesium hydroxide 200 mg; simethicone 25 mg	Chew 2–4 tablets; repeat hourly if symptoms return (12 tablets)
Mylanta Ultimate Strength Liquid	Each 5 mL contains aluminum hydroxide 500 mg; magnesium hydroxide 500 mg	10–20 mL between meals and at bedtime (45 mL)
Mylanta Supreme Liquid	Each 5 mL contains calcium carbonate 400 mg; magnesium hydroxide 135 mg	10–20 mL between meals and at bedtime (90 mL)
Pepto-Bismol Maximum Strength Liquid	Each 15 mL contains bismuth subsalicylate 525 mg	30 mL every 1 hour as required (4 doses or 120 mL)
Pepto-Bismol Original Liquid	Each 15 mL contains bismuth subsalicylate 262 mg	30 mL every 30 minutes to 1 hour as required (8 doses or 240 mL)
Rolaids Regular Strength Antacid Tablets	Calcium carbonate 550 mg; magnesium hydroxide 110 mg	Chew 2–4 tablets as symptoms occur (12 tablets)
Tums Extra Strength 750 Tablets	Calcium carbonate 750 mg	Chew 2–4 tablets as needed for symptoms (10 tablets)
Tums Regular Strength 500 Tablets	Calcium carbonate 500 mg	Chew 2–4 tablets as needed for symptoms (15 tablets)
Children ≤12 Years		
Maalox Children's Relief Chewable	Calcium carbonate 400 mg	*Age 2–5 years:* 1 tablet (3 tablets) *Age 6–11 years:* 2 tablets (6 tablets)
Children's Pepto	Calcium carbonate 400 mg	*Age 2–5 years:* 1 tablet (3 tablets) *Age 6–11 years:* 2 tablets (6 tablets)

[a] Sodium alginate (alginic acid) is listed as an inactive ingredient.

Compared with tablets, liquid antacids usually have a faster onset of action, because they are already dissolved or suspended and provide a maximal surface area for action. Of the tablet dosage forms, the quick-dissolving antacid tablets may provide the most rapid relief of symptoms. The duration of action for all antacids is transient, lasting only as long as the antacid remains in the stomach. The presence of food affects the duration of action of antacids. When administered on an empty stomach, relief can last from 20 to 60 minutes. When taken within 1 hour after a meal, antacids may remain in the stomach for up to 3 hours.[14]

Differences in efficacy, onset, duration, and adverse effects of antacids are determined primarily by the cation, specific salt, and potency. Antacid potency is based on the number of milliequivalents of *acid neutralizing capacity* (*ANC*), defined as the amount of acid buffered per dose over a specified period of time. Factors that contribute to the ANC include product formulation, ingredients, and concentration.[14] As a result, the ANC is product specific; the same number of antacid tablets or equal volumes of different liquid antacids are not necessarily equal in potency.

Most antacids are absorbed minimally into the systemic circulation.[14] Approximately 90% of calcium is converted to insoluble calcium salts; the remaining 10% is absorbed systemically. About 15%–30% of magnesium and 17%–30% of aluminum may be absorbed and then excreted renally; therefore, accumulation may occur in patients with renal insufficiency. Sodium bicarbonate is absorbed readily and is eliminated renally.

Antacids are indicated for the treatment of mild, infrequent heartburn, sour stomach, and acid indigestion. Combination products containing aspirin or acetaminophen are approved by the Food and Drug Administration (FDA) for overindulgence in food and drink and for hangover, although product effectiveness has not been demonstrated. Patients with mild dyspepsia may experience some relief with antacids, but no studies demonstrate their effectiveness for this disorder.[2]

Antacids are administered orally. The effective dose of an antacid varies depending on product ingredients, milliequivalents of ANC, formulation, and the frequency and severity of symptoms. Patients should be instructed to take product-specific recommended doses at the onset of symptoms. Dosing may be repeated in 1–2 hours, if needed, but should not exceed the maximum daily dosage for a particular product (Table 13–4). Patients should be reevaluated if antacids are used more than twice a week or regularly for more than 2 weeks. Frequent antacid users may need to be switched to a longer-acting product, such as an H2RA, an H2RA plus an antacid, or a PPI, or referred to their PCP.

Antacids usually are well tolerated. Adverse effects generally are associated with the cation. The most common adverse effect associated with magnesium-containing antacids is dose-related diarrhea. Diarrhea may be reduced by combining magnesium-containing antacids with aluminum hydroxide. However, when higher dosages of this combination are used, the predominating effect is diarrhea. Magnesium excretion is impaired in patients with renal disease and may result in systemic accumulation of magnesium. Magnesium-containing antacids should not be used in patients with a creatinine clearance of less than 30 mL/minute.[14]

Aluminum-containing antacids are associated with dose-related constipation. Aluminum hydroxide binds dietary phosphate in the GI tract, increasing phosphate excretion in the feces. Frequent and prolonged use of aluminum hydroxide may lead to hypophosphatemia.[14] Chronic use of aluminum-containing antacids in patients with renal failure may lead to aluminum toxicity and should be avoided.

Calcium carbonate may cause belching and flatulence as a result of carbon dioxide production. Constipation occurring during use of calcium antacids has been reported, but there is little evidence to support this adverse effect. Calcium stimulates gastric acid secretion and is hypothesized to cause increased acidity when calcium-containing antacids are used to treat acid-related disorders. The clinical importance of this finding, however, remains uncertain.[14] If renal elimination is impaired, hypercalcemia may occur, and accumulation of calcium may result in the formation of renal calculi. Because many antacids have been reformulated to contain calcium, there is a risk of hypercalcemia when high and frequent dosages of calcium-containing antacids are taken with other calcium supplements or foods such as milk or orange juice with added calcium. The upper limit for calcium intake for adults with normal renal function is 2500 mg/day for ages 19–50 years and 2000 mg/day for those 51 years and older.[15] (See Chapter 23 for a discussion of calcium supplementation.)

Sodium bicarbonate frequently causes belching and flatulence that result from the production of carbon dioxide.[14] The high sodium content (274 mg sodium/gram sodium bicarbonate) may cause fluid overload in patients with congestive heart failure, renal failure, cirrhosis, or pregnancy, and in those on sodium-restricted diets. Patients with normal renal function excrete additional bicarbonate, whereas patients with impaired renal function retain bicarbonate, which may cause systemic alkalosis. A high intake of calcium along with an alkalinizing agent (e.g., sodium bicarbonate, calcium carbonate) may lead to hypercalcemia, alkalosis, irritability, headache, nausea, vomiting, weakness, and malaise (milk–alkali syndrome).[14] Patients who take calcium supplements should avoid using sodium bicarbonate as an antacid. Further, in June 2016, FDA issued a drug safety warning about the risk of serious bleeding with antacid–aspirin products, specifically in the following patient groups:

- Patients 60 years of age or older
- Patients with a history of stomach ulcers or bleeding problems
- Patients using an anticoagulant (i.e., warfarin), systemic steroids, or NSAIDs
- Patients who consume at least 3 alcoholic beverages daily

Although labels for these products already contain warnings about this bleeding risk, FDA continues to receive reports of this safety issue.[16] Table 13–5 lists clinically significant drug–drug interactions.[17–23]

Alginic acid reacts with sodium bicarbonate in saliva to form a viscous layer of sodium alginate that floats on the surface of gastric contents, forming a protective barrier against esophageal irritation. Although alginic acid does not neutralize acid, the combination of alginic acid and antacid may provide better symptomatic relief than the antacid alone.[11] Because evidence supporting alginic acid's efficacy as a single agent is insufficient, FDA has not granted it Category I status. However, alginic acid may be found as an inactive ingredient in several antacid products (Table 13–4). Some antacid products contain simethicone to decrease discomfort related to intestinal gas. (See Chapter 14 for a more detailed description of simethicone.)

Histamine-2 Receptor Antagonists

Cimetidine, ranitidine, famotidine, and nizatidine are approved for nonprescription use (Table 13–6). Nonprescription products containing nizatidine currently are not available in the United States. When used in recommended dosages, the H2RAs are considered interchangeable despite minor differences in potency, onset, duration of symptomatic relief, and adverse effects. H2RAs decrease fasting and food-stimulated gastric acid secretion and gastric volume by inhibiting histamine on the histamine-2 receptor of the parietal cell.[24] Therefore, the H2RAs are effective in relieving fasting and

TABLE 13-5 **Clinically Important Drug–Drug Interactions With Nonprescription Heartburn and Dyspepsia Agents**

Antacid/Acid Reducer	Drug	Potential Interaction	Management/ Preventive Measures
Antacids	Itraconazole, ketoconazole, iron, indinavir, atazanavir	Increased gastric pH may decrease disintegration, dissolution, or ionization of drug leading to decreased absorption.	Separate doses by at least 2 hours.
Antacids	Amphetamines	Absorption of amphetamines is increased.	Separate doses by at least 2 hours.
Antacids	Enteric-coated medications	Increased gastric pH may cause premature breakdown of enteric coating.	Separate doses by at least 2 hours.
Calcium carbonate, magnesium hydroxide, aluminum hydroxide	Levothyroxine	Absorption of levothyroxine is delayed or impaired.	Separate doses by at least 4 hours.
Calcium carbonate, magnesium hydroxide, aluminum hydroxide	Tetracyclines	Absorption of antibiotic is decreased.	Separate doses by at least 4 hours.
Calcium carbonate, magnesium hydroxide, aluminum hydroxide	Fluoroquinolones	Absorption of antibiotic is decreased.	Take antibiotic 2 hours before or 6 hours after taking antacid.
Magnesium hydroxide, aluminum hydroxide	Azithromycin	Absorption of antibiotic is decreased.	Separate doses by at least 2 hours.
Aluminum hydroxide	Isoniazid	Absorption of isoniazid is decreased.	Take isoniazid at least 1 hour before taking antacid.
Sodium bicarbonate	Quinidine	Increased urinary pH may decrease renal excretion of quinidine.	Avoid concurrent use or monitor response to therapy.
Sodium bicarbonate	Salicylates	Increased urinary pH may increase renal excretion of salicylates.	Avoid concurrent use or monitor for decreased response to salicylates.
H2RAs	Nifedipine	Serum concentration of nifedipine is increased.	Monitor for increased effects of nifedipine.
H2RAs, PPIs	Itraconazole, ketoconazole, indinavir, atazanavir, iron sulfate, calcium carbonate	Increased gastric pH may decrease disintegration, dissolution, or ionization of drug leading to decreased absorption.	Avoid concurrent use or monitor response to therapy.
Cimetidine	Phenytoin, warfarin, amiodarone, clopidogrel, theophylline, tricyclic antidepressants, others	Cimetidine inhibits CYP450 3A4, 2D6, 1A2, and 2C9.	Avoid use of cimetidine in patients taking medications metabolized by these CYP enzymes.
PPIs	Diazepam, warfarin, phenytoin, theophylline, tacrolimus	PPI inhibition of CYP2C19 may result in increased concentrations of target drugs.	Avoid concurrent use or check with prescriber.
PPIs	Methotrexate	Concurrent use increases risk of toxicity of methotrexate.	Avoid concurrent use of high-dose methotrexate. Clinically significant toxicity is unlikely with lower weekly doses.
Omeprazole, esomeprazole	Clopidogrel	Inhibition of variants of CYP2C19 reduces conversion of clopidogrel to its active form.	Avoid concurrent use or check with prescriber.
Omeprazole, esomeprazole	Cilostazol	Inhibited metabolism of cilostazol results in increased serum concentration.	Avoid concurrent use. Lansoprazole may be a safer alternative.

Key: CYP = Cytochrome P450; H2RA = histamine-2 receptor antagonist; PPI = protein pump inhibitor.
Source: References 17–23.

TABLE 13-6 **Selected Nonprescription H2RA and PPI Products and Dosage Regimens**

Trade Name	Primary Ingredients	Dosage (maximum daily dosage)
H2RA Products (adults/children ≥12 Years)		
Tagamet HB, various generic	Cimetidine 200 mg	1 tablet with a glass of water (2 tablets)
Pepcid AC, various generic	Famotidine 10 mg	1 tablet with a glass of water (2 tablets)
Pepcid AC Maximum Strength, various generic	Famotidine 20 mg	1 tablet with a glass of water (2 tablets)
Pepcid Complete, various generic	Famotidine 10 mg; calcium carbonate 800 mg; magnesium hydroxide 165 mg	Chew and swallow 1 tablet (2 tablets)
Zantac 75, various generic	Ranitidine 75 mg	1 tablet with a glass of water (2 tablets)
Zantac 150, various generic	Ranitidine 150 mg	1 tablet with a glass of water (2 tablets)
PPI Products (adults ≥18 Years)		
Prilosec OTC, various generic	Omeprazole magnesium 20.6 mg	1 tablet with a glass of water 30 minutes before morning meal; take daily for 14 days (1 tablet)
Zegerid, various generic	Omeprazole 20 mg; sodium bicarbonate 1100 mg	1 capsule with a glass of water 1 hour before morning meal; take daily for 14 days (1 capsule)
Prevacid 24HR, various generic	Lansoprazole 15 mg	1 capsule with a glass of water 30 minutes before morning meal; take daily for 14 days (1 capsule)
Nexium 24HR	Esomeprazole 20 mg	1 capsule with a glass of water 30 minutes before morning meal; take daily for 14 days (1 capsule)

Key: H2RA = Histamine-2 receptor antagonist; PPI = protein pump inhibitor.

nocturnal symptoms. Their bioavailability is not affected by food but may be reduced modestly by antacids. Onset of symptomatic relief with H2RAs is not as rapid as that of antacids, but H2RAs have a longer duration of effect (Table 13–3). Cimetidine is the shortest acting (4–8 hours); ranitidine, famotidine, and nizatidine have a somewhat longer duration of effect. Tolerance to the gastric antisecretory effect may develop when H2RAs are taken daily (versus as needed) and may be responsible for diminished efficacy.[8] Therefore, it is preferable to take an H2RA on an as-needed basis rather than regularly every day. All four H2RAs are eliminated by a combination of renal and hepatic metabolism, with renal elimination being the most important. A reduced daily H2RA dose should be considered in patients with impaired renal function (creatinine clearance <50 mL/minute) and in patients of advanced age.[24]

Nonprescription H2RAs are indicated for the treatment of mild–moderate, infrequent, or episodic heartburn and for the prevention of heartburn associated with acid indigestion and sour stomach. H2RAs are more effective than placebo for relief of mild–moderate heartburn and provide moderate improvement in patients with mild, infrequent uninvestigated dyspepsia.[5] These agents may be used at the onset of symptoms or 30 minutes to 1 hour prior to an event (e.g., meal, exercise) in which heartburn is anticipated. The combination H2RA and antacid product (Pepcid Complete [famotidine plus magnesium hydroxide and calcium carbonate]; Table 13–6) is indicated for patients with postprandial heartburn who have not premedicated with an H2RA. This combination product provides immediate relief and a longer duration of effect. Self-treatment dosing should be limited to no more than 2 times a day. If self-treatment with an H2RA is needed for more than 2 weeks, a medical referral is recommended.

H2RAs are well tolerated and have a low incidence of adverse effects. The most common adverse effects reported with all four H2RAs include headache, diarrhea, constipation, dizziness, and drowsiness. Thrombocytopenia is a rare but serious adverse event associated with all four H2RAs, but this effect is reversible upon discontinuation of the drug. Cimetidine is associated with a weak antiandrogenic effect that, when taken in high doses, may result in decreased libido, impotence, or gynecomastia in men.

Table 13–5 lists drug–drug interactions for H2RAs.

Proton Pump Inhibitors

PPIs are potent antisecretory drugs that relieve heartburn and dyspepsia by decreasing gastric acid secretion. They inhibit hydrogen potassium ATPase (the proton pump), thereby irreversibly blocking the final step in gastric acid secretion and providing a more potent and prolonged antisecretory effect than that of the H2RAs (Table 13–3).[24] The relative bioavailability of PPIs increases with continued daily dosing. Onset of symptomatic relief following an oral dose may occur in 2–3 hours, but complete relief may take 1–4 days. The PPIs are almost completely absorbed after oral administration, regardless of the presence of food.[25]

Omeprazole magnesium 20.6 mg (Prilosec OTC), the first PPI to become available for nonprescription use in the United States (Table 13–6), is available as a delayed-release tablet containing enteric-coated pellets (protection against intragastric degradation) and rapidly dissociates to omeprazole 20 mg. Nonprescription omeprazole is also available as specific pharmacy-branded products. Immediate-release omeprazole (Zegerid) is formulated with omeprazole 20 mg and sodium bicarbonate 1100 mg. The sodium bicarbonate in Zegerid raises intragastric pH, permitting rapid absorption of omeprazole from the duodenum, but there is insufficient evidence to confirm that this action results in a quicker onset of symptomatic relief. Esomeprazole magnesium 22.3 mg (Nexium 24HR) is the S-isomer of omeprazole and is available as a delayed-release capsule. Lansoprazole 15 mg (Prevacid 24HR) is available as a capsule formulation containing enteric-coated granules. Differences in efficacy among the PPIs have not been established. PPI tablets and capsules should not be chewed or crushed, because the enteric coating will be compromised, thus decreasing the effectiveness of the drug.

Nonprescription PPIs are indicated for the treatment of frequent heartburn in patients who have symptoms 2 or more days a week. They are not intended for immediate relief of occasional or acute episodes of heartburn and dyspepsia. Because PPIs inhibit only those proton pumps that are actively secreting acid, they are most effective when taken 30–60 minutes before a meal, preferably before breakfast.[8,25] Self-treatment should be limited to 14 days and no more frequently than every 4 months. If heartburn continues while taking a nonprescription PPI, persists for more than 2 weeks, or recurs within 4 months, a medical evaluation is recommended.

The safety of nonprescription antisecretory medications, when used appropriately, is well established. The most common short-term adverse effects of PPIs are similar to those reported for the H2RAs (i.e., diarrhea, constipation, headache). Chronic acid suppression has the potential to impair natural defenses and to increase the risk of infection.[26–36] Some studies indicate PPI users may have increased susceptibility to community-acquired pneumonia, especially in the first month of therapy.[26] An association of PPI use with enteric infections, such as *Clostridium difficile* and bacterial gastroenteritis, has been shown to be statistically significant in a number of cohort and case-control studies. Patients developing diarrhea or symptoms of gastroenteritis while taking a PPI should stop its use and contact a health care provider (HCP).

An increased risk for hip, spine, and wrist fractures in older patients (>50 years) has been associated with high-dose, long-term (>1 year) PPI therapy.[31–33] Although reduced gastric acid secretion may decrease calcium absorption, longitudinal studies have not found any evidence of a direct effect of PPIs on bone turnover.[32] FDA released a warning concerning the potential for increased risk of fractures with prescription PPIs but subsequently determined that the risk is low with appropriate nonprescription PPI use.[33] Long-term use of PPIs has been correlated with an increase in risk for chronic kidney disease and dementia.[34–36] Rebound acid hypersecretion upon discontinuation of long-term use of PPIs has been reported, but its clinical importance is uncertain.[37] Vitamin B_{12} deficiency, hypomagnesemia, and iron malabsorption have also been described in patients taking PPIs long term (usually >1 year) but not in ambulatory patients taking recommended dosages of nonprescription PPIs short term.[27,28,38] Self-treatment with PPIs should be limited to short-term use at nonprescription doses. Nonprescription PPIs should be used to treat only conditions approved by FDA and listed on the Drug Facts label. Long-term use and ingestion of high doses of acid-suppressing medications should take place only under medical supervision. Table 13–5 lists important drug–drug interactions with PPIs.

Bismuth Subsalicylate

Bismuth subsalicylate (BSS) is indicated for heartburn, upset stomach, indigestion, nausea, and diarrhea. FDA has tentatively determined that BSS is safe and effective for the relief of upset stomach associated with belching and for gas associated with overindulgence in food and drink.[39] It is uncertain how BSS relieves heartburn, but for upset stomach, it is believed to have a topical effect on the stomach mucosa. When used to treat acid-related symptoms, the adult dose of BSS is 262–525 mg every 30 minutes to 1 hour as needed (Table 13–4). BSS is generally not recommended for children and should be avoided in patients with salicylate sensitivities or bleeding risks.[40] Because of the risk of Reye's syndrome, children and teenagers who have or are recovering from chickenpox or influenza-like symptoms should not use this medication.[41] (For a complete discussion of salicylate risk in children, see Chapter 5.) In the past, some nonprescription antacid product line extensions with common trade names were reformulated to contain BSS in place of an antacid, or vice versa. Patients and HCPs should examine the ingredients in an antacid product to determine whether it contains BSS, because these products are periodically reformulated with different antacids and other ingredients. Patients taking bismuth salts should know that bismuth may cause the stool and tongue to turn black. Dark-colored stools may be interpreted as an upper GI bleed, prompting needless medical procedures. (For a complete discussion of BSS, see Chapter 16.)

Product Selection Guidelines

Special Populations

Careful consideration should be given to older patients before recommending self-treatment for new-onset heartburn or dyspepsia. Older patients are more likely to take medications that can contribute to heartburn and dyspepsia. They are also at higher risk for developing complications and may have a more severe underlying disorder. PPIs were added to the 2015 Updated Beers Criteria for Potentially Inappropriate Use of Medications in Older Adults.[42] If self-treatment is appropriate, an assessment should be performed to determine if the patient has renal impairment and to identify potentially problematic medications. Patients with decreased renal function should be cautioned about using aluminum- and magnesium-containing antacids, and if an H2RA is appropriate, the lower dose should be selected. Cimetidine should be avoided because of increased risks for adverse effects and drug–drug interactions. Omeprazole, esomeprazole, and lansoprazole may be used in patients with renal impairment. Sodium bicarbonate should be avoided in patients taking cardiovascular medications.

Antacid selection for eligible patients should be based, in part, on potential adverse effects. For example, if a patient has a tendency toward constipation, a less constipating antacid, such as magnesium hydroxide, may be more appropriate, whereas constipating antacids, such as calcium carbonate, should be avoided.

Children older than 2 years with mild, transient, and infrequent heartburn; acid indigestion; or sour stomach may try children's formulas of calcium carbonate–containing antacids. If symptoms recur or are not resolved quickly, the child should be referred to his or her PCP for further evaluation.[43] Nonprescription antacids containing calcium carbonate are labeled for children ages 2 years and older. If antacids are recommended, an assessment of the child's average daily intake of calcium may help guide the recommendation. The recommended daily intake of calcium for children ages 2–3 years is 700 mg, 4–8 years is 1000 mg, and 9–18 years is 1300 mg.[15] Nonprescription H2RAs are labeled for patients ages 12 years and older, and nonprescription PPIs are indicated for patients ages 18 years or older.

Infrequent and mild heartburn in pregnant women should be treated initially with dietary and lifestyle modifications.[44] Calcium- and magnesium-containing antacids may be used safely if the recommended daily dosages are not exceeded. Special attention should be given to the recommended intake of calcium during pregnancy (1000–1300 mg/day).[15] If a woman is meeting this recommendation, the addition of a calcium-containing antacid may cause her to exceed the upper limit of 2500 mg of calcium per day. H2RAs are considered compatible with pregnancy. Data are limited but suggest there is no increased risk of congenital malformations.[45] Data for use of PPIs during pregnancy are limited. Epidemiologic studies of omeprazole do not demonstrate increased risk of major congenital malformations or other adverse pregnancy outcomes with first-trimester use.[46] The risk associated with lansoprazole also appears to be low.[45] Use of esomeprazole is best avoided because human data are lacking.[45]

(See the Preface for a detailed explanation of pregnancy data.) Pregnant women with frequent and moderate–severe heartburn should be referred for medical evaluation.

Aluminum-, calcium-, or magnesium-containing antacids are considered safe in women who are breastfeeding.[47] The American Academy of Pediatrics considers cimetidine to be compatible with breastfeeding. However, famotidine is less concentrated in the breast milk and may be preferable to cimetidine or ranitidine.[45] Information regarding the use of omeprazole, esomeprazole, and lansoprazole in women who are breastfeeding is insufficient; therefore, lactating patients should not use these medications.[45]

Patient Preferences

Antacids and antisecretory drugs are available in a wide range of prices, flavors, and dosage forms. Once the most appropriate nonprescription medication is determined, the patient should be involved in selecting a product that is affordable, palatable, and practical to administer. Inactive ingredients such as dyes, sodium, and sugar should be considered for patients with allergies, sensitivities, certain medical conditions, or dietary restrictions.

Complementary Therapies

No evidence has shown that any botanical products increase intragastric pH and relieve heartburn. However, peppermint, alone or in combination with other herbs, has been shown in some studies to be useful for dyspepsia. A study of the efficacy of artichoke leaf extract (ALE) for dyspepsia also showed greater improvement of symptoms in the ALE group than in the placebo group.[5] (See Chapter 51 for a more thorough discussion of natural products.)

Assessment of Heartburn and Dyspepsia: A Case-Based Approach

Cases 13–1 and 13–2 illustrate the assessment of patients with heartburn and dyspepsia.

CASE 13-1

Relevant Evaluation Criteria	Scenario/Model Outcome
Collect	
1. Gather essential information about the patient's symptoms and medical history, including	
a. Description of symptom(s) (i.e., nature, onset, duration, severity, associated symptoms)	Patient complains of recurring substernal burning sensation after eating large meals. It occurs 1–2 times a month. The discomfort is rated a 4 on a scale of 1–10 and is associated with a feeling of fullness and occasional burping. Symptoms typically last 3–4 hours after eating.
b. Description of any factors that seem to precipitate, exacerbate, and/or relieve the patient's symptom(s)	Symptoms occur after eating lunch or dinner and often are associated with large meals.
c. Description of the patient's efforts to relieve the symptoms	Patient has tried Alka Seltzer (sodium bicarbonate 1940 mg and citric acid 1000 mg) after meals to help relieve the symptoms. It works quickly but wears off within an hour, and she does not like the burping it causes.
d. Patient's identity	Sonya Majid
e. Patient's age, gender, height, and weight	45 years old, female, 5 ft 6 in., 156 lb
f. Patient's occupation	Writer
g. Patient's dietary habits	Normal balanced diet; drinks one cup of black tea every morning; does not drink alcohol.
h. Patient's sleep habits	Sleeps 7–8 hours a night.
i. Concurrent medical conditions, prescription and nonprescription medications, and dietary supplements	Hypothyroidism: levothyroxine 0.1 mg daily; anxiety/depression: paroxetine 20 mg every evening
j. Allergies	Codeine
k. History of other adverse reactions to medications	None
Assess	
2. Differentiate patient's signs/symptoms, and correctly identify the patient's primary problem(s).	Infrequent postprandial substernal burning is consistent with uncomplicated heartburn.
3. Identify exclusions for self-treatment (Figure 13–2).	None
4. Formulate a comprehensive list of therapeutic alternatives for the primary problem to determine whether triage to a medical provider is required, and share this information with the patient or caregiver.	Options include (1) Refer Sonya to her PCP. (2) Recommend lifestyle modifications. (3) Recommend an OTC antacid and/or acid-reducing product. (4) Take no action.

CASE 13-1 *continued*

Relevant Evaluation Criteria	Scenario/Model Outcome
Plan	
5. Select an optimal therapeutic alternative to address the patient's problem, taking into account patient preferences.	An OTC acid-reducing product should provide relief of symptoms for the desired duration, without undesirable adverse effects. Patient will consider lifestyle modifications.
6. Describe the recommended therapeutic approach to the patient or caregiver.	"Take 20 mg of famotidine 30 minutes prior to meals that may cause heartburn, or when symptoms occur." See directions in Table 13–6.
7. Explain to the patient or caregiver the rationale for selecting the recommended therapeutic approach from the considered therapeutic alternatives.	"Seeing a PCP may not be necessary if adequate relief is experienced and symptoms do not become more severe or frequent. An antacid will not provide long-lasting relief."
Implement	
8. When recommending self-care with nonprescription medications and/or nondrug therapy, convey accurate information to the patient or caregiver.	
a. Appropriate dose and frequency of administration	See Table 13–6.
b. Maximum number of days the therapy should be employed	See the box "Patient Education for Heartburn and Dyspepsia."
c. Product administration procedures	See Table 13–6.
d. Expected time to onset of relief	30 minutes to 1 hour if used after symptoms occur.
e. Degree of relief that can be reasonably expected	Complete prevention of symptoms if used prior to meals, or complete relief of symptoms if used after symptom onset.
f. Most common adverse effects	Adverse effects are uncommon. Some patients report headache, diarrhea, or constipation.
g. Adverse effects that warrant medical intervention should they occur	Moderate–severe diarrhea or symptoms of gastroenteritis
h. Patient options in the event that condition worsens or persists	A PCP should be consulted if symptoms are not resolved satisfactorily, if they increase in frequency or severity, or if alarm symptoms occur (Figure 13–2).
i. Product storage requirements	See the box "Patient Education for Heartburn and Dyspepsia."
j. Specific nondrug measures	"Eat smaller meals and avoid problematic foods. Consider ways to reduce weight." (See the box "Patient Education for Heartburn and Dyspepsia" for other measures.)
Solicit follow-up questions from the patient or caregiver.	"May I take an antacid for immediate relief of symptoms?"
Answer the patient's or caregiver's questions.	"Yes, taking a product that contains calcium carbonate or magnesium hydroxide after symptoms occur will provide quick, short-term relief. Antacids can be taken with famotidine, if needed. An alternative would be to take a combination product that contains both an antacid and an acid reducer."
Follow-up: Monitor and Evaluate	
9. Assess patient response.	Ask Sonya to call or update you on her response to the famotidine, or call Sonya in a week to evaluate her response.

Key: OTC = Over-the-counter; PCP = primary care provider.

CASE 13-2

Relevant Evaluation Criteria	Scenario/Model Outcome
Collect	
1. Gather essential information about the patient's symptoms and medical history, including	
a. Description of symptom(s) (i.e., nature, onset, duration, severity, associated symptoms)	Patient suffers from ongoing upper abdominal discomfort. Patient describes a gnawing pain that causes nausea and fluctuates throughout the day and night. Patient occasionally wakes up in the night with symptoms. Pain severity varies from 2–5 on a scale of 10. Symptoms started about 2 months ago.
b. Description of any factors that seem to precipitate, exacerbate, and/or relieve the patient's symptom(s)	Sometimes worse with food but not always.
c. Description of the patient's efforts to relieve the symptoms	Patient has tried Tums Extra Strength (calcium carbonate 750 mg) with some relief but symptoms return frequently.
d. Patient's identity	Connie Smith
e. Patient's age, gender, height, and weight	68 years old, female, 5 ft 3 in., 165 lb
f. Patient's occupation	Retired teacher
g. Patient's dietary habits	Eats small meals throughout the day.
h. Patient's sleep habits	Averages 6 hours per night.
i. Concurrent medical conditions, prescription and nonprescription medications, and dietary supplements	Osteoarthritis: meloxicam 15 mg daily; hypertension: lisinopril 20 mg daily; hyperlipidemia: atorvastatin 40 mg daily. Takes calcium carbonate 1000 mg with vitamin D 400 IU twice daily and aspirin 81 mg daily.
j. Allergies	NKDA
k. History of other adverse reactions to medications	None
l. Other (describe) _____	Has smoked 15–20 cigarettes/day for the past 50 years. Drinks 2–4 cups of caffeinated coffee daily. Drinks 1 glass of wine 4–5 days a week.
Assess	
2. Differentiate patient's signs/symptoms, and correctly identify the patient's primary problem(s).	Late-onset and ongoing GI symptoms; nocturnal symptoms. Not consistent with uncomplicated heartburn or uncomplicated dyspepsia.
3. Identify exclusions for self-treatment (Figure 13–2).	Nocturnal symptoms and onset after age 45 years indicate medical referral.
4. Formulate a comprehensive list of therapeutic alternatives for the primary problem to determine whether triage to a medical provider is required, and share this information with the patient or caregiver.	Options include (1) Refer Connie to a PCP for a differential diagnosis. (2) Recommend an OTC product with lifestyle modifications. (3) Take no action.
Plan	
5. Select an optimal therapeutic alternative to address the patient's problem, taking into account patient preferences.	Refer the patient to a PCP for a differential diagnosis.
6. Describe the recommended therapeutic approach to the patient or caregiver.	"Call your primary care provider for a medical evaluation."
7. Explain to the patient or caregiver the rationale for selecting the recommended therapeutic approach from the considered therapeutic alternatives.	"You need to see your primary care provider, because your symptoms indicate a more serious medical condition that needs evaluation. Your symptoms suggest a possible ulcer, and the meloxicam and aspirin you take could cause stomach ulcers. OTC therapy is unlikely to be effective or appropriate."

CASE 13-2 *continued*

Relevant Evaluation Criteria	Scenario/Model Outcome
Implement	
8. When recommending self-care with nonprescription medications and/or nondrug therapy, convey accurate information to the patient or caregiver.	Criterion does not apply in this case.
Solicit follow-up questions from the patient or caregiver.	"I thought ulcers would hurt all the time?"
Answer the patient's or caregiver's questions.	"Ulcer symptoms can fluctuate, may be worsened or improved with food, and can wake you up at night. Your PCP may suggest an endoscopic test to make a specific diagnosis."
Follow-up: Monitor and Evaluate	
9. Assess patient response.	Contact Connie in a day or two to ensure that she has contacted her PCP.

Key: GI = Gastrointestinal; NKDA = no known drug allergies; OTC = over-the-counter; PCP = primary care provider.

Patient Counseling for Heartburn and Dyspepsia

Many cases of uncomplicated heartburn and dyspepsia are self-treatable. For optimal outcomes, patients need to understand how to treat symptoms appropriately and when to seek additional care. This information is provided in the box "Patient Education for Heartburn and Dyspepsia." HCPs should screen patients for use of a prescription H2RA or PPI and counsel patients to avoid duplication of therapies.

Evaluation of Patient Outcomes for Heartburn and Dyspepsia

Patients with infrequent heartburn and dyspepsia should obtain symptomatic relief within 5 minutes when treated with an antacid or within 30–45 minutes when treated with an H2RA. Patients taking PPIs may require up to 4 days for complete relief of symptoms, but most patients are asymptomatic within 1 or 2 days. Self-treating patients should be encouraged to contact their PCP or pharmacist to report the effectiveness of therapy and any problems that may arise during treatment (e.g., adverse effects). In some cases, the provider may make a follow-up contact to assess therapeutic outcomes. Patients should be asked to describe the change in frequency and severity of symptoms that occurred after initiation of therapy. Patients should be questioned regarding adverse effects and any new symptoms that may have developed. If the patient reports an inadequate response to therapy, the patient should be reevaluated to determine whether a different therapy is suitable or whether medical referral is necessary. Adverse effects may be managed by adjusting the dose or switching to another product. Patients who develop atypical or alarm symptoms (Figure 13–2) should be referred to their PCP.

PATIENT EDUCATION FOR Heartburn and Dyspepsia

Heartburn and dyspepsia (indigestion) are often self-treatable conditions. Heartburn is characterized by a burning sensation in the chest, usually occurring after meals. Dyspepsia is characterized by discomfort in the upper abdomen. The goals of self-treatment are (1) to provide complete relief of symptoms, (2) to reduce recurrence of symptoms, and (3) to prevent and manage unwanted effects of medications.

Nondrug Measures

- Avoid food, beverages, and activities that may precipitate or increase the frequency and severity of symptoms.
- If possible, avoid the use of medications that may aggravate heartburn or dyspepsia.
- Avoid eating large meals.
- Stop or reduce smoking.
- Lose weight if overweight and not pregnant.
- Wear loose-fitting clothing.
- If nocturnal symptoms are present:
  - Avoid lying down within 3 hours of a meal.
  - Elevate the head of the bed using 6- to 8-inch blocks, or use a foam pillow wedge.

Nonprescription Medications

- Store all medications at 68°F–77°F (20°C–25°C), and protect them from heat, humidity, and moisture. Discard after expiration date.

Antacids

- Antacids (sodium bicarbonate, calcium carbonate, magnesium hydroxide, and aluminum hydroxide) are available alone and in combination with each other and other ingredients.
- Antacids work by neutralizing acid in the stomach.
- Antacids may be used for relief of mild, infrequent heartburn or dyspepsia (indigestion).
- Antacids are usually taken at the onset of symptoms. Relief of symptoms typically begins within 5 minutes.
- Because antacids come in a variety of strengths and concentrations, it is essential to consult the label of an individual product for the correct dose and frequency of administration. Generally antacids should not be used more than 4 times a day, or regularly for more than 2 weeks.
- If symptoms are not relieved with recommended dosages, consult a health care provider.

PATIENT EDUCATION FOR Heartburn and Dyspepsia *(continued)*

- Diarrhea may occur with magnesium- or magnesium/aluminum–containing antacids; constipation may occur with aluminum- or calcium-containing antacids. Consult a health care provider if these effects are troublesome or do not resolve in a few days.
- In children older than 2 years, mild transient and infrequent heartburn; acid indigestion; or sour stomach may be treated with children's products containing calcium carbonate if they are used according to package directions.
- Pregnant women with mild and infrequent heartburn may use calcium- and magnesium-containing antacids safely if recommended daily dosages are not exceeded.
- Patients with kidney dysfunction should consult their primary care provider prior to self-treatment with antacids.
- Patients taking tetracyclines, fluoroquinolones, azithromycin, ketoconazole, itraconazole, iron supplements, or levothyroxine should not take antacids with these medications. (See Table 13–5 for specific information on drug–drug interactions with antacids.)

Histamine-2 Receptor Antagonists (H2RAs)

- H2RAs (cimetidine, famotidine, and ranitidine) may be used to relieve symptoms of or prevent heartburn and indigestion associated with meals.
- H2RAs work by decreasing acid production in the stomach.
- H2RAs are usually taken at the onset of symptoms or 30 minutes to 1 hour before symptoms are expected. Relief of symptoms can be expected to begin within 30–45 minutes after the medication is taken. A combination product that contains both an antacid and an H2RA provides faster relief of symptoms.
- H2RAs generally relieve symptoms for 4–10 hours.
- H2RAs can be taken when needed, up to twice daily for 2 weeks.
- H2RAs should be used for relief of mild–moderate, infrequent, and episodic heartburn and indigestion when a longer effect is needed. Use lower dosages for mild infrequent heartburn and higher dosages for moderate infrequent symptoms.
- If symptoms are not relieved with recommended doses, worsen, or persist after 2 weeks of treatment, consult a primary care provider.
- Adverse effects are uncommon. Consult a health care provider if adverse effects are troublesome or do not resolve within a few days.
- Cimetidine may interact with many medications. Consult a health care provider if you are also taking other medications, including theophylline, amiodarone, a blood thinner such as warfarin or clopidogrel, an antifungal such as ketoconazole, an anticonvulsant such as phenytoin, or an antianxiety medication such as diazepam.

Proton Pump Inhibitors (PPIs)

- Nonprescription PPIs are indicated for mild–moderate frequent heartburn that occurs 2 or more days a week. They are not intended for the relief of mild, occasional heartburn.
- PPIs (omeprazole, esomeprazole, and lansoprazole) work by decreasing acid production in the stomach.
- PPIs should be taken with a glass of water every morning 30 minutes before breakfast for 14 days. Make sure that you take the full 14-day course of treatment.
- Do not take more than 1 tablet a day.
- Complete resolution of symptoms should be noted within 4 days of initiating treatment.
- If symptoms persist, worsen, are not adequately relieved after 2 weeks of treatment, or recur before 4 months has elapsed since treatment, consult your primary care provider.
- Do not crush or chew tablets or capsules because this may decrease the effectiveness of the PPI.
- Adverse effects are uncommon. Consult a health care provider if adverse effects are troublesome or do not resolve within a few days.
- Consult a health care provider if you are also taking other medications, including a blood thinner such as warfarin or clopidogrel, an antifungal such as ketoconazole, an anticonvulsant such as phenytoin, an antianxiety medication such as diazepam, antiretroviral medications, methotrexate, theophylline, tacrolimus, digoxin, or cilostazol.

When to Seek Medical Attention

- Consult your primary care provider if you experience any of the following:
  - Heartburn or dyspepsia (indigestion) that lasts for more than 3 months
  - Heartburn or dyspepsia (indigestion) that occurs with recommended dosages of nonprescription medications
  - Heartburn or dyspepsia (indigestion) that occurs after 2 weeks of continuous treatment with a nonprescription medication
  - Heartburn that awakens you during the night
  - Difficulty or pain on swallowing foods
  - Light-headedness, sweating, and dizziness accompanied by black tarry bowel movements or vomiting of blood or black material
  - Chest pain or shoulder, arm, or neck pain, with shortness of breath
  - Chronic hoarseness, cough, choking, or wheezing
  - Unexplained weight loss
  - Continuous nausea, vomiting, or diarrhea
  - Severe stomach pain

Key Points for Heartburn and Dyspepsia

- ➤ The self-treatment of heartburn and dyspepsia should be limited to mild or moderate symptoms, including postprandial burning in the upper abdomen or centralized abdominal discomfort.
- ➤ Patients with atypical or alarm symptoms (Figure 13–2) should be referred for further evaluation.
- ➤ In children older than 2 years, treatment of mild transient and infrequent heartburn, acid indigestion, or sour stomach symptoms with calcium carbonate–containing antacids should be limited. Prompt referral should be made if symptoms recur or persist.
- ➤ Pregnant women may self-treat mild and infrequent heartburn with calcium- and magnesium-containing antacids.
- ➤ Patients with heartburn should be counseled on nondrug measures, such as the dietary and lifestyle modifications listed in the box "Patient Education for Heartburn and Dyspepsia."
- ➤ Self-treating patients should be advised about the advantages and disadvantages of various antacids and acid-reducing products so they can select a product that is best suited for their needs.
- ➤ Antacids provide temporary relief for mild and infrequent heartburn and dyspepsia. Dosages are product specific because of variability in antacid ingredients and concentrations.

- H2RAs are indicated for mild and infrequent heartburn or dyspepsia. They may be taken at the onset of symptoms or 1 hour prior to an event (e.g., meal, exercise) that may cause symptoms.
- Combining an antacid with an H2RA provides immediate relief of heartburn and a longer duration of action.
- PPIs are indicated for treatment of frequent heartburn (heartburn that occurs ≥2 days a week). PPIs should be used a maximum of 14 days at a time and no more than every 4 months. They are not intended for immediate relief of infrequent symptoms.
- Patients with self-treatable symptoms should be advised to contact their PCP if symptoms worsen or recur after 14 days of effective self-treatment.

REFERENCES

1. Richter JE, Friedenberg FK. Gastroesophageal reflux disease. In: Feldman M, Friedman LS, Brandt LJ, eds. *Sleisenger and Fordtran's Gastrointestinal and Liver Disease.* 9th ed. Philadelphia, PA: Saunders; 2010:705–26.
2. Tack J. Dyspepsia. In: Feldman M, Friedman LS, Brandt LJ, eds. *Sleisenger and Fordtran's Gastrointestinal and Liver Disease.* 9th ed. Philadelphia, PA: Saunders; 2010:183–95.
3. Peery AF, Dellon ES, Lund J, et al. Burden of gastrointestinal disease in the United States: 2012 update. *Gastroenterology.* 2012;143(5):1179–87. doi: 10.1053/j.gastro.2012.08.002.
4. Fujiwara Y, Arakawa T, Fass R. Gastroesophageal reflux disease and sleep disturbances. *J Gastroenterol.* 2012;47(7):760–9. doi: 10.1007/s00535-012-0601-4.
5. Lacy BE, Talley NJ, Locke GR, et al. Review article: current treatment options and management of functional dyspepsia. *Aliment Pharmacol Ther.* 2012;36(1):3–15. doi: 10.1111/j.1365-2036.2012.05128.x.
6. DeVault KR. Symptoms of esophageal disease. In: Feldman M, Friedman LS, Brandt LJ, eds. *Sleisenger and Fordtran's Gastrointestinal and Liver Disease.* 9th ed. Philadelphia, PA: Saunders; 2010:173–81.
7. Ness-Jensen E, Hveem K, El-Serag H, et al. Lifestyle intervention in gastroesophageal reflux disease. *Clin Gastroenterol Hepatol.* 2016;14:175–82. doi: 10.1016/j.cgh.2015.04.176.
8. Katz PO, Gerson LB, Vela MF. Guidelines for the diagnosis and management of gastroesophageal reflux disease. *Am J Gastroenterol.* 2013; 108(3):308–28. doi: 10.1038/ajg.2012.444.
9. Hom C, Vaezi M. Extraesophageal manifestations of gastroesophageal reflux disease. *Gastroenterol Clin N Am.* 2013;42(1):71–91. doi: 10.1016/j.gtc.2012.11.004.
10. Giannini EG, Zentilin P, Dulbecco P, et al. A comparison between sodium alginate and magaldrate anhydrous in the treatment of patients with gastroesophageal reflux symptoms. *Dig Dis Sci.* 2006;51(11):1904–9. doi: 10.1007/s10620-006-9284-0.
11. Kwiatek MA, Roman S, Fareeduddin A, et al. An alginate formulation can eliminate or displace the postprandial "acid pocket" in symptomatic GERD patients. *Aliment Pharmacol Ther.* 2011;34(1):59–66. doi: 10.1111/j.1365-2036.2011.04678.x.
12. Boardman HF, Heeley G. The role of the pharmacist in the selection and use of over-the-counter proton-pump inhibitors. *Int J Clin Pharm.* 2015;37:709–16. doi: 10.1007/s11096-015-0150-z.
13. Prilosec OTC [product monograph]. Proctor and Gamble, Cincinnati, OH. 2016. Available at: http://www.prilosecotc.com/en-us/hcp/prilosec-otc-dosage. Accessed May 1, 2017.
14. Maton PN, Burton ME. Antacids revisited: a review of their clinical pharmacology and recommended therapeutic use. *Drugs.* 1999;57(6):855–70. PMID: 10400401.
15. National Institutes of Health, Office of Dietary Supplements. Dietary supplement fact sheet: calcium. February 11, 2016. Available at: http://dietary-supplements.info.nih.gov/factsheets/calcium.asp. Accessed May 1, 2017.
16. U.S. Food and Drug Administration. FDA Drug Safety Communication: FDA warns about serious bleeding risk with over-the-counter antacid products containing aspirin. Available at: http://www.fda.gov/Drugs/DrugSafety/ucm504328.htm. Accessed May 16, 2017.
17. Ogawa R, Echizen H. Clinically significant drug interactions with antacids. *Drugs.* 2011;71(14):1839–64. doi: 10.2165/11593990-000000000-00000.
18. Plavix (clopidogrel bisulfate tablets) [package insert]. Bridgewater, NJ: Bristol-Myers Squibb/Sanofi Pharmaceuticals Partnership. July 2015. Available at: http://packageinserts.bms.com/pi/pi_plavix.pdf. Accessed May 1, 2017.
19. Fulco PP, Vora UB, Bearman GM. Acid suppressive therapy and the effects on protease inhibitors. *Ann Pharmacother.* 2006;40(11):1974–83. doi: 10.1345/aph.1H022.
20. Frelinger AL 3rd, Lee RD, Mulford DJ, et al. A randomized, 2-period, crossover design study to assess the effects of dexlansoprazole, lansoprazole, esomeprazole, and omeprazole on the steady-state pharmacokinetics and pharmacodynamics of clopidogrel in healthy volunteers. *J Am Coll Cardiol.* 2012;59(14):1304–11. doi: 10.1016/j.jacc.2011.12.024.
21. Suri A, Bramer SL. Effect of omeprazole on the metabolism of cilostazol. *Clin Pharmacokinet.* 1999;37(Suppl 2):53–9. PMID: 10702887.
22. Bezabeh S, Mackey AC, Kluetz P, et al. Accumulating evidence for a drug–drug interaction between methotrexate and proton pump inhibitors. *Oncologist.* 2012;17(4):550–4. doi: 10.1634/theoncologist.2011-0431.
23. Santucci R, Leveque D, Lescoute A, et al. Delayed elimination of methotrexate associated with co-administration of proton pump inhibitors. *Anticancer Research.* 2010;30(9):3807–10.
24. May DB, Rao SSC. Gastroesophageal reflux disease. In Dipiro JT, Talbert RL Yee GC, et al., eds. *Pharmacotherapy: A Pathophysiologic Approach.* 9th ed. New York, NY: McGraw-Hill; 2014:455–70.
25. Hatlebakk JG, Katz PO, Camacho-Lobato L, et al. Proton pump inhibitors: better acid suppression when taken before a meal than without a meal. *Aliment Pharmacol Ther.* 2000;14(10):1267–72. PMID: 11012470.
26. Lambert AA, Lam JO, Paik JJ, et al. Risk of community-acquired pneumonia with outpatient proton-pump inhibitor therapy: a systematic review and meta-analysis. *PLoS ONE.* 2015:10(6):e0128004. doi: 10.1371/journal.pone.0128004.
27. Heidelbaugh JJ, Goldberg KL, Inadomi JM. Overutilization of proton pump inhibitors: a review of cost-effectiveness and risk. *Am J Gastroenterol.* 2009;104(Suppl 2):S27–32. doi: 10.1038/ajg.2009.49.
28. Parikh N, Howden CW. The safety of drugs used in acid-related disorders and functional gastrointestinal disorders. *Gastroenterol Clin North Am.* 2010;39(3):529–42. doi: 10.1016/j.gtc.2010.08.009.
29. Janarthanan S, Ditah I, Adler DG, et al. *Clostridium difficile* associated diarrhea and proton pump inhibitor therapy: a meta-analysis. *Am J Gastroenterol.* 2012;107(7):1001–10. doi: 10.1038/ajg.2012.179.
30. Kwok CS, Arthur AK, Anibueze CI, et al. Risk of *Clostridium difficile* infection with acid suppressing drugs and antibiotics: meta-analysis. *Am J Gastroenterol.* 2012;107(7):1011–9. doi: 10.1038/ajg.2012.108.
31. Gray SL, LaCroix AZ, Larson J, et al. Proton pump inhibitor use, hip fracture, and change in bone mineral density in postmenopausal women: results from the Women's Health Initiative. *Arch Intern Med.* 2010;170(9): 765–71. doi: 10.1001/archinternmed.2010.94.
32. Targownik LI, Lix LM, Leung S, et al. Proton pump inhibitor use is not associated with osteoporosis or accelerated bone mineral density loss. *Gastroenterology.* 2010;138(3):896–904. doi: 10.1053/j.gastro.2009.11.014.
33. U.S. Food and Drug Administration. FDA drug safety communication: possible increased risk of fractures of the hip, wrist and spine with use of proton pump inhibitors. Updated March 23, 2011. Available at: http://www.fda.gov/Drugs/DrugSafety/PostmarketDrugSafetyInformationforPatientsandProviders/ucm213206.htm. Accessed May 1, 2017.
34. Gomm W, von Holt K, Thome F, et al. Association of proton pump inhibitors with risk of dementia: a pharmacoepidemiological claims data analysis. *JAMA Neurol.* 2016;73:410–16. doi: 10.1001/jamaneurol.2015.4791.
35. Lazarus B, Chen Y, Wilson FP, et al. Proton pump inhibitor use and the risk of chronic kidney disease. *JAMA Intern Med.* 2016;176:238–46. doi: 10.1001/jamainternmed.2015.7193.
36. Xie Y, Bowe B, Li T et al. Long-term kidney outcomes among users of proton pump inhibitors without intervening acute kidney injury. *Kidney Int.* 2017;91(6):1482–94. PMID: 28237709.

37. Reimer C, Sondergaard B, Hilsted L, et al. Proton-pump inhibitor therapy induces acid-related symptoms in healthy volunteers after withdrawal of therapy. *Gastroenterology.* 2009;137(1):80–7. doi: 10.1053/j.gastro.2009.03.058.
38. U.S. Food and Drug Administration. FDA drug safety communication: low magnesium levels can be associated with long-term use of proton pump inhibitor drugs (PPIs). March 2, 2011. Available at: http://www.fda.gov/Drugs/DrugSafety/ucm245011.htm. Accessed May 1, 2017.
39. U.S. Food and Drug Administration. Orally administered drug products for relief of symptoms associated with overindulgence in food and drink for over-the-counter human use. Proposed amendment of the tentative final monograph. *Fed Regist.* 2005;70:741–2.
40. Bismuth subsalicylate. Micromedex® Solutions. Greenwood Village, CO: Truven Health Analytics. Available at: http://www.micromedexsolutions.com. Accessed May 1, 2017.
41. U.S. Food and Drug Administration. Labeling of drug preparations containing salicylates. *CFR: Code of Federal Regulations.* Title 21, Part 201, Section 201.314. Updated July 27, 2017. Available at: http://www.ecfr.gov/cgi-bin/text-idx?SID=b1b2224711dc88657752be21f12c574a&mc=true&node=se21.4.201_1314&rgn=div8. Accessed July 31, 2017.
42. American Geriatrics Society 2015 Beers Criteria Update Expert Panel. American Geriatrics Society 2015 updated Beers criteria for potentially inappropriate medication use in older adults. *J Am Geriatr Soc.* 2015;63(11):2227–46. doi: 10.1111/jgs.13702.
43. Hegeland H, Flagstad G, Grotta J, et al. Diagnosing pediatric functional abdominal pain in children (4–15 years old) according to the Rome III Criteria: results from a Norwegian prospective study. *J Pediatr Gastroenterol Nutr.* 2009;49(3):309–15. doi: 10.1097/MPG.0b013e31818de3ab.
44. Phupong V, Hanprasertpong T. Interventions for heartburn in pregnancy. *Cochrane Database Syst Rev.* 2015;9:CD011379. doi: 10.1002/14651858.CD011379.pub2.
45. Briggs GG, Freeman RK. *Drugs in Pregnancy and Lactation.* 10th ed. Philadelphia, PA: Wolters Kluwer Health; 2015.
46. Prilosec® (omeprazole) [package insert]. Wilmington, DE: AstraZeneca LP; 2016.
47. Antacids, oral. LactMed. Bethesda, MD: U.S. National Library of Medicine. Updated September 7, 2013. Available at: http://toxnet.nlm.nih.gov/cgi-bin/sis/htmlgen?LACT. Accessed May 1, 2017.

CHAPTER 14

INTESTINAL GAS

JENNIFER ROBINSON

Intestinal gas–related symptoms and conditions that predispose patients to intestinal gas formation are common, and they may cause considerable discomfort and lifestyle impairment. The most frequent clinical manifestations are *eructation* (belching of swallowed air), *bloating* (uncomfortable fullness, often with abdominal distention, particularly after eating), and *flatulence* (excessive passage of air from the stomach or intestines through the anus). Differentiation of healthy individuals with temporary symptoms from those with a chronic gastrointestinal (GI) disorder or condition such as irritable bowel syndrome (IBS), lactose intolerance, or celiac disease is important in recommending appropriate nonprescription treatment.

The primary categories of nonprescription pharmacologic therapies for intestinal gas symptoms are antiflatulence medications (simethicone, activated charcoal), digestive enzymes (lactase replacement, and α-galactosidase products), and probiotic products (*Bifidobacterium, Lactobacillus, Saccharomyces, Streptococcus thermophiles and other species*).

A significant proportion of the U.S. population is affected by conditions that may be associated with intestinal gas symptoms. Intestinal gas can be caused by lactose malabsorption (affecting 29% of the population), IBS (5%–15%), and other, less common medical conditions such as celiac disease (1%–3% of the general population and 10% of first-degree relatives of the celiac disease population) and pancreatic insufficiency (<1%).[1–4] In the general population, abdominal distention and bloating are reported by approximately 10% and 20% of individuals, respectively, in the United States. More than one-half of symptomatic respondents rated symptoms as moderate–severe; most indicated that symptoms resulted in some limitation in their ability to conduct usual activities, with 10% reporting a reduction in number and/or frequency of such activities by one-half or greater.[5]

Pathophysiology of Intestinal Gas

The pathophysiology of intestinal gas—in this context, gas-related complaints in the GI tract—is poorly understood; however, minor disruptions of normal physiologic processes or bacterial flora of the GI tract appear to play a role. Each time food, liquid, or saliva is swallowed, a small amount of air passes into the stomach. Once in the stomach, swallowed food is mixed with gastric acid, pepsin, and other substances and then churned into small fragments; the resulting liquid–air slurry is then emptied into the small intestine, where most of the absorption of vitamins, minerals, and digestion products (e.g., food-derived monosaccharides, such as glucose) occurs.[6] The rate at which the stomach empties varies, but this process generally takes approximately 1–2 hours. Smooth muscle contractions in the small intestine move the liquid food fragments and air downstream toward the large intestine, where the indigestible liquid waste is mixed with the bacterial flora of the colon. In the colon, most of the remaining liquid is absorbed from a mixture of liquid waste, bacteria, and intestinal gas as it is transported toward the rectum and temporarily stored as stool before a bowel movement occurs. During a bowel movement, stool is eliminated, and intestinal gas is expelled from the rectum as flatus.

Diet, underlying medical conditions, genetics, alterations in intestinal flora, and drugs may precipitate or aggravate symptoms attributable to intestinal gas. Although the exact mechanisms are not fully known, the origin of gas retention and symptoms appears to be affected by alterations in visceral sensitivity and intestinal transit that vary at different physiologic locations along the GI tract.[6]

Certain foods can increase intestinal gas production, leading to bothersome symptoms.[7,8] Dietary sugars (e.g., lactose in dairy products and prepared foods; fructose in fruits, vegetables, candies, soft drinks; sucrose from "table sugar"; glucose from the breakdown of starches) may be incompletely absorbed in the healthy human small intestine. These sugars are the principal substrates for hydrogen gas (H_2) production in the colon. Similarly, other foods can be malabsorbed, including fatty foods; foods rich in complex carbohydrates (e.g., wheat germ, brown rice, bran, corn); and indigestible oligosaccharides (e.g., raffinose, found in asparagus, broccoli, brussels sprouts, cabbage; stachyose, found in black-eyed peas, lima beans, soybeans). These substances remain in the intestinal lumen and are passed into the colon, where they provide a substrate for bacterial fermentation and colonic production of H_2, carbon dioxide (CO_2), and methane (CH_4).[5] Fermentation in the colon is the primary process for generating intestinal gas and is influenced by the type and quantity of foods ingested (Tables 14–1 and 14–2).

Diets high in fiber may lead to bloating and flatulence. With respect to diet and nutrition terminology, recommended intake, and potential benefits associated with fiber are discussed in Chapter 24. Fiber is a valuable component of a balanced diet and may be beneficial in the treatment of constipation (see Chapter 15) and the maintenance of healthy intestinal flora.[9] Soluble fiber absorbs water and stabilizes intestinal contractions; however, soluble fiber supplementation does not appear to decrease GI symptoms.[10] Patients who experience adverse GI effects (bloating, flatulence) from natural fiber preparations (e.g., psyllium) may prefer a soluble semisynthetic fiber supplement (e.g., calcium polycarbophil).[10]

TABLE 14–1 Gas-Producing Foods

Foods Associated With Minimal Gas Production

- Meats: fowl, fish
- Vegetables: lettuce, peppers, avocado, tomato, asparagus, zucchini, okra, olives
- Fruit: cantaloupe, grapes, berries, fruit juice
- Carbohydrates: refined white sugar and flour
- Other: all nuts, eggs, gelatin

Foods Associated With Moderate Gas Production

- Fruits: citrus, apples
- Carbohydrates: refined white sugar and refined white flour

Foods Associated With Major Gas Production

- Vegetables: onions, celery, carrots, brussels sprouts, cucumbers, cabbage, cauliflower, radishes, leeks, parsnips, peas, green salads, beans, potatoes, eggplant
- Fruit: raisins, bananas, apricots, prunes, dried fruit
- Carbohydrates: whole grains, wheat germ, bran, brown rice
- Dairy products: milk, ice cream, cheese (in patients who have trouble digesting lactose; check food labels of processed foods for added lactose or milk-derived ingredients)
- Other: carbonated beverages

Source: References 7 and 8.

The odor attributable to flatulence may be worsened by the ingestion of sulfate-containing foods, such as cruciferous vegetables (e.g., broccoli, cabbage); breads and beers containing sulfate additives; and proteins with a high content of the sulfur-containing amino acids methionine and cysteine (e.g., eggs, macadamia nuts, peanuts, pistachio nuts, red meats). Sulfur-based gases (e.g., hydrogen sulfide [H_2S]), methanethiol, and dimethyl sulfide are produced through the action of sulfate-reducing bacteria.[11] Rating foods by their potential to cause intestinal gas symptoms is difficult, but clinical experience suggests that certain foods are generally more problematic than others (Table 14–1).

Gas-related signs and symptoms may be associated with intake of an excessive amount of air into the upper GI tract with swallowing. Smoking, chewing gum, sucking on hard candies, drinking carbonated beverages, wearing poor-fitting dentures, hyperventilating, or being overly anxious may cause an individual to swallow larger-than-normal amounts of air.[11] Poor eating habits (e.g., gulping food, drinking beverages too rapidly) may cause larger amounts of air to enter the stomach.

A number of medical conditions cause or predispose patients to the formation of intestinal gas. Some conditions (e.g., carbohydrate malabsorption, pancreatic insufficiency) lead to production of an increased amount of gas from bacterial fermentation in the colon. The most common cause of carbohydrate malabsorption is lactase deficiency. Lactase is the enzyme that normally breaks down lactose in the intestinal lumen so that it can be absorbed. Physiologic lactase enzyme activity peaks at birth and starts to decline after the first few months of life as infants are slowly weaned from their mother's milk. The exception to this rule is a genetic modification called *lactase persistence trait* that can be found in descendants of populations that traditionally practice the domestication of cattle. The lactase persistence trait is correlated with the ability to digest and break down lactose-containing foods well beyond infancy. This trait is commonly found in individuals with Northern European ancestry (>90%) and less commonly in descendants of African (5%–20%) or Asian populations (1%).[12] Individuals who lack the lactase persistence trait commonly have a lactase deficiency and experience symptoms of lactose intolerance after consuming dairy products. Approximately 50 million people in the United States are lactose maldigesters and experience symptoms of lactose intolerance on ingestion of dairy products.

In patients with lactase deficiency, the lactase enzyme is not available in sufficient quantities to break down lactose in dairy products before it reaches the colon. In the colon, the malabsorbed lactose remains in the intestinal lumen, where it is available to colonic bacteria for fermentation to H_2 and other substances. Individuals with lactase deficiency experience GI symptoms (e.g., gas pains, bloating, nausea, diarrhea) with exposure to dairy and other foods containing milk or milk-derived carbohydrates (e.g., caramel).[13] Milk-derived protein (e.g., whey powder, caseinate and other lactoproteins) does not cause lactose-associated GI symptoms unless the product is contaminated with a milk-derived carbohydrate (i.e., lactose).

To decrease the risk for development of low bone density and osteoporosis secondary to reduced dietary intake of calcium, patients should be counseled to supplement their diet to achieve the recommended daily intake of 1000–1200 mg of elemental calcium.[14]

Bacterial fermentation in the small intestine resulting from bacterial overgrowth may lead to excessive amounts of intestinal gas. The effects of probiotics on bloating symptoms associated with small bowel bacterial overgrowth and lactose intolerance are uncertain. Research suggests that probiotics help curtail bloating associated with lactose intolerance by producing lactic acid, which improves lactose digestion.[15]

Other conditions such as IBS may predispose affected patients to intestinal gas symptoms. Gas pains and bloating are very common in patients with IBS and may be caused by a number of interrelated factors, including heightened sensation of the GI tract to intestinal stretch (i.e., visceral hypersensitivity), altered intestinal motility, activated intestinal immunity, altered brain–gut interaction, and

TABLE 14–2 Oligosaccharide-Containing Foods Associated With Intestinal Gas Production With Potential Treatment Benefit From α-Galactosidase

Vegetables

Beets
Broccoli
Brussels sprouts
Cabbage
Cauliflower
Corn
Cucumbers
Leeks
Lettuce
Onions
Parsley
Peppers, sweet

Beans

Black-eyed peas
Bog beans
Broad beans
Chickpeas
Lentils
Lima beans
Mung beans
Pinto beans
Red kidney beans

Grains

Barley
Oat bran
Rice bran
Rye
Sorghum grain
Wheat bran
Whole wheat flour

Other

Soy products (soy milk, tofu)
Seed flour (sesame, sunflower)

Source: References 7 and 8.

autonomic dysfunction.[12] Small bowel bacterial overgrowth has been proposed as a unifying theory linking these factors, which has stimulated promising research that aims to further define the relationship between intestinal bacterial overgrowth and the onset of IBS symptoms.[12] Probiotic bacteria (e.g., lactobacilli, saccharomycetes, bifidobacteria) are part of the normal "healthy" flora of the intestinal tract. They are thought to maintain intestinal health through a variety of mechanisms, including shifting the intestinal bacterial content in favor of nonpathologic organisms; producing beneficial substances (e.g., short-chain fatty acids); and acting primarily as carbohydrate-fermenting bacteria, thereby reducing symptoms of intestinal gas (see Chapter 20). Substances such as oligofructose (a "prebiotic") are used as nutrients by the normal intestinal bacterial flora and by probiotic organisms; with use of prebiotics, however, the normal flora produces greater amounts of CO_2, CH_4, and H_2, which may result in increased symptoms of intestinal gas.[5,10]

Intestinal gas symptoms may result from other, less common medical conditions such as celiac disease and diabetic gastroparesis. Patients with celiac disease have an intolerance to gluten (a protein present in wheat, rye, barley, and oats). Intestinal gas symptoms may result from the inflammatory response that occurs in the GI tract after exposure to gluten. Once a diagnosis of celiac disease has been made, and after gluten intolerance has been confirmed with accurate testing, affected patients should follow a strict gluten-free diet, preferably under the supervision of an experienced dietitian.[1] The most common sources of gluten are baked goods containing the causative grains (wheat and oat cereals, noodles, and pastas); however, many other food products (especially processed foods containing thickeners) and some medications contain gluten. Successful adherence to a gluten-free diet requires rigorous label reading, and close scrutiny of the gluten content of foods and prescription and nonprescription medications. In addition, referral to a registered dietitian is encouraged, because *all* gluten must be removed from the diet to avoid symptoms. A number of valuable resources are available for individuals seeking information about celiac disease.[16,17]

A variety of drugs may cause intestinal gas symptoms. These drugs can be categorized broadly by the mechanism of action leading to symptoms caused by physiologic changes: drugs that affect intestinal flora (lactulose, antibiotics); drugs that affect metabolism of glucose and other dietary substances (α-glucosidase inhibitors, including acarbose and miglitol; the biguanides, including metformin); and GI lipase inhibitors (orlistat). Drugs that affect GI motility (narcotics, anticholinergics, calcium channel blockers); drugs that are high in fiber (psyllium) or nonabsorbable polymers (cholestyramine); and drugs that contain or release gas (effervescent solutions such as Alka-Seltzer) may cause intestinal gas symptoms.

Clinical Presentation of Intestinal Gas

Patients with symptoms of intestinal gas complain most commonly of excessive belching, abdominal discomfort or cramping, bloating, and flatulence. Complaints of gas pains and belching are more common than complaints of flatulence. Other, less common symptoms associated with "gaseousness" are nausea; audible bowel sounds (called borborygmi); and dyspepsia or indigestion.

Everyone experiences *belching* ("burping"), especially after eating and drinking. Belching is the easiest way for air to leave the stomach after it is swallowed. Some people experience excessive belching, which may be annoying or embarrassing because of its frequency, intensity, and/or unexpected occurrence. The more frequently a person swallows, the greater the potential for air to enter the stomach. Drinking carbonated beverages or eating food too quickly is an easy way to increase the amount of air that is swallowed inadvertently, which may then cause excessive belching.

Gas pains often are described as a generalized, crampy discomfort associated with gaseousness. Passing gas or having a bowel movement may relieve gas pains. In some patients, symptoms may be brought on by stress or anxiety. In others, the size of a meal may affect onset and severity of gas pains, with larger meals causing more bothersome symptoms. Patients who complain of recurrent gas pains (occurring at least 3 days per month in a 3-month period) that are associated with either diarrhea or constipation may have IBS.[4] Because gas pains can mimic symptoms of other conditions (e.g., biliary colic [and other diseases of the gallbladder and biliary tract], diabetic gastroparesis, peptic ulcer disease, intestinal obstruction, neoplastic disease, pancreatic insufficiency, heart disease), a qualified health care provider should be consulted before initiation of self-management. Patients should be referred to a primary care provider if they are experiencing new-onset, persistent, or frequent and/or severe symptoms. Owing to an increased risk of colorectal cancer after the age of 40 years, patients presenting with new or recurrent gas pains should be referred to their primary care provider. In such cases, the symptoms may be related to an undiagnosed condition, and self-management at that point would be inappropriate. In addition, patients should be referred to a primary care provider for medical evaluation if any of the exclusion criteria for self-management are present (Figure 14–1).

Bloating may be characterized as a sensation of tension or fullness in the abdominal area after eating or as a subjective sensation that the abdomen is larger than normal. Patients with bloating may observe that clothes fit more tightly or are difficult to fit into comfortably. Eating certain foods (especially foods high in fiber) (Tables 14–1 and 14–2), drinking carbonated beverages, eating too rapidly, or eating too much may contribute to bloating. As with chronic gas pains, chronic bloating accompanied by a change in bowel function is suggestive of IBS. Patients with diabetes who complain that their bloating symptoms are accompanied by a sensation of early satiety or fullness after the ingestion of only a small amount of food may be experiencing diabetic gastroparesis and should be referred to their primary care provider.

Most patients who complain of excessive *flatulence* are referring to the unpleasant, uncontrollable, or frequent passage of intestinal gas through the rectum. Passing gas is normal and occurs either consciously or unconsciously between 20 and 40 times a day, even during sleep. Certain foods (especially those that contain fiber, fructose, lactose, or oligosaccharides) (Tables 14–1 and 14–2) are more likely to cause gaseousness, thereby contributing to flatulence. Sorbitol or mannitol from commonly used sweeteners in low-calorie foods and liquid medications can also contribute to flatulence.

Treatment for Intestinal Gas

Treatment Goals

The goals of therapy are (1) to reduce the frequency, intensity, and duration of intestinal gas symptoms and (2) to reduce the impact of intestinal gas symptoms on a patient's lifestyle. Because intestinal gas production is normal and necessary for normal GI function, the complete elimination of intestinal gas is not a realistic or attainable goal.

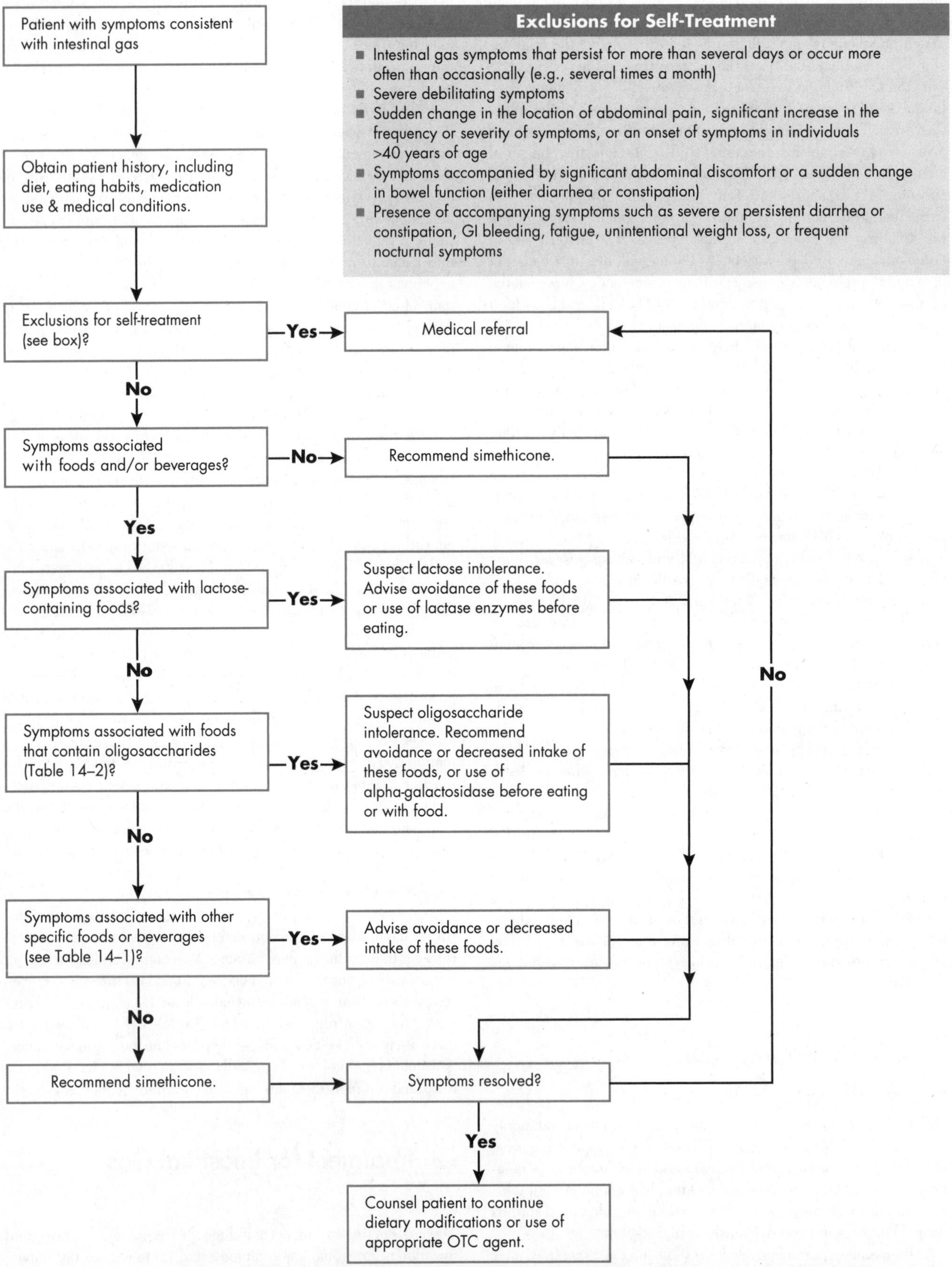
Patient with symptoms consistent with intestinal gas
Exclusions for Self-Treatment
Intestinal gas symptoms that persist for more than several days or occur more often than occasionally (e.g., several times a month)
Severe debilitating symptoms
Sudden change in the location of abdominal pain, significant increase in the frequency or severity of symptoms, or an onset of symptoms in individuals >40 years of age
Symptoms accompanied by significant abdominal discomfort or a sudden change in bowel function (either diarrhea or constipation)
Presence of accompanying symptoms such as severe or persistent diarrhea or constipation, GI bleeding, fatigue, unintentional weight loss, or frequent nocturnal symptoms
Obtain patient history, including diet, eating habits, medication use & medical conditions.
Exclusions for self-treatment (see box)?
Yes
Medical referral
No
Symptoms associated with foods and/or beverages?
No
Recommend simethicone.
Yes
Symptoms associated with lactose-containing foods?
Yes
Suspect lactose intolerance. Advise avoidance of these foods or use of lactase enzymes before eating.
No
Symptoms associated with foods that contain oligosaccharides (Table 14–2)?
Yes
Suspect oligosaccharide intolerance. Recommend avoidance or decreased intake of these foods, or use of alpha-galactosidase before eating or with food.
No
Symptoms associated with other specific foods or beverages (see Table 14–1)?
Yes
Advise avoidance or decreased intake of these foods.
No
Recommend simethicone.
Symptoms resolved?
No
Yes
Counsel patient to continue dietary modifications or use of appropriate OTC agent.

FIGURE 14–1 Self-care for intestinal gas symptoms. Key: GI = Gastrointestinal; OTC = over-the-counter.

General Treatment Approach

Self-treatment for intestinal gas symptoms should begin with an assessment of the patient's history and severity of symptoms, diet, eating habits, medication use, and relevant medical conditions. Most patients will be able to control their symptoms if they understand how the symptoms occur, follow steps to reduce predisposing factors, and make informed decisions regarding the use of nonprescription medications. Identification of the underlying cause of intestinal gas will guide treatment decisions (Figure 14–1). Inquiry into the patient's diet (including a review of the patient's eating habits and the frequency, amount, and type of food and beverages ingested) often can lead to non–drug therapy–based suggestions for reducing the problem. Symptoms that are related to eating habits or diet often will subside quickly once the source of the problem is identified and the necessary changes are made.

Patients for whom symptoms are associated with ingestion of foods containing lactose or oligosaccharides and who have no exclusions for self-treatment (Figure 14–1) may use digestive enzymes (e.g., lactase replacement or alpha-galactosidase products). Although several nonprescription antiflatulence products are available (e.g., activated charcoal, simethicone), their use is largely empirical, and evidence supporting a beneficial effect is limited.

Probiotics (see Chapter 20) maintain GI tract health by protecting against pathologic GI flora; they may be useful for some individuals with intestinal gas complaints.[18] No consensus exists on whether probiotics or prebiotics are beneficial in patients with lactose intolerance or chronic abdominal bloating. Increasing evidence, however, suggests that probiotics may be beneficial for treatment of intestinal gas symptoms in patients with IBS because these agents have favorable effects on the bacterial content of the small intestine and colon.[15,18] The benefit of probiotics may potentially be linked to specific bacterial strains. More research is needed to identify the true value of individual probiotic products.

Exclusions for self-treatment (Figure 14–1) should be reviewed with the patient before recommendation of any therapy. Referral to a primary care provider for further evaluation should be considered for patients with exclusions for self-treatment and for patients whose symptoms persist after initiating simple treatment options (e.g., dietary modification, nonprescription medications).

Nonpharmacologic Therapy

General information for controlling intestinal gas symptoms is provided in Table 14–3.[19] Patients may benefit from changes in eating habits and changes in diet. Reducing the consumption of gas-producing foods (Tables 14–1 and 14–2) may be appropriate, depending on the patient's history. Some people are unable to tolerate gas-producing foods and need to completely avoid such foods. Patients with lactose intolerance either should avoid milk and dairy products or should use lactase replacement products. Low-lactose milk products (e.g., Lactaid Milk, Dairy Ease Milk), fortified soy milk, almond milk, or rice milk products may be used as milk substitutes. Low-lactose milk is a prehydrolyzed milk product (i.e., lactose is already hydrolyzed) and contains the same nutrients as in regular milk, but the product is not entirely lactose-free. Soy milk, almond milk, and rice milk products are lactose-free milk alternatives that are low in fat and may be fortified to include calcium and vitamin D. Similarly, patients who are unable to tolerate foods with a high oligosaccharide content should attempt to reduce their consumption or to remove such foods from the diet.

An understanding of common food choices people make from different cultures, ethnicities, and socioeconomic backgrounds can lead to improved identification of dietary patterns known to contribute to intestinal gas symptoms. This knowledge may allow health care providers to identify and explain, in a culturally sensitive manner, why problematic gas-forming foods are not appropriate options for all patients. Addressing dietary issues with family members may be a better approach for developing healthy eating habits over time, especially for children experiencing intestinal gas symptoms.

TABLE 14-3 Useful Information to Support Patient Self-Management of Intestinal Gas Symptoms

Eating Habit Suggestions

- Avoid the temptation to rush through a meal. Eat and drink slowly in a calm environment.
- Chew food thoroughly.
- Avoid "washing down" solids with a beverage.
- Avoid gulping and sipping liquids, drinking out of small-mouthed bottles or straws, or drinking from water fountains.
- Eliminate pipe, cigar, and cigarette smoking.
- Avoid chewing gum and sucking hard candy, especially those that contain artificial sweeteners (e.g., sorbitol, mannitol).
- Check dentures for proper fit.
- Attempt to be aware of and avoid deep sighing.
- Do not attempt to induce belching or strain to pass gas.
- Do not overload the stomach at any one meal.

Diet

- Keep a food journal for a few days while tracking intestinal gas symptoms.
- Avoid gas-producing foods (Table 14–1).
- Avoid foods with air whipped into them (e.g., whipped cream, soufflés, sponge cake, milkshakes).
- Avoid carbonated beverages (e.g., sodas, beer).
- Avoid caffeinated beverages (e.g., coffee, energy drinks).

Medication Use and Lifestyle Habits

- Avoid long-term or frequent intermittent use of medications intended for relief of cold and allergy symptoms (e.g., anticholinergic antihistamines such as brompheniramine, chlorpheniramine, doxylamine, and diphenhydramine).
- Avoid or minimize the use of drugs affecting GI motility (narcotics and calcium channel blockers).
- Avoid or minimize the use of drugs affecting glucose metabolism (orlistat; α-glucosidase inhibitors, including acarbose and miglitol; and the biguanides, including metformin).
- Avoid or minimize the use of drugs that affect the intestinal flora (lactulose and antibiotics).
- Avoid or gradually increase intake of food or medications that are high in fiber (psyllium).
- Avoid nonabsorbable polymers (cholestyramine).
- Avoid medications that contain or release gas (e.g., Alka-Seltzer).
- Avoid tight-fitting garments, girdles, and belts.
- Do not lie down or sit in a slumped position immediately after eating.
- Develop a regular routine of exercise and rest.

Source: References 7, 8, 19, and Mayo Clinic. Bloating, belching and intestinal gas: how to avoid them. Available at: http://www.mayoclinic.org/diseases-conditions/gas-and-gas-pains/in-depth/gas-and-gas-pains/art-20044739. Accessed June 2, 2017.

Pharmacologic Therapy

Simethicone and activated charcoal may relieve symptoms after intestinal gas has formed. α-Galactosidase and lactase enzymes are taken with foods to prevent gas from forming. Lactase replacement products may be beneficial for reducing intestinal gas and diarrhea associated with lactose intolerance; they are used as digestive aids, allowing individuals with lactose intolerance to incorporate dairy foods into the diet without experiencing intolerable symptoms. Most lactose maldigesters can tolerate some milk (up to 1 cup at a time, so use of these products should be individualized according to the patient's symptoms.

Simethicone

Simethicone (a mixture of inert silicon polymers) is used as a defoaming agent to relieve gas. Simethicone acts in the stomach and intestine to reduce the surface tension of gas bubbles that are embedded in the mucus of the GI tract. As surface tension changes, the gas bubbles are broken or coalesced and then eliminated more easily by belching or passing gas through the rectum.

The U.S. Food and Drug Administration (FDA) considers simethicone to be safe and effective as an antiflatulence agent. In patients with acute, nonspecific diarrhea, the combination of simethicone with loperamide produced quicker relief from gas-related discomfort than either agent alone.[20] However, simethicone's ability to reduce intestinal gas symptoms for all patients with symptoms is questionable.[21] The use of simethicone on a trial basis may be encouraged, because some patients report benefit. The usual adult and pediatric dosages for simethicone are provided in Table 14–4.

Many antacid products contain a combination of simethicone and antacids; therefore, patients should follow the label instructions for dosages of these products. Use of both agents often is unnecessary, however, and the efficacy of such combination products has not been well studied. Furthermore, single-ingredient antiflatulent products (Table 14–5) usually contain a higher concentration of simethicone than that in the combination products. Because simethicone is not absorbed from the GI tract, it has no known systemic adverse effects; its safety has been well documented. Of note, however, simethicone is contraindicated in patients with a known hypersensitivity to simethicone products or with suspected intestinal perforation and obstruction.

Activated Charcoal

Activated charcoal is promoted for relief of intestinal gas; however, it is neither approved nor shown to be effective for this indication.[22] The usual adult dosages for this agent are provided in Table 14–4. The proposed antiflatulent properties of activated charcoal are related to the adsorbent effects of the substance and its potential to facilitate the elimination of intestinal gas from the GI tract. Activated charcoal has been purported to be beneficial for the elimination of malodorous, sulfur-based gases.[22] However, activated charcoal has poor palatability. External devices containing activated charcoal are available to reduce the odor of flatus in patients with ostomies (see Chapter 22).

α-Galactosidase

Another FDA-approved product for use as an antiflatulent is the enzyme α-galactosidase. This enzyme, which is derived from the *Aspergillus niger* mold, hydrolyzes oligosaccharides into their component parts before they can be metabolized by colonic bacteria. α-Glucosidase products are classified as a food. The usual adult and pediatric dosages for this enzyme preparation are provided in Table 14–4.

Because high-fiber foods contain large amounts of oligosaccharides, α-galactosidase is recommended as a prophylactic treatment for intestinal gas produced by high-fiber diets or foods that contain oligosaccharides (Table 14–2). A randomized, double-blind, placebo-controlled trial of α-galactosidase demonstrated that the agent significantly reduced symptoms of intestinal gas in healthy individuals fed oligosaccharide-containing foods.[23]

The safety of α-galactosidase remains to be determined. Although this enzyme has been used in food processing for years and is regarded as safe by FDA, the amount contained in available pharmacologic products is much greater than that in processed foods. Because the enzyme produces galactose, it should not be used by patients with *galactosemia* (an inherited metabolic disorder in which galactose accumulates in the blood because of deficiency of an enzyme that catalyzes conversion of galactose into glucose).

TABLE 14–4 Dosage Guidelines for Products for Self-Management of Intestinal Gas

	Dosage			
Agent	**Adults**	**Children >12 Years**	**Children 2 to ≤12 Years**	**Children <2 Years**
Simethicone	40–125 mg orally after meals and at bedtime, as needed	40–125 mg 4 times daily	40–50 mg 4 times daily	20 mg 4 times daily, as needed
Activated charcoal	500–520 mg orally after meals, as needed; may repeat hourly	Specific guidelines not available	Specific guidelines not available	Specific guidelines not available
α-Galactosidase	300–450 units orally per serving of food	Specific guidelines not available	Specific guidelines not available	Specific guidelines not available
Lactase enzyme	3000–18,000 units orally at first bite of food or drink containing lactose	3000–18,000 units at first bite of food or drink containing lactose	Specific guidelines not available	Specific guidelines not available
Probiotics	Specific guidelines not available	Specific guidelines not available	Specific guidelines not available	Specific guidelines not available

TABLE 14–5 **Selected Antiflatulent Products**

Trade Name	Primary Ingredients
Single-Entity Simethicone Products	
Gas-X Regular Strength Chewable Tablets	Simethicone 80 mg
Gas-X Extra Strength Chewable Tablets	Simethicone 125 mg
Mylanta Gas Maximum Strength Chewable Tablets	Simethicone 125 mg
Gas-X Extra Strength Softgel	Simethicone 125 mg
Gas-X Thin Strips	Simethicone 62.5 mg per edible film strip
Little Remedies for Tummys Gas Relief Drops	Simethicone 40 mg/0.6 mL
Activated Charcoal Products	
Charcoal Plus DS Tablets	Activated charcoal 250 mg
CharcoCaps Capsules	Activated charcoal 260 mg
α-Galactosidase Replacement Products	
Beano Tablets	α-Galactosidase 150 units (1 tablet)
Beano Meltaways Tablets	α-Galactosidase 300 units (1 tablet)
Lactase Replacement Products	
Lactaid Original Strength Caplets	Lactase enzyme 3000 units
Lactaid Chewable Tablets	Lactase enzyme 4500 units
Lactase Fast Act Chewable Tablets	Lactase enzyme 9000 units
Lac-Dose Tablets	Lactase enzyme 3000 units
α-Galactosidase and Lactase Replacement Combo Products	
Beano + Dairy Defense Tablets	α-Galactosidase 300 units + lactase enzyme 9000 units (1 tablet)
Probiotic Products	
Activia Probiotic Yogurt	*Lactobacillus bulgaricus; Streptococcus thermophilus; Bifidobacterium animalis* DN173010 (1×10^8 live bacteria per gram)
Align Digestive Care Probiotic Supplement Capsules	*Bifidobacterium infantis* 35624 (4 mg = 1×10^9 live bacteria)
Culturelle Digestive Health Capsules	*Lactobacillus rhamnosus* (1×10^{10} live bacteria per capsule)
Culturelle Kids Tablets	*Lactobacillus rhamnosus* (2.5×10^9 live bacteria per tablet)
DanActive Probiotic Dairy Drink	*Lactobacillus bulgaricus; Streptococcus thermophilus; Lactobacillus casei* DN-114 001 (1×10^{10} live bacteria per 93 mL)
FloraQ	*Lactobacillus acidophilus; Bifidobacterium; Lactobacillus paracasei; Streptococcus thermophilus* 230 mg (an aggregate with a minimum of 8×10^9 freeze-dried bacteria)
Florastor	*Saccharomyces boulardi* freeze-dried capsules 250 mg
Florastor Kids Granules	*Saccharomyces boulardi* freeze-dried oral granules 250 mg

As noted, α-galactosidase is derived from mold, so allergic reactions are possible in patients allergic to molds.

Lactase Replacement Products

Lactase replacement products are used in patients with lactose intolerance (see Chapter 16). Lactase enzymes break down lactose, a disaccharide, into the monosaccharides glucose and galactose, which are absorbed. Lactase replacement products should be used in patients with lactose intolerance to aid in the digestion of dairy products. No adverse effects are listed for lactase replacement products. The usual adult dose for lactase enzymes is provided in Table 14–4.

Product Selection Guidelines

Special Populations

Several pediatric formulations of simethicone are indicated for the relief of intestinal gas. These products, which contain simethicone 40 mg per 0.6 mL suspension formulation, often are promoted and used to relieve gas associated with colic. However, simethicone has not been found to be superior to placebo for intestinal gas and/or infantile colic.[21] Although its efficacy is questionable, simethicone is not absorbed from the GI tract, and it is considered safe for use in infants and children. No reports linking simethicone to congenital defects have been published to date.[21] Simethicone is considered to be safe for use by nursing mothers.

Safety and efficacy of α-galactosidase products have not been evaluated in infants. However, a small, 52-patient randomized study in children 4–17 years of age found these products to be safe and effective. A large research study would be needed to confirm this result.[23] This product should not be used in pediatric patients younger than 4 years of age but may be safely used in older children. Manufacturers recommend that pregnant or nursing patients consult their primary care provider before using α-galactosidase.

No special population considerations are listed for lactase replacement products. Patients should consult their primary care provider if symptoms continue after using a lactase replacement product, or if symptoms are unusual and seem unrelated to eating dairy products.

Patient Factors

α-Galactosidase and lactase replacement products are used to prevent the onset of symptoms in patients unable to tolerate problematic foods. Patients with gas symptoms who need immediate relief and patients who cannot correlate their symptoms with ingestion of certain foods should use simethicone. Activated charcoal may be an alternative to simethicone for patients with gas symptoms, and it may be beneficial for patients who experience malodorous gas production. Because α-galactosidase produces carbohydrates, patients with galactosemia should avoid its use, and patients with diabetes should consult a health care provider before self-treatment. Patients with lactase maldigestion who experience symptoms of lactose intolerance should consider taking lactase replacement products at the time of exposure to dairy products.

Patient Preferences

Most products for self-management of intestinal gas are available in a variety of strengths and dosage forms. A liquid formulation of simethicone is available for infants. (See Chapter 11, section "Special Populations," for FDA requirements for dispensing devices included in liquid nonprescription products.) Simethicone is available as chewable tablets, softgels, edible filmstrip, and liquid drops. Liquid dosage forms and alternative solid dosage forms are generally more expensive than standard solid oral dosage forms (e.g., tablets, capsules) but may be preferable. Activated charcoal is available in two solid oral dosage forms—tablets and capsules—and in a combination product with simethicone.

α-Galactosidase is available as tablets and as meltaway tablets. No difference in effectiveness between dosage forms has been found, so the choice between dosage forms is left entirely to personal preference and convenience.

Several dosage forms of lactase replacement products are available for patients with lactose intolerance. Some products can be added to milk or dairy products to reduce the amount of lactose in the product, or they can be ingested along with dairy products in an effort to reduce the amount of lactose produced when the food is consumed. Additionally, patients may elect to switch to one of the available milk alternatives (e.g., low-lactose milk, fortified soy milk, almond milk, rice milk).

Complementary Therapies

A variety of probiotic and dietary supplements may be used for GI complaints, including intestinal gas and bloating.[18] The most common formulations for intestinal gas (Table 14–5) are single-bacterium capsules (e.g., *Bifidobacterium infantis*) and capsules containing multiple bacteria (e.g., a combination of *Lactobacillus acidophilus, Lactobacillus paracasei, Lactobacillus rhamnosus, Bifidobacterium,* and *Streptococcus thermophilus*). Functional fermented food products with live active cultures of probiotic species (e.g., kombucha tea, kefir products) are available. In patients with IBS and those with lactose intolerance, limited but increasing evidence suggests that specific probiotics provide temporary relief from GI symptoms.[18] Probiotic bacteria leave the intestine soon after therapy is discontinued. With use of probiotic therapy, daily administration is required to maintain bacterial populations in the intestinal flora. A trial of 14 days is generally recommended for patients embarking on a probiotic regimen. Research shows that probiotics are effective in reducing the incidence of antibiotic-associated diarrhea. More studies are required to identify the probiotic strains that are most efficacious for patients receiving specific antibiotics.[24] (For more information on probiotics, see Chapter 20.)

Herbal carminatives (e.g., fennel, Japanese mint, peppermint, spearmint) are also commonly used for self-management of intestinal gas symptoms.[25] Despite insufficient evidence, these agents are widely used for self-treatment of intestinal gas and IBS.[25,26] Carminatives may reduce the tone of the lower esophageal sphincter and should be minimized or avoided by patients with gastroesophageal reflux disease (see Chapter 13); however, the effect of carminatives on lower esophageal sphincter tone in healthy individuals with intestinal gas symptoms may be less problematic.[27] Fennel can cause photodermatitis, is contraindicated during pregnancy, and enters breast milk in lactating women. If fennel is used, patients should be advised to avoid excessive sunlight and to avoid use during pregnancy and lactation. In addition, coadministration of fennel with ciprofloxacin may lead to reduced ciprofloxacin levels through a chelation mechanism, so doses should be spaced appropriately in patients using both agents.[28]

Assessment of Intestinal Gas Complaints: A Case-Based Approach

When a patient complains of intestinal gas, it is important to try to discern any contributing factors and the duration, severity, and frequency of symptoms (Table 14–6). Behaviors and products that produce relief may provide clues to the underlying cause. A thorough review to identify dietary habits, existing medical problems, and use of prescription and nonprescription medications may provide other clues.

Cases 14–1 and 14–2 are examples of the assessment of two different patients with intestinal gas complaints.

Patient Counseling for Intestinal Gas

Patient counseling is important to ensure the appropriate selection and use of nonprescription medications for self-management of intestinal gas. Patients should be encouraged to keep a food journal in an effort to identify those that are problematic. Avoidance of foods or other substances that cause intestinal gas is the best advice to give patients. The health care provider should explain the proper use of medications for intestinal gas and should warn the patient about possible adverse effects. The box "Patient Education for Intestinal Gas" contains specific information to include in patient counseling.

TABLE 14-6 Differentiation of Intestinal Gas Discomfort and Irritable Bowel Syndrome

Criterion	Intestinal Gas Discomfort	Irritable Bowel Syndrome
Location	Generalized discomfort in the upper, mid-, or lower abdomen	Generalized discomfort, bloating, and/or pain in the lower abdomen or colon
Signs	Eructation (upper abdomen): belching of air; bloating (mid-abdomen): increased abdominal girth; flatulence (lower abdomen, colon): excessive air or other gas in the stomach and intestines	No physical signs of disease; no fever, melena, hematochezia, or signs of other gastrointestinal disorders
Symptoms	Sensation of accumulated intestinal gas; may manifest as minimal physical discomfort but with significant negative psychosocial effects	Vary widely but are commonly described as abdominal pain that is relieved after a bowel movement, is accompanied by either diarrhea or constipation, and usually lasts at least 3 months
Onset	May begin at any age	Begins in early adulthood or, rarely, after the age of 60 years
Etiology	Symptoms commonly believed to be caused by an excessive amount of gas in the stomach (leading to eructation) and intestines (with bloating or flatulence); other causes include lactase deficiency, overgrowth of intestinal bacteria, and excessive air swallowing (aerophagia).	Unknown May result from altered gastrointestinal motility, heightened visceral sensitivity, and/or overgrowth of intestinal bacteria
Exacerbating factors	Diet; underlying medical conditions; and certain drugs (e.g., lactulose, antibiotics, α-glucosidase inhibitors, orlistat, narcotics, anticholinergics, calcium channel blockers, psyllium or cholestyramine, effervescent solutions)	Stress; overeating; problem foods (e.g., alcohol, chocolate, caffeinated beverages, dairy products, sugar-free products that contain sorbitol or mannitol); foods high in fat
Modifying factors	Minimization of exacerbating factors	Minimization of exacerbating factors; primary care provider evaluation and treatment
Location	Generalized discomfort in the upper, mid-, or lower abdomen	Generalized discomfort, bloating, and/or pain in the lower abdomen or colon
Signs	Eructation (upper abdomen): belching of air; bloating (mid abdomen): increased abdominal girth; flatulence (lower abdomen, colon): excessive air or other gas in the stomach and intestines	No physical signs of disease; no fever, melena, hematochezia, or signs of other gastrointestinal disorders
Symptoms	Sensation of accumulated intestinal gas; may manifest as minimal physical discomfort but with significant negative psychosocial effects	Vary widely but commonly described as abdominal pain that is relieved after a bowel movement, is accompanied by either diarrhea or constipation, and usually lasts at least 3 months
Onset	May begin at any age	Begins in early adulthood or, rarely, after the age of 60 years
Etiology	Symptoms commonly believed to be caused by an excessive amount of gas in the stomach (eructation) and intestines (bloating, flatulence); other causes include lactase deficiency, overgrowth of intestinal bacteria, and excessive air swallowing (aerophagia)	Unknown May result from altered gastrointestinal motility, heightened visceral sensitivity, and/or overgrowth of intestinal bacteria
Exacerbating factors	Diet; underlying medical conditions; and certain drugs (e.g., lactulose, antibiotics, α-glucosidase inhibitors, orlistat, narcotics, anticholinergics, calcium channel blockers, psyllium or cholestyramine, effervescent solutions)	Stress; overeating; problem foods (e.g., alcohol, chocolate, caffeinated beverages, dairy products, sugar-free products that contain sorbitol or mannitol); foods high in fat
Modifying factors	Minimization of exacerbating factors	Minimization of exacerbating factors; primary care provider evaluation and treatment

Evaluation of Patient Outcomes for Intestinal Gas

Many patients with intestinal gas have mild–moderate distress, and the discomfort is generally self-limiting, with resolution within 24 hours. Mild–moderate gas and bloating are managed primarily with diet modification, and some relief may be obtained with symptomatic drug therapy. With effective treatment, the patient can expect reduced intensity and duration of gas-related signs and symptoms such as belching, abdominal pain, bloating, and flatulence. Patients who achieve symptomatic relief should be advised to continue self-care measures as needed.

The provider should ask the patient to return or call after 1 week of self-treatment with dietary measures, nonprescription antiflatulents, or digestive enzymes so that outcomes can be assessed. Medical referral is necessary if any of the following occurs before or during treatment:

- Intestinal gas symptoms that are bothersome and or occur more often than occasionally (e.g., 3 times a month) and are associated with diarrhea or constipation

CASE 14-1

Relevant Evaluation Criteria	Scenario/Model Outcome
Collect	
1. Gather essential information about the patient's symptoms and medical history, including	
a. Description of symptom(s) (i.e., nature, onset, duration, severity, associated symptoms)	The patient complains of occasional stomach pain, bloating, and flatulence. She states these symptoms started 4–5 weeks ago and have been progressively getting worse. Symptoms now include diarrhea, nausea, and fatigue.
b. Description of any factors that seem to precipitate, exacerbate, and/or relieve the patient's symptom(s)	The patient states that the symptoms seem to get worse after meals, but the pain is sometimes diffuse, and she cannot identify a cause. Having a bowel movement tends to relieve some of the pain some of the time.
c. Description of the patient's efforts to relieve the symptoms	She has tried several OTC products without much success. These products include simethicone 125 mg 4 times a day and Tums 500 mg 3 times daily.
d. Patient's identity	Lyla Kay
e. Patient's age, gender, height, and weight	48 years old, female, 5 ft 2 in., 185 lb
f. Patient's occupation	Tax attorney
g. Patient's dietary habits	She skips breakfast unless she stops at a coffee stand for a latte and whole wheat muffin. Eats sporadically during the day as her schedule allows. Frequently eats at fast food restaurants or consumes prepackaged meals.
h. Patient's sleep habits	7–8 hours nightly
i. Concurrent medical conditions, prescription and nonprescription medications, and dietary supplements	Depression: citalopram 10 mg once daily; hypertension: lisinopril 20 mg once daily; hyperlipidemia: atorvastatin 20 mg once daily
j. Allergies	Bee stings (anaphylaxis)
k. History of other adverse reactions to medications	None
l. Other (describe) ______	Over the past several months, the patient reports losing 20 pounds without changing her diet or increasing exercise.
Assess	
2. Differentiate patient's signs/symptoms, and correctly identify the patient's primary problem(s) (Table 14–6).	Abdominal symptoms are consistent with intolerance to multiple foods, which suggests the possibility of a lactose intolerance, oligosaccharide intolerance, and possible gluten sensitivity (celiac disease). Fatigue and weight loss support a disorder with a nutritional deficiency component, possibly IBS.
3. Identify exclusions for self-treatment (Figure 14–1).	Unintended weight loss; presence of symptoms for prolonged period; increasing severity of symptoms; onset of symptoms in a patient >40 years of age.
4. Formulate a comprehensive list of therapeutic alternatives for the primary problem to determine whether triage to a health care provider is required, and share this information with the patient or caregiver.	Options include (1) Refer to a PCP or gastroenterologist for a definitive diagnosis. (2) Recommend patient keep a food, stress, and symptom journal. (3) Take no action.
Plan	
5. Select an optimal therapeutic alternative to address the patient's problem, taking into account patient preferences.	Ms. Kay should be referred to a primary care provider or gastroenterologist for a definitive diagnosis.
6. Describe the recommended therapeutic approach to the patient or caregiver.	"You should immediately follow up with your primary care provider or gastroenterologist."
7. Explain to the patient or caregiver the rationale for selecting the recommended therapeutic approach from the considered therapeutic alternatives.	"Available OTC treatment will not adequately address the severity of the current symptoms you have. It is important that you follow up with your primary care provider to identify the cause of your complaints and associated weight loss."

CASE 14-1 *continued*

Relevant Evaluation Criteria	Scenario/Model Outcome
Implement	
8. When recommending self-care with nonprescription medications and/or nondrug therapy, convey accurate information to the patient or caregiver.	Criterion does not apply in this case.
Solicit follow-up questions from the patient or caregiver.	"Is there anything that I can do right now to address my symptoms before getting in to see the doctor?"
Answer the patient's or caregiver's questions.	"You've tried all the products I would recommend, and there is really nothing else that would help at this point. Immediately following up with your primary care provider is the best course of action."
Follow-up: Monitor and Evaluate	
9. Assess patient outcome.	Contact the patient in 1–2 days to ensure she sought medical care and made an appointment.

Key: IBS = Irritable bowel syndrome; OTC = over-the-counter; PCP = primary care provider.

CASE 14-2

Relevant Evaluation Criteria	Scenario/Model Outcome
Collect	
1. Gather essential information about the patient's symptoms and medical history, including	
a. Description of symptom(s) (i.e., nature, onset, duration, severity, associated symptoms)	Patient presents with complaints of bloating with an increased amount of "burping," abdominal discomfort, and flatulence. The symptoms are mild in nature but uncomfortable and embarrassing for the patient.
b. Description of any factors that seem to precipitate, exacerbate, and/or relieve the patient's symptom(s)	Symptoms seem to be worse after eating large meals, especially when ice cream, milk, or other dairy products are consumed. The bloating seems to decrease after episodes of burping or flatulence.
c. Description of the patient's efforts to relieve the symptoms	The patient has tried including one serving of yogurt daily into his diet over the past few weeks with no relief.
d. Patient's identity	Murray Anderson
e. Patient's age, gender, height, and weight	35 years old, male, 6 ft, 240 lb
f. Patient's occupation	Salesman
g. Patient's dietary habits	"Never misses a meal" and enjoys eating fried Southern "comfort foods," ice cream, and soda.
h. Patient's sleep habits	5–7 hours a night
i. Concurrent medical conditions, prescription and nonprescription medications, and dietary supplements	Hypertension: losartan 50 mg, 1 tablet every morning; GERD: omeprazole 20 mg, 1 capsule every morning 30 minutes before eating
j. Allergies	Penicillin (rash)
k. History of adverse reactions to medications	None
Assess	
2. Differentiate patient's signs/symptoms, and correctly identify the patient's primary problem(s).	Patient is currently experiencing intestinal gas and bloating that may be due to potential dietary intolerances.
3. Identify exclusions for self-treatment (Figure 14–1).	None

CASE 14-2 *continued*

Relevant Evaluation Criteria	Scenario/Model Outcome
4. Formulate a comprehensive list of therapeutic alternatives for the primary problem to determine whether triage to a health care provider is required, and share this information with the patient or caregiver.	Options include (1) Refer patient to an appropriate HCP. (2) Recommend self-care with lactose intolerance product (e.g., Lactaid) (3) Recommend self-care until patient can see an appropriate provider. (4) Recommend the patient keep a food journal and decrease the intake of problematic foods. (5) Take no action.
Plan	
5. Select an optimal therapeutic alternative to address the patient's problem, taking into account patient preferences.	Mr. Anderson should take a lactase enzyme whenever he eats more than 4 ounces (120 mL) of dairy. Gas or bloating can be treated with simethicone. He should keep a food journal to identify problematic foods and should avoid large meals and carbonated beverages.
6. Describe the recommended therapeutic approach to the patient or caregiver.	"You should take Lactaid whenever you eat or drink more than 4 ounces (120 mL) of dairy. The Gas-X Extra Strength tablets can be taken with meals or snacks to help with flatulence. You should keep a food journal to identify problematic foods. Avoid eating large meals and drinking carbonated beverages."
7. Explain to the patient or caregiver the rationale for selecting the recommended therapeutic approach from the considered therapeutic alternatives.	"The Lactaid will help with the digestion of dairy products—including yogurt, milk, and ice cream—which should decrease the amount of gas produced. If you do experience an increase in belching, flatulence, or bloating, you can use simethicone, which helps expel gas bubbles formed within your stomach and intestine. By keeping a food journal, reducing your meal size, and avoiding carbonated beverages, you should notice some relief from the bloating you have been experiencing."
Implement	
8. When recommending self-care with nonprescription medications and/or nondrug therapy, convey accurate information to the patient or caregiver.	
a. Appropriate dose and frequency of administration	See Table 14–4.
b. Maximum number of days the therapy should be employed	No maximum, so long as the symptoms are relieved and do not worsen.
c. Product administration procedures	Take the product by mouth.
d. Expected time to onset of relief	Soon after administration
e. Degree of relief that can be reasonably expected	"If your bloating and gas are being caused by lactose intolerance, then the Lactaid should prevent or reduce symptoms."
f. Most common side effects	None
g. Adverse effects that warrant medical intervention should they occur	None
h. Patient options in the event that condition worsens or persists	See Figure 14–1.
i. Product storage requirements	Store in a cool, dry place out of children's reach.
j. Specific nondrug measures	See Table 14–3.
Solicit follow-up questions from the patient or caregiver.	"Can I double the dose of any of the medications for quicker relief?"
Answer the patient's or caregiver's questions.	"No, follow the manufacturer's directions. Additional doses will not provide added benefit."
Follow-up: Monitor and Evaluate	
9. Assess patient outcome.	Ask the patient to call and update you on his response to your recommended treatment; alternatively, you could call him in a week to evaluate his response to the treatment. For the purposes of follow-up, be sure you have the patient's current telephone number on file.

Key: GERD = Gastroesophageal reflux disease; HCP = health care provider.

PATIENT EDUCATION FOR Intestinal Gas

The objectives of self-treatment are (1) to reduce the symptoms of intestinal gas and (2) to reduce the chance of its recurrence. For most patients, carefully following product instructions and the self-care measures listed below will help ensure optimal therapeutic outcomes.

Nondrug Measures

- If possible, avoid foods known to cause intestinal gas.
- Avoid activities known to introduce gas into the digestive system, such as drinking carbonated beverages.

Nonprescription Medications

- Lactase replacement products and α-galactosidase should be taken with foods to prevent intestinal gas from forming.
- Simethicone is used to treat intestinal gas symptoms after onset.

α-Galactosidase

- Do not cook with this product. Add to food after it has cooled, because food temperatures higher than 130°F (55°C) may inactivate the enzyme.
- With drop formulations, add drops to the first bite of problem foods.
- With tablets, swallow, chew, or crumble the recommended number of tablets for consumption with the first bite of problem foods.
- An average meal may contain three servings of a problem food. If needed, use more tablets for larger meals, up to the maximum recommended dose.

Lactase Replacement Products

- Take at first bite of dairy- or lactose-containing food.
- Dosing may vary according to the amount of lactase in the product and the level of lactose intolerance.
- Do not take more than the recommended maximum daily dose.
- Low-lactose milk or fortified soy milk products may also be used to supplement dietary intake of calcium.

Simethicone

- For infants, to ease administration, mix the suspension with 1 ounce of cool water, infant formula, or other liquid.
- Discontinue simethicone if adequate relief is not obtained within 24 hours.

When to Seek Medical Attention

- Seek medical attention if symptoms do not resolve or if they worsen.

- Sudden change in the location of abdominal pain
- Significant increase in the severity or frequency of symptoms
- Sudden change in bowel function (suggestive of IBS)
- Emergence of accompanying signs and symptoms such as severe or persistent diarrhea or constipation; greasy or malodorous stools; GI bleeding (e.g., hematemesis, melena, hematochezia); fatigue; unintentional weight loss; or frequent nocturnal symptoms

Key Points for Intestinal Gas Complaints

- Limit self-treatment for intestinal gas to management of minor symptoms, and identify any exclusions for self-treatment (Figure 14–1).
- Counsel patients on dietary and other measures (Table 14–3) that may reduce the amount of intestinal gas. Certain foods (Tables 14–1 and 14–2) are more likely to cause gas and contribute to symptoms.
- Patients who experience symptoms with ingestion of lactose- or oligosaccharide-containing foods and who have no exclusions for self-treatment may use digestive enzymes (lactase replacement or α-galactosidase products).
- Probiotics or prebiotics may be helpful for patients with lactose intolerance who experience bloating or for patients with bloating associated with irritable bowel syndrome.
- Antiflatulents such as activated charcoal and simethicone may be used, although the available evidence is contradictory regarding the ability of these agents to reduce the amount of intestinal gas formed.
- Referral to a primary care provider for further evaluation should be considered for patients with exclusions for self-treatment and for patients whose symptoms persist after initiation of simple treatment options (e.g., dietary modification, nonprescription medications).

REFERENCES

1. World Gastroenterology Organization global guidelines on celiac disease. *J Clin Gastroenterol.* 2013;47(2):121–6. doi:10.1097/MCG.0b013e31827a6f83.
2. Masoodi M, Mokhtare M, Agah S, et al. Frequency of celiac disease in patients with increased intestinal gas (flatulence). *Glob J Health Sci.* 2016;8(6):147–53. doi:10.5539/gjhs.v8n6p147.
3. Montalto M, Curigliano V, Santoro L, et al. Management and treatment of lactose malabsorption. *World J Gastroenterol.* 2006;12(2):187–91. PMCID:PMC4066025.
4. Brandt LJ, Chey WD, Foxx-Orenstein AE, et al. An evidence-based systematic review on the management of irritable bowel syndrome. *Am J Gastroenterol.* 2009;104(Suppl 1):S1–35. doi:10.1038/ajg.2008.122.
5. Ringel Y, Williams RE, Kalilani L, et al. Prevalence, characteristics, and impact of bloating symptoms in patients with irritable bowel syndrome. *Clin Gastroenterol Hepatol.* 2009;7(1):68–72. doi:10.1016/j.cgh.2008.07.008.
6. Johnson LR. *Gastrointestinal Physiology: Regulation.* 7th ed. Philadelphia, PA: Mosby; 2007:107–26.
7. Greenberger NJ. Overview of GI symptoms: gas-related complaints. In: *Merck Manual Professional Version.* (Gastrointestinal Disorders Sections). Updated March 2016. Available at: https://www.merckmanuals.com/professional/gastrointestinal-disorders/symptoms-of-gi-disorders/gas-related-complaints. Accessed June 2, 2017.
8. Helpful hints for controlling gas (flatus). University of Michigan Health Systems Michigan Bowel Control Program. Available at: https://www.med.umich.edu/fbd/docs/Gas%20reduction%20diet.pdf. Accessed June 2, 2017.
9. Dahl WJ, Stewart ML. Position of the Academy of Nutrition and Dietetics: health implications of dietary fiber. *J Acad Nutr Diet.* 2015;115(11):1861–70. doi:10.1016/j.jand.2015.09.003.
10. Slavin J. Fiber and prebiotics mechanisms and health benefits. *Nutrients.* 2013;5:1417–35. doi:10.3390/nu5041417.

11. Azpiroz F, Malagelada JR. The pathogenesis of bloating and visible distension in irritable bowel syndrome. *Gastroenterol Clin North Am.* 2005; 34(2):257–69. doi:10.1016/j.gtc.2005.02.006.
12. Deng Y, Misselwitz, Dai N, Fox M. Lactose intolerance in adults: biological mechanism and dietary management. *Nutrients.* 2015;7:8020–35. doi: 10.3390/nu7095380.
13. Shaukat A, Levitt MD, Taylor BC, et al. Systematic review: effective management strategies for lactose intolerance. *Ann Intern Med.* 2010;152(12): 797–803. doi:10.7326/0003-4819-152-12-201006150-00241.
14. Beto JA. The role of calcium in human aging. *Clin Nutr Res.* 2015;4:1–8. doi:10.7762/cnr.2015.4.1.1.
15. Lin HC. Small intestinal bacterial overgrowth: a framework for understanding irritable bowel syndrome. *JAMA.* 2004;292(7):852–8. doi:10.1001/jama.292.7.852.
16. Gluten free drugs. Available at: http://www.glutenfreedrugs.com. Accessed March 28, 2016.
17. Celiac Sprue Association (CSA/USA). Available at: http://www.csaceliacs.info. Accessed June 2, 2017.
18. Whelan K, Quigley MM. Probiotics in the management of irritable bowel syndrome and inflammatory bowel disease. *Curr Opin Gastroenterol.* 2013;29(2):184–9. doi:10.1097/MOG.0b013e32835d7bba.
19. Mayer EA. The neurobiology of stress and emotions. *Participate* [quarterly publication of the International Foundation of Functional Gastrointestinal Disorders]. 2010;10(4):2–5.
20. Hanauer SB, DuPont HL, Cooper KM, et al. Randomized, double-blind, placebo-controlled clinical trial of loperamide plus simethicone versus loperamide alone and simethicone alone in the treatment of acute diarrhea with gas-related abdominal discomfort. *Curr Med Res Opin.* 2007;23(5): 1033–43. doi:10.1185/030079907X182176.
21. Hall B, Chesters J, Robinson A. Infantile colic: a systematic review of medical and conventional therapies. *J Paediatr Child Health.* 2012;48(2): 128–37. doi:10.1111/j.1440-1754.2011.02061.x.
22. Suarez FL, Furne J, Springfield J, et al. Failure of activated charcoal to reduce the release of gases produced by the colonic flora. *Am J Gastroenterol.* 1999;94(1):208–12. doi:10.1111/j.1572-0241.1999.00798.x.
23. Nardo GD, Oliva S, Ferrari F, et al. Efficacy and tolerability of alpha-galactosidase in treating gas-related symptoms in children: a randomized, double-blind, placebo controlled trial. *Gastroenterology.* 2013;13:142. doi:10.1186/1471-230X-13-142.
24. Hempel S, Newberry SJ, Maher AR, et al. Probiotics for the prevention and treatment of antibiotic-associated diarrhea: a systematic review and meta-analysis. *JAMA.* 2012;307(18):1959–69. PMID:22570464DOI:10.1001/jama.2012.3507.
25. Merat S, Khalili S, Mostajabi P, et al. The effect of enteric-coated, delayed-release peppermint oil on irritable bowel syndrome. *Dig Dis Sci.* 2010;55:1385–90. doi:10.1007/s10620-009-0854-9.
26. Alam MS, Roy PK, Miah AR, et al. Efficacy of peppermint oil in diarrhea-predominant IBS—a double-blind randomized placebo-controlled study. *Mymensingh Med J.* 2013;22(1):27–30. PMID:23416804.
27. Bulat R, Fachnie E, Chauhan U, et al. Lack of effect of spearmint on lower esophageal sphincter function and acid reflux in healthy volunteers. *Aliment Pharmacol Ther.* 1999;13(6):805–12. PMID:10383511.
28. Brinker FJ. *Herb Contraindications & Drug Interactions: Plus Herbal Adjuncts With Medicines.* 4th ed. Sandy, OR: Eclectic Medical Publications; 2010:227–50.
29. Mayo Clinic. Bloating, belching and intestinal gas: how to avoid them. Available at: http://www.mayoclinic.org/diseases-conditions/gas-and-gas-pains/in-depth/gas-and-gas-pains/art-20044739. Accessed June 2, 2017.

CHAPTER 15

CONSTIPATION

KRISTIN W. WEITZEL AND JEAN-VENABLE "KELLY" R. GOODE

Constipation is a common gastrointestinal (GI) complaint. Although individual bowel habits including stool frequency vary, health care providers (HCPs) generally define *constipation* in adults as occurrence of fewer than 3 bowel movements per week, associated with straining and the difficult passage of hard, dry stools.[1,2] Patients' perceptions of and definitions of normal bowel frequency and constipation vary widely. Clinical descriptions of self-reported constipation may include (1) straining to have a bowel movement; (2) passing hard, dry stools; (3) passing small stools; (4) feeling as though bowel evacuation is not complete; or (5) experiencing decreased stool frequency.[2,3]

Constipation is a common symptom that occurs in male and female patients of all ages. The prevalence in the general population ranges from 2% to 28%.[1,4–6] Constipation is the reason for 2.5 million physician visits per year in the United States, with direct costs of diagnosis and treatment estimated at billions of dollars annually.[7] It is reported more often in women, persons of non-White ancestry, children, and older individuals.[1,4,8] Older adults (>65 years of age) are 5 times more likely to experience constipation than younger adults, and women are more than 3 times as likely as men to be affected.[2] Constipation also is a frequent complaint in late pregnancy and after childbirth.[8] If untreated, constipation can lead to development of hemorrhoids or anal fissures, rectal prolapse, fecal impaction, or other complications.[9]

Pathophysiology of Constipation

All structures shown in Figure 15–1 contribute to the process of digestion. After food is ingested, it is retained in the stomach for approximately 3 hours and then in the small intestine for the same amount of time in individuals with normal gastric motility. Within the stomach, tonic contractions of the stomach wall churn and knead the ingested food, and peristaltic waves move the partially digested matter toward the duodenum.[10]

Once through the stomach, ingested matter enters the small intestine and passes through the large intestine before defecation. Contractions in the small intestine promote movement of nondigestible material into the large intestine. Fecal matter is stored in the sigmoid colon until defecation occurs.[10] The defecation process is controlled by both voluntary and involuntary reflexes. With normal gastric motility, fecal content within the colon triggers an involuntary peristaltic movement that propels fecal matter into the rectum, with consequent relaxation of the internal anal sphincter and subsequently the desire to defecate. Voluntary tightening of the abdominal wall muscles with relaxation of the external anal sphincter then allows stool to pass. When defecating, individuals may use the *Valsalva maneuver,* which entails a forceful increase in intra-abdominal pressure, initiated with an exhalation attempt against a closed glottis, to voluntarily initiate and promote passage of stool. Difficulty passing stool with constipation can lead the affected individual to strain significantly to promote defecation.[10]

Causes of constipation include various medical problems and medications, psychological and physiologic conditions and disturbances (e.g., stress, menopause, dehydration), and lifestyle characteristics. Constipation may stem from either primary or secondary mechanisms, with *primary* constipation characterized as slower-than-normal GI transit time or a defecatory disorder (e.g., pelvic floor dysfunction).[2,6,8] *Secondary* causes of constipation include systemic, neurologic, and psychological disorders and/or structural abnormalities[1–3,5,6] (Table 15–1).

Other factors such as inadequate dietary fiber and fluid intake may also contribute to constipation. Dietary fiber dissolves or swells in the intestinal fluid, which increases fecal bulk to aid in stimulating peristalsis and eliminating stool. A diet that is low in calories, carbohydrates, or fiber may be associated with decreased fecal bulk, with resulting constipation. Inadequate intake of fluids may promote constipation in dehydrated patients.[1] Gravity and normal abdominal muscle tone also contribute to proper bowel function.

Failing to respond to the urge to empty the bowel can eventually lead to constipation. When the urge is ignored or suppressed, rectal muscles can lose tonicity and become less effective, and nerve pathways may stop sending the signal to defecate. Medication-associated constipation can also occur in patients with multiple concomitant medical conditions or therapies (Table 15–2).[2,3,11,12]

Clinical Presentation of Constipation

As noted earlier, constipation is a common complaint. In addition to the patient's report of decreased frequency or difficulty passing stools, presenting manifestations can include anorexia, dull headache, lassitude, low back pain, abdominal discomfort, bloating, flatulence, and psychosocial distress.[1] Occasional bouts of temporary constipation are usually treatable with self-care measures. Constipation continuing over several weeks to months or that complicated by concomitant conditions requires more sustained and aggressive therapy beyond a self-care approach.[13,14]

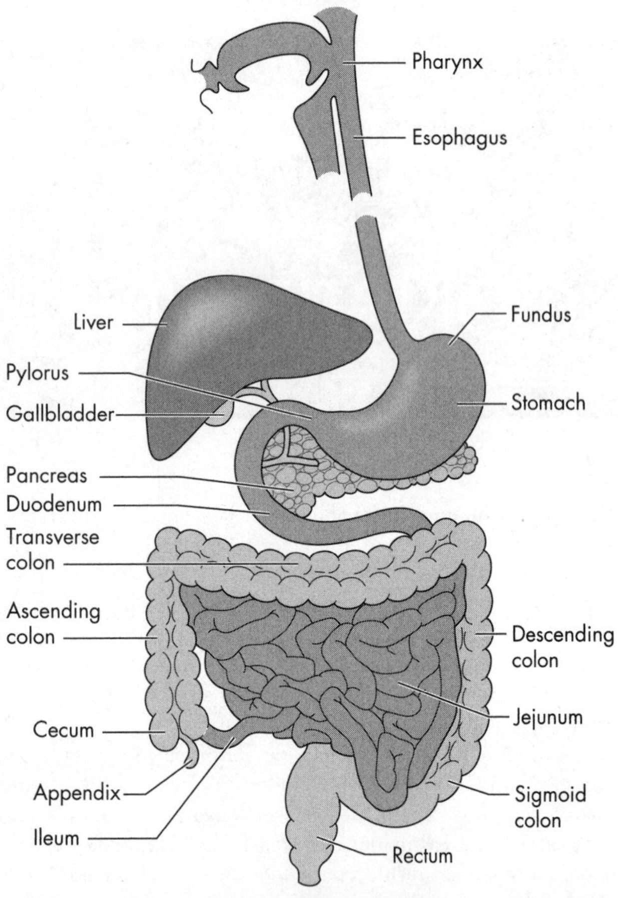

FIGURE 15–1 Anatomy of the digestive system.

TABLE 15–1 Selected Conditions Associated With Constipation

Structural
Colorectal or anorectal injury, inflammation, or damage (e.g., anal fissure)
Pelvic floor disorders
Structural abnormalities (e.g., tumors, hernias, strictures) leading to bowel obstruction
Systemic
Thyroid disorders
Diabetes mellitus
Irritable bowel syndrome
Neurologic disorders
Autonomic neuropathy
Multiple sclerosis
Parkinsonism
Cerebrovascular accidents
Dementia
Psychological
Depression
Eating disorders
Situational stress

Source: References 1–3, 5, and 6.

Long-standing or untreated constipation can lead to complications such as hemorrhoids, anal fissures, or rectal prolapse, fecal impaction, or rectal ulcers. Straining to defecate may cause blood pressure surges or cardiac rhythm disturbances secondary to altered hemodynamics.[9]

Treatment of Constipation

Treatment Goals

The primary goals of treatment are (1) to relieve constipation and reestablish normal bowel function, (2) to establish dietary and exercise habits to help prevent recurrence, and (3) to promote the safe and effective use of laxative products.

General Treatment Approach

Initial management of constipation involves lifestyle changes, such as increasing intake of high-fiber foods, increasing fluid intake, and initiating regular exercise[1–3,8] (Figure 15–2). Pharmacologic intervention can be used if more immediate relief is desired. Laxatives should be selected according to the age and health status of the patient, as well as the mechanism of action of the individual product. U.S. Food and Drug Administration (FDA) labeling for nonprescription products limits their use to short-term (<7 days) treatment without medical referral, which is consistent with the need for medical supervision of chronic constipation treatment.[13,14] Accordingly, patients should not use any nonprescription laxative product for more than 7 days unless the therapy is directed by an HCP. If rectal bleeding occurs at any time during the use of a laxative, or if constipation persists despite an appropriate laxative regimen, the patient should stop use of the laxative and be referred for medical evaluation.[1,15]

Nonpharmacologic Therapy

A balanced diet that incorporates fruits, vegetables, and whole grains helps to prevent constipation. The American Dietetic Association recommends an adult daily dietary fiber intake of 14 g per 1000 kcal, or 25 g for adult women and 38 g for adult men.[16,17] (See Chapter 24 for information on dietary fiber types, sources, intake, and benefits.)

Added fiber increases stool weight and normalizes frequency of bowel movements to 1 movement per day and GI transit time to 2–4 days.[17] This normalization of bowel movement frequency is important: The longer stool is retained in the bowel, the more water is absorbed out of the bowel contents and into the intestinal cells, leading to hard stool consistency and difficulty in passing stool.[17] Patients complaining of constipation should gradually increase their dietary intake of insoluble

TABLE 15–2 Selected Drugs That May Induce Constipation
Analgesics (including nonsteroidal anti-inflammatory drugs)
Antacids (e.g., calcium and aluminum compounds, bismuth)
Anticholinergics (e.g., benztropine, glycopyrrolate)
Anticonvulsants (e.g., carbamazepine, divalproate)
Antidepressants (specifically, tricyclics such as amitriptyline)
Antihistamines (e.g., diphenhydramine, loratadine)
Antimuscarinics (e.g., oxybutynin, tolterodine)
Benzodiazepines (especially alprazolam and estazolam)
Calcium channel blockers (e.g., verapamil, diltiazem)
Calcium supplements (e.g., calcium carbonate)
Diuretics (e.g., hydrochlorothiazide, furosemide)
Hematinics (especially iron)
Hyperlipidemics (e.g., cholestyramine, pravastatin, simvastatin)
Hypotensives (e.g., angiotensin-converting enzyme inhibitors, beta blockers)
Muscle relaxants (e.g., cyclobenzaprine, metaxalone)
Opiates (e.g., morphine, codeine)
Parkinsonism agents (e.g., bromocriptine)
Polystyrene sodium sulfonate
Psychotherapeutic drugs (e.g., phenothiazines, butyrophenones)
Sedative hypnotics (e.g., zolpidem, benzodiazepines, phenobarbital)
Serotonin agonists (e.g., ondansetron)
Sucralfate

Source: References 2, 3, 11, and 12.

fiber (e.g., incorporating more whole grains, wheat bran, fruits, and vegetables into meals) and limit consumption of foods without fiber.[8,17]

If dietary modifications are not effective, patients may use a commercially available fiber supplement. Many newer flavorless and texture-free fiber supplements (e.g., inulin) are classified as dietary supplements (Table 15–3).[8] Other added-fiber supplements (e.g., psyllium, methylcellulose) are bulk-forming laxatives approved by FDA as nonprescription drugs. The pharmacologic effects of FDA-approved fiber supplements have been studied more extensively than for dietary supplement products (see Pharmacologic Therapy). A high-fiber diet or fiber supplement may take 3–5 days or longer to take effect. Significantly increasing dietary fiber may initially lead to erratic bowel frequency, flatulence, and abdominal discomfort. Gradually increasing fiber intake over a period of 1–2 weeks can improve tolerance.[1,8,17] When adding dietary fiber, patients should also increase their fluid intake to approximately 2 L/day. In pregnant and lactating women, an additional 300 mL and 750–1000 mL of fluid, respectively, are recommended.[17]

Behavior modifications (or "bowel training") can also help promote bowel movements. Gastrocolic reflexes are strongest first thing in the morning and 30 minutes after a meal, so attempting a bowel movement at these times promotes defecation consistent with the body's normal physiologic response. Low levels of physical activity have been shown to be associated with increased constipation, so adopting physical activities consistent with a healthy lifestyle in accordance with each patient's capabilities (e.g., with consideration of physical or other limitations) can decrease this risk.[1,18]

Pharmacologic Therapy

The ideal laxative would (1) be nonirritating and nontoxic, (2) act only on the descending and sigmoid colons, and (3) produce a normally formed stool within a few hours. Because no currently available laxative precisely meets these criteria, proper selection of a laxative depends on the underlying cause of the constipation and individual patient factors and preferences. Agents used to treat constipation are classified by mechanism of action and include bulk-forming, hyperosmotic, emollient, lubricant, saline, and stimulant agents (Table 15–4).

Bulk-Forming Agents

Bulk-forming laxatives include products containing methylcellulose, polycarbophil, and psyllium. Use of these agents is the recommended treatment choice in most cases of constipation, because their effects most closely approximate the body's physiologic process.[1,5,8] Available dosage forms include tablets or capsules, powders to be mixed with water or other liquids, and fiber chews, wafers, or "gummies."

The usual time to onset of action for bulk-forming laxatives is 12–24 hours, but onset of effect may be delayed up to 72 hours. These agents are indicated for short-term therapy to relieve constipation and may be useful in (1) patients on low-fiber diets, (2) postpartum women, (3) older adults, and (4) patients with colostomies, irritable bowel syndrome, or diverticular disease. They are also used prophylactically in patients who should avoid straining during a bowel movement. Dosages vary according to the type of product (Table 15–4). Exceeding the recommended dose may lead to increased flatulence or obstruction if appropriate fluid intake is not maintained.

Bulk-forming agents have few systemic adverse effects when used as directed, with abdominal cramping and flatulence most commonly reported. If the dose is not taken with adequate fluid as directed, bulk-forming laxatives may swell in the throat or esophagus, potentially causing choking. Bulk-forming products should be avoided in patients who have swallowing difficulties or esophageal strictures and may be inappropriate for fluid-restricted patients.[19] Because of the danger of fecal impaction or intestinal obstruction, patients with intestinal ulcerations, stenosis, or disabling adhesions should not take bulk-forming products. Patients experiencing chest pain, vomiting, difficulty swallowing, or difficulty breathing after use should seek immediate medical attention.[20] Acute bronchospasm has been associated with accidental inhalation of dry hydrophilic mucilloid, as well as hypersensitivity reactions to psyllium characterized by anaphylaxis.[21] Individuals who are sensitive to inhaled or ingested psyllium should avoid these products.

Calcium polycarbophil can contain up to 150 mg (7.6 mEq) calcium per tablet, which may be clinically relevant in patients at risk for hypercalcemia (e.g., those with renal disease). The sugar content of bulk-forming agents should be considered in patients with diabetes or restricted caloric intake. Although bulk-forming

Exclusions for Self-Treatment

- Marked abdominal pain or significant distention or cramping
- Marked or unexplained flatulence
- Fever
- Nausea and/or vomiting
- Presence of a chronic medical condition that may preclude self-care laxative treatment (e.g., paraplegia or quadriplegia, inflammatory bowel disease, colostomy)
- Daily laxative use (excluding fiber-based therapies)
- Unexplained changes in bowel habits, especially if accompanied by weight loss
- Blood in stool or dark, tarry stool
- Marked change in character of stool (e.g., stool becomes pencil thin)
- Any bowel symptoms that persist >2 weeks or recur over a period of at least 3 months
- Any bowel symptoms that recur after dietary or lifestyle changes, or laxative use
- Inflammatory bowel disease
- Anorexia
- Age < 2 years[a]

[a] Approved age limits for nonprescription laxative products vary. Table 15–4 provides additional guidance for appropriate product selection in pediatrics.
Source: References 1–3 and 8.

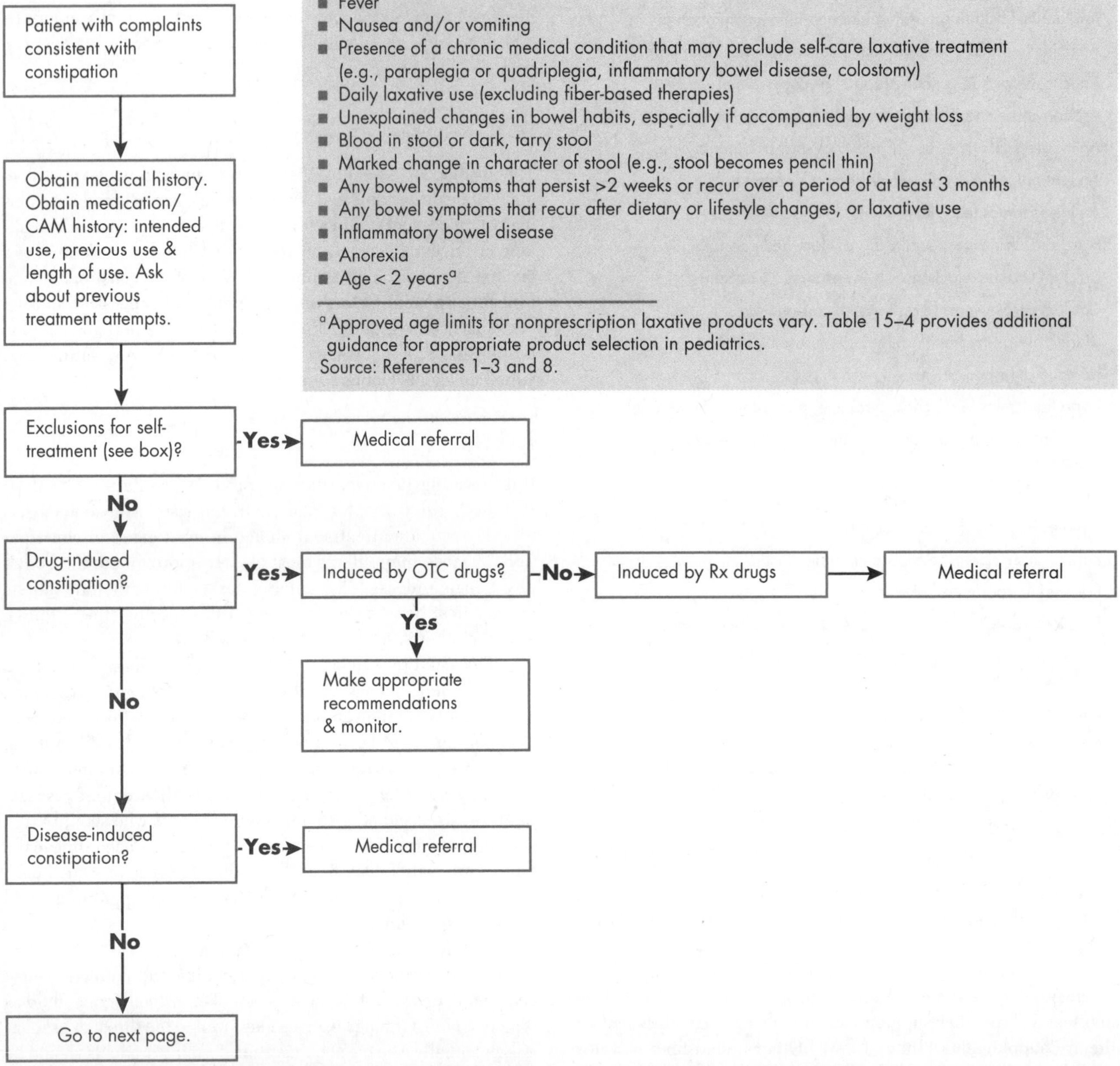

FIGURE 15–2 Self-care for constipation. Key: CAM = Complementary and alternative medicine; OTC = over-the-counter; PCP = primary care provider; PEG = polyethylene glycol; Rx = prescription. (*continued on next page*)

laxatives are not systemically absorbed, they can interfere with the absorption of oral medications as a consequence of physical binding in the GI tract or other mechanisms (Table 15–5).

Hyperosmotic Agents

Hyperosmotic agents include polyethylene glycol 3350 (PEG 3350) and glycerin (Table 15–4). These products contain large, poorly absorbed ions or molecules that draw water into the colon or rectum through osmosis to stimulate a bowel movement.[22]

PEG 3350 is available for self-care use in patients 17 years of age or older. It is supplied as a powder for oral administration and usually is taken as 17 g of powder (approximately 1 capful or 1 packet) mixed into 4–8 ounces of water, once daily as needed. PEG 3350 has minimal systemic absorption, with less than 1% of each dose absorbed and excreted in the urine. PEG 3350 usually produces a bowel movement in 12–72 hours, but onset may take up to 96 hours.

PEG 3350 is safe and effective for the short-term treatment of occasional constipation, with few adverse effects.[23] The most

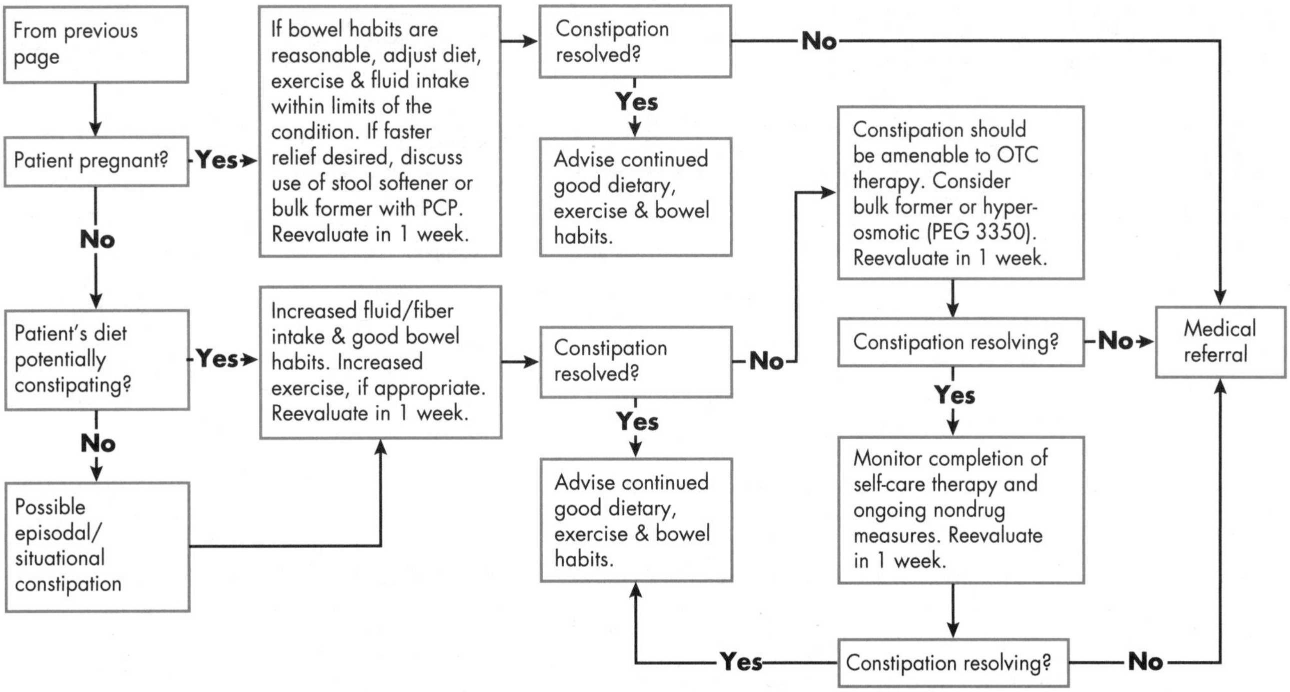

FIGURE 15–2 Self-care for constipation. Key: CAM = Complementary and alternative medicine; OTC = over-the-counter; PCP = primary care provider; PEG = polyethylene glycol; Rx = prescription. (*continued*)

common adverse effects are bloating, abdominal discomfort, cramping, and flatulence. FDA-approved labeling indicates that patients who have renal disease or irritable bowel syndrome should be cautioned to consult their primary care provider before using PEG 3350. No clinically significant drug–drug interactions have been reported with PEG 3350.

TABLE 15–3 **Types of Fiber Supplements**

Type of Fiber	Example(s) of Common Brands
Products Classified as Bulk-Forming Laxatives[a]	
Methylcellulose	Citrucel
Calcium polycarbophil	FiberCon
Psyllium	Metamucil, Konsyl
Products Classified as Dietary Supplements	
Inulin	FiberChoice, Metamucil Clear & Natural
Partially hydrolyzed guar gum	Sunfiber
Powdered cellulose	Unifiber
Wheat dextrin	Benefiber

[a] Products classified as bulk-forming laxatives are FDA-labeled to treat constipation.

Source: Adapted with permission from reference 8.

Glycerin is available as a suppository for lower bowel evacuation (Table 15–4). Glycerin suppositories usually produce a bowel movement within 15–30 minutes and are safe for occasional use in all approved age groups. Adverse effects are limited, although rectal irritation is possible with overdosage. Glycerin suppositories should be avoided in patients with preexisting rectal irritation.

Emollients

Emollients, also called stool softeners, are anionic surfactants that act in the small and large intestine to increase the wetting efficiency of intestinal fluid, facilitating a mixture of aqueous and fatty substances to soften the fecal mass (Table 15–4). They can be used to prevent straining and painful defecation in patients with anorectal disorders or in those who should avoid straining (e.g., with recent abdominal or rectal surgery). Although stool softeners can be taken for occasional constipation, these agents are used more often in combination with a stimulant laxative (e.g., senna, bisacodyl) for opioid-induced constipation.[19,24] (See the box "A Word About Opioid-Induced Constipation.")

Docusate, available as a sodium and a calcium salt, has a time to onset of action of 12–72 hours but may take up to 3–5 days to effect laxation.[8] Although no clinical differences between the salt forms are recognized, availability of docusate sodium in multiple strengths and dosage forms leads to its more frequent use. Docusate sodium is supplied as a capsule or syrup in multiple strengths; docusate calcium is available as a 240 mg capsule. Docusate is not appreciably absorbed from the GI tract and does not hamper absorption of nutrients from the intestinal tract. It is generally well tolerated and has minimal drug

TABLE 15-4 **Dosage Guidelines for Nonprescription Laxative Products[a]**

Agent	Dosage Form/ Strength	Adults/Children ≥12 Years	Children 6 to <12 Years[b]	Children 2 to <6 Years[b,c]
Bulk-Forming Agents				
Methylcellulose	Caplet: 500 mg	2 caplets up to 6 times daily	1 caplet up to 6 times daily	Not recommended for children <6 years, except under advice of a PCP
	Powder: 2 g per heaping tablespoon	Starting dose: 1 rounded tablespoon; increase as needed, 1 rounded tablespoon at a time, up to 3 times daily	Starting dose: 2 level teaspoons; increase as needed, 2 level teaspoons at a time, up to 3 times daily	Not recommended for children <6 years except under advice of a PCP
Calcium polycarbophil	Caplet: 625 mg	2 caplets 1–4 times daily	1 caplet 1–4 times daily	Not recommended for children <6 years, except under advice of a PCP
Psyllium (plantago seeds, ispaghula husks)	Capsule: psyllium husk, 0.52 g	5 capsules with 8 ounces of liquid (swallow 1 capsule at a time), up to 3 times daily	Not recommended for children <12 years except under advice of a PCP	Not recommended for children <6 years except under advice of a PCP
	Powder: 3.4 g psyllium husk per scoop or per packet of "fiber singles" product	1 rounded tablespoon in 8 ounces of liquid, up to 3 times daily	½ of adult dose in 8 ounces of liquid, up to 3 times daily	Not recommended for children <6 years except under advice of a PCP
Hyperosmotic Agents				
Polyethylene glycol 3350	Powder: 17 g per capful	17 g in 4–8 ounces of beverage once daily in adults and children ≥17 years	Not recommended for children <17 years, except under advice of a PCP	Not recommended for children <17 years, except under advice of a PCP
Glycerin	Rectal solid suppository: 2 g	1 suppository, or as directed by a PCP	1 suppository, or as directed by a PCP	Not recommended for children <6 years except under advice of a PCP
	Rectal solid suppository: 1 g (pediatric formulation)	—	—	1 suppository, or as directed by a PCP
	Rectal liquid suppository: 5.6 g glycerin per 5.5 mL	1 suppository, or as directed by a PCP	1 suppository, or as directed by a PCP	Not recommended for children <6 years, except under advice of a PCP
	Rectal liquid suppository: 2.8 g glycerin per 2.7 mL (pediatric formulation)	—	—	1 suppository, or as directed by a PCP
Emollient Agents				
Docusate sodium	Capsules: 50 mg and 100 mg	50–300 mg daily in single or divided doses	50–150 mg daily in single or divided doses	50–150 mg daily in single or divided doses
	Syrup: 60 mg per 15 mL	1–6 tablespoons (15–80 mL) daily, or as directed by a PCP, in single or divided doses (doses must be given in 6–8 ounces of milk or juice to prevent throat irritation)	1–2½ (15–37.5 mL) tablespoons daily, or as directed by a PCP, in single or divided doses (doses must be given in 6–8 ounces of milk or juice to prevent throat irritation)	1–2½ tablespoons (15–37.5 mL) daily, or as directed by a PCP, in single or divided doses (doses must be given in 6–8 ounces of milk or juice to prevent throat irritation)

TABLE 15-4 **Dosage Guidelines for Nonprescription Laxative Products**[a] *(continued)*

Agent	Dosage Form/ Strength	Adults/Children ≥12 Years	Children 6 to <12 Years[b]	Children 2 to <6 Years[b,c]
	Syrup: 50 mg/15 mL (pediatric formulation)	—	1–3 tablespoons (15–45 mL) daily, in single or divided doses (doses must be given in 6–8 ounces of milk or juice to prevent throat irritation)	1–3 tablespoons (15–45 mL) daily, in single or divided doses (doses must be given in 6–8 ounces of milk or juice to prevent throat irritation)
Docusate calcium	Capsule: 240 mg	1 capsule daily for several days, or until bowel movements are normal	Not recommended for children <12 years, except under advice of a PCP	Not recommended for children <6 years, except under advice of a PCP
Lubricant Agent				
Mineral oil[d]	Oral liquid	1–3 tablespoons (15–45 mL); maximum 3 tablespoons (45 mL) in 24 hours	1–3 teaspoons (5–15 mL); maximum 3 teaspoons (15 mL) in 24 hours	Not recommended for children <6 years except under advice of a PCP
		6–15 teaspoons (30–75 mL) per day, or as directed by a PCP	2–5 teaspoons (10–25 mL) per day, or as directed by a PCP	Not recommended for children <6 years except under advice of a PCP
		1 bottle as directed	½ bottle as directed	½ bottle as directed
Saline Laxative Agents				
Magnesium citrate	Liquid: 10 fluid ounces (300 mL)	½–1 bottle (150–300 mL) as directed	⅓–½ bottle (100–150 mL) as directed	Not recommended for children <6 years except under advice of a PCP
Magnesium hydroxide	Liquid: 400 mg/5 mL	2–4 tablespoons (30–60 mL) daily as single or divided doses	1–2 tablespoons (15–30 mL) daily as single or divided doses	Not recommended for children <6 years except under advice of a PCP
	Concentrated liquid: 2400 mg/15 mL	1–2 tablespoons (15–30 mL) daily as single or divided doses	½–1 tablespoon (7.5–15 mL) daily as single or divided doses	Not recommended for children <6 years except under advice of a PCP
	Chewable tablet: 311 mg per tablet	8 tablets once in a 24-hour period, preferably at bedtime, in divided doses or as directed by a PCP	4 tablets once in a 24-hour period, preferably at bedtime, in divided doses or as directed by a PCP	Children 3–5 years: chew 2 tablets once in a 24-hour period, preferably at bedtime, in divided doses or as directed by a PCP Not recommended for children <3 years except under advice of a PCP
	Chewable tablet: 400 mg per tablet (pediatric formulation)	—	3–6 tablets daily in single or divided doses	1–3 tablets daily in single or divided doses
Monobasic sodium phosphate/ dibasic sodium phosphate	Rectal liquid enema: 118 mL	1 bottle, as directed	Not recommended for children <12 years, except under advice of a PCP	Not recommended for children <6 years, except under advice of a PCP
	Rectal liquid enema: 197 mL	1 bottle, as directed	Not recommended for children <12 years, except under advice of a PCP	Not recommended for children <6 years, except under advice of a PCP
	Rectal liquid enema: 59 mL (pediatric formulation)	—	Children 5–11 years: 1 bottle or as directed by a PCP	Children 2–5 years: ½ bottle
Magnesium sulfate (Epsom salt)[d]	Solid: magnesium sulfate USP	2–6 level teaspoons (10–30 g) daily[d]	1–2 level teaspoons (5–10 g) daily[d]	Not recommended for children <6 years except under advice of a PCP

(continued)

TABLE 15-4 **Dosage Guidelines for Nonprescription Laxative Products[a]** *(continued)*

Agent	Dosage Form/ Strength	Adults/Children ≥12 Years	Children 6 to <12 Years[b]	Children 2 to <6 Years[b,c]
Stimulant Agents				
Senna	Tablets: 8.6 mg sennosides	Starting dose: 2 tablets once daily Maximum dose: 4 tablets twice daily	Starting dose: 1 tablet once daily Maximum dose: 2 tablets twice daily	Starting dose: ½ tablet once daily Maximum dose: 1 tablet twice daily
	Tablets or chocolate pieces: 15 mg sennosides	2 tablets or chocolate pieces 1–2 times daily	1 tablet or chocolate piece 1–2 times daily	Not recommended for children <6 years, except under advice of a PCP
	Tablets: 17.2 mg sennosides	Starting dose: 1 tablet once daily Maximum dose: 2 tablets twice daily	Starting dose: ½ tablet once daily Maximum dose: 1 tablet twice daily	Not recommended for children <6 years, except under advice of a PCP
	Pills: 25 mg sennosides	2 pills 1–2 times daily	1 pill 1–2 times daily	Not recommended for children <6 years, except under advice of a PCP
	Liquid[e]: senna concentrate 33.3 mg senna pod concentrate/mL (pediatric formulation [e.g., Fletcher's Laxative for Kids])	—	Age 6–15 years: 2–3 teaspoons (10–15 mL) 1–2 times daily	1–2 teaspoons (5–10 mL) 1–2 times daily
	Liquid[e]: sennosides 1.8 mg sennosides/mL	2–3 teaspoons (10–15 mL) once a day	1–1½ teaspoons (5–7.5 mL) once a day	½–¾ teaspoon (2.5–3.75 mL) once a day
Bisacodyl	Tablets: 5 mg	1–3 tablets (usually 2) once daily	1 tablet daily	Not recommended for children <6 years except under advice of a PCP
	Rectal solid suppository: 10 mg	1 suppository in a single daily dose	½ suppository in a single daily dose	Not recommended for children <6 years except under advice of a PCP
Castor oil[d]	Liquid	1 to a maximum of 4 tablespoons (15–60 mL) in a single daily dose[d]	1 to a maximum of 3 teaspoons (5–15 mL) in a single daily dose[d]	Not recommended for children <6 years except under advice of a PCP

Key: FDA = U.S. Food and Drug Administration; OTC = over-the-counter; PCP = primary care provider.

[a] All doses are based on FDA-labeled instructions and are for oral products, unless indicated otherwise.

[b] All doses for children are listed as those for ages 2 to <6 years or ages 6 to <12 years, unless otherwise indicated in FDA-labeled dosing instructions. In these cases, FDA-labeled age ranges are provided within the table.

[c] No recommended dosages exist for children <2 years of age, except under the advice and supervision of a PCP.

[d] Although magnesium sulfate (Epsom salt) and castor oil are approved as nonprescription laxatives, they are not recommended, because safer, better-tolerated, and well-studied alternatives are available. Self-care use of mineral oil is also discouraged in most cases. See text discussion under Pharmacologic Therapy for specific recommendations on appropriate use of each agent.

[e] Liquid senna products vary in product concentration and dosing, depending on the form of senna. Take care to ensure that patients are following FDA-labeled dosing instructions with use of these products, especially in pediatric patients.

interactions (Table 15–5). Larger-than-recommended doses may result in weakness, sweating, muscle cramps, and irregular heartbeat.

Lubricants

Mineral oil (liquid petrolatum) is the only nonprescription lubricant. Mineral oil softens fecal contents by coating stool and preventing colonic absorption of fecal water. It is available in liquid form for oral or rectal administration (Table 15–4). Mineral oil's time to onset of action is approximately 6–8 hours after oral administration and 5–15 minutes after rectal administration.

The most significant acute safety concern with mineral oil is lipid pneumonia resulting from aspiration into the lungs after an oral dose. Mineral oil should not be taken before lying down and should be avoided in patients at risk for aspiration. FDA labeling

TABLE 15-5 **Clinically Important Drug–Drug Interactions With Nonprescription Laxative Agents**

Laxative Agent	Drug	Potential Interaction	Management/Preventive Measures
Bulk-forming laxatives (e.g., psyllium)	Digoxin, anticoagulants, salicylates and potentially other oral drugs	Interference with drug absorption	Separate dosing of prescription oral medications by at least 2 hours
Docusate salts	Mineral oil	Increased absorption of mineral oil	Avoid concurrent use
Magnesium citrate	Fluoroquinolone and tetracycline antibiotics	Decreased drug absorption	Avoid oral magnesium citrate within 1 to 3 hours of oral tetracyclines or fluoroquinolones
Magnesium hydroxide	Captopril, cefdinir, some oral bisphosphonates, gabapentin, iron salts, nitrofurantoin, phenothiazines, phenytoin, rosuvastatin	Decreased oral bioavailability, and/or rate or extent of drug absorption	Separate dosing by at least 2 hours for most agents
Magnesium hydroxide	Ketoconazole, itraconazole, fluoroquinolone and tetracycline antibiotics, levothyroxine	Decreased drug absorption	Avoid magnesium hydroxide for at least 4 hours before or up to 3 hours after interacting agent
Bisacodyl	Milk products or drugs that raise gastric pH (e.g., proton pump inhibitors)	Premature dissolution of the bisacodyl enteric coating, leading to gastric irritation or dyspepsia	Avoid milk products or interacting drugs within 1 hour before or after bisacodyl

for mineral oil products includes a warning against its use in patients younger than 6 years, pregnant women, bedridden or older adults, and individuals with difficulty swallowing.

Taking larger-than-recommended doses of mineral oil can cause oil leakage through the anal sphincter, anal pruritus (pruritus ani), cryptitis, or other perianal conditions. With repeated and prolonged use of mineral oil, the droplets may reach the mesenteric lymph nodes and may also be present in the intestinal mucosa, liver, and spleen, where they elicit a typical foreign body reaction. Mineral oil may impair the absorption of fat-soluble vitamins A, D, E, and K. Because of these and other safety concerns, potential drug interaction with docusate (Table 15–5), and the availability of better treatment alternatives, use of mineral oil to treat constipation should be avoided if possible.[8]

Saline Laxatives

Saline laxatives include magnesium citrate, magnesium hydroxide, dibasic sodium phosphate, monobasic sodium phosphate, and magnesium sulfate. They are available in liquid or solid form for oral administration and in liquid form for rectal administration (Table 15–4). Saline laxatives draw water into the small and large intestine (oral products) or colon (rectal forms) by osmosis, increase intraluminal pressure, and promote GI motility. Saline laxatives are used to treat constipation or for acute bowel evacuation required before a procedure (e.g., colonoscopy).

Oral magnesium hydroxide is an appropriate agent for treatment of occasional constipation in otherwise healthy patients. When administered at standard doses, magnesium hydroxide produces a bowel movement within 30 minutes to 6 hours of administration.[8]

A WORD ABOUT Opioid-Induced Constipation

Opioid use is common in the treatment of noncancer and cancer pain. Constipation is experienced by approximately 40% of patients taking opioid drugs and is the most common adverse effect with use of these agents. Opioid-induced constipation may prevent patients from receiving appropriate pain-relieving dosages or may cause discontinuation of therapy despite the need for pain relief. Opioids cause constipation by binding to bowel and central nervous system receptors to decrease GI motility and intestinal secretions, leading to longer retention time of fecal matter in the intestines with consequent drying of the stool. Unlike with other opioid-induced adverse effects, patients generally do not develop tolerance to constipation over time. Constipating effects of opioids are dependent on the opioid dose and duration of use.[19,24] Oral opioids generally are more constipating than parenteral agents. Transdermal fentanyl patches are less constipating than oral opioids and may be an option for outpatients requiring chronic opioid therapy.[11,24]

Patients on a chronic opioid regimen will require long-term laxative treatment to prevent and/or treat constipation. Stimulant laxatives (e.g., senna or bisacodyl, with or without docusate) are most commonly recommended.[24] Typically, a stool softener alone is not effective. Polyethylene glycol preparations or other osmotic agents may also be used for prevention and treatment of opioid-induced constipation. Saline laxatives or rectally administered preparations may be needed intermittently for acute evacuation. Bulk-forming laxatives are unlikely to be adequately effective if used alone and may not be tolerated because of fluid restrictions or immobility in some chronic opioid patients (e.g., those under palliative care).[19,24]

Identify patients at risk for opioid-induced constipation to help prevent problems, and provide counseling about nondrug preventive measures. For patients on chronic opioid therapy, emphasize the importance of bowel regimen adherence, and explain the need for long-term laxative therapy with chronic opioid use. If appropriate, suggest alternative opioids (e.g., transdermal fentanyl) that may be less constipating. Educate patients on short-term opioid therapy about constipation, especially those with other risk factors for constipation (e.g., postabdominal surgery, post-childbirth).

Other saline laxatives such as magnesium citrate are more commonly used for acute catharsis (e.g., as preparation for a colonoscopy). With use of saline agents for these purposes, the time to onset of action is 30 minutes–3 hours for oral doses and 2–15 minutes for rectal doses. Although magnesium sulfate (Epsom salt) is labeled for nonprescription use, it should be avoided, because safer laxatives exist.

Adverse effects of saline laxatives may include abdominal cramping, nausea, vomiting, or dehydration. Patients who cannot tolerate fluid loss should not use saline laxatives. In patients who are not on fluid restriction, oral doses of magnesium salts should be followed by at least 8 oz of water to prevent dehydration. If used long-term or at higher-than-recommended doses, saline laxatives containing magnesium can cause electrolyte imbalances, including hypermagnesemia.[8] Magnesium-containing laxatives should be avoided in patients on sodium-, phosphate-, or magnesium-restricted diets and in individuals at increased risk for magnesium toxicity (e.g., newborns, older adults, patients with renal impairment). Pharmacists should also consider potential drug–drug interactions with magnesium-containing laxatives (Table 15–5).

Products containing sodium phosphate can cause hyperphosphatemia, hypocalcemia, and hypernatremia. These should be used with caution in patients with renal impairment, those on sodium-restricted diets, and/or individuals taking medications that may affect serum electrolyte levels (e.g., diuretics).[8] Sodium phosphate products are contraindicated in patients with congestive heart failure. Additionally, rectally administered sodium phosphate should be avoided in patients with megacolon, gastrointestinal obstruction, imperforate anus, or colostomy.[25]

Acute phosphate nephropathy and renal impairment have been reported with use of sodium phosphate products for bowel cleansing. Use of nonprescription oral sodium phosphate solutions is restricted to treatment of constipation only (i.e., not for use as bowel preparations). In 2014, an FDA drug safety communication emphasized the appropriate use of all forms of nonprescription sodium phosphate products by recommending that patients not exceed one dose of these agents in a 24-hour period and advising caution with use in high-risk populations (e.g., age older than 55 years, baseline kidney disease).[25]

Stimulant Agents

Stimulant laxatives are classified according to their chemical structure and pharmacologic activity as anthraquinones (e.g., senna) or diphenylmethanes (e.g., bisacodyl). FDA has deemed formerly available products containing cascara sagrada, casanthranol, and phenolphthalein as "not safe and effective."[26,27] Because some of these unapproved agents are marketed as dietary supplements, they may be available in some pharmacies but should not be recommended as therapeutics. Although rhubarb and aloe were not included in FDA rulings, neither of these very irritating substances should be recommended by pharmacist providers.

Stimulant laxatives (Table 15–4) work primarily in the colon to increase intestinal motility either by local irritation of the mucosa or by a more selective action on the intramural nerve plexus of intestinal smooth muscle. They also increase secretion of water and electrolytes in the intestine.[5] The time to onset of action for senna and bisacodyl is usually 6–10 hours after oral administration, but onset of effect may take up to 24 hours. Bisacodyl suppositories usually take effect 15–60 minutes after administration.

Bisacodyl, administered orally or rectally, is also a component of bowel preparation regimens before colonoscopy or other procedures. Stimulant laxatives often are used in combination with docusate to prevent or treat constipation in patients taking chronic opioids.[19,24] (See the box "A Word About Opioid-Induced Constipation.") Overdoses of stimulants may lead to sudden vomiting, nausea, diarrhea, or severe abdominal cramping and require prompt medical attention.

Major hazards of stimulant laxative use include severe cramping, electrolyte and fluid deficiencies, enteric loss of protein, malabsorption caused by excessive hypermotility and catharsis, and hypokalemia. At very high doses, all stimulants may produce cramping, colic, increased mucus secretion, and in some individuals, excessive evacuation of fluid. Stimulants can be effective but may be overused.[28–31] (See the box "A Word About Laxative Overuse.")

Prolonged use of senna can also cause a harmless, reversible melanotic pigmentation of the colonic mucosa (melanosis coli), which may be seen on sigmoidoscopy, colonoscopy, or rectal

A WORD ABOUT
Laxative Overuse

Identify patients at risk for laxative overuse, such as individuals who do not have symptoms of constipation but inappropriately take laxatives frequently to achieve regular bowel movements (e.g., daily) or a softer soft stool consistency. Other patients may desire to "cleanse the system" of toxins with colon-cleansing regimens that contain laxatives.[28] Factors that contribute to laxative overuse include older age, misconceptions about normal bowel movement frequency, fear of constipation, and comorbid conditions (e.g., eating disorders).[29,30]

Excessive use of laxatives can acutely cause diarrhea and vomiting, fluid and electrolyte losses (especially hypokalemia), and dehydration. Concerns about long-term consequences of chronic stimulant laxative use have been disproved in the literature. Although earlier reports pointed to adverse effects associated with chronic use of stimulant laxatives, recent well-designed clinical trials do not support an increased risk of colonic muscle or nerve damage or colorectal cancer with use of these laxatives.[30,31]

On the other hand, acute adverse effects have been recognized as a potential risk in patients who take large doses of laxatives for purging, colon cleansing, or detoxification purposes. Colon-cleansing preparations are available in many pharmacies and are promoted for a wide range of potential benefits, including removing toxins, losing weight, and preventing disease. No data have emerged to support these claims, and acute overuse of colon-cleansing regimens can cause serious adverse effects. Enemas, colonic irrigation, and "colon hydrotherapy" carry additional risks (e.g., bowel perforation or infection) and are not recommended.[28] If laxative overuse for purging related to anorexia or bulimia is suspected, medical referral for appropriate care is needed.

Educate patients whose misperceptions about the need for a daily bowel movement contribute to unnecessary laxative use. Explain to patients that normal bowel patterns vary and that daily bowel movements are not a physical necessity. Encourage lifestyle changes that can promote regularity, such as increased fluid intake, fiber intake, and physical activity.[30]

Note that chronic laxative use may be appropriate in some patients (e.g., those on a chronic opioid regimen). A thorough medical history can help determine if laxative use and choice are appropriate for individual patients.

biopsy. Senna may color urine pink to red, red to violet, or red to brown, and its presence may affect interpretation of the phenolsulfonphthalein test.

Enteric-coated bisacodyl tablets prevent irritation of the gastric mucosa. These should not be broken, crushed, chewed, or given with agents that increase gastric pH. The administration of bisacodyl tablets within 1 hour of antacids, histamine-2 (H2) receptor antagonists, proton pump inhibitors, or milk results in rapid erosion of the tablet's enteric coating, which may lead to gastric or duodenal irritation.

Although castor oil historically has been viewed as a stimulant laxative, its exact mechanism is unknown.[31] Castor oil acts quickly and has significant laxative effects. Prolonged use of castor oil may result in excessive loss of fluid, electrolytes, and nutrients. Its use in the self-care setting is discouraged, because safer and better-tolerated alternatives are available.[8,19]

Combination Products

Combination laxative products are also available (Table 15–6). Companies attempt to take advantage of multiple mechanisms of action to create a product that better meets the criteria for an ideal laxative. For example, some combination products contain a stimulant and an emollient (e.g., senna with docusate sodium) or a stimulant and psyllium. Other available combination oral products include those with psyllium, bisacodyl, docusate, or another agent as the principal ingredient and glycerin as an adjunctive agent. However, glycerin's contributing effect is likely to be insignificant to the overall laxative action of these products.

Patients should be counseled that combining laxatives can have the potential for greater adverse effects, because a common ingredient in most combination products is a stimulant. If a stimulant and a stool softener are combined, the potential for adverse effects depends largely on the stimulant. However, if a stimulant and a saline are combined, the potential for such effects is enhanced, because both agents have significant effects on the intestine.

Pharmacotherapeutic Comparison

Head-to-head comparison studies of solely nonprescription laxatives are largely lacking because most nonprescription laxative ingredients became available before the current emphasis on comparative evidence. With many products, much of what is practiced has been learned through observation and a common-sense approach. For example, a bulk-forming product should soften the stool by its normal action. Because both a stool softener and a bulk-forming agent take approximately the same length of time to work, a bulk-forming agent may be the correct choice for some patients who require stool softening. Although stimulants and saline-type laxatives have been used widely for self-care, HCPs should recommend a product with the lowest likelihood of untoward effects. Of the available nonprescription agents, PEG 3350 is considered by many professional groups and practitioners to have the strongest evidence for efficacy and safety.[32]

Product Selection Guidelines

In considering the use of any laxative to treat uncomplicated constipation, an important consideration is that normal defecation empties only the rectum and the descending and sigmoid segments of the colon. A bulk-forming laxative exerts its effects in a manner that most closely duplicates this normal physiologic process, and the use of bulking agents often is recommended as the initial treatment choice for self-care for acute constipation. However, bulk-forming laxatives may take up to 72 hours or longer for onset of effect. If faster onset is desired, or if a bulk-forming agent is ineffective or inappropriate, the hyperosmotic PEG 3350 is also considered a first-line agent, in view of its effectiveness and

TABLE 15–6 Selected Nonprescription Laxative Products

Trade Name	Primary Ingredients
Bulk-Forming Laxatives	
Citrucel Powder	Methylcellulose 2 g/heaping tablespoon
Citrucel Sugar Free Powder	Methylcellulose 2 g/heaping tablespoon
FiberCon Caplets	Calcium polycarbophil 625 mg/caplet
Metamucil Smooth Texture, Sugar Free Orange Flavor Powder/Individual Packets	Psyllium fiber 3 g/packet
Emollient Laxatives	
Colace Capsules	Docusate sodium 100 mg/capsule
Lubricant Laxatives	
Fleet Mineral Oil Enema	Mineral oil 100%
Kondremul Emulsion	Mineral oil 55%
Saline Laxatives	
Magnesium Citrate Oral Solution	Magnesium citrate 1.745 g/30 mL
Fleet Enema	Monobasic sodium phosphate 19 g/118 mL; dibasic sodium phosphate 7 g/118 mL
Pedia-Lax Enema	Monobasic sodium phosphate 9.5 g/59 mL; dibasic sodium phosphate 3.5 g/59 mL
Phillips' Milk of Magnesia Suspension	Magnesium hydroxide 400 mg/5 mL
Hyperosmotic Laxatives	
Fleet Glycerin Suppository (adult size)	Glycerin 2 g/suppository
MiraLAX	Polyethylene glycol 3350 17 g/capful
Stimulant Laxatives	
Dulcolax Tablets	Bisacodyl 5 mg/tablet
Senokot Tablets	Sennosides 8.6 mg/tablet
Fletcher's Laxative for Kids	Senna concentrate 33.3 mg/mL
Combination Laxatives	
Senokot-S Tablets	Sennosides 8.6 mg/tablet; docusate sodium 50 mg/tablet

favorable adverse effect profile. If PEG 3350 is unable to produce a satisfactory response, addition of a stimulant (e.g., bisacodyl) should be considered.[6,8,9] In each case, the lowest effective dose should be used, and the dose should be reduced once symptoms subside. Patients who fail to achieve a therapeutic response after 7 days of self-treatment require medical referral.

Special Populations

CHILDREN. Constipation in children is generally defined as a delay or difficulty in bowel movements over a period of 2 weeks or longer; Table 15–4 provides age-based definitions and dosing recommendations for children.[33,34] Constipation affects 16%–37% of children and is the most common cause of abdominal pain in this age group.[15,35] A number of factors can alter bowel habits in children, including unavailability of toilet facilities; emotional distress; febrile illness; chronic medical conditions (e.g., cystic fibrosis, hypothyroidism); family conflict; dietary changes (e.g., switching from human to cow milk); fear of defecation; or a change in daily routine or environment.[33] Children who experience pain from straining to pass stools may further avoid bowel movements or withhold stool, resulting in worsening symptoms and a fear of toileting.[15,33]

Before a laxative product is recommended, the possible causes for constipation should be assessed thoroughly, with consideration of the child's age and any previous laxative use. The route of administration and the taste of oral products are especially significant in children. Laxative use often can be avoided in older children by encouraging them to adhere to suggested dietary guidelines to improve stool regularity.

Evaluation of constipation in children should begin with determination of exclusions for nonprescription therapy (Figure 15–2). Constipation in children may manifest as fecal impaction, and children with suspected impaction (as indicated by abdominal cramping; rectal bleeding; small, semiformed stools; fecal soiling; and/or constipation accompanied by watery diarrhea) should be referred for further evaluation.[15,33]

Mild constipation in children often can be relieved with dietary or behavioral modifications, such as increasing intake of fluid and fruit juices containing sorbitol (e.g., prune, apple, grape) or adding small amounts of barley malt extract or corn syrup to juice or milk.[15,33] Once solid foods are introduced, adding or increasing the amount of high-fiber cereals or grains, vegetables, and fruits to the diet may relieve symptoms of constipation. The recommended dietary fiber intake (in grams) for children older than 2 years should equal or exceed their age plus 5 g/day.[17] Parents or caregivers should establish a regular stooling time for toilet-trained children (usually after a morning meal) and develop a supportive system (e.g., charts, stickers) for positively reinforcing bowel movements. Children should be encouraged to promptly heed the urge to pass a bowel movement, to avoid negative consequences of retaining stool in the rectum (e.g., increased hardening, pain, abdominal distention).[33,34]

If dietary or behavior modifications are insufficient, pharmacologic therapy is indicated (Table 15–4). Nonprescription laxatives approved for self-care in children ranging in age from 2 up to 6 years include oral docusate sodium, magnesium hydroxide, and senna. Rectal use of glycerin, mineral oil, or sodium phosphate products is also approved in this age group. Oral products approved for children 6 up to 12 years of age include methylcellulose, calcium polycarbophil, psyllium powder, docusate sodium, mineral oil, magnesium citrate, magnesium hydroxide, magnesium sulfate, senna, bisacodyl, and castor oil. (See "Pharmacologic Therapy" for recommendations about use of individual agents. See also Chapter 11, section "Special Populations," for FDA requirements for dispensing devices included in liquid nonprescription products.) Oral use of PEG 3350 is not FDA-approved for patients younger than 17 years, but its use in children is increasing. Rectal products approved for children 6 up to 12 years of age include glycerin suppositories, mineral oil, sodium phosphate, and bisacodyl.

If medication is needed for the occasional relief of temporary constipation in children 2 up to 6 years of age, oral docusate sodium or magnesium hydroxide can be recommended first.[15,33] Docusate sodium may be especially helpful if the primary complaint is difficulty passing dry, hard stools. If faster relief is needed, providers can recommend pediatric glycerin suppositories, taking care to ensure that caregivers select the pediatric-size suppositories for this age group (1 g) and understand proper administration technique. Oral senna or magnesium citrate and rectal mineral oil or sodium phosphate enemas should be reserved for use when other treatments fail or at the direction of an HCP.[15,33–36]

In children 6 up to 12 years of age, bulk-forming agents, docusate sodium, or magnesium hydroxide can be recommended for the occasional relief of temporary constipation, with oral stimulants reserved for when other treatments fail.[15,33–36] For faster relief, glycerin or bisacodyl suppositories can be recommended, with mineral oil or sodium phosphate enemas reserved for when other treatments fail, or at the direction of an HCP.[15] Magnesium sulfate (Epsom salt) and castor oil are not recommended, because safer, better-tolerated, and well-studied laxatives are available.

PATIENTS OF ADVANCED AGE. Compared with that in the general adult population, the prevalence of constipation in older adults is higher, with 15%–20% of community-dwelling older patients and up to 50% of nursing home residents reporting constipation.[5] Older adults are at greater risk for constipation because of dietary changes (e.g., reduced caloric, fiber, and/or fluid intake); decreased physical activity; presence of comorbid conditions (e.g., parkinsonism, depression); increased use of medications that cause constipation (e.g., opioids, anticholinergics); and physiologic changes of the body with age (e.g., absorption, distribution, metabolism, excretion).[5,18]

Pharmacists should conduct a complete medication review in older adults to identify potential effects of comorbid conditions and drug therapies (see also Chapter 2). Lifestyle modifications constitute the initial step, including increased fiber and fluid intake, adding prunes or prune juice to the diet, physical activity as tolerated, and bowel training.[5,19] Consideration should be given to fluid or other restrictions that may be associated with comorbid conditions (e.g., congestive heart failure, renal failure).[5]

If medication adjustments and/or lifestyle changes are insufficient, laxative therapy initiated with bulk-forming laxatives as a first step is appropriate. Patients who are dehydrated, very frail, bedridden, or unable to drink adequate fluid to prevent mechanical obstruction or fecal impaction should not use bulk-forming laxatives. If these laxatives cannot be used or do not provide sufficient relief, or if faster onset of effect is desired, PEG 3350 is also used as a first-line option because of its efficacy and tolerability.[5,37] Stool softeners (e.g., docusate) may be helpful in older adults with anal fissures or hemorrhoids that cause painful defecation.[18]

A number of nonprescription laxatives should be avoided or used only with caution in older adults, including mineral oil (associated with increased risk of aspiration) and saline laxatives (with potential for fluid or electrolyte depletion, magnesium toxicity, or drug interactions).[5] Patients of advanced age are sensitive to shifts in fluid and electrolytes, particularly those taking diuretics or with fluid restrictions.[5,18]

Older adults may also require rectal therapy with a suppository or enema, especially if fecal impaction is suspected. Rectal preparations are generally considered to be safe in this age group, although comparative evidence of safety and effectiveness for the various preparations is limited.[5,38] Older adults may be more susceptible to adverse effects with sodium phosphate products, and these agents should be avoided or used with caution in this population (see the box "A Word About Laxative Overuse").[38]

PREGNANCY AND LACTATION. Constipation is common in pregnancy, affecting up to one-third of women throughout pregnancy and in the postpartum period.[39] Contributing factors include compression of the colon by the growing uterus, increasing progesterone levels, low fluid and fiber intake, and the iron and calcium in prenatal vitamin and mineral supplements.[39]

The main goal of treatment in pregnancy is to achieve soft stools without laxative use. Dietary measures (e.g., increasing fiber and fluids) are first-line interventions, with addition of a laxative indicated only after a nondrug approach is determined to be insufficient.[39] Bulk-forming laxatives are recommended initially (taken with plenty of fluid to prevent worsening constipation).[39–41] Docusate may also be used for patients who have primarily dry, hard stools.[41] If needed, short-term use of senna or bisacodyl is considered a low-risk approach in pregnancy.[40,41] Some experts also consider PEG 3350 to be a first-line choice in pregnancy because very little is absorbed systemically.[41] Short-term use of senna or bisacodyl is preferred by some practitioners, however, because more data are available for use of these agents in pregnancy.[39,40] In more severe cases, or when the safety of a laxative product is questionable, consultation with a woman's HCP is recommended before laxative use.

Some laxatives, including castor oil, mineral oil, and saline laxatives, should be used very cautiously or avoided altogether in pregnancy. Castor oil has been associated with uterine contraction and rupture, and mineral oil may impair maternal fat-soluble vitamin absorption. High doses or long-term use of saline laxatives (e.g., magnesium hydroxide) may cause electrolyte imbalances and generally should be avoided.[40,41]

Laxatives may also be used post partum to reestablish normal bowel function. Senna, bisacodyl, PEG 3350, and docusate are considered to be compatible with breastfeeding or to carry a low risk of adverse effects in this setting.[40,42,43] These agents are minimally absorbed or do not accumulate in significant concentrations in breast milk, and no data suggest infant toxicity with their use.[40,42,43] Castor oil and mineral oil, however, should be avoided during breastfeeding.[40]

Patient Factors

Laxative products are available in a wide array of oral dosage forms, which may be useful to improve acceptability of laxatives in children. However, misuse or abuse of laxatives available as chewing gum, wafers, effervescent granules, gummy candy, or chocolate tablets may be more likely. Additionally, the glucose and calorie contents of these dosage forms should be considered in patients with diabetes or calorie restrictions.

Patients with fluid restrictions should avoid bulk-forming laxatives. Patients on sodium-restricted diets should ascertain the sodium content of laxative products (especially saline laxatives).[44] Patients with severely limited mobility (e.g., postoperative patients, older adults) are at increased risk for constipation and may require regular use of stool softeners or laxative products to promote laxation.

Enemas are used routinely to prepare patients for surgery, child delivery, and GI radiologic or endoscopic examinations. The mechanism of laxation with enemas varies by agent. Vegetable oil enemas lubricate and soften fecal matter, whereas tap water, normal saline, and sodium phosphate enemas have osmotic effects. Sodium phosphate enemas are more efficient and effective than tap water, soapsuds, saline, or vegetable oil enemas.

A properly administered enema (Table 15–7) cleans only the distal colon. Improper use or administration may result in adverse effects (e.g., mucosal changes, spasm of the intestinal wall, colonic perforation).

Suppositories containing bisacodyl are used for postoperative, antepartum, and postpartum care and are adequate in preparing for proctosigmoidoscopy. Glycerin suppositories are useful in initiating the defecation reflex in children and in promoting rectal emptying in adults.

Patient Preferences

Palatability and convenience are important considerations with laxative products. Liquid formulations of emollients may be made more palatable if mixed with juices or milk. Mixing gritty, bulk-forming laxative powders (e.g., psyllium) with orange juice instead of water may increase their taste and texture palatability. Patients may also prefer wafer or single-use packets of bulk-forming laxative powders for convenience and ease of use. Patients should be reminded that many fiber products marketed as grit-free, flavor-free, or taste-free may contain ingredients that have not been studied as bulk-forming laxatives and are approved only as dietary supplements (e.g., inulin). Most laxative ingredients are available in some form as generic products. However, patients with a specific dosage form or other preference may need to choose a brand-name product.

Complementary Therapies

Dietary supplements commonly used to treat constipation include flaxseed, aloe, cascara, and probiotics.[45] Evidence supporting the safety and efficacy of these products varies in extent and quality. A single double-blind trial demonstrated the superiority of flaxseed over psyllium in decreasing constipation, bloating, and abdominal pain over a 3-month period in patients with irritable bowel syndrome. However, a much larger body of evidence supports psyllium's effectiveness, and practitioners should not recommend flaxseed on the basis of limited efficacy and safety data.[45]

Although many commercially available stimulant laxatives are derived from plants, patients should be advised to choose FDA-approved products if a stimulant laxative is indicated. FDA has banned the use of aloe and cascara in nonprescription stimulant laxatives, and both agents are classified as generally unsafe and not effective. Senna is available in dietary supplement form, but use of standardized, FDA-approved senna drug products is preferred.

Probiotics are thought to work in constipation through alteration of GI flora, stimulation of motility and peristalsis, and/or

TABLE 15-7 Administration of Enemas and Rectal Suppositories

Enemas

1. If someone else is administering the enema, lie on your left side with knees bent or in the knee-to-chest position (see drawings A and B). The side-lying position (see drawing A) is preferred for children younger than 2 years. If self-administering the enema, lie on your back with knees bent and buttocks raised (see drawing C). A pillow may be placed under the buttocks.
2. If using a concentrated enema solution, dilute solution according to the product instructions. Prepare 1 pint (500 mL) for adults and ½ pint (250 mL) for children.
3. Lubricate the enema tip with petroleum jelly or other nonmedicated ointment/cream. Apply the lubricant to the anal area as well.
4. Gently insert the enema tip 2 inches (recommended depth for children) to 3 inches into the rectum.
5. Allow the solution to flow into the rectum slowly. If you experience discomfort, the flow is probably too fast.
6. Retain the enema solution until definite lower abdominal cramping is felt. (For enema administration in children, the parent/caregiver may have to gently hold the buttocks closed to prevent the solution from being expelled too soon.)

Suppositories

1. Gently squeeze the suppository to determine if it is firm enough to insert. Chill a soft suppository by placing it in the refrigerator for a few minutes, or by holding it under cool running water.
2. Remove the suppository from its wrapping.
3. Dip the suppository in lukewarm water for a few seconds to soften the exterior.
4. Lie on your left side with knees bent or in the knee-to-chest position (see drawings A and B). The side-lying position (see drawing A) is best for self-administration of a suppository. Small children can be held in a crawling position.
5. To ease insertion, relax the buttocks just before inserting the suppository. Gently insert the tapered end of the suppository high into the rectum. If the suppository slips out, it was not inserted past the anal sphincter (the muscle that keeps the rectum closed). In this case, reinsert the suppository correctly.
6. Continue to lie down for a few minutes, and hold the buttocks together to allow the suppository to dissolve in the rectum. (For suppository administration in a child, the parent/caregiver may have to gently hold the buttocks closed.)
7. Try to avoid a bowel movement for up to 1 hour after insertion of the suppository so that the intended action can occur.

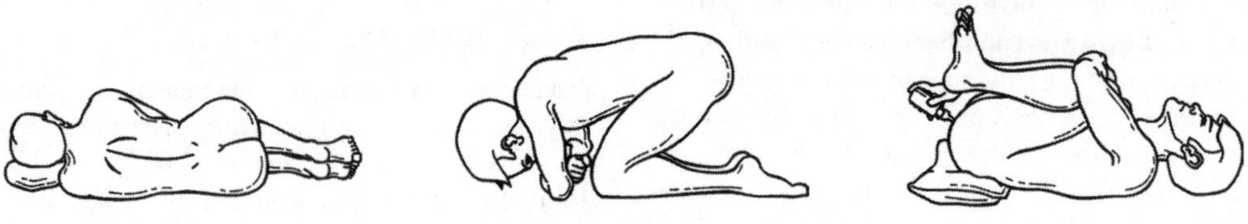

A B C

acceleration of gut transit.[5,46] From a mechanistic or clinical efficacy standpoint, however, the limited evidence available consistently supports use of these agents. A systematic review conducted by Chmielewska and colleagues[47] identified five randomized controlled trials (N = 377) of probiotic supplementation for constipation management. Study results suggested a potential benefit, but the investigators questioned the overall efficacy and clinical relevance of specific study outcomes. Probiotics should be considered investigational for treatment of constipation until additional efficacy and safety evidence are available (see also Chapter 20).[5,46,47]

Assessment of Constipation: A Case-Based Approach

The HCP should obtain as much lifestyle and medical information as possible before making any recommendations for preventing or treating constipation. Appropriate information allows the provider to make rational recommendations that are based on knowledge of the patient, the clinical problem, and available products, as well as on the provider's own judgment and experience. A patient who presents with constipation should initially be evaluated for any signs of significant GI problems that may warrant medical evaluation or in which laxative use is inappropriate (Figure 15–2). Initial assessment should include questions about diet, fluid intake, physical activity, and any underlying pathologic conditions that may produce constipation as a symptom.

Patients should then be questioned regarding the characteristics of bowel movements, including the caliber, color, and texture of stools, as well as frequency of elimination. Additional assessment should include questions about use of medications (both prescription and nonprescription), natural products, and previous laxative use. For patients without a history of constipation, a thorough investigation should be conducted to determine whether an acute case of constipation resulted from new or old disease or from the use of medications. When information is insufficient to assess the cause of the symptoms, or if any doubt exists regarding the patient's disease status, medical referral is appropriate. Cases 15–1 and 15–2 provide sample assessments for patients presenting with constipation.

Patient Counseling for Constipation

Patient education about laxative products is important for all patients (particularly for children and their caregivers and older adults). Before recommending a laxative product, health care providers should inform the patient of available nondrug measures and provide information on proper diet, adequate fluid intake, and reasonable exercise. If a laxative is needed, the provider should explain why a particular type of laxative is appropriate for the present situation, how to use the laxative, when to expect to see results, what adverse effects could occur, and what precautions to take. The box "Patient Education for Constipation" lists specific information to include in patient counseling.

CASE 15-1

Relevant Evaluation Criteria	Scenario/Model Outcome
Collect	
1. Gather essential information about the patient's symptoms and medical history, including	
a. Description of symptom(s) (i.e., nature, onset, duration, severity, associated symptoms)	A mother states her daughter has been constipated for the past 2 weeks. The child has not been able to go to the bathroom and is straining to pass her stool. Her abdomen is also bloated and she is cranky.
b. Description of any factors that seem to precipitate, exacerbate, and/or relieve the patient's symptom(s)	The child recently started preschool and is eating new foods during the day.
c. Description of the patient's efforts to relieve the symptoms	The mother has been giving her daughter prune juice for the last 3 days.
d. Patient's identity	Allison Carter
e. Patient's age, gender, height, and weight	4 years old, female, 3 ft 4 in., 40 lb
f. Patient's occupation	n/a
g. Patient's dietary habits	Eats lots of fruits and vegetables, pasta, pizza, and chicken nuggets.
h. Patient's sleep habits	10 hours
i. Concurrent medical conditions, prescription and nonprescription medications, and dietary supplements	None
j. Allergies	None
k. History of other adverse reactions to medications	None
l. Other (describe) ______	Allison typically has 2–3 bowel movements per day.
Assess	
2. Differentiate patient's signs/symptoms, and correctly identify the patient's primary problem(s).	The patient is experiencing constipation most likely precipitated by her change in routine and environment, and consumption of different food during the day. Constipation in children is common with a change in routine and/or environment.
3. Identify exclusions for self-treatment (Figure 15–2).	None
4. Formulate a comprehensive list of therapeutic alternatives for the primary problem to determine whether triage to a health care provider is required, and share this information with the patient or caregiver.	Options include (1) Refer patient to an appropriate HCP. (2) Recommend nondrug measures: a. Resume a balanced diet with adequate fiber, fruits, and vegetables. b. At a minimum, drink fruit juices with sorbitol. c. Establish a regular stooling time for toilet-trained children (usually after a morning meal), and develop a supportive system (e.g., charts, stickers) for positively reinforcing bowel movements. d. Recommend strategies to prevent future recurrences of constipation. (3) Recommend docusate sodium: capsules 50 mg daily or pediatric liquid 50 mg/15 mL (15 mL) daily to help facilitate resolution of symptoms. (4) Recommend a pediatric glycerin suppository. The glycerin suppository will offer the fastest resolution, if the parent is able and willing to use that dosage form. (5) Recommend magnesium hydroxide chewable tablet 311 mg (2 tablets) or 400 mg (1–2 tablets) at bedtime daily to help facilitate resolution of symptoms. (6) For resolution of the symptoms, recommend senna 8.6 mg sennosides (½ tablet), senna liquid concentrate pediatric formulation 5 mL–10 mL, or liquid sennosides 2.5 mL once daily. A stimulant laxative will also offer fast relief of symptoms.

CASE 15-1 *continued*

Relevant Evaluation Criteria	Scenario/Model Outcome
	(7) Recommend self-care until patient can see an appropriate HCP. (8) Refer patient to an appropriate HCP if the therapeutic option and lifestyle changes do not alleviate symptoms within a week. (9) Take no action.
Plan	
5. Select an optimal therapeutic alternative to address the patient's problem, taking into account patient preferences.	For fast relief of Allison's symptoms, she should be given a stimulant laxative, and her mother should institute the recommended nondrug measures.
6. Describe the recommended therapeutic approach to the patient or caregiver.	The mother should administer senna pediatric liquid concentrate formulation 5 mL (use the supplied measuring cup) once daily for resolution of Allison's symptoms. The medication usually takes effect in about 6–10 hours.
7. Explain to the patient or caregiver the rationale for selecting the recommended therapeutic approach from the considered therapeutic alternatives.	"The senna liquid concentrate pediatric formulation will provide quick relief. Once your child has become used to her new routine and environment, the constipation will most likely resolve. However, it is important to continue a healthy diet with fruits, vegetables, and fiber. It may also be helpful to establish a regular stooling time for toilet-trained children (usually after a morning meal) and to develop a supportive system (e.g., charts or stickers) for positively reinforcing bowel movements."
Implement	
8. When recommending self-care with nonprescription medications and/or nondrug therapy, convey accurate information to the patient or caregiver.	See the box "Patient Education for Constipation."
a. Appropriate dose and frequency of administration	See the box "Patient Education for Constipation."
b. Maximum number of days the therapy should be employed	See the box "Patient Education for Constipation."
c. Product administration procedures	See the box "Patient Education for Constipation."
d. Expected time to onset of relief	"The medication should take effect in 6 to 10 hours."
e. Degree of relief that can be reasonably expected	"The constipation symptoms should be relieved."
f. Most common adverse effects	See the box "Patient Education for Constipation."
g. Adverse effects that warrant medical intervention should they occur	See the box "Patient Education for Constipation."
h. Patient options in the event that condition worsens or persists	See the box "Patient Education for Constipation."
i. Product storage requirements	"Store the medication in a cool, dry place out of children's reach."
j. Specific nondrug measures	See the box "Patient Education for Constipation."
Solicit follow-up questions from the patient or caregiver.	"Can the liquid laxative be mixed in fruit juice or milk to make it easier to give to my daughter?"
Answer the patient's or caregiver's questions.	"No, the senna liquid concentrate pediatric formulation has a root beer flavor to make it easier to administer to children."
Follow-up: Monitor and Evaluate	
9. Assess patient outcome	Ask the mother to call to update you on her daughter's response to your recommendations. Or you could call her in a few days to evaluate the outcome.

Key: HCP = Health care provider.

CASE 15-2

Relevant Evaluation Criteria	Scenario/Model Outcome
Collect	
1. Gather essential information about the patient's symptoms and medical history, including	
a. Description of symptom(s) (i.e., nature, onset, duration, severity, associated symptoms)	The patient says that she is having a very difficult time passing stool. She admits to straining to pass "normal looking" but soft stools. She has only about 1 bowel movement per week. She has been experiencing these symptoms for the past month.
b. Description of any factors that seem to precipitate, exacerbate, and/or relieve the patient's symptom(s)	Patient notes that her problem really started when she broke her ankle in a bicycle accident, and she started taking a pain medication prescribed by her PCP.
c. Description of the patient's efforts to relieve the symptoms	The patient has been using a stool softener for the past 2 weeks.
d. Patient's identity	Margaret Thomas
e. Age, gender, height, and weight	30 years old, female, 5 ft 7 in., 150 lb
f. Patient's occupation	Works for a nonprofit organization.
g. Patient's dietary habits	Usual diet consists of lots of vegetables and salad, pastas, occasional whole-grain breads, meat and fish, caffeinated coffee, diet sodas, and desserts.
h. Patient's sleep habits	Sleeps about 8 hours per night.
i. Concurrent medical conditions, prescription and nonprescription medications, and dietary supplements	Vicodin 7.5 325 mg every 6 hours; docusate 100 mg daily; multivitamin with iron
j. Allergies	None
k. History of other adverse reactions to medications	None
l. Other (describe) ______	She typically has 3–4 bowel movements every week. She takes about 4 Vicodin tablets per day.
Assess	
2. Differentiate patient's signs/symptoms, and correctly identify the patient's primary problem(s).	The patient recently started an opioid medication, Vicodin, which can cause constipation. The patient's constipation appears to be correlated with the start of this medication. The patient takes a multivitamin with iron, which can also contribute to constipation.
3. Identify exclusions for self-treatment (Figure 15–2).	Unexplained changes in bowel habits; bowel symptoms that persist for more than 2 weeks.
4. Formulate a comprehensive list of therapeutic alternatives for the primary problem to determine whether triage to a health care provider is required, and share this information with the patient or caregiver.	Options include (1) Refer patient to an appropriate HCP. (2) Recommend self-care with a nonprescription laxative and nondrug measures. (3) Recommend self-care until patient can see an appropriate HCP. (4) Refer patient to an appropriate HCP if therapeutic option and lifestyle changes do not alleviate symptoms within a week. (5) Take no action.
Plan	
5. Select an optimal therapeutic alternative to address the patient's problem, taking into account patient preferences.	Patient has experienced constipation secondary to the initiation of an opioid medication. She has been experiencing these symptoms for 1 month. She should consult an HCP. However, she should also implement nondrug measures to help prevent constipation and to promote a healthy lifestyle.

CASE 15-2 *continued*

Relevant Evaluation Criteria	Scenario/Model Outcome
6. Describe the recommended therapeutic approach to the patient or caregiver.	"You should consult a health care provider. You should also modify your diet to include more fiber, fruits, and vegetables. You should add a fiber supplement to your diet, and you should increase your fluid intake. Also, you should establish a regular exercise routine once your ankle is healed."
7. Explain to the patient or caregiver the rationale for selecting the recommended therapeutic approach from the considered therapeutic alternatives.	"This option is best because your constipation began after you started your new pain medication, and it has been occurring for a month. Therefore, nonprescription laxative therapy may not be the best choice right now. You should be evaluated by your health care provider."
Implement	
8. When recommending self-care with nonprescription medications and/or nondrug therapy, convey accurate information to the patient or caregiver.	"Even though you need to see your health care provider, you can still implement nondrug measures that promote a healthy lifestyle, such as eating more fiber, fruits, and vegetables, and beginning a regular exercise routine when your ankle is healed. You should consult your health care provider about these measures as well."
Solicit follow-up questions from the patient or caregiver.	"Should I stop taking my pain medication?"
Answer the patient's or caregiver's questions.	"I would discuss this with your primary care provider. It may be time to decrease or stop your pain medication, especially if you are not experiencing severe pain. Your primary care provider may also be able to prescribe a different pain medication that does not cause constipation."
Follow-up: Monitor and Evaluate	
9. Assess patient outcome.	Contact the patient in a day or two to ensure that she made an appointment for further medical care.

PATIENT EDUCATION FOR Constipation

The primary goals of treatment are (1) to relieve constipation and reestablish normal bowel function, (2) to establish dietary and exercise habits to help prevent recurrence, and (3) to promote the safe and effective use of laxative products. For most patients, carefully following the product instructions and the self-care measures listed here will help achieve these goals.

Nondrug Measures

- To promote regular bowel movements, use nondrug strategies such as a high-fiber diet (slowly increase intake to 25–35 g/day), plenty of fluids, and regular exercise.
- Increase dietary fiber by eating foods with whole grains, oats, fruits, and vegetables.
- Avoid constipating foods, such as processed cheeses and concentrated sweets.
- Drink plenty of fluids (six to eight 8-ounce glasses a day) to help soften your stool and move food through your gastrointestinal tract.
- Develop and maintain a routine exercise program. Walking can be helpful if your heart is healthy and if you have no other apparent health risks.
- Establish a regular pattern for bathroom visits. Do not delay in responding to the urge to use the toilet; allow adequate time for elimination in a relaxed, unhurried atmosphere.
- Maintain general emotional well-being and avoid stressful situations.

Nonprescription Medications

- Bulk-forming laxatives (e.g., methylcellulose, psyllium)
- Hyperosmotic laxatives (e.g., polyethylene glycol [PEG] 3350, glycerin)
- Emollient laxatives, or "stool softeners" (e.g., docusate sodium)
- Lubricant laxative (mineral oil)
- Saline laxatives (e.g., magnesium citrate, magnesium hydroxide)
- Stimulant laxatives (e.g., bisacodyl, senna)

Complementary Therapies

- Not routinely recommended for self-treatment of constipation.

Disease Information

- Constipation is usually defined as having fewer than 3 bowel movements per week that involve straining and the difficult passage of dry, hard stools. In most cases, constipation is temporary. Self-treatment of constipation is safe for short-term symptoms in patients without other underlying disorders or conditions.
- You do not need to take laxatives routinely if your bowel habits are interrupted for 1 or 2 days, nor do you need to routinely "clean your system."

Drug Information

Bulk-Forming Laxatives

- Unless a rapid effect is needed (e.g., to clean out the bowel for a diagnostic endoscopic procedure or X-ray study), take a bulk-forming

PATIENT EDUCATION FOR Constipation *(continued)*

laxative. Be sure to drink at least 8 ounces of fluid with each dose to prevent an intestinal blockage. If you have swallowing difficulties, alert your health care provider before taking a bulk-forming laxative.

- If you have diabetes or are on a carbohydrate- or calorie-restricted diet, choose sugar-free bulk-forming agents, if possible. Many bulk-forming agents contain sugar and have a high caloric content per dose.
- Do not give sugar-free bulk-forming products to patients with phenylketonuria.

Hyperosmotic Laxatives

- If you have irritable bowel syndrome, do not take PEG 3350 without the supervision of your primary care provider.
- When using PEG 3350, use the provided cap to measure the dose, or use 1 packet of powder. Mix the powder with 4–8 ounces of a hot, cold, or room-temperature beverage (e.g., water, juice, soda, coffee, tea).
- Consult a primary care provider before using glycerin suppositories if you have previously had a condition that caused rectal irritation.

Emollient Laxatives

- Do not take docusate if you are taking mineral oil unless told to do so by a primary care provider. Taking these together can increase the amount of mineral oil that gets into your body.

Lubricant Laxative

- Although some patients use mineral oil for occasional bouts of constipation, its use in self-care is strongly discouraged because safer agents that work just as well are available.
- Do not give mineral oil to children younger than 6 years, pregnant women, older adults, or bedridden patients without the supervision of a primary care provider. These patients are at a higher risk for adverse effects from mineral oil.
- Do not take mineral oil with emollient laxatives (e.g., docusate). Taking these together can increase the amount of mineral oil that gets into your body.
- To avoid delaying the absorption of foods, nutrients, and vitamins, do not take mineral oil within 2 hours of eating.
- Stop use and consult your health care provider if anal leakage of oil occurs. This may indicate that your dose is too high.

Saline Laxatives

- Take doses with an 8-ounce glass of water, if possible, to prevent dehydration.
- Consult your health care provider before using a saline laxative if you are taking a diuretic ("water pill") for high blood pressure (e.g., hydrochlorothiazide, furosemide), if you are taking other drugs that can cause electrolyte changes, or if you are on a sodium-, phosphate-, or magnesium-restricted diet.
- If you are an older adult, you may be at increased risk for dehydration or electrolyte imbalances with saline laxatives. Consult a health care provider before using these agents.
- Do not use magnesium sulfate (Epsom salt) to treat constipation except under the advice of a primary care provider.

Stimulant Laxatives

- Do not use castor oil to treat constipation except under the advice of a health care provider.
- Do not chew or crush bisacodyl tablets, which may cause stomach discomfort, faintness, and cramps. Do not use bisacodyl within 1 hour after taking an antacid or milk. Doing so can cause the tablet's coating to break down too quickly.

Administration of Medication/Safe Usage

- Read and carefully follow labeled dosage and administration instructions for all laxative products.
- Oral laxatives are available as tablets, capsules, thin-film strips, chewing gum, wafers, effervescent granules, gummy candy, chocolate tablets, and other forms. Choose the best form for you, and consider glucose and caloric content if you have diabetes or calorie restrictions.
- Rectal laxatives (enemas, suppositories) should be used according to administration instructions (Table 15–6).
- If constipation symptoms continue after 7 days of laxative treatment, contact your health care provider.
- Do not give laxatives to children younger than 2 years unless their use is recommended by a primary care provider.
- Take most laxatives at bedtime, especially if more than 6–8 hours will be needed to produce results.
- Do not take any laxatives at doses higher than the recommended amounts.

Warning Signs/Symptoms

- Do not take laxatives if you have marked abdominal pain, nausea, vomiting, significant abdominal distention, cramping, or fever—any of these may be evidence of a more serious condition (e.g., appendicitis).
- Do not take laxatives if you have a sudden change in bowel habits that persists for longer than 2 weeks, because such changes can be a sign of a more serious condition. See your primary care provider for treatment recommendations.
- If rectal bleeding, blood in your stool, or passage of black, tarry stools occurs, see your health care provider. These may be signs of an underlying medical condition.
- If you have kidney or liver disease, heart failure, hypertension, or other conditions requiring sodium, potassium, magnesium, or calcium restriction, do not use laxative products with a maximum daily dose of more than 345 mg (15 mEq) sodium, 975 mg (25 mEq) potassium, 600 mg (50 mEq) magnesium, or 1800 mg (90 mEq) calcium.
- Consult your health care provider before using laxatives if you currently have or have a history of any condition that may affect self-treatment for constipation (e.g., paraplegia or quadriplegia, inflammatory bowel disease, colostomy, megacolon, ileostomy).
- Some laxatives require you to drink a lot of water with each dose. Patients with fluid restrictions should avoid bulk-forming or other laxatives that require abundant fluid intake.

Adverse Effects

- The most common adverse effects of laxatives are abdominal cramping, gas, bloating, and diarrhea.

Interactions

- Avoid taking laxatives within 2 hours of other medications.
- To make sure you avoid any potential drug–drug interactions, alert your health care provider if you are taking anticoagulants (blood thinners), digoxin (a heart medicine), sodium polystyrene sulfonate (a treatment for high potassium levels), or other drugs that need to be maintained at precise levels.

Storage of Medications/Expiration Date/Signs of Instability

- Discard any medications that are outdated, that appear to have been tampered with, or that have an unusual appearance.

Evaluation of Patient Outcomes for Constipation

Once therapy has been selected, treatment effectiveness is determined by how rapidly constipation is relieved and to what degree normal bowel habits have been restored. For acute constipation, dietary changes, exercise, or bulk-forming laxatives may take several days to weeks to provide relief. Most hyperosmotic, saline, or stimulant laxatives will provide relief within 3–72 hours. Enemas can produce evacuation within minutes. If initial treatment of constipation is ineffective, therapy should be repeated according to product-specific directions.

If an adequate response is not achieved after a short period of laxative use (usually within 7 days), assessment of whether the patient needs medical referral is indicated at the follow-up contact. If a laxative must be continued for an extended period, the patient should be referred for further evaluation, because frequent use may be a sign of (1) a more severe form of constipation, (2) a medication adverse effect, or (3) an underlying medical problem.

Key Points for Constipation

- Nonprescription laxative treatment should not be recommended if exclusion criteria for self-treatment are present (Figure 15–2). Patients in whom such exclusions are identified require medical referral.
- Special circumstances and patient characteristics (e.g., pregnancy, age) should be considered in assessing the need for self-medication.
- For most cases of simple constipation, a balanced diet, exercise, and adequate fluid intake are helpful.
- Bulk-forming laxatives and polyethylene glycol (PEG) 3350 taken as directed are first-line laxative choices in most adults, but they may take up to 72 hours to work. Glycerin suppositories or stimulant laxatives provide faster relief, if needed.
- Therapy with any laxative product should be limited to 7 days, unless supervised by a health care provider.
- If rectal bleeding occurs at any time during use of a laxative, or if constipation persists despite therapy, patients should stop using the laxative and consult a health care provider.[15]
- To reduce the potential for drug interactions, patients should avoid taking most laxatives within 2 hours of other medications.

REFERENCES

1. Leung L, Riutta T, Kotecha J, Rosser M. Chronic constipation: an evidence-based review. *J Am Fam Board Med.* 2011;24(4):436–51. doi: 10.3122/jabfm.2011.04.100272.
2. World Gastroenterology Organisation. Constipation: a global perspective. 2010. Available at: http://www.worldgastroenterology.org/constipation.html. Accessed May 13, 2017.
3. Bleser S, Brunton S, Carmichael B, et al. Management of chronic constipation: recommendations from a consensus panel. *J Fam Pract.* 2005;54(8): 691–8. PMID: 16061057.
4. American Gastroenterological Association. Technical review on constipation. *Gastroenterology.* 2013;144(1):219–38. doi: https://doi.org/10.1053/j.gastro.2012.10.028.
5. Gallegos-Orozco JF, Foxx-Orenstein AE, Sterler SM, et al. Chronic constipation in the elderly. *Am J Gastroenterol.* 2012;107(1):18–25. doi: 10.1038/ajg.2011.349.
6. American Gastroenterological Association. Medical position statement on constipation. *Gastroenterology.* 2013;144(1):211–7. doi: http://dx.doi.org/10.1053/j.gastro.2012.10.029.
7. Mugie SM, Benninga MA, Di Lorenzo C. Epidemiology of constipation in children and adults: a systematic review. *Best Pract Res Clin Gastroenterol.* 2011;25(1):3–18. doi: https://doi.org/10.1016/j.bpg.2010.12.010.
8. Berardi R, Chan J. *OTC Advisor: Self-Care for Gastrointestinal Disorders, Module 2.* Washington, DC: American Pharmacists Association; 2010. Available at: http://www.pharmacist.com. Accessed May 13, 2017.
9. National Institute of Diabetes and Digestive and Kidney Diseases (NIDDK). Constipation. Available at: https://www.niddk.nih.gov/health-information/digestive-diseases/constipation. Accessed May 13, 2017.
10. Camilleri M, Murray JA. Diarrhea and constipation. In: Longo DL, Fauci AS, Kasper DL, et al, eds. *Harrison's Principles of Internal Medicine.* 19th ed. New York, NY: McGraw-Hill Professional; 2015:55.
11. Fabel PH, Shealy KM. Diarrhea, constipation, and irritable bowel syndrome. In: DiPiro JT, Talbert RL, Yee GC, et al, eds. *Pharmacotherapy: A Pathophysiologic Approach.* 10th ed. New York, NY: McGraw-Hill Professional; 2017:511.
12. Wald A. Chronic constipation: advances in management. *Neurogastroenterol Motil.* 2007;19(1):4–10. doi: https://doi.org/10.1111/j.1365-2982.2006.00835.x.
13. Jamshed N, Lee ZE, Olden KW. Diagnostic approach to chronic constipation in adults. *Am Fam Physician.* 2011;84(3):299–306. PMID: 21842777.
14. Johanson JF. Review of the treatment options for chronic constipation. *MedGenMed.* 2007;9(2):25. PMCID: PMC1994829.
15. Felt B, Brown P, Coran A, et al. Functional constipation and soiling in children. University of Michigan Health System Guidelines for Clinical Care. 2008. Available at: http://www.med.umich.edu/1info/FHP/practiceguides/newconstipation.html. Accessed May 13, 2017.
16. U.S. Department of Health and Human Services, U.S. Department of Agriculture. 2015–2020 Dietary Guidelines for Americans. 8th Edition. December 2015. Available at: http://health.gov/dietaryguidelines/2015/guidelines/. Accessed May 13, 2017.
17. Slavin JL. Position of the American Dietetic Association: health implications of dietary fiber. *J Am Diet Assoc.* 2008;108(10):1716–31. doi: https://doi.org/10.1016/j.jada.2008.08.007.
18. Mounsey A, Raleigh M, Wilson A. Management of constipation in older adults. *Am Fam Physician.* 2015;92(6):500–4. PMID: 26371734.
19. Ford AC, Talley NJ. Laxatives for chronic constipation in adults. *BMJ.* 2012;345:e6168. doi: https://doi.org/10.1136/bmj.e6168.
20. U.S. Food and Drug Administration. Laxative drug products for over-the-counter human use; psyllium ingredients in granular dosage forms. *Fed Reg.* 2007;72:14669–74.
21. Hoffman D. Psyllium: keeping this boon for patients from becoming a bane for providers. *J Fam Pract.* 2006;55(9):770–2. PMID: 16948959.
22. Seinela L, Sairanen U, Laine T, et al. Comparison of polyethylene glycol with and without electrolytes in the treatment of constipation in elderly institutionalized patients. *Drugs Aging.* 2009;26(8):703–13. doi: 0.2165/11316470-000000000-00000.
23. Ramkumar D, Rao SS. Efficacy and safety of traditional medical therapies for chronic constipation: systematic review. *Am J Gastroenterol.* 2005;100(4): 936–71. doi: https://doi.org/10.1111/j.1572-0241.2005.40925.x.
24. Swegle JM, Logemann C. Management of common opioid-induced adverse effects. *Am Fam Physician.* 2006;74(8):1347–54. PMID: 17087429.
25. U.S. Food and Drug Administration. FDA warns of possible harm from exceeding recommended dose of over-the-counter sodium phosphate products to treat constipation. 2014. Available at: http://www.fda.gov/Drugs/DrugSafety/ucm380757.htm. Accessed May 13, 2017.
26. U.S. Food and Drug Administration. Status of certain additional over-the-counter drug category II and III active ingredients. *Fed Regist.* 2002; 67:31125–7.
27. U.S. Food and Drug Administration. Laxative drug products for over-the-counter human use. *Fed Regist.* 1999;64:4535–40.
28. Acosta RD, Case BD. Clinical effects of colonic cleansing for general health promotion: a systematic review. *Am J Gastroenterol.* 2009;104(11):2830–6. doi: https://doi.org/10.1038/ajg.2009.494.
29. Tozzi F, Thornton LM, Mitchell J, et al. Features associated with laxative abuse in individuals with eating disorders. *Psychosom Med.* 2006;68(3): 470–7. doi: https://doi.org/10.1097/01.psy.0000221359.35034.e7.

30. Muller-Lissner SA, Kamm MA, Scarpignato C, et al. Myths and misconceptions about chronic constipation. *Am J Gastroenterol.* 2005;100(1):232–42. doi: https://doi.org/10.1111/j.1572-0241.2005.40885.x.
31. Kamm MA, Mueller-Lissner S, Wald A, et al. Oral bisacodyl is effective and well-tolerated in patients with chronic constipation. *Clin Gastroenterol Hepatol.* 2011;9(7):577–83. doi: https://doi.org/10.1016/j.cgh.2011.03.026.
32. Horn JR, Mantione MM, Johanson JF. OTC polyethylene glycol 3350 and pharmacists' role in managing constipation. *J Am Pharm Assoc.* 2012;52(3):372–80. doi: https://doi.org/10.1331/JAPhA.2012.10161.
33. Tabbers MM, DiLorenzo C, Berger MY, et al. Evaluation and treatment of functional constipation in infants and children: evidence-based recommendations from ESPGHAN and NASPGHAN. *J Pediatr Gastroenterol Nutr.* 2014;58:258–74. doi: https://doi.org/10.1097/MPG.0000000000000266.
34. Auth MK, Vora R, Farrelly P, et al. Childhood constipation. *BMJ.* 2012; 345:e7309. doi: 10.1136/bmj.e7309.
35. Alper A, Pashankar DS. Polyethylene glycol: a game-changer laxative for children. *J Pediatr Gastroenterol Nutr.* 2013;57(2):134–40. doi: https://doi.org/10.1097/MPG.0b013e318296404a.
36. Pijpers MA, Tabbers MM, Benninga MA, et al. Currently recommended treatments of childhood constipation are not evidence based: a systematic literature review on the effect of laxative treatment and dietary measures. *Arch Dis Child.* 2009;94(2):117–31. doi: 10.1136/adc.2007.127233.
37. Cash BD, Chang L, Sabesin S, et al. Update on the management of adults with chronic idiopathic constipation. *J Fam Pract.* 2007;56(6):S13–20. PMID: 18671930.
38. Fleming V, Wade WE. A review of laxative therapies for treatment of chronic constipation in older adults. *Am J Geriatr Pharmacother.* 2010;8(6): 514–50. doi: https://doi.org/10.1016/S1543-5946(10)80003-0.
39. Vazquez JC. Constipation, haemorrhoids, and heartburn in pregnancy. *BMJ Clin Evid.* February 20, 2008;pii:1411. PMID: 18671930.
40. Mahadevan U, Kane S. Medical position statement on the use of gastrointestinal medications in pregnancy. *Gastroenterology.* 2006;131(1):278–82. doi: https://doi.org/10.1053/j.gastro.2006.04.048.
41. Trottier M, Erebara A, Bozza P. Treating constipation during pregnancy. *Can Fam Physician.* 2012;58(8):836–8.
42. Drug and Lactation Database. National Library of Medicine. Available at: http://toxnet.nlm.nih.gov/cgi-bin/sis/htmlgen?LACT. Accessed May 13, 2017.
43. Sachs HC, Committee on Drugs. The transfer of drugs and therapeutics into human breast milk: an update on selected topics. *Pediatrics.* 2013; 132(3):e796–809.
44. U.S. Food and Drug Administration. Drug labeling: sodium labeling for over-the-counter drugs. Final rule. *Fed Regist.* 2001;76:7743–57.
45. Natural Medicines [database online]. 2017. Available at: https://naturalmedicines.therapeuticresearch.com/. Accessed May 13, 2017.
46. Quigley EM. Probiotics in the management of functional bowel disorders: promise fulfilled? *Gastroenterol Clin North Am.* 2012;41:805–19. doi: https://doi.org/10.1016/j.gtc.2012.08.005.
47. Chmielewska A, Szajewska H. Systematic review of randomized controlled trials: probiotics for functional constipation. *World J Gastroenterol.* 2010;16:69–75. PMCID: PMC2799919.

CHAPTER 16

DIARRHEA

PAUL C. WALKER

Diarrhea is a symptom characterized by an abnormal increase in stool frequency, liquidity, or weight. Although the normal frequency of bowel movements varies with each individual, having more than 3 bowel movements per day is considered abnormal.

Diarrhea may be acute, persistent, or chronic. Acute diarrhea, defined as symptoms lasting less than 14 days, can generally be managed with fluid and electrolyte replacement, dietary interventions, and nonprescription drug treatment. In persistent diarrhea, symptoms last 14 days to 4 weeks. Chronic diarrhea, by definition, lasts more than 4 weeks. Chronic and persistent diarrheal illnesses are often secondary to other chronic medical conditions or treatments and need medical care; therefore, these illnesses are outside the scope of this chapter.

Diarrhea is a common cause of morbidity. Worldwide, approximately 2.5 billion episodes of acute diarrhea occur each year, causing significant morbidity and mortality among all age groups, especially children younger than 5 years of age, in whom it causes 1.9 million deaths annually.[1] Approximately 179 million cases of acute gastroenteritis (irritation of the gastrointestinal [GI] tract commonly caused by viruses or bacteria that often results in diarrhea) occur in the United States each year.[2] The overall prevalence of acute diarrhea is estimated to be 5.1%; the incidence rate is 0.6 episodes per person per year.[3] The prevalence of diarrheal disease is highest in children younger than 5 years and lowest in older adults (ages ≥65 years); prevalence rates are estimated to be 7%–10% for children younger than 5 years and 2%–3% for older adults.[3] Most patients experience diarrheal illness without seeking medical attention; however, in the United States more than 500,000 patients are hospitalized each year, and approximately 5000 deaths result from acute gastroenteritis and its complications.[2]

Pathophysiology of Diarrhea

Table 16–1 highlights some of the common viral, bacterial, and protozoal diarrheas and their treatment. Epidemiologic factors that increase the risk for particular infectious diarrheal diseases or their spread include attendance or employment at daycare centers, occupation as a food handler or caregiver, congregate living conditions (e.g., nursing homes, prisons, multifamily dwellings), consumption of unsafe foods (e.g., raw or undercooked meat, eggs, shellfish), and presence of medical conditions, such as acquired immunodeficiency syndrome (AIDS) or diverticulitis. Acute diarrhea may also be caused by poisoning, medications, intolerance of certain foods, or various non-GI acute or chronic illnesses.

Viral Gastroenteritis

Noroviruses are the most common cause of diarrhea in adults and are rapidly becoming the most common cause in children.[4,5] They cause more than 90% of epidemic viral gastroenteritis and approximately 50% of all-cause epidemic gastroenteritis worldwide.[4] Noroviruses also play a major role in sporadic acute gastroenteritis, accounting for up to 36% of cases.[6] The symptoms, clinical course, and treatment are described in Table 16–1. Although the virus is most often transmitted by contaminated water or food, it can also be transmitted from person to person and through contact with contaminated environmental surfaces. Outbreaks of norovirus gastroenteritis frequently occur in certain populations, such as restaurant patrons, cruise ship passengers, students on college campuses, residents of long-term care facilities and hospitals, military personnel, and immunocompromised patients.

Rotavirus is the most common cause of severe gastroenteritis in infants and young children worldwide. In the United States, prior to widespread rotavirus vaccine administration, approximately 80% of children developed rotavirus gastroenteritis before reaching 5 years of age, and the virus accounted for 30%–50% of all hospitalizations for gastroenteritis in these patients.[7] Two oral vaccines are available to prevent rotavirus gastroenteritis and are recommended for routine use in healthy infants. These vaccines prevent 75%–85% of all rotavirus gastroenteritis and 95%–98% of severe infections, while also substantially reducing the health care burden of rotavirus disease.[7–9] Rotavirus also causes diarrheal disease in adults, although specific epidemiological data are lacking.[10] The virus has been found in 18% of stool specimens of adults presenting to emergency departments with acute gastroenteritis and may account for 3%–5% of adult hospitalizations caused by diarrheal disease.[11,12]

Rotavirus tends to be a seasonal infection, with peaks of gastroenteritis occurring between November and February. It is spread by the fecal–oral route, can cause severe dehydration and electrolyte disturbances, and may result in death. Clinical features are presented in Table 16–1. Other, less frequent viral causes of gastroenteritis include adenoviruses, astroviruses, hepatitis A virus, and sapoviruses.

Bacterial Gastroenteritis

Bacterial pathogens cause approximately 10% of acute diarrheal illnesses in the United States each year; most cases result from foodborne transmission. Pathogens most commonly responsible, in order of decreasing causality, are *Campylobacter* spp.; *Salmonella* spp.; *Shigella* spp.; *Escherichia coli* (including O157:H7,

TABLE 16–1 **Common Infectious Diarrheas and Their Treatment**

Type	Epidemiologic/ Etiologic Factors	Symptoms	Treatment	Usual Prognosis
Viral				
Rotavirus	Infects infants; oral–fecal spread	Onset of 24–48 hours; vomiting, fever, nausea, acute watery diarrhea	Vigorous fluid and electrolyte replacement	Self-limiting, usually lasts 5–8 days
Norovirus	Infects all ages; frequently spread person to person by the fecal–oral route; causes "24-hour stomach flu"	Onset of 24–48 hours; sudden-onset vomiting, nausea, headache, myalgia, fever, watery diarrhea	Fluid and electrolytes	Self-limiting, usually lasts 12–60 hours
Bacterial				
Campylobacter jejuni	Ingestion of contaminated food or water; oral–fecal spread; immunocompromised host	Onset of 24–72 hours; nausea, vomiting, headache, malaise, fever, watery diarrhea	Fluid and electrolytes; in severe or persistent diarrhea, antibiotics may be required[a]	Self-limiting, usually lasts <7 days
Salmonella	Ingestion of improperly cooked or refrigerated poultry and dairy products; immunocompromised host	Onset of 12–24 hours; diarrhea, fever, chills, malaise, myalgia, epigastric pain, anorexia	Fluid and electrolytes for mild cases; antibiotics reserved for complicated cases[b]	Self-limiting
Shigella	Ingestion of contaminated vegetables or water; frequently spread person to person; immunocompromised host	Onset of 24–48 hours; nausea, vomiting, diarrhea, fever	Fluid and electrolytes; antibiotics[c]	Self-limiting, usually lasts ≤7 days
Escherichia coli (enterotoxigenic *E. coli* [ETEC], enteroaggregative *E. coli* [EAEC])	Ingestion of contaminated food or water; recent travel outside the United States or to a U.S. border area	Onset of 8–72 hours; watery diarrhea, fever, abdominal cramps, bloating, malaise, occasional vomiting	Fluid and electrolytes; antibiotics[d]	Self-limiting, usually within 3–5 days
Shiga toxin–producing *E. coli* (STEC), including *E. coli* O157:H7 and non-O157 strains	Ingestion of contaminated food or water; direct person-to-person spread	Onset of 8–72 hours; watery and often bloody diarrhea, abdominal cramps, hemolytic uremic syndrome	Fluid and electrolytes	Self-limiting, usually within 5–10 days
Clostridium difficile	Antibiotic-associated diarrhea leading to pseudomembranous colitis	Onset during or up to several weeks after antibiotic therapy; watery or mucoid diarrhea, high fever, cramping	Fluid and electrolytes; discontinuation of offending agent; antibiotics	Self-limiting; tends to recur
Clostridium perfringens	Ingestion of contaminated food, especially meat and poultry	Onset of 8–14 hours; watery diarrhea without vomiting, cramping, mid-epigastric pain	Fluid and electrolytes	Self-limiting; usually resolves within 24 hours
Staphylococcus aureus	Ingestion of improperly cooked or stored food	Onset of 1–6 hours; nausea, vomiting, watery diarrhea	Fluid and electrolytes	Self-limiting
Yersinia enterocolitica	Ingestion of contaminated food	Onset within 16–48 hours; fever, abdominal pain, diarrhea, vomiting	Fluid and electrolytes; antibiotics may be needed in severe cases	Self-limiting, although diarrhea may persist for up to 3 weeks
Vibrio cholerae	Ingestion of contaminated food, including undercooked or raw seafood; recent travel outside the United States	Onset within 24–48 hours; painless, watery, and often voluminous diarrhea, vomiting	Fluid and electrolytes; antibiotics needed in moderate–severe cases	Self-limiting, although severe, fatal illness may occur

TABLE 16–1 **Common Infectious Diarrheas and Their Treatment** *(continued)*

Type	Epidemiologic/ Etiologic Factors	Symptoms	Treatment	Usual Prognosis
Bacillus cereus	Ingestion of contaminated food	Onset within 10–12 hours; abdominal pain, watery diarrhea, tenesmus, nausea, vomiting	Fluid and electrolytes	Self-limiting
Protozoal				
Giardia intestinalis	Ingestion of water contaminated with human or animal feces; frequently spread person to person; immunocompromised host	Onset of 1–3 weeks; acute or chronic watery diarrhea, nausea, vomiting, anorexia, flatulence, abdominal bloating, epigastric pain	Fluids and electrolytes; antimicrobial therapy[e]	Resolves with treatment
Cryptosporidium spp.	Frequently spread person to person; travel outside the United States; AIDS, immunocompromised host	Onset of 2–14 days; acute or chronic watery diarrhea, abdominal pain, flatulence, malaise	Fluid and electrolytes; antimicrobial therapy[f]	Self-limiting, lasting up to 3 weeks, except in patients with AIDS or other immunosuppressive diseases
Entamoeba histolytica	Travel outside the United States; fecal-soiled food or water; immunocompromised host	Chronic watery diarrhea, abdominal pain, cramps	Fluid and electrolytes; antibiotics[g]	Good, except for immunocompromised host
Isospora belli	Ingestion of contaminated food or water; immunocompromised host	Onset of approximately 1 week; profuse watery diarrhea, malaise, anorexia, weight loss, abdominal cramps	Fluid and electrolytes; antibiotics	Self-limited, remitting in 2–3 weeks

Key: AIDS = Acquired immunodeficiency syndrome.

[a] Empiric therapy with prescription antibiotics (e.g., azithromycin, erythromycin) should be considered for patients with febrile diarrheal illness, especially if moderate–severe invasive disease is suspected, and for patients in whom supportive therapy fails to manage symptoms. Ciprofloxacin and doxycycline have been recommended but are no longer considered first-line therapy, because many *Campylobacter* strains are resistant to these antibiotics.

[b] Antibiotics are not indicated routinely for *Salmonella* gastroenteritis; antibiotic therapy is used in infants and young children who fail to respond to supportive treatment, who do not spontaneously remit, or who are at increased risk of disseminated disease. Antibiotic therapy is also indicated for suspected bacteremia in patients at high risk for this complication. These include patients who appear to be toxic with high fever (>102.2°F [39.0°C]); infants (<3 months); older adult patients (≥65 years); patients with cancer, immunodeficiency (e.g., AIDS), or hemoglobinopathy (e.g., sickle cell disease); immunocompromised patients (including transplant patients and those receiving corticosteroids); patients who are on hemodialysis; and patients with vascular grafts or prosthetic joints. Fluoroquinolones are used for adults; ceftriaxone is used for children. Duration of antimicrobial therapy is usually 7–14 days. Alternatively, azithromycin can be used for 5–7 days.

[c] Empiric prescription antibiotics (fluoroquinolones, if acquired in the United States; ceftriaxone, if acquired in Asia or other areas with a high frequency of antibiotic resistance) should be considered for severely ill and/or medically fragile patients.

[d] Antibiotic treatment with fluoroquinolones, azithromycin, or rifaximin (prescription antibiotics) is given for moderate–severe travelers' diarrhea caused by *E. coli*; mild, self-limited infection can usually be managed symptomatically without antibiotics. Trimethoprim/sulfamethoxazole is no longer an optimal choice because of increasing worldwide resistance. Antibiotic treatment is not recommended for gastroenteritis caused by *E. coli* O157:H7, because the treatment is likely to enhance toxin release and may increase risk for hemolytic uremic syndrome. Antibiotic treatment of traveler's diarrhea has also been associated with increased risk for colonization by extended spectrum β-lactamase–producing Enterobacteriaceae and carbapenemase-producing Enterobacteriaceae.

[e] Self-treatment of giardiasis is not appropriate; metronidazole, nitazoxanide, and tinidazole are effective prescription alternatives for treating giardiasis.

[f] Self-treatment of cryptosporidiosis is not appropriate. Nitazoxanide is the drug of choice for immunocompetent and human immunodeficiency virus (HIV)-negative patients but is not approved for use immunocompromised patients (including HIV-positive patients) and should not be used in this population. Effective antiretroviral therapy is considered to be the best treatment for these patients.

[g] Self-treatment of amebiasis is not appropriate; prescription therapy with metronidazole or tinidazole followed by either paromomycin or iodoquinol is preferred.

Source: Adapted from Riddle MS, DuPont HL, Connor BA. ACG clinical guideline: diagnosis, treatment, and prevention of acute diarrheal infections in adult. *Am J Gastroenterol.* 2016;111(5):602–22. PMID: 25790189; Antimicrobial therapy. *Sanford Guide Web Edition.* 2nd ed. 2016. Available at: https://webedition.sanfordguide.com/. Accessed September 26, 2016; and American Academy of Pediatrics. *Red Book: 2015 Report of the Committee on Infectious Diseases.* 30th ed. Available at: http://aapredbook.aappublications.org/. Accessed May 1, 2017.

non–O157:H7 Shiga toxin–producing *E. coli* [STEC], enterotoxigenic *E. coli* [ETEC], enteroaggregative *E. coli* [EAEC]), diffusely adherent *E. coli* [DAEC], and other diarrheagenic strains); *Staphylococcus* spp.; *Clostridium* spp.; *Yersinia enterocolitica;* and *Bacillus cereus.* In addition, *Aeromonas* spp., *Arcobacter* spp., enterotoxigenic *Bacteroides fragilis, Klebsiella oxytoca, Laribacter hongkongensis,* and *Plesiomonas shigelloides* cause acute diarrhea.[13,14]

Bacteria cause diarrhea through elaboration of enterotoxin (e.g., ETEC, *Staphylococcus aureus*), by attachment and production of localized inflammatory changes in the gut (e.g., EAEC, enteropathogenic *E. coli,* STEC, *Clostridium difficile*), or by directly invading the mucosal epithelial cells (e.g., *Shigella, Salmonella, Yersinia, Campylobacter jejuni,* invasive *E. coli*).[15,16] Patients with diarrhea caused by toxin-producing pathogens have a watery diarrhea, which primarily involves the small intestine. If the large intestine is the primary site of infection, invasive organisms produce a dysentery-like (bloody diarrhea) syndrome characterized by fever, abdominal cramps, tenesmus (straining), and the frequent passage of small-volume stools that may contain blood and mucus. Clinical features of common bacterial diarrheas are presented in Table 16–1.

Enteric infection, most notably bacterial infection caused by *C. jejuni, Shigella, Salmonella,* and diarrheagenic *E. coli,* can cause prolonged bowel dysfunction, including irritable bowel syndrome (IBS), following resolution of the infection. Norovirus and *Giardia intestinalis* may also cause postinfectious IBS. IBS develops in 2%–30% of patients following enteric infection, depending on the causative agent, and is usually diagnosed 1–2 years after an episode of acute bacterial gastroenteritis.[17] The prognosis is favorable for most patients; IBS symptoms resolve 4–8 years after diagnosis. Acute gastroenteritis may also unmask or exacerbate underlying chronic GI diseases, such as celiac disease, Crohn disease, or ulcerative colitis.

Protozoal Diarrhea

Diarrhea may also be caused by protozoa, including *G. intestinalis, Entamoeba histolytica, Isospora belli,* and *Cryptosporidium* spp. Nonprescription therapies are not available to manage diarrhea caused by these pathogens, and self-management is inappropriate.

Foodborne Gastroenteritis

Foodborne transmission of pathogens causes 47.8 million episodes of acute gastroenteritis, 135,000 hospitalizations, and approximately 3000 deaths in the United States each year.[2,18] When pathogens are identified, 59% of these infections are caused by viruses (predominantly noroviruses), 39% by bacteria, and 2% by protozoa.[18] Recent surveillance statistics on the incidence of foodborne illnesses confirm that *Salmonella* and *Campylobacter,* which caused 15.45 and 13.45 cases of illness per 100,000 population in 2012, respectively, are the most frequently diagnosed bacterial pathogens.[19] These are followed by *Shigella* (5.81 cases per 100,000 population), *Cryptosporidium* (2.44 cases per 100,000 population), STEC non-O157 (1.43 cases per 100,000 population), STEC O157:H7 (0.92 cases per 100,000 population), *Vibrio* (0.45 cases per 100,000 population), *Yersinia* (0.28 cases per 100,000 population), and *Listeria* (0.24 cases per 100,000 population).[19] Other causes of foodborne gastroenteritis include *Cyclospora cayetanensis* and rotavirus.

Outbreaks of foodborne bacterial infection have been traced to poor sanitation and manufacturing practices in food production facilities and contamination of foods in various community locations, such as grocery stores and restaurants. Outbreaks of infection have also been associated with specific foods listed in Table 16–2. Therefore, taking a thorough history regarding the patient's food intake 48–72 hours before the onset of diarrhea is essential in identifying a possible cause.

Outbreaks of acute foodborne illness caused by *E. coli* O157:H7 and other STECs are a major public health issue. Toxins produced by these organisms cause an acute bloody diarrhea and may also

TABLE 16–2 Specific Foods Associated With Foodborne Gastroenteritis

Organism	Associated Foods
Shiga toxin–producing *Escherichia coli* (STEC), including *E. coli* O157:H7 and non-O157 strains	Apple cider, unpasteurized
	Bologna
	Clover sprouts, raw
	Eggs
	Gouda cheese
	Ground beef (undercooked)
	Lettuce
	Milk, raw
	Cookie dough, raw, refrigerated prepackaged
	Spinach
Salmonella	Chicken
	Dry dog food[a]
	Eggs
	Ground beef
	Ground turkey
	Jalapeno peppers
	Mangoes
	Melons (e.g., cantaloupe)
	Papayas
	Peanut butter
	Pine nuts
	Pistachio nuts
	Red and black pepper spice
	Yellowfin tuna, raw, scraped, ground
Campylobacter	Milk
	Chicken
Listeria	Hummus
	Melons
	Ricotta cheese
Cyclospora	Raspberries

[a] *Salmonella* infection is a zoonotic disease, i.e., the infection can be transmitted from animals to people, and people have developed *Salmonella* infections after contact with contaminated dry pet food or with an animal that has eaten contaminated dry pet food. Spread is by the fecal–oral route.

Source: Adapted from reference 17.

be associated with serious, potentially fatal systemic complications, such as hemolytic uremic syndrome or thrombotic thrombocytopenic purpura.

Travelers' Diarrhea

Travelers' diarrhea is an acute, secretory diarrhea acquired mainly through ingestion of contaminated food or water. It is usually caused by bacterial enteropathogens; however, a cause may not be identifiable in as many as 40% of cases. ETEC, EAEC, and DAEC are responsible for most cases of travelers' diarrhea.[20–22] ETEC is found in 50%–76% of travelers with diarrhea in various areas around the world.[22] Other important pathogens that cause travelers' diarrhea include *Shigella* spp., *Salmonella* spp., *C. jejuni, Aeromonas* spp., *Plesiomonas* spp., and noncholera *Vibrio;* noroviruses cause 12%–17% of cases.[22] The causative organisms are found most often on foods such as fruits, vegetables, raw meat, seafood, and hot sauces. Pathogens may also be found in the local water, including ice cubes made from local tap water. After ingestion, ETEC produces two plasmid-mediated enterotoxins that cause symptoms; the pathogenic mechanisms underlying diarrhea caused by EAEC are not well understood. The diarrheal disorder caused by these organisms is characterized in Table 16–1. Patients may experience between three and eight (or more) watery stools per day, with symptoms usually subsiding over 3–5 days.

Food-Induced Diarrhea

Food intolerance can provoke diarrhea and may result from a food allergy or ingestion of foods that are excessively fatty or spicy or contain a high amount of dietary fiber or many seeds. Dietary carbohydrates (e.g., lactose, sucrose) are normally hydrolyzed to monosaccharides by the enzyme lactase. If not hydrolyzed, these carbohydrates pool in the lumen of the intestine and produce an osmotic imbalance. The resulting hyperosmolarity draws fluid into the intestinal lumen, causing diarrhea. Lactase activity may be reduced by infectious diarrhea; thus, acute viral diarrhea may cause temporary milk intolerance in patients of all ages. Lactase deficiency resulting from viral gastroenteritis is short-lived, but it is particularly problematic during the first few days of the disease. Infants born with lactase deficiency and adults who develop lactase deficiency are intolerant of cow milk and milk-based products. Lactase enzyme products are effective treatments for some patients (see "Treatment of Diarrhea").

Clinical Presentation of Diarrhea

The most common signs and symptoms of acute infectious diarrheal illnesses are shown in Table 16–1. Variability in the causes of diarrhea makes identification of the pathophysiologic mechanisms difficult. The etiology, and subsequently the pathophysiology, can be determined by conducting a thorough medical history in most cases. However, a complete medical assessment, including clinical laboratory evaluation, may be required to identify the cause in a subset of patients with severe or persistent diarrhea.

Diarrhea can be classified as osmotic, secretory, inflammatory, or motor, depending on the underlying pathophysiologic mechanisms that disrupt normal intestinal function. The common mechanisms of acute diarrhea are osmotic and secretory, whereas motor and inflammatory mechanisms commonly underlie chronic diarrheal illnesses. Table 16–3 correlates the clinical groups and mechanisms with their most common causes.

Bacterial enterotoxins play a role in the pathophysiology of secretory diarrheas. Enterotoxins elaborated by *E. coli* and *Vibrio cholerae* evoke the release of endogenous secretagogues that mediate secretory reflexes, including serotonin, substance P, and vasoactive intestinal peptide. Some enterotoxins, such as cholera toxin, can directly stimulate GI secretomotor neurons to increase intestinal secretion. *Clostridium difficile* enterotoxin A also injures enterocytes and evokes a necroinflammatory response that causes a secretory diarrhea. Although viruses, such as rotavirus, also produce enterotoxins, the role of viral enterotoxins in the disease pathophysiology is uncertain. In addition, inflammatory mediators (e.g., interleukins 1 and 6, prostaglandins, substance P,

TABLE 16-3 **Clinical Classification of Diarrhea**

Type	Mechanism	Common Causes
Osmotic	■ Unabsorbed solutes in intestines increase luminal osmotic load, retarding fluid absorption. ■ Decreased absorption of solutes and fluid can be secondary to brush border damage caused by lactase deficiency or infection. ■ Viral-induced damage to epithelial cells accelerates migration of immature crypt cells to the tip of the villus; altered epithelial turnover also decreases absorption.	Noroviruses, rotaviruses, *Escherichia coli, Campylobacter jejuni,* lactase deficiency, excess magnesium antacid intake
Secretory	■ Stimulation of crypt cells produces net flow of electrolytes and fluids into intestinal lumen. ■ Tumors can secrete GI hormones and peptides that act as secretagogues.	*C. jejuni, Clostridium difficile, E. coli, Salmonella, Shigella, Vibrio,* rotaviruses, *Giardia intestinalis, Cryptosporidium* spp., *Isospora,* ileal resection, thyroid cancer
Inflammatory	■ Impaired fluid absorption and leaking of mucus, blood, and pus into lumen caused by inflammation of intestinal mucosa (e.g., IBD) or bacterial infection (i.e., dysentery).	*C. jejuni, E. coli, Salmonella, Shigella, Yersinia, Entamoeba histolytica,* ulcerative colitis, Crohn disease
Motor	■ Abnormally rapid intestinal transit time reduces contact time between luminal contents and absorptive areas of intestinal wall.	IBS, diabetic neuropathy

Key: GI = Gastrointestinal; IBD = inflammatory bowel disease; IBS = irritable bowel syndrome.

tumor necrosis factor α, platelet-activating factor) evoked by enteric infection stimulate a characteristic GI motility pattern that leads to the urgent defecation associated with diarrhea and causes abdominal cramps.

Stool characteristics give valuable information about the diarrhea's pathophysiology. For example, undigested food particles in the stool suggest disease of the small intestine. Black, tarry stools may indicate upper GI bleeding, and red stools suggest possible lower bowel or hemorrhoidal bleeding or simply recent ingestion of red food (e.g., beets) or drug products (e.g., rifampin). In secretory diarrhea of the small bowel, chloride secretion and inhibition of sodium absorption appear to be the major events; thus, stools will be high in sodium. Passage of many small-volume stools suggests a colonic disorder. Yellowish stools may suggest the presence of bilirubin and a potentially serious pathology of the liver. A whitish tint to the stool suggests a fat malabsorption disease.

Fluid and electrolyte imbalance is the major complication of diarrheal illness. Therefore, assessment of the patient's risk for dehydration and the degree of dehydration present is a key factor in determining the appropriateness of self-care and the need for medical referral. The specific signs and symptoms of dehydration are associated with the severity of the diarrhea, as well as the etiology and degree of fluid and electrolyte losses (Table 16–4).[23]

TABLE 16-4 Assessment of Dehydration and Severity of Acute Diarrhea

	Self-Treatable		Not Self-Treatable
	Minimal or No Dehydration	**Mild–Moderate Dehydration/ Diarrhea**	**Severe Dehydration/ Diarrhea**
Degree of dehydration (% loss of body weight)	<3%	3%–9%	>9%
Signs of dehydration[a]			
Mental status	Good, alert	Normal, fatigued or restless, irritable	Apathetic, lethargic, unconscious
Thirst	Drinks normally, might refuse liquids	Thirsty, eager to drink	Drinks poorly, unable to drink
Heart rate	Normal	Normal to increased	Tachycardia, bradycardia in most severe cases
Quality of pulses	Normal	Normal to decreased	Weak, thready, impalpable
Breathing	Normal	Normal, fast	Deep
Eyes	Normal	Slightly sunken[b]	Deeply sunken[b]
Tears	Present	Decreased[b]	Absent
Mouth and tongue	Moist	Dry	Parched
Skin fold	Instant recoil	Recoil in <2 seconds	Recoil in >2 seconds
Capillary refill	Normal	Prolonged	Prolonged, minimal
Extremities	Warm	Cool	Cold, mottled, cyanotic
Urine output	Normal to decreased	Decreased[b]	Minimal[b]
Number of unformed stools/day	<3	3–5	6–9
Other signs/symptoms	Afebrile, normal blood pressure, no orthostatic changes in blood pressure/pulse	May be afebrile or may develop fever >102.2°F (39.0°C); normal blood pressure; possible mild orthostatic blood pressure/pulse changes with or without mild orthostatic-related symptoms[c]; sunken fontanelle[d]	Fever >102.2°F (39.0°C), low blood pressure, dizziness, severe abdominal pain

[a] If signs of dehydration are absent, rehydration therapy is not required. Maintenance therapy and replacement of stool losses should be undertaken.

[b] Signs and symptoms experienced especially by young children.

[c] Postural (orthostatic) hypotension is defined as a drop in the systolic and/or diastolic pressure of >15–20 mm Hg on movement from a supine to an upright position and may cause lightheadedness, dizziness, or fainting. On rising, the diastolic pressure normally remains the same or increases slightly, and the systolic pressure drops slightly. If the blood pressure drops, the pulse should be checked simultaneously; the pulse rate should increase as blood pressure drops. Failure of the pulse to rise suggests the problem is neurogenic (e.g., diabetic patients with peripheral neuropathy) or that the patient may be taking a beta blocker. The presence of orthostatic hypotension suggests that the patient has lost ≥1 L of vascular volume, and referral for medical care is necessary.

[d] Signs and symptoms of concern for young infants.

Source: Adapted from reference 22.

Children younger than 5 years and adults older than 65 years are at greater risk for complications than other age groups. In the United States, most children recover completely from diarrhea; however, approximately 300–450 children (mostly infants) die annually from complications of acute gastroenteritis.[3,23] Children 2 years of age and younger are more likely to suffer complications that require hospitalization. In newborns, water may make up 75% of total body weight; severe diarrhea may cause water loss equal to 10% or more of body weight. After 8–10 bowel movements within a 24-hour period, a 2-month-old infant could lose enough fluid to cause circulatory collapse and renal failure.

In recent years, deaths from viral and bacterial GI infection have increased most sharply among people 65 years of age and older. Diarrhea in this population is likely to be more severe than in other adults; older adults experience the highest rate of death from enteric infections.

Treatment of Diarrhea

Treatment Goals

The goals of self-treatment of diarrhea are to (1) prevent or correct fluid and electrolyte loss and acid–base disturbance, (2) control symptoms, (3) identify and treat the cause, and (4) prevent acute morbidity and mortality.

General Treatment Approach

Infectious diarrhea is often self-limiting. Initial self-management for adults and children with mild–moderate, uncomplicated diarrhea should focus on fluid and electrolyte replacement by administering commercially available oral rehydration solutions (ORS) in adequate doses (Table 16–5). Simultaneous implementation of oral rehydration and specific dietary measures is appropriate for treating mild–moderate diarrheal illness. Symptomatic control can also be achieved by using nonprescription antidiarrheal drugs, such as loperamide, in carefully selected patients. Patients with uncomplicated acute diarrhea who are otherwise healthy usually improve clinically within 24–48 hours; normal bowel function is often restored in 24–72 hours without additional treatment. If the condition remains the same or worsens after 48 hours of onset, medical referral is necessary to prevent complications. Specific exclusions for self-treatment that require referral for medical evaluation are listed in Figure 16–1.

Diarrhea of any severity in infants younger than 6 months of age; moderate diarrhea in children 2 years of age and younger; and young children who have unusually high fluid output, significant fever, or mental status changes require evaluation by a primary care provider or a health care provider in an emergency department.[23] Severe diarrhea in any patient constitutes a medical emergency and requires immediate referral for medical evaluation and treatment with intravenous (I.V.) fluid therapy. Any patient with stool containing blood or mucus needs medical evaluation.[23,24] Certain medical conditions can increase the risk for dehydration. Referral for medical care should be considered for patients with diabetes, severe cardiovascular or renal diseases, concurrent respiratory tract infection, or multiple unstable chronic medical conditions. Patients with severe abdominal pain or cramping (particularly those >50 years of age), abdominal tenderness, or distention, may have a complicating acute abdominal process, such as ischemic bowel disease, and should be referred for medical evaluation.[25] Immunocompromised patients, such as those receiving cancer treatment, organ transplant recipients, and patients with AIDS, also need medical evaluation, because their diarrhea will often be complicated and difficult to manage.

Self-care during pregnancy is not appropriate. While diarrhea can be a normal physiological occurrence during pregnancy, it may be a symptom of GI infection.[26] *Campylobacter jejuni* and *Salmonella* may cause severe, even fatal maternal infection. Further, *C. jejuni*, *Salmonella*, and *Listeria* are recognized causes of intrauterine infection and perinatal death.[26,27] Pregnant women who develop diarrhea should consult with a primary care provider or an obstetrician.

TABLE 16–5 Selected Oral Rehydration Products

Trade Name	Osmolarity	Calories	Carbohydrate	Electrolytes
CeraLyte 50 Powder Packets	<200 mOsm/L	160 cal/L	Rice starch polymers 40 g/L; sucrose 10 g/L	Sodium 50 mEq/L; chloride 40 mEq/L; citrate 30 mEq/L; potassium 20 mEq/L
CeraLyte 70 Powder Packets	<260 mOsm/L	160 cal/L	Rice starch polymers 40 g/L	Sodium 70 mEq/L; chloride 60 mEq/L; citrate 30 mEq/L; potassium 20 mEq/L
CeraLyte 90 Powder Packets	<260 mOsm/L	160 cal/L	Rice starch polymers 40 g/L	Sodium 90 mEq/L; chloride 80 mEq/L; citrate 30 mEq/L; potassium 20 mEq/L
Enfamil Enfalyte Solution	160 mOsm/L	126 cal/L	Corn syrup solids 30 g/L	Sodium 50 mEq/L; chloride 45 mEq/L; citrate 33 mEq/L; potassium 25 mEq/L
Pedialyte[a]	249 mOsm/L	100 cal/L	Dextrose 20 g/L; fructose 5 g/L	Sodium 45 mEq/L; chloride 35 mEq/L; citrate 30 mEq/L; potassium 20 mEq/L
Pedialyte Freezer Pops[b]	270 mOsm/L	6.25 cal/L	Dextrose 25 g/L	Sodium 45 mEq/L; chloride 35 mEq/L; citrate 30 mEq/L; potassium 20 mEq/L

Key: ORS = Oral rehydration solution.

[a] Many generic products (e.g., store brands) are available.

[b] Product to be used with appropriate maintenance ORS.

Exclusions for Self-Treatment

- Young age (e.g., age <6 months or weight <17.5 lb [8 kg])
- Persistent fever (≥102.2°F [39.0°C] for patients ages ≥6 months)
- Visible blood, pus, or mucus in stool
- High output, including frequent and substantial volumes of diarrhea
- Persistent vomiting
- Signs of severe dehydration
  - Children showing behavioral/mental changes (irritability, apathy, lethargy, unconscious)
  - Children who have not urinated in 8 hours
  - Children who have no tears when crying
  - Orthostatic hypotension
- Severe abdominal pain/distress
- Risk for significant complications, including chronic medical conditions or concurrent illness (see "Assessment of Diarrhea: A Case-Based Approach")
  - Diabetes, severe CVD, renal disease
  - Immunosuppressed patients (e.g., cancer chemotherapy, organ transplant recipients, AIDS), frail patients age ≥65 years
- Pregnancy
- Chronic or persistent diarrhea
- Suboptimal response to ORS already administered

Source: Adapted from references 22–24.

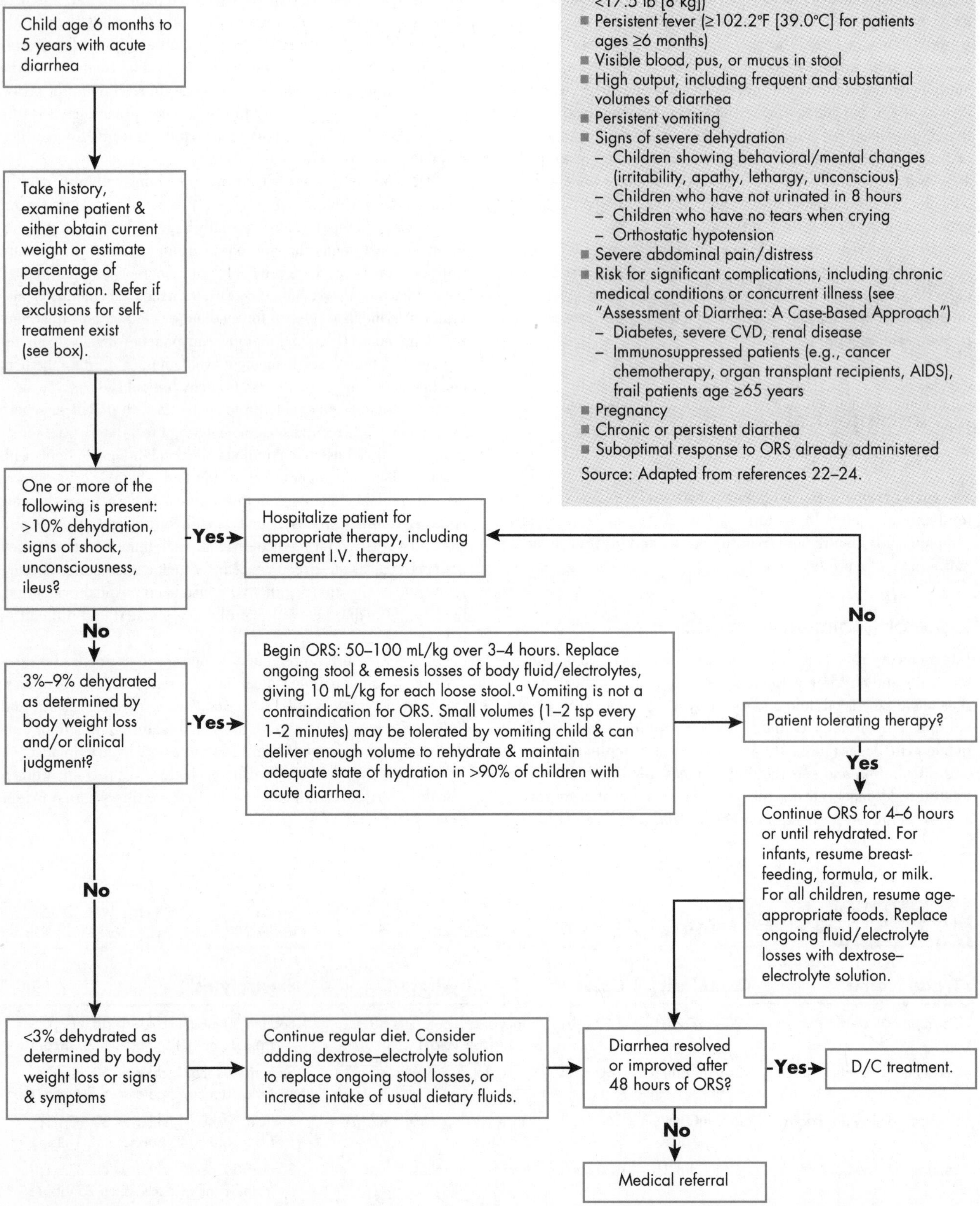

[a] Alternatively: <10 kg BW, give 60–120 mL ORS for each diarrheal stool or vomiting episode; ≥10 kg BW, give 120–240 mL ORS.

FIGURE 16–1 Self-care for acute diarrhea in children 6 months to 5 years. Key: AIDS = Acquired immunodeficiency syndrome; BW = body weight; CVD = cardiovascular disease; D/C = discontinue; I.V. = intravenous; ORS = oral rehydration solution. (Source: Adapted from references 22–24.)

Nonpharmacologic Therapy

Fluid and Electrolyte Management

Rehydration using ORS is the preferred treatment for mild–moderate diarrhea. This approach is as effective as I.V. therapy in managing fluid and electrolytes in children with mild–moderate dehydration secondary to diarrhea. Health care providers can safely recommend an ORS for mild–moderate diarrhea in patients with no exclusions to self-care.

Water absorption in the small intestine is passive and depends on the absorption of electrolytes and selected solutes such as sodium, chloride, glucose, small peptides, and amino acids. As these substances are absorbed, water accompanies their movement to maintain an isotonic state. Sodium ion transport is the primary mechanism controlling water movement. An active sodium–potassium adenosine triphosphatase pump present in enterocytes moves sodium into the cell in exchange for potassium ions. Other transport mechanisms include the sodium–glucose and sodium–amino acid cotransport processes (each of which transports these substances into the enterocytes) and the sodium luminal exchange mechanism. The sodium–glucose cotransport mechanism, in which glucose absorption is coupled with active transport of sodium, is important in the management of diarrhea. Unlike other sodium transport systems, the sodium–glucose cotransport mechanism is not adversely affected by most diarrheal diseases, and hypotonic ORS containing low concentrations of glucose or dextrose (2%–2.5%) can be useful in managing fluid and electrolyte balance. The sugar molecules provide little caloric support but facilitate intestinal sodium and water absorption. Maximal sodium absorption occurs at a molar glucose-to-sodium ratio close to 1.

Depending on the patient's fluid and electrolyte status, oral treatment may be carried out in two phases: rehydration therapy and maintenance therapy. Rehydration over 3–4 hours quickly replaces water and electrolyte deficits to restore normal body composition. In the maintenance phase, electrolyte solutions are given to maintain normal body composition until adequate dietary intake is reestablished. Figures 16–1 and 16–2 outline rehydration and maintenance therapies, including fluid and electrolyte recommendations for children and adults. Although ORS is generally recommended for adults with diarrhea, little evidence supports this use, and ORS may not provide any real benefit to otherwise healthy adults with mild diarrhea who can maintain an adequate fluid intake. For these patients, fluid and electrolyte status can be maintained by increasing intake of fluids such as clear juices, soups, or sports drinks.

A variety of oral rehydration products are available (Table 16–5). Most products are premixed solutions; a few are available as dry powders of glucose and electrolytes that require the addition of water. The premixed products are preferred for use in children, because they are safe and convenient, and improper mixing of dry powders by caregivers has led to fluid and electrolyte complications and injury. All available premixed solutions are equally safe and effective; there is no evidence that one product is clinically superior to another for rehydration. The World Health Organization (WHO) and United Nations Children's Fund (UNICEF) recommend use of an ORS containing 75 mEq/L of sodium.[28] Compared with the previously recommended ORS (which contained 90 mEq/L of sodium), this reduced osmolality ORS significantly reduces the need for unscheduled I.V. therapy, the duration of diarrhea, stool output, and the incidence of vomiting in children with noncholera diarrhea. This ORS is also effective in children and adults with cholera, although transient, asymptomatic hyponatremia may develop in adults. Rehydration solutions available in the United States contain 70–90 mEq/L of sodium; maintenance solutions contain 45–50 mEq/L of sodium.

Some cereal-based products use complex carbohydrates (e.g., rice syrup solids) instead of glucose. Complex carbohydrates are converted into glucose at the intestinal brush border and provide more cotransport molecules while reducing the osmotic load of the ORS. Cereal-based ORS therapy potentially reduces stool volume by 20%–30% in children with cholera, but may not significantly alter stool volume in children with noncholera acute diarrhea.

A variety of common household oral solutions have also been used for oral rehydration and maintenance (Table 16–6). These solutions may be sufficient to manage mild, self-limiting diarrhea in some patients, but they should be avoided if dehydration or moderate–severe diarrhea is present. Unlike commercial ORS, these remedies are not formulated on the basis of the physiology of acute diarrhea. The inappropriately high carbohydrate content and osmolality of these solutions can worsen diarrhea, and their low sodium content can contribute to the development of hyponatremia. Sports drinks may be used in children older than 5 years and adults if additional sources of sodium, such as crackers or pretzels, are used concomitantly. Colas, ginger ale, apple juice, sports drinks, and similar products are not recommended for infants and young children (6 months to 5 years of age) with diarrhea. Tea, another popular household remedy, is also inappropriate for children because of its low sodium content. Chicken broth is not recommended because of its inappropriately high sodium content.

Dietary Management

Oral intake does not worsen diarrhea, and clinically significant nutrient malabsorption is uncommon in acute diarrhea. In fact, during acute diarrhea, patients are able to absorb 80%–95% of dietary carbohydrates, 70% of fat, and 75% of the nitrogen from protein. Furthermore, early refeeding, in combination with maintenance oral rehydration, improves outcomes in children by reducing the duration of the diarrhea, reducing stool output, and improving weight gain. Current guidelines recommend withholding food no longer than 24 hours and encourage the reintroduction of a normal, age-appropriate diet once the patient has been rehydrated, which should take no longer than 3–4 hours to accomplish.[23] Most infants and children with acute diarrhea can tolerate full-strength breast milk and cow milk. The BRAT diet (bananas, rice, applesauce, and toast) is not recommended; it provides insufficient calories, protein, and fat, especially in situations of strict or prolonged use.[23] Patients (or their parents) should be advised to avoid fatty foods, foods rich in simple sugars (e.g., carbonated soft drinks, juice, gelatin desserts) that can cause osmotic diarrhea, spicy foods that may cause GI upset, and caffeine-containing beverages, which can promote fluid secretion and may worsen diarrhea.

There is no evidence that fasting or dietary modification influences outcomes of acute diarrhea in adults; however, the previous recommendations about foods to avoid can be applied if a normal diet is not tolerated.[23]

Preventive Measures

Infectious diarrhea, especially acute viral gastroenteritis, often occurs in congregate living conditions such as daycare centers and nursing homes through person-to-person transmission. Isolating the individual with diarrhea, washing hands, and using sterile techniques are basic preventive measures that reduce the risk of

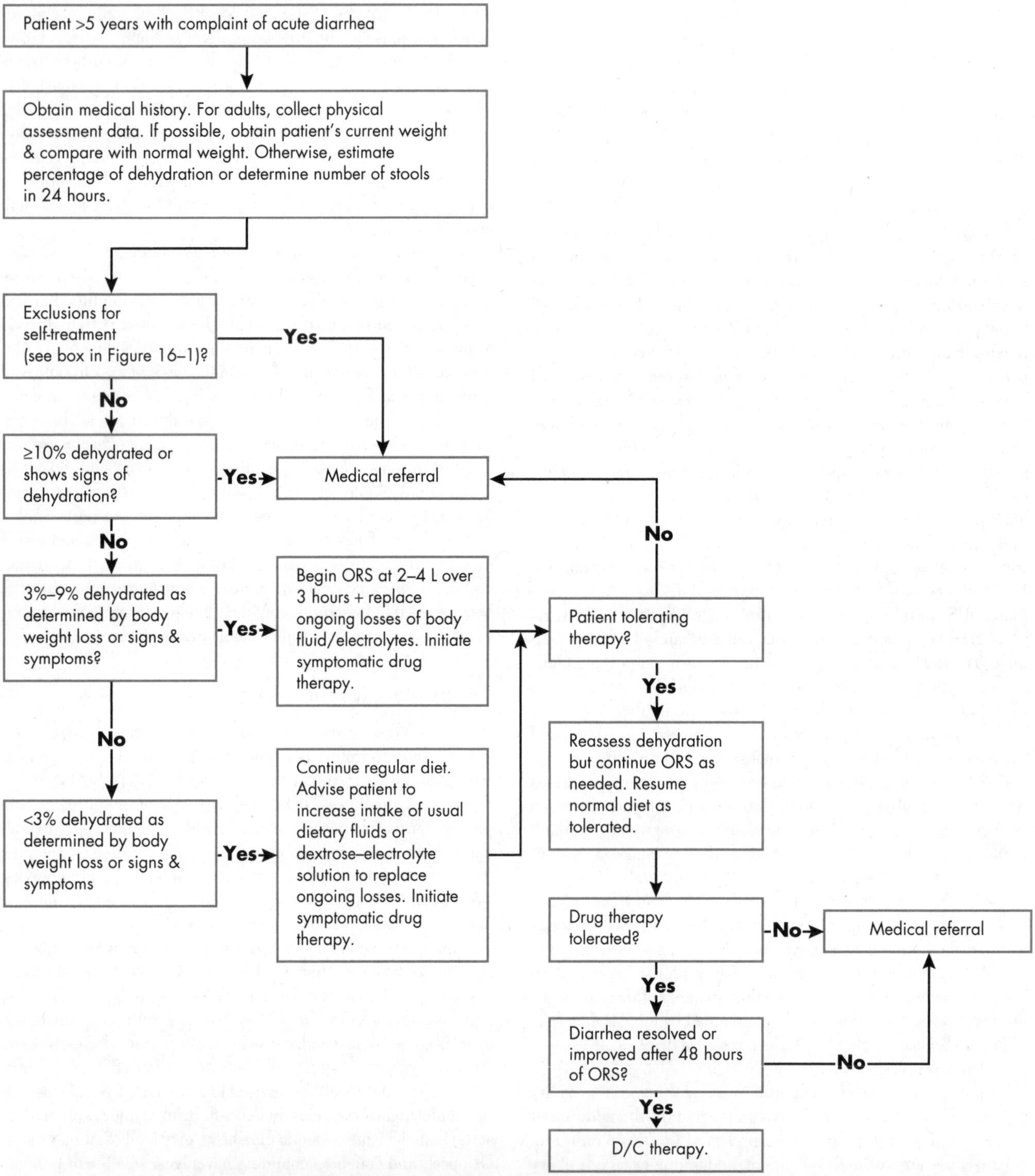

FIGURE 16–2 Self-care for acute diarrhea in children older than 5 years, adolescents, and adults. Key: D/C = Discontinue; ORS = oral rehydration solution.

transmission among such populations and their caregivers. Strict food handling, sanitation, and other hygienic practices help control transmission of bacteria and other infectious agents.

Although short-term bismuth subsalicylate (BSS) prophylaxis is frequently recommended to provide protection against travelers' diarrhea, the Food and Drug Administration (FDA) has deemed that available data are insufficient to support prophylactic use of BSS.[29] However, the American College of Gastroenterology (ACG) has published a guideline on the use of BSS or loperamide to prevent and manage mild–moderate traveler's diarrhea. Unless BSS is contraindicated (e.g., salicylate allergies, patient age, current use of a salicylate product), the recommended dosing is 2.1 g 4 times daily (at meals and bedtime). This regimen may reduce risk by up to 60% and is most effective for trips lasting up to 2 weeks. Neither lower doses nor preventive use in trips lasting longer than 2 weeks has been shown to offer benefit. ACG

TABLE 16–6 **Comparison of Electrolyte and Dextrose Concentrations of Household Fluids**

Clear Liquids	Sodium (mEq/L)	Potassium (mEq/L)	Bicarbonate (mEq/L)	Dextrose (g/L)	Osmolarity (mOsm/L)
Cola	2	0.1	13	50–150 dextrose and fructose	550
Ginger ale	3	1	4	50–150 dextrose and fructose	540
Apple juice	3	20	0	10–150 dextrose and fructose	700
Chicken broth	250	5	0	0	450
Tea	0	0	0	0	5
Gatorade	20	3	3	45 dextrose and other sugars	330
Seven Up	7.5	0.2	0	80 dextrose and fructose	564

recommends dosing of loperamide for a maximum of 48 hours and titration to maximum benefit while attempting to avoid drug-induced constipation. For patients with dysentery, loperamide may still be an option but only if used concomitantly with antibiotics.[30] Antibiotics with reliable activity against endemic enteropathogens (e.g., fluoroquinolones, rifaximin) provide effective prophylaxis. However, prophylactic antimicrobial agents are not currently recommended for most travelers.[29] Prophylactic antibiotics may be considered for short-term travelers who are high-risk hosts (e.g., immunosuppressed patients) or travelers with underlying conditions that may be complicated by diarrheal illness, or for critical trips during which even a short bout of diarrhea could adversely affect the purpose of the trip.[31]

Pharmacologic Therapy

Although most acute, nonspecific diarrhea in the United States is self-limiting, nonprescription antidiarrheal products may provide symptom control and will usually do no harm when used according to label instructions. Table 16–7 lists dosage and administration guidelines for these agents. However, evidence is lacking to show that pharmacologic agents other than loperamide and BSS reduce stool frequency or duration of disease in adults. Table 16–8 lists available trade-name products that contain loperamide and BSS. No antidiarrheal drugs have been shown to significantly improve clinical outcomes of acute, nonspecific diarrhea in infants and children ages 5 years and younger.

Loperamide

Loperamide is a popular, effective, and safe nonprescription antidiarrheal agent. It is a synthetic opioid agonist that lacks central nervous system (CNS) effects, because it is a substrate for P-glycoprotein. P-glycoprotein is an efflux transporter found in many tissues, including the blood–brain barrier. Loperamide is so efficiently removed from the CNS by this efflux transporter that pharmacologically effective concentrations in the CNS are not normally achieved, and the risk of CNS adverse effects is minimized.[32] However, there have been recent reports of overdoses and deaths associated with the misuse and abuse of loperamide as an opioid substitute in individuals addicted to opioids.[33] FDA has also warned that taking high doses of loperamide with potentially interacting medications such as ranitidine, cimetidine (nonprescription and prescription), certain macrolides (erythromycin, clarithromycin), antifungals (itraconazole, ketoconazole), and ritonavir may also increase risk of cardiovascular events.[34] Loperamide produces antidiarrheal effects by stimulating peripheral micro-opioid receptors on the intestinal circular muscles to slow intestinal motility and allow absorption of electrolytes and water. Disruption of cholinergic and noncholinergic mechanisms involved in the regulation of peristalsis may also contribute to this effect. Loperamide also has antisecretory effects that may be mediated through stimulation of GI micro-opioid receptors, inhibition of calmodulin function, and inhibition of voltage-dependent calcium channels.

Loperamide provides symptomatic relief of acute, nonspecific diarrhea. Its therapeutic effects include reduced daily fecal volume, increased viscosity and bulk volume, and reduced fluid and electrolyte loss. It may be used when the patient is afebrile or has a low-grade fever and does not have bloody stools. Nonprescription loperamide is labeled for use in children 6 years of age and older; the product information for prescription loperamide provides directions for use in children as young as 2 years of age. However, use of loperamide in children younger than 6 years is not recommended, because it produces only modest, clinically insignificant effects on stool volume and duration of illness, with an unacceptably high risk of adverse effects, including life-threatening ileus and toxic megacolon.

Loperamide is also indicated for treatment of travelers' diarrhea (in combination with antibiotics) and chronic diarrhea associated with IBS and inflammatory bowel disease, as well as to reduce the volume of discharge from high-output ileostomies. Off-label uses include control of chronic diarrhea secondary to diabetic neuropathy and other conditions, and control of toddler diarrhea (defined as diarrhea of at least 1 month in duration in an otherwise healthy, active, well-nourished child in whom stool examination has revealed no bacterial, viral, or protozoal pathogens). Off-label uses require medical supervision.

At usual doses (Table 16–7), loperamide has few adverse effects other than occasional dizziness and constipation. Infrequently occurring adverse effects include abdominal pain, abdominal distention, nausea, vomiting, dry mouth, fatigue, and hypersensitivity reactions. Loperamide is generally not recommended for use in patients with invasive bacterial diarrhea (enteroinvasive *E. coli*, *Salmonella*, *Shigella*, or *C. jejuni*) or antibiotic-associated diarrhea (*C. difficile*), because it may worsen diarrhea or cause toxic megacolon or paralytic ileus. However, there is no evidence that these complications occur in actual practice when loperamide is used with appropriate antimicrobial therapy. Patients with symptoms suggestive of infection with invasive organisms or antibiotic-associated diarrhea (i.e., fecal leukocytes, high fever, blood or mucus in the stool) require medical evaluation for proper management. If abdominal distention, constipation, or ileus occurs, loperamide should be discontinued.

TABLE 16–7 Recommended Dosages of Nonprescription Antidiarrheal Agents for Acute Diarrhea

Medication	Dosage Forms	Adult Dosages (maximum daily dosage)	Pediatric Dosages	Duration of Use
Loperamide	Caplets (2 mg), liquid (1 mg/7.5 mL)	Caplets: 4 mg initially, followed by 2 mg after each loose stool (not to exceed 8 mg/day) Liquid: 4 mg (30 mL) initially, followed by 2 mg (15 mL) after each loose stool (not to exceed 8 mg/day [60 mL/day])	Consult product instructions; not recommended for children <6 years except under medical supervision 6–8 years (48–59 lb [22–27 kg]): Caplets: 2 mg initially, followed by 1 mg after each loose stool (not to exceed 4 mg/day) Liquid: 2 mg (15 mL) initially, followed by 1 mg (7.5 mL) after each loose stool. Do not give >4 mg (30 mL) in 24 hours 9–11 years (60–95 lb [27–43 kg]): Caplets: 2 mg initially, followed by 1 mg after each loose stool (not to exceed 6 mg/day) Liquid: 2 mg (15 mL) initially, followed by 1 mg (7.5 mL) after each loose stool. Do not give >6 mg (45 mL) in 24 hours.	48 hours
Bismuth subsalicylate	Tablets (262 mg), caplets (262 mg), liquids (262 mg/15 mL, 525 mg/15 mL)	Tablets/caplets: 525 mg every 30–60 minutes up to 4200 mg/day (8 doses/day) Liquid: 262 mg/15 mL strength: 525 mg (30 mL) every 60 minutes up to 240 mL/day (8 doses/day); 525 mg/15 mL strength: 1050 mg (30 mL) every 60 minutes up to 120 mL/day (4 doses/day)	Not recommended for children <12 years except under medical supervision	48 hours
Digestive enzymes (lactase)	Chewable tablets, caplets, liquids	Tablets: 1–3 with first bite of dairy product Capsules: 1–2 with first bite of dairy products Liquid: 5–15 drops placed in or taken with dairy product	Same as adult dosage	Taken with each consumption of dairy product

Very few clinically significant drug–drug interactions are reported for loperamide (Table 16–9). Although loperamide is a substrate for P-glycoprotein and interactions with P-glycoprotein inhibitors (e.g., quinidine, ketoconazole, ritonavir) may result in a 2- to 3-fold increase in loperamide plasma concentrations, these interactions do not appear to cause clinically significant CNS depression or opioid toxicity when loperamide is used in the recommended doses.[32] However, monitoring for loperamide adverse effects when used with a P-glycoprotein inhibitor is recommended.[35] Loperamide is metabolized primarily by cytochrome P450 (CYP)3A4 and CYP2C8. Concurrent administration of loperamide with other substrates for these enzymes (e.g., protease inhibitors, cyclosporine, erythromycin, clarithromycin) may elevate loperamide concentrations, but the effect on loperamide disposition does not appear to be associated with clinically relevant outcomes when taken in the recommended doses.[32,33,35] Loperamide may significantly decrease saquinavir concentrations, and patients receiving saquinavir should be advised not to use loperamide, especially for long periods of time.

Bismuth Subsalicylate

BSS is effective in the treatment of acute diarrhea. BSS reacts with hydrochloric acid in the stomach to form bismuth oxychloride and salicylic acid. Bismuth oxychloride is insoluble and poorly absorbed from the GI tract; less than 1% of the bismuth administered in a dose is absorbed systemically.[36] The salicylate is readily and efficiently absorbed. Both moieties are pharmacologically active. The bismuth moiety exerts direct antimicrobial effects against ETEC and EAEC, *C. jejuni,* and other diarrheal pathogens, whereas the salicylate moiety exerts antisecretory effects that reduce fluid and electrolyte losses. These effects reduce the frequency of unformed stools, increase stool consistency, relieve abdominal cramping, and decrease nausea and vomiting. In travelers' diarrhea, the salicylate appears to be the active moiety. Its antisecretory effects may be mediated by several mechanisms, including inhibition of prostaglandin synthesis, inhibition of intestinal secretion through stimulation of sodium and chloride reabsorption, or disruption of calcium-mediated processes that regulate intestinal ion transport.

TABLE 16–8 Selected Antidiarrheal Products

Trade Name	Primary Ingredients
Loperamide Products	
Imodium A-D Caplets/Imodium EZ Chews (Tablets)	Loperamide HCl 2 mg
Imodium Advanced Caplets/ Chewable Tablets	Loperamide HCl 2 mg; simethicone 125 mg
Imodium A-D Liquid	Loperamide HCl 1 mg/7.5 mL
Bismuth Subsalicylate Products	
Kaopectate Flavored Liquid (Cherry, Peppermint, Vanilla)	Bismuth subsalicylate 262 mg/15 mL (contains 130 mg of salicylate)
Kaopectate Extra Strength Peppermint Flavor Liquid	Bismuth subsalicylate 525 mg/15 mL (contains 236 mg of salicylate)
Kaopectate Antidiarrheal Caplets	Bismuth subsalicylate 262 mg (contains 99 mg of salicylate)
Maalox Total Relief Flavored Liquid (Peppermint, Strawberry)	Bismuth subsalicylate 525 mg/15 mL (contains 232 mg of salicylate)
Pepto-Bismol Caplets	Bismuth subsalicylate 262 mg (contains 99 mg of salicylate)
Pepto-Bismol Cherry Chewable Tablets	Bismuth subsalicylate 262 mg (contains 99 mg of salicylate)
Pepto-Bismol Chewable Tablets (Original, InstaCool Peppermint)	Bismuth subsalicylate 262 mg (contains 102 mg of salicylate)
Pepto-Bismol Liquid (Original, Cherry)	Bismuth subsalicylate 262 mg/15 mL (contains 130 mg of salicylate)
Pepto-Bismol Max Strength Liquid	Bismuth subsalicylate 525 mg/15 mL (contains 236 mg of salicylate)

Note: Pepto-Bismol adult formulations contain bismuth subsalicylate, but the products for children that contain calcium carbonate as the active ingredient are not listed.

The antimicrobial effects of the bismuth moiety have not been shown to be important in the treatment of travelers' diarrhea, although they may play a role in the prophylactic use of this drug. BSS also directly binds to enterotoxins produced by *E. coli* and other diarrheal pathogens; however, the clinical significance of this effect in the treatment of diarrhea is not clear.

BSS is FDA approved for management of acute diarrhea, including travelers' diarrhea, in adults and children 12 years of age and older; it is not recommended for use in young children. BSS is also indicated for indigestion and as an adjuvant to antibiotics for treating *Helicobacter pylori*–associated peptic ulcer disease. Table 16–7 provides dosing information for BSS.

BSS is available in several dosage forms; each contains various amounts of salicylate (Table 16–8). If a patient is taking aspirin or other salicylate-containing drugs, toxic levels of salicylate may be reached even if the patient follows dosing directions on the label for each medication.

Mild tinnitus, a dose-related side effect, may be associated with moderate–severe salicylate toxicity. If tinnitus occurs, the product should be discontinued and the patient referred for medical evaluation. Salicylates may cause adverse effects that are independent of the dose. In susceptible patients, salicylate-induced gout attacks have occurred. Patients who are sensitive to aspirin (i.e., experience asthmatic bronchospasm) should not use BSS.

Because of the risk of Reye's syndrome, children and teenagers who have or are recovering from chickenpox or influenza-like symptoms should not use this product.[37] When using this product, if changes in behavior with nausea and vomiting occur, consult a primary care provider, because these symptoms could be an early sign of Reye's syndrome, a rare but serious illness. Children's Pepto Antacid has been reformulated to contain calcium carbonate as the active ingredient. Unlike other forms of Pepto-Bismol, Children's Pepto Antacid is not associated with Reye's syndrome, but it is not labeled for treatment of diarrhea. (See Chapter 5 for further information.)

Although the oral bioavailability of bismuth from BSS is poor (<1%), BSS has rarely been associated with bismuth-related neurotoxicity. Encephalopathy characterized by slow onset of tremors, postural instability, ataxia, myoclonus, poor concentration, confusion, memory impairment, seizures, visual and auditory hallucinations, psychosis, delirium, depression, and death can occur when bismuth concentrations in the blood exceed 50 mcg/L. Use of BSS in the recommended doses, even for several weeks, such as in prophylaxis for travelers' diarrhea, produces mean blood concentrations well below 50 mcg/L and does not result in bismuth-related neurotoxicity. However, AIDS patients with acute diarrhea may be at particular risk for bismuth encephalopathy, perhaps resulting from altered GI absorption, and should not use BSS.

Harmless black staining of stool (which should not be confused with melena) and darkening of the tongue occur in more than 10% of patients treated with BSS. Bismuth salts react with hydrogen sulfide produced by bacteria in the mouth and colon to form the discoloration. It may be treated by brushing the tongue with a soft-bristled brush or by discontinuing the bismuth product.

Bismuth is radiopaque and may interfere with radiographic intestinal studies. BSS may interact adversely with a number of other drugs, particularly those that potentially interact with aspirin (Table 16–9). The salicylate moiety can increase the risk of toxicity with warfarin, valproic acid, and methotrexate by significantly decreasing plasma protein binding of these drugs in vivo. Salicylate can also increase the plasma concentration of methotrexate by decreasing its renal clearance. The uricosuric effects of probenecid may be inhibited by the salicylate moiety. The bismuth moiety is a trivalent cation and may decrease absorption of other medications, such as tetracycline and quinolone antibiotics, by forming

TABLE 16–9 **Clinically Important Drug–Drug Interactions With Nonprescription Antidiarrheal Agents**

Antidiarrheal	Drug	Potential Interaction	Management/Preventive Measures
Bismuth subsalicylate	Carbonic anhydrase inhibitors (acetazolamide, methazolamide, etc.)[a]	Increased risk for severe metabolic acidosis and/or salicylate toxicity	Avoid high-dose salicylate therapy; if concurrent administration is necessary, monitor closely for toxicity.
Bismuth subsalicylate	Fluoroquinolones (Systemic)	Decreased fluoroquinolone effectiveness	Avoid concurrent use; if concurrent use cannot be avoided, fluoroquinolone should be taken at least 2–3 hours before bismuth subsalicylate dose. Monitor for antibiotic efficacy.
Bismuth subsalicylate	Insulin[b]	Increased risk of hypoglycemia	Monitor glucose levels more frequently and adjust insulin dose, if necessary.
Bismuth subsalicylate	Methotrexate	Increased risk of methotrexate toxicity	Avoid salicylate therapy within 10 days of high-dose methotrexate; if concurrent administration is necessary, monitor closely for toxicity.
Bismuth subsalicylate	Pramlintide	Increased risk of hypoglycemia	Monitor glucose levels more frequently and adjust insulin dose, if necessary.
Bismuth subsalicylate	Probenecid	Increased risk of hyperuricemia	Avoid persistent high-dose salicylate therapy; occasional small doses are not clinically significant.
Bismuth subsalicylate	Sulfinpyrazone	Increased risk of hyperuricemia	Avoid persistent high-dose salicylate therapy; occasional small doses are not clinically significant.
Bismuth subsalicylate	Tamarind	Increased risk of salicylate toxicity	Avoid concurrent use, if possible.
Bismuth subsalicylate	Tetracyclines (systemic)	Decreased tetracycline effectiveness	Avoid concurrent use; if concurrent use cannot be avoided, tetracycline should be taken at least 2–3 hours before bismuth subsalicylate dose. Monitor for antibiotic efficacy.
Bismuth subsalicylate	Warfarin	Increased risk of bleeding	Avoid concurrent use, if possible. Monitor international normalized ratio (INR) closely whenever bismuth subsalicylate is added or discontinued, and adjust warfarin dose as necessary.
Loperamide	Eliglustat	Increased loperamide concentrations with enhanced central effects	Avoid concurrent use. If concurrent use cannot be avoided, monitor for loperamide adverse effects.
Loperamide	Lomitapide	Increased loperamide concentrations with enhanced central effects	Avoid concurrent use. If concurrent use cannot be avoided, monitor for loperamide adverse effects.
Loperamide	Nilotinib	Increased loperamide concentrations with enhanced central effects	Avoid concurrent use. If concurrent use cannot be avoided, monitor for loperamide adverse effects.
Loperamide	Saquinavir	Decreased saquinavir plasma concentrations	Avoid concurrent use.
Loperamide	Simeprevir	Increased loperamide concentrations with enhanced central effects	Avoid concurrent use. If concurrent use cannot be avoided, monitor for loperamide adverse effects.
Loperamide	St. John's wort	Increased risk of delirium with confusion, agitation, and disorientation	Monitor for signs of altered mental status.
Loperamide	Valerian	Increased risk of delirium with confusion, agitation, and disorientation	Monitor for signs of altered mental status.

[a] Although this interaction has not been reported with ocular carbonic anhydrase inhibitors, the possibility of an interaction should be considered.
[b] Including insulin, insulin lispro, insulin aspart, recombinant, insulin glulisine, insulin detemir, insulin degludec.
Source: Adapted from reference 32.

complexes with them in the GI tract. Solid dosage forms of BSS contain calcium carbonate, which may enhance this interaction. When fluoroquinolones are used to treat travelers' diarrhea, the patient should be instructed to discontinue BSS.

Digestive Enzymes

For patients with lactase deficiency who are intolerant of milk products, lactase enzyme preparations (Table 16–10) may be taken with milk or other dairy products to prevent osmotic diarrhea.

Product Selection Guidelines

Table 16–7 provides a quick reference for recommended dosages and durations of therapy for selected antidiarrheal agents. Tables 16–8 and 16–10 list dosage forms and primary ingredients of selected trade-name products.

In May 2011, FDA released final guidance on nonprescription liquid products that include any type of measuring device, such as the dropper packaged with lactase drops.[38] Other devices mentioned include cups, syringes, and spoons. The key points of the guidance are the following recommendations:

- A dosing device be included with all oral liquid nonprescription products.
- The device be calibrated to the dose recommended in the product directions.
- The device be used only with the product in which it is packaged.
- The markings remain visible even when the liquid is in the device.

Special Populations

For young children (≤5 years), self-treatment is limited to treating dehydration with ORS; antidiarrheal medications are not recommended. BSS-containing products should not be used in children and adolescents, especially those recovering from chickenpox or influenza, because of the risk of Reye's syndrome. (See Chapter 5 for further information.)

If diarrhea persists despite oral rehydration therapy, a primary care provider must be consulted.

Older patients (≥65 years) should be strongly cautioned against self-treatment with antidiarrheal medications. Diarrhea in these patients is more likely to be severe or possibly fatal; therefore, these patients should be referred for medical evaluation.

Use of nonprescription antidiarrheals may be inappropriate during pregnancy; therefore, pregnant women should also be referred for medical evaluation before self-treating. (See the Preface for a detailed explanation of the pregnancy data.)

BSS-containing products are contraindicated during pregnancy because of concerns that the salicylate component may inhibit platelet function and, in the third trimester, cause premature closure of the fetal ductus arteriosus. Nursing women should generally avoid BSS.

Patient Factors and Preferences

Selection of antidiarrheal products for older children and adults should be based on factors such as the etiology of the diarrhea (if known), prominent symptoms, potential interactions with prescribed medications, and applicable contraindications. For example, BSS is suggested to be the preferred agent when vomiting is the predominant clinical symptom of acute gastroenteritis. BSS should not be used to treat diarrhea in immunocompromised patients (e.g., AIDS, transplant recipients), because they are at increased risk for bismuth encephalopathy. Preference for a particular dosage form and products requiring fewer doses should also be considered.

Complementary Therapies

Convincing evidence suggests that probiotics, including several *Lactobacillus* species, *Bifidobacterium lactis*, and *Saccharomyces boulardii*, are effective in preventing and treating mild acute, uncomplicated diarrhea, in previously healthy infants and children, especially rotavirus diarrhea and antibiotic-associated diarrhea.[39–43] (See Chapter 20 for discussion of probiotics.) Probiotics release antimicrobial substances in the intestines; produce acids (e.g., lactic acid) and short-chain fatty acids that lower intestinal pH and suppress growth of pathogenic bacteria; enhance mucosal barrier integrity and immune responses; and compete with pathogenic bacteria for intestinal mucosal binding sites. However, their role in moderate–severe diarrhea is not supported conclusively by available evidence.[44]

Probiotics appear to be safe for most patients. Major adverse effects, such as *Lactobacillus* or *Saccharomyces* sepsis, rarely occur. Older, critically ill, and immunocompromised patients and patients with severe bowel diseases are at risk for systemic infection from probiotic use. Recent European evidence-based guidelines for management of acute gastroenteritis in children support the adjunctive use of *Lactobacillus rhamnosus GG* and *S. boulardii* with ORS.[45] The American Academy of Pediatrics has been more conservative, recommending that use of probiotics may be considered in special circumstances, such as for children in long-term health care facilities or care centers.[46] Probiotics are recognized by FDA as dietary supplements or components of functional foods, which limits the health claims that can be made for them, and they should not be recommended for self-treatment or prevention of acute, uncomplicated diarrhea.

Compelling evidence demonstrates that daily zinc supplementation reduces the duration, severity, and persistence of acute

TABLE 16–10 Selected Lactase Enzyme Products

Trade Name	Primary Ingredient
Lactaid Original Caplets	Lactase enzyme 3000 FCC units[a]/caplet
Lactaid Fast Act Caplets	Lactase enzyme 9000 FCC units[a]/caplet
Lactaid Fast Act Chewable Tablets	Lactase enzyme 9000 FCC units[a]/tablet
Lacteeze Children's	Lactase enzyme 3000 FCCLU/tablet
Lacteeze Drops	Lactase enzyme 80 FCCLU/5 drops
Lacteeze Extra Strength Tablets	Lactase enzyme 4000 FCCLU/tablet
Lacteeze Ultra Caplets	Lactase enzyme 9000 FCCLU/tablet
Lactrase Capsules	Lactase enzyme 250 mg/capsule

Key: FCC = Food Chemicals Codex; FCCLU = FCC lactase units.

[a] FCC units are standardized units established by the Food Chemicals Codex, a compendium of internationally recognized standards for purity and identity of food ingredients published by the United States Pharmacopeia.

diarrhea in children younger than 5 years of age, and since 2004, WHO and UNICEF have recommended routine zinc supplementation for children with acute diarrhea for 10–14 days in addition to ORS.[28] Zinc produces antidiarrheal effects by stimulating intestinal water and electrolyte absorption, preventing villous atrophy, and enhancing overall immunity, perhaps in part, through upregulation of T-helper cell (Th1 cell) immune responses, including macrophage activation and cell-mediated immunity. However, most studies showing a benefit were conducted in developing countries where zinc deficiency is prevalent. More recent studies have found zinc supplementation to be of no benefit in developed countries where zinc deficiency is rare; therefore its use is not recommended.[47–49] Zinc supplementation is associated with an increased risk for vomiting.

There is no evidence to substantiate the safety and effectiveness of herbal products and homeopathic remedies in the management of acute diarrheal diseases. Therefore, their use cannot be recommended.

Assessment of Diarrhea: A Case-Based Approach

To evaluate a patient with diarrhea, the health care provider differentiates symptoms and makes clinical judgments. This triage function is based on the patient's responses to questions designed to help determine the cause of the specific signs and symptoms, their characteristics, and their severity (Tables 16–1 and 16–3). The provider should therefore ask the patient about vomiting, high and/or prolonged fever, and other symptoms to determine the patient's susceptibility to complications. Persistent or chronic diarrhea precludes self-treatment and requires immediate medical referral, as does the presence of high fever (>102.2°F [39.0°C]), protracted vomiting, abdominal pain in patients older than 50 years, or blood or mucus in the stool. If none of these significant findings is present, the degree of dehydration should be assessed (Table 16–3); the provider should ask about the nature and amount of fluid intake. Severity of dehydration can be accurately assessed by evaluating changes in body weight. For example, in children, mild dehydration is associated with a 3%–5% loss of body weight, whereas severe dehydration is associated with a loss of more than 9%. However, the patient (or the parent) seldom knows the exact weight before the onset of diarrhea for comparison, and distinguishing between mild and moderate dehydration may be difficult.

The initial assessment of a pediatric patient should also seek to determine plausible causes of the symptoms. The common symptoms of acute gastroenteritis (e.g., vomiting, loose stools, fever) are nonspecific findings associated with many other childhood diseases (e.g., acute otitis media, bacterial sepsis, meningitis, pneumonia, urinary tract infections). This information is a key factor in recommending a proper course of action, which may include self-treatment or referral for medical evaluation. A complete medication history must be assessed before a product is selected.

Physical assessment of a patient with symptoms of diarrhea can provide information useful in assessing the severity of the diarrhea (Table 16–3). Checking skin turgor and moistness of oral mucous membranes will help determine the degree of dehydration. Vital signs (e.g., pulse, temperature, respiration, blood pressure) are important indicators of illness severity and should be routinely measured. Symptoms of moderate–severe dehydration may include postural (orthostatic) hypotension, defined as a drop in the systolic and/or diastolic pressure of greater than 15–20 mm Hg when a patient moves from a supine to an upright position. Normally, the diastolic pressure remains the same or increases slightly and the systolic pressure drops slightly on rising. If the blood pressure drops, the pulse should be checked simultaneously; the pulse rate should increase as blood pressure drops. Failure of the pulse to rise suggests that the problem is neurogenic (e.g., diabetic patients with peripheral neuropathy) or that the patient may be taking a beta blocker. The presence of orthostatic hypotension suggests that the patient has lost 1 L or more of vascular volume, and referral for medical care is necessary.

Cases 16–1 and 16–2 provide examples of assessment of patients with diarrhea.

Patient Counseling for Diarrhea

Patients with diarrhea may focus on the need for a nonprescription medication to stop the frequent bowel movements. The health care provider should remind them that most episodes of acute diarrhea stop after 48 hours and that preventing dehydration is the most important component of treatment. Counseling on the 2-step treatment of dehydration and the need for dietary management should follow. For infants and children, educating parents and caregivers on the appropriate use of an ORS (including appropriate volumes to administer, rates of administration, and use in vomiting) and of dietary management is very important. For patient safety reasons, premixed solutions are preferred. If dry powder ORS is selected, however, the provider should give parents (or caregivers) explicit directions for mixing and verify that they understand the directions. For families with infants, the Centers for Disease Control and Prevention recommends a home supply of ORS, because its early administration at home is vital if hospitalization is to be avoided. If travelers are using ORS dry powder in developing countries, potable water should be used to reconstitute the powder.

If an antidiarrheal product is recommended,

- Review label instructions with the patient or caregiver.
- Calculate an appropriate dosage on the basis of the patient's age and weight, and emphasize the maximum number of doses that can be taken in 24 hours.
- Explain potential drug interactions, adverse effects, contraindications, and the maximum duration of treatment before the patient should seek medical help.

The box "Patient Education for Diarrhea" contains specific information to provide patients.

Evaluation of Patient Outcomes for Diarrhea

Many patients have mild–moderate diarrhea that is generally self-limiting within 48 hours. Mild–moderate diarrhea is managed with oral rehydration therapy, symptomatic drug therapy, and dietary measures. The patient should be monitored for dehydration by measuring body weight, vital signs, and mental alertness. With effective symptomatic treatment, the patient can expect reduced stool frequency and normal consistency of stools, as well as a reduction in generalized symptoms such as lethargy and abdominal pain. As the diarrhea resolves, the patient's appetite will return to normal and the patient can return to a regular diet.

CASE 16-1

Relevant Evaluation Criteria	Scenario/Model Outcome
Collect	
1. Gather essential information about the patient's symptoms and medical history, including	
a. Description of symptom(s) (i.e., nature, onset, duration, severity, associated symptoms)	The patient describes acute-onset diarrhea that started about 36 hours ago. Since it started, she has had 4–5 loose stools per day. She complains of mild–moderate abdominal cramping and 1 episode of vomiting, but she has no other relevant signs or symptoms. She complains of mildly increased thirst and that her mouth is somewhat dry.
b. Description of any factors that seem to precipitate, exacerbate, and/or relieve the patient's symptom(s)	None noted.
c. Description of the patient's efforts to relieve the symptoms	None. She tells you, "I thought it would get better by itself, but it hasn't."
d. Patient's identity	Alice Miller
e. Patient's age, gender, height, and weight	45 years old, female, 5 ft 7 in., 210 lb (95.25 kg)
f. Patient's occupation	Teacher
g. Patient's dietary habits	She eats a well-balanced diet, although she likes dessert; drinks wine and beer several times weekly.
h. Patient's sleep habits	Sleeps 6–7 hours nightly.
i. Concurrent medical conditions, prescription and nonprescription medications, and dietary supplements	Osteoarthritis pain: ibuprofen 200–400 mg, 2–3 times daily, as needed
j. Allergies	NKA
k. History of other adverse reactions to medications	None
l. Other (describe) ______	n/a
Assess	
2. Differentiate patient's signs/symptoms, and correctly identify the patient's primary problem(s) (Table 16–1).	Patient appears to have acute diarrhea, most likely of viral etiology.
3. Identify exclusions for self-treatment (Figure 16–1).	None
4. Formulate a comprehensive list of therapeutic alternatives for the primary problem to determine whether triage to a health care provider is required, and share this information with the patient or caregiver.	Options include (1) Refer Alice to an appropriate HCP. (2) Recommend self-care with a nonprescription antidiarrheal product, such as loperamide, and nondrug measures, such as ORS. (3) Recommend self-care with a nonprescription antidiarrheal product, such as loperamide, and nondrug measures, such as ORS, until patient can see an appropriate HCP. (4) Take no action.
Plan	
5. Select an optimal therapeutic alternative to address the patient's problem, taking into account patient preferences.	Patient has mild–moderate dehydration and no exclusions for self-care. It is appropriate to recommend self-care with a nonprescription antidiarrheal product.
6. Describe the recommended therapeutic approach to the patient or caregiver.	"Loperamide is the preferred treatment for symptomatic relief of your diarrhea. You may continue your regular diet during treatment, but you should increase your intake of your usual fluids to prevent dehydration."
7. Explain to the patient or caregiver the rationale for selecting the recommended therapeutic approach from the considered therapeutic alternatives.	"Nonprescription antidiarrheal products are safe and effective in managing symptoms of acute diarrhea when no fever or signs of serious infection are present."

CASE 16-1 *continued*

Relevant Evaluation Criteria	Scenario/Model Outcome
Implement	
8. When recommending self-care with nonprescription medications and/or nondrug therapy, convey accurate information to the patient or caregiver.	
a. Appropriate dose and frequency of administration	See the box "Patient Education for Diarrhea."
b. Maximum number of days the therapy should be employed	See the box "Patient Education for Diarrhea."
c. Product administration procedures	See the box "Patient Education for Diarrhea."
d. Expected time to onset of relief	Onset of effect is 1–3 hours.
e. Degree of relief that can be reasonably expected	No unformed stools within 48–72 hours of starting loperamide
f. Most common adverse effects	See the box "Patient Education for Diarrhea."
g. Adverse effects that warrant medical intervention should they occur	See the box "Patient Education for Diarrhea."
h. Patient options in the event that condition worsens or persists	See the box "Patient Education for Diarrhea."
i. Product storage requirements	Store in a cool, dry place out of children's reach.
j. Specific nondrug measures	See the box "Patient Education for Diarrhea."
Solicit follow-up questions from the patient or caregiver.	"Would it help if I changed my diet until this resolves?"
Answer the patient's or caregiver's questions.	"Changes to your diet usually are not needed nor are they recommended in mild to moderate diarrheal disease. You may want to avoid fatty foods or foods that aggravate your symptoms, but I would encourage you to eat a normal, healthy diet, because it provides adequate nutrition to help your intestines to heal."
Follow-up: Monitor and Evaluate	
9. Assess patient outcome.	Contact the patient in a day or two to evaluate the response to your recommendations.

Key: HCP = Health care provider; n/a = not applicable; NKA = no known allergies; ORS = oral rehydration solution.

CASE 16-2

Relevant Evaluation Criteria	Scenario/Model Outcome
Collect	
1. Gather essential information about the patient's symptoms and medical history, including	
a. Description of symptom(s) (i.e., nature, onset, duration, severity, associated symptoms)	The patient describes sudden onset of diarrhea with moderate–severe abdominal cramps for the past 4 days. He reports experiencing 3–4 episodes of loose, watery stools per day and notes that his last several stools contained some blood. He also complains of lightheadedness and becomes somewhat dizzy on standing. He has had a fever (maximum 101.1°F [38.4°C]) for the past 2 days.
b. Description of any factors that seem to precipitate, exacerbate, and/or relieve the patient's symptom(s)	None noted.
c. Description of the patient's efforts to relieve the symptoms	The patient has taken acetaminophen for his fever but has not tried anything to relieve his gastrointestinal symptoms.
d. Patient's identity	Charles Austin
e. Patient's age, gender, height, and weight	54 years old, male, 6 ft 11 in., 240 lb (109 kg)
f. Patient's occupation	Computer analyst
g. Patient's dietary habits	Eats a well-balanced diet.
h. Patient's sleep habits	Sleeps 6–7 hours nightly.

CASE 16-2 *continued*

Relevant Evaluation Criteria	Scenario/Model Outcome
i. Concurrent medical conditions, prescription and nonprescription medications, and dietary supplements	Diabetes: Metformin 1000 mg twice daily, sitagliptin 100 mg daily Hypertension: atenolol 50 mg daily, amlodipine 10 mg daily, hydrochlorothiazide 25 mg daily; hyperlipidemia: simvastatin 20 mg daily; cardiac prophylaxis: aspirin 81 mg daily
j. Allergies	NKA
k. History of other adverse reactions to medications	None
l. Other (describe) ______	n/a
Assess	
2. Differentiate patient's signs/symptoms, and correctly identify the patient's primary problem(s) (Table 16–1).	Patient is experiencing acute infectious diarrhea, most likely of bacterial etiology.
3. Identify exclusions for self-treatment (Figure 16–1).	Severe abdominal cramps, blood in the stool, and orthostatic changes (lightheadedness and dizziness on standing) are all exclusions for self-care. Although not an absolute exclusion for self-care, his history of diabetes also warrants consideration.
4. Formulate a comprehensive list of therapeutic alternatives for the primary problem to determine whether triage to a health care provider is required, and share this information with the patient or caregiver.	Options include (1) Refer patient to an appropriate HCP. (2) Recommend self-care with a nonprescription antidiarrheal product, such as bismuth subsalicylate, and nondrug measures, such as ORS. (3) Recommend self-care with a nonprescription antidiarrheal product, such as bismuth subsalicylate, and nondrug measures, such as ORS, until patient can see an appropriate HCP. (4) Take no action.
Plan	
5. Select an optimal therapeutic alternative to address the patient's problem, taking into account patient preferences.	Refer patient to an appropriate HCP, urgent care center, or emergency department for evaluation and treatment.
6. Describe the recommended therapeutic approach to the patient or caregiver.	"You need to seek urgent medical care from your primary care provider, urgent care center, or emergency department right away."
7. Explain to the patient or caregiver the rationale for selecting the recommended therapeutic approach from the considered therapeutic alternatives.	"Your symptoms suggest that your condition is serious. You probably have a bacterial infection that requires prescription antibiotics. No nonprescription remedies are available to treat bloody diarrhea. You also may need intravenous fluids to help with your hydration, and I am concerned that the infection may complicate control of your diabetes."
Implement	
8. When recommending self-care with nonprescription medications and/or nondrug therapy, convey accurate information to the patient or caregiver.	Criterion does not apply in this case.
Solicit follow-up questions from the patient or caregiver.	"Would Imodium help stop the diarrhea?"
Answer the patient's or caregiver's questions.	"Imodium, which is loperamide, should not be used when you have blood in your stool. Given your condition, you should not use any nonprescription medicine and should seek medical attention right away."
Follow-up: Monitor and Evaluate	
9. Assess patient outcome.	Ask patient to call after seeking medical attention to update you on his condition, or obtain his phone number and call him in a few days.

Key: HCP = Health care provider. n/a = not applicable; NKA = no known allergies; ORS = oral rehydration solution.

PATIENT EDUCATION FOR Diarrhea

The primary objective of self-treatment is to prevent excessive fluid and electrolyte losses. For most patients, carefully following product instructions and the self-care measures listed here will help ensure optimal outcomes.

Nondrug Measures

Infants and Children Ages 6 Months to 5 Years

- For mild–moderate diarrhea, indicated by three to five unformed bowel movements per day, give the child or infant an oral rehydration solution (ORS) at a volume of 50–100 mL/kg of body weight over 2–4 hours to replace the fluid deficit. Give additional ORS to replace ongoing losses. Continue to give the solution for the next 4–6 hours or until the child is rehydrated.
- If the child is vomiting, give 1 teaspoon of ORS every few minutes.
- If the child is not dehydrated, give 10 mL/kg or ½–1 cup of the ORS for each bowel movement, or 2 mL/kg for each episode of vomiting. As an alternative, to replace ongoing fluid losses, children weighing less than 22 lb (10 kg) should be given 60–120 mL of ORS for each episode of vomiting or diarrheal stool, and children weighing more than 22 lb (10 kg) should be given 120–240 mL for each episode of vomiting or diarrheal stool.
- After the child is rehydrated, reintroduce food appropriate for the child's age, while also administering an ORS as maintenance therapy.
- If breastfeeding an infant with diarrhea, continue the breastfeeding. If the infant is bottle-fed, consult your primary care provider or pediatrician about replacing a milk-based formula with a lactose-free formula.
- Give children complex carbohydrate–rich foods, yogurt, lean meats, fruits, and vegetables. Do not give them fatty foods or sugary foods. Sugary foods can cause osmotic diarrhea.
- Do not withhold food for more than 24 hours.

Adults and Children Older Than 5 Years

- For mild-moderate dehydration, indicated by a 3%–9% drop in body weight or three to five unformed stools per day, drink 2–4 L of an ORS over 4 hours.
- If not dehydrated, drink ½–1 cup of ORS or fluids after each unformed bowel movement.
- If no medical conditions exist, sports drinks (with salty crackers, etc.), diluted juices, soups, and broths may be consumed until the diarrhea stops.
- Do not withhold food for more than 24 hours.

Nonprescription Medications

- See Table 16–7 for dosages of loperamide and bismuth subsalicylate.

Loperamide

- Note that loperamide can cause dizziness and constipation.
- Nonprescription loperamide is not recommended for children younger than 6 years, except under the supervision of a primary care provider or pediatrician.
- If loperamide is not effective in treating your diarrhea (if no clinical improvement is observed in 48 hours), check with your primary care provider or pharmacist about using a different nonprescription medication. You may have a bacterial diarrhea or pseudomembranous colitis; these conditions require specific antibiotic therapy that loperamide cannot treat.

Bismuth Subsalicylate

- Note that bismuth subsalicylate can cause a dark discoloration of the tongue and stool.
- Do not take this medication if you are taking tetracyclines, quinolones, or medicines for gout (uricosurics).
- Do not give this medication to children younger than 12 years.
- Do not give this medication to children or teenagers who have or are recovering from chickenpox or influenza-like symptoms because of the risk of Reye's syndrome.
- Do not give this medication to patients with acquired immunodeficiency syndrome (AIDS).
- Do not take this medication if you are sensitive to aspirin, have a history of gastrointestinal bleeding, or have a history of problems with blood coagulation.

When to Seek Medical Attention

- If the diarrhea has not resolved after 72 hours of initial treatment, see your primary care provider.
- Monitor for excessive number of bowel movements, signs of dehydration, high fever, or blood in the stool. If any of these complications are present, discontinue bismuth subsalicylate, and consult your primary care provider.

Medical referral is necessary if any of the following signs and symptoms occur before or during treatment: high fever, worsening illness, bloody or mucoid stools, diarrhea continuing beyond 48 hours, or signs of worsening dehydration (e.g., low blood pressure, rapid pulse, mental confusion). Also, medical referral is advised for infants, young children, frail patients of advanced age, pregnant patients, and patients with chronic illness at risk from secondary complications (e.g., diabetes).

Key Points for Diarrhea

- Self-treatment of diarrhea should be limited to patients with mild–moderate acute diarrhea who have minimal, mild, or moderate dehydration. Patients who appear volume depleted, weak, dizzy, febrile (temperature >102.2°F [39.0°C]), or hypotensive should be referred for evaluation.
- ORS is the mainstay of therapy and should be used to rehydrate patients with minimal or mild–moderate dehydration.
- Rehydration should be performed rapidly (i.e., within 3–4 hours). Additional ORS should be given to maintain hydration and replace ongoing fluid losses resulting from diarrheal stools and/or vomiting (Figures 16–1 and 16–2).
- Patients or their caregivers should be instructed how to prepare and administer an ORS.
- Older children and adults may use sports drinks instead of an ORS if additional sources of sodium (e.g., crackers, pretzels) are used concomitantly.
- An age-appropriate, unrestricted diet should be initiated as soon as the patient is rehydrated. Food should be withheld for no more than 24 hours.
- Loperamide and BSS may be used to help control acute diarrhea in carefully selected patients.
- Antibiotic therapy is generally not indicated for patients with acute diarrhea unless it is travelers' diarrhea.

REFERENCES

1. Farthing M, Salam MA, Lindberg G, et al. Acute diarrhea in adults and children: a global perspective. *J Clin Gastroenterol.* 2013;47(1):12–20. doi: 10.1097/MCG.0b013e31826df662.
2. Scallan E, Griccin PM, Angulo FJ, et al. Foodborne illness acquired in the United States—unspecified agents. *Emerg Infect Dis.* 2011;17(1):16–22. doi: 10.3201/eid1701.091101p2.
3. Jones TF, McMillian MB, Scallan E, et al. A population-based estimate of the substantial burden of diarrhoeal disease in the United States; FoodNet, 1996–2003. *Epidemiol Infect.* 2007;135(2):293–301. PMCID: PMC2870567.
4. Patel MM, Hall AJ, Vinje J, et al. Noroviruses: a comprehensive review. *J Clin Virol.* 2009;44(1):1–8. doi: 10.1016/j.jcv.2008.10.009.
5. Payne DC, Vinjé J, Szilagyi PG, et al. Norovirus and medically attended gastroenteritis in U.S. children. *N Engl J Med.* 2013;368(12):1121–30. PMCID: PMC4618551.
6. Patel MM, Widdowson M, Glass RI, et al. Systematic literature review of role of noroviruses in sporadic gastroenteritis. *Emerg Infect Dis.* 2008;14(8):1224–31. PMCID: PMC2600393.
7. Cortese MM, Parashar UD. Prevention of rotavirus gastroenteritis among infants and children: recommendations of the Advisory Committee on Immunization Practices (ACIP). *MMWR Recomm Rep.* 2009;58(RR-2):1–25. PMID: 19194371.
8. Cortese MM, Tate JE, Simonsen L, et al. Reduction in gastroenteritis in United States children and correlation with early rotavirus vaccine uptake from national medical claims databases. *Pediatr Infect Dis J.* 2010;29(6):489–94. doi: 10.1097/INF.0b013e3181d95b53.
9. Flores AR, Szilagyi PG, Auinger P, et al. Estimated burden of rotavirus-associated diarrhea in ambulatory settings in the United States. *Pediatrics.* 2010;125(2):e191–8. doi: 10.1542/peds.2008-1262.
10. Cardemil CV, Cortese MM, Medina-Marion A, et al. Two rotavirus outbreaks caused by genotype G2P[4] at large retirement communities. *Ann Intern Med.* 2012;157(9):621–31. doi: 10.7326/0003-4819-157-9-201211060-00006.
11. Breese JS, Marcys R, Venezia RA, et al. The etiology of severe acute gastroenteritis among adults visiting emergency departments in the United States. *J Infect Dis.* 2012;205(9):1374–81. doi: 10.1093/infdis/jis206.
12. Anderson EJ, Katz BZ, Polin JA, et al. Rotavirus in adults requiring hospitalization. *J Infect.* 2012;64(1):89–95. doi: 10.1016/j.jinf.2011.09.003.
13. Marcos LA, DuPont HL. Advances in defining etiology and new therapeutic approaches in acute diarrhea. *J Infect.* 2007;55(5):385–93. doi: 10.1016/j.jinf.2007.07.016.
14. Kayman T, Abay S, Hizlisoy H, et al. Emerging pathogen *Arcobacter* spp. in acute gastroenteritis: molecular identification, antibiotic susceptibilities and genotyping of the isolated arcobacter. *J Medical Microbiol.* 2012;61 (pt 10):1439–44. doi: 10.1099/jmm.0.044594-0.
15. Schiller LR, Sellin JH. Diarrhea. In: Feldman M, Friedman LS, Brandt LJ, eds. *Sleisenger and Fordtran's Gastrointestinal and Liver Disease.* Vol. 2, 10th ed. New York: Elsevier; 2016:221–41.
16. Hodges K, Gill R. Infectious diarrhea: cellular and molecular mechanisms. *Gut Microbes.* 2010;1(1):4–21. PMCID: PMC3035144.
17. DuPont HL. Gastrointestinal infections and the development of irritable bowel syndrome. *Curr Opin Infect Dis.* 2011;24(5):503–8. doi: 10.1097/QCO.0b013e32834a962d.
18. Scallan E, Hoekstra RM, Angulo FJ, et al. Foodborne illness acquired in the United States—major pathogens. *Emerg Infect Dis.* 2011;17(1):7–15. PMCID: PMC3375761.
19. Centers for Disease Control and Prevention. Preliminary incidence and trends of infection with pathogens transmitted commonly through food—foodborne diseases active surveillance network, 10 U.S. sites, 2006–2014. *MMWR Morb Mortal Wkly Rep.* 2015; 64(18);495–9. PMID: 25974634. Also available at: https://www.cdc.gov/mmwr/preview/mmwrhtml/mm6418a4.htm. Accessed May 1, 2017.
20. Shah N, DuPont HL, Ramsey DJ. Global etiology of travelers' diarrhea: systematic review from 1973 to the present. *Am J Trop Med Hyg.* 2009; 80(4):609–14. PMID: 19346386.
21. DuPont HL. Systematic review: the epidemiology and clinical features of travellers' diarrhoea. *Alimen Pharmacol Ther.* 2009;30(3):187–96. PMID: 19392866.
22. Pareded-Paredes M, Flores-Figueroa J, DuPont HL. Advances in the treatment of travelers' diarrhea. *Curr Gastroenterol Rep.* 2011;13(5):402–7. doi: 10.1007/s11894-011-0208-6.
23. King CK, Glass R, Bresee JS, et al. Managing acute gastroenteritis among children: oral rehydration, maintenance, and nutritional therapy. *MMWR Morb Mortal Wkly Rep.* 2003;52(RR-16):1–16. PMID: 14627948. Available at: https://www.cdc.gov/mmwr/preview/mmwrhtml/rr5216a1.htm. Accessed May 1, 2017.
24. Mims BC, Curry CE. Constipation, diarrhea, and irritable bowel syndrome. In: Chisholm-Burns M, Schwinghammer TL, Wells BG, et al., eds. *Pharmacotherapy Principles and Practice.* 2nd ed. New York: McGraw Medical; 2010:371–86.
25. Wingate D, Phillips SF, Lewis SJ, et al. Guidelines for adults on self-medication for the treatment of acute diarrhoea. *Aliment Pharmacol Ther.* 2001 Jun;15(6):773–82. PMID: 11380315.
26. Zielinski R, Searing K, Deibel M. Gastrointestinal distress in pregnancy: prevalence, assessment, and treatment of 5 common minor discomforts. *J Perinat Neonatal Nurs.* 2015;29(1):23–31. doi: 10.1097/JPN.0000000000000078.
27. Boregowda G, Shehata HA. Gastrointestinal and liver disease in pregnancy. *Best Pract Res Clin Obstet Gynaecol.* 2013;27(6):835–53. doi: 10.1016/j.bpobgyn.2013.07.006.
28. World Health Organization, United Nations Children's Fund. WHO/UNICEF joint statement: clinical management of acute diarrhoea. Available at: http://www.unicef.org/publications/files/ENAcute_Diarrhoea_reprint.pdf. Accessed May 1, 2017.
29. Connor BA; Centers for Disease Control and Prevention. Travelers' diarrhea. Available at: http://wwwnc.cdc.gov/travel/yellowbook/2016/the-pre-travel-consultation/travelers-diarrhea. Accessed May 1, 2017.
30. Riddle MS, Dupont HL, Connor BA. ACG clinical guideline: diagnosis, treatment, and prevention of acute diarrheal infections in adults. *Am J Gastroenterol.* 2016;111(5):602–22.
31. DuPont HL, Ericsson CD, Farthing MJG, et al. Expert review of the evidence base for prevention of travelers' diarrhea. *J Travel Med.* 2009;16(3):149–60. PMID: 19538575.
32. Vandenbossche J, Huisman M, Xu Y, et al. Loperamide and P-glycoprotein inhibition: assessment of the clinical relevance. *J Pharm Pharmacol.* 2010;62(4):401–12. doi: 10.1211/jpp.62.04.0001.
33. Eggleston W, Clark KH, Marraffa JM. Loperamide abuse associated with cardiac dysrhythmia and death. *Ann Emerg Med.* 2017;69(1):83–6. doi: 10.1016/j.annemergmed.2016.03.047.
34. U.S. Food and Drug Administration. FDA Drug Safety Communication: FDA warns about serious heart problems with high doses of the antidiarrheal medicine loperamide (Imodium), including from abuse and misuse. Available at: http://www.fda.gov/Drugs/DrugSafety/ucm504617.htm. Accessed July 21, 2017.
35. Loperamide hydrochloride. Micromedex 2.0. Truven Health Analytics, Greenwood Village, CO. Available at: http://www.micromedexsolutions.com/. Accessed March 9, 2016.
36. Bismuth subsalicylate. Micromedex 2.0. Truven Health Analytics, Greenwood Village, CO. Available at: http://www.micromedexsolutions.com/. Accessed September 25, 2016.
37. U.S. Food and Drug Administration. Labeling of drug preparations containing salicylates. *CFR: Code of Federal Regulations.* Title 21, Part 201, Section 201.314. Updated July 27, 2017. Available at: http://www.ecfr.gov/cgi-bin/text-idx?SID=b1b2224711dc88657752be21f12c574a&mc=true&node=se21.4.201_1314&rgn=div8. Accessed July 31, 2017.
38. U.S. Food and Drug Administration. *Guidance for Industry: Dosage Delivery Devices for Orally Ingested OTC Liquid Drug Products.* Rockville, MD: U.S. Department of Health and Human Services, Food and Drug Administration, Center for Drug Evaluation and Research; May 2011. Available at: https://www.fda.gov/downloads/Drugs/Guidances/UCM188992.pdf. Accessed May 1, 2017.

39. Szajewska H, Guarino A, Hojsak I, et al. Use of probiotics for management of acute gastroenteritis: a position paper by the ESPGHAN Working Group for Probiotics and Prebiotics. *J Pediatr Gastroenterol Nutr.* 2014; 58(4):531–9. doi: 10.1097/MPG.0000000000000320.
40. Floch MH, Walker A, Sanders ME, et al. Recommendations for probiotic use—2015 update. Proceedings and consensus opinion. *J Clin Gastroenterol.* 2015;49(Suppl 1):S69–73. doi: 10.1097/MCG.0000000000000420.
41. Goldin BR, Gorbach SL. Clinical indications for probiotics: an overview. *Clin Infect Dis.* 2008;46(Suppl 2):S96–100. doi: 10.1097/MCG.0000000000000420.
42. Gaundalini S. Probiotics for children with diarrhea: an update. *J Clin Gastroenterol.* 2008;42(Suppl 2):S53–7. doi: 10.1097/MCG.0b013e3181674087.
43. Szajewska H, Skorka A, Dylag M. Meta-analysis: *Saccharomyces boulardii* for treating acute diarrhea in children. *Aliment Pharmacol Ther.* 2007;25(3):257–64. PMID:17269987.
44. Patel R, DuPont HD. New approaches for bacteriotherapy: prebiotics, new-generation probiotics, and synbiotics. *Clin Infect Dis.* 2015;60(Suppl 2): S108–21. PMCID: PMC4490231.
45. Guarino A, Albano F, Ashkenazi S, et al. European Society for Paediatric Gastroenterology, Hepatology, and Nutrition/European Society for Paediatric Infectious Diseases evidence-based guidelines for the management of acute gastroenteritis in children in Europe. *J Pediatr Gastroenterol Nutr.* 2008;46(suppl 2):S81–122. doi: 10.1097/MPG.0b013e31816f7b16.
46. Thomas DW, Greer FR. Clinical report: probiotics and prebiotics in pediatrics. *Pediatrics.* 2010;126:1217–31. doi: 10.1542/peds.2010-2548.
47. Patel A, Mamtani M, Dibley MJ, et al. Therapeutic value of zinc supplementation in acute and persistent diarrhea: a systematic review. *PLoS One.* 2010;5(4):e10386. doi: 10.1371/journal.pone.0010386.
48. Patro B, Golicki D, Szajewska H. Meta-analysis: zinc supplementation for acute gastroenteritis in children. *Aliment Pharmacol Ther.* 2008; 28(6):713–23. PMID: 19145727.
49. Lazzerini M, Ronfani L. Oral zinc for treating diarrhea in children. *Cochrane Database Syst Rev.* 2012;6:CD005436. doi: 10.1002/14651858.CD005436.pub3.

CHAPTER 17

ANORECTAL DISORDERS

JULIANA CHAN

Anorectal disorders involve the perianal canal, anal canal, and/or lower rectum, with symptoms ranging from benign to life-threatening. The most common conditions affecting the anorectal area include hemorrhoids, pruritus ani, anal fistula, anal fissure, or anorectal carcinoma.[1,2] Because these disorders affect the anus, patients may be embarrassed to seek medical attention. Thus, it is imperative for the health care provider to be confident and discrete in reassuring the patient that having these symptoms is nothing to be ashamed of.

Hemorrhoids are common in men and women, and the likelihood of occurrence increases with advancing age.[3] Although epidemiologic data may vary and the true prevalence may be under-reported, 4.4%–12.8% of the general population have hemorrhoids.[4] It is estimated that 1.1 million ambulatory care visits and more than 250,000 hospitalizations are due to hemorrhoids each year.[5] The National Institutes of Health in 2004 reported approximately 2 million prescriptions were obtained to treat hemorrhoids.[5]

Pathophysiology of Anorectal Disorders

Anorectal disorders affect the perianal area (the portion of the skin immediately surrounding the anus), the anal canal, and the lower portion of the rectum (Figure 17–1). The anal canal is about 4 cm long and connects the rectum with the outside of the body.[4] Two different types of epithelia line the anal canal; their junction is defined by the dentate line (also known as the pectinate line). The dentate line divides squamous epithelium from columnar epithelium, thus separating where sensory pain fibers are located in the anal canal. Anorectal disorders occurring below the dentate line may be associated with pain, whereas disorders above the line rarely cause any discomfort.[4] The area proximal to the dentate line contains several longitudinal folds known as the columns of Morgagni. In between and next to these columns are small pockets or crypts containing ducts and glands that may become obstructed and/or cause infections (e.g., abscesses, fistulas).

The external anal sphincter is a voluntary muscle located at the bottom of the anal canal that remains closed under normal conditions to prevent involuntary passage of feces. The internal sphincter is an involuntary muscle innervated by the autonomic nervous system. When the sphincters are relaxed, defecation occurs. In healthy individuals, skin covering the anal canal serves as a barrier against absorption of substances into the body. If the protective barrier breaks, then the absorptive properties of the anal skin may be altered, diminishing the skin's protective capabilities.

The rectum, which lies above the anal canal, is approximately 12–18 cm long and is the terminal portion of the large intestine.[6] The highly vascular rectal mucosa is lined with a semipermeable membrane to protect the body from fecal bacteria. Three hemorrhoidal arteries and their accompanying veins are the most prominent parts of the vasculature. Blood returns to the heart through the hemorrhoidal veins; therefore, rectal medications may be absorbed and enter the systemic circulation without passing through the liver.[6]

Hemorrhoids, a condition that is not curable, are large, bulging, symptomatic conglomerates of inflamed hemorrhoidal vessels that project into the lumen during defecation.[4] With increasing age or poor bowel habits (e.g., prolonged sitting and straining at defecation), muscle fibers weaken and cause the vascular cushions to slide, become congested, bleed, and eventually protrude.[4] Downward pressure during defecation and a high resting anal pressure are common in the development of hemorrhoids.

Internal hemorrhoids originate from the superior hemorrhoidal vein and are located above the dentate line, an area that is covered with columnar epithelium and lacks sensory fibers (Figure 17–1).[4,6] Internal hemorrhoids are graded by severity of prolapse into the anal canal using a grading system[4,7]:

- Grade 1 hemorrhoids enlarge but do not prolapse into the anal canal.
- Grade 2 hemorrhoids protrude into the anal canal and return spontaneously on defecation.
- Grade 3 hemorrhoids protrude into the anal canal on defecation but can be returned to their original position manually.
- Grade 4 hemorrhoids are permanently prolapsed and cannot be reintroduced into the anus.

External hemorrhoids develop from the inferior hemorrhoidal vein and originate below the dentate line. (Figure 17–1).[4,7] These hemorrhoids are visible as bluish lumps at the external or distal boundary of the anal canal (known as the anal verge). The blue color may be caused by thrombosed blood vessels, which cause symptoms ranging from minimal discomfort to severe pain.[4]

Nonhemorrhoidal Anorectal Disorders

Potentially serious nonhemorrhoidal anorectal disorders (e.g., abscesses, fistulas, fissures, neoplasms) may present with hemorrhoid-like symptoms; these disorders should not be self-treated but referred for immediate medical evaluation (Table 17–1).[1,8,9]

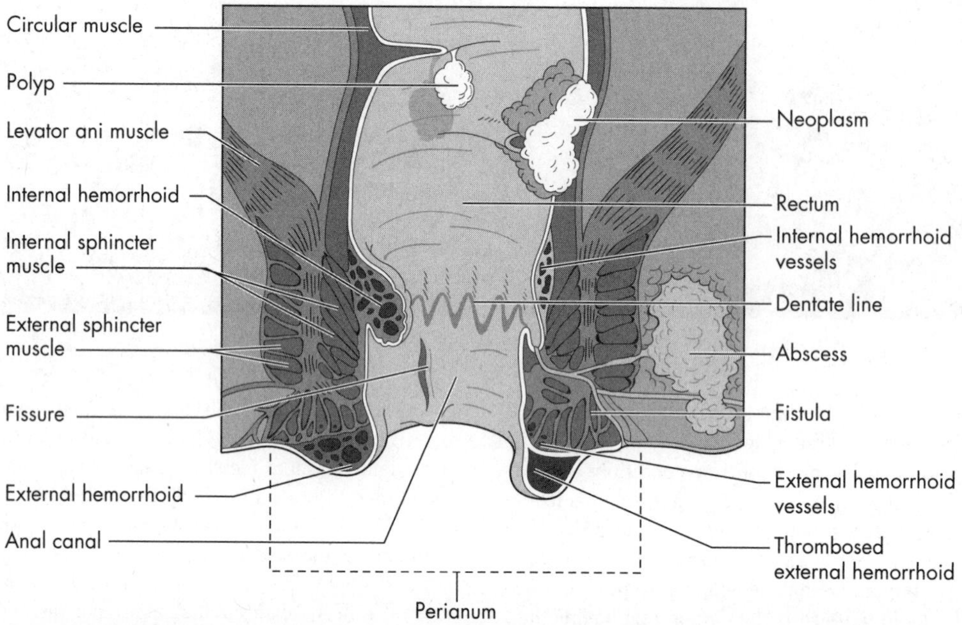

FIGURE 17-1 Disorders of the anorectal canal.

TABLE 17-1 **Nonhemorrhoidal Anorectal Disorders**

Disorder	Definition	Common Signs and Symptoms	Comments
Anal abscess	Collection of pus causing an obstruction of the anal glands, resulting in a bacterial infection	Pain, perirectal swelling, discharge, fever, or chills; pain worsens with sitting and defecation	Possible life-threatening sepsis if not identified and treated promptly
Anal fistula (or groove)	Abnormal internal opening that connects with an external opening (i.e., tube-like appearance between the rectum and anus)	Chronic, persistent drainage; pain; possible bleeding on defecation; perianal itching; stool seeping through external opening	Surgical repair required
Anal fissure	Slit-like ulcer in anal canal resulting from a traumatic tear during passage of stool or explosive diarrhea	Severe or burning pain during and after defecation, lasting several minutes to hours; anal spasms; blood may be seen on toilet tissue	Young, middle-aged individuals; equal in women and men
Anal neoplasms	Include a variety of histologic types classified as epidermoid carcinomas	Rare and usually asymptomatic in 25% of patients; bleeding; changes in bowel habits; anal discharge; anal mass; pain; pruritus; rash	Relatively uncommon, accounting for 1%–2% of all GI malignancies; most are curable, but poor prognosis with anorectal melanomas
Pruritus ani	Itching sensation localized in anorectal area	Persistent itching, scratching in perianal region; more bothersome at bedtime or when patient is not preoccupied	More common in men

Key: GI = Gastrointestinal.

Source: Abramowitz L, Weyandt GH, Havlickova B, et al. The diagnosis and management of haemorrhoidal disease from a global perspective. *Aliment Pharmacol Ther.* 2010 May;31(Suppl 1):1–58. doi: 10.1111/j.1365-2036.2010.04278.x.

Clinical Presentation of Anorectal Disorders

The Food and Drug Administration (FDA) Advisory Review Panel identified signs and symptoms for which a nonprescription anorectal product is indicated.[10] These symptoms include itching, discomfort, irritation, burning, soreness, inflammation, pain, dry anal tissue, and swelling in the perianal area.[10] In contrast, abdominal pain, bleeding, seepage, change in bowel patterns, prolapse, and thrombosis may indicate a more serious condition requiring immediate medical referral (Table 17–2).[8,9]

Treatment of Anorectal Disorders

Treatment Goals

The primary goal of treatment anorectal disorders is to maintain soft stools to prevent straining while having a bowel movement[4,11,12] (see Chapter 15). Additional goals are (1) to alleviate and maintain remission of anorectal symptoms and (2) to prevent complications.

General Treatment Approach

Figure 17–2 presents an algorithm for treating minor anorectal symptoms and lists exclusions for self-treatment. If the symptom is self-treatable, the health care provider may recommend nonpharmacologic measures and a nonprescription agent to treat the symptoms. Patients should be advised to maintain adequate fluid intake and a well-balanced high-fiber diet. Practicing good perianal hygiene and avoiding prolonged sitting on the toilet may also minimize anorectal symptoms.[4,11] Table 17–3 outlines guidelines for applying anorectal products.[13]

Nonpharmacologic Therapy

Nondrug measures for treating anorectal disorders include dietary modifications, surgical interventions, and nonoperative methods.[4,11,14] Patients diagnosed with or suspected of having hemorrhoids should avoid lifting heavy objects and discontinue foods that aggravate symptoms (e.g., alcohol, caffeinated beverages, citrus, fatty foods).[4,14]

Dietary fiber softens stool and may prevent further irritation of symptomatic hemorrhoids and other anorectal disorders. A meta-analysis confirmed that initiating fiber therapy in subjects with grade 1 or grade 2 hemorrhoids improves bleeding and overall symptomatic relief.[4,8,14] Increasing fiber intake to at least 25–40 g/day may permit the passage of softer stools, thus reducing and preventing irritation and straining at defecation.[4,14] Dietary fiber intake should be increased slowly; however, if the intake amount cannot be increased, consider fiber supplements such as psyllium or methylcellulose (see Chapter 15). Additionally, it is important to advise patients to drink an adequate amount of non-caffeinated fluid (1.5–2 L/day) to soften hard stool.[8,14]

Proper bowel habits should be encouraged. Avoiding urges to defecate should be discouraged because doing so may lead to constipation resulting in anorectal discomfort. Avoidance of sitting on the toilet for long periods of time reduces strain and decreases pressure on the hemorrhoidal vessels.[1,8,14] Proper hygiene of the anal area (e.g., cleaning the area regularly and after each bowel movement using mild, unscented soap and water) may relieve anorectal symptoms.[11,15] Commercially available hygienic and lubricated wipes or pads are not recommended as they may be more irritating to the anal area, especially in patients with pruritus ani.[15] Excessive scrubbing should be discouraged to minimize aggravation.[11,15] A nonpharmacologic measure often recommended to promote good anal hygiene, despite the lack of evidence, is sitting in warm water (≤120°F [48.89°C]) in a bathtub or sitz bath (a small bathtub that fits over the toilet rim, available at pharmacies and medical supply vendors) for 10–20 minutes 2–4 times a day.[1,4,16] In a few systematic reviews of randomized controlled trials, no evidence supported the use of sitz baths to relieve pain or assist in wound healing in patients with anorectal disorders, however, health care clinicians commonly recommended this option.[16,17]

Large and prolapsed hemorrhoids (grade 3 or grade 4) often are treated surgically, thus these patients are usually referred to a colorectal specialist for further evaluation.[11,14]

Pharmacologic Therapy

Local anesthetics, vasoconstrictors, protectants, astringents, keratolytics, analgesics, anesthetics, antipruritics, and corticosteroids are commonly used to relieve anorectal symptoms.[10] Certain astringents, protectants, and vasoconstrictors may be used only intrarectally and should be administered with an applicator (i.e., "pile pipe") so that the product may reach the affected area.[10] Suppositories may be considered as another method of administering a drug to the anal area; however, their effectiveness is in question, as suppositories may not "stay in place" after insertion.[18] The remaining agents are for external use only and are not indicated for the relief of anorectal pain, bleeding, seepage, prolapse, or thrombosis.[10] Table 17–4 provides FDA-approved dosages for anorectal drug products.[10]

Local Anesthetics

Local anesthetics are approved for the temporary relief of external anal symptoms (e.g., itching, irritation, burning, discomfort, soreness, and pain); they provide relief by reversibly blocking transmission of nerve impulses (Table 17–4).[10,13] These products should be used with caution, as they may mask the pain of more severe anorectal disorders.[13]

Local anesthetics may produce allergic reactions (e.g., burning itching) that are indistinguishable from the anorectal symptoms. Several cases of contact dermatitis have been reported with hemorrhoidal anesthetics, including benzocaine, dibucaine, and lidocaine.[19–21] Patients who have an allergic reaction to a local anesthetic may try different agents with a different chemical structures (e.g., pramoxine) or avoid use of these agents completely. These preparations must carry a warning stating that allergic reactions may occur.[10] Local anesthetics should be avoided on open sores because they are rapidly absorbed through abraded skin and may cause cardiovascular and central nervous system effects. Accidental oral ingestion of dibucaine-containing anorectal products has been reported in children, resulting in lethargy, seizures, and cardiorespiratory arrest; thus these products should be kept out of children's reach.[10,21,22]

Vasoconstrictors

Topical vasoconstrictors (ephedrine, epinephrine) are structurally related to the endogenous catecholamines epinephrine and norepinephrine. When ephedrine or epinephrine is applied to the anorectal area, stimulation of α-adrenergic receptors in the vascular beds constricts arterioles, producing a modest and transient reduction

TABLE 17-2 Signs and Symptoms of Anorectal Disorders

Sign/Symptom	Definition/Etiology
Usually Self-Treatable	
Itching (pruritus)	Mild stimulation of sensory nerve fibers; associated with many anorectal disorders, including hemorrhoids (typically with a mucoid discharge from prolapsing internal hemorrhoids). Common causes include poor hygiene (e.g., incomplete wiping/cleaning after defecation); diarrhea; parasitic or fungal infections; allergies (e.g., sensitivity to fabrics, soaps, laundry detergents, dyes, perfumes in toilet tissue); anorectal lesions; moisture in anal area. May be secondary to swelling; diet (e.g., caffeinated beverages, chocolate, citrus fruits); oral broad-spectrum antibiotics. Rare cause includes psychogenic origins.
Discomfort	May result from burning, itching, pain, irritation, inflammation, and swelling.
Irritation	Uncomfortable feeling associated with stimulation of sensory nerve fibers.
Burning	Greater degree of irritation of sensory nerve fibers than what is commonly experienced with anal itching; often associated with hemorrhoids; sensation of warmth or intense heat. May be constant or occur only at defecation.
Inflammation	Tissue reaction characterized by heat, redness or discoloration, pain, and swelling; often associated with trauma, allergy, or infection.
Swelling	Temporary enlargement of cells and/or tissue resulting from excess fluid; may be accompanied by pain, burning, and itching.
Requires Medical Referral	
Pain	Intense stimulation of sensory nerve fibers caused by inflammation or irritation. Internal hemorrhoids usually are painless; external hemorrhoids often cause mild pain; acute, severe perianal pain may be from a thrombosed external hemorrhoid. Pain from anal fissure during bowel movement often described as "being cut with sharp glass." Other possible causes of pain include abscess, fistula, or anorectal neoplasm.
Bleeding	Hemorrhoids most common cause of minor bleeds (e.g., from straining or passage of hard stool, or ulceration of perianal skin overlying thrombosed external hemorrhoid). Appears as bright red spots or streaks on toilet tissue, or bright red blood around stool or in toilet. Black or tarry stools (melena) may indicate a possible upper GI bleed (e.g., PUD, erosive esophagitis, or gastric varices). Large amounts of red blood (hematochezia) in toilet bowl indicative of lower GI bleeding (e.g., fissure, IBD, polyps, malignant disease of the colon or rectum). Possible indications of large-volume blood loss include shortness of breath, dizziness, fatigue, or light-headedness, especially upon standing (orthostatic hypotension).
Seepage	Involuntary passage of fecal material or mucus caused by an incompletely closed anal sphincter; may include discharge of pus or feces from a fistula connecting the rectum to the anal canal.
Change in bowel pattern	Unexplained change in bowel frequency or in stool form; may signal serious underlying GI disorder (e.g., IBD) or colorectal cancer.
Prolapse (protrusion)	Protrusion of hemorrhoidal or rectal tissue of variable size into anal canal; usually appears after defecation, prolonged standing, unusual physical exertion, or swelling of hemorrhoidal tissue with loss of muscular support; painless except when accompanied by thrombosis, infection, or ulceration.
Thrombosis	Strangulation of protruded (external) hemorrhoid by anal sphincter, possibly leading to thrombosis; pain is most acute during first 48–72 hours but usually resolves after 7–10 days. Minimal pain with thrombosed internal hemorrhoids; patient likely to be unaware of condition unless sudden change in bowel habits occurs. If a thrombosed hemorrhoid persists, ulcers or gangrene may develop and cause bleeding, especially during defecation.

Key: GI = Gastrointestinal; IBD = inflammatory bowel disease; PUD = peptic ulcer disease.

Source: References 1, 8, 9, and Abramowitz L, Weyandt GH, Havlickova B, et al. The diagnosis and management of haemorrhoidal disease from a global perspective. *Aliment Pharmacol Ther.* 2010 May;31(Suppl 1):1–58. doi: 10.1111/j.1365-2036.2010.04278.x.

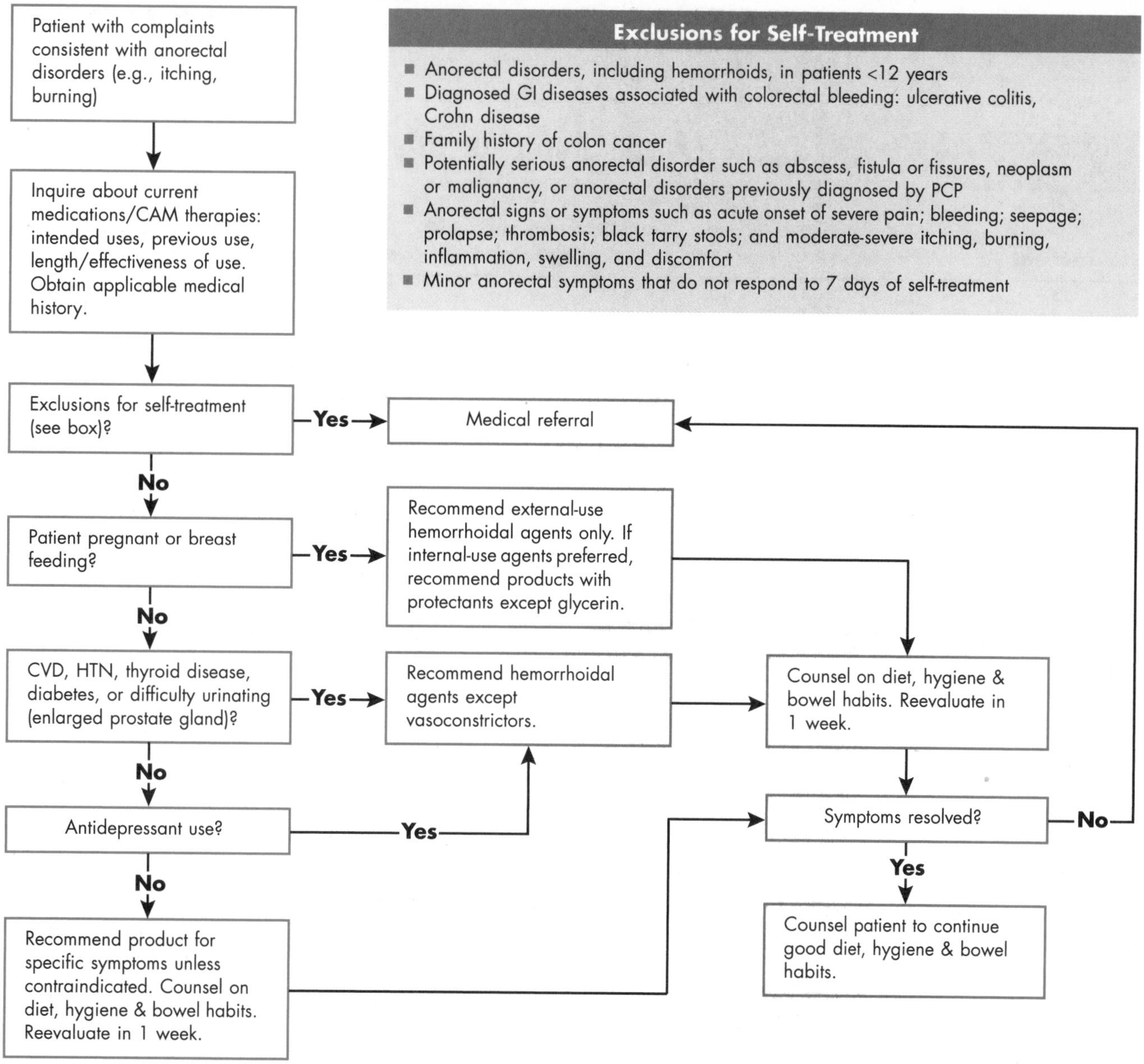
Patient with complaints consistent with anorectal disorders (e.g., itching, burning)
Inquire about current medications/CAM therapies: intended uses, previous use, length/effectiveness of use. Obtain applicable medical history.
Exclusions for Self-Treatment
■ Anorectal disorders, including hemorrhoids, in patients <12 years
■ Diagnosed GI diseases associated with colorectal bleeding: ulcerative colitis, Crohn disease
■ Family history of colon cancer
■ Potentially serious anorectal disorder such as abscess, fistula or fissures, neoplasm or malignancy, or anorectal disorders previously diagnosed by PCP
■ Anorectal signs or symptoms such as acute onset of severe pain; bleeding; seepage; prolapse; thrombosis; black tarry stools; and moderate-severe itching, burning, inflammation, swelling, and discomfort
■ Minor anorectal symptoms that do not respond to 7 days of self-treatment
Exclusions for self-treatment (see box)?
Yes
Medical referral
No
Patient pregnant or breast feeding?
Yes
Recommend external-use hemorrhoidal agents only. If internal-use agents preferred, recommend products with protectants except glycerin.
No
CVD, HTN, thyroid disease, diabetes, or difficulty urinating (enlarged prostate gland)?
Yes
Recommend hemorrhoidal agents except vasoconstrictors.
Counsel on diet, hygiene & bowel habits. Reevaluate in 1 week.
No
Antidepressant use?
Yes
Symptoms resolved?
No
Yes
No
Counsel patient to continue good diet, hygiene & bowel habits.
Recommend product for specific symptoms unless contraindicated. Counsel on diet, hygiene & bowel habits. Reevaluate in 1 week.

FIGURE 17-2 Self-care of hemorrhoids. Key: CAM = Complementary and alternative medicine; CVD = cardiovascular disease; GI = gastrointestinal; HTN = hypertension; PCP = primary care provider.

TABLE 17-3 Guidelines for Applying or Inserting Anorectal Products

- Wash hands before and after application of any anorectal product.
- Empty bladder and bowel before using any anorectal product, if able.
- Clean affected anorectal area after bowel movement with mild, nonmedicated, unscented soap and warm water; rinse thoroughly.
- Clean anorectal area prior to applying products containing aluminum hydroxide gel or kaolin. Be sure to remove any previously used petrolatum-containing or greasy ointment.[a]
- Dry anorectal area gently by patting or blotting with unscented and uncolored toilet tissue or a soft cloth prior to applying product.
- Apply a thin layer to the perianal area and anal canal when using an external anorectal product.
- Insert anorectal products indicated for intrarectal use by using an intrarectal applicator or a finger. Intrarectal applicators are preferred to digital application because an applicator enables the drug product to be applied to the rectal mucosa (which cannot be reached with a finger)
- Clean anorectal applicator per product instructions between uses.
- Ensure that intrarectal applicators have lateral openings and holes in the tip to facilitate anorectal application and coverage of the rectal mucosa.
- Lubricate intrarectal applicator by spreading product around the applicator tip prior to inserting into the anorectal area.
- Avoid using the intrarectal applicator in the anorectal area if it causes additional pain.
- Do not exceed the recommended daily dosage unless directed by a primary care provider.

[a] *Ointment* refers to all semisolid preparations.

Source: References 1, 8, and Gupta PJ. Ano-rectal pathologies encountered under special circumstances. *Acta Chir Iugosl.* 2010;57(3):77–82. PMID: 21066989; and Gupta PJ. Suppositories in anal disorders: a review. *Eur Rev Med Pharmacol Sci.* 2007;11(3):165–70. PMID: 17970232.

TABLE 17-4 **Dosage Guidelines for Anorectal Products**

Ingredient	Concentration per Dosage Unit (%)	Frequency of Use (maximum daily dosage)
Local Anesthetics		
Benzocaine	5–20	Up to 6 times/day (2.4 g)
Benzyl alcohol	1–4	Up to 6 times/day (480 mg)
Dibucaine, dibucaine hydrochloride	0.25–1	Up to 3–4 times/day (80 mg)
Dyclonine hydrochloride	0.5–1	Up to 6 times/day (100 mg)
Lidocaine	2–5	Up to 6 times/day (500 mg)
Pramoxine hydrochloride[a]	1	Up to 5 times/day (100 mg)
Tetracaine, tetracaine hydrochloride	0.5–1	Up to 6 times/day (100 mg)
Vasoconstrictors		
Ephedrine sulfate	0.1–1.25	Up to 4 times/day (100 mg)
Epinephrine hydrochloride/epinephrine	0.005–0.01	Up to 4 times/day (800 mg)
Phenylephrine hydrochloride	0.25	Up to 4 times/day (2 mg)
Protectants		
Aluminum hydroxide gel, cocoa butter, glycerin, hard fat, kaolin, lanolin, mineral oil, white petrolatum, calamine,[c] petrolatum, shark liver oil,[d] zinc oxide,[e] topical starch, white petrolatum, cod liver oil[d]	See footnote b.	Petrolatum/white petrolatum as often as needed; other protectants up to 6 times/day or after each bowel movement
Astringents		
Calamine[c]	5–25	Up to 6 times/day or after each bowel movement
Zinc oxide	5–25	Up to 6 times/day or after each bowel movement
Witch hazel	10–50	Up to 6 times/day or after each bowel movement
Keratolytics		
Alcloxa	0.2–2	Up to 6 times/day
Resorcinol	1–3	Up to 6 times/day
Analgesics, Anesthetics, Antipruritics		
Menthol	0.1–1	Up to 6 times/day
Juniper tar	1–5	Up to 6 times/day
Camphor	0.1–3	Up to 6 times/day
Corticosteroids		
Hydrocortisone	0.25–1	Up to 3–4 times/day

[a] External dosage forms may include aerosol foams, ointments, creams, and jellies (water-miscible base).

[b] Any two, three, or four protectants may be combined, provided that the combined percentage by weight of all protectants in the combination is at least 50% of the final product. Any protectant ingredient included in the combination must be present at a level that contributes at least 12.5% by weight (e.g., 0.25 g of a 2 g dosage unit), except cod liver oil and shark liver oil. If cocoa butter is included in the combination, it must not exceed the concentration limit for calamine,[c] cod liver oil,[d] or shark liver oil.[d]

[c] Calamine not to exceed 25% by weight per dosage unit (based on the zinc oxide content of calamine).

[d] Provided that the product is labeled so that the amount of the product that is used in a 24-hour period represents a quantity that provides 10,000 USP units of vitamin A and 400 USP units of cholecalciferol.

[e] Any product containing calamine or zinc oxide for use as a protectant and/or as an astringent may not have a total weight of zinc oxide exceeding 25% by weight per dosage unit.

Key: USP = United States Pharmacopeia.

Source: Reference 10.

of swelling. These agents are indicated (Table 17–4) for relief of itching, discomfort, and irritation and to shrink and decrease swelling of the hemorrhoidal tissues.[10,13] Ephedrine sulfate and phenylephrine hydrochloride are safe and effective for external and intrarectal use, and epinephrine or epinephrine hydrochloride is approved for external use only.[10]

Adverse effects of ephedrine and epinephrine include increased cardiac rate and contractility, as well as bronchodilation, if absorbed systemically. In contrast, because phenylephrine HCl is structurally related to norepinephrine, effects on the central nervous system and cardiac rhythm are minimal. When used in recommended topical dosages, ephedrine sulfate may cause nervousness, tremors, sleeplessness, nausea, and loss of appetite.[10] Serious adverse effects (e.g., elevation of blood pressure, aggravation of hyperthyroidism, cardiac arrhythmias, irregular heart rate) are less likely to occur with topical than with oral administration.[13] Prolonged use may lead to rebound vasodilatation, anxiety, and (rarely) paranoia. Contact dermatitis may also occur.

Rectally administered vasoconstrictors may attenuate the effects of oral antihypertensive agents and increase blood pressure. Alternatively, the hypertensive effects of vasoconstrictors may be potentiated by monoamine oxidase inhibitors and tricyclic antidepressants. Concomitant use may lead to serious and even lethal outcomes, including cerebral hemorrhage or stroke.[13] Patients with diabetes, thyroid disease, heart disease, hypertension, or difficulty in urination due to an enlarged prostate, as well as those taking antidepressants, antihypertensive agents, or cardiac medications, should not use hemorrhoidal agents with vasoconstrictors without first consulting with their primary care provider.[10,23,24]

Protectants

Protectants are ingredients that provide a physical protective barrier and soften the anal canal by preventing fecal matter from irritating the perianal mucosa.[10] This drug class includes absorbents, adsorbents, demulcents, and emollients. Approved indications for most protectants include the temporary relief of discomfort, irritation, and burning with external and internal hemorrhoids (one exception is glycerin, which is for external use only) (Table 17–4).[10] Protectants are also indicated for providing a protective coating over inflamed anal tissue to prevent tissue drying. Kaolin or aluminum hydroxide gel are indicated for the temporary relief of itching associated with moist anorectal conditions.[10]

Systemic absorption of protectants is minimal; therefore, adverse reactions as a class are uncommon. Lanolin is a natural product obtained from the fleece of sheep, and it may cause allergic reactions.[10] Chemically modified lanolin is available and may be less sensitizing.

A warning statement for aluminum hydroxide gel and kaolin products states that any greasy ointments or petrolatum-based products should be removed prior to applying so that the protectant may adhere properly to the anorectal skin area.[10]

Astringents

Astringents are products that promote coagulation of surface protein in the anorectal skin cells to protect the underlying tissue. Astringents also act to decrease cell volume, making the affected environment drier. To prevent further irritation, astringents form a thin protective layer over the injured mucosal membrane.[10] Astringents listed in Table 17–4 are approved for the temporary relief of itching, irritation, and burning symptoms associated with anorectal disorders.[10] Witch hazel (known as hamamelis water prior to January 1, 1995) is indicated for external use, whereas calamine and zinc oxide may be used for external and internal anorectal disorders.[10]

Adverse effects with the topical use of astringents are uncommon. Upon application, witch hazel may cause a slight stinging sensation from the alcohol used to prepare the compound. Contact dermatitis may occur with witch hazel because it contains a small amount of volatile oil. If calamine or zinc oxide are used for prolonged periods of time (especially for internal anorectal disorders), systemic zinc toxicity (nausea, vomiting, lethargy, and/or severe pain), although rare, may develop.[10]

Keratolytics

Keratolytics are agents that cause desquamation and debridement (or sloughing) of epidermal surface cells. By fostering cell turnover and loosening surface cells, low concentrations of keratolytics may expose the underlying tissue. When other anorectal ingredients are used in combination with keratolytics, they reduce itching and inflammation (Table 17–4).[10] Because mucous membranes do not contain a keratin layer, intrarectal use of keratolytics is not justified and may be harmful.[10,13]

With repeated dosing, the absorption of the keratolytic resorcinol has led to methemoglobinemia, exfoliative dermatitis, death in infants, and myxedema in adults.[13] Other adverse effects range from tinnitus, increased pulse rate, diaphoresis, and shortness of breath to circulatory collapse, unconsciousness, and seizures. Products containing resorcinol must list the following warnings to minimize absorption through abraded mucosal lining and to decrease the potential for systemic toxicity: (1) "Certain persons can develop allergic reactions to ingredients in this product. If the symptoms being treated do not subside, or if redness, irritation, swelling, pain, or other symptoms develop or increase, discontinue use and consult a doctor." (2) "Do not use on open wounds near the anus."[10] Although keratolytics are available in selected anorectal preparations, the potential benefit must be weighed against their potentially serious adverse effects.

Analgesics, Anesthetics, and Antipruritics

Formerly classified as "counterirritants," menthol, juniper tar, and camphor are safe and effective when used for external perianal disorders. These agents (Table 17–4) are approved for the temporary relief of burning, pain, or itching by producing a cool, warm, or tingling sensation.[10] These agents should not be used internally because the rectum has no identifiable nerve fibers. Menthol-containing products must have the following warning: "Certain persons can develop allergic reactions to ingredients in this product. If the symptoms being treated do not subside, or if redness, irritation, swelling, pain, or other symptoms develop or increase, discontinue use and consult a doctor."[10] Extensive application of menthol to the trunk of the body has caused laryngospasm, dyspnea, and cyanosis; therefore, menthol should be used only sparingly.[13] Juniper tar, which contains phenol, should be used sparingly; and it should not be ingested orally because organ failure and cardiac rhythm abnormalities may result.[25] Camphor is readily absorbed through mucous membranes, and it stimulates the central nervous system, which may cause convulsions or death. The latter is seen mostly with accidental oral ingestion, especially in children.[13]

Corticosteroids

Approximately 60% of the topical anorectal agents contains hydrocortisone, which acts as a vasoconstrictor and antipruritic by producing lysosomal membrane stabilization and antimitotic activity.[26]

The onset of action may take up to 12 hours, but the effect has a longer duration than that of most other agents (e.g., local anesthetics). Hydrocortisone, in concentrations of no more than 1%, is the only corticosteroid approved for nonprescription use in anorectal preparations for the temporary relief of minor external anal itching caused by minor irritation or rash.[27] Local adverse effects include rare skin reactions and skin atrophy with prolonged use. Hydrocortisone may mask also the symptoms of bacterial and fungal infections.

Combination Products

Federal regulations state that a nonprescription anorectal product may combine two or more active ingredients; combination products generally are recognized as safe and effective when (1) each active ingredient contributes to the claimed effect; (2) the combination of active ingredients does not decrease the safety or effectiveness of any individual active ingredient; and (3) the combination, when listing adequate directions for use and warning against unsafe use, provides rational, concurrent therapy for a significant proportion of the target population.[10,13] FDA restrictions on combination anorectal products can be found by accessing the *Federal Register*.[10] Use of combination products is reasonable, given that some self-treatable anorectal disorders may have concurrent symptoms. However, a combination of active ingredients has not been shown to be any more effective than a preparation containing a therapeutic amount of a single agent.[10,13] Additionally, restricting the number of ingredients should decrease the risk of interactions and adverse drug reactions.[26]

Product Selection Guidelines

Table 17–5 contains examples of products by category that can be recommended for hemorrhoids.

Knowledge of a patient's medical history, medication profile, and relevant socioeconomic factors is necessary to determine what product to recommend and how an individual may respond to self-treatment. Selection of a product should be based on (1) the type, location, and severity of the anorectal disorder; (2) diseases or significant past medical history; (3) current medications and nutritional supplements and/or herbal products; (4) allergies; (5) ability to apply or insert the medication (considering physical, mental, and emotional limitations); and (6) any other factors that may affect treatment (e.g., diet, daily activities, and the cost of the product).

Special Populations

The most common anorectal disorder in the pregnant population is hemorrhoids.[28,29] Approximately 25% of all pregnant females will complain of hemorrhoids during pregnancy, and this increases to 85% at the time of birth.[28] Pregnant and breastfeeding women should use products recommended for external use; exceptions include protectants (that do not contain glycerin), which may be used internally. Recommending nonpharmacologic interventions, including increasing dietary fiber and fluid intake to minimize constipation, may be of benefit throughout the pregnancy.[28]

Anorectal disorders in children younger than 12 years are not common, and patients should be referred to a specialist for further medical evaluation.[10,29] Because constipation is more common in the older population, these patients may be more prone to hemorrhoids.[29] It is important to note that patients who are older than 40 years and have rectal bleeding or a positive family history of colon cancer should be evaluated for colorectal carcinoma.[29]

TABLE 17–5 Selected Nonprescription Products for Hemorrhoids

Trade Name	Primary Ingredients
Local Anesthetics	
Americaine Ointment[a]	Benzocaine 20%
Nupercainal Hemorrhoidal Ointment	Dibucaine 1%
Tronolane Anesthetic Cream for Hemorrhoids[b]	Pramoxine HCl 1%; zinc oxide 5%
TUCKS Hemorrhoidal Ointment[c]	Pramoxine HCl 1%; zinc oxide 12.5%; mineral oil 46.6%
Vasoconstrictors[d]	
Preparation H Cooling Gel[e]	Witch hazel 50%; phenylephrine HCl 0.25%
Preparation H Suppositories[e]	Phenylephrine HCl 0.25%; cocoa butter 88.4%
Skin Protectants	
Preparation H Ointment[e]	Mineral oil 14%; petrolatum 74.9%; phenylephrine HCl 0.25%
Hydrocortisone Products	
Preparation H Anti-Itch Cream Hydrocortisone 1%[e]	Hydrocortisone 1%
Miscellaneous and Combination Products	
Preparation H Maximum Strength Pain Relief Cream[e]	Glycerin 14.4%; phenylephrine HCl 0.25%; pramoxine HCl 1%; white petrolatum 15%
Preparation H Medicated Wipes[e]	Witch hazel 50%
Preparation H Totables Irritation Relief Wipes[e]	Witch hazel 50%
Preparation H Medicated Wipes for Women[e]	Witch hazel 20%
TUCKS Medicated Cooling Pads[c]	Witch hazel 50%

[a] Source: Prestige Brands website. Available at: http://www.prestigebrands.com/products/skin-care/americaine.html. Accessed May 1, 2017.

[b] Source: Tronolane Anesthetic for Hemorrhoids. Drugs.com. Available at: https://www.drugs.com/mtm/tronolane-anesthetic-for-hemorrhoids.html. Accessed May 1, 2017.

[c] Source: TUCKS website. Available at: http://www.tucksbrand.com. Accessed May 1, 2017.

[d] Source: Preparation H website. Available at: http://www.preparationh.com. Accessed May 1, 2017.

[e] At the time this chapter was written, no U.S. Food and Drug Administration (FDA)-approved nonprescription product contained ephedrine sulfate.

Otherwise, treatment for any special population is similar to treatment of an adult patient.

Patient Factors

FDA does not require comparison trials between combination and individual products; therefore, therapeutic differences are unknown. However, when used to treat anorectal symptoms for the preceding FDA indications, combination products containing approved ingredients in appropriate dosages are most likely therapeutically similar to individual drug products.[10,13] Any perceived differences most likely are related to personal preference for a specific product or dosage form. Using more than one product, or a product containing multiple ingredients, is reasonable because patients may have multiple symptoms that may not be completely treated by one product alone.[10,13]

Medications used to treat anorectal disorders are available in many dosage forms. Creams, suppositories, gels, pastes, liquids, foams, and ointments are primarily used externally. However, the term *ointment* used in this chapter refers to all semisolid preparations designed for intrarectal or external use in the anorectal area for its protectant and emollient properties. Additionally, ointments may be used to provide a vehicle for the safe and efficient delivery of the active ingredients.

Applicators, intrarectal applicators, or the patient's fingers are used to facilitate applying and instilling the anorectal preparations. Although considerable pharmaceutical differences exist among these dosage forms, there do not appear to be clinical differences.[13]

Suppositories are solid dosage forms that deliver drugs into body orifices, typically in the anorectal area.[30] Suppositories should not be recommended as an initial dosage form because they may leave the affected anal region and ascend into the rectum and lower colon when the patient is in an upright position.[13,30] If the patient remains in an upright position after inserting a suppository or ointment, the active ingredients may not distribute evenly over the anal mucosa. Therefore, when inserting the suppository, patients should lie on their left sides with knees bent so that the drug remains in the affected area for at least 15–20 minutes.[18] Suppositories have a relatively slower onset of action than other formulations because the solid dosage form must dissolve to release the active ingredients (see Chapter 15). To prolong retention rates in the anorectal area, some health care providers recommend introducing the base of the suppository first, rather than the tapered end.[30] Also, a suppository that is too soft to administer can be hardened in the refrigerator for at least 30 minutes before use.[30]

Foam products theoretically should provide more rapid release of active ingredients compared with ointments.[13] However, foams are more expensive than ointments and do not offer any advantage. Also, foams may not remain in the affected area, and differences in the size of the foam bubbles may result in different concentrations of the active ingredient.[13]

Complementary Therapies

Dietary supplements used to manage hemorrhoids have been researched poorly, although several have evidence to support their use.[31,32] The combination of diosmin and hesperidin (a micronized purified flavonoid fraction) has been used to stop acute bleeding and decrease symptoms associated with hemorrhoids.[32,33] The mechanism of action is still in question, but animal models suggest this product inhibits prostaglandin and thromboxane mediators, thereby decreasing the inflammation. The combination appears safe when both are taken orally for less than 6 months, with the most common adverse effects being abdominal pain, diarrhea, and gastritis.[32,34,35] Purified diosmin without hesperidin administered orally or topically has been shown to provide benefits in reducing pain, bleeding, and swelling with hemorrhoids.[34] Butcher's broom combined with other dietary supplements (e.g., flavonoids) may also be effective in reducing pain.[34,35] Catechins and epicatechins when used in combination have vasodilation and anti-inflammatory properties, which had been found to be effective in reducing pain, bleeding, and anal itching symptoms associated with hemorrhoids.[32] Horse chestnut seed extract (HCSE) has been used to support the management of hemorrhoids.[35,36] When HCSE is processed properly, it is relatively safe, with adverse effects including itching, nausea, and vomiting. Improperly prepared HCSE preparations may be poisonous and may lead to death.[36] Passionflower has also been used as a topical rinse for the symptoms of hemorrhoids.[37] When used short term and in doses used in foods, it is safe with minimal adverse effects.[37] Pregnant women should avoid taking passionflower by mouth as it may induce uterine contractions.[37]

Assessment of Anorectal Disorders: A Case-Based Approach

To accurately assess whether the anorectal disorder is self-treatable, the health care provider should obtain a thorough description of the patient's signs and symptoms. For self-treatable disorders, the provider should ask questions about the presence of specific diseases (e.g., hypertension, diabetes, benign prostatic hyperplasia, and psychiatric illness); prescription and nonprescription medications; complementary and alternative medicines; and diet, lifestyle, and exercise before recommending self-treatment.

Cases 17–1 and 17–2 illustrate assessment of patients with anorectal disorders.

Patient Counseling for Anorectal Disorders

The most appropriate drug and nondrug measures for treating patient-specific anorectal signs and symptoms should be explained to each patient. Counseling should include dosage and frequency of administration, administration technique, onset of action, possible adverse effects, precautions or warnings, and product storage. Patients should understand when self-care should be discontinued and when to consult a primary care provider. If the topical nonprescription agents do not resolve the anorectal symptoms within 7 days, medical referral is appropriate.[10] Patients should be advised not to exceed the recommended daily dosage unless their primary care provider recommends a higher dosage.[10] The box "Patient Education for Anorectal Disorders" lists specific information to provide patients.

Evaluation of Patient Outcomes for Anorectal Disorders

Self-treatment of anorectal disorders should be limited to minor symptoms. If serious or severe symptoms are present, or if symptoms become progressively worse, advise the patient to contact

CASE 17-1

Relevant Evaluation Criteria	Scenario/Model Outcome
Collect	
1. Gather essential information about the patient's symptoms and medical history, including	
a. Description of symptom(s) (i.e., nature, onset, duration, severity, associated symptoms)	The patient complains of pain and burning after having a bowel movement, which started after giving birth 1 month ago. She also states it is itchy in the anal canal, which sometimes keeps her up at night. Bright red blood is seen on the toilet paper and not in the stool.
b. Description of any factors that seem to precipitate, exacerbate, and/or relieve the patient's symptom(s)	Defecation causes discomfort. Bowel movement causes anal pain. Stool is soft, but she can feel pain during a bowel movement. Drinking water seems to help her symptoms.
c. Description of the patient's efforts to relieve the symptoms	When able to, scratching the anal area seems to relieve symptoms. She notices that her symptoms are less problematic on days she wears dresses.
d. Patient's identity	Monica Price
e. Patient's age, gender, height, and weight	28 years old, female, 5 ft 2 in., 136 lb
f. Patient's occupation	Administrative assistant for accountant
g. Patient's dietary habits	Eats meat, vegetables, fruits, sweets. Lately has a craving for salt and vinegar chips. Fluid intake has been decreased.
h. Patient's sleep habits	3–5 hours nightly
i. Concurrent medical conditions, prescription and nonprescription medications, and dietary supplements	Gave birth 1 month ago; MVI daily, iron daily; docusate sodium twice daily, calcium with vitamin D twice daily
j. Allergies	Penicillin
k. History of other adverse reactions to medications	None
l. Other (describe) _______	Patient had walked 45 minutes every day on a treadmill during pregnancy. Since giving birth, she has not been active.
Assess	
2. Differentiate patient's signs/symptoms, and correctly identify the patient's primary problem(s) (Tables 17–1 and 17–2).	Patient gave birth 1 month ago to a 9.3-lb baby boy, which may have caused the patient's anorectal symptoms including hemorrhoids and pruritus ani.
3. Identify exclusions for self-treatment (Figure 17–2).	None
4. Formulate a comprehensive list of therapeutic alternatives for the primary problem to determine whether triage to a health care provider is required, and share this information with the patient or caregiver.	Options include (1) Recommend self-care with an appropriate OTC anorectal product, and advise on nondrug measures. (2) Recommend self-care with an appropriate OTC anorectal product, and advise on nondrug measures until patient contacts her PCP. (3) Refer patient to her PCP for medical evaluation of her symptoms. (4) Take no action.
Plan	
5. Select an optimal therapeutic alternative to address the patient's problem, taking into account patient preferences.	The second option is the best: self-care and nondrug measures until the patient can contact her PCP. Recommend an external hemorrhoidal agent only. If internal-use agents preferred, recommend products with protectants (except glycerin). Recommend patient increase fluid intake (water), dietary fiber (fruits, vegetables), and, if possible, exercise. Sitz baths used 3 times a day may resolve anorectal symptoms. Encourage patient to wear soft, loose-fitting clothing. Also educate patient to use unscented white toilet paper and wipe anal area delicately.

CASE 17–1 *continued*

Relevant Evaluation Criteria	Scenario/Model Outcome
6. Describe the recommended therapeutic approach to the patient or caregiver.	"Your symptoms, including blood on the toilet paper, may be related to hemorrhoids and anal itching. The hemorrhoids may have developed when you recently gave birth, which puts lots of pressure on the anal area. These changes in your body cause you to have a lot of pressure, especially when you are having a bowel movement, which may produce hemorrhoids. I'm recommending you use a self-care product now; however, you should contact your primary care provider for further evaluation in a few days, if your symptoms do not improve."
7. Explain to the patient or caregiver the rationale for selecting the recommended therapeutic approach from the considered therapeutic alternatives.	"If symptoms do not resolve in a week, seek medical attention. Although your symptoms, including having bowel movement discomfort and anal itching, may be related to hemorrhoids, you should contact your primary care provider for further evaluation. Other conditions also may cause similar symptoms."
Implement	
8. When recommending self-care with nonprescription medications and/or nondrug therapy, convey accurate information to the patient or caregiver.	
a. Appropriate dose and frequency of administration	See Table 17–4.
b. Maximum number of days the therapy should be employed	"Contact your primary care provider if after 7 days the symptoms do not resolve. Be sure to let your primary care provider know what self-care measures you have taken."
c. Product administration procedures	See Table 17–3.
d. Expected time to onset of relief	"The irritation, burning, and discomfort may be relieved within a few days of applying the topical agent as directed." Advise the patient to avoid straining and to drink adequate fluids and eat a healthy diet that is high in dietary fibers. "If required, keep using the stool softener, or add a fiber supplement, as needed. Although the bleeding may stop with treatment, still contact your primary care provider."
e. Degree of relief that can be reasonably expected	"Complete relief of your anorectal symptoms is possible as your body heals from the birthing process."
f. Most common adverse effects	"Most products applied to the anal area are usually well tolerated."
g. Adverse effects that warrant medical intervention should they occur	"If you develop an allergic reaction to the product (redness, swelling, increased irritation, or pain), discontinue use, and contact your primary care provider as soon as possible."
h. Patient options in the event that condition worsens or persists	"If your symptoms worsen, contact your primary care provider as soon as possible."
i. Product storage requirements	"Store medication out of the reach of children and at a controlled room temperature."
j. Specific nondrug measures	"Practice good anal hygiene, use sitz baths, and consider increasing fluid intake. Incorporate an exercise regimen if possible."
Solicit follow-up questions from the patient or caregiver.	"Will this affect my baby if I breastfeed?"
Answer the patient's or caregiver's questions.	"Probably not. If you practice good anal hygiene, use sitz baths, and increase fluid intake and exercise, your breast milk will not be affected. If you decide to use an anorectal product, the amount of product used is minimal so it should not affect the breast milk."
Follow-up: Monitor and Evaluate	
9. Assess patient outcome.	Ask the patient to call to update you on her response to your recommendations. Alternatively, you could call her in a week to evaluate her response and make sure that she touched base with her PCP.

Key: MVI = Multivitamin; OTC = over-the-counter; PCP = primary care provider.

CASE 17-2

Relevant Evaluation Criteria	Scenario/Model Outcome
Collect	
1. Gather essential information about the patient's symptoms and medical history, including	
a. Description of symptom(s) (i.e., nature, onset, duration, severity, associated symptoms)	Patient complains of bleeding in the anal area for the past 5 days. Patient experiences burning, pain, and blood on the toilet paper with each wiping. He has a low-grade temperature (99.9°F [37.2°C], oral). He has had these symptoms before but says there is more pain and blood this time than he had experienced in the past.
b. Description of any factors that seem to precipitate, exacerbate, and/or relieve the patient's symptom(s)	Symptoms are worst when he has his bowel movements. He states that the pain, on a scale of 1–10 (10 being worst), it feels like a 9. He has not changed his soaps or detergents, and he has not changed his diet or exercise.
c. Description of the patient's efforts to relieve the symptoms	The patient has tried topical hydrocortisone cream in the anorectal area without relief for the past 2 days.
d. Patient's identity	Jim Bran
e. Patient's age, gender, height, and weight	34 years old, male, 5 ft 7 in., 156 lb
f. Patient's occupation	Manager at a retail store
g. Patient's dietary habits	Eats healthy meals, including meat, fruits, and vegetables. Eats sweets only on weekends with dinner. Does not drink or smoke.
h. Patient's sleep habits	7–8 hours nightly
i. Concurrent medical conditions, prescription and nonprescription medications, and dietary supplements	Acne diagnosed at age 21; takes MVI daily.
j. Allergies	Penicillin (anaphylactic reaction)
k. History of other adverse reactions to medications	None
l. Other (describe) ______	His father died 25 years ago secondary to colon cancer at the age of 45. His mom is alive and diagnosed with HTN. He has a brother. He is single and has a girlfriend of 8 years.
Assess	
2. Differentiate patient's signs/symptoms, and correctly identify the patient's primary problem(s) (Tables 17–1 and 17–2).	Patient experiences burning, extreme pain, and blood on the toilet paper with each wiping. His underwear is soiled with blood. He states that his diet, fluid, and exercise regimens have not changed. Given that Jim is in his 30s and has a family history of colon cancer, it is possible that he has an oncologic condition.
3. Identify exclusions for self-treatment (Figure 17–2).	Bleeding in the anal area, experiencing pain with each bowel movement. Strong family history of colon cancer.
4. Formulate a comprehensive list of therapeutic alternatives for the primary problem to determine whether triage to a health care provider is required, and share this information with the patient or caregiver.	Options include (1) Recommend self-care with an appropriate OTC anorectal product, and advise on nondrug measures. (2) Recommend self-care with an appropriate OTC anorectal product, and advise on nondrug measures until patient contacts his PCP. (3) Refer patient to his PCP for medical evaluation of his symptoms immediately. (4) Take no action.
Plan	
5. Select an optimal therapeutic alternative to address the patient's problem, taking into account patient preferences.	Patient should consult a health care provider immediately for medical evaluation to rule out bleeding from a source other than a hemorrhoid or anal fissures. He is young and has significant pain with each bowel movement. Patient may have colon cancer, because there is a strong family history of cancer (Figure 17–2).
6. Describe the recommended therapeutic approach to the patient or caregiver.	"You should consult a health care provider for immediate medical evaluation. I'm concerned about your symptoms and your family history."

CASE 17-2 continued

Relevant Evaluation Criteria	Scenario/Model Outcome
7. Explain to the patient or caregiver the rationale for selecting the recommended therapeutic approach from the considered therapeutic alternatives.	"Because you tried using the hydrocortisone cream for 2 days with no relief, the best option is for you to see your primary care provider immediately. You have a strong family history of colon cancer. The signs and symptoms you are complaining about may be symptoms of colon cancer. Please see your primary care provider to have your symptoms evaluated and testing done as soon as possible."
Implement	
8. When recommending self-care with nonprescription medications and/or nondrug therapy, convey accurate information to the patient or caregiver.	Criterion does not apply in this case.
Solicit follow-up questions from the patient or caregiver.	"If I have colon cancer, can it be transmitted to my girlfriend given that we are sexually active?"
Answer the patient's or caregiver's questions.	"No, colon cancer is not transmitted via blood or via sexual contact. She may have other colon cancer risk factors (e.g., a low-fiber diet), but she cannot contract it from you."
Follow-up: Monitor and Evaluate	
9. Assess patient outcome.	Contact the patient in a day or two to ensure that he made an appointment and sought immediate and appropriate medical care.

Key: HTN = Hypertension; MVI = multivitamin; PCP = primary care provider.

PATIENT EDUCATION FOR Anorectal Disorders

The objectives of self-treatment are (1) to relieve specific signs and symptoms and (2) to prevent complications leading to serious problems. The primary goal of treatment is to prevent straining during defecation. For most patients, carefully following product instructions and the self-care measures listed here will help ensure relief of symptoms.

Nondrug Measures

- Maintain hydration and a healthy diet. If experiencing hard stools, straining, or constipation, increase the amount of fiber and fluids in the diet to reduce or prevent straining during bowel movements (see Chapter 15).
- Avoid medications that cause constipation, if possible (see Chapter 15).
- Clean anorectal area after each bowel movement with a moistened, unscented, white toilet tissue or wipe.
- Use a sitz bath, or soak in a bathtub 2–4 times a day, which may help mild anal itching, burning, irritation, and discomfort. Avoid the use of soaps, salts, and oils.

Nonprescription Medications

- Select products containing only the ingredients needed to relieve specific anorectal symptoms.
- See Table 17–3 for guidelines for applying anorectal products.
- See Table 17–4 for recommended dosages of these products.
- Use only selected vasoconstrictors (ephedrine and phenylephrine), protectants (not glycerin), and astringents (calamine and zinc oxide) intrarectally.
- *(If the patient is pregnant)* Use only products approved for external use. If internal use is required, protectants, with the exception of glycerin, may be used.
- *(If the patient has a history of cardiovascular disease, diabetes, hyperthyroidism, hypertension, depression, or difficulty urinating because of prostate problems)* Avoid topical products that contain vasoconstrictors.
- *(If the patient is taking medications for hypertension or depression)* Avoid using any anorectal product containing vasoconstrictors without first consulting your primary care provider.
- Monitor for nervousness, tremor, sleeplessness, nausea, and possible loss of appetite when using an anorectal product containing ephedrine sulfate or phenylephrine.
- Explain that a reduction or relief of symptoms should occur within a few days of self-treatment.
- Review the patient's preferences, especially when the patient may choose from an ointment, cream, or suppository, and when generic products are available.

When to Seek Medical Attention

- Stop using the anorectal product and contact a primary care provider as soon as possible if insertion of a product into the anorectal area causes pain.
- Contact a primary care provider if symptoms worsen, if new symptoms (e.g., bleeding) develop, or if symptoms do not improve after 7 days of self-treatment.
- Discontinue using product and contact a primary care provider at the first occurrence of adverse effects (e.g., a rash; increased itching, redness, burning, or swelling in the anorectal area).
- Discontinue product and contact a primary care provider immediately if allergic or hypersensitivity reactions to the anorectal product develop.

his or her primary care provider. In addition, if alarm signs or symptoms are present, including blood in the stool or severe anal pain, or if symptoms persist beyond 7 days of self-treatment, the patient should be counseled to seek immediate medical attention.[10] If symptoms resolve, the patient should be encouraged to maintain a well-balanced diet, good personal hygiene, and good bowel habits.[13,18]

Key Points for Anorectal Disorders

- Educate patients on limiting self-treatment to minor symptoms such as burning, itching, discomfort, swelling, and irritation.
- Refer patients to their primary care provider when symptoms include anorectal seepage, bleeding, thrombosis, severe pain, fevers, or a change in bowel patterns.
- Advise patients to seek medical attention if their symptoms worsen or do not improve after 7 days of self-treating anorectal symptoms.
- Advise pregnant and breastfeeding women to use only products for external use (except for protectants that do not contain glycerin, which can be used internally).
- Refer parents and caregivers of children younger than 12 years to seek a primary care provider for medical attention.
- Advise patients to select an anorectal product containing the fewest number of ingredients necessary to treat specific symptoms to minimize undesirable effects.
- Instruct patients on the proper use or application of specific anorectal products (Table 17–3).
- Counsel patients on nondrug measures (e.g., dietary measures, perianal hygiene) (see the box "Patient Education for Anorectal Disorders").
- Avoid vasoconstrictors in patients who have conditions such as diabetes, hypertension, cardiac disease, thyroid disease, and enlarged prostate, or who are using antidepressants to avoid the possibility of systemic adverse effects.
- Educate patients on the advantages and disadvantages of various anorectal dosage forms so the best product can be selected for the anorectal symptoms.

REFERENCES

1. Henderson PK, Cash BD. Common anorectal conditions: evaluation and treatment. *Curr Gastroenterol Rep.* 2014 Oct;16(10):408. doi: 10.1007/s11894-014-0408-y.
2. Foxx-Orenstein AE, Umar SB, Crowell MD. Common anorectal disorders. *Gastroenterol Hepatol (N Y).* 2014 May;10(5):294–301. PMCID: PMC4076876
3. National Institute of Diabetes and Digestive and Kidney Diseases (NIDDK). Hemorrhoids. Updated November 2013. Available at: http://www.niddk.nih.gov/health-information/health-topics/digestive-diseases/hemorrhoids/Pages/facts.aspx. Accessed May 1, 2017.
4. Ganz RA. The evaluation and treatment of hemorrhoids: a guide for the gastroenterologist. *Clin Gastroenterol Hepatol.* 2013 Jun;11(6):593–603. doi: 10.1016/j.cgh.2012.12.020.
5. National Institute of Diabetes and Digestive and Kidney Diseases (NIDDK). Digestive diseases statistics for the United States. Updated November 2014. Available at: http://www.niddk.nih.gov/health-information/health-statistics/Pages/digestive-diseases-statistics-for-the-united-states.aspx#8. Accessed May 1, 2017.
6. Barleben A, Mills S. Anorectal anatomy and physiology. *Surg Clin North Am.* 2010;90(1):1–15. doi: 10.1016/j.suc.2009.09.001.
7. Lohsiriwat V. Approach to hemorrhoids. *Curr Gastroenterol Rep.* 2013 Jul;15(7):332. doi: 10.1007/s11894-013-0332-6.
8. Rakinic J, Poola VP. Hemorrhoids and fistulas: new solutions to old problems. *Curr Probl Surg.* 2014 Mar;51(3):98–137. doi: 10.1067/j.cpsurg.2013.11.002.
9. Summers A. Anorectal examination in emergency departments. *Emerg Nurse.* 2013 Apr;21(1):21–6. PMID: 23691894.
10. U.S. Food and Drug Administration. Anorectal drug products for over-the-counter human use. Updated February 16, 2017. *Fed Regist.* Available at: http://www.ecfr.gov/cgi-bin/text-idx?SID=b4ed83742753addbdf5e80a0f25a3f8f&mc=true&node=pt21.5.346&rgn=div5. Accessed May 1, 2017.
11. Summers A. Assessment and treatment of three common anorectal conditions. *Emerg Nurse.* 2013 May;21(2):28–33. PMID: 23802310.
12. Beaty JS, Shashidharan M. Anal fissure. *Clin Colon Rectal Surg.* 2016 Mar;29(1):30–7. doi: 10.1055/s-0035-1570390.
13. U.S. Food and Drug Administration. Anorectal drug products for over-the-counter human use: establishment of a monograph. *Fed Regist.* 1980;45:35576–7.
14. Altomare DF, Giannini I. Pharmacological treatment of hemorrhoids: a narrative review. *Expert Opin Pharmacother.* 2013 Dec;14(17):2343–9. doi: 10.1517/14656566.2013.836181.
15. Ansari P. Pruritus ani. *Clin Colon Rectal Surg.* 2016 Mar;29(1):38–42. doi: 10.1055/s-0035-1570391.
16. Tejirian T, Abbas MA. Sitz bath: where is the evidence? Scientific basis of a common practice. *Dis Colon Rectum.* 2005;48(12):2336–40. doi: 10.1007/s10350-005-0085-x.
17. Lang DS, Tho PC, Ang EN. Effectiveness of the sitz bath in managing adult patients with anorectal disorders. *Jpn J Nurs Sci.* 2011;8(2):115–28. doi: 10.1111/j.1742-7924.2011.00175.x.
18. Gupta PJ. Supportive therapies in ano-rectal diseases—are they really useful? *Acta Chir Iugosl.* 2010;57(3):83–7. PMID: 21066990.
19. Lodi A, Ambonati M, Coassini A, et al. Contact allergy to 'caines' by anti-hemorrhoidal ointments. *Contact Dermatitis.* 1999;41(4):221–2. PMID: 10515104.
20. Ramirez P, Sendagorta E, Floristan U, et al. Allergic contact dermatitis from antihemorrhoidal ointments: concomitant sensitization to both amide and ester local anesthetics. *Dermatitis.* 2010;21(3):176–7. PMID: 20487666.
21. Jovanović M, Karadaglić D, Brkić S. Contact urticaria and allergic contact dermatitis to lidocaine in a patient sensitive to benzocaine and propolis. *Contact Dermatitis.* 2006;54(2):124–6. PMID: 16487290.
22. U.S. Food and Drug Administration. Requirements for child-resistant packaging: requirements for products containing lidocaine or dibucaine. *Fed Regist.* 1995;60:17992–8005. Available at: https://www.gpo.gov/fdsys/pkg/FR-1995-04-10/html/95-8628.htm. Accessed May 1, 2017.
23. Pray WS, Pray GE. Nonprescription products and heart warnings. *US Pharm.* 2011;36(2):12–5.
24. Pray WS. Nonprescription products to avoid with hypertension. *US Pharm.* 2010;35(2):12–5.
25. Koruk ST, Ozyilkan E, Kaya P, et al. Juniper tar poisoning. *Clin Toxicol (Phila).* 2005;43(1):47–9. PMID: 15732446.
26. Havlickova B. Topical corticosteroid therapy in proctology indications. *Aliment Pharmacol Ther.* 2010;31(Suppl 1):19–32. doi:10.1111/j.1365-2036.2010.04278.x.
27. U.S. Food and Drug Administration. External analgesic drug products for over-the-counter human use; amendment of tentative final monograph. *Fed Regist.* 1990;55(39):6932–51. Available at: http://www.fda.gov/downloads/Drugs/DevelopmentApprovalProcess/DevelopmentResources/Over-the-CounterOTCDrugs/StatusofOTCRulemakings/UCM077992.pdf. Accessed May 1, 2017.
28. Zielinski R, Searing K, Deibel M. Gastrointestinal distress in pregnancy: prevalence, assessment, and treatment of 5 common minor discomforts. *J Perinat Neonatal Nurs.* 2015 Jan-Mar;29(1):23–31. doi: 10.1097/JPN.0000000000000078.
29. Gupta PJ. Ano-rectal pathologies encountered under special circumstances. *Acta Chir Iugosl.* 2010;57(3):77–82. PMID: 21066989.
30. Gupta PJ. Suppositories in anal disorders: a review. *Eur Rev Med Pharmacol Sci.* 2007;11(3):165–70. PMID: 17970232.
31. Chauhan R, Ruby K, Dwivedi J. Golden herbs used in piles treatment: a concise report. *Int J Drug Dev Res.* 2012;4(4):50–68. Available at

http://www.ijddr.in/drug-development/6-golden-herbs-used-in-piles-treatment-a-concise-report.php?aid=5095. Accessed May 1, 2017.

32. Aggrawal K, Satija N, Dasgupta G, et al. Efficacy of a standardized herbal preparation (Roidosanal) in the treatment of hemorrhoids: a randomized, controlled, open-label multicentre study. *J Ayurveda Integr Med.* 2014 Apr;5(2):117–24. doi: 10.4103/0975-9476.131732.
33. Misra MC, Parshad R. Randomized clinical trial of micronized flavonoids in the early control of bleeding from acute internal haemorrhoids. *Br J Surg.* 2000;87(7):868–72. PMID: 10931020.
34. Misra MC, Imlitemsu. Drug treatment of haemorrhoids. *Drugs.* 2005; 65(11):1481–91. PMID: 16134260.
35. Gami B. Hemorrhoids—a common ailment among adults, causes & treatment: a review. *Int J Pharm Sci.* 2011;3(Suppl 5):5–12. Available at: http://www.ijppsjournal.com/Vol3Suppl5/2136.pdf. Accessed May 1, 2017.
36. National Center for Complementary and Integrative Health. Horse chestnut. NCCIH Publication No. D321. September 2016. Updated November 30, 2016. Available at: http://nccam.nih.gov/health/horsechestnut. Accessed May 1, 2017.
37. National Center for Complementary and Integrative Health. Passionflower. NCCIH Publication No. D487. September 2016. Updated December 1, 2016. Available at: https://nccih.nih.gov/health/passionflower. Accessed May 1, 2017.
38. Natural Medicines Comprehensive Database. Passionflower. Updated March 3, 2014. Available at: http://naturaldatabase.therapeuticresearch.com/nd/PrintVersion.aspx?id=871. Accessed May 1, 2017.

CHAPTER 18

PINWORM INFECTION

JEFFERY A. GOAD AND EDITH MIRZAIAN

Enterobius vermicularis, commonly referred to as pinworm, seatworm, threadworm, or oxyuriasis, is an intestinal nematode and the primary agent that causes human enterobiasis. This chapter will focus on the detection and management of pinworm infection, because it is the most common worm infestation in the United States. It is also the only helminthic infection for which a nonprescription medication treatment has been approved. This infection is most common in temperate regions of the world; in the United States, pinworms are found with a high prevalence in child care settings and urban areas.[1,2] Although pinworms are a nuisance, the pinworm infection presents little risk to the infected individual or the public.

Pinworm infection may be the most common helminth infection in the United States, with the greatest infection rate in children ages 5–14 years.[3] Enterobiasis is associated with all socioeconomic levels and, in contrast to other helminthic infections, does not affect any particular race or culture. Nearly 50% of all *E. vermicularis* cases occur among individuals who are institutionalized (e.g., in child care facilities or hospitals) and among family members.[3–5]

Pathophysiology of Pinworm Infection

Humans are the only hosts of *E. vermicularis.* Unlike most other worm infections, pinworms do not live in the soil or water and are not transmitted through animal feces. However, animal fur of household dogs and cats may be a carrier of infective eggs.[4] The most common pinworm transmission route is through ingestion of infective eggs by direct anus-to-mouth transfer by fingers or fomites. Reinfection may occur readily, because eggs often are found under fingernails of infected children who have scratched the anal area. Finger sucking may be considered a source of infection, particularly in children with recurring symptoms.[4] Nail biting and nose picking have not been associated with the initial infection; however, they certainly can contribute to reinfection.[6] Embryonated eggs can also be transferred from the perianal region to clothes, bedding, or bathroom fixtures; because of their small size, pinworm eggs sometimes can become airborne in dust and reach the intestinal tract through the nose during breathing.[1,5] Eggs can remain viable outside the intestinal tract and can spread within a microcommunity (e.g., household, school) for 20 days (especially under humid conditions).[7]

After infective eggs are ingested, they may hatch and release larvae in the small intestine. The time lapse between ingestion of the eggs to oviposition (i.e., deposition of eggs) by adult females is approximately 1–2 months.[1] After this period, the adult pinworm emerges as a small, white, thread-like worm with a pin-shaped, pointed tail from which the name is derived (see Color Plates, photograph 6A); its lifespan is approximately 2 months.[3,7] Adult male and female worms inhabit the first portion of the large intestine, or ileocecum, and seldom cause damage to the intestinal wall. The mature female, approximately 8–13 mm in length, usually stores approximately 11,000 eggs in her body (see Color Plates, photograph 6B). After her nocturnal migration down the colon and out the anus, she deposits her sticky eggs in the perianal region and dies shortly afterward. Males are smaller (2.5 mm), live approximately 2 weeks, and do not migrate. If the eggs are not washed off, they hatch within a few hours, and larvae may return to the large intestine through the anus (*retroinfection*). Within 2–6 weeks of egg ingestion, larvae are released and mature into gravid females, thus continuing the cycle indefinitely unless appropriate behavioral and pharmacotherapeutic interventions are instituted.

Rarely, extraintestinal infestations, typically involving the genitourinary tract, may occur, because the pinworms have mistakenly crawled into the urogenital tract.[1] Genitourinary pinworm infections are harder to treat because of the low systemic absorption of antiparasitic agents.[7]

Clinical Presentation of Pinworm Infection

Patients with minor pinworm infections often are asymptomatic. Nocturnal pruritus (perianal or perineal itch) is the most common symptom of enterobiasis.[1] Perianal itching occurs predominantly at night and is caused by an inflammatory reaction to the presence of adult worms and eggs on the perianal skin.[2] Major infestations may produce symptoms ranging from abdominal pain, insomnia, and restlessness, to anorexia, diarrhea, and intractable localized itching.[4,6] Patients with severe symptoms of major infestations and extraintestinal disease should be referred to a primary care provider (PCP) for further evaluation. Before recommending treatment or referral, the pharmacist should ask appropriate assessment questions to rule out diaper dermatitis in children, as well as constipation and hemorrhoids in older patients, because these conditions can also cause inflammation in the rectal region, leading to itching and discomfort.

In addition to physical signs and symptoms, psychological trauma (i.e., pinworm neurosis) to patients and parents can also occur when worms are found near a child's anus. Patients and parents need to be assured that pinworms are common and curable, and that no social stigma is attached to their occurrence.[6]

Scratching to relieve itching from pinworm infection may lead to secondary bacterial infection of the perianal and perineal regions.[7] Helminthic infections in the genital tract may lead to endometritis, salpingitis, tubo-ovarian abscess, pelvic inflammatory disease, vulvovaginitis, and possibly infertility.[7–9] Pinworms may also migrate into the peritoneal cavity and form granulomas. Rarely, they may cause appendicitis in children.[10]

Treatment of Pinworm Infection

Treatment Goals

The goals of self-treatment are (1) to relieve symptoms of pinworm infection and (2) to eradicate pinworms from the patient and the household, thereby preventing reinfection.

General Treatment Approach

The management of pinworm infection and prevention of reinfection includes drug treatment with pyrantel pamoate for the patient and for every household member. Strict hygiene (e.g., washing linens, disinfecting toilet seats) is an integral part of the treatment. Figure 18–1 outlines self-care for this infection and lists exclusions for self-treatment.

Nonpharmacologic Therapy

Once pinworm infection is suspected, the patient or caregiver should follow the nondrug measures in Table 18–1 to minimize family and household infections and reinfections. Children can usually return to school after the first dose of an appropriate antihelminthic agent and after their fingernails are cut and cleaned. Health care providers are in an ideal position to inform patients of behaviors that may increase their risk of helminthic infections.

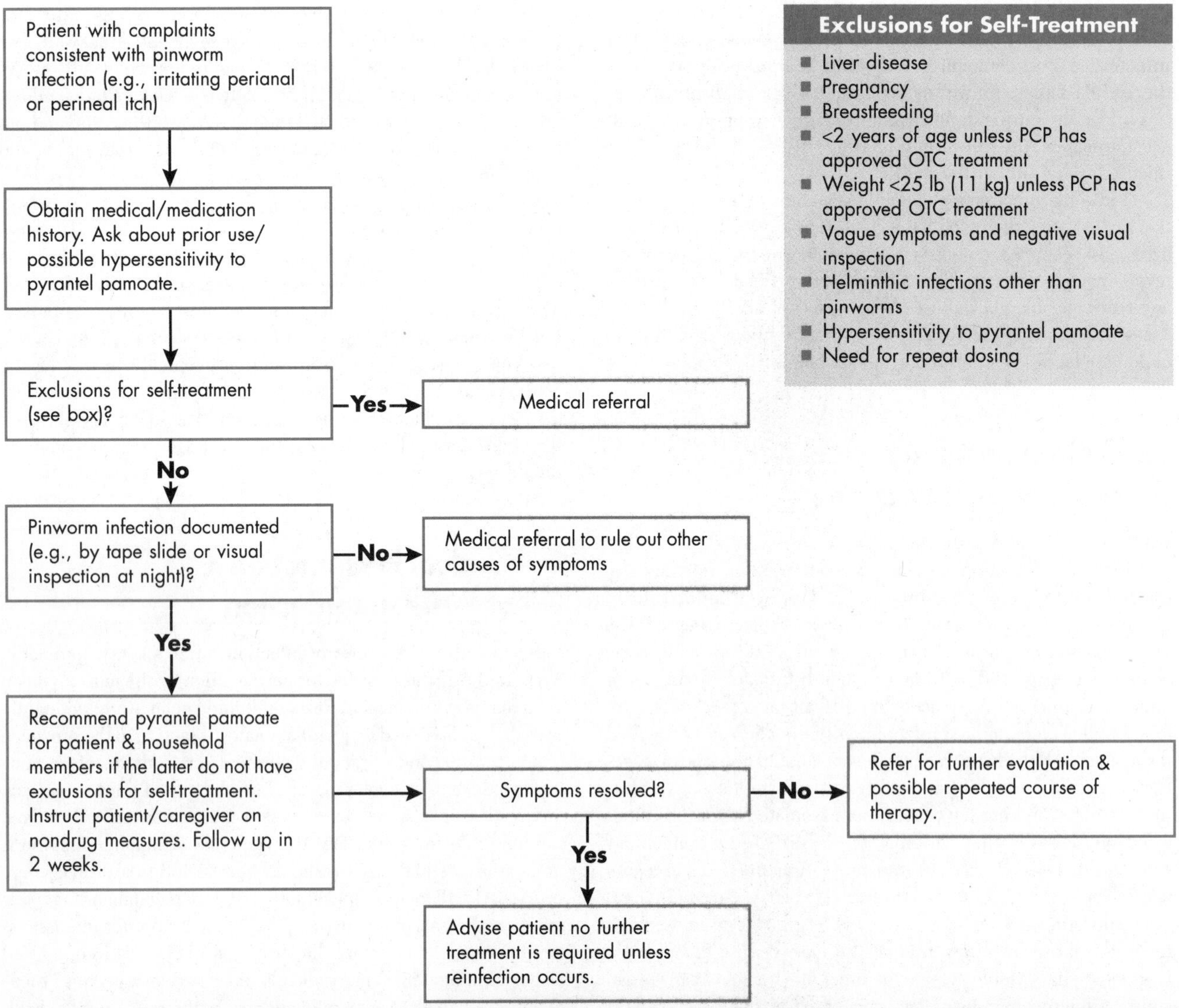

FIGURE 18–1 Self-care for pinworm infection. Key: OTC = Over-the-counter; PCP = primary care provider.

TABLE 18-1 Nondrug and Preventive Measures for Pinworm Infection

- Educate the public in personal hygiene, particularly the need to wash hands before eating or preparing food and after using the toilet. Encourage keeping fingernails short to prevent harboring of eggs and autoinoculation (hand-to-mouth reinfection); discourage biting nails and scratching anal area.
- Eggs are destroyed by sunlight and ultraviolet rays, so ensure that blinds or curtains are open in the affected room to enhance cleaning of the environment.
- Wash bed linens, underwear, bedclothes, and towels of the infected individual and the entire family in hot water daily during treatment. Pinworm eggs are killed by exposure to temperatures of 131°F (55°C) for a few seconds; therefore, the "hot" cycle should be used while washing and drying.
- Bathe daily in the morning; showers (stand-up baths) are preferred over tub baths.
- Change underwear, nightclothes, and bed sheets daily for several days after treatment.
- Clean and vacuum (do not sweep) house daily for several days after treatment of cases. Wet mopping before or instead of vacuuming may limit spread of pinworm eggs into the air.
- Reduce overcrowding in living accommodations.

Source: Heymann D. *Control of Communicable Diseases Manual.* 19th ed. Washington, DC: American Public Health Association; 2008.

Pharmacologic Therapy

Pyrantel Pamoate

Pyrantel pamoate is the only nonprescription medication approved for treatment of pinworm infection. Pyrantel pamoate was first used in veterinary practice as a broad-spectrum drug for pinworms, roundworms, and hookworms. It has become an important drug for treating certain helminthic infections in humans. Pyrantel pamoate has a cure rate of 90%–100% when used for treatment of enterobiasis.[11] This variable cure rate may be a result of the medication's lack of effect on eggs and larvae as well as the eggs' viability for up to 20 days, which may lead to reinfection.

Although this product is readily available in a nonprescription form, helminthic infections other than those caused by pinworms require a medical referral and should be diagnosed and treated by a PCP.

Pyrantel pamoate is a depolarizing neuromuscular agent that paralyzes adult worms, causing them to loosen their hold on the intestinal wall and subsequently be passed out in the stool before they can lay eggs. The drug is poorly absorbed, with 50% excreted unchanged in the feces and about 7% excreted in the urine as unchanged drug and metabolites.[11]

A single oral dose of pyrantel pamoate (liquid, caplet, chewable tablet) is based on the adult or child patient's body weight (11 mg/kg of the pyrantel base). The maximum single dose is 1 g. The recommended dosage is the same for children younger than 2 years or weighing less than 25 lb (11 kg); however, they should not be treated without first consulting a PCP. The product includes a schedule of recommended dosages that is based on a range of body weights. The dose can be repeated in 2 weeks if symptoms do not resolve, because reinfection can occur; however, the repeat dose should be administered only after consultation with a PCP.

Pyrantel pamoate may be taken at any time of the day without regard to meals, and it may be taken or mixed with milk or fruit juice.[11] A special diet or fasting before or after administration is not necessary. The liquid formulation (containing 50 mg/mL of the pyrantel base) should be shaken well before the dose is measured. (See also Chapter 11, section "Special Populations," for FDA requirements for dispensing devices included in liquid nonprescription products.)

Adverse effects are usually mild, infrequent, and transient. The most common adverse effects involve the gastrointestinal (GI) tract and include nausea, vomiting, tenesmus, anorexia, diarrhea, and abdominal cramps.[12] These adverse effects are typically related to expulsion of the helminths from the GI tract. However, patients who experience severe or persistent abdominal symptoms or other adverse effects after taking the first or second dose of this medication should be referred to their PCP for further evaluation. Less common adverse effects such as headache, dizziness, drowsiness, insomnia, rash, fever, and weakness may occur. In very rare circumstances, transient increases in aspartate aminotransferase, ototoxicity, optic neuritis, and hallucinations with confusion and paresthesia have been reported with therapeutic doses.[11]

Patients who do not respond to the recommended doses of pyrantel pamoate should be evaluated further by their PCPs, and the use of prescription products should be considered. Mebendazole (Emverm), recently reintroduced on the market with a new trade name, once was considered by experts to be the drug of choice to treat pinworm infection; however, its efficacy appears to be similar to pyrantel, so it is now considered just another option.[13,14] Some pharmacies still may be able to compound mebendazole. Another available prescription agent for treatment of pinworm infection is albendazole. Albendazole is approved to treat other helminthic infections, but its use to treat pinworms is considered off label by the Food and Drug Administration (FDA). Albendazole is given as a single oral dose (400 mg for patients ages 2 years and older; 200 mg for patients younger than 2 years) with a second available dose that may be repeated at 2 weeks to prevent recurrence caused by reinfection.[2]

Product Selection Guidelines

Pyrantel pamoate is a safe and effective treatment for pinworms. The brands listed in Table 18–2 are comparatively priced and generally less expensive than prescription treatment (e.g.,

TABLE 18-2 Selected Nonprescription Pyrantel Pamoate Products

Trade Name	Primary Ingredient
Pin-X Liquid/Chewable Tablet	Pyrantel pamoate 50 mg/mL (base) and 250 mg/tablet (base)
Pyrantel Suspension	Pyrantel pamoate 50 mg/mL (base)
Reese's Pinworm Caplet	Pyrantel 180 mg (equals 62.5 mg base)
Reese's Pinworm Medicine Liquid	Pyrantel pamoate 144 mg/mL (equals 50 mg/mL base)
Reese's Pinworm Medicine Family Pack	Pyrantel pamoate 144 mg/mL (equals 50 mg/mL base); contains two bottles (each containing 1 fluid ounce) to treat the entire family

mebendazole, albendazole). Pyrantel pamoate is contraindicated in patients with hypersensitivity to the drug. Patients with preexisting liver dysfunction or severe malnutrition should not self-medicate without first consulting their PCPs. Pyrantel pamoate has not been well studied[3,4] in pregnant women; therefore, it should be used during pregnancy only when the benefits clearly outweigh the risks and only under PCP direction.[15] (See the Preface for a detailed explanation of the pregnancy data.) The World Health Organization (WHO) does allow the use of pyrantel pamoate during the second and third trimesters for high-risk patients.[5] However, if symptoms of the infection are compromising the pregnancy, WHO has also concluded that the benefits of treating mothers with this infection outweigh the potential risks to a mother and her unborn child. In addition, the current recommendation is to not withhold treatment while breastfeeding.[3,4] Finally, pyrantel pamoate should not be used in patients younger than 2 years or those weighing less than 25 lb (11 kg), except under the direction of a PCP.

Complementary Therapies

Various home remedies (e.g., applying a combination of garlic paste and petroleum jelly to the anus, ingesting coconut oil and castor oil) and complementary therapies (e.g., white willow bark, green tea, turmeric) have been used to treat pinworm infection. These remedies should not be recommended, because evidence of their efficacy and safety is insufficient to support their use to treat pinworm infections. Because of the high risk of transmission of this infection, patients instead should take nonprescription medications such as pyrantel pamoate or prescription medications that are approved by FDA for pinworm infection.

Assessment of Pinworm Infection: A Case-Based Approach

Before recommending treatment, the provider should explain how to confirm a pinworm infection by any of the following methods: (1) nighttime perianal or perineal itching in a child, (2) visual inspection of the perianal or perineal area for the adult worm, or (3) a cellophane tape or an adhesive paddle test. Adult pinworms and eggs are seldom found in the feces; therefore, looking for worms in the stool is not a reliable way to diagnose enterobiasis.[16] When symptoms of pinworms (e.g., nocturnal perianal, perineal itching) are present in children, nonprescription therapy may be initiated. Other more vague symptoms (e.g., sleep disturbances, GI symptoms) should be evaluated medically before initiating nonprescription therapy. However, asymptomatic disease is common in enterobiasis, and visual inspection may be necessary. To conduct a visual inspection, the parent should inspect the anal area during the night with a flashlight while the child is sleeping or in the very early morning before the child arises. White, thread-like, wriggling worms between 3 and 7 mm in length (about the size of a staple) may be seen. If pinworms are present, treatment should be initiated. Finally, if pinworms are suspected but symptoms are vague and/or visual inspection is negative, a PCP may instruct the patient to obtain a cellophane tape sample. The parent should apply the sticky side of the tape to the perianal area (usually with a tongue depressor) and affix it sticky side down on a glass slide. Commercially available kits, such as the Falcon SWUBE paddles, use a sticky paddle instead of tape to affix to a slide (see Color Plates, photograph 6C). Laboratories usually supply these pinworm paddles to conduct the test. Samples should be taken over 3 consecutive days upon the child's awakening, which may increase the likelihood of detection to around 90%.[6] The samples should then be taken to a PCP for microscopic examination. If the test is positive, treatment of the pinworm infection should be initiated.

Cases 18–1 and 18–2 illustrate the assessment of patients with pinworm infections.

Patient Counseling for Pinworm Infection

Once the decision to treat the pinworm infection with pyrantel pamoate is made, the package insert material should be reviewed with the patient or caregiver. The insert explains the pinworm life cycle, symptoms of pinworm infection, and methods of transmitting the infection. Doses should be calculated for the patient and all family members, and the need to treat the whole family should be emphasized. The patient or caregiver should be advised to implement strict hygienic measures to prevent reinfection or transmission of the infection to other family members (Table 18–1). In addition, it should be explained that the adverse effects of pyrantel pamoate are usually mild and infrequent, but that medical referral may be necessary if more severe effects occur. Patients who experience severe or persistent symptoms after taking this medication should be referred for medical evaluation. Finally, patients should be advised that pinworm infection symptoms (e.g., nocturnal perianal itching) should improve within 2 weeks of treatment and that if symptoms persist or worsen to include systemic symptoms (e.g., abdominal discomfort, insomnia, and/or nervousness), medical referral may be necessary. The box "Patient Education for Pinworm Infection" lists specific information to provide patients.

Evaluation of Patient Outcomes for Pinworm Infection

Patients or caregivers should be instructed to contact their PCPs if anal itching persists beyond 2 weeks, if the itching recurs, or if new symptoms develop. Because of pyrantel pamoate's variable cure rate, a second dose may be required. It should be given 2 weeks after the first dose and only under PCP care. In addition, patients or caregivers should be asked about the implementation of hygienic measures. If these measures are not being followed, their importance for preventing reinfection should be stressed again.

Key Points for Pinworm Infection

- Pinworms are common in the United States and rarely cause significant morbidity.
- Health care providers should be familiar with common helminthic infections, their symptoms, and their treatment.
- A medical referral is necessary when helminths other than pinworms are suspected.
- Although pyrantel pamoate is used in treating other helminthic infections, only pinworm infection should be evaluated for self-treatment with this nonprescription agent.
- Health care providers can aid patients and caregivers in the self-diagnosis, counseling, and self-treatment with nonprescription pinworm medication.

CASE 18-1

Relevant Evaluation Criteria	Scenario/Model Outcome
Collect	
1. Gather essential information about the patients' symptoms, including	
a. Description of symptom(s) (i.e., nature, onset, duration, severity, associated symptoms)	A woman presents to the pharmacy requesting assistance in selecting an OTC product for her family. She reports that her daughter was diagnosed with pinworms by the pediatrician, who recommended an OTC medication to treat the daughter as well as the mother and father. The mother says her daughter has been complaining about perianal itching that gets much worse at night. The mother and her husband have no current symptoms. The mother asks for a liquid formulation, because her daughter is having a hard time learning how to swallow tablets or capsules.
b. Description of any factors that seem to precipitate, exacerbate, and/or relieve the patients' symptom(s)	No precipitating factors
c. Description of the patients' efforts to relieve the symptoms	The parents applied hydrocortisone cream to the child's perianal region for itching, with no relief.
d. Patients' identity	Daughter: Jenny N.; Mother: Theresa N.; Father: Robert N.
e. Patients' age, gender, height, and weight	Daughter: 6 years old, female, 3 ft 6 in., 40 lb (18.2 kg); mother: 36 years old, female, 5 ft. 6 in., 143 lb (65 kg); father: 38 years old, male, 5 ft 11 in., 190 lb (86 kg)
f. Patients' occupation	The father is a mechanical engineer, and his wife is an attorney.
g. Patients' dietary habits	Normal diet
h. Patients' sleep habits	Daughter: frequent awakenings at night caused by perianal itching; parents: normal sleep habits
i. Concurrent medical conditions, prescription and nonprescription medications, and dietary supplements	Daughter: daily children's chewable multivitamin; mother: oral contraceptive, daily multivitamin, fish oil capsule; father: fish oil capsule daily
j. Allergies	Daughter: NKDA; mother: penicillin allergy; father: NKDA
k. History of other adverse reactions to medications	None
l. Other (describe) ______	n/a
Assess	
2. Differentiate patients' signs/symptoms, and correctly identify the patient's primary problem(s).	Jenny is experiencing perianal itching from a pinworm infection, which results in restless sleep at night.
3. Identify exclusions for self-treatment (Figure 18–1).	Patients should be excluded for self-treatment if they (1) are allergic to the OTC product, (2) are younger than 2 years (unless treatment is approved by PCP), (3) weigh less than 25 lb (11 kg) (unless treatment is approved by PCP), or (4) have liver disease. The patients do not have exclusions for self-treatment.
4. Formulate a comprehensive list of therapeutic alternatives for the primary problem to determine whether triage to a medical provider is required, and share this information with the patients or caregiver.	Options include (1) Recommend an appropriate OTC product (e.g., pyrantel pamoate) at appropriate doses for each member of the family, along with nondrug therapies. (2) Recommend that mother and father see their PCP for a prescription medication. (3) Counsel only on environmental control measures. (4) Take no action.
Plan	
5. Select an optimal therapeutic alternative to address the patients' problem, taking into account patient preferences.	OTC treatment with pyrantel pamoate is appropriate for all three patients. The child is not comfortable swallowing tablets or caplets, but she can take chewable tablets or liquid formulations; therefore, pyrantel pamoate is a good choice.

CASE 18-1 *continued*

Relevant Evaluation Criteria	Scenario/Model Outcome
6. Describe the recommended therapeutic approach to the patients or caregiver.	"Both albendazole and pyrantel pamoate are effective in the treatment of pinworms. However, pyrantel pamoate is available without a prescription, and albendazole requires a prescription. Because one of your family members was recently diagnosed with pinworm infection and the medical provider instructed that other family members be treated, pyrantel pamoate is a reasonable option."
7. Explain to the patients or caregiver the rationale for selecting the recommended therapeutic approach from the considered therapeutic alternatives.	"Pinworms are not life threatening and may resolve on their own. However, if the infection is untreated, the infected person (in this case, your daughter) may reinfect herself or infect other family members. She may also experience some complications of infection if she is not treated. Therefore, treatment is recommended. Pyrantel pamoate is a reasonable option because it is available without a prescription; therefore, the other family members do not need to visit a primary care provider, which could have increased the cost of treatment and delayed its initiation. Pyrantel pamoate is also available as a chewable tablet and an oral suspension, which offer flexible dosing based on weight for multiple family members. Other formulations such as tablets and caplets are available, if preferred."
Implement	
8. When recommending self-care with nonprescription medications and/or nondrug therapy, convey accurate information to the patients or caregiver.	
a. Appropriate dose and frequency of administration	• Jenny (daughter) weighs 18.2 kg (40 lb); the dose of pyrantel is 11 mg/kg, so she should receive about 200 mg. She can take 4 mL of the liquid formulation (144 mg/mL equivalent to 50 mg/mL pyrantel base). • Theresa (mother) weighs 65 kg, so she should receive at least 715 mg of pyrantel pamoate (~3 chewable tablets or 15 mL of the liquid formulation). • Robert (father) weighs 86 kg, so he should receive 1000 mg, the maximum dose, of pyrantel pamoate (4 chewable tablets or ~20 mL of the liquid formulation).
b. Maximum number of days the therapy should be employed	"A single dose is usually required. If symptoms persist after 2 weeks, contact your primary care provider for evaluation and, if needed, recommendation for a second dose."
c. Product administration procedures	"Pyrantel pamoate may be taken at any time of day without regard to meals. It may be mixed with milk or fruit juice. If using the oral suspension, shake well before administering." [Note: Prior to administering the medication, the practitioner should verify that other family members who need to be treated do not meet criteria for exclusion for self-treatment. If not, doses will need to be calculated for the other family members.]
d. Expected time to onset of relief	"Relief of symptoms may take several days. The repeat dose should not be administered until 2 weeks have elapsed and should be administered only if recommended by your primary care provider."
e. Degree of relief that can be reasonably expected	"Perianal itching should decrease after several days, with complete pinworm eradication after at least 2 weeks."
f. Most common adverse effects	"Adverse effects are usually mild and may consist of nausea, vomiting, loss of appetite, diarrhea, or abdominal cramps."
g. Adverse effects that warrant medical intervention should they occur	"Severe or persistent abdominal symptoms require medical attention."
h. Patient options in the event that condition worsens or persists	"Contact the appropriate health care provider if any family member's condition worsens, or if, after taking the medication, any family member experiences any severe adverse effects, such as severe or persistent abdominal symptoms." [Note: The practitioner should reinforce to the parents that pinworms are very common and rarely cause serious problems, but that the infection will continue and potentially spread to others if not treated.]

CASE 18-1 *continued*

Relevant Evaluation Criteria	Scenario/Model Outcome
i. Product storage requirements	"Store at room temperature away from direct light with container sealed tightly."
j. Specific nondrug measures	See Table 18–1.
Solicit follow-up questions from the patients or caregiver.	"Should my daughter receive a prescription medication instead because she has an active infection?"
Answer the patients' or caregiver's questions.	"Both the prescription and nonprescription medications are equally effective in treating pinworms. You can use either the prescription medication or the nonprescription pyrantel pamoate, depending on your preferences (such as cost)."
Follow-up: Monitor and Evaluate	
9. Assess patient outcome	You can call the parents in 1–2 weeks to assess the child's response to the medication. If symptoms have resolved, reinforce the importance of hygienic measures. If symptoms persist, another single dose of pyrantel pamoate can be administered but only after reevaluation by the child's pediatrician.

Key: n/a = Not applicable; NKDA = no known drug allergies; OTC = over-the-counter; PCP = primary care provider.

CASE 18-2

Relevant Evaluation Criteria	Scenario/Model Outcome
Collect	
1. Gather essential information about the patient's symptoms, including	
a. Description of symptom(s) (i.e., nature, onset, duration, severity, associated symptoms)	A woman presents to the pharmacy requesting assistance choosing a product to help "slow down the bowels" and a product to help her with intense itching. She says she's had loose stool and generalized abdominal pain for about 10 days. She mentions that her stool has been watery most of the time and that she's noticed tiny white squiggly things on the tissue after wiping. The itching, which began roughly 3 weeks before the diarrhea started, is mostly in her perineal and vaginal area and is worse at night. She also tells you that her grandchildren, whom she visited in another state about a 6 weeks ago, had some symptoms of itching as well and that her daughter was going to take them to see the pediatrician.
b. Description of any factors that seem to precipitate, exacerbate, and/or relieve the patient's symptom(s)	No precipitating factors
c. Description of the patient's efforts to relieve the symptoms	She tried bismuth subsalicylate for 3 days without much relief. She took 3 doses of loperamide, which helped the diarrhea temporarily but did not help the itching. She's tried applying hemorrhoidal ointment and hydrocortisone ointment to the region to help with the itching.
d. Patient's identity	Letty Whitaker
e. Patient's age, gender, height, and weight	61 years old, female, 5 ft 4 in., 132 lb (60 kg)
f. Patient's occupation	Dance instructor
g. Patient's dietary habits	Normal diet; high in fruits, vegetables, and whole grains
h. Patient's sleep habits	Frequent awakenings at night caused by perineal itching
i. Concurrent medical conditions, prescription and nonprescription medications, and dietary supplements	Daily multivitamin; occasional ibuprofen or acetaminophen for pain
j. Allergies	NKDA
k. History of other adverse reactions to medications	None

CASE 18-2 *continued*

Relevant Evaluation Criteria	Scenario/Model Outcome
Assess	
2. Differentiate patient's signs/symptoms, and correctly identify the patient's primary problem(s).	Patient's symptoms, such as perianal itching at night, are consistent with pinworms, but prolonged diarrhea and abdominal pain are unusual symptoms and should be evaluated medically. The appearance of "white squiggly things" on the tissue may indicate the presence of pinworms, but a tape test or a slide test must be done to confirm infection.
3. Identify exclusions for self-treatment (Figure 18–1).	Consider the patient to be excluded from self-treatment if she (1) is allergic to the OTC product, (2) is younger than 2 years (unless treatment approved by PCP), (3) weighs less than 25 lb (11 kg) (unless treatment approved by PCP), (4) has liver disease, (5) is pregnant, (6) is breastfeeding, or (7) has vague symptoms and negative visual inspection.
4. Formulate a comprehensive list of therapeutic alternatives for the primary problem to determine whether triage to a medical provider is required, and share this information with the patient or caregiver.	Options include (1) Recommend an appropriate OTC product at appropriate doses for the patient, along with nondrug therapies. (2) Refer the patient to a PCP for further evaluation, diagnosis, and recommended treatment. (3) Counsel on only environmental control measures. (4) Take no action.
Plan	
5. Select an optimal therapeutic alternative to address the patient's problem, taking into account patient preferences.	Medical evaluation by a PCP is warranted because of the perineal, gastrointestinal, and vaginal symptoms that may require subsequent treatment.
6. Describe the recommended therapeutic approach to the patient or caregiver.	"You should see your primary care provider for further evaluation of your symptoms, appropriate diagnosis, and recommended treatment."
7. Explain to the patient or caregiver the rationale for selecting the recommended therapeutic approach from the considered therapeutic alternatives.	"Because you have no documented pinworm infection, by tape slide, and because you have other symptoms that may be complications of a pinworm infection, self-treatment is not appropriate. Your symptoms may be consistent with pinworm infection, but other possibilities need to be ruled out."
Implement	
8. When recommending self-care with nonprescription medications and/or nondrug therapy, convey accurate information to the patient or caregiver.	"Self-treatment is not appropriate, but you should institute environmental control measures [shown in Table 18–1] and seek medical care."
Solicit follow-up questions from the patient or caregiver.	(1) "What are some of the complications associated with pinworms?" (2) "How are pinworms normally treated?"
Answer the patient's or caregiver's questions.	(1) "If untreated, pinworms could lead to secondary bacterial infections in the perianal and perineal regions. Pinworms can also lead to pelvic inflammatory disease, endometritis, and urinary tract infections. In addition, other possible symptoms associated with pinworm infection include insomnia, restlessness, and anorexia." (2) "Patients may be treated with a single dose of various nonprescription (pyrantel pamoate) or prescription (albendazole) medications. Along with medications, patients must also follow specific nondrug measures to prevent reinfection."
Follow-up: Monitor and Evaluate	
9. Assess patient outcome	Ask the patient to call you in 1 week, or initiate a follow-up call to the patient to assess whether she was evaluated by a PCP and whether her symptoms are improving.

Key: NKDA = No known drug allergies; OTC = over-the-counter; PCP = primary care provider.

PATIENT EDUCATION FOR Pinworm Infection

The objectives of self-treatment are (1) to eradicate pinworms in the infected patient, (2) to prevent reinfection, and (3) to prevent transmission of the infection to others. For most patients, carefully following product instructions and the self-care measures listed here will help ensure optimal therapeutic outcomes.

Nondrug Measures

- See Table 18–1 for nondrug/preventive measures.

Nonprescription Medications

- Read package insert for pyrantel pamoate information carefully; this information will help prevent reinfection or transmission of the infection.
- Consult a primary care provider before giving the medication to a person with liver disease or severe malnutrition, a child who is younger than 2 years and/or weighs less than 25 lb (11 kg), or a woman who is pregnant or breastfeeding, or has vague or rare symptoms and negative visual inspection.
- Treat all household members to ensure elimination of the infection. Medical referral may be necessary if household members meet criteria for exclusion for self-treatment (e.g., malnutrition, pregnancy, liver disease, anemia, age younger than 2 years).
- Take only 1 dose as shown on the dosing schedule included with the product. For adults and children older than 2 years, dosing is the same: 11 mg/kg taken orally. The maximum dose is 1 g.
- Shake the liquid formulation well, and use a measuring spoon to ensure an accurate dose.
- If desired, pyrantel pamoate may be taken with food, milk, or fruit juices on an empty stomach any time during the day. The liquid formulation may be mixed with milk or fruit juice.
- Note that fasting, laxatives, and special diets are not necessary to aid treatment.

When to Seek Medical Attention

Seek medical attention if you experience any of the following:

- Abdominal cramps, nausea, vomiting, anorexia, rash, diarrhea, headache, drowsiness, or dizziness occurs and persists after taking the medication.
- Symptoms of the pinworm infection persist beyond 2 weeks after the initial dose of pyrantel pamoate. A second dose of pyrantel pamoate can be given if symptoms are present beyond 2 weeks, but only if directed to do so by a primary care provider.
- Rare symptoms such as vaginal itching or bleeding, pain upon urination, urinary tract infection, and hives are present.

REFERENCES

1. Wang L, Hwang K, Chen E. *Enterobius vermicularis* infection in schoolchildren: a large-scale survey 6 years after a population-based control. *Epidemiol Infect.* 2010;138(1):28–36. doi:10.1017/S0950268809002660.
2. Stermer E, Sukhotnic I, Shaoul R. Pruritus ani: an approach to an itching condition. *J Pediatr Gastroenterol Nutr.* 2009;48(5):513–6. doi: 10.1097/MPG.0b013e31818080c0.
3. Cappello M, Hotez P. Intestinal nematodes. In: Long S, ed. *Principles and Practice of Pediatric Infectious Diseases* [subscription electronic library]. 4th ed. New York, NY: Churchill Livingstone; 2012. Accessed December 4, 2013.
4. St Georgiev V. Chemotherapy of enterobiasis (oxyuriasis). *Expert Opin Pharmacother.* 2001;2(2):267–75. doi:10.1517/14656566.2.2.267.
5. Centers for Disease Control and Prevention. Parasites—enterobiasis (also known as pinworm infection). Last updated January 10, 2013. Available at https://www.cdc.gov/parasites/pinworm/. Accessed May 3, 2017.
6. Kucik CJ, Martin GL, Sortor BV. Common intestinal parasites. *Am Fam Physician.* 2004;69(5):1161–8. PMID: 15023017.
7. Burkhart CN, Burkhart CG. Assessment of frequency, transmission, and genitourinary complications of enterobiasis (pinworms). *Int J Dermatol.* 2005;44(10):837–40. doi: 10.1111/j.1365-4632.2004.02332.x.
8. Young C, Tataryn I, Kowalewska-Grochowska KT, et al. *Enterobius vermicularis* infection of the fallopian tube in an infertile female. *Pathol Res Pract.* 2010;206(6):405–7. doi:10.1016/j.prp.2009.11.003.
9. Swaim L, Zietz B, Qu Z. An uncommon cause of vaginal bleeding in a child. *Obstet Gynecol.* 2007;110(2 Pt 1):416–20. doi:10.1097/01.AOG.0000268282.68655.30.
10. Arca MJ, Gates RL, Groner JI, et al. Clinical manifestations of appendiceal pinworms in children: an institutional experience and a review of the literature. *Pediatr Surg Int.* 2004;20(5):372–5. doi:10.1007/s00383-004-1151-5.
11. Anthelmintics. In: McEvoy GK, Snow KE, eds. *AHFS Drug Handbook.* STAT!Ref Online Electronic Medical Library. Bethesda, MD: American Society of Health-System Pharmacists; 2010. Accessed November 2, 2010.
12. Bagheri H, Simiand E, Montastruc J-L, et al. Adverse drug reactions to anthelmintics. *Ann Pharmacother.* 2004;38(3):383–8. doi: 10.1345/aph.1D325.
13. Jacobson CC, Abel EA. Parasitic infestations. *J Am Acad Dermatol.* 2007;56(6):1026–43. doi: 10.1016/j.jaad.2006.10.963.
14. Drugs for parasitic infections. *Med Lett Drugs Ther* [online version]. 2013;11(Suppl):e1–31. Available at: http://secure.medicalletter.org/TG-article-143a. Accessed May 2, 2016.
15. Briggs G, Freeman R, Yaffe S. Pyrantel pamoate. In: Briggs G, Freeman R, Yaffe S, eds. *Drugs in Pregnancy and Lactation: A Reference Guide to Fetal and Neonatal Risk.* 8th ed. Philadelphia, PA: Lippincott Williams & Wilkins; 2008.
16. Maguire J. Intestinal nematodes (roundworms). In: Mandell GL, Bennett JE, Dolin R, eds. *Mandell, Douglas, and Bennett's Principles and Practice of Infectious Diseases.* Expert Consult Online Electronic Medical Library. Philadelphia, PA: Churchill Livingston Elsevier; 2010.

CHAPTER 19

NAUSEA AND VOMITING

ADAM C. WELCH

Nausea and vomiting (N/V) symptoms can occur in both adults and children from a variety of circumstances associated with several medical disorders. Common self-care disorders that involve N/V are motion sickness, pregnancy (nausea and vomiting of pregnancy [NVP]), acute viral gastroenteritis, and "upset stomach" (overeating or indigestion). Nonprescription antiemetics can be used to prevent or treat the symptoms of N/V for these disorders. Vomiting accounts for 1.8% of all emergency department visits in the United States. Each year, nearly 2.5 million people, mostly children younger than 15 years, visit an emergency department for vomiting.[1] Accurate data on the epidemiology of N/V are not available, because these symptoms occur in many medical disorders and many individuals do not report these disturbances to a health care provider.

The severity of N/V related to motion sickness is difficult to quantify because of interindividual variability and susceptibility to the condition. Motion sickness rarely occurs in children younger than 2 years. Women and children ages 2–15 years have reported an increased frequency of motion sickness.[2]

The incidence of nausea in early pregnancy is quoted as between 50% and 80%, with rates of vomiting around 50%. Typically these symptoms occur during pregnancy between weeks 6 and 12, but they may persist past 20 weeks in 20% of women.[3] Half of all pregnant women have both N/V, a quarter have nausea only, and it is rare for only vomiting to occur.[4] A very severe form of pregnancy-related vomiting, *hyperemesis gravidarum*, occurs in less than 1% of women and may require rehydration and hospitalization.[5]

The third typically self-treatable cause of N/V is acute viral gastroenteritis. *Viral gastroenteritis* is an inflammation of the stomach and small intestines that commonly presents with acute vomiting and diarrhea.[6] This illness may affect any age group and usually is self-limiting, but pediatric patients may experience serious consequences from dehydration.[7] Gastroenteritis is usually caused by rotavirus and norovirus; it occurs most often in winter[8] (see Chapter 16). The Centers for Disease Control and Prevention (CDC) reports that, in children, rotavirus infections result in approximately 400,000 primary care provider visits, up to 272,000 emergency department visits, and 55,000–70,000 annual hospitalizations, with total costs approximating $1 billion.[9] The rotavirus vaccine is included in the childhood immunization schedule.[10] CDC estimates that 19–21 million cases of acute gastroenteritis each year are caused by norovirus infection, and that norovirus accounts for 50% of all gastroenteritis outbreaks worldwide.[11]

The remaining self-care disorder that involves N/V is indigestion or distention associated with overeating. Limited treatment options for this disorder are discussed in this chapter. A more comprehensive discussion is provided in Chapter 13.

Pathophysiology of Nausea and Vomiting

The pathophysiology of N/V involves both the central nervous system (CNS) and the gastrointestinal (GI) tract. Figure 19–1 shows four different areas of the body that provide input to a complex system of neurons in the medulla oblongata in the brain stem, known as the *vomiting center* (VC): the chemoreceptor trigger zone (CTZ), vestibular apparatus, cerebral cortex, and visceral GI tract afferent nerves.[12–14]

CTZ neurons are outside the blood–brain barrier; therefore, CTZ responds to stimuli from either the bloodstream or the cerebral spinal fluid.[13,14] The vestibular apparatus is located in the bony labyrinth of the temporal lobe. It detects motion and body position, including changes in equilibrium; direct input to VC is through cholinergic pathways. The cerebral cortex system provides VC input through higher cortical centers; this pathway for initiating emesis is the least understood. Sensory input, including sight, smell, anticipation, or memory, may elicit a strong sensation of nausea through the cerebral cortex.[14] Finally, visceral afferent nerve pathways from the GI tract have numerous neurotransmitters that provide VC input. Major neurotransmitters and receptors involved in vomiting include serotonin, dopamine, histamine-1, acetylcholine, opioid, and neurokinin receptors.[12,13]

VC is triggered by different CNS and GI tract stimuli, sending impulses to the salivation center, vasomotor center, respiratory center, and cranial nerves, and then to the pharynx and GI tract, after which nausea and/or vomiting may occur.[14] Table 19–1 lists several stimuli that may elicit N/V; however, many of these are not self-limiting and require medical evaluation and treatment.[12–16] Treatment options should be targeted to the appropriate pathway.[17] Causes discussed in this chapter (motion sickness, pregnancy, viral gastroenteritis, overeating) may be

Editor's Note: This chapter is based on the 18th edition chapter of the same title, written by Stefanie P. Ferreri and Adam C. Welch.

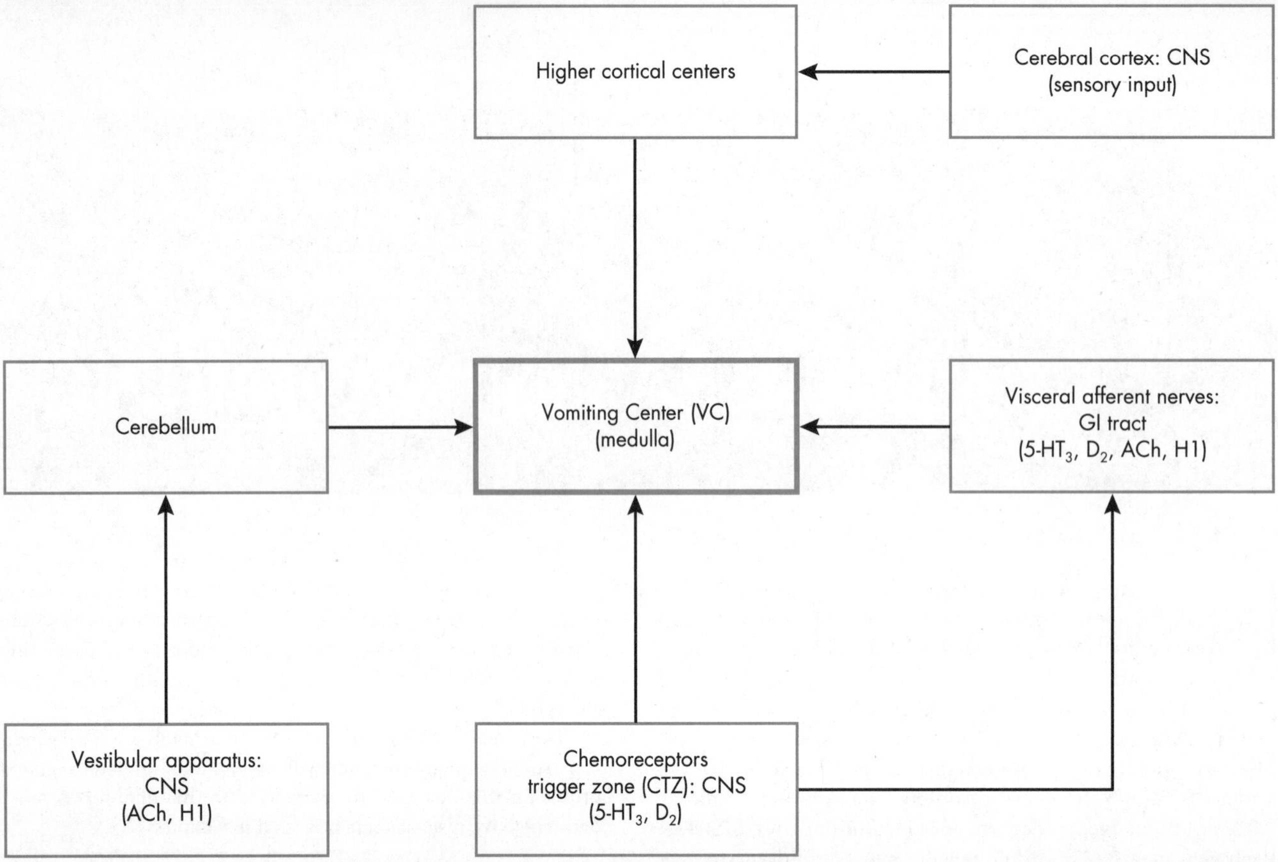

FIGURE 19–1 Vomiting center. Key: ACh = Acetylcholine; CNS = central nervous system; D_2 = dopamine; GI = gastrointestinal; H1 = histamine-1; 5-HT_3 = serotonin.

TABLE 19–1 Primary Causes of Nausea and Vomiting

GI Tract (visceral afferent nerves)	CNS Disorders	Other Disorders
Mechanical Obstruction GI obstruction (e.g., PUD, gastric carcinoma, pancreatic disease); small intestine obstruction **Motility Disorders** Gastroparesis (e.g., diabetes, drug-induced, postviral); chronic intestinal pseudo-obstruction; IBS; anorexia nervosa; idiopathic gastric stasis **Peritoneal Irritation** Appendicitis; bacterial peritonitis; pancreatitis **Infections** Viral gastroenteritis[a] (e.g., norovirus, rotavirus); food poisoning (e.g., toxins from *Bacillus cereus, Staphylococcus aureus, Clostridium perfringens*); hepatitis A or B; acute systemic infections **Topical Gastrointestinal Irritants** Alcohol; NSAIDs; antibiotics, iron	**Vestibular Disorders** Labyrinthitis; Ménière syndrome; motion sickness[a] **Increased Intracranial Pressure** CNS tumor; subdural or subarachnoid hemorrhage; pseudotumor cerebri **Infections** Meningitis; encephalitis **Psychogenic** Anticipatory vomiting; bulimia; psychiatric disorders (anxiety) **Other CNS Disorders** Migraine headache **Irritation of CTZ (medication-induced)** Chemotherapy; opiates; theophylline or digoxin toxicity; antibiotics; radiation therapy; drug withdrawal (e.g., opiates, BDZs)	Cardiac disease (e.g., MI, HF); urologic disease (e.g., stones, pyelonephritis); overeating[a] Diabetes (e.g., DKA); renal disease (e.g., uremia); adrenocortical crisis (e.g., Addison disease); pregnancy[a]

Key: BDZ = Benzodiazepine; CNS = central nervous system; CTZ = chemotrigger receptor zone; DKA = diabetic ketoacidosis; GI = gastrointestinal; HF = heart failure; IBS = irritable bowel syndrome; MI = myocardial infarction; NSAIDs = nonsteroidal anti-inflammatory drugs; PUD = peptic ulcer disease.

[a] Self-treatable or preventable disorders.

Source: References 8, 9, 11, 12, 14, and 15.

self-treatable or prevented with proper patient education. (For nausea secondary to migraines, see Chapter 5.)

Emesis, or vomiting, is thought to be a complicated defense response secondary to a variety of different mechanisms. Retching may occur after subjective feelings of nausea. The abdominal and diaphragmatic musculature may contract or relax, and the associated coordinating circuitry involves other areas, such as the laryngeal or pharyngeal muscles. The epiglottis closes to prevent aspiration, the soft palate is elevated, a retrograde contraction occurs while the gastric fundus relaxes, and the stomach contents move into the esophagus and are expelled as vomiting begins.[14]

Overstimulation of the labyrinth (inner ear) apparatus produces N/V of motion sickness.[18] The three semicircular canals in the labyrinth on each side of the head are responsible for maintaining equilibrium. Postural adjustments are made when the brain receives nerve impulses initiated by the movement of fluid in the canals. Conflicting sensory inputs contribute to motion sickness. Linear and angular movements of the head disrupt a person's perceptions relative to their environment.[18] Individuals differ in their response to motion sickness stimuli, such as flying and boating, but no one is immune. Regardless of the type of stimulus-producing event, motion sickness is easier to prevent than to treat with antiemetics that target the primary neurotransmitters acetylcholine and histamine-1 in the vestibular apparatus.[17] In pregnancy, it is unclear which neurotransmitters are the cause of N/V, because it is thought to be multifactorial.[17] NVP often is undertreated, in part because it is thought to be a natural part of pregnancy.[19]

Intestinal irritation causes N/V secondary to acute gastroenteritis. The visceral afferent nerves are mediated primarily through dopamine, serotonin, acetylcholine, and histamine-1 receptors; therefore, therapy is targeted at those neurotransmitters.[12,14,16,17]

Gut distention and decreased GI emptying may stimulate mechanoreceptors and may be responsible for eliciting N/V related to overeating.[8]

Clinical Presentation of Nausea and Vomiting

Three different processes compose N/V: (1) *nausea* (characterized by a person's subjective feeling of a need to vomit); (2) *retching* (involuntary rhythmic diaphragmatic and abdominal contractions); and (3) *vomiting* (rapid, forceful expulsion of GI tract contents).[12,13,16] Although most cases of N/V are self-limiting, a patient may show signs and symptoms that warrant medical referral. Possible acute complications of vomiting include dehydration, esophageal tears manifested by blood in the vomitus, aspiration, malnutrition, electrolyte and/or acid–base abnormalities, diaphragmatic herniation, and Mallory–Weiss syndrome.[16] Dehydration and electrolyte imbalances are the major concerns associated with vomiting. Signs and symptoms of dehydration include dry mouth, decreased skin turgor, excessive thirst, little or no urination, dizziness, lightheadedness, fainting, and reduced blood pressure.[16] These symptoms warrant medical referral for further evaluation.

In infants and small children, recurrent or protracted N/V (with accompanying diarrhea) may lead to marked dehydration and electrolyte imbalance that should not be ignored. Parents should be educated to recognize signs and symptoms of dehydration, such as dry mucous membranes, decreased skin turgor, irritability, altered mental status, and weight loss (Table 19–2).[20,21] The child should be referred for further evaluation if he or she has any exclusions for self-care of N/V.[6,20]

TABLE 19–2 Signs and Symptoms of Dehydration in Children

- Dry mouth and tongue
- Sunken and/or dry eyes
- Sunken fontanelle
- Decreased urine output (dry diapers for several hours)
- Dark urine
- Fast heartbeat
- Thirst (drinks extremely eagerly)
- Absence of tears when crying
- Decreased skin turgor
- Unusual lethargy, sleepiness, decreased alertness, or irritability
  - "Floppy" body
  - Lightheadedness when sitting or standing up (in older children)
  - Difficulty in waking up the child (may indicate severe dehydration)
- Weight loss
  - Noticeable decrease in abdominal ("tummy") size
  - Clothes or diaper fits loosely
  - <3% body weight loss, indicating minimal or no dehydration
  - 3%–9% body weight loss, indicating mild-moderate dehydration
  - >9% body weight loss, indicating severe dehydration

Source: References 20 and 21.

Treatment of Nausea and Vomiting

Treatment Goals

The goals of treating N/V are (1) to provide symptomatic relief, (2) to identify and correct the underlying cause, (3) to prevent and correct complications, and (4) to prevent future occurrences.

General Treatment Approach

Most acute cases of N/V are self-limiting and will resolve spontaneously. A clear evaluation should be made to determine whether a patient is a candidate for self-treatment. The algorithms in Figures 19–2 and 19–3 outline the self-treatment options and exclusions for self-care of N/V in adults[16,22–24] and children,[20–21] respectively. Severe cases of vomiting can result in dehydration or electrolyte imbalances, which may necessitate further evaluation or hospitalization. Treatment of N/V can involve pharmacologic prescription and nonprescription therapies, as well as nonpharmacologic options. Pharmacologic nonprescription options are limited and include antihistamines. Because most cases of N/V are acute, the nonpharmacologic treatment primarily is directed at correcting dehydration and electrolyte imbalances. Commercial oral rehydration salt (ORS) solutions should be recommended to prevent these complications. These products contain sodium, chloride, potassium, citrate, and a carbohydrate such as glucose or dextrose to restore loss of electrolytes and also restore loss of fluids.

Exclusions for Self-Treatment

- Urine ketones and/or high BG with signs of dehydration in patients with diabetes (may indicate DKA or HHS)
- Suspected food poisoning that does not clear up after 24 hours
- Severe abdominal pain in the middle or right lower quadrant (may indicate appendicitis or bowel obstruction)
- N/V with fever and/or diarrhea (may indicate infectious disease)
- Severe right upper quadrant pain, especially after eating fatty foods (may indicate cholecystitis or pancreatitis)
- Blood in the vomitus (may indicate ulcers, esophageal tears, or severe nosebleed)
- Yellow skin or eye discoloration and dark urine (may indicate hepatitis)
- Stiff neck with or without headache and sensitivity to brightness of normal light (may indicate meningitis)
- Head injury with N/V, blurry vision, or numbness and tingling
- Persons with glaucoma, BPH, chronic bronchitis, emphysema, or asthma (may react adversely to OTC antiemetics)
- Pregnancy (severe symptoms) or breastfeeding
- N/V caused by cancer chemotherapy; radiation therapy; serious metabolic disorders; CNS, GI, or endocrine disorders
- Drug-induced N/V: adverse effects of drugs used therapeutically (e.g., opioids, NSAIDs, antibiotics, estrogens); toxic doses of drugs used therapeutically (e.g., digoxin, theophylline, lithium); ethanol
- Psychogenic-induced N/V: bulimia, anorexia
- Chronic disease-induced N/V: gastroparesis with diabetes; DKA or HHS with diabetes; GERD

Source: References 8, 11, 16, and 19.

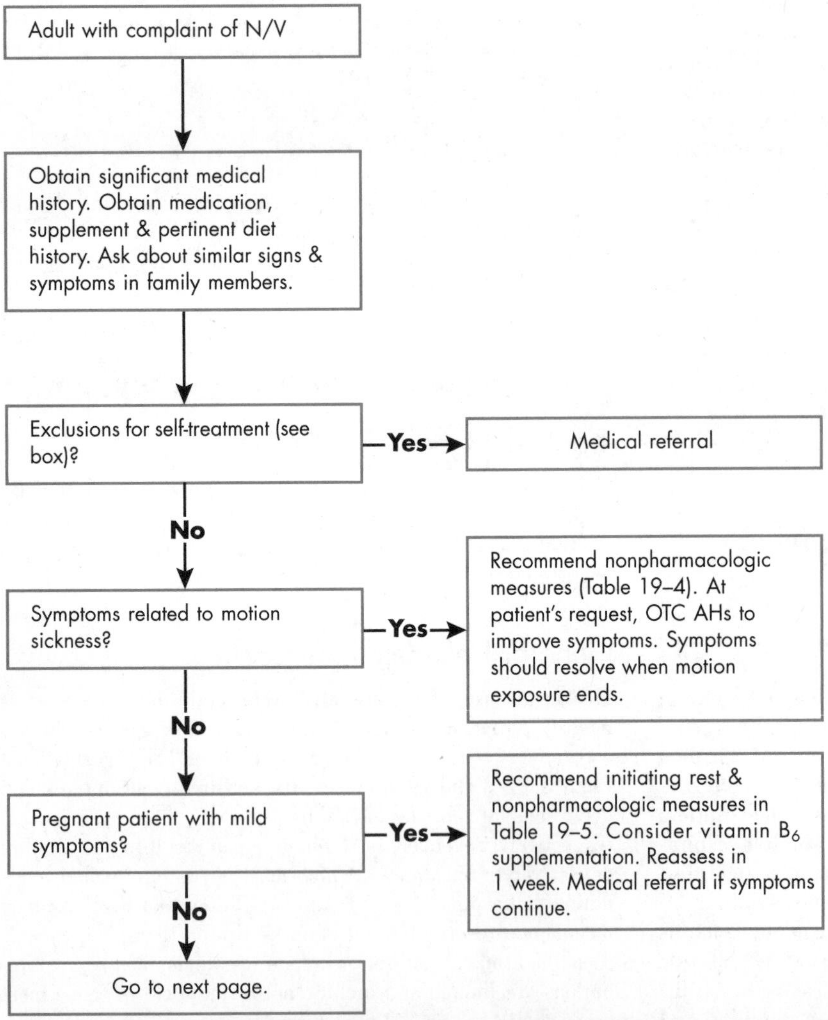
Adult with complaint of N/V
Obtain significant medical history. Obtain medication, supplement & pertinent diet history. Ask about similar signs & symptoms in family members.
Exclusions for self-treatment (see box)?
Yes
Medical referral
No
Symptoms related to motion sickness?
Yes
Recommend nonpharmacologic measures (Table 19–4). At patient's request, OTC AHs to improve symptoms. Symptoms should resolve when motion exposure ends.
No
Pregnant patient with mild symptoms?
Yes
Recommend initiating rest & nonpharmacologic measures in Table 19–5. Consider vitamin B_6 supplementation. Reassess in 1 week. Medical referral if symptoms continue.
No
Go to next page.

FIGURE 19–2 Self-care for N/V in adults. Key: AH = Antihistamine; B_6 = pyridoxine; BG = blood glucose; BPH = benign prostatic hyperplasia; CNS = central nervous system; DKA = diabetic ketoacidosis; GERD = gastroesophageal reflux disease; GI = gastrointestinal; HHS = hyperosmolar hyperglycemic syndrome; H2RA = histamine-2 receptor antagonist; NSAID = nonsteroidal anti-inflammatory drug; N/V = nausea and vomiting; ORS = oral rehydration salt; PCP = primary care provider. (*continued on next page*)

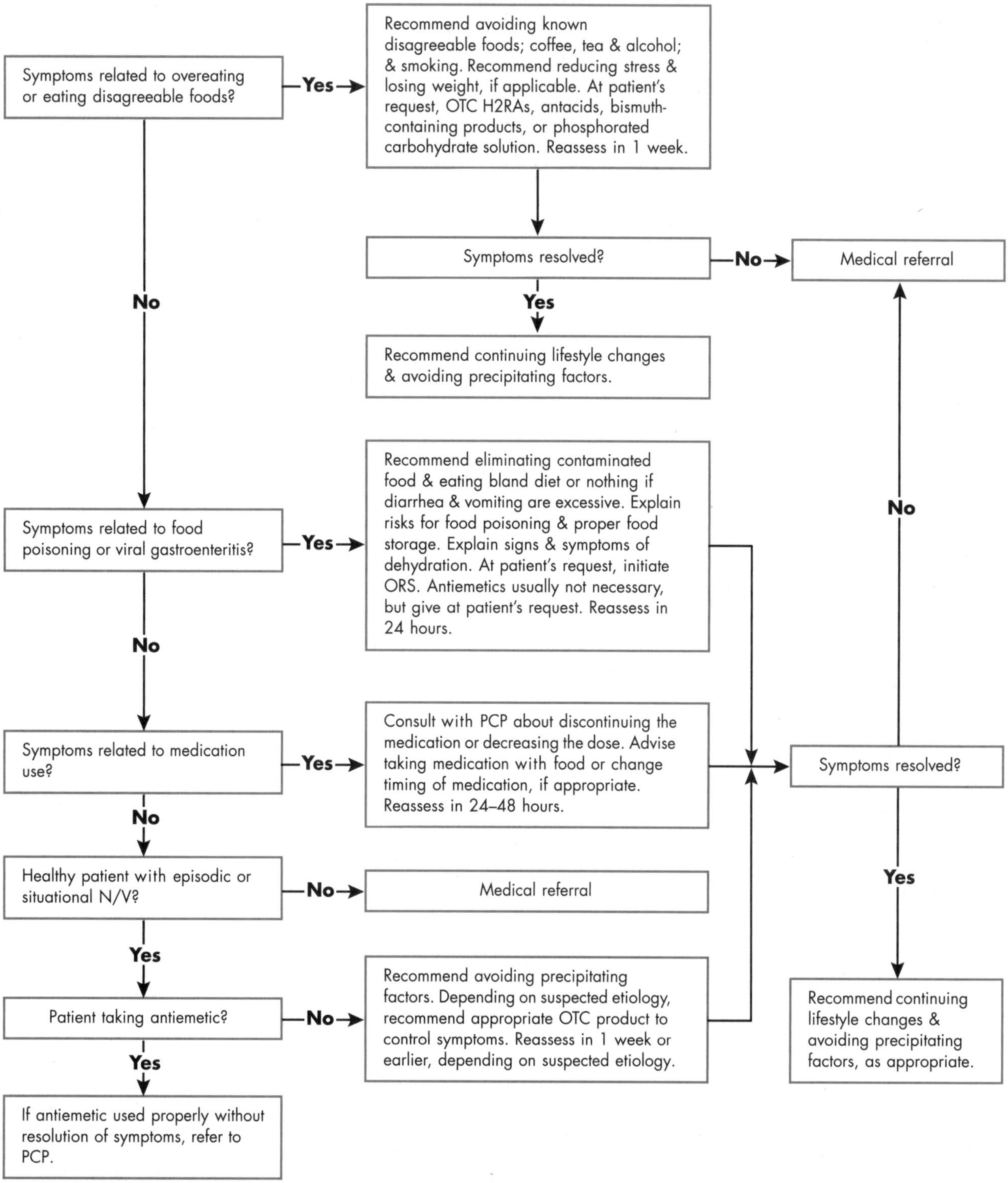

FIGURE 19–2 Self-care for N/V in adults. Key: AH = Antihistamine; B6 = pyridoxine; BG = blood glucose; BPH = benign prostatic hyperplasia; CNS = central nervous system; DKA = diabetic ketoacidosis; GERD = gastroesophageal reflux disease; GI = gastrointestinal; HHS = hyperosmolar hyperglycemic syndrome; H2RA = histamine-2 receptor antagonist; NSAID = nonsteroidal anti-inflammatory drug; N/V = nausea and vomiting; ORS = oral rehydration salt; PCP = primary care provider. *(continued)*

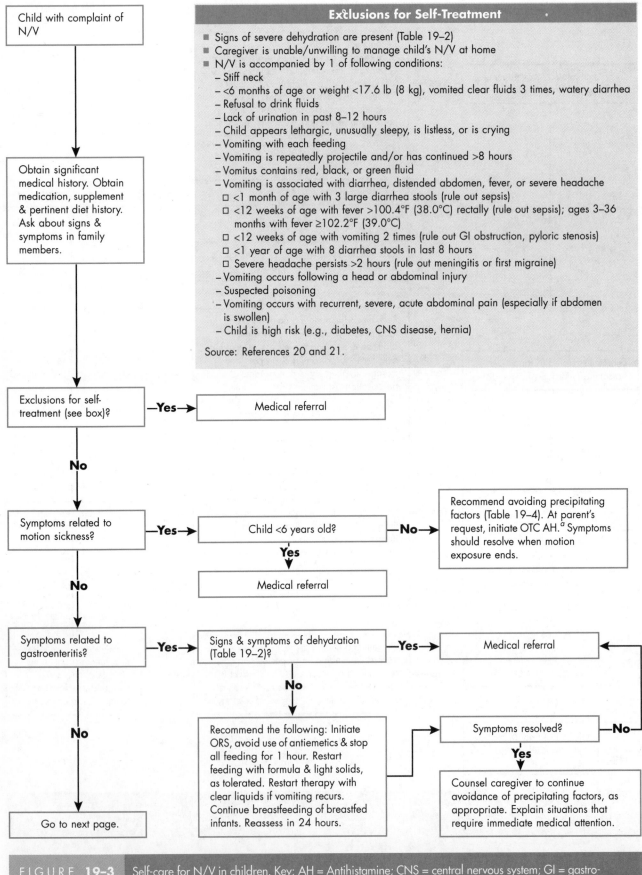

Exclusions for Self-Treatment

- Signs of severe dehydration are present (Table 19–2)
- Caregiver is unable/unwilling to manage child's N/V at home
- N/V is accompanied by 1 of following conditions:
  - Stiff neck
  - <6 months of age or weight <17.6 lb (8 kg), vomited clear fluids 3 times, watery diarrhea
  - Refusal to drink fluids
  - Lack of urination in past 8–12 hours
  - Child appears lethargic, unusually sleepy, is listless, or is crying
  - Vomiting with each feeding
  - Vomiting is repeatedly projectile and/or has continued >8 hours
  - Vomitus contains red, black, or green fluid
  - Vomiting is associated with diarrhea, distended abdomen, fever, or severe headache
    - □ <1 month of age with 3 large diarrhea stools (rule out sepsis)
    - □ <12 weeks of age with fever >100.4°F (38.0°C) rectally (rule out sepsis); ages 3–36 months with fever ≥102.2°F (39.0°C)
    - □ <12 weeks of age with vomiting 2 times (rule out GI obstruction, pyloric stenosis)
    - □ <1 year of age with 8 diarrhea stools in last 8 hours
    - □ Severe headache persists >2 hours (rule out meningitis or first migraine)
  - Vomiting occurs following a head or abdominal injury
  - Suspected poisoning
  - Vomiting occurs with recurrent, severe, acute abdominal pain (especially if abdomen is swollen)
  - Child is high risk (e.g., diabetes, CNS disease, hernia)

Source: References 20 and 21.

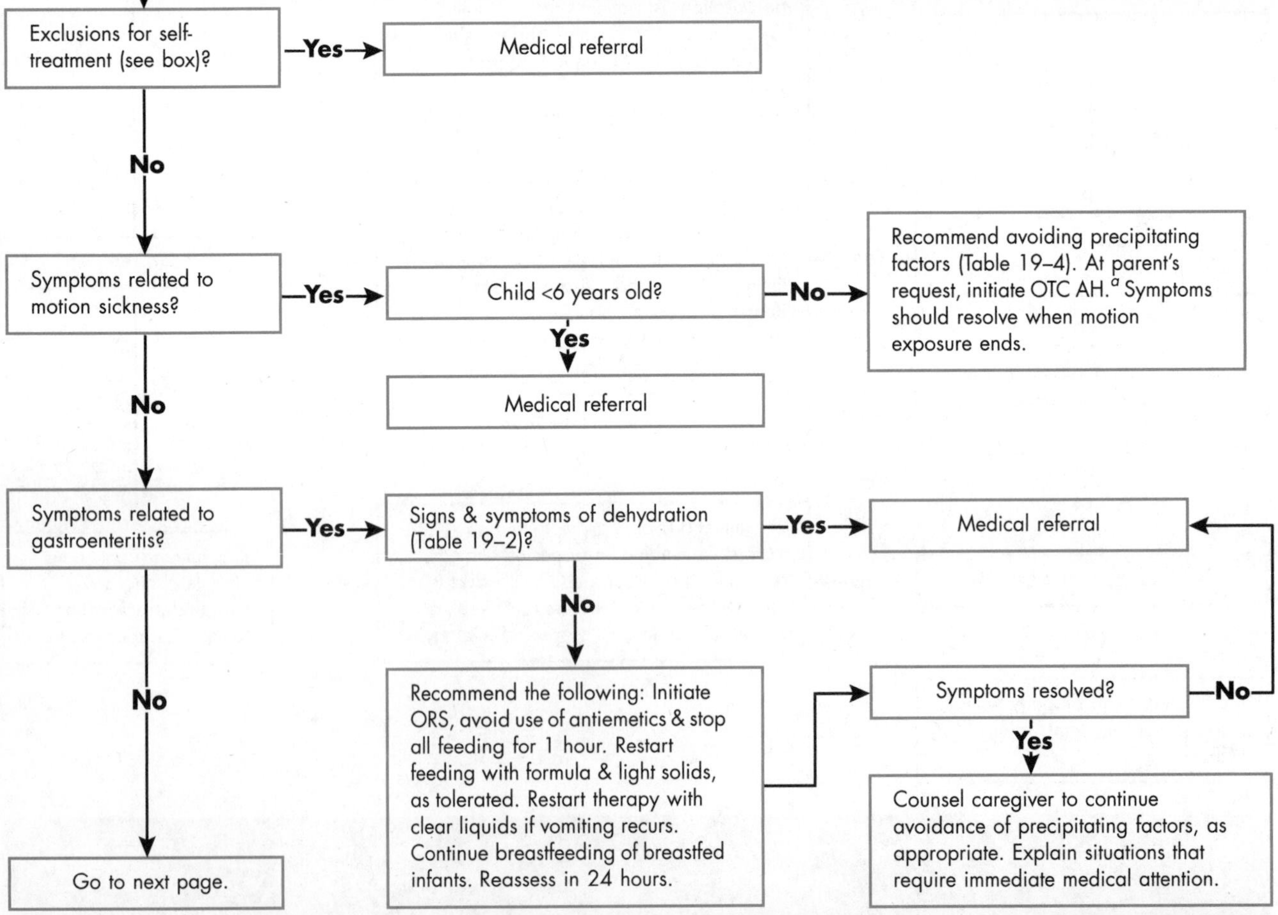
Child with complaint of N/V
Obtain significant medical history. Obtain medication, supplement & pertinent diet history. Ask about signs & symptoms in family members.
Exclusions for self-treatment (see box)?
Yes
Medical referral
No
Symptoms related to motion sickness?
Yes
Child <6 years old?
No
Recommend avoiding precipitating factors (Table 19–4). At parent's request, initiate OTC AH.[a] Symptoms should resolve when motion exposure ends.
Yes
Medical referral
No
Symptoms related to gastroenteritis?
Yes
Signs & symptoms of dehydration (Table 19–2)?
Yes
Medical referral
No
Recommend the following: Initiate ORS, avoid use of antiemetics & stop all feeding for 1 hour. Restart feeding with formula & light solids, as tolerated. Restart therapy with clear liquids if vomiting recurs. Continue breastfeeding of breastfed infants. Reassess in 24 hours.
Symptoms resolved?
No
Yes
Counsel caregiver to continue avoidance of precipitating factors, as appropriate. Explain situations that require immediate medical attention.
No
Go to next page.

FIGURE 19–3 Self-care for N/V in children. Key: AH = Antihistamine; CNS = central nervous system; GI = gastrointestinal; N/V = nausea and vomiting; ORS = oral rehydration salt; PCP = primary care provider. (Source: References 20 and 21.) (*continued on next page*)

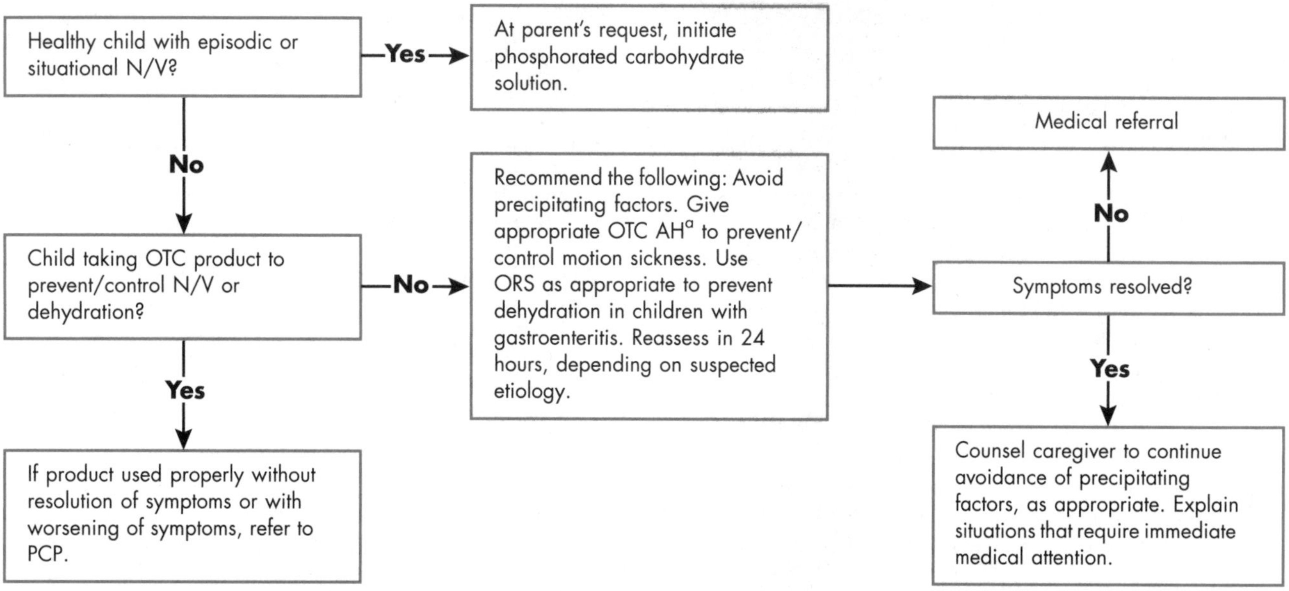

[a] Do not use meclizine in children younger than 12 years.

FIGURE 19–3 Self-care for N/V in children. Key: AH = Antihistamine; CNS = central nervous system; GI = gastrointestinal; N/V = nausea and vomiting; ORS = oral rehydration salt; PCP = primary care provider. (Source: References 20 and 21.) (*continued*)

Nonpharmacologic Therapy

ORS can be used for dehydration associated with vomiting or diarrhea.[25] In cases of vomiting, absorption of fluids may be compromised by continuous emesis in some patients. The World Health Organization (WHO) developed a solution for the treatment of dehydration.[26] ORS used by WHO and the United Nations Children's Fund (UNICEF) has a total osmolarity of 245 mOsm/L and includes 75 mmol/L of carbohydrates, 75 mmol/L of sodium, 20 mmol/L of potassium, 65 mmol/L chloride, and 10 mmol/L of citrate. A simple, glucose-based ORS solution can be made by mixing ½ teaspoon of salt and 6 teaspoons of sugar in 1.06 quarts (1 L) of clean water.[27] In less-developed countries with low health literacy, this formula is roughly explained as a pinch of salt and a handful of sugar. Although glucose-based ORS solution does not contain potassium, supplementation with bananas or orange juice could be given. Osmolarity of the glucose-based ORS solution is higher than that of water and, therefore, is more effective than water alone for rehydration. Commercially available products and the formula for a basic ORS solution are listed in Table 19–3.

Sports drinks, such as Gatorade or Powerade, often do not contain the recommended balance of electrolytes. The preferred ratio of sugar to sodium is 3:1. Original formula Gatorade contains a sugar-to-sodium ratio of 15:1. Dilution of sports drinks with water by the patient may be an option, but it is difficult to achieve accurate sugar-to-sodium ratios, plus sports drinks often are available in multiple formulations. Too much sugar may draw water into the GI tract and facilitate further dehydration. Similarly, sodas, such as

TABLE 19–3 **Selected ORS Solution Therapy**

Solution	Carbohydrate (g/L)	Sodium (mmol/L)	Potassium (mmol/L)	Chloride (mmol/L)	Base (citrate) (mmol/L)
WHO ORS	13.5	75	20	65	30
Enfalyte	30	50	25	45	11
Pedialyte	25	45	20	35	30
Rehydralyte	25	75	20	65	30
Ceralyte 50	40	50	20	40	30

Key: ORS = Oral rehydration salt; WHO = World Health Organization.

Source: Reference 27 and Oral electrolyte mixtures. Drug Facts and Comparisons eAnswers. Facts & Comparisons [database online]. St. Louis, MO: Wolters Kluwer Worldwide; 2016. Available at: http://online.factsandcomparisons.com. Accessed March 31, 2016.

ginger ale or cola, and fruit juices, such as apple, may also contain too much sugar.[20]

The typical dosing of ORS solution varies according to the level of dehydration and the age and weight of the patient. For minimal dehydration, children weighing less than 10 kg should be given 60–120 mL of solution after each vomiting episode; children weighing 10 kg or more should be given 120–240 mL per episode. Mild–moderate dehydration should be treated with 50–100 mL/kg over 3–4 hours. Severe dehydration should be referred to emergency care for intravenous rehydration.[24] Adults should also be rehydrated, but they may gauge their need according to thirst. Replacing 30%–50% of the fluid loss in the first 24 hours is preferred.[16]

Oral rehydration should be offered 10 minutes after the last episode of vomiting and should be offered in small increments. In general, 5 mL of ORS solution may be given to children every 5 minutes, and 15 mL may be given to older children and adults every 5 minutes.[20] Dosage forms such as Pedialyte Freezer Pops may offer the slow administration desired in active vomiting.

Other nonpharmacologic measures, such as those listed in Table 19–4, can also be tried to minimize and prevent motion sickness.[2] Because teratogenicity is a major consideration, many providers are reluctant to prescribe medications for pregnant women. Similarly, many of the medications are excreted in breast milk of lactating women, so nonpharmacologic approaches may be recommended in these populations although such measures are not evidence based[28] (Table 19–5).

Pharmacologic Therapy

Selection of a nonprescription medication for N/V is largely determined by the potential cause.

Nausea Associated With Motion Sickness

Antihistamines are effective and generally safe and well tolerated for N/V related to motion sickness. A detailed description of antihistamines can be found in Chapter 11. Meclizine and diphenhydramine are Food and Drug Administration (FDA)-approved nonprescription agents for the prevention of nausea, vomiting, or dizziness associated with motion sickness. Doxylamine has been used as off-label treatment for nausea. Table 19–6 lists age-specific dosages and maximum daily limits for these antiemetics.[29] Because of their anticholinergic effects, antihistamines may thicken bronchial secretions and should be used with caution in patients with respiratory conditions such as asthma, chronic bronchitis, and emphysema. In addition, the mydriatic effects of antihistamines may exacerbate angle-closure glaucoma. The urinary retention effects of antihistamines may also exacerbate symptoms of benign prostatic hypertrophy. Other adverse effects of nonprescription antihistamines include dry mouth, confusion, dizziness, tremors, and constipation.[17] Drowsiness is also a common adverse effect of antihistamines. Patients should avoid concomitant use of antihistamines with other CNS depressants, such as alcohol, hypnotics, and sedatives. This drowsiness, coupled with the potential for blurred vision, may inhibit the ability to drive safely or operate heavy machinery. Meclizine may be less sedating than doxylamine and diphenhydramine. Paradoxical stimulatory reactions such as insomnia, nervousness, and irritability may occur in some patients. Diphenhydramine is a mild–moderate inhibitor of the cytochrome P450 (CYP) 2D6 enzyme. Therefore, it should be used with caution with other medications metabolized by CYP2D6, such as certain opiates, psychiatric medications, beta blockers, and antiarrhythmics. Some case reports have noted that ultrarapid metabolizers of CYP2D6 may be at a higher risk for this paradoxical excitation. In the United States, approximately 1%–2% of the population are estimated to be ultrarapid metabolizers.[30]

TABLE 19–4 Nonpharmacologic Measures to Prevent Motion Sickness

- Avoid reading during travel.
- Focus the line of vision fairly straight ahead (e.g., seat the patient in a position that allows vision out of the car window).
- Avoid excess food or alcohol before and during extended travel.
- Stay where motion is least experienced (e.g., front of the car; near the wings of an airplane; or midship [midway between bow and stern], preferably on deck).
- Avoid strong odors, particularly from food or tobacco smoke.
- Drive the vehicle if possible.

Source: Reference 2.

TABLE 19–5 Nonpharmacologic Measures to Prevent NVP

- Take a prenatal multivitamin for 3 months prior to conception.
- Before getting out of bed, eat several dry crackers and relax in bed for 10–15 minutes.
- Get out of bed very slowly and do not make any sudden movements.
- Before eating breakfast, nibble on dry toast or crackers.
- Make sure there is plenty of fresh air in the area where meals are prepared and eaten.
- Eat small meals every 1–2 hours to avoid a full stomach.
- Avoid areas of excessive heat or humidity.
- When nauseated, try small sips of carbonated beverages or fruit juices.
- Avoid greasy or fatty foods such as fried foods, gravy, mayonnaise, and salad dressing, as well as spicy or acidic foods (citrus fruits and beverages, tomatoes).
- Avoid sensory stimuli such as odors, noises, or flickering lights.
- Avoid iron-containing supplements.
- Eat dry, bland, and high-protein foods.

Key: NVP = Nausea and vomiting of pregnancy.
Source: References 17 and 28.

Nausea Associated With Food or Beverages

N/V may be associated with overindulgence in food or beverage or consumption of disagreeable foods, and it may present as heartburn, indigestion, and upset stomach. Antacids and histamine-2 receptor antagonists (H2RAs) are approved to relieve symptoms associated with acid indigestion and sour stomach. However, antacids have marginal efficacy for the treatment of N/V secondary to nonulcer dyspepsia. Prolonged and predominant nausea and bloating may be a sign of GI motility dysfunction and may require prescription promotility agents.[31]

TABLE 19–6 **Dosage Guidelines for Nonprescription Antiemetic Antihistamines**[a]

Agent	Dosage (maximum daily dosage): Adults and Children ≥12 Years	Children 6 to <12 Years	Children 2 to <6 Years
Cyclizine	50 mg 30 minutes before travel, then 50 mg every 4–6 hours (200 mg)	25 mg every 6–8 hours (75 mg)	Not recommended
Dimenhydrinate	50–100 mg every 4–6 hours (400 mg)	25–50 mg every 6–8 hours (150 mg)	12.5–25 mg every 6–8 hours (75 mg)
Diphenhydramine	25–50 mg every 6–8 hours (300 mg)	12.5–25 mg every 6–8 hours (150 mg)	Not recommended
Meclizine	25–50 mg 1 hour before travel (50 mg)	Not recommended	Not recommended
Doxylamine[b]	In pregnancy, 10–12.5 mg with or without pyridoxine every 8 hours	Not recommended	Not recommended

[a] Take antihistamines at least 30–60 minutes before travel; then take continuously for the duration of travel.
[b] Off-label use for nausea and vomiting in pregnancy.
Source: References 3, 28, and Nausea and vomiting in infants and children. DynaMed Plus [subscription database online]. EBSCO Health. Updated July 28, 2015. Available at: http://www.dynamed.com/login.aspx?direct=true&site=DynaMed&id=900008. Accessed May 13, 207.

Bismuth subsalicylate may have some benefits for nausea associated with consumption or nonulcer dyspepsia.[32] Bismuth subsalicylate is approved to treat various GI symptoms, including nausea, heartburn, and fullness. In-depth discussion of bismuth subsalicylate can be found in Chapters 13 and 16.

Phosphorated carbohydrate solution (PCS) may also be useful in nausea associated with a food or beverage. This solution is a mixture of dextrose (glucose), levulose (fructose), and phosphoric acid.[33] The hyperosmolar solution is believed to relieve N/V by direct local action on the GI tract wall that may decrease smooth muscle contraction and delay gastric emptying time.[34]

Alternatively, concentrated cola syrup, which also contains the sugars and phosphoric acid that are in PCS, has been used. Because commercially available soda often has a 5:1 water-to-syrup ratio, substituting soda, even if flattened, is not recommended. In adults PCS should be given at 15–30 mL every 15 minutes until distress subsides. Taking more than 5 doses in 1 hour is not recommended. Children 2–12 years can take 5–10 mL every 15 minutes. Dosing should not be diluted, and other fluids should be avoided immediately before or after taking PCS.[33]

Possible adverse effects of PCS are stomach pain and diarrhea. Each 5 mL of PCS contains 3.74 g of total sugar,[35] so caution should be used in patients with diabetes. Similarly, patients with hereditary fructose intolerance should avoid using PCS.

Product Selection Guidelines

Several factors that should be considered in the choice of antiemetic products include whether the patient is pregnant or lactating, the patient is a child or of advanced age, and the patient has any therapeutic limitations, such as hepatic or renal impairment. These factors may affect drug selection and dosing. Furthermore, the product should so be compatible with the patient's lifestyle, concurrent medication use, sensitivity to certain product ingredients such as dyes or fructose, and preference for frequency of dosing. Hence, product selection guidelines should be compatible with special populations and patient factors, such as drug interactions, and should consider patient preferences, such as whether the product is liquid or chewable or contains alcohol (Table 19–7). (See Chapter 11, section "Special Populations," for FDA requirements for dispensing devices included in liquid nonprescription products.)

Special Populations

PREGNANCY. Several nonpharmacologic recommendations can be made to help control NVP. Mild nausea can be prevented by eating frequent small meals and avoiding spicy or fatty foods or sensory stimuli that may provoke symptoms. Bland carbohydrates, such as crackers, and high-protein snacks may be beneficial, especially in the morning. However, there is little published evidence supporting dietary changes for prevention of N/V. In patients with a history of NVP, the American College of Obstetricians and Gynecologists (ACOG) recommends taking a multivitamin for 3 months prior to conception to decrease the severity of NVP.[28] This measure may not be useful if pregnant patients are presenting with nausea, but it may be an option for future preconception counseling.

A Cochrane review published in 2015 found limited strong evidence to support the use of nonprescription antiemetics, such as doxylamine and pyridoxine, for NVP.[3] ACOG recommends pyridoxine with or without doxylamine as first-line pharmacotherapy for NVP.[28] The safety of the combination of pyridoxine and doxylamine in pregnancy is supported by a review of more than 170,000 exposures.[28] Pyridoxine is also excreted in breast milk. Extremely high doses of pyridoxine (600 mg/day) may inhibit prolactin secretion.[36] A combination product was approved in April 2013 as prescription-only.[37] Ginger may be as effective as pyridoxine for treating NVP. (See Chapter 51 for further discussion of this treatment.)

GERIATRIC. Antihistamines should be used with caution in patients of advanced age because of the increased risk of adverse effects. The anticholinergic and sedative effects may not be tolerable in this patient population. The American Geriatrics Society treats these medications as potentially inappropriate and strongly recommends avoiding use of antihistamines in patients of advanced age.[38] In addition, a comprehensive medication review may be necessary in this population to identify and resolve any potential drug-related problems, including drug interactions.

PCS may be used if the patient does not have uncontrolled blood glucose levels or hereditary fructose intolerance. Neither acupressure nor any acustimulation product, such as acupressure bands, should be used in patients with pacemakers. Other

TABLE 19–7 **Selected Nonprescription Antiemetic Products and Common Drug Interactions**

Antiemetic	Drug	Potential Interaction	Management and Prevention Measures
Bismuth subsalicylate	Tetracyclines (tetracycline, doxycycline, minocycline, demeclocycline)	Decreased antibacterial effect caused by impaired absorption	Avoid concurrent administration; take doxycycline 2–3 hours before bismuth subsalicylate.
	Warfarin	Increased risk of bleeding (elevations of INR)	Avoid concurrent use; monitor INR closely near times of administration and discontinuation of bismuth subsalicylate.
	Live vaccines containing varicella or influenza	Increased risk of Reye's syndrome	Avoid concurrent administration with live vaccines.
Antihistamines (cyclizine, doxylamine, dimenhydrinate, diphenhydramine, meclizine)	Anticholinergics (ipratropium, tiotropium)	May increase anticholinergic adverse effects	Monitor for signs of altered mental status, dry skin, dry mouth, constipation, mydriasis, and tachycardia.
	Opioid-related agents (fentanyl, hydrocodone, hydromorphone, methadone, morphine, oxycodone)	May increase sedative adverse effects	Monitor for signs of respiratory suppression, sedation, and hypotension. Consider lower doses of the concomitant agents.
	Bupropion	May lower seizure threshold	Use lowest therapeutic dose of bupropion and increase slowly.
	Donepezil	May lower seizure threshold	Use lowest therapeutic dose of donepezil and increase slowly.
Ginger	Warfarin	Increased risk of bleeding (elevation of INR), possibly seen at higher doses of ginger exceeding 4 g/day	Avoid use of ginger if possible.
Pyridoxine	Altretamine	Reduced anticancer effects of altretamine	Avoid concurrent use.

Key: INR = International normalized ratio.
Source: References 4, 17, and 40.

nonpharmacologic options such as avoiding trigger foods and scents could also be considered.

LACTATION. Antihistamines may adversely affect the mother's milk supply, so nursing mothers should not use these agents. Bismuth subsalicylate should also be used cautiously, according to the American Academy of Pediatrics. Although the bismuth is poorly absorbed, the salicylate is excreted and eliminated slowly in the milk.[39] There is little evidence to support the safety of the use of ginger by lactating women.

PEDIATRIC. In newborns and infants, vomiting may lead rapidly to dehydration and acid–base disturbances. Vomiting is different from simple regurgitation, which is common in infants. Vomiting is distinguished as being more forceful and containing larger amounts of emesis. In newborns, vomiting may be caused by GI tract obstruction. In infants, vomiting may be a sign of gastroesophageal reflux disease (GERD). N/V can occur in children for a variety of reasons, including GI obstruction, CNS abnormalities, and infection.[40]

CDC classifies dehydration in children as mild if less than 3% of body weight is lost, moderate if 3%–9% is lost, and severe if greater than 9% is lost.[20] Moderate–severe cases of dehydration should warrant a medical referral. Mild–moderate cases of dehydration should be treated with oral rehydration therapy as described in this chapter and in Chapter 16. Antihistamines may diminish mental alertness and occasionally produce paradoxical excitation in young children.[29] BSS is not recommended in children or teenagers who have or are recovering from chickenpox or influenza-like symptoms because of the risk of Reye's syndrome.[41] (See Chapter 5 for further information.)

Complementary Therapies

Some evidence supports the use of ginger, pyridoxine (vitamin B_6), and acupressure bands in the treatment of nausea.

Ginger

Ginger (*Zingiber officinale*) has been used for nausea related to pregnancy, motion sickness, and surgery.[42] A 2015 Cochrane review of ginger found limited and inconsistent evidence for its efficacy, although several studies suggested that ginger may be superior to placebo in preventing NVP.[3] The review reported no difference in spontaneous abortion, congenital abnormalities, or other fetal adverse outcomes, although the included studies may have had insufficient power.[3] Other data regarding the safety of the use of ginger in pregnancy are limited. Larger doses of ginger may lead to mild adverse GI effects, including heartburn, diarrhea, and mouth irritation.[43] Some evidence suggests that ginger may have anticoagulant and hypotensive effects. In some countries, such as Finland and Denmark, ginger carries cautionary warnings for its use in pregnancy.[44]

Ginger can be dosed at 250 mg to 2 g per day in 3–4 divided doses although it appears that doses around 1 g/day are more effective than placebo.[43] Ginger may be as effective as pyridoxine for treating N/V. Compared with dimenhydrinate, ginger may cause fewer adverse effects.[45] (See Chapter 51 for an in-depth discussion of ginger.)

Most ginger ale products often are artificially flavored or contain amounts of ginger that are too insignificant to be therapeutic.

Pyridoxine (Vitamin B_6)

Pyridoxine is a water-soluble B vitamin that is important in various metabolic functions, including protein metabolism, hemoglobin synthesis, and neurotransmitter function.[36] The dietary reference intake of pyridoxine in healthy adults is 1.3–2 mg/day. Pyridoxine may be used in NVP. Typical dosing of pyridoxine for nausea is 10–25 mg 3 times a day.

Pyridoxine is generally well tolerated. Large doses (>200 mg/day) of pyridoxine over longer periods of time (>2 months) may result in adverse effects such as peripheral neuropathy, weakness, lethargy, and nystagmus.

Pyridoxine has had mixed results for efficacy in treating N/V. Overall data suggest that pyridoxine is effective.[28] NVP is an off-label indication for pyridoxine.

Acupressure

The use of acupressure involves direct pressure on the pericardium-6 (P6) point on either wrist. The P6 point is located approximately three finger widths from the middle crease of the wrist (see acupuncture-points.org). Pressure can be applied between the two tendons using either the finger or a wristband. Acupressure at P6 may be more effective for preventing postoperative N/V than NVP.[3,46] The "dosing" of acupressure can vary from as needed, to 10 minutes 3 times a day, to continuous pressure. The dosing regimens showed mixed results for efficacy.[47]

Aromatherapy

The use of peppermint oil for the treatment of N/V does not have reliable evidence to support its efficacy. In addition, the use of isopropyl alcohol may be more effective than a saline placebo but less effective than other standard antiemetic medications (both prescription and nonprescription). This lack of efficacy was found in studies that looked at the use of rescue antiemetics for postoperative N/V. Evidence is lacking to support aromatherapy for self-treatment of N/V.[48]

Assessment of Nausea and Vomiting: A Case-Based Approach

Vomiting is a symptom produced not only by benign processes but also by serious illnesses, and it may cause various complications. Physical assessment of the patient may help to determine whether some of the complications of N/V listed in the section "Clinical Presentation of Nausea and Vomiting" have occurred. Physical assessment should include the patient's general appearance, mental status, and volume status, and the presence of any abdominal pain. Evaluation of vital signs such as blood pressure, heart rate, temperature, and weight is also pertinent. Evaluation of concurrent signs and symptoms is useful in determining the potential cause of vomiting. It is also vital to determine whether a toxin could be the cause of the acute onset of vomiting. Therefore, asking about possible ingestion of a toxin, especially in preschoolers and adolescents, is necessary. Detailed information about the patient's medical history related to the GI tract is especially helpful in determining potential causes.

A major concern with vomiting is the loss of fluids and the inability to eat or drink. This situation may result in dehydration and electrolyte disturbances. Self-care is inappropriate for patients with dehydration, severe anorexia, weight loss, or poor nutritional status. Medical evaluation for dehydration should be provided when severe vomiting or diarrhea persists for more than several hours in children or for 48 hours in adults.[16,20,22]

Providers should be aware that some patients might use nonprescription antiemetics to self-treat the early stages of a serious illness. Therefore, to avoid potential additive toxicity, providers should ask patients what they have already used to treat the symptoms. Many patients choose to self-medicate with various nonprescription products to avoid a medical office visit. However, providers should be cautious about recommending self-medication for N/V symptoms and should ask appropriate questions to determine whether medical referral is indicated.

Cases 19–1 and 19–2 are examples of the assessment of patients presenting with vomiting.

Patient Counseling for Nausea and Vomiting

Providers should stress that treatment of N/V must focus on identifying and, if possible, correcting the underlying cause. Patients prone to overeating, eating disorders, or motion sickness should try to avoid behaviors or situations that cause N/V. Patients should be advised that acute vomiting typically requires only symptomatic treatment, because it is usually self-limiting and will resolve spontaneously. If the cause of the symptoms is known and self-treatment is appropriate, proper use of the recommended product should be explained. Patient education should also include information about possible adverse effects, as well as signs and symptoms that indicate further medical attention is warranted. The box "Patient Education for Nausea and Vomiting" lists specific information to provide patients.

Evaluation of Patient Outcomes for Nausea and Vomiting

After a provider has provided information or suggestions for self-management and treatment of N/V, a follow-up assessment of the patient should occur within 24 hours of the initial encounter. A validated assessment tool, established by Rhodes and McDaniel, can be used to monitor symptoms and can be found at http://www.helpher.org/downloads/rhodes-index.pdf.[49] The follow-up should include an assessment of whether the N/V has diminished or abated; whether the patient has any residual related symptoms, such as signs or symptoms of dehydration; whether abnormal vital signs such as tachycardia have returned to normal; and whether the patient is afebrile. If the patient had prolonged N/V (>24–48 hours) or a change in or worsening of symptoms that required immediate referral for medical evaluation, the provider should follow up to determine whether the patient sought medical help and what type of treatment was administered. It is also important for the provider

CASE 19-1

Relevant Evaluation Criteria	Scenario/Model Outcome
Collect	
1. Gather essential information about the patient's symptoms and medical history, including	
a. Description of symptom(s) (i.e., nature, onset, duration, severity, associated symptoms)	Patient has had frequent episodes of nausea for the past 4 days. She has vomited twice in those 4 days. The nausea lasts a few hours during the main part of the day. She has maintained her appetite.
b. Description of any factors that seem to precipitate, exacerbate, and/or relieve the patient's symptom(s)	Symptoms seem to worsen when the patient smells food in the oven and when she wakes up in the morning. She is also nauseated at work.
c. Description of the patient's efforts to relieve the symptoms	The patient eats some dry toast and takes a few sips of ginger ale or water. If she is at home, she will sit quietly with her eyes closed.
d. Patient's identity	Rebecca Forrester
e. Patient's age, gender, height, and weight	28 years old, female, 5 ft 5 in., 135 lb
f. Patient's occupation	Loan officer
g. Patient's dietary habits	Balanced diet with plenty of fruits and vegetables. Patient is able to eat well between nausea episodes.
h. Patient's sleep habits	Averages 7–8 hours per night.
i. Concurrent medical conditions, prescription and nonprescription medications, and dietary supplements	Patient has no chronic conditions. She found out she is 7 weeks pregnant and began a prenatal vitamin. She denies use of dietary supplements.
j. Allergies	Sulfa: rash
k. History of other adverse reactions to medications	Stomach upset with codeine
l. Other (describe) _______	n/a
Assess	
2. Differentiate patient's signs/symptoms, and correctly identify the patient's primary problem(s).	Nausea lasting a few hours during the main part of the day; occasional vomiting. She does not like the smell of certain foods; NVP is likely.
3. Identify exclusions for self-treatment (Figure 19–2).	None
4. Formulate a comprehensive list of therapeutic alternatives for the primary problem to determine whether triage to a health care provider is required, and share this information with the patient or caregiver.	Options include (1) Recommend self-care with – Nondrug strategies (dietary and environmental changes [Table 19–5]) – Acupressure or acustimulation bands – OTC pyridoxine – OTC doxylamine – OTC phosphorated carbohydrate solution – Ginger (2) Recommend lifestyle modifications until an HCP may be consulted. (3) Make a medical referral. (4) Take no action.
Plan	
5. Select an optimal therapeutic alternative to address the patient's problem, taking into account patient preferences.	Because the patient does not appear dehydrated and can drink small amounts of ginger ale and water, and she can tolerate dry toast, encourage her to continue to take sips of liquids and eat toast. She does not have signs/symptoms of dehydration, such as fast heartbeat, decreased skin turgor, noticeable weight loss, or clothes that fit loosely. She can try doxylamine 12.5 mg 3 times a day and vitamin B_6 10 mg 3 times a day. Other nonpharmacologic suggestions in Table 19–5 should be followed. If symptoms persist, she should consult her provider.

CASE 19–1 *continued*

Relevant Evaluation Criteria	Scenario/Model Outcome
6. Describe the recommended therapeutic approach to the patient or caregiver.	"You probably have nausea and vomiting of pregnancy, or NVP. You can take vitamin B_6 orally every 8 hours. In addition, you may add doxylamine 12.5 mg orally every 8 hours. You may also benefit from other nonpharmacologic techniques (Table 19–5), such as continuing to eat dry toast or eating bland foods and crackers in the morning before arising, sleeping in a well-ventilated room, and avoiding strong odors. If you do not feel better, you may want to contact your provider."
7. Explain to the patient or caregiver the rationale for selecting the recommended therapeutic approach from the considered therapeutic alternatives.	"The American College of Obstetricians and Gynecologists state that doxylamine and vitamin B_6, up to 3 tablets daily, may help your symptoms. Because you are able to drink fluids and are not dehydrated, seeking medical care may not be necessary at this time. However, if nausea or vomiting worsens, medical attention for further evaluation is necessary."
Implement	
8. When recommending self-care with nonprescription medications and/or nondrug therapy, convey accurate information to the patient or caregiver.	
a. Appropriate dose and frequency of administration	"Add vitamin B_6 10 mg combined with 12.5 mg of doxylamine (½ of a 25 mg tablet). Doxylamine is available in the United States as a nonprescription sleep aid (doxylamine succinate [Unisom SleepTabs] 25 mg)."
b. Maximum number of days the therapy should be employed	"There are no limits to the number of days that vitamin B_6 and doxylamine can be taken. Nausea associated with pregnancy typically resolves between weeks 16 and 20."
c. Product administration procedures	"Take vitamin B_6 and doxylamine with a small glass of water 3–4 times a day."
d. Expected time to onset of relief/degree of relief that can be reasonably expected	"Expected time to onset of relief and degree of relief are variable for all products and measures."
e. Most common adverse effects	"Vitamin B_6 is not likely to cause any adverse effects. Drowsiness is the most common side effect of doxylamine; therefore, it is important not to drive or operate machinery while taking doxylamine. Other possible adverse effects include dry mouth, dry eyes, nasal congestion, urinary retention, and constipation."
f. Patient options in the event that condition worsens or persists	"Medical attention is necessary if the NVP does not improve or if adverse effects from the nonprescription product occur."
g. Product storage requirements	"Store product at 59°F–86°F."
h. Specific nondrug measures	See Table 19–5 for dietary and other measures.
Solicit follow-up questions from the patient or caregiver.	(1) "Will any of these products hurt my baby?" (2) "What other products could I use instead?"
Answer the patient's or caregiver's questions.	(1) "These products have been used by many other pregnant women and have not caused harm to the mother or baby. Pregnant women have been exposed to these products hundreds of thousands of times without evidence of harm to the baby." (2) "Another product used for nausea during pregnancy is an acupressure band that is worn on the wrists for a short period of time, such as 5 minutes, or throughout the day. Ginger can also be considered. Phosphorated carbohydrate solution may also be tried. If these products do not work, then medical attention is necessary to consider a prescription product for your nausea."
Follow-up: Monitor and Evaluate	
9. Assess patient outcome.	Monitor for episodes of nausea and vomiting.

Key: HCP = Health care provider; n/a = not applicable; NVP = nausea and vomiting of pregnancy; OTC = over-the-counter.

CASE 19-2

Relevant Evaluation Criteria	Scenario/Model Outcome
Collect	
1. Gather essential information about the patient's symptoms and medical history, including	
a. Description of symptom(s) (i.e., nature, onset, duration, severity, associated symptoms)	Patient has had five episodes of nausea, vomiting, and diarrhea in the past 12 hours. The patient seems somnolent and quiet except for violent episodes of vomiting or diarrhea.
b. Description of any factors that seem to precipitate, exacerbate, and/or relieve the patient's symptom(s)	Symptoms worsen when the patient's mother attempts to provide small sips of grape juice.
c. Description of the patient's efforts to relieve the symptoms	Patient's mother tried to get the child to eat a few bites of crackers or drink sips of fluid.
d. Patient's identity	David Smith
e. Patient's age, gender, height, and weight	18 months old, male, 25 inches, 23 lb (26 lb on previous day)
f. Patient's occupation	n/a
g. Patient's dietary habits	Normal healthy diet; consists of cereals, mashed vegetables, pasta, rice, chicken, yogurt, milk, and juice
h. Patient's sleep habits	Up at 7:00 AM; in bed at 7:30 PM; naps for 2 hours from 1–3 PM.
i. Concurrent medical conditions, prescription and nonprescription medications, and dietary supplements	Children's multivitamin with fluoride; patient is up to date on all recommended childhood vaccines, including rotavirus.
j. Allergies	Eggs: stomach upset
k. History of other adverse reactions to medications	None
l. Other (describe) ______	n/a
Assess	
2. Differentiate patient's signs/symptoms, and correctly identify the patient's primary problem(s).	Patient has had several episodes of nausea, vomiting, and diarrhea. The patient appears drowsy and unusually lethargic, and his body appears floppy. The child appears dizzy when he stands up and his abdomen seems somewhat flat. He has had a dry diaper for most of the day. Although the child appears to cry, few tears are noted. Patient appears dehydrated and may have viral gastroenteritis.
3. Identify exclusions for self-treatment (Figure 19–3).	On the basis of his signs/symptoms, patient appears severely dehydrated (Table 19–2).
4. Formulate a comprehensive list of therapeutic alternatives for the primary problem to determine whether triage to a health care provider is required, and share this information with the patient or caregiver.	Options include (1) Recommend that patient's mother administer – OTC ORS solution – OTC phosphorated carbohydrate solution – an acupressure band (2) Recommend that patient's mother administer self-care modalities until a health care provider can be consulted. (3) Refer patient for further medical evaluation. (4) Take no action.
Plan	
5. Select an optimal therapeutic alternative to address the patient's problem, taking into account patient preferences.	David is unable to drink small amounts of fluid or eat small bites of crackers. He also has signs/symptoms of dehydration (appears drowsy and lethargic; has a floppy body, dizziness, flat abdomen; has lost 3 lb, approximately 12% of his body weight since the previous day; has a dry diaper and sheds few tears). On the basis of these signs/symptoms, the patient's mother should immediately take the child for medical evaluation and attempt to administer small sips of ORS solution on the way to the emergency department.
6. Describe the recommended therapeutic approach to the patient or caregiver.	"Your child needs to be seen by a health care provider, because he appears dehydrated. Please have someone drive you and your child to the emergency department at the hospital. On the way, administer 1 teaspoonful of ORS solution, not grape juice, every 1–2 minutes."

CASE 19-2 *continued*

Relevant Evaluation Criteria	Scenario/Model Outcome
7. Explain to the patient or caregiver the rationale for selecting the recommended therapeutic approach from the considered therapeutic alternatives.	"Your child's symptoms (floppy body, flat abdomen, weight loss, dry diaper, few tears) indicate that he is dehydrated. Because he has been unable to drink sufficient fluids or eat anything to counter the dehydration, he needs medical attention."
Implement	
8. When recommending self-care with nonprescription medications and/or nondrug therapy, convey accurate information to the patient or caregiver.	Criterion does not apply in this case.
Solicit follow-up questions from the patient or caregiver.	"Is there a nonprescription medication that might work so that I don't have to take him to the emergency department?"
Answer the patient's or caregiver's questions.	"No. Your child is dehydrated; he needs urgent medical care so that he can feel better and get well."
Follow-up: Monitor and Evaluate	
9. Assess patient outcome.	Monitor for signs of dehydration, including weight loss. Look for normal behaviors and activities.

Key: n/a = Not applicable; ORS = oral rehydration salt; OTC = over-the-counter.

PATIENT EDUCATION FOR

Patient Education for Nausea and Vomiting

The objectives of self-treatment are (1) to improve the symptoms of occasional, self-limited nausea and vomiting (N/V), (2) to identify and correct the underlying cause, (3) to prevent and correct complications of vomiting, and (4) to prevent future occurrences. For most patients, carefully following product instructions and the self-care measures listed here will help ensure optimal therapeutic outcomes.

Nondrug Measures

- To prevent nausea and vomiting of pregnancy (NVP), eat small, frequent meals that are low in fat content. Sleep in a room with fresh air. Also, try eating crackers or a high-protein snack before getting up in the morning. Try lying down to relieve the symptoms once they occur (Table 19–5).
- To prevent motion sickness in young children, place them in a car seat that allows them to look out the windows (Table 19–4). Try acupressure wristbands to prevent motion sickness in adults or older children.
- To prevent nausea associated with overeating, avoid foods or beverages known to cause nausea; consume foods and beverages in moderation.

Nonprescription Medications

Antacids, Histamine-2 Receptor Antagonists (H2RAs), and Bismuth Subsalicylate

- Take antacids, H2RAs (e.g., ranitidine or famotidine), or bismuth subsalicylate for nausea caused by overeating. Follow product instructions for dosages. (See Chapters 13 and 16 for additional information on these medications.)

Phosphorated Carbohydrate Solution

- Take phosphorated carbohydrate solutions for nausea and vomiting associated with upset stomach caused by viral gastroenteritis, food indiscretions, and pregnancy.
- Give 1–2 tablespoonsful (15–30 mL) of the solution to adults at 15-minute intervals until vomiting stops. For children ages 2–12 years old, give 1–2 teaspoonsful (5–10 mL). Do not give more than 5 doses in 1 hour.
- Do not dilute the solution, and do not allow the patient to consume other liquids for 15 minutes after taking a dose.
- Patients with hereditary fructose intolerance should not take this product.
- Patients with diabetes should consult their medical provider before taking this product.

Antihistamines

- Take antihistamines for self-treatment of N/V caused by motion sickness.
- To prevent motion sickness, take antihistamines at least 30–60 minutes before departure. Continue taking the medication during travel. Follow the dosage guidelines in Table 19–6.
- While using antihistamines, avoid driving or operating hazardous machinery or engaging in tasks that require a high degree of mental alertness. Drowsiness is the most common adverse effect of these medications.
- Patients with asthma, narrow-angle glaucoma, obstructive disease of the gastrointestinal or genitourinary tract, or benign prostatic hypertrophy should consult a health care provider before using antihistamines.
- Caution patients that antihistamines may increase the sedative effects of alcohol, tranquilizers, hypnotics, and sedatives. Antihistamines may produce excitability in children or mental confusion in persons of advanced age.
- Do not take oral diphenhydramine products if topical (external) diphenhydramine preparations are being used.

Oral Rehydration Salt (ORS) Solution

- If needed, take an ORS solution to prevent dehydration secondary to vomiting and diarrhea.
- Consider placing ORS solution in the refrigerator to improve taste. Alternatively, the patient can use freezer pops or another dosage form to improve palatability.

When to Seek Medical Attention

- Seek medical attention if there are signs and symptoms of serious dehydration associated with N/V.
- Seek medical attention if vomiting does not stop after 5 doses of a phosphorated carbohydrate solution.

to assess whether he or she needs to provide any further counseling or answer additional questions. The provider should also use this opportunity to provide reassurance and support.

Key Points for Nausea and Vomiting

- N/V are symptoms of an underlying disorder; therefore, treatment should focus on identifying and correcting the underlying cause.
- Nonprescription antiemetic medications are suitable for preventing and controlling the symptoms of occasional self-limiting N/V.
- Overeating, food poisoning, viral gastroenteritis, and motion sickness may cause self-limiting N/V.
- Antacids, nonprescription H2RAs, or PCS may improve symptoms associated with indigestion from overeating.
- Antihistamines are the agents of choice to treat N/V secondary to motion sickness.
- Agents that may be used safely to treat NVP and N/V in all persons 2 years of age and older include acupressure/acustimulation devices and PCS.
- Uncomplicated NVP may be treated with pyridoxine, doxylamine, PCS, ginger, or acupressure/acustimulation devices.
- Loss of fluids and the inability to eat or drink because of N/V may result in dehydration and electrolyte disturbances. This primary complication of N/V should be treated with ORS.
- A patient who presents with complications related to N/V may not be a candidate for self-treatment but instead should be referred for medical evaluation.

REFERENCES

1. Centers for Disease Control and Prevention. *National Hospital Ambulatory Medical Care Survey: 2011 emergency department summary tables.* Available at: http://www.cdc.gov/nchs/data/ahcd/nhamcs_emergency/2011_ed_web_tables.pdf. Accessed May 13, 2017.
2. Brainard A, Gresham C. Prevention and treatment of motion sickness. *Am Fam Physician.* 2014;90(1):41–6. PMID: 25077501.
3. Matthews A, Haas DM, O'Mathúna DP, et al. Interventions for nausea and vomiting in early pregnancy. *Cochrane Database Syst Rev.* 2015;9:CD007575. doi: 10.1002/14651858.CD007575.pub4.
4. Badell ML, Ramin SM, Smith JA. Treatment options for nausea and vomiting during pregnancy. *Pharmacotherapy.* 2006;26(9):1273–87. doi: 10.1592/phco.26.9.1273.
5. Einarson A, Maltepe C, Boskovic R, et al. Treatment of nausea and vomiting in pregnancy—an updated algorithm. *Can Fam Physician.* 2007; 53(12):2109–11. PMCID: PMC2231543.
6. Allen K. The vomiting child: what to do and when to consult. *Aust Fam Physician.* 2007;36(9):684–7. PMID: 17885698.
7. Colletti JE, Brown KM, Sharieff GQ, et al. The management of children with gastroenteritis and dehydration in the emergency department. *J Emerg Med.* 2010;38(5):686–98. doi: 10.1016/j.jemermed.2008.06.015.
8. Metz A. Nausea and vomiting in adults: a diagnostic approach. *Aust Fam Physician.* 2007;36(9):688–92. PMID: 17885699.
9. Centers for Disease Control and Prevention. Prevention of rotavirus gastroenteritis among infants and children. Recommendations of the Advisory Committee on Immunization Practices (ACIP). *MMWR Morb Mortal Wkly Rep.* 2009;58(RR-02):1–25.
10. Committee on Infectious Disease. Prevention of rotavirus disease: updated guidelines for use of rotavirus vaccine. *Pediatrics.* 2009;123:1412–20. doi: 10.1542/peds.2009-0466.
11. Hall AJ, Vinje J, Lopman B, et al. Updated norovirus outbreak management and disease prevention guidelines. *MMWR Recomm Rep.* 2011;60(RR-03):1–15. Available at: http://www.cdc.gov/mmwr/preview/mmwrhtml/rr6003a1.htm. Accessed March 18, 2016.
12. Wilhelm SM, Dehoorne-Smith ML, Kale-Pradhan PB. Prevention of postoperative nausea and vomiting. *Ann Pharmacother.* 2007;41(1):68–78. doi: 10.1345/aph.1H398.
13. DiPiro CV, Ignoffo RJ. Nausea and vomiting. In: DiPiro JT, Talbert RL, Yee GC, et al., eds. *Pharmacotherapy: A Pathophysiologic Approach.* 9th ed. New York, NY: McGraw-Hill Education; 2014. Available at: http://accesspharmacy.mhmedical.com/content.aspx?bookid=689&Sectionid=45310477. Accessed May 13, 2017.
14. Sharkey KA, Wallace JL. Treatment of disorders of bowel motility and water flux; antiemetics; agents used in biliary and pancreatic disease. In: Brunton LL, Chabner BA, Knollmann BC, eds. *Goodman and Gilman's The Pharmacological Basis of Therapeutics.* 12th ed. New York, NY: McGraw-Hill, Inc.; 2011:1323–49.
15. Scorza K, Williams A, Phillips D, et al. Evaluation of nausea and vomiting. *Am Fam Physician.* 2007;76(1):76–84. PMID: 17668843.
16. Quigley EM, Hasler WL, Parkman HP. AGA technical review on nausea and vomiting. *Gastroenterology.* 2001;120(1):263–86. PMID: 11208736.
17. Flake ZA, Linn BS, Hornecker JR. Practical selection of antiemetics in the ambulatory setting. *Am Fam Physician.* 2015;91(5):293–6. PMID: 25822385.
18. Shupak A, Gordon CR. Motion sickness: advances in pathogenesis, prediction, prevention, and treatment. *Aviat Space Environ Med.* 2006; 77(12):1213–23. Available at: http://www.ingentaconnect.com/contentone/asma/asem/2006/00000077/00000012/art00001?crawler=true. Accessed May 13, 2017.
19. Niebyl JR. Nausea and vomiting in pregnancy. *N Engl J Med.* 2010; 363(16):1544–50. doi: 10.1056/NEJMcp1003896.
20. King CB, Glass R, Bresee JS, et al. Managing acute gastroenteritis among children: oral rehydration, maintenance, and nutritional therapy. *MMWR Recomm Rep.* 2003;52(RR-16):1–16. Available at: http://www.cdc.gov/mmwr/PDF/RR/RR5216.pdf. Accessed May 13, 2017.
21. Khanna R, Lakhanpaul M, Burman-Roy S, et al. Diarrhea and vomiting caused by gastroenteritis: diagnosis, assessment and management in children younger than 5 years: summary of NICE guidance. *BMJ.* 2009;338:b1350. doi: https://doi.org/10.1136/bmj.b1350.
22. Mentes JC. Managing oral hydration. In: Boltz M, Capezuti E, Fulmer T, Zwicker D, eds. *Evidence-Based Geriatric Nursing Protocols for Best Practice.* 4th ed. NewYork (NY): Springer Publishing Company; 2012: 419–38.
23. McCarthy FP, Lutomski JE, Greene RA. Hyperemesis gravidarum: current perspectives. *Int J Womens Health.* 2014;6:719–25. doi: 10.2147/IJWH.S37685
24. World Gastroenterology Organisation (WGO). *WGO Global Guidelines: Acute Diarrhea in Adults and Children: a Global Perspective.* February 2012. Available at: http://www.worldgastroenterology.org/UserFiles/file/guidelines/acute-diarrhea-english-2012.pdf. Accessed May 13, 2017.
25. American Academy of Family Physicians (AAFP). Vomiting and diarrhea, treatment. April 2014. Available at: http://familydoctor.org/familydoctor/en/diseases-conditions/vomiting-and-diarrhea/treatment.html. Accessed May 13, 2017.
26. World Health Organization, Global Task Force on Cholera Control. First steps for managing an outbreak of acute diarrhoea. 2010. Available at: http://www.who.int/cholera/publications/firststeps/en/. Accessed May 13, 2017.
27. Rehydration Project. The "simple solution"—homemade oral rehydration salts (ORS) recipe. July 4, 2014. Available at: http://rehydrate.org/solutions/homemade.htm#recipe. Accessed May 13, 2017.
28. American College of Obstetricians and Gynecology. Nausea and vomiting of pregnancy. ACOG Practice Bulletin No. 153. *Obstet Gynecol.* 2015; 126(3):e12–24. doi: 10.1097/AOG.0000000000001048.
29. Antihistamines. Drug Facts and Comparisons eAnswers. St. Louis, MO: Wolters Kluwer; 2016. Available at: http://online.factsandcomparisons.com/. Accessed May 13, 2017.
30. deLeon J, Nikoloff DM. Paradoxical excitation on diphenhydramine may be associated with being a CYP2D6 ultrarapid metabolizer: three case reports. *CNS Spectr.* 2008;13(2):133–5. PMID: 18227744.
31. Loyd RA, McClellan DA. Update on the evaluation and management of functional dyspepsia. *Am Fam Physician.* 2011;83(5):547–52. PMID: 21391521.

32. Talley NJ, Ford AC. Functional dyspepsia. *N Engl J* Med. 2015;373: 1853–63. doi: 10.1056/NEJMra1501505.
33. National Institutes of Health, U.S. National Library of Medicine. Daily Med: Formula EM—dextrose (glucose), levulose (fructose), phosphoric acid solution. Updated June 24, 2016. Available at: https://dailymed.nlm.nih.gov/dailymed/drugInfo.cfm?setid=24d87e9b-58d5-4753-a123-6e1a5336e4ed. Accessed May 13, 2017.
34. Phosphorated carbohydrate solution. Drug Facts and Comparisons eAnswers. St. Louis, MO: Wolters Kluwer; February 2013. Available at: http://online.factsandcomparisons.com. Accessed May 13, 2017.
35. Wellspring Pharmaceutical Corporation. Emetrol. 2015. Available at: http://emetrol.com/otc-nausea-medication/. Accessed May 13, 2017.
36. Pyridoxine hydrochloride (B_6). Drug Facts and Comparisons eAnswers. St. Louis, MO: Wolters Kluwer; September 2014. Available at: http://online.factsandcomparisons.com/. Accessed March 29, 2016.
37. U.S. Food and Drug Administration. Orange book: approved drug products with therapeutic equivalence evaluations. U.S. Department of Health and Human Services; February 2016. Available at: https://www.accessdata.fda.gov/scripts/cder/ob/. Accessed May 13, 2017.
38. The American Geriatrics Society 2015 Beers Criteria Update Expert Panel. American Geriatrics Society 2015 updated Beers criteria for potentially inappropriate medication use in older adults. *J Am Geriatr Soc.* November 2015;63(11):2227–46.
39. Bismuth subsalicylate. Drug Facts and Comparisons eAnswers. St. Louis, MO: Wolters Kluwer; 2016. Available at: http://online.factsandcomparisons.com. Accessed March 29, 2016.
40. Nausea and vomiting in infants and children. DynaMed Plus [subscription database online]. EBSCO Health. Updated July 28, 2015. Available at: https://www.dynamed.com/topics/dmp~AN~T900008. Accessed May 13, 2017.
41. U.S. Food and Drug Administration. Labeling of drug preparations containing salicylates. *CFR: Code of Federal Regulations*. Title 21, Part 201, Section 201.314. Updated July 27, 2017. Available at: http://www.ecfr.gov/cgi-bin/text-idx?SID=b1b2224711dc88657752be21f12c574a&mc=true&node=se21.4.201_1314&rgn=div8. Accessed July 31, 2017.
42. National Center for Complementary and Integrative Health. Ginger. Available at: https://nccih.nih.gov/health/ginger. Accessed May 13, 2017.
43. Ginger. Drug Facts and Comparisons eAnswers. St. Louis, MO: Wolters Kluwer; February 2016. Available at: http://online.factsandcomparisons.com/. Accessed March 28. 2016.
44. Tiran D. Ginger to reduce nausea and vomiting during pregnancy: evidence of effectiveness is not the same as proof of safety. *Complement Ther Clin Pract.* February 2012;18(1):22–5. doi: 10.1016/j.ctcp.2011.08.007.
45. Holst L, Wright D, Haavik S, et al. Safety and efficacy of herbal remedies in obstetrics—review and clinical implications. *Midwifery.* February 2011;27(1):80–86. doi: 10.1186/1472-6882-13-355.
46. Lee A, Chan SKC, Fan LTY. Stimulation of the wrist acupuncture point PC6 for preventing postoperative nausea and vomiting. *Cochrane Database Syst Rev.* 2015;11:CD003281. doi: 10.1002/14651858.CD003281.pub4.
47. Ezzo J, Streitberger K, Schneider A. Cochrane systematic reviews examine P6 acupuncture-point stimulation for nausea and vomiting. *J Altern Complement Med.* 2006;12(5):489–95. doi: 10.1089/acm.2006.12.489.
48. Hines S, Steels E, Chang A, et al. Aromatherapy for treatment of postoperative nausea and vomiting. *Cochrane Database Syst Rev.* 2012;4:007598. doi: 10.1002/14651858.CD007598.
49. Rhodes VA, McDaniel RW. The index of nausea, vomiting, and retching: a new format of the index of nausea and vomiting. *Oncol Nurs Forum.* 1999;26(5):889–94. PMID: 10382187.

CHAPTER 20

PREBIOTICS AND PROBIOTICS

PRAMODINI KALE-PRADHAN AND SHEILA WILHELM

Prebiotics, Probiotics, and the Gut Microbiota

The community of microflora in the gastrointestinal (GI) tract is known as the *enteric microbiota.* The GI tract hosts approximately 300–500 species of commensal bacteria, with concentrations of up to 10^9 colony-forming units (CFUs)/mL in the terminal ileum and 10^{12} CFUs/mL in the colon.[1] In the past 2 decades, the GI microbiome and its role in human health and disease have been explored. The extent of microbiota influence on health maintenance and disease development appears to be significant. Although understanding of the complex interactions between the GI tract and the enteric microbiota remains incomplete, the paradigm of human biology is shifting to embrace the ecology of the individual host, in which transgenomic and epigenomic co-metabolism provide the background for a GI microbiome unique to each person.[2,3] The microbiome is viewed by some researchers as a "superorganism" in a symbiotic relationship with the gut mucosa.[4]

Prebiotics

Prebiotics support the enteric microbiota and typically are substances fermented in the colon. Some types of fiber act as prebiotics. The undigested fiber enters the colon and is fermented by bacteria, primarily bifidobacteria and lactobacilli. Fermentation products, including short-chain fatty acids (acetate, butyrate, and propionate) and lactate, produce an environment favorable to growth of these bacteria. To be considered a prebiotic, fiber must selectively stimulate the growth and/or activity of one or a limited number of health-promoting bacterial species residing in the colon, with consequent benefit to the host.[1,4–6]

Sources and Intake

Inulin-type fructans, including their partial hydrolysis product fructooligosaccharides (FOSs), are the most common prebiotics.[7] They are found in small amounts in asparagus, bananas, chicory, Jerusalem artichoke, leek, onion, soy, and wheat.[6] Inulin-type fructans are isolated from such sources and added to foods to attain concentrations contributing to prebiotic effects. Average intake for adults in the United States is estimated at 2.6 g/day.[7]

Health Effects

Both inulin-type fructans and FOSs significantly increase bifidobacteria concentrations in humans.[7] Doses vary greatly in studies; 5–8 g/day is thought to be adequate for prebiotic effects, and up to 20 g/day is considered an amount that should not cause adverse effects such as bloating, distention, and flatulence.

Beneficial effects of prebiotics supported by some human data include stool bulking and decreased constipation, better absorption of calcium and magnesium, reduced triglycerides in mildly hypercholesterolemic individuals, and stimulation of bifidobacteria growth.[4,7,8] Studies using prebiotics for treatment or prevention of diarrhea have yielded conflicting evidence; results may depend on the underlying causative disorder.[8] It is hypothesized that use of prebiotics results in improved vaccine response, lower rates of GI infections, stimulation of intestinal hormonal peptides, decrease in inflammatory bowel disease symptoms, and reduced tumor growth, possibly as a consequence of changes in the microbiota secondary to prebiotic exposure.[4] Some beneficial effects may be enhanced with *synbiotics,* which are mixtures of both prebiotics and probiotics that together improve host welfare.[6]

Probiotics

Probiotics are nonpathogenic, living microorganisms that have a beneficial effect on host functions when consumed in adequate amounts.[1,6] Probiotics must withstand processing, storage, and delivery of the organism to the host and then survive gastric acidity, bile acid lysis, and pancreatic enzyme digestion.[4,5] Lactic acid–producing bacteria, especially of the genera *Lactobacillus, Bifidobacterium,* and *Streptococcus,* are the most common such microorganisms present in foods and commercial probiotic products and are most often used in investigational studies. Beyond early infancy, these microorganisms do not permanently colonize the GI tract and must be ingested regularly in sufficient quantity to maintain their presence. When a sufficient number of lactic acid–producing bacteria are present, colonization by pathogenic bacteria is reduced and mucosal defenses in the GI tract are enhanced.[4,8,9] Table 20–1 lists possible protective effects of probiotics and postulated mechanisms of action.[1,4–6,8]

Health care providers (HCPs) should use caution when interpreting data, because multiple species and strains of common probiotic bacteria exist, and because effects cannot be extrapolated across species or even across different strains.[6] Dosing may explain variance in treatment response in published studies. The optimal dose for a given probiotic is not known; however, studies showing efficacy typically use a minimum of 10^7 to 10^{10} CFUs per dose or 10^8 to 10^{10} CFUs daily.[6,10] In a dose-ranging study, the probiotic formulation affected the dissolution and the pharmacokinetics of the probiotic, which reduced its efficacy.[11]

TABLE 20–1 **Possible Protective Effects of Probiotics**

Effect of Probiotic	Possible Mechanisms
GI Barrier Function	
Induce production of protective cytokines mediating EC regeneration and inhibiting apoptosis	Action through TLRs; intestinal homeostasis and EC protection that require recognition of commensal bacteria by TLRs
	Induction of IL-6
Redistribute and increase expression of factors involved in maintaining EC tight junctions	Altered protein kinase C signaling
Counteract effects or inhibit production of inflammatory cytokines associated with increased EC permeability	IL-10 upregulation (regulatory cytokine)
	Reduced effect of TNF-α and INF-γ
	Reduce TNF-α production
	Stimulation of IgA secretion
Antimicrobial Activity	
Inhibit growth of potential pathogens	Decreased luminal pH
	Production of bactericidal proteins (bacteriocins)
Inhibit adhesion of pathogenic bacteria to EC	Increased mucin production
	Reduced transepithelial resistance associated with binding of some pathogens
	Competitive exclusion of pathogens from EC surface binding sites due to nonspecific binding associated with the hydrophobic cell surface properties; mucus-binding pili enhance binding to mucosal surface.
	Binding to pathogenic microorganisms, thereby preventing interaction between the microorganism and EC surface
Influence production of cryptdins by Paneth cells	Antibacterial action of cryptdins
Alter virulence	Altered secretion of molecules influencing expression of genes controlling virulence
EC Inflammatory Responses	
Alter EC cytokine production	Downregulation of bacteria-induced protein kinase C and IL-6
	Inhibition of TNF-α–induced IL-8 production
	Downmodulation of genes associated with proinflammatory signal induction
	Attenuation of nuclear factor kappa B activation
Lymphoid Cell	
Enhance antiviral activity	Inhibition of T-cell proliferation
	Induction of macrophages to express increased amounts of inflammatory cytokines and nitric oxide
	Stimulation of granulocyte colony-stimulating factor release by macrophages
	Increased natural killer T-cell activity
Activate macrophages	Increased antigen presentation to B lymphocytes
Regulatory T-Cell Induction	
Increase $CD4^+$ (regulatory) T cells with cell-surface TGF-β (regulatory cytokine)	Monocyte-derived dendritic cells inducing IL-10 production by T cells

Key: EC = Epithelial cell; GI = gastrointestinal; IgA = immunoglobulin A; IL = interleukin; INF = interferon; TGF = transforming growth factor; TLR = Toll-like receptor; TNF = tumor necrosis factor.
Source: References 1, 4–6, and 8.

This finding demonstrates the need to be vigilant in choosing an appropriate probiotic that has been studied for clinical use.

Sources

Many traditional foods from various cultures worldwide are made by bacterial fermentation; such foods contain high concentrations of lactobacilli. Corn, cassava, millet, leafy vegetables (cabbage), and beans commonly serve as basic foodstuffs for fermentation. Fermented foods that are consumed in the United States include brined olives, kimchi (Korean fermented cabbage), miso, sauerkraut, and tempeh; however, the major source of probiotic bacteria in American diets is dairy foods. Many major brands of yogurt contain probiotic bacteria, although FDA does not require that yogurt contain live cultures, and labels do not list the number of viable probiotic organisms. Liquid yogurt drinks (kefir) and cultured fluid milk, such as sweet acidophilus milk and buttermilk, can contain variable amounts of viable organisms; most dairy products, however, provide such bacteria in adequate numbers (10^8 organisms/g).[6] With the current interest in probiotics, new products, whether they are foods enriched with probiotics or dietary supplements of specific probiotic organisms, are appearing regularly, sometimes with limited or no data on microbial strains or species or on the efficacy of the combinations used.

Health Effects

Interest in probiotics increased dramatically over the past decade. Research covers a wide range of disease states and ages. Clinical data are, for the most part, preliminary; however, the use of probiotics is being evaluated for the prevention or treatment of GI disease states, disorders and conditions recognized as cardiovascular risk factors, and metabolic and respiratory syndromes.

Discussed next are indications for probiotics supported by robust evidence. Table 20–2 summarizes these findings and also includes additional indications for probiotics.[1,4,6,12–18] Results may be influenced by the dose, frequency of dosing, and constituent organisms for any individual probiotic product. Most studies have been small and have used preparations of isolated bacteria (classified as nutritional supplements) or foods with added probiotics, rather than foods that naturally contain the beneficial bacteria.

Indications for Prebiotic and Probiotic Use

Inflammatory Bowel Disease

Inflammatory bowel disease (IBD) comprises ulcerative colitis (UC) and Crohn's disease (CD), both of which are relapsing-remitting inflammatory diseases. With both diseases medical management may require costly therapies that are associated with potentially severe adverse effects. It is hypothesized that changes in the gut microbiota contribute to the inflammation within the GI tract.[15] Probiotics may restore the balance in microbiota composition, thereby limiting the inflammatory response. Several strains of probiotics have been evaluated in the treatment of IBD, including *Lactobacillus* spp., *Bifidobacterium* spp., and multispecies products such as VSL#3, which contains four strains of *Lactobacillus* (*Lactobacillus casei, Lactobacillus plantarum, Lactobacillus acidophilus,* and *Lactobacillus delbrueckii* subsp. *bulgaricus*), three strains of *Bifidobacterium* (*Bifidobacterium longum, Bifidobacterium breve,* and *Bifidobacterium infantis*), and one strain of *Streptococcus* (*Streptococcus salivarius* subsp. *thermophilus*).[15,19–21]

According to one meta-analysis, probiotic therapy was better than placebo for reducing symptoms of UC (relative risk [RR] = 1.72 [95% confidence interval (CI) 1.35–2.20]) but not for the induction of remission (RR = 1.56 [95% CI 0.95–2.59]).[20] Continued treatment with probiotics in patients who achieved remission was as effective as continued mesalazine for the prevention of relapses of UC (RR = 0.97 [95% CI 0.78–1.20]). This analysis included studies that used various probiotics. A more specific study investigated the use of *Lactobacillus* GG and VSL#3 in patients with severe UC who required surgical colectomy with an ileoanal anastomosis. After that procedure, symptoms of "pouchitis," or inflammation of the surgically created pouch or artificial rectum, are not uncommon. In this study, *Lactobacillus* GG was no more effective than placebo for relieving acute pouchitis symptoms.[21] VSL#3 performed better than placebo, however, for the maintenance of remission of chronic pouchitis in an analysis of data on 76 of the subjects (RR = 20.24 [95% CI 4.28–95.81]). The findings regarding the prevention of pouchitis with VSL#3 appear to be equivocal. In contrast with reported benefit in UC, CD symptomatology does not appear to be responsive to probiotics (RR = 1.03 [95% CI 0.71–1.48]).[20] Prebiotics such as FOSs, inulin, and lactulose have also been evaluated in the treatment of UC and CD; however, as indicated by the limited data currently available, they do not seem to provide significant symptom reduction.[22]

Irritable Bowel Syndrome

Irritable bowel syndrome (IBS) is a functional gastrointestinal disorder that manifests as a diarrhea- or constipation-predominant syndrome, or as a mixed clinical picture with abdominal pain. The etiology of IBS is not fully elucidated, but one proposed mechanism is that the symptoms may be secondary to an imbalance in the composition of the GI microbiota, with an increase in potentially harmful species (*Clostridium, Escherichia coli, Salmonella, Shigella,* and *Pseudomonas*) and a reduction in beneficial species (*Lactobacillus* and *Bifidobacterium* spp.).[23] In an analysis of data on patients with diarrhea-predominant IBS (IBS-D), constipation-predominant IBS (IBS-C), or mixed IBS symptoms, treatment with *Lactobacillus* was beneficial in both adult and pediatric patients (odds ratio [OR] = 17.62 [95% CI 5.12–60.65] and OR = 3.71 [95% CI 1.05–13.11], respectively).[24] A meta-analysis of data from 23 trials with 2575 subjects who received either single strains or a combination showed benefits of probiotics on global IBS, abdominal pain, bloating, and flatulence scores, with an RR of 0.79 (95% CI 0.70–0.89) for symptoms persisting with probiotics compared with placebo.[25]

Prebiotics support the function of probiotics. It is unclear, however, whether prebiotics alone provide benefit in IBS. As set forth in the American College of Gastroenterology Monograph, prebiotics are not recommended for IBS owing to insufficient evidence.[26]

Hepatic Disorders

In the presence of alcoholic liver disease, consumption of alcohol causes alterations in gut microbiota composition, resulting in endotoxemia and worsening hepatic function.[27] The use of probiotics such as VSL#3, *Lactobacillus* spp., *E. coli* Nissle, and *Bifidobacterium bifidum* is associated with reductions in liver enzyme levels and improvement in Child-Turcotte-Pugh and Model for End-Stage Liver Disease (MELD) scores.[27] In one study, use of VSL#3 was associated with a decrease in rates of hospitalization

TABLE 20-2 Uses of Probiotics

Condition/Disease	Probiotics and Dosages	Comments
Allergy		
Eczema and atopic dermatitis—prevention and treatment	*Lactobacillus rhamnosus* GG: 10^{10} CFUs daily for 2–4 weeks before delivery, then infant administration for 6 months	Conflicting results; several studies show decreased severity; most studies were small. Few studies available with good design and adequate power to support effectiveness for atopic eczema associated with cow milk allergy. Meta-analysis indicated reduced infant eczema with maternal dietary consumption of selected probiotics in the third trimester of pregnancy or during breastfeeding, or with administration to the infant. To help prevent atopic dermatitis in at-risk offspring, probiotic administration to the mother during pregnancy and to the infant for several months after birth, under the supervision of a health care provider, may be of benefit.
Allergic rhinitis[12]	*Lactobacillus* spp. or *Bifidobacterium* spp.: 10^9 CFUs for 4 weeks–12 months	Improves rhinitis quality of life scores
Diarrhea		
Acute, non–antibiotic-associated diarrhea—treatment in pediatric patients and infants	*L. rhamnosus* GG: at least 10^{10} CFUs in 250 mL of oral rehydration solution; 10^{10} to 10^{11} CFUs twice daily for 2–5 days *Lactobacillus reuteri:* 10^{10} to 10^{11} CFUs daily for up to 5 days	Multiple studies and meta-analyses; duration of diarrhea reduced by ~1 day. Evidence is stronger for viral gastroenteritis than for bacterial infection. Timing of administration may be a factor in efficacy. Evidence is stronger for treatment than for prevention.
Antibiotic-associated diarrhea—prevention (not *Clostridium difficile* diarrhea)[13]	*Saccharomyces boulardii:* 4×10^9–2×10^{10} CFUs daily for 1–4 weeks *L. rhamnosus* GG: 6×10^9–4×10^{10} CFUs daily for 1–2 weeks *Lactobacillus acidophilus* + *Lactobacillus bulgaricus:* 2×10^9 CFUs daily for 5–10 days *L. acidophilus* + *Bifidobacterium longum:* 5×10^9 CFUs daily for 7 days *L. acidophilus* + *Bifidobacterium lactis:* 1×10^{11} CFUs daily for 21 days	Multiple studies in both adults and pediatric patients. Some conflicting results; however, literature supports benefit overall.
C. difficile infection[14]	*S. boulardii:* 2×10^{10} CFUs daily for 4 weeks with antibiotic therapy	Meta-analysis shows benefit. Promising role as adjuvant in treatment of recurrent *C. difficile* diarrhea. Current guidelines do not recommend probiotics for prevention or treatment of *C. difficile* diarrhea, owing to limited data.
IBD[15]		
Crohn's disease—induce and maintain remission	*S. boulardii:* 1 g daily for 6 months with concurrent mesalamine	Small clinical studies, some with up to 1 year of follow-up; several randomized, controlled trials with equivocal results. Data are inadequate to establish effectiveness.
Pouchitis—preventing and maintaining remission	VSL#3[a]: 1.8×10^{12} CFUs daily for 9–12 months	Meta-analysis data support probiotics for maintaining remission of chronic pouchitis. Inadequate studies to establish effectiveness for inducing remission or preventing pouchitis.
Ulcerative colitis	*Escherichia coli* Nissle: *Active UC:* 5×10^{10} CFUs twice daily for up to 12 weeks, then 5×10^{10} CFUs daily for up to 12 months *Inactive UC:* 5×10^{10} CFUs daily for 12 weeks *S. boulardii:* *Active UC:* 250 mg 3 times daily for 4 weeks with concurrent mesalamine VSL#3 *Active UC:* 1.8×10^{12} CFUs twice daily for 6 weeks with conventional therapy	Clinical evidence has demonstrated benefit for reducing symptoms but not for inducing or maintaining remission. Some positive studies show efficacy similar to that of anti-inflammatory medications such as mesalamine; however, data are inadequate to establish effectiveness.

TABLE 20-2 **Uses of Probiotics** *(continued)*

Condition/Disease	Probiotics and Dosages	Comments
IBS		
Motility disorders (IBS-D and IBS-C)	VSL#3: 9×10^{11} CFUs daily for 8 weeks *Bifidobacterium infantis:* 10^6–10^{10} CFUs daily for 4 weeks *L. rhamnosus* GG + *L. rhamnosus* LC705 × *Bifidobacterium breve* × *Propionobacterium freudenreichii:* 8–9×10^9 CFUs daily for 6 months	May normalize muscle hypercontractility. Decreased bloating and flatulence in multiple studies; reduced abdominal pain or relief of constipation or diarrhea in some studies; however, there are conflicting results from other studies. Most studies are small and open label. Meta-analyses demonstrate benefit in IBS-D, IBS-C, or mixed IBS symptoms.
Hepatic Disease[16]		
Hepatic encephalopathy	VSL#3: 9×10^{11} CFUs daily for 6 months	VSL #3 significantly reduced the risk of hospitalization for hepatic encephalopathy and Child–Turcotte–Pugh scores in patients with cirrhosis.
Infection		
Helicobacter pylori	*L. rhamnosus* GG: 6×10^9 CFUs twice daily *Bifidobacterium clausii:* 2×10^9 spores 3 times daily *S. boulardii:* 2–4×10^9 CFUs/day *L. reuteri:* 10^8 CFUs/day Kefir: 250 mL twice daily	Probiotic appears to reduce treatment-related side effects. Meta-analyses indicate that probiotics may increase eradication rates when used with antibiotic therapy, especially with previous treatment failure.
Intestinal Permeability		
NEC—prevention	*Bifidobacterium bifidum* NCDO 1453, *L. acidophilus* NCDO 1748: 10^9 CFUs twice daily *L. acidophilus* + *B. infantis:* 10^8 CFUs twice daily *B. infantis* + *B. bifidum* + *Streptomyces thermophilus:* 10^9 CFUs once daily	Strong support for effectiveness in preterm infants; meta-analysis supports supplementation with probiotics in reducing risk of severe NEC and death in premature infants.
Metabolic Disorders		
Cardiovascular risk factors[17]	*Lactobacillus* spp. ± *Bifidobacterium* spp. and/or *S. thermophilus:* 10^6–10^{10} CFUs for 4–16 weeks	Reductions in total cholesterol, low-density lipoproteins, body mass index, and waist circumference were noted.
Diabetes[18]	*Lactobacillus* spp. × *Bifidobacterium* spp. and/or *S. thermophilus:* 10^6–10^9 CFUs for at least 8 weeks	Reduction in fasting plasma glucose was noted with combination probiotics but not with single strains.

Key: CFUs = Colony-forming units; IBD = inflammatory bowel disease; IBS = irritable bowel syndrome; IBS-C = constipation-predominant IBS; IBS-D = diarrhea-predominant IBS; NEC = necrotizing enterocolitis.

[a] VSL#3 contains four lactobacilli strains, three bifidobacteria strains, and *S. thermophilus*. VSL#3 is marketed as a probiotic medical food.

Source: References 1, 4, 6, 12–18, and also Farnworth ER. The evidence to support health claims for probiotics. *J Nutr.* 2008;138:1250s–4s; Floch MH, Walker WA, Guandalini S, et al. Recommendations for probiotic use—2008. *J Clin Gastroenterol.* 2008;42(Suppl 2):S104–8; Minocha A. Probiotics for preventive health. *Nutr Clin Pract.* 2009;24:227–41; and Williams NT. Probiotics. *Am J Health Syst Pharm.* 2010;67:449–58.

for hepatic encephalopathy.[16] Reduced risk of hepatic encephalopathy with probiotic use was also supported by a meta-analysis (OR = 0.42 [95% CI 0.26–0.70]); however, mortality and serum ammonia concentrations were not affected (mortality rate: OR = 0.73 [95% CI 0.38–1.41]; change in serum ammonia level: weighted mean difference [WMD] = −3.67 [95% CI −15.71–8.37]).[28] The current hepatic encephalopathy treatment guidelines do not recommend probiotic use, owing to inadequate evidence, with small sample sizes, open-label studies, varying types and doses of probiotics, and different outcomes.[29] A meta-analysis of data on probiotic use in nonalcoholic fatty liver disease (NAFLD) showed reductions in levels of aspartate transaminase (AST) and alanine transaminase (ALT) (mean difference for AST = −19.77 [95% CI −32.55 to −7.00]; mean difference for ALT = −23.71 [95% CI −33.46 to −13.95]).[30] Addition of probiotics may be considered in NAFLD, but such products are not routinely used owing to insufficient evidence. The prebiotic lactulose, available by prescription only for this use, is a mainstay of therapy for hepatic encephalopathy; management of this clinical entity is beyond the scope of this chapter, however.[29]

Clostridium difficile Infection

Antimicrobials disrupt the normal function and composition of intestinal microbiota. Such changes enable colonization by *Clostridium difficile.* This anaerobic, gram-positive, spore-forming bacillus causes bowel wall inflammation and watery diarrhea. A number of studies have investigated the usefulness of probiotics, administered concurrently with antimicrobials, for primary prevention of *C. difficile* infection (CDI).

A meta-analysis of data from 23 trials with 4213 subjects compared probiotics with placebo for the primary prevention of CDI.[14] CDI occurrence rates were 2.0% in the probiotics group and 5.5% in the control group (RR = 0.36 [95% CI 0.26–0.51]). The results were similar for adult and pediatric subjects, for lower and higher doses, and for different probiotic species. Subjects in the probiotics group exhibited lower rates of abdominal cramping, nausea, fever, soft stools, flatulence, and taste disturbance (RR = 0.80 [95% CI 0.68–0.95]). In many of the trials, probiotics were initiated within 3 days of starting antibiotics and continued for at least the entire duration of antibiotic treatment.[31]

Established CDI treatment guidelines from the Society for Healthcare Epidemiology of America, the Infectious Diseases Society of America, and the American College of Gastroenterology recommend against administering probiotics for prevention of CDI.[32] A survey of the most recent literature, however, revealed that current recommendations are for the use of Bio-K+, a product approved in Canada, containing 5×10^9 CFUs of *L. acidophilus* CL1285 and *L. casei* LBC80R, to prevent nosocomial CDI in hospitalized patients.[33] As the older guidelines are updated, recommendations for use of probiotics to prevent CDI may emerge. At present, however, the limited available data do not support administration of probiotics for the treatment of CDI or prevention of recurrence.[32,33]

Antibiotic-Associated Diarrhea

Diarrheal disease is a common adverse effect of antibiotics and in this context is referred to as *antibiotic-associated diarrhea* (AAD). AAD is due to a disruption of normal intestinal microbiota. Probiotic use may mitigate this disruption. In a pooled analysis of data on 4097 adult and pediatric subjects from 25 trials, probiotics reduced the incidence of AAD (RR = 0.60 [95% CI 0.49–0.72]).[14] Similarly, in an analysis of 22 trials comprising 4155 pediatric patients, probiotics reduced the incidence of AAD (RR = 0.42 [95% CI 0.33–0.53]).[34] No significant effect by type of antibiotic, or by dose (either greater than or less than 10^{10} CFU/day) or duration of probiotic, could be confirmed; in all of the studies, however, the probiotics were given for the duration of antibiotic therapy. Neither of these analyses reported results based on a specific probiotic; rather the results are based on various probiotic regimens. The use of probiotics with antibiotics for the prevention of AAD may be beneficial.

Necrotizing Enterocolitis

Necrotizing enterocolitis (NEC) involves necrosis of the bowel wall with potential perforation, especially in preterm infants with low birth weights, and is associated with increased mortality.[35] Probiotics may be beneficial in reducing the complications of NEC. In a meta-analysis of data from multiple randomized, controlled trials in preterm infants (born before 37 weeks of gestation or weighing less than 2500 g, or both), the use of probiotics for more than 7 days significantly reduced the incidence of severe NEC (in 20 studies comprising 5529 infants: RR = 0.43 [95% CI 0.33–0.56]) and mortality (in 17 studies comprising 5112 infants: RR = 0.65 [95% CI 0.52–0.81]).[31] Probiotics did not affect the development of sepsis (in 19 studies including 5338 infants: RR = 0.91 [95% CI 0.80–1.03]).

In a subgroup analysis based on the type of probiotic evaluated, administration of products delivering *Lactobacillus* organisms or a mixture of two or three probiotic species significantly reduced the incidence of severe NEC (in 5 studies comprising 1955 infants: RR = 0.45 [95% CI 0.27–0.75]; in 9 studies comprising 2807 infants: RR = 0.37 [95% CI 0.25–0.54]), whereas the benefit with use of products delivering *Bifidobacterium* spp. and *S. boulardii* did not reach significance (RR = 0.48 [95% CI 0.16–1.47] and RR = 0.72 [95% CI 0.34–1.55], respectively); however, these strains were evaluated in fewer subjects (409 and 357, respectively), which may have limited the power of the analyses.[35] Another meta-analysis reports similar findings based on 12 cohort studies comprising 10,800 premature infants.[36] The use of probiotics was associated with a reduction in rates of NEC (RR = 0.55 [95% CI 0.39–0.78]) and death (RR = 0.72 [95% CI 0.61–0.85]) but did not affect sepsis rates (RR = 0.86 [95% CI 0.74–1.00]). The use of probiotics in preterm infants appears to prevent severe NEC and to reduce all-cause mortality. *Lactobacillus* single-strain or mixtures of probiotics were most effective, but more studies are needed to determine the efficacy of other strains, as well as optimal dose and duration.

Helicobacter pylori

Helicobacter pylori (*H. pylori*) is an infective organism that colonizes the upper GI tract, causing peptic ulcer disease in susceptible patients.[37] *H. pylori* is also a known carcinogen—hence, patients who test positive for *H. pylori* infection require both antimicrobial treatment and concomitant eradication of the organism. Combination therapy with an antisecretory agent such as a proton pump inhibitor, plus a combination of antibiotics and potentially bismuth, for 7–14 days is currently recommended. Increasing antimicrobial resistance contributes to lower eradication rates, and adverse effects related to combination therapy limit patient tolerance of these regimens.[37] The use of probiotics may have a positive impact on eradication rates and also limit adverse effects.

A meta-analysis of data from 45 randomized controlled trials with 6997 participants showed higher rates of *H. pylori* eradication with 7 days of triple therapy plus probiotics than with triple therapy alone (82.31% and 72.08%, respectively; for eradication: RR = 1.11 [95% CI 1.08–1.15]).[38] Additionally, the rate of adverse effects was much lower with probiotics plus triple therapy than with the triple therapy regimen (21.44% versus 36.27%, respectively; RR = 0.59 [95% CI 0.48–0.71]). Although eradication rates were higher with fewer adverse effects, the addition of probiotics to triple therapy did not have a limiting effect on patient compliance (RR = 0.98 [95% CI 0.68–1.39]). This lack of apparent detriment may be due in part to the short duration of therapy. These findings are consistent with those of another meta-analysis, which evaluated data from 11 studies with 2392 participants.[39] The eradication rates were reported as 83% for 7 days of triple therapy plus probiotics and 73% for 7 days of triple therapy (RR = 1.14 [95% CI 1.07–1.20]). Adverse effects were also similar to those in the aforementioned analysis (RR = 0.65 [95% CI 0.47–0.87]). This analysis also evaluated subgroups based on probiotic strain used. Eradication rates were significant for a number of probiotic strains including *Lactobacillus, Bifidobacterium, Streptococcus,* and *Saccharomyces.* In patients with *H. pylori* infection, therefore, a reasonable option is the addition of probiotics to standard therapy for the duration of the treatment course.

Diabetes

Probiotics have been evaluated for the treatment of diabetes. It has been proposed that probiotics reduce inflammation and prevent pancreatic beta cell destruction, resulting in a reduction of blood glucose.[18] In a meta-analysis of data from eight trials comprising 429 subjects, the subjects using probiotics experienced a significant reduction in fasting plasma glucose (FPG) compared with subjects in the control groups (FPG change = –15.92 mg/dL [95% CI –29.75 to –2.09]).[18] HbA_{1c} was also significantly reduced in the probiotics group in a subgroup analysis of three trials with 158 subjects (HbA_{1c} reduction = 0.54% [95% CI 0.82–0.25]). The use of preparations with multiple strains of probiotics maintained a significant reduction in FPG, whereas the use of single-strain preparations did not (FPG WMD with multiple strains = –35.41 mg/dL [95% CI –51.93 to –18.48]; FPG WMD with single strains = 2.67 mg/dL [95% CI –18.78–24.13]). Additionally, the use of probiotics for 8 weeks resulted in a reduction of FPG, whereas shorter durations of therapy did not (FPG WMD 8 weeks = –20.34 mg/dL [95% CI –35.92 to –4.76]; FPG WMD <8 weeks = –14.29 [95% CI –65.83–37.26]). These results concur with those of a more recent meta-analysis, which reported similar reductions in FPG in subjects receiving probiotics compared with those in the control group.[40] However, the American Diabetes Association Standards of Care do not currently recommend the use of probiotics.[41]

Cardiovascular Risk Factor Modification

Probiotics may play a role in cardiovascular disease by affecting lipid levels. It has been hypothesized that probiotics may assimilate cholesterol during growth, bind cholesterol, disrupt cholesterol micelles, and deconjugate bile salts.[42] In a meta-analysis of data from 13 trials in 485 subjects evaluating probiotics' effects on cholesterol in patients with normal, borderline-high, and high cholesterol, probiotics significantly reduced total blood cholesterol (mean net change = –6.40 mg/dL [95% CI –9.93 to –2.87]).[43] Low-density lipoprotein (LDL) cholesterol was also significantly reduced in the probiotics group (mean net change = –4.90 mg/dL [95% CI –7.91 to –1.90]). Two other recent meta-analyses corroborate these findings.[17,42] Although probiotics significantly decreased total cholesterol and LDL levels, these meta-analyses did not address clinical outcomes. Furthermore, the trials included in the analyses were of short duration, with the longest trial lasting 10 weeks. Dietary probiotics with fermented milk or yogurt but not capsules were found to have a beneficial effect. Probiotics may have a favorable effect on other cardiovascular risk factors. In a meta-analysis comprising 15 studies with 788 subjects, data from a subgroup comprising 234 subjects across four studies reported a significant reduction in BMI with use of probiotics (–0.52 kg/m^2 [95% CI –0.80 to –0.24 kg/m^2]).[17] In a separate subgroup comprising 304 subjects across four studies, waist circumference decreased significantly with probiotic use (–2.11 cm [95% CI –3.54 to –0.68 cm]). More studies are needed to confirm the effectiveness of probiotics regimens as adjunctive therapy to pharmacologic management of cardiovascular disease.

Eczema and Atopic Dermatitis

It has been hypothesized that the gut microbiota plays a role in inflammation and immune dysfunction related to eczema and atopic dermatitis (AD). Probiotics may alter the gut microbiota, thereby affecting this immunologic response. Infants who were exposed to probiotics either indirectly through maternal dietary intake, with consumption of probiotic foods or supplements during the third trimester of pregnancy or while breastfeeding, or directly with postnatal administration of probiotics, or some combination of these, were less likely to develop eczema than were infants without probiotic exposure. Probiotics did not reduce the incidence of other types of allergic diseases in infants in this analysis.[44]

Probiotic use by pregnant mothers or exposure in infants up to 6 months of age was found to significantly reduce the incidence of eczema in children in a meta-analysis of data on 2797 subjects (RR = 0.74 [95% CI 0.67–0.82]).[45]

In a meta-analysis evaluating probiotics for the primary prevention of AD, supplementation with probiotics in 16 studies was protective against the development of AD (OR = 0.64 [95% CI 0.56–0.74]).[46] In subgroup analyses, the protective effects of probiotics were maintained in the general population, as well as in subjects who were at high risk for development of allergies. Administration of prenatal plus postnatal probiotics was effective, whereas probiotics administered only in the prenatal or postnatal period were not. The results did not differ with the probiotic strain used. On the basis of this analysis, probiotics seem to be beneficial for AD prevention if they are administered during the prenatal and postnatal periods in both general and allergy-prone populations. Another meta-analysis of 14 studies evaluated the effects of probiotic supplementation during pregnancy or in infancy on the development of AD.[47] The subjects who received probiotics were less likely to develop AD than those in the control groups (RR = 0.79 [95% CI 0.71–0.88]). The benefits of probiotics were similar whether they were administered only during pregnancy or during pregnancy and in infancy.

Probiotics have also been evaluated for the treatment of AD.[48] A meta-analysis included 25 randomized controlled trials with 1599 total subjects. It reported a significant improvement in the standardized SCORAD (SCORing Atopic Dermatitis) value for all subjects receiving probiotics compared with placebo (WMD = –4.51 [95% CI –6.78 to –2.24]). Probiotics' beneficial effects were seen in two of three age-related subgroups: children 1–18 years old (WMD = –5.74 [95% CI –7.27 to –4.20]) and adults (WMD = –8.26 [95% CI –13.28 to –3.25]). The benefit was not seen in infants younger than 1 year of age (WMD = 0.52 [95% CI –1.59–2.63]). However, conflicting trial data have led the American Academy of Dermatology to not recommend the use of probiotics for these conditions.[49]

For atopy and dermatitis, *Lactobacillus rhamnosus* GG is the most researched and recommended, although *Lactobacillus acidophilus* and *Bifidobacterium lactis* have also shown benefit.[50,51] *Lactobacillus* and *Bifidobacterium* preparations are dosed at 1×10^9 to 10×10^9 CFUs per day, given in divided doses. *S. boulardii* is dosed at 250–500 mg, 2–4 times daily. Trials have investigated multiple species, but *Bifidobacterium*-dominant products are generally preferred in infants because they better match the normal flora in this age group.

Respiratory Syndromes

Probiotics have been assessed in the treatment of allergic rhinitis: An analysis of 23 studies (1919 adult and pediatric subjects) showed that probiotics improved Rhinitis Quality of Life Questionnaire (RQLQ) scores compared with placebo (standard mean difference [SMD] = –2.23 [95% CI –4.07 to –0.4]).[12] The RQLQ metric is a 7-point scale, with lower scores indicating better quality of life. A change of 0.5 point is considered to be a minimally important difference, and a change of 2 or more points represents a great deal of change.[52] The most common strains of probiotics used in this meta-analysis were *Lactobacillus* and *Bifidobacterium*, administered for 4 weeks to 12 months. Although the data appear promising, more studies are needed to permit recommendation of a specific strain and dosing regimen for the treatment of allergic rhinitis.[12]

Probiotics also may be beneficial in the setting of upper respiratory tract infections (URIs). In a meta-analysis of data from 12 trials comprising 3720 subjects ranging from children to older adults, taking probiotics (*Lactobacillus* and *Bifidobacterium*) was associated with a lower risk of developing a URI compared with placebo (OR for developing one URI = 0.53 [95% CI 0.37–0.76]; OR for developing at least three episodes = 0.53 [95% CI 0.36–0.8]).[53] Probiotics also had positive effects on the mean duration of URI episodes (mean difference = –1.89 days [95% CI –2.03 to –1.75]), rate of antibiotics prescribed (OR = 0.65 [95% CI 0.45–0.94]), and common cold–related school absences (OR = 0.10 [95% CI 0.02–0.47]). Adverse effects were similar for probiotics and placebo groups (OR = 0.88 [95% CI 0.65–1.19]), with the most common adverse effects reported as minor GI complaints. Similar findings were reported in an analysis of 11 studies of 2417 pediatric subjects younger than 10 years of age.[54] As with allergic rhinitis, more studies are needed to definitively recommend probiotics for URI.

Safety Considerations for Prebiotic and Probiotic Use

Probiotics may be associated with minor GI adverse effects including cramping, nausea, soft stools, flatulence, and taste disturbance.[55] It has been reported, however, that patients who receive probiotics for treatment of CDI are less likely to experience GI adverse effects than those who do not. Consequently, whether these GI effects are due to the administered probiotic or to the underlying disease state being treated often is difficult to determine.

A concern with the use of probiotic therapy is the development of systemic infection associated with administration of live cultures. At least 50 case reports have described serious infections (e.g., sepsis, endocarditis, fungemia) in immunocompromised patients, in whom the responsible pathogens were infectious organisms consistent with the administered probiotic.[52] Even though probiotic use has become more common, however, an increase in infection risk has not been supported by population-based data on the rates of infections due to commonly administered probiotic strains. Although some data support the use of probiotics in immunocompromised patients, these agents should be avoided because of the reports of systemic infection.[56]

A multicenter randomized, double-blind, placebo-controlled trial, the Probiotics in Pancreatitis Trial (PROPATRIA), assessed the effects of probiotics for the prevention of infectious complications in patients who have acute pancreatitis with a predicted severe course.[57] This trial demonstrated that probiotics had no effect on the rate of infectious complications. However, the mortality rate was more than double in the probiotics group (RR = 2.53 [95% CI 1.22–5.25]). More specifically, bowel ischemia and associated mortality rates were significantly higher in the probiotics group ($P = 0.004$). Therefore, probiotics should be avoided in such severely ill patients. By contrast, no harmful effects have been observed in women in late-stage pregnancy or in breastfeeding infants during long-term use of probiotics.[58] In general, adverse effects secondary to probiotics are mild. In patients with acute illnesses or immunocompromised status, probiotics should be avoided or used with caution.

Assessment and Patient Counseling for Prebiotic and Probiotic Use

Many probiotic preparations containing one or multiple species and wide ranges in the concentration of bacteria are available. HCPs and consumers should be cognizant of these differences when selecting probiotic formulations and should base decisions largely on evidence from clinical trial data and the strains used in these trials. Patients should be counseled to avoid probiotics if they have risk factors for systemic infections or other complications.[55] Recognized risk factors include valvular heart disease, presence of a central venous access port, and immunocompromised status. Premature infants also are at increased risk for the development of adverse effects, and this liability should be weighed against the benefit of preventing NEC. If probiotics are used in conjunction with antibiotics, separating the two for administration is recommended, with scrupulous adherence to manufacturer dosing guidelines.

Cases 20–1 and 20–2 provide examples of assessing a patient's symptoms to determine whether probiotics are appropriate for them to use.

Product quality has been a concern in that some studies found products containing few or no live cultures.[59] Refrigerated products have been recommended as perhaps less likely to have suffered from degrading temperatures. Recent research, however, suggests that nonviable probiotics also may offer beneficial effects similar to those obtained with live cultures.[60] To ensure maximal clinical benefit, HCPs should recommend only the probiotic products used in clinical trials. Because most such products are considered dietary supplements, rather than preparations covered under medication insurance plans, cost may be a consideration for many patients, who need to be aware of the variability in prices for different products.

Key Points for Prebiotic and Probiotic Use

- Prebiotics are fermentable dietary components that selectively stimulate the growth and/or activity of one or a limited number of bacterial species in the colon (typically bifidobacteria and lactobacilli).
- Probiotics are nonpathogenic, living microorganisms that have a beneficial effect on the host when consumed regularly in adequate amounts. They are often present in fermented products derived from milk (yogurt and kefir) or plants (sauerkraut and miso) or are available as manufactured supplements.
- Probiotics have shown beneficial effects in a number of diseases; however, the particular species and strain and the dose necessary for beneficial effects often remain controversial and may vary from condition to condition.

CASE 20-1

Relevant Evaluation Criteria	Scenario/Model Outcome
Collect	
1. Gather essential information about the patient's symptoms and medical history, including	
a. Description of symptom(s) (i.e., nature, onset, duration, severity, associated symptoms)	Patient reports cramping abdominal pain, bloating, and flatulence of 1 week's duration. She reports 8–10 loose and mucus-streaked stools per day for the past couple of weeks. Ms. Smith continues to experience abdominal pain, bloating, and flatulence. Before this 2-week period of symptoms, Ms. Smith notes having 1–2 normal, formed bowel movements daily. Ms. Smith reports similar episodes occurring approximately 14 times over the past year (~1 episode/month).
b. Description of any factors that seem to precipitate, exacerbate, and/or relieve the patient's symptom(s)	Cramping abdominal pain, bloating, and flatulence relieved slightly by defecation. Loose stools respond to loperamide. Symptoms are triggered by specific trigger foods as well as stress.
c. Description of the patient's efforts to relieve the symptoms	Ms. Smith has been avoiding trigger foods, which has reduced the number of episodes she experiences. She takes loperamide for loose stools when they occur. These approaches have not completely relieved her symptoms of abdominal pain, bloating, and flatulence.
d. Patient's identity	Mary Smith
e. Patient's age, gender, height, and weight	52 years, female, 5 ft 2 in., 130 lb (59 kg)
f. Patient's occupation	Elementary school teacher
g. Patient's dietary habits	Eats most foods; avoids specific trigger foods (broccoli, cauliflower).
h. Patient's sleep habits	7 hours per night
i. Concurrent medical conditions, prescription and nonprescription medications, and dietary supplements	Diarrhea-predominant IBS (IBS-D). No other medical conditions. Loperamide OTC 2 mg PO 4 times daily as needed for IBS-D symptoms.
j. Allergies	NKDA
k. History of other adverse reactions to medications	None
l. Other (describe) ______	None
Assess	
2. Differentiate patient's signs/symptoms, and correctly identify the patient's primary problem(s).	Ms. Smith has IBS, which she is treating with loperamide as needed for loose stools.
3. Identify exclusions for self-treatment.	None
4. Formulate a comprehensive list of therapeutic alternatives for the primary problem to determine whether triage to a health care provider is required, and share this information with the patient or caregiver.	Options include (1) Refer Ms. Smith to an appropriate HCP. (2) Recommend self-care with a probiotic. (3) Recommend stress reduction through activities such as yoga or meditation. (4) Take no action.
Plan	
5. Select an optimal therapeutic alternative to address the patient's problem, taking into account patient preferences.	Ms. Smith should incorporate stress-reduction strategies such as yoga or meditation to reduce the number of IBS-D episodes. In addition, Ms. Smith should use a probiotic to manage the symptoms of abdominal pain, bloating, and flatulence that are not relieved by loperamide therapy.

CASE 20-1 *continued*

Relevant Evaluation Criteria	Scenario/Model Outcome
6. Describe the recommended therapeutic approach to the patient or caregiver.	"Probiotic formulations such as VSL#3, which is an oral capsule, should be used to relieve abdominal pain, bloating, and flatulence in IBS. There are a number of other probiotic products available. It is important to choose products that have been studied in patients with IBS-D to ensure the most effective treatment."
7. Explain to the patient or caregiver the rationale for selecting the recommended therapeutic approach from the considered therapeutic alternatives.	"Probiotics were chosen because they help relieve the specific symptoms you are experiencing. Lifestyle modifications that reduce stress are helpful in limiting the number of episodes you experience."
Implement	
8. When recommending self-care with nonprescription medications and/or nondrug therapy, convey accurate information to the patient or caregiver.	"If symptoms continue or worsen after a week, contact your primary care provider."
Solicit follow-up questions from the patient or caregiver.	"Will I get an infection from taking a probiotic since you told me this is a live microorganism?"
Answer the patient's or caregiver's questions.	"In patients like you with a healthy immune system, probiotics are safe to use and will not cause an infection. They are not recommended for patients with weakened immune systems such as those receiving chemotherapy or people who have had an organ transplant."
Follow-up: Monitoring and Evaluation	
9. Assess patient outcome.	Ask the patient to call to update you on her response to your recommendations. Or you could call her in 1 week to evaluate the outcome.

Key: HCP = Health care provider; IBS = irritable bowel syndrome; NDKA = no known drug allergies; OTC = over-the-counter; PO = by mouth.

CASE 20-2

Relevant Evaluation Criteria	Scenario/Model Outcome
Collect	
1. Gather essential information about the patient's symptoms and medical history, including	
a. Description of symptom(s) (i.e., nature, onset, duration, severity, associated symptoms)	Mr. Jones reports severe epigastric pain, especially at night and after eating a spicy or fried meal. His antacids seem to reduce the pain, but it recurs soon after. He also complains of pain with swallowing (dysphagia) and sometimes has difficulty swallowing (odynophagia).
b. Description of any factors that seem to precipitate, exacerbate, and/or relieve the patient's symptom(s)	Mr. Jones' symptoms worsen when he eats spicy or fried foods, or when he is under a lot of stress at work.
c. Description of the patient's efforts to relieve the symptoms	Mr. Jones takes Tums or Mylanta as needed to relieve his symptoms.
d. Patient's identity	Harry Jones
e. Patient's age, gender, height, and weight	42 years, male, 5 ft 10 in., 190 lb (86.4 kg)
f. Patient's occupation	Lawyer
g. Patient's dietary habits	Does not cook for himself; frequently eats at restaurants, including fast food.
h. Patient's sleep habits	5–6 hours nightly
i. Concurrent medical conditions, prescription and nonprescription medications, and dietary supplements	Hypertension treated with hydrochlorothiazide 25 mg PO daily. He also takes Tums 1 tablet and Mylanta 15 mL as needed for dyspepsia.
j. Allergies	NKDA
k. History of other adverse reactions to medications	None
l. Other (describe) ______	None

CASE 20-2 *continued*

Relevant Evaluation Criteria	Scenario/Model Outcome
Assess	
2. Differentiate patient's signs/symptoms, and correctly identify the patient's primary problem(s).	Mr. Jones is presenting with symptoms of dyspepsia, dysphagia, and odynophagia. This clinical picture could be due to GERD, gastritis, PUD due to *H. pylori,* or cancer.
3. Identify exclusions for self-treatment.	Mr. Jones' symptoms include dysphagia and odynophagia, which are two of the alarm symptoms that warrant referral for more invasive testing such as an EGD. The presence of these symptoms excludes him from self-treatment. The other alarm symptoms are bleeding, weight loss, choking, chest pain, and epigastric mass.
4. Formulate a comprehensive list of therapeutic alternatives for the primary problem to determine whether triage to a health care provider is required, and share this information with the patient or caregiver.	Options include (1) Refer patient to an appropriate HCP. (2) Recommend self-care with a probiotic and nonprescription antiulcer medication. (3) Recommend self-care until patient can see an appropriate HCP. (4) Take no action.
Plan	
5. Select an optimal therapeutic alternative to address the patient's problem, taking into account patient preferences.	Refer patient to an appropriate HCP.
6. Describe the recommended therapeutic approach to the patient or caregiver.	"You should consult your primary care provider for treatment."
7. Explain to the patient or caregiver the rationale for selecting the recommended therapeutic approach from the considered therapeutic alternatives.	"Your symptoms of pain and difficulty swallowing require further evaluation. Once a diagnosis is made, we can further recommend appropriate therapies."
Implement	
8. When recommending self-care with nonprescription medications and/or nondrug therapy, convey accurate information to the patient or caregiver.	Criterion does not apply in this case.
Follow-up: Monitor and Evaluate	
9. Assess patient outcome.	Contact the patient in a day or two to ensure he made an appointment and sought medical care.

Key: EGD = Esophagogastroduodenoscopy; GERD = gastroesophageal reflux disease; HCP = health care provider; NKDA = no known drug allergies; PUD = peptic ulcer disease.

➤ Patients should avoid probiotics if they have risk factors for systemic infections or other conditions such as valvular heart disease, presence of a central venous access port, or compromised immune status

REFERENCES

1. Quigley EM. Prebiotics and probiotics; modifying and mining the microbiota. *Pharmacol Res.* 2010;61:213–8. doi: 10.1016/j.phrs.2010.01.004.
2. Li M, Wang B, Zhang M, et al. Symbiotic gut microbes modulate human metabolic phenotypes. *Proc Natl Acad Sci U S A.* 2008;105:2117–22. doi: 10.1073/pnas.0712038105.
3. Muegge BD, Kuczynski J, Knights D, et al. Diet drives convergence in gut microbiome functions across mammalian phylogeny and within humans. *Science.* 2011;332:970–4. doi: 10.1126/science.1198719.
4. Vieira AT, Teixeira MM, Martins FS. The role of probiotics and prebiotics in inducing gut immunity. *Front Immunol.* 2013;4:445. doi: 10.3389/fimmu.2013.00445.
5. Charalampopoulos D, Rastall RA. Prebiotics in foods. *Curr Opin Biotechnol.* 2012;23:187–91. doi: 10.1016/j.copbio.2011.12.028.
6. Guarner F, Khan AG, Garisch J, et al. World Gastroenterology Organisation Global Guidelines: probiotics and prebiotics October 2011. *J Clin Gastroenterol.* 2012;46:468–81. doi: 10.1097/MCG.0b013e3182549092.
7. Roberfroid MB. Inulin-type fructans: functional food ingredients. *J Nutr.* 2007;137:2493s–502s. PMID: 17951492.
8. Boirivant M, Strober W. The mechanism of action of probiotics. *Curr Opin Gastroenterol.* 2007;23:679–92. doi: 10.1097/MOG.0b013e3282f0cffc.
9. Nagpal R, Kumar A, Kumar M, et al. Probiotics, their health benefits and applications for developing healthier foods: a review. *FEMS Microbiol Lett.* 2012;334:1–15. doi: 10.1111/j.1574-6968.2012.02593.x.

10. Saavedra JM. Use of probiotics in pediatrics: rationale, mechanisms of action, and practical aspects. *Nutr Clin Pract.* 2007;22:351–65. doi: 10.1177/0115426507022003351.
11. Whorwell PJ, Altringer L, Morel J, et al. Efficacy of an encapsulated probiotic *Bifidobacterium infantis* 35624 in women with irritable bowel syndrome. *Am J Gastroenterol.* 2006;101:1581–90. doi: 10.1111/j.1572-0241.2006.00734.x.
12. Zajac AE, Adams AS, Turner JH. A systematic review and meta-analysis of probiotics for the treatment of allergic rhinitis. *Int Forum Allergy Rhinol.* 2015;5:524–32. doi: 10.1002/alr.21492.
13. Kale-Pradhan PB, Jassal HK, Wilhelm SM. Role of *Lactobacillus* in the prevention of antibiotic-associated diarrhea: a meta-analysis. *Pharmacotherapy.* 2010;30:119–26. doi: 10.1592/phco.30.2.119.
14. Goldenberg JZ, Ma SS, Saxton JD, et al. Probiotics for the prevention of *Clostridium difficile*-associated diarrhea in adults and children. *Cochrane Database Syst Rev.* 2013;5:CD006095. doi:10.1002/14651858.cd006095.pub3.
15. Jonkers D, Penders J, Masclee A, Pierik M. Probiotics in the management of inflammatory bowel disease: a systematic review of intervention studies in adult patients. *Drugs.* 2012;72:803–23. doi: 10.2165/11632710-000000000-00000.
16. Dhiman RK, Rana B, Agarwal S, et al. Probiotic VSL#3 reduces liver disease severity and hospitalization in patients with cirrhosis: a randomized, controlled trial. *Gastroenterology.* 2014;147:1327–37 e3. doi: 10.1053/j.gastro.2014.08.031.
17. Sun J, Buys N. Effects of probiotics consumption on lowering lipids and CVD risk factors: a systematic review and meta-analysis of randomized controlled trials. *Ann Med.* 2015;47:430–40. doi: 10.3109/07853890.2015.1071872.
18. Zhang Q, Wu Y, Fei X. Effect of probiotics on glucose metabolism in patients with type 2 diabetes mellitus: a meta-analysis of randomized controlled trials. *Medicina.* 2016;52:28–34. doi: 10.1016/j.medici.2015.11.008.
19. Durchschein F, Petritsch W, Hammer HF. Diet therapy for inflammatory bowel diseases: the established and the new. *World J Gastroenterol.* 2016;22:2179–94. doi: 10.3748/wjg.v22.i7.2179.
20. Fujiya M, Ueno N, Kohgo Y. Probiotic treatments for induction and maintenance of remission in inflammatory bowel diseases: a meta-analysis of randomized controlled trials. *Clin J Gastroenterol.* 2014;7:1–13. doi: 10.1007/s12328-013-0440-8.
21. Singh S, Stroud AM, Holubar SD, et al. Treatment and prevention of pouchitis after ileal pouch-anal anastomosis for chronic ulcerative colitis. *Cochrane Database Syst Rev.* 2015;11:CD001176. doi: 10.1002/14651858.cd001176.pub3.
22. Wasilewski A, Zielinska M, Storr M, Fichna J. Beneficial effects of probiotics, prebiotics, synbiotics, and psychobiotics in inflammatory bowel disease. *Inflamm Bowel Dis.* 2015;21:1674–82. doi: 10.1097/MIB.0000000000000364.
23. Distrutti E, Monaldi L, Ricci P, Fiorucci S. Gut microbiota role in irritable bowel syndrome: new therapeutic strategies. *World J Gastroenterol.* 2016;22:2219–41. doi: 10.3748/wjg.v22.i7.2219.
24. Tiequn B, Guanqun C, Shuo Z. Therapeutic effects of *Lactobacillus* in treating irritable bowel syndrome: a meta-analysis. *Intern Med.* 2015;54:243–9. doi: 10.2169/internalmedicine.54.2710.
25. Ford AC, Quigley EM, Lacy BE, et al. Efficacy of prebiotics, probiotics, and synbiotics in irritable bowel syndrome and chronic idiopathic constipation: systematic review and meta-analysis. *Am J Gastroenterol.* 2014;109:1547–61. doi:10.1038/ajg.2014.202.
26. Ford AC, Moayyedi P, Lacy BE, et al. American College of Gastroenterology monograph on the management of irritable bowel syndrome and chronic idiopathic constipation. *Am J Gastroenterol.* 2014;109(Suppl 1):S2–26. doi:10.1038/ajg.2014.187.
27. Li F, Duan K, Wang C, et al. Probiotics and alcoholic liver disease: treatment and potential mechanisms. *Gastroenterol Res Pract.* 2016;2016:5491465. doi:10.1155/2016/5491465.
28. Xu J, Ma R, Chen LF, et al. Effects of probiotic therapy on hepatic encephalopathy in patients with liver cirrhosis: an updated meta-analysis of six randomized controlled trials. *Hepatobiliary Pancreat Dis Int.* 2014;13:354–60. doi:10.1016/S1499-3872(14)60280-0.
29. Vilstrup H, Amodio P, Bajaj J, et al. Hepatic encephalopathy in chronic liver disease: 2014 Practice Guideline by the American Association for the Study of Liver Diseases and the European Association for the Study of the Liver. *Hepatology.* 2014;60:715–35. doi:10.1002/hep.27210.
30. Ma YY, Li L, Yu CH, et al. Effects of probiotics on nonalcoholic fatty liver disease: a meta-analysis. *World J Gastroenterol.* 2013;19:6911–8. doi:10.3748/wjg.v19.i40.6911.
31. Lau CS, Chamberlain RS. Probiotics are effective at preventing *Clostridium difficile*-associated diarrhea: a systematic review and meta-analysis. *Int J Gen Med.* 2016;9:27–37. doi: 10.2147/IJGM.S98280.
32. Ollech JE, Shen NT, Crawford CV, Ringel Y. Use of probiotics in prevention and treatment of patients with *Clostridium difficile* infection. *Best Pract Res Clin Gastroenterol.* 2016;30:111–8. doi:10.1016/j.bpg.2016.01.002.
33. Goldstein EJ, Johnson S, Maziade PJ, et al. Pathway to prevention of nosocomial *Clostridium difficile* infection. *Clin Infect Dis.* 2015;60(Suppl 2):S148–58. doi:10.1093/cid/civ142.
34. McFarland LV, Goh S. Preventing pediatric antibiotic-associated diarrhea and *Clostridium difficile* infections with probiotics: a meta-analysis. *World J Meta-Anal.* 2013;1:102–20. doi:10.13105/wjma.v1.i3.102.
35. AlFaleh K, Anabrees J. Probiotics for prevention of necrotizing enterocolitis in preterm infants. *Evid Based Child Health.* 2014;9:584–671. doi: 10.1002/ebch.1976.
36. Olsen R, Greisen G, Schroder M, Brok J. Prophylactic probiotics for preterm infants: a systematic review and meta-analysis of observational studies. *Neonatology.* 2016;109:105–12. doi:10.1159/000441274.
37. Chey WD, Wong BC; Practice Parameters Committee of the American College of Gastroenterology. American College of Gastroenterology guideline on the management of *Helicobacter pylori* infection. *Am J Gastroenterol.* 2007;102:1808–25. doi:10.1111/j.1572-0241.2007.01393.x.
38. Zhang MM, Qian W, Qin YY, et al. Probiotics in *Helicobacter pylori* eradication therapy: a systematic review and meta-analysis. *World J Gastroenterol.* 2015;21:4345–57. doi:10.3748/wjg.v21.i14.4345.
39. Li BZ, Threapleton DE, Wang JY, et al. Comparative effectiveness and tolerance of treatments for *Helicobacter pylori*: systematic review and network meta-analysis. *BMJ.* 2015;351:h4052. doi:10.1136/bmj.h4052.
40. Samah S, Ramasamy K, Lim SM, Neoh CF. Probiotics for the management of type 2 diabetes mellitus: a systematic review and meta-analysis. *Diabetes Res Clin Pract.* 2016;118:172–82. doi:10.1016/j.diabres.2016.06.014.
41. Standards of Medical Care in Diabetes—2016: Summary of Revisions. *Diabetes Care.* 2016;39(Suppl 1):S4–5. doi:10.2337/dc16-S003.
42. Shimizu M, Hashiguchi M, Shiga T, et al. Meta-analysis: effects of probiotic supplementation on lipid profiles in normal to mildly hypercholesterolemic individuals. *PloS One.* 2015;10:e0139795. doi:10.1371/journal.pone.0139795.
43. Guo Z, Liu XM, Zhang QX, et al. Influence of consumption of probiotics on the plasma lipid profile: a meta-analysis of randomised controlled trials. *Nutr Metab Cardiovasc Dis.* 2011;21:844–50. doi:10.1016/j.numecd.2011.04.008.
44. Cuello-Garcia CA, Brozek JL, Fiocchi A, et al. Probiotics for the prevention of allergy: a systematic review and meta-analysis of randomized controlled trials. *J Allergy Clin Immunol.* 2015;136:952–61. doi:10.1016/j.jaci.2015.04.031.
45. Mansfield JA, Bergin SW, Cooper JR, Olsen CH. Comparative probiotic strain efficacy in the prevention of eczema in infants and children: a systematic review and meta-analysis. *Milit Med.* 2014;179:580–92. doi:10.7205/MILMED-D-13-00546.
46. Panduru M, Panduru NM, Salavastru CM, Tiplica GS. Probiotics and primary prevention of atopic dermatitis: a meta-analysis of randomized controlled studies. *J Eur Acad Dermatol Venereol.* 2015;29:232–42. doi:10.1111/jdv.12496.
47. Pelucchi C, Chatenoud L, Turati F, et al. Probiotics supplementation during pregnancy or infancy for the prevention of atopic dermatitis: a meta-analysis. *Epidemiology.* 2012;23:402–14. doi:10.1097/EDE.0b013e31824d5da2.
48. Kim SO, Ah YM, Yu YM, et al. Effects of probiotics for the treatment of atopic dermatitis: a meta-analysis of randomized controlled trials. *Ann Allergy Asthma Immunol.* 2014;113:217–26. doi:10.1016/j.anai.2014.05.021.
49. Sidbury R, Tom WL, Bergman JN, et al. Guidelines of care for the management of atopic dermatitis: Section 4. Prevention of disease flares and use of adjunctive therapies and approaches. *J Am Acad Dermatol.* 2014;71(6):1218–33. doi:10.1016/j.jaad.2014.08.038.

50. Betsi GI, Papadavid E, Falagas ME. Probiotics for the treatment or prevention of atopic dermatitis: a review of the evidence from randomized controlled trials. *Am J Clin Dermatol.* 2008;9:93–103. doi:10.2165/00128071-200809020-00002.
51. Gerasimov SV, Vasjuta VV, Myhovych OO, Bondarchuk LI. Probiotic supplement reduces atopic dermatitis in preschool children: a randomized, double-blind, placebo-controlled, clinical trial. *Am J Clin Dermatol.* 2010;11:351–61. doi:10.2165/11531420-000000000-00000.
52. Juniper EF, Riis B, Juniper BA. Development and validation of an electronic version of the Rhinoconjunctivitis Quality of Life Questionnaire. *Allergy.* 2007;62:1091–3. doi:10.1111/j.1398-9995.2007.01370.x.
53. Hao Q, Dong BR, Wu T. Probiotics for preventing acute upper respiratory tract infections. *Cochrane Database Syst Rev.* 2015;2:CD006895. doi:10.1002/14651858.CD006895.pub3.
54. Araujo GV, Oliveira Junior MH, Peixoto DM, Sarinho ES. Probiotics for the treatment of upper and lower respiratory-tract infections in children: systematic review based on randomized clinical trials. *J Pediatr (Rio J).* 2015;91:413–27. doi:10.1016/j.jped.2015.03.002.
55. Doron S, Snydman DR. Risk and safety of probiotics. *Clin Infect Dis.* 2015;60(Suppl 2):S129–34. doi:10.1093/cid/civ085.
56. Liong MT. Safety of probiotics: translocation and infection. *Nutr Rev.* 2008;66:192–202. doi:10.1111/j.1753-4887.2008.00024.x.
57. Besselink MG, van Santvoort HC, Buskens E, et al. Probiotic prophylaxis in predicted severe acute pancreatitis: a randomised, double-blind, placebo-controlled trial. *Lancet.* 2008;371:651–9. doi:10.1016/S0140-6736(08)60207-X.
58. Rautava S, Kainonen E, Salminen S, Isolauri E. Maternal probiotic supplementation during pregnancy and breast-feeding reduces the risk of eczema in the infant. *J Allergy Clin Immunol.* 2012;130:1355–60. doi:10.1016/j.jaci.2012.09.003.
59. Temmerman R, Scheirlinck I, Huys G, Swings J. Culture-independent analysis of probiotic products by denaturing gradient gel electrophoresis. *Appl Environ Microbiol.* 2003;69:220–6. doi:10.1128/AEM.69.1.220-226.2003.
60. Asama T, Kimura Y, Kono T, et al. Effects of heat-killed *Lactobacillus kunkeei* YB38 on human intestinal environment and bowel movement: a pilot study. *Benef Microbes.* 2016;7:337–44. doi:10.3920/BM2015.0132.

CHAPTER 21

POISONING

WENDY KLEIN-SCHWARTZ AND BARBARA INSLEY CROUCH

Poisoning is the leading cause of injury death in the United States, surpassing motor vehicle traffic deaths and deaths from firearms, and it is a major public health problem.[1–3] Drug related morbidity is also significant.

Nonprescription medications pose a risk for adverse effects and poisoning among all age groups, but especially those at the extremes of age. Acetaminophen is one of the leading nonprescription pain relievers. It is also a leading cause of poisoning reported to U.S. poison control centers for both unintentional and intentional poisonings. More than 600 products containing acetaminophen are on the market; thus, misunderstanding their use and unintended misuse is common for all ages.[4–6] The Acetaminophen Awareness Coalition, whose members include the American Pharmacists Association, the National Association of Boards of Pharmacy, and the National Community Pharmacists Association, launched a website (www.knowyourdose.org) to educate patients and consumers about how to use acetaminophen correctly. Several initiatives to promote safe acetaminophen use include converting pediatric liquid acetaminophen preparations to one standardized concentration and highlighting the ingredient acetaminophen on nonprescription labels.

Restrictions and label changes on pediatric cough and cold preparations have led to a reduction in pediatric unintentional poison exposures and emergency department visits.[7–9] Use of nonprescription cough and cold medications to get high remains an issue identified through the Monitoring the Future study, with 4.6% of 12th graders indicating they used these medications in the past year.[10] Most poisonings in young children are unintentional, whereas poisonings in other age groups may be unintentional or intentional (e.g., suicide attempts, substance abuse, medication misuse). The majority of poisonings are a result of ingestion of a substance, but poisonings may also occur after a toxin is inhaled or comes in contact with the skin and eyes. Bites and envenomations are other potential sources of toxin exposures. First aid for poisonings focuses on minimizing the extent of the exposure and stemming the progression or development of toxicity.

Poison control centers are 24-hour resources for poison information, clinical toxicology consultation, and poison prevention education. They are staffed around the clock with pharmacists, nurses, physicians, and physician's assistants who have additional training in clinical toxicology. The centers are available for consultation with health care providers (HCPs) as well as with the public. The entire United States and its territories are covered by a network of poison control centers. A poison control center should be contacted for assessment and treatment of poisonings, as well as for educational materials on poison prevention. Figure 21–1 shows the nationwide poison control center number and logo.

In 2014, a total of 56 poison control centers serving the United States and territories reported 2,165,142 cases to the National Poison Data System of the American Association of Poison Control Centers.[11] The majority of poison exposures (47.7%) occur in children younger than 6 years, of which 88.7% involve children ages 3 years and younger.[11] Nonprescription and prescription medications are frequently responsible for potentially toxic exposures reported to poison control centers. Nonprescription products such as analgesics, cough and cold preparations, topical preparations, vitamins, and antihistamines are among the most common substances ingested by young children. The large number of nonprescription medications involved in pediatric exposures reflects the common use and availability of these products in the home. Other common substances involved in poison exposures in children younger than 6 years include cosmetics and personal care products, cleaning substances, foreign bodies or toys, pesticides, and plants.

Nearly 70% of poison exposures reported to poison control centers are managed on site, usually in a residence. Only 12.7% of children younger than 6 years are managed in a health care facility, and major effects or fatal outcomes occurred in 1.1%.[11] Calls to poison control centers involving unintentional poison exposures to pharmaceuticals in children younger than 6 years that resulted in a health care facility visit increased 22% between 2001 and 2008.[12] Poison control centers are cost-effective and have a favorable cost-to-benefit ratio.[13] A significant portion of the cost savings results from home observation, as well as from the reduction of unnecessary emergency medical transport and treatment costs. Poison control center consultation results in shorter length of hospital stay and lower charges for patients who require hospitalization.[14,15] A policy analysis group reviewed the existing literature on the cost savings associated with use of a poison control center; the group estimated medical care savings and reduced productivity loss of $13.39 per year per dollar of poison control center funding.[16] A study of pediatric poison exposures treated in a tertiary children's hospital found that 18.6% of visits were for nontoxic exposures that could have been managed on site by the poison control center. Children with nontoxic exposures were more likely to be covered by Medicaid or no insurance (73%) and had a mean charge of $286 per patient.[17] HCPs are encouraged to work closely with their local poison control centers to ensure the most appropriate, cost-effective care of the poisoned patient.

Consumers and/or HCPs can also use an online/smart phone app to assist them in deciding whether to call their poison

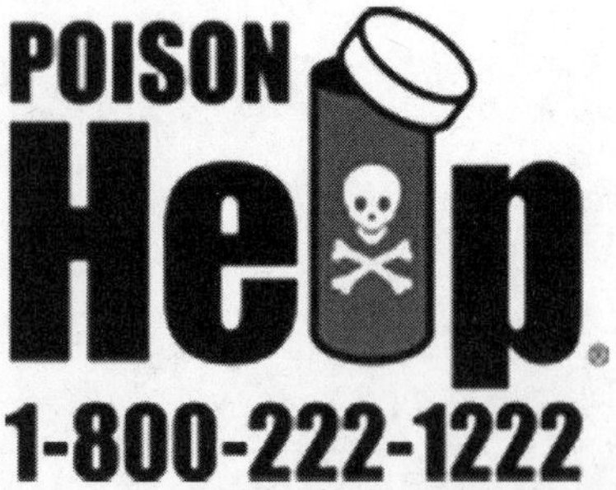

FIGURE 21–1 Nationwide toll-free telephone number to access a poison control center. (Source: Reprinted with permission from the American Association of Poison Control Centers, Alexandria, Virginia.)

center. For those who prefer to use an online/smart phone resource, this tool can be useful and cost-effective. WebPoisonControl.org is a free application that was launched in December 2014. To date, more than 9000 public cases have been logged, and in 73.3% of cases, it was determined to be safe to treat the event at home.[18] In 24.5% of the cases, the user was referred to the poison control center, and in 2.1% of cases, the user was referred directly to an emergency department. A survey of users demonstrated that more than 91% thought the tool was quick and easy to use. Another online resource launched in 2017 is poisonhelp.org. Other web/smart phone apps may be available in the near future.

Unintentional childhood poisonings remain a common cause of injury-related morbidity, requiring significant expenditures of health care dollars for inpatient and outpatient care. Unintentional poisonings are one of the leading causes of injury-related hospitalizations in preschool children; however, fatalities among preschoolers have declined significantly since the early 1970s. According to a recent analysis of the National Electronic Injury Surveillance System–All Injury Program (NEISS–AIP), an estimated 58,000 children younger than 6 years are evaluated in emergency departments annually for unintentional medication-related exposures.[19] Hospitalization or specialized medical care was required in nearly 16% of cases. The most common categories of medications were acetaminophen, cough and cold medications, antidepressants, and nonsteroidal anti-inflammatory drugs (NSAIDs).

The National Safety Council reported 50 deaths caused by unintentional poisoning in children younger than 5 years in 2013.[20] Only 34 of the 1835 fatalities reported by poison control centers in 2014 involved children younger than 6 years.[11] Medications and illicit drugs (excluding ethanol) were the primary substances responsible for fatalities. Child-resistant closures (CRCs) legislated through the Poison Prevention Packaging Act (PPPA) of 1970 help prevent unintentional poisonings. CRCs have been responsible for a decline in pediatric fatalities from prescription and nonprescription medications.[21] Although CRCs have improved child safety, exemptions to the law allow dispensing medications without CRCs.[22] An analysis of NEISS data revealed that an estimated 55% of nonfatal poisonings in children younger than 5 years treated in an emergency department involved a product regulated by the PPPA.[23] Whereas CRCs may reduce unintentional pediatric poisoning, use of nonstandard liquid measuring devices and caregiver misinterpretation of nonprescription medication labels increase the risk for pediatric poisoning. Further work is needed to improve the format and content of nonprescription labels to improve caregiver understanding of the medication and dosing instructions.[24–26]

Clinical Presentation of Poisoning

Poisons can affect every organ system. Signs and symptoms of poisoning can range in severity from mild to life threatening. For some drugs, toxicity after overdose is similar to the drug's adverse effect profile with therapeutic use. For example, ibuprofen overdose is characterized primarily by nausea, vomiting, and abdominal pain. Patients with diphenhydramine overdose may exhibit sedation or stimulation (e.g., agitation, hallucinations), tachycardia, hypertension, dry mouth, and dilated pupils from the drug's antimuscarinic properties. Overdoses of other drugs, such as aspirin, result in multiorgan system effects including gastrointestinal (GI), central nervous system, metabolic, cardiovascular, pulmonary, and hematologic toxicity. A lack of symptoms immediately after a poison exposure does not preclude toxicity. Patients may be asymptomatic initially, but they can develop severe toxicity hours after ingestion of some sustained-released or enteric-coated products or products that delay gastric emptying or slow GI motility (e.g., antihistamines). For other drugs (e.g., acetaminophen) and some chemicals (e.g., methanol, acetonitrile), clinical effects are delayed while the substance is metabolized to active or toxic metabolites. The time course of acetaminophen overdose is related to formation and covalent binding of a toxic metabolite to hepatic cells. As a result, a relatively mild initial clinical course characterized by nausea, vomiting, anorexia, and malaise can be followed by severe hepatic and renal toxicity 3–5 days later. Keep in mind that symptoms may be due to causes other than poisoning. Regardless of the cause of symptoms, if symptoms are serious enough, they warrant medical attention.

Treatment of Poisoning

Most unintentional poison exposures in small children result in minimal, if any, adverse effects and require no treatment other than observation. Although self-treatment may be appropriate, HCPs, caregivers, and patients are encouraged to seek counsel from the nearest poison control center before attempting any treatment.

Treatment Goals

The primary goal of home or prehospital therapy is to prevent absorption of toxins or stem the progression of toxicity, thus minimizing morbidity and mortality.

General Treatment Approach

The first step in assessing a potential poison exposure is to determine whether the patient has symptoms and whether the exposure puts the patient at risk of toxicity. Many exposures are, in fact, nontoxic or minimally toxic, because either the substance has a very low inherent toxicity or the amount consumed is too low to cause toxicity. A decision regarding the option for self-treatment depends on the reason or circumstance of the poison exposure, toxicity of the agent, and general health status of the patient. Self-treatment should be considered only if the ingestion is unintentional and the potential for toxicity is assessed as minor. Any inadvertent exposure to a toxin that potentially can result in moderate–severe toxicity, as well as all intentional exposures, should be referred immediately to a hospital. If the patient exhibits potentially life-threatening clinical effects (e.g., coma, convulsions, syncope), transportation to an emergency department should be arranged immediately through the emergency 911 system. Additional exclusions for self-treatment can be found in Figure 21–2. Hospital care includes observing the patient, supporting vital functions (e.g., airway, breathing, circulation), preventing absorption, enhancing elimination, and using antidotes.

Suicide is a serious public health problem in the United States. Intentional ingestions of medications often are a cry for help. Individuals who are trying to harm themselves or are abusing or misusing drugs on purpose are not always truthful about what they ingested. It is important to be vigilant and recognize when someone has taken a medication purposefully and to refer them immediately for evaluation in an emergency department.

The majority of individuals who do not require immediate hospital referral are managed with on-site observation only and no specific treatment.[11] In some instances, the approach is to attenuate the exposure by irrigation or prevention of further absorption. The nonprescription drug activated charcoal may prevent or reduce the absorption of some ingested substances. However, its routine use is not recommended without consultation with a poison control center. In the past, ipecac syrup, nonprescription cathartics, or both were recommended to induce vomiting or decrease absorption of substances by facilitating their

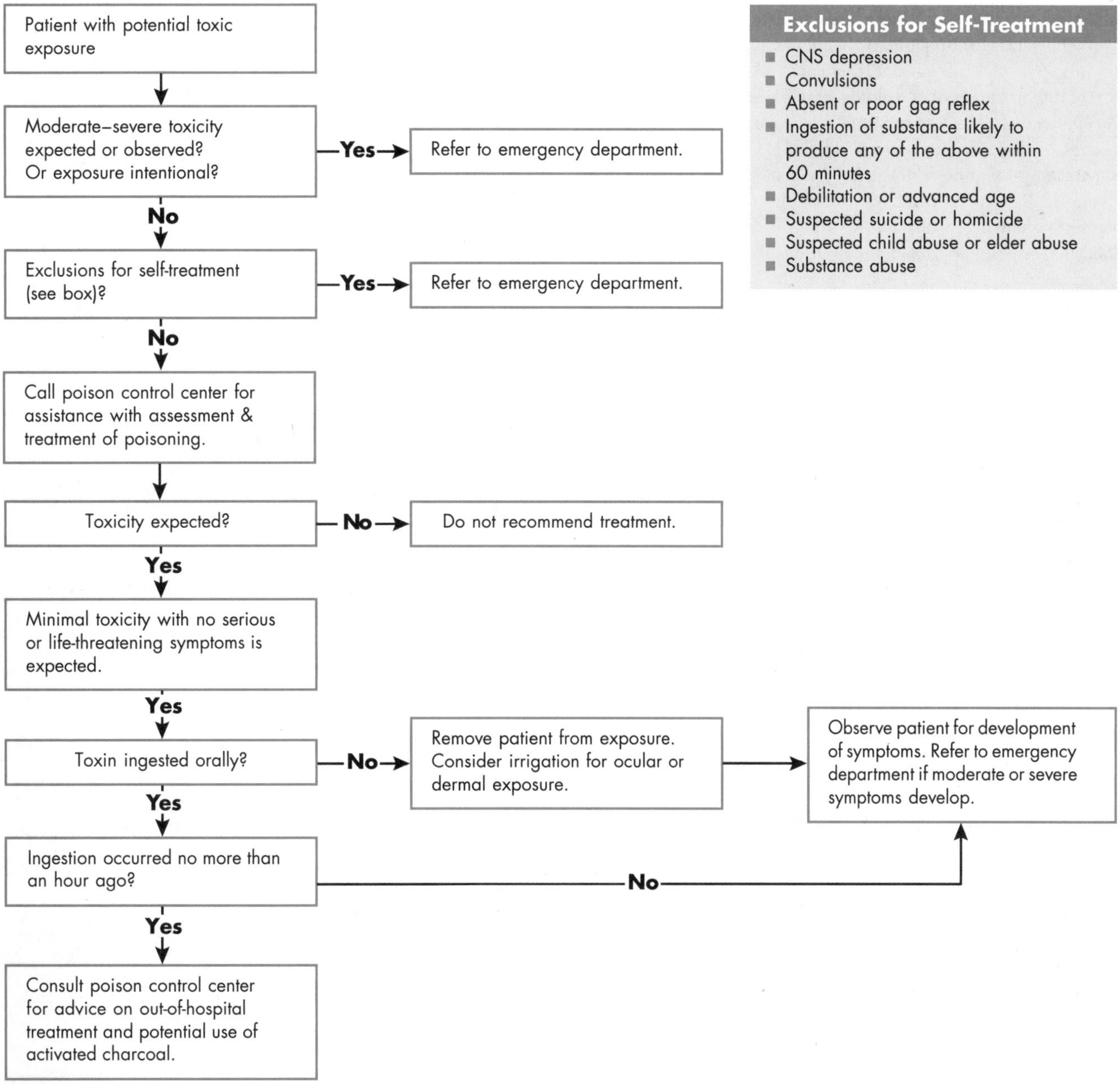

FIGURE 21–2 Self-care for poisoning. Key: CNS = Central nervous system.

elimination through the GI tract. However, ipecac syrup is no longer available, and cathartics by themselves are not beneficial in the treatment of a poisoned patient. Figure 21–2 outlines self-care for exposure to poisons.

Nonpharmacologic Therapy

Inhalation exposures are managed by removing the patient from the toxic fumes to fresh air. Irrigation may be beneficial to decrease the contact time of a chemical with the skin or mucosal surface. Skin surfaces should be washed with soap and water (usually twice) to decrease the contact time of a chemical exposure, taking care to include nail beds and hair when appropriate. Irrigation of the eye with water should be initiated immediately after an ocular exposure to a chemical or drug not intended for ocular use (e.g., inadvertent ocular administration of an otic preparation). If an irritating chemical has been swallowed, administration of a small amount of fluids may decrease the contact time of the chemical with the mucosal surface. Neutralization after a chemical contacts skin or eyes or for ingested substances is not recommended.

Administration of oral fluids after ingestion of a drug is not recommended. The administration of a large amount of fluids should be discouraged, because the fluids are likely to result in spontaneous vomiting, which is risky in some situations. The fluids theoretically may facilitate dissolution of a solid dosage form, thereby enhancing its absorption. Administering fluids after drug ingestions should be considered for drugs that are known to have a high risk of esophageal impaction, such as bisphosphonates, or those that may cause renal injury owing to dehydration, such as ibuprofen or other NSAIDs. Manually stimulating the gag reflex at the back of the throat with either a blunt object or a finger may induce vomiting, but this practice is not recommended and can lead to soft palate injury.

Pharmacologic Therapy

Activated charcoal, an adsorbent, and ipecac syrup, an emetic, are the only approved self-treatments for ingested poisons. Ipecac syrup does not improve outcomes of poisoned patients and its use should be avoided.[27] Although the Code of Federal Regulations still states that ipecac syrup is considered the emetic of choice for certain poisoning scenarios, ipecac syrup is no longer commercially available as a nonhomeopathic product.[28] Therefore, it is no longer a viable option for self-treatment of poisoning. However, some internet sources that provide instructions on how to induce vomiting still list ipecac as an option. Pharmacists should recommend that existing supplies in the home be discarded and encourage consultation with a poison control center regarding first-aid recommendations for poisoning. Controversy surrounds the use of activated charcoal as a self-treatment, given the lack of evidence that it improves outcome and its poor tolerability.

Treatment With Activated Charcoal

Activated charcoal is a tasteless, gritty, fine, black insoluble powder made from the pyrolysis of various organic materials.[29] Its large surface area of 950–2000 m^2/g makes activated charcoal a highly effective adsorbent.[29]

Activated charcoal has been shown to adsorb a large number of commonly ingested drugs and many other toxic agents. These substances are bound in the internal surface of the pores of the charcoal particle, thereby preventing their absorption. Activated charcoal is not absorbed from the GI tract. As the ratio of activated charcoal to toxin increases, the proportion of bound toxin increases.[29] Highly ionized substances, such as potassium and lithium, are poorly adsorbed by activated charcoal. Activated charcoal does not bind well to alcohols or glycols (e.g., ethanol, methanol, ethylene glycol), hydrocarbons, mineral acids and alkali, heavy metals (e.g., iron, lead, arsenic), or cyanide (Table 21–1).

TABLE 21–1 Contraindications to GI Decontamination With Activated Charcoal as Self-Treatment

Category	Inclusion Criteria	Recommendation
Patient condition	Coma, convulsions, syncope, airway or breathing problems, blood pressure or pulse irregularities, hallucinations, and severe agitation; history of bariatric surgery	Refer to hospital for evaluation.
Reason or circumstance	Intentional self-harm, substance abuse, malicious intent	Refer to hospital for medical and psychiatric or social service evaluation.
Ingestion of low-viscosity hydrocarbons and terpenes	Gasoline, kerosene, mineral seal oil (furniture polish), naphtha (lighter fluid), pine oil (cleaners), turpentine (paint removers), mineral oil	Contact poison control center.
Ingestion of caustic substances	Methacrylic acid (artificial nail primers), sodium silicate and carbonate (automatic dishwashing detergents), sulfuric acid (automotive battery, drain cleaners, toilet bowl cleaners), sodium hydroxide (drain cleaners, oven cleaners, hair relaxers), hypochlorites (bleach, pool chlorine), thioglycolates (hair relaxers), hydrofluoric acid (rust removers), hydrochloric acid (toilet bowl cleaner)	Contact poison control center.
Ingestion of substances not adsorbed by charcoal	Ethanol (alcoholic beverages, colognes, mouthwashes, aftershaves, hand sanitizers), isopropyl alcohol (rubbing alcohol), methanol (windshield washer fluid), ethylene glycol (antifreeze), ionized substances (potassium), metals (iron, lithium, lead, arsenic), cyanide (potassium cyanide, acetonitrile artificial nail remover, laetrile)	Contact poison control center.

Key: GI = Gastrointestinal.

The presence of food in the GI tract may reduce the efficacy of activated charcoal.

Activated charcoal is approved by the Food and Drug Administration for use as an emergency antidote in the treatment of an ingested poison. Home use of activated charcoal should never include more than 1 dose. The usual dose of activated charcoal is approximately 1 g/kg (Table 21–2).[29] This dose provides an estimate of the amount (rounded to the nearest full or half-full bottle) of activated charcoal to administer,. Activated charcoal is available premixed either with water or with water and carboxymethylcellulose. Activated charcoal combined with sorbitol is also available to improve palatability and to act as a cathartic, shortening transit time of the activated charcoal complex through the GI tract and preventing constipation; however, most activated charcoal products marketed specifically for home use do not contain sorbitol. Examples of nonprescription activated charcoal products are Actidose-Aqua or Liqui-Char with or without sorbitol; they generally are available at strengths of 15 g/72 mL, 25 g/120 mL, and 50 g/240 mL. Activated charcoal slurries are prone to settling, so they should be shaken vigorously before administration. Activated charcoal is also available as a powder for reconstitution into an oral suspension just before use; this product should be stirred thoroughly or shaken vigorously after water is added. Flavoring agents have been used to try to increase the palatability of activated charcoal. Activated charcoal capsules marketed as a dietary supplement for GI symptoms or other ailments should not be used to manage poisonings, because the surface area of charcoal in these products is too small to effectively adsorb toxins.

The most common adverse effects of activated charcoal are vomiting and black stools. Vomiting occurs in 12%–20% of patients receiving activated charcoal.[29] One-fifth of children younger than 18 years who were given activated charcoal for poisoning vomited a median time of 10 minutes after initiation of charcoal administration. More serious complications, such as pulmonary aspiration and GI obstruction, are associated more often with administration of multiple doses of activated charcoal.

Activated charcoal is contraindicated in patients in whom the GI tract is not anatomically (e.g., following caustic injury) or functionally (e.g., ileus) intact. Following bariatric surgery, patients may not tolerate charcoal or may need smaller, more frequent doses. Activated charcoal is also contraindicated in patients at high risk for aspiration without airway protection (Table 21–1). Activated charcoal should not be administered after ingestion of substances that it does not adsorb unless the presence of other ingestants that are adsorbed by charcoal is suspected.

TABLE 21–2 Activated Charcoal Dosing Information

Age	Dose
0–12 months[a]	10–25 g
1–12 years	25–50 g
>12 years	25–100 g

[a] Used primarily in a health care setting in this age group.

Source: Reference 29.

Pharmacotherapeutic Considerations for Activated Charcoal

Studies have demonstrated that the effectiveness of GI decontamination decreases significantly with increasing time interval since ingestion. For most overdoses, GI decontamination with activated charcoal should be performed early, usually within an hour of the ingestion.[30–32]

There is no convincing evidence that activated charcoal improves patient outcomes, and its utility in adults who intentionally overdose has been questioned, particularly in patients with mild–moderate poisoning.[32,33] In some subgroups of patients with severe poisoning, activated charcoal may be beneficial; however, these poisonings should not be self-treated.[32] A position statement by the American Academy of Clinical Toxicology and the European Association of Poisons Centres and Clinical Toxicologists concluded that activated charcoal may be considered for a potentially toxic amount of a poison ingested up to 1 hour before treatment. There are insufficient data to support or exclude use of charcoal when poison ingestion occurred more than 1 hour previously.[29] The majority of studies on which the position statement was based were conducted in a controlled research or hospital environment.

Although activated charcoal is available as a nonprescription drug, it is not available in most homes, nor is it routinely recommended for home use by poison control centers. HCPs should consult their poison control center to determine whether to promote routine availability of activated charcoal in the home.

Sometimes activated charcoal is given in the home setting to provide early prehospital GI decontamination in patients who subsequently are transported to an emergency department. Data on prehospital administration provide insight into the potential difficulty in administering activated charcoal in the home. A study of prehospital emergency medical technicians or paramedics reported that charcoal was not given to 15.4% of patients in whom administration was attempted; in 71% of these cases the reason was patient refusal.[34]

Consideration of home use of activated charcoal requires addressing the following questions: What are the benefits? Will children drink it at home? Does home administration shorten the interval between the overdose and charcoal administration? Is it safe to give at home?[35] Eldridge et al.[35] cited two studies (21 children total) that questioned whether activated charcoal can be administered successfully at home after researchers found that most children did not drink a full dose administered by parents. Three other studies (217 children total) reported that a full dose was administered in 64% of children and a partial dose was ingested in 16% of 157 children.[35] While a full dose of charcoal may not be necessary for poison ingestions of very low dosage (e.g., dosage in milligrams rather than grams), it is important to weigh the risks and benefits. Problems with these studies include reliance on parent reports and lack of validation of the accuracy of the amount of charcoal administered.

Home administration shortens time to administration of charcoal.[35,36] When administered at home, charcoal generally is given within the desired 1 hour. Consideration should be given to the relative benefit of parents administering charcoal to children before their arrival at the emergency department compared with the risk associated with possible delay in emergency department treatment if charcoal was administered earlier.

To date, experience with home administration of activated charcoal has shown that it is relatively safe. GI effects have been reported, with the main adverse effect being vomiting. Before an HCP recommends use of activated charcoal, a poison control center should be consulted.

Assessment of Poisoning: A Case-Based Approach

After obtaining the history of the exposure to a poison and performing an initial assessment of the patient's condition, the HCP must decide whether to refer the patient directly to an emergency treatment facility, to manage him or her at home, or not to recommend any specific treatment. Clearly patients with serious clinical effects including altered mental status (e.g., stupor, coma, seizures, agitation, hallucinations), respiratory distress, or changes in cardiovascular status (e.g., syncope, hypotension) are not candidates for self-care and should be transported immediately to the emergency treatment facility. Alternatively, recognizing nontoxic or minimally toxic exposures that can be managed outside a health care facility is an essential component of self-treatment of poisoning. Involving the poison control center in this triage and treatment decision is important. because poison control centers have considerable experience managing poisoned patients and specialized resources that are not usually available to providers. The nationwide toll-free poison control center number, 800-222-1222, connects callers to the center that serves their area (Figure 21–1).

Self-treatment at home is primarily intended for unintentional poison exposures in children younger than 6 years in whom no or, at most, minimal toxicity is expected. In addition, unintentional inhalation or skin or eye exposures in any age group, with possible minimal toxicity, often can be self-treated.

If an individual inquires about purchasing activated charcoal, the pharmacist must determine whether these drugs are being purchased for an acute situation, in which case the poison control center should be contacted to assess the appropriateness of self-treatment. The poison control center will need information about the patient (age, weight, medical history, whether the patient is currently experiencing clinical effects), the toxin (name of the toxin, dose, route of exposure, time since exposure), and what treatment, if any, has already been administered.

Cases 21–1 and 21–2 provide examples of assessment of patients who have been poisoned.

Patient Counseling for Poisoning

After patients are removed from toxic fumes, they should be counseled about when to seek medical attention (e.g., difficulty breathing, worsening or persistent symptoms). In the home or other nonindustrial setting, fumes often are soluble, irritant gases (e.g., chlorine), so clinical effects are evident immediately and usually resolve soon after exposure stops. Patients should also be counseled about ventilating the room to disperse the vapor. If the exposure resulted from mixing products such as bleach and ammonia, the patient should be warned not to mix household products in the future. If carbon monoxide is suspected, the patient should be instructed to have the source turned off or removed (e.g., malfunctioning furnace, stove, vehicle). The poison control center should be contacted to assess the severity and expected duration of clinical effects in symptomatic patients and the possibility of delayed onset in asymptomatic patients. Home carbon monoxide detectors are important home safety devices, and homeowners should be encouraged to install them to prevent or minimize carbon monoxide exposures.

Patients with eye exposures should be counseled on how to irrigate the eye at home under the faucet. Contact lenses should be removed before irrigation. Instructions should include running the water at room temperature and at a low pressure. Irrigating the eyes in the shower or using a clean cup to pour water into the eyes may be an easier alternative in children. Placing a damp washcloth on the eye or irrigating with small-volume nonprescription eyewashes is ineffective. Finally, eye drops, including topical vasoconstrictors, should not be used after irrigation. Patients with skin exposures should be counseled to remove clothing, if necessary, and to wash affected areas thoroughly. For eye and skin exposures, counseling should stress the importance of immediate irrigation or washing of the affected area.

If the poison control center in a region recommends activated charcoal for home use, pharmacies in that area should stock the appropriate product, and pharmacists should educate parents that activated charcoal should never be used without first consulting a poison control center staff member. Patients who purchase activated charcoal for immediate use following the recommendation of a poison control center should be counseled to ensure appropriate drug use, including provision of instructions on preparation (depending on the formulation). The pharmacist should also explain potential adverse effects, as well as signs and symptoms that indicate medical attention should be sought.

Counseling older adults on self-managing their medications can prevent poisonings and adverse drug reactions. Polypharmacy may place older adults at risk for errors relating to dose, dosage regimen, and possibly administration techniques. Educating them about the potential for interactions, including drug–drug, drug–food, and drug–alcohol, is important. They should be reminded to seek advice before mixing nonprescription or herbal products with prescription medications. Counseling older adults should emphasize the importance of ongoing communication with their HCPs to ensure both efficacy and safety of their medication regimen.

Patients who are taking multiple prescriptions and using a regular pill minder should be advised to purchase a locking pill minder if they are around young children. When loading the device, they should place a paper or cardboard underneath the pill minder to catch stray tablets or capsules that might fall on the floor. Pharmacists can also prevent therapeutic 10-fold error types of poisonings by always dispensing 1 mL oral syringes for prescription medications that are dosed in infants at less than 1 mL, such as metoclopramide. The box "Patient Education for Toxic Exposures" lists specific information to provide parents, caregivers, or patients.

Counseling should include providing the nationwide toll-free number for the poison control center (Figure 21–1) and promoting poison prevention practices, including purchase of nonprescription drugs and household products with child-resistant packaging. However, caregivers should be reminded that CRCs are not childproof; even products with CRCs should be stored up and out of reach of small children and preferably in a locked cabinet. The Up and Away campaign (www.upandaway.org) is a new initiative developed by PROTECT, a public–private initiative (Preventing Overdoses and Treatment Errors in Children Taskforce) in partnership with the Centers for Disease Control and Prevention.

CASE 21-1

Relevant Evaluation Criteria	Scenario/Model Outcome
Collect	
1. Gather essential information about the patient's symptoms and medical history, including	
a. Description of symptom(s) (i.e., nature, onset, duration, severity, associated symptoms)	A mother asks the pharmacist about treatment options for her previously healthy 13-year-old daughter, who ingested a handful of acetaminophen 325 mg tablets after they got into an argument. The now empty bottle of 325 mg acetaminophen originally contained 100 tablets and none remain. However, the bottle was purchased approximately 1 year ago, and it is not known how many tablets were used by other family members prior to ingestion by the daughter. The ingestion happened 1 hour ago. The daughter vomited 1 time and appears pale.
b. Description of any factors that seem to precipitate, exacerbate, and/or relieve the patient's symptom(s)	The mother stuck her finger down the back of her daughter's throat to induce vomiting.
c. Description of the patient's efforts to relieve the symptoms	n/a
d. Patient's identity	Samantha Jones
e. Patient's age, gender, height, and weight	13 years old, female, 5 ft 1 in., 101.4 lb (46 kg)
f. Patient's occupation	n/a
g. Patient's dietary habits	Normal
h. Patient's sleep habits	Sleeps approximately 7 hours a night during the school week and 12 hours a night on weekends.
i. Concurrent medical conditions, prescription and nonprescription medications, and dietary supplements	Healthy, takes no medications.
j. Allergies	No known allergies
k. History of other adverse reactions to medications	None
l. Description of other medications or products in the vicinity	No other medications or products are available.
Assess	
2. Differentiate patient's signs/symptoms, and correctly identify the patient's primary problem(s).	Acute intentional overdose of acetaminophen; total amount ingested is unknown. It is possible that Samantha's vomiting and pallor are related to the acetaminophen.
3. Identify exclusions for self-treatment (Figure 21–2).	This is a suspected suicide attempt, which is an exclusion from self-treatment.
4. Formulate a comprehensive list of therapeutic alternatives for the primary problem to determine whether triage to a health care provider is required, and share this information with the patient or caregiver.	Options include (1) Refer to emergency department for possible GI decontamination and evaluation. (2) Contact the poison control center for recommendations. (3) Have her mother administer an OTC treatment to decrease absorption at home. (4) Have her mother administer oral fluids to dilute the acetaminophen. (5) Take no action.
Plan	
5. Select an optimal therapeutic alternative to address the patient's problem, taking into account patient preferences.	Refer to the emergency department for evaluation and treatment.
6. Describe the recommended therapeutic approach to the patient or caregiver.	The mother should be directed to immediately take her daughter to the closest emergency department for evaluation and treatment.
7. Explain to the patient or caregiver the rationale for selecting the recommended therapeutic approach from the considered therapeutic alternatives.	"Samantha has tried to hurt herself and it is not safe to treat her at home. Take Samantha immediately to the closest emergency department."

CASE 21-1 *continued*

Relevant Evaluation Criteria	Scenario/Model Outcome
Implement	
8. When recommending self-care with nonprescription medications and/or nondrug therapy, convey accurate information to the patient or caregiver.	Criterion does not apply in this case.
Solicit follow-up questions from the patient or caregiver.	"I have activated charcoal at home. Should I give it to her to be on the safe side?"
Answer the patient's or caregiver's questions.	"No, do not give activated charcoal. She has already vomited and is at risk for vomiting and aspirating the activated charcoal."
Follow-up: Monitor and Evaluate	
9. Assess patient outcome.	n/a

Key: GI = Gastrointestinal; n/a = not applicable; OTC = over-the-counter.

CASE 21-2

Relevant Evaluation Criteria	Scenario/Model Outcome
Collect	
1. Gather essential information about the patient's symptoms and medical history, including	
a. Description of symptom(s) (i.e., nature, onset, duration, severity, associated symptoms)	A mother asks the pharmacist about treatment options for her previously healthy 2-year-old daughter, who was found with an open ibuprofen bottle. The now empty bottle of 200 mg ibuprofen originally contained 50 tablets and 42 had been used previously. The ingestion happened 1 hour ago. The child vomited once but is otherwise asymptomatic. The mother states that the child vomited 15 minutes ago, and the mother saw 1 partially dissolved tablet in the vomit.
b. Description of any factors that seem to precipitate, exacerbate, and/or relieve the patient's symptom(s)	n/a
c. Description of the patient's efforts to relieve the symptoms	The mother gave the child some juice to drink after she vomited.
d. Patient's identity	Lily Smith
e. Patient's age, gender, height, and weight	2 years old, female, 32 in., 22 lb (10 kg)
f. Patient's occupation	n/a
g. Patient's dietary habits	She ate lunch 2 hours before the exposure.
h. Patient's sleep habits	It is close to her nap time.
i. Concurrent medical conditions, prescription and nonprescription medications, and dietary supplements	Healthy; takes no medications.
j. Allergies	NKDA
k. History of other adverse reactions to medications	None
l. Describe other medications or products in the vicinity______	No other medications or products are available.

CASE 21-2

Relevant Evaluation Criteria	Scenario/Model Outcome
Assess	
2. Differentiate patient's signs/symptoms, and correctly identify the patient's primary problem(s).	Acute unintentional overdose of ibuprofen. Although mom saw a partially dissolved tablet, one should assume that close to 8 tablets were ingested. Therefore, Lily ingested 8 ibuprofen 200 mg; total dose of 1.6 g or 160 mg/kg.
3. Identify exclusions for self-treatment (Figure 21–2).	Lily vomited once but is now asymptomatic. She has taken a larger than therapeutic but minimally toxic dose of ibuprofen. There are no exclusions for self-treatment.
4. Formulate a comprehensive list of therapeutic alternatives for the primary problem to determine whether triage to a health care provider is required, and share this information with the patient or caregiver.	Options include (1) Contact the poison control center for recommendations regarding whether to refer Lily to an emergency department for possible GI decontamination and evaluation. (2) Have her mother administer an OTC treatment to decrease absorption at home. (3) Have her mother administer oral fluids to dilute the ibuprofen. (4) Take no action.
Plan	
5. Select an optimal therapeutic alternative to address the patient's problem, taking into account patient preferences.	The poison control center should be contacted immediately. The center will determine whether it is safe to manage the child at home.
6. Describe the recommended therapeutic approach to the patient or caregiver.	No specific therapy is needed at this time. Doses under 200 mg/kg can be managed at home. The poison control center recommends that Lily remain at home.
7. Explain to the patient or caregiver the rationale for selecting the recommended therapeutic approach from the considered therapeutic alternatives.	"Lily has ingested a larger than therapeutic dose of ibuprofen but not enough to require treatment at a hospital. Ibuprofen can cause stomach upset, so it is not unexpected that she vomited. Give Lilly something to drink, and call back if she has any further vomiting or other stomach-related symptoms."
Implement	
8. When recommending self-care with nonprescription medications and/or nondrug therapy, convey accurate information to the patient or caregiver.	Criterion does not apply in this case.
Solicit follow-up questions from the patient or caregiver.	"I have activated charcoal at home. Should I give it to her to be on the safe side?"
Answer the patient's or caregiver's questions.	"No, do not give activated charcoal. She has not taken a toxic dose. If the dose had been toxic, we would recommend that she be treated in a hospital."
Follow-up: Monitor and Evaluate	
9. Assess patient outcome.	Ask Lily's mother to call you if Lily vomits again or has a stomachache or diarrhea. Reassure the mother that Lily will be fine.

Key: GI = Gastrointestinal; n/a = not applicable; NKDA = no known drug allergies; OTC = over-the-counter.

PATIENT EDUCATION FOR Toxic Exposures

The objectives of self-treatment are (1) to minimize exposure and reduce development of toxicity by removing the patient to fresh air, irrigating the skin or eyes, or preventing absorption of potentially toxic agents in the gastrointestinal (GI) tract and (2) to treat patients with minimally toxic ingestions at home under the supervision of a poison control center. For most patients, carefully following the self-care measures listed here will help ensure optimal therapeutic outcomes.

Treatment

- For eye exposures, immediately irrigate with water for 10–15 minutes.
- For skin exposures, immediately wash with soap and water.
- For inhalation exposures, immediately remove the patient to fresh air.

When to Seek Medical Attention

- Referral to an emergency department by contacting 911 directly is appropriate if the patient
  - Is lethargic or comatose or is having convulsions or hallucinations
  - Has decreased respirations or is having difficulty breathing
  - Has abnormal blood pressure or pulse
  - Has taken medications that may produce a rapid decline in consciousness or convulsions

Evaluation of Patient Outcomes for Poisoning

Patients who have inhaled potentially toxic fumes or spilled or splashed a substance on their skin or in their eyes should be reassessed for symptoms after irrigation of the affected area or removal to fresh air. If clinical effects are minimal and resolve within a relatively short period of time (e.g., <30 minutes), the patient may be observed at home. If symptoms persist or worsen, the patient should be referred to a primary care provider or the emergency department, depending on the severity of symptoms and immediacy of need for medical evaluation. The poison control center can facilitate the referral to the appropriate health care facility and provide treatment recommendations to the HCP.

Patients who receive activated charcoal should be contacted afterward at least once to determine whether any symptoms related to the exposure have developed. The time of the call depends on what substance was ingested, how rapidly it is absorbed, and when symptoms would be anticipated. If clinical effects develop and are minor, the patient may be observed at home. If more significant effects develop, the patient should be referred to an emergency department for treatment. If the poison control center recommended self-treatment with activated charcoal, the center staff should remain involved in subsequent decisions regarding the appropriateness of continued home treatment of these patients.

Key Points for Poisoning

- Poison exposures are a common cause of pediatric and adult injury.
- Individuals who purposely misuse, abuse, or use medications as a means of self-harm are not candidates for self-care and should be referred for medical care urgently.
- Medication errors are a common cause of drug-related toxicity, especially in extremes of age (infants and older adults).
- Minimizing the duration or limiting the extent of the exposure is the rationale for most self-treatment practices.
- There are no data demonstrating that self-treatment for poisoning with activated charcoal improves patient outcomes. It should be used only upon recommendation of a poison control center.
- Self-treatment should be considered only for unintentional poison exposures that are likely to cause no or minimal toxicity (i.e., no serious or life-threatening symptoms; Figure 21–2).
- HCPs should consult with the poison control center for guidance on patient assessment and on decisions for the appropriateness of self-treatment.
- Referral directly to the poison control center should be considered for complicated cases, including those with unclear patient histories or lacking specific product or toxin information, and to ensure case follow-up.
- All patients who exhibit potentially life-threatening clinical effects (e.g., seizures, coma) should be referred to an emergency department through the emergency 911 system.

REFERENCES

1. Centers for Disease Control and Prevention, National Center for Injury Prevention and Control. 10 Leading causes of injury deaths by age group highlighting violence-related injury deaths, United States—2014. Available at: http://www.cdc.gov/injury/images/lc-charts/leading_causes_of_injury_deaths_violence_2014_1040w760h.gif. Accessed May 14, 2017.
2. Centers for Disease Control and Prevention, National Center for Health Statistics. NCHS data on drug poisoning deaths. Updated March 2016. Available at: http://www.cdc.gov/nchs/data/factsheets/factsheet_drug_poisoning.htm. Accessed May 14, 2017.
3. Rossen LM, Bastian B, Warner M, et al. Drug poisoning mortality. United States 1999–2015. National Center for Health Statistics 2017. Available at: https://www.cdc.gov/nchs/data-visualization/drug-poisoning-mortality/. Accessed May 14, 2017.
4. Shone LP, King JP, Doane C, et al. Misunderstanding and potential unintended misuse of acetaminophen among adolescents and young adults. *J Health Comm.* 2011;16(Suppl 3):256–67. doi: 10.1080/10810730.2011.604384.
5. King JP, Davis TC, Bailey SC, et al. Developing consumer-centered, nonprescription drug labeling. A study in acetaminophen. *Am J Prev Med.* 2011;40(6):593–8. doi: 10.1016/j.amepre.2011.02.016.
6. Wolf MS, King J, Jacobson K, et al. Risk of unintentional overdose with non-prescription acetaminophen products. *J Gen Intern Med* 2012;27(12):1587–93. doi: 10.1007/s11606-012-2096-3.
7. Klein-Schwartz W, Sorkin JD, Doyon S. Impact of the voluntary withdrawal of over-the-counter cough and cold medications on pediatric ingestions reported to poison centers. *Pharmacoepidemiol Drug Saf.* 2010;19(8):819–24. doi: 10.1002/pds.1971.
8. Mazer-Amirshahi M, Reid N, van den Anker J, et al. Effect of cough and cold medication restriction and label changes on pediatric ingestions reported to United States Poison Centers. *J Pediatr* 2013;163(5):1372–6. doi: 10.1016/j.jpeds.2013.04.054.
9. Hampton LM, Nguyen DB, Edwards JR, et al. Cough and cold medication adverse events after market withdrawal and label revision. *Pediatrics.* 2013;132(6):1047–54. doi: 10.1542/peds.2013-2236.

10. National Institute on Drug Abuse. Monitoring the Future 2015 Survey Results. Last updated December 2015. Available at: https://www.drugabuse.gov/related-topics/trends-statistics/infographics/monitoring-future-2015-survey-results. Accessed May 14, 2017.
11. Mowry JB, Spyker DA, Brooks DE, et al. 2014 Annual report of the American Association of Poison Control Centers' National Poison Data System (NPDS): 32nd annual report. *Clin Toxicol.* 2015;53(10):962–1146. doi: 10.3109/15563650.2015.
12. Bond GR, Woodward RW, Ho M. The growing impact of pediatric pharmaceutical poisoning. *J Pediatr.* 2012;160(2):265–70. doi: 10.1016/j.jpeds.2011.07.042.
13. Galvao TF, Silva EN, Silva MT, et al. Economic evaluation of poison centers: a systematic review. *Int J Technol Assess Health Care.* 2012;28(2):86–92. doi: 10.1017/S0266462312000116.
14. Vassilev ZP, Marcus SM. The impact of a poison control center on the length of hospital stay for patients with poisoning. *J Toxicol Environ Health A.* 2007;70(2):107–10. doi: 10.1080/15287390600755042.
15. Kostic MA, Oswald J, Gummin DD, et al. Poison center consultation decreases hospital length of stay and inpatient charges. *Clin Toxicol.* 2010;48:605. doi: 10.3109/15563650.2010.493290.
16. The Lewin Group. *Final Report on the Value of the Poison Control System.* Alexandria, VA: American Association of Poison Control Centers; 2012. Available at: https://aapcc.s3.amazonaws.com/files/library/Value_of_the_Poison_Center_System_FINAL_9_26_2012_--_FINAL_FINAL_FINAL.pdf. Accessed May 14, 2017.
17. Polivka BJ, Casavant M, Baker SD. Factors associated with healthcare visits by young children for nontoxic poisoning exposures. *J Community Health.* 2010;35(6):572–8. doi: 10.1007/s10900-010-9243-8.
18. Litovitz T, Benson BE, Smolinske S. webPOISONCONTROL: can poison control be automated? *Am J Emerg Med.* 2016;34(8):1614–9. doi: 10.1016/j.ajem.2016.06.018.
19. Schillie SF, Shehab NE, Thomas KE, et al. Medication overdoses leading to emergency department visits among children. *Am J Prev Med.* 2009;37(3):181–7. doi: 10.1016/j.amepre.2009.05.018.
20. National Safety Council. *Injury Facts 2015 Edition.* Itasca, IL: National Safety Council; 2015.
21. Rodgers GB. The safety effects of child-resistant packaging for oral prescription drugs. Two decades of experience. *JAMA.* 1996;275(21):1661–5. doi:10.1001/jama.1996.03530450051032.
22. U.S. Consumer Product Safety Commission. *Poison Prevention Packaging: A Guide for Healthcare Professionals.* Washington, DC: U.S. Consumer Product Safety Commission; 2005, Publication 384. Available at: https://www.cpsc.gov/s3fs-public/384.pdf. Accessed May 14, 2017.
23. Franklin RL, Rodgers GB. Unintentional childhood poisonings treated in United States hospital emergency departments: national estimates of incident cases, population-based poisoning rates, and product involvement. *Pediatrics.* 2008;122(6):1244–51. doi: 10.1542/peds.2007-3551.
24. Yin HS, Parker RM, Wolf MS, et al. Health literacy assessment of labeling of pediatric nonprescription medications: examination of characteristics that may impair parent understanding. *Academ Pediatrics.* 2012;12(4):288–96. doi: 10.1016/j.acap.2012.02.010.
25. Wallace LS, Keenum AJ, DeVoe JE, et al. Women's understanding of different dosing instructions for a liquid pediatric medication. *J Ped Health Care.* 2012;26(6):443–50. doi: 10.1016/j.pedhc.2011.06.006.
26. Lokker NL, Sanders L, Perrin EM, et.al. Parental misinterpretations of over-the-counter pediatric cough and cold medication labels. *Pediatrics.* 2009;123:1464–71. doi: 10.1016/j.pedhc.2011.06.006.
27. Hojer J, Troutman WG, Hoppu K, et al. Position paper update: ipecac syrup for gastrointestinal decontamination. *Clin Toxicol (Phila).* 2013;51(3):134–39. doi: 10.3109/15563650.2013.770153.
28. U.S. Food and Drug Administration. Ipecac syrup; warnings and directions for use for over-the-counter sale. CFR: Code of Federal Regulations, Title 21, Part 201, Section. 201.308. Last updated September 21, 2016. Available at: http://www.accessdata.fda.gov/scripts/cdrh/cfdocs/cfcfr/CFRSearch.cfm?fr=201.308. Accessed May 14, 2017.
29. Chyka PA, Seger D, Krenzelok EP, et al.; American Academy of Clinical Toxicology; European Association of Poisons Centers and Clinical Toxicologists. Position paper: Single-dose activated charcoal. *Clin Toxicol (Phila).* 2005;43(2):61–87. doi: 10.3109/15563659709162569.
30. Albertson TE, Owen KP, Sutter ME, et al. Gastrointestinal decontamination in the acutely poisoned patient. *Int J Emerg Med.* 2011;4:65. doi: 10.1186/1865-1380-4-65.
31. Juurlink DN. Activated charcoal for acute overdose: a reappraisal. *Brit J Clin Pharmacol.* 2016;81(3):482–7. doi: 10.1111/bcp.12793.
32. Isbister GK, Kumar VV. Indications for single-dose activated charcoal administration in acute overdose. *Curr Opin Crit Care.* 2011;17(4):351–7. doi: 10.1097/MCC.0b013e328348bf59.
33. Olson KR. Activated charcoal for acute poisoning: One toxicologist's journey. *J Med Toxicol.* 2010;6(2):190–8. doi: 10.1007/s13181-010-0046-1.
34. Alaspaa AO, Kuisma MJ, Hoppu K, et al. Out-of-hospital administration of activated charcoal by emergency medical services. *Ann Emerg Med.* 2005;45(2):207–12. doi: 10.1016/j.annemergmed.2004.07.448.
35. Eldridge DL, Van Eyk J, Kornegay C. Pediatric toxicology. *Emerg Med Clin North Am.* 2007;15(2):283–308. doi:10.1016/j.emc.2007.02.011.
36. Lapus RM. Activated charcoal for pediatric poisonings: the universal antidote? *Curr Opin Pediatr.* 2007;19(2):216–22. doi: 10.1097/MOP.0b013e32801da2a9.

CHAPTER 22

OSTOMY CARE AND SUPPLIES

JOAN LERNER SELEKOF AND SHARON WILSON

An *ostomy* is an opening or outlet through the abdominal wall created surgically for the purpose of eliminating waste. The opening is usually made by bringing a portion of the bladder, colon, small intestine, or ureter through the abdominal wall. The opening of the ostomy is called the *stoma* (the Greek word for "mouth").

The establishment of an ostomy, whether temporary or permanent, to replace normal elimination anatomy may be a dramatic, life-changing event. The health care provider is a crucial resource for the reassurance, support, and education needed by the patient and family. Fostering an understanding of improvements in surgical procedures, ostomy supplies, and outcomes can help allay much of the patient's fear and anxiety. The goal in ostomy care is to enable resumption of the previous lifestyle as much as possible—to be a person, not a patient. In encounters with health care providers, the person with an ostomy will notice their reaction to the presence of the stoma. Any negative response—even unconscious signals such as a hurried interaction or avoidance of eye contact—may contribute to the patient's difficulties with altered self-image related to the ostomy, so special care should be taken to convey acceptance and knowledgeability about various aspects of stoma management.

More than 700,000 Americans are currently living with an ostomy.[1] Ostomy surgery is performed on people of all ages and for many conditions, both acquired and congenital. When medically advisable, the current trend in ostomy surgery is a laparoscopic approach. Laparoscopic surgery is a type of minimally invasive surgery that uses smaller-scale instruments, placed through minor incisions, with the assistance of video camera technology. Patients report experiencing less pain, quicker recovery, and less scarring than with traditional ostomy surgery.

Indications for Ostomies

Ostomies may be permanent or temporary, and ostomy surgery is performed in all age groups, ranging from neonates to older adults. Reasons for needing an ostomy include congenital anomalies (e.g., imperforate anus, Hirschsprung disease), inflammatory bowel disease (i.e., ulcerative colitis and Crohn's disease), familial polyposis, cancer, radiation damage, pressure ulcers, trauma, and any other need to divert the urinary or fecal stream.[2,3] The type of ostomy depends on the condition being treated.

The two most common disorders leading to *ileostomy* surgery are (1) ulcerative colitis, which affects the large intestine and rectum, and (2) Crohn's disease, which may involve any part of the gastrointestinal (GI) tract. Other conditions that may result in an ileostomy include traumatic injury, cancer, familial polyposis, and necrotizing enterocolitis.

The most common reasons for *colostomy* surgery are (1) cancer of the colon or rectum, (2) diverticulitis, and (3) traumatic injury. Other indications include obstruction of the colon or rectum, genetic malformation, radiation colitis, and loss of anal muscular control. In some cases, a temporary colostomy may be placed to protect areas of the colon that have been surgically repaired. Healing of diseased or damaged bowel may take several weeks, months, or years, but eventually the colon and the rectum are reconnected and bowel continuity is restored. Figure 22–1 shows the location of various types of colostomies.

Urinary diversions, or *urostomies,* are created to correct bladder dysfunction or to restore functionality after bladder loss, which can be secondary to cancer, neurogenic bladder, genetic malformation, or interstitial cystitis.

Types of Ostomies

The three basic types of ostomies are (1) ileostomy, (2) colostomy (the most common type), and (3) urostomy (see Color Plates, photographs 7A–I). Each type of ostomy has several variations, depending on the location of the stoma, the reason for the surgical procedure, or whether the procedure will maintain urinary or fecal continence.

Ileostomy

An ileostomy is surgically created by bringing a portion of the ileum through the abdominal wall (see Color Plates, photograph 7A). Initially, the discharge is liquid, but as the ileum adapts, it assumes some of the absorptive functions of the colon and the discharge may become semisoft. The discharge is continuous and contains intestinal enzymes that may irritate the peristomal skin.

Several types of continent ileostomies have been devised (see Color Plates, photograph 7B). Typically, an internal pouch is created from the ileum, and an intussusception (a slipping of a length of intestine into an adjacent portion) of the bowel is used to create a "nipple" that renders the patient continent for stool and flatus. The pouch is periodically emptied by inserting a catheter through the nipple, which is attached to the skin usually in the right lower abdominal quadrant, into the pouch. At first, the pouch holds approximately 75 mL, but it stretches with use, so that at

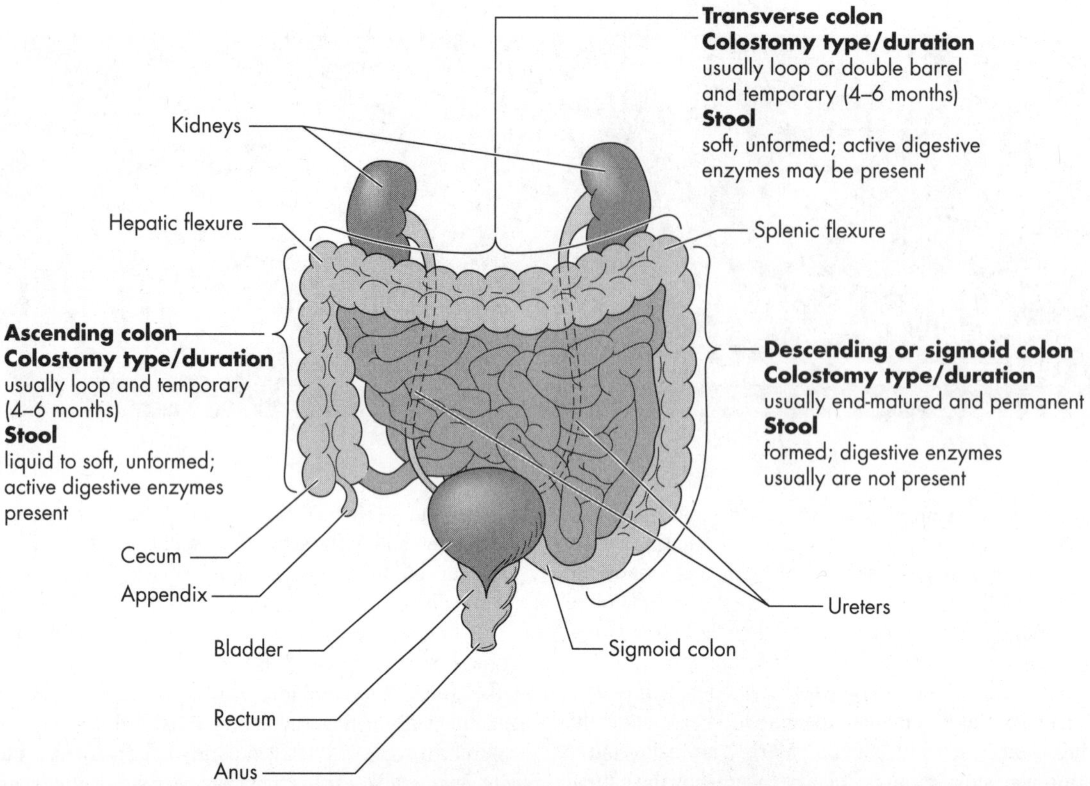

FIGURE 22-1 Anatomic drawing of the lower digestive and urinary tracts depicting location and permanence of colostomies. (Source: Adapted with permission from *Am J Nurs.* 1977;77:443.)

6 months postoperatively, it may hold 600–800 mL and can be drained 3–5 times daily. Patients do not need to wear an external pouching system, but they often use a gauze pad or stoma cap over the opening.

The restorative proctocolectomy (S pouch or J pouch) with ileoanal reservoir spares the rectum in patients with ulcerative colitis or familial polyposis. The colon is removed and the diseased mucosa is stripped from the rectum, and an internal pouch is created from the ileum. The distal end of the small intestine is stapled or hand sewn to the remaining rectal tissue. The sphincter is preserved, and ostomy pouching systems are unnecessary. However, a patient undergoing this procedure may have a temporary stoma (for approximately 3–6 months) placed to protect the healing pouch. After ileoanal reservoir surgery, bowel movements will be more frequent, and the patient may experience perianal skin irritation.

Colostomy

A colostomy is created by bringing a portion of the colon through the abdominal wall. The discharge may be semisoft, paste-like, or formed, depending on the portion of bowel used (Figure 22–1).

Ascending colostomies are uncommon. The ascending colon is retained, but the rest of the large bowel is removed or bypassed (see Color Plates, photograph 7C). The stoma is usually on the right side of the abdomen. The discharge is similar to that with an ileostomy—semisoft—and a pouch must be worn at all times.

The *transverse* colon is the site of most temporary colostomies (Figure 22–1). A loop of the transverse colon is lifted through the abdominal incision, and a rod or bridge (which is removed within 1–2 weeks) is placed under the loop to give it support while the stoma heals. The discharge is usually semiliquid or very soft and contains digestive enzymes.

Loop colostomies have one large opening but two tracts (see Color Plates, photograph 7D). The proximal tract discharges fecal material, and the distal tract secretes small amounts of mucus. A pouching system must be worn at all times. A person with a loop colostomy may also pass a minimal amount of stool or mucus through the rectum. This is a normal occurrence.

For a *double-barrel transverse* colostomy, the bowel is completely divided by bringing both the proximal end and the distal end through the abdominal wall and then suturing them to the skin (see Color Plates, photograph 7E). The distal stoma may also be called the mucous fistula.

Descending and *sigmoid* colostomies are fairly common; generally the stoma is on the left side of the abdomen (see Color Plates, photograph 7F). The fecal discharge has a paste-like consistency and at times may consist of formed stool. This type of colostomy may be regulated by irrigation; therefore, a pouching system may or may not be needed. However, many patients prefer a pouch to irrigation. Not everyone with a descending or sigmoid colostomy is a good candidate for irrigation or prefers irrigation. Factors to consider in making the decision to irrigate include the presence or absence of stomal complications and the patient's normal stooling pattern, psychomotor ability, and willingness to commit the time required to properly irrigate the ostomy.

Urinary Diversions

Urinary diversion surgery creates an alternative route for discharge of urine through an opening in the abdominal wall. Urinary stomas should function immediately after surgery. The broad term for a urinary diversion is *urostomy.*

The *ileal conduit* is the most common type of urinary diversion (see Color Plates, photograph 7G). After the bladder is removed, ileal or colon conduits are created by implanting the ureters into an isolated loop of bowel; one end of the bowel loop is sutured, and the distal end is brought to the surface of the abdomen. The stoma looks similar to an ileostomy or colostomy stoma. A pouching system must be worn continuously. Mucous shreds will be present in the urine when the small intestine or the large intestine is used to create the diversion (see Color Plates, photograph 7H). Because the ileum is used to create an ileal conduit, some people incorrectly refer to the ileal conduit as an ileostomy. Clarification of the type of effluent (stool or urine) will help in selecting the correct type of pouch.

In an *ureterostomy,* one or both ureters are detached from the bladder and brought to the outside of the abdominal wall, where a stoma is created. This procedure is used less frequently because the ureters tend to narrow unless they have been dilated permanently because of previous disease (see Color Plates, photograph 7I).

A *cystostomy* is performed when blockage or narrowing of the urethra occurs. Urine is diverted from the bladder to the abdominal wall. A pouch must be worn continuously. An infant with a cystostomy may wear diapers instead of a pouch.

The *continent urinary diversion* is available for selected patients, but its use requires that certain criteria be met. An Indiana pouch is a type of continent urostomy in which a pouch is created from part of the cecum and ileum, with a portion of the ileum brought through the abdominal wall to create a stoma. The ureters are attached to the cecum pouch. The remaining ileum is reattached to the colon for normal digestive flow. The ileocecal valve is left intact and becomes part of the continence mechanism, preventing urine from exiting the pouch. The internal pouch is emptied by inserting a catheter into the stoma to drain the urine. Patients are usually placed on a strict schedule for catheterizing the stoma often enough to avoid leakage. The new pouch may hold up to 600 mL of urine. An external pouching system is not necessary. Most patients wear a gauze pad or stoma cap.

The orthotopic neobladder is a rebuilt bladder. The small intestine is used to create a pouch, and the pouch is then attached to the native urethra. This procedure allows patients to void using their urethra, but voiding relies on use of the abdominal muscles to empty the neobladder.

Management of Ostomies

Management Goals

The ideal ostomy pouching system should be leak-proof, odor-proof, comfortable, easily manipulated, inconspicuous, safe, and as inexpensive as possible. The patient with an ostomy has lost a normal body function, and an appropriately selected pouching system assists in managing that loss. In a functional context, it becomes almost a part of the body. Nevertheless, especially during the first several weeks or months after surgery, patients and their families often find discussing ostomy needs difficult or embarrassing.

The ostomy industry is highly specialized and rapidly changing as researchers and manufacturers try to improve designs, resulting in a wide range of choices. Pouch selection is extremely personal and is based on the patient's specific needs and abilities and on the cost of the system.

General Management Approach

Adult and adolescent patients must be taught self-care skills to manage the ostomy, including (1) sizing the stoma, (2) cutting a pouch or skin barrier to fit the stoma (or selecting a precut pouch or barrier), (3) cleaning the skin, (4) applying paste (caulking) or powder if necessary, (5) applying the pouch, (6) removing the pouch, and (7) emptying the pouch. Patients must be prepared for effluent from the stoma at any time.

Patients are most likely to achieve optimal outcomes if a pouching system is properly fitted (Figure 22–2) and if the stoma is cared for appropriately. In interactions with persons with an ostomy, the health care provider should always be aware of the sensitive nature of the topic and ensure that privacy is respected during all encounters. Failure to provide a comfortable environment in which to discuss problems, concerns, and alternatives may cause patients to avoid such discussions, with less-than-optimal outcomes. Follow-up assessment and care may be accomplished through a telephone call or scheduled appointment or during the patient's routine visits to purchase supplies or medications.

Frequent changes in the pouching system and accessories should signal a potential problem, as should the use of multiple products intended for the same purpose. In many cases, patients may be referred to a primary care provider or a wound, ostomy, and continence (WOC) nurse for follow-up evaluation and treatment of problems identified by a health care provider. Complications such as impotence; peristomal hernia; and stenosis, prolapse, retraction, or peristomal skin injury warrant medical referral. In some cases, however, self-care is appropriate, particularly with experienced ostomy patients.

The presence of an ostomy and its location in the GI or urinary system should always be noted in the patient's profile, to minimize medication-related risks. It is helpful to maintain a record of current and past ostomy products that the patient has used and any problems that the patient has experienced. This information can be helpful in making future recommendations.

Types of Ostomy Pouches

The surgical technique used to create the stoma influences the pouching system required, the complexity of the pouching procedure, and the risks of stomal (e.g., necrosis, stenosis, hernia) and peristomal complications. In the past, most ostomy pouches were reusable. The advantages of reusable pouching systems were their durability, availability in numerous configurations, and relatively low cost. Their disadvantages were that they required cleaning before each use, were heavy, tended to retain odor, and often required a separate skin barrier.

Ostomy patients are now fitted with odor-proof, lightweight, disposable pouching systems. The health care provider measuring the stoma should cut to the skin stoma junction. Most pouches

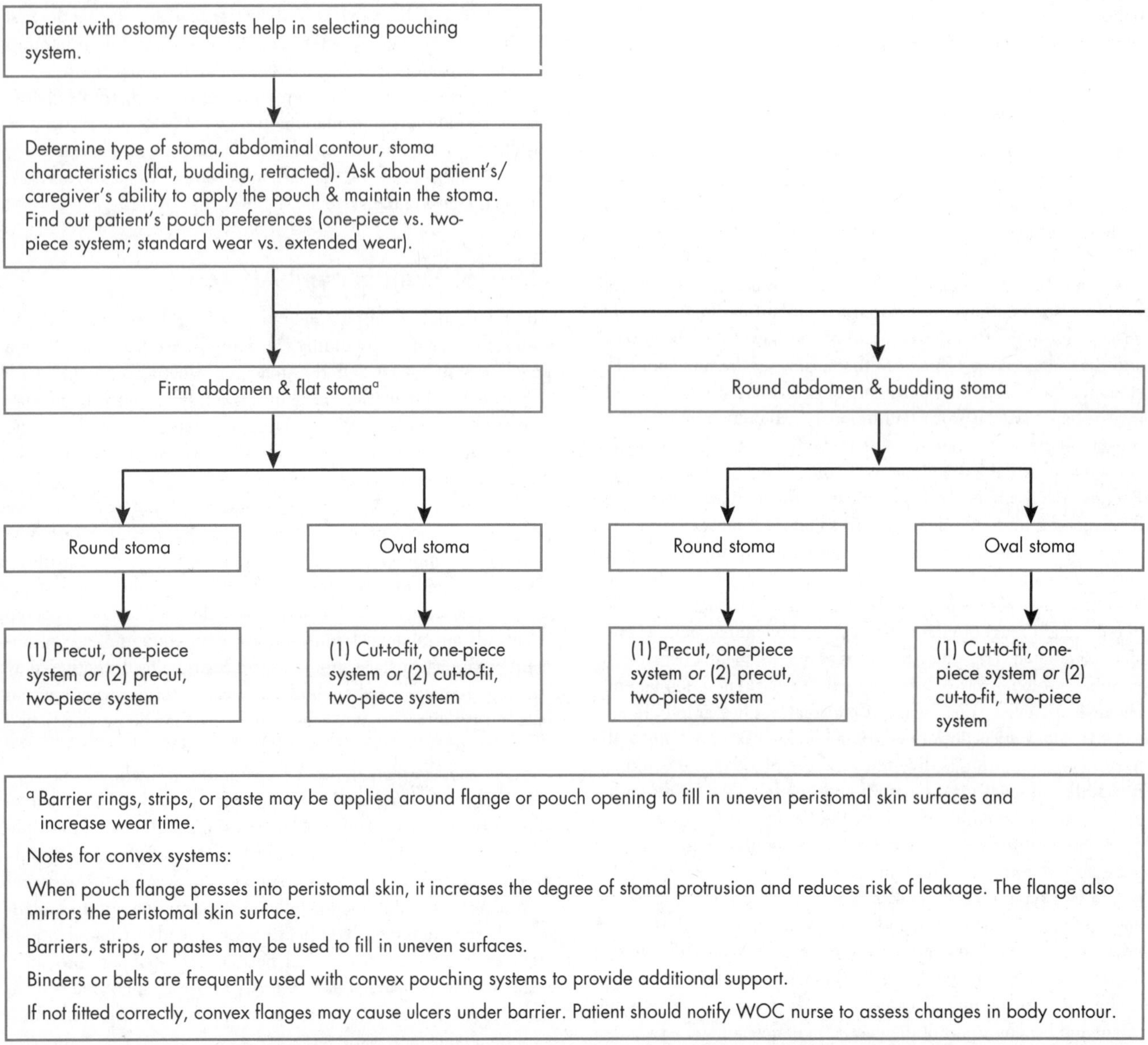
Patient with ostomy requests help in selecting pouching system.
Determine type of stoma, abdominal contour, stoma characteristics (flat, budding, retracted). Ask about patient's/caregiver's ability to apply the pouch & maintain the stoma. Find out patient's pouch preferences (one-piece vs. two-piece system; standard wear vs. extended wear).
Firm abdomen & flat stoma[a]
Round abdomen & budding stoma
Round stoma
Oval stoma
Round stoma
Oval stoma
(1) Precut, one-piece system or (2) precut, two-piece system
(1) Cut-to-fit, one-piece system or (2) cut-to-fit, two-piece system
(1) Precut, one-piece system or (2) precut, two-piece system
(1) Cut-to-fit, one-piece system or (2) cut-to-fit, two-piece system
[a] Barrier rings, strips, or paste may be applied around flange or pouch opening to fill in uneven peristomal skin surfaces and increase wear time.
Notes for convex systems:
When pouch flange presses into peristomal skin, it increases the degree of stomal protrusion and reduces risk of leakage. The flange also mirrors the peristomal skin surface.
Barriers, strips, or pastes may be used to fill in uneven surfaces.
Binders or belts are frequently used with convex pouching systems to provide additional support.
If not fitted correctly, convex flanges may cause ulcers under barrier. Patient should notify WOC nurse to assess changes in body contour.

FIGURE **22-2** Selection of ostomy pouching system. Key: WOC = Wound, ostomy, and continence. (*continued on next page*)

incorporate a solid skin barrier in each flange or one-piece pouch, which eliminates the need for a separate skin barrier. Disposable equipment is available in one- and two-piece systems (Figure 22–3). The one-piece system, in which the skin barrier and the pouch are available in one piece, is easy to apply, especially for patients with impaired manual dexterity. In the two-piece system, the skin barrier is separate from the pouch. This design provides ready access to the flange and allows changing the pouch, if desired, without removal of the flange from the skin. The flange is easy to apply and is generally more pliable and adaptable to different abdominal contours.

One- and two-piece pouching systems are also available for young children. Although pouches are available for infants, some ostomies are managed with a diaper. If a diaper is used, care must be taken to avoid skin irritation from a caustic effluent. Moisture barrier ointments and creams are required for neonates and infants who are only diapered. The decision to diaper or pouch is based on the location of the stoma, the type and amount of effluent, and the child's activity level. Once the child is crawling or exploring, it is difficult to keep stool contained in a diaper.

Both one- and two-piece pouch systems are available in drainable, high-output, closed-end, and urostomy styles. Drainable styles are used when bowel regulation cannot be established; they allow for easy and frequent emptying. A closed-end system requires the wearer to remove and discard the pouch when it is almost full. Closed-end systems are used by patients who have regulated colostomies, have one or two formed bowel movements within 24 hours, or routinely irrigate the ostomy to remove output. Urostomy systems allow a constant output of urine and easy emptying throughout the day through a narrow valve opening. At night, most urostomy patients connect their pouch to dependent drainage to prevent overfilling of the pouch.

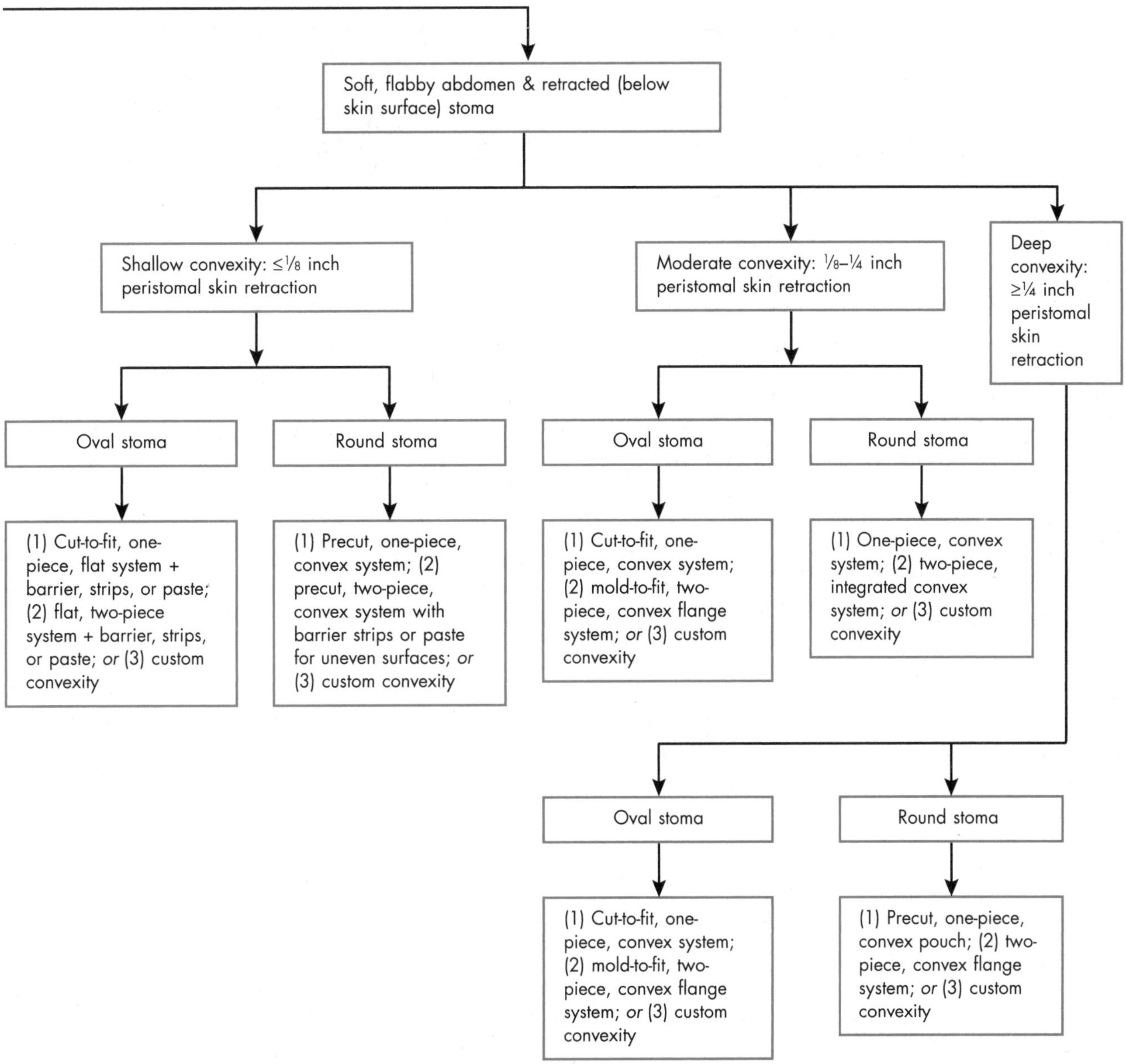

FIGURE 22-2 Selection of ostomy pouching system. Key: WOC = Wound, ostomy, and continence. *(continued)*

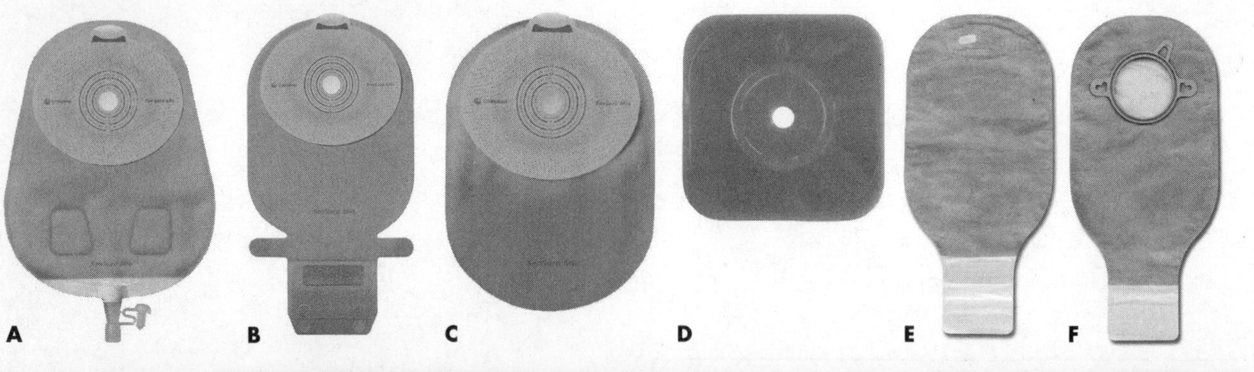

FIGURE 22–3 Sample ostomy appliances: **A**, Coloplast SenSura Mio urostomy pouch; **B**, Coloplast SenSura Mio drainable pouch; **C**, Coloplast SenSura Mio closed-end pouch; **D–F**, Hollister New Image two-piece pouching system with Lock'n Roll closure, pouch and flange views, respectively. (Source: **A–C** reprinted with permission from Coloplast, Minneapolis, MN; **D–F** reprinted with permission from Hollister Incorporated, Libertyville, IL.)

Fitting and Application

Pouches are available in transparent and opaque styles and in various sizes. The pouch opening may be cut to fit or presized. Other options in skin barriers include a flat or convex skin barrier. When convex barriers are indicated, they are available with round, oval, or moldable openings.

Measuring the stoma to determine the proper fit of a pouch is an important part of ostomy care. The diameter of the round stoma is measured at the base, where the mucosa meets the skin; this area is considered the widest measurement. Oval stomas should be measured at their widest and narrowest diameters. A stoma may swell if the adhesive fits too tightly or slips, or if the patient falls or experiences a hard blow to the stoma. It is important to periodically reassess the size for proper fitting.

Other considerations in fitting the pouch include the patient's body contour, stoma location, presence of any skin creases and scars, and ostomy type. The lack of uniformity in types of ostomies and ostomy equipment makes it difficult to give standard instructions for application. In addition, the stoma and the contour of the surrounding area change over time, necessitating continuous adjustments to pouches and accessories. In general, when a flange is used, the opening should be cut to fit the skin-stoma junction. A WOC nurse is an excellent source of assistance in custom-fitting these pouching systems.

Wear Time

The pouch should be emptied when it is one-third to one-half full, to prevent leakage. With a two-piece system, the closed-end pouch is simply removed from the flange and thrown away. Patients who want to save on pouch costs may use the two-piece drainable system and alternate the use of two pouches. The full pouch is removed and replaced by a second pouch; the first pouch is then emptied, washed, and reused when the second pouch is changed. One-piece, closed-end systems are removed and disposed of once or twice daily; those that can be drained can be left in place for as long as they are comfortable and there is no leakage. The flange and skin barrier may be left in place for 3–7 days, depending on the condition of the skin and skin barrier. Average wear time is 4 days.

The skin barrier is constructed from a material called a *hydrocolloid.* The hydrocolloid softens in the presence of moisture. As the hydrocolloid softens, less adhesive is present to secure the seal. Accordingly, a person with a high liquid output or very moist skin (as from heavy perspiration) may find that the skin barrier must be changed in 3–4 days. A person with solid to semisolid stool may be able to wear the skin barrier longer than 4 days. Although activities such as swimming or playing tennis may decrease the wear time of the pouch, this decreased time should not discourage participation in physical activities. New pouch adhesives can effectively keep the system in place during these activities. Because water will not enter the stoma, it is not necessary to cover it while bathing or showering. The patient does not need to cover a continent stoma when swimming. However, the pouching system can be secured with waterproof tape (e.g., Hy-Tape, Pink Tape) by taping around the edges of the wafer/flange to prevent leakage of output from the stoma.

Product Selection Guidelines

The selection of products must be tailored to the patient's activity level and, if present, specific disabilities. Some systems require manipulation that a patient with arthritis may not be able to perform. Special products are also available to assist patients who have poor vision. In general, patients with visual or physical impairments will do best with one-piece systems because these systems have precut pouches and require minimal manipulation. Waterproof materials or a stoma cover should be included with the system. Table 22–1 lists ostomy manufacturers, with addresses for websites that detail all available products and product information. No particular device will prevent patients who are confused from touching and dislodging the pouching system (e.g., patients with Alzheimer disease). It may be helpful to dress these patients in garments that make it difficult for them to reach the pouch. Dressing infants in one-piece clothing will help prevent them from exploring and pulling off their pouches.

TABLE 22–1 **Sources of Ostomy Support, Products, and Information**

Organization/Manufacturer	Telephone Number	Website
American Cancer Society	800-ACS-2345	www.cancer.org
Colo-majic Liners	866-611-6028	www.colomajic.com
Coloplast	800-533-0464	www.coloplast.com
ConvaTec	800-422-8811	www.convatec.com
Crohn's and Colitis Foundation of America, Inc.	800-343-3637	www.ccfa.org
Cymed Ostomy Company	800-582-0707	www.cymed-ostomy.com
C&S Ostomy Pouch Covers	877-754-9913	www.cspouchcovers.com
Dansac (importer: Incutech, Inc.)	800-699-4232	www.incutech.com; www.dansac.dk
Hollister, Inc.	800-323-4060	www.hollister.com
Hy-Tape Corporation	800-248-0101	www.hytape.com
International Ostomy Association	N/A	www.ostomyinternational.org
Kem-Osto EZ-Vent	888-562-8802	www.kemOnline.com
Marlen Manufacturing	276-292-9196	www.marlenmfg.com
Nu-Hope Laboratories, Inc.	800-899-5017	www.nu-hope.com
Options Ostomy Support/Barrier, Inc.	800-736-6555	www.options-ostomy.com
Ostomysecrets	877-613-6246	www.ostomysecrets.com
Rally 4 Youth		www.rally4youth.org
Schena Ostomy Technologies	239-263-9957	www.ostomyezclean.com
Safe n' Simple	248-214-4877	www.SnS-medical.com
Stealth Belt	800-237-4491	www.stealthbelt.com
Stoma Guard	800-814-4195	www.sto-med.com
The Parthenon Company, Inc.	800-453-8898	www.parthenonInc.com
Torbot Group, Inc.	800-545-4254	www.torbot.com
United Ostomy Associations of America, Inc.	800-826-0826	www.uoaa.org
■ Continent Diversion Network ■ GLO Network—Gay/Lesbian/Bisexual Ostomates and their partners ■ Pull-Thru Network		■ www.uoaa.org/forum/viewforum.php?f=8 ■ www.glo-uoaa.org ■ www.pullthrunetwork.org
United Ostomy Association of Canada, Inc.	416-595-5452; 888-969-9698 (Canadian residents only)	www.ostomycanada.ca
Wound, Ostomy and Continence Nurses Society (WOCN)	888-224-WOCN (9626)	www.wocn.org

Ostomy Accessories

Belts

Special elastic belts that attach to various pouching systems provide additional support. However, not all ostomy patients need to wear belts. Indications for their use are a deeply convex flange, short pouch-wearing time, high activity level (especially in children), heavy perspiration, and personal preference. Some patients may find that wearing a belt for just a few hours after changing the pouch helps the adhesive to "cure" without undue disturbance, thereby increasing wear time and decreasing the risk of leakage. Belts that are too tight may cause skin ulcers. To be effective, the belt must be kept even with the belt hooks. If the belt slips up around the waist, this annoyance may contribute to poor adherence, and a moving belt may possibly cut the stomal tissue. Women may find that pantyhose and a panty support are excellent alternatives to a belt.

Many belts contain latex, so the patient should be asked about a latex allergy before a belt is recommended.

Skin Barriers, Powders, and Pastes

Skin barriers, powders, and pastes are available to address specific skin problems (Table 22–2). Skin barriers are intended to protect the skin immediately adjacent to the stoma from stoma discharge and to serve as a means of attaching a pouching system. They correct imperfections in the skin surface, allowing the pouching system to fit securely. Powders are used on weeping skin to absorb excessive moisture and support healing, but excessive powder must be dusted off or sealed with a no-sting liquid skin

TABLE 22-2 Selected Ostomy Skin Barriers, Adhesives, Adhesive Removers, Belts, Powders, Cleaners, and Air Vent System

Product	Description
Hollister Adapt Lubricating Deodorant	Available in 8-ounce bottle or 8 mL packs. Facilitates emptying of pouch by providing lubrication
Coloplast Brava: rings, strips, strip paste	Moldable strips/paste to fill in uneven surfaces
ConvaTec AllKare Adhesive Remover Wipes	Helps prevent skin damage by easing removal of all adhesives; has oily residue; skin should be washed after use
ConvaTec AllKare Protective Barrier Wipes	Thin film protects against skin stripping; excellent liquid skin barrier for adhesives, tapes, and self-adhesive dressings
ConvaTec Eakin Cohesive Seals	Moldable, double-sided adhesive seals designed to help prevent skin damage; absorbs moisture and forms a gel to further protect skin; adheres to moist, sore skin; suitable for all types of ostomies (especially hard-to-fit stomas); can be used with pastes and all skin barriers and pouching systems
ConvaTec Stomahesive Paste	Pectin product; helps prevent leakage and skin irritation by filling in uneven surfaces; new easy-to-squeeze tube
ConvaTec Stomahesive Powder	Pectin base; light dusting applied to denuded skin to promote healing
Hollister Adapt Barrier Rings, Strips, Paste	Custom (molded, shaped, and stacked) convex barrier rings; barrier strips can mold and stack; paste in easy-to-squeeze tube
Hollister Medical Adhesive	Improves adhesive contact between skin and barrier
Hollister M9 Cleaner/Decrystallizer	Cleans urinary drainage systems; pH-balanced and nonacidic
Hollister M9 Odor Eliminator	Available in spray or drops, scented or unscented; is an enzyme that helps to neutralize odor
Hollister Adapt Powder	Light dusting applied to denuded skin to promote healing
Hollister Universal Remover Wipes	Removes adhesives and barriers; available as spray and wipes
KEM Air VENT System (OSTO-EZ-VENT)	Quickly and easily releases gas buildup in ostomy pouches
Nu-Hope Barrier Rings and Strips	Karaya/pectin; moldable rings and strips
Nu-Hope Cement	Natural rubber; hexane; excellent adherence for difficult pouching
Nu-Hope Support Belt	Standard 2⅜-inch opening; 3- to 9-inch widths; customized belts available; provides excellent support to prevent parastomal herniation; prolapse overbelt and custom openings available
Smith & Nephew Adhesive Remover	Helps prevent skin damage by easing removal of all adhesives
Torbot Skin Cement	4-ounce can; natural rubber; hexane; excellent adherence for difficult pouching
3M No Sting Wipes	Does not contain alcohol; thin film protects against skin stripping; excellent liquid skin barrier for adhesives, tapes, and self-adhesive dressings

preparation before pouch application. Pastes (which are not a glue but have a paste-like consistency) are used to seal the area around the stoma and to fill creases in the skin. Pastes produce a flat surface for application of other skin barriers and can be used to caulk the edge of the skin barrier.

Solid skin barriers are preattached to the pouch (one-piece system) or provided separately (two-piece system) and may be custom-cut (sizable) or precut (presized). Some manufacturers will custom-cut the barriers; typically, however, the patient or the WOC nurse modifies the barrier to fit the stoma. The opening in the skin barrier should match the size and shape of the patient's stoma. To apply a skin barrier, the patient should place a bead of skin barrier paste either around the stoma or directly on the inside edge of the skin barrier and then apply the skin barrier to dry, wrinkle-free skin, pressing the skin barrier around the stoma to improve its adherence. Newer moldable seals and rings are now available from major manufacturers.

Solid skin barriers may melt if exposed to high temperatures. Therefore, during the summer and especially when traveling, the solid skin barrier should be put in an insulated box (ice is not required) to minimize the risk of melting. Pouches should not be left in a vehicle during the day, unless it is in a completely shaded location and the outside temperature is not extremely high.

Absorbent Gel Packets and Flakes

Absorbent gel packets and flakes (e.g., Ileosorb, Par-Sorb) dissolve as the pouch fills, turning the liquid effluent into a gel. They reduce noise caused by sloshing of stomal fluids, control odor, prevent peristomal skin irritation, and prevent leakage, especially at night while the patient sleeps.

Cleansing and Special Skin Care Products

Cleansing of the stoma and surrounding skin is best done with plain water. If soap is used, it should be rinsed off thoroughly, and the skin should be dried before a new pouching system is applied. Use of moisturizers and products containing lanolin, petrolatum, or oils should be avoided because they prevent the pouching system from adhering to the skin.

Adhesives

Adhesives, in the form of cements or tapes, may be used by some patients to keep the pouch in place. Hypoallergenic tape may be used to support the pouch. A strip may be applied across the top, bottom, and sides of the flange, with half on the flange and half on the skin. Waterproof tape may be used during swimming or bathing. Solvents are available to remove adhesive residue; however, solvents or adhesive removers must be removed from the skin before application of the new pouching system.

Irrigating Sets

Irrigating sets can be used to maintain control of output without the use of a pouch in patients with colostomies who are candidates for irrigation. Irrigation is similar to performing an enema at the site of the stoma. Approximately 1000 mL of lukewarm tap water is instilled into the bowel through a cone inserted in the stoma. The bowel then expands, causing peristalsis, with subsequent elimination of waste through the stoma. A good candidate for irrigation is an adult patient who has a colostomy distal to the splenic flexure; does not have a history of irritable bowel syndrome or a disability; has good mentation, manual dexterity, and appropriate bathroom facilities (running water); and is not undergoing chemotherapy or radiation therapy. For the process to be safe and effective, the patient should use a colostomy irrigation set, rather than a standard enema set.

Frequency of irrigation depends somewhat on the patient's normal bowel habits. The recommended approach is to irrigate at the same time every day and eventually to regulate irrigation to every other day. Establishing the irrigation regimen takes approximately 6 weeks. After achieving good control, the patient may wear a security pouch or a piece of gauze, a stoma cover, or a cap over the stoma. Irrigation is not necessary for health; it is merely one method of colostomy management. Patients should use this procedure only if desired and instructed in technique by a WOC nurse or a primary care provider.

TABLE 22-3 Effects of Food on Stoma Output

Foods That Thicken Stool	Applesauce; bananas; bread; buttermilk; cheese; marshmallows; milk; pasta, boiled; peanut butter, creamy; potatoes; pretzels; rice; tapioca; toast; yogurt
Foods That Loosen Stool	Beer and other alcoholic beverages; chocolate; dried or string beans; fried foods; greasy foods; highly spiced foods; leafy green vegetables (lettuce, broccoli, spinach); prune or grape juice; raw fruits (except bananas); raw vegetables, fruit juices, milk
Foods That Cause Stool Odor	Asparagus; beans; cabbage-family vegetables (cabbage, brussels sprouts, broccoli, cauliflower); cheese; eggs; fish; garlic; onions; some spices; turnips
Foods That Cause Urine Odor	Asparagus; seafood; some spices
Foods That Combat Urine Odor	Buttermilk; cranberry juice; yogurt
Foods That Cause Gas	Beans (dried, string, or baked); beer; cabbage-family vegetables (cabbage, brussels sprouts, broccoli, cauliflower); carbonated beverages; corn; cucumbers; dairy products; mushrooms; onions; peas; radishes; spinach; spicy foods
Foods That Color Stool	Beets; berries; chocolate; fats; fish; meat (large amounts of red meat); milk; red gelatin; vegetables

Source: References 4 and 5.

Deodorizers

If needed, deodorizers are available as liquids or tablets. Liquid concentrates, which are available as companion products with most ostomy pouches, can be placed directly into the pouch to neutralize odor. DevKo external tablets may also be placed into the pouch to decrease odor. Derifil internal deodorant tablets (active ingredient is 100 mg chlorophyllin copper complex sodium) also may be used. The purpose of such deodorizers is to lessen the odor during pouch emptying; no odor should be detectable when the pouch is on and adequately sealed.

Changes in Diet

Diet does not generally play an important role in ostomy management. Most patients can eat their usual diet, including all of the foods they ate before surgery if they chew everything well. A diet low in fiber is advisable for the first 6 weeks after surgery, however, to allow the intestine to heal and the swelling to resolve. The usual diet can be resumed after that time.

The effects of various foods on ostomy output are summarized in Table 22–3. Patients with a urostomy may want to avoid foods that cause urine odor. Patients with colostomies, especially those who irrigate, should avoid foods that cause loose stools. (This problem varies among individual patients.) Because they have no control over passage of gas, patients with a fecal ostomy may prefer to reduce their intake of gas-forming foods. Products such as alpha-D-galactosidase may be used to control gas (see Chapter 14). Patients with ileostomies are more prone to intestinal obstruction from high-fiber foods eaten in large quantities or eaten exclusive of other foods (Table 22–4).[4,5] Thoroughly chewing high-fiber foods and eating them in small amounts and with other types of food will help prevent food blockage. The patient should be instructed on how to manage a food blockage. Table 22–5 lists signs and symptoms of blockage; Table 22–6 summarizes its management.

Complications of Ostomies

Persons with ostomies may experience both psychological and physical complications. The health care provider should be prepared to address these complications or to refer patients to their primary care provider or to a WOC nurse. These nurse specialists are often based in hospitals or home health care agencies. The United Ostomy Associations of America is an organization that provides peer support for patients. Before surgery, patients should receive a thorough explanation that describes what procedure will be performed, what to expect during the postsurgical recovery

TABLE 22-4 **High-Fiber Foods**[a]

Apple skins	Hot dogs
Apricots	Mushrooms
Asparagus	Nuts
Beans and lentils	Oranges and orange rinds
Bologna	Pineapples
Bran	Popcorn
Celery	Potato peels
Chinese vegetables	Raisins
Coconut	Raw vegetables
Corn	Sausage
Dried figs	Seeds
Grapefruit	Shrimp
Grapes	Tomatoes

[a] To be consumed cautiously by persons with ileostomies.
Source: References 4 and 5.

period, and what pouching and supplies will be used. Presented next is a review of potential complications that can be used to assist patients seeking advice after their surgery.

Psychological Complications

Some patients anticipating ostomy surgery fear that they will not be able to continue their former job, participate in sports, perform sexually, or have children. These patients need reassurance that an ostomy rarely impairs the ability to carry out such activities. Contacting the local United Ostomy Associations of America is of utmost importance in assisting with the rehabilitation of these patients; both providers and patients are encouraged to utilize the support of this organization. Patients may also wish to find a local WOC nurse. Before and after ostomy surgery, appropriate education and counseling on ostomy care will provide needed information and support. Literature is available from all of the major ostomy product manufacturers, the United Ostomy Associations of America, and the American College of Surgeons.

TABLE 22-5 **Signs and Symptoms of Intestinal Obstruction**

Partial Obstruction	Complete Obstruction
Watery output with foul odor	Absence of output (urine and fecal)
Cramping abdominal pain	Severe cramping pain
Abdominal distention (possible)	Abdominal distention
Stomal swelling (possible)	Stomal swelling
Nausea and vomiting (possible)	Nausea and vomiting
	Decreased pulse rate
	Fever (possible)

Source: Reference 4.

TABLE 22-6 **Conservative Management of Food Blockage**

1. Sit in warm tub bath to relax abdominal muscles.
2. Massage the peristomal area while in the knee-to-chest position to attempt dislodgement of fibrous mass.
3. If stoma is swollen, remove pouch and replace with a pouch that has a larger stoma opening.
4. If able to tolerate fluids (i.e., not vomiting) and passing stool, increase intake of fluid and electrolytes, but avoid solid foods. Drink one glass of liquid each time pouch is emptied. Juices such as grape juice exert a mild cathartic effect.
5. If vomiting, not passing stool, or both, do not take liquids or solid food orally.
6. Notify a primary care provider or WOC nurse if any of the following is noted:
   - Stool output stops (complete blockage).
   - Conservative measures (listed above) fail to resolve symptoms.
   - Signs of partial obstruction persist (Table 22–5).
   - Inability to tolerate fluids or replace fluids and electrolytes develops.
   - Signs and symptoms of fluid and electrolyte imbalance (Table 22–7) develop.

Source: Reference 4. Key: WOC = Wound, ostomy, and continence.

Physiologic Complications

The major physiologic consequence of a GI ostomy is fluid and electrolyte imbalance. This is most problematic in patients with a liquid or semisoft stoma discharge, such as with ileostomies or ascending and transverse colostomies. Patients with these types of ostomies must maintain adequate fluid intake to compensate for loss of the absorptive function of the colon and for absence of ileocecal valve function. Patients with ileostomies lose approximately 500–1000 mL of fluid daily through the stoma, whereas those with a normally functioning colon lose 100–200 mL daily.[3] During common illnesses, patients with ileostomies, especially infants, are particularly vulnerable to fluid and electrolyte imbalance caused by vomiting and diarrhea. Caregivers and patients should be counseled regarding common signs and symptoms of a fluid and electrolyte imbalance (Table 22–7).[4,5]

Because the GI tract is the site of nutrient absorption, some patients with ostomies may experience deficiencies. For example, iron and vitamins D_2 and D_3 are absorbed in the small intestine; riboflavin is absorbed in the upper GI tract; vitamin B_{12} is absorbed in the terminal ileum; phytonadione is absorbed in the proximal small intestine; menadione is absorbed in the distal small intestine; and calcium, pyridoxine, pantothenic acid, biotin, choline, inositol, carnitine, vitamins C and E, and thiamine (vitamin B_1) are absorbed in various sites within the intestinal tract (specific sites have not been identified). Vitamin A deficiency may be seen in persons with disease of the terminal ileum (e.g., Crohn's disease). Hypophosphatemia and hypomagnesemia are present in people with calcium deficiency caused by malabsorption. In addition, copper deficiency, which interferes with the absorption of iron, has been reported in patients who have undergone intestinal bypass surgery. Folic acid absorption requires interaction with enzymes present in the upper part of the jejunum; therefore, absorption of folic acid takes place predominantly in the proximal part of the small intestine.[6–9]

The effect of ostomy surgery on absorption of vitamins and minerals has not been well studied; however, patients with ileostomies

TABLE 22-7 **Signs and Symptoms of Fluid and Electrolyte Imbalance**

Adults	Infants
Increased thirst	Depressed fontanel
Dry mouth and mucous membranes	Lethargy
Orthostatic hypotension	Sunken eyes
Decreased urine volume	Weak cry
Increased urine concentration (dark in color)	Decreased frequency of wet diapers
Sunken eyes	Increased urine concentration (dark in color)
Extreme weakness	
Flaccid muscles	
Diminished reflexes	
Muscle cramps (abdominal and leg)	
Lethargy	
Tingling or cramping in feet and hands	
Confusion	
Nausea and vomiting	
Shortness of breath	

Source: References 4 and 5.

or colostomies should be monitored for signs and symptoms of deficiencies.

Patients with a urostomy, an ileostomy, or an ascending colostomy require adequate daily intake of fluid to prevent the precipitation of crystals or kidney stones in the urine. In addition, they may be at increased risk for gallbladder stone formation. Patients with a urostomy should adjust their diet to produce acidic urine, thereby reducing the risk of infection and crystal formation around the stoma. Cranberry products have been studied in the prevention of recurrent urinary tract infections. Evidence does not support the use of cranberry products for the treatment of such infections, however.[10–15] (See Chapter 51 for an in-depth discussion of cranberry.)

Systemic Complications

Constipation is caused by the regular use of constipating analgesics or other medications or may be a result of the patient's eating habits. Constipation may be a problem in patients with descending and sigmoid colostomies. Treatment depends on the cause and may include dietary changes or medication adjustment. Patients experiencing problems with constipation should be encouraged to avoid the foods listed in Table 22–3 that can thicken the stool.[4,5]

Certain foods can cause diarrhea in ostomy patients (Table 22–3).[4,5] Gut pathology (e.g., ulcerative colitis, Crohn's disease, *Clostridium difficile* colitis) or obstruction caused by a food bolus can also cause diarrhea. Medications, influenza, and food poisoning are other potential causes. Diarrhea is a special problem in patients with ileostomies and ascending colostomies because the associated bowel changes cause impaired fluid and electrolyte reabsorption. Patients with chronically loose stools may wish to use an absorptive agent (e.g., Ileosorb, Par-Sorb) designed for use in the pouch. Absorptive agents do not correct the problem; they merely assist in coping with the problem. Increased fiber (e.g., Metamucil, Citrucel) may be used to help correct diarrhea in patients with a colon. Antidiarrheals may be ordered to slow transit time and decrease output. Of note, an unexpected high or decreased output or no output in a patient with an ileostomy may represent a partial small-bowel obstruction. In such instances, the patient needs to seek emergency medical attention.

Intestinal gas may be related to food. Eliminating foods that cause gas from the diet may solve the problem (Table 22–3). Oral simethicone to reduce gas production or use of pouches with gas filters may be helpful. Odor is not normal except when the pouching system is changed or emptied. Otherwise, odor may be an indication of poor hygiene, leakage, or failure to properly connect the pouch to the skin barrier. The health care provider should review proper care and connection of the pouching system with patients who are concerned about odor. Oral deodorants that will act in the digestive system to eliminate odors from digested foods are discussed in the section Deodorizers.

Local Complications

The mucosa of the normal stoma is shiny, moist, and either pink or red. The stoma does not contain nerve fibers, so it does not transmit pain or other sensations. In an adult, the mature stoma size is approximately ⅛–3 inches, depending on the portion of the bowel or urinary tract used. The stoma gradually shrinks after surgery and reaches its permanent size within 6 weeks.

Skin irritation around the stoma can result from prolonged contact of stoma effluent. Ostomy pouching systems and accessories can also irritate skin as a consequence of poor fit or from the materials used in their composition. The peristomal skin may look weepy or erythematous, with papules and macules evident. The Ostomy Skin Tool (OST) is a new standardized peristomal skin assessment tool that was developed by WOC nurses in concert with an ostomy manufacturing company. This tool has three clinical parameters: discoloration, erosion, and tissue overgrowth.[16] The patient may use a skin powder or a barrier wipe to protect the skin, although a properly fitting pouching system should be the first priority.

Denuded peristomal skin is caused by erosion of the epidermis by digestive enzymes. The eroded or denuded epidermis including that incurred when the pouch is applied may bleed, and it is painful to the touch. Denudation of peristomal skin occurs when an improper pouch is worn, when the pouch opening is too big or too small, or when the pouch has leaked and not been promptly replaced. These problems can allow the output to come in contact with the skin. The output with ileostomies is particularly irritating to skin. The patient should be referred to a WOC nurse or primary care provider for treatment. Once a cause for the denuded skin is identified and the underlying problem corrected, a skin barrier powder may be applied to the peristomal skin before the pouch is applied. A skin barrier powder may be a pectin- or karaya-based powder, which absorbs skin moisture and provides a dry surface. A liquid skin barrier may be used over the powder so that the pouching system can adhere. This beneficial effect is called "crusting." The pouch should be changed more often to reduce the risk of further irritation. Treatment should be continued until intact skin has been restored.

Contact dermatitis is characterized by burning, stinging, pruritus (itching), and red or denuded skin. This complication usually results from an allergic reaction to the pouching system or an accessory. A patch test will identify the allergen in patients who have a history of allergy, a reaction to adhesive tape, eczema, or psoriasis, as well as in those who have very fair skin. Patients exhibiting sensitivity may need to change products. A fabric pouch cover may be helpful if the allergy is to the pouch itself. Special precautions are necessary in patients with a latex allergy. On request, manufacturers will provide written information regarding the natural latex rubber content of their products and packaging (see the specific manufacturer's website). In some products, the latex source is a dry, natural latex rubber, which is used to seal blister packs that contain nonlatex products.

Alkaline dermatitis (encrustation) may occur in patients with urinary diversions because of the alkaline nature of the output. The stoma or peristomal skin may feel gritty, like sandpaper. Alkaline dermatitis, which renders the stoma extremely friable, is a common cause of blood in the pouch. A cloth soaked with a solution of one-third white vinegar to two-thirds water should be applied to the involved area for 5–10 minutes at least once weekly before the pouching system is put on. Patients who use a two-piece system can apply the solution as often as 3–4 times daily. The vinegar may cause the stoma to blanch, but blanching is not indicative of damage. The two-piece pouching system allows the wearer to remove the pouch for access to the stoma if this is involved in the encrustations.

Treatment for alkaline dermatitis is acidification of the urine. Patients should avoid alkaline ash foods, such as citrus fruits and juices; paradoxically, these foods are acidic when consumed but generate an alkaline output. Increasing fluid intake to between 2 and 3 quarts daily may also reduce alkalinity. Use of a urinary appliance with an antireflux feature is recommended because this design prevents urine from contacting the skin when the patient is lying down.

Hyperplasia (an overgrowth of skin) occurs when the pouch opening is too large. There is no pain in the early stages, but later the affected skin cells multiply, causing agonizing pain. The condition resembles a mucosal polyp and may also be called *hyperkeratosis* or *pseudoverrucous lesion.* Treatment entails ensuring that the pouch has the correct opening size and that the seal is secure. The seal is achieved with paste, paste strips, or a moldable seal or skin barrier ring that will mold into the irregular surfaces. Other management approaches include cauterization using silver nitrate sticks and/or surgical removal.

Mechanical injury may result from a poorly fitting appliance or skin barrier, attempts to care for a stoma in a location with difficult access, or wearing tight-fitting clothing. A poorly fitting pouching system can be corrected or avoided by measuring the stoma before each purchase of supplies, selecting a skin barrier of the proper size, and adjusting the size of the skin barrier opening, if necessary. The opening should be cut to fit the skin stoma junction. New "moldable flanges" should fit at the mucocutaneous junction. Patients who exhibit signs of mechanical injury should be encouraged to contact a WOC nurse.

Skin stripping refers to inadvertent sloughing or removal of the top layer of skin around the stoma. The skin around the stoma may be irritated from use of a strong adhesive or removal of the skin barrier in a rough manner. An important principle in stoma management is that for removal of the skin barrier, the skin is pushed away from the barrier, rather than pulling the barrier away from the skin. Adhesive removers are useful in preventing skin damage if the stoma is new or the peristomal skin is fragile. After use of adhesive removers, the peristomal skin must be cleaned to remove all adhesive remover residue, which may cause blistering, irritation, or ineffective adhesion of a new pouching system.

Stenosis, or narrowing, of the stoma results from the formation of scar tissue. Excessive scarring usually is secondary to improper surgical construction, postoperative ischemia, active disease, or alkaline stomatitis or dermatitis. Although mechanical dilation of the opening is often advocated to prevent or palliate this problem, the only cure is surgical revision of the stoma.

Excessive sweating under the pouch can lead to skin changes associated with decreased wearing time and development of monilial (candidal) infection. A skin sealant or cement plus a belt may be necessary to hold the pouching system in place. Purchasing or making a cover or bib to keep the pouch material from touching the skin can alleviate discomfort from perspiration underneath the collection pouch.

Folliculitis, an inflammation of the hair follicles, is characterized by redness at the base of the hair follicles around the stoma. Aggressive removal of any adhesive around the stoma can remove hairs, resulting in irritation and infection. Using an electric razor to clip the areas on which adhesive will be applied may help prevent folliculitis. Because folliculitis is related to an overgrowth of staphylococci on the skin, the use of an antibacterial wash should be considered; in some advanced cases, use of an oral antibiotic may be considered.

Infections are not more frequent in patients with ostomies, with the possible exceptions of patients with Crohn's disease, diabetes, or diverticular rupture, or those undergoing radiation treatment or chemotherapy. In some cases, however, infections may arise under the pouching system. Candidal infection may be a problem in patients who wear a pouch continuously. A dark, warm, moist environment promotes the growth of *Candida* organisms. The primary symptoms are pruritus (itching) and rash. If the infection is allowed to continue unchecked, the skin will become denuded, the pouching system will not stick, and additional skin irritation will result from contact with the output.

Minor candidal infections may be treated with nystatin powder or 2% miconazole powder. Excessive powder should be brushed off before the pouch is applied. Antifungal preparations are generally used with every pouch change for 1 week after the skin has become clear. In treatment of candidal infections, it is important to ascertain whether the patient is taking antibiotics. Any antibiotic, but especially a broad-spectrum agent, changes the flora of the skin, and the entrenched *Candida* can become difficult to eradicate. Therefore, in patients with an ostomy being treated with antibiotics, it is often helpful to continue using nystatin powder or 2% miconazole powder for 1 month after all signs of candidal infection are gone.[17,18]

If the skin is indurated, swollen, and red, an abscess may be present, which may necessitate incision and draining. Culture and susceptibility testing should be performed, and an appropriate antibiotic should be prescribed for topical use, systemic use, or both. Patients should be encouraged to contact a WOC nurse for assistance.

Peristomal hernia is a protrusion of the colon or ileum through a defect in the fascia in the area around the stoma. It usually occurs if the abdominal wall is weak or the stoma was placed lateral to the rectus muscle. The patient may complain of a bulge when standing or sitting, pain, pouching difficulties, leakage, and peristomal skin irritation. Modification of the pouching system or technique may help to alleviate some of the symptoms of a peristomal hernia. An ostomy support belt or binder may be used to provide comfort and possibly prevent further herniation. The patient should be referred to the WOC nurse for a plan of care. Surgery may be required if pain at the site increases, the degree of herniation worsens, or signs of stoma obstruction develop.

Fistula is an abnormal opening between two internal organs, or from inside the body extending to the skin. Enterocutaneous fistulas (an opening between the intestine and skin) can occur in patients with or without an ostomy. This complication is most often a manifestation of Crohn's disease. Other causes include cancer, abscess formation, foreign body retention, radiation damage, tuberculosis, and traumatic injury. If a fistula has excessive drainage, an ostomy pouching system may be applied to contain the drainage and prevent the skin from becoming denuded.

Prolapse is a telescoping of the bowel through the stoma. This problem results when the opening in the abdominal wall is too large. Women with ileostomies may experience prolapse of the ileostomy during pregnancy. Other causes include inadequate fixation of the bowel to the abdominal wall, poorly developed fascial support, and increased abdominal pressure associated with tumors, coughing, or crying (the last being of special concern in infants). The danger of prolapse is in the resulting decrease in blood supply to the bowel outside the abdominal cavity.

A prolapse may be reduced by having the patient lie supine (on the back) and applying continuous pressure on the most distal part of the stoma. Once the prolapse is reduced, use of a rigid pouching system should be avoided because of the risk of strangulation of the stoma. The patient should apply a flexible pouch with a resized opening while lying on the back. A support belt may also be used. Surgical correction may be required if the stomal tissue becomes purple or ecchymotic or if the prolapse persists.

Retraction, a recession of the stoma to a subnormal length at or below skin level, is caused by several factors. Active Crohn's disease and weight gain may lead to such changes to the skin surface. If the retraction is not severe, use of a convex pouching system and an elastic belt may be adequate. In other cases, surgical correction may be required.

Organic impotence in men is secondary to a radical resection of the rectum or bladder, which results in disruption of nerves and vascular supply to the genitalia. Male patients who are impotent should be referred to a urologist for evaluation and treatment.

Medication Absorption Challenges for Ostomies

An understanding of the absorption characteristics of medications is important to optimize their effectiveness in patients with ostomies. The upper portion of the small intestine is the major absorptive site for many medications. However, certain preparations rely on an intact colon for drug absorption.[18,19] Both prescription and nonprescription medications should be reviewed to assess the best formulation for the patient. Potential drug interactions and adverse effects should be addressed in the drug therapy plan. Table 22–8 lists some general drug management principles for patients with colostomies, ileostomies, and urostomies.[18,19]

Drug Absorption

Patients with ostomies should be instructed to check the pouch for undissolved tablets or tablet fragments whenever they take solid oral medications. If the absorptive areas of the intestine have been altered, coated or sustained-release preparations may pass through the intestinal tract without being absorbed, potentiating drug failure.[20] Some medications are also contained within a wax matrix (e.g., Slow K) from which the active drug leaches as the tablet moves through the GI tract. In addition to the noted challenges with drug absorption, Table 22–9 lists a broad selection of medications with the potential to cause adverse effects, which vary with different dosage forms.[21–33]

Antibiotics

In general, antibiotics may alter the normal flora of the intestinal tract, causing diarrhea or fungal infection of the skin surrounding the stoma.

TABLE 22-8 General Drug Management Principles

Type of Ostomy	General Management
Ileostomy, colostomy	Avoid sustained-release, extended-release, and enteric-coated medications or those that contain a wax matrix. Liquid, crushed, and chewable preparations are preferred.
Ileostomy, colostomy	Do not crush medications before first consulting an appropriate health care provider.
Ileostomy, colostomy	Check pouch for undissolved tablets to monitor drug absorption.
Ileostomy, colostomy, urostomy	Review medication plans for potential drug interactions and/or adverse effects.
Ileostomy, colostomy, urostomy	Alert patients to medication-induced color changes to urine and/or stool.

Source: References 18 and 19.

Sulfa Drugs

Sulfa drugs should be used with caution in ostomy patients, because crystallization in the kidney occurs more often in the setting of fluid imbalance. To minimize this problem, patients with ostomies should increase their fluid intake.

Diuretics

Diuretics can increase the amount of fluids and electrolytes lost through urostomies, thereby adding to the losses already inherent with ileostomies. Diuretics should be used with caution. Frequent monitoring of fluid balance and serum electrolytes is required.

Laxatives

Because of the risk of electrolyte imbalance and dehydration, ileostomy patients should never use laxatives unless these agents have been prescribed. Patients with colostomies may use laxatives, but only under close supervision. If constipation is an issue, the primary care prescriber may recommend a stool softener.

Antacids

Products that contain calcium may cause stone formation in patients with urostomies. Magnesium-based products can cause diarrhea in patients with ileostomies. If patients have problems with constipation, they should avoid aluminum-based antacids, which can also cause constipation.

Urine and Stool Discoloration

Some medications can cause color changes in the urine and/or feces. These events can be unsettling to an uninformed patient, leading to unnecessary anxiety. Table 22–10 lists common medications that cause color changes.[34–37] The health care provider should discuss these possible changes with the patient in developing the drug therapy plan.

TABLE 22-9 **Potential Effects of Selected Prescription Drugs in Patients With Ostomies**

Drug Class	Type of Ostomy	Potential Effects
Histamine-1 (H1) receptor antagonists	Ileostomy, colostomy, urostomy	No problems have been reported with cetirizine, loratadine, or fexofenadine.
Anti-inflammatory agents	Ileostomy	NSAIDs are associated with GI irritation and bleeding. Use with caution in patients with history of GI ulceration or bleeding and in those with inflammatory bowel disease (COX-2 inhibitors may have lower risk profile).
		No problems have been reported with Celecoxib.
Opiates	Colostomy	Tramadol's opiate agonist activity can cause constipation, by similar mechanism for opiates such as oxycodone.
		Liquids, IR products, or patches are preferred to avoid erratic absorption associated with ER products.
Selective serotonin reuptake inhibitors	Ileostomy	No problems have been reported with sertraline, citalopram, or fluoxetine.
		Hyponatremia and diarrhea have been reported with paroxetine, requiring close monitoring of fluid and electrolyte status.
Antipsychotics	Colostomy, ileal conduit	Constipation has been reported with olanzapine and clozapine and can occur with all anticholinergic drugs.
		Reported delayed lithium toxicity requires close monitoring of serum levels in patients with ileal conduits.
Antidiabetic agents	Ileostomy	Possible dose-related GI effects are related to variable absorption of metformin, a weak base primarily absorbed in the small intestine. Some patients have experienced increased stoma output, requiring a change in their antidiabetic regimen.
		No problems have been reported with other antidiabetic agents.
Anticonvulsants	Ileostomy	Erratic absorption has been reported with enteric-coated and SR products.
		Use of liquids or IR products is generally recommended.
Antilipidemics	Ileostomy, colostomy, urostomy	No problems have been reported with use of HMG-CoA reductase inhibitors.
Cardiac/antihypertensive drugs	Ileostomy	Fluid and electrolyte abnormalities are common with diuretics.
		Careful monitoring is recommended during use of ACE inhibitors.
		Hyperkalemia may be a particular problem.
GI medications	Ileostomy, colostomy	Diarrhea is associated with all PPIs, requiring careful monitoring of fluid and electrolyte status.
		No problems have been reported with H2RAs.
		Avoid laxatives in patients with ileostomies owing to risk of severe fluid and electrolyte disturbances.
Antimicrobial agents	Ileostomy, urostomy, colostomy	Altered normal bowel flora and diarrhea related to broad-spectrum antibiotics can be a significant problem for patients with ileostomies.
		High doses of ciprofloxacin are associated with alkaline urine; if used, urinary acidification to avoid bacterial overgrowth in urostomy patients requires close monitoring.
Other drugs	End-jejunostomy, ileostomy	Some reports of drug failure are associated with malabsorption of warfarin in patients with short-bowel syndrome.
		Length of the functionally intact proximal small bowel is important in cyclosporine dosing; if liquid formulation or I.V. administration is required, more frequent monitoring is recommended.
		Variable volume of distribution and increased clearance of gentamicin have been reported in patients with ileostomies, possibly necessitating more frequent monitoring.
		Highly variable bioavailability of digoxin (depends on length of remaining bowel) requires monitoring for drug failure.

Key: ACE = Angiotensin-converting enzyme; COX-2 = cyclooxygenase-2; ER = extended release; GI = gastrointestinal; HMG-CoA = hydroxymethylglutaryl coenzyme A; H2RAs = histamine-2 receptor antagonists; IR = immediate release; I.V. = intravenous; NSAID = nonsteroidal anti-inflammatory drug; PPI = proton pump inhibitor; SR = sustained release.

Source: References 20–33.

TABLE 22–10 Selected Drugs That Discolor Feces and Urine

Drugs That Discolor Feces

Black
- Acetazolamide
- Aluminum hydroxide
- Aminophylline
- Amphetamine
- Amphotericin B[a]
- Anticoagulants[a]
- Aspirin[a]
- Barium
- Bismuth
- Chloramphenicol
- Chlorpropamide
- Cholestyramine
- Corticosteroids
- Cyclophosphamide
- Cytarabine
- Ethacrynic acid
- Fluorouracil
- Hydralazine
- Iodide-containing drugs
- Iron
- Levodopa
- Melphalan
- Methotrexate
- Nitrates
- Nonsteroidal anti-inflammatory drugs[a]
- Phenylephrine
- Potassium salts[a]
- Procarbazine
- Sulfonamides
- Tetracycline
- Thallium
- Theophylline
- Thiotepa[a]

Blue
- Chloramphenicol
- Manganese dioxide
- Methylene blue

Gray
- Colchicine

Green
- Indomethacin
- Iron
- Medroxyprogesterone

Green-Gray
- Oral antibiotics

Orange-Red
- Phenazopyridine
- Rifampin
- Rifapentine

Orange-Brown
- Rifabutin

Pink-Red
- Anticoagulants[a]
- Aspirin
- Barium
- Cefdinir[b]
- Clofazimine
- Nonsteroidal anti-inflammatory drugs[a]
- Tetracycline syrup

White or Speckled
- Aluminum hydroxide
- Barium
- Oral antibiotics

Yellow or Yellow-Green
- Senna

Drugs That Discolor Urine

Black
- Ferrous salts
- Phenacetin
- Senna

Blue or Green
- Amitriptyline
- Cimetidine (injection)
- Flutamide
- Indomethacin
- Magnesium salicylate
- Methocarbamol
- Methylene blue
- Mitoxantrone
- Promethazine (injection)
- Propofol (injection)
- Triamterene

Dark
- Aminosalicylic acid
- Chloroquine
- Metronidazole
- Nitrofurantoin
- Phenacetin
- Primaquine

Orange
- Chlorzoxazone
- Dantrolene
- Entacapone
- Warfarin

Orange-Red
- Phenazopyridine
- Rifampin

Pink-Red
- Phenothiazines
- Phenytoin

Purplish Red
- Chlorzoxazone

Red
- Carbidopa/levodopa
- Daunorubicin
- Dimethylsulfoxide
- Doxorubicin
- Idarubicin

Red-Brown
- Aloe
- Levodopa
- Phenytoin
- Quinine
- Warfarin

Violet
- Senna

Yellow
- Aloe
- Riboflavin
- Tolcapone
- Sulfasalazine
- Vitamin B_{12}

Yellow-Brown
- Cascara
- Nitrofurantoin
- Primaquine
- Senna
- Sulfonamides

Yellow-Orange
- Sulfasalazine
- Vitamin A

Yellow-Pink
- Cascara
- Aspirin

Key: GI = gastrointestinal.

[a] Discoloration may be caused by bleeding.

[b] Discoloration caused by nonabsorbable complex between cefdinir or metabolites and iron in the GI tract.

Source: References 34–37.

Dietary Supplements

Herbal products are not regulated by the U.S. Food and Drug Administration (FDA) because they are considered dietary supplements. Moreover, not all ingredients contained in a product are listed on the label. Herbal supplements can interact with medications and cause a variety of adverse effects. Patients with ostomies who desire to use herbal agents should do so only under medical supervision.

Assessment of Patients with Ostomies: A Case-Based Approach

In most cases, ostomy surgery necessitates the use of a pouching system designed to collect the waste material normally eliminated through the bowel or bladder. Because the specific circumstances dictating the need for an ostomy and the resultant surgical outcomes are highly variable, one patient may benefit from a particular type of pouch or accessory, whereas another may develop problems with the same products. Moreover, a patient's needs may change over time. A pouching system or accessory that previously produced ideal outcomes may no longer be appropriate because of changes in body contour caused by aging, pregnancy, weight gain or loss, or concurrent medical conditions. As the rate of obesity continues to rise, so do the challenges for health care providers caring for the special needs of that ostomy population.

Patients scheduled for ostomy surgery often are apprehensive about how the operation will proceed, how to manage the ostomy, and how they will be perceived by others. Both pre- and postoperatively, the person's self-image is typically threatened, with a detrimental effect on self-esteem. Therefore, special efforts should be made during the assessment to ensure privacy, to establish a trusting relationship, and to bolster the patient's confidence in subsequent self-management.

Cases 22–1 and 22–2 illustrate assessment of two different patients with established ostomies.

Patient Counseling for Ostomy Care

The pharmaceutical care needs of a patient with an ostomy include procurement and distribution of ostomy supplies and selection of appropriate products. Monitoring the ostomy self-management regimen and counseling the patient and family on special needs (e.g., skin care, diet, fluid intake, drug therapy) are other important components of ostomy care.

Counseling of the person with an ostomy should be done in a sensitive and caring manner. A common postsurgical issue is disturbance in the person's self-image, with consequent damage to self-esteem; therefore, in assisting patients with ostomy needs, special care must be taken to avoid verbal or facial expressions that might convey negative feelings regarding the necessary maintenance procedures. Peer support can be especially helpful for the ostomate population. Patients should be provided with contact information for local and national ostomy associations and a list of product manufacturers that can supply information about product use (Table 22–1). Further assistance can be obtained from a WOC nurse in the patient's geographic area (www.wocn.org). The

CASE 22-1

Relevant Evaluation Criteria	Scenario/Model Outcome
Collect	
1. Gather essential information about the patient's symptoms and medical history, including	
a. Description of symptom(s) (i.e., nature, onset, duration, severity, associated symptoms)	The patient's stoma-related symptoms began during the summer when she was at the beach and perspired a lot.
b. Description of any factors that seem to precipitate, exacerbate, and/or relieve the patient's symptom(s)	She has experienced pruritus (itching) and rash underneath her ileostomy appliance for the past week, and now the affected skin is becoming denuded and weepy. Her pouch has started to leak more often. She usually wears this pouching system for 3–4 days, but now she can keep it on for only 24 hours.
c. Description of the patient's efforts to relieve the symptoms	The patient applied pectin-based powder before appliance changes, but her symptoms have not resolved.
d. Patient's identity	Alexis Jones
e. Patient's age, gender, height, and weight	32 years old, female, 5 ft 6 in., 130 lb
f. Patient's occupation	Web designer
g. Patient's dietary habits	MNT diet for diabetes
h. Patient's sleep habits	n/a
i. Concurrent medical conditions, prescription and nonprescription medications, and dietary supplements	Glucophage 500 mg twice daily, Flovent 220 mg 2 puffs twice daily, albuterol 2 puffs every 6 hours as needed. The patient underwent ileostomy 2 years earlier for control of severe ulcerative colitis.
j. Allergies	Aspirin
k. History of other adverse reactions to medications	None
l. Other (describe) ______	n/a

CASE 22-1 *continued*

Relevant Evaluation Criteria	Scenario/Model Outcome
Assess	
2. Differentiate patient's signs/symptoms, and correctly identify the patient's primary problem(s).	Since the summer, Ms. Jones has developed a rash and itching. The rash appears to be caused by rash around the stoma caused by moisture. The patient's diabetes is another related factor.
3. Identify exclusions for self-treatment.	None
4. Formulate a comprehensive list of therapeutic alternatives for the primary problem to determine whether triage to a medical provider is required, and share this information with the patient or caregiver.	Options include (1) Refer the patient to a WOC nurse. (2) Recommend application of 2% miconazole powder to affected area with each pouch change. (3) If 2% miconazole is not effective, have the patient see her provider for a prescription for nystatin powder to apply to the affected area with each pouch change. (4) Take no action.
Plan	
5. Select an optimal therapeutic alternative to address the patient's problem, taking into account patient preferences.	OTC treatment with a powder containing 2% miconazole is appropriate for Ms. Jones. She should also change her pouching system more frequently.
6. Describe the recommended therapeutic approach to the patient or caregiver.	"You can use a nonprescription powder containing 2% miconazole to treat the rash and itching. You should change your pouching system more often and apply the powder with each change to prevent these symptoms from occurring again."
7. Explain to the patient or caregiver the rationale for selecting the recommended therapeutic approach from the considered therapeutic alternatives.	"Seeing a WOC nurse or your provider is very important to treat this situation."
Implement	
8. When recommending self-care with nonprescription medications and/or nondrug therapy, convey accurate information to the patient or caregiver.	"Wash peristomal skin per your usual routine. Apply 2% miconazole powder sparingly, and massage it into the peristomal skin. Dust off excess powder. A protective barrier wipe, such as 3M No Sting Skin Prep, may be applied to enhance the pouch seal. Apply the pouch. Use the miconazole powder with each pouch change until 1 week after the rash has resolved. You should change the appliance every other day until the rash clears; then you can return to twice-weekly appliance change. If rash and itching continue, consult a WOC nurse or your primary care provider."
Solicit follow-up questions from the patient or caregiver.	"How long should I continue using the 2% miconazole or the nystatin powder?"
Answer the patient's or caregiver's questions.	"Use for 1 week after rash has resolved. You may use it as needed if the rash develops again."
Follow-up: Monitor and Evaluate	
9. Assess patient outcome.	Ask the patient to call and update you within 1 week. If the itching has not subsided, have her schedule an appointment with the WOC nurse.

Key: MNT = Medical nutrition therapy; n/a = not applicable; WOC = wound, ostomy, and continence.

CASE 22-2

Relevant Evaluation Criteria	Scenario/Model Outcome
Collect	
1. Gather essential information about the patient's symptoms and medical history, including	
a. Description of symptom(s) (i.e., nature, onset, duration, severity, associated symptoms)	Patient has developed leakage from his colostomy pouching system in the past few weeks. He also noticed redness, denuded skin, and a bulge around the stoma. Pain at the site is also distressing for the patient.
b. Description of any factors that seem to precipitate, exacerbate, and/or relieve the patient's symptom(s)	Since his surgery 1 year ago, the patient has gained 20 pounds. He usually changes his pouch twice a week, but now he has to change it every day and continues to have leakage and peristomal redness.
c. Description of the patient's efforts to relieve the symptoms	Patient applied skin barrier powder and skin sealant to protect skin, but he continues to have skin irritation and leakage.
d. Patient's identity	Kevin Smith
e. Patient's age, gender, height, and weight	60 years old, male, 5 ft 11 in., 175 lb
f. Patient's occupation	Retired engineer
g. Patient's dietary habits	High-fiber diet with junk food
h. Patient's sleep habits	n/a
i. Concurrent medical conditions, prescription and nonprescription medications, and dietary supplements	Nasonex 2 spray in each nostril once daily or 1 spray in each nostril once daily. Mr. Smith developed rectal cancer 2 years ago. After radiation treatment and chemotherapy, he underwent a colostomy.
j. Allergies	Latex
k. History of other adverse reactions to medications	None
l. Other (describe) ______	Patient has been nervous about family issues and has been constantly eating, which has increased his weight.
Assess	
2. Differentiate patient's signs/symptoms, and correctly identify the patient's primary problem(s).	Leakage, pain, and denuded skin around his stoma are caused by abdominal creases from increased weight and documented peristomal hernia.
3. Identify exclusions for self-treatment.	None
4. Formulate a comprehensive list of therapeutic alternatives for the primary problem to determine whether referral to a medical provider is required, and share this information with the patient or caregiver.	Options include (1) Refer Mr. Smith to a WOC nurse for further assessment and treatment. (2) Recommend use of a skin barrier powder to improve peristomal skin, followed by application of a skin sealant. (3) Recommend use of a barrier ring with pouching system. Patient should be fitted with a hernia belt, which will provide support. (4) Take no action.
Plan	
5. Select an optimal therapeutic alternative to address the patient's problem, taking into account patient preferences.	Assessment of the stoma and skin indicates that a barrier ring and appropriate pouch are needed, as well as a hernia belt for support. Upon further discussion, Mr. Smith says he prefers a one-piece pouch with belt over a two-piece pouch.
6. Describe the recommended therapeutic approach to the patient or caregiver.	"Because you have developed a hernia, a belt for support is needed. Treat skin around the stoma with a skin barrier powder, such as Stomahesive powder, and a skin sealant, such as 3M No Sting Skin Prep, before applying the pouch with barrier ring. Change the pouching system every 2 days until the peristomal skin is free of burning and is no longer denuded; then resume pouch changes twice a week."

CASE 22-2 *continued*

Relevant Evaluation Criteria	Scenario/Model Outcome
7. Explain to the patient or caregiver the rationale for selecting the recommended therapeutic approach from the considered therapeutic alternatives.	"Pouch leakage and denuded skin will decrease with proper follow-up with a WOC nurse to modify your pouching technique. The bulge will be less prominent when wearing a hernia support belt. Contact the local chapter of the United Ostomy Associations of America for peer support to help you improve your self-esteem and body image." (See Table 22–1.)
Implement	
8. When recommending self-care with nonprescription medications and/or nondrug therapy, convey accurate information to the patient or caregiver.	
a. Appropriate dose and frequency of administration	See Figure 22–3 and Table 22–2 for proper pouching and skin accessories.
b. Maximum number of days the therapy should be employed	"Change pouch twice a week."
c. Product administration procedures	"Wash peristomal skin as usual. Apply thin layer of powder. Massage powder into skin well and dust off excess powder. Apply skin sealant before applying the pouch with barrier ring."
d. Expected time to onset of relief	"With proper skin care and hernia belt for support, leakage and skin excoriation should decrease within 24 hours. You will notice a decrease in the burning sensation."
e. Degree of relief that can be reasonably expected	"You should notice a decreased intensity of symptoms within 24–48 hours."
f. Most common adverse effects	"Some ostomates have had an allergic reaction to the powder or pouch adhesive."
g. Adverse effects that warrant medical intervention should they occur	"Consult a WOC nurse if burning, stinging, or local irritation occurs."
h. Patient options in the event that condition worsens or persists	"Consult a WOC nurse or your primary care provider if leakage or burning continues after 1 week of treatment."
i. Product storage requirements	"Store pouch away from heat."
j. Specific nondrug measures	"Change pouch every 2 days until peristomal skin is clear."
Solicit follow-up questions from the patient or caregiver.	"What happens if I can't lose weight, I develop more creases, and my stoma retracts more?"
Answer the patient's or caregiver's questions.	"Consult a WOC nurse; you may need another type of pouching system. In addition, obesity is now epidemic; consult a nutritionist for a proper diet program."
Follow-up: Monitor and Evaluate	
9. Assess patient outcome.	Ask the patient to call you at the next pouch change to ensure that no further leakage has occurred and that the skin has improved. If the leakage continues, have the patient call the WOC nurse.

Key: n/a = Not applicable; WOC = wound, ostomy, and continence.

following self-help books should also be recommended to patients with ostomies:

- Barrie B. *Second Act.* New York, NY: Scribner; 1997.
- Benirschke R. *Alive & Kicking.* San Diego, CA: Rolf Benirschke Enterprises; 1999.
- Benirschke R. *Embracing Life.* San Diego, CA: Rolf Benirschke Enterprises; 2009.
- Benirschke R. *Great Comebacks.* San Diego, CA: Rolf Benirschke Enterprises; 2002.
- Elsagher B. *I'd Like to Buy a Bowel Please! Ostomy A to Z.* Andover, MN: Expert Publishing; 2006.
- Elsagher B. *If the Battle Is Over Why Am I Still in Uniform? Humor as a Survival Tactic to Combat Cancer.* Andover, MN: Expert Publishing; 2005.
- Kupfer B, Foley-Bolch K, Kasouf MF, et al. *Yes We Can.* Worchester, MA: Chandler House Press; 2000.
- Ruggieri P. *Colon & Rectal Cancer. A Patient's Guide to Treatment.* Omaha, NE: Addicus Books; 2001.
- Taylor J. *Pretty Girl Blues.* PGB Publishing; 2013. Available at: http://www.prettygirlblues.com/PurchasePGB.html.

The person with an ostomy must adapt to many challenges in everyday life. Supporting the patient's involvement in the various

PATIENT EDUCATION FOR Ostomy Care

The objectives of self-care for ostomies are (1) to understand how the stoma functions and to maintain an effective ostomy management regimen; (2) to identify and implement proper techniques for use of the pouching system and accessories, and to avoid complications that result from improper use; and (3) to reduce the risk of other types of complications. For most patients, carefully following the product instructions and the self-care measures listed here will help to ensure optimal therapeutic outcomes.

Pouching System Selection and Use

- Use only the type of pouching system recommended for your type of ostomy.
- If your system no longer fits well, consult your WOC nurse or primary care provider before changing to a different type of pouching system.
- Do not consider skin irritation to be inevitable; identify the cause and correct and treat the irritation as soon as it occurs.
- If possible, identify the cause for leakage around the pouching system and correct the problem immediately. Consult your WOC nurse or primary care provider if you cannot determine the cause.
- Establish a routine for ostomy care. Keep the routine simple; use as few accessories as possible.

Effects of Medication Use

- Sustained- or extended-release medicines may undergo erratic absorption because of the altered postsurgical anatomy, which makes their effect unpredictable. These medications should be used with caution. Coated medications, as well as sustained- or extended-release medications, should not be crushed or chewed.
- Use caution when taking antibiotics and diuretics. Antibiotics can cause diarrhea or fungal infections of the skin around the stoma. Diuretics can cause dehydration or electrolyte imbalance in people with ileostomies.
- Use caution when taking laxatives, antidiarrheals, or other medications that alter gastrointestinal motility. Laxatives can increase fecal output in people with ileostomies, whereas antidiarrheals decrease the fecal output.
- Know which medications will discolor the urine or feces (Table 22–10).

When to Seek Medical Attention

- Consult your WOC nurse or primary care provider about using nonprescription medications to treat diarrhea or constipation. Return for reevaluation of the problem after 1 week of self-treatment.
- See your WOC nurse if you experience any of the following complications:
  - Depression and anxiety
  - Sexual dysfunction
  - Abdominal pain
  - Narrowing of the stoma
  - A bulge near the stoma
  - An extension of the bowel through the stoma
  - Recession of the stoma margins to a subnormal length
  - Bleeding from or around the stoma
  - Pain from touching the skin around the stoma or applying the appliance
  - Overgrowth of the skin around the stoma

Key: WOC = Wound, ostomy, and continence.

aspects of self-care and in the development of health care plans will help to alleviate much of the fear and anxiety often associated with living with an ostomy. Expression of any problems and concerns should be encouraged, so that the patient's ability to achieve self-treatment objectives can be better assessed. Health care providers or managers should also consider patients' special needs for conditions unrelated to the ostomy. The box Patient Education for Ostomy Care lists specific information for patient counseling.

Key Points for Ostomy Care

- Patients with ostomies may experience both psychological and physical complications after ostomy surgery. Specific issues should be addressed, with referral as needed to the primary care provider, WOC nurse, and/or United Ostomy Associations of America.
- The objectives of self-care for an ostomy are to understand how the stoma functions, to maintain an effective ostomy management regimen, to identify and implement proper techniques for use of the pouching system and accessories, to avoid complications that result from improper use, and to reduce the risks of other complications.
- Patients should be advised about the effects of food on stomal output and the need to monitor for signs and symptoms of dehydration.
- The selection of an appropriate pouching system depends on the patient's body contour, manual dexterity, and type of ostomy.
- The ideal ostomy pouching system should be leak-proof, odor-proof, comfortable, and easy to use. Providers can assist the patient in achieving these outcomes.
- Patients should be counseled on the effects of medications:
  - Use of liquid, crushed, or chewable medications is preferable.
  - Coated or sustained-release medications should be used with caution, because if the GI tract has been shortened or its function otherwise altered, full absorption may not occur. Most tablets should not be crushed or chewed.
- Caution is warranted with use of antibiotics and diuretics. Antibiotics can cause diarrhea or fungal infections of the skin around the stoma. Diuretics can cause dehydration or electrolyte imbalance in patients with ileostomies.
- Laxatives, antidiarrheals, or other medications that alter GI motility should be used with caution. Laxatives can increase fecal output in patients with ileostomies, whereas antidiarrheals decrease the fecal output.

REFERENCES

1. Increasing Awareness of and Recognizing the Life-Saving Role of Ostomy Care and Prosthetics in the Daily Lives of Hundreds of Thousands of People in the United States. Senate Resolution 95. 112th Congress (2011–2012). March 8, 2011. Available at: https://www.congress.gov/bill/112th-congress/senate-resolution/95/text. Accessed May 29, 2017.
2. Wise B, McKenna C, Gavin G, et al. *APSNA Nursing Care of the General Pediatric Surgical Patient.* Gaithersburg, MD: Aspen Publishers; 2000.
3. Wound, Ostomy and Continence Nurses Society. *WOCN Best Practice for Clinicians Series: Management of the Patient with a Fecal Ostomy.* Mount Laurel, NJ: Wound, Ostomy and Continence Nurses Society; 2010.

4. Colwell JC, Goldberg MT, Carmel JE. *Fecal & Urinary Diversions: Management Principles.* St. Louis, MO: Mosby; 2004.
5. Krenta KS. *Living with Confidence after Ileostomy Surgery.* Princeton, NJ: ConvaTec/Bristol-Myers-Squibb; 2003.
6. Hillman RS. Hematopoietic agents: growth factors, minerals, and vitamins. In: Hardman JG, Limbird LE, eds. *Goodman and Gilman's The Pharmacological Basis of Therapeutics.* 10th ed. New York, NY: McGraw-Hill; 2001:1487–517.
7. Marcus R. Agents affecting calcification and bone turnover: calcium, phosphate, parathyroid hormone, vitamin D, calcitonin, and other compounds. In: Hardman JG, Limbird LE, eds. *Goodman and Gilman's The Pharmacological Basis of Therapeutics.* 10th ed. New York, NY: McGraw-Hill; 2001:1715–43.
8. Marcus R, Coulston AM. Water-soluble vitamins: the vitamin B complex and ascorbic acid. In: Hardman JG, Limbird LE, eds. *Goodman and Gilman's The Pharmacological Basis of Therapeutics.* 10th ed. New York, NY: McGraw-Hill; 2001:1753–71.
9. Marcus R, Coulston AM. Fat-soluble vitamins: vitamins A, K, and E. In: Hardman JG, Limbird LE, eds. *Goodman and Gilman's The Pharmacological Basis of Therapeutics.* 10th ed. New York, NY: McGraw-Hill; 2001:1773–91.
10. Wang CH, Fang CC, Chen NC, et al. Cranberry-containing products for prevention of urinary tract infections in susceptible populations: a systemic review and meta-analysis of randomized controlled trials. *Arch Intern Med.* 2012;172(13):988–96. doi: 10.1001/archinternmed.2012.3004.
11. Wang P. The effectiveness of cranberry products to reduce urinary tract infections in females: a literature review. *Urol Nurs.* 2013;33(1):38–45. PMID: 23556378.
12. Bailey DT, Dalton C, Daugherty J, Tempesta MS. Can a concentrated cranberry extract prevent recurrent urinary tract infections in women? A pilot study. *Phytomedicine.* 2007;14(4):237–41. doi: 10.1016/j.phymed.2007.01.004.
13. Jepson RG, Williams G, Craig JC. Cranberries for preventing urinary tract infections. *Cochrane Database Syst Rev.* 2012;10:CD001321. doi: 10.1002/14651858. CD001321.pub5.
14. Wing DA, Rumney PJ, Preslicka CW, et al. Daily cranberry juice for the prevention of asymptomatic bacteriuria in pregnancy: a randomized, controlled pilot study. *J Urol.* 2008;180(3):1367–72. doi: 10.1016/j.juro.2008.06.016.
15. McMurdo ME, Argo I, Phillips G, et al. Cranberry or trimethoprim for the prevention of recurrent urinary tract infections? A randomized controlled trial in older women. *J Antimicrob Chemother.* 2009;63(2):389–95. doi: 10.1093/jac/dkn489.
16. Haugen V, Ratliff C. Tools for assessing peristomal skin complications. *J Wound Ostomy Continence Nurs.* 2013;40(2):131–4. doi: 10.1097/WON.0b013e31828001a7.
17. Aly R, Forney R, Bayes C. Treatment for common superficial fungal infections. *Dermatol Nurs.* 2001;13(2):91–9. PMID: 11917313.
18. Carmel J, Colwell J, Goldberg M, eds. *WOCN Core Curriculum: Ostomy Management.* Philadelphia, PA: Wolters Kluwer; 2016.
19. Ward N. The impact of intestinal failure on oral drug absorption: a review. *J Gastrointest Surg.* 2010;14(6):1045–51. doi: 10.1007/s11605-009-1151-9.
20. Severijnen R, Bayat N, Bakker H, et al. Enteral drug absorption in patients with short small bowel. *Clin Pharmacokinet.* 2004;43(14):951–62. PMID: 15530127.
21. McEvoy GK, ed. *AHFS Drug Information 2009.* Bethesda, MD: American Society of Health-System Pharmacists; 2009.
22. Tewari A, Ward RG, Sells RA, et al. Reduced bioavailability of cyclosporine A capsules in a renal transplant patient with partial gastrectomy and ileal resection. *Ann Clin Biochem.* 1993;30(Pt 6):587–9.
23. Gaskin TL, Duffull SB. Enhanced gentamicin clearance associated with ileostomy fluid loss. *Aust N Z J Med.* 1997;27(2):196–7.
24. Ritchie HA, Duggull SB. Another case of high gentamicin clearance and volume of distribution in a patient with high output ileostomy. *Aust N Z J Med.* 1998;28(6):212–3.
25. Al-Habet S, Kinsella HC, Rogers HJ, et al. Malabsorption of prednisolone from enteric-coated tablets after ileostomy. *BMJ.* 1980;281(6244):843–4. PMCID: PMC1714295.
26. Owens JP, Mirtallo JM, Murphy CC. Oral anticoagulation in patients with short-bowel syndrome. *Drug Intell Clin Pharm.* 1990;24(6):585–9. PMID: 2113745.
27. Lutomski DM, LaFrance RJ, Bower RH, et al. Warfarin absorption after massive small bowel resection. *Am J Gastroenterol.* 1985;80(2):99–102. PMID: 3970008.
28. Chen JP. Ileostomy and ramipril-induced acute renal failure and shock. *Heart Lung.* 2007;36(4):298–9. doi: 10.1016/j.hrtlng.2006.10.006.
29. Brophy DF, Ford SL, Crouch MA. Warfarin resistance in a patient with short bowel syndrome. *Pharmacotherapy.* 1998;18(3):1375–6. PMID: 9620117.
30. Roberts R, Sketris IS, Abraham I, et al. Cyclosporine absorption in two patients with short-bowel syndrome. *Drug Intell Clin Pharm.* 1988;22 (7–8):570–2. 3416741.
31. Lavi E, Rivkin L, Carmon M, et al. Clozapine-induced colonic obstruction requiring surgical treatment. *Isr Med Assoc J.* 2009;11(6):385–6. PMCID: PMC2719458.
32. Knoben JE, Anderson PO. *Handbook of Clinical Drug Data.* 7th ed. Hamilton, IL: Drug Intelligence Publications; 1998.
33. Alhasso A, Bryden AA, Neilson D. Lithium toxicity after urinary diversion with ileal conduit. *BMJ.* 2000;320(7241):1037. PMCID: PMC27345.
34. Allen J, Burson SC. Drug discoloration of the urine. Document 150907. *Pharm Lett.* 1999:15(9):150907.
35. *Physicians' Desk Reference Electronic Library.* Montvale, NJ: Medical Economics; 2003.
36. Fecal discoloration induced by drugs, chemicals, and disease states. Drug Consults. Micromedex 2.0. Englewood, CO: Thomson Reuters; April 14, 2010.
37. Urine discoloration—drug and disease induced. Drug Consults. Micromedex 2.0. Englewood, CO: Thomson Reuters; November 20, 2007.

section

VI

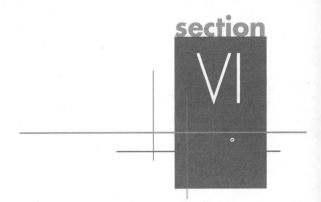

NUTRITION AND NUTRITIONAL SUPPLEMENTATION

CHAPTER 23

ESSENTIAL AND CONDITIONALLY ESSENTIAL NUTRIENTS

MARY M. BRIDGEMAN AND CAROL J. ROLLINS

Vitamin and mineral supplements represent one of the largest and most widely used nonprescription product categories in the United States. Multivitamin/mineral (MVM) products account for one-sixth of all dietary supplement sales and 40% of all purchases for vitamin and mineral supplements in 2014.[1] Annual U.S. sales data for all dietary supplements in 2014 was an estimated $36.7 billion, including $14.3 billion for all vitamin- and mineral-containing supplements, encompassing an estimated $5.7 billion for MVMs.[1] More than one-third of the U.S. population uses a MVM supplement on a routine basis, and use has increased over the past 25 years.[2,3] Nutrition experts agree that foods are the preferred source of vitamins and minerals and that most individuals can easily meet their daily requirements by eating a balanced diet. Experts agree less about the extent to which the U.S. population consumes such a diet. The lack of overt symptoms of nutritional deficiency in this country supports the position that most Americans receive adequate intake of vitamins and minerals from dietary sources; however, concern is growing that subclinical deficiencies may be contributing to chronic diseases. Similarly, there are concerns that the presence of medical comorbidities and use of certain chronic medications may precipitate nutritional deficits, either by preventing adequate intake or absorption of essential nutrients (i.e., those the human body cannot make) or by creating a situation in which nutrients that are not usually essential now become essential (i.e., conditionally essential nutrients). These concerns emphasize the importance of encouraging the selection of nutrient-dense foods throughout the life cycle and recognition of the need to recommend appropriate nutritional supplementation for individuals at risk for deficiency.

According to the Dietary Supplement Health and Education Act (DSHEA) of 1994, dietary supplements, including vitamins, minerals, and MVM preparations, are not drugs and thus are not intended to prevent, cure, diagnose, treat, or mitigate disease. Health-conscious consumers, however, often seek nutritional supplements as a means to prevent and self-treat a myriad of actual or perceived health ailments; commonly cited reasons for use include to maintain overall health and improve health status.[4] Marketing claims and natural product enthusiasts encourage these self-care behaviors by promoting use of nutrient supplementation, often in doses well above established tolerable upper limits.[5] However, the issue of who will benefit from or be harmed by the use of nutritional supplements and the necessity of supplementation in a nutrient-replete individual is unresolved. Regular use of supplements can help some people meet their recommended dietary requirements; however, a potential risk exists that some users will exceed the tolerable upper intake levels of some nutrients.[5] Currently, little to no available evidence supports the use of supplements for cancer prevention; in fact, evidence suggests the potential for increased cancer risk with use of certain nutrients at higher doses for prolonged periods of time.[6,7] Further, the National Institutes of Health–sponsored State-of-the-Science Conference concluded that insufficient evidence exists to support routine use of MVM supplements for primary prevention of chronic diseases.[8]

Beyond the risk of toxicity, one of the greatest dangers of food fads, use of multiple supplements, and large doses of single vitamins is that some people use them in place of sound medical care. The lure of marketing or the desire to self-treat may attract desperate or uninformed patients who have serious illnesses, thereby placing them at greater risk because they delay seeking appropriate medical attention. Furthermore, drug–nutrient interactions can be significant, yet they are often overlooked as part of the patient's medical history. For these reasons, practitioners should be well aware of the potential use—as well as the benefits and risks—of various nutrient supplements.

Epidemiology and Etiology of Nutritional Deficiencies

Although overt nutrient deficiency is rare in the United States, the prevalence of subclinical nutrient deficiencies is unknown. Specific patient populations may be at higher risk of deficient nutrient intakes because of pathophysiologic, physiologic, metabolic, behavioral, or economic situations (Table 23–1).[9,10] Because foods contain numerous other compounds that are important for health maintenance and disease prevention, health care professionals play an important role in educating patients on choices of nutrient-dense food before vitamin and/or mineral supplementation is recommended. (See Chapter 24 for further discussion of dietary components.)

Pathophysiology of Nutritional Deficiencies

A comprehensive discussion of the pathophysiology of vitamin and mineral deficiencies is outside the scope of this chapter. The reader is referred to standard medical and nutrition textbooks for such information.

TABLE 23-1 Factors Contributing to Nutritional Deficiency

- Inadequate dietary intake resulting from substance abuse, poverty, eating disorders, dementia, or restrictive diets
- Consumption of energy-dense but nutrient-poor foods
- Poor dentition, swallowing difficulty, or xerostomia
- Loss of taste, smell, or sight perception
- Decreased absorption resulting from cystic fibrosis, short bowel syndrome, Roux-en-Y gastric bypass, gastric hypochlorhydria, or chronic diarrhea
- Inability to buy or prepare meals because of tremor, fatigue, or arthritic pain
- Anorexia caused by reduced physical activity, social isolation, pain, disease, or depression
- Lack of knowledge about balanced nutrition
- Increased losses, as with hemodialysis therapy
- Inadequate synthesis
- Abnormal metabolism, as with alcoholism or certain genetic polymorphisms
- Increased metabolic requirements resulting from severe injury, infection, trauma, pregnancy, or prolonged physical exercise
- Medications affecting judgment, coordination, memory, appetite, nutrient absorption, gastric pH, or gastrointestinal tract function

Clinical Presentation of Nutritional Deficiencies

A vitamin deficiency may evolve in several stages, and clinical signs may not be present until prolonged and significant deficiency occurs (Table 23–2).[10] Attributing clinical symptoms to a single nutrient deficiency is difficult, as symptoms may overlap and reflect multiple rather than individual nutrient deficiencies. Signs and symptoms of specific vitamin and mineral deficiencies are discussed in the individual micronutrient sections later in the chapter.

Globally speaking, poor nutrition increases the risks of chronic disease, infection, and complications associated with reproduction, acute illness, surgery, and chemotherapy. For the pediatric population, growth, development, and learning may be compromised. For adults, poor nutrition over a lifetime can exacerbate the aging process, causing earlier morbidity and mortality. Balanced nutrition (with varied food choices providing adequate protein and appropriate calories, vitamins, and minerals) is essential for health through all stages of the life cycle.

Nutrient Supplementation

Vitamin and mineral supplements should be used as *adjuncts* to a balanced diet, not as substitutes for nutritious food. Although nutritional supplements can be obtained without a prescription and are typically self-prescribed, they are complex agents with specific indications. Medical assessment should precede their use, especially if daily intakes exceed the dietary reference intakes (DRIs) for a specific nutrient. Furthermore, patients should be reminded that vitamins and minerals are often better absorbed from food sources than from supplements. Practitioners may refer patients to a registered dietitian for personalized counseling on diet modification as well as nutritional supplementation.

Nutritional supplement use is intended to prevent nutritional deficiencies, replenish compromised nutrient stores, or maintain the present nutritional status. Nonprescription nutritional supplements are not intended for the self-treatment of vitamin deficiencies.

If a patient's diet is not providing micronutrients in the daily required amount for normal growth and function, supplementation with vitamins and minerals may be appropriate, provided the patient has no underlying pathology or contraindication to use. A once-daily MVM formulation providing no more than 100% of the DRIs should suffice in most cases. Patients should be reminded that healthy individuals derive no established benefit from supplementing nutrients in doses above the DRI; in addition, tolerable upper limits (ULs) for daily use should not be exceeded without medical supervision.

Practitioners should counsel patients regarding the potential disparity between a product's actual contents and its label. The potential for labeling inaccuracy exists because, despite U.S. regulations requiring that the actual content of a vitamin or mineral supplement be greater than or equal to the product's labeling (to account for shelf-life losses and differences between manufacturer product batches), dietary supplements are not assessed for compliance or standardization by any government agency.[11] Unlike prescription drugs, dietary supplements do not require proof of safety or efficacy before being marketed, and inspection for production under good manufacturing practices has not been required since passage of the DSHEA in 1994. However, the United States Pharmacopeia (USP) provides a Dietary Supplement Verification Program that allows product labeling with the USP mark if the tested product meets specific requirements, including verification of the product's ingredients and amounts; effective disintegration and dissolution for absorption; absence of harmful contaminants; and safe, sanitary, well-controlled manufacturing.[12] Practitioners should advise patients to look for the USP mark on vitamin and mineral supplement labels. However, if no brand with the USP mark can be found for a specific product, consider a brand whose other products bear a USP mark. Because of the high cost of verification, manufacturers typically seek the USP mark only for their best-selling products.

The best method for avoiding nutritional deficiencies is to consume a balanced diet each day that includes foods from sources high in several essential nutrients. To guide consumers in selecting a balanced diet while allowing individual preferences, the U.S. Department of Health and Human Services and the U.S Department of Agriculture released the reference *Dietary Guidelines for Americans, 2015–2020.*[13] In these guidelines, consumers are advised to regularly choose a variety of nutrient-dense foods in moderate portion sizes, as exemplified in the *MyPlate* figure (Figure 23–1). Each food group represented on *MyPlate* provides a significant source of essential nutrients. For example, the dairy group is a major source of calcium, whereas the fruit and vegetable groups are sources of fiber and the primary sources of antioxidant vitamins. By selecting a

TABLE 23-2 Stages in Evolution of Vitamin Deficiency

1. Inadequate nutrient delivery, synthesis, or absorption
2. Depletion of nutrient stores
3. Biochemical changes
4. Physical manifestations of deficiency
5. Morbidity and mortality

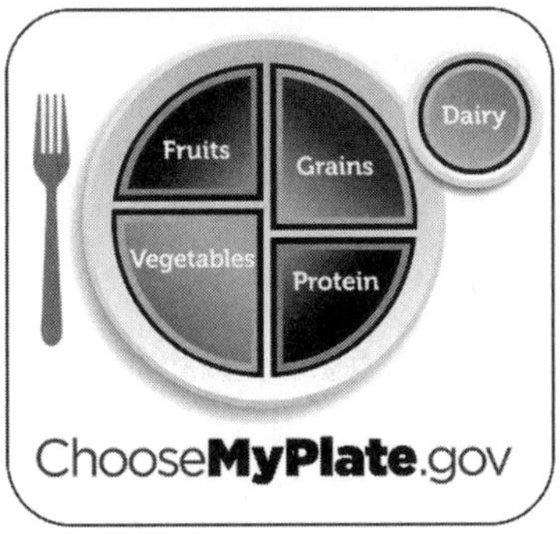

FIGURE 23–1 *MyPlate.* (Source: Image from www.choosemyplate.gov.)

variety of foods within the various groups and eating the appropriate number of servings from each food group daily, consumers can "balance" their diet relative to essential and conditionally essential nutrients. *MyPlate* is an evidence-based tool that is both user friendly and comprehensive for assessing the need for nutrient supplementation. When performing a nutritional assessment and determining the need for multivitamin supplementation, practitioners should inquire about the patient's intake from these food groups.[13]

Although situations exist in which high doses of specific vitamins and minerals are reported to be of therapeutic benefit, megavitamin enthusiasts' claims have not been confirmed objectively. To the contrary, as noted earlier, some clinical trials have suggested potential harm from supplementation originally claimed to be beneficial. These results are described within the individual micronutrient sections.

Vitamins and minerals that have therapeutic value in the treatment of medical conditions (e.g., niacin therapy for hyperlipidemia) are being used as drugs rather than as supplements for disease prevention or health maintenance. Deficiency states should be treated under medical supervision. Furthermore, in many cases, prolonged ingestion of megadoses of vitamin and mineral supplements has not been evaluated in large-scale clinical trials for safety and efficacy. Some vitamins (e.g., A, D, niacin, pyridoxine) and minerals (e.g., iron, fluoride) are known to be toxic in high doses. Therefore, practitioners should caution patients against initiating high-dose self-medication with any nutrient without proper medical supervision.

Vitamins

Vitamins are nutrients that cannot be synthesized in the body in sufficient quantities and must be obtained through the diet. Conditionally essential vitamins have adequate endogenous production in most circumstances, but there are disorders (e.g., cardiovascular disease) that require dietary intake of these conditionally essential vitamins to meet requirements. Vitamins are used as both dietary supplements and therapeutic agents to treat deficiencies or other pathologic conditions.

DRIs have replaced the traditional recommended dietary allowances (RDAs) as reference values of daily nutrient intake recommended by the Food and Nutrition Board of the Institute of Medicine of the National Academies (Tables 23–3 and 23–4).[14,15] The DRIs include four reference categories: estimated average requirements (EARs), RDAs, adequate intakes (AIs), and tolerable upper intake levels (ULs). EARs are values obtained after a careful review of the literature on specific nutrients. The EARs provide nutrient intake values that are estimated to meet the requirements of half of the healthy individuals in a specific gender and age group. The RDA is defined as the amount of a nutrient needed per day for maintenance of good health. This value is set at 2 standard deviations above the EAR as an estimate of daily nutrient intake sufficient to meet the requirements of nearly all (97%–98%) healthy individuals of a specified age group and gender. AIs are used as recommended intakes for nutrients for which inadequate scientific data exist to establish an EAR with confidence. Finally, the ULs are the highest dose of nutrient intake that may be consumed daily without risk of adverse effects in the general population. ULs are based on current literature, but they are not available for all nutrients (Table 23–5).[14,15] DRIs should be used as guidelines for nutritional assessment in healthy individuals; adjustment for strenuous physical activity or the presence of disease may be necessary. As nutritional supplements, vitamins are usually dosed at 50%–150% of the DRI values. Practitioners should advise caution for use of high-dose supplements (> 200% of the DRI) without medical supervision. As therapeutic agents, vitamins should be recommended only for specific evidence-based medical indications.

The Food and Drug Administration (FDA) has published a less comprehensive set of values to be used for food and dietary supplement labeling.[16] Nutrients are listed as a percentage of daily value (%DV). These values are based on the recommended intakes for a 2000-calorie diet for adults older than 18 years. The vitamin or mineral supplement label includes a box with the heading "Supplement Facts." In addition to information on serving size and servings per container, the label lists all required nutrients that are present in the dietary supplement in significant amounts and the %DV, if a reference has been established. It also lists all other dietary ingredients that are present in the product (including botanicals and amino acids) for which no %DV has been established. The %DV is based on DRI values for adults and for children ages 4 years and older, unless the product is designed for children younger than 4 years or for women who are pregnant or lactating.

Frequently, "natural" vitamin products are supplemented with synthetic vitamins. For example, because the amount of vitamin C that can be acquired from rose hips (the fleshy fruit of a rose) is relatively small, synthetic vitamin C is added to prevent too large a tablet size. However, this addition may not be noted on the label, and the price of the partially natural product is often considerably higher than that for the completely synthetic—but equally effective—product. Patients should be informed that the body cannot distinguish between a vitamin molecule derived from a synthetic source and one derived from a natural source, and that most synthetic vitamins are equal to the more expensive "natural" vitamins.

Fat-Soluble Vitamins

Two broad categories of vitamins exist: fat-soluble and water-soluble. Vitamins A, D, E, and K are fat-soluble vitamins. They are soluble in lipids and are usually absorbed into the lymphatic system before passing into general circulation. Their absorption is facilitated by bile. These vitamins are stored in body tissues, so ingestion of excessive quantities may be toxic. Fat-soluble vitamins, in general, come from similar dietary sources, including

TABLE 23-3 Dietary Reference Intakes (DRIs): Recommended Dietary Allowances and Adequate Intakes, Vitamins Food and Nutrition Board, Institute of Medicine, National Academies

Life Stage Group	Vitamin A (μg/day)[a]	Vitamin C (mg/day)	Vitamin D (IU/day)[b,c]	Vitamin E (mg/day)[d]	Vitamin K (μg/day)	Thiamin (mg/day)	Riboflavin (mg/day)
Infants							
0–6 mo	400*	40*	**400**	4*	2.0*	0.2*	0.3*
6–12 mo	500*	50*	**400**	5*	2.5*	0.3*	0.4*
Children							
1–3 y	**300**	**15**	**600**	**6**	30*	**0.5**	**0.5**
4–8 y	**400**	**25**	**600**	**7**	55*	**0.6**	**0.6**
Males							
9–13 y	**600**	**45**	**600**	**11**	60*	**0.9**	**0.9**
14–18 y	**900**	**75**	**600**	**15**	75*	**1.2**	**1.3**
19–30 y	**900**	**90**	**600**	**15**	120*	**1.2**	**1.3**
31–50 y	**900**	**90**	**600**	**15**	120*	**1.2**	**1.3**
51–70 y	**900**	**90**	**600**	**15**	120*	**1.2**	**1.3**
>70 y	**900**	**90**	**800**	**15**	120*	**1.2**	**1.3**
Females							
9–13 y	**600**	**45**	**600**	**11**	60*	**0.9**	**0.9**
14–18 y	**700**	**65**	**600**	**15**	75*	**1.0**	**1.0**
19–30 y	**700**	**75**	**600**	**15**	90*	**1.1**	**1.1**
31–50 y	**700**	**75**	**600**	**15**	90*	**1.1**	**1.1**
51–70 y	**700**	**75**	**600**	**15**	90*	**1.1**	**1.1**
>70 y	**700**	**75**	**800**	**15**	90*	**1.1**	**1.1**
Pregnancy							
14–18 y	**750**	**80**	**600**	**15**	75*	**1.4**	**1.4**
19–30 y	**770**	**85**	**600**	**15**	90*	**1.4**	**1.4**
31–50 y	**770**	**85**	**600**	**15**	90*	**1.4**	**1.4**
Lactation							
14–18 y	**1200**	**115**	**600**	**19**	75*	**1.4**	**1.6**
19–30 y	**1300**	**120**	**600**	**19**	90*	**1.4**	**1.6**
31–50 y	**1300**	**120**	**600**	**19**	90*	**1.4**	**1.6**

Life Stage Group	Niacin (mg/day)[e]	Vitamin B_6 (mg/day)	Folate (μg/day)[f]	Vitamin B_{12} (μg/day)	Pantothenic Acid (mg/day)	Biotin (μg/day)	Choline (mg/day)[g]
Infants							
0–6 mo	2*	0.1*	65*	0.4*	1.7*	5*	125*
6–12 mo	4*	0.3*	80*	0.5*	1.8*	6*	150*
Children							
1–3 y	**6**	**0.5**	**150**	**0.9**	2*	8*	200*
4–8 y	**8**	**0.6**	**200**	**1.2**	3*	12*	250*

TABLE 23-3 Dietary Reference Intakes (DRIs): Recommended Dietary Allowances and Adequate Intakes, Vitamins Food and Nutrition Board, Institute of Medicine, National Academies *(continued)*

Life Stage Group	Niacin (mg/day)[e]	Vitamin B_6 (mg/day)	Folate (μg/day)[f]	Vitamin B_{12} (μg/day)	Pantothenic Acid (mg/day)	Biotin (μg/day)	Choline (mg/day)[g]
Males							
9–13 y	**12**	**1.0**	**300**	**1.8**	4*	20*	375*
14–18 y	**16**	**1.3**	**400**	**2.4**	5*	25*	550*
19–30 y	**16**	**1.3**	**400**	**2.4**	5*	30*	550*
31–50 y	**16**	**1.3**	**400**	**2.4**	5*	30*	550*
51–70 y	**16**	**1.7**	**400**	**2.4**[h]	5*	30*	550*
>70 y	**16**	**1.7**	**400**	**2.4**[h]	5*	30*	550*
Females							
9–13 y	**12**	**1.0**	**300**	**1.8**	4*	20*	375*
14–18 y	**14**	**1.2**	**400**[i]	**2.4**	5*	25*	400*
19–30 y	**14**	**1.3**	**400**[i]	**2.4**	5*	30*	425*
31–50 y	**14**	**1.3**	**400**[i]	**2.4**	5*	30*	425*
51–70 y	**14**	**1.5**	**400**	**2.4**[h]	5*	30*	425*
>70 y	**14**	**1.5**	**400**	**2.4**[h]	5*	30*	425*
Pregnancy							
14–18 y	**18**	**1.9**	**600**[i]	**2.6**	6*	30*	450*
19–30 y	**18**	**1.9**	**600**[i]	**2.6**	6*	30*	450*
31–50 y	**18**	**1.9**	**600**[i]	**2.6**	6*	30*	450*
Lactation							
14–18 y	**17**	**2.0**	**500**	**2.8**	7*	35*	550*
19–30 y	**17**	**2.0**	**500**	**2.8**	7*	35*	550*
31–50 y	**17**	**2.0**	**500**	**2.8**	7*	35*	550*

Note: This table (taken from the DRI reports; see www.nap.edu) presents recommended dietary allowances (RDAs) in **bold type** and adequate intakes (AIs) in regular type followed by a single asterisk (*). Both RDAs and AIs may be used as goals for individual intake. RDAs are set to meet the needs of almost all (97%–98%) individuals in a group. For healthy breast-fed infants, AI is the mean intake. AI for other life stage and gender groups is believed to cover the needs of all individuals in the group, but lack of data or uncertainty in the data prevents being able to specify with confidence the percentage of individuals covered by this intake.

[a] As retinol activity equivalents (RAEs). 1 RAE = retinol 1 mcg, beta-carotene 12 mcg, alpha-carotene 24 mcg, or beta-cryptoxanthin 24 mcg. To calculate RAEs from retinol equivalents (REs) of provitamin A carotenoids in foods, divide REs by 2. For preformed vitamin A in foods or supplements and for provitamin A carotenoids in supplements, 1 RE = 1 RAE.

[b] Cholecalciferol 1 mcg = vitamin D 40 IU.

[c] In the absence of adequate exposure to sunlight.

[d] As alpha-tocopherol. Alpha-tocopherol includes RRR-alpha-tocopherol, the only form of alpha-tocopherol that occurs naturally in foods, and the 2R-stereoisomeric forms of alpha-tocopherol (RRR-, RSR-, RRS-, and RSS-alpha-tocopherol) that occur in fortified foods and supplements. It does not include the 2S-stereoisomeric forms of alpha-tocopherol (SRR-, SSR-, SRS-, and SSS-alpha-tocopherol), also found in fortified foods and supplements.

[e] As niacin equivalents (NE). Niacin 1 mg = tryptophan 60 mg; 0–6 months = preformed niacin (not NE).

[f] As dietary folate equivalents (DFE). 1 DFE = food folate 1 mcg = folic acid 0.6 mcg from fortified food or as a supplement consumed with food = supplement 0.5 mcg taken on an empty stomach.

[g] Although AIs have been set for choline, insufficient data exist to assess whether a dietary supply of choline is needed at all stages of the life cycle; the choline requirement may be met by endogenous synthesis at some of these stages.

[h] Because 10%–30% of people of advanced age may malabsorb food-bound B_{12}, those older than 50 years should meet their RDA mainly by consuming foods fortified with B_{12} or a supplement containing B_{12}.

[i] In view of evidence linking folate intake with neural tube defects in the fetus, all women capable of becoming pregnant should consume folate 400 mcg from supplements or fortified foods, in addition to intake of food folate from a varied diet.

[i] RDA assumes that women will continue consuming folic acid 400 mcg from supplements or fortified food until their pregnancy is confirmed and they enter prenatal care, which ordinarily occurs after the end of the periconceptional period, the critical time for formation of the neural tube.

Source: Reprinted with permission from references 14 and 15.

TABLE 23-4 Dietary Reference Intakes (DRIs): Recommended Dietary Allowances and Adequate Intakes, Select Elements Food and Nutrition Board, Institute of Medicine, National Academies

Life Stage Group	Calcium (mg/day)	Chromium (μg/day)	Copper (μg/day)	Fluoride (mg/day)	Iodine (μg/day)	Iron (mg/day)
Infants						
0–6 mo	200*	0.2*	200*	0.01*	110*	0.27*
6–12 mo	260*	5.5*	220*	0.5*	130*	**11**
Children						
1–3 y	**700**	11*	**340**	0.7*	**90**	**7**
4–8 y	**1000**	15*	**440**	1*	**90**	**10**
Males						
9–13 y	**1300**	25*	**700**	2*	**120**	**8**
14–18 y	**1300**	35*	**890**	3*	**150**	**11**
19–30 y	**1000**	35*	**900**	4*	**150**	**8**
31–50 y	**1000**	35*	**900**	4*	**150**	**8**
51–70 y	**1000**	30*	**900**	4*	**150**	**8**
>70 y	**1200**	30*	**900**	4*	**150**	**8**
Females						
9–13 y	**1300**	21*	**700**	2*	**120**	**8**
14–18 y	**1300**	24*	**890**	3*	**150**	**15**
19–30 y	**1000**	25*	**900**	3*	**150**	**18**
31–50 y	**1000**	25*	**900**	3*	**150**	**18**
51–70 y	**1200**	20*	**900**	3*	**150**	**8**
>70 y	**1200**	20*	**900**	3*	**150**	**8**
Pregnancy						
14–18 y	**1300***	29*	**1000**	3*	**220**	**27**
19–30 y	**1000***	30*	**1000**	3*	**220**	**27**
31–50 y	**1000***	30*	**1000**	3*	**220**	**27**
Lactation						
14–18 y	**1300***	44*	**1300**	3*	**290**	**10**
19–30 y	**1000***	45*	**1300**	3*	**290**	**9**
31–50 y	**1000***	45*	**1300**	3*	**290**	**9**

Life Stage Group	Magnesium (mg/day)	Manganese (mg/day)	Molybdenum (μg/day)	Phosphorus (mg/day)	Selenium (μg/day)	Zinc (mg/day)
Infants						
0–6 mo	30*	0.003*	2*	100*	15*	2*
6–12 mo	75*	0.6*	3*	275*	20*	**3**
Children						
1–3 y	**80**	1.2*	**17**	**460**	**20**	**3**
4–8 y	**130**	1.5*	**22**	**500**	**30**	**5**
Males						
9–13 y	**240**	1.9*	**34**	**1250**	**40**	**8**
14–18 y	**410**	2.2*	**43**	**1250**	**55**	**11**

TABLE 23-4 Dietary Reference Intakes (DRIs): Recommended Dietary Allowances and Adequate Intakes, Select Elements Food and Nutrition Board, Institute of Medicine, National Academies *(continued)*

Life Stage Group	Magnesium (mg/day)	Manganese (mg/day)	Molybdenum (μg/day)	Phosphorus (mg/day)	Selenium (μg/day)	Zinc (mg/day)
19–30 y	**400**	2.3*	**45**	**700**	**55**	**11**
31–50 y	**420**	2.3*	**45**	**700**	**55**	**11**
51–70 y	**420**	2.3*	**45**	**700**	**55**	**11**
>70 y	**420**	2.3*	**45**	**700**	**55**	**11**
Females						
9–13 y	**240**	1.6*	**34**	**1250**	**40**	**8**
14–18 y	**360**	1.6*	**43**	**1250**	**55**	**9**
19–30 y	**310**	1.8*	**45**	**700**	**55**	**8**
31–50 y	**320**	1.8*	**45**	**700**	**55**	**8**
51–70 y	**320**	1.8*	**45**	**700**	**55**	**8**
>70 y	**320**	1.8*	**45**	**700**	**55**	**8**
Pregnancy						
14–18 y	**400**	2.0*	**50**	**1250**	**60**	**12**
19–30 y	**350**	2.0*	**50**	**700**	**60**	**11**
31–50 y	**360**	2.0*	**50**	**700**	**60**	**11**
Lactation						
14–18 y	**360**	2.6*	**50**	**1250**	**70**	**13**
19–30 y	**310**	2.6*	**50**	**700**	**70**	**12**
31–50 y	**320**	2.6*	**50**	**700**	**70**	**12**

Note: This table presents recommended dietary allowances (RDAs) in **bold type** and adequate intakes (AIs) in regular type followed by a *single* asterisk (*). Both RDAs and AIs may be used as goals for individual intake. RDAs are set to meet the needs of almost all (97%–98%) individuals in a group. For healthy breastfed infants, AI is the mean intake. AI for other life stage and gender groups is believed to cover the needs of all individuals in the group, but lack of data or uncertainty in the data prevents the ability to specify with confidence the percentage of individuals covered by this intake.

Source: Reprinted with permission from references 14 and 15.

dietary fats and oils, milk products, and egg yolks (Table 23–6).[13,17] Deficiencies occur when fat intake is limited or fat absorption is compromised. Disease states that may cause malabsorption of fat-soluble vitamins include celiac disease, cystic fibrosis, obstructive jaundice, hepatic cirrhosis, bariatric surgical procedures, and short-bowel syndrome. These deficiencies may also be precipitated by drugs that affect lipid absorption, such as cholestyramine, which binds bile acids, thereby hindering lipid emulsification; orlistat, which inhibits gastric and pancreatic lipases in the intestinal lumen; and mineral oil, which is an unabsorbed oil that increases fecal loss of fat-soluble vitamins. Potential drug–nutrient interactions are listed in Table 23–7. A daily multivitamin supplement is recommended by the manufacturer for those taking orlistat; Chapter 27 provides a more comprehensive discussion of the use of orlistat for weight loss.

Vitamin A

The designation *vitamin A* refers to a large group of compounds that includes the retinoids (e.g., retinol) and the carotenoids (e.g., alpha-carotene, beta-carotene). Biochemical changes occur in some of these compounds during absorption in the intestine to form active vitamin A. Other compounds (e.g., the carotenoids, lutein, lycopene) are not converted to active vitamin A but have other health-promoting properties. These compounds can be found in dark green vegetables and red, orange, or deep yellow vegetables and fruits.

In healthy adults, more than 90% of the body's supply of vitamin A is stored in the liver. Because of this generous reserve, the risk of deficiency during short-term periods of inadequate intake or fat malabsorption is minimal. Infants and young children, however, are more susceptible to vitamin A deficiency because they have not established the necessary reserves.

FUNCTION. Vitamin A is essential for normal growth and reproduction, normal skeletal and tooth development, and proper functioning of most organs of the body (notably, the specialized functions of the eye involving the conjunctiva, retina, and cornea). Vitamin A is thus indicated in preventing and treating symptoms of vitamin A deficiency, such as xerophthalmia (dry eye) and nyctalopia (night

TABLE 23-5 Adult Tolerable Upper Intake Levels of Selected Micronutrients

Nutrient	Tolerable UL (mg/day)
Vitamin A	3
Vitamin D	0.1 (4000 IU/day)
Vitamin E	1000
Vitamin C	2000
Folate	1
Niacin	35
Vitamin B_6	100
Choline	3500
Calcium	3000 mg/day (9–18 years of age)
	2500 mg/day (19–50 years of age)
	2000 mg/day (>50 years of age)
Iron	45
Magnesium	350
Phosphorus	4000 (9–70 years of age)
	3000 (>70 years of age)
Copper	10
Fluoride	10
Iodine	1.1
Manganese	11
Molybdenum	2
Selenium	0.4
Zinc	40

Key: UL = Upper limit.
Source: Reference 14.

blindness). Synthesis of the glycoproteins necessary to maintain normal epithelial cell mucous secretions also requires vitamin A. This mucosal barrier is vital to the body's defense against bacterial infections in the upper respiratory system.

DEFICIENCY. Vitamin A deficiency is rare in well-nourished populations. However, an estimated 250,000–500,000 children worldwide develop blindness each year because of vitamin A deficiency.[18] Conditions such as celiac or Crohn's disease, pancreatic disorders, cancer, tuberculosis, pneumonia, and prostate disease, as well as therapy with corticosteroids, may cause excessive excretion of vitamin A. Fat malabsorption may impair vitamin A absorption; in the United States, vitamin A deficiency occurs more often from diseases of fat malabsorption than from malnutrition.

One of the earliest symptoms of vitamin A deficiency is night blindness.[18] Other characteristic clinical findings include follicular hyperkeratosis, loss of appetite, impaired taste and smell, and impaired equilibrium. Some of these findings may be masked by concurrent deficiencies of other nutrients. The drying and hyperkeratinization of the skin caused by the disruption of vitamin A–dependent epithelial integrity predisposes patients to infections.

DOSING AND DAILY REQUIREMENTS. Vitamin A is indicated for use in the treatment and prevention of vitamin A deficiency.[19] The patient's estimated dietary intake of vitamin A is needed to determine a nontoxic dose for supplementation.

The DRI values for vitamin A are measured in micrograms of retinol activity equivalents (RAEs; Table 23–8).[14] The Food and Nutrition Board recommends RAEs as a way to determine the amounts of carotenoids absorbed, as well as their degree of conversion to vitamin A in the body. RAEs replace the former designation of retinol equivalents (REs) used to calculate total vitamin A values from various dietary sources.

The DRI values for vitamin A are listed in Table 23–3.[14] The UL of 3 mg vitamin A daily in adults has been established on the basis of congenital birth defect risks and liver abnormalities associated with vitamin A toxicity.[14] Evidence suggests high-dose vitamin A intake, even that below the established UL, may be associated with an increased risk of bone fractures.[20]

Clearly, if the practitioner determines vitamin A supplementation is appropriate, a nonprescription multivitamin containing no more than the DRI value of vitamin A can be recommended as self-care until the patient can be fully evaluated; under medical supervision, doses may be considerably higher.[14] Preferably, a significant percentage of total vitamin A content should be contributed by beta-carotene because beta-carotene intake is not associated with the risk of fractures or vitamin A toxicity. Beta-carotene's improved safety profile may be related to limitations in its absorption and conversion to retinol.[20] However, the increased cancer risk associated with beta-carotene supplementation in those who smoke should be kept in mind (see "Safety Considerations" section). High-dose vitamin A or beta-carotene therapy should never be undertaken without close medical supervision.

SAFETY CONSIDERATIONS. Because vitamin A is stored in the body, high doses of it can lead to a toxic syndrome known as hypervitaminosis A. The potential for hypervitaminosis A increases as patients consume multiple sources containing vitamin A: a multivitamin for eye health, another for cancer prevention, and potentially another one or two for skin disorders and wound healing. Long-term administration of vitamin A is unlikely to cause toxicity when administered at doses less than 10,000 IU per day of retinol or equivalents; however, the risk for toxicity may increase in individuals with chronic renal or liver disease, and in those with low body weight, protein malnutrition, alcohol consumption, or vitamin C deficiency.[19] Headache is a predominant symptom, and it may be accompanied by diplopia (double vision), nausea, vomiting, vertigo, fatigue, or drowsiness. Treatment consists of discontinuing vitamin A supplementation, which should result in complete recovery. Although beta-carotene toxicity is not likely, eating large amounts of carrots in the daily diet may result in carotenemia, which can produce a yellow skin hue. Pregnant women or women of childbearing age should avoid vitamin A doses above the DRI because of the teratogenic risk. For this reason, women of childbearing age should carefully evaluate the total vitamin A content of all dietary supplements and fortified foods consumed regularly. These patients should be reminded not to take other dietary supplements when a prescription prenatal vitamin is dispensed.

The potential role of vitamin A as a cancer-preventing antioxidant prompted two large randomized controlled trials to evaluate supplementation in current or former smokers at risk of developing lung cancer. In these trials, either no benefit to supplementation or greater risks of lung cancer, cardiovascular disease, or death in those receiving supplementation were identified.[21,22] Such trials confirm that vitamin supplementation cannot provide the same health benefits as a diet rich in fruits and vegetables.

TABLE 23-6 Food Sources Rich in Selected Nutrients

Vitamin	Food Sources
Fat-Soluble Vitamins	
Vitamin A	Liver, milk fat, egg yolk, yellow and dark green leafy vegetables, apricots, cantaloupe, peaches, carrots
Vitamin D	Vitamin D–supplemented milk, egg yolk, liver, salmon, tuna, sardines, milk fat
Vitamin E	Wheat germ, vegetable oils, margarine, green leafy vegetables, milk fat, egg yolks, nuts
Vitamin K	Liver, vegetable oil, spinach, kale, cabbage, cauliflower
Water-Soluble Vitamins	
Vitamin C	Green and red peppers, broccoli, spinach, tomatoes, potatoes, strawberries, citrus fruit, kiwi
Vitamin B_{12}	Liver, meat, poultry, oysters, clams, dairy products
Folate	Liver, lean beef, wheat, whole-grain cereals, eggs, fish, dry beans, lentils, green leafy vegetables
Niacin	Lean meats, fish, liver, poultry, many grains, eggs, peanuts, milk, legumes
Pantothenic acid	Eggs, kidney, liver, salmon, yeast, some present in all foods
Vitamin B_6	Meats, cereals, lentils, legumes, nuts, egg yolk, milk
Riboflavin	Meats, poultry, fish, dairy products, green leafy vegetables, enriched cereals and breads, eggs
Thiamin	Legumes, whole-grain and enriched cereals and breads, wheat germ, pork, beef
Biotin	Liver, egg yolk, mushrooms, peanuts, milk, most vegetables, bananas, yeast
l-Carnitine	Dairy products, meat
Choline	Egg yolk, cereal, fish, meats
Minerals	
Calcium	Dairy products, sardines, clams, oysters, turnip greens, mustard greens
Iron	Liver, meat, egg yolk, legumes, whole or enriched grains, dark green vegetables, shrimp
Magnesium	Whole-grain cereals, tofu, nuts, legumes, green vegetables
Phosphorus	Milk, meat, poultry, fish, seeds, nuts, egg yolk
Chromium	Liver, fish, clams, meats, whole-grain cereals, milk, corn oil
Cobalt	Organ meats, oysters, clams, poultry, milk, cream, cheese
Copper	Liver, shellfish, whole grains, cherries, legumes, poultry, oysters, chocolate
Manganese	Vegetables, fruits, nuts, legumes, whole-grain cereals
Molybdenum	Legumes, cereals, dark green leafy vegetables, organ meats, milk
Selenium	Meat, grains, onions, milk
Silicon	Cereal products, root vegetables
Vanadium	Shellfish, mushrooms, parsley, dill seed, black pepper
Zinc	Oysters, shellfish, liver, beef, lamb, pork, legumes, milk, wheat bran

Source: References 13 and 17.

Vitamin D (Calciferol)

A number of chemical compounds are associated with vitamin D activity. Cholecalciferol (vitamin D_3) is the naturally occurring form of vitamin D that is synthesized in the skin from endogenous or dietary cholesterol on exposure to ultraviolet radiation (sunlight). Ergocalciferol (vitamin D_2), which is used as a food additive, differs only slightly in structure from cholecalciferol. Metabolic activation of vitamin D requires hydroxylation by both the liver and the kidneys. The metabolite, 25-hydroxycholecalciferol (calcidiol), is formed by the liver and then hydroxylated by the kidneys to its active form, 1,25-dihydroxycholecalciferol (calcitriol). Therefore, either renal or hepatic dysfunction may result in clinical manifestations of vitamin D deficiency, including hypocalcemia unresponsive to nonprescription vitamin D supplementation. These patients require a hydroxylated vitamin D preparation available only by prescription.

FUNCTION. Vitamin D, which has properties of both a hormone and a vitamin, is necessary for the proper formation of bone and for mineral homeostasis. It is closely involved with the activity of parathyroid hormone, phosphate, and calcitonin in maintaining homeostasis of serum calcium levels. Adequate vitamin D intake and supplementation used in conjunction with sufficient calcium, not vitamin D alone, may reduce the risk of bone fractures and falls in postmenopausal women with osteoporosis when dosed according to clinical evidence.[23,24] Other nonskeletal effects (e.g., reduced overall mortality and risk of diabetes, cancer, multiple sclerosis,

TABLE 23-7 Micronutrient–Drug and Micronutrient–Micronutrient Interactions

Micronutrient	Drug/Micronutrient	Effect	Precautionary Measures
Vitamins			
Vitamins A, E (large doses)	Warfarin	Increased anticoagulation and risk of bleeding	Take only recommended U.S. DRIs.
Vitamins A, E, D, K, C	Cholestyramine, colestipol, orlistat, or mineral oil	Decreased vitamin absorption	Avoid prolonged use of cholestyramine, colestipol, orlistat, or mineral oil.
Vitamin D	Phenytoin, carbamazepine, barbiturates	Increased metabolism of vitamin D	Ensure adequate dietary intake of vitamin D.
	Corticosteroids	May impair metabolism of vitamin D	Ensure adequate dietary intake of vitamin D.
Vitamin K	Broad-spectrum antibiotics (long-term therapy)	Vitamin K deficiency induced by decreased gut flora	Ensure adequate dietary intake of vitamin K.
	Warfarin	Decreased anticoagulation	Keep daily intake of vitamin K consistent.
	Vitamin E (large doses)	Antagonizes function of vitamin K	Avoid chronic supplementation with high-dose vitamin E.
	Vitamin A (large doses)	May interfere with vitamin K absorption	Avoid chronic supplementation with high-dose vitamin A.
Vitamin B_{12}	Metformin, colchicine, anticonvulsants, ascorbic acid supplements, gastric acid lowering agents, tetracyclines, and long-term use of antibiotics	Potential decreased absorption of cyanocobalamin	Clinical significance is unknown.
Folic acid	Phenytoin and possibly other related anticonvulsants (chronic use)	Possible inhibition of folic acid absorption, leading to megaloblastic anemia; subsequent increased folic acid supplementation may decrease serum phenytoin levels and complicate seizure control	Monitor for megaloblastic anemia. Consult with neurologist regarding supplementation, if possible. Patient should report use of any dietary supplement to their neurologist.
	Trimethoprim	Weak folic acid antagonism; decreased activity/effectiveness; rare occurrence of megaloblastic anemia in patients with low folic acid level at onset of trimethoprim therapy	Monitor for megaloblastic anemia.
	Pyrimethamine (large doses)	Possible megaloblastic anemia	Monitor for megaloblastic anemia.
	Methotrexate	Folic acid antagonism; decreased activity/effectiveness	Monitor use of folic acid in patients on maintenance regimens for psoriasis or rheumatoid arthritis.
	Sulfasalazine	Decreased folic acid absorption when these agents are administered together	Separate dosing of these agents.
Niacin	Oral hypoglycemic agents; Sulfinpyrazone and probenecid	Decreased hypoglycemic effects; possible inhibited uricosuric effects	Monitor blood glucose with regular finger sticks.
Vitamin B_6	Isoniazid	Pyridoxine antagonism, manifested as perioral numbness resulting from peripheral neuropathy	Routinely take 50 mg/day of pyridoxine hydrochloride with isoniazid, or 10 mg of pyridoxine for each 100 mg of isoniazid.
	Phenobarbital and phenytoin	Decreased serum drug levels	Consider monitoring levels in patients taking high-dose pyridoxine.
	Levodopa	Levodopa antagonism; decreased effectiveness	Avoid supplemental pyridoxine or, if possible, substitute levodopa-carbidopa for levodopa.

TABLE 23-7 Micronutrient–Drug and Micronutrient–Micronutrient Interactions *(continued)*

Micronutrient	Drug/Micronutrient	Effect	Precautionary Measures
Minerals			
Calcium	Iron, zinc, magnesium	Inhibited nutrient absorption caused by high calcium intake	Separate dosing by at least 2 hours.
	Corticosteroids	Inhibited calcium absorption from gut; increased bone fractures and osteoporosis	Consider calcium supplementation.
	Aluminum-containing antacids, phosphates, cholestyramine	Decreased calcium absorption	Separate dosing by at least 2 hours.
	H2RAs, proton pump inhibitors	Decreased absorption of calcium carbonate, which requires an acidic environment	Consider calcium citrate supplementation.
	Levothyroxine	Reduced drug absorption	Separate dosing by 4 hours.
	Tetracyclines, fluoroquinolones	Decreased antibiotic absorption	Separate dosing by 2 hours before or 6 hours after the antibiotic.
	Phenytoin, carbamazepine, phenobarbital	Decreased calcium absorption by increasing metabolism of vitamin D	Consider calcium and vitamin D supplementation.
Magnesium	Tetracyclines, fluoroquinolones	Decreased antibiotic absorption	Separate dosing by 2 hours before or 6 hours after the antibiotic.
	Levothyroxine	Reduced drug absorption	Separate dosing by 4 hours.
Phosphorus	Sucralfate or antacids containing magnesium, calcium, or aluminum	Decreased absorption of phosphorus	Ensure adequate intake of dietary phosphorus.
Iron	Antacids	Decreased iron solubility and absorption	Separate dosing by at least 2 hours.
	Tetracyclines, fluoroquinolones	Decreased antibiotic and iron absorption	If concurrent administration is medically necessary, take tetracycline or fluoroquinolone 2 hours before or 6 hours after taking iron.
	Levothyroxine	Decreased drug absorption	Separate dosing by 4 hours.
Trace Elements			
Copper	Zinc, high-dose vitamin C	Copper antagonism	Micronutrients may compete for absorption and utilization; ensure supplements are administered in balanced doses, or monitor for signs of deficiency.
Fluoride	Magnesium, aluminum, calcium	Decreased effect and absorption of fluoride	Separate supplementation by at least 2 hours.
Iodine (potassium iodide)	Lithium salts	Possible additive hypothyroid effects	Monitor thyroid function tests.
Zinc	Copper	Possible decreased copper levels	High-dose, prolonged zinc supplementation may require copper supplementation.
	Tetracyclines, fluoroquinolones	Possible decreased antibiotic absorption	Separate dosing by 2 hours before or 6 hours after the antibiotic.

Key: DRI = Dietary reference intake; H2RA = histamine-2 receptor antagonists.

TABLE 23-8 Retinol Activity Equivalents

1 retinol activity equivalent	= 1 retinol equivalent
	= 1 mcg retinol
	= 12 mcg beta-carotene
	= 24 mcg alpha-carotene
	= 24 mcg beta-cryptoxanthin
	= 3.33 IU vitamin A activity from retinol
	= 10 IU vitamin A activity from beta-carotene

risk of allergies and asthma) have been evaluated in controlled clinical trials with varying results.[25] Recent clinical data suggest that vitamin D deficiency may be associated with increased risk of cardiovascular diseases, including hypertension, coronary artery disease, and cardiomyopathy.[26] Vitamin D supplementation may be associated with reduced mortality in heart failure patients, although much of this literature is derived from retrospective database review rather than prospective clinical investigation.[27] Regarding cancer risks, practitioners should advise individuals to avoid excess supplementation, because some people may show greater risk of breast, esophageal, prostate, and pancreatic cancers.[25,28] Additional controlled trials are needed to confirm the health benefits, risks, and role of vitamin D supplementation for specific patient populations. Further, as data on vitamin D supplementation and the role of serum level monitoring continue to evolve, dosing recommendations for prescription-only vitamin D formulations that are based on serum monitoring may be considerably higher.

DEFICIENCY. Vitamin D deficiency may result from inadequate intake; gastrointestinal (GI) diseases (e.g., hepatobiliary disease, malabsorption, chronic pancreatitis); chronic renal failure; inadequate sunlight exposure or dark skin pigmentation; hereditary disorders of vitamin D metabolism; obesity or gastric bypass therapy; or long-term therapy with antiepileptic medications (e.g., phenytoin, carbamazepine, primidone). Older patients' aging skin may not synthesize vitamin D efficiently, and the converting process that takes place in the liver and kidneys may also be compromised. The altered physiologic actions—in addition to older patients' reduced sun exposure, absorption, and dietary intake of vitamin D—leave the elderly at increased risk of vitamin D deficiency.

The signs and symptoms of vitamin D deficiency are reflected as calcium abnormalities, specifically those involved with bone formation. Vitamin D deficiency also has been associated with muscle weakness, an increased risk of falls, an increased risk of cardiovascular disease and certain cancers, and psychiatric disorders.[28] However, caution is advised since an "association" does not indicate causation.

The classic vitamin D deficiency state is rickets; osteoporosis with increased risk of fractures also occurs. Vitamin D increases calcium and phosphate absorption from the small intestine, mobilizes calcium from bone, permits normal bone mineralization, improves renal reabsorption of calcium, and maintains serum calcium and phosphorus levels. As serum calcium levels fall, compensatory mechanisms (e.g., increased secretion of parathyroid hormone) become activated in an attempt to restore serum calcium homeostasis. Long-term increases in parathyroid hormone secretion ultimately lead to secondary hyperparathyroidism. If physiologic mechanisms fail to make the appropriate adjustments in calcium and phosphorus levels, demineralization of bone ensues to maintain essential plasma calcium levels. During growth, demineralization leads to a failure of bone matrix mineralization, widening of the epiphyseal plate from weight load on softened bone structures, and deformed joints. In adults, such demineralization may lead to severe osteomalacia.

The incidence of rickets in the United States is low but not absent. Rickets is most likely to occur in children who abstain from milk and in infants breast-fed by mothers who receive an inadequate intake of vitamin D.

DOSING AND DAILY REQUIREMENTS. Most people obtain the AI for vitamin D from dietary sources and from exposure to sunlight (Table 23–3). People who are regularly exposed to sunlight will generally have no dietary requirement for vitamin D. However, substantial segments of the U.S. population receive limited sunlight exposure, especially during the winter months. Regular use of sunscreen is broadly encouraged to prevent skin cancer, but that protection limits vitamin D synthesis in the skin and warrants careful consideration of vitamin D intake from dietary sources. Milk and milk products are the major sources of preformed dietary vitamin D in the United States, because milk is routinely supplemented with 100 IU (2.5 mcg) of vitamin D per cup.

Vitamin D is FDA approved for the treatment of hypocalcemia and hypophosphatemia associated with hypoparathyroidism. Prescription vitamin D analogues (e.g., calcitriol) are FDA approved for the treatment of secondary hyperparathyroidism in patients with chronic renal failure.[19]

If the practitioner determines that vitamin D supplementation is appropriate based on poor dietary intake or inadequate exposure to sunlight, a multivitamin supplement containing cholecalciferol (vitamin D_3) 15–20 mcg (600–800 IU) taken daily may be recommended. Some evidence suggests that vitamin D intake of up to 25 mcg (1000 IU) daily may have health benefits. The current UL for vitamin D is 100 mcg (4000 IU) daily, although this value may be increased in the future.[14] Data gathered from the recent upswing in use of prescription-only high-dose (50,000 IU weekly) vitamin D supplements suggests such doses are safe and necessary to achieve adequate serum concentrations. However, these high doses should not be recommended for self-care without further evaluation.

SAFETY CONSIDERATIONS. Taking more than the UL of vitamin D daily may lead to adverse effects, including anorexia, hypercalcemia, soft tissue calcification, kidney stones, renal failure, and increased risk of certain types of cancer.[14,15] Patients receiving doses above the UL (e.g., those who have rickets or low serum concentrations) should be under medical supervision and closely monitored for these adverse effects.

Vitamin E (Tocopherol)

The term *vitamin E* refers to the tocopherols and the tocotrienols, compounds that occur naturally in plants.

FUNCTION. Vitamin E functions primarily as an antioxidant, protecting cellular membranes from oxidative damage or destruction. This process may be aided by selenium and vitamin C. Vitamin E may also have a role in heme biosynthesis, steroid metabolism, and collagen formation.

Vitamin E supplements, often combined with other antioxidants, have been promoted for treatment of numerous diseases (e.g., atherosclerosis, diabetes, cancer, Parkinson's disease, Alzheimer's disease). These recommendations are often based on observational studies in which regular intake of fruits and vegetables rich in antioxidants have shown beneficial effects in health maintenance and prevention of disease. However, clinical trials have suggested a lack of benefit with vitamin E supplementation in reducing the risks of multiple conditions, including cardiovascular events or mortality, stroke, cancer, diabetes, and Alzheimer's disease.[29–31] On the contrary, antioxidant supplementation that includes vitamin E may be associated with an increased risk of congestive heart failure in certain populations, increased risk of hemorrhagic stroke in adults, and an increased risk of fetal loss when given to prevent preeclampsia.[31–33]

Practitioners should remember that vitamin supplementation is not necessarily benign and has not shown benefit over a well-balanced diet, especially when taken in excess of the DRI.

DEFICIENCY. Vitamin E deficiency is extremely rare but may occur in two groups: premature infants with very low birth weight and patients who do not absorb fat normally. For example, neurologic abnormalities responsive to supplemental vitamin E have been reported in some patients with biliary disease and cystic fibrosis. Vitamin E deficiency has also been associated with symptoms of peripheral neuropathy, intermittent claudication, muscle weakness, and hemolytic anemia.

DOSING AND DAILY REQUIREMENTS. The RDA for vitamin E is reported as milligrams of alpha-tocopherol.[14] However, most food and nutrient supplement labels list vitamin E content in international units (IU). (Note: 1 mg of alpha-tocopherol vitamin E is equivalent to 1.49 IU.)

The average diet contains approximately 3–15 mg/day of vitamin E; therefore, large doses in excess of the DRI are not necessary unless the patient is experiencing fat malabsorption. The FDA-approved use of vitamin E is for prevention and treatment of hemolytic anemia associated with deficiency.[19]

Vitamin E requirements may vary in proportion to the amount of polyunsaturated fatty acids in the diet. The polyunsaturated fatty acid content of the U.S. diet has increased, and the plant oils responsible for the increase are rich in tocopherol. The lack of evidence of deficiency at the present intake supports the current adult RDA of 15 mg/day; the UL for vitamin E is 1000 mg daily.[14]

SAFETY CONSIDERATIONS. Potential risks associated with vitamin E supplementation are described in the preceding section.

Vitamin K

Phytonadione (vitamin K_1) is present in many vegetables. Menaquinone (vitamin K_2) is a product of colonic bacterial metabolism. Menadione (vitamin K_3) is a synthetic compound that is 2–3 times as potent as the natural vitamin K.

FUNCTION. Vitamin K has important roles in normal physiology. First, it promotes the synthesis of clotting factors II, VII, IX, and X in the liver. Second, it activates these factors, along with the anticoagulation proteins C and S. The clotting factors remain inactive in the liver in the presence of warfarin or in the absence of vitamin K. When vitamin K is administered, normal activity of the clotting factors resumes. Third, vitamin K is necessary for the activation of osteocalcin, which appears to play a role in bone mineralization and the prevention of osteoporosis.[34]

DEFICIENCY. The DRI value for vitamin K is 90–120 mcg/day for adults, depending on age and gender.[14] The microbiologic flora of the normal gut synthesizes enough menaquinone to supply a significant part of the body's requirement for vitamin K. Therefore, the incidence of deficiency among healthy, well-nourished individuals is low. Interference with bile production or secretion may contribute to vitamin K deficiency, because vitamin K absorption in the small intestine requires bile. Malabsorption syndromes and bowel resections may decrease vitamin K absorption. Liver disease may also cause symptoms of vitamin K deficiency if hepatic production of the prothrombin clotting factor is decreased. Other potential causes of deficiency include intestinal disease or resection and chronic, broad-spectrum antibiotic therapy. Deficiency may be evidenced by unusual bleeding and demonstrated by a prolonged prothrombin time (PT). Comparisons of lower and higher dietary intake of vitamin K indicate increased risk of osteoporotic fractures with lower intake; however, well-designed trials are needed to confirm this association.[34]

DOSING AND DAILY REQUIREMENTS. The DRI values for vitamin K are listed in Table 23–3; a UL for vitamin K has not been established.[14] Vitamin K_1 (phytonadione) is FDA approved for use in neonates at birth (1 dose of 1 mg) to prevent hemorrhage. This dose is necessary because placental transport of vitamin K is low, and the neonate has yet to acquire the intestinal microflora that produce the vitamin. Other approved uses include the prevention and treatment of hypoprothrombinemia caused by drug-induced deficiency and the treatment of hemorrhage.[19]

Consistent dietary intake of vitamin K (70–140 mcg/day) does not usually interfere with warfarin anticoagulant activity. However, sudden changes in the dietary or supplemental intake of vitamin K can significantly alter the patient's PT and international normalized ratio (INR).

SAFETY CONSIDERATIONS. Even in large amounts over an extended period, vitamin K does not produce toxic manifestations. However, the vitamin K content of MVM products should be evaluated for anyone receiving warfarin for anticoagulation.

Water-Soluble Vitamins

Vitamin C, the B-complex vitamins (riboflavin, thiamin, B_6, B_{12}, niacin, pantothenic acid, biotin, folic acid), and the vitamin-like compound, choline, are classified as water-soluble vitamins. These vitamins are generally not stored in the body, and excessive quantities tend to be excreted in the urine. Therefore, daily intake of these vitamins is desirable for optimal health. Thiamin, riboflavin, niacin, vitamin B_6, and pantothenic acid are involved in cellular energy production and utilization, and they may support synthesis of amino acids, fatty acids, cholesterol, steroids, and glucose.[35] Biotin may support fat and carbohydrate metabolism, whereas folate, vitamin B_{12}, choline, and riboflavin are involved with homocysteine metabolism; folate is also a critical co-factor in deoxyribonucleic acid (DNA) synthesis. All B-complex vitamins come from similar dietary sources (Table 23–6), so individuals presenting with symptoms of deficiency in one B-complex vitamin may also be at risk of deficiency in others. A listing of select drug–micronutrient interactions with the water-soluble vitamins is included in Table 23–7.

Vitamin C (Ascorbic Acid)

Vitamin C is the most easily destroyed of all the vitamins because of its sensitivity to heat, oxygen, and alkaline environments. It is a relatively simple compound with powerful antioxidant activity that serves to protect the capillary basement membrane. Vitamin C has been called the "fresh food" vitamin; most of the daily vitamin C intake is derived from vegetables and fruit sources.

FUNCTION. Vitamin C is necessary for the biosynthesis of hydroxyproline, a precursor of collagen, osteoid, and dentin. This vitamin also assists in the absorption of nonheme iron from food by reducing the ferric iron in the stomach to ferrous iron. However, use of vitamin C supplementation with iron is generally not necessary for patients with normal gastric acidity who are taking adequate doses of iron.

Large doses of vitamin C (500–1000 mg/day) have been promoted to prevent and treat the common cold. However, such claims are largely unsupported by well-designed controlled clinical studies.[18,36] Consumption of 5 servings or more of fruits and vegetables daily (≥200 mg vitamin C) has been associated with a lower incidence of cancer, heart disease, stroke, and certain eye diseases.[37] However, currently available data are inadequate to support vitamin C supplementation above the DRI for the prevention or treatment of these chronic conditions.[36]

DEFICIENCY. Characteristics of vitamin C deficiency include fatigue, capillary hemorrhages and petechiae, swollen hemorrhagic gums, and bone changes. Deficiency may also impair wound healing. Profound dietary deficiency can eventually lead to scurvy, producing widespread capillary hemorrhaging and a weakening of collagenous structures.

Scurvy is rare in the United States because it develops only with chronically inadequate consumption of vitamin C. Infants who are fed artificial formulas without vitamin supplements may develop symptoms of scurvy. In adults, however, scurvy occurs after 3–5 months of a diet free of vitamin C.

DOSING AND DAILY REQUIREMENTS. Practitioners are rarely confronted with overt symptoms of vitamin C deficiency. Only 10 mg/day of vitamin C prevents scurvy; a normal diet containing fresh fruits and vegetables contains many times this amount. The DRI values for vitamin C are listed in Table 23–3. Supplementation of 100–125 mg/day has been recommended for smokers, because higher daily ascorbic acid losses were observed in these individuals.[36] The UL for vitamin C is 2 g/day.[14]

Most adult multivitamin supplements contain 60–100 mg of vitamin C, an appropriate amount to consume if supplements are required. A daily dose greater than 400 mg is rarely indicated, and excess intake is excreted in the urine. In patients with a severe vitamin C deficiency, as evidenced by clinical signs of scurvy, 100–300 mg/day of vitamin C for at least 2 weeks is recommended to replenish body stores.[19] Infants who do not have vitamin C supplements in their formula should receive 40–50 mg/day; infants who are breast-fed by well-nourished mothers will receive a sufficient amount. If a supplement is warranted for an adult, practitioners may recommend a multivitamin product containing 60–200 mg of vitamin C to be taken once a day. Vitamin C is FDA approved for use in the prevention and treatment of scurvy and to acidify the urine.[19]

SAFETY CONSIDERATIONS. The practitioner is urged to weigh the relative risks and benefits of ascorbic acid therapy. A short-term trial of ascorbic acid with medical supervision may be warranted to promote wound healing in potentially deficient patients. Megadoses, however, may cause nausea, stomach cramps, diarrhea, and nephrolithiasis. Ascorbic acid toxicity can also lead to hemolysis in patients deficient in glucose 6-phosphate dehydrogenase. Rebound scurvy has occurred in infants whose mothers took megadoses of vitamin C during pregnancy. Vitamin C in doses of 1 g/day with 400 IU of vitamin E resulted in an increased risk of fetal loss or perinatal death when given as prenatal supplementation.[33] Patients with diabetes mellitus, recurrent renal calculi, or renal dysfunction should also avoid prolonged use of high-dose vitamin C supplementation.

Vitamin B_{12} (Cyanocobalamin)

Vitamin B_{12}, the most complex vitamin molecule, exists in several forms, all of which contain the element cobalt. The term *vitamin B_{12}* refers to all cobalamins that have vitamin activity in humans. Cyanocobalamin, the common pharmaceutical form of the vitamin, is the most stable of the cobalamins.

FUNCTION. Vitamin B_{12} is active in all cells, especially those in the bone marrow, the central nervous system (CNS), and the GI tract. It is also involved in fat, protein, and carbohydrate metabolism. A cobalamin coenzyme functions in the synthesis of DNA and in the synthesis and transfer of single-carbon units (e.g., the methyl group in the synthesis of methionine and choline). Vitamin B_{12} participates in methylation reactions and cell division, usually in concert with folic acid. Vitamin B_{12} is necessary for the metabolism of folates; therefore, folate deficiency may be observed as a feature of vitamin B_{12} deficiency. Vitamin B_{12} also is necessary for the metabolism of lipids and the formation of myelin.

Vitamin B_{12} has been studied in relation to elevated levels of homocysteine, an amino acid that requires vitamins B_{12}, B_6, and folate as cofactors for metabolism. Hyperhomocysteinemia has been identified as an independent risk factor for cardiovascular disease. Supplementation with folate, vitamin B_6, and vitamin B_{12} has been shown to reduce plasma homocysteine levels. However, this has not been proven to lower the risk of major coronary or major vascular events in individuals at increased risk for cardiovascular disease.[38]

DEFICIENCY. Vitamin B_{12} is found almost exclusively in animal protein; healthy individuals without dietary restriction rarely experience vitamin B_{12} deficiency. The body stores enough vitamin B_{12} in the liver that a deficiency would take approximately 3 years to develop. Vitamin B_{12} deficiency may be caused by poor absorption or utilization, an increased requirement, or excretion of this vitamin. Absorption is a complex process with about 99% of absorption occurring via an active process (Figure 23–2). In patients with conditions that affect absorption (e.g., those with ileal diseases, intestinal resection, gastrectomy), the reabsorption phase of the enterohepatic cycle is affected, and deficiency may occur. Patients older than 50 years are at increased risk of vitamin B_{12} deficiency that results from reduced gastric acidity and the associated decrease in release of food-bound vitamin B_{12}. Reduced intestinal motility, achlorhydria, and use of gastric acid–lowering agents in this patient population contribute to bacterial overgrowth in the small intestine, resulting in more microorganisms utilizing available vitamin B_{12}.[39] In addition, atrophic gastritis is a condition that affects 10%–30% of older adults, and it can result in macrocytic anemia due to inadequate release of vitamin B_{12} from foods or to inadequate production of gastric intrinsic factor (pernicious anemia). For these reasons, vitamin B_{12} supplementation from either fortified foods or a dietary supplement is recommended for this age group.

Long-term treatment with metformin can induce malabsorption of vitamin B_{12}, thereby contributing to the development of vitamin B_{12} deficiency.[40] In fact, vitamin B_{12} deficiency has been reported after as little as 3 months of metformin therapy.[41]

Vegetarians who do not consume any animal products (including infants breast-fed by vegetarian mothers) also are at risk for developing vitamin B_{12} deficiency. Vitamin B_{12} supplementation should be encouraged for these patients.

Vitamin B_{12} is necessary for the maintenance of myelin, and deficiency states produce many neurologic symptoms (e.g., paresthesia, peripheral neuropathy, unsteadiness, poor muscular coordination, mental confusion, agitation, hallucinations, overt psychosis). Other symptoms of vitamin B_{12} deficiency mimic those of folate deficiency and are manifested in organ systems with rapidly duplicating cells. Effects on the hematopoietic system result in macrocytic anemia, whereas GI effects include glossitis and epithelial changes occurring along the entire digestive tract.

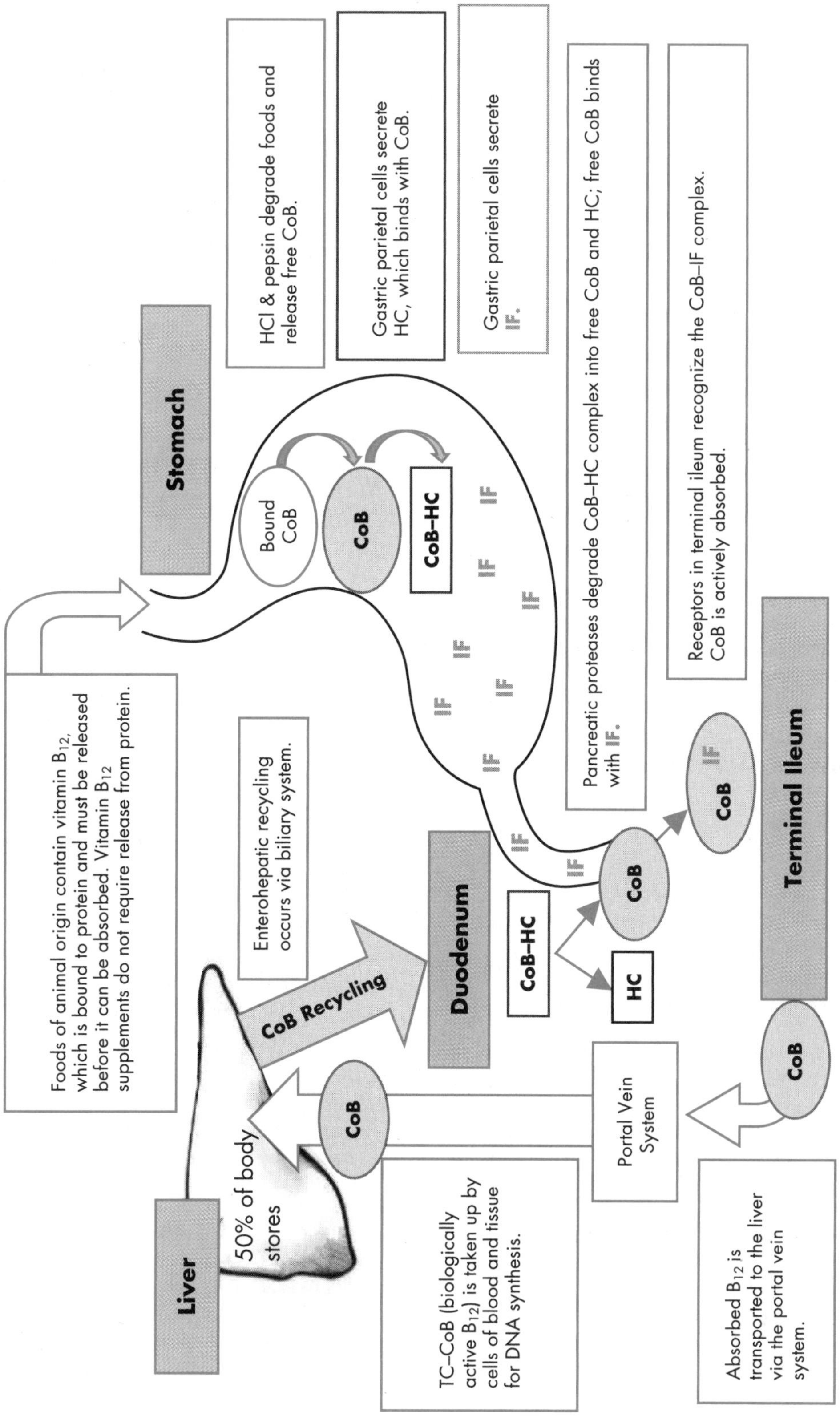
Foods of animal origin contain vitamin B_{12}, which is bound to protein and must be released before it can be absorbed. Vitamin B_{12} supplements do not require release from protein.
Stomach
HCl & pepsin degrade foods and release free CoB.
Gastric parietal cells secrete HC, which binds with CoB.
Gastric parietal cells secrete IF.
Bound CoB
CoB
CoB–HC
IF
Pancreatic proteases degrade CoB–HC complex into free CoB and HC; free CoB binds with IF.
Receptors in terminal ileum recognize the CoB–IF complex. CoB is actively absorbed.
Enterohepatic recycling occurs via biliary system.
CoB Recycling
Duodenum
HC
Terminal Ileum
Liver
50% of body stores
Portal Vein System
TC–CoB (biologically active B_{12}) is taken up by cells of blood and tissue for DNA synthesis.
Absorbed B_{12} is transported to the liver via the portal vein system.

FIGURE 23-2 Vitamin B_{12} homeostasis. Key: CoB = Cobalamin; Hc = haptocorrin; HCl = hydrochloride; IF = intrinsic factor; TC = transcobalamin.

Practitioners should caution patients that accurate diagnosis of a suspected anemia requires laboratory assessment of the complete blood cell count with differential and potentially other laboratory parameters Anemia resulting from a folic acid deficiency should be treated with folic acid; pernicious anemia and vitamin B_{12} deficiency should be treated with vitamin B_{12}; and iron-deficiency anemia should be treated with iron. Practitioners should avoid use of a "shotgun" antianemia preparation that contains multiple hematinic factors.

DOSING AND DAILY REQUIREMENTS. The DRI values for vitamin B_{12} are listed in Table 23–3; a UL has not been established for vitamin B_{12}.[14] Oral forms can be used if the deficiency is caused by inadequate intake; high-dose oral supplementation is appropriate for most deficiencies caused by malabsorption. Intramuscular or deep subcutaneous administration is sometimes used but is seldom required, because the small percentage of a high dose absorbed by passive mechanisms does not require intrinsic factor, and the binding of vitamin B_{12} in the terminal ileum can achieve adequate concentrations in the body to meet requirements. Vitamin B_{12} is FDA approved for use in the treatment of pernicious anemia and vitamin B_{12} deficiency. Other approved uses include supplementation during periods of increased requirements (e.g., pregnancy, thyrotoxicosis, hemorrhage, malignancy, liver disease, kidney disease).[19] Patients who have undergone bariatric surgery (e.g., gastric bypass, gastric sleeve) require lifelong vitamin B_{12} supplementation to prevent deficiency.

Hydroxocobalamin, a prescription-only product equal in hematopoietic effect to cyanocobalamin, may be appropriate for some patients. It is more extensively bound to proteins at the site of injection and in plasma, making renal excretion slower and prolonging the duration of action.

SAFETY CONSIDERATIONS. Excessive doses have not resulted in toxicity; however, nondeficient patients taking large quantities of the vitamin have reported no benefit.

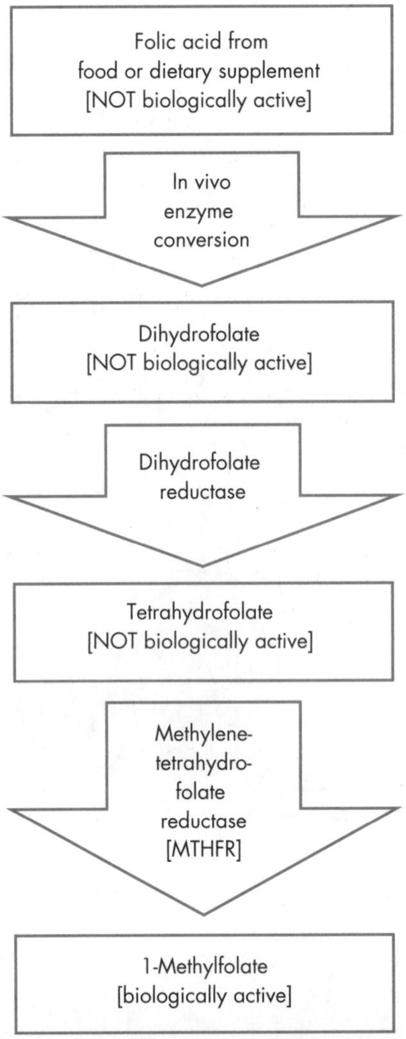

FIGURE 23–3 Folate activation pathway.

Folic Acid (Pteroylglutamic Acid, Folate)

FUNCTION. Folate is essential for cell division, DNA production, and brain and spinal cord development. It is also used in the metabolism of various amino acids. *Folic acid* refers to the synthetic version of this vitamin found in nutritional supplements and in fortified foods; *folate* refers to the naturally occurring form found only in food sources.

Folates are present in a wide variety of food sources and are heat-labile; the folic acid content of food depends on how the food is processed. Many commercially prepared carbohydrate foods (e.g., breads, pasta) are fortified with folic acid. Folic acid, whether contained in a nutritional supplement or consumed through dietary sources, is not biologically active and must undergo in vivo enzymatic conversion to the usable form (Figure 23–3).[42] A significant percentage of the population may have a genetic polymorphism of MTHFR that results in inadequate enzyme activity and inability to convert folic acid to its active form.[43] This genetic variance has major implications for pregnant women, because folic acid supplementation in patients with this polymorphism is not effective at reducing the risk of neural tube defects.[42] Other genetic defects in folate metabolism may lead to abnormalities in homocysteine metabolism (leading to elevated homocysteine levels), which has been associated with neural tube defects.[44] Folate deficiency is closely linked with deficiency of other water-soluble vitamins. Further, low plasma concentrations of folate, vitamin B_6, and vitamin B_{12} have been associated with elevated concentrations of homocysteine, which may increase the risk of cardiovascular disease. Folate supplementation may reduce elevated serum homocysteine concentrations, although this effect has not translated into improved cardiovascular outcomes.[41]

DEFICIENCY. The requirements for folic acid are related to metabolic rate and cell turnover, and increased amounts of folic acid are needed during pregnancy, lactation, and infancy. Infection, hemolytic anemia, blood loss (in which red blood cell production must be increased to replenish blood supply), and hypermetabolic states (e.g., hyperthyroidism) also increase folic acid requirements. Because folic acid deficiency has been associated with an increased risk of neural tube defects in newborns, supplementation for all women of childbearing age is recommended.

Causes of folic acid deficiency include alcoholism, malabsorption, food faddism, and liver disease. Iatrogenic causes are associated with administration of certain medications, including dihydrofolate reductase inhibitors (e.g., methotrexate, trimethoprim), anticonvulsants, and sulfasalazine.[19]

Deficiency of folic acid results in impaired cell division and protein synthesis. Symptoms of folic acid deficiency include sore mouth, diarrhea, and CNS symptoms (e.g., irritability, forgetfulness). The most common laboratory-identified feature of folic acid deficiency is megaloblastic anemia (an anemia characterized by large erythroblasts circulating in the blood).

Because vitamin B_{12} is essential for the metabolism of folates, a megaloblastic anemia responsive to folic acid administration is a feature of vitamin B_{12} deficiency. Folic acid given without vitamin B_{12} to patients with inadequate intrinsic factor (pernicious anemia) or vitamin B_{12} deficiency would correct the anemia but would not stop the damage to the CNS (characterized by lack of coordination, impaired sense of position, and various behavioral disturbances). Because folic acid can mask the signs—but not the progression—of vitamin B_{12} deficiency, patients should receive an appropriate medical evaluation for the cause of anemia rather than an empiric vitamin supplement.

DOSING AND DAILY REQUIREMENTS. The DRI values for folic acid are listed in Table 23–3. Folate is FDA approved for use in the treatment of megaloblastic anemias caused by folate deficiency. Folate is also approved for prevention of neural tube defects of the newborn.[19]

All women of childbearing age should consume synthetic folic acid at a dose of 400 mcg/day from fortified foods and/or dietary supplementation in addition to the folate obtained from food sources.[14]

Individuals known to have a polymorphism in MTHFR should receive a prescription vitamin containing biologically active derivatives of folic acid, available in forms such as l-methylfolate, 5-methyltetrahydrofolate calcium salt, and (6S)-5-methyltetrahydrofolate glucosamine salt.[42]

The supplemental dose of folic acid for correction of a deficiency in adults is usually 1 mg/day, particularly if the deficiency occurs with conditions that may increase the folate requirement or suppress red blood cell formation (e.g., pregnancy, hypermetabolic states, alcoholism, hemolytic anemia). Doses larger than the UL of 1 mg/day are not necessary, except in some life-threatening hematologic diseases. Maintenance therapy for deficiencies may be stopped after 1–4 months if the diet contains at least one fresh fruit or vegetable daily. For chronic malabsorption diseases, folic acid treatment may be lifelong, and parenteral doses may be required.

SAFETY CONSIDERATIONS. Folic acid toxicity is virtually nonexistent because of its water solubility and rapid excretion. Doses up to 15 mg/day have been given without toxic effect. The UL is set to minimize the risk of masking vitamin B_{12} deficiency. Several drugs, when taken chronically, may increase the need for folic acid (Table 23–7).

Niacin (Nicotinic Acid)

The physiologically active form of niacin is niacinamide. Niacin and niacinamide are constituents of the coenzymes nicotinamide adenine dinucleotide (NAD) and nicotinamide adenine dinucleotide phosphate (NADP).

FUNCTION. The niacin coenzymes are electron transfer agents; that is, they accept or donate hydrogen in the aerobic respiration of all body cells. Niacin is a unique vitamin, because humans can synthesize it from dietary tryptophan, with about 60 mg of tryptophan being equivalent to 1 mg of niacin. Most individuals receive about 50% of their niacin requirement from tryptophan-containing proteins and the rest as preformed niacin or niacinamide.

DEFICIENCY. The classic and only described niacin deficiency state is pellagra. Pellagra is rare, occurring most often in alcoholics, poorly nourished persons of advanced age, and individuals on diets that severely restrict sources of niacin. It may also occur in areas where large quantities of corn are consumed, as some of the niacin found in corn is bound to undigestible constituents, making it unavailable for absorption. Other causes of pellagra include isoniazid therapy and decreased tryptophan conversion, as in Hartnup disease and carcinoid tumors.

Clinical findings of niacin deficiency include the "three D's" of dermatitis, diarrhea, and dementia, often accompanied by neuropathy, glossitis (beefy red tongue), stomatitis, and proctitis. Patients manifest a characteristic rash with well-demarcated lesions of hard, cracked skin with blackish pigmentation that is crusty and scaly. Lesions occur primarily on sun-exposed areas, including dorsal surfaces of the hands, arms and feet, on the neck (Casal necklace), and face. Secondary infections may occur in such lesions. The entire GI tract is generally affected, with atrophy of the epithelium. Inflammation of the small intestine may be associated with episodes of occult bleeding and/or diarrhea.

DOSING AND DAILY REQUIREMENTS. The DRI values for niacin are listed in Table 23–3. The recommended UL for this vitamin in adults is 35 mg/day.[14]

Niacin requirements are increased after a severe injury, infection, or burn, or when the patient has an acute illness; has substantially increased caloric expenditure or dietary caloric intake; or has a low tryptophan intake (e.g., a low-protein diet, high intake of corn as a staple in the diet). Both niacin and niacinamide are FDA approved for the prevention and treatment of pellagra. Niacin, but not niacinamide, is also approved for adjunctive treatment of hyperlipidemia and hypercholesterolemia.[19]

Niacin or niacinamide, 150–500 mg daily in divided doses, is used to treat pellagra. Daily dosages of 1–2 grams 3 times per day, up to 8 g/day, of niacin (*not* niacinamide) are used to treat hypercholesterolemia and hyperlipidemia. Niacin increases beneficial high-density lipoprotein cholesterol and decreases concentrations of potentially harmful triglycerides, total cholesterol, and low-density lipoprotein cholesterol by mechanisms unrelated to its function as an essential micronutrient. However, such high-dose niacin therapy should not be undertaken as self-care; close medical supervision is required because of potentially serious drug-induced toxicity, primarily hepatic toxicity.

SAFETY CONSIDERATIONS. Niacinamide is associated with little toxicity; conversely, niacin toxicity can involve GI symptoms (e.g., nausea, vomiting, diarrhea), hepatotoxicity, skin lesions, tachycardia, and hypertension. Patients should be forewarned that therapeutic doses of niacin may cause flushing and a sensation of warmth, especially around the face, neck, and ears. This reaction, which is prevalent upon initiation of therapy, may be diminished with aspirin 325 mg or ibuprofen 200 mg taken 30–60 minutes before the niacin dose, provided no contraindications exist. Alternatively, the extended-release formulation may cause less flushing but has a greater risk of gastric and hepatic side effects. Itching or tingling and headache may also occur with niacin supplementation. These effects will usually subside or decrease in intensity within 2 weeks of continued therapy. If niacin causes GI upset, it should be taken with meals.

Because of the adverse GI effects, high doses of niacin are contraindicated in patients with gastritis or peptic ulcer disease. Niacin can provoke the release of histamine, so its use in patients with asthma should be undertaken carefully. Niacin may also impair liver function, disturb glucose tolerance, and cause hyperuricemia. Patients prescribed therapeutic doses of this nutrient must be monitored regularly for potential adverse effects.

Vitamin B_6 (Pyridoxine)

This water-soluble vitamin exists in three forms: pyridoxine (vitamin B_6), pyridoxal, and pyridoxamine. Although all three forms are equally effective in nutrition, pyridoxine hydrochloride is the form most often used in vitamin formulations.

FUNCTION. Vitamin B_6 serves as a cofactor for more than 60 enzymes, including decarboxylases, synthetases, transaminases, and hydroxylases. It is important in heme production and in the metabolism of homocysteine. As previously stated, hyperhomocysteinemia is a potential risk factor for cardiovascular disease, and it has been shown to respond particularly to folic acid supplementation but also to vitamin B_6. Whether the impact of these nutrients on homocysteine levels results in improved clinical outcomes has yet to be determined.[37] Limited data support a role of vitamin B_6 in treatment of migraine headache and nausea of pregnancy; however, use of vitamin B_6 in these conditions is generally undertaken as part of an overall plan under medical supervision rather than as strict self-care. Vitamin B_6 has also been suggested as a potential treatment of carpal tunnel syndrome, premenstrual syndrome (PMS), and depression; clinical research evidence for use of vitamin B_6 for these ailments is inadequate.[45]

DIETARY SOURCES. See Table 23–6. Cooking destroys some vitamin B_6.

DEFICIENCY. Causes of vitamin B_6 deficiency include alcoholism, severe diarrhea, food faddism, malabsorptive syndromes, drugs (isoniazid and penicillamine), and genetic diseases (cystathioninuria and xanthurenic aciduria).

The symptoms of severe vitamin B_6 deficiency in infants include irritability and convulsive disorders. Medical referral is indicated, and treatment with vitamin B_6 hydrochloride generally normalizes the electroencephalogram and resolves clinical symptoms. Symptoms in adults whose diets are deficient in vitamin B_6 or who have been given a vitamin B_6 antagonist are difficult to distinguish from symptoms of niacin and riboflavin deficiencies. These symptoms include pellagra-like dermatitis; oral lesions; peripheral neuropathy; scaliness around the nose, mouth, and eyes; and dulling of mentation. Serious deficiency symptoms include convulsions, peripheral neuritis, and sideroblastic anemia.

DOSING AND DAILY REQUIREMENTS. DRI values for vitamin B_6 are listed in Table 23–3. The FDA-approved use of this vitamin is for treatment of vitamin B_6 deficiency, including drug-induced deficiency as seen with isoniazid.[19] Daily doses up to 250 mg of vitamin B_6 have been used in the treatment of hyperhomocysteinemia.[38] However, the UL for this vitamin is 100 mg/day for adults.[14]

Treatment of sideroblastic anemia requires 50–200 mg/day of pyridoxine hydrochloride to aid production of hemoglobin and erythrocytes. Several vitamin B_6–dependent inborn errors of metabolism have been shown to respond to large doses of vitamin B_6.

SAFETY CONSIDERATIONS. Vitamin B_6 may be toxic in high doses. A severe sensory neuropathy similar to that observed with the deficiency state has been reported when gram quantities were taken to relieve symptoms of PMS. Similar symptoms have been reported in women taking doses as small as 50 mg/day for PMS. Recovery occurred slowly upon withdrawal of vitamin B_6.

High daily doses of vitamin B_6 (200–600 mg) inhibit prolactin. Prenatal vitamins, which contain 1–10 mg per dosage unit, do not appear to have a significant antiprolactin effect.

Thiamin (Vitamin B_1)

Thiamin is a water-soluble, B-complex vitamin available in oral tablet and injectable dosage forms.

FUNCTION. Thiamin's active form, thiamin pyrophosphate (formerly known as cocarboxylase), plays a vital role in the oxidative decarboxylation of pyruvic acid; in the formation of acetyl coenzyme A (CoA), which enters the Krebs cycle; and in other important biochemical conversion cycles. Thiamin is necessary for myocardial function, nerve cell function, and carbohydrate metabolism. The amount of thiamin required increases with increased carbohydrate consumption.

DIETARY SOURCES. Dietary sources highest in thiamin are listed in Table 23–6. The thiamin content of food can be destroyed by heat, oxidation, and an alkaline environment but is stable through frozen storage.

DEFICIENCY. The primary causes of thiamin deficiency are generally inadequate diet, alcoholism, malabsorptive syndromes, prolonged diarrhea, chronic furosemide therapy, increased requirements (e.g., pregnancy), and food faddism.

Thiamin deficiency in the United States is found primarily in alcoholics. Not only is their diet often nutritionally deficient, but alcohol ingestion also impairs thiamin absorption and transport across the intestine, and increases the rate of thiamin diphosphate destruction. Thiamin deficiency, also known as beriberi, may present with neuromuscular symptoms such as peripheral neuritis, weakness, and Wernicke's encephalopathy. Cardiac dysfunction may also be observed, possibly accompanied by edema, tachycardia on minimal exertion, enlarged heart, and electrocardiographic abnormalities.

DOSING AND DAILY REQUIREMENTS. The DRI values for thiamin are listed in Table 23–3. Symptomatic patients are preferably treated with intravenous thiamin. However, long-term supplementation may be recommended for patients at continued risk of deficiency, including alcoholic patients and those prescribed high-dose furosemide therapy. The FDA-approved use of thiamin is for the treatment of thiamin deficiency.[19]

SAFETY CONSIDERATIONS. The kidney easily clears excessive thiamin intake, and oral doses of 500 mg have been found to be nontoxic.

POTENTIAL DRUG–NUTRIENT INTERACTIONS. Diuretics have been shown to increase the urinary excretion of thiamin. Therefore, patients on chronic diuretic therapy (e.g., those with congestive heart failure or hypertension) may be at risk of subclinical thiamin deficiency and associated cardiovascular complications. Recommending supplementation with 100% of the DRI for this vitamin is reasonable.[46]

Pantothenic Acid, Riboflavin (Vitamin B_2), and Biotin (Vitamin H)

Other water-soluble B-complex vitamins include pantothenic acid, riboflavin, and biotin. All of these nutrients serve a variety of roles in the metabolism and conversion of carbohydrate and other macronutrients into sources of energy for numerous metabolic processes.

FUNCTIONS. Pantothenic acid is a cofactor for numerous biological reactions necessary for energy synthesis. Pantothenic acid is a precursor of CoA, a product that is active in many biological reactions and plays a primary role in cholesterol, steroid, and fatty acid synthesis. Pantothenic acid is important for acetylation reactions and the formation of citric acid for the Krebs cycle, and it is crucial in the intraneuronal synthesis of acetylcholine. This nutrient also is important in gluconeogenesis; synthesis and degradation of fatty acids; synthesis of sterols, steroid hormones, and porphyrins; and in the release of energy from carbohydrates.

Riboflavin is a water-soluble vitamin essential for cellular growth and maintenance of vision, mucous membranes, skin, nails, and hair. Riboflavin is a constituent of two coenzymes: flavin adenine dinucleotide and flavin mononucleotide. It is involved in numerous oxidation and reduction reactions, including the cytochrome P450 reductase enzyme system involved in drug metabolism.

Biotin is necessary for various metabolic functions, including carbohydrate, fat, and amino acid metabolism; several biotin-dependent enzymes are known to exist.

DEFICIENCY. Because pantothenic acid, riboflavin, and biotin are contained in many foods, deficiency states are rare and hard to detect. In malabsorption syndromes, it is difficult to distinguish pantothenic acid deficiency symptoms from those of other nutrient deficiencies. Symptoms of pantothenic acid deficiency include somnolence, fatigue, cardiovascular instability, abdominal pain, and paresthesia of hands and/or feet followed by hyperreflexia and muscular weakness in the legs. Administration of pharmacologic doses of pantothenic acid reverses these symptoms and has even been used to eliminate burning feet syndrome.

As with pantothenic acid, riboflavin deficiency, although rare, may be caused by inadequate intake, alcoholism, or malabsorptive syndromes. Deficiency of this vitamin may occur in association with other vitamin B-complex deficiency states (e.g., pellagra) or during pregnancy. Early signs of riboflavin deficiency may involve ocular symptoms, as the eyes become light sensitive and easily fatigued. The patient may develop blurred vision; itching, watering, sore eyes; and corneal vascularization, which causes a bloodshot appearance of the eye. Clinical findings of more advanced deficiency include stomatitis, seborrheic dermatitis, and magenta tongue.

Deficiency states of biotin are rare but appear to result in symptoms of nausea, vomiting, lassitude, muscle pain, anorexia, anemia, and depression. Dermatitis, a grayish color of the skin, and glossitis may be among the physical findings; hypercholesterolemia and cardiac abnormalities may also occur. Biotin deficiency in humans can be caused by ingesting a large number of raw egg whites. Raw egg whites contain avidin, a protein that binds biotin, thereby preventing its absorption. Individuals undergoing a rapid weight-loss program with intense caloric restriction and those with chronic malabsorption may not obtain adequate biotin and should receive supplementation, generally as part of an MVM supplement.

DOSING AND DAILY REQUIREMENTS. AI and DRI values for these vitamins are listed in Table 23–3; there is no established UL for pantothenic acid.[14] The need for riboflavin appears to increase during periods of increased cell growth, such as during pregnancy and wound healing. Its absorption is enhanced when taken with food. The FDA-approved use of riboflavin is in the prevention and treatment of riboflavin deficiency.[19] No UL has been determined for this vitamin.

SAFETY CONSIDERATIONS. Pantothenic acid, riboflavin, and biotin are generally considered nontoxic, even in large doses. The use of riboflavin typically causes a yellow-orange fluorescence or discoloration of the urine. Patients who report this effect should be reassured that this color is normal. No known toxic concentration is associated with pantothenic acid, riboflavin, or biotin. Adverse effects have not been reported with biotin therapy.

Vitamin-Like Compounds and Pseudovitamins

Vitamin-like compounds, or pseudovitamins, are substances that have a chemical structure very similar to that of vitamins but lack the usual physiologic or biochemical actions. That is, they are not essential for specific body functions of growth, maintenance, and reproduction.

Choline

Choline is contained in most living cells and in foods. It is usually present in the form of phosphatidylcholine, commonly known as lecithin, and in several other phospholipids found in cell membranes. Intestinal mucosal cells and pancreatic secretions contain enzymes capable of splitting phospholipids to release choline. Choline is also found in sphingomyelin and is highly concentrated in nervous tissue.

Choline is found in food sources and is also synthesized in the body. Therefore, choline most likely is not a vitamin. Choline is obtained from the diet as either choline or lecithin. Food sources are listed in Table 23–6; Table 23–3 lists DRI values. An average diet furnishes ample choline daily. The recommended UL for choline is 3.5 g/day.[14]

FUNCTION. Choline, a precursor in the biosynthesis of acetylcholine, is an important donor of methyl groups used in the biochemical formation of other substances in vivo. It can be biosynthesized in humans. Furthermore, choline and inositol are considered to be lipotropic agents (i.e., agents involved in the mobilization of lipids). They have been used to treat fatty liver and abnormal fat metabolism, but their efficacy has not been established.

DEFICIENCY. A deficiency state has not been identified in humans, possibly because choline is readily available in the diet and is synthesized in the body.

SAFETY CONSIDERATIONS. The administration of large doses of lecithin has been associated with sweating, GI distress, vomiting, and diarrhea.

Minerals

Minerals constitute about 4% of body weight. These micronutrients are present in the body in a diverse array of organic compounds (e.g., phosphoproteins, phospholipids, hemoglobin, thyroxine). They function as constituents of many enzymes, hormones, vitamins, and inorganic compounds (e.g., sodium chloride, potassium chloride, calcium, phosphorus) that are present as free ions. Different body tissues contain various quantities of different minerals. For example, bone has a high content of calcium, phosphorus, and magnesium, whereas soft tissue has a high quantity of potassium. Minerals are involved in regulating cell membrane permeability, osmotic pressure, and acid–base and water balance. In addition, certain ions act as the mediators of action potential conduction and neurotransmitter action.

A well-balanced diet is required to maintain proper mineral balance. Optimal mineral intake values for humans are still imprecise; only AIs are available for trace element minerals such as chromium, fluoride, and manganese. Table 23–4 lists the DRIs for select elements and minerals, and Table 23–6 includes dietary sources of the minerals discussed in this chapter. Possible adverse effects of long-term ingestion of high-dose mineral supplements are often unknown, and high doses of one mineral can decrease the bioavailability of other minerals and vitamins. Practitioners should be aware of select drug–nutrient interactions and mineral deficiencies that may be precipitated by certain medications (Table 23–7).

Calcium

The most abundant cation in the body is calcium (about 1200 grams). Approximately 99% of calcium is present in the skeleton, and the remaining 1% is present in extracellular fluid, intracellular structures, and cell membranes. Calcium is a major component of bones and teeth. The calcium content in bone is continuously undergoing a process of resorption and formation. In people of advanced age, the resorption process predominates over formation, and a decrease in calcium absorption efficiency results in a gradual loss of bone density that leads to osteoporosis. This effect can be minimized by encouraging optimal calcium and vitamin D intake throughout the life cycle and by encouraging regular participation in weight-bearing exercise.

Function

Calcium activates a number of enzymes and is required for acetylcholine synthesis. Calcium increases cell membrane permeability, aids in vitamin B_{12} absorption, regulates muscle contraction and relaxation, and catalyzes several steps in the activation of plasma-clotting factors. Calcium also is necessary for the functional integrity of many cells, especially those of the neuromuscular and cardiovascular system.

Dietary Sources

Teenagers experiencing rapid growth and bone maturation need to consume adequate calcium through dairy products (especially milk) or through a nutritional supplement. Most adults can easily meet calcium RDAs by incorporating dairy products into their diets daily. Each 8-ounce serving of nonfat milk contains about 300 mg of calcium. As an alternative, calcium supplements are usually well tolerated in daily doses of less than 2 g. Table 23–9 lists selected calcium supplements.

Practitioners should evaluate the dietary intake of calcium (including calcium-fortified foods) before recommending daily calcium supplementation. Calcium fortification is found in numerous nontraditional sources (e.g., juices, breads, breakfast bars). To optimize calcium absorption, patients should avoid co-ingestion with bran, whole-grain cereals, or high-oxalate foods (e.g., cocoa, soybeans, spinach); for those using a supplement, a product co-formulated with vitamin D may be recommended if vitamin D intake from other sources is inadequate.

Deficiency

Decreased calcium concentrations may have profound and diverse consequences, including convulsions, tetany, behavioral and personality disorders, mental and growth retardation, and bone deformities (the most common being rickets in children and osteomalacia in adults). Changes that occur in osteomalacia include softening of bones, rheumatic-type pain in the bones of the legs and lower back, general weakness with difficulty walking, and spontaneous fractures. Common causes of hypocalcemia and associated skeletal disorders include malabsorptive syndromes; hypoparathyroidism; vitamin D deficiency; renal failure with impaired activation of vitamin D; long-term anticonvulsant therapy (with increased breakdown of vitamin D); and decreased dietary intake of calcium, particularly during periods of growth, pregnancy, and lactation, and among people of advanced age.

TABLE 23–9 Selected Nonprescription Calcium Supplements

Trade Name	Primary Ingredients Per Serving
Caltrate 600+D Tablets	Elemental calcium 600 mg (as carbonate); vitamin D 200–800 IU (depending on formulation)
Citracal Maximum+D3 Caplets	Elemental calcium 630 mg (as citrate); vitamin D 500 IU
Tums Regular Strength Chewable Tablets	Elemental calcium 400 mg (as carbonate)
Viactiv Calcium plus D Soft Chews	Elemental calcium 500 mg (as carbonate); vitamin D 500 IU; vitamin K 40 mcg

Dosing and Daily Requirements

Oral calcium supplements are FDA approved for use in the treatment and prevention of calcium deficiency, which may result in rickets, osteomalacia, or osteoporosis. Other FDA-approved uses include treatment of acid indigestion and hyperphosphatemia associated with end-stage renal disease.[19] The recommended UL for calcium is 2–3 g/day for individuals older than 1 year.[15]

Recommendations for calcium intake are based on elemental calcium content, not the calcium salt. Because labels can be misleading, practitioners should be familiar with the many salt forms and the different percentages of calcium in each, including carbonate (40%), citrate (21%), lactate (13%), gluconate (9%), and phosphate salts (23%–39%).[47] Calcium carbonate and calcium phosphate salts are insoluble in water and should be taken with meals to enhance absorption, which is optimal in a low pH. Patients requiring supplementation who have achlorhydria or who are on chronic therapy with histamine-2 antagonists or proton pump inhibitors may benefit most from taking one of the water-soluble salt formulations (e.g., calcium citrate), which are absorbed more readily in basic environments.

The small intestine controls calcium absorption. Patients ingesting relatively low amounts of calcium absorb proportionately more calcium than those with adequate intake; patients taking large amounts of calcium excrete more as fecal calcium. Optimal absorption occurs with individual doses of 500 mg or less; therefore, patients taking more than 500 mg of supplemental calcium should be encouraged to take calcium in divided doses.[15] In conjunction with adequate calcium and vitamin D intake, weight-bearing exercise is essential in maintaining bone mass.

Safety Considerations

Calcium in doses greater than 3 g/day can be harmful. Large amounts taken as dietary supplements or antacids can lead to high levels of calcium in the urine and to the formation of renal stones; development of the latter may result in permanent renal damage. Development of hypercalcemia is possible (particularly in patients taking concomitant high-dose vitamin D preparations) and is associated with anorexia, nausea, vomiting, constipation, and polyuria. Increased deposition of calcium in soft tissue can also occur with hypercalcemia. The U.S. Preventive Services Task Force (USPSTF) is more conservative regarding calcium intake and recommends that daily calcium intake not exceed 1000 mg.[48] USPSTF's recommendation is based on the fact that insufficient evidence exists to determine whether calcium supplementation can reduce fractures in community-dwelling adults and on concerns that high-dose supplementation may increase the risk of adverse effects.

The relationship between dietary and supplemental calcium intake and increased cardiovascular disease risk has caused much controversy and uncertainty in the medical community over the past several years. According to results of a prospective study, supplemental calcium intake at a dose greater than 1000 mg/day was associated with an increased risk of death from heart disease in men.[49] Supplemental calcium intake at any dose in women, on the other hand, was not found to correlate with increased risk of cardiovascular disease, heart disease, or cerebrovascular death in this trial. Moreover, dietary calcium intake was found to be unrelated to increased risk of cardiovascular death in either men or women, underscoring the importance of dietary calcium intake over supplemental calcium use. The study was conducted in 388,229 men and women ages 50–71 years and was designed to evaluate the effects of both dietary and supplemental calcium intake on mortality from cardiovascular disease, heart disease, and stroke. Results from a post hoc analysis of the Women's Health Initiative dataset also identified no increased risks of myocardial infarction, coronary heart disease, total heart disease, stroke, or overall cardiovascular disease in postmenopausal women receiving 1000 mg/day elemental calcium carbonate plus 400 IU/day of vitamin D_3.[50] Clearly, more information is necessary to further elucidate the correlations between calcium supplementation and cardiovascular disease risk. Patients considering calcium supplementation should undergo a complete dietary and lifestyle evaluation to determine the possible risks and benefits of supplementation with this mineral.

Calcium intake has also been suggested to influence risk of prostate cancer. In fact, three trials have found an increased risk for prostate cancer with calcium intakes greater than 1500 mg daily from either supplements or dietary sources.[51] Recommending calcium intakes closer to the DRI/RDA for those at risk of prostate cancer is reasonable until further evidence clarifies this association.

Practitioners should counsel patients about potential constipation associated with calcium supplementation and the importance of adequate hydration, dietary fiber, and physical activity in preventing this side effect.

Iron

Iron is widely available in the U.S. diet. Iron absorption from the intestinal tract is controlled by the body's need for iron, the intestinal lumen conditions, the food source of iron, and the other components of the meal (e.g., the meal's vitamin C content).

Function

Iron plays an important role in oxygen and electron transport. In the body, it is either functional or stored (Figure 23–4).

Dietary Sources

Dietary iron is available in two forms: heme and nonheme iron. Heme iron is found in meats and is reasonably well absorbed. Nonheme iron (e.g., that found in enriched grains and dark green vegetables) constitutes most of the dietary iron but is poorly absorbed. Therefore, the published values of iron content in foods are misleading because the amount absorbed depends on the nature of the iron. Although specific ways to calculate the iron absorption from a given meal exist, the available iron content of foods is often estimated by assuming that about 10% of the total iron (heme plus nonheme) is absorbed if no iron deficiency exists. In the iron-deficient state, iron absorption improves, so as much as 20% may be absorbed and utilized from an average diet. However, this estimate is not valid in the absence of heme iron. Less iron is absorbed from vegetarian diets.

Ingested nonheme iron (which is mostly in the form of ferric hydroxide) is solubilized in gastric juice to ferric chloride, then reduced to the ferrous form, and finally chelated to substances such as ascorbic acid, sugars, and amino acids. Chelates have a low molecular weight and can be solubilized and absorbed before they reach the alkaline medium of the distal small intestine, where precipitation may occur. When released at the spleen, liver, bone marrow, intestinal mucosa, and other iron storage sites, the iron is combined with apoferritin to form ferritin or hemosiderin (Figure 23–4). As needed, ferritin is released into the plasma, where it is oxidized to the ferric state and bound to a beta globulin to form transferrin. Iron is used in all cells of the body; however, most of it is incorporated into the hemoglobin of red blood cells.

Deficiency

The major source of iron loss is through blood loss (e.g., hemorrhagic loss, menstruation). Iron is also lost from the body by the sloughing of skin cells and GI mucosal cells, and by excretion in urine, sweat, and feces. Excess iron loss may result in iron deficiency. Early symptoms of iron deficiency are vague. Although pallor and easy fatigability may be associated with iron deficiency, they can be attributed to other causes and are nonspecific findings. Other signs and symptoms of iron-deficiency anemia include split or "spoon-shaped" nails, sore tongue, angular stomatitis, and dyspnea on exertion. Coldness and numbness of the extremities may also be reported. Hypochromic microcytosis, as evidenced by a decreased mean corpuscular volume and low hemoglobin concentration (decreased mean corpuscular hemoglobin concentration), characterizes iron deficiency on laboratory assessment.

Iron-deficiency anemia is a widespread clinical problem and the most common form of anemia in the United States. Although it causes few deaths, it does contribute to poor health and suboptimal performance. Iron deficiency results from inadequate intake (e.g., inadequate diet, malabsorption) or increased demands (e.g., pregnancy and lactation, growth, blood loss, treatment with erythropoietic stimulating agents). Because normal iron losses through the urine, feces, and skin are minimal, and because the majority of total body iron is efficiently stored and conserved (recycled), iron deficiency caused by poor diet or malabsorption develops very slowly over the course of several months.

Despite fortification of flour and educational efforts regarding proper nutrition, iron deficiency remains a problem, especially during the following four life periods:

- During childhood (younger than 2 years): Children obtain low iron content from cow's milk.
- During adolescence: In addition to blood loss during menses, young women experience rapid growth, which entails an expanding red cell mass and the need for iron in myoglobin.
- During and after pregnancy: Women face the expanding blood volume of pregnancy, the demands of the fetus and placenta, and the blood loss of childbirth.
- During later years: Persons of advanced age (i.e., 65 years or older) often consume inadequate dietary iron, demonstrate compromised absorption caused by achlorhydria, and experience an increased incidence of GI tract blood loss resulting from malignancy, gastric ulceration, or use of nonsteroidal anti-inflammatory drugs (NSAIDs). However, the prevalence of elevated iron stores may be significantly greater than the prevalence of iron deficiency in this age group. Therefore, absent a confirmed diagnosis of iron-deficiency anemia, routine supplementation is not recommended for this age group.

Supplemental iron may be warranted for women with heavy or prolonged menstrual blood loss or for individuals who frequently donate blood. Iron may also be indicated during recovery from disease- and injury-associated blood loss (e.g., peptic ulcer disease, esophageal varices, cancer, traumatic injury such as motor vehicle accidents). In addition, infants being fed human milk may need supplemental iron beginning between the ages of 4–6 months if iron-rich foods are not introduced into the diet.

Chronic use of drugs such as salicylates, NSAIDs, corticosteroids, or anticoagulants may cause drug-induced blood loss. This effect may be the result of direct irritation of the gastric mucosa or these drugs' tendency to cause increased bleeding. Iron

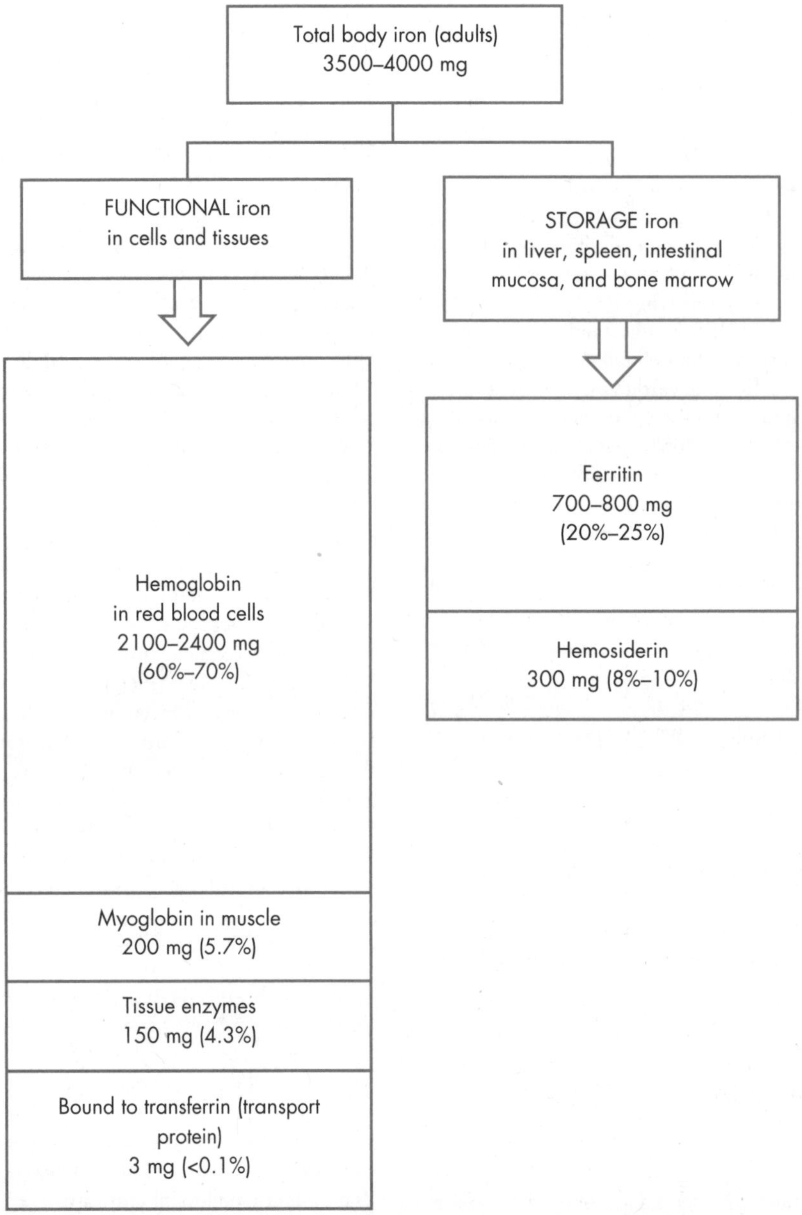

FIGURE 23–4 Iron distribution in the body.

supplementation should be used cautiously, if at all, in patients at high risk for GI bleeding.

Dosing and Daily Requirements

Because of the GI side effects associated with oral iron supplementation, the UL for elemental iron has been set at 45 mg/day for adults.[14] Oral iron supplements are FDA approved for the prevention and treatment of iron-deficiency anemia.[19]

When iron supplementation is appropriate, the practitioner will need to evaluate which iron product is best. The choice should be based on how well the iron preparation is absorbed and tolerated, the amount of elemental iron per dose, and product price. Because ferrous salts are absorbed 3 times more efficiently than ferric salts, an iron product of the ferrous group is usually appropriate. Ferrous sulfate is the standard against which other iron salts are compared.

Ferrous sulfate contains 20% elemental iron, or about 65 mg in a 325 mg tablet. In patients with iron deficiency, 20% of the elemental iron (12 mg) may be absorbed. Maximum incorporation of iron into red blood cells and replacement of stores is supported by 36–48 mg of elemental iron daily; thus, the usual therapeutic dose for treating iron deficiency is 2–4 (325 mg) ferrous sulfate tablets daily for 3 months. Inadequate response or worsening symptoms during this time indicate the patient should consult a primary care provider. In cases of severe or chronic iron deficiency, when serious medical conditions have been ruled out, continuous maintenance doses of 3–4 (325 mg) ferrous sulfate tablets daily for 3–6 months should normalize hemoglobin and replace iron stores (in the absence of ongoing bleeding).

Table 23–10 lists comparison data on various iron salts.[52] Ferrous salts may be given in combination with ascorbic acid to improve iron absorption. If necessary, the practitioner can

TABLE 23–10 **Common Nonprescription Oral Iron Formulations**

Iron Formulation	Typical Dose	Percent Elemental Iron	Comparison Data
Ferrous sulfate	325 mg/tablet	20% (65 mg/tablet)	The gold standard for supplementation; available in multiple dosage forms; extensive history of use; proven effective; and economical. Delayed-release and enteric-coated products may improve tolerability, but iron absorption may be reduced.
Ferrous fumarate	60 mg/tablet	33% (20 mg/tablet)	No advantage over ferrous sulfate; however, may be better tolerated for some individuals.
Ferrous gluconate	225 mg/tablet	12% (27 mg/tablet)	No advantage over ferrous sulfate; however, may be better tolerated for some individuals.

Source: Reference 52.

encourage that iron be taken with fruit or juice high in ascorbic acid or with a vitamin C supplement. Combination products with iron and ascorbic acid are also available, but these products can be expensive, and the dose of vitamin C is often inadequate. Chemicals that may decrease iron absorption include phosphates in eggs and milk, carbonates, oxalates, tannins, and phytates in cereals.

Safety Considerations

All iron products tend to irritate the GI mucosa and may produce nausea, abdominal pain, constipation, and (less frequently) diarrhea. These adverse effects may be minimized by reducing the dose or by giving iron with meals; however, food may decrease the amount of iron absorbed by as much as 50%. Practitioners may want to recommend that iron be initiated on an empty stomach; they should instruct the patient to change this routine and take the iron with food, if GI side effects occur.

A frequent side effect of iron therapy is constipation. This adverse effect has prompted the formulation of iron products that also contain a stool softener (e.g., docusate). During iron therapy, stools commonly have a black, tarry appearance because of the presence of unabsorbed iron in the feces. Unfortunately, this symptom may also indicate GI blood loss and a serious medical problem. Medical evaluation is indicated if an underlying GI condition is suspected, or if a history of GI disease exists. If the stool does not darken somewhat during iron therapy, however, the iron product may not have disintegrated properly or released the iron.

Iron must be dispensed and stored in a child-resistant container. Accidental poisonings with iron occur most often in children, who are attracted to the sugar-coated, colored tablets or who may accidentally overdose on chewable multivitamins containing iron. Such poisoning is considered a medical emergency, and any accidental ingestion of iron should be referred for evaluation by a medical provider or to a Poison Control Center. The clinical outcome depends on the speed and adequacy of treatment.

Symptoms of acute iron poisoning include abdominal pain, vomiting, diarrhea, electrolyte imbalances, and shock. In later stages, cardiovascular collapse may occur, especially if the cause has not been properly recognized and treated as a medical emergency. Treatment of iron toxicity may begin immediately at home after consultation with a Poison Control Center or local emergency department.

Magnesium

Magnesium is essential for all living cells. It is the second most plentiful cation of intracellular fluids and the fourth most abundant cation in the body. About 2000 mEq magnesium are present in an average 70 kg adult, with about 50% of this amount in the bone, about 45% as an intracellular cation, and about 1%–5% in the extracellular fluid.

Function

Magnesium is required for normal bone structure formation and the proper function of more than 300 enzymes, including those involved with adenosine triphosphatase (ATP)–dependent phosphorylation, protein synthesis, and carbohydrate metabolism. Extracellular magnesium is critical to both the maintenance of nerve and muscle electrical potentials and the transmission of impulses across neuromuscular junctions.

Magnesium tends to mimic calcium in its effects on the CNS and skeletal muscle. Magnesium deficiency blunts the normal response of the parathyroid glands to hypocalcemia. Therefore, tetany, caused by a lack of calcium, cannot be corrected with calcium unless hypomagnesemia is also corrected. Similarly, magnesium deficiency impairs the transport of potassium into cells; therefore, hypokalemia cannot be corrected in the presence of magnesium deficiency.

Dietary Sources

Individuals who consume fresh foods regularly should not develop magnesium deficiency because all unprocessed foods contain magnesium (albeit in widely varying amounts). Processing (during which the germ and outer layers of cereal grains are removed) results in significant loss of available magnesium.

Deficiency

Deficiency states are usually caused by GI or renal losses. Examples include malabsorptive syndromes, acute or chronic diarrhea, steatorrhea, and drug-induced magnesium wasting in the urine, as seen with alcohol abuse, diuretic therapy, long-term use of proton pump inhibitors, calcineurin inhibitors (e.g., cyclosporine, tacrolimus) and nephrotoxins (e.g., amphotericin B). Symptoms of magnesium deficiency may include neuromuscular irritability, increased CNS stimulation, delirium, and convulsions.

Dosing and Daily Requirements

Oral magnesium supplements are FDA approved for use in the treatment and prevention of hypomagnesemia.[19] The recommended UL for magnesium is 350 mg/day for older children and adults.[14]

Safety Considerations

No evidence is available to suggest that oral intake of magnesium is harmful to individuals with normal renal function, although diarrhea may occur with large doses. Hypermagnesemia can occur with overzealous use of magnesium sulfate (Epsom salts) or magnesium hydroxide (milk of magnesia) as a laxative, or with use of magnesium-containing antacids in patients with severe renal failure. Hypermagnesemia may cause diminished deep tendon reflexes and varying degrees of muscle weakness, lethargy, and sedation. These effects may progress to stupor and coma, especially at high serum concentrations. Cardiovascular symptoms may include hypotension and dysrhythmia.

Phosphorus

Phosphorus is present throughout the body, but approximately 85% of the body's store is located in bone. Phosphorus is present in nearly all foods, especially protein-rich foods and cereal grains (Table 23–6).

Function

Phosphorus is essential for many metabolic processes. It serves as an integral structural component of the bone matrix as calcium phosphate, and it is a functional component of phospholipids, carbohydrates, nucleoproteins, and high-energy nucleotides. Plasma phosphate levels are under the tight biologic control of parathyroid hormone, calcitonin, and vitamin D. DNA and RNA structures contain sugar–phosphate linkages. Cell membranes contain phospholipids, which regulate the transport of solutes into and out of the cell. Many metabolic processes depend on phosphorylation. The adenosine diphosphate (ADP)–ATP system (which provides a mechanism for the storage and release of energy for use in all of the body's metabolic processes) involves phosphorus compounds. Additionally, an important buffer system of the body consists of inorganic phosphates.

Calcium and phosphorus have a reciprocal relationship. Both minerals are regulated partially by parathyroid hormone. Secretion of parathyroid hormone stimulates an increase in serum calcium levels through increased bone resorption, gut absorption, and reabsorption in renal tubules. Parathyroid hormone also causes a decrease in the reabsorption of phosphate by the kidney. Therefore, when serum calcium is high, serum phosphate is generally low, and vice versa.

Deficiency

Because nearly all foods contain phosphorus, deficiency states usually do not occur unless induced. For example, patients receiving aluminum hydroxide as an antacid for prolonged periods may exhibit hypophosphatemia, characterized by weakness, anorexia, malaise, pain, and bone loss. Aluminum binds dietary phosphorus, forming insoluble and poorly absorbed complexes.

Dosing and Daily Requirements

The FDA-approved use for phosphorus is to alleviate signs and symptoms of deficiency.[19] The recommended UL for phosphorus is 4 g/day for older children and most adults.[14]

Safety Considerations

GI side effects (e.g., diarrhea, stomach pain) have been reported with oral supplementation of phosphate salts.

Trace Elements

Trace elements, which are present in minute quantities in plant and animal tissue, are considered essential for numerous physiologic processes. A subset of trace elements, the "ultratrace" elements, has an estimated dietary requirement of less than 1 mg/day. Zinc and manganese are trace elements. The essential ultratrace minerals include arsenic, boron, cobalt, copper, chromium, iodine, molybdenum, nickel, selenium, and silicon. Lithium and vanadium possibly are essential minerals, but further study is required. Bromine, cadmium, fluorine, lead, and tin are not considered essential. The trace and ultratrace element content of foods typically reflects the content of the soil in which the food was grown. One of the best defenses against deficiencies is to consume foods from a variety of geographically diverse regions.

For the purpose of this chapter, a detailed review of the elements copper, fluoride, iodine, and zinc will be included; these particular trace elements may need to be supplemented in individuals with specialty needs. The reader is referred to more comprehensive references for detailed description of the functions, daily requirements, and safety concerns of other trace and ultratrace elements not included in this discussion. Tables 23–4 and 23–5 provide a summary of DRIs and ULs for select trace elements, and Table 23–6 lists food sources of these nutrients.

Copper

Copper ions exist in two states: the cuprous ion and the cupric ion (a potent oxidizing agent). Copper is similar to zinc in the complexes it forms with a number of the same chelating agents. Copper is found in virtually all tissues of the body, but concentrations are highest in the liver, brain, heart, and kidney.

Function

Copper is essential for the proper structure and function of the CNS, and it plays a major role in iron metabolism. Ceruloplasmin, one of the copper metalloenzymes, is especially important in converting absorbed ferrous iron to transported ferric iron. Other copper-containing enzymes are cytochrome oxidase, dopamine beta-hydroxylase, and superoxide dismutase.

Deficiency

Copper deficiency is uncommon in humans, with a few notable exceptions. Deficiencies have been observed in premature infants; in severely malnourished infants fed milk-based, low-copper diets; following Roux-En-Y gastric bypass in individuals who do not consume a supplement; and in patients receiving parenteral nutrition with inadequate copper.

One of the prominent features of copper deficiency is neurologic symptoms with gait disturbances, particularly impaired proprioception and vibration sense. Ataxia, myelopathy, optic neuritis, polyneuropathy, and demyelination can occur. In deficiency states, iron absorption is impaired, typically resulting in hypochromic anemia, and spontaneous rupture of major vessels may also be observed.

Dosing and Daily Requirements

For protection against possible hepatotoxicity, the recommended UL for copper is 10 mg/day for adults.[14]

Safety Considerations

Copper sulfate doses in excess of 250 mg produce vomiting.

Wilson's disease is an inborn error of metabolism resulting in copper retention. These individuals must avoid any copper supplementation. Wilson's disease results in CNS, kidney, and liver damage. Acute symptoms of copper toxicity include nausea, vomiting, diarrhea, hemolysis, convulsions, and GI bleeding. Symptoms respond to treatment with penicillamine.

Supplementation should be avoided in patients with severe hepatic dysfunction or cholestasis, as biliary clearance of copper may be compromised.

Fluoride

Available therapeutic forms of fluoride include sodium fluoride, acidulated phosphate fluoride, and stannous fluoride. Sodium fluoride contains about 45% fluoride ion, whereas stannous fluoride contains about 24% fluoride ion.

Function

Fluoride occurs normally in bones and tooth enamel as a calcium salt. Intake of small amounts has been shown to reduce tooth decay markedly, presumably by making the enamel more resistant to the erosive action of acids produced by bacteria in the oral cavity.

Dietary Sources

Fluoride is present in soil and water, but the content varies widely from region to region. Most municipal water supplies are fluoridated to 1 ppm of fluoride, a level that has been shown to be safe and to reduce dental caries in children by nearly 50%. Estimates of fluoride intake from food, beverages, and water vary greatly, depending on the presence of fluoridated drinking water.

Deficiency

Fluoride deficiency states in humans, other than potential dental decay, have not been described.

Dosing and Daily Requirements

The recommended UL for this trace element is 10 mg/day for older children and adults.[14]

Fluoride is FDA approved for use in the prevention of dental caries.[19] Fluoride is a normal constituent of the diet, given that it occurs in soils, water supplies, plants, and animals. All sources of fluoride should be evaluated before supplementation is recommended for children whose home water supply is low in fluoride. Children may obtain fluoride from other water sources (e.g., day care, school) or from other beverages that may contain varying amounts of fluoride (e.g., soft drinks, juices, bottled water).[53]

Sodium fluoride is available by prescription as oral tablets and solutions, topical solutions, and gels, as well as in combination products. Nonprescription topical rinses containing fluoride 0.01%–0.02% (e.g., sodium fluoride) and gels containing 0.4% stannous fluoride (e.g., Gel-Kam) are rinsed or brushed onto the teeth to reduce sensitivity and prevent dental cavities.

Safety Considerations

Excessive fluoride can be toxic. Acute toxicity should not result from the low levels present in drinking water but may result from the administration of excessive doses of fluoride supplements. Because acute toxicity affects the GI system and the CNS, it can be life threatening. Symptoms include salivation, GI distress, muscle weakness, tremors, and (rarely) seizures. Because fluoride binds calcium, symptoms of calcium deficiency (including tetany) may also be seen. Eventually, respiratory and cardiac failure may occur. All accidental ingestions of fluoride in children should be referred for evaluation by a medical practitioner or Poison Control Center, as fluoride intoxication may be fatal. Treatment includes precipitation of the fluoride by using gastric lavage with calcium hydroxide 0.15% solution, intravenous administration of dextrose and saline for hydration, and treatment with calcium to prevent tetany.

Chronic fluoride toxicity is manifested as changes in the structure of bones and teeth. Tooth enamel, if still under development, acquires a mottled appearance consisting of white, patchy plaques occurring with pitting brown stains. Prolonged ingestion of water that contains greater than 2 ppm of fluoride has resulted in a significant incidence of mottling. Extremely large doses (e.g., 20–80 mg/day) have resulted in chalky, brittle bones that tend to fracture easily, a condition known as crippling skeletal fluorosis.

Iodine

The thyroid gland contains about one-third of the iodine in the body, stored in the form of a complex glycoprotein, thyroglobulin. The only known function of thyroglobulin is to provide thyroxine and triiodothyronine, hormones that regulate the metabolic rate of cells, thereby influencing physical and mental growth, nervous and muscle tissue function, circulatory activity, and nutrient utilization.

Function

Iodine is an essential micronutrient required to synthesize thyroxine and triiodothyronine. High concentrations of iodine inhibit the release of these hormones.

Dietary Sources

The primary dietary source of iodine is iodized salt, which contains 1 part of sodium or potassium iodide per 10,000 parts (0.01%) of salt. A dose of about 95 mcg of iodine can be obtained from about one-fourth teaspoon of salt (1.25 g). In the United States, most of the table salt sold is iodized; however, salt used in food processing and for institutional use is not. Additional dietary sources of iodine include saltwater fish and shellfish. Produce may also be a source of iodine; the iodine content of produce reflects that of the soil in which it was grown.

Deficiency

A moderate iodine deficiency can lead to thyroid hypertrophy, resulting in goiter; severe deficiency results in hypothyroidism. The consumption of foods from diverse locations and the addition of iodide to table salt have essentially eliminated goiter as a health problem in the United States.

Dosing and Daily Requirements

Because of the fortification of salt, the iodine content of typical diets in the United States is still well above the DRI values for adults (Table 23–4). Iodine supplements are unwarranted for most individuals. Potassium iodide is available as a tablet, syrup, and solution, and it is included in various combination products.

Safety Considerations

Some individuals are allergic to iodine or organic preparations containing iodine and may develop a rash. Symptoms of chronic iodism (iodine intoxication) may include an unpleasant taste and burning in the mouth or throat, along with soreness of the teeth or gums. Increased salivation, sneezing, eye irritation, and eyelid swelling can occur. In addition, prolonged use of iodine supplementation can result in hypothyroidism.[18] A UL of 1.1 mg/day in adults has been recommended.[14]

Zinc

Zinc is an integral part of at least 70 metalloenzymes, including carbonic anhydrase, lactic dehydrogenase, alkaline phosphatase, carboxypeptidase, aminopeptidase, and alcohol dehydrogenase.

Function

Zinc is a cofactor in the synthesis of DNA and RNA. It is involved in the mobilization of vitamin A from the liver and in the enhancement of follicle-stimulating hormone and luteinizing hormone. Zinc is essential for normal cellular immune functions, spermatogenesis, and normal testicular function. It also is important in the stabilization of membrane structure.

The divalent ion is most commonly found and used in the body. Zinc has a relatively rapid turnover rate. The balance between zinc absorption from the small intestine and excretion through feces is efficiently regulated by the body. Vegetarians may require higher amounts of zinc, because diets high in fiber and phytates hinder zinc absorption.

Dietary Sources

Most dietary zinc (about 70%) is derived from animal products (Table 23–6).

Deficiency

Zinc deficiency is not widespread in the United States. Marginally low zinc values have been associated with birth defects, growth retardation in children, and slow wound healing in adults. Additional symptoms include immunologic abnormalities, impaired taste and smell, delayed sexual maturation, hypogonadism, hypospermia, and dermatitis.

Malabsorptive syndromes, infection, major surgery, alcoholism, pregnancy, lactation, and high-fiber diets rich in phytates predispose individuals to zinc deficiency. Zinc depletion is relatively rare but may be seen in patients on long-term parenteral nutrition and in patients with GI tract abnormalities (e.g., fistulas; prolonged, severe diarrhea).

Zinc deficiencies adversely affect DNA, RNA, carbohydrate, and protein catabolism. Iron supplements decrease zinc absorption just as zinc supplements decrease iron absorption, likely through competition for the same transport system. If these minerals are taken with a meal, the adverse interaction is less pronounced. In patients with impaired wound healing, zinc supplementation may be marginally beneficial.

Dosing and Daily Requirements

Typical Western diets supply 10–15 mg of zinc per day. Because only 10%–40% of zinc is absorbed from the GI tract, ingestion of zinc sulfate 220 mg (50 mg of elemental zinc) will supply 5–20 mg of zinc. Treatment of suspected deficiencies usually involves short-term administration of elemental zinc. Patients with large GI losses through fistulas, ostomies, or stool require larger supplemental doses of zinc. At doses above 40 mg elemental zinc per day, copper deficiency may be induced. Therefore, the UL for elemental zinc is 40 mg daily in adults if therapy with zinc is going to be long term.[14] Absorption of zinc supplements may be reduced when taken with foods high in calcium or phosphorus.

Zinc has been evaluated in numerous studies as a potential treatment for the common cold. However, zinc formulations and doses have varied, and trial results have been conflicting. Insufficient evidence exists at this time to recommend zinc supplementation for the treatment or prevention of the common cold.[54]

Safety Considerations

Because ingestion of 2 g or more of zinc sulfate has resulted in GI irritation and vomiting, zinc should be taken with food. Zinc also is toxic; however, the emetic effect that occurs after consumption of large amounts may minimize problems with accidental overdose. Reported signs of zinc toxicity in humans include vomiting, dehydration, poor muscle coordination, dizziness, and abdominal pain.

Multivitamin and Multimineral Supplements

Multivitamin and multimineral supplements, as previously described, are not intended to supplant a healthy, balanced diet but rather to augment dietary sources and support general health. Specific nutrients of concern for inadequate intake (shortfall nutrients) specified by the *Dietary Guidelines for Americans 2015–2020* include vitamin A, vitamin D, vitamin E, vitamin C, folate, calcium, magnesium, and potassium, with iron also being a concern in adolescent and premenopausal females. Of these vitamins, calcium, vitamin D, and potassium are of particular concern, given direct evidence of adverse health effects associated with inadequate daily intake and deficiency.[13] However, MVM supplements do not target these or any specific nutrients; rather, they provide a broad range of micronutrients. When such a product is being evaluated for an individual, the practitioner should consider recommending a preparation that contains the basic and essential vitamins and minerals, including the following: vitamins C, B_1 (thiamin), B_2 (riboflavin), B_3 (niacin), B_6 (pyridoxine), B_9 (folic acid), B_5 (pantothenic acid), A, E, D_2 or D_3 (cholecalciferol), and K, as well as biotin, potassium, iodine, selenium, borate, zinc, calcium, magnesium, manganese, molybdenum, and beta carotene.

The multitude of different nonprescription multivitamin products that are available warrant further consideration of an individual's age and gender to ensure selection of a formulation that is most likely to meet individual nutritional needs. Most multivitamins formulated for women ages 18–50 years contain increased amounts of iron and folic acid to prevent anemia related to menstrual blood loss and neural tube defects in those of childbearing age. Multivitamins formulated for men younger than 50 generally contain higher amounts of certain vitamins and less iron. Finally, senior multivitamins formulated for individuals older than age 50 may contain more calcium and certain B vitamins (e.g., B_6, B_{12}) but do not contain iron. Individuals should be reminded to refer to the product labeling for directions for use and not to exceed the recommended intake.

Assessment of Nutritional Adequacy: A Case-Based Approach

Assessing an individual's nutritional status is difficult in the ambulatory environment. Clinical impressions are often erroneous, because the stages between well-nourished and poorly nourished states are not readily evident. However, guidelines may help provide a more objective assessment of an individual's nutritional status. Practitioners should exercise good observational skills, know which questions yield helpful information (see cases for examples of questions), and know which population groups tend to be at risk for particular deficiencies. By asking key questions, the practitioner may detect cultural, physical, environmental, and social conditions that suggest inadequate vitamin intake. The more specific the information obtained from the individual, the more helpful the practitioner can be in determining the need for nutritional supplementation. Questions about the absence of different food types in the diet and about previous treatment of similar symptoms also may be important.

Although most nutritional assessment measures are beyond the scope of routine pharmacy practice, the pharmacist can observe the physical status of the patient. For example, an individual's fingernails may indicate malnutrition if the nails are not lustrous and are dark at the upper ends. The texture, amount, and appearance of hair may indicate the patient's nutritional status. The eyes (particularly the conjunctiva) may indicate vitamin A and iron deficiencies. The mouth may show stomatitis, glossitis, or hypertrophic or pale gums. Poor dentition may limit the foods that an individual is able to eat, thereby compromising intake from certain food groups, such as protein. Visible goiter, poor skin color and texture, obesity or thinness relative to bone structure, and the presence of edema may also indicate malnutrition. The pharmacist should be able to recognize overt but nonspecific symptoms of vitamin and mineral deficiencies for which prompt referral to a primary care provider may be crucial. Additionally, pharmacists should refer individuals at risk for nutritional deficiency or with increased metabolic demands (e.g., older persons, chronic alcohol abusers, pregnant and lactating women) for appropriate medical evaluation as necessary.

Checking a patient's medication history is important because of the number of potential drug–micronutrient interactions (Table 23–7). Practitioners also are responsible for referring patients with a suspected serious illness to a primary care provider. Just as nutritional deficiencies may lead to disease, disease may lead to nutritional deficiencies. Patients may present with one or more deficiencies, which may be very difficult to identify. Rarely in the United States do practitioners encounter patients with severe deficiencies resulting in diseases such as scurvy, pellagra, or beriberi. However, milder forms of malnutrition may be seen.

Cases 23–1 and 23–2 are examples of the assessment of patients with nutritional inadequacy.

CASE 23-1

Relevant Evaluation Criteria	Scenario/Model Outcome
Collect	
1. Gather essential information about the patient's symptoms and medical history, including	
a. Description of symptom(s) (i.e., nature, onset, duration, severity, associated symptoms)	Patient inquires about information received from a friend that recommends supplementation with various vitamins to help prevent cancer. She indicates that she currently takes a women's multivitamin–multimineral each day along with her prescription medications.
b. Description of any factors that seem to precipitate, exacerbate, and/or relieve the patient's symptom(s)	n/a
c. Description of the patient's efforts to relieve the symptoms	n/a
d. Patient's identity	Maggie Patrick
e. Patient's age, gender, height, and weight	63 years old, female, 5 ft 3 in., 130 lb
f. Patient's occupation	Middle school teacher; widow
g. Patient's dietary habits	Eats alone most of the time: typically cereal, milk, and juice or fruit for breakfast; soup or sandwich for lunch; easy meals for dinner (e.g., frozen dinners with protein, starch, vegetable). Often meets a few friends for lunch on Saturday.
h. Patient's sleep habits	n/a
i. Concurrent medical conditions, prescription and nonprescription medications, and dietary supplements	Patient has a history of gastroesophageal reflux disease and high blood pressure. Every morning she takes pantoprazole 40 mg; the combination hydrochlorothiazide/lisinopril 12.5/20 mg; and 1 women's multivitamin/multimineral tablet. For occasional headaches, she takes acetaminophen 325 mg.
j. Allergies	Sulfa
k. History of other adverse reactions to medications	n/a
Assess	
2. Differentiate patient's signs/symptoms, and correctly identify the patient's primary problem(s).	The patient's age and dietary habits may warrant consideration of a multivitamin supplement. However, no evidence to date supports the use of multivitamins to completely negate cancer risk.
3. Identify exclusions for self-treatment.	None

CASE 23-1 *continued*

Relevant Evaluation Criteria	Scenario/Model Outcome
4. Formulate a comprehensive list of therapeutic alternatives for the primary problem to determine whether triage to a medical provider is required, and share this information with the patient or caregiver.	Options include (1) Assess the client's perceived need for the nutrient supplements. (2) Evaluate dietary intake from food groups, encouraging at least 5 servings of produce, 3 servings of low-fat dairy products, 2 servings of protein, and 6 servings of whole-grain food sources daily. (3) Discuss which nutrients may need supplementation based on the patient's patterns of dietary intake, age, and special requirements. Evaluate the women's multivitamin/multimineral product for adequacy while avoiding intakes above the UL. (4) Discuss the lack of data and potential harm associated with mega doses of vitamins. (5) Take no action.
Plan	
5. Select an optimal therapeutic alternative to address the patient's problem, taking into account patient preferences.	Regular intake of a well-balanced diet that includes fruit, vegetables, whole grains, and low-fat dairy and lean protein sources is recommended for patients with high blood pressure. A multivitamin/mineral supplement that includes vitamin B_{12} and a balance of other nutrients would be reasonable for this older patient who prefers simple, easy meals and is on chronic acid suppression therapy. She should also be evaluated for adequate calcium and vitamin D intake.
6. Describe the recommended therapeutic approach to the patient or caregiver.	"A nutrient-rich diet, as described, has been shown to be beneficial in the prevention of many diseases, including hypertension and cancer. You can achieve this diet by (1) adding a fruit or a vegetable to your midday meal or as a snack, (2) choosing whole-grain breads and cereals, and (3) looking for healthy frozen meals and soups as opposed to those with much hidden fat and salt. It would be reasonable to continue a daily multivitamin/multimineral supplement to ensure you are meeting daily nutritional needs; however, it would be best to change to an "over 50" product designed for persons over 50 years of age. Your current women's formula contains too much iron for you. If you are not regularly consuming dairy products, calcium and vitamin D supplementation is recommended. Check your intake from supplemented products, such as some orange juice brands, and the multivitamin as well."
7. Explain to the patient or caregiver the rationale for selecting the recommended therapeutic approach from the considered therapeutic alternatives.	"There is no evidence that vitamin supplements, in the absence of deficiency, can completely reduce cancer risk. When selecting a multivitamin, be sure to compare the level of supplementation of each nutrient, including calcium and vitamin D, with its DRI. Additional supplementation in excess of the DRI is often unnecessary unless specifically recommended by your primary care provider or other health care provider."
Implement	
8. When recommending self-care with nonprescription medications and/or nondrug therapy, convey accurate information to the patient or caregiver.	
a. Appropriate dose and frequency of administration	"Consider one USP-approved senior multivitamin/multimineral supplement daily that contains no more than 100% of DRI for nutrients."
b. Maximum number of days the therapy should be employed	n/a
c. Product administration procedures	"You may take your multivitamin with your current medications in the morning. However, check with your pharmacist about taking your vitamin with any newly prescribed medications."

CASE 23-1 *continued*

Relevant Evaluation Criteria	Scenario/Model Outcome
Solicit follow-up questions from the patient or caregiver.	"What about antioxidant vitamins? Do they prevent cancer?"
Answer the patient's or caregiver's questions.	"Data from well-designed trials do not support antioxidant supplementation for the prevention or treatment of cancer. In fact, some trials have suggested potential harm is associated with supplementation of vitamins A, E, and C, selenium, and other nutrients in relation to cancer risk. Therefore, dosing of these nutrients above the DRI cannot be recommended at this time."
Follow-up: Monitor and Evaluate	
9. Assess patient outcome.	Enquire about patient's compliance with multivitamin recommendations and dietary modification. If necessary, reinforce the recommendations.

Key: DRI = Dietary reference intake; n/a = not applicable; UL = upper intake level; USP = United States Pharmacopeia.

CASE 23-2

Relevant Evaluation Criteria	Scenario/Model Outcome
Collect	
1. Gather essential information about the patient's symptoms and medical history, including	
a. Description of symptom(s) (i.e., nature, onset, duration, severity, associated symptoms)	Patient approaches the pharmacy counter seeking a recommendation. She reports her friend recently fell and "broke her hip." She wants to start a calcium/vitamin D supplement because she read that such supplements can reduce fracture risk.
b. Description of any factors that seem to precipitate, exacerbate, and/or relieve the patient's symptom(s)	n/a
c. Description of the patient's efforts to relieve the symptoms	n/a
d. Patient's identity	Irene Allen
e. Patient's age, gender, height, and weight	68 years old, female, 5 ft 1 in., 95 lb
f. Patient's occupation	Financial records clerk
g. Patient's dietary habits	Eggs, juice, and tea with milk for breakfast; soup or a sandwich for lunch; easy-to-prepare microwavable meals for dinner
h. Patient's sleep habits	n/a
i. Concurrent medical conditions, prescription and nonprescription medications, and dietary supplements	Patient suffers from high blood pressure, varicose veins, heartburn, and insomnia. Each morning, Mrs. Allen takes enalapril 2.5 mg. At bedtime, she takes zolpidem 5 mg as needed. She takes omeprazole 20 mg (nonprescription) with lunch on most work days but often skips it on the weekend.
j. Allergies	NKA
k. History of other adverse reactions to medications	Family history of glaucoma and osteoporosis
Assess	
2. Differentiate patient's signs/symptoms, and correctly identify the patient's primary problem(s).	According to recent warnings, use of chronic acid suppressive medications can reduce dietary calcium uptake and potentially increase fracture risk. Furthermore, given Mrs. Allen's family history of osteoporosis and small size, she may warrant further medical evaluation.
3. Identify exclusions for self-treatment.	None

CASE 23-2 *continued*

Relevant Evaluation Criteria	Scenario/Model Outcome
4. Formulate a comprehensive list of therapeutic alternatives for the primary problem to determine whether triage to a medical provider is required, and share this information with the patient or caregiver.	Options include (1) Focus on potential drug–nutrient interactions in counseling about need for calcium supplementation. (2) Discuss the role of balanced nutrition as the ideal route of taking vitamins and minerals. Identify nutritional needs unique to this client and where supplementation may be recommended. (3) Refer Mrs. Allen for medical evaluation and osteoporosis screening. Given her age, body habitus, family history of osteoporosis, and chronic use of acid suppressive therapy, she may be at an increased risk of osteoporosis and bone fracture. (4) Take no action.
Plan	
5. Select an optimal therapeutic alternative to address the patient's problem, taking into account patient preferences.	Assess the client's perceived need for the nutrient supplements. Evaluate dietary intake from food groups, encouraging at least 5 servings of produce, 3 servings of low-fat dairy products, 2 servings of protein, and 6 servings of whole-grain food sources daily.
6. Describe the recommended therapeutic approach to the patient or caregiver.	Discuss the vitamin and mineral content of the various supplements and compare the total intake with each nutrient's DRI. "For a woman of your age, a daily calcium and vitamin D intake of 1200 mg and 800 IU, respectively, is indicated. Speak with a health care provider about your potential risk for osteoporosis and fracture."
7. Explain to the patient or caregiver the rationale for selecting the recommended therapeutic approach from the considered therapeutic alternatives.	"Calcium and vitamin D supplementation alone may not be sufficient intervention to reduce your risk of fracture from a fall if you have underlying osteoporosis. Further, chronic use of omeprazole may further increase this risk and complicate management. Calcium absorption from both dietary and supplement forms may be affected by stomach acid production; suppression of acid with medications such as omeprazole may result in impaired calcium absorption. Alternative forms of calcium are available for supplementation; however, asking your PCP whether continued use of acid suppressive therapy is warranted."
Implement	
8. When recommending self-care with nonprescription medications and/or nondrug therapy, convey accurate information to the patient or caregiver.	Criterion does not apply in this case.
Follow-up: Monitor and Evaluate	
9. Assess patient outcome.	Enquire about the patient's compliance with multivitamin recommendations and dietary modifications. If necessary, reinforce the recommendations

Key: DRI = Dietary reference intake; n/a = not applicable; NKA = no known allergies; PCP = primary care provider.

Patient Counseling for Nutrient Supplementation

The public is often exposed to exaggerated and fraudulent claims concerning vitamin products. The practitioner should keep up with medical and pharmaceutical literature and should not support or appear to support claims until they are substantiated by reliable clinical studies. Patients inquiring about such claims should be educated regarding increased potential risk with nontraditional use of vitamins.

Patients purchasing a nonprescription liquid dietary supplement should be instructed on its proper use and storage, including dilution and preparation techniques. In addition, the practitioner should counsel the patient on possible adverse effects (e.g., diarrhea, constipation).

The box "Patient Education for Nutritional Deficiencies" lists specific information to provide patients. The practitioner could also refer the consumer to websites and printed literature that provide evidence-based recommendations for vitamin and mineral supplementation, such as those listed in the reference section of

PATIENT EDUCATION FOR
Nutritional Deficiencies

The objective of self-treatment is to prevent nutritional deficiencies or to maintain present nutritional status. For most patients, carefully following product instructions and the self-care measures listed here will help ensure optimal therapeutic outcomes.

Vitamins, Minerals, and Trace Elements

- To ensure proper nutrition, eat a varied diet as recommended in *MyPlate* (Figure 23–1). Vitamin supplements are not a substitute for a well-balanced diet.
- Carefully read labels on all vitamin and mineral preparations before taking them. Note the quantity of vitamins and minerals required to meet the DRI, or dietary reference intake, values.
- Do not take doses of vitamins and minerals higher than the recommended DRIs. High doses of vitamins or minerals may be dangerous and should not be taken indiscriminately.
- Take vitamin and mineral supplements with meals if you experience gastrointestinal symptoms.
- Women of childbearing age should take 400 mcg of supplemental folic acid in addition to a well-balanced diet. This has been shown to reduce the risk of neural tube defects in the fetus.
- Be aware that iron supplements or vitamins with iron may turn the stool black. This occurrence is not a cause for alarm, unless it is associated with other symptoms consistent with a gastrointestinal bleed.
- As with any medicine, store vitamin and combination vitamin/mineral supplements out of the reach of children, especially if the product contains iron. Teach children that vitamins are drugs and potential poisons and therefore cannot be taken indiscriminately.
- Be aware that therapeutic use of niacin-containing products (but not niacinamide) may cause a flushing, itching, or tingling sensation, which should decrease in intensity with continued therapy. Taking an aspirin or nonsteroidal anti-inflammatory drug 30–60 minutes before taking niacin may help decrease these effects.
- Do not self-medicate if you suspect a vitamin deficiency; consult a health care practitioner instead.

this chapter. Referral to a registered dietitian (RD) or registered dietitian nutritionist (RDN) should be considered for patients with evidence of nutritional deficiencies.

Evaluation of Patient Outcomes for Nutritional Adequacy

Nutritional therapy should involve a diet that is based on *MyPlate* and possibly the use of nutritional supplements. The practitioner should advise patients to return 30 days after implementing nutritional therapy (or sooner if symptoms worsen). Patients whose symptoms have worsened should be referred to a primary care provider. Patients whose symptoms have improved while taking nutritional supplements should be encouraged to eat a healthful diet and not to rely on supplements as the primary source for vitamins and minerals.

Key Points for Nutritional Adequacy

- The benefits of a varied, balanced diet in terms of health maintenance and disease prevention have been demonstrated repeatedly. However, the same benefits have not been observed when suboptimal dietary intake is augmented with vitamin and mineral supplementation.
- Practitioners can assess the variety of a patient's food choices by comparing the patient's typical food pattern to that recommended in *MyPlate*. The practitioner may refer patients to a an RD or RDN for personalized and more complete counseling on diet modification and nutritional supplementation.
- Overt vitamin or mineral deficiencies are rare in this country; however, subclinical deficiencies may be contributing to chronic disease.
- The need, if any, for vitamin, mineral, or multivitamin/multimineral supplementation should be based on the practitioner's assessment of the patient's dietary intake, metabolic requirements, absorptive capability, and potential drug–micronutrient interactions. However, supplementation should rarely exceed 100% of the DRI. Clinical trials continue to reveal unanticipated health risks with megadoses of various micronutrients.

REFERENCES

1. National Institutes of Health, Office of Dietary Supplements. Dietary supplement fact sheet: multivitamin/multimineral supplements. Available at: https://ods.od.nih.gov/factsheets/MVMS-HealthProfessional/#en3. Accessed May 1, 2017.
2. Gahche J, Bailey R, Burt V, et al. Dietary supplement use among U.S. adults has increased since NHANES III (1988–1994). *NCHS Data Brief.* 2011(61);61:1–8. PMID: 21592424.
3. Bailey RL, Gahche JJ, Lentino CV, et al. Dietary supplement use in the United States, 2003–2006. *J Nutr.* 2011;141(2):261–6. doi: 10.3945/jn.110.133025.
4. Bailey RL, Gahche JJ, Miller PE, et al. Why US adults use dietary supplements. *JAMA Intern Med.* 2013;173:355–61. doi: 10.1001/jamainternmed.2013.2299.
5. Troppmann L, Gray-Donald K, Johns T. Supplement use: is there any nutritional benefit? *J Am Diet Assoc.* 2002;102(6):818–25. PMID: 12067048.
6. Martínez ME, Jacobs ET, Baron JA, et al. Dietary supplements and cancer prevention: balancing potential benefits against proven harms. *J Natl Cancer Inst.* 2012;104(10):732–9. doi: 10.1093/jnci/djs195.
7. U.S. Preventive Services Task Force. *Routine Vitamin Supplementation to Prevent Cancer and CVD: Preventive Medication.* Rockville, MD: Agency for Healthcare Research and Quality; February 2014. Available at: http://www.uspreventiveservicestaskforce.org/uspstf/uspsvita.htm. Accessed May 1, 2017.
8. Coates PM, Dwyer JT, Thurn AL. Introduction to State-of-the-Science Conference: multivitamin/mineral supplements and chronic disease prevention. *Am J Clin Nutr.* 2007;85(1):255S–6S.
9. Ward E. Addressing nutritional gaps with multivitamin and mineral supplements. *Nutr J.* 2014;13:72. doi: 10.1186/1475-13-72.
10. Wells JL, Dumbrell AC. Nutrition and aging: assessment and treatment of compromised nutritional status in frail elderly patients. *Clin Intervent Aging.* 2006;1(1):67–79. PMCID: PMC2682454.
11. Yetley EA. Multivitamin and multimineral dietary supplements: definitions, characterization, bioavailability, and drug interactions. *Am J Clin Nutr.* 2007;85(Suppl):269S–76S.
12. U.S. Pharmacopeial Convention. USP verified dietary supplements. Available at: http://www.quality-supplements.org/verified-products/verified-products-listings. Accessed May 1, 2017.

13. U.S. Department of Health and Human Services and U.S. Department of Agriculture. *Dietary Guidelines for Americans 2015–2020.* 8th ed. December 2015. Available at: http://health.gov/dietaryguidelines/2015/guidelines/. Accessed May 1, 2017.
14. National Agricultural Library, United States Department of Agriculture. DRI tables and application reports. Available at: https://www.nal.usda.gov/fnic/dri-tables-and-application-reports. Accessed May 1, 2017.
15. Institute of Medicine of the National Academies. Dietary reference intakes for calcium and vitamin D. Available at: https://www.nap.edu/catalog/13050/dietary-reference-intakes-for-calcium-and-vitamin-d. Accessed May 1, 2017.
16. U.S. Food and Drug Administration, Guidance for industry: a food labeling guide. Available at: http://www.fda.gov/Food/GuidanceRegulation/GuidanceDocumentsRegulatoryInformation/LabelingNutrition/ucm064928.htm. Accessed May 1, 2017.
17. Centers for Disease Control and Prevention, National Center for Environmental Health, Division of Laboratory Sciences. Second National Report on Biochemical Indicators of Diet and Nutrition in the U.S. population, 2012. Available at: http://www.cdc.gov/nutritionreport/. Accessed May 1, 2017.
18. World Health Organization. Nutrition. Micronutrient deficiencies: vitamin A deficiency. Available at: http://www.who.int/nutrition/topics/vad/en/. Accessed May 1, 2017.
19. DRUGDEX® System (electronic version). Truven Health Analytics, Ann Arbor, Michigan, USA. Available at: http://www.micromedexsolutions.com/. Accessed May 1, 2017.
20. Feskanich D, Singh V, Willett W, et al. Vitamin A intake and hip fractures among postmenopausal women. *JAMA.* 2002;287(1):47–54. PMID: 11754708.
21. The Alpha-Tocopherol, Beta Carotene Cancer Prevention Study Group. The effect of vitamin E and beta carotene on the incidence of lung cancer and other cancers in male smokers. *N Engl J Med.* 1994;330(15):1029–35. doi:10.1056/NEJM199404143301501.
22. Goodman GE, Thornquist MD, Balmes J, et al. The Beta-Carotene and Retinol Efficacy Trial: incidence of lung cancer and cardiovascular disease mortality during 6-year follow-up after stopping beta-carotene and retinol supplements. *J Natl Cancer Inst.* 2004;96(23):1743–50. doi:10.1093/jnci/djh320.
23. Avenell A, Gillespie WJ, Gillespie LD, et al. Vitamin D and vitamin D analogues for preventing fractures associated with involutional and post-menopausal osteoporosis. *Cochrane Database System Rev.* 2009;2:CD000227. doi: 10.1002/14651858.CD000227.pub3.
24. Fosnight S, Zafirau W, Hazelett S. Vitamin D supplementation to prevent falls in the elderly: evidence and practical considerations. *Pharmacotherapy.* 2008;28(2):225–34. doi: 10.1592/phco.28.2.225.
25. Thacher TD, Clarke BL. Vitamin D insufficiency. *Mayo Clin Proc.* 2011; 86(1):50–60. doi: 10.4065/mcp.2010.0567.
26. Vacek JL, Vanga SR, Good M, et al. Vitamin D deficiency and supplementation and relation to cardiovascular health. *Am J Cardiol.* 2012;109(3): 359–63. doi: 10.1016/j.amjcard.2011.09.020.
27. Gotsman I, Shauer A, Zwas DR, et al. Vitamin D deficiency is a predictor of reduced survival in patients with heart failure; vitamin D supplementation improves outcomes. *Eur J Heart Fail.* 2012;14(4):357–66. doi: 10.1093/eurjhf/hfr175.
28. Toner C, Davis C, Milner J. The vitamin D and cancer conundrum: aiming at a moving target. *J Am Diet Assoc.* 2010;110:1492–500. doi: 10.1016/j.jada.2010.07.007.
29. Lee IM, Cook NR, Gaziano JM, et al. Vitamin E in the primary prevention of cardiovascular disease and cancer: the Women's Health Study: a randomized controlled trial. *JAMA.* 2005;294:56–65. doi:10.1001/jama.294.1.56.
30. Issac MG, Quinn R, Tabet N. Vitamin E for Alzheimer's disease and mild cognitive impairment. *Cochrane Database Syst Rev.* 2008;3:CD002854. doi: 10.1002/14651858.CD002854.pub3.
31. Schurks M, Glynn RJ, Rist PM, et al. Effects of vitamin E on stroke subtypes: meta-analysis of randomized controlled trials. *BMJ.* 2010;341:c5702. doi: 10.1136/bmj.c5702.
32. Bjelakovic G, Nikolova D, Gluud LL, et al. Antioxidant supplements for prevention of mortality in healthy participants and patients with various diseases. *Cochrane Database Syst Rev.* 2008;2:CD007176. doi: 10.1002/14651858.CD007176. Available at: http://www.thecochranelibrary.com/view/0/index.html.
33. Xu H, Perez-Cuevas R, Xiong X, et al. An international trial of antioxidants in the prevention of preeclampsia (INTAPP). *Am J Obstet Gynecol.* 2010;202(3):239.e1–10. doi: 10.1016/j.ajog.2010.01.050.
34. Pearson DA. Bone health and osteoporosis: the role of vitamin K and potential antagonism by anticoagulants. *Nutr Clin Pract.* 2007;22(5):517–44. PMID:17906277.
35. National Academies Press. The B Vitamins and Choline: Overview and Methods. In: Dietary References Intakes for Thiamin, Riboflavin, Niacin, Vitamin B6, Folate, Vitamin B 12, Pantothenic Acid, Biotin, and Choline. Available at: https://fnic.nal.usda.gov/sites/fnic.nal.usda.gov/files/uploads/27-40_150.pdf. Accessed May 1, 2017.
36. Lykkesfelt J, Poulsen HE. Is vitamin C supplementation beneficial? Lessons learned from randomized controlled trials. *Br J Nutr.* 2010; 103(9):1251–9. doi: 10.1017/S0007114509993229.
37. Jacob RA, Sotoudeh G. Vitamin C function and status in chronic disease. *Nutr Clin Care.* 2002;5(2):47–9. PMID:12134712.
38. Clarke R, Halsey J, Lewington S, et al. Effects of lowering homocysteine levels with B vitamins on cardiovascular disease, cancer, and cause-specific mortality: meta-analysis of 8 randomized trials involving 37,485 individuals. *Arch Intern Med.* 2010;170(18):1622–31. doi: 10.1001/archinternmed.2010.348.
39. Dharmarajan TS, Adiga GU, Norkus EP. Vitamin B12 deficiency: recognizing subtle symptoms in older adults. *Geriatrics.* 2003;58(3):30–8. PMID:12650116.
40. de Jager J, Kooy A, Lehert P, et al. Long term treatment with metformin in patients with type 2 diabetes and risk of vitamin B-12 deficiency: randomized placebo controlled trial. *BMJ.* 2010;340:c2181. doi: 10.1136/bmj.c2181.
41. Fuhrman MP. Identifying your patient's risk for a vitamin deficiency. *Nutr Clin Pract.* 2001;16:S8–11.
42. Greenberg JA, Bell SJ, Guan Y, et al. Folic acid supplementation and pregnancy: more than just neural tube defect prevention. *Rev Obstet Gynecol.* 2011;4(2):52–9. PMCID: PMC3218540.
43. Greenberg JA, Bell SJ. Multivitamin supplementation during pregnancy: emphasis on folic acid and L-methylfolate. *Rev Obstet Gynecol.* 2011;4(3/4):126–7. PMCID: PMC3250974.
44. Whitehead AS, Gallagher P, Mills JL. A genetic defect in 5,10 methylenetetrahydrofolate reductase in neural tube defects. *QJM.* 1995;88(11): 763–6. PMID: 8542260.
45. Bender DA. Non-nutritional uses of vitamin B6. *Br J Nutr.* 1999;81(1): 7–20. PMID: 10341670.
46. Suter PM, Vetter W. Diuretics and vitamin B1: are diuretics a risk factor for thiamin malnutrition? *Nutr Rev.* 2001;58:319–23. PMID: 11127971.
47. Straub DA. Calcium supplementation in clinical practice: a review of forms, doses, and indications. *Nutr Clin Prac.* 2007;22(3):286–96. PMID: 17507729.
48. U.S. Preventive Health Task Force, Understanding Task Force Recommendations: Vitamin D and Calcium Supplementation to Prevent Fractures. Available at: http://www.uspreventiveservicestaskforce.org/uspstf12/vitamind/vitdfact.pdf. Accessed May 1, 2017.
49. Xiao Q, Murphy RA, Houston DK, et al. Dietary and supplemental calcium intake and cardiovascular disease mortality: The National Institutes of Health-AARP Diet and Health Study. *JAMA.* 2013;173(8):639–46. doi: 10.1001/jamainternmed.2013.3283.
50. Prentice RL, Pettinger MB, Jackson RD, et al. Health risks and benefits from calcium and vitamin D supplementation: Women's Health Initiative clinical trial and cohort study. *Osteoporos Int.* 2013;24(5):567–80. doi: 10.1007/s00198-012-2224-2.
51. U.S. Department of Health and Human Services, Agency for Healthcare and Research Quality. Vitamin D and calcium: systematic review of health outcomes. Available at: https://www.ahrq.gov/downloads/pub/evidence/pdf/vitadcal/vitadcal.pdf. Accessed May 1, 2017.
52. National Institutes of Health, Office of Dietary Supplements. Dietary supplement fact sheet: iron. Available at: https://ods.od.nih.gov/factsheets/Iron-HealthProfessional/. Accessed May 1, 2017.
53. Centers for Disease Control and Prevention. FAQs for dental fluorosis. Available at: http://www.cdc.gov/fluoridation/safety/dental_fluorosis.htm. Accessed May 1, 2017.
54. Singh M, Das RR. Zinc for the common cold. *Cochrane Database Syst Rev.* 2011;2:CD001364. doi: 10.1002/14651858.

CHAPTER 24

FUNCTIONAL AND MEAL REPLACEMENT FOODS

CAROL J. ROLLINS

Foods serve many purposes in our lives. Foremost is their role in survival: foods provide us with sustenance to maintain metabolism and be physically active. Scientific research suggests that foods also affect health and wellness, and consumers are aware of these findings. In a 2013 survey of 1005 adults selected to reflect the American population, 90% believed health benefits other than basic nutrition are associated with certain foods.[1] Americans also report making changes to improve the healthfulness of their diet, including making an effort to eat more fruits and vegetables (87%) and more foods that contain whole grains (75%).[2] Decisions about purchasing foods and beverages are influenced by healthfulness (61%) slightly more than convenience (53%). The perception of healthfulness depends on a number of factors, including nutrition knowledge, claims or information about health benefits of a food, attitudes and beliefs regarding health and susceptibility to disease, and trust of the information source.[3] Regardless of other influences, taste (87%) continues to dominate purchasing decisions, followed by price (73%).[2] Lack of time to plan and prepare meals leads health-conscious consumers to seek convenient methods to optimize nutrition for wellness and health promotion, including fast yet healthy alternatives to traditional "sit-down" meals. In addition, more individuals who have conditions or impairments that affect their ability to obtain adequate nutrients through a regular diet are living independently, and they may seek convenient methods to supplement or replace conventional meals.

Although dietitians are the recognized food and nutrition experts, all health care providers (HCPs) should be aware of the role that foods may play in an overall plan to improve or maintain health, especially foods that have benefits beyond their basic nutrients or that help patients reach nutrient goals when healthy meals are not readily available or cannot be ingested. (See Chapter 23 for discussion of basic nutrition.) This chapter provides an introduction to foods used for their potential health benefits (*functional foods*), as well as foods intended to replace regular meals (*meal replacement foods*).

Drugs, Dietary Supplements, and Foods

The Food and Drug Administration (FDA) is charged with regulating drugs, dietary supplements, and foods (see Chapter 4). *Foods* are substances used "primarily for taste, aroma, or nutritive value."[4] Specific FDA regulations pertain to food safety and labeling. FDA requires that all regulated foods provide assurance in advance (premarket) that ingredients are safe and that claims are substantiated, truthful, and not misleading. Particular forms or uses of foods, such as infant formulas (see Chapter 26) and medical foods, are required to meet additional criteria to ensure the safety of somewhat vulnerable groups.

FUNCTIONAL FOODS

As defined by FDA, functional foods (FF) blur the distinction between drugs and foods, much as dietary supplements did until 1994 when the Dietary Supplement Health and Education Act (DSHEA) established a distinct regulatory scheme for dietary supplements.[4] The term *functional food* is not officially sanctioned by FDA, and there is no legal definition or regulatory category for FF. A specific FF may be regulated as a drug or in one of several subcategories of food depending on its intended use and labeling.[4,5] This lack of validation of products makes it difficult to determine sales figures and market estimates; however, the global market for FF was estimated at $50 billion annually a few years ago.[6] Projections of annual growth in FF vary widely, from 5% to 30% depending on country and product type.[6] Contemporary U.S. health care reforms that mandate preventive care and the field of nutrition economics will likely fuel the growth of FF as their role in dietary recommendations and public health policy, including as a primary care option, increases.[7]

HCPs should be familiar with FF to fully evaluate their patients' diets in relation to preventive and proactive lifestyle changes that modify risks for chronic diseases. In addition, as a trusted source of information, HCPs may influence a patient's acceptance of foods with health benefits.[3] Unfortunately, making evidence-based decisions related to the use of FF can be difficult, because few randomized controlled trials have been conducted, and because for many studies, only a small number of subjects are enrolled. Epidemiologic studies generally rely on people recalling their food intake, which obscures true associations between selected food components and disease risk. If researchers are to translate the epidemiology of dietary patterns into clinical interventions, they need a detailed look at specific diets from certain geographic regions that have low and very low incidence of the major chronic diseases, along with detailed quantification and qualification of dietary phytochemical content.[8] Interactions between dietary components must also be considered as contributing to beneficial effects of specific foods and dietary patterns.[9] Other factors to consider include the use of biomarkers and the nutrigenomic and epigenomic effects of dietary phytochemicals in whole foods as bioactive food components in individuals.[10] The large number of compounds that can arise from a basic chemical structure (e.g., a flavonoid) to produce distinctive effects further complicates the task of identifying active compounds within foods, because a specific food within a given category (e.g., citrus) may not lead to the same outcome relative to health or disease mitigation.[11] This daunting complexity makes it challenging to design and conduct clinical trials aimed at prevention of disease. Isolating the food component and administering it as a dietary supplement rather than as an FF, as is done in many clinical studies, simplifies study design and reduces interactions among food components. Unfortunately, available data do not support this approach, because multiple-constituent dietary phytochemicals in the matrix of plant-based whole foods appear to be safer and more effective than single and multiple constituent high-dose dietary supplements.[9,12–14] Associations between FF or bioactive food components and health maintenance or disease prevention usually show an RR (relative risk) of <2.[15] In a traditional medical toxicology model, in which exposures are generally large doses of a single component, an RR <2 is considered weak. In contrast, nutritional exposures are broad based and occur in small doses of multiple-component mixtures within whole foods over a prolonged time. An RR of 1.5 should be ranked as "strong" for such exposures. Given the limitations of available data and the potential for complex interactions between FF and bioactive food components, lifestyle factors, and genetics, the evaluation of FF requires examination of the totality of evidence, including that from biological models and multiple types of research (preclinical, epidemiologic, clinical, translational).[15] Dietary phytochemical patterns in whole foods and functional dietary patterns have become leading areas for FF science and functional nutrition in current research programs; these patterns will become more important in future research as understanding of these areas evolve.[14,15] To compare results or combine results for analysis, researchers must include preparation methods and sources of FF (whole food, isolated component, dietary supplement) in study reports.

"Health benefits beyond those of basic nutrition" is a broad definition of *FF*, encompassing unmodified whole foods (fruits, vegetables, whole-grain products) and designer foods such as purple carrots.[4,5] A somewhat narrower definition used by the International Life Sciences Institute restricts *FF* to "unmodified foods with naturally occurring bioactive components."[5] Examples include tomatoes, for their lycopene content, and soybeans, which provide isoflavones. The Institute of Medicine (IOM) Food and Nutrition Board restricts the definition of *FF* to "those foods in which the concentration of one or more ingredients has been altered to enhance the food's contribution to a healthful diet."[4,5] This definition includes foods enriched or fortified with nutrients, phytochemicals, or botanical products, including foods such as orange juice with added calcium. Elements isolated from nontraditional food sources and added to traditional foods, such as stanol esters added to margarine-type spreads, also fit this definition of FF. From the viewpoint in current biomedical paradigms, plant-based foods are considered functional because of the synergy in dietary phytochemicals.[7,14]

Categories of Foods Classified as Functional Foods

FF typically fit into one of five categories on the basis of statutory definitions and regulatory guidelines for health claims on food labels:

1. Foods associated with health claims recognized by FDA
2. Foods that carry structure or function claims
3. Foods for special dietary use
4. Medical foods
5. Certain conventional foods

HCPs should have a basic understanding of these categories, because the need for medical supervision varies by category. All labeling claims require prior approval by FDA; however, the required level of supporting science varies depending on the category under which FF are marketed (i.e., greater supporting science is required for medical foods than for structure–function claims).

Foods With Health Claims

Health claims characterize the relationship between a substance (food, food component, dietary ingredient, dietary supplement) and a disease or health-related condition.[4,5,16] (See Chapters 50 and 51 for discussion of dietary supplements.) Only claims about reduction of disease risk are allowed; no claim about "diagnosis, cure, mitigation, or treatment of disease" can be made. Three types of health claims can be made for conventional foods: authorized, authoritative, and qualified. Each type of claim is associated with specific levels of supportive data and specified labeling criteria. *Authorized* health claims require publication of an FDA regulation after an extensive review of the scientific literature, along with significant scientific agreement that the food/nutrient and disease relationship is well established. Of the health claims allowed for foods, authorized claims undergo the most thorough FDA review. The exact wording of the claim statement is not specified, but the statement appearing on the food label must meet specific criteria.

Statements for authorized health claims cannot quantify the degree of risk reduction, and either the term *may* or *might* must be used to qualify the relationship between a food or dietary component and a disease. The label must state that the disease or health-related condition depends on many factors, implying that diet is not the only consideration in disease management. It also must indicate that the benefit related to a disease or health-related condition is part of a total dietary pattern; thus, the need for an overall healthy diet is reinforced. No health claims are permitted for foods containing more than 13 g of fat, 4 g of saturated fat, 60 mg of cholesterol, or 480 mg of sodium per reference amount customarily consumed (RACC); up to double these amounts are allowed for main dishes and meal products.[16,17] The *RACC* is typically 1 serving as defined on the product label. Health claims cannot be indicated for children younger than 2 years. Table 24–1 lists authorized health claims, requirements for foods listing these health claims, and sample statements that might be used on a food label.[4,5,16,17]

The manufacturer can make certain health claims for foods, food components, or dietary ingredients (but not dietary supplements) by notifying FDA after the agency receives a statement from an authoritative scientific body of the U.S. government that has responsibility to protect public health or to conduct research related to human nutrition; this type of health claim is called an

TABLE 24-1 **Authorized and Authoritative Health Claims**

Health Claim	Requirements for Foods	Sample Claim Statement Containing Required Components	Selected Foods Meeting Claim Requirements
Authorized Health Claims			
Calcium—osteoporosis [Calcium and vitamin D—osteoporosis]	High in calcium [high in calcium and vitamin D] Bioavailable Phosphorus content no more than calcium content	Adequate calcium throughout life, as part of a well-balanced diet, may reduce the risk of osteoporosis. Adequate calcium and vitamin D, as part of a well-balanced diet along with physical activity, may reduce the risk of osteoporosis.	Milk Orange juice with added calcium
Sodium—hypertension	Low sodium	Diets low in sodium may reduce the risk of high blood pressure, a disease associated with many factors.	Fruits and vegetables, canned or frozen with no added salt, fresh
Dietary fat—cancer	Low fat "Extra lean" fish and game meat	Development of cancer depends on many factors. A diet low in total fat may reduce the risk of some cancers. (Cannot specify types of fats or fatty acids that may be related to risk of cancer.)	Fruits and vegetables, fresh, frozen, or canned Most cereals Nonfat and low-fat milk and dairy products
Dietary saturated fat and cholesterol—risk of coronary heart disease	Low saturated fat Low cholesterol Low fat "Extra lean" fish and game meat	While many factors affect heart disease, diets low in saturated fat and cholesterol may reduce the risk of this disease.	Fruits and vegetables, fresh, frozen, or canned Most cereals Nonfat and low-fat milk and dairy products
Fiber-containing grain products, fruits, and vegetables—cancer	Grain product, fruit, or vegetable containing dietary fiber Low fat Good source of dietary fiber without fortification	Low-fat diets rich in fiber-containing grain products, fruits, and vegetables may reduce the risk of some types of cancer, a disease associated with many factors. (Cannot specify types of dietary fiber that may be related to risk of cancer.)	Fruits and vegetables, fresh, frozen, or canned Whole-grain breads, cereals, and pasta Brown rice
Fruits, vegetables, and grain products that contain fiber, particularly soluble fiber—risk of coronary heart disease	Fruit, vegetable, or grain product containing fiber Low saturated fat Low cholesterol Low fat Minimum of 0.6 g soluble fiber per RACC without fortification Soluble fiber content provided on the label	Diets low in saturated fat and cholesterol and rich in fruits, vegetables, and grain products that contain some types of dietary fiber, particularly soluble fiber, may reduce the risk of heart disease, a disease associated with many factors.	Fruits and vegetables, fresh, frozen, or canned Whole-grain breads, cereals, and pasta Brown rice
Fruits and vegetables—cancer	Fruit or vegetable Low fat Good source of vitamin A or C, or dietary fiber without fortification	Low-fat diets rich in fruits and vegetables (foods that are low in fat and may contain dietary fiber, vitamin A, or vitamin C) may reduce the risk of some types of cancer, a disease associated with many factors. [X food is high in vitamin A, vitamin C, and/or is a good source of fiber.]	Broccoli Berries Green beans Carrots Cantaloupe Citrus fruits Most dark green leafy vegetables
Folate—neural tube defects	Contains at least 40 mcg folate per serving Foods in conventional form that are a good source without fortification Contains not more than the RDI for vitamin A as retinol, or preformed vitamin A or D Amount of folate must be in the nutrition label	Healthful diets with adequate folate may reduce a woman's risk of having a child with a brain or spinal cord defect.	Most dark green leafy vegetables (see Chapter 23)

(continued)

TABLE 24-1 **Authorized and Authoritative Health Claims** *(continued)*

Health Claim	Requirements for Foods	Sample Claim Statement Containing Required Components	Selected Foods Meeting Claim Requirements
Dietary noncarcinogenic carbohydrate sweeteners—dental caries	Sugar-free Eligible substances listed in 21 CFR 101.80; examples include xylitol, sorbitol, mannitol, maltitol, isomalt, isomalulose, lactol, hydrogenated starch hydrolysates, hydrogenated glucose syrups, erythritol, d-tagatose, and sucralose Does not lower plaque pH below 5.7 when fermentable carbohydrate is present	Frequent between-meal consumption of foods high in sugars and starches promotes tooth decay. The sugar alcohols in [name of food] do not promote tooth decay. Short claim for small packages: Does not promote tooth decay.	Many "dietetic" sugar-free products marketed for people with diabetes Many low-calorie products marketed for weight loss
Soluble fiber from certain foods—risk of coronary heart disease	Low saturated fat Low cholesterol Low fat Includes one or more: (1) an eligible source of whole oat or barley with ≥0.75 g soluble fiber per RACC, (2) Oatrim containing ≥0.75 g beta-glucan per RACC, (3) psyllium husk containing ≥1.7 g soluble fiber per RACC Amount of soluble fiber per RACC must be declared in the nutrition label	Soluble fiber from foods such as [name of soluble fiber source (optional—name of food product)], as part of a diet low in saturated fat and cholesterol, may reduce the risk of heart disease. A serving of [name of food product] supplies [X] grams of the [necessary daily dietary intake for the benefit] soluble fiber from [name of soluble fiber source] necessary per day to have this effect. Foods with a psyllium seed husk health claim must also bear a statement on the label concerning the need to consume adequate fluids and that it should not be taken by those with difficulty swallowing.	Rolled oats, oatmeal Whole oats cold cereals Whole oat flour Oat bran Barley (whole grain, dry milled barley) Cereals with added psyllium
Soy protein—risk of coronary heart disease[a]	Contains ≥6.25 g soy protein per RACC Low saturated fat Low cholesterol Low fat, unless fat is from whole soybeans (no added fat)	Example 1: Foods containing 25 g of soy protein a day, as part of a diet low in saturated fat and cholesterol, may reduce the risk of heart disease. A serving of [name of food] supplies [X] grams of soy protein. Example 2: Diets low in saturated fat and cholesterol that include 25 g of soy protein a day may reduce the risk of heart disease. One serving of [name of food] provides [X] grams of soy protein.	
Plant sterol/stanol esters—risk of coronary heart disease	Spreads and salad dressings must contain ≥0.65 g plant sterol esters per RACC Spreads, salad dressings, and snack bars must contain ≥1.7 g plant stanol esters per RACC Low saturated fat Low cholesterol	Example 1: Foods containing at least 0.65 g per serving of plant sterol esters, eaten twice a day with meals for a total intake of at least 1.3 g, as part of a diet low in saturated fat and cholesterol, may reduce the risk of heart disease. A serving of [name of food] supplies [X] grams of vegetable oil sterol esters. Example 2: Diets low in saturated fat and cholesterol that include 2 servings of foods that provide a daily total of at least 3.4 g of plant [vegetable oil] stanol esters in two meals may reduce the risk of heart disease. A serving of [name of food] supplies [X] grams of plant [vegetable oil] stanol esters. Spreads and salad dressings with > 13 g fat per 50 g of product must include a statement "see nutrition information for fat content."	Margarine spreads with added sterol/stanol esters Orange juice with added sterol/stanol esters Nonfat milk with added sterol/stanol esters

TABLE 24-1 **Authorized and Authoritative Health Claims** *(continued)*

Health Claim	Requirements for Foods	Sample Claim Statement Containing Required Components	Selected Foods Meeting Claim Requirements
Authoritative Health Claims[b]			
Whole-grain foods—risk of heart disease and certain cancers (Docket No. 199P-2209)	Must contain ≥51% whole-grain ingredients by weight per RACC Low fat Must meet specified dietary fiber content: 3 g/RACC of 55 g; 2.8 g/RACC of 50 g; 2.5 g/RACC of 45 g; 1.7 g/RACC of 35 g	Diets rich in whole-grain foods and other plant foods and low in total fat, saturated fat, and cholesterol may reduce the risk of heart disease and some types of cancer.	Low-fat whole-grain breads and cereals Whole-grain cereals and pasta Brown rice
Whole-grain foods with moderate fat content—risk of heart disease (Docket No. 03Q-0547)	Same as above (Docket No. 199P-2209) except "low fat" is omitted	Diets rich in whole-grain foods and other plant foods and low in total fat, saturated fat, and cholesterol may help reduce the risk of heart disease	Moderate-fat whole-grain breads and cereals
Potassium—risk of high blood pressure and stroke (Docket No. 2000Q-1582)	Good source of potassium Low sodium Low total fat Low saturated fat Low cholesterol	Diets containing foods that are a good source of potassium and that are low in sodium may reduce the risk of high blood pressure and stroke.	Many fruits and vegetables (see Chapter 23)
Fluoridated water—reduced risk of dental caries (Docket No. 2006Q-0418)	Total fluoride > 0.6–1 mg/L Bottled water must meet standards of identity and quality (21 CFR 165.110) Excludes bottled water for infants	Drinking fluoridated water may reduce the risk of dental caries [or tooth decay].	Bottled water containing fluoride
Saturated fat, cholesterol, and trans fat—reduced risk of heart disease (Docket No. 2006Q-0458)	Low saturated fat Low cholesterol Quantity of trans fat on label and <0.5 g trans fat per RACC Total fat < 6.5 g	Diets low in saturated fat and cholesterol, and as low as possible in trans fat, may reduce the risk of heart disease.	Fruits and vegetables, fresh, frozen, or canned Most cereals Nonfat and low-fat milk and dairy products
Substitution of saturated fat in the diet with unsaturated fatty acids—reduced risk of heart disease (Docket No. 2007Q-0192)	Low fat Low cholesterol	Replacing saturated fat with similar amounts of unsaturated fats may reduce the risk of heart disease. To achieve this benefit, total daily calories should not increase.	Baked goods using polyunsaturated oils rather than butter or hydrogenated oils

Key: CFR = Code of Federal Regulations; RACC = reference amount customarily consumed (usually 1 serving as listed on label); RDI = recommended dietary intake.

[a] Soy protein content of foods is available from the Agricultural Research Service, U.S. Department of Agriculture (USDA). Nutrient Data Laboratory [database online]. [Search for "standard reference."] Available at: http://www.nal.usda.gov/fnic/foodcomp/search. Accessed July 7, 2017.

[b] Wording in the sample claim statement for authoritative claims is required by the Food and Drug Administration.

Source: References 4 and 16–19.

authoritative claim.[4,16] The National Institutes of Health, the Centers for Disease Control and Prevention, and the National Academy of Sciences are sources for authoritative claims. Significant scientific evidence supports such health claims, although FDA itself does not complete an extensive review of the data. Authoritative health claims currently recognized by the FDA and required wording for the claims statement are listed in Table 24–1.[4,16,17]

The third type of health claim is a qualified claim. *Qualified health claims* are appropriate for use when evidence of health benefits of a food, food component, or dietary supplement is still emerging; scientific research supporting the claim tends to be limited or preliminary; and the "significant scientific agreement" level of evidence required for authorized and authoritative health claims cannot be met. Table 24–2 lists qualified claims and specific "qualifying" terms required by FDA to indicate that evidence for the claim is limited.[4,5,18–20] Labeling guidance issued by FDA for qualified health claims intermixes information regarding labeling of dietary supplements and conventional foods.[18] Chapter 50 provides further discussion of qualified health claims and labeling.

Foods With Structure–Function Claims

Structure–function claims indicate the effect that consuming the product has on a body structure or function. These claims are commonly associated with dietary supplements but can also appear on food labels. Structure–function claims differ from health claims in that FDA validation or authorization is not required before their use; however, prior notification of FDA regarding the claim is required. In addition, structure–function claims cannot make reference regarding reduced risk of disease, because such a reference would place the product under regulation as a drug.[4,5,16,21] For example, a probiotic yogurt marketed as preventing or treating diarrhea is considered a drug; however, if the label instead claims to "improve digestion," it is considered an acceptable structure–function claim. Other examples of structure–function claims include statements that the product builds strong bones, supports the immune system, improves memory, maintains intestinal flora, improves strength, and promotes urinary tract health. Foods carrying a structure–function claim are considered FF; they are not considered dietary supplements when they are represented as a conventional food. For instance, margarine-type spreads with added stanol esters are a food, and the stanol ester is considered a food additive. However, dietary supplements in food form (drinks and bars) that are labeled and marketed as dietary supplements are regulated as dietary supplements (see Chapter 50). Distinguishing FF from dietary supplements therefore can be confusing.

Foods for Special Dietary Use

Foods for special dietary use, as defined by FDA, include foods used to supply particular dietary needs, or to supplement or fortify the usual diet, and are marketed as such; they do not meet general dietary needs (see Chapter 23).[4,16] Particular dietary needs may exist because of physical, physiologic, pathologic, or other conditions, such as disease, convalescence, pregnancy, lactation, underweight, overweight, infancy, or the need for sodium restriction. Foods intended for use as the only nutrient source in the diet and those intended to supplement the diet by increasing total dietary intake of a specific ingredient (vitamin, mineral, other nutrient) are also considered to meet a particular dietary need. These foods are subject to general labeling requirements for foods, and medical supervision of their use is not required. By some definitions, foods for special dietary use are considered FF; however, this approach to marketing FF is seen in the food supply much less frequently than is structure–function labeling.

Medical Foods

Medical foods were first defined in the *Federal Register* in 1973; they were represented by an infant formula for patients with phenylketonuria, which had previously been regulated as a drug.[4] The Orphan Drug Act Amendments of 1988 also define medical foods and require that specific criteria be met before their use and distribution. These foods are to be recommended or prescribed by a physician and used under continued medical supervision; however, many are not prescription-only products in the same manner as prescription drugs, because they can be sold without a physician's written order. Medical foods do not occur naturally; rather, they are specially formulated and processed to meet *distinctive nutritional requirements* of the disease or condition for which they are intended.[4] Distinctive requirements for a select medicinal component in the food (or the food product as a whole) must be established by prior medical evaluation on the basis of recognized scientific principles. HCPs should be able to distinguish between medical foods that require physician supervision and products that can be safely used as "nutritional self-care" by the public. (See the "Medical Foods and Meal Replacement Foods" section of this chapter for further discussion of medical foods.)

Conventional Foods

Conventional foods that do not fit into any of the preceding four categories can also be classified as FF. Research on conventional FF comes from contemporary medical ethnobiology and ethnopharmacy, with the foundation being ethnic or traditional foods associated with health benefits in various cultures and supported by epidemiologic studies. For example, long-standing systems of traditional FF use in Asia are linked epidemiologically to some of the lowest cancer rates in the world and to very low incidence of other chronic diseases.[22,23] The strength of evidence supporting a functional role for such foods is typically weak–moderate, and clinical trials tend to be lacking; therefore, even a qualified health claim often cannot be supported at this time.[5] However, other foods are known to contain specific compounds for which molecular functional nutrition and pharmacology studies have been conducted. Studies of dietary phytochemicals and fish oils have revealed a variety of specific phytochemicals and marine zoochemicals (e.g., EGCG, resveratrol, curcumin, EPA, DHA) that modulate several molecular targets at the same time and can serve collectively as agents for chronic disease prevention and health preservation.[13,24–26] Table 24–3 provides examples of conventional foods and the components likely responsible for their role as FF, and Table 24–4 lists examples of functional components and typical food sources.[5,7,9–11,15,27–30] Figure 24–1 shows the narrowing cascade of knowledge from an extensive array of plants on earth to the few phytochemicals identified as health modifiers; the figure also serves as an indicator of the extensive research needed to fully understand the potential of FF in health.[11–13,23,26,29]

TABLE 24-2 **Qualified Health Claims for Conventional Foods**[a]

Food/Nutrient[b]	Disease/ Condition	Level of Evidence	Comments
Claims Related to Cardiovascular Disease			
Omega-3 fatty acids: EPA and DHA (Docket No. 2003Q-0401, 09/08/2004)	CHD	Supportive but not conclusive research	Total fat, saturated fat, cholesterol, and sodium maximum limits apply. Fish may not exceed 16 g total fat per RACC unless a statement to see nutrition information for total fat content is included with the health claim.
Walnuts (Docket No. 2002P-029, 03/09/2004)	Heart disease	Supportive but not conclusive research	1.5 ounces of whole or chopped walnuts per day
Nuts (Docket No. 2002P-0505, 07/14/2003)	Heart disease	Supportive but not conclusive research	Limited to almonds, hazelnuts, peanuts, pecans, some pine nuts, pistachio nuts, walnuts; 1.5 ounces per day. Nut-containing products must contain >11 g acceptable nuts and <13 g total fat.
Monounsaturated fat from olive oil (Docket No. 2003Q-0559, 11/01/2004)	CHD	Limited and not conclusive evidence	Suggested intake of about 2 tablespoons (23 g) daily; replaces a similar amount of saturated fat and does not increase the total number of calories.
Unsaturated fatty acids from canola oil (Docket No. 2006Q-0091, 10/06/2006)	CHD	Limited and not conclusive evidence	Suggested intake of about 1.5 tablespoons (19 g) daily; replaces a similar amount of saturated fat and does not increase the total number of calories.
Corn oil and corn oil–containing products (Docket No. 2006P-0243, 03/26/2007)	Heart disease	Very limited and preliminary evidence	Suggested intake of about 1 tablespoon (16 g) daily; replaces a similar amount of saturated fat and does not increase the total number of calories.
100% whey-protein partially hydrolyzed infant formula (Docket No. FDA-2009-Q-0301, 05/24/2011)	Atopic dermatitis	Very little to little scientific evidence, uncertain	Healthy infant, not exclusively breastfed, with family history of allergy, fed the formula from birth to 4 months, claim for reduced atopic dermatitis up to 3 years of age
Claims Related to Cancer Risk			
Green tea (Docket No. 2004-Q-0427, 02/24/2011)	Cancer	Highly unlikely to reduce risk, very little scientific evidence	Breast cancer and prostate cancer studies were evaluated.
Tomatoes, tomato sauce (Docket No. 2004-Q-0201, 11/08/2005)	Prostate, ovarian, gastric, and pancreatic cancers	Unlikely, uncertain, or little scientific evidence	Few studies; major study limitations and conflicting results; ½–1 cup per week for prostate cancer; twice weekly for ovarian cancer
Psyllium husk (Docket No. FDA-2013-Q-0167, 06/24/2014)	Diabetes	Very little scientific evidence	Claim for reduced risk of diabetes Psyllium husk must not be present in trivial amounts, although FDA does not specify a minimum amount; psyllium husk must be >95% pure to minimize potential allergenicity.
High-amylose resistant starch	Diabetes	Limited to little scientific evidence	Claim for reduced risk of type 2 diabetes

Key: CHD = Coronary heart disease; DHA = docosahexaenoic acid; EPA = eicosapentaenoic acid.

[a] Includes only claims related to conventional foods.

[b] Docket number is given first and followed by the date of enforcement or discretion letter.

Source: References 4, 5, 16, 18, 20, and 27.

TABLE 24-3 **Examples of Conventional Foods Classified as Functional Foods**

Food	Functional Component	Potential Health Benefit	Comments
Apples	Flavonols, phenols, proanthocyanidins, soluble fiber (pectin)	Decreased risk of certain types of cancer; improved glucose and cholesterol concentrations; may contribute to maintenance of heart health	Recommend one a day but quantity for health benefit is not defined.
Bananas, ripe	Prebiotics, FOS	Decreased hypertension and hypercholesterolemia	Weak evidence exists for 3–10 g/day.
Berries; cherries	Anthocyanidins	Antioxidant functions; may contribute to healthy immune system	Recommend ½–1 cup per day, but amount for health benefit is not defined.
Cinnamon	Proanthocyanidins	May contribute to maintenance of urinary tract and heart health	Weak evidence exists; amount for health benefit is not well researched.
Citrus fruits	Ascorbic acid, zeaxanthin, limonene	Decreased risk of ARMD; decreased cancer risk	Weak–moderate evidence exists for ARMD with 6 mg/day as lutein; rodent studies involved limonene and cancer.
Cocoa, chocolate	Flavonols	Antioxidant functions, decreased risk of coronary heart disease	Dark chocolate appears to be most effective.
Corn	Lutein, zeaxanthin, free stanols/sterols	Decreased risk of ARMD; may decrease risk of CHD	Weak–moderate evidence exists for 6 mg/day as lutein; health claim pertains to stanol/sterol esters added to foods.
Cranberry juice	Proanthocyanidins	Decreased UTI from decreased adherence of bacteria to cell walls; may also prevent adhesion of plaque-forming bacteria in the mouth	Moderate evidence exists for 300 mL/day to decrease UTI (58% reduction in bacteriuria in 150 elderly women in the first randomized controlled trial [1994]).
Cruciferous vegetables: broccoli, brussels sprouts, cauliflower, cabbage	Glucosinolates, indoles, isothiocyanates (sulphoraphane), organosulfur compounds, thiols	Decreased risk of certain types of cancer	Weak–moderate evidence exists for greater than ½ cup/day.
Dairy products, including some cheese	Conjugated linoleic acid	Decreased risk of breast cancer; possible role in improved body composition	Weak evidence exists for breast cancer link; animal studies suggest role in decreased body fat; necessary amount for health effects is not determined.
Dairy products, fermented (acidophilus milk, buttermilk, kefir, yogurt)	Probiotic organisms (lactobacilli, bifidobacteria)	Maintenance of GI tract health; decreased colon cancer risk; decreased cholesterol	See Chapter 20 for discussion of probiotics.
Eggs (yolk)	Lutein, zeaxanthin	Decreased risk of ARMD	Weak–moderate evidence exists for 6 mg/day as lutein.
Eggs, enriched with DHA	DHA	Decreased risk of CHD; increased HDL cholesterol	Chickens are fed fish oils or algae as a source of DHA.
Fatty fish (wild salmon, herring)	Omega-3 fatty acids	Decreased triglycerides and risk of heart disease, including fatal and nonfatal MI	Recommend 2 meals/week containing fatty fish; supportive but not conclusive evidence exists per qualified health claim.
Flax	Phytoestrogens (lignans), alpha-linolenic acid	Decreased risk of CHD by decreasing cholesterol and platelet aggregation; weak estrogenic activity may decrease hormone-related cancers; maintenance of a healthy immune system; alpha-linolenic acid may contribute to maintenance of visual function	Weak evidence exists for CHD association; very weak evidence exists for cancer risk; amounts necessary for health benefit from flax are not defined.

TABLE 24-3 Examples of Conventional Foods Classified as Functional Foods *(continued)*

Food	Functional Component	Potential Health Benefit	Comments
Garlic	Organosulfur compounds, thiols	Decreased total and LDL cholesterol; may decrease the risk of gastric cancer; promotes healthy immune function	Weak–moderate evidence exists for approximately 1 fresh clove daily for cholesterol; epidemiologic evidence for decreased cancer is equivocal; considerable variation exists in the amount of active compounds for available products.
Grapes, red and black	Anthocyanidins, phenolic compounds	Antioxidant functions; decreased CV risk	Epidemiologic evidence suggests inverse association with CV disease risk.
Grape juice	Resveratrol	Decreased risk of MI caused by decreased platelet aggregation	Moderate–strong evidence exists for 8–16 ounces/day.
Greens: spinach, kale, collards	Lutein, zeaxanthin	Decreased risk of ARMD	Weak–moderate evidence exists for 6 mg/day as lutein.
Jerusalem artichoke	Prebiotics, FOS	Decreased hypertension; decreased hypercholesterolemia	Weak evidence exists for 3–10 g/day.
Meat (beef, lamb, turkey) and milk	Conjugated linoleic acid	Antitumor effect proposed; possible role in improved body composition	Suppression of cancer cell growth in rat studies; animal studies suggest role in decreased body fat; necessary amount for health effects is not determined.
Onions, leeks, scallions	Organosulfur compounds, thiols	Decreased total and LDL cholesterol	Weak–moderate evidence exists.
Onion powder	Prebiotics, FOS	Decreased hypertension; decreased hypercholesterolemia	Weak evidence exists for 3–10 g/day.
Rye	Phytoestrogens (lignans)	May contribute to maintenance of heart health and healthy immune system	Amounts necessary for health benefit from rye are not defined.
Tea, black	Polyphenols, flavonoids	Decreased risk of CHD	Evidence is not conclusive.
Tea, green	Catechins (epigallocatechin-3-gallate, epigallocatechin, epicatechin-3-gallate, epicatechin)	Decreased risk of certain types of cancer; improved CV health; weight control	Qualified health claim evaluation concluded it is highly unlikely that green tea (not specifically catechins) reduces risk for cancer; evidence for prevention of CV disease and obesity is weak (intake estimates of >4 cups/day).
Tomatoes and processed tomato products	Lycopene	Antioxidant that efficiently decreases singlet oxygen in biological systems; possible decreased risk of certain cancers (prostate) and MI	Evidence based on inverse associations of tissue lycopene and cancers or MI is weak; qualified health claim evaluation concluded that it is unlikely or uncertain that tomatoes or sauce (not specifically lycopene) reduces risks.
Tree nuts	Monounsaturated fatty acids, vitamin E	Decreased risk of CHD	Moderate evidence exists for 1–2 ounces/day; some nuts have qualified health claim.

Key: ARMD = Age-related macular degeneration; CHD = coronary heart disease; CV = cardiovascular; DHA = docosahexaenoic acid; FOS = fructooligosaccharides; GI = gastrointestinal; HDL = high-density lipoprotein; LDL = low-density lipoprotein; MI = myocardial infarction; UTI = urinary tract infection.

Source: Adapted from references 5, 7, 9–11, 15, and 27–30.

TABLE 24-4 Examples of Functional Flavonoid Components in Conventional Foods

Functional Component (Subclass of Flavonoids)	Dietary Phytochemicals	Food Source	Potential Health Benefit
Anthocyanins	Cyanidin Delphinidin Malvidin	Red, blue, and purple berries and grapes; cherries; potatoes; purple sweet potatoes; blue corn; rhubarb; plums	Augment cellular antioxidant defenses; may contribute to maintenance of brain function
Flavones	Hesperetin Naringenin	Citrus fruits and juices	Neutralize free radicals, which may damage cells; augment cellular antioxidant defenses
Flavonols	Isorhamnetin Kaempferol Myricetin Quercetin	Apples, berries, broccoli, kale, tea, onions (scallions, yellow onions; onions have highest flavonol content)	Neutralize free radicals, which may damage cells; augment cellular antioxidant defenses
Flavanols (monomers)	Catechin Epicatechin Epigallocatechin ECG EGCG	Teas (green and white), chocolate, grapes, berries, apples	May contribute to maintenance of heart health
Flavanols (polymers)	Proanthocyanidins Theaflavins Thearubigins	Teas (oolong and black), chocolate, apples, berries, red grapes	May contribute to maintenance of heart health and urinary tract health

Key: ECG = Epicatechin-3-gallate; EGCG = epigallocatechin-3-gallate.
Source: Adapted from references 4, 5, and 27.

Protective Effects of Functional Foods

Functional Foods and Biomarkers: Epigenomics and Chemoprevention

The disposition of dietary phytochemicals is similar to that of drugs and xenobiotics to the extent that the phytochemicals can be studied with respect to their individual pharmacokinetics and pharmacodynamics.[30] Pharmacokinetic studies suggest that variations in disease risk or preventive efficacy of certain dietary phytochemicals may be at least partially related to genetic polymorphisms in metabolism that result in altered enzyme activity; thus, the same phytochemical may have different pharmacodynamic effects in different individuals. It is unclear if genetic polymorphisms contribute to the beneficial effects associated with fiber, prebiotics, and probiotics, or whether these effects have a great association with changes that alter the environment within the gastrointestinal (GI) tract and thereby affect the types of organisms that thrive in the GI tract. It is possible that phytochemicals, fibers, and prebiotics interact with the genetic polymorphisms or with the genetics, in general, of the probiotic organisms to induce the benefits associated with these FF components. (See Chapter 20 for discussion of probiotics.) Because of such complexities, common biomarkers used to monitor a condition or health risk may be inadequate to establish a link between a phytochemical, fiber, prebiotic, or probiotic and each component's clinical end point. The IOM developed a framework for the qualification of risk biomarkers that recommends evaluation of the relationship between the clinical end point and the risk biomarker as well as evidence that the intervention affecting the risk biomarker is concomitantly linked to the clinical end point.[22,30] Linking biomarkers for health and disease to *epigenomics* (defined as heritable changes in gene expression that occur without a change in DNA sequence)[26] is a major challenge in FF research.[10]

Fiber

Fiber is a component of FF that has been widely studied for associations with potential health benefits. *Fiber* consists of dietary components that humans cannot digest, including plant cell walls; nonstarch polysaccharides from seaweed, microorganisms, or seed husks (psyllium); resistant starches; and nondigestible oligosaccharides.[31] The terms *dietary fiber* and *functional fiber* are related to dietary reference intakes (see Chapter 23) and distinguish between sources of fiber.[31,32] However, because of the heterogenic composition of these substances, dietary fiber has no chemical definition, and until 2016, FDA regulations had no established definition for its use.[33] Based on the IOM definition, *total fiber* is the sum of dietary and functional fiber.[31] In their amendment to food labeling regulations, FDA determined that "total fiber" should be used on food labels, rather than listing dietary fiber and functional fiber separately. *Dietary fiber* is defined by the IOM as "nondigestible carbohydrates and lignin that are naturally occurring (intrinsic and intact) in plants"; FDA added "and insoluble carbohydrates (with 3 or more monomeric units)" to its definition.[31,33] Per the IOM definition, *functional fiber* is defined as "isolated nondigestible carbohydrates that have

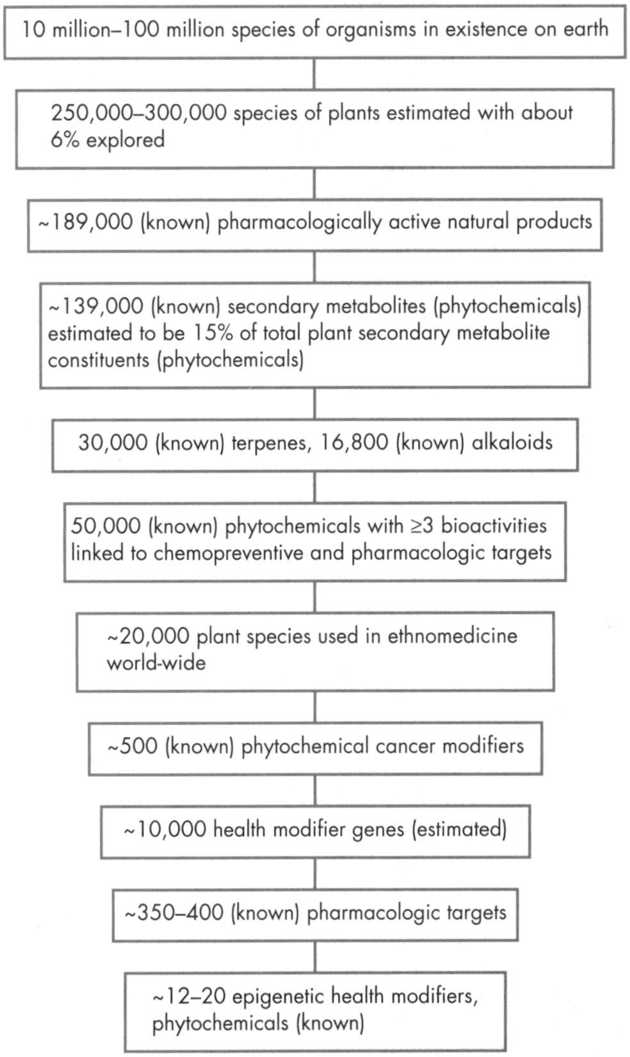
10 million–100 million species of organisms in existence on earth
250,000–300,000 species of plants estimated with about 6% explored
~189,000 (known) pharmacologically active natural products
~139,000 (known) secondary metabolites (phytochemicals) estimated to be 15% of total plant secondary metabolite constituents (phytochemicals)
30,000 (known) terpenes, 16,800 (known) alkaloids
50,000 (known) phytochemicals with ≥3 bioactivities linked to chemopreventive and pharmacologic targets
~20,000 plant species used in ethnomedicine world-wide
~500 (known) phytochemical cancer modifiers
~10,000 health modifier genes (estimated)
~350–400 (known) pharmacologic targets
~12–20 epigenetic health modifiers, phytochemicals (known)

FIGURE 24–1 Cascade of knowledge from plants to phytochemicals to health modifiers. (Source: Adapted from references 13, 23, 26, and 29.)

beneficial physiologic effects in humans, including fiber extracted or modified from plants or animal sources"; FDA also included "synthetic non-digestible carbohydrates (with 3 or more monomeric units)" in the regulation. Through a rigorous science review, FDA identified isolated or synthetic non-digestible carbohydrates that were determined to have health benefits and to meet the agency's new definition of fiber, provided a document with data used to determine fibers that did not meet the new definition, and published draft guidance regarding information that should be submitted for a scientific evaluation to prove other purified or isolated fibers meet the agency's definition of fiber.[34–36]

FDA evaluated the literature for 26 fibers that were determined to not meet the agency's definition of fiber.[35] The final report included background information and various physiologic effects reported for the fibers, such as effects on blood cholesterol, blood glucose, laxation or bowel function, and mineral absorption. Only 7 of these fibers were deemed to meet FDA requirements for fiber and were listed in the Code of Federal Regulation.[34] Two of the fibers, beta-glucan soluble fiber and psyllium husk, already had in place authorized health claims related to the risk of coronary heart disease.[15,16,34] The other recognized fibers included cellulose, guar gum, pectin, locust bean gum, and hydroxypropylmethylcellulose. Numerous products currently considered fiber by many manufacturers were not included in the FDA rule, leading to submission of a large number of comments to the agency and a suggestion that the current guidance on fiber requires major revision.[37] At this time, however, more rigorous research will be required to have such "fibers" added to the list of FDA-recognized fibers. Research should include the effects of extracting fiber from cell walls, because the effects may differ from those of in situ fiber owing to altered chemical and physical properties. Viscosity and fermentability were not included in FDA's definition for fiber, although these factors may have important correlates with health effects.[38,39] The terms *soluble fiber* and *insoluble fiber,* as used here, remain pervasive in both professional and nonprofessional literature, and FDA regulations require listing the number of grams of soluble or insoluble fiber on the nutrition label if a claim for fiber is included on the product.[34]

Recommended and Actual Intake

Adequate intakes (AIs) for total fiber published by IOM range from 21–38 g/day, with amounts for women and older people being lower than those for men and younger people.[32] (See Chapter 23 for general information on AIs.) Values for AIs are based on usual caloric intake in each age group and 14 g of dietary fiber per 1000 calories, which appears to be the amount needed to promote heart health.[31,40] Unfortunately, actual mean fiber intake is only about 15–18 g/day; little progress toward meeting the goals has been made over the past 2 decades.[41–43]

Soluble and Insoluble Fibers

Soluble fibers typically undergo substantial degradation and fermentation in the colon; negligible degradation and fermentation occur with most insoluble fibers. Table 24–5 outlines food components, food sources, and functional fiber sources typically associated with soluble and insoluble fibers. The food sources listed are good to excellent sources of fiber based on tests previously accepted for identifying fiber content[43]; however, not all fibers listed in the table are recognized in the new FDA regulations for nutrient labeling.[17]

Methods of Increasing Fiber Intake

Table 24–6 lists ideas for increasing fiber content in the diet. Caution is advised for the use of fiber-containing products in patients with poor GI motility or underlying GI dysfunction, including narcotic-associated dysmotility. Inadequate fluid intake may also contribute to GI distress from a high-fiber diet. It is advisable to gradually increase fiber, because a sudden increase can cause bloating, gas, and, occasionally, diarrhea. A reasonable approach is to add 1 or 2 servings of foods that are abundant in fiber (Table 24–5) to the diet every few days until the goal for fiber intake is reached. Reading ingredient labels is essential to ensure adequate fiber content, especially for breads and cereals, in which a *whole* grain should be the first ingredient listed.

TABLE 24-5 Components and Sources of Soluble and Insoluble Fiber[a]

	Soluble Fiber	Insoluble Fiber
Food component	Pectins, gums, mucilages, algal substances, some hemicellulose	Cellulose, lignin, most hemicellulose
Food sources with ≥2.5 g of total fiber per serving[b]	Cereals: oat bran (uncooked, ⅔ cup), oatmeal (cooked, 1 cup) Fruits: apples and pears with skin on, oranges (1 medium), figs and prunes (3 small) Vegetables: broccoli, carrots, cauliflower, corn, kale and other greens, dark green or loose leaf lettuce, peas, squash, zucchini (cooked, ¾–1 cup)	Bran and whole-grain (corn, rye, wheat) products: bran cereals (dry cereal, ⅓–1 cup), brown rice (cooked, 1 cup), whole-wheat bread (2 slices) Dried beans: lima, kidney, pinto, white (cooked, ¼–½ cup) Dried peas: green, split (cooked, ¼–½ cup)
Functional fiber sources	Beet fiber, FOS, guar gum (galactomannan, Benefiber), inulin, karaya gum, konjac mannan, locust bean gum, pectin, psyllium (ispaghula seed husk)	Calcium polycarbophil, methylcellulose, powdered cellulose, soy polysaccharide (also has significant soluble fiber effects)

Key: FOS = Fructooligosaccharides.

[a] Not all fibers listed in the table are recognized by the Food and Drug Administration in regulations for nutrient labeling.

[b] Serving size shown in parentheses. The food sources listed are good (2.5–4.9 g of fiber per serving) to excellent (5 g or more of fiber per serving) sources of total dietary fiber and are listed under the heading that exemplifies their predominant health effects.[43]

TABLE 24-6 Methods for Increasing Fiber in the Diet

- Eat breads containing whole-wheat grain, whole-wheat flour, or other whole grains as the first ingredient on the label. These products should replace breads from refined flours that do not include whole grains.
- Replace part of refined-grain (non–whole-grain) cereals with whole-grain cereal for individuals who prefer refined cereals; or mix very high fiber cereals into a favorite brand of cereal.
- Eat oatmeal as a hot breakfast cereal, or select a cold cereal with oats or whole grain as the primary ingredient.
- Sprinkle bran on cereal, yogurt, or other foods.
- Eat brown rice, whole-wheat pasta, and whole-grain crackers rather than white rice and products from refined grains.
- Add fruit to breakfast cereals, breads, yogurt, and salads.
- Select recipes that use whole-grain flours, and/or add rolled oats to baked goods.
- Select recipes for baked goods that include apples, applesauce, carrots, pumpkins, or other fruits or vegetables as a significant ingredient.
- Add kidney, garbanzo, navy, or other beans to salads and soups, including canned soups. Rinse and drain canned beans to reduce components prone to cause intestinal gas.
- Serve fruit and/or vegetable salads with picnic lunches instead of potato chips.
- Serve canned beans (black, kidney, white, baked) as an alternative protein source.
- Eat fresh or dried fruit for snacks and desserts; frozen and canned fruits can also be used.
- Use a low-fat refried bean dip or hummus with whole-wheat baked tortilla chips for snacks.
- Eat fruits and vegetables, including potatoes, with the skin on.
- Select snack or meal replacement bars containing at least 2.5 g of fiber per serving.
- Include "finger food" vegetables (carrots, celery, cauliflower pieces, broccoli flowerets) in lunch boxes and as snacks.
- For children, make animal or other fun shapes from vegetables pieces.
- Eat nuts and/or seeds for snacks, or add to mixed dishes, salads, breads, and cereals.

Benefits of Fiber

The generally accepted benefits of fiber are laxation effects, normalization of blood lipid concentrations, and attenuation of blood glucose response.[35,36,38,43] These benefits are the accepted measures of efficacy that are required for label claims of fiber content in Canada and that will be required in the United States when new labeling regulations become effective in 2018.[32,33] Benefits of fiber, such as cancer risk reduction and weight control, have been suggested in humans; however, results are limited and conflicting.

Laxation

Stool characteristics associated with *laxation,* or improved bowel function, include increased stool bulk, weight, and water content; decreased stool transit time and normalization of stool frequency to once daily; reduced symptoms of constipation; and an overall improvement in ease of defecation. Epidemiologic studies strongly support the positive role of fiber from whole grains, fruits, and vegetables in laxation. Insoluble fiber has been associated most frequently with improved laxation, although evidence also indicates some soluble fibers have similar effects. The role of functional fibers in laxation is well accepted, and adequate scientific evidence exists to support FDA approval of some fibers as nonprescription bulking agents for treatment of *occasional* constipation, as discussed in Chapter 15. Studies supporting the efficacy of bulk-forming fibers in *chronic* constipation are less certain and tend to be of intermediate to low quality.

Normalization of Blood Lipid Concentrations

Data on reduced risk of coronary heart disease (CHD) are sufficient for certain fibers to support an FDA-authorized health claim[4,5,16] (Table 24–1). Multiple epidemiologic studies have reported a reduced risk of CHD or cardiovascular disease (CVD) with high dietary fiber intake and/or fiber-rich foods. The relationship appears to hold over many years and across ethnic groups. Table 24–7 summarizes data related to risk of CHD from several large, well-designed prospective epidemiologic studies with longer-term follow-up and pooled data studies.[31,40,44–49]

TABLE 24-7 Summary of Selected Studies Related to Fiber and Risk of CHD and Improved Glucose Control

Study Name and Population Characteristics[a]	Follow-Up Time (Years)	Results/Conclusions
Nurse's Health Study[31,44]: cohort design; >65,000 women; ages 37–64 years	10	*CHD:* Inverse relationship between dietary fiber intake and risk of CHD only for dietary fiber from cereal sources, not fruits and vegetables; cereal fiber intake averaging 7.7 g/day reduced risk of CHD by 34%, compared with average intake of 2.2 g/day; RR 0.77 with higher fiber intake; 19% decrease in risk for CHD events per 10 g/day increase in dietary fiber and a 37% decrease per 5 g increase in cereal fiber.
		Glucose: RR type 2 diabetes 2.5 for high-GL/low-cereal-fiber diet (<2.5 g/day), compared with low-GL/high-cereal-fiber diet (>5.8 g/day); more frequent intake of dark breads, whole-grain breakfast cereals, and brown rice was associated with decreased likelihood of developing diabetes.
Nurses' Health Study, type 2 diabetes subgroup[45]: cohort design; 7822 women; ages 37–64 years	Up to 26 (70,102 person-years[b])	*CVD:* RR CVD-specific mortality 0.65 for highest fifth of bran intake after multivariate adjustment. RR all-cause mortality 0.75 for highest fifth of bran intake.
Health Professionals' Follow-Up Study[31,44]: cohort design; >42,000 men; ages 40–75 years	6–12	*CHD:* RR fatal CHD 0.45 and RR total MI 0.59 in those averaging 28.9 g dietary fiber per day, compared with those averaging 12.5 g/day; stronger association with cereal fiber than with fruits and vegetables; 19% decrease in risk of MI per 10 g/day increase in dietary fiber and a 29% decrease per 10 g/day increase in cereal fiber.
		Glucose: RR type 2 diabetes 2.17 for high-GL/low-cereal-fiber diet (<2.5 g/day), compared with low-GL/high-cereal-fiber diet (>5.8 g/day).
Iowa Women's Health Study[31,44]: cohort design; nearly 36,000 women, postmenopause	6	*CHD:* About one-third decrease in risk of fatal CHD with ≥1 serving/day of whole grains, compared with those with little whole-grain intake; risk decreased with fiber from cereals, not fruits and vegetables; decreased likelihood of mortality from ischemic heart disease with more frequent intake of dark (whole-grain) bread and whole-grain breakfast cereals.
		Glucose: Inverse relationship of insoluble fiber intake from cereals and risk of diabetes; no relationship to fruit, vegetable, legume intake; RR diabetes 0.79 for median intake of 20.5 servings/week of whole-grain products, compared with median of 1 serving/week.
Iowa Women's Health Study[46]: cohort design; 27,312 women, postmenopause; ages 55–69 years	17	*CVD/CHD:* Inverse relationship between total whole-grain intake and mortality from CVD and CHD. After multivariate adjustment, RR mortality from CVD and CHD 0.73 and 0.72, respectively, for consuming >19 g/week versus rarely to never consuming whole-grain products. Participants were free of CVD at baseline.
Cardiovascular Health Study, fiber intake analysis[40]: cohort design; 3588 men and women; ages ≥65 years (average 72 at baseline)	8.6	*CHD/CVD:* Cereal fiber intake was inversely associated with incident CVD. Hazard ratio 0.79 (21% lower risk) in highest quintile of fiber intake versus lowest quintile. The difference was seen with about 4.6 g fiber/day (2 slices whole-grain bread). Lower risk predominantly with fiber in dark bread (whole-wheat, rye, pumpernickel). Fruit and vegetable fiber intake was not associated with incident CVD. Participants were free of known CVD at baseline.
Alpha-tocopherol, beta-carotene cancer prevention study[31]: nearly 22,000 men; ages 50–69 years	6	*CHD:* RR CHD 0.84 for those averaging 34.5 g dietary fiber/day, compared with those averaging 16.1 g/day with fiber intake adjusted to 2000 calories; high-fiber intake: 12.9 g/1000 cal; low-fiber intake: 5.9 g/1000 cal.
Pooled data, prospective cohort studies[40]: total of 91,058 men and 245,186 women in 10 studies; ages 35–98 years	6–10	*CHD:* RR for all coronary events 0.86 (14% decrease) and RR 0.73 (27% decrease) for coronary death for each 10 g/day increment of total dietary fiber. For cereal fiber, RR 0.9 for all coronary events and RR 0.75 for death; for fruit fiber, RR 0.84 and 0.7; for vegetable fiber, RR 1.00 for all coronary events and death. Similar results for men and women.
Japanese Collaborative Cohort Study for Evaluation of Cancer Risks[40,48]: 58,730 men and women; ages 40–79 years	14.3	*CHD:* Fiber intake from fruit and from cereal but not vegetables was inversely related to CHD mortality. Overall CHD risk was 0.79 for highest quintile of fiber versus lowest. The association for insoluble fiber was stronger than for soluble fiber. All participants were Japanese.
Atherosclerosis Risk in Communities (ARIC) Study, subset with retinal vascular caliber measurements[44]: 10,659 men and women; ages 45–64 years	6	*CVD–retinal vascular caliber:* Inverse dose–response relationship between wider retinal arteriolar caliber/narrower venular caliber and fiber from all sources and from cereal fiber but not from vegetable fiber. Wider retinal arteriolar caliber and narrower venular caliber provide an objective measurement associated with lower CVD risk. Participants included whites and African Americans.

(continued)

TABLE 24-7 **Summary of Selected Studies Related to Fiber and Risk of CHD and Improved Glucose Control** *(continued)*

Study Name and Population Characteristics[a]	Follow-Up Time (years)	Results/Conclusions
Atherosclerosis Risk in Communities (ARIC) Study[44]: 12,251 men and women: 9529 whites and 2722 African Americans; ages 45–64 years	9	*Glucose:* Inverse relationship with 1 g/day of cereal fiber intake and risk of diabetes in both African American and white subgroups, but statistically significant only in whites; no relationship to fruit and legume intake in either subgroup. Participants were free of diabetes at baseline.
Insulin Resistance Atherosclerosis Study (IRAS), subgroup with carotid sonograms[47]: 1178 men and women; ages 40–69 years	5	*CVD–carotid artery intimal medial thickness (IMT) and IMT progression:* Inverse relationship between whole-grain intake and common carotid artery IMT and IMT progression. Carotid IMT is an objective measure related to atherosclerosis; IMT progression is associated with subsequent cardiovascular events. Multiethnic participants with a relatively high proportion of ethnic minority at 26%.
Finnish Mobile Clinic Health Examination Survey[40,44]: 2286 men and 2030 women; ages 40–69 years	10	*Glucose:* Inverse relationship of cereal fiber intake and risk of DM (cereal fiber predominantly from rye; little wheat).
Nurses' Health Studies: NHS-I and NHS-II[40]: cohort design; total 161,737 women; NHS-I: 73,327, ages 37–64 years; NHS-II: 88,410, ages 26–46 years	12–18	*Glucose:* For each 40 g increment in whole-grain intake, multivariate analysis indicated RR for DM of 0.54 (NHS-I) and 0.64 (NHS-II). BMI accounted for 42% and 57% of the association with RR after adjusting for BMI of 0.7 and 0.83, respectively, for NHS-I and NHS-II.
Black Women's Health Study[49]: cohort design; 40,078 black women with no prior history of diabetes or CVD; ages 21–69 years	8	*Glucose:* Inverse relationship between cereal fiber intake and diabetes (IRR 0.82). Risk of diabetes was 18% less for highest quintile of cereal fiber intake compared with lowest quintile. GId associated with risk of diabetes (IRR 1.23) for the highest quartile versus lowest. Stronger associations for BMI <25.

Key: BMI = Body mass index; CHD = coronary heart disease; CVD = cardiovascular disease; DM = diabetes mellitus; GId = glycemic index; GL = glycemic load; IMT = intimal medial thickness; IRR = incident rate ratio; MI = myocardial infarction; RR = relative risk.

[a] Number of participants included in the analysis is not always the entire study population; meta-analyses may include subsets of data from more than one trial.

[b] One person-year is equivalent to one person followed for 1 year.

Source: References 31, 40, and 44–49.

The key to fiber's ability to lower cholesterol and reduce CHD risk appears to be consuming an adequate quantity of highly viscous fiber, primarily from whole-grain cereal (oats, barley, rye) and beans (legumes), or from guar gum, pectin, and psyllium. Fruit fiber may have a beneficial effect relative to CHD/CVD, but the association is less clear. Vegetable fiber does not appear to be associated with reduced risk of CHD/CVD.

Attenuation of Blood Glucose Response

Multiple large, well-designed prospective epidemiologic and cohort studies with longer-term follow-up have reported an association between consumption of fiber and attenuation of blood glucose, improved insulin response, and/or reduced risk of diabetes, as summarized in Table 24–7.[31,40,44–49] The overall conclusion from these studies is that an inverse relationship exists between risk of diabetes and intake of dietary fiber. Intake of cereal fiber appears to be most frequently related to improved glucose control and/or reduced risk of diabetes; foods most likely to provide a positive effect include cereal grains such as oats, barley, and rye. Some legumes (beans), fruits, and vegetables, as well as guar gum and pectin, may also have a beneficial effect on glucose control. Evidence suggests that nonviscous fibers, such as wheat bran, have little effect on glycemic control.

Weight Loss and Maintenance

Epidemiologic studies show a lower body mass in participants who eat a high-fiber diet and greater incidence of obesity in those with low intake of dietary fiber.[31,40] Interventional studies show mixed results with high-fiber diets and weight loss, although there is an association of less weight gain over time with higher intake of whole grains.[48] Research suggests that fiber intake may influence body weight through various mechanisms, such as delayed gastric emptying, prolonged small bowel transit time and subsequent effects on peptides associated with satiety and gut function, activation of the ileal break, and stimulation of colonic cells, resulting in production of appetite-regulating hormones.[50]

Assessment of Functional Food Use: A Case-Based Approach

FF play a role in preventing disease and optimizing health. For patients who have mild signs of or are at risk for CHD, these foods may be a viable alternative to pharmacotherapy, as Case 24–1 illustrates.

CASE 24-1

Relevant Evaluation Criteria	Scenario/Model Outcome
Collect	
1. Gather essential information about the patient's symptoms and medical history, including	
a. Description of symptom(s) (i.e., nature, onset, duration, severity, associated symptoms)	Patient has no symptoms; she recently had a health assessment at work and was told that she is at risk of coronary heart disease because of her family history. She says she does not feel sick, but she does not want to end up taking a "bunch of pills everyday" like her mother and oldest brother. She wants to do what she can to avoid heart disease and is particularly interested in "functional foods" because of a healthy lifestyle program she recently watched.
b. Description of any factors that seem to precipitate, exacerbate, and/or relieve the patient's symptom(s)	n/a
c. Description of the patient's efforts to relieve the symptoms	n/a
d. Patient's identity	Maria Bracamonte
e. Patient's age, gender, height, and weight	28 years old, female, 5 ft 5 in., 195 lb
f. Patient's occupation	Third-grade teacher
g. Patient's dietary habits	Eats breakfast most mornings: typically a cup of coffee and cereal bar from home or a fast food English muffin with egg and bacon. Lunch: usually has a sandwich with potato chips and soft drink from the cafeteria. Afternoon snack: typically has a candy bar or granola bar. Dinner: Usually has meat (beef, pork, or chicken mostly) and fish every once in a while when someone has gone fishing; potatoes or pasta most nights; fresh, frozen, or canned vegetable four to five times per week; sweet dessert (cake, pie, baked goods) or ice cream five to six times a week; typically has a soft drink with dinner and occasionally an alcoholic drink.
h. Patient's sleep habits	Usually sleeps about 8 hours per night.
i. Concurrent medical conditions, prescription and nonprescription medications, and dietary supplements	None; birth control pill and multivitamin with folate
j. Allergies	NKDA
k. History of other adverse reactions to medications	None
l. Other (describe) ______	n/a
Assess	
2. Differentiate patient's signs/symptoms and correctly identify the patient's primary problem(s).	Mrs. Bracamonte has no signs/symptoms of disease but wants to follow a preventive strategy of a healthy diet.
3. Identify exclusions for self-treatment.	None
4. Formulate a comprehensive list of therapeutic alternatives for the primary problem to determine whether triage to a health care provider is required, and share this information with the patient or caregiver.	Options include (1) Refer Mrs. Bracamonte to her PCP for a more thorough assessment of heart disease and evaluation of her risk. (2) Refer Mrs. Bracamonte to a registered dietitian for comprehensive nutritional assessment and counseling. (3) Inform Mrs. Bracamonte of foods that have health claims associated with reduced risk of heart disease. (4) Take no action.

CASE 24-1 *continued*

Relevant Evaluation Criteria	Scenario/Model Outcome
Plan	
5. Select an optimal therapeutic alternative to address the patient's problem, taking into account patient preferences.	A combination of the options is appropriate. (1) Provide basic information and counseling related to functional foods with health claims associated with heart disease. Emphasize authorized and authoritative health claims (Table 23–1), because these have strong scientific evidence supporting the claim. The limited evidence for qualified claims and structure–function claims can be presented along with a discussion of where they fit, if at all, in the patient's overall plan. (2) Refer Mrs. Bracamonte for cholesterol screening (or perform screening in the pharmacy) and assessment for heart disease. (3) Refer Mrs. Bracamonte to a dietitian if she wants/needs more than basic counseling on nutrition, or have her request a referral from her PCP (may be necessary for insurance coverage). (4) Weight control and heart disease should be discussed with Mrs. Bracamonte, or these issues should be suggested as part of her discussion with her PCP or a dietitian.
6. Describe the recommended therapeutic approach to the patient or caregiver.	"A number of foods with health claims are associated with decreased risk of heart disease. For several foods, there is significant scientific agreement regarding their potential benefits. Using these foods in place of some of your current foods may reduce your risk of heart disease. However, it would also be helpful to know what your risks are, including your cholesterol level."
7. Explain to the patient or caregiver the rationale for selecting the recommended therapeutic approach from the considered therapeutic alternatives.	"Given your family history, you should have your cholesterol checked periodically and be evaluated for other risk factors for heart disease. Your weight is a risk factor for heart disease for you." "I can provide you with basic information on foods that have health claims related to heart disease and that may be of benefit in maintaining heart health. Dietitians are the food and nutrition experts; they can do a comprehensive assessment of your diet and provide more in-depth dietary counseling if you want that."
Implement	
8. When recommending self-care with nonprescription medications and/or nondrug therapy, convey accurate information to the patient or caregiver.	(1) "Decrease the saturated fat and cholesterol in your diet. No more than 10% of your calories should come from saturated fat, and you should keep cholesterol in your diet at no more than 300 mg cholesterol a day, but less is better. When you use milk, you might want to try 1% milk; most people find that to be more acceptable than nonfat (skim) milk, and it is lower in fat than 2% milk. Or you could try soy milk. Low-fat yogurt is also another good calcium source and is usually tolerated by people with lactose intolerance." (2) "Eat fruits, vegetables, and grain products that contain fiber, particularly soluble fiber. Replace white breads and pasta with whole grain. Total dietary fiber should be at least 25 g/day." [AI for women 19–50 years of age] (3) "You can also get soluble fiber from oat bran, rolled oats, or whole oat flour in certain foods, or from barley. Incorporate these products into the diet as replacement for breads and cereals that are not whole grain." (4) "Soy protein, 25 g/day, and a diet low in saturated fat and cholesterol also help to reduce the risk of heart disease. However, for many people, the major changes in diet needed to eat this much soy are very difficult to make, especially if all family members are not committed to the changes."

CASE 24-1 *continued*

Relevant Evaluation Criteria	Scenario/Model Outcome
	(5) "Plant sterol and stanol esters also help to reduce the risk of heart disease. Total intake is at least 1.3 g/day of sterol esters or 3.4 g/day of stanol esters, as part of a diet low in saturated fat and cholesterol. You usually need to eat the products at least twice a day to get the recommended amount. Some margarines and orange juice have added plant sterol/stanol esters." (6) "The health benefits of eating whole-grain foods overlap somewhat with that for "grain products that contain fiber" (#2) but does not specify "particularly soluble fiber." Insoluble fibers are also important in health. Look for whole grains, such as whole wheat, as the first ingredient on labels." "To make these health claims, foods must generally contain a certain amount of the desired component. Check food labels for these claims and for ingredient amounts." "There are also other foods that are considered healthy but do not yet have strong evidence to suggest they help to reduce the risk of heart disease. Therefore, the health claims may not be as effective or the claims might be changed if new studies are reported. Because the following foods are otherwise healthy foods when used in moderation, they can still be safely incorporated into your diet." (1) "Walnuts and several other types of nuts: 1.5 ounces a day; remember that nuts are a concentrated source of calories, so use judiciously." (2) "Omega-3 fatty acids: specifically eicosapentaenoic acid (EPA) and docosahexaenoic acid (DHA), found in salmon, lake trout, herring, and other oily fish." (3) "Monounsaturated fats from olive oil: 23 g/day (2 tablespoons) in place of a similar amount of saturated fat. A number of salad dressings and a few soft margarines now include olive oil." (4) "Canola oil, unsaturated fatty acids: 19 g/day (1.5 tablespoons) in place of a similar amount of saturated fat. Some cooking oil, a number of salad dressings, a few soft margarines, and some baked goods include canola oil."
Solicit follow-up questions from the patient or caregiver.	(1) "Are there any things I need to be aware of as I add these foods into my diet?" (2) "Are there any side effects from changing my diet?" (3) "Where can I find more information on dietary changes and diet plans to prevent heart disease?" (4) "May I use dietary supplements instead of changing to functional foods? Most information on the internet is advertising for dietary supplements."
Answer the patient's or caregiver's questions.	(1) "These foods should replace other foods in your diet so that the total calories do not increase. The more 'healthful' fats must replace saturated fats and not increase the total fat intake. You will need to read food labels carefully to be sure you are getting whole grains, low saturated fats, low cholesterol, and sterol/stanol esters in the product. Also look for the amount of soy or soluble fiber." (2) "Rapid increases in fiber content of the diet can cause gas and bloating, so it is best to gradually increase the fiber in your diet. Replace 1–2 servings of white bread and pasta with whole-grain products every few days until the refined foods are totally replaced. Also add extra fiber by gradually replacing the low-fiber cereals with a whole-grain cereal or oatmeal. Fruits and vegetables can be increased gradually as well to replace snacks and desserts. Be sure to drink plenty of water when eating a high-fiber diet."

CASE 24-1 *continued*

Relevant Evaluation Criteria	Scenario/Model Outcome
	(3) "The Food and Drug Administration website (www.fda.gov) includes information on health claims and food labels that you might find helpful. You could consider making an appointment with a registered dietitian, who could help develop some menus that incorporate foods you like and provide more specific plans for substituting healthier foods. Your health insurance plan may contract with a dietitian for coverage. If not, the Academy of Nutrition and Dietetics can provide the name(s) of private consultants and the contact information for a dietitian. The phone number for referrals is on their website (www.eatright.org)."
	(4) "In general, foods are better than supplements. Many studies have shown beneficial effects from a diet containing fiber-rich foods and whole grains but not with isolated supplements. Psyllium, found in products like Metamucil, fits criteria for a health claim related to soluble fiber and risk of congestive heart disease, and could be used to increase soluble fiber. It also has the added benefit of reducing constipation, as do fibers from whole grains."
Follow-up: Monitor and Evaluate	
9. Assess patient outcome.	"May we talk about the changes you have made in your diet when you pick up your prescription refills next month?"

Key: AI = Adequate intake; n/a = not applicable; NKDA = no known drug allergies; PCP = primary care provider.

MEDICAL FOODS AND MEAL REPLACEMENT FOODS

Traditional medical foods include products developed for patients with inborn errors of metabolism ("metabolics"). Product descriptions are available on manufacturer websites and may be available from the federally funded Special Supplemental Nutrition Program for Women, Infants, and Children (WIC), because this program is often involved in distribution of products and patient monitoring. Enteral nutrition formulas, specialty formulas in particular, may meet the definition of a medical food; however, many are better classified as food for "special dietary use," because they are readily available without medical supervision and are marketed directly to consumers as regular foods, often as meal replacement products. Enteral formulas are typically semisynthetic liquid formulas intended for oral consumption or administration through a feeding tube. Certain liquid diets designed for use in medically supervised very-low-calorie diets or bariatric programs are classified as medical foods. Various puddings, shakes, and other solid or semisolid food forms specially formulated and processed to meet *distinctive* nutritional requirements of the disease or condition for which they are intended can also be classified as medical foods. Both liquid and solid medical foods replace regular meals or enhance nutrient intake to meet the distinctive nutritional requirements of patients. However, these products are also frequently used to meet general nutritional needs.

HCPs involved with self-care counseling should determine when a product is used as a medical food to meet truly distinctive nutritional requirements, as determined by scientific studies, and when it is used as meal replacement or enhancement to meet *general* nutritional requirements. Foods intended to meet general nutritional requirements (see Chapter 23) do not need medical oversight and can be used safely for self-care. In contrast, FDA regulations state that use of medical foods requires recommendation or prescription by a physician or other authorized prescriber *and* ongoing medical supervision.[4,16] When enteral formulas are used to meet general nutritional requirements, however, third-party providers may refuse to cover the cost under insurance benefits, leaving patients with self-care responsibility.

Enteral Formula Uses

Tube Feeding

Enteral formulas are best known as complete nutritional replacements for patients requiring a feeding tube to meet their nutritional needs, such as stroke patients with severe dysphagia. Patients who cannot, should not, or will not take adequate nutrients by mouth are candidates for tube feeding and should be under medical care; tube feeding is not a condition conducive to safe and effective self-care. Unfortunately, little if any support is provided by most suppliers of adult enteral formulas in today's health care environment, even if the formula itself is covered by insurance benefits. Patients in this situation may benefit from referral to a Certified Nutrition Support Clinician (CNSC) or Board Certified Nutrition Support Pharmacist (BCNSP) if they are experiencing any difficulty with their feedings. For information related to tube feeding, the reader is referred to one of the many specialized references available; to the Oley Foundation (www.oley.org), a consumer-oriented organization for support of individuals requiring intravenous or tube feeding; or to the American Society for

TABLE 24-8 Enteral Formula Characteristics Consistent With Need for Medical Supervision

Characteristic	Examples
Protein as peptides and/or free amino acids	Peptamen, Crucial, Vital
Alteration of the amino acid content by addition of individual amino acids, such as glutamine, arginine, or branch-chain amino acids	Juven, Impact, Perative
Addition of specific fatty acids to alter the inflammatory response	Oxepa
Addition of significant amounts of medium-chain triglycerides to alter absorption	Portagen, Enfaport
High percentage (>50%) of calories from fat	Pulmocare, Nutren Pulmonary
Very high protein content (≥25% of calories as protein)	Nutren Replete, Promote
Intended for patients with organ failure	Nepro, NutriRenal, NutriHep

Parenteral and Enteral Nutrition (ASPEN). In addition to topics related to enteral and parenteral nutrition, the ASPEN website (www.nutritioncare.org) contains literature and other resources related to malnutrition.

Many enteral preparations are currently available. Most formulas provide nutritional support consistent with general dietary guidelines and are safe for use in self-care. Formulas intended for patients with impaired digestion and those designed for specific metabolic or clinical conditions require oversight by an HCP. Characteristics that are likely to result in the use of a formula as a true medical food requiring medical supervision are listed in Table 24–8, along with a few representative products. The patient's overall health condition also influences the need for medical supervision. For example, formulas with >25% of its calories from protein should be used with medical supervision in patients with compromised renal function, but there is less concern of adverse effects when these products are used occasionally by people with "normal" renal function.

Supplementation of Nutrition Intake

Liquid food preparations, including enteral products initially developed for tube feeding, are frequently used as oral supplements and are frequently marketed directly to consumers as supplements to the usual diet and as convenience foods to meet general nutrient goals, most commonly protein, calories, or both. Older adults tend to be a major target for such products because of changes related to aging (Table 24–9) that may contribute to reduced oral intake and increased risk of malnutrition.[51–54] Products are also marketed as "meal replacement" alternatives that are healthier than eating "fast foods" or skipping meals and that serve as a method of portion control. Individuals participating in sports activities are targeted for selective products (see Chapter 25).

TABLE 24-9 Changes With Aging and Other Factor That May Contribute to Poor Oral Intake and Malnutrition

Gastrointestinal Tract Changes

Reduced taste threshold

Motility dysfunction of lower esophageal sphincter

Slowed gastric emptying

Reduced gastric acid production

Decreased number and density of nerve fibers in the myenteric plexus

Impaired renewal and regeneration of intestinal epithelial tissue

Decreased number of Brunner glands in the duodenum resulting in a lower pH, which impairs pancreatic enzyme function

Colonic motility dysfunction resulting in either constipation or fecal incontinence

Structural changes of the pancreas

Decreased pancreatic lipase

Reduced gut-associated lymphoid tissue (GALT) immune response

Changes That Affect Protein Requirement and Intake

Reduced anabolic response to ingested protein

Impaired antiproteolytic response to insulin

High splanchnic protein extraction

Increased inflammatory and catabolic conditions

Other Factors

Poor appetite

Edentulousness

Self-reported poor health

Hospitalization

Source: Adapted from References 51–54.

Oral nutritional supplements (ONS) benefit hospitalized patients who are undernourished at baseline and reduce hospital readmissions.[52,54,55] A systematic review and meta-analysis conducted in the United Kingdom reported a reduction in readmissions from 33.8% to 23.9% with use of ONS compared with standard care; the number needed to treat was 10.[54] Benefit from routine ONS use at home or for those who are well nourished in any setting is more difficult to demonstrate. However, the prevalence of malnutrition among community-dwelling older adults living in industrialized nations is reported to range from 7% to 35%, depending on the criteria used to define malnutrition and the settings included.[53] Among chronically ill community-dwelling patients in the United States, 10% have disease-associated malnutrition.[56] The cost of community-based disease-associated malnutrition in the United States is estimated to be $157 billion based on 2010 dollars, with more than 75% of the cost associated with increased morbidity. In addition, evidence is mounting for the need for higher protein intake among all older adult patients to maintain physical function and mitigate risk for sarcopenia, osteoporosis, and impaired immune response.[52] Unfortunately, physicians typically receive minimal training in nutrition, and malnutrition is often not addressed until patients are significantly malnourished. Patients and families may, therefore, seek self-care alternatives, including ONS, to improve nutritional intake and mitigate or prevent malnutrition. Growing evidence indicates that ONS can be useful to prevent malnutrition.[52,54,55] These ONS products may or may not be complete (i.e., contain all necessary nutrients, including vitamins and trace elements) and balanced (i.e., contain appropriate ratio of nutrients) in their nutritional content. Users of such products should be cautious to ensure that their overall diet is complete and balanced.

Classification of Enteral Nutrition Products

Enteral products are classified as polymeric formulas, oligomeric formulas, and modular components. In addition, a growing segment of meal supplement and meal replacement products, including beverages, bars, and puddings, are designed to assist in meeting nutrient goals within an appropriate caloric intake.

Polymeric Formulas

Polymeric formulas are used most often. They are for individuals with normal digestive capability and contain macronutrients in the form of intact (whole) proteins, carbohydrates, and fatty acids or oils. Most individuals who require alternative nutrition support will tolerate and do well with standard polymeric formulas. The standard formulas usually (1) are 1 kcal/mL unless concentrated to provide less free water; (2) contain a macronutrient composition typical of the American diet (carbohydrate: 45%–70%; protein: 10%–18%; and fat: 20%–40%); and (3) are isotonic to slightly hypertonic (300–450 mOsm/kg); however, the osmolality of flavored products often range from 500 to 700 mOsm/kg. Polymeric formulas are listed as being generally safe for self-care when taken orally (Table 24–10).

Oligomeric Formulas

Oligomeric products require minimal digestion and are also known as predigested, peptide, or elemental formulas. They contain free amino acids, hydrolyzed or partially hydrolyzed protein, and less complex carbohydrates. These formulas frequently alter the fat content to improve absorption in patients with impaired absorption. They are rarely consumed orally because of very poor palatability. In general, oligomeric formulas require medical supervision.

Modular Products

Modular products supplement a single macronutrient. Examples include protein powder; medium-chain triglyceride oil; emulsified oils; and powdered, flavorless glucose polymers. These products can be incorporated into food to increase protein and calorie content. For example, a protein powder may benefit an older adult who is having difficulty meeting protein requirements with his or her usual oral diet.

Specialty Formulas

Specialty formulas may be either polymeric or oligomeric. They are designed to optimize the nutrient intake and improve disease management for patients with specific disease states such as renal insufficiency, diabetes mellitus, hepatic dysfunction, and carbon dioxide–retaining pulmonary dysfunction. The use of specialty formulas is controversial, because data supporting improved outcomes are minimal. In general, use of specialty formulas requires medical supervision. Consultation with a registered dietitian, CNSC, or BCNSP may be warranted.

Some specialty formulas, such as certain pulmonary and diabetic formulas, alter the ratio of fat and carbohydrate but contain no special dietary components. Although technically such products are medical foods, most individuals who use them could

TABLE 24–10 Examples of Meal Replacement Products/Liquid Formulas Suitable for Self-Care[a]

Product Name	Energy (kcal/mL)	Protein (g [% kcal])	CHO (g [% kcal])	Fat (g [% kcal])	Fiber (g)	Comments
Routine Formula						
Boost	240 (1.0)	10 (17)	41 (67)	4 (16)	None	Hypertonic
Ensure	250 (1.06)	9 (14)	40 (64)	6 (22)	None	Hypertonic
Jevity 1 Cal	250 (1.06)	10.4 (17)	6.5 (54)	8.2 (29)	3.4	Fiber from soy; isotonic
Routine Formula With Extra Protein						
Boost High Protein Drink	240 (1.0)	15 (24)	33 (55)	6 (21)	None	
Ensure High Protein	230 (0.97)	12 (21)	31 (55)	6 (24)	None	
Routine Concentrated (High-Calorie) Formula						
Boost Plus	350 (1.5)	14 (16)	45 (50)	14 (34)	None	
Ensure Plus	350 (1.5)	13 (15)	51 (57)	11 (28)	None	
Jevity 1.5 Cal	355 (1.5)	15 (17)	51 (54)	11.8 (29)	5.3 (75% I; 25% S; 10 g FOS)	Osmolite 1.5 Cal has similar nutrient profile without fiber.

TABLE 24-10 Examples of Meal Replacement Products/Liquid Formulas Suitable for Self-care[a] *(continued)*

Product Name	Energy (kcal/mL)	Protein (g [% kcal])	CHO (g [% kcal])	Fat (g [% kcal])	Fiber (g)	Comments
Diabetic Formula[b]						
Boost Glucose Control	250 (1.06)	14 (22)	20 (35)	12 (43)	3.5 (I: 0.9; S: 2.6; FOS)	Complex CHO including tapioca starch
Glucerna 1.2 Cal	285 (1.2)	14.2 (20)	27 (35)	14.2 (45)	3.8 (I, S, FOS: 2.4)	Higher omega-3 fat content than many routine formulas; 1 and 1.5 cal versions are available.
Nutren Glytrol	250 (1.0)	11.3 (18)	25 (40)	11.9 (42)	3.8 (I: 1.3; S: 2.5)	Amylase starch (low glycemic index)
Pulmonary Formula[c]						
Pulmocare	355 (1.5)	14.8 (17)	25 (28)	22 (55)	None	High-fat content
Nutren Pulmonary	375 (1.5)	17 (18)	25 (27)	23.7 (55)	None	High-fat content
Other Meal Replacements and Supplements						
Ensure Clear	200 (0.61)	7 (20)	43 (80)	None		6.7-ounce serving package; clear liquid; not intended as sole source of nutrition
Carnation Breakfast Essentials (powder for mixing)	220 (0.8)	13 (23)	39 (74)	0.5 (3)	<1	Put 1 packet in 1 cup fat free milk for 9-ounce serving; mixing with 2% or whole milk would increase number of calories as fat. Can mix with soy milk or reduced lactose milk.
Carnation Ready to Drink	220 (0.8)	14 (24)	31 (57)	5 (19)		
Glucerna Shake	200 (0.84)	10 (20)	26 (48)	7 (32)	3	Fiber is from FOS and soy polysaccharide; not for tube feeding; product not intended as sole source of nutrition.
Modular Components						
Beneprotein	25	6 (100)	None	None	None	Listed content per 7 g packet or 1 scoop
ProMod Liquid Protein	100	10 (40)	14 (60)	None	None	Listed content per ounce
Benecalorie	330 (7.5)	7 (9)	None	33 (91)	None	Listed content per 1.5-ounce serving (44 mL). Product is a modular component; add to enteral formula or foods to increase calories.

Key: CHO = Carbohydrate; FOS = fructooligosaccharides; I = insoluble fiber; S = soluble fiber.

[a] Amounts are for an 8-ounce serving unless otherwise indicated.

[b] Use sparingly for self-care, because the fat content is relatively high compared with that in studies of high-fat/low-carbohydrate diets and is higher than that recommended by general dietary guidelines. In accordance with recommendations from the American Diabetes Association (www.ada.org; see American Diabetes Association, Bantle JP, Wylie-Rosett J, et al. Nutrition recommendations and interventions for diabetes: a position statement of the American Diabetes Association. *Diabetes Care.* 2008;31(Suppl 1):S61–78), monounsaturated fatty acid content tends to be higher than in many standard formulas, and saturated fat content is low.

[c] Use sparingly for self-care, because the fat content is higher than that recommended by general dietary guidelines.

Note: The most current and detailed information is available at manufacturer websites, including Abbott Nutrition (www.abbottnutrition.com) and Néstle Nutrition (www.ensure.com/products).

replace a few meals per week with little concern for adverse effects. However, individuals must be encouraged to limit their use of these products unless otherwise advised by their primary care provider or a provider who specializes in nutritional management of their condition. They should advise their primary care provider when they use these products, because management of the underlying disease itself requires medical oversight. Table 24–10 includes a few examples of pulmonary and diabetic formulas.

Product Use for Self-Care

All products recommended for self-care, whether initially marketed for tube feeding or intended for oral ingestion, should contain basic nutrition labeling, including serving size, calories, protein, fat, and other components consistent with food labeling so that nutrient intake can be determined in the same manner as with regular foods. Many formulas are available in a variety of flavors to reduce taste fatigue; slight differences in nutrient content may be noted among the flavors.

Administration and Monitoring Guidelines for Enteral Nutrition

For products taken orally, the individual should be encouraged to vary flavors to avoid taste fatigue and to consume the product after an attempt to eat a well-balanced meal or a between-meal snack. Chilling may improve palatability. Once opened, the container should be kept refrigerated to prevent bacterial growth, and all open or prepared products should be discarded after 24 hours.

When products are given as tube feeding, medical supervision is recommended. Enteral nutrition practice recommendations are available at the ASPEN website (www.nutritioncare.org). Referral to a nutrition support provider may be appropriate. Medical referral is appropriate for individuals who develop diarrhea, nausea, or abdominal distention when taking meal replacement formulas. Formula-related diarrhea is an osmotic diarrhea that usually stops within 24 hours of discontinuing the formula; diarrhea that persists longer is unlikely to be caused by the formula per se. Lactose intolerance is seldom an issue with enteral formulas, because most formulas, except powders prepared with milk, are lactose-free. Other products not intended for tube feeding, however, may contain lactose. High-fat products can delay gastric emptying, resulting in nausea and/or abdominal bloating.

Food–Medication Interactions

Interactions between medications and enteral formulas often are complex and poorly understood. Interactions involving a formula component have the potential to occur with either oral administration or feeding tube administration. The HCP is advised to consult specialty references for a more complete list and explanation of such interactions. Although controversial, general practice for certain medications (including phenytoin, carbamazepine, warfarin) is to withhold the tube feeding formula for 1 or 2 hours before and after administering the medication, especially when therapeutic levels are not achieved with typical doses. It is reasonable to suggest this same precaution of separating the drug by 1 or 2 hours when formula is taken by mouth and to advise supervision of the medication response by a primary care provider. Vitamin K content of the formula should also be checked for individuals on warfarin. Although most formulas provide no more vitamin K than that of a typical diet, a few contain amounts that could interfere with anticoagulation. Manufacturers' websites, such as those listed in the footnotes of Table 24–10, provide detailed, up-to-date information on the nutrient content of formulas.

Other Medical Food and Meal Replacement Food

In recent years, several medical foods have become available for a range of common diseases treated in the ambulatory care setting (Table 24–11). Foods used in weight-loss and bariatric programs are also medical foods that require medical supervision when used as intended because of the significant risks associated with rapid weight loss. Meal replacement foods such as Slim Fast, Weight Watchers, and Jenny Craig products are not medical foods. They can be used safely without medical supervision to help control portion size and to balance nutrient intake; however, they should be used as part of an overall weight-loss plan (see Chapter 27).

Assessment of Enteral Nutrition and Meal Replacements: A Case-Based Approach

The first step in assessing the type of meal replacement (or supplement) to recommend is to determine whether the individual has any of the exclusions for self-care listed in Table 24–12. If self-care is appropriate, the provider should ascertain the reason for a meal replacement or supplement so that the most appropriate product can be selected. For instance, an older adult with early satiety may benefit from a concentrated formula that provides 1.5 or 2 kcal/mL, whereas a young person wanting a meal supplement for use with weight lifting may benefit from a higher protein formula. The selected formula should be appropriate to meet the individual's specific nutritional needs according to health status while avoiding excessive or contraindicated macronutrients and micronutrients.

TABLE 24–11 Medical Foods for Common Conditions

Condition	Product (Manufacturer)
Alzheimer disease	Axona (Accera Inc.)
Depression	Deplin (Pamlab)
Depression-associated sleep disorders	Sentra PM (Targeted Medical Pharma)
Irritable bowel syndrome	VSL#3 (probiotic; Sigma-Tau Pharmaceuticals)
Osteoarthritis	Limbrel (Primus Pharmaceuticals)
Osteopenia/osteoporosis	Fosteum (Primus Pharmaceuticals)
Pain and inflammation	Theramine (Targeted Medical Pharma)
Ulcerative colitis	VSL#3 (probiotic; Sigma-Tau Pharmaceuticals)

TABLE 24–12 Exclusions for Self-Care With Enteral Formulas

Condition	Example/Comment
Organ dysfunction requiring diet modification	Renal insufficiency requiring restriction of protein and electrolytes eliminated through the kidneys (potassium, phosphorus, magnesium).
Gastrointestinal dysfunction	Poor motility: Dietary modification may be required to avoid bowel obstructions; enteral formula may be appropriate under the supervision of a PCP or nutrition specialist; use for self-care is not appropriate.
	Reduced absorption: Hydrolyzed protein, modified fats, and/or relatively simple carbohydrates may be necessary for adequate absorption; monitoring for nutrient deficiencies is required.
	Dysphagia: Referral for medical evaluation is required.
	Bariatric surgery: Medical supervision is required; recommendations of a PCP or nutrition specialist should be followed.
Significant unintended weight loss	Refer for medical evaluation to determine the etiology.
	Life-threatening fluid and electrolyte abnormalities can occur when refeeding these individuals; medical supervision and monitoring are required.
Disease state affected by diet, such as diabetes mellitus, chronic obstructive pulmonary disease	Enteral formula may be appropriate to meet nutritional requirements; use should be under the supervision of a PCP or nutrition specialist; use for self-care is not appropriate.

Key: PCP = Primary care provider.

Meal replacement products can have efficacy for the treatment of many health concerns. Traditionally, meal replacement has been considered a therapeutic intervention needed to maintain adequate nutrition in malnourished patients; to completely replace nutritional intake in patients with a physical limitation that interferes with nutritional intake (e.g., dysphagia); or to precisely control intake of specific dietary components (calories for obesity and phenylalanine in phenylketonuria). Increasingly, nutrition products are used as lifestyle choices of self-directed therapy. This practice is particularly true of the meal replacement products used by working individuals who are too busy to prepare or eat a proper meal or who perceive these products as healthier alternatives to fast foods.

Case 24–2 illustrates assessment of a patient with who seeks a food/liquid meal product for Alzheimer disease.

CASE 24–2

Relevant Evaluation Criteria	Scenario/Model Outcome
Collect	
1. Gather essential information about the patient's symptoms and medical history, including	
a. Description of symptom(s) (i.e., nature, onset, duration, severity, associated symptoms)	Alzheimer dementia symptoms, progressive. Patient is easily frustrated and demanding of attention. Patient's daughter describes him as being very forgetful and showing more signs of Alzheimer dementia in the past month. At the Alzheimer family support meeting last week, she heard about a new food/liquid meal that is helpful in slowing the disease's progression, and she is requesting this product for her father.
b. Description of any factors that seem to precipitate, exacerbate, and/or relieve the patient's symptom(s)	n/a
c. Description of the patient's efforts to relieve the symptoms	Patient is currently taking a combination product containing donepezil and memantine (changed 2 months ago from donepezil). He also takes a multivitamin/mineral supplement.
d. Patient's identity	Tom Lambert
e. Patient's age, gender, height, and weight	79 years old, male, 6 ft 1 in., 150 lb
f. Patient's occupation	Retired banker

CASE 24-2 *continued*

Relevant Evaluation Criteria	Scenario/Model Outcome
g. Patient's dietary habits	Usually takes two meals daily and a couple of snacks. Must be reminded to eat and encouraged to eat more than one food off his plate; sometimes he refuses to eat anything.
h. Patient's sleep habits	Sleeps about 6 hours at night but also naps during the day.
i. Concurrent medical conditions, prescription and nonprescription medications, and dietary supplements	Hydrochlorothiazide for hypertension; multivitamin/mineral supplement
j. Allergies	Codeine; sulfa (rash)
k. History of other adverse reactions to medications	Ataxia with metronidazole
l. Other (describe) _______	n/a
Assess	
2. Differentiate patient's signs/symptoms and correctly identify the patient's primary problem(s).	Patient's daughter is requesting a medical food for use in Alzheimer dementia.
3. Identify exclusions for self-treatment (Table 24-12).	Medical foods require medical supervision.
4. Formulate a comprehensive list of therapeutic alternatives for the primary problem to determine whether triage to a health care provider is required, and share this information with the patient or caregiver.	Options include (1) Refer patient to his PCP to discuss use of the medical food and to obtain a prescription. (2) Recommend self-care with a general supplement to improve nutrient intake. (3) Take no action.
Plan	
5. Select an optimal therapeutic alternative to address the patient's problem, taking into account patient preferences.	Patient's daughter should consult with her father's PCP regarding the medical food.
6. Describe the recommended therapeutic approach to the patient or caregiver.	"You are requesting a product that requires medical supervision for use. The pharmacy can order the product for you once you have discussed this with your father's physician and you have a prescription."
7. Explain to the patient or caregiver the rationale for selecting the recommended therapeutic approach from the considered therapeutic alternatives.	"In addition to verifying that your father has medical supervision for using the product, a prescription may make the product eligible for coverage by your father's insurance."
Implement	
8. When recommending self-care with nonprescription medications and/or nondrug therapy, convey accurate information to the patient or caregiver.	Criterion does not apply in this case.
Solicit follow-up questions from the patient or caregiver.	"Do you know how this product works, and could I just change what I cook for my father rather than getting a prescription? I thought this product would also help with his calorie intake: he has lost about 25 pounds in the last couple months, because he often refuses to eat at mealtime. He will drink a milk shake when I'm home to make one for him in the afternoon, but I'm at work most afternoons. Is there a nonprescription product that I could use instead that would also increase his daily calories?"
Answer the patient's or caregiver's questions.	"The product for Alzheimer disease is based on a specific type of fat that is absorbed and metabolized differently than the typical oils found in the grocery store. It must be given in an appropriate amount with a proper balance of other nutrients to achieve the desired effect. Your father's weight loss is concerning and should be evaluated by his primary care provider to be certain the weight loss is related only to not eating enough; it could be related to a medical condition that requires treatment."

CASE 24-2 *continued*

Relevant Evaluation Criteria	Scenario/Model Outcome
Follow-up: Monitor and Evaluate	
9. Assess patient outcome.	"Let me know when you have discussed these issues with your father's primary care provider. If you decide to try the medical food for Alzheimer disease, I can order the product once you obtain the necessary prescription. If you want more information on the product, you can also check the product manufacturer's website (www.about-axona.com). The Alzheimer's Association website (www.alz.org) also has information on current research, alternative therapies, and their evaluation of various types of products marketed for Alzheimer disease. "A prescription is not required for most liquid meal products intended to supplement calories, and I can help you select a product if your father's primary care provider thinks his weight loss is primarily due to inadequate food intake. You may also want to ask your father's primary care provider about a nutrition consult, because a dietitian or nutrition support specialist could provide a more complete nutritional assessment as well as more comprehensive recommendations related to his diet."

Key: PCP = Primary care provider.

Patient Counseling for Enteral Nutrition and Meal Replacements

Advancements in enteral products and home infusion therapy are allowing more people with serious, even terminal, illnesses to be cared for at home. Enteral products are also appropriate for ambulatory patients with metabolic or digestive diseases and for individuals who want to ensure adequate nutrition for their life stage. Providers serve a pivotal role in helping patients to use the product best suited for their nutritional needs and to use it under medical supervision when appropriate. The box "Patient Education for Enteral and Meal Replacement Products" lists specific information to provide patients and caregivers.

Key Points for Functional and Meal Replacement Foods

- ➤ The definition of FF typically includes "health benefits beyond those of basic nutrition."
- ➤ Health claims are statements describing an association between a food, food component, dietary ingredient, or dietary supplement and the risk of a disease or health-related condition.
- ➤ Authorized and authoritative health claims meet the significant scientific agreement level of evidence. These claims should be routinely incorporated into counseling for lifestyle changes associated with health benefits and, when

PATIENT EDUCATION FOR Enteral and Meal Replacement Products

The objective of self-treatment is to provide the appropriate amounts and types of specific micronutrients and macronutrients to meet the individual's nutritional needs. For most individuals, the product instructions and self-care measures listed here will help ensure optimal therapeutic outcomes.

- Typical products provide 1 Cal/mL; higher-calorie products are available if you must limit your fluid intake or can drink only a small amount at a time.
- When drinking the formula, take about ½–1 can at a time. You can drink the formula at room temperature, but it may taste better if chilled or semifrozen as a slush-type drink.
- Varying the flavor of the formula may reduce taste fatigue.
- For tube feeding, the product should be used as directed by your primary care or nutrition care provider. The Oley Foundation (www.oley.org) provides consumer information on tube feeding.
- Keep opened containers refrigerated and covered to prevent bacterial growth; discard all remaining prepared products after 24 hours. Unopened product can be stored at room temperature.
- Use of meal replacement products as the sole or primary source of nutrition for more than a short time (2–3 weeks) requires medical supervision and should be discussed with your primary care provider. Periodic laboratory testing may be appropriate to detect electrolyte abnormalities in this situation.

When to Seek Medical Attention

- Monitor blood glucose (sugar) levels if you have diabetes or have had high blood glucose levels. Talk to your primary care provider if your blood glucose levels are high or low.

appropriate, as part of an overall plan for management of diseases associated with these claims.

- Qualified health claims do not meet the significant scientific agreement level of evidence; a claim statement must include language that indicates the qualified nature of the health claim.
- Structure–function claims lack the significant scientific agreement level of evidence and make no association between the product and the risk of a disease or health-related condition; they do not require validation or authorization by FDA.
- HCPs should understand the limitations of qualified health claims and structure–function claims. When counseling for lifestyle changes, the limited scientific evidence for these claims should be clearly delineated so individuals can understand the role, or lack thereof, for these products in a healthy lifestyle.
- Foods for special dietary use meet particular dietary needs related to physical, physiologic, pathologic, or other conditions, such as disease, convalescence, pregnancy, lactation, underweight, overweight, infancy, or need for sodium restriction, or these foods supplement or fortify the usual diet. They are subject to general labeling requirements for foods and do not require use under medical supervision.
- Medical foods are specially formulated and processed to meet distinctive nutritional requirements (established by medical evaluation based on recognized scientific principles) of the disease or condition for which they are intended. These foods are to be recommended and used under medical supervision.
- Conventional foods classified as FF are typically associated with health benefits in epidemiologic studies; evidence supporting a functional role for these foods is weak–moderate, with clinical trials often lacking.
- Fiber is associated with improved laxation, cholesterol reduction, satiety, and probably glucose control for select fiber sources.
- Enteral nutrition products may be classified as medical foods; however, many polymeric enteral formulas are readily available and can often be used safely as a meal replacement product.
- Specialty enteral formulas should be used with medical supervision, not for self-treatment.
- Semisynthetic liquid formulas intended for oral consumption may or may not be complete and balanced nutritional products.
- Nutrient content of meal replacement products should be considered in evaluating dietary intake to ensure the overall dietary content is complete and balanced.

REFERENCES

1. International Food Information Council. Functional foods consumer survey results: consumer insights to help Americans step up to the (functional foods) plate. Available at: http://www.foodinsight.org/blogs/2013-functional-foods-consumer-survey-results-consumer-insights-help-americans-step-functional. Accessed July 7, 2017.
2. International Food Information Council. Food and health survey: consumer attitudes toward foods safety, nutrition and health. Available at: http://www.foodinsight.org/2012_Food_Health_Survey_Consumer_Attitudes_toward_Food_Safety_Nutrition_and_Health. Accessed July 7, 2017.
3. Mogendi JB, DeSteur H, Gellynck X, Makokha A. Consumer evaluation of food with nutritional benefits: a systematic review and narrative synthesis. *Int J Food Sci Nutr.* 2016;67(4):355-371. doi: 10.3109/09637486.2016.1170768. Available at: http://dx.doi.org/10.3109/09637486.2016.1170768. Accessed July 7, 2017.
4. Pew Initiative on Food and Biotechnology. Applications of biotechnology for functional foods. Washington, DC: Pew Charitable Trusts; 2007. Available at: http://www.pewtrusts.org/en/research-and-analysis/reports/0001/01/01/application-of-biotechnology-for-functional-foods. Accessed July 7, 2017.
5. Academy of Nutrition and Dietetics. Position of the Academy of Nutrition and Dietetics: functional foods. *J Acad Nutr Diet.* 2013;113(8):1096–103. doi: 10.1016/j.jand.2013.06.002.
6. Caselli M, Cassol F, Calo G, et al. Actual concept of "probiotics": is it more functional to science or business? *World J Gastroenterol.* 2013;19(10):1527–40. doi: 10.3748/wjg.v19.i10.1527. Available at: https://www.ncbi.nlm.nih.gov/pmc/articles/PMC3602470/. Accessed July 7, 2017.
7. Wijnkoop-Lenoir I, Jones PJ, Milner J, et al. Nutrition economics: food as an ally of public health. *Br J Nutr.* 2013;109(5):777–84. doi: 10.1017/S0007114512005107.
8. Panagiotakos DB, Polychronopoulous E. The role of the Mediterranean diet in the epidemiology of metabolic syndrome: converting epidemiology to clinical practice. *Lipid Health Dis.* 2005;4:7–12. doi: 10.1186/1476-511X-4-7.
9. Padayachee A, Day L, Howell K, Gidley MJ. Complexity and health functionality of plant cell wall fibers from fruits and vegetables. *Crit Rev Food Sci Nutr.* 2017;57(1):59–81. doi: 10.1080/10408398.2013.850652. Available at: http://dx.doi.org/10.1080/10408398.2013.850652. Accessed July 7, 2017.
10. Ong TP, Moreno FS, Ross SA. Targeting the epigenome with bioactive foods components for cancer prevention. *J Nutrigenet Nutrigenomics.* 2011;4(5):275–92. doi: 10.1159/000334585.
11. Cirmi S, Ferlazzo N, Lombardo GE, et al. Chemopreventative agents and inhibitors of cancer hallmarks: may *Citrus* offer new perspectives? *Nutrients.* 2016;8:698-736. doi: 10.3390/nu8110698. Available at: https://www.ncbi.nlm.nih.gov/pmc/articles/PMC5133085/. Accessed July 7, 2017.
12. Gul K, Singh AK, Jabeen R. Nutraceuticals and functional foods: the foods for the future world. *Crit Rev Food Sci Nutr.* 2016;56(16):2617–27. doi: 10.1080/10408398.2014.903384. Available at: http://dx.doi.org/10.1080/10408398.2014.903384. Accessed July 7, 2017.
13. Baker CB, Rodriquez E. New models in translational phytotherapy: dietary phytochemicals in functional nutrition management and pharmaconutrition. *Pharmaceut Biol.* 2012;5(2):642–9.
14. Son TG, Camandola S, Mattson MP. Hormetic dietary phytochemicals. *Neuromolecular Med.* 2008;10(4):236–46. doi: 10.1007/s12017-008-8037-y.
15. Navia J, Byers T, Djordjevic D, et al. Integrating the totality of food and nutrition evidence for public health decision making and communication. *Crit Rev Food Sci Nutr.* 2010;50(Suppl 1):1–8. doi: 10.1080/10408398.2010.526825.
16. U.S. Food and Drug Administration, Center for Food Safety and Applied Nutrition. Food ingredients, packaging, and labeling: labeling and nutrition. Health claims meeting significant scientific agreement (SSA). Updated December 16, 2016. Available at: http://www.fda.gov/Food/IngredientsPackagingLabeling/LabelingNutrition/ucm2006876.htm. Accessed July 7, 2017.
17. U.S. Food and Drug Administration, Center for Food Safety and Applied Nutrition. Guidance for industry: a food labeling guide (11. Appendix C: health claims). Updated August 20, 2015. Available at: https://www.fda.gov/Food/GuidanceRegulation/GuidanceDocumentsRegulatoryInformation/LabelingNutrition/ucm064919.htm. Accessed July 7, 2017.
18. U.S. Food and Drug Administration, Office of Nutritional Products, Labeling, and Dietary Supplements. Summary of qualified health claims subject to enforcement discretion. Update December 14, 2014. Available at: http://www.fda.gov/Food/IngredientsPackagingLabeling/LabelingNutrition/ucm073992.htm. Accessed July 7, 2017.
19. U.S. Food and Drug Administration, Center for Food Safety and Applied Nutrition. Guidance for industry: A food labeling guide (12. Appendix D:

qualified health claims). Updated August 20, 2015. Available at: https://www.fda.gov/food/guidanceregulation/guidancedocumentsregulatoryinformation/labelingnutrition/ucm064923.htm. Accessed July 7, 2017.

20. Balentine D for Office of Nutrition and Food Labeling, Center for Food Safety and Applied Nutrition. Response to petition for a health claim for high-amylose maize starch (containing type-2 resistant starch) and reduced risk of type 2 diabetes mellitus (Docket No. FDA-2015-Q-2352). Posted December 13, 2016. Available at: https://www.regulations.gov/docket?D=FDA-2015-Q-2352. Accessed July 7, 2017.
21. U.S. Food and Drug Administration, Center for Food Safety and Applied Nutrition. Label claims for conventional foods and dietary supplements. Updated April 11, 2016. Available at: https://www.fda.gov/Food/IngredientsPackagingLabeling/LabelingNutrition/ucm111447.htm. Accessed July 7, 2017.
22. Combs GF Jr., Trumbo PR, McKinley MG, et al. Biomarkers in nutrition: new frontiers in research and application. *Ann NY Acad Sci.* 2013;1278:1–10. doi: 10.1111/nyas.12069.
23. Kato H. Nutrigenomics: the cutting edge and Asian perspectives. *Asian Pacific J Clin Nutr.* 2008;17(1):12–5. Available at: http://apjcn.nhri.org.tw/SERVER/APJCN/17/s1/12.pdf. Accessed July 7, 2017.
24. Pezzuto JM, Venkatasubramanian V, Hamad M, et al. Unraveling the relationship between grapes and health. *J Nutr.* 2009;139(9):1783S–7S. PMCID: PMC2728694. Available at: https://www.ncbi.nlm.nih.gov/pmc/articles/PMC2728694/. Accessed July 7, 2017.
25. Lordan S, Ross RP, Stanton C. Marine bioactives as functional food ingredients: potential to reduce the incidence of chronic diseases. *Mar Drugs.* 2011;9(6):1056–100. doi: 10.3390/md9061056.
26. Reuter S, Gupta S, Park B, et al. Epigenetic changes induced by curcumin and other natural compounds. *Genes Nutr.* 2011;6(2):93–108. PMCID: PMC3092901. Available at: https://www.ncbi.nlm.nih.gov/pmc/articles/PMC3092901/. Accessed July 7, 2017.
27. International Food Information Council Foundation. Functional foods. July 2011. Available at: http://www.foodinsight.org/Content/3842/Final%20Functional%20Foods%20Backgrounder.pdf. Accessed July 7, 2017.
28. International Food Information Council Foundation. Functional food fact sheet: antioxidants. *Food Insight.* October 15, 2009. Available at: http://www.foodinsight.org/Resources/Detail.aspx?topic=Functional_Foods_Fact_Sheet_Antioxidants. Accessed July 7, 2017.
29. Baker, CB. Traditional functional foods for the chemoprevention of chronic diseases: phytopharmacological concepts in food synergy. In: Martirosyan D, Abate N, eds. *Functional Foods for Chronic Diseases: Diabetes and Related Diseases.* Vol 5. Richardson, TX: Food Science Publisher; 2010:343–4.
30. Lampe JW. Interindividual differences in response to plant-based diets: implications for cancer risk. *Am J Clin Nutr.* 2009;89(5):1553S–7S. doi: 10.3945/ajcn.2009.26736D. Available at: https://www.ncbi.nlm.nih.gov/pmc/articles/PMC2677005/. Accessed July 7, 2017.
31. Food and Nutrition Board, Institute of Medicine, National Academy of Sciences. Dietary, functional, and total fiber. In: *Dietary Reference Intakes for Energy, Carbohydrates, Fiber, Fat, Protein and Amino Acids (Macronutrients).* Washington, DC: National Academies Press; 2005: 339–421. Available at: http://www.nap.edu/openbook.php?record_id=10490&page=339. Accessed July 7, 2017.
32. Food and Nutrition Board, Institute of Medicine, National Academy of Sciences. Summary tables, dietary reference intakes. Recommended intakes for individuals, total water and macronutrients. In: *Dietary Reference Intakes for Energy, Carbohydrates, Fiber, Fat, Protein and Amino Acids.* Washington, DC: National Academies Press; 2002:1324. Available at: https://live-up.co/wp-content/uploads/2015/09/Dietary-Reference-Intake-for-Energy-Carbohydrate-Fiber-Fat-Fatty-Acids-Colesterol-Protein-and-Amino-Acids.pdf. Accessed July 7, 2017.
33. U.S. Food and Drug Administration. Food labeling: revision of the nutrition and supplement facts labels, final rule. *Fed Regist.* May 27, 2016;81(103):33742 (Docket No. FDA-2012-N-1210). Available at: https://www.gpo.gov/fdsys/pkg/FR-2016-05-27/pdf/2016-11867.pdf. Accessed July 7, 2017.
34. U.S. Food and Drug Administration. Nutrition labeling of food. CFR: Code of Federal Regulations Title 21, Chapter 1, Subchapter B, Part 101, Subpart A, 101.9: CFR 101.9(c)(6)(i). Updated June 30, 2017. Available at: https://www.ecfr.gov/cgi-bin/text-idx?SID=3b4d97544079845f3160253cb50cc0b4&mc=true&node=se21.2.101_19&rgn=div8. Accessed July 7, 2017.
35. U.S. Food and Drug Administration, Office of Nutrition and Food Labeling, Center for Food Safety and Applied Nutrition. *Science Review of Isolated and Synthetic Non-Digestible Carbohydrates.* November 2016. Available at: https://www.fda.gov/downloads/Food/IngredientsPackagingLabeling/LabelingNutrition/UCM529049.pdf. Accessed July 3, 2017.
36. U.S. Food and Drug Administration, Center for Food Safety and Applied Nutrition. Scientific evaluation of the evidence on the beneficial physiological effects of isolated or synthetic non-digestible carbohydrates submitted as a citizen petition (21 CFR 10.30): Guidance for industry. November 2016. Available at: https://www.fda.gov/Food/GuidanceRegulation/GuidanceDocumentsRegulatoryInformation/ucm528532.htm. Accessed July 7, 2017.
37. NUTRA ingredients-usa.com. Schultz H. Groups call for deep revision or outright rejection of FDA fiber guidance. February 15, 2017. Available at: http://www.nutraingredients-usa.com/Regulation/Groups-call-for-deep-revision-or-outright-rejection-of-FDA-fiber-guidance. Accessed July 7, 2017.
38. Kendall CWC, Esfahani A, Jenkins DJA. The link between dietary fibre and human health. *Food Hydrocolloids.* 2010;24:42–8.
39. Chutkan R, Fahey G, Wright WL, et al. Viscous versus nonviscous fiber supplements: mechanisms and evidence for fiber-specific health benefits. *J Am Acad Nurse Pract.* 2012;24(8):476–87. doi: 10.1111/j.1745-7599.2012.00758.x.
40. Bernstein AM, Titgemeier B, Kirkpatrick K, et al. Major cereal grain fibers and psyllium in relation to cardiovascular health. *Nutrients.* 2013;5(5):1471–87. doi: 10.3390/nu5051471. Available at: https://www.ncbi.nlm.nih.gov/pmc/articles/PMC3708330/. Accessed July 7, 2017.
41. King DE, Mainous AG III, Lambourne CA. Trends in dietary fiber intake in the United States, 1999–2008. *J Acad Nutr Diet.* 2012;112(5):642–8. doi: 10.1016/j.jand.2012.01.019.
42. Hoy MK, Goldman JD. Fiber intake of the US population. What we eat in America, NHANES 2009-2010. Beltsville, MD: U.S. Department of Agriculture, Agricultural Research Service, Beltsville Human Nutrition Research Center, Food Surveys Research Group; September 2014. Food Surveys Research Group Dietary Data Brief No. 12. Available at: https://www.ars.usda.gov/ARSUserFiles/80400530/pdf/DBrief/12_fiber_intake_0910.pdf. Accessed July 7, 2017.
43. International Food Information Council Foundation. Fiber fact sheet. November 24, 2008. Available at: http://www.foodinsight.org/Content/6/FINAL%20IFICFndtnFiberFactSheet%2011%2021%2008.pdf. Accessed July 7, 2017.
44. Parillo M, Riccardi G. Diet composition and the risk of type 2 diabetes: epidemiological and clinical evidence. *Br J Nutr.* 2004;92(1):7–19. doi: 10.1079/BJN20041117.
45. He M, van Dam RM, Rimm E, et al. Whole-grain, cereal fiber, bran, and germ intake and the risks of all-cause and cardiovascular disease-specific mortality among women with type 2 diabetes mellitus. *Circulation.* 2010;121(20):2162–8. PMCID: PMC2886277. Available at: https://www.ncbi.nlm.nih.gov/pmc/articles/PMC2886277/. Accessed July 7, 2017.
46. Jacobs DR, Anderson LF, Blomhoff R. Whole-grain consumption is associated with a reduced risk of noncardiovascular, noncancer death attributed to inflammatory diseases in the Iowa Women's Health Study. *Am J Clin Nutr.* 2007;85:1606–14. Available at: http://ajcn.nutrition.org/content/85/6/1606.full.pdf. Accessed July 7, 2017.
47. Mellen PB, Liese AD, Tooze JA, et al. Whole-grain intake and carotid artery atherosclerosis in a multiethnic cohort: the Insulin Resistance Atherosclerosis Study. *Am J Clin Nutr.* 2007;85(6):1495–502. PMID: 17556684.
48. Ye EQ, Chacko SA, Chou EL, et al. Greater whole-grain intake is associated with lower risk of type 2 diabetes, cardiovascular disease, and weight gain. *J Nutr.* 2012;142(7):1304–13. doi: 10.3945/jn.111.155325.
49. Krishnan S, Rosenberg L, Singer M, et al. Glycemic index, glycemic load, and fiber intake and risk of type 2 diabetes in US black women. *Arch Intern Med.* 2007;167(21):2304–9. doi: 10.1001/archinte.167.21.2304.

50. Kristensen M, Jensen MG. Dietary fibers in the regulation of appetite and food intake. Importance of viscosity. *Appetite.* 2011;56(1):65–70. doi: 10.1016/j.appet.2010.11.147.
51. Soenen S, Rayner CK, Jones KL, Horowitz M. The ageing gastrointestinal tract. *Curr Opin Clin Nutr Metab Care.* 2016;19:12–8. doi: 10.1097/MCO.0000000000000238.
52. Bauer J, Biolo G, Cederholm T et al. Evidence-based recommendations for optimal dietary protein intake in older people: a position paper from the PROT-AGE study group. *JAMDA.* 2013;14:542–59. doi: 10.1016/j.jamda.2013.05.021. Available at: http://dx.doi.org/10.1016/j.jamda.2013.05.021. Accessed July 7, 2017.
53. van der Pols-Vijlbrief R, Wijnhoven HAH, Schaap LA et al. Determinants of protein-energy malnutrition in community-dwelling older adults: a systematic review of observational studies. *Ageing Res Rev.* 2014;18:112–31. doi: 10.1016/j.arr.2014.09.001. Available at: http://dx.doi.org/10.1016/j.arr.2014.09.001. Accessed July 7, 2017.
54. Stratton RJ, Hebuterne X, Elia M. A systematic review and meta-analysis of the impact of oral nutritional supplements on hospital readmissions. *Ageing Res Rev.* 2013;12:884–97. doi: 10.1016/j.arr.2013.07.002. Available at: https://doi.org/10.1016/j.arr.2013.07.002. Accessed July 7, 2017.
55. Milne AC, Potter J, Vivanti A, Avenell A. Protein and energy supplementation in elderly people at risk from malnutrition. *Cochrane Database Syst Rev.* 2009;2:CD003288.
56. Snider JT, Linthicum MT, Wu Y et al. Economic burden of community-based disease-associated malnutrition in the United States. *J Parent Enteral Nutr.* 2014(Suppl 2);38:77S-85S. doi: 10.1177/0148607114550000.

CHAPTER 25

SPORTS NUTRITION AND PERFORMANCE-ENHANCING NUTRIENTS AND SUPPLEMENTS

MARK NEWNHAM

Competing athletes exercise at various levels. Recreationally active individuals may spend 5–10 hours or more per week in physical activity, and diet alone should meet their nutritional needs. By comparison, high-volume intense training for 10–20 hours or more per week may require specific nutritional intake to maintain or enhance performance.[1] This chapter provides an introduction to the effects of products that contain macronutrients and nutritional supplements on physical activity and performance for both the recreational athlete and the more aggressive competitor. Food supplements and natural products are marketed as ergogenic aids to athletes and active people for three primary purposes: (1) to improve strength and power, (2) to prolong the duration of exercise by providing fuel for continued effort, and (3) to replace water and electrolytes lost from sweat, which in turn prevent dehydration and support normal muscle contractions. Readers are referred to two guidelines for detailed discussions on this topic: (1) the International Society of Sports Nutrition (ISSN) Exercise and Sport Nutrition Review[1] and (2) a joint statement of the Academy of Nutrition and Dietetics, the Dietitians of Canada, and the American College of Sports Medicine (referred to as the Academy in the remainder of this chapter) guidelines for Nutrition and Athletic Performance (referred to as Academy guidelines in the remainder of this chapter).[2] Sports nutrition is a complex field. Highly competitive and elite athletes who seek advice about sport specific nutrition or ergogenic aids should be referred to a clinical dietitian with a subspecialty in Sports Nutrition.

Popularity of Sports Nutrition Products

Sports nutrition products and performance-enhancing supplements have gained wide acceptance in both highly trained athletes and mildly to moderately active individuals. Increasing numbers of consumers are choosing sports nutrition products as lifestyle alternatives to traditional beverages and snacks. In 2015, the sports nutrition market was estimated to reach $16 billion in sales worldwide.[3] The market segment includes traditional carbohydrate and electrolyte sports drinks, along with energy drinks with supplemental caffeine; recovery drinks; and other nutrient-enhanced soft drinks, juices, and waters. The market for solid forms includes meal replacement bars and easy-to-digest carbohydrate gels. Tablets, capsules, and powders that contain macronutrients, electrolytes, and herbal supplements are included in the supplement market.

FDA, NCAA, Antidoping Agencies, and Regulation of Performance-Enhancing Supplements

The Food and Drug Administration (FDA) does not approve dietary supplements or validate claims of performance enhancement. Reports of nutritional supplement misbranding are common.[4,5] *Misbranding* occurs when products contain an ingredient not listed on the nutrition facts and ingredients label, or when products contain amounts other than the stated quantity of a labeled ingredient. Unlabeled doping substances, including stimulants and anabolic steroids, were found in 19% of vitamin and creatine supplements submitted for voluntary testing by Olympic athletes in 2002.[4] An even higher percentage of misbranding was reported in black market supplements confiscated by Norwegian authorities and tested by the Norwegian Control Doping Laboratory.[5] Of the 296 products seized, 80% contained prohibited substances, including anabolic-androgenic steroids, glucocorticoids, antiestrogens, cannabinoids, and other drugs.

The World Anti-Doping Agency states clearly in their Anti-Doping Code that "*Athletes* are responsible for any *Prohibited Substance* or its *Metabolites* or *Markers* found to be present in their *Samples*."[6] A positive test results in a violation regardless of the athlete's intent or the package label, even when the source can be traced to a nutritional supplement.[6] Nutritional products are tested at independent laboratories such as ConsumerLab.com, which provides reports for a fee. A list of banned substances and antidoping resources is available at these websites: www.usantidoping.org (U.S. Anti-Doping Agency), www.wada-ama.org (World Anti-Doping Code), and www.consumerlab.com (Consumer Lab.com). Chapter 50 provides a more detailed discussion of dietary supplement regulation.

Dietary supplements and prescription drugs are used and shared among college and high school athletes, possibly for performance gains. In 2013, the National Collegiate Athletic Association (NCAA) surveyed 21,000 athletes who participated in sports at division I, II, and III levels.[7] The NCAA survey reported high rates of nutritional supplement use, including a 28.6% rate for using an energy booster (e.g., energy drinks, energy shots) in the previous 12 months. Other observations include a 42% use of protein supplements and a 14% use of creatine. The NCAA survey also reported that amphetamine use increased from 3.7% in 2009 to 4.6% in 2013. Friends, teammates, and relatives continue to be a common source of unprescribed amphetamines. Reports of amphetamine swapping are concerning, because these activities are illegal and show a willingness to break the law to improve sports or academic performance.

High school athletes are also exposed to nutritional supplements and may have access to prescription medications that affect performance.[8] A survey of American high school athletes published in 2007 noted a high rate of nutritional supplement use: 62.1% used a daily multivitamin, 31.2% used energy drinks, 21.8% used protein powders, and 12.2% used creatine. Among female athletes, 18.6% of seniors reported using a "fat burner" to lose weight. Among male students, 5.9% reported using an anabolic steroid. High school athletes reported greater use of these substances compared with college-age students; therefore, education on the safe and effective use of nutritional intervention, supplements, and performance-enhancing products is needed as early as the high school level.

The American Academy of Pediatrics (AAP) has determined that the average child engaged in routine physical activity should drink water. AAP has taken the position that carbohydrate-containing sports drinks are not necessary and that caffeine-containing "energy drinks" should not be consumed by children and adolescents.[9]

Macronutrient Use for Athletic Performance—Basic Concepts

Macronutrients (carbohydrates, fats, proteins) play pivotal roles in athletic performance and muscle development, but each type of macronutrient has unique properties and use. Even during competition, the primary drive is to preserve muscle glycogen for "fight or flight" responses. Four primary concepts explain sports nutrition macronutrient intake and its contribution to energy provision for athletic performance. First, when not exercising, macronutrient intake is stored for later use. Second, during exercise, stored macronutrients are used slowly according to the exerciser's aerobic capacity to burn fats rather than glycogen, thus preserving glycogen. Fatty-acid oxidation is the primary fuel for aerobically intense activity. Third, muscle glycogen is depleted slowly at lower intensities or when the athlete is aerobically adapted to use fats. By comparison, muscle glycogen is depleted rapidly at high intensities, particularly when the athlete is trained to use carbohydrates as fuel or expects carbohydrate availability during the event. Finally, at the highest intensities, an anaerobic energy system contributes energy from muscle phosphocreatine directly to depleted adenosine diphosphate (ADP), permitting restoration of muscle adenosine triphosphate (ATP).

Humans are biologically designed to maintain a full reserve of glycogen as an immediate energy source for short-duration, high-intensity activity, such as fight or flight. At the lowest level of exercise intensity, a walking state, calorie utilization per minute is minimal, with 80% of the calories obtained from fatty-acid oxidation and the remaining 20% from carbohydrates.[10,11] As exercise intensity increases from walking to aerobic jogging, calorie consumption per minute increases, and fatty-acid oxidation continues to provide about 80% of the fuel.[10,11] Conversion of fatty acids to energy is slow and rate limited, and the conversion rate varies from athlete to athlete. Fatty-acid oxidation is increased by low carbohydrate availability in the diet and by adaptation to aerobic physical exercise.[12] No proposed ergogenic supplements consistently improve the rate of fatty-acid metabolism.[1,2] A detailed discussion of fatty-acid metabolism is beyond the scope of this chapter and can be found elsewhere.[11,12]

Second, calories burned per minute from fat are limited and reach a plateau; therefore, athletic performance is impaired without additional calories from other sources such as carbohydrates[10,11] At the intensity of a fast run, such as a 10-km running race, fatty-acid oxidation cannot meet all of the energy requirement, and carbohydrate utilization is added to the energy derived from fats. At this level of intensity, carbohydrate utilization increases to 50% of total calorie expenditure.[13] The rate reaches 80%–90% for sprint events (200 meters).[13] Progression of exercise intensity from walking to running to sprinting is seen in many sports, and some sports, such as soccer and field hockey, have a combination of extreme high-intensity effort intermixed with efforts at a more aerobic pace. The oxidation of fatty acids is the predominant fuel until exercise intensity requires the faster energy conversion from carbohydrates.

Third, glycogen depletion is an intensity and durational concept. Marathon runners refer to muscle glycogen depletion as "hitting the wall." A similar term, "bonking," references the cognitive and mental attention deficits athletes can experience when glycogen depletion leads to hypoglycemia. Limited storage capacity exists for glucose as glycogen within the liver and skeletal muscle; an average 150-pound individual stores only about 2000 total calories of glycogen. High-intensity exercise over time depletes glycogen stores.[10,11,14] Muscle glycogen is burned initially, and as this resource is depleted, the liver releases glucose from stored glycogen to maintain serum glucose levels. When both muscle and liver glycogen stores are depleted, serum glucose decreases and athletic performance declines. Sudden drops in blood glucose levels affect the athlete's mental acuity, attention, and focus.[10,11] Endurance athletes slow to an aerobic effort in which fatty-acid mobilization predominates, but they are less competitive at that rate of intensity. Athletes participating in sports that require high cognitive skill, such as shooting sports, archery, and automobile racing, experience lower performance and brain activity as their serum glucose levels decrease.[1,2] The rate of glycogen depletion is dependent on the intensity and duration of exercise, as well as the fitness level of the athlete.[10,11] Endurance runners can deplete muscle glycogen in about 2–2.5 hours at a marathon run training pace; they do not require carbohydrate intake unless they exercise for that duration or longer at lower intensities (see the section "Carbohydrate-Based Products" for recommended carbohydrate intake).[1,2] Carbohydrate intake during the race can delay the onset of muscle glycogen depletion when running at the higher intensity of a marathon race pace. The same runners may deplete glycogen in 60 minutes when running at the faster intensity of a 10-kilometer run, but they generally do not require carbohydrate supplements, because they complete the event in less time (30–40 minutes) than it takes to deplete muscle glycogen.[1,2] Team sports such as football, lacrosse, field hockey, and basketball have official game time durations of 60 minutes or less, as well as time-outs, half-times, and player substitutions that allow for periods of aerobic recovery. For these sports and durations, glycogen depletion is not expected to occur unless the athlete is consistently on the field playing at a high intensity. Compared with undertrained athletes, very fit athletes adapt over time to a state of efficient fatty-acid utilization and require less glycogen; their carbohydrate stores are available in later stages of events.[10,11]

A fourth concept is that the highest intensity sports, those requiring short bursts of power lasting less than 30 seconds to 1 minute, use the phosphagen system and energy stored primarily as ATP.[15] Examples include track and field events and weight lifting. Energy stored in phosphate bonds is depleted in a matter of seconds and then regenerates with rest. This energy system is discussed further in the section "Creatine." Intermittent high-intensity sports such as football, soccer, basketball, tennis, and ice hockey use both very short (phosphagen and ATP) energy systems and intermediate (glycogen) systems over the competition range of 30–60 minutes.

Sports Nutrition Market Basics

The sports nutrition market was developed for well-trained athletes competing at high intensities for long durations. College football players may exercise for 4 hours daily and exceed 20 hours of exercise per week. These athletes may need to provide fuel during exercise to delay or prevent glycogen depletion, or they may require rapid muscle glycogen restoration between morning and afternoon practices. Sports drinks can be consumed during practice or competition and have replaced the concept of carbohydrate loading prior to long-duration events. Most marathon runners and triathletes consume carbohydrates during the event.[1,2] Sports products also contain electrolytes to prevent deficiencies from sweat loss.

By comparison, moderate physical activity such as daily exercise for health and wellness usually occurs at a lower intensity and typically lasts 60 minutes or less per day.[1,2] Glycogen depletion is unlikely for recreational athletes, even if they exercise 7 hours per week; consequently, carbohydrate- and electrolyte-containing sports products are unnecessary for health and wellness athletes or sedentary individuals who do not participate in prolonged exercise.[1,2]

Carbohydrate-Based Products

Carbohydrate-based sports nutrition products contain monosaccharides (glucose and fructose) as well as the disaccharide sucrose (glucose + fructose); these sugars provide rapid absorption and availability of carbohydrates. Maltodextrin (glucose + glucose as a polymer) is used in endurance formulas and is marketed as having slower absorption; maltodextrin is also tasteless, which is preferred by many athletes. Lactose (glucose + galactose), or milk sugar, can also be used as a recovery fuel after exercise.[1,2]

The Academy guidelines recommend 30–60 grams of carbohydrate intake per hour of continued exercise beyond 60 minutes.[2] This recommendation translates to 8–15 g of carbohydrates or 4–8 ounces of a sports drink every 15 minutes. Most sports nutrition drinks contain 6%–8% carbohydrates for optimal absorption and gastrointestinal (GI) tolerance.[1,2] The amount of carbohydrates is small and should be used rapidly during continuing exercise; however, the fluid volume is relatively large. Energy gel packets are lighter and easier to carry, but they contain 20%–25% carbohydrate and should be consumed with water for dissolution. These products should be used in practice and under simulated competition so that the athlete can learn how they tolerate a product. Research suggests that pre-exercise carbohydrate consumption may stimulate the release of insulin and result in hypoglycemic symptoms and reduced performance in some athletes, whereas others experience improved performance.[16] Ultra endurance athletes require very large intake of calories to meet energy expenditure rates even though their exercise intensity is lower. This allows for longer durations (24 hours or longer) of continuous exercise. These athletes have trained to tolerate greater amounts of food during sustained exercise. Their food choices include energy-dense fats as well as protein and carbohydrate. The various carbohydrate forms (i.e., drinks, gels, bars) do not differ in their effectiveness, although individual tolerances to various forms may differ. However, the amount of water and electrolytes and the specific sugar sources do vary. Bars and gels are lighter and easier to carry than an equivalent amount of calories in the form of a sports drink; however, these bars and gels require a water source for proper dissolution, absorption, and GI tolerance. In addition, compared with sports drinks, the bars tend to contain other macronutrients, such as fats, proteins, and vitamins, making them better suited for lower intensity exercise or exercise that does not have as much jostling, such as cycling. Bars are also appropriate for recovery after exercise.

Although the original intent of these products was to provide fuel on the go, the market has evolved to provide meal replacements for active people in a hurry. These products are misunderstood by the public as healthier than soft drinks, candy bars, or even regular meals, despite their high sugar and caloric content. Health care providers (HCPs) should be prepared to read and interpret the nutrition label with patients and to calculate total calories if the package offers multiple servings. These products are not required by active adults or children who exercise 60–90 minutes in any one session.[2,9] Recreational athletes and sedentary individuals should be discouraged from using these products before, during, or after exercise that lasts less than 90 minutes.[2,9] The Academy and AAP recommend eating a meal after exercise as a suitable glycogen recovery method.[2,9] Examples of bars, gels, and drinks are presented in Table 25–1.

Fats: Triglyceride-Containing Products

Fats are an important source of energy, fat-soluble vitamins, and essential fatty acids for athletes, and their consumption should not be restricted.[2] The timing of fat intake may be important.[2] Long-chain triglycerides, found in typical fats and oils, should be avoided in sports nutrition products used 1–2 hours before and during exercise, because they tend to slow gastric emptying and may cause discomfort, bloating, and GI intolerance during intense exercise. Medium-chain triglycerides (MCTs) are packaged into sports drinks and powders to provide an alternative fuel to glucose and to reduce muscle glycogen utilization.[12] The moderate length (8–12 carbons) of MCTs results in absorption from the GI tract directly into the bloodstream, allowing more rapid utilization than with long-chain triglycerides, which are absorbed through the lymphatic system. Some MCT beverages are marketed to strength and conditioning athletes on low-carbohydrate diets. Clinical data in athletes suggest that MCTs are utilized metabolically within 30 minutes of ingestion, but no data show improved performance or muscle glycogen sparing (Table 25–1).[12]

Protein Products for Muscle Mass Gain

Athletes and those who exercise according to health standard recommendations may train with weights or their own body weight to maintain or build muscle. This approach allows the exerciser to perform their sport, improve performance, and prevent chronic disease such as sarcopenia and osteoporosis. Many athletes believe they need to consume large quantities of protein to provide substrates for muscle development. Dietary sources of protein include meat and dairy; vegetarian sources such as legumes, beans, and nuts; and prepackaged protein sources, such as protein powders, amino acid supplements, and various protein-containing bars, gels, and drinks.

Many variables affect nutrient requirements; however, compared with the less active general population, athletes who exercise for 10 or more hours per week have increased protein and calorie

TABLE 25-1 **Sports Nutrition Products**[a]

	Serving Size	Energy (kCal)	Carbohydrate (g)	Sugar (g)	Protein (g)	Fat (g)	Sodium (mg)	Potassium (mg)
Electrolyte Drinks and Wafers (low calorie)[b]								
Gatorade G2 Low Cal	12 ounces	30	7	7	0	0	160	45
Nuun Active Tablet	16 ounces, 1 wafer	10	1	1	0	0	360	100
Powerade Zero	12 ounces	0	0	0	0	0	150	35
Propel Flavored Water	12 ounces	0	0	0	0	0	160	40
Zym Endurance Tablet	16 ounces, 1 wafer	8	0	0	0	0	300	100
Energy Drinks (carbohydrates, electrolytes)[c]								
Accelerade	31 g 1 scoop 12 ounces water	120	21	20	5	1	210–220	65–90
Cytomax	25 g 1 scoop 12 ounces water	90	22	12	0	0	120	60
Gatorade Thirst Quencher	12 ounces	80	21	21	0	0	160	45
Powerade	12 ounces	80	22–21	21–20	0	0	150	35
Recovery Drinks (carbohydrates, proteins, electrolytes, hydration)[d]								
Endurox R4	74 g 2 scoops 12 ounces water	270–280	52	38–40	13	1–1.5	210–220	150–190
Gatorade Recover	11 ounces	270	45	21	20	1	330	540
IsoPure ZeroCarb	20 ounces	160	0	0	40	0	50–80	45–60
Milk, Low Fat, Chocolate Flavor	½ pint 236 mL	140	25	24	7	1	190	382
Muscle Milk, Chocolate Flavor	11 ounces	130	7	0	20	1	240	790

Energy Gels (carbohydrates, electrolytes)[e]								
Accel Gel	1 packet	100	20	13	5	0	100–115	No data
CarbBoom	1 packet	110	26	2–3	0	0	50–55	45-60
Clif Shot (Chocolate)	1 packet	110	22	12	0	0	60	80
Gu	1 packet	100	20–25	5–6	0	0–2	40–65	35–60
Hammer Gel	1 packet	80–90	21–22	2–4	0	0	20–35	10–25
Energy/Recovery Bars (carbohydrates, proteins, fats, electrolytes)[f]								
Balance Bar Original	1 bar	180–210	20–22	14–18	13–15	6–7	110–200	120–320
Cliff Bar	1 bar	230–240	42–44	16–25	9–10	3.5–7	125–240	180–280
Luna Bar	1 bar	180–190	25–28	11–13	8–10	4.5–7	115–210	90–160

[a] Composition per serving. In a brand-name product that is available in different flavors and formulations, the quantity of nutrients differs slightly among the product line extensions. (See product nutrition label or the manufacturer's website for the most current information.)

[b] Intended as a healthy, low-calorie alternative to carbohydrate sports drinks. For rehydration and electrolyte replacement following exercise time of 1 hour or less when glycogen depletion is not a concern. Performance benefits are unproven.

[c] Intended for use during exercise to provide carbohydrates for energy and glycogen sparing, as well as electrolytes and water for rehydration.

[d] Intended for use after exercise of prolonged duration when glycogen depletion is expected.

[e] Intended for use during exercise to provide electrolytes as well as carbohydrates for energy and glycogen sparing. Require a water source for proper dissolution and absorption. Not intended for rehydration.

[f] Intended for post-exercise recovery after exercise of prolonged duration when glycogen depletion is expected. Can serve as a meal replacement product. Often contain added vitamins and minerals.

requirements.[17] The Academy guidelines recommend protein intake of 1.2–2.0 g/kg/day in highly active adults who participate in endurance exercise and in those who are attempting to increase body mass; this recommendation is in addition to an increased overall caloric intake to meet higher metabolic demands.[2] The Academy no longer offers a specific kcal/kg/day target but rather uses a complicated formula to calculate an individual's energy availability, where energy intake and energy expenditure are balanced with the athlete's goals for body image and energy training. The Academy desires to calculate the athletes planned exercise expenditure to allow proper balance with energy intake.[2] Readers are encouraged to review the Academy guidelines for a more detailed understanding.[2] By comparison, the ISSN guidelines recommend 25 kcal/kg/day for a sedentary population and 25–35 kcal/kg/day for a population who chooses a moderate exercise duration of 90–120 minutes weekly.[1] Competitive athletes training 15–30 hours per week may expend 600–1200 kcal per hour of intense exercise. This increased volume of energy expenditure may require up to 50–80 kcal/kg/day.[1]

Athletes attempting to gain muscle mass may require an increased total calorie intake to balance their increased energy needs from exercise and to provide protein for muscle building.[2] Athletes who wish to build muscle should be educated not to exceed reasonable total calorie goals, because energy intake that exceeds energy expenditure may lead to an accumulation of body fat, defeating the intent of a lean physical appearance. Anecdotal evidence of athletes ingesting 2.0–2.5 g/kg/day of protein has been reported despite lack of data supporting its effectiveness.[2,17,18] The marketplace offers a large number of protein supplements that provide specific protein sources, namely essential amino acids or branched-chain amino acids (BCAAs). ISSN and the Academy guidelines indicate that simple adjustments to the athlete's diet can provide sufficient protein to meet dietary intake goals for increasing muscle mass.[1,2,17] There is insufficient evidence to support packaged protein supplements or specific amino acid mixtures as more effective for increasing body mass than eating whole foods that contain equal amounts of high-quality protein.[1,2,17,18] The Academy recognizes that the use of protein supplements may be reasonable for their convenience.[2]

Clinical Evidence of Protein Needs for Muscle Building

Muscle protein is in a constant state of synthesis and breakdown. Resistance exercise induces changes in muscle that effectively stimulate muscle remodeling and growth, provided the diet offers an adequate quality and timing of protein for that growth.[17,18] The process is slow and requires repeated exercise stimulus, optimal nutrition, and several months to observe weight gain. Protein intake recommendations from the Academy and ISSN are similar (1.2–2.0 and 1.4–2.0 g/kg/day, respectively).[1,2,17] ISSN recommends that individuals participating in strength/power exercise consume protein at the higher end of the range. Well-designed studies of protein intake at 2 g/kg/day and greater have not resulted in consistent increases in lean body mass, compared with the control group, and indicate only increased protein oxidation for energy.[17,18] ISSN recommends that the athlete consume a high-quality protein source within the time frame of their exercise stimulus.[17] Theories that support protein intake before, during, and immediately after exercise are discussed in detail elsewhere, but protein intake within 30 minutes after exercise may be optimal for tolerance and convenience.[1,2,17] The ISSN position is that the protein source should include BCAAs from either whole-food sources or a whey protein supplement.[17] The Academy makes no recommendation for post-exercise protein intake but references that intakes of 50–100 g of protein ingested during the recovery period may improve the recovery of static force and dynamic power indices.[2]

Adverse Effects of Protein Supplement Use and Diets With High-Protein Intake (>2 g/kg/day)

The Academy and ISSN have concluded that protein intake up to 2.0 g/kg/day is effective and safe in healthy exercising adults.[1,2,18] They have similarly concluded that insufficient evidence is available to support the claim that high-protein diets exceeding 2.0 g/kg/day are unsafe in the same healthy population.[1,2,18] Concerns over kidney damage and bone osteoporosis have been speculated but remain unfounded.[18] Minor side effects, such as GI distress and diarrhea, have been reported. GI distress may be related to the osmolality of the final product as mixed by the athlete or by individual athlete tolerance to the product. More concerning are case reports of hypertension, abdominal pain, hepatitis, and renal insufficiency that have been reported in military servicemen who reported using protein supplements, although the quantity and duration of protein intake are not reported.[19] The quantity of protein supplement contents, compared with the food-label ingredients, is regularly tested and reported on websites such as ConsumerLab.com. The most recent tests of protein powders found the quantity of protein present was consistent with the label value but did report variations between test and label values for sodium and cholesterol content for a few products.[20]

Water and Electrolytes

Water and electrolytes are essential to performance. A *critical water deficit,* defined as a 2% decrease in total body weight, can affect physical and mental performance.[21] Dehydration results in increased physical strain, as measured by elevations in core body temperature, heart rate, and perceived exertion. The greater the body water deficit, the greater is the strain for a given task. Dehydration can also affect cognitive performance, such as mental concentration and focus on skilled tasks. A greater amount of dehydration (3%–5% body weight) does not appear to affect anaerobic performance and muscle strength.[21] Readers are referred to the position statement of the American College of Sports Medicine for guidelines and detailed discussion of this topic.[21]

Dehydration involves water loss and electrolyte concentrations as separate issues. Athletes generate heat from exercise-related muscle contractions in proportion to the intensity and duration of exercise. This heat generation is transferred to the blood and then to the body core. Blood circulation through peripheral blood vessels and the skin allows radiant heat exchange with the environment. Fluid and electrolyte loss as sweat onto the skin surface facilitates evaporative cooling. Environmental conditions such as temperature, humidity, air motion, helmets, and layers of clothing influence the success of evaporative cooling. If sweat-related water and electrolyte losses are not replaced, the athlete experiences dehydration.

The significance of dehydration depends on environmental conditions, exercise intensity, and its duration. For example, compared with a recreational runner, an elite marathon runner may demonstrate a higher sweat rate, as measured by sweat loss per hour, but both athletes will have similar total sweat losses for the event owing to the prolonged time that the recreational athlete needs to complete the event. By comparison, when practicing under identical conditions, American football players have significantly greater sweat rates than those of soccer players.[21] A greater sweat rate may be related to the layers of clothing and use of helmets, which contribute to greater heat accumulation and greater sweat and electrolyte losses, while preventing evaporative cooling.[21] The risk of dehydration in any sport is further influenced by twice-daily practice sessions, which may not allow adequate time between sessions for water and electrolyte replacement.[2]

Health Conditions Related to Hydration and Electrolytes

Hydration can affect health through water loss or water gain (overdrinking) and can affect serum sodium levels sufficiently to endanger health. In general, dehydration is more common, but overhydration resulting in hyponatremia can be equally life-threatening. Signs of dehydration include fatigue, confusion, irritability, and increased risk of heat illness with symptoms of muscle cramps, heat exhaustion, heat stroke, and exertional rhabdomyolysis.[21] Rhabdomyolysis has been reported as a result of dehydration, heat stress, and novel training. *Novel training* involves the introduction of new exercise patterns in athletes who have not been acclimated to the new exercise, such as military recruits at boot camp or high school students attending preseason football camps.

Prevention of Dehydration

Meal consumption is an important aspect of maintaining optimal hydration status between exercise sessions.[2,21] Eating promotes fluid intake and retention of water, provided the meal is a sufficient source of sodium.[21] Water alone is sufficient for rehydration during events lasting 60 minutes or less.[2,9] Sports drinks can provide water and electrolytes after exercise, but when assessed 24 hours after a 60-minute or less workout, the drinks have not proven superior to the consumption of a meal and water after exercise.[1,2,21]

Hyponatremia Risk From Drinking Excessive Free Water

Most laboratory-based studies of dehydration have occurred on stationary treadmills in climate-controlled rooms with little-to-no convective airflow to help sweat evaporation.[21] Because of such studies, athletes have been taught to drink as much water as possible to prevent dehydration. However, liberal water intake has been called into question, particularly for endurance athletes, following clinical observations of weight gain, severe hyponatremia, cerebral edema, and death in athletes who consumed water without added electrolytes during athletic events lasting longer than 4 hours.[21–23] Improved water availability to athletes competing in marathons has not resulted in fewer athletes seeking medical care after races.[22,23] The original research was directed at elite-level athletes competing for 60–150 minutes who consumed small sips of water while running very fast and generating significant body heat and high sweat rates. Unfortunately, this description does not apply to average athletes, who complete the same marathon races at a much slower pace, generate less heat accumulation, and have lower sweat rates.

Observations from actual marathon race conditions resulted in an advisory statement from the International Marathon Medical Directors Association (IMMDA).[23] Heat production by athletes is significantly affected by their effort (the combination of duration and intensity or speed of the exercise); therefore, a 10-km race effort will generate more heat than a marathon effort (42.2 km). Average athletes run slower than elite athletes; therefore, average athletes are at less risk of heat illness and have more time to consume water at aid stations. The result is that clinical hyponatremia occurs more frequently in non-elite athletes, particularly women, who require more than 4 hours to finish a marathon, and in long-course triathletes who require 13–17 hours to complete their events.[21–23] IMMDA recommendations suggest that fluid consumption in athletes' drinks be based on the trigger of actual thirst, rather than on a set volume of fluid intake. As the athletes' thirst increases, they can increase fluid intake from sips of water to a calculated sweat rate. IMMDA strongly recommends that the athlete choose an electrolyte replacement drink instead of free water to avoid the risk of hyponatremia when competing in events that last 4 hours or longer.[23]

Athletes competing for 2 or more hours can determine their individual sweat rates by observing their total body weight before and after prolonged exercise. For example, an athlete who takes a 2-hour run on a hot afternoon may drop 2 kg in body weight. Each kilogram change in body weight would be associated with a 1000-mL water deficit, suggesting that the athlete has lost 2000 mL of water. This athlete can target a drinking rate of 1000 mL per hour, or 240 mL (8 ounces) every 15 minutes, during prolonged exercise.

Providing athlete education before the event and electrolyte-containing sports drinks during the event reduces hyponatremia cases in triathletes[23] but not in experienced marathon runners.[21–23] Other factors are likely involved. For example, clinical observations indicate exercise-induced hyponatremia may increase with concurrent use of nonsteroidal anti-inflammatory drugs (NSAIDs) in marathon runners[23] and long-course triathletes.[24] An exact mechanism is unknown; however, NSAIDs may interfere with normal prostaglandin-mediated regulation of glomerular filtration and renal blood flow. Triathletes with significant hyponatremia were observed to have elevated nitrogen and potassium levels, suggestive of reduced glomerular filtration.[24]

Postural hypotension, rather than heat-related illness or dehydration, has been recognized as a health risk in endurance running that is not directly related to fluid intake. When athletes cross the finish line, the sudden decrease in leg muscle contractions allows pooling of blood in the legs and decreased venous return. The resulting decrease in cardiac output may leave the brain under-perfused with oxygenated blood, causing the athlete to black out.[23] Athletes should continue walking past the finish line to prevent this reaction. Only athletes demonstrating a rectal temperature higher than 104°F (40°C) should be treated for heat illness.[23]

Carbonated and Oxygen-Enhanced Water

Available research does not substantiate a performance benefit of oxygenated water or carbonated water in humans.[21,25] Dissolved gases can accumulate and cause GI distress and bloating, resulting in decreased total fluid consumption.[21] Oxygenated water claims to have 30% or higher dissolved oxygen; however, when packed in plastic bottles, it may contain no more dissolved oxygen than tap water, and 12 ounces of oxygenated water in glass bottles contains less oxygen than a single breath of room air.[25]

Electrolytes and Water Without Added Carbohydrates

Several carbohydrate-free products that offer water, electrolytes, and vitamins have been developed; they contain an artificial sweetener to replace most or all carbohydrates typically found in a carbohydrate-containing sport drink. Low-calorie carbohydrate-containing sports drinks provide as little as 3 g of carbohydrates per 8-ounce serving, or just 10 kcal, contrasting with 11–18 g of carbohydrates and 50–80 kcal per 8-ounce serving of most carbohydrate-containing sports drinks. These low-calorie and no-calorie electrolyte waters have not been evaluated for performance benefits. An alternative to carbohydrate-containing sports drinks is artificially sweetened electrolyte drinks, but they offer no more performance benefits than water does, other than the observation that a small amount of added sweetness to sodium may improve the absorption rate of water and the volume of fluid consumed.[2,21]

Electrolytes, Carbohydrates, and Water

Addition of carbohydrates to sports drinks benefits athletes competing longer than 60–90 minutes by replacing muscle glycogen lost during periods of intense or prolonged effort. Carbohydrate supplementation during exercise provides exercising muscles with fuel for energy while allowing muscles to conserve stored carbohydrate energy as glycogen. This strategy of providing fuel during exercise at a rate of 30–60 g/hour for events lasting longer than 60 minutes has been shown to prolong the time to exhaustion in football and soccer players, as well as in long-distance endurance athletes such as runners and cyclists.[2] Carbohydrate-containing sport drinks appropriate for consumption during exercise provide 6%–7% carbohydrate. To meet the target of 30–60 g of carbohydrate per hour, the athlete would drink 500–1000 mL per hour. Many triathletes and runners use a combination of carbohydrate-containing drinks and gels or chews, which must be consumed with water or another fluid to assist in dissolution and absorption of the carbohydrate.

Electrolytes, Carbohydrates, Protein, and Water

Several sports nutrition drinks combine an electrolyte–carbohydrate solution with added protein. The protein is added to provide an additional metabolic fuel for ATP production.[26,27] These products are marketed to endurance athletes competing at aerobic intensities for long durations, including marathon runners (2.5–5 hours), long-distance triathletes (2–17 hours), and adventure racers (12 hours to 5 days). Only a few studies have compared carbohydrate-only and carbohydrate with added protein groups. The studies that have carefully controlled equal caloric consumption in the groups have shown equivalent performance effects on cycling exercise duration. [26,27] However, the group that drank the carbohydrate–protein solution had significantly lower creatine phosphokinase levels and perceived muscle soreness the next day. Unfortunately, these studies did not measure cycling performance on subsequent days and cannot show an association between performance and the observed muscle soreness.[26,27]

Although ready-to-drink options exist, some protein-containing drinks are powders that require reconstitution and can release significant amounts of gas when mixed with water. Bubbles and foam appear in the hydrated powder, which can influence GI tolerance in athletes. Protein-containing sports drinks should be introduced during the training regimen so that athletes can determine their tolerance to the products and the products' impact on performance before the drinks are used during an event. Because hydrolysis can affect stability of some proteins once they are mixed with water, athletes should not hydrate protein-containing dry-powder drinks the night before an event. Optimal protein potency and effect may require athletes to carry unmixed powder and add water during the event, a potentially unsafe practice. For example, athletes could lose control of their bicycle when reconstituting powder in triathlon events. Once mixed, all sports drinks should be consumed or stored in the refrigerator within 2 hours to prevent bacterial growth.

Pre-exercise Nutrition and Hydration

The Academy guidelines recommend that a hydration fluid of 5–10 mL/kg of body weight be consumed 2–4 hours before exercise.[2] For example, a 59-kilogram athlete would consume 295–590 mL of fluid prior to exercise. This allows time for the excretion of excess fluid in the urine before exercise begins. Hyperhydration with glycerol increases the risk of needing to void during competition, provides minimal performance advantage, and is discouraged.[21,28]

The timing of pre-exercise carbohydrates is controversial. Eating a meal prior to exercise or competition can affect the athlete's performance through GI intolerance and the body's metabolic response to the meal. Athletes are encouraged to allow several hours between a meal and exercise to allow for digestion and absorption of the meal.[2] Carbohydrate intake prior to exercise is intended to ensure optimal muscle glycogen for competition. However, studies of pre-exercise carbohydrate intake have had varied effects on performance.[29,30] Carbohydrate intake before exercise can provide energy for sustained effort and improve performance in some athletes but impair performance in others.[29,30] Carbohydrate intake before exercise is known to stimulate insulin release and inhibit fatty-acid oxidation. The athlete becomes less dependent on fatty-acid oxidation and more dependent on carbohydrate energy sources. As exercise intensity or duration increases, the athlete can deplete glycogen and consequently risk hypoglycemia and performance impairment if additional carbohydrate doses are not provided during the event.[30]

The Academy guidelines state that optimal performance depends on individually determined distribution of macronutrient intake prior to exercise because of variations in athlete size, the energy demands of different sports, overall daily calorie needs, and the timing of macronutrient intake prior to the practice or event. Individual athletes should consider nutrition a part of their training regimen and should practice the timing, quality, and quantity of intake to become familiar with their own tolerance and timing.

Nutrition and Hydration During Exercise

As detailed previously, for competitions lasting longer than 60–90 minutes, athletes are recommended to determine a sweat rate by measuring their pre- and post-exercise body weights. A reasonable goal is to drink 16–24 fluid ounces of a sports drink for every 0.5 kg of body weight loss during exercise.[2] The Academy guidelines recommend consuming 30–60 g of carbohydrate (from food and/or fluids) per hour during exercise to maintain blood glucose levels.[2] These rates are adjustable according to an athlete's tolerance. A carbohydrate drink concentration of 6%–8% is recommended, because concentrations greater than 8% are associated with adverse GI effects.[2]

Post-exercise Nutrition and Recovery Drinks

Goals of post-exercise recovery nutrition are to rehydrate, restore muscle glycogen, and provide protein to repair muscle damage and synthesize new muscle tissue, thereby preparing the athlete for another period of activity. The choice of recovery nutrition depends on how much time is available until the next session of intense activity. When recovery time between bouts of exercise is 4 hours or greater, the Academy recommends that an athlete consume a balanced meal or snack after exercise for glycogen restoration, optimal rehydration, and correction of electrolyte imbalances.[2] Several studies have compared a carbohydrate-only sports nutrition drink with consuming a glass of low-fat milk containing an equal number of calories from low concentrations of fat, carbohydrate, and protein.[31–33] Consumption of low-fat milk was associated with greater hydration, lower urine output, and improved weight replacement after exercise.[31] In addition, low-fat milk was associated with a longer time to exhaustion in subsequent exercise sessions.[32,33] Milk is an effective after-exercise meal and is better for recovery than a carbohydrate-only sports drink. Readers are advised to avoid confusing low-fat and skim milk with products such as Muscle Milk, which is advertised as a nondairy product despite containing milk protein isolate, and calcium and sodium caseinates from milk. Compared with low-fat or skim milk, each serving of Muscle Milk contains considerably more calories in the form of added fats and high-glycemic-index carbohydrate. When recovery time is less than 4 hours, drinking a carbohydrate sports drink improves muscle glycogen recovery better than drinking water. The sooner the carbohydrate is consumed after exercise, the sooner muscle glycogen is replaced. The Academy guidelines recommend carbohydrate consumption of 1.0–1.2 g/kg/hour for the first 4 hours after a glycogen-depleting exercise.[2]

Safety and Efficacy of Specific Ergogenic Supplements

This section discusses evidence that supports the safety and efficacy of specific nutritional supplements and micronutrients for sports performance, namely herbs, plant extracts, antioxidants, and other supplements purported to improve sports performance. These nutritional supplements are marketed as "foods" and are not regulated as drugs by FDA. These foods are not required to provide safety and efficacy data in humans to prove their effectiveness on the playing field, nor do they require testing to prove their labeled contents. Readers are reminded of previous evidence of misbranding and the frequent inclusion of substances banned by antidoping agencies in these products.[4–6] They are also referred to Table 25–2[1,2,34–46] for a list of substances for which available evidence does not support claimed effectiveness. Athletes should take extreme caution when using nutritional supplements to enhance sports performance: misbranding of these supplements may lead to doping infractions and serious adverse effects and deaths have been reported from supplement use.

Caffeine and Caffeine-Supplemented Energy Drinks

Caffeine supplementation has shown effects in some, but not all, anaerobic resistance exercises (weight lifting).[47] Pre-exercise caffeine doses of 2 mg/kg have improved duration of endurance exercise but not measured oxygen uptake.[47] Caffeine has no effect on high-intensity sprints or on agility tests,[48,49] although it does improve alertness in very-long-duration endurance races, such as 24-hour bicycle races, because it may counteract sleep deprivation. Caffeine doses affecting sports performance (2–6 mg/kg) are similar to doses that can be obtained from foods and beverages that are unrelated to exercise or performance. Doses exceeding 9 mg/kg do not add benefit.[48] Incidental exposure to caffeine is common, and complete avoidance is unrealistic. WADA does not list caffeine as a problematic substance, and many questions regarding the effective use of caffeine for ergogenic benefit are still unanswered.

> The class of products labeled as providing "energy" is broad and increasingly popular, although the vast majority of consumption is recreational and unrelated to sports.[3,48] Although the composition of sports drinks is similar to that of energy drinks (EDs) and energy shots (ESs), the latter contain caffeine in addition to water and electrolytes. EDs may contain carbohydrates or be labeled as "calorie free." They usually contain a blend of other nutrients and herbal additives such as taurine or guarana that are proposed to affect exercise performance or mental performance during exercise. These additives have not been proven to affect sports performance or weight loss.[48]

EDs are not without a risk of unintended adverse effects. The additional caloric load may affect blood glucose and insulin levels and consequently promote weight gain.[48] EDs have been associated with tooth decay, demonstrating a faster rate of enamel loss than available sports drinks.[49] Limits on the amount of caffeine present in EDs are not enforced within the United States at this time. Caffeine content may range from 100–286 mg per serving, whereas Canada has limited EDs to 180 mg per drink.[48] This quantity of caffeine is similar to a 16-ounce serving of coffee. Users are cautioned to consider the possible adverse effects from cumulative daily doses of caffeine. In addition to GI intolerance, adverse effects include insomnia, nervousness, tachycardia, tremors, and anxiety. A recent clinical observation in healthy college-age adults showed that a single dose of an ES can increase systolic and diastolic blood pressure by 5 mm Hg from baseline, although none of the healthy subjects were reported to have reached a level of prehypertension.[50] More severe adverse effects from EDs are prompting emergency department visits and are related to indiscriminate use of EDs, often with other illicit drugs or alcohol.[51] AAP has concluded that children and school-age athletes should not consume EDs or ESs and that they have no place in sports competition.[9] In addition, the use of EDs and ESs by sedentary children may promote unintentional weight gain and increased body mass index.[52] ISSN further states that diabetics and individuals with preexisting cardiovascular, neurologic, or metabolic disorders should avoid these products.[48] Avoiding the use of EDs and ESs for sports performance is generally appropriate advice for any age group.

Creatine

Creatine is the most widely used ergogenic aid among athletes, and it has the most consistent data.[15,53] Creatine, a naturally occurring substance, is synthesized in the body by the combining of arginine and glycine, or it is absorbed intact after ingestion of red meats and fish.[15,53] Creatine is found in all skeletal muscle as free creatine or high-energy phosphorylated creatine (PCr). PCr

TABLE 25-2 Selected Products Marketed as Ergogenic Supplements

Ingredient	Marketed Claim	Conclusion/Evidence
Antioxidants[1,2,34]	Antioxidants claim to be able to reduce oxidative stress from exercise and/or to speed recovery following exercise. Many antioxidants have been included in sports nutrition supplements, including alpha-lipoic acid, carotenoids, glutathione, n-acetylcysteine, ubiquinones (coenzyme Q10), vitamin B complex, vitamin C, and vitamin E.	Evidence does not support an effect on reducing oxidative damage or enhancing performance. Frequent exercise is associated with an enhanced antioxidant system.
Arginine[35]	Arginine has been promoted to improve muscle building and cardiovascular functioning through the production of nitrous oxide, which causes cardiac vasodilatation and increased oxygen delivery to the heart.	Evidence does not support an effect on performance enhancement.
BCAAs (branch-chain amino acids)[1,2,35,36]	BCAAs are isoleucine, leucine, and valine. Skeletal muscle cells use BCAAs to supply energy during exercise. Supplementation may reduce fatigue and increase exercise time to exhaustion by reducing serum levels of l-tryptophan and its effect on serotonin levels in the brain.	Evidence does not consistently support an effect on endurance performance.
Carnitine[2]	Carnitine is an essential cofactor for the transport of long-chain fatty acids into the mitochondria. Product is proposed to improve fatty acid oxidation, fat burning, and oxygen absorption as well as to reduce lactic acid accumulation.	Evidence does not support an effect on performance.
Chromium[2]	Chromium is marketed to enhance carbohydrate utilization in the body, promoting fat burning and dietary protein sparing for muscle building. Product is marketed to improve endurance and strength.	Evidence does not support an effect on performance.
Citrulline[2]	l-Citrulline is a metabolic precursor to arginine. Citrulline is not affected by first-pass hepatic metabolism and is converted by the kidneys to arginine. Product is proposed to improve oxygen consumption and time to exhaustion in treadmill running.	Evidence does not support an effect on performance.
Conjugated linoleic acid (CLA)[2]	CLA is promoted to endurance athletes as a thermogenic aid, body fat reducer, and ergogenic aid that enhances fat metabolism. CLA may increase cardiac risk by lowering high-density lipoprotein and increasing lipoprotein(a) concentrations.	Evidence does not support an effect on performance or body composition.
Cordyceps sinensis[37,38]	*Cordyceps sinensis* is used in Chinese medicine to treat lung disease and fatigue. Products claim that this mushroom can decrease oxygen consumption and improve endurance. Product is frequently combined with *Rhodiola*. Available research published in English is limited and does not show a performance benefit.	Evidence does not consistently support an effect on performance.
Eleuthero[39]	Extracts of Siberian ginseng have been reported to affect cardiorespiratory performance, fat metabolism, and improved endurance.	Evidence does not support an effect on performance.
Ginseng[40]	Extracts of *Panax ginseng* have been reported to improve lactate clearance and delay the onset of fatigue.	Evidence does not support an effect on performance.
Glycerol[2,41]	Glycerol is reported to act as an osmotic agent to promote hyperhydration prior to exercise, therefore reducing the risk of dehydration from intensive exercise in the heat.	Evidence does not support an effect on performance.
Hydroxy-methylbutyrate (HMB)[2,35,42]	Beta-HMB is a metabolite of leucine metabolism, purported to decrease muscle protein breakdown after a workout and to increase protein synthesis. HMB has also been proposed to improve aerobic performance.	Evidence does not consistently support an effect on performance. Untrained individuals appear to receive greater benefit than trained individuals.
Lecithin[43]	Lecithin is a source of choline and a precursor to acetylcholine. Decreased plasma choline and acetylcholine levels have been reported in marathon runners. Supplementation of lecithin before a marathon does prevent the decline in serum acetylcholine levels but does not affect finishing times.	Evidence does not support an effect on performance.
Rhodiola sp.[36,44–46]	*Rhodiola rosea* and *Rhodiola crenulata* are Chinese herbs used to stimulate the nervous system, improve aerobic work performance, and reduce fatigue. *Rhodiola* is reported to improve oxygenation at high altitudes and to elevate the lactate threshold. Endurance athletes have seen 1%–2% reductions in cycling time trials and running events.	Evidence suggests small improvements in endurance exercise that are minimal enough to question the herbs' performance value.

functions as an energy buffer, transferring a phosphate group to ADP, thereby rapidly regenerating ATP during periods of exercise. Skeletal muscle contains limited amounts of energy stored as ATP at rest; exercise depletes this stored ATP energy quickly. The body must oxidize macronutrients through the Krebs cycle to restore ADP to the high-energy ATP state for continuous or repeated efforts. PCr transfers its energy to ADP in seconds, acting as a secondary fuel. However, the total amount of PCr energy in muscles lasts for only 20–30 seconds.[15,53]

Performance gains with creatine are limited to laboratory-based studies of short bursts of anaerobic activity lasting 30 seconds or less. Creatine supplementation attenuates normal decreases in the force associated with repeated work applications.[15,53] For example, a weight lifter performs three sets of a bench press, with a goal of 10 lifts, or repetitions, per set. The lifter takes 30 seconds of rest between each set. Ordinarily, the lifter may be able to move a planned amount of weight for 10 repetitions in the first set, 8 repetitions in the second set, and only 6 repetitions in the third set. The decreasing number of lifts is called *attenuation* and is related to decreased energy (ATP) in the muscles. Creatine can improve the amount of ATP energy available to lift the weight; the same athlete may complete more repetitions in each subsequent set (e.g., 10, 10, and 8 repetitions rather than 10, 8, and 6).[15,53] Similar improvements in maximum weight lifted in a single lift have also been reported.[15,53] Creatine is useful for athletic events that require repeated, short, explosive bursts of power, such as sprinting and jumping seen in American football, soccer, and track and field events. By comparison, creatine does not benefit athletes in sports that require more than 20–30 seconds of high-intensity activity. Aerobic activities as short as 800-meter (2-minute) and 1600-meter (5-minute) runs on a track have not shown performance benefits.[53]

Current evidence does not support that creatine can induce structural changes in muscle fibers. The muscles may be larger and weigh more, owing to the presence of creatine and water in complex with creatine. The athlete may gain mass and appear stronger in the gym, but this change is dependent on maintenance supplementation. Short-term studies show a return to normal muscle creatine concentrations and depletion of the extra PCr energy upon cessation of creatine supplementation. Creatine itself does not appear to cause permanent alteration of muscle fiber types.[54,55] Poor study design and inappropriate statistical analysis affect interpretation of existing studies. An observation of increased satellite cells after 8 weeks of supplementation was not validated after 12 weeks or confirmed after cessation of supplement use.[54] A similar observation of increased myosin heavy chain expression and increased type IIx muscle fibers was not properly compared between groups or confirmed as a permanent change by reassessment after cessation of use and washing out of the supplement.[55]

Loading doses of creatine are not required if performance benefits are not desired within 10–14 days.[53] A maintenance dose of 5–6 g/day is adequate to boost muscle creatine levels and is associated with fewer GI adverse effects. If an immediate improvement in strength is required, benefits can be detected in 5 days following a loading dose of creatine at 20 g/day (or 0.3 g/kg/day).[53] This loading dose is usually divided into 4 doses to reduce GI adverse effects of stomach upset and nausea. Nausea may be related to osmotic effects or to malabsorption. Muscle cramping has been reported, but dehydration and heat-related illness have not been associated with long-term studies of creatine supplementation.[53] Creatine supplements have been reported to be misbranded and to contain substances banned by antidoping agencies.[4]

All athletes should be discouraged from using creatine supplements until regulated testing is required. They should be encouraged to seek natural creatine sources from food rather than from supplements. When the athlete insists on using creatine, HCPs can assist the athlete by recommending that creatine be used only as long as necessary (e.g., maintaining supplementation only during the competitive season). No reason exists to continue the supplements during the off season. HCPs should also recommend appropriate additional hydration during creatine exposure, because creatine is a protein that is filtered through the kidneys. If an athlete becomes significantly dehydrated, it is best to temporarily hold creatine use until proper fluid balance is restored.

Dimethylamylamine, Geranium Seeds, and Extracts

Dimethylamylamine (DMAA), also known as methylhexanamine, was previously marketed as a sympathomimetic to treat nasal congestion. DMMA has recently appeared in nutritional supplements; product labeling claims include increased muscle mass and reduced body weight, and imply that the chemical was derived from a natural source, such as geranium stems or extract. These products are associated with multiple cases of cardiac toxicity, acute hepatic failure, liver transplant, and death from cardiogenic shock.[56,57] One report indicated 29 cases of hepatic failure, with 40% of cases requiring hospitalization. Twenty-four of these individuals reported use of a DMAA-containing supplement in the 60 days prior to hepatic injury. Twelve of these individuals reported no other supplement intake besides the DMAA-containing supplement.[56]

Ephedra and Pseudoephedrine

Pseudoephedrine is available without a prescription but, even when taken temporarily for appropriate medical reasons, its use may be troublesome for elite athletes because of random drug testing. Urine concentrations of pseudoephedrine greater than 150 mcg/mL are flagged as prohibited use by WADA. No evidence supports performance enhancement with pseudoephedrine at nonprescription doses (120 mg/day).[58] However, at 2.5 mg/kg, a dose roughly 5 times the recommended nonprescription dose, one study of 7 runners showed an average 6-second improvement in 1500-meter time.[59] Reports that ephedra was associated with hypertension, cardiac arrhythmias, and seizures in otherwise healthy young adults were used to determine that ephedra was unsafe for human consumption, and ephedrine alkaloids were banned from U.S. markets in 2004.[60] No data support ephedra as useful for athletic performance.[58] Athletes and consumers should be aware that plant alkaloids related to ephedra may appear in nutritional supplements (e.g., ma huang, Mormon tea, some weight-loss supplements). Ephedra is available in foreign markets and through internet sales.

Steroidal Precursors and Aromatization Inhibitors

The Anabolic Steroid Control Act of 2004 classified hormone substances that are pharmacologically related to testosterone as legend, or prescription-only, drugs. Dehydroepiandrosterone (DHEA) and androstenedione, prohormone precursors to testosterone, were sold as nutritional supplements prior to passage of the act, but they are now identified as misbranded ingredients in nutritional supplements sold through the internet.[5] Well-designed studies demonstrated significant elevations in estradiol and estrone, but no elevations in serum testosterone, in men who took the supplements.[61] Aromatase inhibitors prevent the conversion of testosterone to estrone, and their use is specifically prohibited by the antidoping agencies. Many body-building supplements claim to include substances such as *Tribulus terrestris* that act as aromatase inhibitors. No data support these claims; however, some supplements have been misbranded with the legend drug tamoxifen.[5] Products that suggest that they boost testosterone or provide aromatase inhibition should not be recommended as performance-enhancing supplements.

Stacking

Sports nutrition products often combine several agents into a single product, a process known as "stacking." Many products include individual vitamins, minerals, metabolites, amino acids, or herbal supplements. Some product labels claim improved endurance and muscle strength or reduction of oxidative stress related to exercise. Ingredients with insufficient data to support a clear positive effect on performance are reviewed in Table 25–2.[1,2,34–46]

Assessment of Performance-Enhancing Nutrients: A Case-Based Approach

Performance enhancers run the gamut from electrolyte solutions to energy bars to herbal supplements. To help someone select a product, the HCP should determine the type of exercise or physical activity in which the individual engages, the intensity and duration of activity, and any products previously tried. The individual should also be asked about any ill effects experienced after physical activity or after using a performance enhancer.

Cases 25–1 and 25–2 illustrate basic assessment of individuals who wish to use a performance-enhancing product.

Sales of sports nutrition products designed to enhance or improve performance are increasing every year. The most common self-treatments are use of creatine to improve muscle power and administration of carbohydrates during exercise to preserve

CASE 25–1

Relevant Evaluation Criteria	Scenario/Model Outcome
Collect	
1. Gather essential information about the patient's symptoms and medical history, including	
a. Description of symptom(s) (i.e., nature, onset, duration, severity, associated symptoms)	Carlos is a second-string running back for his high school football team. He wishes to gain muscle mass and body weight to improve his performance and durability on the football field. His teammates are using supplements to provide protein after morning weight-lifting practice and afternoon football practice. The most commonly used supplements are protein shakes made from powder and Muscle Milk. Carlos plays 15 minutes of game time with no change in his intensity. He does not experience a decline in effort during the course of the game.
b. Description of any factors that seem to precipitate, exacerbate, and/or relieve the patient's symptom(s)	He has gained 6 pounds since starting a weight-lifting program 3 months earlier without modifying his diet. He started to use protein supplements last month but has seen no change in his body weight or strength.
c. Description of the patient's efforts to relieve the symptoms	Protein supplements are expensive. He pays for the supplements with money from his after-school job, but this expense is decreasing his savings to help pay for a college education. He has also brought peanut butter and crackers to eat after morning workouts, because he knows peanuts are a source of protein.
d. Patient's identity	Carlos Hernandez
e. Patient's age, gender, height, and weight	16 years old, male, 5 ft 9 in., 165 lb (75 kg)
f. Patient's occupation	High school student
g. Patient's dietary habits	Carlos and his family own a restaurant that serves food common to their Hispanic culture. They eat healthy salads, rice, and beans although much of their food is fried. Carlos eats dinner at the restaurant and often eats leftover food for breakfast.
h. Patient's sleep habits	Carlos sleeps 6–7 hours on school nights. He works in the family restaurant after school and completes his homework between 8 and 11 pm. He is back at school at 7 am for morning weight lifting.

CASE 25-1 *continued*

Relevant Evaluation Criteria	Scenario/Model Outcome
i. Concurrent medical conditions, prescription and nonprescription medications, and dietary supplements	A preseason medical examination identified no issues. Carlos's blood pressure and fasting glucose levels are normal, and he takes no medications or supplements.
j. Allergies	NKA
k. History of other adverse reactions to medications	None
Assess	
2. Differentiate patient's signs/symptoms, and correctly identify the patient's primary problem(s).	Carlos is a healthy young man with normal weight for his height and normal muscle mass. He desires to build muscle and put on weight to improve his performance in sports.
3. Identify exclusions for self-treatment.	None
4. Formulate a comprehensive list of therapeutic alternatives for the primary problem to determine whether triage to a medical provider is required, and share this information with the patient or caregiver.	Options include (1) Carlos can choose to take no action other than optimization of training. Regular weight-lifting sessions over an extended period of time (≥3 months) are associated with weight gain and improvement in muscle strength without the need for supplements or additional protein intake. (2) Carlos can consider increasing his muscle mass naturally by optimizing his dietary intake of protein with healthy food choices, rather than a nutrition supplement. (3) Carlos can continue to purchase protein supplements for use as a breakfast replacement and for post-workout protein. (4) Carlos can be referred to a dietitian for a complete evaluation of his dietary requirements and recommendations for their appropriate intake.
Plan	
5. Select an optimal therapeutic alternative to address the patient's problem, taking into account patient preferences.	Carlos will adjust his dietary selections to optimize his dietary protein intake.
6. Describe the recommended therapeutic approach to the patient or caregiver.	"You can adjust your food consumption to optimize protein intake and build muscle strength naturally, without having to rely on a packaged nutrition supplement. Keep a record of your protein intake for review and recommendations."
7. Explain to the patient or caregiver the rationale for selecting the recommended therapeutic approach from the considered therapeutic alternatives.	"A diet that includes intact protein will provide protein for muscle building and recovery after intensive workouts. It will also provide a natural source of creatine and the amino acids arginine and glutamine from which the body can build creatine."
Implement	
8. When recommending self-care with nonprescription medications and/or nondrug therapy, convey accurate information to the patient or caregiver.	
a. Appropriate dose and frequency of administration	"The Academy recommends an intake of 1.2–2.0 g/kg/day of protein to optimize muscle building. You weigh 75 kg, so your target intake is 90–150 g per day. The Academy recommends that the protein dose be divided (0.3 g/kg/dose) and consumed at regular intervals. Consuming a small amount of protein within 30 minutes after exercise is optimal to support building muscle."
b. Maximum number of days the therapy should be employed	"An athlete starting a new training program can benefit from an increase in protein intake to help establish a positive nitrogen balance and to build muscle. It is reasonable to boost protein intake to 1.2–2.0 g/kg/day (150 g/day) for 3–4 months and then reduce intake to a maintenance level. Athletes who have been training for several months can maintain their muscle mass and a neutral nitrogen balance with 1.4 g/kg/day of protein intake during maintenance training."

CASE 25-1 *continued*

Relevant Evaluation Criteria	Scenario/Model Outcome
c. Product administration procedures	"The Academy recommends that the athlete consume a small amount of protein (0.3 g/kg/day) within 30 minutes after the completion of intense physical exercise, because protein has been associated with improved muscle building. A simple snack such as 8–12 ounces of skim milk with a 4-ounce serving of chicken or tuna would meet this requirement. Adding a protein dose after each workout would add 45 g (0.6 g/kg/day) to your normal diet and should be adequate for your protein needs. You should consider maintaining a diet journal of your meals and snacks. This information can be assessed later to determine an estimated protein intake and make further recommendations, including referral to a registered dietitian or registered dietitian nutritionist for a more thorough evaluation of your requirements."
d. Expected time to onset of relief	"Performance benefits from intense training can be measured in as little as 2–3 weeks. By comparison, measuring an increase in total body weight may require 2 months or more. The best way for you to assess the gains from your dietary plan is to record your muscle strength gains from training."
e. Degree of relief that can be reasonably expected	"How much gain in muscle mass will help your performance is difficult to measure. Individual performance gains vary. The position of running back is a skill position and depends heavily on other team members to perform their roles well for optimal success."
f. Most common adverse effects	"The adverse effects from small increases in dietary protein intake are minimal. Gastrointestinal discomfort such as bloating, cramping, and diarrhea have been reported. Be sure to drink plenty of fluids to allow the nitrogen waste from the protein to be eliminated through your kidneys."
g. Adverse effects that warrant medical intervention should they occur	"During any period of increased training, you should always tell your coach if you are not feeling well. Any signs of heat illness, muscle cramping, or pain on urination should be reported immediately."
h. Patient options in the event that condition worsens or persists	n/a
i. Product storage requirements	"Most food sources of protein require refrigeration to avoid spoiling and possible bacterial growth on the food. Store your lunches or protein snacks in a cooler or refrigerator if you will not be eating all the food within 2 hours."
Solicit follow-up questions from the patient or caregiver.	"Why isn't a creatine supplement recommended for me although many of my friends are using it?"
Answer the patient's or caregiver's questions.	"The protein available from dietary meat sources will contain a sufficient amount of creatine to meet your needs. As an athlete, you should be aware that dietary supplements may not contain the labeled quantity of protein. Supplements may also be misbranded with performance-enhancing chemicals. It is important, particularly for the high-school athlete, to prepare for competition by achieving appropriate training and experience to reach his or her personal best effort. Using an artificial substance to enhance athletic potential is not as great a victory as reaching it on your own."
Follow-up: Monitor and Evaluate	
9. Assess patient outcome.	Contact the patient within 2–3 weeks to review his diet intake to ensure that he has adjusted his diet appropriately. Consider referral to an RD or RDN if there are additional questions related to Carlos' diet and nutritional requirements.

Key: n/a = Not applicable; NKA = no known allergies; RD = registered dietitian; RDN = registered dietitian nutritionist.

CASE 25-2

Relevant Evaluation Criteria	Scenario/Model Outcome
Collect	
1. Gather essential information about the patient's symptoms and medical history, including	
a. Description of symptom(s) (i.e., nature, onset, duration, severity, associated symptoms)	The patient is an active-duty military member, and is an enthusiastic weight lifter. He has been lifting for 5 years and has reached a plateau in weight lifting. Because he has been unable to improve his lifted weight for the last year, he decided to try some nutrition supplements that claim he will become leaner and stronger. He has asked for a review of his supplements for safe use after experiencing new-onset adverse effects that include abdominal pain, ankle edema, and soreness of the pectoral major muscle on his right side.
b. Description of any factors that seem to precipitate, exacerbate, and/or relieve the patient's symptom(s)	He spends 8 hours a week in the gym, splitting time between upper body and lower body exercise. He reports increasing symptoms of discomfort in the pectoralis muscle group. He reports that he can feel a lump when he massages the muscle. The symptoms are new and began in the last few weeks.
c. Description of the patient's efforts to relieve the symptoms	He has been taking a number of supplements at the recommendation of other soldiers and a personal trainer.
d. Patient's identity	John Wilkins
e. Patient's age, gender, height, and weight	22 years old, male, 6 ft 1 in., 215 lb
f. Patient's occupation	Active military
g. Patient's dietary habits	Eats well at home and prepares healthy meals for his lunch breaks.
h. Patient's sleep habits	Works the day shift and spends his late afternoon in the gym. Generally asleep by 10 pm. Awakens daily at 6 am to go to work.
i. Concurrent medical conditions, prescription and nonprescription medications, and dietary supplements	Has no medical conditions. Creatine 5 g/day, conjugated linoleic acid 770 mg/day, and testosterone booster 2 capsules twice a day. The testosterone booster is labeled to contain a proprietary blend of common vitamins, saw palmetto, *Tribulus terrestris,* and resveratrol.
j. Allergies	NKA
k. History of other adverse reactions to medications	None reported.
Assess	
2. Differentiate patient's signs/symptoms, and correctly identify the patient's primary problem(s).	John's most concerning symptom is that of a lump near his pectoral muscle group. The location puts this lump near his breast, which increases concern. John also complains of abdominal pain that could be an adverse effect of the new supplements that he is taking
3. Identify exclusions for self-treatment.	John should be referred to his HCP for an evaluation of this lump. The temporal association with the use of a supplement labeled to increase testosterone would increase the urgency of this recommendation.
4. Formulate a comprehensive list of therapeutic alternatives for the primary problem to determine whether triage to a medical provider is required, and share this information with the patient or caregiver.	Options include (1) Refer patient to his HCP to evaluate the presence of a lump near his breast. (2) John should discontinue the use of his supplements until further investigation. (3) John does not require performance benefits for competition, and any benefits from these unproven supplements do not outweigh the risk from adverse effects or misbranding. (4) John should consider optimization of his diet for healthy protein sources.

CASE 25-2 *continued*

Relevant Evaluation Criteria	Scenario/Model Outcome
Plan	
5. Select an optimal therapeutic alternative to address the patient's problem, taking into account patient preferences.	John will stop his supplements until he undergoes medical evaluation by a medical professional.
6. Describe the recommended therapeutic approach to the patient or caregiver.	"The lump in your pectoral muscle group should be evaluated by a health care provider. If your provider thinks it is safe for you to continue weight lifting, you can increase the amount of protein in your diet to help build muscle mass."
7. Explain to the patient or caregiver the rationale for selecting the recommended therapeutic approach from the considered therapeutic alternatives.	1. "The presence of lump near the breast of any patient, man or woman, should require further investigation by a health care provider." 2. "Nutritional supplements containing the testosterone precursors androstenedione and DHEA have demonstrated increases in serum estrone in men. The Food and Drug Administration removed these supplements from the market, although misbranding of supplements with these banned substances is still reported." 3. "There is no compelling indication to use these supplements, because none have demonstrated improvements in sports performance." 4. "Optimization and timing of dietary protein intake using whole sources of protein can provide the necessary elements for muscle gain."
Implement	
8. When recommending self-care with nonprescription medications and/or nondrug therapy, convey accurate information to the patient or caregiver.	"*Tribulus terrestris* often is labeled as an aromatase inhibitor, but there is no data to support its inclusion in supplements. The mechanism of saw palmetto is unknown but it may be anti-androgenic; resveratrol does not appear to inhibit aromatase. CLA has not demonstrated any effect on performance despite the product's claims."
a. Appropriate dose and frequency of administration	• "The Academy guidelines recommend a target protein amount of 1.2–2.0 g/kg/day for gaining muscle mass. Any additional protein is consumed for energy." • "Consider taking 30 g of protein within 30 minutes after resistance training exercise. This dose of protein is associated with improved recovery and muscle building." • "Small doses of protein can be obtained from convenient dietary sources, such as nuts, legumes, beans, skim milk, Greek yogurt and tofu."
b. Maximum number of days the therapy should be employed	"Clinical studies of muscle building and weight gain have shown that 2–3 months of training stimulus and good nutrition are typically required to show sustained weight gains."
c. Product administration procedures	n/a
d. Expected time to onset of relief	n/a
e. Degree of relief that can be reasonably expected	"The abdominal pain could be related to supplement use. CLA is an omega-6-polyunsaturated fatty acid and has been associated with gastrointestinal discomfort. If the CLA is the cause of your abdominal discomfort, that should improve within a few days. Creatine has also been associated with abdominal cramping."
f. Most common adverse effects	"Choosing dietary protein sources rather than using packaged supplements should minimize the risk of side effects."
g. Adverse effects that warrant medical intervention should they occur	"In the future, if you return to supplement use and the abdominal cramping persists, you should stop the supplements, including creatine. Similarly, if you observe a urine color that is significantly darker than usual or has a new foul odor, first assess your hydration status. If the urine changes are persistent with proper hydration, you will want to follow up with your primary care provider."

CASE 25-2 *continued*

Relevant Evaluation Criteria	Scenario/Model Outcome
h. Patient options in the event that condition worsens or persists	"If you observe a dark urine that is not improving from proper hydration, you can elect to reduce the protein in your diet for a few days. If the color, or odor persists, then consider seeing your primary care provider."
i. Product storage requirements	"Most food sources of protein require refrigeration."
Solicit follow-up questions from the patient or caregiver.	"I have read that creatine is natural and safe. Do you think that use of creatine could also be related to my symptoms?"
Answer the patient's or caregiver's questions.	"Creatine is a naturally occurring compound found in red meats and fish. Choosing natural sources of creatine from dietary protein is ideal, particularly when dealing with unintended adverse effects. Creatine supplements have not proven to be more effective than natural dietary creatine in building muscle mass. In addition, misbranding of nutrition supplements has occurred, either by intentional or unintentional causes. You should use natural protein sources when possible. If you choose to use a supplement, at least narrow your choice of supplement to a product that has undergone quality assurance testing by an independent lab."
Follow-up: Monitor and Evaluate	
9. Assess patient outcome.	Contact the patient within 1 week to determine whether he has made an appointment with his physician.

Key: CLA = Conjugated linoleic acid; DHEA = dehydroepiandrosterone; HCP = health care provider; n/a = not applicable; NKA = no known allergies.

muscle glycogen and prolong time to fatigue across all sports. Several herbal supplements claim to enhance performance, but evidence to support these claims is currently lacking. Although these natural herbal products are touted as safe, evidence suggests that some may have detrimental effects on long-term health by altering cardiovascular risk, levels of high-density lipoprotein, and levels of natural, sex-determined hormones.

Patient Counseling for Performance-Enhancing Nutrients

The quest for enhanced physical performance has resulted in serious health consequences for some athletes. Clinical studies of many botanical and hormonal dietary supplements touted as performance-enhancing products reveal significant adverse effects and little or no enhancement in physical performance. HCPs should discourage use of performance-enhancing products, because none except creatine has been found to be effective. The box "Patient Education for Performance-Enhancing Nutrients" lists specific information to provide individuals.

Registered dietitians with national board certification as Certified Specialist in Sports Dietetics are uniquely qualified to assist athletes of all levels in evaluating their nutritional needs and to work with them on their hydration, and the quality, quantity, and timing of foods and supplements for optimal performance. Sports dietitians can be found at the Sports, Cardiovascular and Wellness Nutrition Web site (www.scandpg.org).

Key Points for Sports Nutrition and Performance-Enhancing Nutrients

- Training regularly and eating a well-balanced diet are consistently shown to benefit sports performance and activity. Most athletes do not require sports nutrition products.
- Despite marketing claims, the benefits of most performance-enhancing nutritional products and ergogenic aids are unproven, and several may be unsafe.
- Misbranding of nutritional supplements has occurred and can lead to unintentional safety risks and to positive results on screening tests performed by antidoping agencies.
- Most sports nutrition drinks, gels, and bars are significant sources of carbohydrate calories. AAP has developed a position that these carbohydrate and energy drinks should not be used in adolescents and children. They should similarly be avoided in adults who are not engaging in prolonged bouts of exercise (>60–90 minutes).
- Dehydration can significantly affect performance. However, no evidence supports sports nutrition drinks as beneficial when used during events lasting 60 minutes or less. For activity longer than 60 minutes, electrolytes in carbohydrate-containing sports drinks are encouraged and may enhance fluid absorption.
- Sports nutrition drinks containing carbohydrates and electrolytes can prolong the time to fatigue (glycogen depletion) in events or practice lasting 60–90 minutes or longer and, therefore, may be considered when exercise duration is anticipated to exceed this duration.

PATIENT EDUCATION FOR

Patient Education for Performance-Enhancing Nutrients

The objective in selecting a performance enhancer is to choose a product that is safe and appropriate for the type, intensity, and duration of the physical activity. Following the recommendations of a primary care provider (PCP) and other health care providers, as well as carefully following product instructions and the self-care measures listed here, will help ensure optimal therapeutic outcomes.

Muscle Glycogen Preservation

- Carbohydrate-containing sports drinks contain one or more forms of sugar and the electrolytes sodium and potassium. These drinks are optimal for practice or training sessions that last longer than 90 minutes and are generally not needed during the first 60–90 minutes of training. Small doses repeated every 15–20 minutes may be necessary for sustained energy over longer events to maintain glucose levels for performance energy, thereby delaying the time to fatigue.
- Athletes with diabetes should seek the advice of a PCP or sports dietitian before beginning an exercise program to ensure that they are prepared to avoid hypoglycemia while exercising.
- Note that sports bars often contain other macronutrients, such as fats and proteins. Many of these bars are more appropriate for after-exercise recovery than for use during athletic events. If a well-balanced meal is unavailable within 2 hours of exercise, many of these bars may be an appropriate after-exercise fuel replenishment source. (Table 25–1 lists specific products.)
- Long-chain triglycerides can cause discomfort and bloating during intense exercise; therefore, avoid consuming meals that contain large amounts of fat at least 2 hours before exercise.

Enhancement of Muscle Mass

- Athletes do not need to exceed the recommended daily intake of 2.0 g of protein per kilogram of body weight to increase body mass. Available data indicate that higher intakes do not produce additional muscle mass or strength.
- Athletes who ingest high amounts of protein, either through their foods or protein supplements, should discuss this practice with their PCP or sports dietitian. Blood urea nitrogen and serum creatinine levels may be monitored to ascertain whether high-protein intake is affecting kidney function.

Hydration and Electrolytes

- For athletes exercising less than 60–90 minutes, water intake alone is sufficient to complete the exercise.
- Athletes exercising longer than 60 minutes may consider incorporating a carbohydrate- and electrolyte-containing sports drink into the exercise program for optimal performance.
- Endurance athletes exercising for 4 hours and longer are discouraged from drinking only free (regular) water owing to the risk of dilutional hyponatremia. Exercise of this duration (e.g., marathon running, long-distance triathlons) will require electrolyte and carbohydrate replacement for optimal performance.
- Athletes should not target a set quantity of water to consume during exercise; rather, they should drink according to the trigger of thirst. Slower runners and walkers exercising in cool conditions can consume water at a lower rate (sips), whereas faster and heavier athletes and those exercising in heat and humidity should be prepared to drink a large volume. Individual calculations of sweat rate for fluid needs during exercise and an additional calculation for recovery fluids can be made to better meet the athlete's needs.
- Athletes should consume 6–12 ounces of plain water if exercise lasts less than 60 minutes. If exercise lasts longer than 60 minutes, they should consider a carbohydrate- and electrolyte-containing sports drink. (See *Fluid Tips for Training and Competition*, available at http://arizona.openrepository.com/arizona/bitstream/10150/146640/1/az1387-2006.pdf.)
- Carbonated water may cause gastrointestinal distress and bloating; avoid drinking carbonated water before or during an athletic event.

Ergogenic Supplements

- Little or no clinical evidence supports the performance-enhancing claims of most herbal supplements. Quality concerns, misbranding, and contamination with heavy metals have occurred with sufficient frequency to suggest that risk outweighs benefit and that supplements should be avoided.
- Creatine may help increase muscle strength and power in events that require short bursts of power, but gastrointestinal discomfort may occur. To avoid this problem, do not take loading doses. The same benefits occur within 7–14 days of taking a daily maintenance dose of 5 g/day. Maintain proper hydration to assist in the elimination of metabolic waste and to avoid dehydration.
- Long-term use of creatine has no known benefit. The strength improvements of creatine are not maintained and will "wash out" to baseline when the supplement is stopped. Athletes should consider optimizing their nutritional intake rather than using creatine.

➤ To minimize the risk of dehydration or hyponatremia caused by the intake of salt-free fluids, athletes exercising for very long periods of time should use sports drinks that contain electrolytes and carbohydrates rather than using plain water.

➤ Creatine supplementation can increase muscle phosphocreatine concentrations, thus increasing the amount of stored energy in muscles. Phosphocreatine can lend its high-energy phosphate bond to ADP to rapidly restore ATP, allowing increased power for single and repeated activities for 30 seconds or less.

➤ Pseudoephedrine is monitored by the U.S. Anti-Doping Agency, and athletes subject to testing for banned substances should be warned of any product containing pseudoephedrine. A similar warning should be given for any cough and cold product that includes a sympathomimetic amine as a decongestant, such as oxymetazoline nasal spray.

REFERENCES

1. Kreider RB, Wilborn CD, Taylor L, et al. ISSN exercise & sport nutrition review: research & recommendations. *J Int Soc Sports Nutr.* 2010;7:7. Available at: http://jissn.biomedcentral.com/articles/10.1186/1550-2783-1-1-1/. Accessed May 15, 2017. doi: 10.1186/1550-2783-7-7.
2. Travis DT, Erdman KA, Burke LM, et al. Position of the Academy of Nutrition and Dietetics, Dietitians of Canada, and the American College of Sports Medicine: nutrition and athletic performance. *J Acad Nutr Diet.* 2016;116:501–528. doi: 10.1016/j.jand.2015.12.006.
3. Daniells S. NUTRA ingredients-usa.com. Protein powders: The heavy weight in the $16 bn sports nutrition market. September 17, 2015. Available at: http://www.nutraingredients-usa.com/Markets/Protein-powders-the-heavyweight-in-the-16bn-sports-nutrition-market/. Accessed May 15, 2017.
4. deHon O, Coumans B. The continuing story of supplements and doping infractions. *Br J Sports Med.* 2007;41(11):800–5. doi: 10.1136/bjsm.2007.037226.

5. Hullstein IR, Malerod-Fjeld H, Dehnes Y, et al. Black market products confiscated in Norway 2011–2014 compared to analytical findings in urine samples. *Drug Test Anal.* 2015;7:1025–9. doi: 10.1002/dta.1900.
6. World Anti-Doping Agency. *World Anti-Doping Code* 2015. Available at: https://www.wada-ama.org/sites/default/files/resources/files/wada-2015-world-anti-doping-code.pdf/. Accessed May 15, 2017.
7. National College Athletic Association. *National Study of Substance Use Trends among NCAA College Student-Athletes: Final Report.* Indianapolis, IN: The National Collegiate Athletic Association; July 2014. Available at: http://www.ncaa.org/sites/default/files/Substance%20Use%20Final%20Report_FINAL.pdf/. Accessed May 15, 2017.
8. Hoffman JR, Faigenbaum AD, Ratamess NA, et al. Nutritional supplementation and anabolic steroid use in adolescents. *Med Sci Sport Exerc.* 2008;40(1):15–24. doi: 10.1249/mss.0b013e31815a5181.
9. American Academy of Pediatrics Committee on Nutrition and the Council on Sports Medicine and Fitness. Clinical report—sports drinks and energy drinks for children and adolescents: are they appropriate? *Pediatrics.* 2011;127(6):1182–9. doi: 10.1542/peds.2011-0965.
10. Coyle EF. Physical activity as a metabolic stressor. *Am J Clin Nutr.* 2000;72(Suppl):512S–20S. PMID: 10919953.
11. Coyle EF. Substrate utilization during exercise in active people. *Am J Clin Nutr.* 1995;61(4 Suppl):968S–79S. PMID: 7900696.
12. Howowitz JF, Klein S. Lipid metabolism during endurance exercise. *Am J Clin Nutr.* 2000;72(2 Suppl):558S–63S. PMID: 10919960.
13. Spencer MR, Gastin PB. Energy system contribution during 200- to 1500-m running in highly trained athletes. *Med Sci Sport Exerc.* 2001: 33(1);157–62. PMID: 11194103.
14. Burke LM, Hawley JA. Fat and carbohydrate for exercise. *Curr Opin Clin Nutr Metab Care.* 2006;9(4):476–81. doi: 10.1097/01.mco.0000232911.69236.3b.
15. Bemben MG, Lamont HS. Creatine supplementation and exercise performance. *Sports Med.* 2005;35(2):107–25. PMID: 15707376.
16. Foster C, Costill DL, Fink WJ. Effects of preexercise feedings on endurance performance. *Med Sci Sport Exerc.* 1979;11(1):1–5. PMID: 582616.
17. Campbell B, Kreider RB, Ziegenfuss T, et al. International Society of Sports Nutrition position stand: protein and exercise. *J Int Soc Sports Nutr.* 2007;4:8. Available at: https://jissn.biomedcentral.com/articles/10.1186/1550-2783-4-8/. Accessed May 15, 2017. doi: 10.1186/1550-2783-4-8.
18. Tipton KD. Efficacy and consequences of very-high-protein diets for athletes and exercisers. *Proc Nutr Soc.* 2011;70:205–14. doi: 10.1017/S0029665111000024.
19. Hughes J, Shelton B, Hughes B. Suspected dietary supplement injuries in special operations soldiers. *J Spec Oper Med.* 2010;10:14–24.
20. Protein Powders and Drinks Review. Consumer Lab.com. Updated Jun 10th, 2016. Available at: https://www.consumerlab.com/reviews/Protein_Powders_Shakes_Drinks_Sports/NutritionDrinks/#quality/. Accessed May 15, 2017.
21. American College of Sports Medicine, Sawka MN, Burke LM, et al. American College of Sports Medicine position stand: Exercise and fluid replacement. *Med Sci Sport Exerc.* 2007;39(2):377–90. doi: 10.1249/mss.0b013e31802ca597.
22. Almond CS, Shin AY, Fortescue EB, et al. Hyponatremia among runners in the Boston marathon. *N Engl J Med.* 2005;325(15):1550–6. doi: 10.1056/NEJMoa043901.
23. Hew-Butler T, Verbalis JG, Noakes TD. Updated fluid recommendation: position statement from the International Marathon Medical Directors Association (IMMDA). *Clin J Sport Med.* 2006;16(4):283–92.
24. Wharham PC, Speedy DB, Noakes TD, et al. NSAID use increases the risk of developing hyponatremia during an ironman triathlon. *Med Sci Sports Exerc.* 2006;38(4):618–22. doi: 10.1249/01.mss.0000210209.40694.09.
25. Hampsom NB, Pollock NW, Piantadosi CA. Oxygenated water and athletic performance. *JAMA.* 2003;290(18):2408–9. doi: 10.1001/jama.290.18.2408-c.
26. Valentine R, Saunders MJ, Todd MK, et al. Influence of carbohydrate-protein beverage on cycling endurance and indices of muscle disruption. *Int J Sport Nutr Exerc Metab.* 2008;18(4):363–78. PMID: 18708686.
27. Toone RJ, Betts JA. Isocaloric carbohydrate versus carbohydrate-protein ingestion and cycling time-trial performance. *Int J Sport Nutr Exerc Metab.* 2010;20(1):34–43. PMID: 20190350.
28. van Rosendal SP, Osborne MA, Fassett RG, et al. Physiological and performance effects of glycerol hyperhydration and rehydration. *Nutr Rev.* 2009;67(12):690–705. doi: 10.1111/j.1753-4887.2009.00254.x.
29. Ke rsick C, Harvey T, Stout J, et al. International Society of Sports Nutrition position stand: nutrient timing. *J Int Soc Sports Nutr.* 2008;5:17. doi: 10.1186/1550-2783-5-17. Available at: http://jissn.biomedcentral.com/articles/10.1186/1550-2783-5-17/. Accessed May 15, 2017.
30. Jeukendrup AE, Killer SC. The myths surrounding pre-exercise carbohydrate feeding. *Ann Nutr Metab.* 2010;57(Suppl 2):18–25. doi: 10.1159/000322698.
31. Shirreffs SM, Watson P, Maughan RJ. Milk as an effective post-exercise rehydration drink. *Br J Nutr.* 2007;98(1):173–80. doi: 10.1159/000322698.
32. Pritchett K, Bishop P, Pritchett R, et al. Acute effects of chocolate milk and a commercial recovery beverage on post exercise recovery indices and endurance cycling performance. *Appl Physiol Nutr Metab.* 2009; 34(6):1017–22. doi: 10.1139/H09-104.
33. Thomas K, Morris P, Stevenson E. Improved endurance capacity following chocolate milk consumption compared with 2 commercially available sport drinks. *Appl Physiol Nutr Metab.* 2009;34(1):78–82. doi: 10.1139/H08-137.
34. Fisher-Wellman K, Bloomer RJ. Acute exercise and oxidative stress: a 30 year history. *Dyn Med.* 2009;8:1–25. doi: 10.1186/1476-5918-8-1.
35. Flakoll P, Sharp R, Levenhagen D, et al. Effect of beta-hydroxy-beta-methylbutyrate, arginine and lysine supplementation on strength, functionality, body composition, and protein metabolism in elderly women. *Nutrition.* 2004;20(5):445–51. doi: 10.1016/j.nut.2004.01.009.
36. Cheuvront SN, Carter R, Kolka MA, et al. Branched-chain amino acid supplementation and human performance when hypohydrated in the heat. *J Appl Physiol.* 2004;97(4):1275–82. doi: 10.1152/japplphysiol.00357.2004.
37. Parcell AC, Smith JM, Schulthies SS, et al. Cordyceps sinensis (CordyMax Cs-4) supplementation does not improve endurance exercise performance. *Int J Sport Nutr Exerc Metab.* 2004;14(2):236–42. PMID: 15118196.
38. Colson SN, Wyatt FB, Johnston DL, et al. Cordyceps sinensis- and Rhodiola rosea-based supplementation in male cyclists and its effect on muscle tissue oxygen saturation. *J Strength Cond Res.* 2005;19(2):358–63. doi: 10.1519/R-15844.1.
39. Goulet ED, Dionne IJ. Assessment of the effects of Eleutherococcus senticosus on endurance performance. *Int J Sport Nutr Exerc Metab.* 2005; 15(1):75–83. PMID: 15902991.
40. Engels H, Fahlman MM, Wirth JC. Effects of ginseng on secretory IgA, performance and recovery from interval exercise. *Med Sci Sports Exerc.* 2003;35(4):690–6. doi: 10.1249/01.MSS.0000058363.23986.D2.
41. Nelson JL, Robergs RA. Exploring the potential ergogenic effects of glycerol hyperhydration. *Sports Med.* 2007;37(11):981–1000. PMID: 17953468.
42. Wilson JM, Fitschen PJ, Campbell B, et al. International Society of Sports Nutrition position stand: beta-hydroxy-beta-methylbutyrate (HMB). *J Int Soc Sports Nutr.* 2013;10:6. doi: 10.1186/1550-2783-10-6. Available at: http://jissn.biomedcentral.com/articles/10.1186/1550-2783-10-6/. Accessed May 15, 2017.
43. Buchman AL, Awal MA, Jenden D, et al. The effect of lecithin supplementation on plasma choline concentrations during a marathon. *J Am Coll Nutr.* 2000;19(6):768–70. PMID: 11194530.
44. De Bock K, Eijnde BO, Ramaekers M, et al. Acute Rhodiola rosea intake can improve endurance exercise performance. *Int J Sport Nutr Exerc Metab.* 2004;14(3):298–307. PMID: 15256690.
45. Earnest CP, Morss GM. Effects of a commercial herbal-based formula on exercise performance in cyclists. *Med Sci Sports Exerc.* 2004;36(3):504–9. PMID: 15076794.
46. Chen C, Hou C, Bernard JR, et al. Rhodiola crenulata- and Cordyceps sinesis-based supplement boosts aerobic exercise performance after short-term high altitude training. *High Alt Med Biol.* 2014;15:371–9. doi: 10.1089/ham.2013.1114.
47. Davis JK. Caffeine and anaerobic performance: ergogenic value and mechanism of action. *Sports Med.* 2009;39(10):813–32. doi: 10.2165/11317770-000000000-00000.

48. Campbell B, Wilborn C, LaBounty P, et al. International Society of Sports Nutrition position stand: energy drinks. *J Int Soc Sports Nutr.* 2013;10(1): 1–16. doi: 10.1186/1550-2783-10-1.
49. Jain P, Hall-may E, Golabek K, et al. A comparison of sports and energy drinks—Physiochemical properties and enamel dissolution. *Gen Dent.* 2012;60:190–7.
50. Kurtz AM, Leong J, Anand M, et al. Effects of caffeinated versus decaffeinated energy shots on blood pressure and heart rate in healthy young volunteers. *Pharmacotherapy.* 2013;33(8):779–86. doi: 10.1002/phar.1296.
51. Field AE, Sonneville KR, Falbe J, et al. Association of sports drinks with weight gain among adolescents and young adults. *Obesity.* 2014;22: 2238–43. doi: 10.1002/oby.20845.
52. Howland J, Rohsenow JR. Risks of energy drinks mixed with alcohol. *JAMA.* 2013;309(3):245–6. doi: 10.1001/jama.2012.187978.
53. Terjung RL, Clarkson P, Eichner ER, et al. American College of Sports Medicine consensus statement. The physiological and health effects of oral creatine supplementation. *Med Sci Sport Exerc.* 2000;32(3):706–17. PMID: 10731017.
54. Olsen S, Aagaard P, Kadi F, et al. Creatine supplementation augments the increase in satellite cell and myonuclei number in human skeletal muscle induced by strength training. *J Physiol.* 2006;573(Pt 2):525–34. doi: 10.1113/jphysiol.2006.107359.
55. Willoughby DS, Rosene J. Effects of oral creatine and resistance training on myosin heavy chain expression. *Med Sci Sport Exerc.* 2001;33(10): 1674–81. doi: 10.1249/01.MSS.0000069746.05241.F0.
56. Centers for Disease Control and Prevention. Notes from the field: acute hepatitis and liver failure following the use of a dietary supplement intended for weight loss or muscle building, May–October 2013. *MMWR Morb Mortal Wkly Rep.* 2013;62(40):817–9. PMID: 24113901.
57. Eliason MJ, Eichner A, Cancio A, et al. Case reports: death of active duty soldiers following ingestion of dietary supplements containing 1,3-dimethylamylamine (DMAA). *Mil Med.* 2012;12:1455–9. PMID: 23397688.
58. Shekelle PG, Hardy ML, Morton SC, et al. Efficacy and safety of ephedra and ephedrine for weight loss and athletic performance: a meta analysis. *JAMA.* 2003;289(12):1537–45. doi: 10.1001/jama.289.12.1537.
59. Hodges K, Hancock S, Currell K, et al. Pseudoephedrine enhances performance in 1500m runners. *Med Sci Sports Exerc.* 2006;38(2):329–33. doi: 10.1249.01.mss.0000183201.79330.9c.
60. Centers for Disease Control and Prevention. Adverse events associated with ephedrine containing products–Texas, December 1993–September 1995. *MMWR Morb Mortal Wkly Rep.* 1996;45(32):689–93. PMID: 8772203.
61. Hoffman JR, Kraemer WJ, Bhasin S, et al. Position stand on androgen and human growth hormone use. *J Strength Cond Res.* 2009;23(5 Suppl): S1–S59. doi: 10.1249.01.mss.0000183201.79330.9c.

CHAPTER 26

INFANT NUTRITION AND SPECIAL NUTRITIONAL NEEDS OF CHILDREN

M. PETREA COBER

Human milk is most physiologically suited to infants and is their optimal milk source up to the age of 12 months. The American Academy of Pediatrics (AAP) recommends that human milk be used as the sole source of nutrition for infants during the first 6 months of life. For infants whose mothers choose not to breastfeed, the nutritional quality, safety, and convenience of infant formulas make such products an appropriate alternative. Variations among formulas allow for product selection to meet a specific infant's nutritional needs, along with considerations of palatability, digestibility, nutrient sources, convenience, and cost.

In the area of infant nutrition, an important role for today's pharmacist is as an additional information resource for parents or other caregivers to promote successful breastfeeding. In addition, in consultation with the child's parents and primary care provider (PCP), the pharmacist also can evaluate indications, advise on formula selection, and help ensure its appropriate use. This service requires in-depth knowledge about infant and child nutrition needs, breastfeeding issues and practices, and commercially prepared infant and pediatric formulas, including differences in formula composition and specific uses for therapeutic formulas.

Some children may require specialized enteral formulas after the age of 1 year because of various disease states and conditions. Familiarity with these products and their appropriate use is essential to allow the pharmacist to answer related caregiver questions, facilitate their procurement, and perform triage for associated complications.

Organ Maturation and Infant Growth

Knowledge of the development of the gastrointestinal (GI) tract and the kidney is crucial to understanding infant nutrition. Different aspects of maturation are reflected in physiologic parameters and events of digestive function, as reviewed in this section.

In clinical practice, monitoring growth and growth rate using World Health Organization (WHO) growth charts is important for assessing the infant for possible abnormal or unhealthy growth. WHO growth charts are recommended for use in children younger than 24 months of age, and the Centers for Disease Control and Prevention (CDC) growth charts are recommended for use in children 24 months and older.[1]

Gastrointestinal Maturation

By the completion of 27 weeks gestational age, all segments of the fetal GI tract are formed and display some physiologic function. From 28 weeks gestational age, however, maximal GI tract growth and differentiation occurs. Therefore, premature infants—those born before 37 weeks of gestation—often have reduced GI tract function, especially those born before 32 weeks. Transition from intrauterine nutrition delivered through the maternal–fetal unit (i.e., the placenta) to extrauterine nutrition derived from mother's milk or infant formula requires the maturation of many physiologic processes. These processes include effective sucking, swallowing, gastric emptying, intestinal peristalsis, and defecation; salivary, gastric, pancreatic, and hepatobiliary secretions; and intestinal brush border enzymes and transport systems (Table 26–1).[2]

Nutritive sucking develops at approximately 33–34 weeks of gestation. In term infants, a mature, efficient pattern of sucking is seen within a few days after birth. In premature infants, an immature, inefficient pattern may persist for a month or longer. Infants born before they attain a gestational age of 34 weeks cannot coordinate sucking, swallowing, and breathing and may therefore require tube feedings for several weeks to months until these reflexes mature. Liquid nutrition is appropriate for all infants until complex tongue movements and swallowing reflexes mature. Maturation of these reflexes typically occurs by the age of 4–6 months, and it is at this time that solid foods can be safely added to the infant's diet.[2] For infants born prematurely, corrected gestational age should be used to determine these developmental milestones. *Corrected gestational age* is calculated by adding the chronologic age of the patient to the gestational age at birth. Once premature infants reach 40 weeks corrected gestational age, their growth and developmental parameters are assessed using an age adjusted for gestational age (i.e., chronologic age in weeks minus number of weeks premature). For example, if a patient is born at 23 weeks' gestational age and is currently 25 weeks old, the corrected gestational age would be 48 weeks, with a maturation age of 2 months (or 8 weeks) corrected age. The patient would therefore be developmentally equivalent to a term infant at 2 months of age.

Early in life, frequent feedings (every 2–3 hours) are necessary, because the stomach capacity of a term newborn with a birth weight greater than 2500 g (5 pounds 8 ounces) is only 20–90 mL. Gastric capacity increases to 90–150 mL by 1 month of age, at which time longer periods between feedings are possible, enabling the infant to sleep for longer periods of time (i.e., through the night). Human milk empties more rapidly from the stomach than infant formula; therefore, human milk–fed infants typically eat more often than their formula-fed peers.

In term infants, gastric acid and pepsin secretion peak in the first 10 days of life, decrease between 10 and 30 days of life, and then increase to adult levels by the age of 3 months. In premature

TABLE 26-1 Gastrointestinal Maturation

Function	Weeks of Gestation When First Detectable	Comments
Sucking and swallowing	16	16 weeks: swallowing of amniotic fluid
		26 weeks: sucking
		33–35 weeks: mature, coordinated sucking, swallowing, and breathing
Gastric motility and secretion	20	Gastric emptying delayed in first few days of life; affected by caloric density, carbohydrate concentration, pathologic conditions
Intestinal motility	20	26–30 weeks: disorganized contractile activity
		30–34 weeks: repetitive groups of contractions
		34–35 weeks: more mature migrating motor complexes

Digestion and Absorption

Important Factors	Weeks of Gestation When First Detectable	Proportion of Adult Values
Protein		
Enterokinase	24–26	30 weeks: 20%
		Term: 10%–25%
Hydrochloric acid	At birth	30 weeks: <20%
		Term: <30%
		First 3 months: 50%
Peptidases	<12	30 weeks: 15%
		Term: nearly 100%
Trypsinogen/chymotrypsinogen	20	Term: 10%–60%
Amino acid transport	ND	Term: nearly 100%
Macromolecule absorption	ND	Term: nearly 100%
Fat		
Lingual lipase	30	Term: nearly 100%
Pancreatic lipase	16–20	Term: 5%–10%
Bile acids	22	32 weeks: 25%
		Term: 50%
Medium-chain triglyceride uptake	ND	100% (absorption occurs in the stomach)
Long-chain triglyceride uptake	ND	Term: 10%–90%
Carbohydrate		
Pancreatic alpha-amylase	22–30	Term: 0%
		6 months of age: secretion begins
Salivary alpha-amylase	16	30 weeks: 0%
		Term: 10%–20%
Lactase	10	28–34 weeks: 30%
		Term: nearly 100%
Monosaccharide absorption	11–19	Term: glucose absorption: 50%–60%

Key: ND = Not determined.

Source: Reference 2; and Kleinman RE, Kamin DS. Gastrointestinal development. In: Baker SS, Baker RD, Davis AM, eds. *Pediatric Nutrition Support*. Sudbury, MA: Jones & Bartlett; 2007:15–27.

infants, basal acid output is lower than that in term infants but increases with postnatal age. Milk in the infant's stomach causes a sharp increase in the pH of the gastric contents and a slower return to lower pH values than in older children and adults. Gastric acidity in the newborn is unsuitable for optimal pepsin action. Therefore, little protein digestion occurs in the stomach, because of this low pepsin activity. The extent of protein absorption, however, is similar to that seen in children and adults. Amino acids and peptides produced by protein digestion are absorbed passively or by active transport mechanisms that reach adult capacity by the age of 14 weeks.

Premature and full-term infants can digest most carbohydrates, because the production of intestinal enzymes such as sucrase, maltase, isomaltase, and glucoamylase is sufficiently mature at birth. Lactase activity increases relatively late in fetal life and begins to decline after the age of 3 years, especially in African American children and those of Asian ancestry. By adulthood, approximately 15% of Whites, 40% of Asian Americans, and 85% of African Americans are deficient in intestinal lactase.[3] Pancreatic amylase secretion does not reach adult levels until the age of approximately 1 year. Salivary amylase may help compensate for this relative lactase and amylase deficiency in early infancy. Despite this relative lactase deficiency, most term and preterm infants tolerate lactose-containing formulas, with negligible unabsorbed carbohydrate output in the stool. Unabsorbed lactose that enters the colon undergoes bacterial fermentation (colonic salvage) to short-chain fatty acids, thereby creating an acidic environment that favors growth of acidophilic bacterial flora (lactobacilli) and suppresses growth of more pathogenic organisms. This acidity also promotes water absorption and prevents osmotic diarrhea. Because of the relative abundance of glucoamylase compared with lactase in the premature infant's intestine, glucose polymers are digested and absorbed better than lactose is.[2]

Newborns exhibit low concentrations of pancreatic lipase and slow rates of synthesis of bile acid. Both pancreatic lipase and bile acids are important for fat absorption. The rate of bile acid synthesis increases throughout gestation and with increasing postnatal age. The bile acid pool in a premature infant is one-fourth that in an adult, whereas a term infant's is one-half that in an adult. However, fat malabsorption is not a major problem in preterm or term infants, because of the presence of lingual and gastric lipases. Infants born earlier than 34 weeks' gestation, however, may exhibit steatorrhea.

Intestinal length also may affect nutrient absorption. At birth, a term infant's small intestine is approximately 270 cm (106 inches) long. From 28 weeks gestational age, the intestinal length approximately doubles. Infants born prematurely, therefore, have less small intestine and consequently a decreased surface area for absorption. Adult intestinal length of 4–5 m (13–16.5 feet) is reached by the age of approximately 4 years.

Kidney Maturation

Maturation of the kidney also is important in nutrition because it determines the ability of the kidney to excrete a solute load. Glomerular filtration begins around week 9 of fetal life; however, kidney function does not appear to be necessary for normal intrauterine homeostasis, because the placenta serves as the major excretory organ. After birth, the rate of glomerular filtration increases until growth stops, toward the end of the second decade of life. Even after correction for body surface area, the glomerular filtration rate in children does not approximate adult values until the third year of life.

Growth

Birth weight is determined primarily by maternal prepregnancy weight and pregnancy weight changes. The average birth weight of a term infant is approximately 3500 g (7 pounds 8 ounces). Premature infants are categorized by birth weight as follows: *low-birth-weight* infants weigh less than 2500 g (5 pounds 8 ounces); *very low-birth-weight* infants weigh less than 1500 g (3 pounds 4 ounces); *extremely low-birth-weight infants* weigh less than 1000 g (2 pounds 3 ounces); and so-called *micropreemies* weigh less than 750 g (1 pound 10 ounces).

Water weight loss (6%–10% of body weight) occurs immediately after birth over a period of 1–2 weeks and is followed by an average weight gain of 1%–2% of birth weight daily (25–35 g/day in term infants) during the first 4 months and then 15 g/day over the next 8 months. Most term infants double their birth weight by 4–6 months of age and triple it by 12 months. Premature infants may reach these milestones sooner than predicted by their corrected gestational age. From the age of 2 years to approximately 10 years, the growth rate is fairly constant at approximately 2.3 kg (5 pounds) each year. Growth velocity increases, and a major growth spurt occurs during adolescence. Height shows a growth pattern similar to that of weight; most infants increase their length by 50% in the first year, 100% in the first 4 years, and 300% by the age of 13 years. Changes in body composition accompany height and weight changes. Most notably, total body water decreases as adipose tissue increases. Total body water accounts for approximately 90% of total body weight at 24 weeks of gestation, 70% at term, and 60% by 1 year of age.

Normal values for weight, length/height, and head circumference (until 3 years of age) in infants and children generally are expressed in terms of percentile-for-age; the reference standards most commonly used are WHO growth standards for infants and children younger than 2 years of age and the CDC growth charts developed by the National Center for Health Statistics (NCHS) for children 2 years of age and older. In 2006, representatives from CDC, the National Institutes of Health (NIH), and AAP met to discuss the use of the recently released WHO growth standards in the United States. Three primary benefits of WHO growth standards for infants and children younger than 2 years of age were cited as the reason for their use in the United States: (1) establishing growth of the breast-fed infant as the norm for growth, (2) providing a better description of physiologic growth in infancy, and (3) basing information on a high-quality study designed explicitly for creating growth charts. For children 2 years of age and older, the CDC growth charts should still be used, because the methods used to create both the CDC and WHO growth charts were similar for 2- to 5-year-olds, and WHO growth charts represent only children up to 5 years of age.[1] Charts can be downloaded free of charge on the CDC website (www.cdc.gov/growthcharts). The infant charts are intended for use in term infants. In premature infants, growth parameters should be plotted on these charts using an age corrected for gestational age, as discussed previously, until the age of 24 months for weight and length/height and 24–36 months for head circumference. Charts for premature infants younger than 40 weeks' gestational age and children with certain pathologic conditions (e.g., cerebral palsy, Turner syndrome) are available and should be used when appropriate. These specialized growth charts can be found on various websites, including those for the Kennedy Krieger Institute for children with disorders of the brain and spinal cord, such as cerebral palsy (www.kennedykrieger.org), and the Turner Syndrome Society of the United States (www.turnersyndrome.org). Specialized growth charts are no longer recommended by the AAP guidelines for children with Down syndrome, and standard charts for age should be used in this population.[4] Some experts, however, advocate for the continued use of such charts that have recently been updated.[5]

The most commonly used charts for premature infants are either the Fenton charts or the Babson and Benda charts (available at www.ucalgray.ca/fenton/2013chart or www.biomedcentral.com/1471-2431/3/13, respectively). Most infants' growth parameters will fall between the 2nd and 98th percentiles on the gender-specific weight-for-age, length/height-for-age, weight-for-length, and head circumference-for-age charts. In children younger than 2 years of age, a recumbent length measurement is obtained in the primary care office, whereas in children 2 years of age or older, a standing height is measured. Most children grow along a percentile established shortly after birth, but spurts and plateaus are common. *Failure to thrive* is defined as a fall of 2 or more growth percentiles from a previously established percentile in 6 months or less. If growth is not progressing as expected, particularly in the first year of life, when growth should be rapid, the infant's diet and other potential contributory factors (e.g., environment, diseases, syndromes) should be evaluated. Satisfactory growth is the most sensitive indicator of whether nutritional needs are being met.

For children 2 years and older, body mass index (BMI)-for-age charts can be useful in assessing obesity risk. BMI, a measure of body weight adjusted for height, is a useful tool to assess body fat. BMI is calculated as weight in kilograms divided by height in meters squared. In 2005, the American Medical Association, in collaboration with the Health Resources and Services Administration and the CDC, convened an expert committee charged with revising these recommendations. The committee's nomenclature changes were intended to make it easier to discuss children's weight issues with parents and children and to effect the transition to adult assessments. These new recommendations state that a child whose BMI is at or above the 85th percentile but below the 95th percentile or 30 kg/m^2, whichever is smaller, should be classified as "overweight." A child whose BMI is at or above the 95th percentile or 30 kg/m^2, whichever is smaller, should be classified as "obese."[6] In 2011–2012, 7.1% of infants and toddlers from birth to 2 years of age had BMIs at or above the 97th percentile on WHO growth charts, whereas 17% of children and adolescents 2–19 years of age in 2011–2014 had values at or above the 95th percentile on the CDC growth charts.[7,8] In 2011–2012, 31.8% had values at or above the 85th percentile for BMI-for-age growth on the CDC growth charts. The prevalence of obesity in children and adolescents 2–9 years of age has not statistically changed since 2008–2009 (16.8% in 2008–2009 versus 17.2% in 2013–2014). The incidence of obesity still remains high. However, the proportion of obesity prevalence differs among various ethnic groups, with 21.9% of Hispanics, 19.5% of non-Hispanic Blacks, 14.7% of non-Hispanic Whites, and 8.6% of non-Hispanic Asians between 2 and 19 years of age classified as obese.

A BMI below the 5th percentile is indicative of underweight. In applying these definitions, however, the pharmacist should keep in mind that because of the way the growth charts were developed, values for 5% of normally growing and healthy children will fall below the 5th percentile and those for another 5% will fall above the 95th percentile on the weight-for-age or height-for-age charts. These children should not be branded as "malnourished" and "obese," respectively.

Energy Requirements and Growth

Acceptable growth is achievable only with adequate intake, absorption, and utilization of energy, protein, carbohydrates, minerals, and vitamins. The Food and Nutrition Board of the National Research Council has established dietary reference intakes (DRIs) as reference values for nutrient intake sufficiency and safety. The DRIs for micronutrients are discussed in detail in Chapter 23 and tables in that chapter list the current established recommended dietary allowances (RDAs) and adequate intakes (AIs) for healthy infants and children. Table 26–2 lists the DRIs of macronutrients for healthy infants and children.[9] Children with various diseases and syndromes may have different needs. An example is the need for "catch-up" calories in infants and children recovering from failure to thrive. Calorie requirements for catch-up growth are often 1.25 times those of age-matched peers, depending on the degree of catch-up growth needed. In patients with fat malabsorption (e.g., patients with cystic fibrosis or other cause of pancreatic insufficiency, bile acid deficiency, or short bowel syndrome), calories for catch-up growth may be 1.5 times or more those of age-matched peers.

Energy requirements vary with age and clinical condition. Total energy expenditure is a combination of basal energy needs, the energy required to digest food (thermic effect of feeding, also called "specific dynamic action of food"), thermoregulation, and activity. Estimates of energy requirements for infants and children are based on meeting total energy expenditure plus promoting growth. An infant's energy requirement is higher in relation to body mass than that of an adult or older child because of the rapid growth experienced during infancy. Estimated energy requirements for term infants and children are shown in Table 26–2.[9] Although no RDA has been established, premature infants require as much as 120–150 kcal/kg/day or more for adequate growth.

Infant Nutritional Standards

An amendment to the Food, Drug, and Cosmetic Act (Infant Formula Act of 1980, amended 1986) gives the U.S. Food and Drug Administration (FDA) the authority to revise nutrient levels for infant formulas, establish quality control, and require adequate labeling. FDA sets specifications for minimum amounts of 29 nutrients and maximum amounts of 9 of those nutrients. All formulas marketed in the United States must meet these requirements. Parents should be cautioned against using any infant formula not manufactured in the United States. FDA alerts have warned of the dangers of using infant formulas from China whose contents fall well below FDA standards. Formulas granted exemption from FDA-established nutrient specifications must be labeled for use in infants with specific indications, such as inborn errors of metabolism, low birth weight, or other unusual medical problems or dietary needs. A list of exempt formulas can be obtained at the FDA website (www.fda.gov). In addition, FDA has published guidance documents to clarify certain requirements for industry on labeling of infant formula, including nutrient content claims, health claims and qualified health claims, and requirements for preparation directions and a statement regarding the need to add or not add water. The September 2016 guidance document is available at http://www.fda.gov/FoodGuidances.

TABLE 26-2 Dietary Reference Intakes of Macronutrients for Full-Term Infants and Children[a,b]

Nutrient	0–6 Months	7–12 Months	1–3 Years	4–8 Years	9–13 Years
Energy[c] (kcal/day)	M: 570 F: 520	M: 743 F: 676	M: 1046 F: 992	M: 1742 F: 1642	M: 2279 F: 2071
Protein[c] (g/kg/day)	1.5	1.5[d]	1.1[d]	0.95[d]	0.95[d]
(g/day)	9.1	13.5[d]	13[d]	19[d]	34[d]
Carbohydrate (g/day)	60	95	130[d]	130[d]	130[d]
Water (L/day)[e]	0.7	0.8	1.3	1.7	M: 2.4 F: 2.1
Fat (g/day)	31	30	ND	ND	ND
Alpha-linolenic acid (g/day)	0.5	0.5	0.7	0.9	M: 1.2 F: 1
Linoleic acid (g/day)	4.4	4.6	7	10	M: 12 F: 10
Fiber (g/day)	ND	ND	19	25	M: 31 F: 26

Key: AI = Adequate intake; DRI = dietary reference intake; F = female; M = male; ND = not determined; RDA = recommended dietary allowance.

[a] Expressed as AIs unless noted otherwise.

[b] DRIs have not been established for premature infants.

[c] Estimated requirements; include needs associated with growth (i.e., energy expenditure plus energy deposition). The assumed normal body weight and length used for the DRIs are as follows: 0–6 months: 6 kg, 62 cm; 7–12 months: 9 kg, 71 cm; 1–3 years: 12 kg, 86 cm; 4–8 years: 20 kg, 115 cm; and 9–13 years: 36 kg, 144 cm for males, 37 kg, 144 cm for females.

[d] Expressed as RDA.

[e] Water from all sources including formula, human milk, foods, beverages, and drinking water.

Source: Reference 9.

Components of a Healthy Diet

Infants require the same dietary components as for adults: fluid, carbohydrates, proteins, fats, and micronutrients. However, the desired proportions of these components in the infant diet differ from those recommended for adults.

Fluid

Water is an important part of an infant's diet, in that it makes up a larger proportion of the infant's body weight than that of older children or adults. The Holliday–Segar method is most often used to estimate maintenance water needs: 100 mL/kg/day for the first 10 kg of body weight, plus 50 mL/kg/day for each kilogram between 10 and 20 kg, and 20 mL/kg/day for each kilogram over 20 kg. Body surface area also may be used to estimate daily fluid requirements; fluid requirements are approximately 1500 mL/m^2/day. These methods, however, will underestimate the needs of premature infants, whose requirements are in general much higher (i.e., 120–170 mL/kg/day, or as high as 200 mL/kg/day based on specific patient circumstances). Adequate water intake in the first 6 months of life can be derived from human milk or formula. Both contain sufficient amounts of water, so the normal, healthy infant does not need supplemental water. At the age of 6–12 months, when solid foods are introduced, water intake remains high, because most infant foods contain at least 60%–70% more water than other foods, and formula or human milk intake should still be high.

Renal excretion, evaporation from the skin and lungs, and, to a lesser extent, elimination of feces are the major routes of fluid loss. Increased water loss caused by diarrhea, fever, or unusually rapid breathing, particularly in concert with decreased water intake, may result in significant dehydration and electrolyte imbalance and must be offset by fluid intake in excess of maintenance needs.

Carbohydrates

An AI for carbohydrates has been established for infants (Table 26–2).[9] Under normal circumstances, an infant can efficiently use a diet with 40%–50% of total calories from a carbohydrate source. Carbohydrate intake should be balanced with adequate fat intake to allow proper neurologic development. A carbohydrate-free diet is generally undesirable because it may lead to metabolic modifications favoring fatty acid breakdown, dehydration, and tissue protein and cation loss. However, children with seizure disorders may receive an essentially carbohydrate-free diet—the ketogenic diet—because these metabolic effects may facilitate seizure control. Use of a ketogenic diet should be under the direct, strict supervision of a physician along with a registered dietitian or other qualified health care provider (HCP).

Lactose, the primary carbohydrate source in human milk and most milk-based formulas, is hydrolyzed to its monosaccharide components, glucose and galactose, by gastric acid and lactase. Congenital lactase deficiency is a rare type of lactose intolerance resulting from an inborn error of metabolism. Infants born prematurely, before the maturation of significant lactase activity (before approximately 36 weeks' gestation), are relatively lactase-deficient. Secondary lactase deficiency is a temporary reduction in intestinal lactase caused by gastroenteritis or significant malnutrition. Because of low lactase activity, infants with congenital lactase deficiency, premature infants, and infants recovering from diarrhea or severe malnutrition may be unable to completely metabolize the lactose found in human milk or milk-based infant formulas, with consequent development of lactose intolerance resulting in diarrhea, abdominal pain or distention, bloating, gas, and cramping.

Fiber intake is of considerable interest because in adults, high-fiber diets have been associated with the prevention of diverticular disease, colon cancer, and coronary heart disease. (See Chapter 24 for further discussion of fiber.) AAP has recommended a daily fiber intake calculated using the following equation: fiber (g/day) = age (in years) plus 5. Age-plus-10 g/day is also thought to be a safe intake.[10] An AI for fiber for infants 0–12 months of age has not been established. Infants rarely require fiber to maintain normal bowel function. Starting from the age of 6–12 months, however, whole cereals, green vegetables, and legumes typically are introduced to provide a source of fiber in the infant's diet. The fiber AI for older children is shown in Table 26–2. Adult values are reached by the teenage years.

Protein and Amino Acids

The most recent revision of the DRIs established new AIs for protein in term infants and children (Table 26–2).[9] Total body protein increases by an average of 3.5 g/day in the first 4 months of life and by 3.1 g/day over the next 8 months, representing an overall increase in body protein composition from 11% to 15% of total body weight.

A specific protein's amino acid composition (i.e., chemical makeup) also is important. Amino acids are classified as essential (or indispensable), nonessential, or conditionally essential. The amino acids cysteine, histidine, isoleucine, leucine, lysine, methionine, phenylalanine, threonine, tryptophan, tyrosine, and valine are considered essential for infants because the human body cannot synthesize them from other amino acid and carbohydrate precursors. In the neonate and young infant, immature biochemical pathways for synthesis or conversion of amino acids may prevent adequate synthesis for normal growth and development.

Taurine is an especially important amino acid in infancy. Quantities in human milk are high, and all infant formulas are supplemented during the manufacturing process to provide the same margin of physiologic safety as that provided by human milk.[11] Taurine is not an energy source and is not used for protein synthesis, but it serves as a cell membrane protector by attenuating toxic substances (e.g., oxidants, secondary bile acids, excess retinoids) and acting as an osmoregulator. Additionally, the conjugation of bile acids requires taurine. Taurine deficiency can result in reduced bile acid secretion, leading to accumulation of toxic bile acids, retinal dysfunction, slow development of auditory brainstem-evoked response in preterm infants, and poor fat absorption in preterm infants and children with cystic fibrosis. These conditions can be improved with taurine supplements.

Despite similar amino acid densities and milk intakes in formula-fed and human milk–fed infants, serum concentrations of some amino acids measured in formula-fed infants tend to exceed those measured in human milk–fed infants; however, both groups exhibit comparable growth. The protein content of human milk adjusts to a growing infant's needs, but the high protein needs of preterm infants are not completely met by early human milk. Fortification with commercially available powders or liquids is required for the preterm infant to achieve reasonable amino acid profiles and to meet requirements for expected growth rates. In evaluating the adequacy of an infant's protein intake, it is important to consider not only the absolute amount of protein ingested but also the *linear growth velocity,* (i.e., rate of linear growth over a defined period of time), the quantity of nonprotein calories and other nutrients necessary for protein synthesis, and the quality of the protein itself.

Fat and Essential Fatty Acids

Fat is the most calorically dense component in the diet, providing 9 kcal/g, compared with 4 kcal/g for both protein and carbohydrates. Fat accounts for approximately 50% of the nonprotein energy in both human milk and infant formula. Infant feeding choices, especially fat and calorie intake, are increasingly being linked to obesity and other diseases (e.g., diabetes, cardiovascular disease [CVD]) in adulthood. Despite these concerns, children younger than 2 years (the time of most rapid growth and development requiring high-energy intakes) should not receive a fat- or cholesterol-restricted diet unless medically prescribed. Children between 12 months and 2 years of age who are at increased risk for development of CVD because of a family history of obesity, dyslipidemia, or CVD may be candidates for reduced-fat milk products.[12] AAP supports this position, with attention to appropriate fat intake, on account of the recognized need for adequate fatty acids for normal neurologic development and adequate calories for growth.[12] Parents of children with or without hypercholesterolemia should be encouraged to adopt a diet that contains no more than 30% of total calories from fat, with 7%–10% of calories from saturated fats and dietary cholesterol (≤300 mg/day).[12]

The diet must also contain small amounts of the two essential polyunsaturated fatty acids (PUFAs): linolenic acid, an omega-3 (n-3) fatty acid, and linoleic acid, an omega-6 (n-6) fatty acid. These fatty acids are precursors for the n-3 and n-6 long-chain PUFAs: docosahexaenoic acid (DHA) and arachidonic acid (ARA), respectively. Essential fatty acid deficiency, rarely seen in the United States, can manifest as increased metabolic rate, failure to thrive, hair loss, dry flaky skin, thrombocytopenia, and impaired wound healing. Because of substantial fat stores, overt clinical manifestations of essential fatty acid deficiency generally are delayed for weeks in older children and adults; however, rapid onset (within days) may occur in premature infants with inadequate linoleic acid in their diets. Linoleic acid represents the bulk of PUFAs in infant formulas. Generally, an intake of linoleic acid equal to 1%–2% of total dietary calories is adequate to prevent essential fatty acid deficiency; 3%–7% is the amount found in human milk. AIs for the essential PUFAs are shown in Table 26–2.[9]

Historically, infant formulas contained only the precursor PUFAs: linoleic and linolenic acid. Nowadays, most infant formulas are supplemented during manufacturing with DHA and ARA. In fact, more than 60 countries permit the addition of these fatty acids to infant formulas. AAP has not taken an official stand on whether infant formulas should be supplemented with DHA and ARA. However, the current European recommendations supported by the World Association of Perinatal Medicine, the Early Nutrition Academy, and the Child Health Foundation are for the addition of 0.2%–0.5% DHA to all infant formulas.[13] These long-chain PUFAs, which are abundant in human milk but not in cow milk, are not considered essential but are thought to provide extra nutritional benefits. Increased amounts of DHA beyond what is currently being added to term infant formulas to mimic term human milk levels are being recommended for some preterm infants.[14,15] DHA is important in both brain and eye development; the direct role of ARA is less clear. However, supplementation of DHA without ARA may lead to ARA deficiency and possible growth suppression.[16]

Whether the addition of DHA and ARA to infant formulas improves visual and cognitive function remains controversial. Some studies have shown benefit for visual function, cognitive and behavioral development, and growth with DHA and ARA supplementation in infants; other studies have shown no differences in supplemented versus control infants.[17–19] Benefits such as decreasing allergies and a reduced incidence of common respiratory illnesses have also been suggested, but studies have had mixed results.[20–22] No adverse effects have been noted in infants receiving DHA- and ARA-supplemented formulas; however, two studies in which the formula was supplemented with only DHA reported growth suppression, stressing the importance of supplementation with both DHA and ARA.[19] Several studies have examined the long-term benefits, particularly cognitive, of DHA supplementation and have not found sustained benefits.[23,24] However, significant benefits were observed in selected cognitive components in a more recent study conducted in children 3–6 years of age.[25]

FDA has issued a "generally recognized as safe" (GRAS) notification to Martek Biosciences Corporation for its patented plant-based fatty acid blends DHASCO (DHA-rich single cell oil), extracted from *Crypthecodinium cohnii*, and ARASCO (ARA-rich single cell oil), extracted from *Mortierella alpine*, which are currently used to supplement infant formulas during manufacturing.

Some evidence also indicates that maternal diet can affect fatty acid concentrations in the infant, both in utero and during lactation for human milk–fed infants, but supplementation has not shown to significantly improve neurodevelopmental outcomes, visual acuity, or growth and only weakly favors supplementation.[26] Many prenatal vitamins, as both prescription (e.g., Nexa Plus, Duet DHA Balanced) and nonprescription (e.g., Similac Prenatal, various store brands) products, currently are available, with an additional softgel capsule containing either DHA or DHA with eicosapentaenoic acid (EPA). The sources of DHA and EPA range from fish-based products to plant-derived sources. Enfamil Expecta Prenatal, softgel capsules containing 200 mg DHA, is marketed as a non–fish-based (algae) supplement for pregnant and lactating women to increase maternal dietary DHA and potentially increase DHA concentrations in their infants. These capsules may have less aftertaste than other sources of DHA. Additionally, selecting "burpless" products and freezing the product before administration may help to decrease the aftertaste of the fish-derived products. Routine supplementation during pregnancy and lactation remains controversial and should be discussed with an HCP.

Micronutrients

DRIs for term infants (given as AIs if defined or as RDAs if AIs are not defined) for vitamins and minerals, including trace elements, are shown in Tables 23–3 and 23–4 in Chapter 23. Precise needs are difficult to define and depend on energy, protein, and fat intakes as well as absorption and nutrient stores. Infant formulas are supplemented with adequate amounts of vitamins and minerals to meet the needs of most term and premature infants when the appropriate formula is chosen. Similar to protein fortification, human milk must be fortified to meet the micronutrient needs of most premature infants. Appropriate supplementation is included in the discussion of specific milks and formulas.

Infant Food Sources

Human milk– and cow milk–based formulas are the primary food sources for most infants in the United States. Soy protein–based formulas and goat milk are alternatives. A variety of formulas are available to feed infants with special nutritional needs, including those unable to consume a regular oral diet, those with inborn errors of metabolism, and those with various malabsorptive conditions. Most infants and children receive either human milk or an enteral formula by mouth; however, some children will receive these through feeding tubes such as naso- or orogastric, nasoduodenal, gastrostomy, or jejunostomy tubes. A discussion of these feeding techniques is beyond the scope of this chapter. For more information on enteral feeding tubes and potential complications, please see the following websites: www.nutritioncare.org and www.oley.org.

Human Milk

Both WHO and AAP recommend that infants be breastfed without supplemental foods or liquids for approximately the first 6 months (i.e., exclusive breastfeeding).[27–29] Breastfeeding initiation rates worldwide have increased steadily since 1990, with the rate at hospital discharge increasing from a low of 24.7% in 1971 to 80% in 2012. However, in 2012, the reported rates of any breastfeeding in infants 6 and 12 months of age were only 51% and 29%, respectively. Sociodemographic factors affect breastfeeding rates. Black women are less likely than White, Hispanic, and Asian women to breastfeed. Poor, unmarried, and poorly educated women are also less likely to breastfeed their infants. Table 26–3a shows breastfeeding rates worldwide for infants born in 2012 based on various ethnicities.[30–32]

Because breastfeeding is a major public health issue, breastfeeding goals were included in *Healthy People 2020: National Health Promotion and Disease Prevention Objectives,* the national plan to improve the health of the American people.[33] Objectives of *Healthy People 2020* are provided in Table 26–3b, including data from 2011 (the year of last official reporting of information). All values showed improvement from the 2006 baseline levels (www.healthypeople.gov). AAP recommends support for breastfeeding through the first year of life. The AAP policy statement on breastfeeding and the use of human milk was updated in 2012 and includes reinforcement of breastfeeding and human milk as the reference normative standards for infant feeding and nutrition and reaffirmation of the recommendation to exclusively breastfeed for 6 months, followed by continued breastfeeding for 1 year or longer as mutually desired by mother and infant. AAP cautions that medical contraindications to breastfeeding are rare in the United States (e.g., positive maternal human immunodeficiency virus [HIV] serostatus, need for maternal medication not compatible with breastfeeding). Moreover, AAP recommends (1) the use of WHO growth charts to avoid mislabeling of infants as underweight and with failure-to-thrive status, (2) hospital initiatives to encourage and support the initiation and sustaining of exclusive breastfeeding, (3) support by pediatricians as advocates of breastfeeding, and (4) acknowledgment of the economic benefits to society of breastfeeding.[28]

TABLE 26-3 **Breastfeeding Rates**

a. Worldwide Depending on Ethnicity

	All Ethnic Groups (%)	Asian (%)	Black (%)	Hispanic (%)	White (%)
Breastfeeding at					
Any time after birth	—	83	66	82	83
6 months	51	66	35	51	56
12 months	29	42	17	27	32

b. U.S. Data Comparison With *Healthy People 2020* Goals

	Healthy People 2020 Goals (%)	U.S. Rate, 2011 (%)
Breastfeeding at		
Birth	82	79
6 months	61	49
1 year	34	27
Exclusive breastfeeding at		
3 months	46	41
6 months	25	19
Formula supplementation within first 2 days of life	14	19

Source: References 30–33.

Breastfeeding not only offers an optimal source of nutrition for the infant but also provides other benefits, such as improved mother–child bonding and advantages for the infant's general health, growth, and development. Strong evidence indicates that a human milk–based diet decreases the incidence and severity of various infections (e.g., nonspecific gastrointestinal tract infections, respiratory tract infections, otitis media) in infants and necrotizing enterocolitis in premature infants.[28] Other proposed benefits of human milk include decreased rates of sudden infant death syndrome, type 1 and type 2 diabetes, leukemia, overweight, obesity, hypercholesterolemia, asthma, atopic dermatitis, eczema, celiac disease, and childhood inflammatory bowel disease. Breastfeeding also has been associated with slightly enhanced performance on tests of cognitive development; however, the effect of genetic and socioenvironmental factors on intelligence is difficult to measure separately from that of breastfeeding.[28] For premature infants, improvement is also seen in clinical feeding tolerance, quicker attainment of full enteral feeding, and more favorable neurodevelopmental outcomes. With these benefits in mind, AAP recommends use of human milk for all preterm infants. If the mother's own milk cannot be provided, pasteurized donor milk, term or preterm as appropriate, should be used.[28]

Besides enhanced mother–child bonding, maternal benefits of breastfeeding include decreased postpartum bleeding, more rapid uterine involution, decreased menstrual blood loss, increased spacing between children, earlier return to prepregnancy weight, decreased risk of breast and ovarian cancer, decreased risk of rheumatoid arthritis, and decreased rates of hip fracture and osteoporosis in the postmenopausal period.

A savings of more than $13 billion per year ($3.7 billion in direct and indirect pediatric health costs, with $10.1 billion in premature death from pediatric diseases) could be realized if 90% of mothers in the United States would exclusively breastfeed for 6 months. If only 80% chose to exclusively breastfeed for 6 months, $10.5 billion per year would be saved. More important, 911 deaths annually would be prevented if a 90% exclusive breastfeeding rate was achieved (741 deaths with an 80% achievement rate).[34,35] In the business environment, the case for breastfeeding is an economic one. For every $1 a business spends on creating and supporting lactation support programs at the business site, a $2–$3 return on investment is achieved.[36] An economic analysis of estimated direct health care costs for diarrhea, lower respiratory tract infections, and otitis media in the first year of life found that costs for infants who were never breastfed were $300 more than for infants exclusively breastfed for at least 3 months.[37]

Many unanswered questions regarding the protective effects of breastfeeding remain: What is the duration of protection after breastfeeding has been discontinued? What influence does maternal age have on the protective effect? How great is the interactive effect of social and demographic variables? How does the addition of solid foods (complementary feeding) to the diet of a human milk–fed infant influence the protective effect? What consequence does partial formula feeding have for the protective effect? Well-designed studies are needed to answer these questions.

The impact of the use of breast pumps also should be considered. The 2005–2007 Infant Feeding Practices Study II (IFPS II) assessed the use of expressed human milk among breastfeeding mothers of infants between the ages of 1.5 and 4.5 months.[38] Of these mothers, 85% had expressed their own milk sometime during their child's infancy, and 5.6% of mothers had exclusively fed their infants expressed human milk. As with breastfeeding rates in general, the use of expressed human milk is more common among women with a higher level of education and a higher household income. The primary reason reported in IFPS II for the use of expressed human milk is the ability to have someone else feed the infant, allowing many mothers to continue to provide breast milk while working outside of the home. Unfortunately, the use of expressed human milk is not always an elective decision. When women express milk for nonelective reasons (i.e., to alleviate sore nipples, to increase milk supply, or to allow later feedings when the baby is unable to nurse owing to sickness or when the mother is working), a concern is that breastfeeding duration may be adversely affected. Mothers thought to be less likely to continue to breastfeed, with consequent shorter duration of human milk feedings for their infants, include those who are pumping because of either employment or a recognized difficulty with infant feeding at the breast.[39]

Although breast milk pumping can provide many of the same benefits to infant and mother, some potential problems have been noted. If an electric breast pump is used improperly, the mother can incur mastitis, pain, trauma, and nipple wounds. With respect to the infant, the expressed milk can become contaminated with bacteria if it is expressed or stored improperly.[40] Recommendations and protocols for handling and storing human milk have been established by CDC and the Academy of Breastfeeding Medicine.[41,42] Storing human milk in nonglass containers can destroy some key milk components, and storing milk at either refrigerator or freezer temperatures can reduce levels of key milk components (i.e., vitamin C, lipids, and immunologic cells). Finally, the composition of human milk changes throughout a single feeding and with the infant's age. For example, most mothers who pump their milk breast-feed the infant first and then express the remainder for later use. This method separates the foremilk, which is high in carbohydrate content, from the hindmilk, which is high in fat content. Such separation of the macronutrient components within a feeding of mother's milk can lead to adverse gastrointestinal effects in the infant, such as diarrhea. Well-designed research is needed in this area to assess the true impact of the use of breast pumps on maternal health and infant nutrition.[38]

Very few contraindications to the use of human breast milk have been recognized. In developed countries, such as the United States, one reason for women not breastfeeding is a maternal diagnosis of HIV infection, which can be transmitted through human milk. Women with HIV-seropositive status in underdeveloped countries, however, are encouraged to breastfeed, because the risk of infant morbidity and death with formula use (from inadequate sanitation or refrigeration and illiteracy-associated errors in preparation) is greater than the risk of HIV transmission.[28] Other reasons for not breastfeeding in women in developed countries, either temporarily or permanently, include the following medical disorders and conditions: classic galactosemia, active untreated tuberculosis, human T cell lymphotropic virus type I or II infection, presence of a herpes simplex lesion on the breast (although use of the other breast may be possible), and the use of drugs not compatible with breastfeeding. Several excellent textbooks provide information regarding the use of drugs during lactation and pregnancy (e.g., Briggs' *Drugs in Pregnancy and Lactation*, Hale's *Medications & Mother's Milk;* see also the Preface of this book for a detailed explanation of the pregnancy data).

In addition, a comprehensive database of available information on drugs in lactation (LactMed) is maintained by the National Library of Medicine (http://toxnet.nlm.nih.gov/cgi-bin/sis/htmlgen?LACT) and is currently recommended as a definitive source by AAP.[43] Further questions can be directed to the poison control center hotline (800-222-1222) or the National Breastfeeding Helpline (800-994-9662) or website (http://www.womenshealth.gov/breastfeeding/).

The overall risk of an adverse reaction to a drug in a breastfed infant depends on the concentration in the infant's blood and the effects of the drug on the infant (http://www.infantrisk.com/content/drug-entry-human-milk). Feeding immediately before the mother's dose may help minimize exposure, because the concentration in milk is likely to be lowest toward the end of the dosing interval. This may not be true for lipid-soluble drugs. Alternating breast and bottle feedings or pumping and discarding breast milk is an option if the need for a particular drug is short term.

In the United States and other countries, human milk donor banks have been established, with 24 member banks in the Human Milk Banking Association of North America (HMBANA) and 5 sites in various stages of development. Another source of human donor milk is preparations available from private companies such as Prolacta Bioscience: human milk from carefully screened, unpaid donors undergoes Holder pasteurization to eliminate potential viral and bacterial contaminants while maintaining most of the milk's unique immunologic factors.[44,45] It is estimated that approximately 50% of the immunoglobulin A (IgA) is lost in processing; however, because cow milk contains no IgA at all, infants who receive donor human milk still benefit from its presence at lower levels. The cost is approximately $4 per ounce plus shipping and handling. More information about donor milk banks, including how to be a donor or receive donor milk, can be obtained on the HMBANA and Prolacta websites (www.hmbana.org and www.prolact.com, respectively). A positive impact on decreased rates of necrotizing enterocolitis, a severe inflammation of the intestinal mucosa, with the use of donor milk when maternal human milk is either unavailable or insufficient has recently been shown for very low-birth-weight infants.[46]

Cow Milk

Cow milk is the primary nutrient source for commercially prepared milk-based infant formulas. In both human and cow milk, more than 200 constituent factors have been identified in the fat- and water-soluble fractions. Estimates of the major nutrients contained in pooled mature human milk and whole cow milk are listed in Table 26–4.

Whole Cow Milk

Whole cow milk is not suitable for providing nutrition to infants younger than 1 year. Because of the low concentration and poor bioavailability of iron, a whole cow milk–based diet has been associated with iron-deficiency anemia.[47,48] Sensitivity to dietary proteins, most commonly cow or soy milk proteins, can manifest as occult GI bleeding, further increasing the risk of anemia. In the past decade, convincing evidence has accumulated to indicate that iron deficiency impairs psychomotor development and cognitive function in infants, even with relatively mild anemia. Milk protein intolerance and/or allergy can also result in rash, wheezing, diarrhea, vomiting, colic, and anaphylaxis when whole cow milk is used. Moreover, when whole cow milk is fed with solid food, infants receive unnecessarily high intakes of protein and electrolytes, resulting in a high renal solute load (RSL)[49] (Table 26–5). The implications of a high RSL are discussed later in the chapter. The current position of the AAP Committee on Nutrition (AAP-CON) is that iron-fortified infant formula is the

TABLE 26-4 Average Composition of Mature Human Milk and Whole Cow Milk

Component	Mature Human Milk[a]	Whole Cow Milk
Water (mL/100 mL)	87.1	87.2
Energy		
(kcal/100 mL)	65–70	66–68
(kcal/oz)	19.5–21	19–20
Protein (g/100 mL)	0.9	3.3–3.4
Whey-casein ratio	72:28	18:82
Alpha-lactalbumin (g/100 mL)	0.326	0.1
Alpha-lactoglobulin (g/100 mL)	—	0.4
Lactoferrin (g/100 mL)	0.194	Trace
Secretory IgA (g/100 mL)	0.1	Trace
Albumin (g/100 mL)	0.04	0.04
Fat (g/100 mL)	3.9	3.4–3.8
Carbohydrate (g/100 mL)	6.7–7.2[b]	4.7–4.8[c]
Minerals		
Calcium (mg/L)	200–250	1200
Phosphorus (mg/L)	120–140	960
Calcium-phosphorus ratio	2:1	1.3:1
Sodium (mg/L)	120–250	500
Potassium (mg/L)	400–550	1560
Chloride (mg/L)	400–450	1020
Magnesium (mg/L)	30–35	120
Vitamins		
Vitamin A (international units/L)	1333–3000[d]	1000
Thiamin (mcg/L)	200	300
Riboflavin (mcg/L)	400–600	1750
Niacin (mg/L)	1.8–6	0.8
Pyridoxine (mg/L)	0.09–0.31	0.5
Pantothenate (mg/L)	2–2.5	3.6
Folic acid (mcg/L)	80–140	50
Biotin (mcg/L)	5–9	35
Vitamin B_{12} (mcg/L)	0.5–1	4
Vitamin C (mg/L)	100	17
Vitamin D (international units/L)	13.2	24
Vitamin E (international units/L)	0.0045–0.012	0.4–0.9
Vitamin K (mcg/L)	2–3	5
Trace Minerals		
Chromium (mcg/L)	45–55	20
Manganese (mcg/L)	3	20–40
Copper (mg/L)	0.2–0.4	100

TABLE 26-4 **Average Composition of Mature Human Milk and Whole Cow Milk** *(continued)*

Component	Mature Human Milk[a]	Whole Cow Milk
Zinc (mg/L)	1–3	3.5
Iodine (mcg/L)	150	80
Selenium (mcg/L)	7–33	5–50
Iron (mg/L)	0.3–0.9	0.46
Fluoride (mcg/L)	4–15	—

Key: IgA = Immunoglobulin A.

[a] ≥28 days post partum.

[b] As lactose, glucose, and oligosaccharides.

[c] As lactose.

[d] As both retinol and carotenoids.

Source: Picciano MF. Representative values for constituents of human milk. In: Schanler RJ, ed. Breastfeeding 2001, part 1: the evidence for breastfeeding. *Pediatr Clin North Am.* 2001;48:263–4; Committee on Nutrition, American Academy of Pediatrics. Appendix R. In: Kleinman RE, Greer FR, eds. *Pediatric Nutrition.* 7th ed. Elk Grove Village, IL: American Academy of Pediatrics; 2014:1431–2.

only acceptable alternative to human milk. The use of cow milk is not recommended during the first year of life.[50]

Reduced-Fat Cow Milk

Consumption of reduced-fat cow milk, such as skim milk (0.1% fat), low-fat milk (1% fat), and reduced-fat milk (2% fat), has been advocated to prevent obesity and atherosclerosis as part of a "heart-healthy diet." However, when the low-fat diet recommended for adults is imposed on children younger than 2 years of age, it puts them at risk for failure to thrive and impaired neurologic development. Infants who receive a major percentage of their caloric intake from reduced-fat milk may receive an exceedingly high protein intake and an inadequate intake of essential fatty acids. The maximum protein concentration allowed by FDA in infant formulas is 4.5 g/100 kcal, but skim milk and 2% milk provide approximately 8–10 g/100 kcal and 7–10 g/100 kcal, respectively. Therefore, using reduced-fat cow milk for infant nutrition will provide an unbalanced percentage of calories supplied from protein, fat, and carbohydrates.

Per unit volume, skim milk has a slightly higher potential RSL (PRSL) than that of whole cow milk (Table 26–5). The solute concentration is further increased by water loss during processing. Reduced-fat milk is not recommended during episodes of diarrhea because of the possibility of hypertonic dehydration. As stated earlier, AAP does not recommend the use of low-fat diets during the first 2 years of life, except in children between 12 months and 2 years of age with a family history of CVD.

TABLE 26-5 **Potential Renal Solute Load (PRSL) for Selected Milks and Infant Formulas**

Milk/Formula	PRSL mOsm/L	PRSL mOsm/100 kcal
Human milk	93	14
Milk-based formula	135–260	20–39
Soy protein–based formula	160	24
Whole cow milk	308	46
Skim cow milk	326	93
FDA upper limit	277	41
Beikost[a]	153	23

Key: FDA = U.S. Food and Drug Administration; PRSL = potential renal solute load.

[a] *Beikost* is foods other than milk or formula.

Source: References 7 and 49.

Evaporated Milk

Evaporated milk is a sterile, convenient source of cow milk with standardized concentrations of protein, fat, and carbohydrate. However, it is not recommended for infant feeding.

Goat Milk

Although goat milk is the primary milk source for more than 50% of the world's population, it is rarely used in the United States for infants with intolerance to cow milk. The use of goat milk is not recommended by AAP.[51] Goat milk is commercially available in powdered and evaporated forms. It contains primarily medium- and short-chain fatty acids, so the fat is more readily digested than that in cow milk. Unfortified goat milk is not recommended during infancy because it is deficient in folate and low in iron and vitamin D. The evaporated and powdered whole milk forms of Meyenberg goat milk, however, are supplemented with vitamin D and folic acid. Because goat milk is not a complete formula, vitamin supplementation is required if it is used for infant nutrition.

Commercial Infant Formulas

When provision of human milk to an infant is not possible (e.g., lack of maternal supply, positive maternal HIV serostatus, maternal medication contraindicated with breastfeeding) or not desired by the mother, then commercially supplied infant formulas are an acceptable alternative (Table 26–6). Differences in palatability, digestibility, sources of nutrients, convenience of administration, and cost among these formulas allow for individualization to the infant's special nutrient needs and the family's resources.

Formula Properties

The International Formula Council is a voluntary, nonprofit trade association composed of the five companies that manufacture and market infant formulas and adult nutritionals: Abbott Nutrition, Mead Johnson Nutrition, Nestlé Infant Nutrition, Perrigo Nutritionals, and Pfizer Nutrition. This association has established guidelines requiring liquid formulations to be free of all viable pathogens, including spores, and other organisms that may cause product degradation. In addition, infant formula constituents must meet certain concentrations to ensure optimum nutrition. Guidelines have been established to ensure safety and efficacy of infant formulas.

Microbiologic Safety

Manufacturers sterilize liquid formulas using heat treatment, and the product is free of microbes so long as the container remains intact. Powdered formulas are not required or guaranteed to be sterile; however, coliforms and other pathogens are absent, and levels of contamination with other microorganisms are below acceptable government standards. If clinically significant microbiologic contamination occurs, an infant ingesting the formula could develop diarrhea with subsequent fluid and electrolyte losses. In 2002, FDA issued an alert after the death of an infant in a neonatal intensive care unit after consumption of powdered formula contaminated with *Enterobacter sakazakii* (now referred to as *Cronobacter*) at the manufacturing site. Information regarding potential contamination can be found on the CDC website (www.cdc.gov/features/cronobacter).

Risk for infection after exposure to contaminated formula is likely to depend on a number of factors, including immune status. Accordingly, for premature and immunocompromised infants, use of ready-to-feed or liquid concentrates is recommended unless no suitable alternative to a powdered formula is available.

Physical Characteristics

Infant formulas are emulsions of edible oils in aqueous solutions, but fat separation rarely occurs. If it does, shaking the container usually will redisperse the fat. Redispersion may not happen if stabilizers are lacking or if the formula was stored beyond its shelf life. Liquid infant formulas may contain thickening agents, stabilizers, and emulsifiers to provide uniform consistency and prolong stability. Protein agglomeration may occur, however, if storage time is excessive. Evidence of such agglomeration ranges from development of a slightly grainy consistency through increased viscosity and gel formation to eventual protein precipitation. Agglomeration and separation do not affect a formula's safety or nutritional value; however, the formula's appearance may deter caregivers from using it.

Caloric Density

The standard caloric density for infant formulas is 20 kcal/oz, or approximately 67 kcal/100 mL, which mimics the historical average caloric density of human milk. One recent exception is selected standard infant formulas manufactured by Abbott Nutrition, which, if prepared according to standard preparation instructions, provide 19 kcal/oz, or approximately 65 kcal/100 mL (Table 26–6). According to the manufacturer, this change is the result of more recent information indicating that the caloric density of term breast milk is closer to 19 kcal/oz (www.nutritionnews.abbott). A healthy term infant should have no difficulty consuming enough formula to meet both energy (calorie) and fluid needs with this caloric density. Premature, malnourished, volume-restricted (e.g., for cardiac or liver disease or from poor oral feeding), or severely ill infants may require more calories (130–150 kcal/kg/day or higher) or formulas with higher caloric densities (e.g., 22, 24, 27 kcal/oz) to meet their energy needs. Infant formulas with caloric densities significantly lower or higher than 20 kcal/oz are regarded as therapeutic formulas to be used in managing special clinical conditions (Tables 26–6 and 26–7). Concentrated formulas should be used only under close medical supervision, especially with monitoring for dehydration caused by the reduction in free water consumed.

Osmolality and Osmolarity

Osmolality is the preferred term for reporting the osmotic activity of infant formulas. Osmolality represents the number of osmoles of solute per kilogram of solvent (Osm/kg). Any dietary component soluble in water contributes to osmolality. Osmolality is directly related to the concentration of molecular or ionic particles in the solution (i.e., amino acids, small peptides, electrolytes, and simple sugars) and inversely proportional to the concentration of water in the formula. The osmolality of human milk is approximately 295 mOsm/kg; osmolality of standard-caloric-density formulas is 200–300 mOsm/kg.

The *osmolarity* of an infant formula may be expressed as the concentration of solute per unit of total volume of solution, or as the number of osmoles of solute per liter of solution (Osm/L). The osmolarity of human milk is approximately 273 mOsm/L. Formulas for infants should have osmolarities no higher than 400 mOsm/L. Unless the formula is very concentrated, there is no meaningful difference between osmolality and osmolarity of infant formulas.

The osmolality of a formula increases with increasing caloric density. The relationship between osmolality and caloric density is reasonably linear within the range of caloric concentrations usually fed to infants. Thus, if the osmolality of a 20 kcal/oz formula is known, the same formula with any other caloric density can be calculated, assuming a direct proportion between osmolality and caloric density. For example, if a 20 kcal/oz formula has an osmolality of 283 mOsm/kg, then the same formula concentrated to 24 kcal/oz would have an osmolality of approximately 340 mOsm/kg.

No clinically meaningful differences in osmolality have been noted for the various 20 kcal/oz, ready-to-use formulas in common

TABLE 26-6 Selected Formulas for Infants and Children

Trade Name [form] (Mfr)	Kilocalories[a] (per ounce)	Protein[a] (g/L) (C:W ratio)	Protein Source(s)	Carbohydrate[a] (g/L)	Carbohydrate Source(s)	Fat[a] (g/L)	Fat Source(s)	MCTs (% fat kcal)	Iron[a] (mg/L)
Infant Formulas									
Milk-Based Formulas									
Enfamil Premium Infant[b] [C,P,R] (MJ)	20	13.5 (40:60)	Nonfat milk, whey protein concentrate	76.4	Lactose, galacto-oligosaccharides, polydextrose	35.8	Vegetable oil (palm olein, coconut, soy, and high oleic sunflower oils), DHA, ARA, linoleic acid, linolenic acid, soy lecithin	—	12.2
Enfamil Gentlease[c] [P,R] (MJ)	20	15.6 (40:60)	Partially hydrolyzed nonfat milk and whey protein concentrate (soy)	69.7	Corn syrup solids	35.6	Vegetable oil (palm olein, soy, coconut, and high oleic sunflower oils), DHA, ARA, linoleic acid, linolenic acid	—	12.2
Stage 1 Gerber Good Start Gentle[d,e] [C,P,R] (G)	20	14.9 (0:100)	100% whey protein partially hydrolyzed concentrate (milk)	78.5	Corn maltodextrin (30%), lactose (70%), galacto-oligosaccharides	34.5	Vegetable oil (palm olein, soy, coconut, high oleic safflower or sunflower oils), DHA, ARA, linoleic acid, linolenic acid, soy lecithin	—	10.1
Similac Advance[f,g] [C,P,R] (A)	19/20	13.3/14	Nonfat milk, whey protein concentrate	69.2/75.7	Lactose, galacto-oligosaccharides	36.2/36.5	Vegetable oil (soy, coconut, high oleic safflower or sunflower oils), DHA, ARA, linoleic acid, linolenic acid, soy lecithin	—	12.2
Similac Advance Organic [P,R] (A)	20	14.1	Organic nonfat milk	71	Organic malto-dextrin, organic sugar, fructo-oligosaccharides	38.3	Organic high oleic sunflower, organic soy, and organic coconut oils, DHA, ARA	—	12.2

(continued)

TABLE 26-6 Selected Formulas for Infants and Children *(continued)*

Trade Name [form] (Mfr)	Kilocalories[a] (per ounce)	Protein[a] (g/L) (C:W ratio)	Protein Source(s)	Carbohydrate[a] (g/L)	Carbohydrate Source(s)	Fat[a] (g/L)	Fat Source(s)	MCTs (% fat kcal)	Iron[a] (mg/L)
Soy Protein–Based Therapeutic Formulas									
Enfamil ProSobee [C,P,R] (MJ)	20	16.9	Soy protein isolate, L-methionine, taurine	71.6	Corn syrup solids	35.8	Vegetable oils (palm olein, soy, coconut, and high oleic sunflower oils), DHA, ARA, linoleic acid, linolenic acid	—	12.2
Stage 1 Gerber Good Start Soy[e] [C,P,R] (G)	20	16.9	Enzymatically hydrolyzed soy protein isolate, L-methionine, taurine	75.1	Corn maltodextrin (79%), sucrose (21%)	34.5	Vegetable oils (palm olein, soy, coconut, and high oleic safflower or sunflower oils), DHA, ARA, linoleic acid, linolenic acid, soy lecithin	—	12
Similac Soy Isomil[g] [C,P,R] (A)	19/20	15.8/16.6	Soy protein isolate, L-methionine	67/69.7	Corn syrup solids, sugar, fructo-oligosaccharides	35.1/36.9	High oleic safflower, soy, and coconut oils; DHA, ARA	—	12.2
Similac Expert Care for Diarrhea [R] (A)	20	18	Soy protein isolate, L-methionine	68.3 (6 g/L of dietary fiber)	Corn syrup, sugar	36.9	Soy, coconut oils	—	12.2
Other Therapeutic Infant Formulas									
Enfamil A.R. [P,R] (MJ)	20	16.9	Nonfat milk	76.4	Rice starch, lactose, maltodextrin, galacto-oligosaccharides, polydextrose	34.5	Vegetable oils (palm olein, soy, coconut, and high oleic sunflower oils), DHA, ARA, linoleic acid, linolenic acid	—	12.2
Similac Sensitive [C,P,R]/Similac For Spit Up [P,R] (A)	19/20 (depending on formulation)	13.5 (13.8)[f]/ 14.5	Milk protein isolate	71.4 (70.7)[f]/75.1	Maltodextrin, sugar, glacto-oligosaccharides/ additional, rice starch	34.7 (34.7)[f]/ 36.5	High oleic safflower, soy, and coconut oils; DHA, ARA, soy lecithin	—	12.2
Similar Total Comfort [P,R] (A)	19	14.9	Whey protein hydrolysate	70.07	Corn syrup solids, sugar, galacto-oligosaccharides	34.7	High oleic safflower, soy, coconut, DHA, ARA, soy lecithin	—	12.2
Similac PM 60/40 [P] (A)	20	15 (40:60)	Whey protein caseinate, sodium caseinate	69	Lactose	37.9	High oleic safflower, soy, and coconut oils	—	4.7

Nutramigen[h] [C,R] (MJ)	20	18.9	Casein hydrolysate, L-cystine, L-tyrosine, L-tryptophan, taurine	69.6	Corn syrup solids, modified corn starch	35.8	Vegetable oils (palm olein, soy, coconut, and high oleic sunflower oils), DHA, ARA, linoleic acid, linolenic acid	—	12.2
Pregestimil [P,R]/ Pregestimil 24 [R] (MJ)	20/24	18.9/22.5	Casein hydrolysate (milk), L-cystine, L-tyrosine, L-tryptophan, L-carnitine, taurine	68.9/82	Corn syrup solids, modified corn starch	37.8/45	MCT, soy, corn, and high oleic vegetable oils (sunflower/safflower); DHA, ARA, linoleic acid, linolenic acid	55	12.2/14.5
Similac Expert Care Alimentum [P,R] (A)	20	18.6	Casein hydrolysate, L-cystine, L-tyrosine, L-tryptophan	69	Corn maltodextrin, sugar	37.5	High oleic safflower, MCT, and soy oils; DHA, ARA	33	12.2
PurAmino DHA & ARA [P] (MJ)	20	18.9	Free L-amino acids	71.6	Corn syrup solids, modified tapioca starch	35.8	MCT, vegetable oil (soy and high oleic sunflower oils), DHA, ARA, linoleic acid, linolenic acid	9	12.2
Gerber Extensive HA[d] [P] (A)	20	17.6	100% whey, extensively hydrolyzed	73.7	Maltodextrin (90%), potato starch (10%)	34.5	MCT, soy, high oleic sunflower, high 2-palmitic vegetable oils; CITREM[i], DHA, ARA, linoleic acid, linolenic acid	49	12
EleCare (for Infants) [P] (A)	20	20.9	Free amino acids	72.3	Corn syrup solids	32.4	High oleic safflower, MCT, and soy oils; DHA, ARA	33	9.9
Neocate Infant DHA&ARA [P] (Nut)	20	18.9	Free L-amino acids	73	Corn syrup solids	34.5	MCT, high oleic sunflower, and canola oils; DHA, ARA	33	10.1
Enfaport [R] (MJ)	30	36	Calcium and sodium caseinates (milk)	100	Corn syrup solids	55	MCT and soy oils, DHA, ARA, linoleic acid, linolenic acid, soy lecithin	84	18.3
RCF[j,k] [C] (A)	20	20.3	Soy protein isolate, L-methionine, taurine	68.2	None in actual product	35.8	High oleic safflower, soy, and coconut oils; soy lecithin	—	12.2
3232A[j,l] [P] (MJ)	20	18.9	Casein hydrolysates (milk), L-cystine, L-tyrosine, L-tryptophan, L-carnitine, taurine	90.5	Modified tapioca starch	28.3	MCT and corn oils, soy lecithin	85	12.5

(continued)

TABLE 26-6 **Selected Formulas for Infants and Children** *(continued)*

Trade Name [form] (Mfr)	Kilocalories[a] (per ounce)	Protein[a] (g/L) (C:W ratio)	Protein Source(s)	Carbohydrate[a] (g/L)	Carbohydrate Source(s)	Fat[a] (g/L)	Fat Source(s)	MCTs (% fat kcal)	Iron[a] (mg/L)
Formulas for Premature Infants: Initial Feeding									
Enfamil Premature 20 Cal [R] (MJ)	20	22 (40:60)	Nonfat milk, whey protein concentrate	73	Corn syrup solids, lactose	34	MCT, soy, and high oleic sunflower oils; DHA, ARA, linoleic acid, linolenic acid	40	12.2
Similac Special Care 20 with Iron [R] (A)	20	20.3	Nonfat milk, whey protein concentrate	69.7	Corn syrup solids, lactose	36.7	MCT, soy, coconut oils; DHA, ARA, soy lecithin	50	12.2
Gerber Good Start Premature 20 [R] (G)	20	20 (0:100)	100% enzymatically hydrolyzed whey protein isolate	71	Lactose (50%), maltodextrin (50%)	35	MCT, high oleic oils (sunflower or safflower), soy oils; DHA, ARA, linoleic acid, linolenic acid	40	12
Enfamil Premature 24 Cal [R]/Enfamil Premature 24 Cal High Protein [R] (MJ)	24	27/29 (40:60)	Nonfat milk, whey protein concentrate	88/85	Corn syrup solids, lactose	41	MCT, soy, and high oleic sunflower oils; DHA, ARA, linoleic acid, linolenic acid	40	14.6
Similac Special Care 24 with Iron [R]/ Similac Special Care 24 High Protein [R] (A)	24	24.3/26.8	Nonfat milk, whey protein concentrate	83.6/81	Corn syrup solids, lactose	44.1	MCT, soy, coconut oils; DHA, ARA, soy lecithin	50	14.6
Gerber Good Start Premature 24 [R]/Gerber Good Start Premature 24 High Protein [R] (G)	24	24/29 (0:100)	100% enzymatically hydrolyzed whey protein isolate	85/79	Lactose (50%), maltodextrin (50%)	42	MCT, high oleic (sunflower or safflower), soy oils; DHA, ARA, linoleic acid, linolenic acid	40	15
Enfamil Premature 30 Cal [R] (MJ)	30	33 (40:60)	Nonfat milk, whey protein concentrate	109	Maltodextrin	51	MCT, soy, and high oleic sunflower oils; DHA, ARA, linoleic acid, linolenic acid, soy lecithin	40	18.3

Similac Special Care 30 with Iron [R] (A)	30	30.4	Nonfat milk, whey protein concentrate	78.4	Corn syrup solids, lactose	67.1	MCT, soy, coconut oils; DHA, ARA, soy lecithin	50	18.3
Gerber Good Start Premature 30 [P] (G)	30	30 (0:100)	100% enzymatically hydrolyzed whey protein isolate	107	Lactose (50%), maltodextrin (50%)	53	MCT and high oleic sunflower oils; DHA, ARA, linoleic acid, linolenic acid	40	18
Formulas for Premature Infants: Transition or Postdischarge									
Enfamil EnfaCare [P,R] (MJ)	22	21 (40:60)	Nonfat milk, whey protein concentrate	77	Powder = corn syrup solids, lactose Liquid = maltodextrin, lactose	39	High oleic sunflower, soy, MCT, and coconut oils; DHA, ARA, linoleic acid, linolenic acid	20	13.3
Similac Expert Care NeoSure [P,R] (A)	22	20.8	Nonfat milk, whey protein concentrate	75.1	Corn syrup solids, lactose	40.9	Soy, high oleic safflower, MCT, and coconut oils; DHA, ARA, soy lecithin	25	13.4
Older Infant/Toddler Milk-Based Formulas									
Stage 2 Gerber Good Start Gentle[d,e] [P] (G)	20	12.9 (0:100)	100% whey protein partially hydrolyzed concentrate (milk)	80.5	Lactose (70%), maltodextrin (30%), galacto-oligosaccharides	34.5	Palm olein, soy, coconut, and high oleic safflower or sunflower oils; DHA, ARA, linoleic acid, linolenic acid, soy lecithin	—	14
Go & Grow by Similac[f] [P] (A)	19	16.9	Nonfat milk	67.6	Lactose, sucrose, galacto-oligosaccharides	35	High oleic safflower, soy, and coconut oils; DHA, ARA	—	30%[m]
Enfagrow Toddler Transitions [P,R] (MJ)	20	17.6 (80:20)	Nonfat milk	73	Corn syrup solids, lactose, galacto-oligosaccharides	35.8	Vegetable oils (palm olein, soy, coconut, and high oleic sunflower oils), DHA, ARA, linoleic acid, linolenic acid	—	10.1
Enfagrow Toddler Transitions-Gentlease [P] (MJ)	20	17.6	Partially hydrolyzed nonfat milk, whey protein concentrate solids (soy)	70.9	Corn syrup solids, galacto-oligosaccharides	35.8	Vegetable oils (palm olein, soy, coconut, and high oleic sunflower oils), DHA, ARA, linoleic acid, linolenic acid	—	13.5

(continued)

TABLE 26-6 **Selected Formulas for Infants and Children** *(continued)*

Trade Name [form] (Mfr)	Kilocalories[a] (per ounce)	Protein[a] (g/L) (C:W ratio)	Protein Source(s)	Carbohydrate[a] (g/L)	Carbohydrate Source(s)	Fat[a] (g/L)	Fat Source(s)	MCTs (% fat kcal)	Iron[a] (mg/L)
Soy-Based Products									
Enfagro Toddler Transitions Soy [P] (MJ)	20	22.3	Soy protein isolate, L-methionine, taurine	79.7	Corn syrup solids	29.7	Vegetable oils (palm olein, soy, coconut, high oleic sunflower oils), DHA, ARA, linoleic acid, linolenic acid, soy lecithin	—	13.5
Stage 3 Gerber Good Start Soy [P] (G)	20	18.9	Enzymatically hydrolyzed soy protein isolate, L-methionine, taurine	73.7	Corn maltodextrin (79%), sucrose (21%)	33.8	Vegetable oils (palm olein, soy, coconut, high oleic safflower or sunflower oils), DHA, ARA, linoleic acid, soy lecithin	—	14
Go & Grow by Similac Sensitive [P] (A)	19	16.9	Milk protein isolate, taurine	67.6	Corn syrup, sugar, galacto-oligosaccharides	33.8	High oleic safflower, soy, and coconut oils; DHA, ARA	—	30%[m]
Children's Formulas									
PediaSure (Grow & Gain)/ PediaSure Enteral Formula [R] (A)	30	29.5	Milk protein concentrate, soy protein isolates	139.2	Corn maltodextrin, sugar, short-chain fructo-oligosaccharides	38	High oleic safflower, soy, and canola oils; soy lecithin	—	15%[n]
PediaSure 1.5 Cal [R] (A), vanilla	45	59.1	Milk protein concentrate	160.3	Corn maltodextrin	67.5	High oleic safflower, soy, and MCT oils; soy lecithin, DHA	15	11.4
PediaSure with Fiber[o]/ PediaSure Enteral Formula with Fiber[o] [R] (A)	30	29.5	Milk protein concentrate, soy protein isolates	139.2 (12.6 g/L of dietary fiber[o])	Corn maltodextrin, sugar, short-chain fructo-oligosaccharides, soy fiber	38	High oleic safflower and soy oils; soy lecithin, DHA	—	15%[n]
PediaSure 1.5 Cal with Fiber[o] [R] (A), vanilla	45	59.1	Milk protein concentrate	164.6 (12.7 g/L of dietary fiber with 6.3 g/L of scFOSs[o])	Corn maltodextrin	67.5	High oleic safflower, soy, and MCT oils; soy lecithin, DHA	15	11.4
Nutren Junior [R]/Nutren Junior with Fiber[p] [R] (Nes)	30	30 (50:50)	Milk protein concentrate, 50% whey protein concentrate	110 (3.8 g/L of insoluble fiber and 2.2 g/L of soluble fiber as PreBio)[p]	Maltodextrin, sugar; fiber product also contains pea fiber, fructo-oligosaccharides, inulin	49.6	Soybean, canola, and MCT oils (coconut and/or palm kernel oils); soy lecithin	20	14

Boost Kid Essentials [R] (Nes)	30	29.2	Sodium and calcium caseinates, whey protein concentrate	133.3	Maltodextrin, sugar	37.5	High oleic sunflower, soybean, and MCT oils; soy lecithin	20	11.3
Boost Kid Essentials 1.5 [R]/Boost Kid Essentials 1.5 with Fiber [R] (Nes)	45	42	Sodium and calcium caseinates, whey protein concentrate	163.8 (7.4 g/L of fiber)	Maltodextrin, sugar	75	MCT, soybean, and sunflower oils; soy lecithin	10	11.3
Compleat Pediatric [R] (Nes)	30	38	Chicken, sodium caseinate, and pea puree	132 (6.8 g/L of Nutrisource Fiber)	Corn syrup, green pea and green bean puree, peach puree, cranberry juice, maltodextrin	39	Canola and MCT oils (coconut and/or palm kernel); hydroxylated soy lecithin	20	14
Carnation Breakfast Essentials [R] (Nes)	30	41.7	Milk protein concentrate, soy protein isolate	170.8	Corn syrup, sugar	16.7	Vegetable oil (high oleic sunflower and corn), soy lecithin	—	18.75
Other Therapeutic Formulas—Older Infants, Toddler, and Pediatric Formulations									
Neocate Splash [R] (Nut), unflavored	30	30	Free L-amino acids	105	Maltodextrin, sugar	51	High oleic sunflower oil, MCT (palm kernel/coconut), and canola oils	35	15
E028 Splash [R] (Nut), flavored	30	24.9	Free L-amino acids	146	Maltodextrin, sugar	35	Fractionated coconut, canola, and high oleic sunflower oils	35	7.6
EleCare Jr [P] (A), flavored or unflavored	30	31	Free amino acids	106.7	Corn syrup solids	49.1	High oleic safflower, MCT, and soy oils	33	18
Neocate Junior [P] (Nut), flavored or unflavored	30	33	Free L-amino acids	104	Corn syrup solids	50	MCT, refined vegetable oils (palm kernel and/or coconut, canola, and high oleic safflower oils)	35	16
Peptamen Junior [R] (Nes)	30	30 (0:100)	Enzymatically, hydrolyzed whey protein (milk)	136	Maltodextrin, sugar, corn starch, guar gum, sucralose	38.4	MCT (coconut and/or palm kernel oil), soybean, and canola oils; soy lecithin	60	14
Peptamen Junior 1.5[P] [R] (Nes), flavored or unflavored	45	45	Enzymatically, hydrolyzed whey protein (milk)	180 (6 g/L of PreBio[P] fiber)	Maltodextrin, corn starch, fructo-oligosaccharides, inulin, guar gum	68	MCT (coconut and/or palm kernel oils), soybean, and canola oils; soy lecithin	60	21
Peptamen Junior Fiber with PreBio[P] [R] (Nes)	30	30 (0:100)	Enzymatically, hydrolyzed whey protein (milk)	136 (7.4 g/L of fiber[P])	Maltodextrin, sugar, corn starch, pea fiber, fructo-oligosaccharides, inulin	38.4	MCT (coconut and/or palm kernel oils), soybean, and canola oils; soy lecithin	60	14

(continued)

TABLE 26-6 Selected Formulas for Infants and Children *(continued)*

Trade Name [form] (Mfr)	Kilocalories[a] (per ounce)	Protein[a] (g/L) (C:W ratio)	Protein Source(s)	Carbohydrate[a] (g/L)	Carbohydrate Source(s)	Fat[a] (g/L)	Fat Source(s)	MCTs (% fat kcal)	Iron[a] (mg/L)
Pediasure Peptide 1.0 Cal [R] (A), unflavored	30	30	Whey protein hydrolysate, hydrolyzed sodium caseinate	134 (3 g/L of dietary fiber, 3 g/L of scFOSs[o])	Corn maltodextrin, short-chain fructo-oligosaccharides	40.5	Structured lipid (inter-esterified canola, MCT); MCT and canola oils; soy lecithin	60	14
Pediasure Peptide 1.5 Cal [R] (A), flavored (vanilla)	45	45.1	Whey protein hydrolysate, hydrolyzed sodium caseinate	201 (4.6 g/L of dietary fiber, 4.6 g/L of scFOSs[o])	Corn maltodextrin, short-chain fructo-oligosaccharides	60.8	Structured lipid (inter-esterified canola, MCT); MCT and canola oils; soy lecithin	60	21
Vivonex Pediatric [P] (Nes)	24	24	100% free L-amino acids	126	Maltodextrin, modified corn starch	23.2	MCT (coconut and/or palm kernel oil), soybean oils	70	10
Portagen [P] (MJ)	30	35.9	Sodium caseinate	116.3	75% corn syrup solids, 25% sugar	48.6	MCT and corn oils, soy lecithin	87	19

Key: A = Abbott Nutrition; ARA = arachidonic acid; C = concentrate; C:W = casein-whey ratio; DHA = docosahexaenoic acid; G = Gerber; MCTs = medium-chain triglycerides; mfr = manufacturer; MJ = Mead Johnson Nutrition; Nes = Nestlé Nutrition; Nut = Nutricia North America; P = powder; R = ready-to-feed; scFOSs = short-chain fructo-oligosaccharides.

Note: Federal regulations require nutrient values to be reported as intakes per 100 kcal. These intakes can be found on the manufacturer's website. Values per liter of formula are provided for ease of calculation. Changes are made periodically in formula composition; for the most up-to-date information, refer to the manufacturer's website.

[a] When powder is prepared to achieve the stated caloric density.

[b] Available as newborn formulation [R, P] with C:W ratio of 20:80. Provides sufficient vitamin D (400 international units) in minimum volume of 27 fl oz.

[c] Has ⅕ the lactose content of standard milk-based formula.

[d] Contains *Bifidus* BL (*Bifidobacterium lactis*), which is similar to probiotics found in human milk.

[e] Standard product available as non–genetically modified organism (GMO)–based.

[f] Product available as non–GMO–based option.

[g] Product content depends on formulation (i.e., ready-to-feed, powder, or concentrate).

[h] Powder form available as Nutramigen with Enflora LGG.

[i] Product contains CITREM (citric acid esters of mono- and diglycerides).

[j] When carbohydrate is added as directed to make a 20 kcal/oz concentration. For RCF: 54 g of carbohydrate + 12 fl oz water + 13 fl oz of RCF to yield 26 fl oz. For 3232A: 81 g of 3232A + 59 g carbohydrate per quart prepared.

[k] Marketed as the only infant formula available for the ketogenic diet.

[l] Potential option for infants with disaccharidase deficiencies

[m] Percentage of daily value for children 1–4 years of age.

[n] Percentage of daily value for 2000 kcal/day diet.

[o] Prebiotic Nutraflora scFOSs are short-chain fructo-oligosaccharides that provide fuel for beneficial bacteria in the digestive tract to help support a healthy immune system.

[p] PreBio is a unique blend of fructo-oligosaccharides and inulin. These compounds may increase colonic mucosal integrity and permeability, promote potentially beneficial bacteria, and improve colonic absorption of water and electrolytes.

Source: Abbott Nutrition (www.abbottnutrition.com); Gerber (medical.gerber.com); Mead Johnson Nutrition (www.meadjohnson.com); Nestlé Healthcare Nutrition (http://www.nestlehealthscience.us); and Nutricia North America (www.nutricia-na.com). Accessed September 26, 2016.

TABLE 26-7 Indications for Therapeutic Infant Formulas[a]

Problem/Indication	Suggested Therapeutic Formulas	Comments
Allergy or sensitivity to cow milk or soy protein	EleCare (for Infants), Neocate Infant DHA & ARA, Nutramigen, PurAmino DHA & ARA, Pregestimil, Similac Expert Care Alimentum, Gerber Extensive HA	Protein hydrolysate or free amino acid formula is best. Up to 50% cross-sensitivity between cow milk and soy protein allergies is possible.
Biliary atresia, cholestatic liver disease	EleCare (for Infants), Enfaport, Pregestimil, Similac Expert Care Alimentum	Impaired digestion and absorption of long-chain fats; higher percentage of MCTs may improve absorption.
Carbohydrate intolerance (severe)	3232A, RCF	Carbohydrate-free A patient-tolerated carbohydrate source is added gradually (e.g., dextrose, glucose, sucrose, fructose).
Cardiac disease	No therapeutic formula generally necessary	Low electrolyte content (Similac PM 60/40) is indicated if infant has renal insufficiency. Electrolyte supplementation may be needed in patients receiving diuretics. Calorically dense, standard formulas often used in cases of failure to thrive and for volume restriction.
Celiac disease	EleCare (for Infants), Neocate Infant DHA & ARA, Nutramigen, PurAmino DHA & ARA, Pregestimil, Similac Expert Care for Diarrhea	Advance to standard formulas as intestinal epithelium returns to normal; diet must be gluten-free.
Chylothorax or chylous ascites	Enfaport	High MCT intake decreases flow through the lymphatic system.
Constipation	No therapeutic formula necessary	Continue routine formula; increase water; refer cases of severe constipation.
Cystic fibrosis	EleCare (for Infants), Pregestimil, Similac Expert Care Alimentum, Gerber Extensive HA	Impaired digestion and absorption of long-chain fats; cow milk–based formula or human milk may be used with appropriate pancreatic enzyme supplementation. Enzyme supplementation may be required even with predigested therapeutic formulas; soy protein–based formulas are contraindicated.
Diarrhea, chronic nonspecific	Enfamil ProSobee, Nutramigen, Similac Soy Isomil, Stage 1 Gerber Good Start Soy	Trial of lactose-free cow milk or soy protein–based formula may be needed; avoid fruit juices.
Diarrhea, intractable	3232A, EleCare (for Infants), PurAmino DHA & ARA, Pregestimil, RCF, Similac Expert Care Alimentum	Hydrolyzed protein is needed because of impaired digestion of intact protein, long-chain fats, and disaccharides. Similac Expert Care Alimentum contains sucrose and may not be appropriate for all cases.
Diarrhea, antibiotic-associated	Similac Expert Care for Diarrhea	Contains added dietary fiber from soy and was specifically formulated for infants with diarrhea secondary to antibiotics; use short term until diarrhea resolves.
Failure to thrive	No therapeutic formula generally necessary; EleCare (for Infants), Pregestimil, Similac Expert Care Alimentum	Most cases related to inadequate intake. Start with standard formula; may need more calorically dense formula for catch-up growth; change to predigested formula only if malabsorption is present.
Galactosemia	Enfamil ProSobee, Nutramigen, Pregestimil	Formulas without lactose or sucrose; cow and human milk are contraindicated.
Gastroesophageal reflux	Enfamil A.R., Similac For Spit-Up	In otherwise healthy children, start with standard formula thickened with rice cereal. (Start with 1–2 teaspoons per ounce of formula and increase to a maximum of 1 tablespoon per ounce as tolerated.) Thickening formula with rice cereal increases the caloric density, may cause constipation, results in delivery of less volume, and usually requires enlarging the nipple. Some infants may have an allergic-type reaction to rice cereal; oatmeal may be used in such cases. Attempt small, frequent feedings; avoid using products like Thick-It and SimplyThick to thicken formula (these products are intended for patients with dysphagia or swallowing difficulties); use more calorically dense formula if decreased volume or catch-up growth is needed.

(continued)

TABLE 26-7 Indications for Therapeutic Infant Formulas[a] *(continued)*

Problem/Indication	Suggested Therapeutic Formulas	Comments
Hepatitis without liver failure	No therapeutic formula necessary	Impaired digestion or absorption of long-chain fats is uncommon.
Hepatitis with liver failure	EleCare (for Infants), Enfaport, Pregestimil, Similac Expert Care Alimentum	Digestion or absorption of long-chain fats may be impaired.
Increased ostomy output	Similac Expert Care for Diarrhea	Improve consistency in term infants without malabsorption (e.g., Hirschsprung disease, imperforate anus, necrotizing enterocolitis, intestinal atresias)
Lactose intolerance (primary or secondary)	Enfamil ProSobee, Similac Soy Isomil, Stage 1 Gerber Good Start Soy	Remove lactose from diet; use lactose-free formula.
Necrotizing enterocolitis (during recovery or postresection)	EleCare (for Infants), Neocate Infant DHA & ARA, Pregestimil, Similac Expert Care Alimentum	Impaired digestion or absorption requires a hydrolysate or free amino acid formula.
Prematurity	Fortified human milk (preferred); Enfamil Premature 20 Cal, Similac Special Care 20 with Iron, Gerber Good Start Premature 20, or transition infant formula (Enfamil EnfaCare or Similac Expert Care NeoSure)	Human milk fortifier needed; transition formula (see Suggested Therapeutic Formula(s) column) can be added to human milk to increase caloric density after hospital discharge to home (1 tsp/90 mL milk makes 24 kcal/oz).
Renal insufficiency	Similac PM 60/40	Formula is low phosphate, low PRSL.

Key: MCT = Medium-chain triglyceride.

[a] Products are listed alphabetically. List is not all-inclusive; other products may be acceptable.

Source: Abbott Nutrition (www.abbottnutrition.com); Mead Johnson Nutrition (www.meadjohnson.com); Gerber (www.medical.gerber.com); Nestlé Healthcare Nutrition (www.nestlehealthscience.us); and Nutricia North America (www.nutricia-na.com). Accessed May 15, 2017.

use. In addition, when concentrated products are diluted to yield a formula providing 20 kcal/oz, no meaningful difference in osmolality is seen relative to the similar ready-to-use product. However, directions for diluting concentrated and powdered formulas must be followed exactly. Soy protein–based formulas have somewhat lower osmolalities than milk-based formulas because of the difference in carbohydrate source.

Potential Renal Solute Load

The PRSL is the solute load derived from the diet that must be excreted by the kidney if the amino acids from protein digestion are not used for growth or eliminated by nonrenal routes. The PRSL of an infant formula can be calculated using the following equation: PRSL (mOsm) = N/28 + sodium + chloride + potassium + $\text{phosphorus}_{(\text{available})}$, where N is the total nitrogen in milligrams, and concentrations of sodium, chloride, potassium, and $\text{phosphorus}_{(\text{available})}$ (P_a) are expressed in millimoles (or milliosmoles), typically measured per liter of formula. The P_a is assumed to be the total phosphorus content except in soy-based formulas, in which it represents only two-thirds of the total phosphorus. Table 26–5 lists PRSLs for various milks and infant formulas compared with the FDA-recommended upper PRSL limit.[49] Excretion of 1 mOsm of ingested solute requires 1 mL of water intake. Standard 20 kcal/oz infant formulas supply approximately 1.5 mL of water per kilocalorie ingested, an adequate amount of water to provide usual needs. Accordingly, when the infant is healthy, the PRSL generally is not a factor; however, during illnesses associated with water loss, such as vomiting, diarrhea, and fever, or in infants with compromised renal function or diabetes insipidus, the formula's PRSL becomes a factor in maintaining fluid balance. Feeding a formula with a high PRSL (i.e., high protein content or concentrated to more than 24 kcal/oz) may produce a hypertonic urine, leading to increased renal water losses and dehydration.

Types, Uses, and Selection of Commercial Infant Formulas

Standard formulas for term infants are milk-based, or milk-based with added whey protein (whey-predominant). Other formulas are available for infants and children with specific dietary needs and should be used only under medical supervision.

Milk-Based Formulas

Milk-based formulas (Table 26–6) are prepared from nonfat cow milk, vegetable oils, and added carbohydrate (lactose). The added carbohydrate is necessary because the ratio of carbohydrate to protein in nonfat cow milk solids is less than desirable for infant formulas. The most widely used vegetable oils are corn, coconut, safflower, sunflower, palm olein, and soy. Replacement of the butterfat with vegetable oils allows for better fat absorption. Although Similac Sensitive and Similac Total Comfort are milk-based formulas, they contain sucrose with corn maltodextrin, rather than lactose, as the carbohydrate source and may be used for infants with lactose intolerance. Enfamil Gentlease and Stage 1 Gerber Good Start Soothe contain decreased lactose amounts (20% and 30%, respectively) when compared with the relevant product line's standard milk-based formulas, and both are marketed for infant colic.

Therapeutic Formulas

Therapeutic infant formulas are used for infants with conditions requiring dietary adjustment and should be used with medical supervision, rather than being self-selected by parents. Table 26–7 lists indications for various therapeutic formulas, including soy protein–based, casein-based, casein hydrolysate–based, and whey hydrolysate–based formulas, and low-electrolyte and low-mineral formulas. Formulas intended for use by premature infants and those formulated specifically for children 1–10 years of age also are considered therapeutic formulas.

PRETHICKENED MILK-BASED FORMULAS. Enfamil A.R. and Similac For Spit-Up were developed specifically for infants with gastroesophageal reflux. These iron-fortified formulas contain rice starch. Before ingestion, the viscosity of Enfamil A.R. or Similac For Spit-Up is much lower than that of a standard infant formula thickened with rice cereal. Therefore, these formulas flow better through a nipple than standard infant formula thickened with rice cereal. Once they are ingested, however, the viscosity increases dramatically in the stomach's acidic pH, reaching a viscosity equal to that for the combination of standard infant formula plus rice cereal. This effect may be minimized in infants receiving a histamine-2 receptor antagonist (e.g., ranitidine, famotidine) or proton pump inhibitor (e.g., omeprazole, lansoprazole, pantoprazole, esomeprazole) for treatment of their gastroesophageal reflux, if the gastric pH is greater than 5.4. Also, Similac For Spit-Up is a lactose-free formula. Neither Enfamil A.R. nor Similac For Spit-Up is recommended for use in premature infants, because neither product will adequately meet their nutritional needs, especially for protein, calcium, and phosphorus. In May 2011, FDA cautioned parents against using thickening agents such as SimplyThick and Thick-It in premature infants because of reports of associated necrotizing enterocolitis. This cautionary statement was expanded to apply in infants of all ages in September 2012 (www.fda.gov).

SOY PROTEIN–BASED FORMULAS. Despite relatively few true indications for soy protein–based formulas, approximately 20% of formulas sold in the United States are soy protein–based, suggesting that these formulas are being selected by parents rather than being prescribed by HCPs.[33,37] Soy protein–based formulas (Table 26–6) contain a soy isolate fortified with L-methionine; none contain lactose. Soy formulas are a safe and nutritionally sound alternative for achieving normal growth and development in infants who are not fed human milk, who do not tolerate cow milk–based formula, or whose parents choose such products for other reasons (e.g., to follow a vegetarian diet). However, because soy formulas have insufficient amounts of calcium, phosphorus, and vitamin D for meeting the increased needs of some children, they are not recommended for infants weighing less than 1800 g. Additionally, even after the infant attains a weight of 1800 g, these formulas may not be adequate to provide optimal growth and prevent osteopenia of prematurity in the long term.[52]

Food allergy develops in infants because the immature digestive and metabolic processes may not be completely effective in converting dietary proteins into nonallergenic amino acids. Cow milk protein allergy occurs in 2%–3% of infants and is defined as symptomatology involving the respiratory tract (wheezing), skin (rash), or GI tract (diarrhea and bloody stools) that resolves when cow milk is removed from the diet. The disappearance of symptoms may take up to 2 weeks. To confirm a cow milk allergy, two separate challenges of reintroduction of cow milk are conducted during a symptom-free period; reappearance of the symptoms on both tests is diagnostic. Symptoms of cow milk protein intolerance generally regress within 3–4 years in most children.

Soy protein–based formulas are appropriate for infants with lactose intolerance resulting from lactase deficiency and with documented immunoglobulin E (IgE)–mediated allergy to cow milk protein. However, infants with cow milk protein–induced enteropathy or enterocolitis are also frequently sensitive to soy protein (with cross-sensitivity rates of up to 50%); therefore, AAP-CON recommends protein hydrolysate formulas for these infants.[52] Most infants suspected of having adverse reactions to milk-based formulas have not experienced life-threatening manifestations. These infants appear to tolerate soy protein–based formulas, which are less expensive and better-tasting than the protein hydrolysate formulas. Routine use of soy protein–based formulas has no proven value in prevention of atopic disease.[53] Some infants with moderate–severe gastroenteritis will exhibit intolerance to lactose and sucrose because of a temporary lactase and sucrase deficiency. After rehydration, however, most infants with diarrhea can be managed by continuing their usual nutrition regimen, whether milk-based or soy protein–based.

In addition, soy protein–based formulas are not recommended for infants with cystic fibrosis, because these children do not use soy protein adequately, will lose substantial nitrogen in their stools, and are prone to the development of hypoproteinemia or even anasarca (generalized infiltration of fluid into subcutaneous connective tissue). Formula-fed infants with cystic fibrosis do well nutritionally when given an easily digested formula that contains semi-elemental protein and medium-chain triglycerides (MCTs) (e.g., a casein hydrolysate–based formula). However, studies have shown that infants with cystic fibrosis grow equally well on a regular cow milk–based formula and on human milk so long as adequate pancreatic enzyme supplementation is given.[54]

RCF (historically, Ross Carbohydrate Free) is a soy protein–based formula that contains no carbohydrates and is currently marketed as the only infant formula available for patients requiring the ketogenic diet. Use of this formula is limited to infants unable to tolerate the type or amount of carbohydrates in human milk or infant formulas. A carbohydrate source (sucrose, dextrose, fructose, or glucose polymers) is added gradually in increasing amounts to improve carbohydrate tolerance over time.

CASEIN HYDROLYSATE–BASED FORMULAS. Protein in casein hydrolysate–based formulas is supplied by enzymatically hydrolyzed, charcoal-treated casein, rather than by whole protein. Available products include Pregestimil, Nutramigen, and Similac Expert Care Alimentum (Table 26–6). These formulas are classified as semielemental and contain nonantigenic polypeptides with molecular masses less than 1200 daltons; therefore, they can be fed to infants who are sensitive to intact milk protein. Casein hydrolysate–based formulas are supplemented with L-cysteine, L-tyrosine, and L-tryptophan, because the concentrations of these amino acids are reduced during the charcoal treatment.

Carbohydrate sources in casein hydrolysate–based formulas vary and include corn syrup solids, modified corn and tapioca starch, corn maltodextrin, and sucrose (Table 26–6). Glucose polymers found in corn syrup solids, modified corn starch, or corn maltodextrin are particularly useful in infants who have malabsorption disorders and are frequently intolerant of high concentrations of lactose, sucrose, and glucose. In addition, glucose polymers contribute little to the total osmolar load. Low osmolality is an advantage in intestinal disorders in which the osmolar load of disaccharide- or glucose-containing elemental diets may not be tolerated. The formula 3232A is an extensively hydrolyzed casein–based formula with added amino acids that is intended, like RCF, to be used with small amounts of added carbohydrate to gradually improve tolerance. This product contains modified tapioca starch and fat, 85% of which is MCTs.

Hydrolysate formulas usually contain modified fat sources. MCTs are typically included because they do not require emulsification with bile and are more easily digested and absorbed than long-chain fats. Shorter-chain fatty acids and MCTs are directly absorbed into the portal system, not into the lacteals of the lymphatic system. In addition, MCTs enhance the absorption of long-chain triglycerides and do not require carnitine for transport into the mitochondria, where oxidation and energy production occur. MCTs cannot be the sole source of dietary fat, however, because they do not provide essential fatty acids—an important consideration in prevention of essential fatty acid deficiency. Pregestimil and Similac Expert Care Alimentum contain DHA and ARA as long-chain fatty acids. Diarrhea can result from MCT malabsorption caused by overfeeding or intestinal mucosal disease.

Use of casein hydrolysate–based formulas for allergy prophylaxis is controversial. The AAP policy statement on hypoallergenic formulas notes that infants at high risk for development of allergy identified by a strong family history (in both parents or in one parent and a sibling) may benefit from a hypoallergenic formula, but studies are not conclusive.[52] Currently, no evidence has emerged to support the use of hydrolysate formulas for treating colic, irritability, or gastroesophageal reflux. Although these problems are common in infants, they are rarely a result of an IgE-mediated allergic reaction to cow milk protein.

Extensively hydrolyzed casein formulas are less palatable than standard formulas. If the formula is rejected by the infant when first offered, it should be tried again after a few hours. These products are designed to provide a sole source of nutrition for infants up to 4–6 months of age and a primary source of nutrition for children up to 12 months of age, when indicated. Extended use of hydrolysate formulas as a sole source of nutrition in children older than 6 months requires close medical supervision and monitoring.

WHEY HYDROLYSATE–BASED FORMULAS. Enzymatically hydrolyzed whey protein is another protein source used in infant formulas. Infants who have GI intolerance to cow milk but are not allergic to it often tolerate whey hydrolysate–based formula. This product, Stage 1 Gerber Good Start Gentle, is promoted as having a pleasant taste, smell, and appearance. It may be better accepted than casein hydrolysate–based formulas, which parents and infants find differ noticeably from cow milk– and soy protein–based formulas in both appearance and taste. No specific indications are recognized for these products, so they may be chosen according to parent, patient or program preference.

AMINO ACID–BASED FORMULAS. Occasionally, infants are intolerant of even hydrolyzed casein and require a free amino acid–based formula. Neocate Infant DHA & ARA, EleCare (for infants), and PurAmino DHA & ARA contain 100% free amino acids and are considered hypoallergenic. They are used for infants with cow milk protein allergy, multiple food protein allergies, or intolerance to casein hydrolysate formulas.

HIGH MCT FORMULAS. Enfaport and Portagen are unique formulas because of their high MCT content (i.e., 84% and 87% of the fat, respectively). They also contain higher concentrations of both lipid- and water-soluble vitamins than those found in casein hydrolysate–based formulas. The higher concentrations of MCTs and vitamins in these formulas help compensate for the impaired digestion and absorption of long-chain fats in patients with pancreatic insufficiency (e.g., cystic fibrosis) or bile acid deficiency (e.g., biliary atresia, cholestatic jaundice) and those who have undergone intestinal resection. Another use is to decrease lymphatic flow in patients with lymphatic anomalies such as chylothorax and chylous ascites. Enfaport can be used as the sole dietary source for infants, whereas Portagen can be used as the sole dietary source for children and adults or can be given as a beverage to be consumed with each meal as a supplement. Children with fat malabsorption who receive Portagen are at risk for development of essential fatty acid deficiency. Linoleic acid (e.g., corn or safflower oil, Microlipid) can be given in the diet, either by mixing with the formula or delivered by syringe through a feeding tube, to prevent essential fatty acid deficiency.

LOW PRSL FORMULAS. Similac PM 60/40 is an infant formula with lower mineral (potassium and phosphorus) and protein (1.5 g/100 mL) content and, consequently, lower PRSL than in standard infant formulas. It is most appropriately used for infants with renal insufficiency. Similac PM 60/40 also contains less calcium and iron than standard infant formulas; supplementation of these minerals may be necessary.

PREMATURE INFANT FORMULAS. The current AAP recommendation is for all premature infants to receive maternal human milk or donor human milk.[28] Nutrient intake can be inadequate in human milk–fed premature infants, however, because unfortified human milk does not meet the needs of this population. Because of their increased nutrient needs and somewhat decreased ability to consume an adequate volume, premature infants (especially those born before 34 weeks' gestation) often need feedings providing a higher caloric density, as well as increased protein, calcium, phosphorus, and other nutrients. The nutritional goal for a preterm infant is to achieve a postnatal growth rate approximating the intrauterine growth rate of a normal fetus of the same corrected gestational age.

No commercially available formula is completely satisfactory for premature infants. Formulas for premature infants (Table 26–6) share features such as whey-predominant proteins, carbohydrate mixtures of lactose and corn syrup solids, and fat mixtures containing both MCTs and long-chain triglycerides. They differ in electrolyte, vitamin, mineral, protein, and caloric content. When given in sufficient volume, these formulas promote adequate growth in preterm infants. An isotonic osmolality (approximately 300 mOsm/kg of water) is maintained at a caloric density of 24 kcal/oz or 80 kcal/100 mL.

Calcium and phosphorus are crucial to the development and maintenance of the human skeleton. In addition, calcium and phosphorus are integral components of many biochemical reactions. Calcium requirements are affected by protein and phosphorus intake in that these nutrients interact with the renal tubular reabsorption of calcium. Calcium-to-phosphorus weight ratios vary significantly for human milk (2:1) and cow milk (1.2:1). This ratio also varies in commercial infant formulas. Formulas designed for term infants will not meet the calcium and phosphorus needs of premature infants. For these infants, the additional calcium and phosphorus found in premature infant formulas is necessary for normal bone growth and mineralization. Typical amounts of calcium and phosphorus found in 20 kcal/oz infant formulas are 112–122 mg calcium/100 mL and 61–68 mg phosphorus/100 mL for preterm formulas versus 53–65 mg calcium/100 mL and 28–36 mg phosphorus/100 mL for term formulas. Human milk fed to premature infants requires calcium and phosphorus supplementation with either a human milk fortifier or addition of a transitional premature formula, as discussed later.

Nutrient-enriched transition or postdischarge formulas are designed specifically to provide for continued catch-up growth in premature infants after hospital discharge. Similac Expert Care NeoSure and Enfamil EnfaCare (both milk-based formulas) contain MCTs as part of the fat source. The caloric (22 kcal/oz), protein, vitamin, and mineral content of these formulas exceed those of standard term formulas but are less than those of 24 kcal/oz premature infant formulas. Use of these formulas in preterm infants until 9 months of postnatal age results in greater linear growth, weight gain, and bone mineral content than that achieved with the use of standard, term infant formulas.[55]

HUMAN MILK FORTIFIERS. Mothers who give birth to premature infants produce milk that is higher in protein, sodium, potassium, chloride, and iron, and possibly other nutrients than the milk of mothers who deliver at full term. However, these nutrients decline to the amounts found in mature human milk by 4–8 weeks after delivery. From 28 weeks gestational age, the fetus receives 125–150 mg of calcium and 65–80 mg of phosphorus daily, with 80% being deposited in bone during this time. Without supplementation, human milk, whether preterm or mature, cannot supply that amount of calcium and phosphorus, which are needed to prevent osteopenia of prematurity. Human milk must therefore be fortified for premature infants to achieve adequate growth.[56]

Commercial products have been developed to supplement the nutrient content of human milk to meet the needs of most preterm infants. Enfamil Human Milk Fortifier Acidified Liquid, Similac Special Care 30 with Iron, Similac Human Milk Fortifier Concentrated Liquid, Similac Human Milk Fortifier Hydrolyzed Protein Concentrated Liquid, and Prolact+ H^{2}MF all are liquids that add nutrients to human milk without displacing a significant amount of volume. Enfamil Human Milk Fortifier Acidified Liquid, Similac Special Care 30 with Iron, Similac Human Milk Fortifier Concentrated Liquid, and Similac Human Milk Fortifier Hydrolyzed Protein Concentrated Liquid are made from cow milk supplemented with whey protein to provide a whey:casein ratio of 60:40 and a fat mixture to provide MCTs. When added to human milk, fortifiers increase the osmolality by only 10–36 mOsm/kg. Prolact+ H^{2}MF is made from concentrated 100% human milk. It provides extra protein, calories, vitamins, and minerals and is specifically indicated for preterm infants weighing less than 1250 g. This product does not meet all nutritional goals, however, because it is human milk–based, necessitating added vitamin and mineral supplementation (e.g., vitamin D, iron). Table 26–8 summarizes the composition of the human milk fortifiers. Studies support adequate weight gain and nutrient retention in infants when either fortified human milk or commercial preterm formulas are ingested.[57] However, human milk has been shown to provide various immunologic benefits, as well as to improve the intelligence quotient (IQ) in infants born small for gestational age and very low-birth-weight infants.[58] The use of these products will result in weight gain equivalent to that with intrauterine growth rates in most premature infants. Product selection will therefore be dictated by cost and clinical preference.

These products are expensive. Enfamil Human Milk Fortifier Acidified Liquid costs approximately $2.62 per vial, and one vial is generally added to each 25 mL of human milk to yield a 24 kcal/oz concentration. Moreover, this product comes only in cartons of 100–200 vials. Similac Special Care 30 with Iron costs as much as $0.90 per ounce and, when added in equal parts (2 ounces of human milk to 2 ounces of Similac Special Care 30 with Iron), yields a 25 kcal/oz concentration. Similac Human Milk Fortifier Concentrated Liquid and Similac Human Milk Fortifier Hydrolyzed Protein Concentrated Liquid both come in 5 mL packets, and addition of one packet to 50 mL of human milk yields a 22 kcal/oz concentration. When 5 mL is added to 25 mL of human milk, a 24 kcal/oz concentration is obtained. These two products differ primarily in the amount of additional protein provided and cost approximately $0.95/5 mL packet and are available as 6 boxes of 24 packets each (total 144 packets). Prolact+ H^{2}MF is the most expensive, at a cost of approximately $6.25/mL, and the addition of 20 mL of Prolact+4 H^{2}MF to 80 mL of human milk is required to yield a 24 kcal/oz concentration. The strongest evidence supporting the financial benefit of human milk as a sole source of nutrition is in relation to decreased incidence of necrotizing enterocolitis.[46,59] Once the infant is ready for discharge from the hospital or has reached a weight of 2.5 kg, one of the transition or postdischarge formulas can be added to human milk to increase the caloric density (1 teaspoon of powder added to 90 mL of formula yields 24 kcal/oz) and to promote delivery of other nutrients. Assessment of vitamin and mineral composition should be determined before discharge to ensure that no further supplementation is required.

METABOLIC FORMULAS. Infants with various inherited inborn errors of metabolism require specific formulas tailored to their particular condition and must be under the care of a specialist, usually a pediatric endocrinologist or geneticist. Information about these formulas is available on the various manufacturers' websites. These formulas, as well as formulas intended for use in low-birth-weight infants or in patients with specific medical conditions or dietary needs, are classified by FDA as *exempt formulas,* which means they are exempt from FDA nutrient content and labeling requirements.[60]

CONCENTRATED FORMULAS. A child with caloric needs exceeding normal requirements may be given concentrated formula under medical supervision. A few ready-to-use formulas made from cow milk are available in a caloric density of 22 or 24 kcal/oz (Table 26–6). Various concentrations can be prepared from liquid concentrates or powders by varying the amount of water added (Tables 26–9 and 26–10). Increasing caloric density by adding less water also increases delivery of all nutrients, including protein and electrolytes, and decreases free water delivery. Increased concentration of protein and electrolytes (i.e., PRSL) in conjunction with decreased fluid intake may result in dehydration and electrolyte imbalances. Careful monitoring of the infant's fluid intake and output, weight, serum electrolytes, blood urea nitrogen, serum creatinine, and urine specific gravity and osmolality is recommended, especially on initiation of the concentrated formula.

Modular macronutrient components (Table 26–11) can be added to either human milk or infant formula and are available as alternatives to concentrated formulas. Adding carbohydrates as glucose polymers can result in diarrhea. Protein supplementation may increase the PRSL. Fat may be added as MCTs (MCT Oil, Nestlé Nutrition; Liquigen, Nutricia) or Microlipid (Nestlé Nutrition) for infants with fat malabsorption or intolerance. Microlipid is an emulsion made from safflower oil that provides long-chain fatty acids and mixes well with formula. Addition of fat to milk or formula can lead to diarrhea, steatorrhea, delayed gastric emptying, vomiting, and gastroesophageal reflux. Adding modular components is more expensive and time-consuming than simply concentrating the formula; these components should be reserved for situations in which a single nutrient is needed or further concentration of the formula is not appropriate.

TABLE 26-8 **Human Milk Fortifiers**

Component	Enfamil Human Milk Fortifier Acidified Liquid[a]	Similac Special Care with Iron 30[b]	Similac Human Milk Fortifier Concentrated Liquid[c]	Similac Human Milk Fortifier Hydrolyzed Protein Concentrated Liquid[c]	Prolact+4 H²MF[d]
Calories	30	60	6.85	7	28
Protein (g)	2.2	1.8	0.349	0.5	1.2
Fat (g)	2.3	4	0.266	0.21	1.8
Carbohydrates (g)	<1.2	4.6	0.807	0.75	1.8
Vitamin A (international units)	1160	750	197	197	61
Vitamin D (international units)	188	90	34.9	35	26
Vitamin E (international units)	5.6	2.4	0.973	1	0.4
Vitamin K (mcg)	5.7	7.2	2.43	2.4	<0.2
Thiamin (mcg)	184	150	47.9	48	4
Riboflavin (mcg)	260	372	123	74	15
Vitamin B_6 (mcg)	140	150	49.4	50	4.1
Vitamin B_{12} (mcg)	0.64	0.33	0.0825	0.13	0.05
Niacin (mg)	3.7	3	1.044	0.98	0.0524
Folic acid (mcg)	31	22.2	6.82	7	5.4
Pantothenic acid (mg)	0.92	1.14	0.309	0.31	0.0748
Biotin (mcg)	3.4	22.2	7.57	5.8	—
Vitamin C (mg)	15.2	22.2	7.71	7.7	<0.2
Calcium (mg)	116	108	35.1	30	103
Phosphorus (mg)	63	60.8	20	17	53.8
Magnesium (mg)	1.84	7.2	2.16	2.1	4.7
Iron (mg)	1.76	1.1	0.107	0.11	0.1
Zinc (mg)	0.96	0.9	0.304	0.31	0.7
Manganese (mcg)	10	7.2	2.12	2.2	<12
Copper (mcg)	60	150	14.7	15	64
Iodine (mcg)	—	3.6	0.47	0.4	—
Selenium (mcg)	—	2	0.204	0.2	—
Sodium (mg)	27	25.8	5.39	5	37
Potassium (mg)	45.2	77.4	20.7	21	50
Chloride (mg)	28	48.6	13.4	13	29

Note: Changes are made periodically in human milk fortifier composition; for the most up-to-date information, refer to the manufacturer's website.

[a] Amount per 4 vials; generally mixed with 100 mL human milk to yield 120 mL, with a caloric density of 24 kcal/oz.

[b] Amount per 60 mL; generally mixed with 60 mL human milk to yield 120 mL, with a caloric density of 25 kcal/oz.

[c] Amount per 5 mL; 5 mL packet with 50 mL human milk to yield 55 mL, with a caloric density of 22 kcal/oz, or 5 mL packet with 25 mL human milk to yield 30 mL, with a caloric density of 24 kcal/oz.

[d] Amount per 20 mL of Prolact + 4; generally mixed with 80 mL human milk to yield 100 mL, with a caloric density of 24 kcal/oz. Nutrient contribution from Prolact + 4 based on target values for macronutrients and minerals and on averages of three lots for vitamins.

Source: Abbott Nutrition (www.abbottnutrition.com); Mead Johnson Nutrition (www.meadjohnson.com); and Prolacta Bioscience (www.prolacta.com). Accessed July 4, 2016.

TABLE 26-9 Dilution of Concentrated Liquid Infant Formulas[a]

Caloric Concentration Desired (kcal/oz)	Liquid Formula Concentrate (oz)	Added Water (oz)
20	1	1
22 (actual 21.8)	3	2.5
24	3	2
26–27 (actual 26.7)	3	1.5
28–29 (actual 28.6)	5	2

[a] Commercial concentrates of infant formula generally contain 40 kcal/oz before dilution with water.

TABLE 26-10 Dilution of Powdered Term Infant Formulas[a]

Caloric Concentration Desired (kcal/oz)	Formula Powder (scoop)[b]	Added Water (oz)
20	1	2
24	3	5
28	4	5.5
28	7	10.0

[a] Powdered infant formulas generally contain 44 kcal per one level, unpacked scoop before dilution. If a large volume of formula is to be prepared, add powder necessary to supply desired calories; then add water to achieve the final volume desired. Directions for preparation may vary; check manufacturer's information.

[b] Historically, the conversion of 1 scoop = 1 tablespoon of powder has been used. However, this scoop-equivalent measurement varies between powders. For improved accuracy, parents and caregivers should be instructed always to use the manufacturer's provided scoop for preparing formula products.

TODDLER FORMULAS. Toddler formulas (see under Older Infants/Toddler Milk-Based Formulas in Table 26–6) (e.g., Stage 2 Gerber Good Start Gentle, Go & Grow by Similac, Enfagrow Toddler Transitions) are designed for infants and children 9–24 months of age. AAP, however, has stated that these formulas offer no nutritional advantages; standard formulas are appropriate for infants up to 12 months of age.[47]

FORMULAS FOR CHILDREN 1–13 YEARS OF AGE. Nutritionally complete, isotonic, virtually lactose-free enteral formulas designed for young children who cannot tolerate a normal diet or eat solid food are available (see under Children's Formulas in Table 26–6) (e.g., PediaSure [Grow & Gain], Nutren Junior, Boost Kid Essentials). Flavored products contain sucrose, have a pleasant taste, and can be used as oral supplements. These formulas are also appropriate to use as tube feedings regardless of delivery mode (e.g., gastric, duodenal, jejunal). They contain adequate amounts of calcium,

TABLE 26-11 Modular Additives

Additive[a] (Mfr)	Nutrient(s) Provided	Amount of Nutrient(s)	Calories
Polycal (Nut)	Maltodextrin	Per 5 g scoop: carbohydrate ~5 g	~20 kcal/scoop
Beneprotein (Nes)	Whey protein isolate (milk), soy lecithin	Per 7 g scoop or packet: protein 6 g	25.2 kcal/scoop
Procel (GHP)	Whey protein concentrate (milk), soy lecithin	Per 6.6 g scoop: protein 5 g; fat 0.5 g	26 kcal/scoop
Microlipid (Nes) (liquid)	Long-chain fats (safflower oil)	Per mL: fat 0.5 g	4.5 kcal/mL
MCT Oil (Nes) (liquid)	MCTs (coconut/palm kernel oils)	Per mL: fat 0.93 g	7.7 kcal/mL
Liquigen (Nut) (liquid)	MCTs (50%, palm kernel/coconut oils)	Per mL: fat 0.5 g	4.5 kcal/mL
Super Soluble Duocal (Nut)	MCT (35%, coconut/palm kernel oils), hydrolyzed cornstarch, vegetable oils (corn and coconut)	Per tablespoon: carbohydrate 6.2 g; fat 1.9 g	25 kcal/scoop 42 kcal/tablespoon
Benecalorie (Nes) (liquid)	Calcium caseinate (milk); high oleic sunflower oil	Per 1.5 ounces: protein 7.2; fat 33.75 g	7.5 kcal/mL
ProMod Liquid Protein (A) (liquid)	Hydrolyzed beef collagen	0.33 g protein/mL	3.3 kcal/mL
Liquid Protein Fortifier (A) (liquid)	Casein hydrolysate	0.17 g protein/mL	0.67 kcal/mL

Key: A = Abbott Nutrition; GHP = Global Health Products; MCT = medium-chain triglycerides; Mfr = manufacturer; Nes = Nestlé Nutrition; Nut = Nutricia North America.

[a] Products listed are powders unless specified otherwise.

Source: Abbott Nutrition (www.abbottnutrition.com); Global Health Products (globalhp.com); Nestlé Healthcare Nutrition (www.nestlehealthscience.us); and Nutricia North America (www.nutricia-na.com). Accessed September 26, 2016

phosphorus, iron, and vitamin D for this age group; the amounts contained in adult enteral products typically are inadequate.

Several therapeutic formulas have also been developed for children 1–13 years of age (Table 26–6). Peptamen Junior and Pediasure Peptide are peptide-based, semielemental formulas. Vivonex Pediatric, Neocate Junior, Neocate Splash (unflavored), E028 Splash (a flavored, nutritionally complete drink), and EleCare Jr are amino acid–based elemental formulas. These products are intended for use in children with altered digestive or absorptive capabilities caused by a number of conditions, including severe protein allergy and eosinophilic esophagitis (Table 26–7). Another area of infant feeding and nutrition of increasing popularity is home-prepared blenderized diets and whole food formulas (e.g., Pediatric Compleat, Nourish, Liquid Hope). A discussion of these feeding modalities is beyond the scope of this chapter.

Nutritional Problems in Infancy

GI problems, especially diarrhea, can occur with the use of infant formulas, as well as with human milk or any food. Tooth decay and nutritional deficiencies are other potential problems.

Diarrhea

Diarrhea can lead to failure to thrive (chronic) and dehydration (acute). Infants are particularly susceptible to dehydration because of their high metabolic rate and relatively higher ratio of surface area to weight and height. Fluid depletion by diarrhea or vomiting may quickly (within 24 hours) produce severe dehydration with fluid and electrolyte imbalances, shock, and possible death. A potential formula-related cause of diarrhea and vomiting is the improper dilution of a concentrated liquid or powdered formula or the incorrect addition of a modular product.

If diarrhea develops, the pharmacist should ascertain the severity and duration, stool frequency, and formula preparation method. If the diarrhea appears to be severe (i.e., with many more stools per day than normal) or has continued for more than 72 hours, or if the infant is clinically ill (exhibiting fever, lethargy, anorexia, irritability, dry mucous membranes, or decreased urine output), referral for medical attention is warranted. (Diarrhea is discussed in Chapter 16.)

Mild diarrhea will usually resolve without the need for medical intervention, but the infant should be observed closely for signs of dehydration. Temporarily discontinuing usual dietary intake is not recommended except during a 4- to 6-hour period of oral rehydration if the infant is dehydrated. Oral electrolyte replacement solutions manufactured especially for infants (e.g., Pedialyte, Enfamil Enfalyte) may be used for short-term replacement of fluid and electrolyte losses in mild-to-moderate dehydration to augment fluid intake, but these solutions should not replace formula or human milk intake.[61] Prevention of dehydration by replacement of ongoing losses with a glucose-electrolyte solution in liquid or frozen form is the best intervention for diarrhea in infants and children.

Lactose-free formulas or a lactose-free diet may be considered for infants and children with moderate-severe diarrheal illness, but full-strength lactose-containing formulas, human milk, or a regular diet can be used in most infants. Parents should be advised that diarrhea is likely to continue for 3–7 days regardless of the type of formula, and seeking medical consultation is advised if a sudden increase in stool output occurs with resumption of feeding.[61]

Other Gastrointestinal Issues

Adverse GI effects of formula include mechanical obstruction (inspissated milk curds) and hypersensitivity to specific milk protein. Cow milk intolerance is associated most often with an inability to digest lactose or milk proteins. Hyperosmolar formulas may adversely affect premature infants during the early neonatal period and may be a contributing factor in the development of necrotizing enterocolitis. For this reason, initiation of feedings in these infants is most often done with unfortified human milk or a 20 kcal/oz premature infant formula. Typically, after the infant has reached an intake of 80–100 mL/kg/day of enteral feedings, the caloric density can be advanced, but a recent study suggests that earlier fortification at 20 mL/kg/day to improve the provision of protein is possible.[50,62] Initiation and advancement of formula for premature infants should occur under medical supervision and are not appropriate for self-care.

Tooth Decay

"Baby bottle" tooth decay can occur in children who are bottle-fed beyond the typical weaning period (1 year) and who go to sleep with a bottle. It also can occur if the infant is allowed to sip on a bottle or from a training cup frequently during the day. Caries can be seen in children younger than 2 years and may involve the maxillary incisors, maxillary and mandibular first molars, or maxillary and mandibular canines. Restorative dentistry is often required, leading to the potential for difficulty in speech development. Methods for prevention once teeth start to erupt include substituting plain water for carbohydrate-containing formula or other drinks given in a bottle until the infant is weaned from the bottle, encouraging the use of a cup for high-sugar drinks such as juice, using either infant juices that contain a higher proportion of water or standard juices diluted with additional water, ensuring adequate fluoride intake, cleaning the baby's mouth at least once daily, and weaning from breast or bottle by the age of 12 months.[63] Going to sleep with a bottle should be actively discouraged for all infants.

Nutritional Deficiencies or Toxicities

Generally, age- and condition-appropriate commercial infant formulas are nutritionally adequate and safe for most infants and children. Nutritional deficiencies reported historically with commercial infant formulas are unlikely today with appropriate supplementation procedures and technological advances in processing.

Because of a concern about possible aluminum contamination of infant formulas, the Food and Agriculture Organization of the United Nations has identified a provisional tolerable aluminum intake of 1 mg/kg/day. Aluminum in toxic amounts can interfere with cellular and metabolic processes in the nervous system as well as negatively affect bone and liver tissues.[64] Aluminum toxicity is primarily a concern in patients with decreased or immature renal function, such as premature infants, and in those receiving intravenous therapies. If an infant were to ingest as much as 200 mL/kg/day of a formula known to have the highest aluminum content, the amount of aluminum received per day would still be less than 0.5 mg/kg/day. The highest aluminum concentrations in infant formulas (500–2400 mg/L) have been reported for soy protein–based formulas, because plants readily absorb aluminum from soil.

Infant Formula Preparation

Most formulas are available as a ready-to-use liquid or as a liquid concentrate or powder for reconstitution mixed with water. Ready-to-use formulas should *never* be diluted. They are convenient but usually more expensive. By contrast, concentrated liquids *must* be diluted, typically by mixing equal amounts of water and concentrated liquid (e.g., a 13-ounce can of formula with a 13-ounce can of water) to prepare a 20 kcal/oz formula (Table 26–10). Powdered term and preterm transition or postdischarge formulas provide a measuring scoop in the can and require addition of 1 unpacked, level scoop of powder to each 2 ounces of water for a 20 kcal/oz term formula and a 22 kcal/oz preterm postdischarge formula. Directions for preparation may vary between products, and the caregiver should always prepare the formula according to the manufacturer's or health care professional's directions. If the family is given alternative directions from those printed on the can, these should be given in writing and explained thoroughly to the caregiver. Directions should be provided in the appropriate language for non–English-speaking patients. Before use, infant formula containers should be inspected for the expiration date and damage. Unopened formula containers, cans, or bottles can be stored at room temperature but must not be subjected to extreme temperature changes.

Preparation Techniques

Each infant formula has specific instructions for preparation, and most formulas have symbols on the containers that can be used as guidelines in preparing formula. Because infants may be more susceptible to infection, various sterilization methods have been recommended for infant formula preparation. Table 26–12 reviews sterilization methods for different types of formulas. Studies have shown that the "clean" method of preparing formula (i.e., not boiling the water) is as safe as terminal sterilization (i.e., boiling the water); therefore, some providers do not recommend boiling water. WHO and AAP currently recommend that all water for formula preparation be boiled because of reports of municipal water supply contamination in some areas. If well or pond water is used or if the area is prone to flooding, the water must be boiled.[65,66] If tap water is used, cold water should be run for at least 2 minutes before use to clear any lead that might be in the pipes and decrease lead exposure. If bottled water is used in infant formula preparation, it should be treated the same as for tap or well water (i.e., it is boiled and cooled before use) unless the water is labeled as sterile.

Table 26–12 provides handling instructions and recommendations for storage of infant formulas once the original container has been opened. Expressed human milk should be stored in glass or plastic airtight containers, refrigerated, and used within 24–48 hours. Human milk can be frozen, preferably in the rear of the freezer compartment, for up to 2 weeks if the freezer compartment is inside the refrigerator, for up to 3–6 months when the freezer has a separate door from the refrigerator, and for up to 6–12 months in a −4°F (−20°C) freezer (https://www.cdc.gov/breastfeeding/recommendations/handling_breastmilk.htm). Frozen milk should be rapidly thawed by holding the container under tepid running water or placing it in a tepid water bath. Thawed human milk should always be used within 24 hours of thawing and never refrozen.

Adverse Effects of Improperly Prepared and/or Administered Formulas

As stated previously, the failure to properly dilute a concentrated infant formula can result in a hypertonic solution that could result in adverse effects of diarrhea and dehydration. In extreme cases, the ingestion of an overly concentrated formula can lead to hypernatremic dehydration (induced by water deficit), metabolic acidosis, and renal failure. Excessive formula dilution can lead to water intoxication that can result in irritability, hyponatremia, coma, brain damage, or death. Such a situation may occur when a caregiver misunderstands the instructions for preparing a concentrated formula, dilutes a ready-to-use formula, or tries to make the baby's formula last longer by diluting it.

Parents or other caregivers may have questions about how much infant formula their child should receive. Typically, a HCP at the hospital will have given parents feeding instructions before mother and infant are discharged home. When a formula change is made after hospital discharge, however, adequate information may not be provided in some health care settings. Generally, the required daily formula intake depends on an infant's age and weight and individual considerations such as the need for catch-up growth (Table 26–13). During the first year of life, a normal healthy formula-fed term infant usually eats every 3–5 hours (average of 4 hours). Small or weak infants may eat every 2–3 hours, because they have smaller stomach capacity or shorter gastric emptying time, or tire easily during feedings. Breastfed infants or those receiving human milk from a bottle also will nurse or eat more often, reflecting that human milk empties from the stomach more rapidly than formula.

Most term infants will tolerate longer intervals between feedings of up to 4 hours by the age of 3–4 weeks. Premature infants may continue to require frequent feedings past 6–8 weeks of age, depending on birth weight, corrected gestational age, and growth. Some infants begin to stop nighttime feedings after the age of 1–2 months, whereas others take as long as 4–6 months. The process is highly variable and may depend more on the weight attained than on a specific age; most infants are able to sleep through the night when they reach approximately 11 pounds.

The amount of formula offered to a bottle-fed infant should be consistent with the DRI for energy according to age and weight (Table 26–2). Table 26–13 lists typical quantities of feedings for various age groups. The infant should be fed on demand and not forced to take more formula than is desired at any one feeding. If the infant finishes a bottle and still seems hungry, more formula should be offered. Parents should also be aware that a newborn typically loses weight (mostly water) during the first week of life, but by 2 weeks of age, the infant should be gaining weight. Healthy weight gain usually indicates that the infant is receiving an appropriate amount of formula. WHO standardized growth charts are used to determine whether an infant is growing appropriately. Weight, length/height, and head circumference should be determined at each medical visit.

Both underfeeding and overfeeding are potential problems. Infants who like to "graze" all day can take in too much milk and gain too much weight. However, this behavior also can be a sign of inadequate intake in breast-fed infants, with consequent failure to thrive. Other problems associated with overfeeding are regurgitation, gastroesophageal reflux, vomiting, loose stools, constipation, and colic. Spitting up a small amount of formula, even after every feeding, is usually not a cause for concern. If an infant is regurgitating or vomiting significant amounts, a primary care provider should be consulted. Bilious emesis (with green-tinged vomitus) is always a reason to immediately consult the child's primary care provider.

Loose stools are normal for some infants, especially those receiving human milk or hydrolyzed formulas. A loose stool

TABLE 26-12 Sterilization Method for Infant Formula Preparation

General Preparation

- Always wash hands before preparing formula or handling bottles and nipples; repeat washing if interrupted.
- Sterilize bottles and other equipment (e.g., glass measuring cup, spoons, nipples, rings, disks) separately from the formula.[a] Many pediatricians and other primary care providers now consider the use of a dishwasher with a heated drying cycle as adequate for sterilization of infant feeding supplies.
- Using tongs, place all equipment in a deep pan or sterilizer, cover all equipment with cold tap water, bring to a boil, and continue boiling for 5 minutes.
- Tap and bottled water should be heated until it reaches a rolling boil, allowed to continue to boil for 1–2 minutes, and then allowed to cool to room temperature. Boiling for a longer period of time may concentrate impurities (e.g., lead) in the water.
- Using tongs, remove all items from the pan or sterilizer and place on a clean towel. Place bottles and nipples on the towel with their open ends facing down.

Concentrated Liquid Formula

- For cans, wash top of can with hot water and detergent, rinse in hot running water, and dry. Shake can well and open it with a clean punch-type can opener.
- For bottles, the protective cap must be removed. Shake bottle well and open.
- Mix appropriate amounts of concentrated liquid and sterilized water (according to product label or health care provider instructions). For accuracy, use a measuring cup for all measurements of formula and water.
- Pour formula into sterilized bottles; place nipples, rings, and disks on bottles.
- Tightly cover any unused formula and store in refrigerator. Use formula within 48 hours of preparation or discard.

Powdered Formula

- Wash top of can with hot water and detergent, rinse in hot running water, and dry.
- Open can and mix appropriate amounts of powder and sterilized water (according to product label or health care provider instructions). For accuracy, use the scoop provided or a dry measuring cup for all measurements.
- Pour formula into sterilized bottles; place nipples, rings, and disks on the bottles.
- Tightly cover any unused formula and store in the refrigerator. Use formula within 48 hours of preparation.
- Cover any formula remaining in the can with the plastic top. Write the date on the opened can. Store in a cool, dry place for up to 1 month.

Ready-to-Use Formula

Ready-to-Use Cans

- Wash top of can with hot water and detergent, rinse in hot running water, and dry.
- Shake can well, and open it with a clean punch-type can opener.
- Add the amount of formula needed for a single feeding to one sterilized bottle or to the number of bottles needed for a full day's feedings.
- *Do not add water.*
- Prepared bottles and any formula left in the can should be tightly covered and refrigerated for up to 48 hours after the can was opened.

Ready-to-Use Bottles

- The protective cap must be removed, and a sterile nipple must be screwed onto the bottle before feeding.
- Shake each bottle well to ensure mixing of formula.

All Types of Formulas

- Warm bottle to desired temperature by immersing in hot water bath or holding under hot running water.
- Heating bottles in the microwave is not recommended.
- Never boil or overheat formula.
- Shake each bottle well before feeding infant.
- Test formula temperature before feeding infant.
- After feeding, discard any formula left in bottle, and immediately rinse bottle and nipple in cool water.

[a] If disposable bottle liners are used, only nipples, rings, and screw tops of bottles need to be sterilized; the bottle liners provided by the manufacturer are sterile.

consistency also may be the result of an improperly concentrated formula or overfeeding. Rarely, loose stools may be the result of the administration of contaminated formula as mentioned previously. The contaminated formula results in pathologic changes in the gut leading loose stools. Human milk–fed infants may have only 1 stool every 1–3 days; however, some infants will have 10–12 stools each day. Formula-fed infants usually have 1–3 stools per day. *Diarrhea,* defined as increased stool volume and frequency that differ from the usual volume and frequency, warrants medical attention when it persists for more than 3 days or when the infant appears dehydrated. Constipation is rare in human milk– or formula-fed infants; it most often results from inadequate formula (fluid) intake. Severe or prolonged constipation with straining and blood streaks on the stool warrants a visit to the primary care provider.

TABLE 26-13 **Average Age-Appropriate Number of Daily Feedings and Volume per Feeding**

Age	Average Number of Daily Feedings	Average Volume per Feeding (oz)
Birth–2 weeks	6–10	2–3
2 weeks–1 month	6–8	4–5
1–3 months	5–6	5–6
3–4 months	4–5	6–7
4–12 months	3–4	7–8

Product Selection Guidelines

For healthy, term infants, a milk-based formula with or without added whey protein is indicated, except in patients who require a therapeutic formula. Recommendations for a formula should be based on ease of preparation or administration, the parent's or caregiver's ability to follow product directions, parental attitudes and preferences, sanitary conditions and availability of refrigeration facilities, and cost. Before assisting parents in selecting a therapeutic formula, the pharmacist should determine that a primary care provider recommended the formula.

For many parents, cost may be a critical factor in formula selection. Concentrated liquids and powders typically are less expensive than ready-to-use products. Convenience is also a consideration. The preparation of powdered and concentrated liquid formulas requires more manipulative functions and more attention to clean technique. The formula selected should be one that is well tolerated by the infant, convenient for parents and caregivers, and priced to fit the family's budget. To simplify formula preparation away from home, parents can select products available in unit-of-use packaging for ready-to-use liquids, or they can place a powder packet or powder in an empty bottle and add water whenever needed.

The federal grant program Special Supplemental Nutrition Program for Women, Infants, and Children (WIC) helps ensure that all infants, children (up to 5 years of age), and pregnant, postpartum, and breastfeeding women have access to adequate nutrition. State health departments and other agencies regulate and allocate funds in the federal grant program (i.e., almost $5.9 billion in FY2016). Formula and preventive services are subsidized for eligible participants but often require a prescription and previous authorization. More than 7.2 million persons received WIC benefits each month in 2016, most of them infants and children.[67]

Vitamin and Mineral Supplementation

Routine multivitamin and mineral supplementation is generally unnecessary for most formula- or human milk–fed term infants. However, some infants may be at risk for deficiency and require supplementation. Cases of vitamin D–deficiency rickets continue to be reported in the United States, and the prevalence of iron-deficiency anemia among children 1–3 years of age is 2.1% in the general population.[48,68] Accordingly, particular care is warranted to ensure that children in this age group get adequate dietary iron. AAP does not, however, endorse routine iron supplementation in children 1–3 years of age unless the child's diet is low in iron-containing foods.[48]

Vitamin and mineral supplementation may be needed for preterm and human milk–fed infants whose nutrition is inadequate[69–71] (Table 26–14). These infants and those with other nutritional deficiencies, malabsorptive and other chronic diseases, rare vitamin-dependent conditions, inborn errors of vitamin or mineral metabolism, or deficiencies related to the intake of certain medications will need medically supervised vitamin and mineral supplementation.

Human Milk–Fed, Full-Term Infants

The healthy, full-term, human milk–fed infant requires little to no special supplementation for the first 4–6 months of life except for vitamin D and iron. AAP recommends vitamin D supplementation (400 international units per day) for all human milk–fed infants unless they are weaned to at least 1000 mL/day of vitamin D–fortified formula. Risk factors for vitamin D deficiency include higher birth order (third child or later), dark skin, cultural factors that minimize maternal skin exposure to sunlight, and delayed intake of dairy products in the infant or mother because of intolerance or other factors.[72] Mothers should be encouraged to maintain a balanced diet and to drink three to five 8-ounce glasses of milk each day while breastfeeding. If the mother cannot tolerate milk because of lactose intolerance, lactose digestion aids (e.g., Lactaid, Dairy Ease, various store brands) and lactose-free milk are available. Mothers who do not drink milk should be encouraged to increase vitamin D and calcium intake through other dietary sources or by taking supplements. Furthermore, if the infant is showing signs or symptoms of being excessively colicky, the primary care provider should consider a "milk" sensitivity. If sensitivity is confirmed, the breastfeeding mother should decrease her dairy consumption and seek nondairy sources of calcium and vitamin D. Some primary care providers recommend complete removal of dairy products from the diet, whereas others suggest a more moderate approach that allows foods such as yogurt and cottage cheese.

Human milk–fed infants rarely develop iron-deficiency anemia before the age of 4–6 months.[48] Although the iron concentration in human milk averages only 0.3–0.5 mg/L, the form of iron is well absorbed. At the age of 4–6 months and beyond, the iron stores in infants fed human milk exclusively may become exhausted, requiring a supplemental source. The addition of iron-enriched foods such as fortified infant cereals will usually meet needs, or alternatively, an iron supplement (as elemental iron at a dosage of 2 mg/kg/day) can be given. A more recent study, however, indicates an association between increased duration of breastfeeding and decreased iron stores in the body.[73] Term infants who are small for gestational age are likely to have higher requirements, but the necessity for supplementation in this population is unclear.

The first iron-enriched food introduced into the infant's diet typically is infant cereal. Bioavailability of the large-particle, electrolytic iron powder used to fortify dry infant cereals is substantially less than that of ferrous sulfate iron used in milk- or soy protein–based formulas. Cereals also contain potent inhibitors of iron absorption and constitute an unreliable source of iron sufficient to prevent deficiency for infants who receive minimal iron from other sources. With iron-fortified, wet-packed cereal and fruit combinations marketed in jars, the iron sulfate is not exposed to oxygen until the jar is opened; therefore, iron

TABLE 26–14 Guidelines for Use of Vitamin and Mineral Supplements in Healthy Infants[a]

Age Group	Multivitamin/Mineral	Vitamin D[b]	Vitamin E	Folate	Iron[c]
Full-Term Infants					
Human milk–fed	0	+	0	0	±
Formula-fed	0	±[d]	0	0	0
Preterm Infants					
Human milk–fed[e]	+	+	0	0	+
Formula-fed[e]	+	+	0	0	+
Older Infants (>6 Months)					
Normal	0	0	0	0	±
High-risk[f]	+	0	0	0	±

Key: + = Supplement usually indicated; ± = supplement sometimes indicated; 0 = supplement not usually indicated.

[a] Not shown is vitamin K for newborn infants and fluoride in areas with insufficient fluoride in drinking water supply (Table 26–15).

[b] All infants should have a minimum daily intake of 400 international units of vitamin D beginning during the first few days of life; this intake should be continued throughout childhood and adolescence.

[c] Iron-fortified formula and infant cereals are more convenient and reliable sources of iron than a supplement.

[d] Supplement typically is indicated if infant is receiving less than 1000 mL/day of formula. An exception is Enfamil Premium Newborn, which is indicated for use from birth to the age of 3 months and provides 400 international units of vitamin D in 810 mL (27 fluid ounces).

[e] Multivitamin supplements (plus added folate) are needed primarily when calorie intake is below approximately 300 kcal/day or when the infant weighs less than 2.5 kg; vitamin D should be supplied at least until the age of 6 months in human milk–fed infants. Iron should be started by the age of 2 months.

[f] Multivitamin/mineral preparations including iron are preferred to supplements containing iron alone.

Source: References 9 and 69–71.

absorption is improved. Consuming fruit juices and other products containing ascorbic acid along with iron-fortified cereals has been shown to enhance iron absorption.[74]

Formula-Fed, Full-Term Infants

Full-term infants who consume adequate amounts of an iron-fortified, milk-based formula do not need vitamin and mineral supplementation in the first 6 months of life. An iron-fortified formula is preferred to ensure adequate iron stores for growing infants. Infants fed iron-fortified formulas do not demonstrate a difference in stool consistency, fussiness, colic, or regurgitation compared with infants fed low-iron formulas. Vitamin and mineral supplements are not needed for infants older than 6 months who receive a diet consisting of formula and increasing amounts of infant and table foods. A multivitamin with minerals may be needed, however, if the infant is at special nutritional risk secondary to a metabolic syndrome or other medical condition.

Preterm Infants

Preterm infants fed with either human milk or formula need vitamin and mineral supplementation. Their nutrient needs are greater than those of full-term infants because of their more rapid growth rate, inability to ingest an adequate volume of formula or human milk, decreased intestinal absorption, and lower body stores. Often these infants require a multivitamin supplement to provide the equivalent of the recommended intakes for full-term infants while receiving maternal breast milk, inadequate daily volume totals (~1000 mL/day), or certain formulas (e.g., Similac Alimentum), or prior to reaching a body weight of 2.5 kg.

Premature infants are especially susceptible to iron-deficiency anemia because of their marginal iron stores at birth. Without iron supplementation or receipt of blood transfusions for clinically significant low hemoglobin/hematocrit, iron stores will be depleted by the age of 2 months, in contrast with depletion at 4–6 months in full-term infants.

Originally the AAP/CON recommendations included supplementation with elemental iron at a dosage of 2 mg/kg daily for premature infants with birth weights between 1500 and 2500 g once they are 2 months old or have doubled their birth weight.[48,55] AAP now recommends that preterm infants who receive human milk should receive elemental iron supplementation (2–6 mg/kg/day) earlier, within 1 month, through 12 months of age. If these preterm infants are switched from human milk to formula, they will most likely not require iron supplementation once they are consuming 150 mL/kg/day. Recent reports, however, have shown that approximately 14% of preterm infants receiving appropriate formula will still need a supplement at 4–8 months of age because of decreased iron stores.[48] To prevent such diminished stores, some clinicians advocate even earlier initiation of iron supplementation in preterm infants born at less than 30 weeks of gestational age by starting supplementation as early as 2 weeks of chronological age with elemental iron doses of 2–4 mg/kg/day.[75] Infants receiving erythropoietin should receive elemental iron 6 mg/kg daily. To minimize the possibility of hemolytic anemia related to insufficient vitamin E absorption, iron supplements should be withheld until the preterm infant is several weeks old. However, with adequate vitamin E supplementation in the formula, the risk of hemolytic anemia is minimal.

Supplementation of calcium, phosphorus, and vitamin D in preterm infant formulas is necessary to ensure adequate bone mineralization and to prevent osteopenia and rickets. The prevention of severe bone disease in preterm infants appears to depend on both high oral intakes of calcium and phosphorus and the intake of at least 400 international units (12.5 mg) of vitamin D per day.[55] Therefore, preterm infants should receive specialized formulas, tailored to their needs, containing appropriate amounts of calcium, phosphorus, and vitamin D. Depending on the volume of formula consumed, vitamin D supplementation may be necessary, along with a premature formula, to provide 400–800 international units/day. Additionally, if patients are receiving either furosemide for congestive heart failure or bronchopulmonary dysplasia or phenobarbital for seizure disorders, increased vitamin D supplementation may be required.[76]

Fluoride Supplementation

When used appropriately, fluoride is both safe and effective in preventing and controlling dental caries. Fluoride helps prevent dental decay by reducing the solubility of enamel, limiting the ability of bacteria to produce acid, and promoting remineralization. Systemic fluoride, such as that obtained from fluoridated water, primarily provides a topical benefit to teeth: Fluoride is secreted from the salivary glands, for near-constant contact with tooth surfaces.[77] In 2014, CDC reported that 75% of the U.S. population for which the water supply comes from a community water system receive adequate fluoride.[78]

Fluoride supplementation currently is not recommended from birth to the age of 6 months. Furthermore, the recommended supplementation for children 6 months to 6 years of age whose drinking water is inadequately fluoridated and who do not receive adequate fluoride from other sources has been decreased from previous recommendations because of an increased incidence of fluorosis.[79] Fluorosis, which affects approximately 22% of U.S. children, is manifested in the dentition as changes ranging from minor white lines running across the teeth to a very chalky appearance resulting from too much fluoride. Infants who are being fed powdered or concentrated formula should be given fluoride supplements only if the community's drinking water, or bottled water used for making formula, contains less than 0.3 ppm of fluoride. Bottled water is often free of fluoride, and its use for reconstituting formula mandates appropriate supplementation. Table 26–15 can be used to determine the proper fluoride supplementation for a child, depending on the fluoride level in the drinking water. Ready-to-use formulas are manufactured with defluoridated water and contain less than 0.3 ppm of fluoride. The primary care provider may recommend a fluoride supplement for infants not receiving adequate fluoride.

TABLE 26–15 Recommended Fluoride Supplementation

	Supplementation (mg/day)[a] Indicated for Fluoride Concentration in Drinking Water		
Age Group	**<0.3 ppm**	**0.3–0.6 ppm**	**>0.6 ppm**
Birth–6 months	0	0	0
6 months–3 years	0.25	0	0
3–6 years	0.50	0.25	0
6–16 years	1.00	0.50	0

[a] Sodium fluoride 2.2 mg contains fluoride 1 mg.

Source: References 72, 73, 77, and 79; and Rozier RG, Adair S, Graham F, et al. Evidence-based clinical recommendations on the prescription of dietary fluoride supplements for caries prevention. *J Am Dent Assoc.* 2010;141(12):1480–9. Available at: http://jada.ada.org/article/S0002-8177(14)60477-3/pdf. Accessed May 15, 2017.

Assessment of Infant Nutrition: A Case-Based Approach

Body weight, length (height), and head circumference are the growth standards for determining whether infants are receiving the appropriate nutrients, are digesting and absorbing ingested nutrients, or both. If an infant appears to be underweight or underdeveloped, the pharmacist should advise the parent to take the infant to a primary care provider for evaluation.

The pharmacist's primary role is to provide information about breastfeeding and infant formula products, including assistance with product selection and preparation instructions.

Cases 26–1 and 26–2 are examples of assessment of infant nutrition in two different patients.

CASE 26–1

Relevant Evaluation Criteria	Scenario/Model Outcome
Collect	
1. Gather essential information about the patient's symptoms and medical history, including	
a. Description of symptom(s) (i.e., nature, onset, duration, severity, associated symptoms)	Braydon Smith's mother is worried because he spits up formula after every feeding, almost always with a little force. Although some emesis has occurred since birth, the amount and frequency have increased over the past few days. Mrs. Smith thinks he seems colicky, often crying from "gas pains." Braydon has always been a "good burper," so his mother feels that his gas pains are not related to too much air in his stomach. The infant appears well hydrated, and according to his mother, he has no fever.

Relevant Evaluation Criteria	Scenario/Model Outcome
b. Description of any factors that seem to precipitate, exacerbate, and/or relieve the patient's symptom(s)	Emesis occurs only after feedings. Braydon appears to be more comfortable after each episode of emesis. Irritability associated with gas pains appears to be relieved by simethicone.
c. Description of the patient's efforts to relieve the symptoms	Braydon's mother has been giving him simethicone for gas. Nothing specific has been done for the emesis.
d. Patient's identity	Braydon Smith
e. Patient's age, gender, length/height, and weight	3 weeks, male, 22 in., 10 lb 2 oz (4.6 kg)
f. Patient's dietary habits	Braydon was receiving primarily breast milk until 3 days ago, when his mother switched him to formula because of inadequate breast milk supply. The infant's feedings were changed to Enfamil Infant. Per Mrs. Smith's report, the formula is being mixed to a standard 20 kcal/oz concentration according to the instructions on the container. The infant takes approximately 180 mL (6 ounces) every 3 hours. No extra water or juice is given during the day.
g. Patient's sleep habits	Braydon has not yet started sleeping through the night.
h. Concurrent medical conditions, prescription and nonprescription medications, and dietary supplements	Braydon is a healthy term infant without any significant medical conditions or past medical history. His mother is currently giving him simethicone 20 mg up to 4 times a day as needed for apparent gas pains. She says that she usually gives approximately 2–3 doses per day.
i. Allergies	NKA
j. History of other adverse reactions to medications	None
k. Other (describe) ______	n/a
Assess	
2. Differentiate patient's signs/symptoms, and correctly identify the patient's primary problem(s).	Primary problem: emesis with feedings Secondary problem: increased intestinal gas
3. Identify exclusions for self-treatment.	Bloody or bilious emesis Signs of dehydration: sunken fontanelle, dry mucous membranes, decreased number of wet diapers, dark urine, decreased oral intake
4. Formulate a comprehensive list of therapeutic alternatives for the primary problem to determine whether triage to a medical provider is required, and share this information with the patient or caregiver.	Options include (1) Refer Braydon for immediate medical attention/PCP management. (2) Review preparation of infant formula with Mrs. Smith. (3) Monitor Braydon's symptoms and recommend nondrug measures only. (4) Recommend a medication alone or combined with nondrug measures. (5) Take no action.
Plan	
5. Select an optimal therapeutic alternative to address the patient's problem, taking into account patient/caregiver preferences.	Braydon's current feeding schedule, 180 mL of 20 kcal/oz of formula every 3 hours, provides 209 kcal/kg/day in a volume of 313 mL/kg/day. Both exceed the usual recommended intakes for a healthy term newborn (Tables 26–2 and 26–12). Because the emesis and gas pain have increased since Braydon's transition from breast milk to infant formula, Braydon most likely is not tolerating the volume of the formula provided every 3 hours. Unlike when Braydon was breastfed, the formula provided in a bottle can be visually seen by the caregiver, and the infant is often encouraged to complete ingestion of the bottle contents. If the caregiver is providing an excessive volume of formula, the infant may consume the entire volume but may regurgitate the additional quantity owing to a much smaller tolerated gastric volume. Additionally, Braydon may benefit from a slow-flow nipple to regulate the flow of milk. Explain the correlation between the increased emesis and volume of formula provided. Recommend that Mrs. Smith contact Braydon's PCP to discuss appropriate advancement of infant formula as he grows. If Braydon continues to have problems after a change in formula, his mother should follow up with his PCP for further management.

CASE 26-1 *continued*

Relevant Evaluation Criteria	Scenario/Model Outcome
6. Describe the recommended therapeutic approach to the patient or caregiver.	"The increased emesis and gas pain are caused by an excessive volume of formula provided every 3 hours. A smaller volume of infant formula at each feeding should relieve Braydon's symptoms. If the symptoms persist after the change in volume, Braydon should be seen again by his primary care provider."
7. Explain to the patient or caregiver the rationale for selecting the recommended therapeutic approach from the considered therapeutic alternatives.	"Because the symptoms started (or acutely worsened) with the change from breast milk to infant formula and the caloric density but not the volume of the infant formula is appropriate for a healthy term infant, excessive volume of formula at each feeding is the most likely cause of Braydon's emesis and irritability. If the volume is the major issue, changing the volume should produce relief of symptoms within several days."
Implement	
8. When recommending self-care with nonprescription medications and/or nondrug therapy, convey accurate information to the patient or caregiver.	
a. Product storage requirements	"Infant formula should be used soon after mixing or kept tightly covered in the refrigerator and used within 24 hours of preparation. If the infant has already consumed some of the formula out of the bottle, the rest should either be consumed within 1 hour or discarded. See product information for any specific storage requirements."
b. Specific nondrug measures	n/a
Solicit follow-up questions from the patient or caregiver.	"What if Braydon continues to have emesis and gas pain after seeing the primary care provider and decreasing the volume of formula provided?"
Answer the patient's or caregiver's questions.	"From the history, it sounds like Braydon might be receiving too much formula at each feeding. If he receives less volume at each feeding, his emesis and gas pains should noticeably lessen. If a change in volume does not help relieve his symptoms, his primary care provider will further assess his gastrointestinal intolerance."
Follow-up: Evaluate and Monitor	
9. Assess patient outcome.	Ask Mrs. Smith to call in 2–3 days to update you on Braydon's response to your recommendations, or you could call her in 2–3 days to evaluate the response. If no improvement has occurred, ensure that she has made an appointment with Braydon's PCP for further evaluation.

Key: GI = Gastrointestinal; n/a = not applicable; NKA = no known allergies; PCP = primary care provider.

CASE 26-2

Relevant Evaluation Criteria	Scenario/Model Outcome
Collect	
1. Gather essential information about the patient's symptoms and medical history, including	
a. Description of symptom(s) (i.e., nature, onset, duration, severity, associated symptoms)	Annie Adams is a healthy-appearing 4-month-old, term infant. Her mother comes to the pharmacy today because she is wondering if she should start to give Annie vitamins because she is exclusively breastfed. Her pediatrician suggested this at her recent well child checkup. Mrs. Adams asks specifically if she should have Annie take Poly-Vi-Flor, which her friend's 11-month-old son takes since he is still breastfeeding.

CASE 26-2 *continued*

Relevant Evaluation Criteria	Scenario/Model Outcome
b. Description of any factors that seem to precipitate, exacerbate, and/or relieve the patient's symptom(s)	None
c. Description of the patient's efforts to relieve the symptoms	n/a
d. Patient's identity	Annie Adams
e. Patient's age, gender, length/height, and weight	4 months (born at 40 weeks' gestational age), female, 25 in., 15 lb 2 oz (6.9 kg)
f. Patient's occupation	n/a
g. Patient's dietary habits	Mrs. Adams is still on maternity leave. Annie is exclusively breastfed, eating approximately every 3–4 hours during the day.
h. Patient's sleep habits	She sleeps from 10 PM to 6 AM.
i. Concurrent medical conditions, prescription and nonprescription medications, and dietary supplements	Annie is a healthy term infant with no preexisting medical conditions. She currently takes no prescription or nonprescription medications and no dietary supplements.
j. Allergies	NKA
k. History of other adverse reactions to medications	None
l. Other (describe) ______	n/a
Assess	
2. Differentiate patient's signs/symptoms, and correctly identify the patient's primary problem(s).	Potential for vitamin D and iron deficiency due to age and exclusive breast milk diet. No current need exists for fluoride supplementation, because the patient is younger than 6 months of age.
3. Identify exclusions for self-treatment.	None
4. Formulate a comprehensive list of therapeutic alternatives for the primary problem to determine whether triage to a medical provider is required, and share this information with the patient or caregiver.	Options include (1) Refer this patient to the PCP. (2) Recommend a nonprescription multivitamin with iron but without fluoride supplementation. (3) Take no action.
Plan	
5. Select an optimal therapeutic alternative to address the patient's problem, taking into account patient/caregiver preferences.	Recommend a standard infant multivitamin containing ferrous sulfate.
6. Describe the recommended therapeutic approach to the patient or caregiver.	"Your primary care provider suggested a multivitamin since Annie is now 4 months of age and is exclusively breastfed. I would recommend a standard infant multivitamin containing ferrous sulfate."
7. Explain to the patient or caregiver the rationale for selecting the recommended therapeutic approach from the considered therapeutic alternatives.	"Term infants have approximately a 4- to 6-month store of iron reserves in their bodies. Human milk is very low in iron but meets most infants' needs for the first 4–6 months. Moreover, Annie's need for adequate vitamin D currently exceeds the amount provided in breast milk. Annie is younger than 6 months old, so she currently does not require fluoride supplementation, which is present in Poly-Vi-Flor. For these reasons, your primary care provider suggested you start giving a daily multivitamin containing iron."
Implement	
8. When recommending self-care with nonprescription medications and/or nondrug therapy, convey accurate information to the patient or caregiver.	
a. Appropriate dose and frequency of administration	"Infant multivitamin with iron (e.g., Enfamil Poly-Vi-Sol with Iron Drops) 1 mL by mouth daily."
b. Maximum number of days the therapy should be employed	"Until recommended to discontinue per Annie's primary care provider."
c. Product administration procedures	"Measure liquid using the dropper that comes with the medication and have Annie swallow the liquid."

CASE 26-2 *continued*

Relevant Evaluation Criteria	Scenario/Model Outcome
d. Expected time to onset of relief	n/a
e. Degree of relief that can be reasonably expected	n/a
f. Most common side effects	"Adverse effects are rare, but gastrointestinal symptoms are possible. Give the iron drops with food if these effects occur."
g. Side effects that warrant medical attention	"Contact a health care provider if signs of an allergic reaction, such as a rash or trouble breathing, occur after a dose is given."
h. Patient's/caregiver's options in the event that condition worsens or persists	n/a
i. Product storage requirements	"Keep medication in a tightly secured container away from any extreme temperature and out of children's reach."
j. Specific nondrug measures	n/a
Solicit follow-up questions from the patient or caregiver.	"What do I do if Annie spits out a dose of the multivitamin product?"
Answer the patient's or caregiver's questions.	"If Annie spits out a dose of the multivitamin product, do not try to give the dose again. The medication is not so vital that it must be given each day for a medical condition, and Annie could potentially receive too much iron if given multiple doses. Be aware of the potential for the multivitamin product to stain clothing."
Follow-up: Monitor and Evaluate	
9. Assess patient outcome.	Ask Mrs. Adams mother to call after 1 week with an update on her response to your recommendations for Annie, or you could call her in a week to evaluate Annie's response.

Key: n/a = Not applicable; NKA = no known allergies; PCP = primary care provider.

Patient Counseling for Infant Nutrition

The number and variety of infant formulas available may bewilder some parents. Once the formula type recommended or prescribed by the baby's primary care provider is known, the parents can be directed to the appropriate product. If the parents need further assistance with product selection, the pharmacist can make a recommendation to accommodate their preferences. At these encounters, the parents should demonstrate that they know how to properly prepare their baby's formula and how much formula to give at each feeding. The box "Patient Education for Infant Nutrition" lists specific information to include in patient counseling for parents and caregivers. In addition, families who may qualify for the WIC program but are not enrolled can be advised of its availability and benefits.

Key Points for Infant Nutrition and Special Nutritional Needs of Children

- Human milk is the optimal food for infants younger than 12 months of age, and its use should be encouraged for nearly all infants. When breastfeeding or provision of human milk is not possible or desired, commercial infant formulas provide a safe, nutritionally adequate substitute.
- Commercial formulas are available in a variety of types to meet the needs of most infants, as well as children with special nutritional needs, such as those with a feeding tube.
- Therapeutic formulas designed for infants and children with altered requirements dictated by disease or other conditions, including prematurity, vary in content and are not generically equivalent. These formulas should be used under medical supervision and are not self selected.
- Accurate preparation of formula is critical to ensure optimal nutritional outcomes. Parents and caregivers should be counseled on proper preparation techniques.
- Some infants will require vitamin and/or mineral supplementation when their needs are not adequately met by their formula intake.
- Parents should be referred to a PCP if the child has persistent vomiting or if at any time the emesis fluid is bilious (green-tinged).
- Parents should be referred to a PCP if the child has diarrhea lasting more than 3 days, especially if dehydration develops, if the child looks clinically ill, or if blood is present in the stool.

PATIENT EDUCATION FOR Infant Nutrition

Optimal nutrition is critical in infants and children to ensure normal growth and development. Parents who carefully follow product instructions for formula preparation and the measures listed here will help ensure optimal nutrition-related outcomes.

- Check unopened formula containers for damage. Do not use products if the container is significantly dented or if the expiration date has passed.
- When preparing formula from powder or liquid concentrate, carefully follow instructions for dilution to the desired caloric density (Tables 26–8 and 26–9). If the formula is too concentrated, the baby may have diarrhea or become dehydrated. If it is too dilute, the baby can become water-intoxicated, which can lead to irritability, seizures, coma, or brain damage.
- When preparing formula from powder or liquid concentrate, follow the technique for aseptic processing and sterilization. Be sure to sterilize the bottles (or use sterile liners) and other equipment, and boil the water used to make the formula (Table 26–11).
- When preparing ready-to-use formulas, do not add water to the formula. Follow the instructions in Table 26–11. Be sure to sterilize the bottles (or use sterile liners) and other equipment.
- Use prepared or opened ready-to-use formula within 48 hours. Keep refrigerated.
- Feed your baby according to the frequency and quantities listed in Table 26–12 unless instructed otherwise by the baby's primary care provider. Paying careful attention to your infant's hunger and fullness cues is important to avoid over- and underfeeding. Discuss any concerns with your infant's primary care provider.
- Heating formula in a microwave is not recommended. However, if formula or human milk is warmed in a microwave, follow these instructions to prevent a container explosion incident or scalds or burns to the baby's mouth:
  - Remove the bottle's lid to allow heat to escape.
  - Heat only 4 ounces or more of refrigerated milk; do not thaw frozen human milk in a microwave. Place frozen human milk in a tepid water bath to thaw.
  - Heat 4 ounces of refrigerated formula on full power for no longer than 30 seconds; heat 8 ounces of refrigerated formula for 45 seconds.
  - After heating the formula, replace the nipple assembly and invert the bottle a minimum of 10 times.
  - Test the formula's temperature by putting a few drops on your tongue or the top part of your hand or the back of the wrist. Do not feed the baby the formula unless it feels cool to the touch.

When to Seek Medical Attention

- Seek medical attention if
  - Your baby is regurgitating or vomiting significant amounts of formula. A small amount of spitting up is normal. Projectile vomiting or bilious emesis (with green-tinged vomitus) always warrants immediate medical attention.
  - Your baby has severe diarrhea or diarrhea that persists for more than 3 days.
  - Your baby appears dehydrated (e.g., decreased number of wet diapers, dark urine, limp body tone, no tears, lethargic appearance).
  - Your baby's stools have blood in them.

REFERENCES

1. Grummer-Strawn LM, Reinold C, Krebs NF; Centers for Disease Control and Prevention (CDC). Use of World Health Organization and CDC growth charts for children aged 0–59 months in the United States. *MMWR Recomm Rep.* 2010;59(RR-9):1–15. PMID: 20829749. Available at: http://www.cdc.gov/mmwr/pdf/rr/rr5909.pdf. Accessed May 15, 2017.
2. Committee on Nutrition, American Academy of Pediatrics. Development of gastrointestinal function. In: Kleinman RE, Greer FR, eds. *Pediatric Nutrition.* 7th ed. Elk Grove Village, IL: American Academy of Pediatrics; 20014:15–40.
3. Lentze MJ, Branski D. Disorders of malabsorption—enzyme deficiencies. In: Kliegman RM, Stanton BF, St. Geme JW, et al., eds. *Nelson Textbook of Pediatrics.* 20th ed. Philadelphia, PA: Elsevier Science; 2016:1835.
4. Bull MJ; Committee on Genetics. Health supervision for children with Down syndrome. *Pediatrics.* 2011;128(2):393–406. doi: 10.1542/peds.2011-1605. Available at: http://pediatrics.aappublications.org/content/128/2/393.full.pdf+html. Accessed May 15, 2017.
5. Zemel BS, Pipan M, Stallings VA, et al. Growth charts for children with Down syndrome in the United States. *Pediatrics.* 2015;136(5):e1204-11. doi: 10.1542/peds.2015-1652. Available at: http://pediatrics.aappublications.org/content/pediatrics/early/2015/10/21/peds.2015-1652.full.pdf. Accessed May 15, 2017.
6. Krebs NF, Himes JH, Jacobson D, et al. Assessment of child and adolescent overweight and obesity. *Pediatrics.* 2007;120(Suppl 4):S193–228. doi: 10.1542/peds.2007-2329D. Available at: http://pediatrics.aappublications.org/content/120/Supplement_4/S193.full.pdf+html. Accessed May 15, 2017.
7. Ogden CL, Carroll MD, Kit BK, et al. Prevalence of childhood and adult in the United States, 2011–2012. *JAMA.* 2014;311(8):806–14. doi: 10.1001/jama.2014.734. Available at: http://jama.jamanetwork.com/article.aspx?articleid=1832542. Accessed May 15, 2017.
8. Ogden CL, Carroll MD, Lawman HG, Fryar CD, et al. Trends in obesity prevalence among children and adolescents in the United States, 1988–1994 through 2013–2014. *JAMA.* 2016;315(21):2292–9. doi: 10.1001/jama.2016.6361.
9. Institute of Medicine, Food and Nutrition Board, Standing Committee on the Scientific Evaluation of Dietary Reference Intakes. *Dietary Reference Intakes for Energy, Carbohydrate, Fiber, Fat, Fatty Acids, Cholesterol, Protein, and Amino Acids.* Washington, DC: National Academy Press; 2005. Available at: http://www.nap.edu. Accessed May 15, 2017.
10. Committee on Nutrition, American Academy of Pediatrics. Carbohydrate and dietary fiber. In: Kleinman RE, Greer FR, eds. *Pediatric Nutrition.* 7th ed. Elk Grove Village, IL: American Academy of Pediatrics; 2014: 387–406.
11. Heird WC. Taurine in neonatal nutrition—revisited. *Arch Dis Child Fetal Neonatal Ed.* 2004;89(6):473–4. doi: 10.1136/adc.2004.055095.
12. National Heart, Lung, and Blood Institute. Expert Panel on Integrated Guidelines for Cardiovascular Health and Risk Reduction in Children and Adolescents: summary report. *Pediatrics.* 2011;128(Suppl 5): S213–56. doi: 10.1542/peds.2009-2107C. Available at: http://pediatrics.aappublications.org/content/128/Supplement_5/S213.full.pdf. Accessed May 15, 2017.
13. Koletzko B, Lien E, Agostoni C, et al. The roles of long-chain polyunsaturated fatty acids in pregnancy, lactation and infancy: review of current knowledge and consensus recommendations. *J Perinat Med.* 2008;36(1):5–14. doi: 10.1515/JPM.2008.001.
14. Lapillonne A, Groh-Wargo S, Gonzalez GHL, et al. Lipid needs of preterm infants: updated recommendations. *J Pediatr.* 2013;162(3 suppl): S37–47. doi: 10.1016/j.jpeds.2012.11.052.
15. Delplanque B, Gibson R, Koletzko B, et al. Lipid quality in infant nutrition: current knowledge and future opportunities. *J Pediatr Gastroenterol Nutr.* 2015;61(1):8–17. doi: 10.1097/MPG.0000000000000818. Available at: http://journals.lww.com/jpgn/Fulltext/2015/07000/Lipid_Quality_in_Infant_Nutrition___Current.6.aspx. Accessed May 15, 2017.
16. Breanna JT. Arachidonic acid needed in infant formula when docosahexaenoic acid is present. *Nutr Rev.* 2016;74(5):329–36. doi: 10.1093/nutrit/nuw007.

17. Koletzko B, Lien E, Agostoni C, et al. The roles of long-chain polyunsaturated fatty acids in pregnancy, lactation and infancy: review of current knowledge and consensus recommendations. *J Perinat Med.* 2008;36(1):5–14. doi: 10.1515/JPM.2008.001.
18. Simmer K, Patole SK, Rao SC. Long chain polyunsaturated fatty acid supplementation in infants born at term. *Cochrane Database Syst Rev.* 2008;1:CD000376. doi: 10.1002/14651858.CD000376.pub3. Available at: http://www.thecochranelibrary.com/view/0/index.html. Accessed May 15, 2017.
19. Schulzke SM, Patole SK, Simmer K. Long-chain polyunsaturated fatty acid supplementation in preterm infants. *Cochrane Database Syst Rev.* 2011; 2:CD000375. doi: 10.1002/14651858.CD000375.pub4. Available at: http://onlinelibrary.wiley.com/doi/10.1002/14651858.CD000375.pub4/epdf. Accessed May 15, 2017.
20. Atwell K, Collins CT, Sullivan TR, et al. Respiratory hospitalization of infants supplemented with docosahexaenoic acid as preterm neonates. *J Paediatr Child Health.* 2013;49(1):E17–22. doi: 10.1111/jpc.12057. Available at: http://onlinelibrary.wiley.com/doi/10.1111/jpc.12057/pdf. Accessed May 15, 2017.
21. Lapillonne A, Pastor N, Zhuang W, et al. Infants fed formula with added long chain polyunsaturated fatty acids have reduced incidence of respiratory illnesses and diarrhea during the first year of life. *BMC Pediatr.* 2014; 14:168. doi: 10.1186/1471-2431-14-168. Available at: http://bmcpediatr.biomedcentral.com/articles/10.1186/1471-2431-14-168. Accessed May 15, 2017.
22. Foiles AM, Kerling EH, Wick JA, et al. Formula with long-chain polyunsaturated fatty acids reduces incidence of allergy in early childhood. *Pediatr Allergy Immunol.* 2016;27(2):156–61. doi: 10.1111/pai.12515. Available at: http://onlinelibrary.wiley.com/doi/10.1111/pai.12515/epdf. Accessed May 15, 2017.
23. Beyerlein A, Hadders-Algra M, Kennedy K, et al. Infant formula supplementation with long-chain polyunsaturated fatty acids has no effect on Bayley development scores at 18 months of age—IPD meta-analysis of 4 large clinical trials. *J Pediatr Gastroenterol Nutr.* 2010;50(1):79–84. doi: 10.1097/MPG.0b013e3181acae7d. Available at: http://journals.lww.com/jpgn/pages/articleviewer.aspx?year=2010&issue=01000&article=00020&type=abstract. Accessed May 15, 2017.
24. Qawasmi A, Landeros-Weisenberger A, Leckman JF, et al. Meta-analysis of long-chain polyunsaturated fatty acid supplementation of formula and infant cognition. *Pediatrics.* 2012;129(6):1141–9. doi: 10.1542/peds.2011-2127. Available at: http://pediatrics.aappublications.org/content/129/6/1141.full.pdf. Accessed May 15, 2017.
25. Colombo J, Carlson SE, Cheatham CL, et al. Long-term effects of LCPUFA supplementation on childhood cognitive outcomes. *Am J Clin Nutr.* 2013;98(2):403–12. doi: 10.3945/ajcn.112.040766. Available at: http://ajcn.nutrition.org/content/98/2/403.full.pdf+html. Accessed March 17, 2017.
26. Delgado-Noguera MF, Calvache JA, Bonfill Cosp X, et al. Supplementation with long chain polyunsaturated fatty acids (LCPUFA) to breastfeeding mothers for improving child growth and development. *Cochrane Database Syst Rev.* 2015;7:CD007901. doi: 10.1002/14651858.CD007901.pub3. Available at: http://onlinelibrary.wiley.com/doi/10.1002/14651858.CD007901.pub3/abstract. Accessed May 15, 2017.
27. World Health Organization. *Global Strategy for Infant and Young Child Feeding.* Geneva, Switzerland: World Health Organization; 2003. Available at: http://apps.who.int/iris/bitstream/10665/42590/1/9241562218.pdf?ua=1&ua=1. Accessed May 15, 2017.
28. Section on Breastfeeding, American Academy of Pediatrics. Breastfeeding and the use of human milk. *Pediatrics.* 2012;129(3):e827–41. doi: 10.1542/peds.2011-3552. Available at: http://pediatrics.aappublications.org/content/129/3/e827.full.pdf+html. Accessed May 15, 2017.
29. Horta BL, Victora CG. Long-term effects of breastfeeding: a systematic review. Geneva, Switzerland: World Health Organization; 2013. Available at: http://apps.who.int/iris/bitstream/10665/79198/1/9789241505307_eng.pdf. Accessed May 15, 2017.
30. McDowell MM, Wang CY, Kennedy-Stephensen J. Breastfeeding in the United States: findings from the National Health and Nutrition Examination Surveys, 1999–2006. Hyattsville, MD: National Center for Health Statistics; 2008. NCHS Data Brief, No. 5. Available at: http://www.cdc.gov/nchs/data/databriefs/db05.pdf. Accessed May 15, 2017.
31. Centers for Disease Control and Prevention. Breastfeeding among US children born 2002–2012: CDC National Immunization Surveys. Centers for Disease Control and Prevention, Atlanta, GA; July 2015. Available at: http://www.cdc.gov/breastfeeding/data/NIS_data/index.htm. Accessed May 15, 2017.
32. Centers for Disease Control and Prevention. Breastfeeding report card—United States, 2014. Centers for Disease Control and Prevention, Atlanta, GA; August 2015. Available at: http://www.cdc.gov/breastfeeding/pdf/2014BreastfeedingReportCard.pdf. Accessed May 15, 2017.
33. U.S. Department of Health and Human Services. *Healthy People 2020: National Health Promotion and Disease Prevention Objectives.* Washington, DC: U.S. Government Printing Office; 2010. Available at: http://www.healthypeople.gov/2020/default.aspx. Accessed May 15, 2017.
34. Batrick M. Breastfeeding and the U.S. economy. *Breastfeed Med.* 2011; 6:313–8. doi: 10.1089/bfm.2011.0057. Available at: http://online.liebertpub.com/doi/pdf/10.1089/bfm.2011.0057. Accessed May 15, 2017.
35. Bartick M, Reinhold A. The burden of suboptimal breastfeeding in the United States: a pediatric cost analysis. *Pediatrics.* 2010;125(5): e1048–56. doi: 10.1542/peds.2009-1616. Available at: http://pediatrics.aappublications.org/content/125/5/e1048.pdf. Accessed May 15, 2017.
36. Tuttle DR, Siavit WI. Establishing the business case for breastfeeding. *Breastfeed Med.* 2009;4(suppl 1):S59–62. doi: 10.1089/bfm.2009.0031.
37. Ball TM, Bennett DM. The economic impact of breastfeeding. *Pediatr Clin North Am.* 2001;48(1):253–62. PMID: 11236730.
38. Rasmussen KM, Geraghty SR. The quiet revolution: breastfeeding transformed with the use of breast pumps. *Am J Public Health.* 2011;101(8): 1356–9. doi: 10.2105/AJPH.2011.300136. Available at: http://www.ncbi.nlm.nih.gov/pmc/articles/PMC3134520/pdf/1356.pdf. Accessed May 15, 2017.
39. Felice JP, Cassano PA, Rasmussen KM. Pumping human milk in the early postpartum period: its impact on long-term practices for feeding at the breast and exclusively feeding human milk in a longitudinal survey cohort. *Am J Clin Nutr.* 2016;103(5):1267–77. doi: 10.3945/ajcn.115.115733. Available at: http://ajcn.nutrition.org/content/103/5/1267.full.pdf+html. Accessed May 15, 2017.
40. Haiden N, Pimpel B, Assadian O, et al. Comparison of bacterial counts in expressed breast milk following standard or strict infection control regimens in neonatal intensive care units: compliance of mothers does matter. *J Hosp Infect.* 2016;92(3):226–8. doi: 10.1016/j.jhin.2015.11.018. Available at: http://www.sciencedirect.com/science/article/pii/S0195670115005241. Accessed May 15, 2017.
41. Academy of Breastfeeding Medicine Protocol Committee, Eglash A. ABM clinical protocol #8: human milk storage information for home use for full-term infants. *Breastfeed Med.* 2010;5(3):127–30. doi: 10.1089/bfm.2010.9988. Available at: http://online.liebertpub.com/doi/abs/10.1089/bfm.2010.9988?url_ver=Z39.88-2003&rfr_id=ori%3Arid%3Acrossref.org&rfr_dat=cr_pub%3Dpubmed&. Accessed May 15, 2017.
42. Centers for Disease Control and Prevention. Proper handling and storage of human milk. March 4, 2010. Available at: https://www.cdc.gov/breastfeeding/recommendations/handling_breastmilk.htm. Accessed May 15, 2017.
43. Sachs HC; Committee on Drugs. The transfer of drugs and therapeutics into human breast milk: an update on selected topics. *Pediatrics.* 2013;132(3):e796–809. doi: 10.1542/peds.2013-1985. Available at: http://pediatrics.aappublications.org/content/132/3/e796. Accessed May 15, 2017.
44. Moro GE. Processing of donor human milk. *J Pediatr Gastroenterol Nutr.* 2015;61(Suppl 1):S6–7. doi: 10.1097/01.mpg.0000471453.93544.ef. Available at: http://journals.lww.com/jpgn/Citation/2015/09001/V__Processing_of_Donor_Human_Milk.9.aspx. Accessed May 15, 2017.
45. Bloom BT. Safety of donor milk: a brief report. *J Perinatol.* 2016; 36(5):392–3. doi: 10.1038/jp.2015.207.
46. Kantorowska A, Wei JC, Cohen RS, et al. Impact of donor milk availability on breast milk use and necrotizing enterocolitis rates. *Pediatrics.* 2016;137(3):1–8. doi: 10.1542/peds.2015-3123. Available at: http://pediatrics.aappublications.org/content/137/3/e20153123.pdf. Accessed May 15, 2017.
47. Committee on Nutrition, American Academy of Pediatrics. Formula feeding of term infants. In: Kleinman RE, Greer FR, eds. *Pediatric Nutrition.* 7th ed. Elk Grove Village, IL: American Academy of Pediatrics; 2014:61–82.

48. Baker RD, Greer FR; Committee on Nutrition, American Academy of Pediatrics. Diagnosis and prevention of iron deficiency and iron-deficiency anemia in infants and young children (0–3 years of age). *Pediatrics.* 2010;126(5):1040–50. doi: 10.1542/peds.2010-2576. Available at: http://pediatrics.aappublications.org/content/126/5/1040. Accessed May 15, 2017.
49. Fomon SJ. Potential renal solute load: considerations related to complementary feedings of breastfed infants. *Pediatrics.* 2000;106(5 Suppl): 1284. PMID: 11061831. Available at: http://pediatrics.aappublications.org/content/pediatrics/106/Supplement_4/1284.full.pdf. Accessed May 15, 2017.
50. Shah SD, Dereddy N, Jones TL, Dhanireddy R, et al. Early versus delayed human milk fortification in very low birth weight infants—a randomized controlled trial. *J Pediatr.* 2016;174:126–31.e1. doi: 10.1016/j.jpeds.2016.03.056.
51. Basnet SI, Schneider M, Gazit A, et al. Fresh goat's milk for infants: myths and realities—a review. *Pediatrics.* 2010;125(4):e973–7. doi: 10.1542/peds.2009-1906.
52. Bhatia J, Greer F; American Academy of Pediatrics Committee on Nutrition. Use of soy protein-based formulas in infant feeding. *Pediatrics.* 2008;121(5):1062–8. doi: 10.1542/peds.2008-0564. Available at: http://pediatrics.aappublications.org/content/121/5/1062.full.pdf+html. Accessed May 15, 2017.
53. Greer FR, Sicherer SH, Burks AW; American Academy of Pediatrics Committee on Nutrition; American Academy of Pediatrics Section on Allergy and Immunology. Effects of early nutritional interventions on the development of atopic disease in infants and children: the role of maternal dietary restriction, breastfeeding, timing of introduction of complementary foods, and hydrolyzed formulas. *Pediatrics.* 2008;121(1): 183–91. doi: 10.1542/peds.2007-3022. Available at: http://pediatrics.aappublications.org/content/121/1/183.full.pdf+html. Accessed May 15, 2017.
54. Ellis L, Kalnias D, Corey M, et al. Do infants with cystic fibrosis need a protein hydrolysate formula? A prospective, randomized, comparative study. *J Pediatr.* 1998;132(2):270–6. doi: http://dx.doi.org/10.1016/S0022-3476(98)70444-5.
55. Committee on Nutrition, American Academy of Pediatrics. Nutritional needs of preterm infants. In: Kleinman RE, Greer FR, eds. *Pediatric Nutrition.* 7th ed. Elk Grove Village, IL: American Academy of Pediatrics; 2014:83–122.
56. Underwood MA. Human milk for the premature infant. *Pediatr Clin North Am.* 2013;60(1):189–207. doi: 10.1016/j.pcl.2012.09.008.
57. Reis BB, Hall RT, Schanler RJ, et al. Enhanced growth of preterm infants fed a new powdered human milk fortifier: a randomized, controlled trial. *Pediatrics.* 2000;106(3):581–8. doi: 10.1542/peds.106.3.581.
58. Slykerman RF, Thompson JM, Becroft DM, et al. Breastfeeding and intelligence of preschool children. *Acta Paediatr.* 2005;94(7):832–7. doi: 10.1080/08035250510031601.
59. Ganapathy V, Hay JW, Kim JH. Costs of necrotizing enterocolitis and cost-effectiveness of exclusively human milk-based products in feeding extremely premature infants. *Breastfeed Med.* 2012;7(1):29–37. doi: 10.1089/bfm.2011.0002. Available at: http://online.liebertpub.com/doi/pdf/10.1089/bfm.2011.0002. Accessed May 15, 2017.
60. U.S. Food and Drug Administration, Center for Food Safety and Applied Nutrition. Exempt infant formulas marketed in the United States by manufacturer and category. October 2, 1015. Available at: http://www.fda.gov/Food/GuidanceRegulation/GuidanceDocumentsRegulatoryInformation/InfantFormula/ucm106456.htm. Accessed May 15, 2017.
61. Centers for Disease Control and Prevention. Managing acute gastroenteritis among children: oral rehydration, maintenance, and nutritional therapy. *MMWR Morb Mortal Wkly Rep.* 2003;52(RR-16):1–20. Available at: http://www.cdc.gov/mmwr/PDF/rr/rr5216.pdf. Accessed May 15, 2017.
62. Brown JV, Embleton ND, Harding JE, McGuire W. Multi-nutrient fortification of human milk for preterm infants. *Cochrane Database Syst Rev.* 2016;5:CD000343. doi: 10.1002/14651858.CD000343.pub3. Available at: http://onlinelibrary.wiley.com/doi/10.1002/14651858.CD000343.pub3/epdf. Accessed May 15, 2017.
63. Caufield PW, Griffen AL. Dental caries: an infectious and transmissible disease. *Pediatr Clin North Am.* 2000;47(5):1001–20. PMID: 11059347.
64. Committee on Nutrition, American Academy of Pediatrics. Aluminum toxicity in infants and children. *Pediatrics.* 1996;97(3):413–6. PMID: 8604282. Available at: http://pediatrics.aappublications.org/content/97/3/413.full.pdf+html?sid=35eaebf7-76d7-45b5-8313-a0602cc7052f. Accessed May 15, 2017. [Guideline reaffirmed by AAP in January 2004.]
65. Committee on Environmental Health and Committee on Infectious Diseases. Drinking water from private wells and risks to children. *Pediatrics.* 2009;123(6);1599–605. doi: 10.1542/peds.2009-0751. Available at: http://pediatrics.aappublications.org/content/123/6/1599.full.pdf+html. Accessed May 15, 2017. [Guideline reaffirmed by AAP in January 2013].
66. World Health Organization; Food and Agriculture Organization of the United Nations. *Safe Preparation, Storage and Handling of Powdered Infant Formula: Guidelines. 2007.* Geneva, Switzerland: World Health Organization; 2007. Available at: http://www.who.int/foodsafety/publications/micro/pif_guidelines.pdf. Accessed May 15, 2017.
67. U.S. Department of Agriculture, Food and Nutrition Service. WIC: the Special Supplemental Nutrition Program for Women, Infants and Children. Updated March 10, 2017. Available at: http://www.fns.usda.gov/wic. Accessed May 15, 2017.
68. Abrams SA; Committee on Nutrition. Calcium and vitamin D requirements of enterally fed preterm infants. *Pediatrics.* 2013;131(5):e1676–83. doi: 10.1542/peds.2013-0420. Available at: http://pediatrics.aappublications.org/content/131/5/e1676.full.pdf+html. Accessed May 15, 2017.
69. Committee on Nutrition, American Academy of Pediatrics. Trace elements. In: Kleinman RE, Greer FR, eds. *Pediatric Nutrition.* 7th ed. Elk Grove Village, IL: American Academy of Pediatrics; 2014:467–94.
70. Committee on Nutrition, American Academy of Pediatrics. Fat-soluble vitamins. In: Kleinman RE, Greer FR, eds. *Pediatric Nutrition.* 7th ed. Elk Grove Village, IL: American Academy of Pediatrics; 2014:495–516.
71. Committee on Nutrition, American Academy of Pediatrics. Water-soluble vitamins. In: Kleinman RE, Greer FR, eds. *Pediatric Nutrition.* 7th ed. Elk Grove Village, IL: American Academy of Pediatrics; 2014:517–34.93.
72. Wagner CL, Greer FR; American Academy of Pediatrics Section on Breastfeeding; American Academy of Pediatrics Committee on Nutrition. Prevention of rickets and vitamin D deficiency in infants, children, and adolescents. *Pediatrics.* 2008;122(5):1142–52. doi: 10.1542/peds.2008-1862. Available at: http://pediatrics.aappublications.org/content/122/5/1142.full.pdf+html. Accessed May 15, 2017.
73. Maguire JL, Salehi L, Birken CS, et al. Association between total duration of breastfeeding and iron deficiency. *Pediatrics.* 2013;131(5);e1530. doi: 10.1542/peds/2012-2465.
74. Lynch SR, Stoltzfus RJ. Iron and ascorbic acid: proposed fortification levels and recommended iron compounds. *J Nutr.* 2003;133(9):2978S–84S. PMID: 12949396. Available at: http://jn.nutrition.org/content/133/9/2978S.full.pdf+html. Accessed May 15, 2017.
75. Tudehope D, Fewtrell M, Kashyap S, et al. Nutritional needs of the micropreterm infant. *J Pediatr.* 2013;162(3 Suppl):S72–80. doi: 10.1016/j.jpeds.2012.11.056.
76. Ruppe MD. Medications that affect calcium. *Endocr Pract.* 2011;17 (Suppl 1):26–30. doi: 10.4158/EP10281.RA.
77. Committee on Nutrition, American Academy of Pediatrics. Nutrition and oral health. In: Kleinman RE, Green FR, eds. *Pediatric Nutrition.* 7th ed. Elk Grove Village, IL: American Academy of Pediatrics; 2014:1167–86.
78. Centers for Disease Control and Prevention. 2014 water fluoridation statistics. March 3, 2016. Available at: http://www.cdc.gov/fluoridation/statistics/2014stats.htm. Accessed May 15, 2017.
79. Centers for Disease Control and Prevention. Recommendations for using fluoride to prevent and control dental caries in the United States. *MMWR Morb Mortal Wkly Rep.* 2001;50(RR-14):1–59. doi: 10.1177/003335491513000408. Available at: http://www.cdc.gov/mmwr/PDF/rr/rr5014.pdf. Accessed May 15, 2017.

CHAPTER 27

OVERWEIGHT AND OBESITY

SARAH J. MILLER AND SHERRILL BROWN

Obesity rates in the United States have increased dramatically since the mid-1970s. Overweight and obesity are significant, because they are associated with increased morbidity from various conditions, including cardiovascular diseases (CVD), type 2 diabetes, gallbladder disease, osteoarthritis, and several cancers.[1] In the United States, increasing concern centers on overweight and obesity in children and adolescents.

The National Health and Nutrition Examination Surveys (NHANES) of the U.S. population have tracked prevalence of overweight and obesity in adults from 1960 to the present. These surveys have demonstrated a marked increase in obesity in both men and women across all age and ethnic groups. More than one-third of U.S. adults are currently obese (Figure 27–1).[2] Increases in obesity prevalence appear to have slowed for both females and males for the period 2003–2012.[3] Figure 27–1 also illustrates the changes in prevalence of overweight across recent NHANES surveys. These have remained fairly stable.[2] More males than females fall into the overweight but not obese category, whereas more females than males are obese.[2]

Prevalence of obesity during childhood and adolescence is also concerning (Figure 27–2).[2] Increases in obesity in children also appear to have slowed over the period 2003–2014.[3] NHANES data from 2011 to 2014 indicate that 17% of youth ages 2–19 years are obese.[2,3]

The economic impact of overweight and obesity is substantial. The Institute of Medicine estimates that obesity-related illness costs about $190 billion, accounting for more than 20% of annual health spending in the United States.[4] Quantification of costs that are directly due to obesity is difficult, because many comorbidities of obesity have other etiologies.

Americans spend billions of dollars on weight-control products and services annually. Use of nonprescription or dietary supplement weight-loss products is common. Health care providers (HCPs) should be knowledgeable in discussing benefits as well as limitations and potential harm of weight-loss products, and they should be comfortable in recommending effective nonpharmacologic lifestyle changes, such as diet and exercise. If patients need additional strategies, the HCP may then refer them for consideration of prescription weight-loss therapies or weight-loss surgery.

Clinical Indicators of Overweight and Obesity

The 2013 systematic review *Managing Overweight and Obesity in Adults*, prepared by the United States Department of Health and Human Services, defines overweight and obesity in adults by body mass index (BMI), a parameter that takes into account both height and weight.[1] The U.S. Preventive Services Task Force (USPSTF) on screening for and management of obesity also recommends the use of BMI for screening of obesity.[5] Table 27–1 illustrates BMI values for individuals of various heights and weights and also provides equations for calculation of BMI. *Overweight* is defined in adults as a BMI of 25–29.9 (kg/m^2) and *obesity* as a BMI of 30 or greater.

Exclusive use of BMI as an indicator of overweight and obesity has limitations, because it does not consider extreme variation in body composition. Very muscular individuals, for example, may be classified by BMI as overweight or obese when, in fact, they are not carrying excessive adipose tissue. Alternatively, some people with BMI in the desirable range may have less than optimal muscle mass and high levels of body fat. Some of these individuals may be classified as "metabolically obese normal weight," with increased insulin resistance, hypertriglyceridemia, and a predisposition to type 2 diabetes and CVD.[6] Finally, the optimal BMI range for minimizing the risk of obesity-related CVD may differ among ethnic groups.[3] For example, BMI values that indicate increased risk for some Asian populations may be lower than those for other ethnic groups.[3] The so-called "obesity paradox," that is, some epidemiological studies indicate that being overweight or mildly obese appears to confer survival benefit in some CVD, remains controversial; the most recent meta-analysis does not support this contention.[7]

The importance of the distribution of body fat to risk of morbidity and mortality has long been recognized. Central fat around the waist and deep visceral adipose surrounding internal organs are associated with greater health risk than inert subcutaneous adipose in regions such as the buttock or thigh. Fat cells in the viscera of the abdomen are associated with chronic inflammation, which in turn can contribute to chronic diseases such as CVD, type 2 diabetes, and cancer.[8] Men with waist circumference greater than 40 inches and women with waist circumference greater than 35 inches are often considered at increased relative risk of type 2 diabetes and CVD. The USPSTF recommendations suggest that waist circumference may be an alternative to BMI in some populations.[5] In an effort to better identify and address obesity and its related risks, HCPs are strongly encouraged to take measurements of height, weight, and waist circumference; these physical assessment techniques can be realistically accomplished, even in a busy clinical setting.

Metabolic syndrome is characterized by the presence of certain metabolic risk factors and has been associated with increased risk of coronary artery disease, other vascular diseases, and type 2

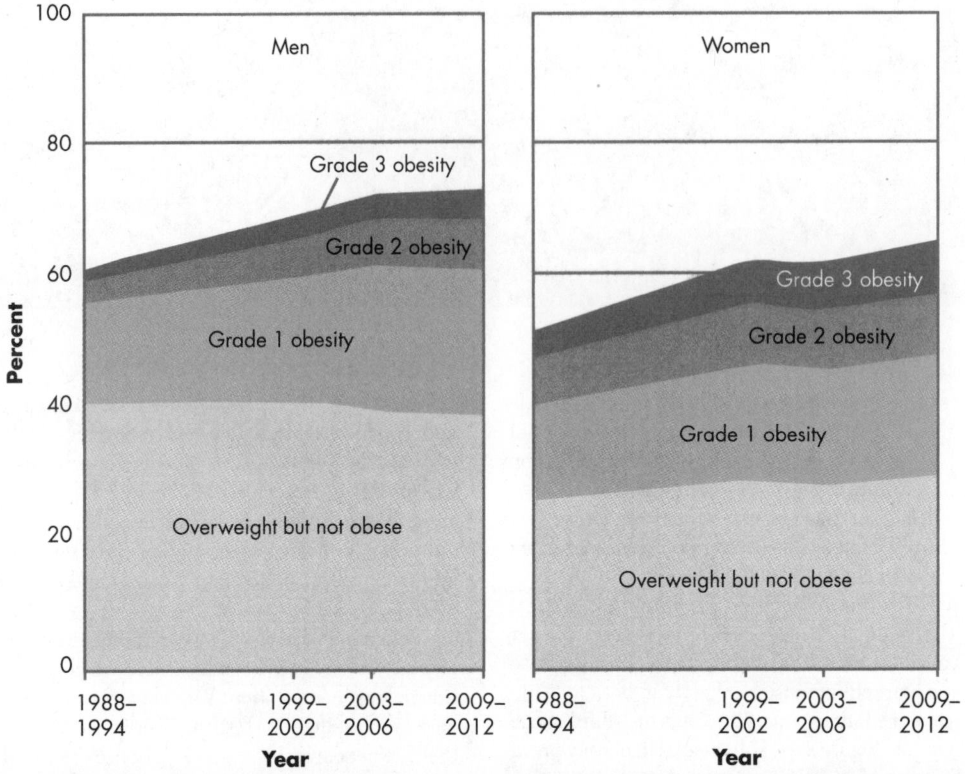

FIGURE 27-1 Overweight and obesity among adults 20 years of age and older. (Source: Reference 2.)

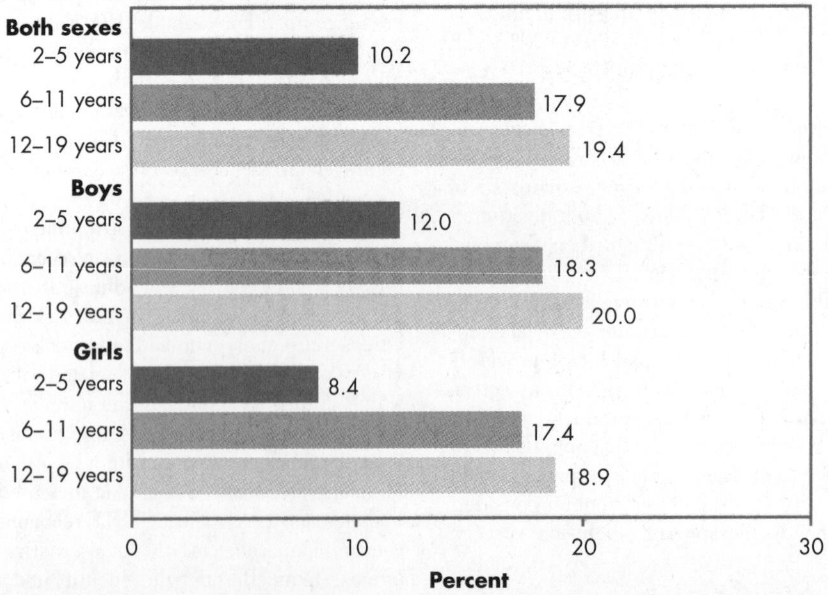

FIGURE 27-2 Obesity among children. (Source: Reference 2.)

TABLE 27-1 BMI Corresponding to Height and Body Weight[a]

	BMI (kg/m²)[b,c]													
	19	20	21	22	23	24	25	26	27	28	29	30	35	40
Height (inches)	**Body Weight (pounds)**													
58	91	96	100	105	110	115	119	124	129	134	138	143	167	191
59	94	99	104	109	114	119	124	128	133	138	143	148	173	198
60	97	102	107	112	118	123	128	133	138	143	148	153	179	204
61	100	106	111	116	122	127	132	137	143	148	153	158	185	211
62	104	109	115	120	126	131	136	142	147	153	158	164	191	218
63	107	113	118	124	130	135	141	146	152	158	163	169	197	225
64	110	116	122	128	134	140	145	151	157	163	169	174	204	232
65	114	120	126	132	138	144	150	156	162	168	174	180	210	240
66	118	124	130	136	142	148	155	161	167	173	179	186	216	247
67	121	127	134	140	146	153	159	166	172	178	185	191	223	255
68	125	131	138	144	151	158	164	171	177	184	190	197	230	262
69	128	135	142	149	155	162	169	176	182	189	196	203	236	270
70	132	139	146	153	160	167	172	181	188	195	202	207	243	278
71	136	143	150	157	165	172	179	186	193	200	208	215	250	286
72	140	147	154	162	169	177	184	191	199	206	213	221	258	294
73	144	151	159	166	174	182	189	197	204	212	219	227	265	302
74	148	155	163	171	179	186	194	202	210	218	225	233	272	311
75	152	160	168	176	184	192	200	208	216	224	232	240	279	319
76	156	164	172	180	189	197	205	213	221	230	238	246	287	328

Key: BMI = Body mass index.

[a] To determine BMI, find the height in the left-hand column; then move across the row to a given weight. The number above the weight column is the BMI for that height and weight.

[b] BMI calculations: weight (kg)/height (m²) or (weight [lb]/height [in.²]) × 703.

[c] BMI 30–34.9 known as Class I obesity; BMI 35–39.9 known as Class II obesity; BMI ≥ 40 known as Class III obesity.

diabetes. Patients with three or more of the following are said to have metabolic syndrome:

- Waist circumference greater than 40 inches in men or 35 inches in women (numbers may vary among different ethnicities)
- Serum triglycerides of 150 mg/dL or greater
- High-density lipoprotein (HDL) cholesterol less than 40 mg/dL in men or less than 50 mg/dL in women
- Blood pressure level of 130 mm Hg systolic or 85 mm Hg diastolic or higher
- Fasting serum glucose of 100 mg/dL or greater

Individuals with metabolic syndrome are likely to demonstrate insulin resistance and may benefit more from weight loss for reduced morbidity and mortality than would overweight or obese individuals without the syndrome. In addition, increased muscle mass is associated with improved insulin sensitivity. Therefore, physical activity resulting in increased muscle mass may result in improved insulin sensitivity even in the absence of weight loss.

Some evidence suggests that the correlation between obesity and CVD is not as strong as it once was, perhaps because of improvements in medical care for CVD and its risk factors. However, this reduction in obesity-related CVD mortality has been accompanied by an increase in obesity-associated disability, perhaps because people are becoming overweight or obese at earlier ages or because they are living longer. Some evidence supports cardiorespiratory fitness as an independent determinant of mortality in overweight and obese individuals (i.e., the concept that being fat but fit carries significantly lower risk than being fat and unfit).[6]

The Endocrine Society has published guidelines for obesity in children and adolescents that are based on Centers for Disease Control and Prevention growth charts.[9] These guidelines define a BMI "percentile for age" between the 85th and 95th percentiles as *overweight* and 95th percentile or greater as *obese.*

Pathophysiology of Overweight and Obesity

Weight gain is, to some extent, a reflection of energy intake exceeding energy expenditure. A pound of adipose tissue represents about 3500 calories (kcal) of energy. An excessive intake of only

10 kcal/day over the level of energy expenditure could result in a gain of approximately 1 pound of fat in a year's time. However, the physiology of energy intake and expenditure is complex and involves numerous body systems, including the hypothalamic–pituitary axis, autonomic nervous system, central nervous system, endocrine system, gastrointestinal (GI) tract, and adipose tissue.

Both genetic and environmental factors are important in the etiology of overweight and obesity, and there is a complex interplay between these factors. The rapid increase in obesity over the past few decades argues for a strong environmental role. Increased portion sizes and caloric intakes are undoubtedly contributing to recent trends in obesity rates. Today's lifestyle and environment are likely modulating genetic expression of obesity in many individuals. For example, recent studies have shown that higher intakes of sugar-sweetened beverages and fried foods may predispose individuals with certain genetic traits to risk for developing obesity.[10,11] However, consumers should be cautioned about commercial weight management programs offering genetic analysis as part of their packages: these programs may be beneficial, but currently their marketing overstates the evidence for their proven utility.

Researchers studying obesity have identified several different hormones and proteins potentially involved in energy balance.[12] Studies are ongoing to determine whether excesses, deficiencies, or resistance to specific substances are related to weight homeostasis. Leptin is a hormone secreted by adipose tissues; studies indicate resistance to leptin may be a factor in obesity. Other compounds of research interest include neuropeptide Y, ghrelin, and melanocortins. An in-depth discussion of this topic is beyond the scope of this chapter.

Environmental factors contributing to recent increases in obesity include decreased physical activity coupled with increased food availability and consumption, especially calorie-dense foods. Guidelines for regular moderate physical activity are met by only a minority of adult Americans.[13] About half of adolescents meet neither aerobic or muscle-strengthening activity guidelines.[14] Initiation of even modest amounts of exercise by sedentary individuals can have multiple health benefits, including maintenance of current weight instead of continued weight gain.

Significant increases in portion sizes of food and increased sedentary working hours may be environmental factors contributing to increasing rates of obesity. (See Chapter 23 for a discussion of a healthy diet and *MyPlate*.)

Another factor of interest as a possible etiology of overweight and obesity is sleep duration.[15] Several mechanisms have been postulated and studied regarding this association.[15] Sleep deprivation has been associated with decreased leptin and increased ghrelin levels in some studies; these hormonal alterations could lead to increased appetite. People who do not sleep well or who sleep for only short durations each night may engage in more sedentary screen-based activities (e.g., television and computer viewing), which may encourage unhealthy snacking.

Still another concept in the etiology of obesity relates to the gut microbiome.[16] Lean and obese individuals have been found to have different proportions of certain bacteria. Furthermore, these proportions have been shown to change with weight loss. These findings may lead to investigation of prebiotics, probiotics, and antibiotics as tools for weight maintenance and weight loss. (See Chapter 20 for a discussion of prebiotics and probiotics.)

Some medications can lead to weight gain.[17] There is clear evidence that the majority of the second-generation antipsychotics contribute to significant weight gain and related metabolic disorders. Older antidepressants (tricyclics and monoamine oxidase inhibitors) are associated with modest weight gain. Although some of the selective serotonin reuptake inhibitor antidepressants have been touted as producing weight loss, this loss is usually short lived, and weight gain can eventually occur. Other important groups of medications contributing to significant weight gain are hormonal contraceptives, systemic corticosteroids, certain anticonvulsants, certain sulfonylureas, thiazolidinediones, and insulins. The latter three groups are noteworthy because patients with type 2 diabetes placed on these medications frequently are already overweight.

Obesity and Chronic Health Problems

Overweight and obesity are associated with myriad chronic health problems.[1] Many of these problems improve with even modest weight loss. Obese individuals experience more difficulties in performing activities of daily living, such as walking several flights of stairs or bending and kneeling.

Obesity is closely associated with cerebrovascular disease. Overweight and obesity are associated with both hemorrhagic and ischemic stroke.[1] Both fatal and nonfatal stroke risk increases with increasing BMI.[1] Overweight and obesity have been linked to increased risk for hypertension, dyslipidemia, coronary artery disease, and arrhythmias.[18] Prevalence of hypertension begins to increase at relatively low levels of overweight. Weight loss in obese individuals is associated with significant reductions in blood pressure.[1]

There is a correlation between increasing BMI and increasing triglyceride and low-density lipoprotein (LDL) cholesterol levels. Beneficial HDL cholesterol levels tend to be lower in both men and women with higher BMI values. Even modest weight loss of 3–8 kg can have a beneficial effect on blood lipid levels.[19]

The relationship between overweight and obesity and type 2 diabetes is well documented. Visceral adiposity (high waist circumference) has been shown to be a risk factor for development of type 2 diabetes. Individuals who are initially insulin resistant, typically evidenced by high plasma triglycerides and low HDL cholesterol, are most likely to benefit from weight loss for reduced morbidity and mortality. Modest weight loss is effective in improving blood glucose control in patients with type 2 diabetes and preventing development of type 2 diabetes in those at risk.[1,19]

Negative attitudes exist toward obese people, leading to social stigmatization and discrimination. Overweight children may develop psychosocial difficulties stemming from compromised peer relationships.[20]

Obesity appears to increase the risk for a number of other diseases, including gallbladder disease, nonalcoholic fatty liver disease, osteoarthritis, sleep apnea, asthma, certain types of cancer, and disorders of female reproduction.[1] Obesity is a risk factor for hyperuricemia and gout.[1] Overweight is believed to contribute to a significant proportion of certain cancers and increased mortality from cancer.[1] Of particular concern are cancers with a hormonal basis such as cancers of the breast, prostate, or endometrium, as well as cancers of the colon, rectum, and gallbladder. Hypertension and gestational diabetes are more likely in obese women who become pregnant.

Management of Overweight and Obesity

Management Goals and General Management Approach

The three major approaches to weight management are adoption of a healthy lifestyle (i.e., diet and exercise habits), pharmacologic therapy (nonprescription and prescription medications, dietary supplements), and bariatric surgery. A combination of these approaches may sometimes be used. Treatment goals of weight loss can be classified into three main categories: (1) improvement in comorbid condition and chronic diseases associated with overweight and obesity, such as type 2 diabetes and CVD; (2) improvement in psychological health and feelings of well-being; and (3) cosmetic benefit.

For many individuals, losing weight or maintaining weight loss is a lifelong challenge. Successful weight loss and maintenance of loss require significant behavioral modification. Pharmacologic therapy using nonprescription agents should be only a short-term measure unless a primary care provider (PCP) supervises therapy. Long-term use of prescription therapies under the care of a PCP may be an option for patients with a BMI of 30 or higher or a BMI of 27 or higher with comorbid conditions.[19] However, pharmacologic interventions often result in only modest weight loss that is regained after drug discontinuation. Bariatric surgery may be considered for patients with a BMI of 40 or higher or a BMI of 35 or higher with comorbid conditions, including hypertension, hyperlipidemia, and type 2 diabetes.[19] This surgery is effective for helping many patients to achieve weight loss, although success following surgery also requires lifestyle changes. The procedures carry their own significant risks.

Many chronic diseases and conditions improve with weight loss. However, weight-loss goals set by many individuals are unrealistic and based on cosmetic rather than health benefit. Weight loss (and maintenance of that loss) of 5%–10% of initial weight can have positive benefits in individuals with hypertension and type 2 diabetes. Guidelines prepared by the American Heart Association/American College of Cardiology/The Obesity Society state that the initial goal of weight loss is to reduce body weight by about 5%–10% over 6 months.[19] If this goal is achieved and further weight loss is indicated, it can be attempted. The first 10% loss carries the greatest health benefits; it is also easiest to attain, because a decreased basal metabolic rate often causes weight loss to plateau after about 6 months. In many patients, it is more important to maintain the 10% weight loss than to pursue further weight loss, and most patients find weight maintenance to be more difficult than the initial modest weight loss. An approach often overlooked may be to prevent further weight gain in individuals who have slowly but steadily gained weight over a period of years. Figure 27–3 is a guide for the HCP in recommending weight-loss measures.

Nonpharmacologic Therapy (Lifestyle Intervention)

Dietary modification or restriction is the mainstay of weight-loss therapy. Physical activity is less effective in producing weight loss initially but is important in maintaining weight loss and improving overall fitness. The term *lifestyle intervention* describes a strategy of dietary change, physical activity, and behavior therapy.[1] One major key to weight loss and maintenance of that loss is implementing lifestyle interventions that are sustained over a long period of time. Lifestyle intervention programs should be included in pharmaceutical care services.

Dietary Change

Dietary change is the most commonly used weight-loss strategy. Diet strategies include caloric restriction; changes in dietary proportions of fat, protein, and carbohydrate; use of macronutrient substitutes (i.e., sugar and fat substitutes); and changes in timing or frequency of meals. Short-term success for many methods has been documented; however, data on longer-term effectiveness and safety are less encouraging. Weight loss at the end of relatively short-term programs can exceed 10% of initial body weight. However, there is a strong tendency to regain weight. A relatively small portion of participants do maintain weight loss over more extended periods. The National Weight Control Registry tracks individuals who have maintained weight loss of at least 30 pounds for at least 1 year.[21] To initially lose weight, individuals in this registry used a variety of methods; about half were self-directed and half were some type of program. Most individuals reported maintaining weight loss through a combination of a low-calorie, low-fat diet and exercise.

Even small changes in dietary patterns can have a positive effect. Cutting portion sizes, switching to water or diet soda rather than sugar-sweetened beverages, using smaller plates for meals, and keeping healthy snacks such as fruits and vegetables on hand are useful, sustainable strategies. Trying to eat foods with low energy density (i.e., low calories per weight of food) may be helpful, because these foods tend to promote satiety. Because these are long-term lifestyle changes, patients should be encouraged to make these realistic, smaller changes, rather than opt for the more radical fad diets that are difficult to adhere to long term. (See Chapter 23 for more details about healthy diets.)

Caloric Restriction

Daily caloric allowances for moderately active individuals vary with age, gender, and body weight. The U.S. population suffers from "portion distortion" and needs to relearn appropriate food portion sizes based on age and activity levels. Daily caloric intake allowances for an average 30-year-old man (BMI = 18.5–25; height, 5 ft 11 in.) in a temperate climate range from approximately 2400–3000 kcal/day, depending on activity level. Corresponding figures for an average 30-year-old woman (BMI = 18.5–25; height, 5 ft 5 in.) are approximately 1800–2400 kcal/day.[22] These figures are lower for older adults and higher for younger adults. Caloric requirements for women increase during pregnancy and lactation (see Chapter 23).[23] Self-initiated weight loss during pregnancy is not recommended.

A diet that is individually planned and seeks to create a deficit of 500 kcal/day or more should be an integral part of any weight-loss program.[1] A low-calorie diet (LCD) of approximately 1200–1800 kcal/day may involve a structured commercial program, or it may involve guidelines for selecting conventional foods, including careful attention to portion sizes. Initial weight loss on an LCD is typically 1–2 pounds per week. A very-low-calorie diet (VLCD) of 800 or fewer calories per day should be conducted and monitored under medical supervision and accompanied by high-intensity lifestyle intervention.[1] VLCDs are frequently administered as liquid formulas given several times a day. Although weight loss with

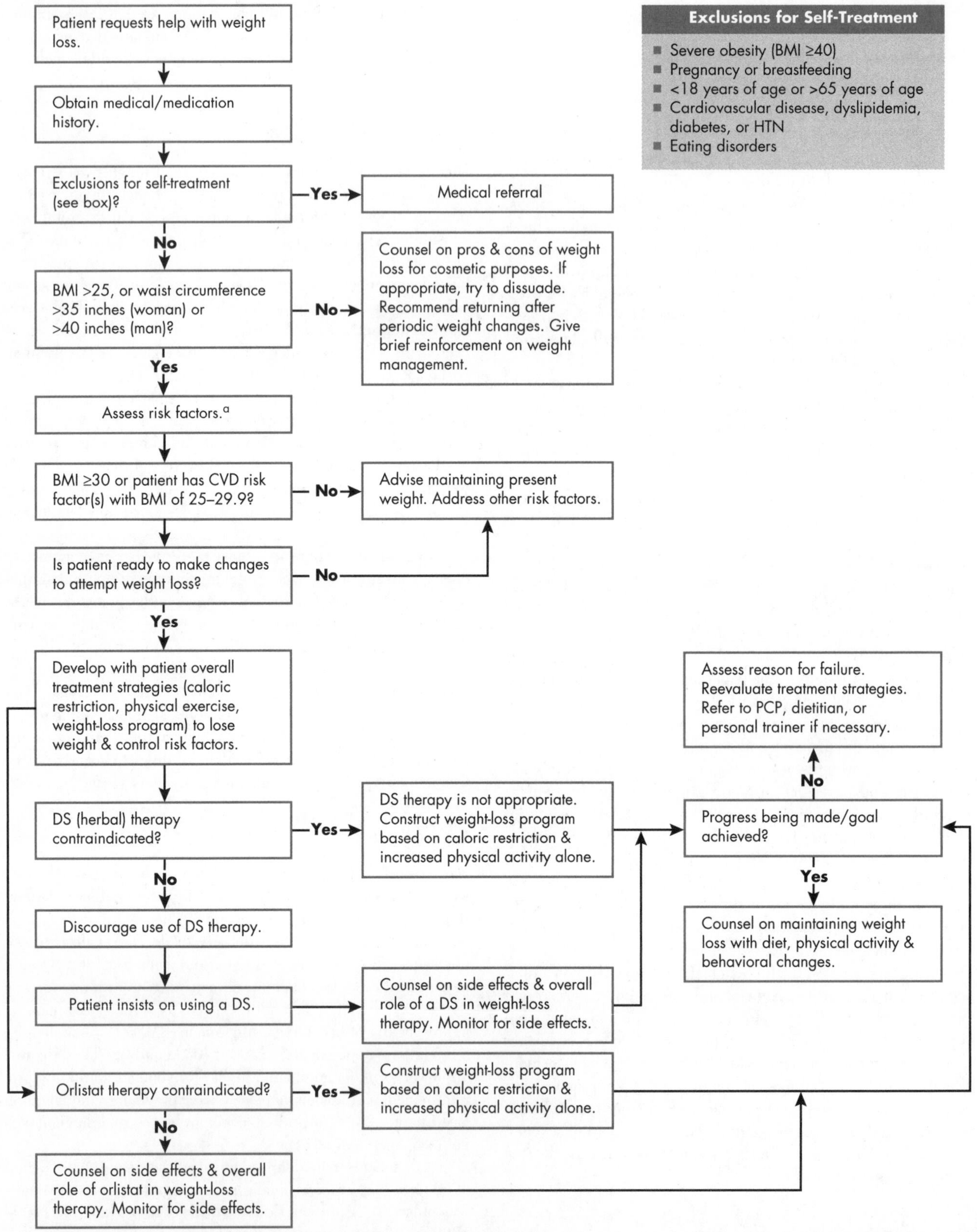
Patient requests help with weight loss.
Obtain medical/medication history.
Exclusions for self-treatment (see box)?
Yes
Medical referral
No
BMI >25, or waist circumference >35 inches (woman) or >40 inches (man)?
No
Counsel on pros & cons of weight loss for cosmetic purposes. If appropriate, try to dissuade. Recommend returning after periodic weight changes. Give brief reinforcement on weight management.
Yes
Assess risk factors.ᵃ
BMI ≥30 or patient has CVD risk factor(s) with BMI of 25–29.9?
No
Advise maintaining present weight. Address other risk factors.
Is patient ready to make changes to attempt weight loss?
No
Yes
Develop with patient overall treatment strategies (caloric restriction, physical exercise, weight-loss program) to lose weight & control risk factors.
DS (herbal) therapy contraindicated?
Yes
DS therapy is not appropriate. Construct weight-loss program based on caloric restriction & increased physical activity alone.
No
Discourage use of DS therapy.
Patient insists on using a DS.
Counsel on side effects & overall role of a DS in weight-loss therapy. Monitor for side effects.
Orlistat therapy contraindicated?
Yes
Construct weight-loss program based on caloric restriction & increased physical activity alone.
No
Counsel on side effects & overall role of orlistat in weight-loss therapy. Monitor for side effects.
Assess reason for failure. Reevaluate treatment strategies. Refer to PCP, dietitian, or personal trainer if necessary.
No
Progress being made/goal achieved?
Yes
Counsel on maintaining weight loss with diet, physical activity & behavioral changes.
Exclusions for Self-Treatment
Severe obesity (BMI ≥40)
Pregnancy or breastfeeding
<18 years of age or >65 years of age
Cardiovascular disease, dyslipidemia, diabetes, or HTN
Eating disorders

[a] Risk factors for cardiovascular disease, as defined by AHA/ACC/TOS, include diabetes, prediabetes, hypertension, dyslipidemia, and waist circumference >35 inches (88 cm) in women or >40 inches (102 cm) in men.

FIGURE **27–3** Self-care of overweight and obesity. Key: ACC = American College of Cardiology; AHA = American Heart Association; BMI = body mass index; CVD = cardiovascular disease; DS = dietary supplement; HTN = hypertension; PCP = primary care provider; TOS = The Obesity Society.

VLCDs over 12–16 weeks is typically double that of LCDs, long-term results are generally no better. A multivitamin and multimineral preparation should be recommended to patients consuming fewer than 1200 kcal/day for prolonged periods.

Altered Proportions of Food Groups

The most commonly recommended diets for weight loss are reduced-calorie diets emphasizing decreased fat intake, particularly decreased saturated fat. The 2010 Dietary Guidelines for Americans recommended a diet supplying no more than 35% of total calories from fat, of which no more than 10% of total calories come from saturated fat [13] The 2015–2020 Dietary Guidelines still recommend a diet low in saturated fat but do not state a ceiling for percentage of overall fat in the diet.[23] A low-fat diet alone is inadequate for weight loss; the diet must also reduce total calories.

Very-low-fat vegetarian diets in the context of other lifestyle changes have been advocated. Although such programs can result in regression of coronary atherosclerosis and improvement of endothelial function in some patients with moderate–severe coronary heart disease, their applicability to larger populations remains questionable with regard to compliance.[24] Dietary fats must be carefully chosen for a very-low-fat diet to prevent essential fatty acid deficiency. Such diets increase triglyceride levels and lower HDL cholesterol in the short term because of the high carbohydrate content.

There is a spectrum of popular high-protein, higher-fat, and low-carbohydrate diets. Some contain very low amounts of carbohydrates (approximately 5%–15% of total calories; e.g., Atkins diet) and are ketogenic, whereas others are considered moderate-carbohydrate diets (approximately 35%–50% of calories from carbohydrate; e.g., Zone diet). People often start out on the ultralow form of the diet and transition to a more moderate form. Part of the success of low-carbohydrate diets may lie in the fact that they simplify food choices, thus facilitating dietary adherence.

Very-low-carbohydrate diets prevent elevated insulin levels that promote storage of body fat. Much of the weight loss seen with these diets is a result of decreased caloric intake from avoiding high-carbohydrate foods. Initial weight loss partially results from a diuretic effect and glycogen depletion. Low-carbohydrate diets result in significant weight loss over 6–24 months. Long-term effects of these diets on CVD risk are still largely speculative.[1] Low-carbohydrate diets generally have more favorable effects on triglycerides and HDL cholesterol levels, whereas low-fat diets have more favorable effects on LDL and total cholesterol.[1] Potential adverse effects of low-carbohydrate diets include lack of essential nutrients, such as potassium, calcium, and magnesium. High-protein foods consumed in large quantities on these diets could increase uric acid levels and precipitate gout, although this problem has not been common in studies with up to a year of follow-up. High animal protein content promotes calcium excretion in the urine that could be deleterious to bone health. Restriction of fruits, vegetables, whole grains, and milk products could increase an individual's risk of various cancers by depleting essential vitamins, minerals, and fiber and could also lead to constipation. High-protein content may predispose individuals to dehydration and hyperfiltration by the kidneys, leading to eventual kidney damage, particularly in diabetic patients. Headache, muscle weakness, and fatigue are other adverse events reported by some individuals on low-carbohydrate diets. Several published randomized trials of these diets demonstrated relative safety of the low-carbohydrate, higher-fat, high-protein diets for 6–24 months, with greatest weight loss seen in the first 6 months.[25] In the Women's Health Initiative trial, reduction of total fat intake for 8 years did not reduce risk for CVD.[26] This finding may be related to the observation that, when compared with fat-restricted diets, carbohydrate-restricted diets have more favorable effects, not only on triglyceride and HDL cholesterol levels, but also on small dense LDL cholesterol mass.[26]

Low-glycemic-index food products are promoted commercially. *Glycemic index* refers to the amount of blood glucose rise seen over a set period of time after ingestion of a standardized amount of a food. Many high-carbohydrate, low-fat diets exhibit a high glycemic index. By making carbohydrate choices carefully, a lower glycemic response can be obtained. Low-glycemic-index diets would promote satiety, prevent large fluctuations in insulin concentrations, and might help maintain insulin sensitivity. Studies have not consistently supported the usefulness of low-glycemic-index diets in weight control, and the methods used to classify foods with this system are controversial.

Use of Food Additives

Some patients may use food additives such as artificial sweeteners and fat substitutes to reduce caloric intake. Although theoretically the use of these agents should help decrease caloric intake, the existing data are conflicted as to the beneficial effects of these products. Table 27–2 outlines information related to sugar and fat substitutes.

Meal Replacement Therapy

Diets that use meal replacement foods typically involve replacing up to 2 meals a day with a liquid drink, snack bar, or measured frozen meal, with the dieter encouraged to eat a "reasonable" third meal each day. The main advantage to this approach is portion control. Products typically contain about 200–300 kcal per serving and are low fat, although low-carbohydrate options are also available. The challenge with this approach is that dieters enter their third meal extremely hungry and may consume excessive calories by overeating at this time. Early weight loss with these products, part of which may be a result of low sodium content leading to water loss, can give a psychological boost to adhere to the program. Meal replacement products are discussed further in Chapter 24.

Commercial Weight-Loss Programs

Structured commercial weight-loss programs such as Weight Watchers, Jenny Craig, and Take Off Pounds Sensibly (TOPS) are very popular in the United States. Women tend to gravitate to these programs more than men do. Participation in structured commercial programs may be expensive if participants are required to purchase program-specific tools as well as specially packaged snacks or meals. The success seen with these programs is likely at least partially due to the social support that develops with periodic meetings. Online tools such as diet and exercise diaries and support groups are increasingly available; these resources may be less expensive than community-based structured commercial programs.

Physical Activity

Encouragement of physical activity for preventing overweight and obesity is an important public health strategy for all age groups,

TABLE 27-2 **Common Sugar and Fat Substitutes**

Substitute (Selected Trade Name)	Comments
Sugar Substitutes	
Monk fruit extract[a] (Nectresse)	Products may contain very small amounts of other natural sweeteners such as erythritol, molasses, and sugar
Saccharin (Sweet'n Low)[a]	Has bitter taste; has been replaced largely by newer sweeteners
Aspartame (NutraSweet)[a]	Contains phenylalanine, therefore, contraindicated in patients with phenylketonuria; not for use in cooking or baking as heat breaks it down into free amino acids, which impart a bitter taste
Fructose	Nutritive sweetener and should not be viewed as sugar free; insulin not required for fructose utilization in the body; contains approximately 10 calories when supplied in an amount providing the equivalent of about 1 teaspoon of sucrose
Sorbitol	Nutritive sweetener and should not be viewed as sugar free; does not cause tooth decay, but can cause osmotic diarrhea when ingested in large quantities; contains approximately 10 calories when supplied in an amount providing the equivalent of about 1 teaspoon of sucrose
Xylitol	Nutritive sweetener and should not be viewed as sugar free; does not cause tooth decay; contains approximately 10 calories when supplied in an amount providing the equivalent of about 1 teaspoon of sucrose
Acesulfame potassium (Sweet One)[a]	May be substituted for sucrose in cooking; may be combined with aspartame, because some people detect a metallic aftertaste with acesulfame potassium alone
Sucralose (Splenda)[a]	May be used in cooking
Neotame[a]	Chemically similar to aspartame; may be used in cooking
Cyclamates[a]	Banned by FDA in 1969 because of association with cancer in animals; applicability of this finding to humans has been challenged; remains available in many countries
Stevia (Truvia)[a]	Approved in United States as of 2008 as a food additive in a specific purified form
Fat Substitutes[b]	
Microparticulated protein (Simplesse)	Used in frozen desserts, salad dressing; unstable if heated
Soluble fiber (Oatrim)	Derived from oats and designed to replace fat in meats, cheeses, baked goods, and frozen desserts
Sucrose polyester (Olean)	Also known as olestra; is not absorbed; can cause malabsorption of fat-soluble vitamins; GI adverse effects can be seen with ingestion of large quantities; can be used for cooking and frying

Key: FDA = Food and Drug Administration; GI = gastrointestinal.

[a] Can be labeled as noncaloric based on FDA labeling regulations; cyclamates no longer approved by FDA for use as sugar substitute.

[b] Use of these fat substitutes in food products in place of fat typically decreases caloric content of the foods by about half, unless extra sugars are added into the products.

including children. The U.S. Department of Health and Human Services outlines the physical activity recommendations shown in Table 27–3.[27] For older adults, regular exercise can reduce functional declines that occur with aging.

Increased physical activity is an important component of weight-loss therapy and is even more important in weight maintenance after weight loss. Patients who regularly exercise may, in general, be more committed to a healthy lifestyle. Exercise builds muscle, which has a higher metabolic rate than a corresponding amount of fat. Weight loss that can be achieved by an exercise program is modest; combining a reduced-calorie diet with increased physical activity produces greater weight loss and reduction in abdominal fat than either approach alone. Patients who have restrictions as to types of exercise should have a medical evaluation before starting an exercise regimen. Regardless of concomitant diseases, current recommendations call for men older than age 40 and women older than age 50 to undergo a medical evaluation before starting an exercise program.

For sedentary patients, a walking program is often a good place to begin. A pedometer or other inexpensive activity tracker may be an aid to increasing activity in some individuals. Patients can start by walking 30 minutes each day for 3 days a week, building up to at least 60 minutes of moderate-intensity physical activity most days of the week. The 60-minute activity periods can be accrued in multiple smaller increments throughout the day with similar benefit. Patients should be encouraged to participate in activities that they enjoy and are therefore more likely to continue.

Behavioral Therapy

Behavioral therapy used in combination with other strategies, such as diet, exercise, and medications, can improve the outcome of weight-loss programs. Behavioral interventions are most effective when patients participate in sessions at least once or twice a month.[5] Behavioral therapy may be administered in either an individual or group setting by professionals or lay leaders. Remote

TABLE 27-3 Physical Activity Recommendations[a]

Children and Adolescents

Aerobic: ≥60 minutes of moderate or vigorous aerobic activity a day, including vigorous activity at least 3 days a week

Muscle and bone: strengthening physical activity should occur at least 3 times a week

Adults

Aerobic: 150 minutes of moderate aerobic activity or 75 minutes of vigorous physical activity a week, performed in ≥10-minute episodes[b]

Muscle: strengthening activities involving major muscle groups should occur at least twice a week

[a] As proposed by the U.S. Department of Health and Human Services' *2008 Physical Activity Guidelines for Americans*.[27]

[b] More activity than is outlined here is necessary to promote weight loss in most individuals. Exercise should be used in combination with dietary restriction to promote weight loss.

coaching and mobile technologies are increasingly being explored as less expensive methods for encouraging adherence to lifestyle modifications.

Behavioral techniques include the following[28]:

- Environmental modification: do not have high-calorie foods readily available, thus avoiding problem foods altogether; be vigilant in reading food labels and identifying reasonable food portions.
- Thought-pattern modification: set reasonable, specific, proximate goals; identify and plan for potential obstacles.
- Self-efficacy: maintain an optimistic and positive approach.
- Social support: rely on family, friends, and HCPs.

Public Health Initiatives

In an era when federal and state governments bear an increasing percentage of the cost of health care in the United States, interest in public health initiatives to decrease overweight and obesity has increased. Efforts by all levels of government to require dietary information in restaurant menus, to limit portion sizes of sugar-sweetened beverages, to eliminate trans-fat content in commercial foods, and to levy taxes on certain unhealthy foods are just a few examples of initiatives that have been considered or actually implemented. Many schools have banned the sale of sugar-sweetened beverages and high-fat snacks on their premises. These measures are controversial, and positive benefits on public health are not consistently shown at this time.

Pharmacologic Therapy

Pharmacologic therapy is generally not recommended for weight loss. In recent years, many more weight-loss products have been removed from the market for safety reasons than were approved. The ideal weight-loss drug, which would provide fast and permanent weight loss with no adverse effects, does not exist despite the billions of research and consumer dollars spent on weight-loss products every year.

Guidelines for obesity and overweight management only recommend weight-loss medications as adjunct therapy to lifestyle interventions in patients with either a BMI greater than or equal to 30 kg/m^2 or a BMI greater than or equal to 27 kg/m^2 with concomitant diseases or risk factors.[19] The most recent guidelines on overweight and obesity treatments did not specifically address medication therapy for weight management because of the scarcity of medications approved for chronic management of obesity. Since the publication of the updated guidelines, additional medications have been approved for weight loss and could be considered for adjunct therapy in patients with a BMI of 30 kg/m^2 or higher or in patients with a BMI of 27 kg/m^2 or higher with comorbidities.[19] These guidelines should apply to all weight-loss products (prescription or nonprescription drugs, or dietary supplements) although nonprescription orlistat (Alli) can be used in patients with a BMI of at least 25 kg/m^2, as discussed in the following section. Weight-loss medications and supplements should be used in conjunction with lifestyle intervention and should be continually assessed for efficacy, safety, and tolerability.

Status of Nonprescription Weight-Loss Products

Since 1991, FDA has banned more than 100 weight-control ingredients in nonprescription drug products, including phenylpropanolamine, ephedrine, aloe, and cascara sagrada.[29] Ephedrine alkaloids are contained in several botanicals, including sea grape, yellow horse, joint fir, popotillo, ma huang, and country mallow. Although these products are banned from sale in the United States, other substances that may pose similar risks are still included in dietary supplements and are often found as components of weight-loss products.

From 2013 to 2015, FDA sent warning letters to several manufacturers of products containing BMPEA (beta-methylphenethylamine), DMBA (1,3-dimethylbutylamine), and DMAA (1,3-dimethylamylamine).[30–32] FDA does not consider BMPEA, DMBA, and DMAA to meet the legal definition of dietary ingredient, primarily because these substances are not from botanical sources, regardless of the manufacturers' claims. FDA warns consumers to avoid products containing these ingredients because of potentially dangerous adverse effects, such as hypertension and cardiovascular problems.

Dietary supplements are distinct entities from nonprescription drugs. They include herbal and other products meant to supplement the diet and are regulated under the Dietary Supplement Health and Education Act of 1994 (see Chapter 50).

The majority of drugs currently considered safe and efficacious for weight loss have prescription-only status and include benzphetamine (Didrex), diethylpropion (Tenuate), methamphetamine (Desoxyn), orlistat (Xenical), phendimetrazine (Bontril), phentermine (Ionamin), phentermine/topiramate (Qsymia), lorcaserin (Belviq), naltrexone/bupropion (Contrave), and liraglutide (Saxenda). Sibutramine (Meridia) was removed from the U.S. market in October 2010. The reader is directed to standard references for more information about these drugs.

Orlistat was approved by FDA as a prescription weight-loss medication (Xenical) in 1999 and as a nonprescription weight-loss medication (Alli) in 2007.[33] The prescription strength of orlistat (120 mg) is approved for use in patients ages 12 years and older; however, the nonprescription strength (60 mg) is approved only for patients 18 years and older.

Orlistat aids in weight loss by decreasing absorption of dietary fats. It inhibits gastric and pancreatic lipases and specifically reduces absorption of fat by inhibiting hydrolysis of triglycerides.[34]

It is recommended for use along with a reduced-calorie, low-fat diet and exercise program. The labeling for the prescription product states that the drug is indicated for obese patients with a BMI of at least 30 kg/m^2 or for patients with a BMI of 27 kg/m^2 or higher who also have risk factors such as diabetes, hypertension, or dyslipidemia. The labeling for the nonprescription product simply states that the drug is indicated for use in overweight adults, which by the standard definition would be individuals with a BMI of at least 25 kg/m^2.[34]

The recommended dosage of prescription-strength orlistat is 120 mg taken 3 times a day before meals containing fat; at this dosage, it inhibits dietary fat absorption by about 30%.[34] The nonprescription form of the drug is recommended at a dosage of 60 mg taken 3 times a day before meals containing fat; its inhibition of fat absorption is approximately 25%.[35] With either dosage of orlistat, the risk of greasy diarrhea increases as the amount of fat increases in a meal. Because of its mechanism of action, the drug need not be given with a fat-free meal.

Most studies have used the 120 mg dosage in combination with a reduced-calorie diet and have reported modest weight losses, especially during the first 6 months of therapy. This dosage may also be useful for weight-loss maintenance following initial weight loss. In one of the few full-text studies published with the 60 mg nonprescription dose, weight loss after 16 weeks in the active drug group was significantly greater than in patients receiving placebo (3.05 kg versus 1.90 kg; $P < 0.001$).[36] The nonprescription product labeling notes that most patients lost 5–10 pounds (about 2–5 kg) over 6 months in clinical trials.[37] Patients receiving orlistat have had significantly greater reductions in LDL cholesterol and blood pressure compared with placebo.[34] Effects on lipid levels may be independent of weight loss, whereas the changes in blood pressure are probably largely due to weight loss. Orlistat 120 mg has been shown to be effective in preventing and delaying development of type 2 diabetes over a 4-year period in patients with impaired glucose tolerance.[38]

Orlistat may decrease absorption of fat-soluble vitamins (A, D, E, and K). It is recommended that patients taking this medication take a multivitamin once daily at bedtime or separated by at least 2 hours from an orlistat dose. Orlistat is minimally absorbed and therefore exhibits little systemic toxicity. Common GI adverse effects are caused by the increased fat present in the GI tract and include flatulence with oily spotting, loose and frequent stools, fatty stools, and fecal urgency and incontinence. Decreasing the amount of ingested fat can minimize these effects. These adverse effects are expected to be less common with the nonprescription dosage, and they generally improve within a few weeks of initiating therapy.

Drug interactions with orlistat are unlikely because of the drug's limited absorption. Table 27–4 lists potential or documented drug interactions with orlistat. Patients with malabsorption disorders should avoid taking orlistat, and patients with a history of thyroid disease, cholelithiasis, nephrolithiasis, or pancreatitis should consult their PCP before taking orlistat. Both the prescription and nonprescription strengths of orlistat contain warnings of potential liver injury. These warnings are based on rare cases of severe liver injury with orlistat, including one case associated with the nonprescription strength. There has also been concern about a potential association between orlistat and development of breast and colon cancers, but FDA concluded there was no causal relationship between orlistat and cancer.[39]

Nonprescription orlistat may be useful as an adjunct to lifestyle changes in helping patients lose modest amounts of weight. Results will be more favorable when this agent is combined with a reduced-calorie, low-fat diet and increased physical activity. Orlistat has the ability to help change people's eating habits. Rather than suppressing the appetite, an effect that goes away once the drug is discontinued, orlistat helps people choose food with less fat content, resulting in fewer adverse effects. Once orlistat is discontinued, these people should be able to continue to make these healthier food choices. Patients should be aware that the GI adverse effects of the medication are likely to be exacerbated by concomitant ingestion of a low-carbohydrate, high-fat diet. There is some concern that this nonprescription agent may be misused, particularly by adolescents; it would be prudent for HCPs to watch for adolescents purchasing this medication.

Orlistat is rated pregnancy category X and is contraindicated in pregnancy because weight loss offers no potential benefit to a pregnant woman and may result in fetal harm.[34] (See the Preface for a detailed explanation of the pregnancy data.) It is not known if orlistat is excreted into human milk. Caution should be exercised when orlistat is administered to a nursing mother. The safety and effectiveness of the nonprescription orlistat product have not been established for patients younger than 12 years of age. Clinical studies of orlistat did not include sufficient numbers of patients ages 65 years and older to determine whether they respond differently from younger patients. No dosage adjustment is recommended in patients with renal or hepatic dysfunction.

TABLE 27–4 Potential Drug–Drug Interactions With Orlistat

Drug	Interaction
Cyclosporine	Reductions in cyclosporine concentration may be seen.
Fat-soluble vitamins	Absorption of these vitamins may be decreased.
Levothyroxine	Levothyroxine concentrations may be decreased, leading to hypothyroidism.
Warfarin	Malabsorption of vitamin K may lead to over anticoagulation.
Amiodarone	Starting oral amiodarone during orlistat therapy may result in decreased concentrations of amiodarone.
Antiepileptic drugs	Orlistat could decrease concentrations of various antiepileptic drugs.

Source: Reference 34.

Use of Inappropriate Medications for Weight Loss

Individuals seeking to lose weight will sometimes turn to inappropriate, potentially dangerous methods to induce loss, such as using laxatives or diuretics. The risks associated with laxatives and diuretics are discussed in Chapter 15 and Chapter 9, respectively.

Reformulated Weight-Loss Products

Since FDA banned ephedra-containing dietary supplements, many manufacturers have started including bitter orange (*Citrus aurantium*) in weight-loss medications, often in combination with sources of caffeine such as cola nut (*Cola acuminata* or *Cola nitida*), guarana (*Paullinia cupana* or *Paullinia sorbilis*), or maté (*Ilex paraguariensis*). Bitter orange contains synephrine, which is structurally similar to epinephrine, and octopamine, which is similar to norepinephrine. Bitter orange is touted as a safe alternative to ephedra in many herbal weight-loss products. Although adrenergic effects of synephrine and octopamine have the potential for appetite suppression and lipolysis, these products have the same potential health risks as ephedra. In a study with healthy adults, single doses of *C. aurantium* increased heart rate and blood pressure significantly compared with placebo. However, those effects may be due to the combination of *C. aurantium* with caffeine and other stimulants in the multicomponent product used in the study.[40] Clinical trials of *C. aurantium* for weight loss have failed to support efficacy for this indication.

Numerous nonprescription weight-loss products list multiple ingredients, many of which are herbal extracts with varying active ingredients, together with vitamins and minerals. Many of these ingredients lack any scientific evidence for usefulness in weight loss. To confuse matters further, many of the herbal extracts are listed by their common or not-so-common names (e.g., bitter orange, Seville orange, and sour orange are all common names for *C. aurantium*). Many products do not list the botanical name, making it difficult to determine exactly what the herbal product contains. The majority of these products have not been clearly demonstrated to be effective or safe, and many have been associated with serious adverse effects. HCPs are advised to carefully review the labels of all dietary supplement weight-loss products to determine the risk for adverse reactions and drug–supplement interactions.

Complementary Therapies

A summary of botanicals commonly used in weight-loss supplements is provided in Table 27–5.[41–44] Chapter 51, "Natural Products" provides an in-depth discussion of the more common dietary

TABLE 27–5 Complementary Therapies Commonly Used for Weight Loss

Agent	Risks
Stimulants, Energy Boosters, and Thermogenic Aids	
Bitter orange (*Citrus aurantium*)	Synephrine may cause hypertension, cardiovascular toxicity, myocardial infarction, stroke, and seizure.
Caffeine: Cola nut (*Cola acuminata, Cola nitida*); green tea (*Camellia sinensis*); guarana (*Paullinia cupana, Paullinia sorbilis*); maté (*Ilex paraguariensis*)	Caffeine may cause GI distress, nausea, dehydration, headaches, insomnia, nervousness, anxiety, muscle tension, heart palpitations, hypertension, addiction, decreased appetite, and vertigo; avoid in patients with gastric ulcers.
	Use with caution in patients with renal disease, panic disorder, hyperthyroidism, anxiety, or susceptibility to spasm; use only under medical supervision in patients with peptic ulcers, cardiovascular disease, or blood-clotting abnormalities; discontinue use at least 24 hours before surgery; may alter effects of anticoagulant medications.
Forskolin (*Coleus forskohlii*)	Forskolin is generally well tolerated.
Fat and Carbohydrate Modulators	
Chromium	Chromium is generally well tolerated at low doses.
	Rhabdomyolysis and renal failure may occur with large doses.
	May cause mood and sleep changes, headaches, and cognitive and perception dysfunction.
	Evidence of benefit of chromium picolinate is inconsistent and controversial.
Cinnamon (*Cinnamomum* spp.)	Cinnamon is usually well tolerated.
	Allergic reactions, such as dermatitis and gingivitis, may occur with external application and with use of flavored chewing gums, mints, or toothpastes.
Conjugated linoleic acid (CLA)	CLA causes GI upset.
Garcinia or brindleberry (*Garcinia cambogia*)	Garcinia may cause GI distress with high doses; not recommended in patients with diabetes or dementia.
Green coffee	Green coffee is generally well tolerated. Green coffee extract contains caffeine (see Caffeine, listed above).
Green tea (*Camellia sinensis*)	See Caffeine, listed above.
Licorice (*Glycyrrhiza glabra*)	Pseudoaldosteronism, hypertension, and hypokalemia may occur.

(continued)

TABLE 27-5 Complementary Therapies Commonly Used for Weight Loss *(continued)*

Agent	Risks
Pyruvate	GI upset may occur.
Turmeric or curcumin	Curcumin causes GI upset. Increased bleeding risk may occur with high doses of curcumin.
Appetite Suppressants and Satiety Promoters	
Damiana (*Turnera diffusa*)	Damiana may cause diarrhea, headache, insomnia, and hallucinations.
Glucomannan (*Amorphophallus konjac*)	Risks are similar to those of plantain, listed below.
Guar gum (*Cyamopsis tetragonolobus*)	Risks are similar to those of plantain, listed below.
Hoodia (*Hoodia gordonii*)	No risks are reported.
Plantain or psyllium (*Plantago lanceolata, Plantago major, Plantago psyllium, Plantago arenatia*)	Flatulence, GI distress, nausea, and vomiting may occur; plantain may interact with lithium or carbamazepine.
Fat Absorption Blockers	
Chitosan	Chitosan is generally well tolerated; may cause GI upset, flatulence, nausea, increased stool bulk, constipation; may exhibit cross-sensitivity in patients with shellfish allergies.
Green coffee	See comments under Fat and Carbohydrate Modulators, listed above.
Raspberry ketones extract (*Rubus idaeus*)	No reliable information about adverse effects of raspberry extract is available. The active ingredient is structurally similar to phenylephrine; see Bitter Orange, listed above.
Carbohydrate Absorption Blockers	
Ginseng (*Panax* sp.)	Ginseng may cause nervousness, excitation, inability to concentrate, estrogenic effects, Stevens–Johnson syndrome, allergy, and hypoglycemic effects; may interact with several drugs including warfarin, digoxin, alcohol, and phenelzine.
Laxatives and Diuretics	
Cascara sagrada (*Rhamnus purshiana*)	Abdominal pain, cramps, and diarrhea may occur; chronic use can lead to potassium depletion, disturbed heart function, and muscle weakness; avoid in patients taking digoxin or potassium-depleting diuretics.
Dandelion (*Taraxacum officinale*)	Avoid use in patients with allergies to ragweed, marigolds, etc. (Asteraceae/Compositae family); contraindicated in patients with gallbladder or bile-duct obstruction, or with bowel obstruction or pus in the pleural cavity.
Miscellaneous	
Calcium	Constipation, nausea, and vomiting may occur; possibly effective when ingested as naturally occurring calcium in foods, but not when used as a dietary supplement.
Guggul (*Commiphora mukul*)	GI distress, diarrhea, nausea, and skin rash may occur; use only under medical supervision in patients with hyperthyroidism; may alter effects of thyroid medications, cholesterol-lowering medications, anticoagulants, antiplatelet medications, propranolol, and diltiazem.
Willow bark (*Salix alba*)	Willow bark is a salicin source; no risks reported when taken orally.

Key: GI = Gastrointestinal.

Source: References 41–44. (See also Chapter 51 for additional related information.)

supplements. Many of these supplements also contain vitamins and minerals, presumably to ensure adequate intake of these essential nutrients by patients on low-caloric diets. In addition, the majority of these supplements contain multiple ingredients with several purported actions, although the advertising claims frequently focus on one solitary ingredient or action or both. To further complicate the problem, many of the supplements contain "proprietary blends." Ingredients of proprietary blends must be listed, but their amounts do not have to be specified. It is important to note, however, that none of these ingredients have sufficient scientific evidence to support their usefulness in weight loss. Broadly speaking, the ingredients of weight-loss supplements can be categorized as outlined in Table 27–6.

Herbal laxatives and diuretics are often included in multiple-ingredient dietary supplements marketed for weight loss. For example, "dieter's" or "slimming" teas contain a variety of botanical laxatives and diuretics. Diuretics, whether herbal or drug, may result in an initial transient weight loss, but this effect lasts only a few days. Herbal or drug laxatives typically act in the colon and, therefore, will not decrease caloric absorption in the small intestine, which is the primary site of food absorption. Many of these botanicals are stimulant laxatives that should be used for only 1–2 weeks at a time. Prolonged use may lead to electrolyte imbalances and dependence on the laxative for regular bowel movements (*cathartic colon*), as discussed in Chapter 15.

Herbal sources of caffeine often have been used in combination with ephedra and willow bark (as a source of salicin) for weight loss because of purported synergistic effects. This combination is often referred to as a "fat-burning stack" or "ECA" (ephedrine-caffeine-aspirin), with claims of additive thermogenic or heat-producing effects.[43,44] However, adverse reactions to these products, either alone or in combination, range from relatively mild symptoms, such as headache, nervousness, and hypertension, to more severe reactions, such as stroke, myocardial infarction, and sudden death. In several cases, significant adverse events occurred in otherwise healthy young or middle-aged adults, and many occurred following consumption of relatively low doses for short periods.[43,44]

Economically Motivated Adulteration

Although adulteration of medications is not a new concept, it is of increasing concern in the dietary supplement industry. A working definition of *economically motivated adulteration* proposed by FDA is the "fraudulent, intentional substitution or addition of a substance in a product for the purpose of increasing the apparent value of the product or reducing the cost of its production, i.e., for economic gain."[45] One example of economically motivated adulteration is a hoodia weight-loss product that was found to contain material derived from cacti and actually contained no hoodia.[46] FDA tracks tainted supplements; the most common issue related to weight-loss supplements is the undisclosed inclusion of sibutramine, a prescription weight-loss medication that was voluntarily withdrawn from U.S. and Canadian markets because of an increased risk of heart attack and stroke in patients with concomitant CVD.[47] For example, in 2015, FDA issued warnings about bee pollen weight-loss supplements that were found to contain sibutramine and/or phenolphthalein, a laxative that is not approved in the United States.[48] Economic adulteration, whether intentional or unintentional, is of particular concern in the weight-loss dietary supplement industry, because increasing numbers of cases that had the potential to cause serious adverse events are appearing in the literature.

Assessment of Overweight and Obesity: A Case-Based Approach

When HCPs are asked to recommend a weight-loss method or product, they should determine the patient's motivation for weight loss. The reason may be immediately obvious for some patients; others may want to lose a few pounds to improve their appearance or to enhance their perception of good health. To assess the patient, the HCP should measure the patient's waist circumference and calculate the patient's BMI. The HCP should review the patient's current medication history (prescription and nonprescription) and also ask about use of herbal products and other dietary supplements. Family history of overweight and obesity

TABLE 27–6 Categories of Ingredients in Weight-Loss Dietary Supplements

Category	Purported Mechanism	Selected Ingredients
Stimulants/energy boosters/thermogenic aids	Increase basal metabolism, increase energy, counteract fatigue	Caffeine, bitter orange
Fat and carbohydrate modulators	Alter fat or carbohydrate metabolism, resulting in decreased body fat mass and increased lean muscle mass	Green tea, chromium, garcinia
Appetite suppressants and satiety promoters	Reduce caloric intake by suppressing appetite or promoting satiety	Guar gum, glucomannan, psyllium
Fat absorption blockers	Block intestinal absorption of dietary fat	Chitosan
Carbohydrate absorption blockers	Block intestinal absorption of dietary carbohydrate	Kidney bean extract, mung bean extract
Cortisol blockers	Block stress-induced release of cortisol to avoid cortisol-induced increased appetite and fat storage	Beta-sitosterol, phosphatidylserine, theanine
Laxatives	Promote weight loss by increasing fecal loss	Cascara sagrada, psyllium
Diuretics	Promote weight loss by increasing urination and fluid loss	Dandelion, caffeine

should be assessed and eating habits queried (food types, number of meals and their timing).

The HCP should assess what weight-loss strategies were used previously and whether the attempts were successful. Part of this assessment also includes any dietary counseling or physical activity training the patient may have received in the past. The patient's support system should be considered; support from family and friends is a critical component for success. Similarly, cultural backgrounds should be considered, because cultural and social factors have a strong effect on food decisions. Such factors should not be seen as insurmountable obstacles. The HCP can serve an important role to motivate and encourage the patient in weight loss.

Using all information obtained during the assessment, the HCP can decide whether weight loss is appropriate and, if warranted, can help select the type, intensity, and duration of a weight-loss program. Patients with significant comorbid conditions in addition to obesity should be discouraged from using dietary supplements. Individuals within the normal height and weight range who want to lose weight for other reasons (e.g., improved appearance, sense of well-being) should be advised about the difficulty of the task and the potential adverse physical and psychological effects; often these individuals can be refocused to engage in healthy exercise activities that will attain the results they are seeking.

Cases 27–1 and 27–2 illustrate assessment of patients who seek assistance with weight control.

Patient Counseling for Overweight and Obesity

The objectives for counseling patients who want to lose weight are to foster realistic goals for weight loss while also promoting a healthy restricted-calorie diet and increased physical activity. The ultimate goal for the patient is to achieve a healthy weight and maintain that weight over the long term. For patients unable to lose weight, the objective is to prevent further weight gain. The box "Patient Education for Overweight and Obesity" lists specific information for patients.

Evaluation of Patient Outcomes for Overweight and Obesity

Successful weight loss generally requires a lifelong approach that combines healthy eating and exercise patterns. Realistic weight-loss intervals might be loss of 5%–10% of the initial weight over

CASE 27-1

Relevant Evaluation Criteria	Scenario/Model Outcome
Collect	
1. Gather essential information about the patient's symptoms and medical history, including	
a. Description of symptom(s) (i.e., nature, onset, duration, severity, associated symptoms)	Patient has been overweight since middle school. He gained a lot of weight to play football in high school and never lost most of this weight after he stopped playing. His obese status does not significantly affect his ability to perform activities of daily living.
b. Description of any factors that seem to precipitate, exacerbate, and/or relieve the patient's symptom(s)	Patient is a lawyer and eats when stressed, particularly when he is preparing for trial.
c. Description of the patient's efforts to relieve the symptoms	Patient has tried various diet and exercise programs over the past 20 years. The demands of his job generally have thwarted these efforts after a few weeks.
d. Patient's identity	Ronald Godwin
e. Patient's age, gender, height, and weight	45 years old, male, 5 ft 11 in., 240 lb
f. Patient's occupation	Attorney
g. Patient's dietary habits	Usually eats a bagel or cold cereal and milk for breakfast. Usually eats out or eats a sandwich delivered to the office for a working lunch. Because he often works long into the night, he frequently orders in pizza or Chinese food for dinner, or he waits until he gets home late at night and fixes a quick frozen dinner or other easy-to-prepare meal.
h. Patient's sleep habits	Goes to bed late and gets up early; averages about 5.5 hours of sleep per night during the week and 7–8 hours on the weekends.
i. Concurrent medical conditions, prescription and nonprescription medications, and dietary supplements	Takes lisinopril for hypertension, which is currently well controlled. Takes ibuprofen occasionally for aches and pains, and famotidine for heartburn.
j. Food/drug allergies	NKA
k. History of other adverse reactions to medications	None
l. Other (describe) ______	Plays pickup basketball most Saturdays.

CASE 27-1 *continued*

Relevant Evaluation Criteria	Scenario/Model Outcome
Assess	
2. Differentiate patient's signs/symptoms, and correctly identify the patient's primary problem(s).	Patient's BMI is 34, placing him in the obese category (Table 27–1). Poor dietary habits, inadequate sleep, and lack of exercise probably contribute.
3. Identify exclusions for self-treatment (Figure 27–3).	None identified.
4. Formulate a comprehensive list of therapeutic alternatives for the primary problem to determine whether triage to a health care provider is required, and share this information with the patient or caregiver.	Options include (1) Refer Ronald to a dietitian and personal trainer for diet and exercise advice, respectively. (2) Refer Ronald to reputable websites such as myfitnesspal.com for tracking food intake and exercise, and for advice on both. (3) Refer Ronald to a support group such as Weight Watchers. (4) Counsel Ronald on diet and exercise. (5) Recommend a dietary supplement for weight loss. (6) Recommend orlistat. (7) Take no action.
Plan	
5. Select an optimal therapeutic alternative to address the patient's problem, taking into account patient preferences.	The patient chooses to try nonprescription orlistat while also trying to improve his diet by enrolling in a local program that provides healthy dinners for a fee, with delivery of 7 meals per week that can be frozen until use. He also agrees to try to make healthier choices when ordering lunch at work. He commits to using the stairs at work and in the parking garage, when possible, instead of using the elevator. He is encouraged to share these resolutions with coworkers and to try to enlist others in making healthier lunch choices.
6. Describe the recommended therapeutic approach to the patient or caregiver.	"Take orlistat up to 3 times a day before meals that contain fat. Skip the dose if a meal contains no fat."
7. Explain to the patient or caregiver the rationale for selecting the recommended therapeutic approach from the considered therapeutic alternatives.	"Orlistat should not be used as the sole method for weight loss, but it should be combined with a lower-calorie diet and increased physical activity."
Implement	
8. When recommending self-care with nonprescription medications and/or nondrug therapy, convey accurate information to the patient or caregiver.	
a. Appropriate dose and frequency of administration	"Take 60 mg of orlistat up to 3 times a day."
b. Maximum number of days the therapy should be employed	"The biggest weight loss is usually seen within the first 6 months of therapy. Decreased serum cholesterol and blood pressure may accompany weight loss."
c. Product administration procedures	"Take orlistat before eating meals that contain fatty foods. Spreading dietary fat across 3 meals a day, plus minimizing the amount of dietary fat, should help minimize gastrointestinal adverse effects, such as oily discharge and gas. Taking a multivitamin supplement at bedtime (separately from orlistat) is recommended, because orlistat can cause malabsorption of fat-soluble vitamins."
d. Expected time to onset of relief	"Some weight loss should occur within 2 weeks of initiating orlistat therapy, especially if you follow the diet and exercise regimens."
e. Degree of relief that can be reasonably expected	"Loss of 5–10 pounds during the first 6 months of therapy is a common outcome. Larger weight loss may be seen if you achieve significant changes in eating and exercise patterns."
f. Most common adverse effects	"You may experience flatulence, oily spotting, loose and frequent stools, fatty stools, fecal urgency, and fecal incontinence. These can be minimized by decreasing dietary fat; they also tend to decrease with time."
g. Adverse effects that warrant medical intervention should they occur	"Because of rare reports of liver toxicity, you should contact your primary care provider immediately if itching of skin, yellow eyes or skin, dark urine, or loss of appetite occurs."

CASE 27-1 *continued*

Relevant Evaluation Criteria	Scenario/Model Outcome
h. Patient options in the event that condition worsens or persists	"Consult a dietitian or personal trainer for diet and exercise advice. Consult your primary care provider about prescription therapy for weight loss."
i. Product storage requirements	None
j. Specific nondrug requirements	"Dietary caloric restriction and exercise are of greatest importance in losing weight. Adding stair climbing is a great idea, because once it becomes a habit, it should be sustainable. Find other exercise that is enjoyable. Consider getting a desk that can accommodate you in either the standing or sitting position, and try standing during some of your computer work. Attempt to reduce stress and, thus, stress eating. Keep healthy snacks such as fruits and vegetables in the house. Too little sleep has been associated with increased body weight, so sleep hygiene measures may be helpful." (See Chapter 46.)
Solicit follow-up questions from the patient or caregiver.	"Can I double the dose of medication if weight loss slows?"
Answer the patient's or caregiver's questions.	"Dosage above 60 mg up to 3 times a day should be attempted only under the supervision of a primary care provider."
Follow-Up: Monitor and Evaluate	
9. Assess patient outcome.	Ask Ronald to weigh himself twice a week and to record these values. He should return to you in a month to show you his progress and to discuss his diet and exercise regimen. A weight loss of a few pounds over the first month should be considered a success.

Key: BMI = Body mass index; NKA = no known allergies.

CASE 27-2

Relevant Evaluation Criteria	Scenario/Model Outcome
Collect	
1. Gather essential information about the patient's symptoms and medical history, including	
a. Description of symptom(s) (i.e., nature, onset, duration, severity, associated symptoms)	Patient is concerned about his weight. He has been considered overweight since kindergarten. His mother is encouraging him to lose weight before starting high school in the fall.
b. Description of any factors that seem to precipitate, exacerbate, and/or relieve the patient's symptom(s)	Patient tends to eat sugary foods after school to cope with being teased by classmates for his weight.
c. Description of the patient's efforts to relieve the symptoms	Patient has tried to lose weight in the past, mostly at his mother's urging. However, these attempts resulted in little weight loss, because the patient began hiding his eating from his parents.
d. Patient's identity	James Krist
e. Patient's age, gender, height, and weight	14 years old, male, 5 ft 7 in., 200 lb
f. Patient's occupation	Ninth-grade student
g. Patient's dietary habits	He eats cereal and nonfat milk for breakfast. He takes his lunch to school, usually a peanut butter and jelly sandwich and carrot sticks, but he also buys candy, potato chips, and soda from the vending machine. He has dinner with the family every night. Often he snacks in his bedroom in the evening.
h. Patient's sleep habits	Averages about 7–8 hours a night.
i. Concurrent medical conditions, prescription and nonprescription medications, and dietary supplements	None
j. Food/drug allergies	NKA

CASE 27-2 *continued*

Relevant Evaluation Criteria	Scenario/Model Outcome
k. History of other adverse reactions to medications	None
l. Other (describe) ______	Patient participates in physical education classes at school every day. He has no other regular exercise activity. Both parents and his younger brother are overweight.
Assess	
2. Differentiate patient's signs/symptoms, and correctly identify the patient's primary problem(s).	Patient's BMI is 31.3 kg/m^2, placing him above the 95th BMI percentile for age and, thus, in the obese category. The patient's current weight status places him at increased risk for type 2 diabetes, high cholesterol, hypertension, sleep apnea, and orthopedic problems during adolescence and adulthood unless he normalizes his weight. Having daily sodas, regularly consuming fatty and salty snacks, and having minimal physical activity are contributing to his weight problem.
3. Identify exclusions for self-treatment (Figure 27–3).	Age younger than 18 years is an exclusion for self-treatment.
4. Formulate a comprehensive list of therapeutic alternatives for the primary problem to determine whether triage to a health care provider is required, and share this information with the patient or caregiver.	Options include (1) Refer James to a PCP for a health screen. (2) Refer James to a dietitian and personal trainer for diet and exercise advice, respectively. (3) Recommend nonprescription orlistat. (4) Recommend a dietary supplement weight-loss product. (5) Take no action.
Plan	
5. Select an optimal therapeutic alternative to address the patient's problem, taking into account patient preferences.	Refer the patient to a PCP for a health screen.
6. Describe the recommended therapeutic approach to the patient or caregiver.	"Your primary care provider may refer you to a dietitian and/or personal trainer, or the provider could also offer prescription-strength orlistat."
7. Explain to the patient or caregiver the rationale for selecting the recommended therapeutic approach from the considered therapeutic alternatives.	"You need to see your provider to determine whether a diet and exercise program is appropriate. Healthy eating habits and exercise are the mainstays of successful weight loss, and these should be a lifelong goal." "Seeing a counselor who may be able to help you identify your personal barriers to weight loss and strategies for making successful long-term lifestyle changes may be helpful."
Implement	
8. When recommending self-care with nonprescription medications and/or nondrug therapy, convey accurate information to the patient or caregiver.	Criterion does not apply in this case.
Solicit follow-up questions from the patient or caregiver.	"Is there a nonprescription medication that might work?"
Answer the patient's or caregiver's questions.	"No nonprescription medications are approved or appropriate to recommend in a patient younger than age 18 without referral from a primary care provider."
Follow-up: Monitor and Evaluate	
9. Assess patient outcome.	Contact the patient in a day or two to ensure he made an appointment and sought medical care.

Key: BMI = Body mass index; NKA = no known allergies; PCP = primary care provider.

PATIENT EDUCATION FOR Overweight and Obesity

The objectives of self-treatment are (1) to foster realistic weight-loss and exercise goals, (2) to maintain a healthy weight, and (3) to prevent further weight gain. Carefully following the self-care measures listed here, together with continued adherence to a safe and effective weight-loss program, will help ensure optimal therapeutic outcomes.

Objectives of Self-Treatment: Prevention of Health Risks of Obesity

- Health risks related to overweight and obesity include the following:
  - Coronary heart disease
  - Type 2 diabetes
  - Sleep apnea
  - Elevated serum triglycerides and dyslipidemia
  - Hypertension
  - Stroke
  - Gallbladder disease
  - Osteoarthritis
  - Certain types of cancers

Nondrug Treatment Guidelines

- Focus on small, gradual changes in eating and exercise patterns.
- Maintain realistic goals for weight loss and increased activity levels.
- Eat a low-calorie balanced diet.
- Eat meals at the table, and do nothing else while eating (no television, etc.).
- Set a regular eating schedule, and avoid skipping meals.
- Eat slowly and enjoy the food.
- Put down your fork or spoon between bites.
- Try to leave some food on your plate each time you eat.
- Wait 5 minutes before going back for extra helpings of food.
- Remove serving dishes from the table after the first servings have been made.
- Leave the table, or at least clear food from the table after eating.
- Use smaller plates so moderate servings do not appear too small.
- Start a meal with a broth-based soup (low salt) to help you feel fuller.
- Strive to consume at least 5 servings a day of fruits and vegetables.
- Keep on hand healthful snacks such as fruits and vegetables, low-fat cheese and yogurt, and frozen fruit juice bars.
- Drink at least 8 glasses of noncaloric beverages each day to help you feel full.
- When you experience a craving, try doing something else, such as going for a walk; cravings generally pass within minutes.
- Shop for food immediately after a meal, and use a prepared list.
- Gradually increase your activity level, with the goal of engaging in 60 minutes of moderate-intensity physical activity most days of the week.
- Increase your lifestyle activity: walk and stand more, climb stairs, and park farther from your destination.
- Limit the amount of time spent watching television, playing video games, or using the internet.
- Keep a diary of your weight, physical activity, and caloric intake so you can see your progress and success.

Drug Management Guidelines

- Avoid taking nonprescription drugs and supplements marketed for weight loss, with the exception of orlistat. They are not proven to work, and they can cause significant adverse effects.
- If you do decide to take one of these products, make sure to notify your primary care provider and pharmacist so you can be adequately followed for potential adverse effects and drug interactions.
- Both prescription and nonprescription formulations of orlistat are available; be sure you do not take both forms concurrently.

6 months, or 1–2 pounds per week. The patient should be counseled that weight management is a lifelong process and that regain after loss is typical if good lifestyle habits are not continued. During any weight-loss program, the patient should be monitored for healthy eating and exercise patterns, and, at a minimum, blood pressure should be routinely measured. More extensive physical examinations and laboratory measures may be indicated, particularly in patients with comorbid conditions such as hypertension or type 2 diabetes. Follow-up with patients attempting weight loss should be encouraged, preferably monthly or more frequently. In addition to measuring weight at follow-up visits, the HCP should explore eating habits and exercise patterns with the patient, especially if weight loss is not being achieved. The HCP should also reexamine the goals that were set and follow up on the patient's progress, with new goals or modifications set as appropriate. Referral to a dietitian or personal trainer may be helpful. Following weight loss, emphasis should be placed on the importance of maintaining the weight loss by continuing healthful dietary and exercise habits. Referral for pharmacologic therapy or consideration of bariatric surgery may be an option for patients with more significant obesity who fail to lose weight through lifestyle interventions.

Key Points for Overweight and Obesity

- A reasonable goal for weight loss in most overweight and obese subjects is a 5%–10% loss over 6 months.
- Although this amount of weight loss may not result in the cosmetic effect desired by the dieter, it is associated with a reduction in risk for chronic disease.
- The safest approach to losing weight entails combining a reduced-calorie diet with increased physical activity.
- Physical activity typically needs to be something the dieter enjoys if it is to be sustained over long periods of time.
- A key to sustained weight loss is modification of behavior related to eating and exercise.
- If nonprescription or dietary supplement products for weight loss are used, they should be continuously assessed for efficacy, safety, and tolerance. All HCPs should be informed of the product(s) used. Labels of nonprescription or dietary supplement weight-loss products should be carefully reviewed to determine the risk for adverse reactions and drug–supplement interactions.

REFERENCES

1. Managing overweight and obesity in adults. Systematic evidence review from the obesity expert panel, 2013. Washington, DC: National Heart, Lung, and Blood Institute; 2013. Available at: http://www.nhlbi.nih.gov/sites/www.nhlbi.nih.gov/files/obesity-evidence-review.pdf. Accessed May 30, 2017.
2. National Center for Health Statistics. *Health, United States, 2014.* Hyattsville, MD: U.S. Department of Health and Human Services, Centers for Disease Control and Prevention, National Center for Health Statistics; 2014. DHHS Publication No. 2015–1232. Available at: http://www.cdc.gov/nchs/data/hus/hus14.pdf. Accessed May 30, 2017.
3. Prevalence of obesity among adults and youth, United States, 2011–2014. National Center for Health Statistics data brief, 219, November 2015. Available at: https://www.cdc.gov/nchs/data/databriefs/db219.pdf. Accessed May 30, 2017.
4. Institute of Medicine, National Academy of Sciences. Accelerating progress in obesity prevention. Solving the weight of the nation. 2012. Available at: http://www.nationalacademies.org/hmd/Reports/2012/Accelerating-Progress-in-Obesity-Prevention.aspx. Accessed May 30, 2017.
5. Moyer VA, on behalf of the U.S. Preventive Services Task Force. Screening for and management of obesity in adults: U.S. Preventive Services Task Force recommendation statement. *Ann Intern Med.* 2012;157(5):373–8. doi: 10.7326/0003-4819-157-5-201209040-00475.
6. Florez H, Castillo-Florez S. Beyond the obesity paradox in diabetes: fitness, fatness, and mortality. *JAMA.* 2012;308(6):619–20. doi: 10.1001/jama.2012.9776.
7. The Global BMI Mortality Collaboration. Body-mass index and all-cause mortality: individual-participant-data meta-analysis of 239 prospective studies in four continents. *Lancet.* 2016;388(10046):776–86. doi: 10.1016/S0140-6736(16)30175-1. Epub 2016 Jul 13. Available at: http://www.thelancet.com/journals/lancet/article/PIIS0140-6736(16)30175-1/fulltext. Accessed May 30, 2017.
8. Dulloo AG, Montana JP. Body composition, inflammation and thermogenesis in pathways to obesity and the metabolic syndrome: an overview. *Obes Rev.* 2012;13(Suppl 2):15. doi: 10.1111/j.1467-789X.2012.01032.x.
9. August GP, Caprio S, Fennoy I, et al. *Prevention and Treatment of Pediatric Obesity.* Chevy Chase, MD: Endocrine Society; 2008. Available at: https://www.endocrine.org/~/media/endosociety/Files/Publications/Clinical%20Practice%20Guidelines/FINAL-Standalone-Pediatric-Obesity-Guideline.pdf. Accessed May 30, 2017.
10. Qi Q, Chu AY, Kang JH, et al. Sugar-sweetened beverages and genetic risk of obesity. *New Engl J Med.* 2012;367(15):1387–96. doi: 10.1056/NEJMoa1203039.
11. Qi Q, Chu AY, Kang JH, et al. Fried food consumption, genetic risk, and body mass index: gene-diet interaction analysis in three US cohort studies. *BMJ.* 2014;348:g1610. doi: 10.1136/bmj.g1610.
12. Loh K, Herzog H, Shi YC. Regulation of energy homeostasis by the NPY system. *Trends Endocrinol Metab.* 2015;26(3):125–35. doi: 10.1016/j.tem.2015.01.003.
13. U.S. Department of Agriculture, U.S. Department of Health and Human Services. *Dietary Guidelines for Americans, 2010.* 7th ed. Washington, DC: U.S. Government Printing Office; 2010. Available at: http://health.gov/dietaryguidelines/2010/. Accessed May 30, 2017.
14. Song M, Carroll DD, Fulton JE. Meeting the 2008 physical activity guidelines for Americans among U.S. youth. *Am J Prev Med.* 2013;44(3):216–22. doi: 10.1016/j.amepre.2012.
15. Leger D, Bayon V, de Sanctis A. The role of sleep in the regulation of body weight. *Mol Cell Endocrinol.* 2015;418(Pt 2):101–7. doi: 10.1016/j.mce.2015.06.030.
16. Gerard P. Gut microbiota and obesity. *Cell Mol Life Sci.* 2016;73(1):147–62. doi: 10.1007/s00018-015-2061-5.
17. Domecq JP, Prutsky G, Leppin A, et al. Clinical review: drugs commonly associated with weight change: a systematic review and meta-analysis. *J Clin Endocrinol Metab.* 2015;100(2):363–70. doi: 10.1210/jc.2014-342118.
18. Chrostowska M, Szyndler A, Hoffmann M, et al. Impact of obesity on cardiovascular health. *Best Pract Res Clin Endocrinol Metab.* 2013;27(2):147–56. doi: 10.1016/j.beem.2013.01.00419.
19. Jensen MD, Ryan DH, Apovian CM, et al. 2013 AHA/ACC/TOS Guideline for the management of overweight and obesity in adults: a report of the American College of Cardiology/American Heart Association Task Force on Practice Guidelines and The Obesity Society. *Circulation.* 2014;129(Suppl 2);S102–38. doi: 10.1161/01.cir.0000437739.71477.ee. Available at: http://circ.ahajournals.org/content/early/2013/11/11/01.cir.0000437739.71477.ee.full.pdf. Accessed May 30, 2017.
20. Pulgaron E. Childhood obesity: a review of increased risk for physical and psychological comorbidities. *Clin Ther.* 2013;35(1):A18–32. doi: 10.1016/j.clinthera.2012.12.014.
21. The National Weight Control Registry Web site. The National Weight Control Registry. Available at: http://www.nwcr.ws. Accessed May 30, 2017.
22. Food and Nutrition Board, Institute of Medicine. *Dietary Reference Intakes for Energy, Carbohydrate, Fiber, Fat, Fatty Acids, Cholesterol, Protein, and Amino Acids (Macronutrients).* Washington, DC: National Academies Press; 2002. http://www.nap.edu/books/0309085373/html. Accessed May 30, 2017.
23. U.S. Department of Agriculture, U.S. Department of Health and Human Services. *Dietary Guidelines for Americans, 2015-2020.* 8th ed. Washington, DC. U.S. Government Printing Office; 2015. Available at: http://health.gov/dietaryguidelines/2015/guidelines/. Accessed May 30, 2017.
24. Dod HS, Bhardwal R, Sajja V, et al. Effect of intensive lifestyle changes on endothelial function and on inflammatory markers of atherosclerosis. *Am J Cardiol.* 2010;105(3):362–7. doi: 10.1016/j.amjcard.2009.09.038.
25. Hession M, Rolland C, Kulkarni U, et al. Systematic review of randomized controlled trials of low-carbohydrate vs. low-fat/low-calorie diets in the management of obesity and its comorbidities. *Obes Rev.* 2009;10(1):36–50. doi: 10.1111/j.1467-789X.2008.00518.x.
26. Volek JS, Fernandez ML, Feinman RD, et al. Dietary carbohydrate restriction induces a unique metabolic state positively affecting atherogenic dyslipidemia, fatty acid partitioning, and metabolic syndrome. *Prog Lipid Res.* 2008;47(5):307–18. doi: 10.1016/j.plipres.2008.02.003.
27. U.S. Department of Health and Human Services. *2008 Physical Activity Guidelines for Americans.* Washington, DC: U.S. Department of Health and Human Services; 2008. ODPHP Publication No. U0036. Available at: http://www.health.gov/paguidelines. Accessed May 30, 2017.
28. Thompson WG, Cook DA, Clark MM, et al. Treatment of obesity. *Mayo Clin Proc.* 2007;82(1):93–101. doi: 10.4065/82.1.93.
29. U.S. Food and Drug Administration. Clean-up of ineffective ingredients in OTC drug products [news release]. November 7, 1990. Available at: http://pinch.com/skin/docs/FDA-OTC-ingredients-ban. Accessed May 30, 2017.
30. U.S. Food and Drug Administration. BMPEA in dietary supplements. April 27, 2015. Available at: http://www.fda.gov/Food/DietarySupplements/ProductsIngredients/ucm443790.htm. Accessed May 30, 2017.
31. U.S. Food and Drug Administration. DMAA in dietary supplements. July 16, 2013. Available at: http://www.fda.gov/Food/DietarySupplements/ProductsIngredients/ucm346576.htm. Accessed May 30, 2017.
32. U.S. Food and Drug Administration. DMBA in dietary supplements. April 28, 2015. Available at: https://www.fda.gov/food/dietarysupplements/productsingredients/ucm444719.htm. Accessed May 30, 2017.
33. U.S. Food and Drug Administration. Orlistat (marketed as Alli and Xenical) Information. Available at: https://www.fda.gov/Drugs/DrugSafety/PostmarketDrugSafetyInformationforPatientsandProviders/ucm180076.htm. Accessed May 30, 2017.
34. Xenical [prescribing information]. Genentech USA, South San Francisco, CA; August 2015. Available at: http://www.gene.com/download/pdf/xenical_prescribing.pdf. Accessed May 30, 2017.
35. GlaxoSmithKline. Alli. Frequently asked questions. 2015. Available at: https://www.myalli.com/faqs/. Accessed May 30, 2017.
36. Anderson JW, Schwartz SM, Hauptman J, et al. Low-dose orlistat effects on body weight of mildly to moderately overweight individuals: a 16-week, double-blind, placebo-controlled trial. *Ann Pharmacother.* 2006;40(10):1717–23. doi: 10.1345/aph.1H234.
37. Glaxo Smith Kline. Alli orlistat label. 2007. Available at: http://www.accessdata.fda.gov/drugsatfda_docs/label/2007/021887lbl.pdf. Accessed February 4, 2017.
38. Mancini MC, Halpern A. Orlistat in the prevention of diabetes in the obese. *Vasc Health Risk Manag.* 2008;4(2):325–36. PMCID: PMC2496972.
39. U.S. Food and Drug Administration. Re: Docket No. 2006P-0154/CP1 and SUP1. February 7, 2007. Available at: http://www.fda.gov/ohrms/dockets/dockets/06p0154/06P-0154-pdn0001.pdf. Accessed May 30, 2017.

40. Haller CA, Benowitz NF, Jacob P III. Hemodynamic effects of ephedra-free weight-loss supplements in humans. *Am J Med.* 2005;118(9):998–1003. doi: 10.1016/j.amjmed.2005.02.034.
41. Ulbright CE. *Natural Standard Herb & Supplement Guide: An Evidence-Based Reference.* 1st ed. Maryland Heights, MO: Mosby; 2010:799–823.
42. Hasani-Ranjbar S, Nayebi N, Larijani B, et al. A systematic review of the efficacy and safety of herbal medicines used in the treatment of obesity. *World J Gastroenterol.* 2009;15(25):3073–85. PMCID: PMC2705729.
43. Egras AM, Hamilton WR, Lenz TL, Monaghan MS. An evidence-based review of fat modifying supplemental weight loss products. *J Obes.* 2011; 2011. pii: 297315. doi: 10.1155/2011/297315. Epub 2010 Aug 10. Available at: http://dx.doi.org/10.1155/2011/297315. Accessed May 30, 2017.
44. Dwyer JT, Allison DB, Coates PM. Dietary supplements in weight reduction. *J Am Diet Assoc.* 2005;105(5 Suppl 1):S80–6. doi: 10.1016/j.jada.2005.02.028.
45. U.S. Food and Drug Administration. Addressing Challenges of Economically-Motivated Adulteration. [PowerPoint presentation] May 2009. Available at: http://www.fda.gov/downloads/NewsEvents/MeetingsConferencesWorkshops/UCM163631.ppt. Accessed May 30, 2017.
46. U.S. Food and Drug Administration. Economically Motivated Adulteration in the Dietary Supplement Market Place. [PowerPoint presentation, n.d.] Available at: http://www.fda.gov/downloads/NewsEvents/Meetings-ConferencesWorkshops/UCM163645.ppt. Accessed May 30, 2017.
47. U.S. Food and Drug Administration. Tainted supplements marketed as dietary supplements_CDER. Available at: http://www.accessdata.fda.gov/scripts/sda/sdNavigation.cfm?sd=tainted_supplements_cder. Accessed May 30, 2017.
48. U.S. Food and Drug Administration. Some bee pollen weight loss products are a dangerous scam. July 25, 2015. Available at: http://www.fda.gov/forconsumers/consumerupdates/ucm401676.htm. Accessed May 30, 2017.

COLOR PLATES

Color Illustration Contributors

Allergan, Inc.

Lawrence R. Ash

Umberto Benelli (eyeatlas.com)

Jean A. Borger

Richard C. Childers

Stanley Cullen

emedicine.com, Inc.

Jeffery A. Goad

Alfred C. Griffin (deceased)

Harold L. Hammond

Hollister Incorporated

Christopher Huerter

Thomas C. Orihel

Joan Lerner Selekof

R. Gary Sibbald

George Yatskievych

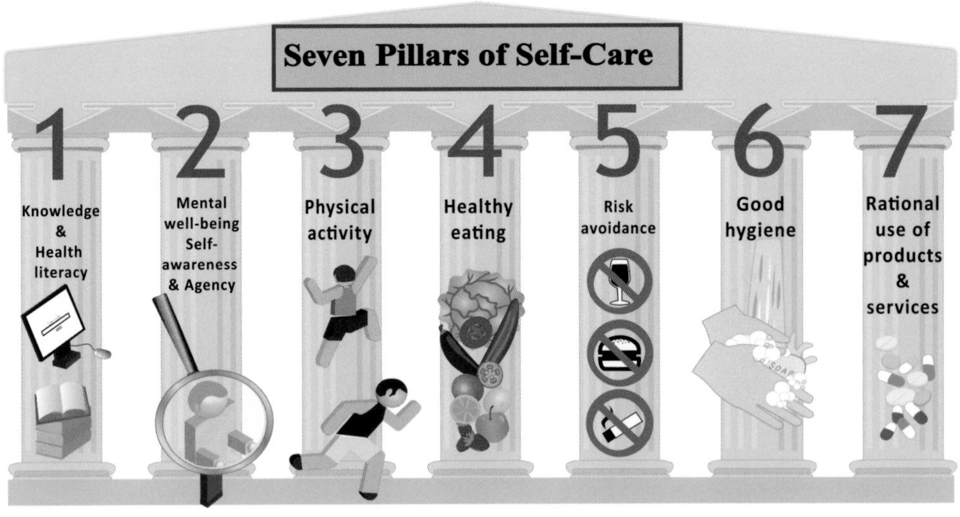

1

1 The seven pillars of self-care illustrate the broad scope of self-care, as defined by the International Self-Care Foundation. (See Chapter 1, Table 1–1, for discussion of the seven elements.) (Adapted with the permission of the International Self-Care Foundation.)

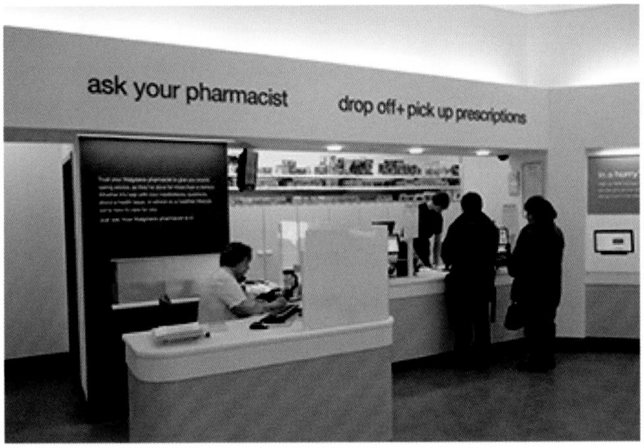

2A

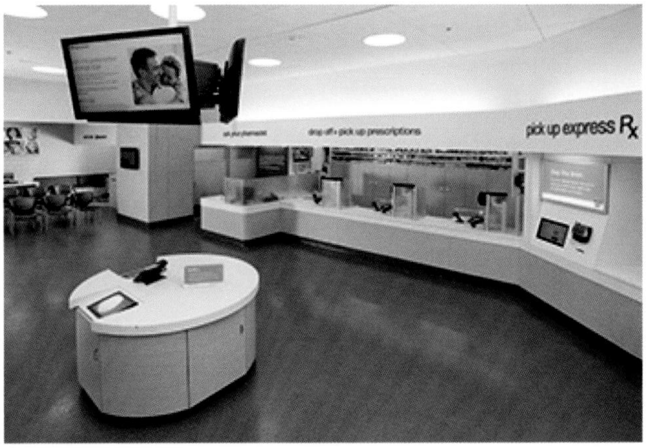

2B

2A, B Walgreens and other pharmacies have changed pharmacy design and operations to improve accessibility and visibility of pharmacists (see Chapter 1). At several Walgreens pharmacies, pharmacists work at desks in front of the pharmacy. (Photographs courtesy of Walgreens.)

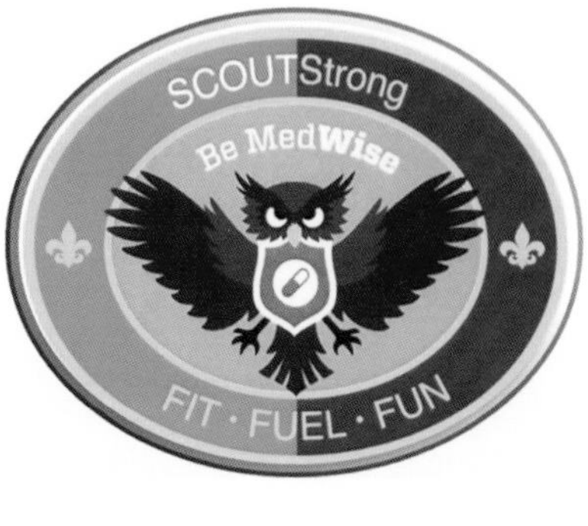

3

3 Boy Scouts and Venturers ages 11–17 years can earn the SCOUT-Strong Be MedWise award after they complete four lessons on safe and responsible nonprescription medication use. The award is sponsored by a partnership between the National Council on Patient Information and Education (NCPIE) and the Boy Scouts of America (see Chapter 1). (Photograph of badge used with the permission of the Boy Scouts of America.)

4 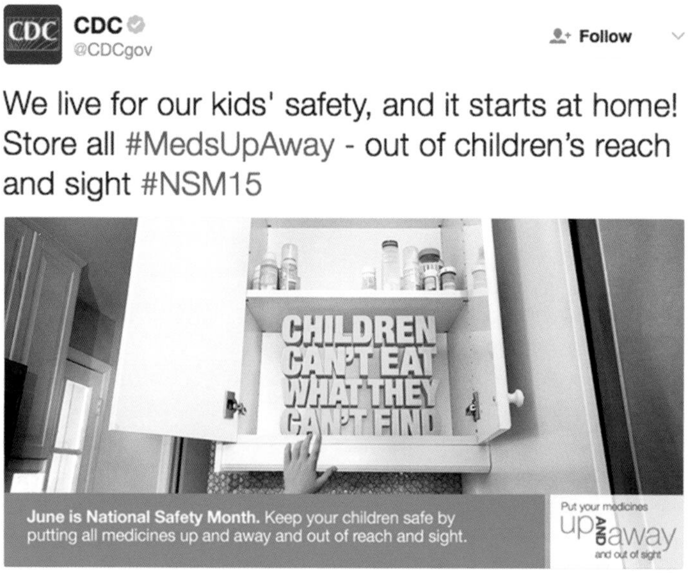

4 The Up and Away project, a collaborative effort by public health agencies, private sector companies, professional organizations, consumer and patient advocates, and academic experts, has developed strategies to keep children safe from unintentional medication overdoses (see Chapter 1).

5 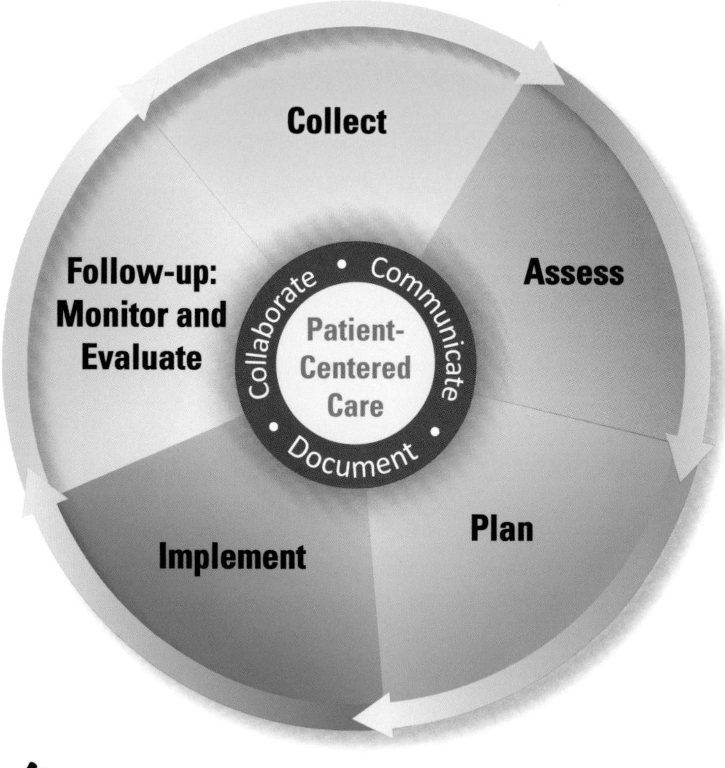

Pharmacists' Patient Care Process

Pharmacists use a patient-centered approach in collaboration with other providers on the health care team to optimize patient health and medication outcomes.

Using principles of evidence-based practice, pharmacists:

Collect
The pharmacist assures the collection of the necessary subjective and objective information about the patient in order to understand the relevant medical/medication history and clinical status of the patient.

Assess
The pharmacist assesses the information collected and analyzes the clinical effects of the patient's therapy in the context of the patient's overall health goals in order to identify and prioritize problems and achieve optimal care.

Plan
The pharmacist develops an individualized patient-centered care plan, in collaboration with other health care professionals and the patient or caregiver that is evidence-based and cost-effective.

Implement
The pharmacist implements the care plan in collaboration with other health care professionals and the patient or caregiver.

Follow-up: Monitor and Evaluate
The pharmacist monitors and evaluates the effectiveness of the care plan and modifies the plan in collaboration with other health care professionals and the patient or caregiver as needed.

APhA
Improving medication use.
Advancing patient care.

5 The Pharmacists' Patient Care Process was developed by the Joint Commission of Pharmacy Practitioners to provide a consistent process in the delivery of patient care across the profession (see Chapter 2).

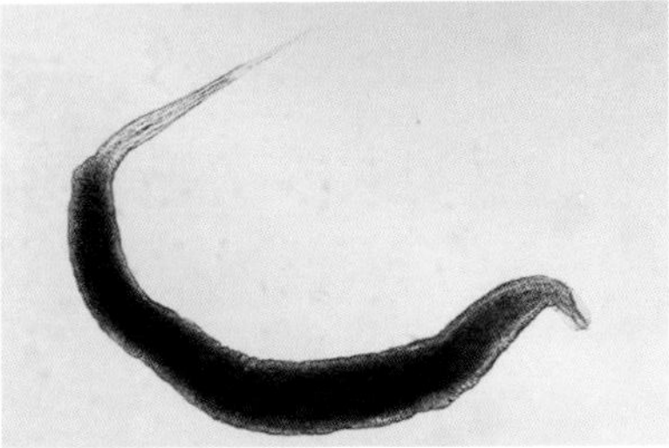

6A

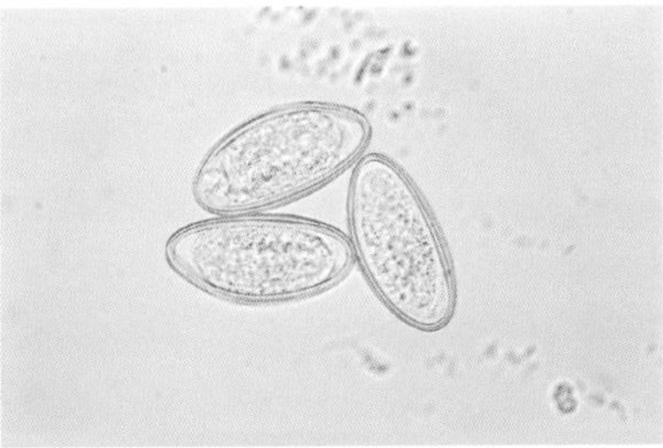

6B

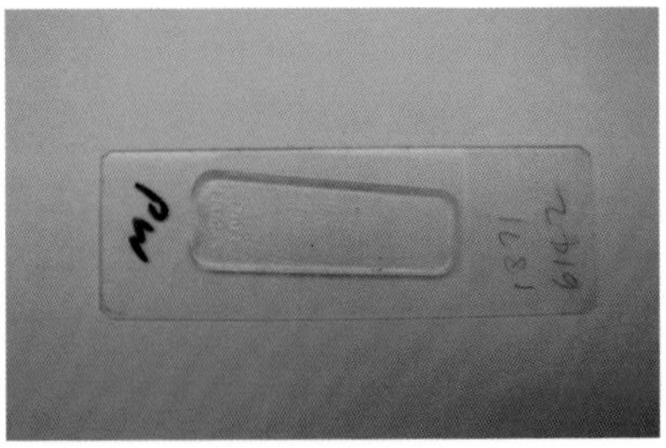

6C

6A, B, and C **Pinworm infection,** the most common worm infestation in the United States, is caused by ingestion of pinworm eggs from fecally contaminated hands, food, clothing, or bedding. **A,** The adult pinworm is a small (1-cm long), white, thread-like worm with a pin-shaped, pointed tail. **B,** The mature female stores approximately 11,000 eggs in her body, which she deposits in the perianal region of the host, usually at night. Reinfection occurs when the hatched larvae return to the large intestine or when eggs are transferred from the anus to the mouth and swallowed. **C,** Commercial pinworm detection kits use a sticky paddle, instead of tape, to affix the adult pinworm to a slide, which is then examined microscopically (see Chapter 18). (Photographs 6A and B courtesy of Lawrence R. Ash, PhD, and Thomas C. Orihel, PhD, © 1997, *Atlas of Human Parasitology.* 4th ed. Chicago: ASCP Press; 1997. Photograph 6C courtesy of Jeffery A. Goad, PharmD, University of Southern California, School of Pharmacy, Los Angeles, © 2003.)

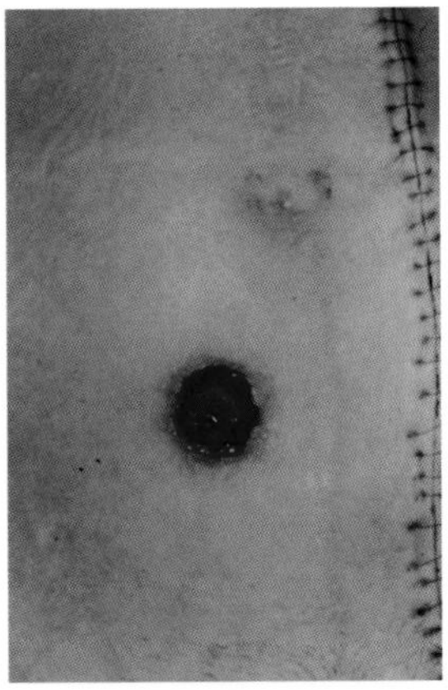

7A

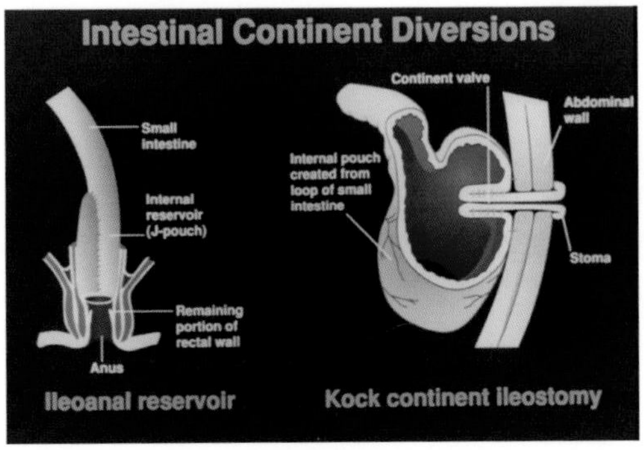

7B

7A–B There are three major types of ostomies: ileostomy, colostomy, or urinary diversion. **A,** In an ileostomy, a portion of the ileum is brought through the abdominal wall. **B,** The two most common types of continent ileostomies are the ileoanal reservoir and the Kock continent ileostomy. The ileoanal reservoir is created by stripping diseased mucosa from the rectum, creating an internal pouch from the ileum, and pulling the distal end of the pouch through the rectum and attaching it. In the Kock continent ileostomy, an internal pouch is created from the ileum and an intussusception of the bowel is used to create a "nipple."

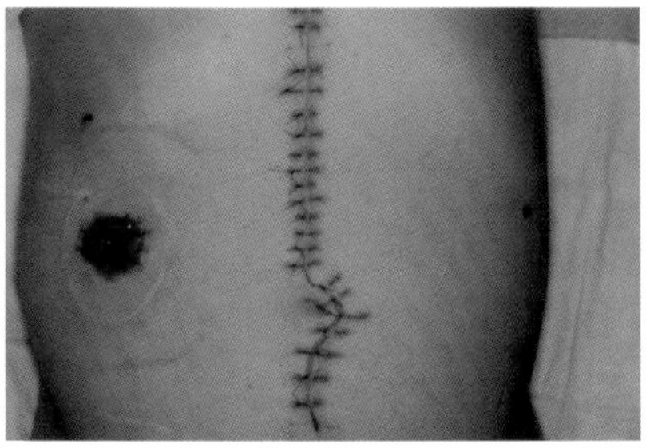

7C

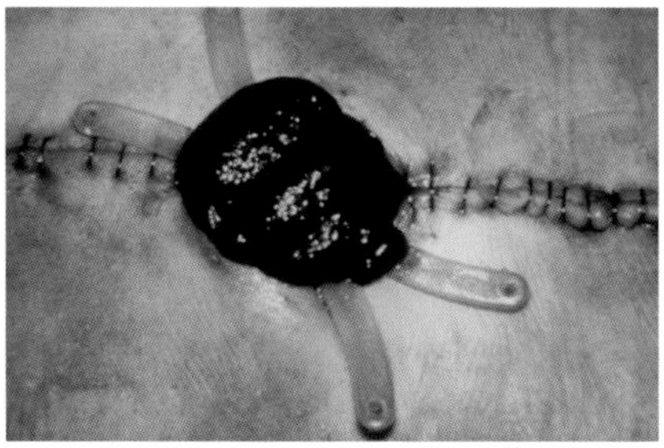

7D

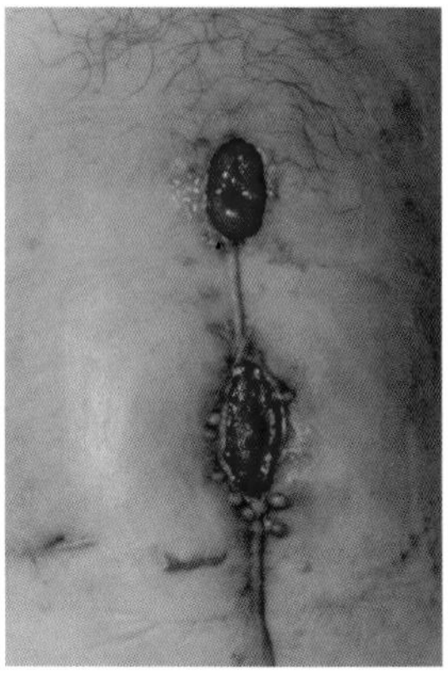

7E

7C–F Colostomies are located on the ascending, transverse, or descending/sigmoid colon. **C,** Ascending colostomies are uncommon. The ascending colon is retained, but the rest of the large bowel is removed or bypassed. The stoma is usually on the right side of the abdomen. The transverse colon is the site of most temporary colostomies. A loop of the transverse colon is lifted through the abdominal incision, and a rod or bridge is placed under the loop to give it support. **D,** Loop colostomies have one large opening, but two tracts. The proximal tract discharges fecal material; the distal tract secretes small amounts of mucus. **E,** In a double-barrel transverse colostomy, the bowel is completely divided by bringing both the proximal end and the distal end through the abdominal wall and suturing them to the skin. **F,** Descending and sigmoid colostomies are fairly common and generally are on the left side of the abdomen.

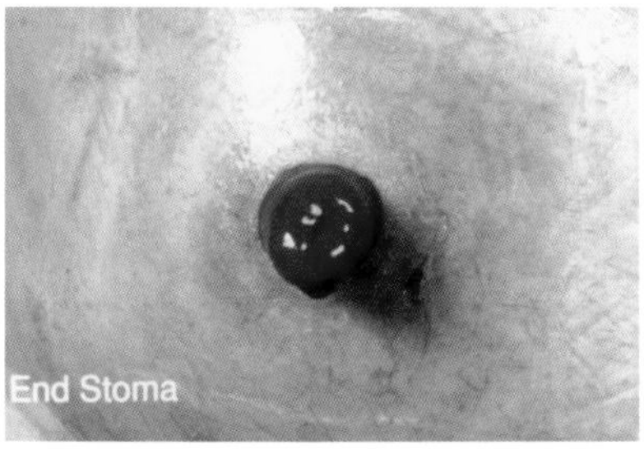

7F

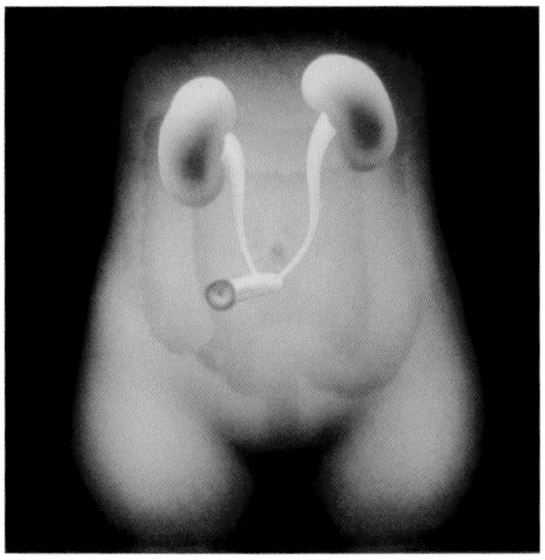

7G

7G–I Urinary diversion surgery diverts the urinary stream through an opening in the abdominal wall. **G,** In the ileal conduit, the most common type of urinary diversion, ileal and colon conduits are created after removal of the bladder by implanting the ureters into an isolated loop of bowel, the distal end of which is brought to the surface of the abdomen. **H,** Mucous shreds will be present if the bowel is used to create the diversion. **I,** In a ureterostomy, one or both ureters are detached from the bladder and brought to the outside of the abdominal wall, where a stoma is created. This procedure is used less frequently because the ureters tend to narrow unless they have been dilated permanently by previous disease (see Chapter 22). (Copyrighted photographs 2B, D, and G courtesy of Hollister Incorporated, Libertyville, Illinois. Copyrighted photographs 2A, C, E, F, H, and I courtesy of Joan Lerner Selekof, BSN, CWOCN, University of Maryland Medical Center, Baltimore, Maryland.)

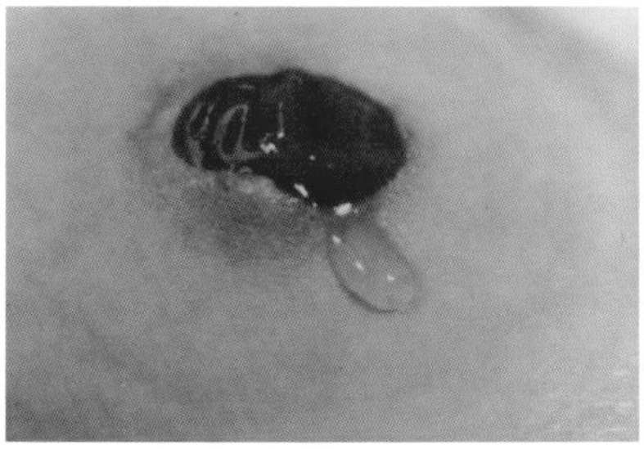

7H

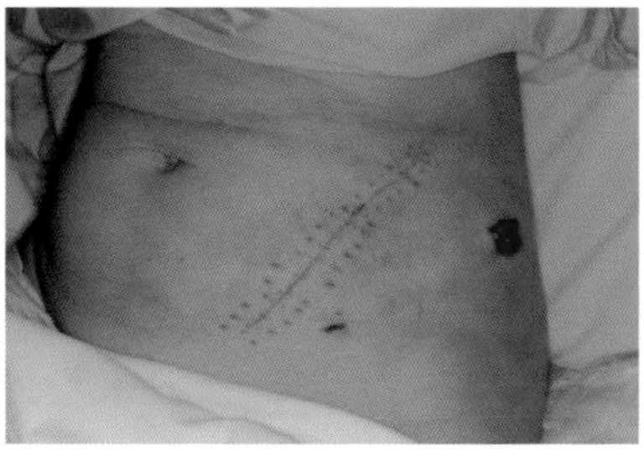

7I

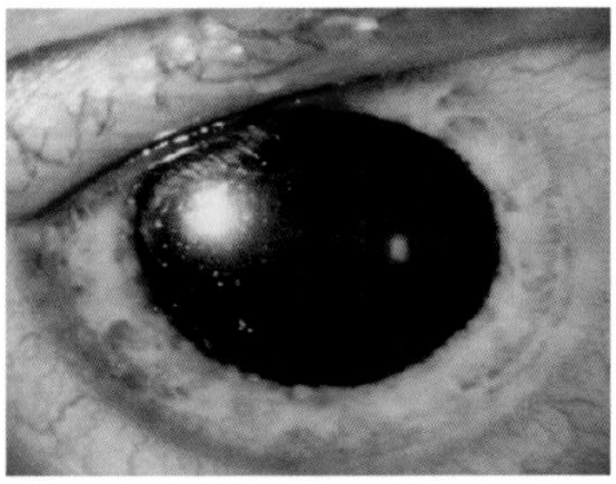

8

8 Severe dry eye can result from failure to properly diagnose and treat dry eye diseases. Severe damage to eye tissue, particularly the corneal surface, can occur (see Chapter 28). (Photograph courtesy of Allergan, Inc., Irvine, California.)

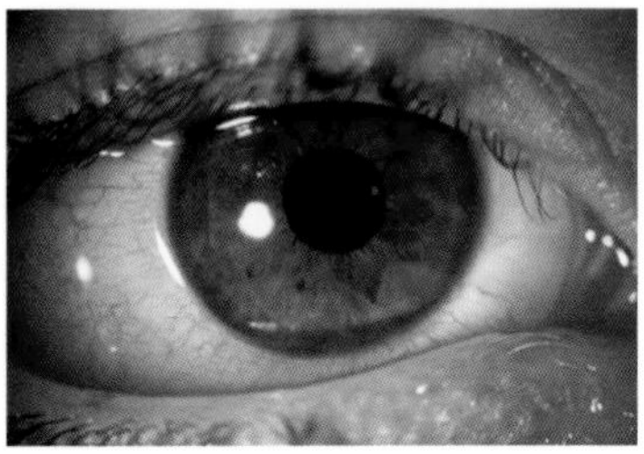

9

9 Allergic conjunctivitis is characterized by itchy, red eyes with a watery discharge. Vision is usually not impaired, but it may be blurred because of excessive tearing (see Chapter 28).

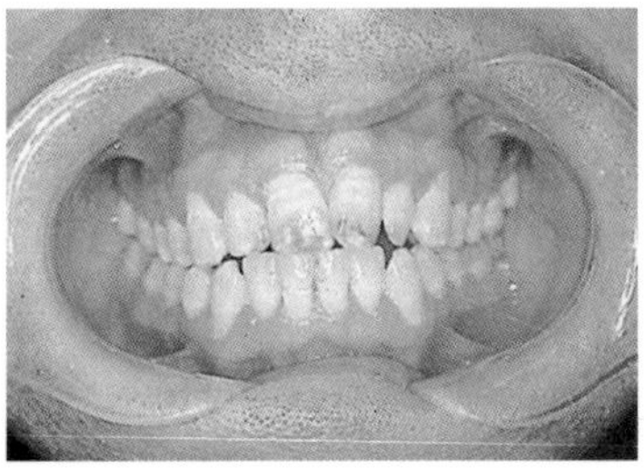

10

10 Dental fluorosis (mottled enamel) can develop during the time of tooth formation in children who receive higher than optimal intake of fluoride. Discoloration of the teeth varies, depending on the level of fluoride in the water, and ranges from white flecks or spots to brownish stains, small pits, or deep irregular pits that are dark brown in color (see Chapter 31).

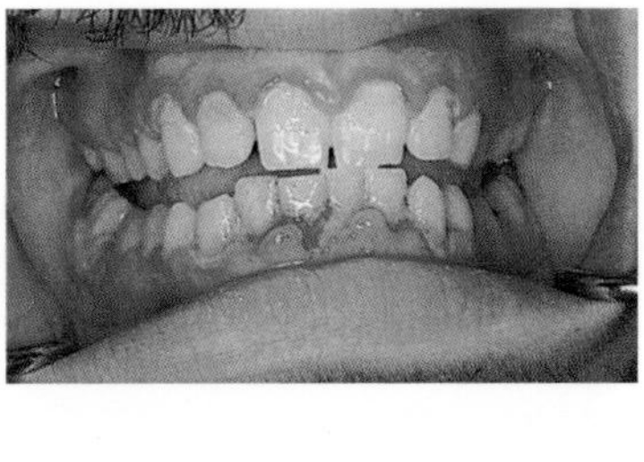

11

11 Chronic gingivitis, an asymptomatic inflammation of the gingivae (gums) at the necks of the teeth, is an early stage of periodontitis and is usually caused by poor oral hygiene. The gingivae are erythematous (red) and may have areas that appear swollen and glossy. In addition, mild bleeding may occur during toothbrushing (see Chapter 31).

12 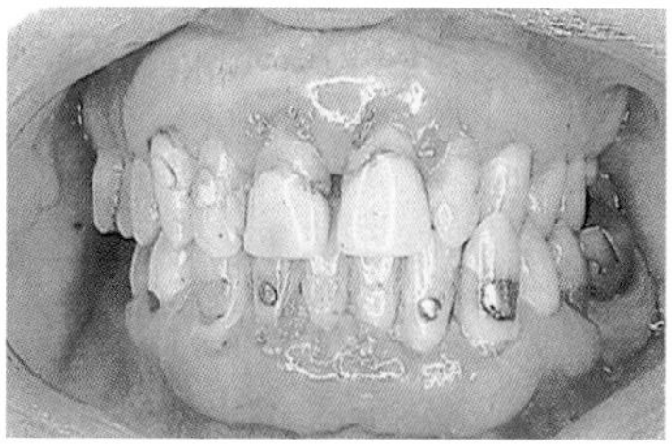

12 Chronic periodontitis (pyorrhea), an inflammation of the tissues surrounding the teeth, including the gingivae, periodontal ligaments, alveolar bone, and the cementum (bony material covering the root of a tooth), is caused by plaque accumulation resulting from poor oral hygiene. The gingivae may be erythematous and swollen, and may recede from the necks of the teeth. The condition is not painful and usually is accompanied by halitosis, loosening of the teeth, and mild bleeding during toothbrushing (see Chapter 31).

13 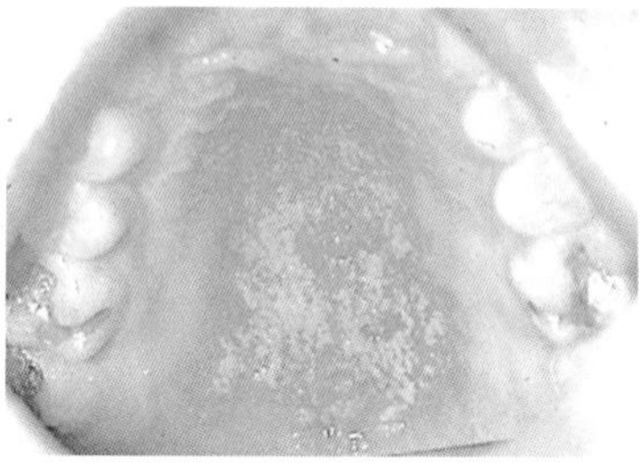

13 Candidiasis (candidosis, moniliasis, thrush), an infection caused by overgrowth of *Candida albicans,* tends to occur in people with debilitating or chronic systemic disease or those on long-term antibiotic therapy. Candidiasis commonly manifests as a whitish-gray to yellowish, soft, slightly elevated pseudomembrane-like plaque on the oral mucosa; the plaque is often described as having a milk curd appearance. If the membrane is stripped away, a raw bleeding surface remains. A dull, burning pain is often present (see Chapters 31 and 32).

14 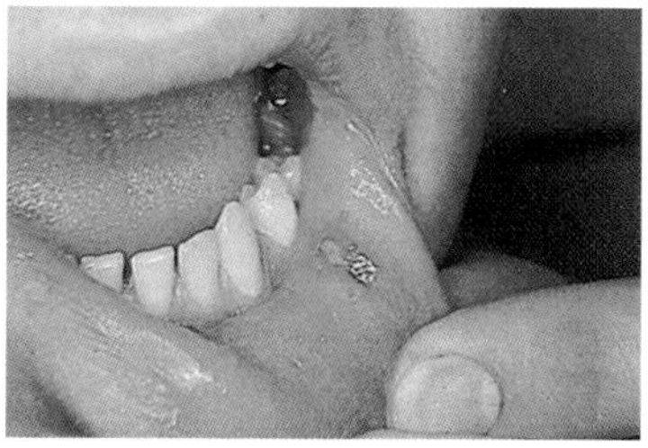

14 Recurrent aphthous ulcers (canker sores) are recurrent, painful, single, or multiple ulcerations of bacterial origin. The central ulceration is sharply demarcated, often has a gray to grayish-yellow surface of necrotic debris, and is surrounded by an erythematous margin (see Chapter 32).

15 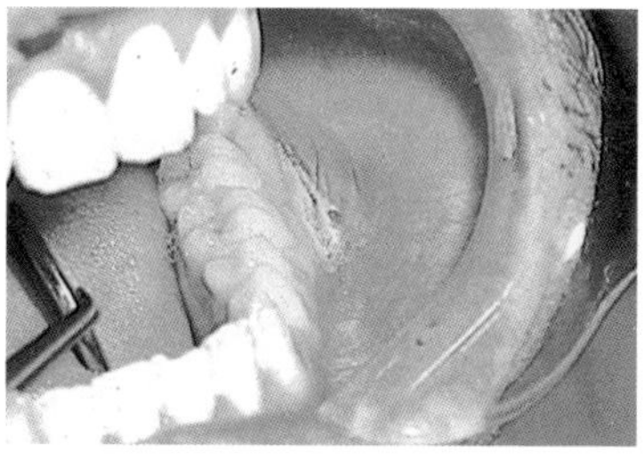

15 Aspirin burn results from the topical use of aspirin to relieve toothache. An aspirin tablet is placed against the tooth, where it is held in place by pressure from the buccal (cheek) mucosa. The mucosa becomes necrotic and is characterized by a white slough that rubs away, revealing a painful ulceration (see Chapter 32).

16 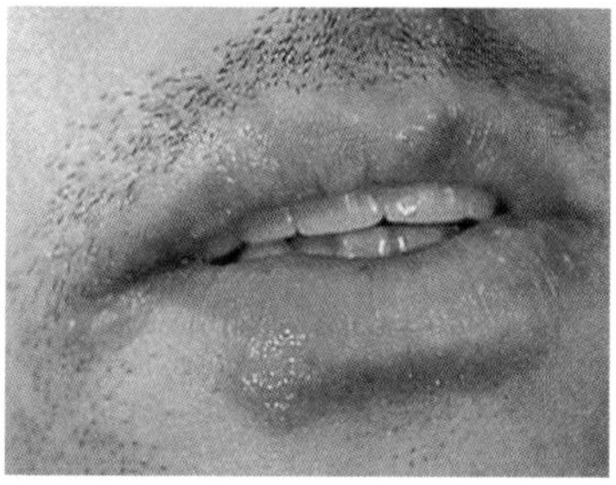

16 Herpes simplex lesions of the mouth and the eye usually start as a small cluster of vesicles (tiny blisters) that subsequently heal over with a serosanguineous (blood-tinged) crust. Local stinging, burning, and pain often herald the onset of lesions. Eye involvement should always be referred to an ophthalmologist (see Chapter 32).

17A
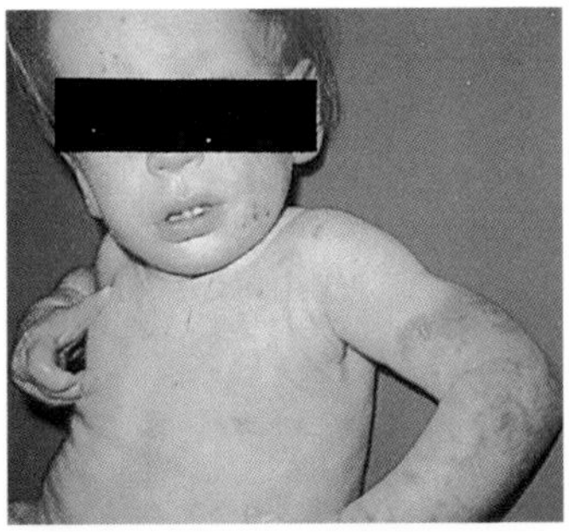

17B
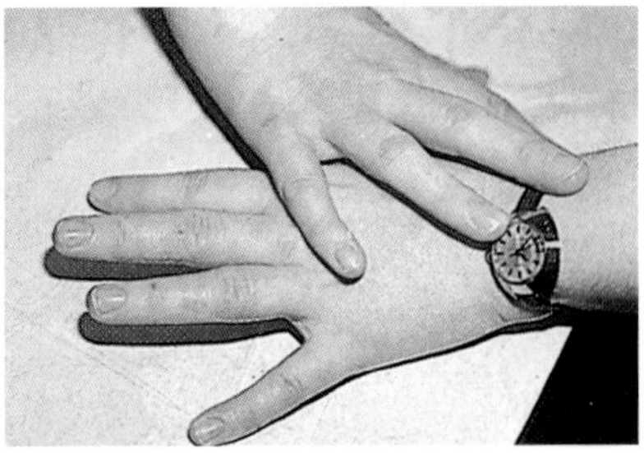

17C
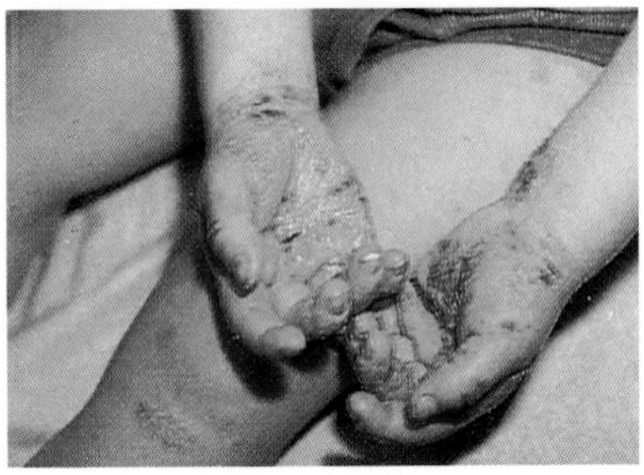

17A, B, and C Atopic dermatitis (eczema) is an inflammatory condition that occurs **(A)** on the extensor surface of the elbows and knees during the first year of life and then **(B)** involves predominantly the flexors. **C,** The hands, feet, and face are often involved as well. The dermatitis is characterized by erythema, scale, increased skin surface markings, and crusting; secondary infection is common (see Chapter 33).

18
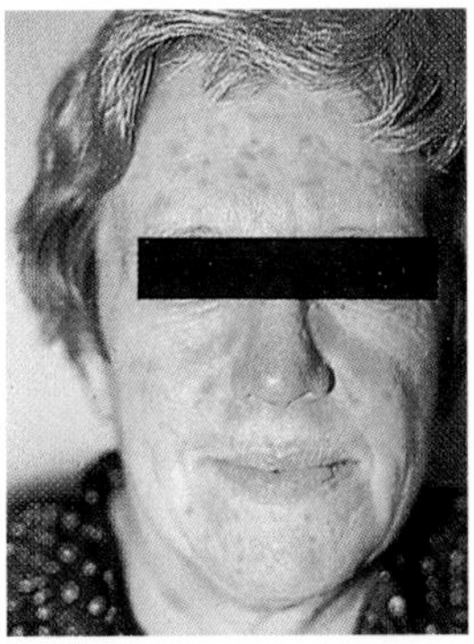

18 Seborrheic dermatitis is a red scaling condition of the scalp, midface, and upper midchest of adults. This dermatitis is marked by characteristic greasy, yellowish scaling and is associated with erythema (see Chapter 34).

19A
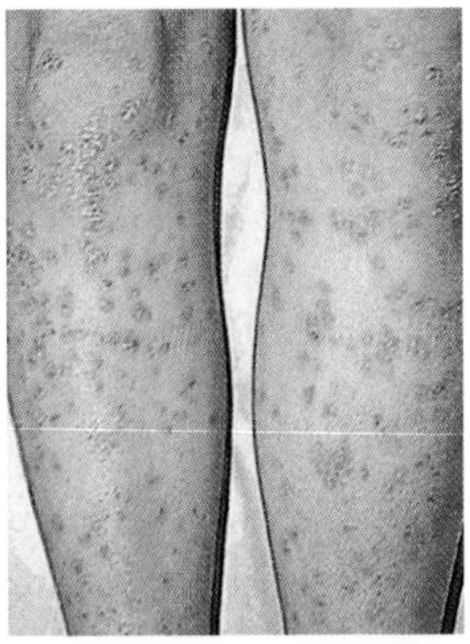

19B
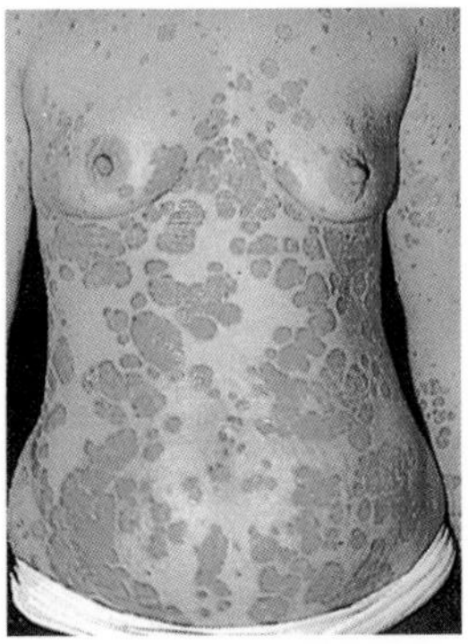

19C
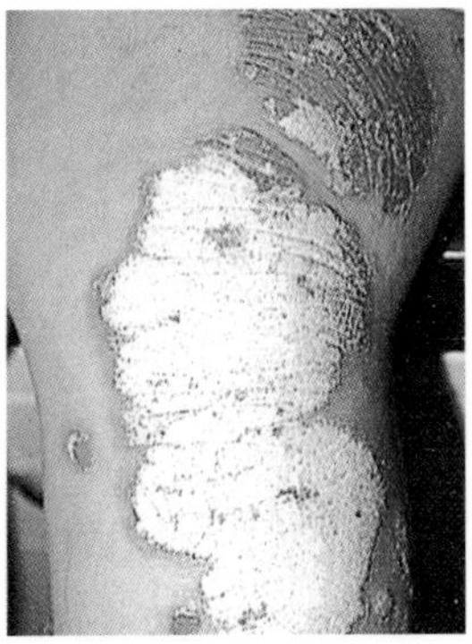

19A, B, and C Psoriasis is a scaling condition in which erythematous plaques (red raised areas) are covered by a thick adherent scale. The borders of the lesions are well developed and vary from guttate (very small drop-shaped plaques) to much larger plaques: (**A**) guttate, (**B**) medium-size plaques, (**C**) large plaques (see Chapter 34).

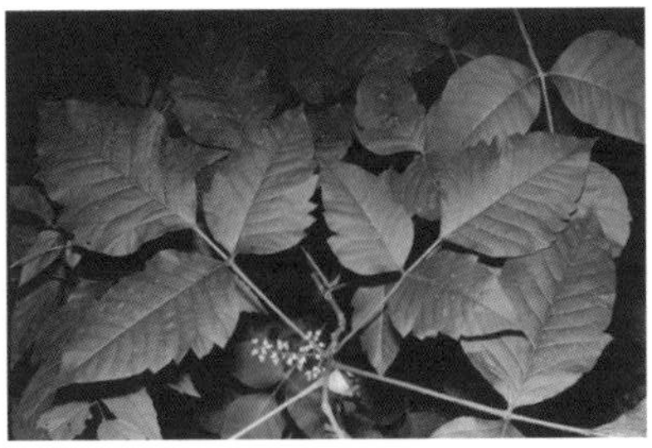
20A

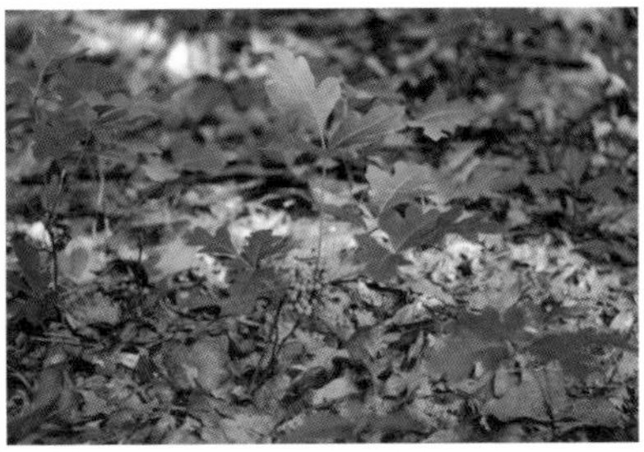
20B

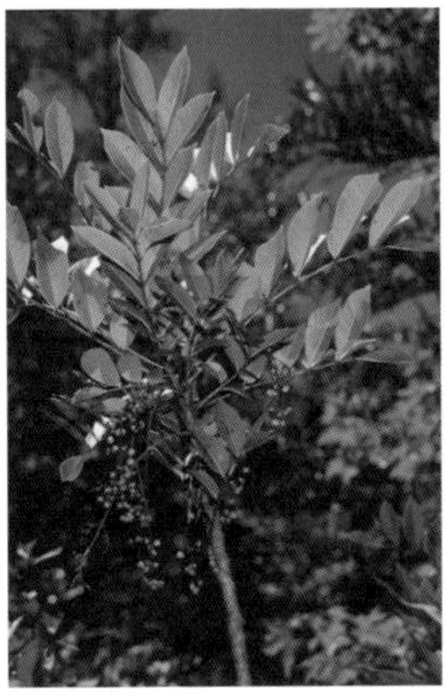
20C

20A, B, and C Poison ivy, oak, and sumac account for the majority of plant-induced allergic contact dermatitis. **A,** In the United States, poison ivy is the most common of the three plants. It usually grows as a scrambling shrub or a climbing hairy vine that often grows up poles, trees, and building walls. Its leaves are usually large, broad, and spoon-shaped. **B,** Two species of poison oak are indigenous to the United States; both possess leaves with unlobed edges that look similar to those of oak trees. Eastern poison oak (*Toxicodendron toxicarium*) commonly displays three leaflets, whereas Western poison oak (*Toxicodendron diversilobum*) has between 3 and 11 leaflets per stem. Poison oak usually grows as a shrub capable of reaching heights of 131 feet (40 meters). **C,** Poison sumac (*Toxicodendron vernix*) grows in remote areas of the eastern one third of the United States in peat bogs and swampy areas. It grows as a shrub or small tree and attains a height of about 9.8 feet (3 meters). Its pinnate leaves have smooth edges that come to a tip and may be almost 16 inches (40 cm) in length. The leaves are odd numbered, ranging between 7 and 13 leaflets (see Chapter 35). (Photographs courtesy of George Yatskievych, PhD, Missouri Botanical Garden, St. Louis, © 2000.)

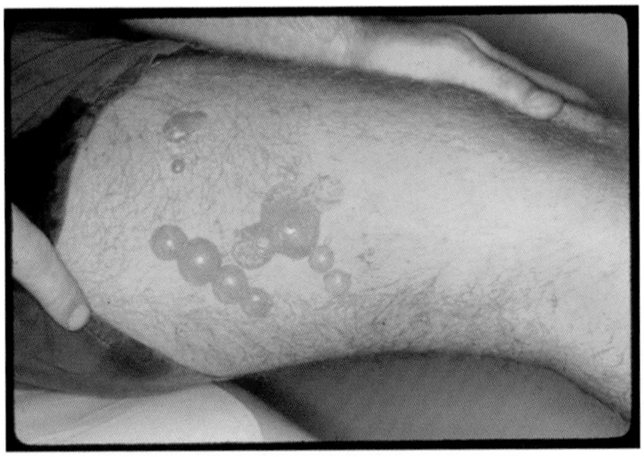
21A

21A, B, and C Poison ivy dermatitis is often associated with **(A)** fluid-filled vesicles (blisters) or bullae, depending on a person's sensitivity. **B,** Streaks of vesicles that correspond to the points of urushiol contact from the damaged plant are highly suggestive of poison ivy exposure. **C,** Oozing and weeping of the vesicular fluid occur for several days, until the affected area develops crusts and begins to dry. Similar reactions can also be caused by poison oak and poison sumac (see Chapter 35). (Photographs courtesy of Christopher Huerter, MD, Creighton University Medical Center, Omaha, Nebraska, © 2002.)

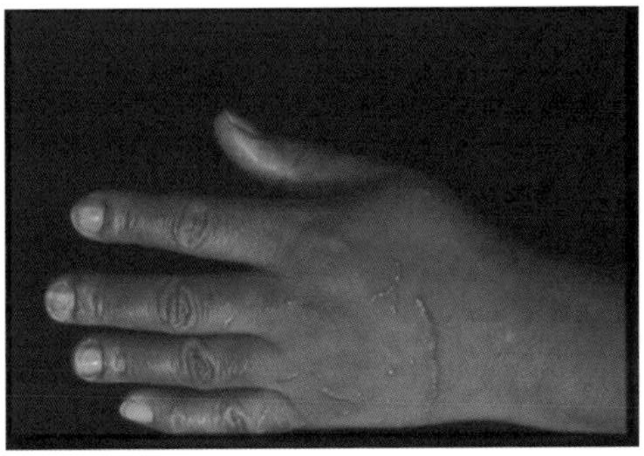
21B

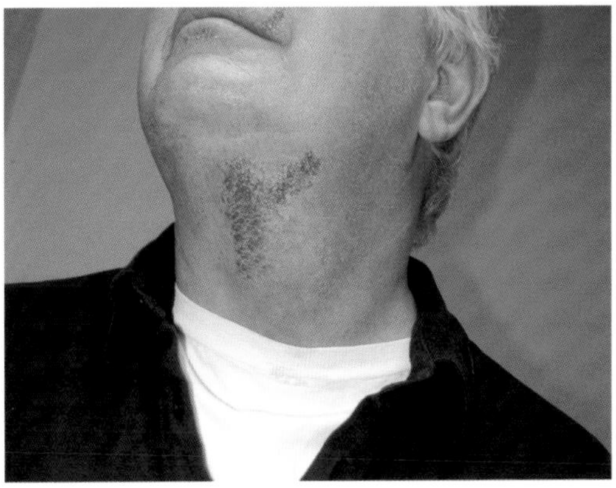
21C

22 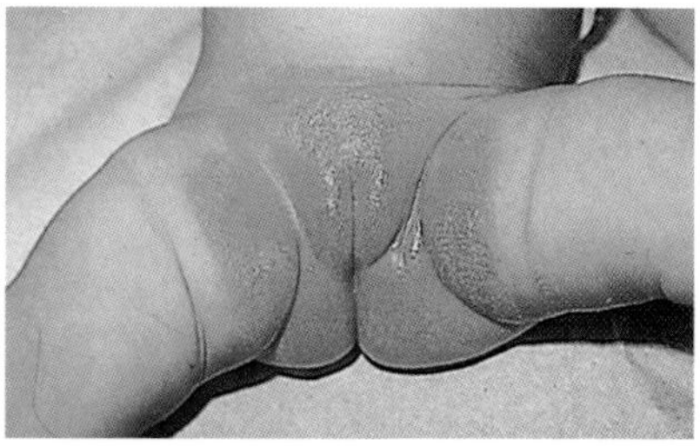

22 Diaper dermatitis presents as erythema of the groin (crease area around the genitals) and is common in infants. The case shown here was caused by a contact allergen. Contact irritants, such as urine and feces, and secondary bacterial and yeast infections may also cause problems in this area (see Chapter 36). (Photograph reprinted with permission from emedicine.com, Inc., © 2003.)

23 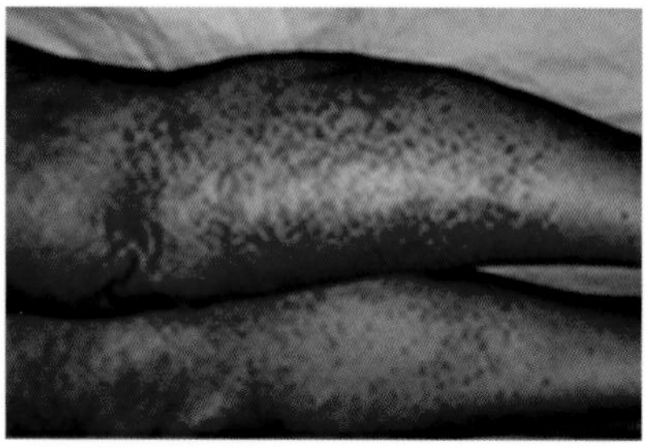

23 Miliaria rubra (heat rash) is an obstruction of sweat glands. Superficial involvement results in only tiny vesicles (blisters) appearing on the skin surface (miliaria crystallina). When deeper inflammation is present, the surrounding erythema is characteristic of miliaria rubra (see Chapter 36). (Photograph reprinted with permission from emedicine.com, Inc., © 2003.)

24 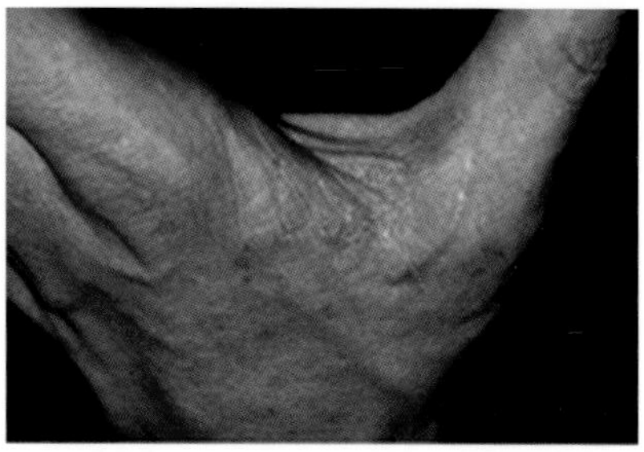

24 Scabies is caused by a small mite that burrows under the superficial skin layers. Small linear blisters that cause intense itching can be seen between the finger webs, on the inner wrists, in the axilla, around the areola (nipple) of the breast, and on the genitalia (see Chapter 37). (Photograph reprinted with permission from emedicine.com, Inc., © 2003.)

25 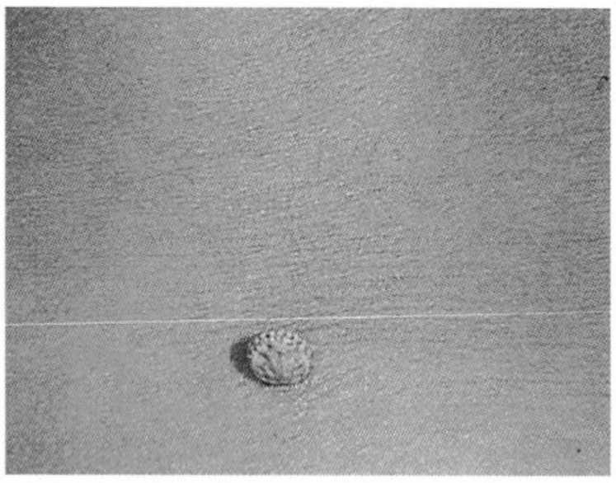

25 Ticks can attach to human skin and burrow into superficial skin layers. With careful examination, the back of the organism is usually visible on the skin surface. Ticks are vectors of several systemic diseases (see Chapter 37).

26A 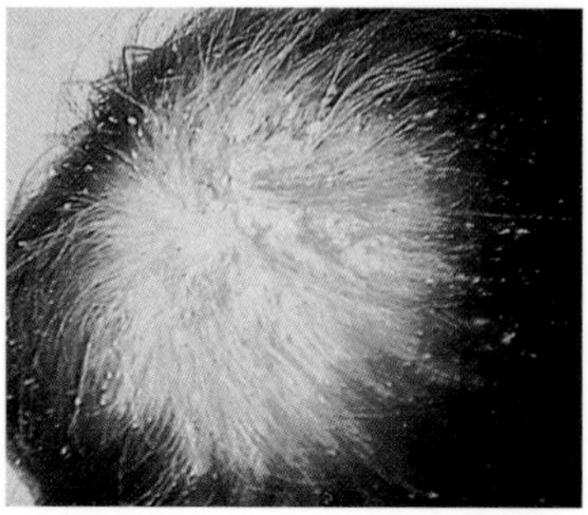

26B 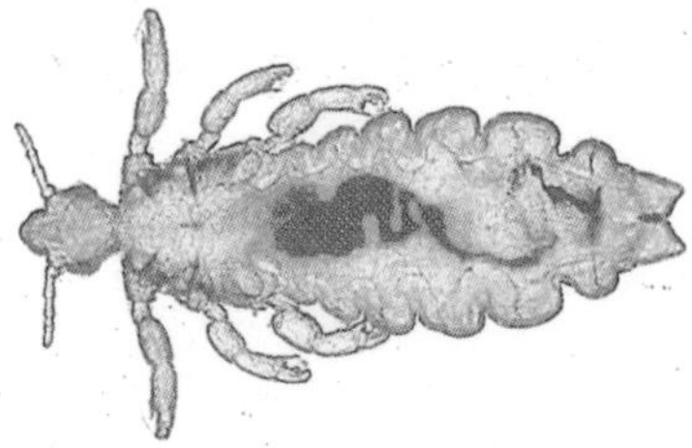

26A and B Pediculosis humanus capitis is a louse infestation of the scalp. **A,** Examination of the scalp hair in this infestation shows tiny nits (eggs) attached to the hair shaft. **B,** The organism shown is only occasionally seen (see Chapter 37).

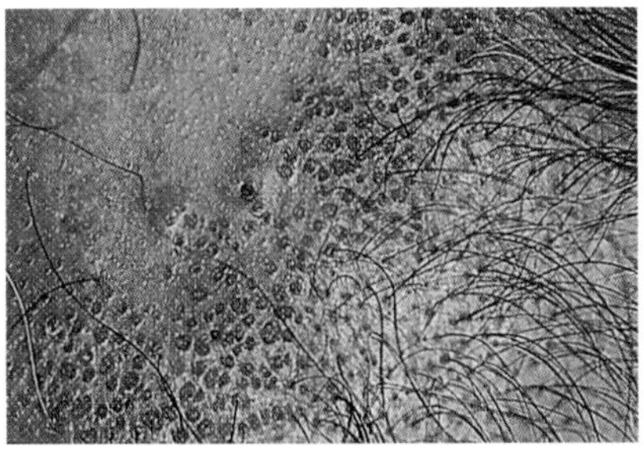

27

27 Comedonic acne (noninflammatory) occurs when follicles become plugged with sebum, forming a comedone on the surface. The black color is caused by oxidation of lipid and melanin, not dirt as is commonly believed (see Chapter 38).

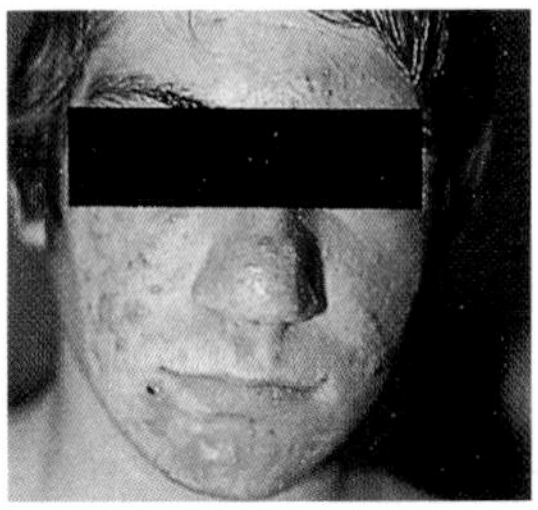

28

28 Pustular acne (inflammatory) presents as inflamed papules that are formed when superficial hair follicles become plugged and rupture at a deeper level. Superficial inflammation results in pustules; deep lesions cause large cysts to form with possible resultant scarring (see Chapter 38).

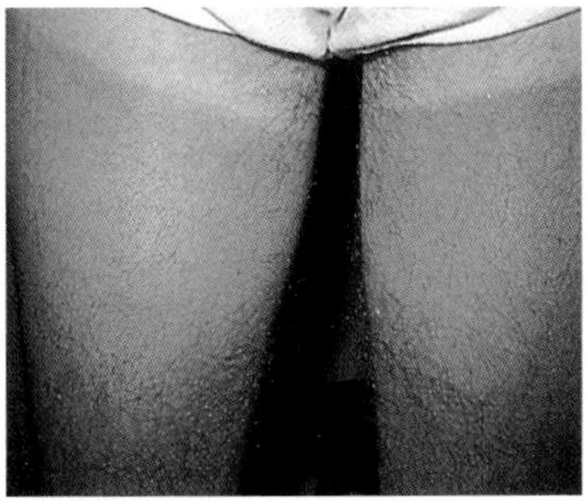

29

29 Sunburn presents as an erythema that occurs after excessive sun exposure; severe burns can result in large blister formation. Proper sunscreen application can provide photoprotection for susceptible patients (see Chapters 39 and 41).

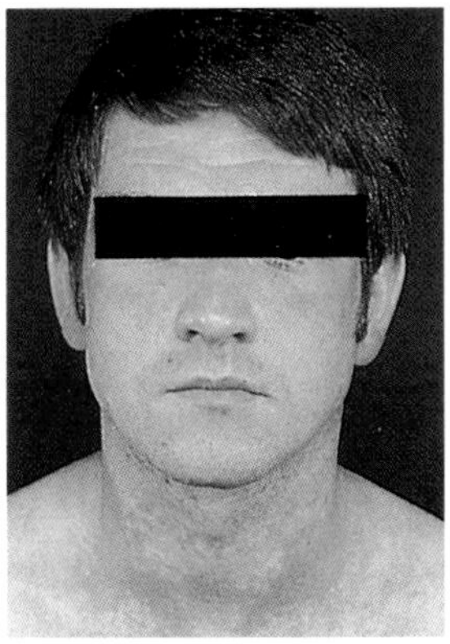

30

30 Drug-induced photosensitivity is a reaction that occurs on sun-exposed surfaces of the head, neck, and dorsum (back) of the hands. The erythema does not occur on photoprotected areas, such as under the nose and chin, behind the ears, and between the fingers (see Chapters 39 and 41).

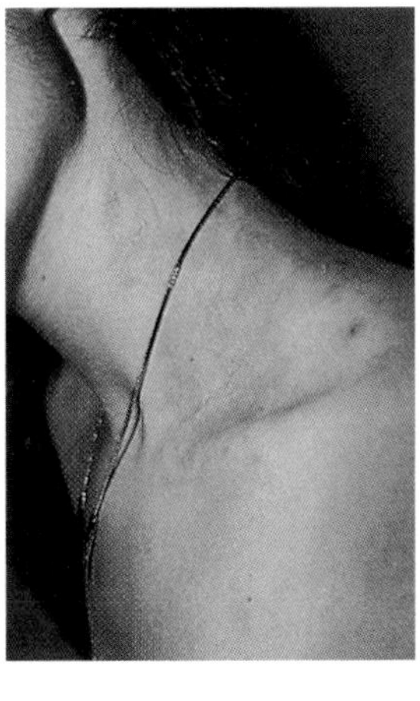

31

31 Cosmetic-induced photosensitivity can be caused by ingredients in certain topical colognes and perfumes. This reaction produces a local erythema that leaves characteristic postinflammatory pigmentation (see Chapters 39 and 41).

32 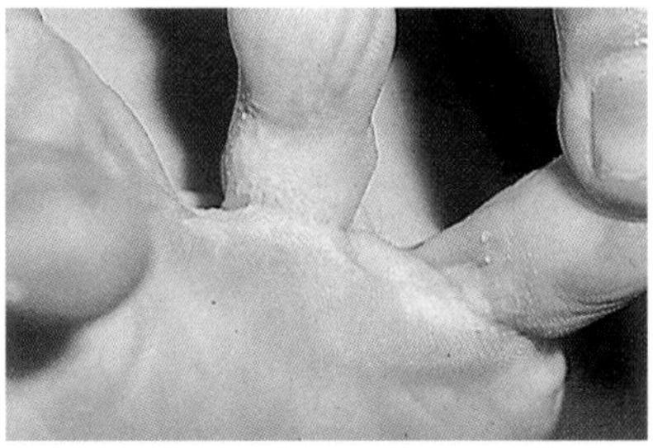

32 Tinea pedis infection of the toes characteristically starts between the fourth and fifth web space and spreads proximally. Scaling can progress to maceration with resultant small fissures (see Chapter 42).

33 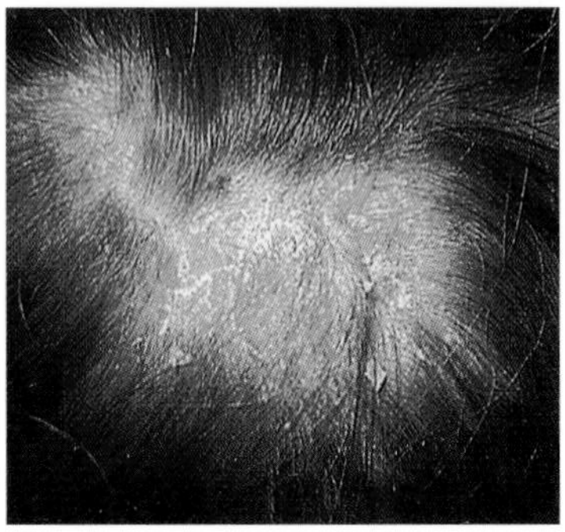

33 Tinea capitis, a fungal infection of the scalp, is marked by scale on the scalp with local breaking or loss of hair; erythema (redness) is usually not observed (see Chapter 42).

34 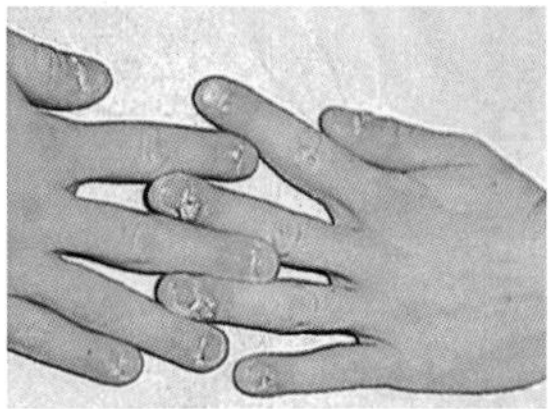

34 Common warts are viral-induced lesions that present as localized rough accumulations of keratin (hyperkeratosis) containing many tiny furrows. If the wart's surface is pared, small bleeding points can be seen (see Chapter 43).

35 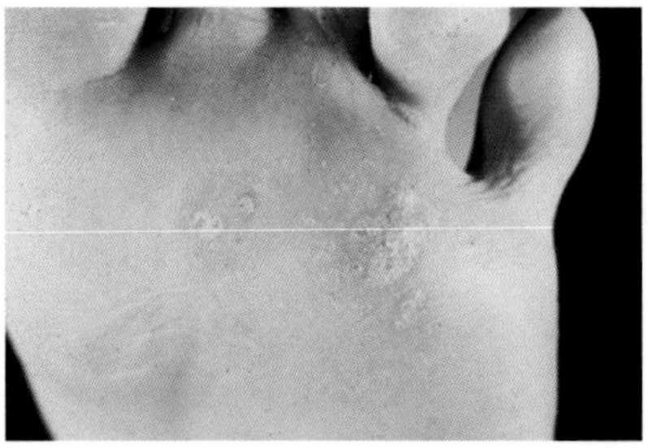

35 Plantar warts, caused by a viral infection, are often found on the plantar surface of the foot and present with hard, localized accumulations of keratin. The punctate bleeding points seen when the lesions are pared distinguish plantar warts from calluses (see Chapter 43). (Photograph reprinted with permission from emedicine.com, Inc., © 2003.)

36 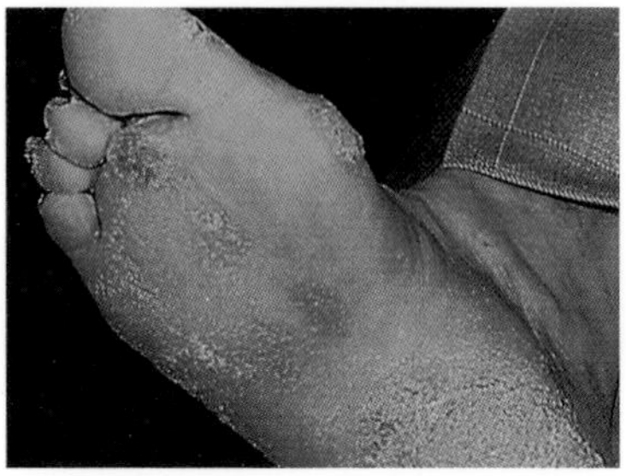

36 Calluses are thickened scales that often form on joints and weight-bearing areas. A callus on the plantar surface of the foot is shown here (see Chapter 44).

section

VII

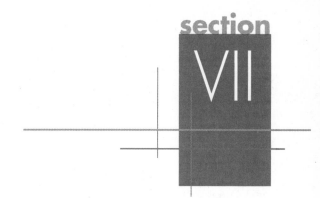

OPHTHALMIC, OTIC, AND ORAL DISORDERS

CHAPTER 28

OPHTHALMIC DISORDERS

RICHARD G. FISCELLA AND MICHAEL K. JENSEN

The nonprescription ophthalmic products market consists of preparations that treat a wide range of disorders. Limited population-based data are available on the epidemiology of these disorders. People with ocular conditions are commonly seen in the primary care provider's office, the hospital emergency department, the eye care practitioner's office, or the pharmacy. Ocular discomfort associated with dry eye disease may be the most common condition for which nonprescription ophthalmic products can be used. In the United States, dry eye disease may affect as many as 5 million people ages 50 years and older.[1–5]

Many common conditions that cause ocular discomfort are minor and self-limiting. In some instances, however, relatively minor symptoms may be associated with severe, potentially vision-threatening conditions. Health care providers should be well versed in eye anatomy and physiology (as well as in common ocular conditions and disorders) so that they can offer the best possible guidance for patients who want help choosing between self-treatment and professional medical care.

Self-treatable ophthalmic disorders primarily are those affecting the eyelids; a few disorders and conditions involving the eye surface, however, may also be responsive to self-treatment. The latter group includes dry eyes, allergic conjunctivitis, corneal edema of known etiology, presence of loose foreign debris, minor ocular irritation, and use of an artificial eye requiring cleaning and lubricating. *Careful assessment is important,* especially with current symptoms, to rule out more complicated disorders or conditions that may necessitate referral to an eye care specialist.

Role of Eye Anatomy in Ocular Drug Pharmacokinetics

The external location of the eye, with concomitant exposure of vulnerable tissues, makes it susceptible to environmental and microbiologic contamination. The eye has many natural defense mechanisms to protect it against contamination, however, and the eyelid is one of its major protective elements (Figure 28–1).

The *eyelids* consist of a multilayer tissue comprising an external skin covering and an internal thin, mucocutaneous epithelial layer called the palpebral conjunctiva. The middle layer of the eyelid contains glandular tissue and muscles for lid movement. This specialized glandular tissue, along with conjunctival goblet cells, secretes the bulk of nonstimulated tears.

The eyelids primarily protect the anterior surface of the eye and, through the blink reflex, spread the tears produced by the glandular tissue over the ocular surface. The lids force the flow of tears toward the nose and into the drainage canals located in the upper and lower eyelids that form what is known as the puncta. The drainage canals converge, forming the lacrimal sac between the inner eyelid and the nose. The lacrimal sac is drained by a canal opening just below the inferior turbinate of the nasal cavity. A highly vascularized epithelium lines the lacrimal drainage system, and absorption into the systemic circulation along this pathway is the means by which topically administered eye medications can produce systemic effects.[2,3,6]

The *tear layer* keeps the ocular surface lubricated, provides a mechanism for removing debris that touches the ocular surface, and has potent antimicrobial activity conferred by specific enzymes and a number of immunoglobulin proteins (including the most prevalent, immunoglobulin A). The tear layer is a complex, multilayer film. The outer, lipid layer maintains the optical properties of the eye and reduces evaporation. The middle, aqueous layer is largely responsible for the wetting properties of the tear film. The inner, mucinous layer allows the outer lipid and middle aqueous layers to maintain constant adhesion across the cornea and conjunctiva. Abnormalities within any one of the tear layers can result in ocular discomfort.

Tears are produced at a rate of 1–2 µL/minute, with a turnover of approximately 16% of the total volume each minute.[2,3] As much as 25% of the total tear volume is lost to evaporation.[2,3] An ambient tear volume of approximately 7–10 µL is found on the ocular surface at any given moment.[2,3] During episodes of ocular irritation, reflex tearing is stimulated by the lacrimal gland found underneath the outer portion of the upper eyelid, and tear production increases to greater than 300% of the nonstimulated production rate.[2,3] Reflex tearing occurs immediately on instillation of a drug into the eye, diluting the drug's concentration. Drug penetration into the eye is reduced because of this increase in tear production and lacrimal drainage, sufficient to release teardrops that fall down the cheek. Studies have shown that as much as 90% of an instilled dose of a drug administered to the eye may be lost.[2,3,6]

The visible external portion of the eye is composed of the normally white, noninnervated sclera, and the normally clear, innervated cornea. The *sclera* is a tough, collagenous layer that gives the eye rigidity and encases the internal eye structures. The visible sclera is covered by two epithelial layers: the episclera and the bulbar conjunctiva. The bulbar conjunctiva is contiguous with the palpebral conjunctiva at the junction between the eyelid and the ocular surface (the fornix). The episcleral and bulbar conjunctival layers (which contain the vascular and lymphatic systems of the anterior eye surface) are the affected tissues in eye redness from ocular irritation or inflammation.

The *cornea,* aspherical in contour, consists of vascular tissue that is the principal refractive element of the eye. The cornea is

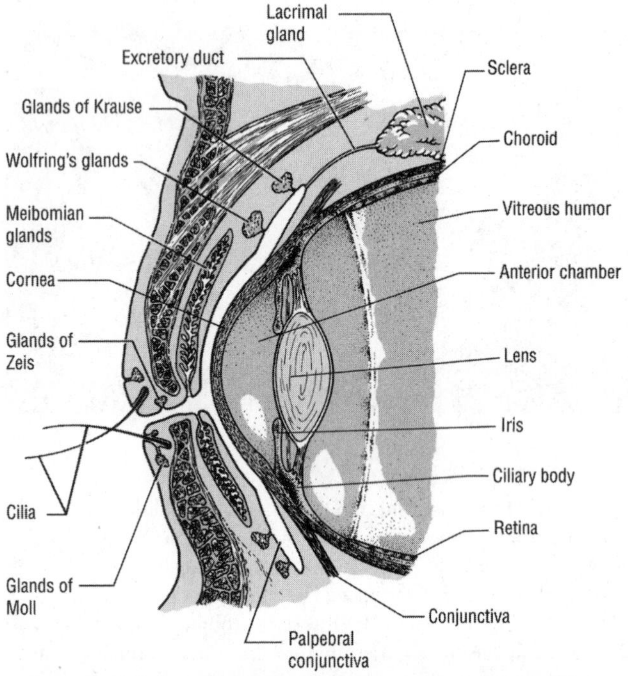

FIGURE **28-1** Anatomy of the eyelid and eye surface.

approximately 12 mm wide and 0.5 mm thick and comprises five distinct layers. The pharmacokinetics of ocularly administered drugs is mediated by three of these layers: the outermost epithelium layer, the middle and most abundant stromal layer, and the innermost endothelial layer. The corneal epithelium is lipophilic and facilitates the passage of fat-soluble drugs. However, if a drug is too lipophilic, it may become trapped in the corneal epithelium. This epithelial sequestering is often the rate-limiting step in absorption of medication into the anterior chamber. The corneal stroma is hydrophilic and allows the passage of water-soluble drugs.

Damage to the corneal epithelium may often increase drug absorption rates. Comparative studies with intact and compromised epithelium have shown that drug penetration into the aqueous humor may be increased as much as threefold in corneas with compromised epithelium.[7] Corneal epithelium can be compromised by trauma, routine contact lens wear, topical ocular anesthetics, preservatives, and thermal or ultraviolet (UV) light exposure.

Directly behind the cornea is the *anterior chamber,* a cavity filled with aqueous humor. The aqueous humor maintains the normal intraocular pressure (IOP) and provides nutritional support for the cornea and crystalline lens. The aqueous humor is produced by the ciliary body and is drained from the anterior chamber through the uveoscleral tract and the trabecular meshwork. The *trabecular meshwork,* which is located at the junction of the cornea and iris, accounts for approximately 80%–90% of aqueous drainage from the anterior chamber. The *uveoscleral tract* (located posterior to the iris and comprising the sclera, ciliary body, and choroid areas) accounts for approximately 10%–20% of aqueous drainage, although this percentage may vary with age and disease state.

During episodes of internal eye inflammation, inflammatory cells may block the drainage system, causing the IOP to rise. Increased IOP is one of the most significant risk factors for primary open-angle glaucoma. Similarly, during episodes of primary angle-closure glaucoma, the iris physically blocks the trabecular meshwork, which also results in an increase in IOP. Dilating the pupil with mydriatic drugs may precipitate an acute angle-closure attack. These attacks often occur as the pupil is returning to its normal state several hours after the mydriatic drug has been instilled. Any agent with anticholinergic or dilating effects has the potential to cause angle closure. The most common symptoms are blurred or hazy vision with halos around lights, brow ache, or headache, often accompanied by nausea and vomiting. These symptoms are severe enough to cause affected persons to visit their eye care providers.

The visible, colored portion of the eye, the *iris,* is located in the anterior segment of the eye, behind the cornea. It functions in much the same way as with an aperture on a camera by regulating the amount of light striking the retina. The central opening in the iris is the *pupil.* The pupillary diameter is controlled by two opposing muscles within the iris: the sphincter and the dilator. The sphincter muscle runs along circular arcs parallel to the pupillary border and exerts a miotic (closing) effect through parasympathetic stimulation. The dilator muscles are radial from the pupillary border and exert a mydriatic (opening) effect through sympathetic stimulation. Prostaglandins released by the iris during episodes of inflammation may affect the sphincter muscle, resulting in constriction of the pupil.

The *ciliary body* is bordered anteriorly by the iris and is continuous posteriorly with the choroid. In addition to producing aqueous humor, the ciliary body participates in focusing the optical apparatus (lens) for near viewing—a process known as accommodation. During episodes of ocular inflammation, the ciliary muscle may go into spasm, resulting in fluctuating vision and pain. Therefore, inhibition of the ciliary muscle (cycloplegia) with anticholinergic agents is a frequently used approach to treatment of internal ocular inflammation.

The *vitreous cavity,* located in the posterior segment of the eye, is the largest portion of the eye and is filled with vitreous humor. Floating spots in the visual field, or "floaters," have their origin here. Floaters are deposits of various shapes, sizes, and motility in the vitreous humor; they may be related to degenerative changes in gel that is normally transparent. Problems in this area are not amenable to self-treatment and require professional evaluation because of the possibility of concurrent retinal problems.

The *retina* is responsible for the initial processing and transmission of light signals. A number of inflammatory conditions of the retina can occur, and most are associated with prominent symptoms. Some, however, cause relatively mild symptoms, mimicking common irritative conditions. Trauma, even minor, may cause the retina to separate from its underlying layer (the pigment epithelium), resulting in retinal detachment. The retinal pigment epithelium provides vital "electrical" support to the retina. Macular degeneration, the leading cause of blindness in the United States, is directly related to atrophy in the pigment epithelium and choroidal neovascularization. Diabetic retinopathy and diabetic macular edema are also major causes of vision loss.

DRY EYE DISEASE

Pathophysiology and Clinical Presentation of Dry Eye

Dry eye disease is among the most common disorders affecting the anterior eye.[1] Most often associated with the aging process (especially in postmenopausal women), dry eye can also be the result of lid or corneal defects, loss of lid tissue turgor, Sjögren syndrome, Bell's palsy, thyroid disorder–related eye disease, various collagen diseases (e.g., rheumatoid arthritis), and some ocular and systemic medications.[7–13] Dry eye disease often is classified into mild, moderate, and severe categories (Table 28–1). Patients who have undergone refractive surgery may complain of transient dry eyes for weeks to months after the procedure. This effect usually is mild if it does occur, but it can be more pronounced in some patients. Drugs with anticholinergic properties (e.g., antihistamines, antidepressants), decongestants, diuretics, and beta blockers are some of the more common pharmacologic agents that may cause dry eye. The condition may be exacerbated by allergens or other environmental conditions (e.g., dry or dusty working situations), or by exposure to heating and air conditioning systems that reduce relative humidity, thereby increasing the evaporation of tears.

Dry eye disease is characterized by a normal-appearing white sclera or a mildly red eye, often associated with patient complaints of a sandy, gritty feeling or a sensation that something is in the eye. Contrary to what the name suggests, dry eye disease often may manifest with excessive tearing initially. Abnormalities in the tear layer cause less-than-optimal lubrication of the ocular surface, with subsequent inadequate tear production and initiation of a vicious circle. Without proper and timely diagnosis and treatment, dry eye disease can eventuate in severe damage to ocular tissues, particularly the corneal surface (see Color Plates, photograph 8). Evidence demonstrates that dry eye disease can be linked to a T cell–mediated inflammatory process, which can respond to treatment with immunomodulatory agents (e.g., cyclosporine).[8–11]

TABLE 28-1 Treatment Recommendations for Dry Eye Disease by Severity Level

Mild

Education, environmental modifications

Elimination of offending topical or systemic medications

Aqueous enhancement using artificial tear substitutes, gels/ointments

Eyelid therapy (warm compresses and eyelid hygiene)

Treatment of contributing ocular factors such as blepharitis or meibomianitis

Moderate

Same as for mild disease, plus the following:

Anti-inflammatory agents (topical cyclosporine and corticosteroids, systemic omega-3 fatty acid supplements)

Punctal plugs

Spectacle side shields and moisture chambers

Severe

Same as for mild–moderate disease, plus the following:

Systemic cholinergic agonists

Systemic anti-inflammatory agents

Mucolytic agents

Autologous serum tears

Contact lenses

Correction of eyelid abnormalities

Permanent punctal occlusion

Tarsorrhaphy

Source: Adapted from the American Academy of Ophthalmology Preferred Practice Guidelines, available at http://www.AAO.org.

Treatment of Dry Eye Disease

Treatment Goals

The goal in treating dry eye disease is to alleviate the dryness of the ocular surface, thereby relieving the symptoms of irritation and preventing possible corneal and noncorneal tissue damage. Although dry eye disease has also been referred to as "dysfunctional tear syndrome" and "keratoconjunctivitis sicca," a recent report of the International Dry Eye Workshop (DEWS) accepted *dry eye disease* as the most appropriate term.[1,9] The DEWS report, in conjunction with a Delphi panel paper and the recently published preferred practice patterns from the American Academy of Ophthalmology, has introduced a severity scale and an accompanying set of guidelines for treatment of dry eye disease.[9–11]

General Treatment Approach

The primary modality of self-treatment for dry eye disease is the use of ocular lubricants. With mild-moderate dry eye disease, however, treatment may also include other pharmacologic and nonpharmacologic recommendations, including patient education, environmental modifications, eyelid-specific therapies, elimination of offending topical or systemic medications, and use of systemic omega-3 fatty acid supplements (e.g., flaxseed oil) (Table 28–1). The availability of synthetic chemicals suitable for topical application to the eye led to the development of various solutions, so-called artificial tears, to help alleviate dryness of the ocular surface.

Artificial tear products vary by viscosity in accordance with the ingredients used in their preparation. Increasing the viscosity of a product results in a more prolonged ocular contact time and greater resistance to tear dilution. Mild cases of dry eye disease may show improvement with less viscous products, whereas more severe cases may require more viscous products. Bland (i.e., nonmedicated) ophthalmic ointments (e.g., petrolatum) or gels constitute another type of ocular lubricant. Because ointment preparations tend to cause blurred vision, they typically are reserved for use only at bedtime or for severe cases of dry eye. As with ointments, the more viscous the tear drops are, the greater their blurring effect becomes. Vitamin A preparations are also available for treating dry eye disease.

Nonpharmacologic measures (e.g., application of warm compresses, discontinuing any offending agents, maintaining good eyelid hygiene) may also increase eye comfort for patients with this disorder. Dietary supplementation with omega-3 oils or flaxseed oil in the normal doses recommended by the manufacturer is thought to improve lid function, possibly because the products have some anti-inflammatory properties.[9–11]

Eye care providers treat the most severe cases of dry eye disease with punctal plugs, which occlude the lacrimal drainage system to increase the available tear pool. New understanding of the underlying pathophysiology of dry eye disease suggests potential benefit from treatment with topical cyclosporine.[8,11] Whereas patients with mild dry eye disease may require relief of only ocular surface dryness, patients with moderate–severe disease may benefit from a combined approach incorporating immunomodulating agents (e.g., topical cyclosporine in conjunction with ocular surface lubrication). Accordingly, signs and symptoms suggestive of moderate-severe dry eye disease dictate referral to an eye care specialist.

Nonpharmacologic Therapy

The primary nondrug measure in self-care for dry eye disease is avoiding environments that increase evaporation of the tear film. If possible, patients should avoid dry or dusty places. Using humidifiers or repositioning workstations away from heating and air conditioning vents may help alleviate dry eye symptoms. In addition, avoiding prolonged use of computer screens and wearing eye protection (e.g., sunglasses, goggles) in windy, outdoor environments may further help alleviate dry eye problems.

Pharmacologic Therapy

Nonmedicated ointments are commonly used in treating minor ophthalmic disorders, including dry eye. Because ointments can cause blurred vision (resulting in severe vision limitations), combination therapy using artificial tears and nonmedicated ointments usually is recommended. Gels offer some clinical advantage in that they disturb vision less compared with ointments and are tolerated better by the patient. The effectiveness of retinol solutions for treating dry eye remains speculative.

Artificial Tear Solutions

Although many advances have been made in elucidating the mechanisms involved in tear film formation, the role of tears in maintaining a normal conjunctival and corneal surface is still not completely understood. Lubricants that are formulated as artificial tear solutions consist of preservatives, inorganic electrolytes to achieve tonicity and maintain pH, and water-soluble polymeric systems. The lubricating agents in artificial tear products are similar in palliative effect in that they all provide ocular lubrication, but buffering agents, preservatives, pH, and other formulation components may vary (Table 28–2). The newer artificial tear substitutes have important properties, including the ability to stabilize the tear film, protect the corneal and conjunctival cells, reduce tear evaporation with the combination of lipids, and enhance wound healing and lubrication of the ocular surface.[1–3]

One class of ophthalmic vehicles or ocular lubricants, in their commonly used ophthalmic formulation concentrations, is the substituted cellulose ethers, which include hydroxypropyl methylcellulose 0.3%–0.8% and carboxymethylcellulose (CMC) 0.5% and 1.0%. CMC 1% is often classified as a "gel" because of higher viscosity. These solutions are colorless and vary in viscosity depending on the grade and concentration of the cellulose ether. Polyvinyl alcohol (PVA) 1.4%, povidone 0.6%–2.0%, polyethylene glycol 400, propylene glycol 0.3%–0.6%, and glycerin 0.5%–1.0% are other vehicles commonly used as ocular lubricants.[14–21] Carbomer polymers (e.g., Carbopol 980) are often added as inactive ingredients but may contribute to increasing viscosity, providing the "gel" component of artificial tears (e.g., GenTeal Severe Dry Eye). Sodium hyaluronate is also classified as an inactive ingredient, although some researchers believe that it may promote healing of the corneal epithelium.[14]

Combining drugs with these vehicles increases overall viscosity, with consequent enhancement of the drugs' action. The increased viscosity retards drainage of the active ingredient from the eye, thereby increasing the retention time of the active drug and enhancing bioavailability at the external ocular tissues. These effects generally are not accompanied by irritation or toxicity to the ocular tissues. Similar to the cellulose ethers, PVA also enhances stability of the tear film without causing ocular irritation or toxicity.

Povidone has surface-active properties similar to those of cellulose ethers. This compound is believed to form a hydrophilic layer on the corneal surface, mimicking natural conjunctival mucin. This mucomimetic property has firmly established the role of povidone as an artificial tear formulation. Because this agent promotes wetting of the ocular surface, mucin- and aqueous-deficient dry eyes appear to benefit from its use.

An example of the most commonly recommended and newer products on the market is Refresh Optive Advanced Lubricant Eye Drops, which contains glycerin (0.9%), polysorbate 80 (0.5%), CMC 0.5%, boric acid, castor oil, erythritol, levocarnitine, and carbomer copolymer type A. This product is reported to be a lipid-based, triple-action preparation that helps lubricate and hydrate dry eyes and protects against evaporation of natural tears. Another product, Soothe, is an artificial tear solution that contains a lipid restorative layer, which provides a barrier to prevent loss of the aqueous component of the tears.

Many Systane products combine lubricants such as propylene glycol and/or polyethylene glycol with a gelling and polymer system. Hydroxypropyl guar binds to the hydrophobic corneal surface, forming a glycocalyx or gel-like environment that stays in contact with the ocular surface for a longer period of time. Systane is said to create an ocular shield, allowing epithelial repair that promotes patient comfort and relief of symptoms. Refresh Optive, a combination of CMC and glycerin, is believed to help protect the corneal epithelium through an osmotic protective effect.

Studies have shown that formulations of artificial tear products without preservatives are less likely than those with preservatives to irritate the ocular surface.[7,10,13] Providers and patients should be aware, however, that nonpreserved products should be discarded immediately after being opened and used. This precaution is needed because the remaining product in the opened container can become contaminated, potentially causing infection if applied to the ocular surface.

In most mild cases of dry eye disease, the patient instills drops of artificial tears once or twice a day, typically on arising in the morning and/or before retiring at night (Table 28–3).[11] A regimen of at least twice-daily drops is a good starting point. The viscosity of the drops and amount used can then be adjusted according to the patient's clinical response. For more severe cases, the dosage can be increased to 3–4 times daily. If the patient's clinical needs and response to therapy indicate the need for more frequent use, these solutions may be given as often as hourly. In many cases, use of artificial tears may be continued indefinitely, depending on patient response. Preservative-free products or those with less toxic preservatives (e.g., Purite [sodium perborate]) (see Ophthalmic Preservatives) are preferred in patients with moderate–severe dry eye disease or those who are sensitive to such agents.

Federal Drug Administration (FDA) has warned the public about eye drop bottles that have loose plastic safety seals or tamper-evident rings (i.e., collar or band), located below the bottle cap, that may fall onto the eye when the product is used. These devices are supposed to stay connected to the bottle neck. Some of these safety seals have dropped into consumers' eyes when the bottle was tilted or squeezed. These rings or seals should not be removed because of the potential to contaminate the tip of the dropper. FDA is in the process of identifying all relevant products and will require a revision to the packaging design that recommends a tamper-evident ring.[22]

Use of ocular lubricants requires balancing the number of instillations (i.e., drops) per day with the viscosity of the recommended solution and the presence of a preservative; as the daily dosage increases, toxicity from preservatives becomes more likely.[7,13,16]

TABLE 28-2 **Commonly Used Nonprescription Ophthalmic Lubricants**

Trade Name	Primary Ingredients
Artificial Tear Solutions	
Bion Tears[a]	Hydroxypropyl methylcellulose 0.3%, dextran 70 0.1%
Clear Eyes Contact Lens Relief Drops	Sorbic acid 0.25%, EDTA 0.1%, NaCl, hydroxypropyl methylcellulose, glycerin
GenTeal Lubricant Eye Drops, Mild and Mild to Moderate	Hydroxypropyl methylcellulose, boric acid, phosphonic acid, NaCl, sodium perborate
Moisture Eyes[b]	Propylene glycol 1%, glycerin 0.3%, BAK 0.01%
Murine Tears Lubricant	Povidone 0.6%, PVA 0.5%, BAK
Nature's Tears Eyemist	Hydroxypropyl methylcellulose 2906 0.4%, KCl, NaCl, sodium phosphate, BAK 0.01%, EDTA
Ocucoat Lubricating[b]	Hydroxypropyl methylcellulose 0.8%, dextran 70 0.1%, BAK 0.01%
Preservative-Free Moisture Eyes[a]	Propylene glycol 0.95%, boric acid, NaCl, KCl, sodium borate, EDTA
Refresh	PVA 1.4%, povidone 0.6%
Refresh Optive	CMC 0.5%, glycerin 0.9%, Purite[c], boric acid, calcium chloride, magnesium chloride, KCl, levocarnitine, erythritol
Refresh Optive Sensitive PF	CMC sodium 0.5%, glycerin 0.9%, boric acid, calcium chloride, erythritol, levocarnitine, magnesium chloride, KCl, water (purified), sodium borate, NaCl
Refresh Optive Sensitive PF Advanced	CMC sodium 0.5%, glycerin 1%, polysorbate 80, 0.5%, boric acid, castor oil, erythritol, levocarnitine, carbomer copolymer type A, purified water, Purite; may also contain hydrochloric acid, sodium hydroxide
Refresh Plus[a]	CMC sodium 0.5%
Refresh Tears	CMC sodium 0.5%, Purite[c]
Soothe	Restoryl (Drakeol-15 1.0% and Drakeol-35 4.5%), polysorbate 80 0.4%, octoxynol 40, NaCl, sodium phosphate, EDTA, polyhexamethylene biguanide preservative
Systane Lubricant Eye Drops	PEG-400 0.4%, propylene glycol 0.3%, boric acid, calcium chloride, hydroxypropyl guar, magnesium chloride, polyquaternium preservative, KCl, NaCl, zinc chloride, water
Tears Naturale Forte	Dextran 70 0.1%, hydroxypropyl methylcellulose 0.3%, glycerin 0.2%, polyquaternium 1 0.001%, NaCl, KCl, sodium borate
Tears Naturale Free[a]	Hydroxypropyl methylcellulose 0.3%, dextran 70 0.1%
Tears Naturale II	Hydroxypropyl methylcellulose 0.3%, dextran 70 0.1%, Polyquad 0.001%
Tears Plus	PVA 1.4%, povidone 0.6%, chlorobutanol 0.5%
TheraTears PF[a]	CMC 0.25%
Nonmedicated Ointments	
Refresh Lacri-Lube[a]	White petrolatum 57.3%, mineral oil 42.5%, lanolin alcohols
Refresh Lacri-Lube S.O.P.	White petrolatum 56.8%, mineral oil 42.5%, lanolin alcohols, chlorobutanol 0.5%
Bausch and Lomb Preservative Free Moisture Eyes PM	White petrolatum 80%, mineral oil 20%
Refresh P.M.[a]	White petrolatum 56.8%, mineral oil 41.5%, lanolin alcohols
Tears Renewed[a]	White petrolatum, light mineral oil
Nonmedicated Gels	
GenTeal Lubricant Eye Gel	Hydroxypropyl methylcellulose 0.3%, sodium perborate 0.028%, carbopol 980, phosphoric acid, sorbitol
TheraTears Gel	CMC 1%, KCl, sodium bicarbonate, NaCl, sodium phosphate

Key: BAK = Benzalkonium chloride; CMC = carboxymethylcellulose; EDTA = ethylenediaminetetraacetic acid; KCl = potassium chloride; NaCl = sodium chloride; PEG = polyethylene glycol; PVA = polyvinyl alcohol.

[a] Preservative-free product.

[b] Preservative-free formulation available.

[c] Stabilized oxychloro complex.

TABLE 28-3 **Administration Guidelines for Eyedrops**

1. If you have difficulty determining whether eyedrops have been successfully instilled into your eye, refrigerate the solution before administering it—the cold drops on the eye surface are easily detected. Do not refrigerate suspensions, however. Always check the expiration date.
2. Wash hands thoroughly. Wash areas of the face around the eyes. Contact lenses should be removed unless the product is designed specifically for use with contact lenses.
3. Tilt head back. When administering drops to children, have the patient lie down before placing drops in the eyes.
4. Gently grasp lower outer eyelid below lashes, and pull eyelid away from eye to create a pouch.
5. Place dropper over eye by looking directly at it, as shown in the drawing.

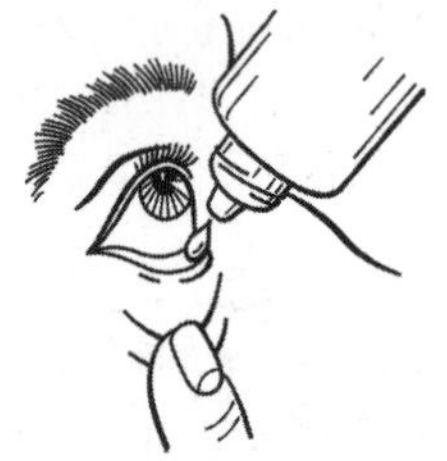

6. Just before applying a single drop, look up.
7. As soon as the drop is applied, release the eyelid slowly. Close eyes gently for 3 minutes and position the head downward as though looking at the floor (using gravity to pull the drop onto the cornea). Minimize blinking or squeezing of the eyelid.
8. Use a finger to put gentle pressure over the opening of the tear duct.
9. Blot excessive solution from around the eye.
10. If multiple medications are indicated, wait at least 5 minutes before instilling the next drop. This pause helps ensure that the first drop is not flushed away by the second and that the second drop is not diluted by the first.
11. If using a suspension, shake well before instilling. If using the suspension with another dosage form, place the suspension drop last, because it has prolonged retention time in the tear film.
12. If both drop and ointment therapy are indicated, instill the drops at least 10 minutes before the ointment so that the ointment does not present a barrier to the drops' penetration of the tear film or cornea.

Although PVA is compatible with many commonly used drugs and preservatives, certain compounds (e.g., sodium bicarbonate, sodium borate, the sulfates of sodium, potassium, zinc) can thicken or gel solutions containing PVA. For example, sodium borate is found in some extraocular irrigating solutions or irrigants and may react with contact lens wetting solutions that contain PVA.[17] Therefore, health care providers must be cautious when recommending solutions containing PVA.

Nonmedicated Ophthalmic Ointments

The primary ingredients in commercial nonprescription ophthalmic ointments (Table 28–2) are white petrolatum 60% (which contains a lubricant and an ointment base), mineral oil 40% (which helps the ointment melt at body temperature), and lanolin (which facilitates incorporation of water-soluble medications and also prevents evaporation).

The principal advantage of nonmedicated (bland) ointments is their longer retention time in the eye, which appears to enhance the integrity of the tear film. Therefore, mucin- and aqueous-deficient eyes can benefit from the application of lubricating ointments.

Ointment formulations usually are administered twice daily (Table 28–4). However, depending on the patient's clinical needs and therapeutic response, ointments may be administered as often as every few hours or only occasionally, as needed. Many patients prefer to instill the ointment at bedtime to keep the eyes moist during sleep and to help prevent morning symptoms of dry eye.

Because of the viscosity of the melted ointment base in the tear film, many patients complain of blurred vision with use of these products. This problem usually can be managed by decreasing the amount of ointment instilled or by administering the ointment at bedtime. Providers should routinely counsel patients about the blurred vision associated with eye ointments.

Ointment preparations generally are nonirritating, but preservatives can be toxic to ocular tissues. Some patients develop hypersensitivity reactions, which may prompt them to discontinue therapy. Changing to a single-use and/or preservative-free formulation (e.g., Systane Nighttime, Soothe Nighttime, Refresh PM) may eliminate symptoms associated with preservative-containing ointments. Preservative-free products are particularly helpful for use in long-term treatment. As a rule, pharmacists should recommend preservative-free, nonmedicated ointments for the treatment of dry eye to avoid the potential problems associated with preservatives.

TABLE 28-4 **Administration Guidelines for Eye Ointments**

1. Wash hands thoroughly. Wash areas of the face around the eyes.
2. If both drop and ointment therapy are indicated, instill the drops at least 10 minutes before the ointment so that the ointment does not present a barrier to the drops' penetration of the tear film or cornea.
3. Tilt head back.
4. Gently grasp lower outer eyelid below lashes, and pull eyelid away from eye, as shown in the drawing.

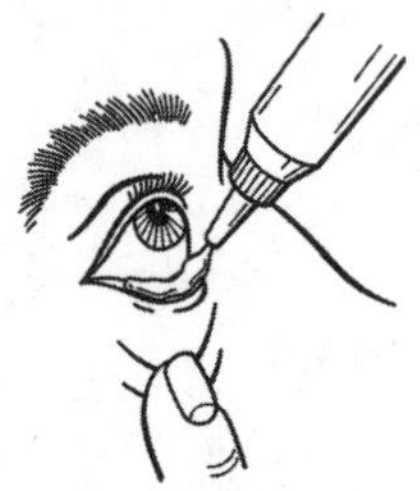

5. Place ointment tube over eye by looking directly at it.
6. With a sweeping motion, place a strip of ointment, one-fourth to one-half inch wide, inside the lower eyelid by gently squeezing the tube, but avoid touching the tube tip to any tissue surface.
7. Release the eyelid slowly.
8. Close eyes gently for 1–2 minutes.
9. Blot excessive ointment from around the eye.
10. Vision may be blurred temporarily. Avoid activities that require good visual ability until vision clears.

Formulation Considerations for Ocular Lubricants and Other Ophthalmic Products

Ocular lubricants and other nonprescription ophthalmic products are formulated to reduce the stinging, burning, and other adverse effects commonly associated with some conventional ophthalmic drugs. With these products, lack of (or minimal) ocular discomfort on instillation is a major advantage, deriving from carefully controlled pH and the presence of buffers, tonicity adjusters, and preservative systems; patients are therefore more likely to adhere to recommended self-treatment regimens. Drug vehicle and preservative systems are among the most important inactive ingredients of these products. Other commonly used vehicles are dextran 70, gelatin, glycerin, hydroxyethylcellulose, methylcellulose, polyethylene glycol, and propylene glycol. Various other ingredients often are included as excipients (i.e., agents to improve tolerability and solubility of artificial tears).

Ophthalmic Preservatives

Preservatives are incorporated into multidose ophthalmic products. These components are intended to destroy or limit the growth of microorganisms inadvertently introduced into the product. Surfactants, one of two distinct groups of preservatives, are usually bactericidal, meaning they disrupt the bacterial plasma membrane. Of the quaternary surfactants, benzalkonium chloride (BAK) and benzethonium chloride are preferred by many manufacturers because of their stability, excellent antimicrobial activity, and long shelf-lives. Unfortunately, these agents can have toxic effects on both the tear film and the corneal epithelium.[7,18,19] Long-term use of topical products containing BAK can lead to damage of conjunctival and corneal epithelial cells. Complications associated with BAK include allergy, fibrosis, dry eye disease, and increased risk of failure of glaucoma surgery.[7,20] Although only a small percentage of patients with dry eye disease experience BAK toxicity, this drawback may become quite problematic for those exhibiting symptoms. Polyquad, a high-molecular-weight quaternary compound, does not bind to contact lenses and may be less toxic than BAK.

Chlorhexidine is useful as an antimicrobial agent in the same range of concentrations as for BAK, yet it is used at lower concentrations in commercial ophthalmic formulations. Because it does not alter corneal permeability to the same extent as with BAK, chlorhexidine is not as toxic to the eye.

The second distinct group of preservatives includes the metals mercury and iodine, their derivatives, and alcohols. With the mercury-based preservatives, patients who become sensitized to thimerosal can develop contact blepharitis or conjunctivitis after several weeks of exposure and must discontinue the use of products that contain it. These products are rapidly disappearing from the marketplace.

Chlorobutanol is less effective than BAK as an antimicrobial preservative and, in fact, tends to break down in bottles during prolonged storage.[17,18] However, prolonged use of chlorobutanol does not appear to produce allergic reactions. This preservative often is used in 0.5% concentrations and has both antifungal and antibacterial properties.

Methylparaben and propylparaben, both *p*-hydroxybenzoic acid derivatives, have a long history of use in some ophthalmic medications (especially in artificial tears and nonmedicated ointments). However, these preservatives are unstable at high pH and can sometimes induce allergic reactions.

Ethylenediaminetetraacetic acid (EDTA) is a chelating agent that preferentially binds and sequesters divalent cations. EDTA assists the action of thimerosal, BAK, and other agents. EDTA can sometimes induce contact allergic reactions.[17,18]

Sodium perborate (e.g., GenAqua), which has been used extensively as a tooth-bleaching agent, has found a new use as an ophthalmic preservative. The first of two so-called disappearing preservatives, sodium perborate dissociates on contact with the eye to form hydrogen peroxide, which in turn rapidly dissociates to oxygen and water. The amount of hydrogen peroxide formed is so small that it does not produce eye irritation. The second disappearing preservative, a stabilized oxychloro complex (e.g., Purite, OcuPure), is also designed to dissociate on contact with the eye. After exposure to long-wavelength UV light, Purite breaks down quickly to water and sodium chloride. These disappearing preservatives have the advantage of microbial protection while potentially limiting preservative toxicity.

Other, less commonly used ophthalmic preservatives include cetylpyridinium chloride, phenylethyl alcohol, sodium propionate, and sorbic acid.

Ophthalmic Excipients

Other useful excipients are antioxidants, wetting agents, buffers, and tonicity adjusters. Antioxidants prevent or delay deterioration of products that are exposed to oxygen. Wetting agents reduce surface tension, allowing the drug solution to spread more easily over the ocular surface. Buffers are added to help maintain a pH range of 6.0–8.0, thereby preventing ocular discomfort on product instillation. Tonicity adjusters allow the medication to be isotonic with the physiologic tear film. Products in the sodium chloride equivalence range of 0.9%–1.2% are considered isotonic; use of these products helps limit ocular irritation and tissue damage. Solutions in the tonicity range of 0.6%–1.8% usually cause no discomfort when placed on the human eye. Hypertonic solutions used for corneal edema are not well tolerated.

Product Selection Guidelines

In recent years, artificial tear preparations have been introduced in preservative-free formulations and, more recently, in disappearing-preservative formulations. These preparations are beneficial for patients who are sensitive to preservatives such as BAK and thimerosal, those who use drops frequently, and those with compromised corneas. Products such as GenTeal (Mild to Moderate or Moderate to Severe), Refresh Optive, Refresh Tears, and lubricant gels such as Systane Lubricant Eye Gel and Tears Again Liquid Gel, are uniquely formulated to allow the preservative to rapidly dissociate into nontoxic components on the ocular surface. True preservative-free artificial tear preparations (e.g., Refresh Optive Advanced Preservative Free, Soothe Preservative Free, Blink Tears Preservative Free) are available in a variety of unit-dose dispensers. Some of these products are formulated to provide electrolyte support to the damaged surface epithelium of the eye. Preservative-free formulations not only are more expensive than preserved artificial tear solutions but are also easily contaminated by the patient during use. Therefore, patients must follow strict hygienic procedures for self-administration and should discard any unused product immediately after opening and using it.

Clinical results and patient acceptance remain the final criteria for determining a product's efficacy in the treatment of patients with dry eye. Of importance, no single formulation has yet been identified that will universally relieve clinical signs and symptoms while maintaining patient comfort and acceptance.[16,17]

If symptoms do not subside after 72 hours of treatment, the patient should be encouraged to seek professional assessment from an eye care provider.

ALLERGIC CONJUNCTIVITIS

Pathophysiology and Clinical Presentation of Allergic Conjunctivitis

The list of antigens that can cause ocular allergy is virtually endless, but the most common allergens include pollen, animal dander, and topical eye preparations. Patients with ocular allergy will often report seasonal allergic rhinitis, as well. Allergic conjunctivitis is characterized by a red eye with watery discharge (see Color Plates, photograph 9). The hallmark symptom of ocular allergy is *pruritus* (itching). Vision usually is not impaired but may be blurred because of excessive tearing. Contact lenses should not be used until the allergic symptoms resolve.[23]

Treatment of Allergic Conjunctivitis

Treatment Goals

The goals in treating allergic conjunctivitis are (1) to remove or avoid the allergen, (2) to limit or reduce the severity of the allergic reaction, (3) to provide symptomatic relief, and (4) to protect the ocular surface.[23]

General Treatment Approach

Questioning the patient about exposure to allergens may help identify the offending substance. Removal or avoidance of the responsible allergen is the best treatment, but nonprescription ocular lubricants, ocular decongestants, ocular decongestant/antihistamine preparations, ocular antihistamines/mast cell stabilizers, oral antihistamines, and cold compresses will help relieve symptoms.[24–28]

Nonpharmacologic Therapy

In addition to removing and/or avoiding exposure to the offending allergen, applying cold compresses to the eyes 3–4 times per day will help reduce redness and itching. Other important measures for avoiding the allergic response include checking the pollen count, keeping doors and windows closed, running air conditioning, using air filters, and so on. If eyes are itchy, cool compresses often help relieve some symptoms.[24,29] Sunglasses will provide shielding from the wind and allergens for many patients if used while outside.

Pharmacologic Therapy

The first-line treatment of allergic conjunctivitis is to instill artificial tears as needed (see Treatment of Dry Eye). Artificial tears may help to wash out the allergens and provide some symptom relief.[23,24] If symptoms persist, the patient should switch to an ophthalmic antihistamine/mast cell stabilizer product. The reclassification of a product from prescription to nonprescription status has been a very favorable improvement for the treatment of allergic conjunctivitis. Ketotifen fumarate 0.025% (e.g., Zaditor, Alaway) is very safe and can be used in individuals ages 3 years and older; it is dosed twice daily and is very effective in relieving the signs and symptoms of allergic conjunctivitis. Although a definite time period of treatment has not been well studied, these antihistamine/mast cell stabilizer products have been used for many years in patients, depending on symptoms. An oral antihistamine can be added to the second treatment option, if needed. Medical referral is indicated if symptoms do not resolve after 72 hours of appropriate treatment.

Other nonprescription ophthalmic products designated specifically for treatment of allergic conjunctivitis include decongestants (often in combination with antihistamines) and, more recently, the antihistamine/mast cell stabilizer combination. (See Chapter 11 for discussion of systemic nonprescription antihistamines and topical corticosteroids.)

Ophthalmic Decongestants/Alpha-Adrenergic Agonists

Four decongestants are available in nonprescription strength for topical application to the eye: phenylephrine, naphazoline, tetrahydrozoline, and oxymetazoline. Decongestants reduce ocular redness by acting as local vasoconstrictors. In nonprescription ophthalmic products, phenylephrine is available in a concentration of 0.12% or lower. Higher concentrations of phenylephrine (2.5% and 10%) are prescription products and are often used for pupillary dilation. Naphazoline, tetrahydrozoline, and oxymetazoline are chemically classified as imidazoles. As Table 28–5 shows, these agents are available as solutions in a variety of concentrations.

Phenylephrine acts primarily on alpha-adrenergic receptors of the ophthalmic vasculature to constrict conjunctival vessels, thereby reducing eye redness. Similar to phenylephrine, the imidazoles have greater alpha- than beta-receptor activity and are therefore clinically useful in constricting conjunctival blood vessels. These agents have only minimal effect on the underlying vessels of the episclera and sclera. Vasoconstrictors are effective in constricting conjunctival vessels, with consequent reduction in redness, vascular congestion, and eyelid edema, but they do not diminish the allergic response.[24–28,30] Table 28–6 lists dosages of ophthalmic decongestants.

When used as directed, ocular decongestants generally do not induce ocular or systemic adverse effects. However, presence of these products in households with young children and the use of such agents in this age group are risk factors that require patient education for prevention of adverse events. Ingestion of these products can result in coronary emergencies and death. When used excessively or for other than brief periods, ocular decongestants have the potential to produce rebound conjunctival hyperemia (i.e., rebound redness due to conjunctival congestion), allergic conjunctivitis, and allergic blepharitis.[25] Accordingly, they should not be used for more than 72 hours. Rebound congestion appears to be less likely with topical ocular use of naphazoline or tetrahydrozoline than with use of oxymetazoline or phenylephrine. Rebound congestion may be experienced within a few days of initiating treatment, and a case was reported within 8 hours of use.[25] Patients with apparent rebound congestion should be referred to an eye care provider for differential diagnosis and management.

Indiscriminate use of decongestants in an irritated eye can induce papillary dilation and may precipitate angle-closure glaucoma in eyes that have narrow anterior chamber angles. Use of these products in angle-closure glaucoma is contraindicated, and

TABLE 28-5 Commonly Used Nonprescription Ophthalmic Products Containing Decongestants, Antihistamines, and/or Astringents

Trade Name	Primary Ingredients
Decongestant Eyedrop Products	
All Clear	Naphazoline 0.012%, PEG 300 0.2%, BAK 0.01%, EDTA
Clear Eyes	Naphazoline HCl 0.012%, glycerin 0.2%, BAK
Clear Eyes Itchy Eye Relief	Naphazoline 0.012%, BAK, EDTA, zinc sulfate 0.25%, glycerin 0.2%
Murine Plus for Dry Eyes	Tetrahydrozoline HCl 0.05%, povidone 0.6%, PVA 0.5%, BAK
Naphcon	Naphazoline HCl 0.012%, BAK 0.01%
Opti-Clear	Tetrahydrozoline 0.05%, BAK 0.01%, boric acid, EDTA, sodium borate, NaCl
Tetrasine Extra	Tetrahydrozoline 0.05%, PEG 400 1.0%, EDTA, BAK
Visine Advanced Relief	Tetrahydrozoline HCl 0.05%, PEG 400 1.0%, povidone 1.0%, BAK 0.01%, dextran 70, 1.0%
Visine Original	Tetrahydrozoline HCl 0.05%, BAK 0.01%
Antihistamine/Mast Cell Stabilizer Eyedrop Products	
Zaditor, Alaway	Ketotifen 0.025%, BAK 0.01%, glycerol, sodium hydroxide and/or hydrochloric acid, purified water
Antihistamine/Decongestant Eyedrop Products	
Naphcon A	Pheniramine maleate 0.3%, naphazoline HCl 0.025%, BAK 0.01%
Opcon-A	Pheniramine maleate 0.315%, naphazoline HCl 0.02675%, hydroxypropyl methylcellulose 0.5%, BAK 0.01%
Visine-A	Pheniramine maleate 0.3%, naphazoline HCl 0.025%, BAK 0.01%
Decongestant/Astringent Eyedrop Products	
Clear Eyes ACR	Naphazoline HCl 0.012%, zinc sulfate 0.25%, glycerin 0.2%, BAK
Zincfrin	Phenylephrine HCl 0.12%, zinc sulfate 0.25%, BAK 0.01%

Key: BAK = Benzalkonium chloride; EDTA = ethylenediaminetetraacetic acid; NaCl = sodium chloride; PEG = polyethylene glycol; PVA = polyvinyl alcohol.

[a] Preservative-free formulation.

TABLE 28-6 Dosage Guidelines for Nonprescription Ophthalmic Decongestants and Antihistamines

Agent	Nonprescription Concentration (%)	Dosage	Duration of Action (hours)	Duration of Use
Decongestant Products[a]				
Phenylephrine	0.12	1–2 drops up to 4 times/day	0.5–1.5	72 hours
Naphazoline	0.1, 0.12, 0.02, 0.03	1–2 drops up to 4 times/day	3–4	72 hours
Oxymetazoline	0.025	1–2 drops every 6 hours	4–6	72 hours
Tetrahydrozoline	0.05	1–2 drops every 4 hours	1–4	72 hours
Antihistamine/Mast Cell Stabilizer[b]				
Ketotifen	0.025	1 drop every 8–12 hours	8–12	>72 hours
Decongestant/Antihistamine Products[a]				
Naphazoline/pheniramine	0.025 (naphazoline) 0.3 (pheniramine)	1–2 drops 3–4 times/day	3–4	72 hours
Naphazoline/antazoline	0.05 (naphazoline) 0.5 (antazoline)	1–2 drops 3–4 times/day		72 hours

[a] U.S. Food and Drug Administration. Ophthalmic drug products for over-the-counter human use: final monograph. *Fed Regist.* 1958;53(43):7076–92.

[b] Zaditor [product insert]. Novartis Pharmaceuticals Corporation, East Hanover, NJ.

providers should counsel patients with angle-closure glaucoma against using these products in treating allergic conjunctivitis.

Some patients may experience epithelial xerosis (abnormal dryness) from prolonged topical instillation of ocular decongestants, which may exacerbate the symptoms of irritation, pain, and dryness associated with allergic conjunctivitis.

Ocular decongestants should be used cautiously by patients with systemic hypertension, arteriosclerosis, other cardiovascular diseases, or diabetes. Adverse cardiovascular events are also possible when these agents are used in patients with hyperthyroidism.[26] Because of these possible adverse reactions, patients should not use phenylephrine and other ocular decongestants as ocular irrigants. During pregnancy, women should use ocular decongestants sparingly, if at all. Use of solutions that have been stored at high temperatures may cause ocular reactions and severe mydriatic responses on instillation. In such cases, if signs or symptoms do not resolve within 72 hours, the patient should see an eye care provider.

Ophthalmic Antihistamines and Ophthalmologic Antihistamines/Mast Cell Stabilizers

Two nonprescription antihistamines are available for topical ophthalmic use: pheniramine maleate and antazoline phosphate. Although these antihistamines are effective alone, nonprescription products containing them also contain a decongestant. The two combinations are pheniramine/naphazoline and antazoline/naphazoline (Table 28–5).

Pheniramine and antazoline are in different antihistamine classes, but both act as specific histamine-1 receptor antagonists.[27] Topical antihistamines are used for rapid relief of symptoms associated with seasonal or atopic conjunctivitis. Using a decongestant with either of these topical antihistamines has receptor been shown to be more effective than using either agent alone.[28–30]

Ketotifen fumarate is a combination ophthalmic antihistamine/mast cell stabilizer. It has very potent H-1 receptor-antagonist activity, thereby preventing acute histamine-mediated allergy symptoms. The mast cell stabilization activity inhibits mast cell degranulation, preventing the release of inflammatory mediators, including histamine. Ketotifen also inhibits eosinophils, which in turn inhibits the release of late-phase mediators. Ketotifen provides relief within minutes, its effects may last up to 12 hours from a single dose, and it does not contain a vasoconstrictor.[24,28] It is therefore a very safe product, raising no concerns for vasoconstrictor overuse.

Table 28–6 provides dosages of the antihistamine combination products. Burning, stinging, and discomfort on instillation are the most common side effects of ophthalmic antihistamines.[24,28,30]

Ophthalmic antihistamines have anticholinergic properties and may cause pupillary dilation. This effect is seen most commonly in people with light-colored irises or compromised corneas (e.g., contact lens wearers).[27] In susceptible patients, pupillary dilation can lead to angle-closure glaucoma. Therefore, these drugs are contraindicated in people with a known risk for angle-closure glaucoma.[27] Sensitivity to any of the components is another contraindication.

Product Selection Guidelines

After artificial tear solutions, ketotifen is the second safest and most effective product for the treatment of allergic conjunctivitis. Introduction of this agent in 2006 represents the greatest improvement in the nonprescription treatment of allergic eye disease in many years. The twice-daily dosing and the safety of this product for children ages 3 years and older make it the primary therapeutic agent for self-treatment of signs and symptoms of allergic conjunctivitis.

Although product-to-product comparisons are available for decongestant and antihistamine ophthalmic products, reaching definitive conclusions regarding clinical comparisons of the available nonprescription ocular decongestants is difficult. Naphazoline 0.02%, however, is an excellent choice for nonprescription therapy of mild-moderate conjunctivitis of environmental, viral, or noninfectious origin, because it can be soothing, reduces redness, and does not mask signs of infection if used for 72 hours or less.[24,27,28,30]

Because rebound congestion appears to be less likely after topical ocular use of naphazoline or tetrahydrozoline, these agents should generally be recommended over phenylephrine or oxymetazoline.

Complementary Therapies

The homeopathic product known as Similasan Eye Drops #2 is indicated for relief from itching and burning caused by allergic reactions. The active homeopathic ingredients are Apis, Euphrasia, and Sabadilla. The efficacy of this formulation has not been established in controlled clinical trials.

CORNEAL EDEMA

Pathophysiology and Clinical Presentation of Corneal Edema

Corneal edema may occur from a variety of conditions, including overwear of contact lenses, surgical damage to the cornea, and inherited corneal dystrophies. The edematous area of the cornea often is confined to the epithelium. Because the accumulated fluid distorts the optical properties of the cornea, subjective perception of halos or starbursts around lights (with or without reduced vision) is a hallmark symptom of corneal edema. An eye care provider must diagnose this disorder before self-treatment is attempted.

Treatment of Corneal Edema

Treatment Goals

The goal in treating corneal edema is to draw fluid from the cornea, thereby relieving the associated symptoms.

General Treatment Approach

Once the initial diagnosis is established, patients can use topical hyperosmotic formulations to treat corneal edema. Of the topical ophthalmic hyperosmotic agents available, only sodium chloride can be obtained without a prescription in both solution and ointment formulations (Table 28–7). Sodium chloride is available as a 2% or 5% solution and as a 5% ointment. First-line treatment is instillation of a 2% solution 4 times per day. If symptoms persist for more than 1–2 weeks, nighttime use of a 5% hyperosmotic ointment should be added to the regimen.[31] If symptoms do not abate after 1–2 weeks of the augmented treatments, the patient should switch to a 5% hyperosmotic solution and continue nighttime use of the ointment. If symptoms still persist without relief after another 1–2 weeks, medical referral is necessary.[31]

TABLE 28–7 Commonly Used Miscellaneous Nonprescription Ophthalmic Products

Trade Name	Primary Ingredients
Hyperosmotics	
AK-NaCl Ointment[a]	NaCl 5%, lanolin oil, mineral oil, white petrolatum
Muro 128 Solution 2%	NaCl 2%, hydroxypropyl methylcellulose 2906, methylparaben 0.046%, propylparaben 0.02%, propylene glycol, boric acid
Muro 128 Solution 5%	NaCl 5%, boric acid, hydroxypropyl methylcellulose 2910, propylene glycol, methylparaben 0.023%, propylparaben 0.01%
Muro 128 Ointment[a]	Mineral oil, white petrolatum, lanolin
Irrigant Solutions	
Bausch and Lomb Eye Wash	Sodium borate, boric acid, NaCl, sorbic acid 0.1%, EDTA 0.025%
Bausch and Lomb Eye Wash Eye Irrigating Solution	Boric acid, sodium borate, NaCl; preserved with benzalkonium chloride 0.01% in purified water
Collyrium for Fresh Eyes	Boric acid, sodium borate, BAK
Eye Stream	Sodium acetate 0.39%, sodium citrate 0.17%, sodium hydroxide and/or hydrochloric acid, BAK
Walgreens Sterile Soothing Eye Wash Eye Irrigating Solution	Boric acid, sodium borate, NaCl, hydrochloric acid, sodium hydroxide, edetate disodium (0.025%); preserved with asorbic acid in purified water
Prosthesis Lubricant/Cleaner	
Enuclene Solution	Tyloxapol 0.25%, hydroxypropyl methylcellulose 0.85%, BAK 0.02%
TheraTears SteriLid Eyelid Cleanser	Water, PEG-80, sorbitan laurate, sodium trideceth sulfate

Key: BAK = Benzalkonium chloride; EDTA = ethylenediamine tetraacetic acid; NaCl = sodium chloride; PEG = polyethylene glycol.
[a] Preservative-free formulation.

Pharmacologic Therapy

Hyperosmotics

Hyperosmotic agents increase the tonicity of the tear film, promoting movement of fluid from the cornea to the more highly osmotic tear film. Normal tear flow mechanisms then eliminate the excessive fluid. Many patients with mild–moderate corneal epithelial edema may experience subjective improvement in comfort and vision after appropriate use of these medications.

Usually, 1 or 2 drops of the solution are instilled every 3–4 hours (Table 28–3). The ointment formulation, however, requires less frequent instillation and is usually reserved for use at bedtime to minimize symptoms of blurred vision (Table 28–4). Because vision associated with corneal edema is often worse upon awakening, several instillations of the solution during the first few waking hours may be helpful.

In general, sodium chloride 5% in ointment form is the most effective product for reducing corneal edema and improving vision, but it tends to cause stinging and burning. For that reason, patients often prefer the 2% solution for long-term therapy. Hypertonic saline is nontoxic to the external ocular tissues, and allergic reactions are rare.[31]

The most important contraindication to the use of topical hyperosmotic sodium chloride is traumatic injury of the corneal epithelium. In such cases, this agent must not be given to treat associated corneal edema. The intact corneal epithelium permits only limited permeability to inorganic ions; therefore, an absent or compromised corneal epithelium will result in increased corneal penetration of the hyperosmotic product, reducing its osmotic effect.[31] If the history or physical appearance of the eye suggests a damaged corneal epithelium, the affected person should be referred to an eye care provider immediately. It is essential to warn patients against preparation of homemade saline solutions for use in the eye because of the associated risk of infection.

LOOSE FOREIGN SUBSTANCES IN THE EYE

Pathophysiology and Clinical Presentation of Loose Foreign Substances in the Eye

Despite the protective effect of the eyelids, foreign substances often contact the ocular surface. The immediate symptoms are pain and watering (tearing). If exposure to the substance causes only minor irritation, with no abrasion of the eye surface, self-treatment is appropriate.[32]

Treatment for Loose Foreign Substances in the Eye

Treatment Goals

The goal in treatment for loose foreign substances in the eye is to remove the irritant by irrigating the eye. If a known foreign substance is a fragment of wood or metal, prompt attention from an eye care provider is imperative because of the potential for penetrating injuries.

General Treatment Approach

If reflex tearing does not remove the foreign substance, the eye may need to be flushed. Lint, dust, and similar materials usually can be removed by rinsing the eye with sterile specific eyewash preparations (irrigants). Outside of a medical setting, loose particles can be washed away by flushing the eyes with copious amounts of water from a sink faucet or even a garden hose. If needed, nonmedicated ophthalmic petrolatum ointment can be applied at bedtime.[32] Ophthalmic petrolatum provides prolonged duration of protection, and the associated blurry vision does not pose a problem when the patient is sleeping.

Pharmacologic Therapy

Ocular Irrigants

An ocular irrigant is used to cleanse ocular tissues while maintaining their moisture; these solutions must be physiologically balanced with respect to pH and osmolality. Because the tissues that the irrigant contacts obtain nutrients (e.g., immunoglobulins, mucins) elsewhere, the role of irrigants is primarily to clear away unwanted materials or debris from the ocular surface. To reduce risk of contamination, patients should use ocular irrigants only on a short-term basis, and they should be alert to any further signs or symptoms that may point to other pathologic processes involving the eye. All ophthalmic irrigating solutions are available without a prescription (Table 28–7).

In the eye care provider's office, irrigating solutions come in handy after certain clinical procedures, and they are often used to wash away mucous or purulent exudates from the eye. They are also administered in the hospital setting to clean out eyes between changes of ocular dressings.

Ocular irrigants should not be used for open wounds in or near the eyes. Although irrigating solutions may be used to wash out the eyes after contact lens wear, they have no particular value as contact lens wetting, cleansing, or cushioning solutions.

If the patient experiences unremitting eye pain, changes in vision, or continued redness or irritation of the eye, or if the ocular condition persists or worsens, evaluation by an eye care provider should be strongly encouraged. Irrigants may be packaged with an eyecup; however, because contamination of the eyecup is possible, it should never be used by anyone to rinse the eye.

MINOR EYE IRRITATION

Pathophysiology and Clinical Presentation of Minor Eye Irritation

Nonallergic, minor eye irritation can be caused by a loose foreign substance in the eye, contact lens wear, or exposure of the eye to wind, sun (e.g., during snow skiing without protective eye goggles), smog, chemical fumes, or chlorine. Redness of the eye is a common sign of minor irritation. In cases of snow blindness (i.e., temporary overexposure to light from the reflection off the snow), other burns from UV light, or arc welder's burns, common additional symptoms include pain and the feeling of "sand in the eyes."

Treatment of Minor Eye Irritation

Minor irritation often responds well to artificial tear solutions or nonmedicated ointments (see Treatment of Dry Eye Disease).

Zinc sulfate, a mild astringent, may be recommended for temporary relief of minor ocular irritation. The dosage is 1–2 drops up to 4 times daily.

The homeopathic product known as Similasan Eye Drops #1 is marketed to relieve dryness and redness caused by smog, contact lens wear, and other factors. The active homeopathic ingredients are Belladonna, Euphrasia, and Mercurius sublimatus. Controlled clinical trials have not demonstrated the efficacy of this formulation in the treatment of dry eye disease. This product is not approved by the FDA.

CHEMICAL BURN

Pathophysiology and Clinical Presentation of Chemical Burn

Chemical burns may occur from exposure to alkalis (e.g., oven cleaners, cement, lye), acids (e.g., battery acid, vinegar), detergents, and various solvents and irritants (e.g., tear gas, Mace). Chemical burns range in degree from mild to severe, depending on the inciting agent and/or exposure time. Patients complain of pain, irritation, photophobia, and tearing. Signs will vary according to the severity of injury. With less severe chemical burn injury, clinical signs include superficial *punctate keratitis* (small pinpoint loss of epithelial cells in the cornea), perilimbal ischemia, chemosis, hyperemia, eyelid edema, hemorrhages, and concomitant first- or second-degree burns of the lid and outer skin. With more severe chemical burn injury, signs include corneal edema and opacification, anterior chamber inflammation, increased IOP, and retinal toxicity from scleral penetration. Alkali burns are more penetrating and potentially more damaging to eye tissues than acid burns. Alkali burns often are more resistant to irrigation and are associated with greater tissue destruction when they penetrate into the deeper (stromal) layers of the cornea. If the burns are more superficial and only several layers of the corneal epithelium have been affected, the cells should be replenished within approximately 24 hours.[32]

Emergency Treatment of Chemical Burn

Emergency treatment includes immediate copious irrigation with sterile ocular irrigants (Table 28–7), or with tap water if nothing else is available. Irrigation must be continued until an eye care specialist can be seen; if irrigation is stopped prematurely, residual material that may still be under the lid or in the inferior cul-de-sac may cause the pH of the tear film to revert to either acidic or alkaline.[32] Further treatment after irrigation may include the use of cycloplegic agents, topical antibiotics, and analgesics. In more severe cases, if significant inflammation of the anterior chamber or cornea is present, topical steroids may be prescribed. Antiglaucoma medications are also used if the IOP is elevated. Follow-up treatment by an eye care provider is required to prevent development of conjunctival adhesions and corneal complications. Chemical burns are considered ophthalmic emergencies, and patients with a history or clinical manifestations consistent with such injury should be referred to an eye care specialist or emergency department physician immediately.

ARTIFICIAL EYES

Besides the obvious aesthetic benefits, clearing dried mucus or fluid secretions from the surfaces of artificial eyes eliminates a potential medium for bacterial growth. A sterile, isotonic buffered solution containing tyloxapol 0.25% and BAK 0.02% is available especially for cleaning and lubricating ophthalmic prostheses. The primary method of preventing bacterial growth is routine hygiene with mild, nonallergenic soap and water.

Tyloxapol is a surfactant that softens solid matter on the prosthesis, and BAK aids tyloxapol in wetting the artificial eye. The solution is used in the same manner as for ordinary artificial tears. With the artificial eye in place, 1–2 drops of solution should be applied 3–4 times daily. In addition, the solution can be used as a cleanser to remove oil or mucus deposits; in this case, the artificial eye is removed and then rubbed between the fingers and thumb and rinsed with tap water before reinsertion.

CONTACT DERMATITIS

Pathophysiology and Clinical Presentation of Contact Dermatitis

Contact dermatitis of the eyelid can be a reaction to either an allergen or an irritant. Causes of contact dermatitis include a change in cosmetics or soap, exposure to eye medications, and contact with other foreign substances. The involvement of both eyelids suggests allergy, because both eyes are often exposed. Common clinical manifestations include swelling, scaling, or redness of the eyelid, along with profuse itching. Sunburn of the eyelids and UV burn to the cornea (e.g., with recent sun exposure from beach or ski outings without eye protection) should be ruled out.

Treatment of Contact Dermatitis

Questioning the patient about the use of eye medications or new personal care products (e.g., eyeliner, eye shadow) may help identify the offending substance quickly. Discontinuing use of the suspected product is the best treatment. If swelling of the eyelid is marked, nonprescription oral antihistamines (e.g., diphenhydramine) along with application of cold compresses 3–4 times per day will help reduce the inflammation and itching.

Assessment of Ophthalmic Disorders: A Case-Based Approach

For patients who have not seen an eye care provider, the pharmacist or the primary care provider must determine whether the ophthalmic disorder is self-treatable or requires medical referral. Great care must be taken in assessing a patient with a new-onset, acute problem. Ocular inflammation and irritation can be caused by many disorders and conditions, some of which can be treated safely and effectively with nonprescription ophthalmic products. These products are used primarily to relieve minor symptoms of burning, stinging, itching, and watering. FDA has suggested that self-treatment may be indicated for tear insufficiency, corneal edema, and external inflammation or irritation.

Cases 28–1 and 28–2 are examples of the assessment of two different patients presenting with ophthalmic disorders.

Table 28–8 describes the major features of disorders that require medical referral. Any self-treated condition that does not resolve within 72 hours necessitates referral to an eye care provider for further assessment.

Patient Counseling for Ophthalmic Disorders

Before counseling a patient with an ophthalmic disorder, the health care provider should carefully consider the nature and extent of ocular involvement. Patients with acute ocular disease must receive a prompt, definitive diagnosis (including baseline visual acuity) before the provider can consider the appropriateness of nonprescription therapy. Some acute conditions (which may or may not involve ocular pain or blurred vision) can be appropriately treated with nonprescription agents, but a recent diagnosis from an eye care provider can give additional reassurance and confidence in recommending such treatment. Although the cost-effectiveness of ophthalmic care can be greatly improved through the use of nonprescription agents, severe visual impairment—including blindness—can be a serious clinical and medicolegal complication if referral for definitive diagnosis and treatment is delayed. After careful consideration of the patient's history, the primary care provider should always counsel patients on the indications for and limitations of self-treatment. The algorithms in Figures 28–2 and 28–3 can assist providers in recommending the

CASE 28-1

Relevant Evaluation Criteria	Scenario/Model Outcome
Collect	
1. Gather essential information about the patient's symptoms and medical history, including	
a. Description of symptom(s) (i.e., nature, onset, duration, severity, associated symptoms)	Patient was recently diagnosed with seasonal allergies to tree pollen. Since then she has been using a nasal steroid for her symptoms. Her nasal symptoms have subsided. However, she says that she is still has itchy eyes.
b. Description of any factors that seem to precipitate, exacerbate, and/or relieve the patient's symptom(s)	Symptoms usually occur during the spring when trees start to bud. Her allergy specialist recently told her that she is especially allergic to maple trees. She has three mature maples at her residence.
c. Description of the patient's efforts to relieve the symptoms	Decongestant eyedrops marketed to "get the red out" do not appear to give her any relief from her ocular symptoms.
d. Patient's identity	Kalina Cooper
e. Patient's age, gender, height, and weight	36 years old, female, 5 ft 6 in., 125 lb
f. Patient's occupation	Real estate agent
g. Patient's dietary habits	Normal healthy diet with occasional social drinking; works out on treadmill 4 times weekly.
h. Patient's sleep habits	Sleep schedule varies according to how busy she is at work.
i. Concurrent medical conditions, prescription and nonprescription medications, and dietary supplements	Seasonal allergies (spring): fluticasone propionate 1–2 sprays in each nostril daily until tree pollen count is less than 2.5 grains/m^3; tetrahydrozoline eyedrops 3–4 times daily in both eyes.
j. Allergies	Seasonal allergies to trees
k. History of other adverse reactions to medications	None
l. Other (describe) _______	n/a
Assess	
2. Differentiate patient's signs/symptoms, and correctly identify the patient's primary problem(s).	Patient is experiencing ocular pruritus that is not being controlled by her current therapy.
3. Identify exclusions for self-treatment (Table 28–8 and Figure 28–2).	None
4. Formulate a comprehensive list of therapeutic alternatives for the primary problem to determine whether triage to a health care provider is required, and share this information with the patient or caregiver.	Options include (1) Refer Mrs. Cooper to an eye care provider (optometrist or ophthalmologist). (2) Suggest that Ms. Cooper discontinue her topical decongestant eyedrops and switch to ketotifen topical drops twice daily. (3) Take no action.
Plan	
5. Select an optimal therapeutic alternative to address the patient's problem, taking into account patient preferences.	The patient prefers to discontinue her decongestant drops and start the new ocular antihistamine.
6. Describe the recommended therapeutic approach to the patient or caregiver.	"Instill 1 drop of the ketotifen eyedrops twice daily in both eyes, as described in Table 28–3. Supplement throughout the day with the artificial tear product as much as you desire; however, wait at least 5 minutes after instilling the ketotifen eyedrops."
7. Explain to the patient or caregiver the rationale for selecting the recommended therapeutic approach from the considered therapeutic alternatives.	"You may not need to see an eye care provider if you follow the administration guidelines in Table 28–3."
Implement	
8. When recommending self-care with nonprescription medications and/or nondrug therapy, convey accurate information to the patient or caregiver.	
a. Appropriate dose and frequency of administration	See Table 28–6.
b. Maximum number of days the therapy should be employed	See Table 28–6.

CASE 28–1 *continued*

Relevant Evaluation Criteria	Scenario/Model Outcome
c. Product administration procedures	See Table 28–3.
d. Expected time to onset of relief	See Table 28–6.
e. Degree of relief that can be reasonably expected	"Complete symptom control should be possible. Some minor symptoms likely will appear from time to time."
f. Most common adverse effects	"Burning, stinging, and discomfort may occur on instillation of the drops."
g. Adverse effects that warrant medical intervention should they occur	"If the eye pain worsens and the redness continues, see your eye care provider."
h. Patient options in the event that condition worsens or persists	"An eye care provider should be consulted if the condition does not improve, or if irritation and pain become intolerable."
i. Product storage requirements	"Store under room temperature and away from heat and light. Observe product expiration date."
j. Specific nondrug measures	"Remove and/or avoid exposure to the offending allergen (e.g., check pollen count, keep doors and windows closed, run air conditioning, use air filters). In addition, apply cold compresses to the eyes 3–4 times a day to help reduce redness and itching."
Solicit follow-up questions from the patient or caregiver.	(1) "If my eyes still bother me, may I use the drops that I was using previously to get the red out?" (2) "Also, my spouse has tobramycin/dexamethasone eyedrops that he used previously, and they seemed to help him very quickly. May I try his eyedrops?"
Answer the patient's or caregiver's questions.	(1) "No. The 'get-the-red-out' eyedrops actually can cause more ocular redness (rebound hyperemia) and eye dryness." (2) "No. The tobramycin/dexamethasone drops (steroid and antibiotic) can cause significant eye complications, such as secondary infection, glaucoma, and cataract."
Follow-up: Monitor and Evaluate	
9. Assess patient outcome.	Inform the patient to feel free to contact you if she has any further questions.

Key: n/a = Not applicable.

CASE 28–2

Relevant Evaluation Criteria	Scenario/Model Outcome
Collect	
1. Gather essential information about the patient's symptoms and medical history, including	
a. Description of symptom(s) (i.e., nature, onset, duration, severity, associated symptoms)	The patient explains that he fell asleep this afternoon while sunbathing by a pool and burned the skin on his eyelids. His eyelids appear very swollen, with evidence of blistering. He is having trouble opening his eyes wide enough to see. He is also experiencing excessive tearing. The redness and pain subsided when he applied a wet cloth to his eyes, now but they seem to be getting worse. He would like assistance choosing a product that might help relieve his symptoms.
b. Description of any factors that seem to precipitate, exacerbate, and/or relieve the patient's symptom(s)	The patient mentions he experiences pain and excessive tearing when he tries to open his eyes enough to see.
c. Description of the patient's efforts to relieve the symptoms	He has taken 2 ibuprofen tablets for the pain, but they are not giving him much relief.

CASE 28-2 *continued*

Relevant Evaluation Criteria	Scenario/Model Outcome
d. Patient's identity	Mark Wastl
e. Patient's age, gender, height, and weight	20 years old, male, 6 ft 2 in., 195 lb
f. Patient's occupation	College student
g. Patient's dietary habits	Fast food for breakfast and lunch, healthy evening meal at his fraternity house
h. Patient's sleep habits	7 hours a night
i. Concurrent medical conditions, prescription and nonprescription medications, and dietary supplements	None; occasional upset stomach relieved by calcium carbonate
j. Allergies	None
k. History of other adverse reactions to medications	None
l. Other (describe) _______	Patient is an avid swimmer; swims 4 times per week.
Assess	
2. Differentiate patient's signs/symptoms, and correctly identify the patient's primary problem(s).	Mr. Wastl has a thermal burn of the eyelids and surrounding ocular tissue.
3. Identify exclusions for self-treatment.	See Table 28–8.
4. Formulate a comprehensive list of therapeutic alternatives for the primary problem to determine whether triage to a health care provider is required, and share this information with the patient or caregiver.	Options include (1) Take no action (2) Apply cold compresses as needed to control pain. (3) Seek medical care.
Plan	
5. Select an optimal therapeutic alternative to address the patient's problem, taking into account patient preferences.	Initially, Mr. Wastl did not want to see an eye care specialist; after being presented with a brief description of thermal burns, emphasizing that such burns could lead to complications such as scarring and infection, he said he would go right away.
6. Describe the recommended therapeutic approach to the patient or caregiver.	The patient needs to see an eye care specialist immediately. In the meantime, he should use cold compresses to alleviate the pain.
7. Explain to the patient or caregiver the rationale for selecting the recommended therapeutic approach from the considered therapeutic alternatives.	"Seeing an eye care provider is the best option. This practitioner can determine how much damage has been done and if additional treatment is required, and can also recommend a topical treatment for your eyelids."
Implement	
8. When recommending self-care with nonprescription medications and/or nondrug therapy, convey accurate information to the patient or caregiver.	Criterion does not apply in this case.
Solicit follow-up questions from the patient or caregiver.	"Is there anything I should do to prevent this in the future?"
Answer the patient's or caregiver's questions.	"In the future, wear sunglasses and avoid falling asleep during sun exposure."
Follow-up: Monitor and Evaluate	
9. Assess patient outcome.	Ask the patient to call office to report the results of the eye care provider's examination and treatment.

TABLE 28–8 Differentiation of Ophthalmic Disorders/Conditions That Necessitate Medical Referral

Disorder/ Condition	Potential Signs/Symptoms	Complications	Treatment Approach
Blunt trauma	Ruptured blood vessels, bleeding into eyelid tissue space, swelling, ocular discomfort, facial drooping	Internal eye bleeding, secondary glaucoma, detached retina, periorbital bone fracture (blowout fracture)	Medical referral is appropriate.
Foreign particles trapped/ embedded in the eye	Reddened eyes, profuse tearing, ocular discomfort	Corneal abrasions/scarring, chronic red eye, intraocular penetration from metal striking metal at high speeds	Medical referral for removal of particles is appropriate.
Ocular abrasions	Partial/total loss of corneal epithelium, blurred vision, profuse tearing, difficulty opening eye	Risk of bacterial/fungal infection with eye exposure to organic material, corneal scarring, anterior chamber rupture	Medical referral is appropriate.
Infections of eyelid/ eye surface	Red, thickened lids, scaling, ocular discharge and matting of the lashes	Scarring of lids, dry eye, corneal abrasion or scarring, loss of vision, hordeolum (stye), chalazion (risk of malignancy), and blepharitis (loss of lashes, corneal irritation)	Medical referral is appropriate.
Eye exposure to chemical splash, solid chemical, or chemical fumes	Reddened eyes, watering, difficulty opening eye	Scarring of eyelids and eye surface, loss of vision	To prevent/reduce scarring of eyelids from chemical burns, flush eye immediately for at least 10 minutes, preferably with sterile saline or water. If neither is available, flush with tap water. After flushing eye, arrange immediate transportation to an emergency facility. No recommendation is noted for chemical neutralization.
Thermal injury to eye (welder's arc)	Reddened eyes, pain, sensitivity to light	Corneal scarring, secondary infection	Medical referral for definitive care (including possible eye patching) is appropriate.
Bacterial conjunctivitis	Reddened eyes with purulent, colored (mucous) discharge, ocular discomfort, eyelids stuck together on awakening	Typically self-limited, with resolution in 2 weeks	Medical referral for treatment with topical antibiotics to clear infection more quickly is appropriate; some infections require systemic antibiotic treatment.
Viral conjunctivitis	Reddened eyes with watery, clear or white discharge, ocular discomfort, hyperemia, matting of the lashes	Typically self-limited, with resolution in 2 or 3 weeks	Medical provider will monitor for corneal involvement. Treatment with topical decongestants to provide comfort is appropriate; cold compresses can be applied.
Chlamydial conjunctivitis	Watery or white or yellow mucous discharge, ocular discomfort, low-grade fever, possible blurred vision	Scarring	If infection with *Chlamydia* spp. is known or suspected, or if symptoms are too vague to rule out viral or allergic conjunctivitis, medical referral is mandatory.

Source: Reference 32.

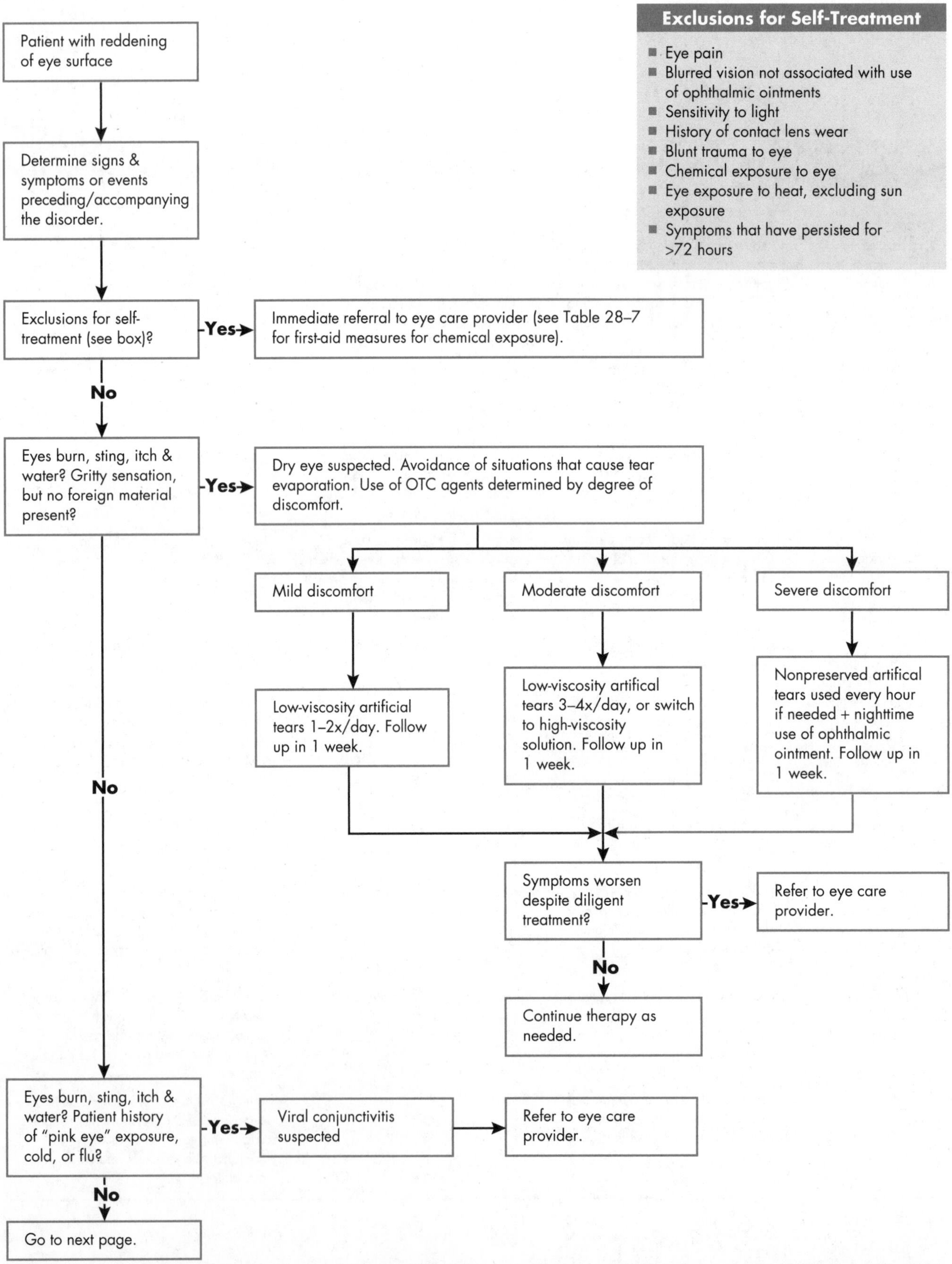

FIGURE 28–2 Self-care for eye surface disorders. Key: AH = Antihistamine; D/C = discontinue; MCS = mast cell stabilizer; OTC = over-the-counter.

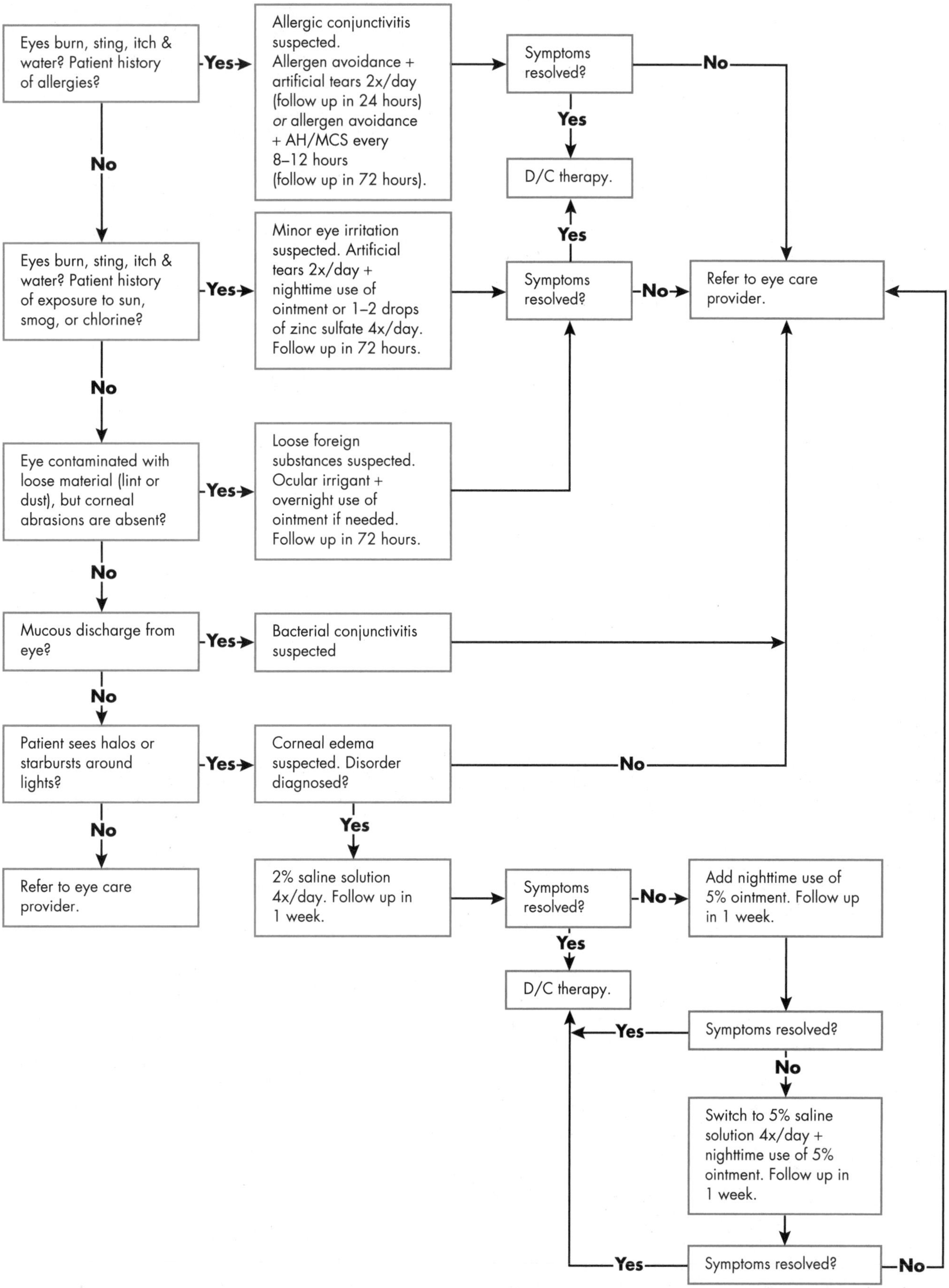

FIGURE 28–2 Self-care for eye surface disorders. Key: AH = Antihistamine; D/C = discontinue; MCS = mast cell stabilizer; OTC = over-the-counter. (*continued*)

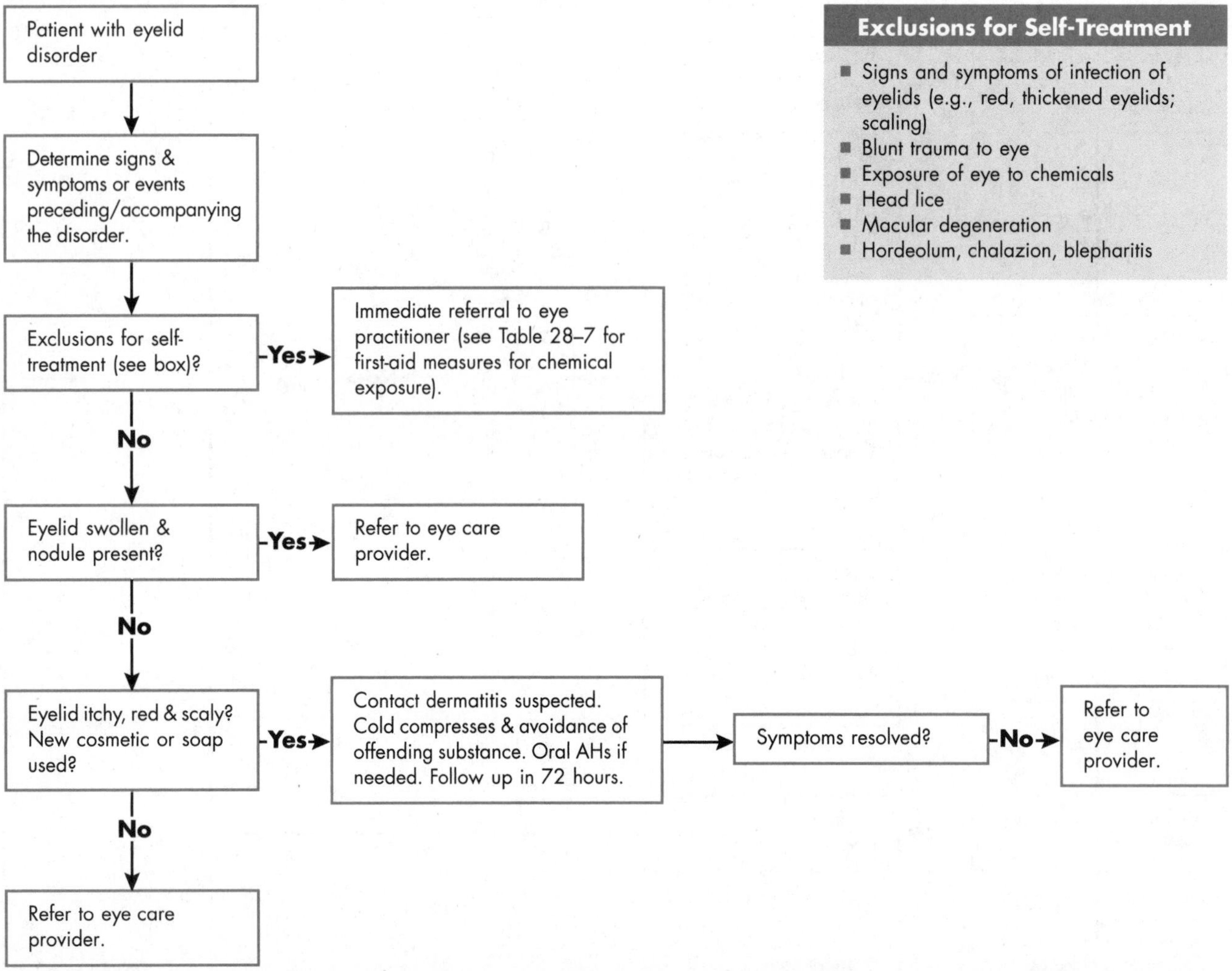

Exclusions for Self-Treatment

- Signs and symptoms of infection of eyelids (e.g., red, thickened eyelids; scaling)
- Blunt trauma to eye
- Exposure of eye to chemicals
- Head lice
- Macular degeneration
- Hordeolum, chalazion, blepharitis

FIGURE **28–3** Self-care for eyelid disorders. Key: AH = Antihistamine; D/C = discontinue.

appropriate measures for self-treatable disorders of the eye surface and eyelid, respectively.

Numerous nonprescription ophthalmic products for treating minor ocular irritations are available for self-administration by the patient with minimal or no supervision. These products are also adequate for treating certain clinical conditions diagnosed by primary care providers or eye care specialists. First-line therapy should always include counseling on nonpharmacologic treatment. These treatments alone frequently are sufficient to relieve the ocular symptoms or are necessary as an adjunct to the ophthalmic drug therapy.

Proper drug instillation technique is critical if the target tissue (the eye) is to receive the maximum benefit from the medication. Ophthalmic solutions and ointments are often used incorrectly. Carefully instructing patients in the proper self-administration procedures can help ensure maximum safety and effectiveness of these agents. Appropriate patient education and counseling must accompany dispensing of any ophthalmic product.

Although drug adverse effects and interactions are rare with topically applied ophthalmic products, the potential for such effects is well recognized. Accordingly, patients should be advised of the specific adverse effects, including the clinical signs of drug toxicity or allergy, associated with the products they are using.

The health care provider must actively assist patients in selecting the appropriate product, which will enhance compliance, minimize or avoid adverse effects, and reduce the attendant costs of therapy. The other major considerations in making therapeutic recommendations are whether the person has sensitivity to one of the product constituents, whether the product can be used with contact lenses, and whether the product has the potential to wash out prescription ophthalmic drugs the patient may be using. With the exception of ophthalmic antihistamines and decongestants, little product-to-product comparative research has been done for nonprescription ophthalmic preparations. Accordingly, therapy recommendations should be made on the basis of the patient's diagnosis and the products the patient is using. The box "Patient Education for Ophthalmic Disorders" lists specific information to provide in patient counseling.

Evaluation of Patient Outcomes for Ophthalmic Disorders

Patients who self-treat for allergic conjunctivitis, dry eyes, loose foreign substances in the eye, or minor eye irritation should see an eye care provider if symptoms persist after 72 hours of appropriate

PATIENT EDUCATION FOR Ophthalmic Disorders

The objectives of self-treatment are (1) to relieve the symptoms of minor ophthalmic disorders using appropriate nonprescription products or nondrug measures and (2) to use nonprescription products as directed for adjunctive treatment of ophthalmic disorders diagnosed by an eye care provider. For most patients, carefully following product instructions and the self-care measures listed here will help ensure optimal therapeutic outcomes.

- Remove the offending agent/irritant responsible for your ocular condition or disease.
- If *blunt trauma* to the eye occurs, visit an eye care specialist for further evaluation as soon as possible.
- If you have *dry eye disease* and the ophthalmic lubricants used for initial treatment are not effective, ask your eye care provider or pharmacist about the following treatment options: increasing the dosage, switching to a product with increased viscosity, and/or switching to a preservative-free product (Table 28–2).
- When treating *allergic conjunctivitis,* do not exceed the recommended dosages for ophthalmic antihistamine/mast cell stabilizer, decongestant, or antihistamine/decongestant products (Tables 28–5 and 28–6). Consult an eye care provider if symptoms persist after 72 hours of treatment.
- Discard or replace eyedrop bottles 30 days after the sterility safety seal is opened. The manufacturer's expiration date does not apply once the seal is broken.
- If *eye exposure to chemicals* occurs, irrigate the eye continuously for 10 minutes with copious amounts of water or an eye irrigant (Table 28–7) and seek immediate eye care.
- If *loose foreign substances* such as lint, dust, or pollen enter the eye, flush the substance from the eye using an ocular irrigant or water (Table 28–7).
- If a *foreign object or substance* becomes embedded in the eye or trapped under the eyelid, see an eye care provider for removal. Continued presence of the substance could lead to an eye infection or tissue damage.
- Consult an eye care provider before self-treating *corneal edema.* If hyperosmotic solutions (Table 28–7) are recommended, follow the recommended dosages even though the product may sting. Continued utilization of these products will depend on the eye care professional's recommendations.
- Note that taking ophthalmic vitamin supplements for macular degeneration along with general multivitamins may result in gastrointestinal upset or vitamin toxicity.
- If *contact dermatitis of the eyelid* occurs, wash the affected areas, identify the cause of the reaction, and try to avoid future contact with the substance. Consult an eye care provider if symptoms persist after 72 hours of use of oral antihistamines.

treatment. Dry eye disease is often a chronic disorder, requiring regular use of ophthalmic lubricants. Patients with corneal edema should consult an eye care provider if the symptoms persist or worsen despite adherence to the recommended treatment regimen for the causative disorder.

Symptoms of contact dermatitis should resolve quickly once exposure to the offending substance is terminated. If symptoms persist after 72 hours of antihistamine use, the patient should see an eye care provider.

Key Points for Ophthalmic Disorders

- The pharmacist is well positioned in the community to treat and triage ophthalmic pathology or to recommend self-management with one or more nonprescription drugs.
- Many ophthalmic products are available to manage the symptoms of minor acute or chronic disorders and conditions of the eye and eyelid.
- Familiarity with the pathophysiology of certain ocular conditions and proficiency in the assessment of patients who present with such conditions will allow the pharmacist to optimize the safe, appropriate, effective, and economical use of nonprescription drugs to manage selected conditions of the eye and eyelid.
- Nonprescription ophthalmic products should be used only in cases of minor pain or discomfort. If the nature of the problem is in doubt, the pharmacist should refer the patient for medical care.
- Nonprescription ocular medications should not be recommended to patients who have demonstrated an allergy to any of the active ingredients, preservatives, or other excipients in the product.
- Patients who are already using a prescription ophthalmic product should use nonprescription products only after consulting with an eye care provider or a pharmacist.
- Patients with narrow anterior chamber angles or narrow-angle glaucoma should not use topical ocular decongestants because of the risk of angle-closure glaucoma.
- Drug administration should be conservative in patients with hyperemic conjunctiva because of the potential for increased systemic drug absorption and the risk of adverse effects.
- The lowest concentration and conservative dosage frequencies should be used, especially for ocular decongestants; overuse should be avoided.
- Ophthalmic products frequently are used incorrectly; therefore, counseling on appropriate application of products is crucial.

REFERENCES

1. Lemp M. Advances in understanding and managing dry eye disease. *Am J Ophthalmol.* 2008;146(3):350–6. doi:10.1016/j.ajo.2008.05.016.
2. Dartt D. Formation and function of tear film. In: Levin L, Nilsson S, Verhoeve J, eds. *Adler's Physiology of the Eye.* 11th ed. Edinburgh, UK: Elsevier; 2011:350–62.
3. Pflugfelder SC. Tear dysfunction and the cornea: LXVII Edward Jackson Memorial Lecture. *Am J Ophthalmol.* 2011;152(6):900–9.e1. doi: 10.1016/j.ajo.2011.08.023.
4. Salomon-Ben Zeev M, Miller D, Latkany R. Diagnosis of dry eye disease and emerging technologies. *Clin Ophthalmol.* 2014;8:581–90. doi: 10.2147/OPTH.S45444.
5. Bartlett JD, Keith MS, Sudharshan L, Snedecor SJ. Associations between signs and symptoms of dry eye disease: a systematic review. *Clin Ophthalmol.* 2015;9:1719–30. doi:10.2147/OPTH.S89700.
6. Flach AJ. Proposed mandate for instructions and labeling regarding the use of eye drops. *Arch Ophthalmol.* 2009:127:1207–10. doi: 10.1001/archophthalmol.2009.259.
7. Tressler CS, Beatty R, Lemp MA. Preservative use in topical glaucoma medications. *Ocul Surf.* 2011;9:140–58. PMID: 21791189.
8. Stern ME, Beurman RW, Fox RI, et al. The pathology of dry eye: the interaction between the ocular surface and lacrimal glands. *Cornea.* 1998;17(6):584–9. PMID: 9820935.

9. Lemp MA, Daudouin C, Baum J, et al. The definition and classification of dry eye disease: report for the Definition and Classification Subcommittee of the International Dry Eye Workshop (2007). *Ocul Surf.* 2007;5(2):75–92, 163–78. PMID: 17508116.
10. Behrens A, Doyle JJ, Stern L, et al. Dysfunctional tear syndrome: a Delphi approach to treatment recommendations. *Cornea.* 2006;25(8):900–7. PMID: 17102664.
11. American Academy of Ophthalmology. Dry Eye Syndrome: Preferred Practice Patterns. 2013. Available at: http://www.AAO.org. Accessed March 5, 2016.
12. She Y, Li J, Xiao B, et al. Evaluation of a novel artificial tear in the prevention and treatment of dry eye in an animal model. *J Ocul Pharm Ther.* 2015;31:525–30. doi: 10.1089/jop.2015.0042.
13. Fraunfelder FT, Sciubba JJ, Mathers WD. The role of medications in causing dry eye. *J Ophthalmol.* 2012;2012:285851. doi: 10.1155/2012/285851.
14. Smith RE. The tear film complex. Pathogenesis and emerging therapies for dry eyes. *Cornea.* 2015;24:1–7.
15. Wegener AR, Meyer LM, Schonfeld C. Effect of viscous agents on corneal density in dry eye disease. *J Ocul Pharm Ther.* 2015;31:504–8. doi: 10.1089/jop.2014.0157.
16. Moshirfar M, Pierson K, Hanamaikai K, et al. Artificial tears potpourri: a literature review. *Clin Ophthalmol.* 2014;8:1419–33. doi: 10.2147/OPTH.S65263.
17. Pensyl CD. Preparations for dry eye and ocular surface disease. In: Bartlett JD, Jaanus SD, eds. *Clinical Ocular Pharmacology.* 5th ed. Boston, MA: Butterworth-Heinemann; 2007:263–78.
18. Fiscella R, Burstein NL. Ophthalmic drug formulations. In: Bartlett JD, Jaanus SD, eds. *Clinical Ocular Pharmacology.* 5th ed. Boston, MA: Butterworth-Heinemann; 2007:17–37.
19. Whitson JT, Petroll WM. Corneal epithelial cell viability following exposure to ophthalmic solutions containing preservatives and/or antihypertensive agents. *Adv Ther.* 2012;29:874–88. doi: 10.1007/s12325-012-0057-1.
20. Debbasch C, Brignole F, Pisella PJ, et al. Quaternary ammoniums and other preservatives' contribution in oxidative stress and apoptosis on Chang conjunctival cells. *Invest Ophthalmol Vis Sci.* 2001;42(3):642–52.
21. Simmons PA, Carlisle-Wilcox C, Vehige JG. Comparison of novel lipid-based eye drops with aqueous eye drops for dry eye: a multicenter, randomized controlled trial. *Clin Ophthalmol.* 2015;9:657–64. PMCID: PMC4404875.
22. U.S. Food and Drug Administration. FDA warns consumers about potential risks of using eye drops packaged in bottles with loose safety seals. March 15, 2016. Available at: https://www.fda.gov/Drugs/DrugSafety/ucm490693.htm. Accessed June 8, 2017.
23. Bielory L. Ocular allergy overview. *Immunol Allergy Clin North Am.* 2008;28:1–23. doi:10.1016/j.iac.2007.12.011.
24. Bielory L. Ocular allergy treatment. *Immunol Allergy Clin North Am.* 2008;28:189–224. doi:10.1016/j.iac.2007.12.001.
25. Soparkar CN, Wilhelmus KR, Koch DD, et al. Acute and chronic conjunctivitis due to over-the-counter ophthalmic decongestants. *Arch Ophthalmol.* 1997;115(1):34–8. PMID: 9006422.
26. Portello JK. Mydriatics and mydriolytics. In: Bartlett JD, Jaanus SD, eds. *Clinical Ocular Pharmacology.* 5th ed. Boston, MA: Butterworth-Heinemann; 2007:113–23.
27. Adamczyk DT, Jaanus SD. Antiallergy drugs and decongestants. In: Bartlett JD, Jaanus SD, eds. *Clinical Ocular Pharmacology.* 5th ed. Boston, MA: Butterworth-Heinemann; 2007:245–61.
28. O'Brien T. Allergic conjunctivitis: an update on diagnosis and management. *Curr Opin Allergy Clin Immunol.* 2013;13:543–49. doi:10.1097/ACI.0b013e328364ec3a.
29. Bilkhu PS, Wolffsohn JS, Naroo SA, et al. Effectiveness of nonpharmaoclogic treatment for acute seasonal allergic conjunctivitis. *Ophthalmology.* 2014;21:72–8. doi: 10.1016/j.ophtha.2013.08.007.
30. Slonim CB, Boone R. The ocular allergic response: a pharmacotherapeutic review. *Formulary.* 2004;39:213–22.
31. Jaanus SD. Antiedema agents. In: Bartlett JD, Jaanus SD, eds. *Clinical Ocular Pharmacology.* 5th ed. Boston, MA: Butterworth-Heinemann; 2007: 279–81.
32. Khare GD, Symons RCA, Do DV. Common ophthalmic emergencies. *Int J Clin Pract.* 2008;62(11):1776–84. PMID: 19143862.

CHAPTER 29

PREVENTION OF CONTACT LENS–RELATED DISORDERS

ALEDA M.H. CHEN AND ANDREW M. STRAW

An estimated 40.9 million people use contact lenses in the United States, and more than $7 billion is spent annually worldwide on contact lenses. Soft contact lenses, introduced in 1971, provide greater comfort than rigid lenses and account for 90% of lens purchases. In 2015, U.S. consumers spent $2.7 billion on soft contact lenses.[1] The newest soft lens material, known as silicone hydrogel, continues to dominate this market category, being favored by 54% of soft lens wearers worldwide[2] and by 68% in the United States.[1]

The types of lenses prescribed vary markedly among countries. Gas-permeable (GP) lenses account for approximately 20% of prescribed contact lenses in some countries, such as Germany, Austria, Switzerland, and the Netherlands, and for 82% in Slovenia,[2] whereas only 11% of contact lenses prescribed in the United States are of the GP type.[1]

As many as 50% of contact lens wearers experience complications; however, this number varies widely by type of lens, wearing schedule, and adherence to the prescribed care regimen.[3] Contact lenses, even when expertly fitted, induce local changes that alter ocular tissues and affect corneal metabolism. The prevention of contact lens–related disorders requires that both patients and health care providers (HCPs) understand the proper prescribing, fitting, and care regimens associated with safe contact lens wear. Failure to follow optimal practices can greatly increase the chance for development of corneal infection (ulcers) and other ocular conditions that may result in permanent eye damage and blindness. Preventive measures aimed at improving patient hygiene and appropriate contact lens care, as well as adherence to recommended replacement frequency schedules, will reduce the overall risk of contact lens complications.[4] Fortunately, most complications from contact lens wear are reversible, if attended to promptly. Approximately 23%–33% of patients discontinue wearing their contact lenses periodically or permanently, with lens discomfort or dryness cited as the most common reason.[5–7] Silicone hydrogel contact lenses have the lowest discontinuation rates,[6] and proper care and fitting of lenses can help eliminate discomfort and encourage patients to continue wearing their lenses.

The fitting and dispensing of contact lenses, traditionally the sole domain of optometrists and ophthalmologists, have undergone dramatic changes in recent years. The Fairness to Contact Lens Consumers Act, passed by Congress in 2003, requires that contact lens prescribers release a copy of the contact lens prescription to the patient at the conclusion of the fitting process, whether or not it is requested.[8] This act allows the patient to purchase prescribed contact lenses and related supplies from any of various authorized sources, including pharmacies.

The availability of contact lenses from nonprofessional sources such as department stores, mail-order services, or internet websites raises potential health and safety issues. In accordance with the Fairness Act, after presentation of a valid prescription, contact lenses can be dispensed by any person or agency, who may or may not have basic training in eye care, that complies with state and local business statutes; typically the statutes contain no stipulations for such training or for professional or technical licensing in health care. Moreover, recent research has shown that individuals who purchase contact lenses from internet sources are less likely to adhere to recommended lens care,[9,10] which is particularly concerning because online sales of eyeglasses and contact lenses continue to increase.[1]

As detailed in this chapter, fitting and dispensing contact lenses involve more than specifying parameters for the lenses themselves. Additional considerations of importance include patient education regarding adherence to requirements of lens care systems, wearing schedules, and lens replacement schedules. Patient education also should incorporate proper lens handling and the signs and symptoms of complications as other essential aspects of a successful wear regimen. Another concern is enforcement of expiration dates for lens prescriptions.

Use of Contact Lenses

Most people can wear one or more types of contact lenses without problems if certain precautions are taken. In a few cases, use of contact lenses is contraindicated.

Indications for Contact Lenses

Indications for the use of contact lenses include the correction of refractive errors such as myopia (nearsightedness), hyperopia (farsightedness), astigmatism, and presbyopia. Astigmatism occurs when dissimilar curvatures of the refractive surface of the eye result in a blurred image. GP lenses or toric soft lenses can be used to correct astigmatism.

The benefits of contact lens wear are widely known and include the convenience of freedom from eyeglasses, no obstruction to vision from eyeglass frames, no fogging of lenses caused by sudden temperature changes, improved optics and clarity of vision, wider peripheral field of vision, equal image sizes when refractive disparity exists between eyes, and better function during sports activities or exercise. Perhaps a significant reason for choosing contact lenses is the perceived improvement in self-image and personal appearance.[11]

The decision to wear contact lenses rather than eyeglasses is sometimes based on therapeutic necessity or cosmetic interest. For example, in patients with keratoconus (a corneal dystrophy causing a gradual protrusion of the central cornea), satisfactory vision is usually unattainable with ordinary eyeglasses but can be achieved with rigid contact lenses, which can favorably reshape the curvature of the cornea. Another example of therapeutic necessity is the use of soft contact lenses as "bandage" lenses in the case of severe corneal abrasions. Other, less common indications for contact lenses include aphakia (absence of the natural lens of the eye), corneal scarring, and disfigured eyes. In the first two conditions, patients typically see better with contact lenses, and for patients with disfigurement, tinted prosthetic soft contact lenses may improve cosmetic appearance by rendering defects from a variety of conditions virtually unnoticeable. Additionally, some patients utilize "special effects" contact lenses for cosmetic or occupational purposes, such as costume-related events, theatrical productions, or expression of personal style. These lenses often have a tint that hides the natural eye color and may add unique features to the appearance of the eye.

Contraindications and Warnings for Contact Lens Wear

Certain patients are poor candidates for contact lens wear—they either cannot or should not wear contact lenses. Contraindications are often based on lifestyle as well as on medical history. The following are relative contraindications that should be considered on an individual basis before the patient is fitted for contact lenses:

- Monocular vision. In persons with vision in only one eye, the risk of complications such as inflammation or infection that can permanently scar the cornea in the seeing eye must be weighed against the need for optimal visual correction. Overnight wear of lenses should absolutely be avoided.
- Presence of an active pathologic process involving the lids, cornea, or conjunctiva. Such conditions include blepharitis, corneal infections (i.e., herpes, keratitis, *Staphylococcus aureus* infection, *Pseudomonas* infection), and conjunctivitis. Conjunctivitis associated with common colds or chronic allergic conditions such as hay fever and asthma also may make contact lens wear extremely uncomfortable or impossible.
- Presence of dry eye (keratitis sicca), except for use of "bandage" soft contact lenses for protection. Although this condition presents obvious difficulties for successful lens wear, it has been recognized that some patients with severe dry eye actually benefit from the use of bandage soft contact lenses to protect the ocular surface. In general, however, lens wearers who have insufficient tear production, a deficiency or excess of mucin, or excessive lipid production and those who spend time in excessively dry environments may be unable to use contact lenses successfully. Poor blink rate or "incomplete" blinking (where the eyelid does not completely close) also may contribute to difficulty with lens wear. Postmenopausal women may experience higher rates of dry eye, precluding successful contact lens wear.
- Pregnancy or use of oral contraceptives. The fluid-retaining effects of estrogen may lead to edema of the cornea, which will alter corneal topography and affect the fit of contact lenses.
- Diabetes. Patients with diabetes are advised against use of continuous-wear contact lenses because of the retarded healing processes and reduced corneal sensitivity associated with this disease. These considerations probably are of lesser significance with daily-wear lenses, which often may be used unless specific problems arise (e.g., inflammation, infection, abstasion).
- Eye medications requiring frequent dosing (e.g., for treatment of glaucoma). The preservatives in multidose bottles can bind to soft contact lenses, with potential toxicity to the corneal epithelium.
- Personal habit, vocation, or hobby that is not conducive to lens wear (e.g., smoking, exposure to chemically toxic environments). Occupational conditions that may prohibit the wearing of contact lenses include exposure to wind, glare, molten metals, irritants, dust and particulate matter, fur, dander, feathers, sand, tobacco smoke, and chemicals and chemical fumes. Certain chemical fumes may be particularly hazardous because of the potential for concentration of irritants under a rigid lens or inside a soft lens. With lenses on the eye, contact of such substances with the cornea is potentially prolonged, which can lead to corneal toxicity.
- Medications that cause discoloration of bodily fluids. Rifampin, used in therapy for tuberculosis, is a common offender.
- Activity (e.g., frequent air travel) that entails moving from a low to a high altitude. Such changes in altitude may induce hypoxia, with consequent edema of the cornea, or metabolic deficiency, resulting in irritation and corneal abrasions.
- A pattern of abusing lens wear or multiple episodes of ocular complications. The patient's medical history should be reviewed to identify potential problems.
- Inability to care for contact lenses appropriately. This restriction typically affects pediatric patients who are not properly supervised and older or impaired persons who lack the cognitive skills or dexterity to handle contact lenses.

Soft Versus Rigid Contact Lenses

The three major categories of contact lenses are soft (hydrophilic), rigid gas-permeable (i.e., GP), and rigid non–gas-permeable (polymethylmethylacrylate [PMMA]). PMMA lenses—often known as "hard" contact lenses—are rarely used today owing to their lack of oxygen permeability and are not discussed in this chapter. Soft and GP lenses are composed of single or multiple plastic monomers; soft lens materials contain water but GP lens materials do not. Soft lenses are popular because of their excellent initial comfort on insertion. Rigid lenses, by contrast, have always provided the best optics, with consequent superior visual acuity. In the contact lens area of clinical practice, use of the term "hard lenses" during patient counseling is no longer acceptable, because it creates a stigma about optimal lens designs for individual needs. Therefore, rigid lenses should simply be referred to as "gas-permeable lenses." Table 29–1 provides a comparison of soft and GP lenses. Table 29–2 compares the advantages and disadvantages of soft and GP contact lenses with regard to lens properties, ease of care and handling, potential associated complications, and other characteristics.

Hydrophilic (Soft) Contact Lenses

First introduced in 1971, soft contact lenses have become the lens of choice from the standpoint of HCPs and patients alike. In the United States alone, soft contact lenses represent almost 90% of all contact lens prescriptions.[1] Once limited by poor reproducibility and limited parameter availability, soft contact lenses are

TABLE 29-1 Comparison of Contact Lens Characteristics

Lens Properties	Lens Type: Soft	Lens Type: Gas-Permeable
Lens Characteristics		
Rigidity	0	+++
Durability	+	++
Oxygen transmission	++	+++
Chemical adsorption	+++	0
Optical Quality		
Visual acuity	+	+++
Correction of astigmatism	Toric	Yes
Photophobia	+	++
Spectacle blur	0	++
Convenience		
Comfort	+++	++
Adaptation period	Days	Weeks
Continuous wear	Yes	Yes
Intermittent wear	Yes	No

Key: PMMA = Polymethylmethylacrylate; + = degree to which the characteristic is present; 0 = the characteristic is not present.

now available in any spherical or cylindrical power, and they can correct for presbyopia, myopia or hyperopia, and astigmatism. The equilibrium point of hydration of soft lenses may be adversely influenced by several variables, including temperature, oxidative reactions of lens care solutions, hyper- or hypotonicity, and pH.[12]

In 1986, the U.S. Food and Drug Administration (FDA) classified soft hydrogel contact lenses into four categories according to water content and ionic properties: low water nonionic, high water nonionic, low water ionic, and high water ionic. Soft contact lenses with less than 50% water content are considered to be in the low-water category. Less reactive surfaces are called nonionic, and more reactive materials are called ionic.[1] Most eye care providers prescribe nonionic soft contact lenses because of the lenses' inherent chemical ability to deter the formation of charged protein and lipid deposits. Originally, soft contact lenses were intended to be cleaned and disinfected daily and replaced on a yearly basis. Compliance was poor because patients opted for convenience over ocular health by not following prescribed daily care regimens, by not replacing lenses until after years of wear, and by sleeping overnight while wearing lenses, in some cases without appropriate lens care for weeks at a time. Contact lens complications such as corneal edema, neovascularization, and ocular infiltrates were observed. Oxygen deprivation, or hypoxia, was known to be a significant factor in many of these complications. The oxygen transmissibility of contact lenses is described by the term Dk/t,[12] where D represents gas diffusion, k is the solubility coefficient, and t the contact lens oxygen transmissibility. A higher Dk/t value allows more oxygen to pass through the lens. As the water content increases, so does the k value, along with oxygen permeability. However, permeability also depends on lens thickness.

Tighter quality control and refinement of manufacturing techniques have led to improved lens reproducibility and to the advent of disposable soft contact lenses. Disposable lenses represent the fastest-growing segment of the soft lens market. A true disposable soft contact lens is worn once and replaced without interval cleaning, implying that it is worn continuously for the recommended period. The advantage of having a fresh, clean lens available on a regular basis appealed to many patients, and this hygienic benefit has lessened the incidence of complications from a soiled lens, such as contact lens–associated papillary conjunctivitis. With disposable contact lenses, the traditional yearly replacement schedule no longer applies: These soft lenses are replaced monthly. However, some patients use soft contact lenses that are replaced biweekly or daily. Silicone hydrogel materials have contributed to the ability to have continuous wear lenses.

HCPs were hopeful that frequent lens replacement would improve general lenswear hygiene and negate the negative effects of biofilm development on the surface of lenses. Many also believed that silicone hydrogel materials would effectively eliminate inflammatory and infectious complications of contact lens wear, including microbial keratitis, by removing the effects of hypoxia on the corneal epithelium. Although years of clinical use have shown that these materials do in fact diminish the hypoxic effect of lens wear, such as redness, limbal neovascularization, and microcystic edema, they have failed to eliminate infectious and inflammatory complications.[13] One study showed identical rates of microbial keratitis for overnight wear of silicone hydrogel materials and use of lenses composed of older materials.[14] FDA, however, continues to allow two different continuous-wear schedules that are lens-specific to remain in effect. The first is 6 continuous days and nights of wear, with the lens being discarded on day 7, as implemented during the early days of continuous wear. For some of the most permeable materials, FDA approves 30 nights of continuous wear, followed by replacement of the lens. Patients should be made aware that the continuous wear of contact lenses has clearly been shown to be the greatest risk factor for the most devastating consequences of lens wear, primarily microbial keratitis. Even though lenses are approved for 30 nights of continuous wear, some patients may not be able to tolerate wearing them for this length of time. None of the soft contact lenses on the market, including the silicone hydrogel types, can prevent or protect the eye from inflammatory and infectious complications. The importance of patient education regarding adherence to lens care regimens, wearing and replacement schedules as well as awareness of more serious signs and symptoms cannot be overemphasized to ensure safe contact lens wear.

Even a disposable, continuous-wear lens can be used only on a daily-wear basis, and patients should replace lenses at the prescribed interval. When used on a daily-wear basis, these lenses must be cleaned and disinfected regularly. Patients looking to optimize convenience without exposing themselves to the risk of continuous wear should be directed toward daily disposable lenses. Daily disposables have the following advantages: (1) each lens is sterile before removal from its package for immediate insertion into the eye; (2) no cleaning regimen is necessary because the lens is discarded after wear for a day; (3) deposit formation is minimal; and (4) lens-related problems, such as giant papillary conjunctivitis or allergic reactions to lens care solutions, occur less frequently.

TABLE 29–2 **Advantages and Disadvantages of Soft and Gas-Permeable (GP) Contact Lenses**

Soft Contact Lenses	GP Contact Lenses
Advantages	
Excellent initial lens comfort	Excellent optics for optimal visual acuity
Rapid adaptation; well suited to intermittent lens wear	Correction of nearly all forms of refractive error
Correction of nearly all forms of refractive error	Improved vision for conditions with irregular corneas
Ease of fitting	Fit customized to individual patient
Ease of care	Economical
Trapping of foreign material under the lens unlikely	Lower incidence of inflammatory/infectious complications
Low likelihood of dislodging or falling out; well suited to use in sports activities	
Can be tinted for cosmetic or prosthetic purposes (many lenses have light tints to improve visibility when handling)	
Disadvantages	
Less successful vision correction—achievement of excellent visual acuity not possible in all patients	Longer initial adaptation period
Fluctuations in vision due to variability in lens hydration with prolonged wear and changes in ambient temperature and humidity	Capable of trapping foreign material beneath the lens, causing discomfort
Lens fitting not customized to the patient's eye	May dislodge from the eye
Greater likelihood of complications, especially from hypoxia	More difficult to fit
Fragility and ripping (or tearing) of lenses during handling	Subjective flare around the periphery that may be noticed at night, particularly with large pupils
Susceptibility of lenses to adverse effects of preservatives in ophthalmic products	
Lack of surface markers on lens to verify correct eye once packaging is removed, with no means of distinguishing between lenses for left and right eyes	

Hydrophilic Lens Fitting

Unlike with rigid contact lenses, which typically are custom-designed, the parameters of the most commonly used soft contact lenses are predetermined by the manufacturer and are proprietary in nature. Often, the lens diameter and base curve are limited to one or two choices at most, providing little flexibility for adjusting fit. Thus, if a lens does not fit correctly or causes some other complication, another lens design must be tried. Some exceptions are available, and custom soft lenses with a specified diameter, base curve, and power can be ordered.

Hydrophilic Contact Lenses as Therapeutic Devices

Aside from the cosmetic use of contact lenses, hydrophilic lenses have found wide application in the treatment of ocular disease and are being investigated for potential use as ocular drug delivery devices. Of note, hydrophilic lenses are employed as an "eye bandage" to protect the cornea and to promote corneal reepithelialization after corneal injury or various corneal surgical procedures. Four soft contact lenses are currently approved by FDA for use therapeutically as such bandage lenses in the treatment of corneal abrasions and other ocular surface problems. It is important to counsel patients who are prescribed contact lenses for this purpose to be diligent in cleaning and disinfecting the lenses.[14,15]

Gas-Permeable Contact Lenses

Rigid contact lenses preceded soft lenses in the market but were quickly surpassed because of one primary factor: patients have greater initial awareness of rigid lenses on the eye. In terms of optical quality, rigid lenses are far superior to soft lenses. However, patients are willing to sacrifice clarity for comfort. In defense of rigid lenses, initial discomfort can dissipate over several weeks as adaptation occurs and nerve endings on the inner surface of the eyelids become desensitized to the presence of the lens.

Rigid GP lenses are made from monomer components of hydrophobic plastic compounds that allow oxygen to diffuse through the lens.[16] Advantages of GP lenses over soft contact lenses include increased oxygen transmissibility, reduced lipophilicity (e.g., less contamination from the environment), and sharper vision. These lenses also have less surface reactivity, thereby decreasing tear film deposits.[16] Other advantages of GP lenses over soft contact lenses include fewer adverse inflammatory or infectious consequences. When properly cared for, GP lenses are durable and can be reused repeatedly for months to years before replacement is necessary, making them more economical than soft lenses. Surface scratches and deposits can be removed with powerful cleaners or in-office polishing machines. The disadvantages of GP lenses include lesser surface wettability; a negative surface charge, which can attract lysozymes and other positively charged deposits; and greater mass, which can affect lens fit, depending on the type of GP lens.

GP lenses are the lens of choice for dealing with complicated corneal disease such as keratoconus, corneal scarring from disease or trauma, and transplanted corneas or those with high astigmatism. Unlike soft lenses, which drape over the surface of the cornea, even if it is irregular, GP lenses create a new refracting surface, with a tear layer filling the gap between lens and cornea. GP lenses are available in a wide range of designs, including toric lenses for astigmatism and bifocals for presbyopia. Although far more limited in terms of choice, some GP materials are also FDA-approved for either 7 or 30 days of continuous wear, depending on the material.

Gas-Permeable Lens Fitting

Most providers who prescribe contact lenses agree that compared with soft lenses, fitting GP lenses requires a higher level of both art and science. Unlike soft lenses, GP lenses are not mass-manufactured but rather are custom-designed and manufactured on demand, requiring the optometrist to provide the parameters of diameter, base curve, power, and material to order a lens.

Specialty Contact Lenses

Numerous companies manufacture soft contact lenses. The product offerings of many companies overlap to address the most common myopic, hyperopic, and astigmatic refractive errors. Many companies sell prepackaged, mass-produced lenses that consumers can buy in bulk with a prescription. Some offer customized lenses to address unusual needs. Several companies promote materials that absorb ultraviolet light. Corrective, tinted lenses are available for easier handling and for cosmetic purposes. Translucent tints facilitate handling by increasing the visibility of the lens and also enhance eye color. Opaque lenses cover the iris and hide its natural color. These lenses may also be used as a prosthesis to mask corneal scarring. By contrast, all GP lenses are custom made by laboratories that often use proprietary, computer-generated lens designs. These unique designs are aimed at specialty needs such as keratoconus, post–corneal transplantation use, scarred corneas, post–refractive surgery use, aphakia, or high astigmatism.

Two specialty lenses worth mentioning are lenses for presbyopia and hybrid lenses. *Presbyopia* is the loss of accommodation in the aging eye, typically beginning around the age of 40 years, requiring the addition of plus power (i.e., adjustment for farsightedness) to improve the clarity of vision at a near reading distance. It affects individuals who are nearsighted or farsighted or who have an astigmatism. Presbyopia is not to be confused with cataracts, another common cause of visual loss, which are marked by reduced clarity in the crystalline lens and usually are attributable to long-term oxidation and genetic predisposition. Presbyopes are projected to be the single largest group of contact lens wearers by 2018, at 28%.[17] In eyeglasses, a separate portion of the spectacle lens at the bottom of the lens provides this additional plus power for reading (bifocal glasses). This change in power is more difficult to accomplish with contact lenses. A common method of correcting presbyopia with contact lenses is monovision, a technique that uses standard lenses, fitted to the dominant eye corrected for distance and to the other eye corrected for near vision. Monovision can be effective, but it can affect depth perception, intermediate-distance vision, and night driving. Today, multifocal contact lenses are being designed to provide binocular vision for patients, which provides a smooth transition among the near, intermediate, and far zones of the lens. The practitioner should discuss the options with the patient to determine what would work best for personal preferences or lifestyle requirements.[17,18]

A *hybrid contact lens* is a unique contact lens that combines GP and soft lens materials in the same lens. The overall advantages of this lens are excellent optics through the GP portion of the lens, improved comfort from the soft lens portion, greater oxygen permeability (compared with an earlier version of the lens), and the ability to deal with astigmatism and irregular corneas (e.g., keratoconus and corneal transplant). The disadvantages are expense, difficulty with insertion and removal, longer fitting time, and complications of lens wear. The care of these lenses follows the patterns described for soft contact lenses in later sections.

Formulation Considerations for Lens Care Products

The manufacturing and marketing of contact lenses are regulated by the FDA ophthalmic devices division.[19] Patients who wear contact lenses should use only lens care products that have been approved by FDA for use with their specific contact lenses.

The basic considerations for a well-formulated contact lens solution include pH, viscosity, isotonicity with tears, stability, sterility, and provisions for maintaining sterility (bactericidal action). The pH range of comfort is not well defined because although normal tear pH is 7.4, tear pH varies among individual patients. In theory, a weakly buffered solution that can readily adjust to any tear pH is best, because highly buffered solutions can cause significant discomfort, or even ocular damage, when they are instilled. As with therapeutic ophthalmic solutions, however, the stability of the solution takes precedence over comfort. Accordingly, many contact lens solutions are formulated with pH values above or below 7.4. These systems are weakly buffered and usually are well tolerated by the eye. Solutions from different manufacturers should not be mixed because a precipitate may form.[3,20] For instance, a product containing alkaline borate buffers will form a gummy, gel-like precipitate on lenses if mixed with a wetting solution containing polyvinyl alcohol. Furthermore, solutions containing a cationic preservative such as chlorhexidine, polyquaternium-1, or polyaminopropyl biguanide should not be mixed with solutions containing an anionic preservative such as sorbic acid; this combination, too, will cause a precipitate to form.

Soft Contact Lens Care

The goals of cleaning a contact lens are (1) to remove debris from the lens surface, (2) to prevent the accumulation of proteins from the tear layer on the lens, and (3) to disinfect the lens of organisms that can bind to the lens surface and potentially lead to infection. Lens disinfection is a crucial step, although all steps must be completed on a daily basis or after each wearing period to avoid ocular complications.[21] The basic care regimen for soft lenses (Figure 29–1) differs from that for GP lenses.

Since the early days of contact lens use, separate solutions have been available for each step of cleaning, rinsing, disinfecting, storing, and protein removal. These include surfactants for cleaning the lens surface, saline solution for rinsing, disinfecting agents for sterilization, and enzymes for protein removal, in addition to wetting drops for use while lenses are on the eye. To improve convenience and compliance, multipurpose products are

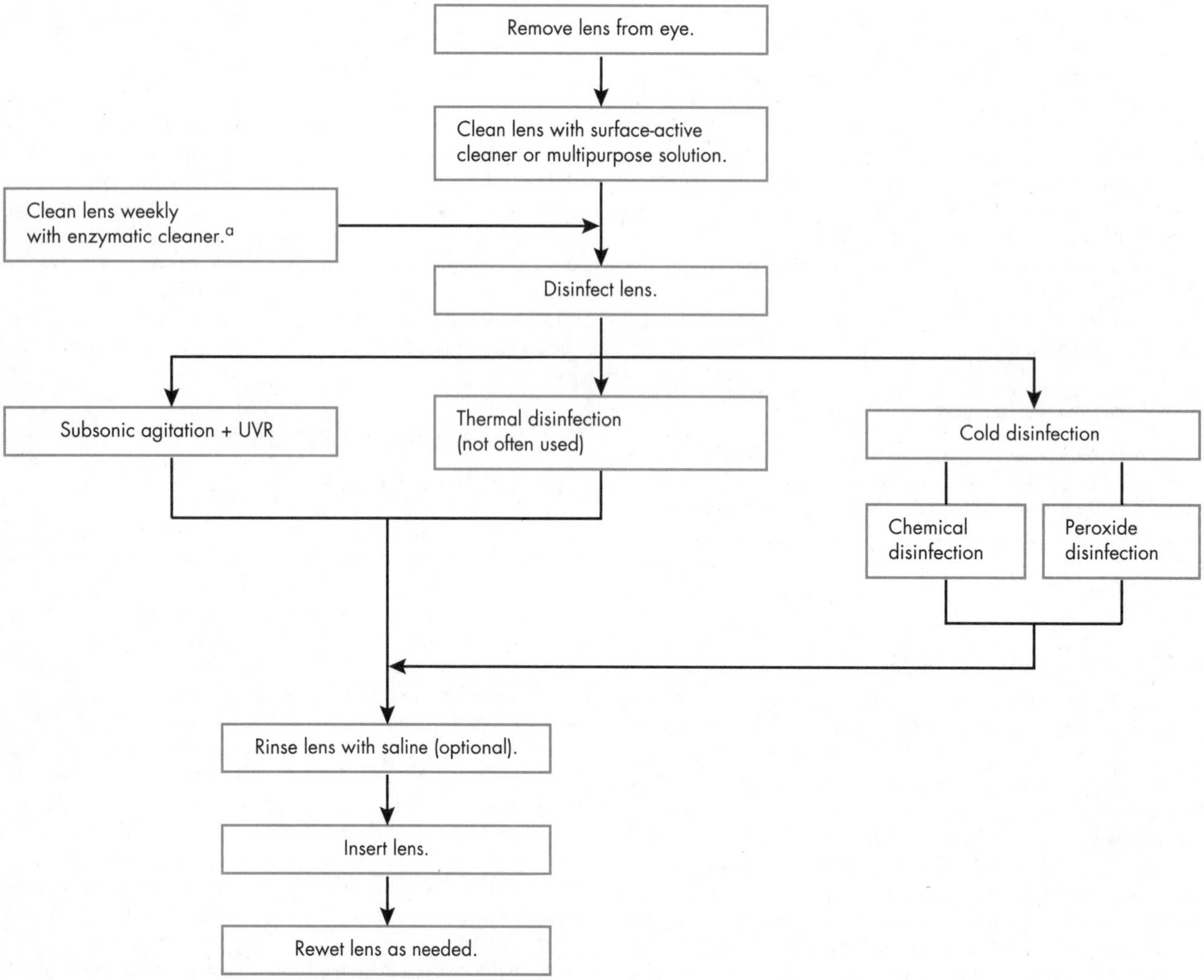

[a] Step is not necessary for planned replacement or disposable lenses.

FIGURE 29–1 Self-care for soft lenses. Key: UVR = Ultraviolet radiation.

available that combine these active ingredients in a biocompatible solution buffered for pH balance for use directly in the eye. Some of these solutions also contain demulcents to increase lubrication and comfort of the eye.

Tables 29–3 and 29–4 present detailed steps for cleaning soft contact lenses.

Soft Lens Disinfection

The lens care regimen must be built primarily around the use of a disinfecting system. In patient education, emphasis must be placed on hand hygiene and adherence to the manufacturer's requirements for each disinfecting system, while stressing the minimum soaking time for disinfection.

Preservatives

The most important point in a consideration of contact lens disinfection regards the preservatives that are used both to keep multiuse solutions sterile and to disinfect the lens. Daily use of the

TABLE 29–3 **General Cleaning Procedures for All Lens Types**

- Wash hands with noncosmetic soap and rinse them thoroughly before handling lenses.
- Clean contact lenses only with commercially manufactured products made specifically for that type of lens. Homemade cleansers can scratch and contaminate the lenses or cause eye irritation or injury.
- Do not mix contact lens care products from different manufacturers unless an eye care provider confirms that the products are compatible.
- During cleaning, check lenses for scratches, chips, or tears and for the presence of foreign particles, warping, or discoloration. Also, ensure that lenses are clean and thoroughly rinsed of cleaner. Any residual impurities could cause eye discomfort.
- When cleaning a lens, rub it in a back-and-forth, rather than a circular, direction, even if using a no-rub solution.
- Discard cleansers and other lens care products if the labeled expiration date has passed.

TABLE 29–4 Specific Cleaning Procedures for Soft Lenses

- Clean regular soft lenses daily with a surface-active cleaner. Clean continuous-wear soft lenses with a surface-active cleaner after each wearing.
- Wash hands before handling your lenses.
- Place several drops of a cleaning product on the lens; gently rub the lens with the tip of the forefinger against the palm of the opposite hand, for 20–30 seconds, even if using a no-rub product, to ensure removal of protein deposits.
- Avoid cutting the lens with a fingernail or scratching the lens surface with grit or dirt on the hands.
- Rinse lenses with a sterile isotonic buffered solution. Never use tap water, because it is not isotonic and contains harmful microorganisms.
- Clean lenses at least weekly (or every day if using a daily product) with enzymatic cleaners, either separately from disinfection or as part of the disinfecting process.
- When combining enzymatic cleaning and disinfecting of the lenses as one step, see Tables 29–6 and 29–7 for the appropriate products.
- Discard any enzyme cleaner that is discolored.

same bottle of any contact lens solution over a long period of time increases the risk of bacterial contamination. The solution must therefore contain a bactericidal agent that is both effective over the long term and nonirritating to the eye with daily use. Despite the presence of preservatives, once opened, any contact lens solution not used within the recommended time frame on the label, typically 1–3 months, must be discarded. Patients should be directed to write the date on which the container is opened on the outside of the bottle.[22]

Edetate disodium and sorbic acid are the most commonly used preservatives in saline, daily cleaners, and wetting drops for contact lenses; benzalkonium chloride is used less frequently. Polyquaternium and polyhexamethylene biguanide are the preservatives used most commonly as disinfecting agents for soft contact lens solutions; both are recognized as effective antimicrobial agents.[22,23]

Disinfecting Methods

FDA recommends disinfecting soft contact lenses before each reinsertion.[21,22] Chemical-based disinfection is by far the most popular (Table 29–5). Thermal, or heat, disinfection is no longer a viable method of caring for soft contact lenses. The alternative is an electronic system, PuriLens, that uses subsonic ultrasound agitation for cleaning and high-intensity ultraviolet (UV) light for disinfection. However, one study suggests that additional antimicrobial agents may be needed because some bacteria may survive the UV disinfection process.[24,25]

In chemical disinfection, lenses are stored for a specified period (usually 4–6 hours) in a solution containing bactericidal agents that are compatible with soft lens materials. Two basic chemical disinfection methods are available in the United States. The first is based on the original chemical disinfecting solutions, which consisted of antimicrobial preservatives at sufficient concentration in storage solutions composed primarily of saline.[22,26] These original disinfecting solutions contained chlorhexidine and thimerosal, both of which induce sensitivity reactions in many soft lens wearers.[26,27] To sidestep this limitation, manufacturers are

TABLE 29–5 Guidelines for Disinfecting Gas-Permeable and Soft Lenses

Chemical Disinfection with Hydrogen Peroxide

- Using the cup provided with the hydrogen peroxide product, soak lenses for the length of time specified by the manufacturer. Do not use lens cups or cases that came with other products.
- To disinfect and neutralize in one step, place platinum catalytic disk in lens case and leave the disk there until time to replace it. Add hydrogen peroxide, place lenses in the case, and leave for at least 6 hours.
- Never place neutralizing solution in a lens case with a catalytic disc. An unwanted chemical reaction may occur, or a gummy residue may form on the disc.
- Before inserting lenses in the eyes, make sure the hydrogen peroxide is completely neutralized by carefully following product instructions.
- Rinse lenses thoroughly with saline before inserting them.

Chemical Preservative Disinfection

- Store lenses for the prescribed period of time (usually a minimum of 4 hours) in a preservative disinfecting solution that is appropriate for the lens type.
- If you experience irritation, remove lenses and rinse them thoroughly with saline to remove any disinfecting solution.
- If not wearing lenses for prolonged periods after chemical disinfection, store the cleaned lenses in an appropriate multipurpose contact lens solution and change out the multipurpose solution in the storage container daily.

Combination Enzyme Cleaning and Disinfection

- When combining enzyme cleaning and disinfecting of the lenses as one step, select products compatible with your disinfecting system.
- Add appropriate solution (hydrogen peroxide or chemical disinfecting product) to the storage case of the disinfecting system.
- Place the lenses in the case and then add appropriate enzymatic cleaner.
- Follow directions for the appropriate disinfecting system listed previously.
- Rinse lenses thoroughly with saline to remove residual enzymes.

currently marketing solutions with less-sensitizing disinfectants for soft contact lens care. Such antimicrobial preservatives include quaternary ammonium compounds (e.g., polyquaternium-1), biguanides (e.g., polyhexanide, polyaminopropyl biguanide), and amidoamine (e.g., myristamidopropyl dimethylamine), which are touted as being much less toxic or allergenic than their predecessors. Some of these agents, however, also may be less effective, especially against fungi and protozoa.[27]

The second chemical disinfection method uses hydrogen peroxide as the antimicrobial agent. Soft lenses are placed in purified hydrogen peroxide, and disinfection occurs with the liberation of oxygen from peroxide. Household hydrogen peroxide solution should not be used; its pH is too low, and it may discolor lenses. After disinfection is completed, the peroxide is neutralized to trace levels by a neutralizing tablet that contains a delayed-release catalase or by the catalytic action of a platinum disc.[28]

One potential disadvantage of hydrogen peroxide disinfection is that patients may mistakenly insert the lens directly from the peroxide solution without neutralization. Patients must be warned not to perform a final rinse with the disinfecting solution before inserting their lenses, as they might do with a multipurpose chemical system. Emphasis on the neutralization step is critical. A peroxide-soaked lens placed on the eye will cause a toxic keratitis with symptoms of pain, photophobia, and redness. In this event, the patient should immediately remove the lens and flush the eye copiously with sterile saline solution or, if this is not available, even tap water. If symptoms do not abate, the patient should consult an eye care provider.[28] Of note, the catalytic disc used with some systems must be replaced every 3 months. Any sensation of discomfort or burning experienced by the user when inserting contact lenses that have been disinfected with hydrogen peroxide is likely to mean incomplete neutralization and the need to replace the disc. Patients must also be instructed that once disinfection of contact lenses with a hydrogen peroxide system is completed, the remaining liquid is nonpreserved and is not suitable for prolonged storage (maximum of 7 days). Bacterial contamination may occur after that time. Hydrogen peroxide systems are not recommended for patients who wear lenses intermittently and leave their lenses in neutralized solution for extended days of storage. Patients with these wear habits should be advised to switch solutions after each peroxide cleaning to a multipurpose solution, or to change to daily disposable contact lenses.

Although the catalytic disc systems require only one step, the disinfection and neutralization processes take 6 hours, which decreases the system's flexibility and rules out morning use. Clear Care, Clear Care Plus with HydraGlyde, and PeroxiClear are all peroxide systems approved by FDA for use with silicone hydrogel materials. Enzymatic cleaner may be added weekly for protein removal.

Oxysept UltraCare is a catalase-based system. With this product, the user adds a delayed-release neutralizing tablet at the beginning of the 6-hour disinfecting cycle. Disinfection and neutralization then occur at the appropriate time intervals. This tablet contains catalase and cyanocobalamin; the latter ingredient turns the solution pink, reminding the user that the tablet has been added.[29] The tablet is coated with hydroxypropyl methylcellulose, which helps lubricate the eye if the lens is not rinsed again between disinfection and insertion. A separate daily cleaning step is required. An enzymatic cleaner may be added weekly for protein removal (Table 29-6).

Patients who choose Oxysept UltraCare should be familiar with the following specific considerations for use of this peroxide disinfecting system:

- This product requires a minimum of 6 hours for complete disinfection of the lenses and neutralization of the peroxide.
- The neutralizing tablet should not be crushed or used if cracks in the coating are evident, because the tablet will start neutralizing the peroxide before adequate disinfection occurs.
- Pliagel, used for surface-active cleaning, can leave a film on the lenses and lens cup if it is not carefully rinsed off the lenses before peroxide disinfection. This film may result in foaming and overflow of the peroxide–neutralizer solution. If this occurs, lenses should be rinsed more carefully, or another surface-active cleaner should be used.
- The user should clean the lens case once a week. For this procedure, lenses are removed from the case if they are not being worn, and the case is then filled with fresh Oxysept UltraCare disinfection solution and the cap is tightened. Of note, a neutralization tablet is not used. The cup is turned upside down to allow the solution to bathe the upper portion of the cup and cap. The case is soaked in this manner until lenses need to be disinfected. The solution is replaced for the next disinfection cycle.
- Before lenses are to be inserted in eyes, the case should be turned upside down to ensure full neutralization of all residual disinfecting solution in the case. Then the lenses can be removed from the case and inserted.

When counseling a patient about the best disinfecting method to use, the primary care provider should consider the patient's ability or reliability in adherence to the lens care regimen, wearing schedule, and convenience. Peroxide-based systems provide excellent disinfection against many organisms and essentially eliminate solution sensitivity issues. They are not well suited, however, for intermittent wear of disposable lenses or to adoption by the careless user, who may inadvertently instill peroxide in the eye. If the patient has a history of sensitivity reactions to lens solutions or is unsure whether sensitivity exists, it is best to recommend a product containing one of the nonsensitizing preservatives.

Multipurpose Products

Initially, manufacturers recommended three separate products for the cleaning, removal of protein deposits, and disinfection of soft contact lenses. More recently, a trend toward use of multipurpose solutions for all of these functions has emerged, in attempt to simplify lens care and improve adherence to optimal wear regimens. The original sequence for cleaning and disinfecting contact lenses was to rub, rinse, and soak the lens overnight. However, with promotion of the "no-rub" technique by manufacturers of multipurpose solutions, patients often are confused about proper lens care.[30,31] Several studies have demonstrated that in regard to multipurpose solution, a no-rub technique does not adequately remove protein and other deposits and cosmetics compared with active rubbing of the lens with the fingertip. To reduce risk of infection, irritation, and other complications, proper rub, rinse, and soak technique should be recommended with use of all multipurpose solutions. This recommendation is shared by FDA, the American Optometric Association, and the American Academy of Ophthalmology.[21]

The newest multipurpose solutions were made with both disinfection and comfort in mind featuring two significant chemical preservatives and agents to improve wettability. Biotrue contains hyaluronan, which adheres to the lens and acts as a moisturizing agent. OptiFree PureMoist is set apart from its predecessors in that it contains increased concentrations of preservatives and a different surfactant (polyoxyethylene-polyoxybutylene) to improve wettability. RevitaLens OcuTec solution contains the preservative alexidine, which provides broad antimicrobial coverage and is often found in mouthwashes. Table 29–6 compares products made specifically for use with soft contact lenses.[32]

Reactions to solutions should always be considered in the differential diagnosis in attempts to discern the cause of patient symptoms or findings of surface irritation during an eye examination. Most if not all of the chemicals listed as preservatives can cause irritation to the epithelium.[33] If symptoms are related to solution use, possible remedies are to use a final saline rinse before lens insertion or to change to another formulation of multipurpose solution that uses a different preservative. Another alternative for patients who are sensitive to chemical-based care systems is the PuriLens system, as discussed earlier.

Cleaning Products

Daily use of separate cleaners and protein removal products, in addition to use of multipurpose solutions, generally is not necessary

TABLE 29-6 Selected Products for Use With Soft Lenses

Trade Name	Disinfectants/Preservatives	Other Ingredients
Surface-Active Cleaning Solutions		
Sensitive Eyes Daily Cleaner	Sorbic acid 0.25%, EDTA 0.5%	Hydroxypropyl methylcellulose, sodium chloride, borate buffer, poloxamine
Sof/Pro 2 Sterile Extra Strength Daily Cleaner	None	Purified water, isopropyl alcohol 15.7%, poloxamer 407, amphoteric 10
Sereine Extra Strength Daily Cleaner	None	Purified water, isopropyl alcohol 15.7%, poloxamer 407, amphoteric 10
Combination Hydrogen Peroxide Disinfecting Solutions and Rinsing/Neutralizing Products		
Clear Care	Hydrogen peroxide 3%	0.79% sodium chloride, phosphoric acid, phosphate buffer, Pluronic 17R4
Clear Care Plus	Hydrogen peroxide 3%	Phosphonic acid, sodium chloride 0.79%, phosphate buffer, Pluronic 17R4, EOBO-21-polyethylene-polyoxybutylene
Oxysept UltraCare	Hydrogen peroxide 3%	Sodium stannate, sodium nitrate, phosphates
PeroxiClear	Hydrogen peroxide 3%	Phosphonic acid, potassium chloride, propylene glycol, carbamide, poloxamer 181, citrate and phosphate buffer
Preserved Saline Solutions		
Sensitive Eyes Plus Saline	Sorbic acid 0.1%, EDTA	Sodium chloride, borate buffer
Preservative-Free Saline Products		
PuriLens Solution[a]	None	Isotonic, buffered saline
Rewetting/Lubricating Solutions		
Blink Contacts Lubricant Eye Drops	Stabilized oxychloro complex 0.005% (OcuPure)	Purified water, sodium hyaluronate, sodium chloride, potassium chloride, calcium chloride, magnesium chloride, boric acid
Complete Lubricating and Rewetting Drops	Polyhexamethylene biguanide 0.0001%, EDTA	Purified water, sodium chloride, tromethamine, hydroxypropyl methylcellulose
Clerz Plus Lens Drops	Polyquaternium-1 0.001%, EDTA 0.05%	Sodium chloride, citrate buffer, Clens 100, Tetronic 1304
Opti-Free Express Rewetting Drops	Polyquaternium-1 0.001%, EDTA 0.05%	Citric acid, sodium citrate, sodium chloride
Opti-Free Lubricant Eye Drops	Polyquaternium-1 0.001%, EDTA	Propylene glycol 0.6%, boric acid, dimyristoyl phosphatidylglycerol, hydroxypropyl guar, mineral oil, polyoxyl 40 stearate, sorbitan tristearate, sorbitol, purified water
ReNu Rewetting Drops	Sorbic acid 0.15%, EDTA 0.1%	Boric acid, poloxamine, sodium chloride
Renu MultiPlus Lubricating and Rewetting Drops	Sorbic acid 0.1%, EDTA 0.1%	Povidone, boric acid, potassium chloride, sodium borate, sodium chloride
Sensitive Eyes Rewetting Drops	Sorbic acid 0.1%, EDTA 0.025%	Boric acid, sodium borate, sodium chloride
Multipurpose Solutions		
Biotrue	Polyaminopropyl biguanide (PHMB) 0.00013%, polyquaternium 0.0001%, edetate disodium	Hyaluronan, sulfobetaine, poloxamine, boric acid, sodium borate, sodium chloride
Complete Multi-Purpose Solution Easy Rub Formula	Polyhexamethylene biguanide 0.0001%, EDTA	Purified water, phosphate buffer, poloxamer 237, sodium chloride, potassium chloride
OPTI-FREE Express	Polyquaternium-1 0.001%, myristamidopropyl dimethylamine 0.0005%, EDTA	Sodium citrate, sodium chloride, citric acid, citrate buffer, aminomethypropanol, Tetronic 1304

(continued)

TABLE 29-6 **Selected Products for Use With Soft Lenses** *(continued)*

Trade Name	Disinfectants/Preservatives	Other Ingredients
OPTI-FREE PureMoist	Polyquaternium-1 0.001%, myristamidopropyl dimethylamine 0.0006%, EDTA	Sodium citrate, sodium chloride, boric acid, sorbitol, aminomethylpropanol, Tetronic 1304, EOBO-41
OPTI-FREE Replenish	Polyquaternium-1 0.001%, myristamidopropyl dimethylamine 0.0005%	Sodium citrate, sodium chloride, sodium borate, propylene glycol, Tetronic 1304, nonanoyl ethylenediaminetriaceticacid
Renu Fresh	Polyaminopropyl biguanide 0.0001%, EDTA	Hydroxyalkylphosphonate, boric acid, poloxamine, sodium borate, sodium chloride
Renu Sensitive	Polyaminopropyl biguanide 0.00005%, EDTA	Sodium chloride, sodium borate, boric acid, poloxamine
RevitaLens Ocutec	Alexidine dihydrochloride 0.00016% Polyquaternium-1 0.0003%, EDTA	Boric acid, sodium borate decahydrate, Tetronic 904, sodium citrate, sodium chloride

Key: EDTA = Ethylenediaminetetraacetic acid.
[a] To be used only with the PuriLens UV System.

with disposable lenses that will be discarded after a few weeks of wear. These products should be recommended if patients have longer replacement schedules (>1 month) or demonstrate rapid formation of heavy deposits on lenses. The nature of deposits varies, but they generally consist of proteins and lipids from lacrimal secretions.

Soft lens cleaning solutions generally contain a nonionic detergent, a wetting agent, a chelating agent, buffers, preservatives, and, in some cases, polymeric cleaning beads. Cleaning with a surface-active cleaner can be done daily or, in the case of continuous-wear lenses, each time they are removed from the eyes. In addition to surfactants, some products contain mild abrasives that aid in the removal of lens deposits. Patients who have difficulty removing deposits from their lenses will benefit from this type of cleaner. These products should be shaken before use. Care should be taken to ensure that no residue from the cleaning solution remains on the lens before insertion. Some surface-active cleaners (e.g., Bausch + Lomb Sensitive Eyes Daily Cleaner) have a lower viscosity and may be good choices for patients who have difficulty completely rinsing the cleaner off their lenses.

Although the surface-active cleaners generally are quite effective in removing lipid deposits, they remove tenacious protein debris less successfully. Enzymatic cleaners constitute an additional cleaning aid that can solve this problem. These enzymes hydrolyze polypeptide bonds of protein and dissolve the protein deposits. For the enzyme solution to work properly, however, the lens must be cleaned with a surface-active cleaner first; enzymes are ineffective on debris that covers or is mixed with protein.

Enzymatic cleaners are recommended according to the disinfection system used by the patient. Ultrazyme and Unizyme are used weekly with hydrogen peroxide cleaning systems.[34] These products can be placed in the peroxide solution, thereby cleaning and disinfecting lenses at the same time. Table 29–7 lists characteristics of available enzymatic products.

Saline Solutions

A common source of confusion among patients is the use of saline solutions in lieu of disinfecting agents. At one point, isotonic normal saline was the basic solution used for rinsing, thermally disinfecting, and storing soft contact lenses.[27] It is now recognized, however, that saline used alone lacks disinfecting properties, and the HCP should direct the patient toward a suitable multipurpose or hydrogen peroxide solution.

Saline still has a use as a final rinsing agent before insertion, especially for patients who experience eye irritation from the chemicals in multipurpose solutions. Prepared saline is available in either preserved or preservative-free forms. Sorbic acid–preserved products are commonly promoted for sensitive eyes and appear to be acceptable to most wearers. Several preservative-free saline solutions are also available but must be used within 30 days if they are in a multiuse bottle. Patients using nonpreserved saline should be counseled that only aerosolized solutions can be used to rinse lenses just before insertion into the eye. Multipurpose nonpreserved saline (e.g., Unisol 4) should never be used to rinse lenses just before insertion, unless the bottle is new and has not been opened. Once

TABLE 29-7 **Enzymatic Contact Lens Cleaners With Disinfectant Properties**

Trade Name	Active Ingredient	Concurrent Use With Chemical Preservative Disinfection	Concurrent Use With Hydrogen Peroxide Disinfection
Ultrazyme Tablets	Subtilisin A	No	Yes
Unizyme Tablets	Subtilisin A	No	Yes

these products have been opened, they should be used only if a disinfection step will be performed before insertion. Patients should avoid using other forms of saline, such as intravenous normal saline or saline nasal sprays, because these products usually are too acidic for use with soft contact lenses. Patients should not try to make their own saline solution, because it can become easily contaminated and cause infections.

Rewetting Solutions

Because dryness and discomfort with contact lens wear are common, additional lubricating or wetting drops are often recommended for use during lens wear. Exposing lenses to wind and high temperature also causes some dehydration, even with the lens in the eye. These accessory solutions permit lubricating and rewetting and, in some cases, cleaning of the soft lens while on the eye. Patients should be directed toward products specific for use with contact lenses, to avoid drops preserved with benzalkonium chloride. Preservative-free lubricating drops are also a good alternative. The associated discomfort is sometimes relieved by 1 or 2 drops of rewetting solution. To minimize contamination, the tip of the applicator bottle should not touch the eye, eyelid, or any other surface.

Generic Solutions

Many generic versions of brand-name solutions are now available. Of note, however, patients who choose to buy generic (e.g., mass merchandiser–labeled) multipurpose lens solutions may be purchasing older, potentially obsolete formulas. Mass merchandisers generally acquire older formulations of nationally known brands of multipurpose solutions and then market them under their private label. In addition, the composition of a particular generic formulation can vary because the generic brand stores submit bids to manufacturers two or three times per year. Generally, patients should not use generic brands unless they carefully read the label and compare all ingredients with those of the product that was recommended by their eye care or other provider. Manufacturers are not required to use the same name for generic and brand-name ingredients, so comparing formulations may be difficult.[35]

Product Incompatibility

Several incompatibilities may occur during mixing of soft lens products. Most manufacturers test for compatibility within their own product lines; however, compatibility with other manufacturers' products is usually not determined. Generally, chemical disinfecting solutions should not be used interchangeably or concurrently, as discussed earlier.

Product Selection Guidelines

Table 29–6 lists examples of products designed specifically for soft contact lenses.

Insertion and Removal

Table 29–8 provides instructions for inserting and removing soft lenses.

Gas-Permeable Lens Care

The care of GP contact lenses follows the same general guidelines as for soft lenses, but the solutions for GP and soft lenses are not interchangeable. The patient's eye care provider will recommend various products and regimens for the particular GP lens type, and lens wearers should be advised against substituting other products for those specifically recommended.

Rigid lens care involves the steps of cleaning, disinfecting, soaking, and wetting (Figure 29–2), which should be performed each time the lenses are removed from the eye, for optimal lens care. Modern solutions combine these steps in various formulations. Because GP lenses are replaced less frequently, allowing more time for deposits to accumulate, separate solutions for daily cleaning and protein removal are still popular. Oxidation systems (hydrogen peroxide) can also be used, but heat disinfection should not be used with GP lenses. Rinsing with tap water also is not recommended because of microorganisms in the water.[36] Tables 29–3, 29–5, 29–7, and 29–9 specify proper cleaning and disinfecting procedures for rigid contact lenses.

TABLE 29–8 Insertion and Removal of Soft Lenses

Insertion

- Wash your hands with noncosmetic soap and rinse thoroughly; dry hands with a lint-free towel.
- Remove one lens from its storage container.
- Rinse the lens with saline solution to dilute any preservatives left from disinfection (optional).
- Place the lens on the top of a finger, and examine it to be sure it is not inside out. This determination can be made by means of the "taco test": Gently fold the lens at the apex (not the edges) between your thumb and forefinger. The edges should look like a taco shell with the edges pointed inward. If the edges roll out, the lens is inverted and must be reversed.
- Examine the lens for cleanliness. If necessary, clean it and rinse again.
- Place the lens on the eye using the procedure described for GP lenses (Table 29–11).
- Repeat all steps with the other lens.

Removal

- Before removing the lenses, wash hands with a noncosmetic soap; rinse hands thoroughly and dry them with a lint-free towel.
- Using the right middle finger, pull down the lower lid of the right eye. Touch the right index finger to the lens and slide the lens off the cornea, as shown in drawing A.
- Using the index finger and thumb, grasp the lens and remove it (drawing B).
- Repeat the procedure for the left eye.

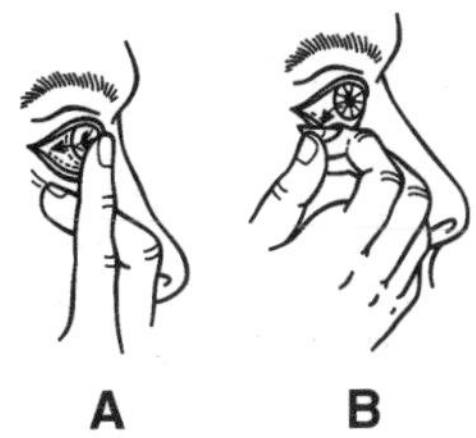

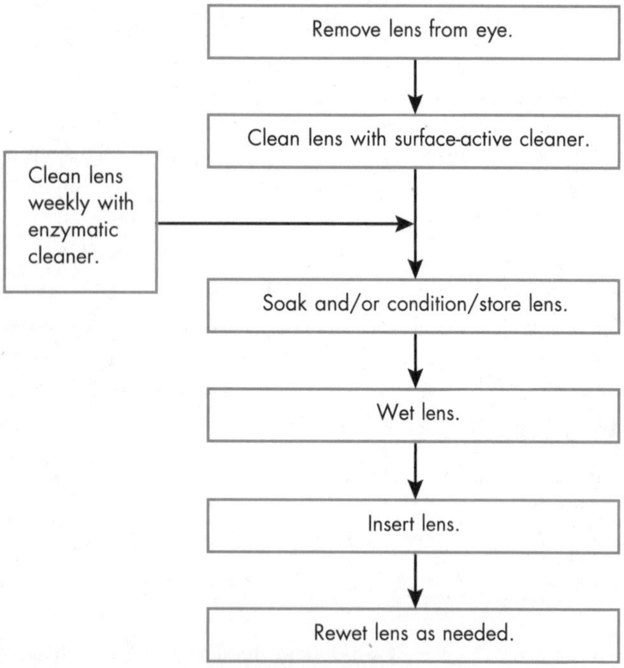

FIGURE 29-2 Self-care for gas-permeable lenses.

Product Selection Guidelines

With the abundance of combination wetting–disinfection solutions now on the market, the appropriate lens care regimen for GP lenses is fairly straightforward. Patients wearing GP lenses should be advised to purchase a surface-active cleaning product, an enzymatic product, and a conditioning or soaking solution, depending on the type of lens worn. A rewetting or reconditioning product should also be recommended. Table 29–10 lists examples of products for use with GP lenses.

TABLE 29-9 Specific Cleaning Procedures for Gas-Permeable (GP) Lenses

- Use the cleansing, soaking, and conditioning products recommended by your eye care provider for care of your lenses.
- If you are unsure of your lens type, ask the eye care provider about proper cleaning procedures.
- Upon removal of the lens, apply an appropriate cleaning solution to both lens surfaces. Then rub the lens with the tip of the forefinger against the palm of the opposite hand, using a back-and-forth motion, to avoid chipping an edge, which may occur if the lens is cleaned between the forefinger and the thumb. Do not apply too much pressure. If debris is still on the lens, soak a cotton swab in the surfactant cleaner, and use the swab to clean the lens.
- Soak and store the lenses in a soaking or conditioning solution recommended by the eye care provider for the specified amount of time. Rewet lenses before inserting them in the eyes.
- Enzymatic cleaning may also be recommended by your eye care provider and is typically performed weekly.

Source: Reference 36.

Cleaning Solutions

Cleaning solutions are used more often for GP lenses because of the longer wear time before disposal Accumulated residue, primarily proteinaceous debris and lipids from tears and glandular secretions, acts as a growth medium for bacteria. If not routinely removed by daily cleaning, the residue may harden to form coatings or tenacious deposits that create an irregular surface on the lens. Decreased visual acuity and shorter toleration time are likely consequences of a cloudy lens created by this residue. Cleaners formulated for tenacious deposits contain silica gel, which acts to mechanically break the adhesive bonds that have formed between the lens and the deposits. Homemade cleaning solutions should never be used, owing to the potential risk of scratching, contaminating, or damaging the lens.

Soaking Solutions

Soaking solutions are used to store rigid contact lenses after removal and during insertion of the lens in the eye. The solution maintains lenses in a constant state of hydration for maximum comfort and visual acuity, and it aids in removing deposits that accumulate on the lenses during wear. If lenses are allowed to dry out during overnight storage, accumulated deposits are more difficult to remove with normal cleaning.

An ideal soaking solution performs the following functions: (1) it converts the hydrophobic lens surface to a hydrophilic surface by means of a uniform film that does not easily wash away; (2) it increases comfort by providing cushioning and lubrication between the contacting surfaces; (3) it places a viscous coating on the lens to protect it from oil on the fingers during insertion; and (4) it stabilizes the lens on the fingertip to ease insertion, particularly for individuals with poor manual dexterity or unsteady hands. Cellulose gum derivatives are often used in such solutions, but they do not promote uniform wetting of a rigid lens; therefore, polyvinyl alcohol is also often used to decrease surface tension.

Because GP lenses that contain high levels of silicone have decreased surface wettability, *conditioning solutions* are generally used instead of soaking solutions to aid in the formation of a cushioning tear layer. A conditioning solution is essentially a specially formulated wetting solution that enhances wettability of the lens, increases wearing comfort, and disinfects the lens. Saliva should never be used to wet contact lenses because it can lead to infection by many pathogens.

Rewetting Solutions

Rewetting solutions are intended to clean and rewet the contact lens while it is in the eye. These solutions depend on the use of surfactants to loosen deposits; removal is assisted by the natural cleaning action of blinking. Although these products function well to recondition the lens, the cornea benefits more if the lens is actually removed, cleaned, and rewetted. Removing the lens for even a brief time allows the cornea to be resurfaced with a new proteinaceous or mucinaceous layer.

To maintain sterility in rewetting products, preservative levels are carefully selected. Higher levels do not necessarily result in increased effectiveness and may lead to impaired wetting or corneal irritation because of the adsorption of preservatives onto the lens. Most rewetting agents are preserved, multidose products. Patients who use these products frequently should be encouraged to use products that contain preservatives such as oxychloro complex or perborates. Patients should be informed that preserved artificial tears and rewetting agents are different; most preserved artificial tears are incompatible with contact lenses.[37]

TABLE 29–10 Selected Products for Use With Gas-Permeable Lenses

		Function							
Manufacturer	**Product**	**Wetting**	**Daily Cleaner**	**Weekly Cleaner**	**Soaking**	**Cleaning/ Soaking**	**Wetting/ Soaking**	**Lubricant**	**Preservative(s)**
Abbot Medical Optics	Blink Contacts							X	None
Alcon	Clear Care					X			None
	Clear Care Plus				X	X	X	X	None
	Clerz Plus Lens Drops						X	X	EDTA, polyquaternium-1 0.001%
Bausch + Lomb	Boston Advance Comfort Formula Conditioning Solution						X		EDTA, chlorhexidine, polyaminy-lpropyl biguanide
	Boston Advance Cleaner		X						None
	Boston Conditioning Solution		X		X		X		EDTA, chlorhexidine
	Boston Cleaner Original Formula		X						None
	Boston Simplus Multi-Action Solution	X	X		X	X	X	X	Chlorhexidine, polyaminopropyl biguanide
	Boston One Step Liquid Enzymatic Cleaner			X					None
	Boston Rewetting Drops							X	EDTA, chlorhexidine
Lobob	Cleaner		X						
	Optimum Extra Strength Cleaner		X						
	Soaking Solution				X				EDTA, benzalkonium chloride
	Optimum Wetting/Rewetting	X						X	Benzyl alcohol
	Wetting Solution	X							EDTA, benzalkonium chloride
	Optimum Cleaning, Disinfecting, Storage		X			X			Benzyl alcohol
Menicon	Unique pH	X			X	X	X	X	Poly quaternium-1 0.001%
	Progent Protein Remover			X					None
	Wetting and Rewetting	X							EDTA, sorbic acid, benzyl alcohol
	MeniCare CDS		X			X			EDTA, benzyl alcohol

Key: EDTA = Ethylenediaminetetraacetic acid.

TABLE 29–11 **Insertion and Removal of Gas-Permeable Lenses**

Insertion

- After washing your hands, remove one lens from the lens storage case, rinse it with fresh conditioning or soaking solution, and inspect it for cleanliness and signs of damage (cracks or chips).
- If a wetting or conditioning solution is being used, place a few drops on the lens.
- Place the lens on the top of the index finger, as shown in drawing A.
- Place the middle finger of the same hand on the lower lid and pull it down (drawing B).
- With the other hand, use a finger to lift the upper lid, and then place the lens on the eye (drawing C).
- Release the lids and blink.
- Check vision immediately to see if the lens is in the proper position.
- If vision is blurred, blink three or four times. If vision is still blurred, the lens may be off center, on the wrong eye, or dirty.
  - Instill 1–3 drops of rewetting or reconditioning drops into the eye.
  - If vision is not improved, remove the lens, place several drops of wetting or conditioning solution onto both surfaces, and reinsert lens.
- Repeat all steps with the other lens.

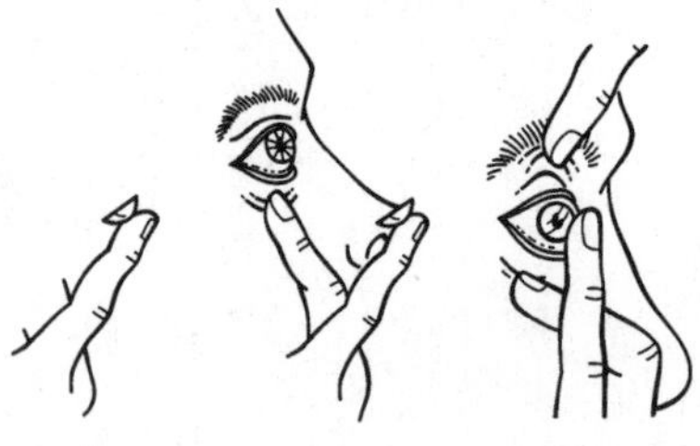

A B C

Removal

- Before removing the lenses, wash hands with a noncosmetic soap; rinse hands thoroughly and dry them with a lint-free towel.
- Before removing the lens, fill the storage cases with soaking or conditioning solution.
- Remove the top from the cleaning solution.
- Place a hand (or a towel) under the eye.
- Use one of the following methods to remove the lens from the eye.

Two-Finger Method of Removing Lenses

- Place the tip of the forefinger of one hand on the middle of the upper eyelid by the lashes, as shown in drawing D.
- Place the forefinger of the other hand on the center of the lower lid margin (drawing D).
- Push the lids inward and then together, as shown in drawing E. The lens should pop out.
- If the lens becomes displaced onto only the white part of the eye, recenter the lens and try again.

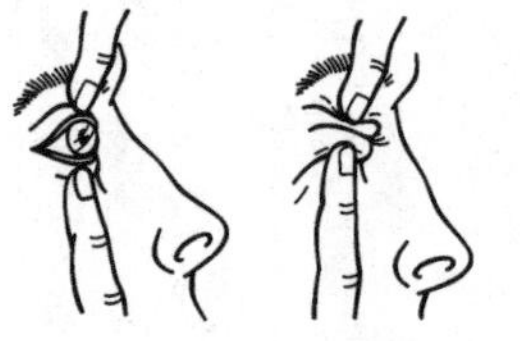

D E

Temporal Pull/Blink Method of Removing Lenses

- Place an index finger on the temporal edge of the lower and upper lids. Initially, widen the eyelids a little (drawing F).
- Stretch the skin outward and slightly upward without allowing the lid to slide over the lens. Blink briskly, as shown in drawing G. The lens will pop out because of the pressure of the eyelids at the top and bottom of the lens. Blinking facilitates removal after the lids have been tightened around the lens.

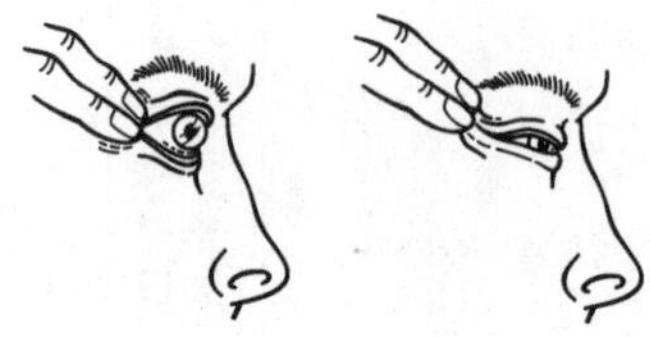

F G

Enzymatic Solutions

As the silicone content of GP lenses increases, so does the amount of protein adherence. Silicone acrylate lenses have an active surface that promotes the binding of tear constituents. Protein deposits on a lens will decrease the oxygen permeability and may contribute to wear discomfort. If daily cleaning is not sufficient, lenses of this type should be cleaned with an enzymatic product once weekly.[36] Omission of this cleaning step may result in the need for professional polishing or replacement of the lens.

Insertion and Removal

Wearers of GP lenses should be counseled to follow proper insertion and removal procedures (Table 29–11).

Lens Storage Case

Patient education on the care of all contact lenses must include discussion of the proper care and cleaning of the contact lens storage case as well as the lens material. A dirty lens case can be contaminated with a biofilm that will attract pathogens and increase the risk of infection. The lens case should be cleaned daily. After lens insertion, the case (and case lid, if separate) must be emptied, rinsed with the same disinfecting solution, wiped, and air-dried between uses.[38] Tap water should not be used. All added solutions should be discarded daily. The case should not be used if cracked and should be replaced periodically, at least every 3 months.[36,38]

Follow-up Care

Follow-up care is essential for the long-term success of contact lens wear. The minimum recommendation is 1 year between provider visits in the case of uncomplicated lens wear. These visits allow the prescriber to evaluate the integrity of the lenses worn and the condition of the cornea. Patient education content on the wearing schedule, replacement frequency, and lens-care regimen should also be reviewed. Regular contact lens follow-up care is an important aspect of prevention of contact lens complications.

Contact Lens–Related Problems

Both soft and GP contact lenses provide good vision and safe, comfortable wear over years of use, provided that they are fitted properly and patients adhere to correct care regimens. Unfortunately, complications of contact lens wear have not been eradicated despite advances in material, lens design, and solutions. In general, soft contact lens wearers tend to have more complications because less tear exchange occurs beneath the lens and because wear times are longer, including overnight. Problems with GP lenses tend to be related to improper fit. Although occasional symptoms of mild redness and discomfort are common with contact lens wear, eye care providers should be familiar with more severe symptoms that may herald significant complications, including threats to sight. Whenever a patient presents with signs or symptoms that are believed to be related to contact lens wear, discontinuing lens wear is recommended until the underlying cause is diagnosed and treated. Therefore, every patient should have eyeglasses to wear as a backup for contact lenses.

Evaluation of a contact lens–related problem should begin with a thorough history of the problem. During the patient interview, the eye care provider should determine what types of eye problems are present and how long the patient has been experiencing them. Ascertaining whether the patient has a previous history of eye problems and identifying current medications will give a general sense of the etiology and urgency of the presenting problem. This information also will help to determine whether the problem is related to noncompliance with care regimens or to drug–lens interactions. Determining which type of contact lenses a patient is wearing and how long the patient has worn them is crucial in assessing problems that are related to improper lens care or deteriorated lenses. Patients should be asked to describe how they care for their lenses, which lens care products they use, and whether they have recently changed products.

Unfortunately, mild and severe complications of lens wear manifest with similar symptoms that overlap and vary in degree. For example, mild redness and irritation in both eyes occurring at the end of the day for several weeks or months are likely to reflect dryness that might resolve with a change in lens material, wearing schedule, or lubricating drops. However, a patient who presents with acute symptoms of marked, sectoral redness in one eye, accompanied by photophobia and pain that started 1 day earlier, suggests a more severe problem such as a corneal ulcer.

The following signs and symptoms are common manifestations of lens-related problems:

- *Itching.* Patients are usually not allergic to lens materials, but they may have an allergy to solutions. Itching may also be a sign of allergic conjunctivitis unrelated to lens wear.
- *Blurred vision.* Mild blurring may suggest wrong lens power, lenses switched between eyes, lenses placed on the eye inside out, or debris buildup on the lens. Blurring also accompanies problems with the ocular surface, such as superficial keratitis, corneal abrasion, and corneal edema associated with infiltration or ulceration.
- *Redness.* Redness can occur as a response to numerous insults. The degree of redness typically, but not always, corresponds to the severity of the problem. Mild, diffuse redness can accompany end-of-day dryness, whereas severe redness, especially sectoral, can indicate a corneal problem. Ocular decongestants reduce the mild conjunctival hyperemia associated with prolonged lens wear. On cessation of use of these topical agents, however, a rebound hyperemia can result, especially with use for longer than 72 hours. Therefore, routine use of these products should be avoided, and if symptoms persist, the patient should be referred to an eye care provider.
- *Pain.* Pain is a significant finding because it is likely to be related to pathology involving the eye's corneal nerve endings. Mild discomfort or irritation is not uncommon among wearers of all types of contact lenses. It may be related to the material, lens fit, or a torn or dirty lens. Severe pain or deep aching of the eye can signify corneal abrasions, infiltrates, or ulcers and typically persists even after removal of the lens. These latter symptoms are likely to represent urgent, sight-threatening conditions, and referral to an eye care provider is essential.
- *Fogging.* Misty or smoky vision can be caused by coatings or deposits on lens surfaces or by poor wetting of the lens while on the eye.
- *Photophobia (light sensitivity).* Similar to pain, photophobia suggests complications with the cornea or may be a symptom of iritis. This symptom necessitates referral to an eye care provider.
- *Excessive tearing.* Corneal nerves can start a feedback loop that promotes tearing; therefore, irritation to the corneal surface, such as a torn or dirty lens, will increase tearing.
- *Flare.* Point sources of light that have a sunburst or streaming quality can be caused by inadequate optic zone size or decentration of a poorly fitting lens.
- *Lens falling out of the eye.* Improper fit is usually the cause; however, even properly fitted rigid lenses may occasionally slide off the cornea or be blinked out of the eye. Soft lenses that dry out on the eye may move excessively and dislocate.
- *Squinting.* This effect is caused by excessive movement of a lens or by a poorly fitted lens. The wearer will squint as an unconscious maneuver to center the optical portion of the lens over the pupil. Squinting may also indicate improper lens power.

Redness, discomfort, and dryness are the most common ocular complaints and the leading causes of discontinuing lens wear. Even with brand new contact lenses, mere presence of the lens disrupts the tear film and alters the environment of the anterior ocular surface, with corresponding clinical effects. A change in lens material or solution, alteration of lens fit, or use of lubricating drops usually leads to symptomatic improvement.

By contrast, microbial keratitis (leading to corneal ulceration) is the most serious complication of contact lens wear. The HCP should be alert for signs and symptoms of this condition including blurred vision, redness, pain, light sensitivity, and watering that often worsen even after discontinuation of lens wear. A white infiltrate visible on the cornea requires urgent referral for evaluation by an eye care provider. Removal of contact lenses and prompt treatment are crucial to improve outcomes.

Overall, distinguishing common lens wear–associated complaints from signs of more severe inflammatory or infectious complications can be challenging. Considerations include whether one or both eyes are involved, the duration and severity of symptoms, and whether symptoms are isolated or found in conjunction with others. Even experienced HCPs have difficulty distinguishing inflammatory from infectious complications. Timely referral to an eye care provider is indicated if the clinical findings suggest more than lens wear–associated symptoms.

Precautions for Contact Lens Wear

Adverse Effects of Drugs

Many undesired effects have been reported when a patient who wears contact lenses ingests, applies, or encounters certain drugs (Table 29–12). Wearers of soft hydrophilic contact lenses should

TABLE 29-12 Drug–Contact Lens Interactions

Changes in Tear Film or Production

Decreased Tear Volume

Alcohol
Anticholinergic agents
Antihistamines
Antipsychotics
Beta blockers
Benzodiazepines
Botulinum toxin type A (Botox)
Conjugated estrogens
Diuretics/thiazides
Histamine-2 (H_2) receptor antagonists
Oral contraceptives
Pain relievers—ibuprofen, acetaminophen-containing products
Phenothiazines
Proton pump inhibitors
Retinoids
Selective serotonin reuptake inhibitors
Sildenafil citrate
Statins
Timolol (topical)
Tricyclic antidepressants
Vardenafil HCl

Increased Tear Volume

Cholinergic agents
Garlic (dietary supplement)
Reserpine

Changes in Lens Color (Primarily With Soft Lenses)

Diagnostic dyes (i.e., fluorescein)
Epinephrine (topical)
Fluorescein (topical)
Nicotine
Nitrofurantoin
Phenazopyridine
Phenolphthalein
Phenothiazines
Phenylephrine
Rifampin
Sulfasalazine
Tetracycline
Tetrahydrozoline (topical)

Changes in Tear Tonicity

Pilocarpine (8%)
Sodium sulfacetamide (10%)

Lid/Corneal Edema

Chlorthalidone
Clomiphene
Conjugated estrogens
Oral contraceptives
Primidone

Ocular Inflammation/Irritation

Diclofenac (topical ophthalmic)
Garlic (dietary supplement)
Gold salts
Isotretinoin
Salicylates

Changes in Refractivity (Induction of Myopia)

Acetazolamide
Sulfadiazine
Sulfamethizole
Sulfamethoxazole
Sulfisoxazole

Changes in Pupil Size

Pupillary Dilation

Anticholinergic agents
Antidepressants
Antihistamines
CNS stimulants
Kava
Phenothiazines

Pupillary Miosis

Opiates

Miscellaneous Drug Effects

Digoxin—increased glare
Sedative-hypnotics/muscle relaxants—decreased blink rate
Ribavirin—cloudy lenses
Topical ciprofloxacin/prednisolone acetate—precipitate

Key: CNS = Central nervous system.

Source: Adapted with permission from Engle JP. Contact lens care. *Am Druggist.* 1990;201:5465. Updated with information from references 39 and 42.

be particularly cautious about exposure of the lenses to chemicals. These chemicals, many of which penetrate and bind with the lens material, can come from cosmetics, environmental pollutants, and ophthalmic and systemic products. The health care provider must be fully cognizant of these potential drug-induced problems to counsel patients effectively.

Topical Medications

In general, patients should be counseled not to place any ophthalmic solution, suspension, gel, or ointment into the eye when contact lenses are in place. A nonprescription ophthalmic product that is not specifically designed for compatibility with contact lenses also should not be used when lenses are in the eye. Soft lenses can absorb chemical compounds from topically administered ophthalmic products.[39] Topical administration of ophthalmic drugs also may have physiologic consequences or may modify pharmacologic responses to drugs. The use of solutions that may be considered benign, such as artificial tears, may reduce tear breakup time and alter the distribution of the mucoid, aqueous, and lipid components of tears, perhaps causing initial discomfort on instillation of the drops.[39] A topical drug administered while soft lenses are in place may have an exaggerated pharmacologic effect. The soft lens may absorb the drug and either release it over time, creating a sustained-release dosage form, or bind it tightly so that none of it is released into the eye. Furthermore, the presence of any kind of contact lens may increase the amount of time the medication is in contact with the eye. Finally, increased drug absorption may occur secondary to a compromised corneal epithelium from contact lens wear.[39] The only exceptions to this rule are products specifically formulated to be used with contact lenses, such as rewetting drops, or those products that an eye care provider has specifically recommended for use with contact lenses.

After a drug solution has been instilled into the eye, insertion of a lens must wait until the solution has cleared from the lower eyelid's precorneal (conjunctival) pocket (approximately 5 minutes). Ideally, when topical ophthalmic ointments, gels, or suspensions are being used, the lenses should not be worn at all.

Airborne Drugs and Particulate Matter

Some drugs that are present in indoor air may damage lenses, so HCPs should be cautious with prescribing medications that are administered by inhalation for contact lens wearers. Similarly, lens wearers who have been exposed to a large amount of cigarette smoke have discovered a brown discoloration and nicotine deposits on their lenses. Other particulate matter, such as pollen, animal dander, sawdust, or sand, may also create issues for contact lens wearers.

Systemic Medications

Use of a systemic medication often has far-reaching and unanticipated effects aside from the expected pharmacodynamic actions. Perhaps the most common manifestation of ocular-related systemic drug toxicity is found among contact lens users who develop ocular discomfort or irritation and contact lens intolerance while using a particular systemic drug. Contact lens wearers often present with complaints of new-onset eye dryness or irritation and intolerance to contact lens wear and request a nonprescription product to provide symptomatic relief. Although such symptoms are similar to those arising with other, more common underlying problems, such as improper contact lens hygiene, health care professionals should always consider the pharmacology of specific systemic medications as well as potential relationships between medication initiation and onset of symptoms.[39]

The effects of medications on the eye vary by drug class.[39] As a general rule, compounds with anticholinergic effects can reduce tear volume and induce dry eye, with or without concomitant loss of accommodation and blurry vision.[40] Other classes of drugs, such as hormones (most notably birth control pills), may also alter tear volume and the shape of the corneal surface, resulting in blurring and contact lens intolerance. Some systemic medications are secreted into tears and may interact with the component material of the (primarily soft) lens. For example, rifampin will stain both lenses and tears orange. Drugs and dietary supplements such as gold salts and garlic are secreted into the tears, with consequent ocular irritation. Other drugs may affect tear production, the refractive properties of the eye, the shape of the cornea, or the actual lens (Table 29–12). Some medications may influence the size of the pupil, leading to complaints of glare or flare when lenses are in place. Visual performance may be diminished, especially in patients who wear multifocal lenses or GP lenses, for which pupil size may determine placement of the reading segment or the optic zone of the lens, respectively.[41,42]

Use of Cosmetics

Patients who wear contact lenses should choose—and use—cosmetics with care. The patient should insert lenses before applying makeup and should avoid touching the lens with eyeliner or mascara applicators. Cosmetics, moisturizers, and makeup removers with an aqueous base should be used, because oil-based products may cause blurred vision and irritation if they are deposited on the lens. Water-based products are preferable, and when possible, users should choose makeup that has been specifically formulated for contact lens wearers. Lens wearers should avoid loose powders (e.g., face, eye) and instead use pressed or cream-based products, if available. Water-resistant mascara (as opposed to waterproof mascara, which requires an oil-based remover) should be applied only to the very tips of the lashes. Eyeliners should never be applied inside the eyelid margin; the liner material can clog glands in the eyelid and contaminate the contact lens. Eye makeup products should be discarded and replaced at least every 3 months.[43]

Aerosol products, in particular, must be used with caution: users should close the eyes when applying the product and step out of the mist before opening the eyes. Nail polish, hand creams, and perfumes also should be applied only after the lenses have been inserted. Men often contaminate their lenses with hair preparations and spray deodorants. Lens wearers should be reminded to take special care to clean the hands thoroughly before handling their lenses. Soaps that contain cold cream or deodorants should be avoided.[43]

Corneal Hypoxia and Edema

An adequate supply of oxygen is available only if the cornea is continuously bathed with oxygenated tears. During blinking, metabolic byproducts from the surface epithelium are flushed from under the contact lenses, and oxygen is brought in as the lenses move sequentially toward and away from the cornea. Even when properly fitted, however, both rigid and soft lenses can produce a progressive hypoxia of the cornea while the lenses are in place, especially in individuals who have a low blink frequency or exhibit incomplete blinking.

Corneal Abrasions

Corneal abrasions are surface defects in the epithelial layer of the cornea. The causes of these abrasions range from poorly fitted lenses or simple overwear to the entrapment of foreign bodies under the lens. The cornea is sensitive to abrasion, so blepharospasm (reflexive lid closure), tearing, and rubbing of the affected eye occur immediately. However, rubbing the eye while the lens remains in place can cause more extensive damage and must be avoided. All instances of suspected corneal abrasion require referral for evaluation by an eye care provider.

Fortunately, the pain associated with corneal abrasion usually is worse than the damage sustained. The epithelium regenerates quickly; most minor epithelial defects generally heal within 12–24 hours. The lens should be left out for 2–7 days. The wearer may then proceed to use a modified break-in schedule suggested by the eye care provider.

Exclusions for Self-Care

When lens care is appropriate but the lenses are old or, in the case of hard lenses, chipped or scratched, the patient should see an eye care provider for replacement lenses. Other situations that require referral are suspected vision changes, deep aching of the eyes, occurrence of the last eye examination more than 1 year previously, and a suspected interaction between the lenses and systemic medications. Patients experiencing lens problems that are related to the medical conditions or other factors discussed in the section "Contraindications and Warnings for Contact Lens Wear" also should be referred for further evaluation.

Cases 29–1 and 29–2 illustrate the assessment of two different patients with contact lens–related problems.

CASE 29-1

Relevant Evaluation Criteria	Scenario/Model Outcome
Collect	
1. Gather essential information about the patient's symptoms and medical history, including	
a. Description of symptom(s) (i.e., nature, onset, duration, severity, associated symptoms)	Patient complains of a "fogginess" in both eyes that is not present when she wears her glasses, as well as dry, itchy eyes. She reports that this has been going on for the past week, but it typically occurs toward the end of each month. She wears monthly disposable soft contact lenses and has been wearing the current pair for 3 weeks. She reports changing her lenses on the first of each month and does not sleep in them. The patient's lens care regimen includes soaking the lenses daily by topping off the solution in the case using whatever multipurpose solution is on sale at the store. She also reports she does not rub or rinse the contact lenses daily.
b. Description of any factors that seem to precipitate, exacerbate, and/or relieve the patient's symptom(s)	Patient reports that she experiences less itching and redness when she first starts wearing a new pair of contact lenses.
c. Description of the patient's efforts to relieve the symptoms	Patient has not tried anything.
d. Patient's identity	Esther Smith
e. Patient's age, gender, height, and weight	30 years old, female, 5 ft 6 in., 120 lb
f. Patient's occupation	Administrative assistant
g. Patient's dietary habits	n/a
h. Patient's sleep habits	The patient gets about 6 hours of sleep per night.
i. Concurrent medical conditions, prescription and nonprescription medications, and dietary supplements	Ethinyl estradiol 0.035 mg and norgestimate 0.25 mg, with one menstrual cycle every 84 days
j. Allergies	NKA
k. History of other adverse reactions to medications	None
l. Other (describe) ______	Nonsmoker, social alcohol use on the weekends
Assess	
2. Differentiate patient's signs/symptoms, and correctly identify the patient's primary problem(s).	Discomfort due to poor contact lens hygiene and care, as well as premature contact lens wear, but the problem also could be due to oral contraceptive use.
3. Identify exclusions for self-treatment.	Potential exclusion with oral contraceptive use. This possibility needs to be ruled out.

CASE 29-1 *continued*

Relevant Evaluation Criteria	Scenario/Model Outcome
4. Formulate a comprehensive list of therapeutic alternatives for the primary problem to determine whether triage to a health care provider is required, and share this information with the patient or caregiver.	Options include (1) Refer the patient to an eye care provider. (2) Recommend self-treatment. (3) Take no action.
Plan	
5. Select an optimal therapeutic alternative to address the patient's problem, taking into account patient preferences.	Recommend using proper contact lens care and hygiene.
6. Describe the recommended therapeutic approach to the patient or caregiver.	"Your symptoms suggest that you are not using an appropriate care regimen for your contacts. Topping off the solution can increase the risk of infection, and not rinsing or rubbing your lenses daily can allow buildup of proteins on your lens, leading to fogginess. Also, using any solution that is on sale is not advisable, because it may not contain the same ingredients as in the brand your eye care provider recommended."
7. Explain to the patient or caregiver the rationale for selecting the recommended therapeutic approach from the considered therapeutic alternatives.	"Fogginess is a common contact lens complaint. Your symptoms are present only when you wear the contact lenses toward the end of the month when appropriate contact lens care has not been used. This is likely to be a self-care issue and does not require that you see an eye care provider at this time."
Implement	
8. When recommending self-care with nonprescription medications and/or nondrug therapy, convey accurate information to the patient or caregiver.	
a. Appropriate dose and frequency of administration	"Discard and use new contact lens multipurpose solution daily. Rinse and rub contact lenses to remove proteins daily for at least 20 seconds. Use the recommended contact lens solutions from your eye care provider."
b. Maximum number of days the therapy should be employed	"Perform appropriate lens care daily."
c. Product administration procedures	"If your symptoms do not resolve, then return to your contact lens specialist for a refitting appointment and other options."
d. Expected time to onset of relief	"Symptoms should resolve within the next day."
e. Degree of relief that can be reasonably expected	"The fogginess should disappear with proper cleaning."
f. Most common adverse effects	n/a
g. Adverse effects that warrant medical intervention should they occur	"Fogginess that does not go away warrants medical attention."
h. Patient options in the event that condition worsens or persists	"See your eye care provider if the fogginess persists even after proper cleaning of the lenses, because your oral contraceptive could instead be causing the problem."
i. Product storage requirements	"Solution should be stored at room temperature in a dry place. The contact lens case should be allowed to air dry while contact lenses are not in it."
j. Specific nondrug measures	n/a
Solicit follow-up questions from the patient or caregiver.	"What if I don't want to have to do this every day?"
Answer the patient's or caregiver's questions.	"You can call your eye care provider and discuss some options. The provider could potentially change your prescription to daily disposable contact lenses."
Monitor: Follow-up and Evaluate	
9. Assess patient outcome.	"Please call me and let me know how everything is going and if these suggestions worked for you or if you have any more questions."

Key: n/a = Not applicable; NKA = no known allergies.

CASE 29-2

Relevant Evaluation Criteria	Scenario/Model Outcome
Collect	
1. Gather essential information about the patient's symptoms and medical history, including	
a. Description of symptom(s) (i.e., nature, onset, duration, severity, associated symptoms)	Patient complains of pain and aching in his left eye. He reports he initially woke up with this several mornings ago and thought it would go away, but the pain has become a bit worse. Yesterday, he did not wear his contact lenses all day to see if that would help. He follows all of his eye care provider recommendations for cleaning and use of his GP contact lenses. He reports that his last eye exam was more than a year and a half ago.
b. Description of any factors that seem to precipitate, exacerbate, and/or relieve the patient's symptom(s)	Patient reports that not wearing contact lenses helps.
c. Description of the patient's efforts to relieve the symptoms	The patient has not tried anything to help the situation other than not wearing contact lenses yesterday.
d. Patient's identity	Roger Chavez
e. Patient's age, gender, height, and weight	50 years old, male, 6 ft 5 in., 200 lb
f. Patient's occupation	Engineer
g. Patient's dietary habits	Patient eats a balanced diet.
h. Patient's sleep habits	Patient has to work long hours, but he gets about 6 hours of sleep per night.
i. Concurrent medical conditions, prescription and nonprescription medications, and dietary supplements	Patient has high cholesterol and takes atorvastatin 10 mg. No other conditions requiring medication. He does take a multivitamin daily.
j. Allergies	Penicillin
k. History of other adverse reactions to medications	None
l. Other (describe) ______	Patient is a nonsmoker and drinks socially.
Assess	
2. Differentiate patient's signs/symptoms, and correctly identify the patient's primary problem(s).	Corneal abrasion, contact lens–induced
3. Identify exclusions for self-treatment.	Possible corneal abrasion caused by overwear, possible poor fit, or a chip or scratch in the lens
	Pain that does not subside with removal of contact lenses
4. Formulate a comprehensive list of therapeutic alternatives for the primary problem to determine whether triage to a health care provider is required, and share this information with the patient or caregiver.	Options include (1) Refer the patient to eye care provider.
Plan	
5. Select an optimal therapeutic alternative to address the patient's problem, taking into account patient preferences.	Inform patient that he needs to get immediate care from his eye care provider or go to a hospital emergency department to identify the extent of the problem. The patient should not use self-care treatment at this time.
6. Describe the recommended therapeutic approach to the patient or caregiver.	"Your symptoms suggest that you have injured your eye, and you need to go to either your eye care provider or a hospital emergency department immediately."
7. Explain to the patient or caregiver the rationale for selecting the recommended therapeutic approach from the considered therapeutic alternatives.	"Self-care treatment is not recommended for your condition, and no nonprescription products are currently available to treat these problems. You need to go to either your eye care provider or the emergency department immediately to prevent any permanent damage, such as vision loss."

CASE 29-2 *continued*

Relevant Evaluation Criteria	Scenario/Model Outcome
Implement	
8. When recommending self-care with nonprescription medications and/or nondrug therapy, convey accurate information to the patient or caregiver.	Criterion does not apply in this case.
Solicit follow-up questions from the patient or caregiver.	"It is a really busy week at work. Do you think I can wait until this evening to contact my eye care provider?"
Answer the patient's or caregiver's questions.	"No, you need to be seen by your eye care provider or an emergency department physician immediately. You could suffer permanent damage to your eye if it is not treated immediately."
Monitor: Follow-up and Evaluate	
9. Assess patient outcome.	"Please call me and let me know how everything worked out. Also, in the future, feel free to contact me with any questions you may have."

Key: GP = Gas-permeable.

Patient Counseling for Prevention of Contact Lens–Related Disorders

Patient education on lens insertion and removal should always be provided at the time lenses are fitted. Patients should also be instructed on proper care techniques, with a specific recommendation for a lens care system. Often the prescriber's advice to use a particular product is ignored, and patients select products by price alone, especially with the availability of generic solutions. Similar product labels and lack of standardized labeling lead to further confusion. Patients often ask whether it matters which solution they use. The correct answer is that it does matter, because incompatible solutions can be the cause of contact lens complications. Lens care products typically are formulated for use with either soft or gas-permeable lenses and, with a few exceptions, should not be used interchangeably. The box "Patient Education for Prevention of Contact Lens–Related Disorders" outlines the care regimen for each type of contact lens.

PATIENT EDUCATION FOR Prevention of Contact Lens–Related Disorders

The objective of contact lens care is to prevent lens-related problems such as abrasions or infections of the cornea. For most patients, following the prescribed lens care regimen, product instructions, and self-care measures listed here will help ensure trouble-free use of contact lenses.

General Care Instructions for Most Contact Lens Types

- See Table 29–3. Wash hands with noncosmetic soap and rinse them thoroughly before handling or caring for contact lenses.
- Each time contact lenses are removed, clean, rinse, and disinfect them before wearing them again.
- Gently rub both surfaces of the contact lens, rinse thoroughly, and soak lenses overnight in the recommended solution according to the eye care provider's instructions.
- For care of your lenses, use only those contact lens products recommended by the prescribing eye care provider.
- Do not change brands or products unless instructed to do so by the eye care provider. (Not all care systems are alike, and some may not be compatible with the contact lenses prescribed.)
- Do not top off a storage solution in the case after the solution has been used.
- Replace soaking or disinfecting solutions in the lens case after each use.
- Store contact lenses in fresh disinfecting solution overnight for the minimum soaking time recommended by the manufacturer to provide adequate disinfection.
- If lenses are worn intermittently, check and replace the solution weekly; consider daily disposable lens wear.
- Discard open bottles of solution if not used within the recommended time frame after being opened. Refer to the package labeling for individual products because "use within" time frames range from 1 up to 3 months, depending on the product. Write the date of first use of the solution on the outside of the bottle.
- Store contact lenses in a proper lens case when not in use. Clean the contact lens case daily by rubbing with a disinfecting solution and allowing the case to air dry.
- Replace the contact lens case every 3 months.
- Saline solution is used only to rinse lenses; saline will not clean or disinfect contact lenses and should not be used as a storage solution.
- Do not use tap water to rinse contact lenses or to clean cases. Never store lenses in tap water.
- Do not place contact lenses in your mouth to clean or lubricate the lens. This practice can result in eye infections.
- To prevent contamination, do not touch dropper tips or the tips of lens care product containers.
- While wearing lenses, use only ophthalmic solutions specifically formulated for contact lens use.
- Avoid swimming, showering, bathing in hot tubs, or rafting or other activities in natural bodies of water while wearing contact lenses unless external eye protection, such as watertight goggles, is used.

PATIENT EDUCATION FOR Prevention of Contact Lens–Related Disorders *(continued)*

- Follow prescribed wearing and replacement schedules.
- Avoid exposing contact lenses to extreme temperatures.
- Avoid use of oily cosmetics while wearing lenses. Bath oils or soaps with an oil or a cream base may leave a film on the hands that will be transferred to the lenses. Apply cosmetics after inserting contact lenses.
- To avoid mixing up the lenses, always insert or remove the same lens first. Check hard lenses for a dot in the lens periphery that identifies right from left.
- If the lenses are not comfortable after insertion or vision is blurred, check to see if they are on the wrong eyes or are inside out (inverted).
- To avoid damaging lenses, either apply aerosol cosmetics and deodorants well before lens insertion or keep eyes closed until the air is completely clear of spray particles.
- Except for prescription continuous-wear lenses, do not wear lenses while sleeping.
- To avoid excessive dryness of the eyes, do not wear lenses while sitting under a hair dryer, overhead fans, or air ducts.
- When lenses are worn outside on windy days, protect the eyes from soot and other particles, which may become trapped under the lens and scratch the cornea, by wearing sunglasses or other protective eyewear.
- Use eye protection in industry, sports, or any other occupation or hobby associated with the potential for eye damage.
- Do not insert lenses in red or irritated eyes. If the eyes become irritated while lenses are being worn, remove the lenses until the irritation subsides. If irritation or redness does not subside, consult an eye care provider.
- If an eye infection is suspected, see an eye care provider immediately.

Care Instructions for Soft Lenses

- See Tables 29–3 and 29–4 for guidelines on cleaning and disinfecting soft lenses.
- Handle soft lenses carefully because they are very fragile and can be torn easily.
- Remove these lenses before instilling any ophthalmic preparation not specifically intended for concurrent use with soft contact lenses. Wait at least 20–30 minutes before reinserting the lenses, unless directed otherwise by an eye care provider.
- Do not wear lenses when a topical ophthalmic ointment is being used.
- Do not wear soft contact lenses in the presence of irritating fumes or chemicals.

Care Instructions for GP Lenses

- See Tables 29–3 and 29–9 for guidelines on cleaning GP lenses.
- Do not use tap water to rinse off cleaner or to rewet lenses. If exposure to tap water occurs, disinfect lenses before inserting them in the eyes.
- See Table 29–5 for guidelines on using disinfecting systems.

Care Instructions for Continuous-Wear Lenses (GP or Soft)

- Remove mascara before sleeping because it can flake off during sleep, with particles becoming trapped underneath the lens.
- If a lens appears to be lost on awakening, check to see whether the lens was displaced within the affected eye. Soft lenses can fold over on themselves and get lodged underneath the top or bottom eyelid.
- Each morning, check eyes carefully for unusual or persistent redness, discharge, or pain. If redness does not abate within 45 minutes, or if discharge or pain is present, remove the lens and call your eye care provider.
- Check vision after inserting lenses. (Some hazy vision is normal on awakening because of the corneal hypoxia that develops overnight.) Apply a few drops of rewetting solution to improve hydration of the lens and help correct the hypoxia. If the problem is not resolved, remove lenses, clean them, and reinsert. If vision is not improved within an hour, remove lenses and call your eye care prescriber.

Key Points for Prevention of Contact Lens–Related Disorders

- Following the prescribed lens care program is the best strategy for avoiding lens wear–related problems.
- The health care provider should explain the care regimen for the patient's particular lens type and emphasize that the patient should use only the products recommended for the prescribed lenses.
- Instructions on avoiding practices or situations that can cause eye irritation or lens damage are also important in educating the patient about successful wearing of contact lenses:
  - Used contact lens solutions should not be "topped off" or reused.
  - Even when using "no-rub" solutions, patients should be counseled to rub and rinse contact lenses to fully remove protein deposits.
- Patient counseling should identify signs and symptoms that indicate the need for medical care. Patients should be informed that if eye redness or pain or blurry vision occurs during wear of any form of contact lens, they should immediately remove the lens and see an eye care provider for evaluation before reinserting the lens.

REFERENCES

1. Nichols JJ. Annual report: contact lenses 2015. *Contact Lens Spectr.* January 2016. Available at: http://www.clspectrum.com/articleviewer.aspx?articleID=113689. Accessed May 30, 2017.
2. Morgan PB, Woods CA, Tranoudis IG, et al. International contact lens prescribing in 2015. *Contact Lens Spectr.* January 2016. Available at: http://www.clspectrum.com/articleviewer.aspx?articleID=113690. Accessed May 30, 2017.
3. Forister JF, Forister EF, Yeung KK, et al. Prevalence of contact lens-related complications: UCLA contact lens study. *Eye Contact Lens.* 2009;35(4): 176–80. doi: 10.1097/ICL.0b013e3181a7bda1.
4. Yeung KK, Forister JF, Forister EF, et al. Compliance with soft contact lens replacement schedules and associated contact lens-related ocular complications: UCLA contact lens study. *Optometry.* 2010;81(11):598–607. doi: 10.1016/j.optm.2010.01.013.
5. Richale K, Sinnott LT, Skadahl E, et al. Frequency of and factors associated with contact lens dissatisfaction and discontinuation. *Cornea.* 2007;26(2):168–74. doi: 10.1097/01.ico.0000248382.32143.86
6. Dumbleton K, Woods CA, Jones LW, Fonn D. The impact of contemporary contact lenses on contact lens discontinuation. *Eye Contact Lens.* 2013; 39(1):93–9. doi: 10.1097/ICL.0b013e318271caf4.
7. Hickson-Curran S, Chalmers RL, Riley C. Patient attitudes and behaviour regarding hygiene and replacement of soft contact lenses and storage cases. *Cont Lens Anterior Eye.* 2011;34(5):207–15. doi: 10.1016/j.clae.2010.12.005.
8. Federal Trade Commission. FTC issues final rule implementing Fairness to Contact Lens Consumers Act. June 29, 2004. Available at: http://www.ftc.gov/opa/2004/06/contactlens.htm. Accessed May 30, 2017.

9. Fogel J, Zidile C. Contact lenses purchased over the Internet place individuals potentially at risk for harmful eye care practices. *Optometry.* 2008;79(1):23–35. doi: 10.1016/j.optm.2007.07.013.
10. Wu Y, Carnt N, Stapleton F. Contact lens user profile, attitudes, and level of compliance to lens care. *Cont Lens Anterior Eye.* 2010;33(4):183–8. doi: 10.1016/j.clae.2010.02.002.
11. Pesudovs K, Garamendi E, Elliott DB. A quality of life comparison of people wearing spectacles or contact lenses or having undergone refractive surgery. *J Refract Surg.* 2006;22(1):19–27.
12. Jones L. Modern contact lens materials: a clinical performance update. *Contact Lens Spectr.* September 2002. Available at: http://www.clspectrum.com/issues/2002/september-2002/modern-contact-lens-materials-a-clinical-performa. Accessed May 30, 2017.
13. DeNaeyer GW. Soft lens material choices and selection. *Contact Lens Spectr.* May 2012. Available at: http://www.clspectrum.com/issues/2012/may-2012/soft-lens-material-choices-and-selection. Accessed May 30, 2017.
14. DeNaeyer GW. Therapeutic applications of contact lenses. *Contact Lens Spectr.* May 2010. Available at: http://www.clspectrum.com/articleviewer.aspx?articleID=104223. Accessed May 30, 2017.
15. Gromacki S. The case for bandage soft contact lenses: a primer on the use of these therapeutic lenses to serve and protect the corneas of our patients. *Rev Cornea Contact Lenses.* January 2012. Available at: http://www.reviewofcontactlenses.com/content/d/soft_lenses/c/32147. Accessed May 30, 2017.
16. Del Pizzo N. Gas permeable (GP) contact lenses. December 2015. Available at: http://www.allaboutvision.com/contacts/rgps.htm. Accessed May 30, 2017.
17. Dzurinko V, Quinn TG, Woods J. Today's multifocal opportunity. *Contact Lens Spectr.* Updated February 2012. Available at: http://www.clspectrum.com/article.aspx?article=106665. Accessed May 30, 2017.
18. Morgan PB, Efron N. Contact lens correction of presbyopia. *Cont Lens Anterior Eye.* 2009;32(4):191–2. doi: 10.1016/j.clae.2009.05.003.
19. U.S. Food and Drug Administration. Device classification. Available at: http://www.fda.gov/MedicalDevices/DeviceRegulationandGuidance/Overview/ClassifyYourDevice/default.htm#determine. Accessed May 30, 2017.
20. Mayers M. The dangers of mixing solutions. *Rev Cornea Contact Lenses.* January 2011. Available at: http://www.reviewofcontactlenses.com/content/c/26326/. Accessed May 30, 2017.
21. U.S. Food and Drug Administration. Ensuring safe use of contact lens solution. Available at: http://www.fda.gov/forconsumers/consumerupdates/ucm164197.htm. Updated February 26, 2016. Accessed May 30, 2017.
22. Ward MA. Soft contact lens care products. *Contact Lens Spectr.* July 2003. Available at: http://www.clspectrum.com/articleviewer.aspx?articleid=12384. Accessed May 30, 2017.
23. Rolando M, Crider JY, Kahook MY. Ophthalmic preservatives: focus on polyquarternium-1. *Expert Opin Drug Deliv.* 2011;8(11):1425–38. doi: 10.1517/17425247.2011.617736.
24. Hwang TS, Hyon JY, Song JK, et al. Disinfection capacity of PuriLens contact lens cleaning unit against Acanthamoeba. *Eye Contact Lens.* 2004;30(1):42–3. doi: 10.1097/01.ICL.0000102296.62871.E4.
25. Choate W, Fontana F, Potter J, et al. Evaluation of the PuriLens contact lens care system: an automatic care system incorporating UV disinfection and hydrodynamic shear cleaning. *CLAO J.* 2000;26(3):134–40.
26. Smick KL. The evolution of dual disinfection: where we are today. *Rev Cornea Contact Lenses.* January 2011. Available at: http://www.reviewofcontactlenses.com/content/c/26327/. Accessed May 30, 2017.
27. Gromacki SJ, Ward MA. Understanding contemporary contact lens care products. *Contact Lens Spectr.* June 2013. Available at: http://www.clspectrum.com/articleviewer.aspx?articleID=108437. Accessed May 30, 2017.
28. Gromacki SJ. Hydrogen peroxide contact lens disinfection, part 1. *Contact Lens Spectr.* May 2012. Available at: http://www.clspectrum.com/issues/2012/may-2012/contact-lens-care-compliance. Accessed May 30, 2017.
29. Gromacki SJ. Hydrogen peroxide contact lens disinfection, part 2. *Contact Lens Spectr.* September 2012. Available at: http://www.clspectrum.com/articleviewer.aspx?articleID=107417. Accessed May 30, 2017.
30. Pauline C, Cheng SY, Chan WY, Yip WK. Soft contact lens cleaning: rub or no-rub? *Ophthalmic Physiol Opt.* 2009;29:49–57. doi: 10.1111/j.1475-1313.2008.00606.x.
31. Zhu H, Bandara MB, Vijay AK, et al. Importance of rub and rinse in use of multipurpose contact lens solution. *Optom Vis Sci.* 2011;88(8):967–72. doi: 10.1097/OPX.0b013e31821bf976.
32. Ward MA. MPS dual disinfection trends. *Contact Lens Spectr.* November 2011. Available at: http://www.clspectrum.com/articleviewer.aspx?articleID=106332. Accessed March 30, 2016.
33. Bowling EL. Laying the groundwork for successful lens wear. *Contact Lens Spectr.* June 2011. Available at: http://www.clspectrum.com/articleviewer.aspx?articleID=105671. Accessed May 30, 2017.
34. White P. *2015 Contact Lenses and Solutions Summary.* July 2015 (supplement). Available at: http://www.clspectrum.com/class. Accessed May 30, 2017.
35. Schacet JL. Taking charge of patients' solution selections. *Rev Cornea Contact Lenses.* January 2012. Available at: http://www.reviewofcontactlenses.com/content/c/32146/. Accessed May 30, 2017.
36. Bennett ES, Heiting G. Caring for gas permeable contact lenses. Available at: http://www.allaboutvision.com/contacts/carergplens.htm. Updated October 2015. Accessed May 30, 2017.
37. Ward MA. Approved GP wetting drops. *Contact Lens Spectr.* January 2011. Available at: http://www.clspectrum.com/articleviewer.aspx?articleID=105082. Accessed May 30, 2017.
38. Ward MA. GP contact lens care pearls. *Contact Lens Spectr.* October 2012. Available at: http://www.clspectrum.com/articleviewer.aspx?articleID=107511. Accessed May 30, 2017.
39. Silbert JA. Medications and contact lens wear. *Contact Lens Spectr.* May 2002. Available at: http://www.clspectrum.com/articleviewer.aspx?articleid=12149. Accessed May 30, 2017.
40. Dartt DA. Neural regulation of lacrimal gland secretory processes: relevance in dry eye diseases. *Progr Retin Eye Res.* 2009;28(3):155–77. doi: 10.1016/j.preteyeres.2009.04.003.
41. Elton M. Care and advice for contact lens wearers. *Pharm J.* 2010;285:235–8.
42. Bowling E. Which oral meds cause dry eye? *Rev Cornea Contact Lenses.* June 2011. Available at: http://www.reviewofcontactlenses.com/content/d/dry_eye/c/28762/. Accessed May 30, 2017.
43. Ward MA. Contact lenses and makeup contamination. *Contact Lens Spectr.* February 2013. Available at: http://www.clspectrum.com/articleviewer.aspx?articleID=107943. Accessed May 30, 2017.

CHAPTER 30

OTIC DISORDERS

VERONICA T. BANDY

Ear complaints are common. Ear disorders affect pediatric and geriatric patients with greater frequency than in the adult patient population. Otic disorders are responsible for approximately 1.5% of ambulatory care visits each year.[1] The National Health and Nutrition Examination Survey (NHANES) found self-reported rates of 15% for excessive cerumen and up to 3% for impacted cerumen among adolescents 12–19 years of age.[2] Excessive or impacted cerumen can affect up to 10% of children, 5% of adults, and greater than 30% of the geriatric population. Excessive cerumen is one of the most common causes of transient hearing loss in all age groups.[3–5] Approximately 12 million patients will visit their primary care provider annually because of cerumen impaction, and approximately 8 million cerumen removal procedures will be performed.[5]

Self-treatment with nonprescription medications and complementary therapies should be restricted to external ear disorders, which include disorders of the auricle and the external auditory canal (EAC). Excessive cerumen and water-clogged ears are self-treatable EAC disorders for which the U.S. Food and Drug Administration (FDA) has approved nonprescription otic medications. Other self-treatable disorders of the auricle include atopic dermatitis, seborrhea and psoriasis, and allergic and contact dermatitis. Chapters 33, 34, and 35, respectively, provide detailed discussions of the etiology and treatment of these disorders.

Diseases of the head and neck can cause referred pain, which the patient often perceives as originating from the ear. The health care provider (HCP) must attempt to determine the cause of pain before recommending self-treatment or medical referral. This chapter first briefly examines the anatomy of the ear and pathophysiology of ear disorders and then reviews associated nonprescription therapies for excessive or impacted cerumen and water-clogged ears. Next, an approach to the assessment of self-treatable otic disorders is described, with relevant case studies, followed by sections on patient counseling and evaluation of patient outcomes.

Pathophysiology of Otic Disorders

The anatomy of the ear is conducive to certain types of otic disorders, especially in children; therefore, an overview of its anatomic features is included in this discussion of common otic disorders. The external ear consists of the auricle (also called the pinna), the EAC (Figure 30–1), and the tympanic membrane (eardrum), which separates the external ear from the middle ear.[6] The auricle is composed of cartilage with a closely apposed thin layer of highly vascular skin. Adipose (fatty) subcutaneous tissue, which insulates blood vessels elsewhere in the body, is absent except in the lobe. The lobe has fewer blood vessels and is composed primarily of fatty tissue. The triangular piece of cartilage in front of the ear canal adjacent to the cheek is called the tragus.

The EAC consists of an outer cartilaginous portion, which makes up one-third to one-half of its length, plus an inner body, or osseous, portion.[6] The canal ends in a blind cul-de-sac ("dead end"). The EAC in children is shorter, straighter, and flatter than in adults, in whom the canal tends to lengthen and form an S shape.[7] At the same time, the eustachian tube (part of the inner ear) in adults lengthens downward as it enters the nasal cavity. This conformation helps to promote drainage and inhibits aspiration of pharyngeal and nasal contents into the middle ear, which may help to explain why children have middle ear infections more often than adults do.[8]

The skin that covers the auricle is especially susceptible to bleeding when scratched because of the lack of flexibility usually afforded by a subcutaneous layer of fat and the generous blood supply to the area.[9] The skin is highly innervated, resulting in a disproportionate degree of otalgia (ear pain) relative to any inflammation present. Skin farther along the course of the EAC is thicker and contains apocrine and exocrine glands as well as hair follicles.[6,7] The skin in the canal is continuous with the outer layer of the tympanic membrane.

Oily secretions from the exocrine glands mix with the milky, fatty fluid from the apocrine glands to form cerumen, which appears on the surface of the skin in the outer half of the EAC. Cerumen lubricates the canal, traps dust and foreign materials, and provides a waxy, waterproof barrier to the entry of pathogens.[7] It also contains various antimicrobial substances, such as lysozymes, and it has an acidic pH, which also aids in inhibition of bacterial and fungal growth.

The canal skin is shed continuously and mixes with cerumen. The debris-laden cerumen slowly migrates outward with jaw movements (such as chewing and talking). This migration serves as a process of self-cleaning.[5] Cerumen may appear dry and flaky or have an oily and pastelike consistency. Color varies from individual to individual; it can be honey-colored to light gray or tan and may darken on exposure to air.[10]

The natural defenses of the ear canal include the skin layer with its protective coating of cerumen, an acidic pH (<6.5), and hairs that line the outer half of the canal. Together they protect

Editor's Note: This chapter is based on the 18th edition chapter of the same title, written by Judith B. Summers Hanson.

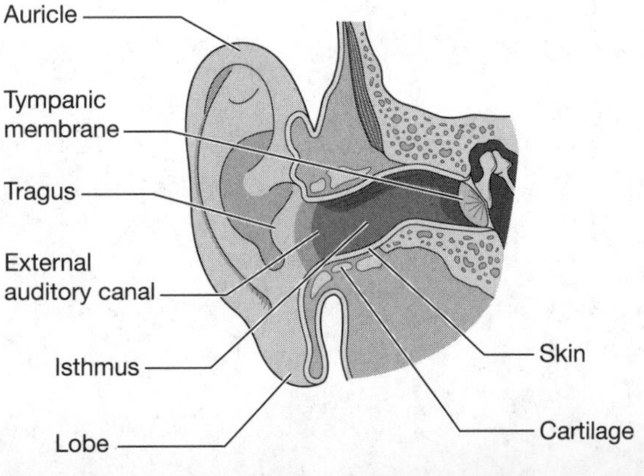

FIGURE 30–1 Anatomy of the auricle and external ear.

against injury from foreign material and infection. Important information for the provider to convey in patient counseling is the normal role and function of cerumen.

Because the EAC forms a blind cul-de-sac, it is especially prone to collecting moisture. Its dark, warm, moist environment is ideal for fungal and bacterial growth. In the preinflammatory stage, moisture, local trauma, or both remove the lipid layer covering the skin. Local trauma from fingernails, cotton-tipped swabs, or other items inserted into the canal can abrade the skin, allowing pathogens to enter. Because a normal, healthy ear canal is impervious to potentially pathogenic organisms, skin integrity generally must be interrupted before such microorganisms can produce infection. Trauma to the ear from thermal injuries, sports injuries, ear piercing, and poorly fitting or improperly cleaned ear devices or hearing aids can contribute to the breakdown of the EAC's natural defenses.[7] When involving the ear, dermatologic skin disorders, such as contact dermatitis, seborrhea, psoriasis, and malignancies, may also compromise these defenses.[6]

Viral illnesses such as the common cold and upper respiratory infections can contribute to the breakdown of natural defenses of the middle and inner ear, especially in children, who are very susceptible to middle ear infections after such illnesses. Because the eustachian tube in a child is shorter and angled flatter than that in an adult, presumably nasopharyngeal secretions can easily be aspirated and accumulate in the middle ear, leading to proliferation of bacteria with increased risk of disease in this age group.[8] Holding back or trying to stifle a sneeze can force secretions into the middle ear and therefore should be strongly discouraged, even in adults.

EXCESSIVE OR IMPACTED CERUMEN

Cerumen is a naturally occurring substance that assists in the defense of the external ear canal. A common myth that all earwax should be removed by cleaning may lead to excessive attempts at clearing the ear canal, with consequent damage to the EAC if done improperly.[5]

Pathophysiology of Excessive or Impacted Cerumen

A variety of factors can cause disruption of the normal flow of cerumen toward the outer EAC. Anatomic variations such as narrowing or irregular shape of the EAC, presence of excessive hair, irritation from foreign objects that are used to assist in amplification or blocking of sound (e.g., hearing aids, ear plugs), use of cotton-tipped swabs, or atrophy of the ceruminous glands with increasing age can lead to impaction of cerumen.[11-13] Recent research suggests that hearing aid use does not increase the likelihood of cerumen impaction, but more studies are needed to refute this belief. Inappropriate methods of removal of excessive or impacted cerumen can lead to damage to the EAC or tympanic membrane and may result in otitis media.[14]

Clinical Presentation of Excessive or Impacted Cerumen

The symptom of sensation of ear fullness or dull pain may be associated with excessive or impacted cerumen. Patients may present with one or more common symptoms, including discomfort, itching, hearing loss, tinnitus, dizziness, ear fullness, vertigo, cough, and hearing aid malfunction or feedback (if worn).[3,5,15] Impacted cerumen can have negative effects on hearing and cognition in elderly patients.[12,16,17]

Treatment for Excessive or Impacted Cerumen

Treatment Goals

The goal of treating excessive or impacted cerumen is to remove the cerumen using safe and effective products while preventing potential adverse events. Appropriate use of cerumen removal treatments can be expected to eliminate signs and symptoms of excessive or impacted cerumen and other associated symptoms. The provider should assist the patient to choose a product that is cost-effective and readily administered at home.

General Treatment Approach

Therapeutic interventions include the use of cerumen-softening agents with or without irrigation. Manual removal of cerumen is an option for HCPs with the proper skills and instrumentation, but caution is warranted in such removal attempts by the patient, which are associated with greater risk of damage to the ear canal (e.g., skin laceration).[11] The updated clinical practice guidelines state that if the presence of excessive cerumen is asymptomatic that active management is not required. Manual removal of cerumen is stated as optional rather than recommended treatment.[5]

The ear wax–softening agent should be instilled into the ear for the appropriate amount of time, followed by rinsing with warm water, often done using a bulb syringe. Drying of the ear canal can be hastened by gently towel-drying the outer ear structures or with use of a handheld blow dryer.[18] The algorithm presented in Figure 30–2 outlines the appropriate self-treatment approach for excessive or impacted cerumen; exclusions for self-treatment are listed as well.

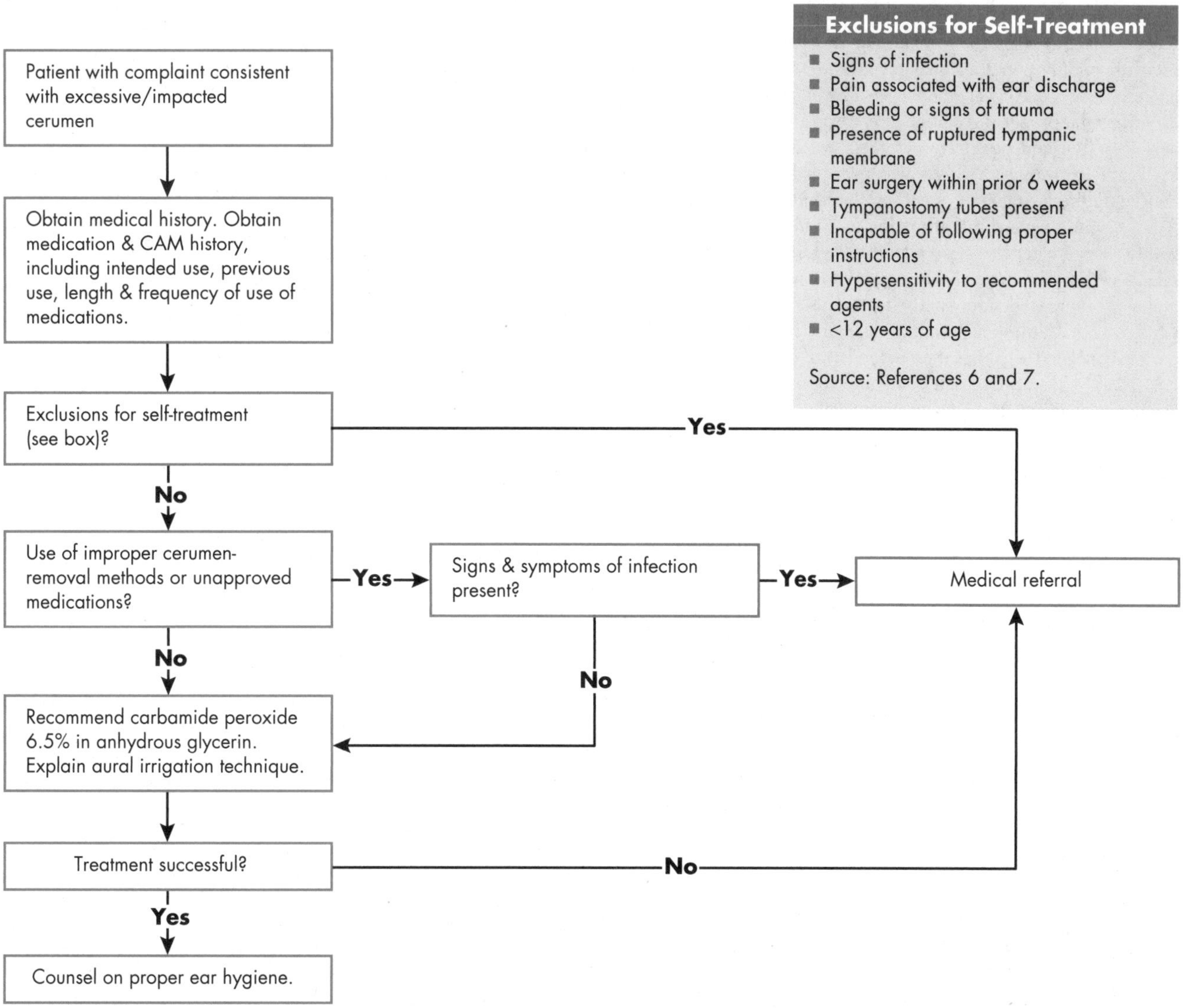

FIGURE 30-2 Self-care for excessive/impacted cerumen. Key: CAM, complementary and alternative medicine.

Nonpharmacologic Therapy

Earwax should be removed only when it has migrated to the outermost portion of the EAC. The nonpharmacologic method of removing cerumen is with a curette (e.g., Clinere Ear Cleaners). Such devices should be used with caution, however; appropriate training is recommended.[5] The use of cotton-tipped swabs for ear cleansing may be associated with an increase in cerumen impaction with occlusion of the ear canal and is not recommended for use by clinical practice guidelines.[5,14]

Pharmacologic Therapy

Care should be taken in attempting removal of cerumen from the EAC. If patients experience pain or bleeding after repeated attempts to remove excessive cerumen, or if their symptoms persist, they should be immediately referred to an HCP. If tympanic membrane rupture is suspected, referral to an HCP is warranted, and nonprescription treatment should not be attempted.[5,11] Currently the only FDA-approved nonprescription ear wax–softening agent is carbamide peroxide 6.5% in anhydrous glycerin.[19] HCPs have also used water-based agents (acetic acid, docusate sodium, hydrogen peroxide, or saline) or oil-based agents (almond oil, olive oil, or mineral oil), but these agents are no more effective than carbamide peroxide.[3,6,20]

Carbamide Peroxide

Carbamide peroxide 6.5% in anhydrous glycerin is FDA-approved for use in the removal of hardened or impacted cerumen within the EAC. It can be used alone or in conjunction with warm water irrigation to remove the loosened cerumen. This product can be used in children 12 years of age and older or in adults. Use in patients younger than 12 years of age should be done only under the advice of a physician.

For correct administration, 5–10 drops of the solution are instilled into the affected ear(s), with care taken to prevent the tip of the applicator from entering the ear canal. Care is also warranted to prevent contact of the solution with the eyes during administration. The solution should remain in the ear canal for several minutes (up to 15 minutes) for effective softening of excessive earwax. As carbamide peroxide is exposed to moisture, hydrogen peroxide and oxygen are slowly released, resulting in a weak antibacterial effect and mechanical loosening of cerumen. (Table 30–1 describes the proper instillation of eardrops.) Anhydrous glycerin acts to soften and penetrate cerumen to aid in the loosening of excessive ear wax. Anhydrous glycerin is widely used as a solvent and vehicle that has both emollient and humectant properties.[21] Any cerumen remaining after treatment may be removed with gentle, warm-water irrigation administered with a rubber otic bulb syringe.[22] Earwax removal syringes are now widely marketed, with claims of increased safety and effectiveness compared with bulb ear syringes. Caution is essential to ensure that the syringe tip is correctly placed and that the device is not overinserted into the EAC (Table 30–2). Use of a home oral jet irrigator in the ears is not recommended. The high-pressure water jet from the irrigator, as well as associated introduction of large amounts of moisture into the ear canal, may lead to development of otitis externa, perforated tympanic membrane, localized painful injury, vertigo, otitis media, or tinnitus.[3]

Carbamide peroxide may be used twice daily for up to 4 days. Patients should contact a primary care provider if symptoms persist after 4 days of use, if adverse effects develop, or if the presence of infection is suspected. Reported adverse effects include pain, rash, irritation, tenderness, redness, discharge, and dizziness.[23]

Docusate Sodium

Docusate sodium is classified as an emollient and has been used off-label to soften earwax by topical application in the ear canal.[21] Although providers have used docusate sodium for impacted cerumen, studies are conflicting on its efficacy compared with that of other products.[3,24] Results with use of docusate for this purpose are variable, and this agent is not FDA-approved to soften excessive or impacted cerumen.

Hydrogen Peroxide

Hydrogen peroxide can be a source of nascent oxygen when exposed to moisture and can also function as a weak antibacterial agent.[23] Hydrogen peroxide 3% has been used topically to cleanse abrasions and to flush the ear canal when softening or removing earwax.[4,24] Because hydrogen peroxide solutions contain water, overuse may predispose the ear to infection from tissue maceration caused by excessive water left in the canal. This product is not FDA-approved to treat excessive/impacted cerumen.

Olive Oil (Sweet Oil)

Olive oil is used as an emollient and a demulcent and has been used as a home remedy to soften earwax.[19,21] This product is not FDA-approved to treat excessive or impacted cerumen.

Product Selection Guidelines

Table 30–3 lists examples of cerumen-softening and other otic products. No nonprescription cerumen-softening agents are approved for patients younger than 12 years. No special consideration is necessary for use of these agents in pregnant, lactating, or geriatric patients.

TABLE 30–1 Guidelines for Administering Eardrops

1. Wash your hands with soap and warm water; then dry them thoroughly.
2. Carefully wash and dry the outside of the ear with a damp washcloth, taking care not to get water in the ear canal. Then dry the ear.
3. Warm eardrops to body temperature by holding the container in the palm of your hand for a few minutes. Do not warm the container in hot water or microwave. Instilling hot eardrops can cause ear pain, nausea, or dizziness.
4. If the label indicates, gently shake the container to mix contents.
5. Tilt your head (or have the patient tilt the head) to the side, as shown in drawing A. Or lie down with the affected ear up, as shown in drawing B. Use gentle restraint, if necessary, for an infant or a young child.
6. Open the container carefully. Position the dropper tip near, but not inside, the ear canal opening. Do not allow the dropper to touch the ear, because it could become contaminated or injure the ear. Eardrop bottles must be kept clean.
7. Pull your ear (or the patient's ear) backward and upward to open the ear canal (drawing A). If the patient is a child younger than 3 years, pull the ear backward and downward (drawing B).
8. Place the proper dose or number of drops into the ear canal. Replace the cap on the container.
9. Gently press the small, flat skin flap (tragus) over the ear canal opening to force out air bubbles and push the drops down the ear canal.
10. Stay (or keep the patient) in the same position for the length of time indicated in the product instructions. If the patient is a child who cannot stay still, the primary care provider may tell you to place a clean piece of cotton gently into the child's ear to prevent the medication from draining out. Use a piece large enough to remove easily, and do not leave it in the ear longer than 1 hour.
11. Repeat the procedure for the other ear, if needed.
12. Gently wipe excess medication off the outside of the ear, using caution to avoid getting moisture in the ear canal.
13. Wash your hands to remove any medication.

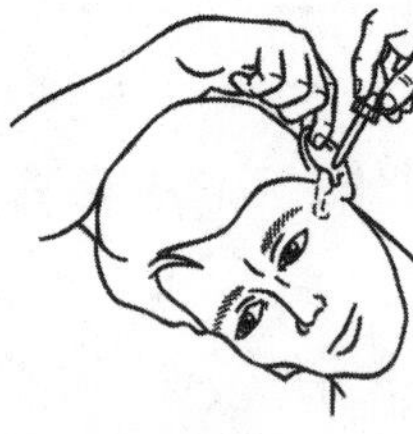

A

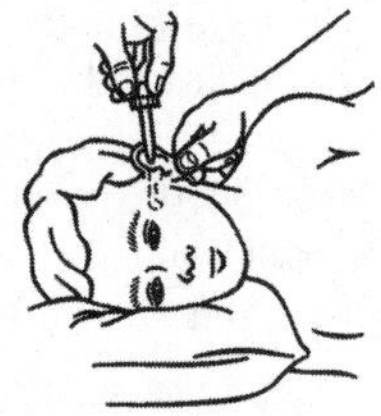

B

Source: *APhA Special Report: Medication Administration Problem Solving in Ambulatory Care.* Washington, DC: American Pharmaceutical Association; 1994:9.

TABLE 30-2 Guidelines for Removing Excessive or Impacted Cerumen

Ceruminolytics

1. Place 5–10 drops of the cerumen-softening solution into the ear canal, and allow it to remain for at least 15 minutes, as described in Table 30–1.
2. Perform this procedure daily for no longer than 4 consecutive days.

Irrigation Technique

The use of ceruminolytics and irrigation together may improve overall removal of impacted cerumen. The ceruminolytic agent is administered first. Then follow the irrigation technique as described below, paying special attention to cautionary instructions.

1. Prepare a warm (not hot) solution of plain water or other solution as directed by your primary care provider. Eight ounces of solution should be sufficient to clean out the ear canal.
2. To catch the returning solution, hold a container under the ear being cleaned. An emesis basin is ideal because it fits the contour of the neck. Tilt the head slightly toward the side of the ear being cleaned.
3. Gently pull the earlobe down and back to expose the ear canal, as shown in drawing A.
4. Place the open end of the syringe into the ear canal with the tip pointed slightly upward toward the side of the ear canal (drawing A). Do not aim the syringe to the back of the ear canal. Make sure that the syringe does not obstruct the outflow of solution.
5. Squeeze the bulb gently—not forcefully—to introduce the solution into the ear canal and to avoid rupturing the eardrum. (Note: Only health care professionals trained in aural hygiene should use forced water spray irrigators [e.g., Waterpik] to remove cerumen.)
6. Do not let the returning solution come into contact with the eyes.
7. If pain or dizziness occurs, remove the syringe and do not resume irrigation until a health care provider is consulted.
8. Make sure all water is drained from the ear to avoid predisposing to infection from presence of excessive moisture (water-clogged ears).
9. Rinse the syringe thoroughly before and after each use, and let it dry.
10. Store the syringe in a cool, dry place (preferably, in its original container) away from hot surfaces and sharp instruments
11. If cerumen still remains, consult your primary care provider.

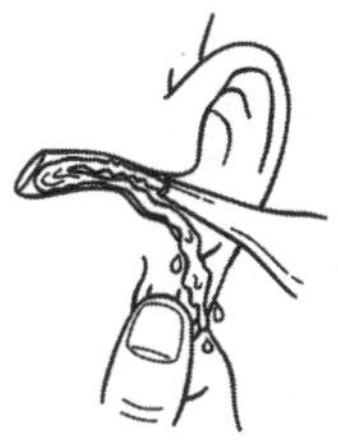

A

Source: Adapted with permission from *Ohio Clin.* 1996;14(5):10.

TABLE 30-3 Selected Products for Otic Disorders

Trade Name	Primary Ingredients
Cerumen-Softening Products	
Auro Ear Drops	Carbamide peroxide 6.5%; anhydrous glycerin
Debrox Earwax Removal Aid Kit	Carbamide peroxide 6.5%; glycerin; packaged with or without syringe
Ear Wax Removal Complete Kit	Carbamide peroxide 6.5%; glycerin; packaged with sterile saline spray, ear plugs and ear cleaning tool
Murine Ear Wax Removal	Carbamide peroxide 6.5%; glycerin; packaged with or without syringe
Ear-Drying Products	
Auro-Dri Drops	Isopropyl alcohol 95%; anhydrous glycerin
Swim Ear Drops	Isopropyl alcohol 95%; anhydrous glycerin
Botanical and Homeopathic Products	
Similasan Ear Wax Relief	Causticum HPUS 12X; Graphites HPUS 15X; Lachesis HPUS 12X; Lycopodium HPUS 12X
Highlands Earache Drops	Belladonna 30C HPUS; Calcarea Carbonica 30C HPUS; Lycopodium 30C HPUS; Pulsatilla 30C HPUS; Sulphur 30C HPUS

Key: HPUS = *Homeopathic Pharmacopeia of the United States.*

Complementary Therapies

A number of ear cleaning tools are on the market. Examples are Ototek Loop and Clinere Ear Cleaners. These products are intended to be reusable and are marketed for manual earwax removal. The Ototek loop is for use in persons 16 years of age or older, and according to the product instructions, it can be inserted into the EAC until the guard reaches the outer ear. The Clinere Ear Cleaners are marketed only to clean the area at the entrance of the EAC.[25,26] Caution is indicated with use of any product intended for insertion into the EAC, because of the associated risk of trauma to canal skin or the tympanic membrane.

A homeopathic remedy proposed to remove excessive cerumen is the use of ear candles. A hollow candle is inserted in the ear canal and the external protrusion is then lit on fire. It is hypothesized that the burning of the candle creates a negative pressure with enough force to draw cerumen from the EAC and into the hollow area of the candle. Two reports, including a review of articles, found this method to be ineffective and potentially dangerous, occasionally causing patient burns and deposition of candle wax into the EAC.[27,28] FDA posted a consumer alert and video warning advising against the use of such products.[29] Clinical practice guideline recommends not to use ear candles.[5] For patients who inquire about this practice, it is important to emphasize the associated risks, because these candles can still be purchased on the internet. Despite the continued availability of these herbal and homeopathic products, no published studies have documented their safety and effectiveness (Table 30–3). (See Chapters 51 and 52 for more information on complementary therapies.)

WATER-CLOGGED EARS

Water-clogged ears constitutes a disorder that is defined as the retention of water within the EAC. This water retention can lead to hearing impairment, localized discomfort, or a sensation of fullness in the ear canal. Water-clogged ears should not be confused with externa otitis or swimmer's ear. Currently, no nonprescription FDA-approved products are available for the treatment of externa otitis. Only isopropyl alcohol 95% in anhydrous glycerin 5% base as the active ingredient is approved as an ear-drying aid. FDA-approved labeling for ear-drying products is limited to statements that may include "dries water in the ears and relieves water-clogged ears after swimming, showering, bathing, washing the hair." Any misleading statements would be considered misbranding.[30,31] Of note, these products are approved only to aid in ear drying after such activities and not for prevention of moisture accumulation or treatment of an inflammatory process.

Pathophysiology of Water-Clogged Ears

A few specific host and environmental factors are recognized to contribute to the presence of excessive moisture within the ear canal. Physical or anatomic changes within the ear canal, such as excessive hair growth and narrowing of the canal, may lead to wax or debris buildup, which in turn can lead to retention of moisture. Overproduction or the absence of cerumen can also lead to moisture retention. Excessive moisture may become trapped within the ear from sweating, high humidity, or swimming.[31]

Clinical Presentation of Water-Clogged Ears

The presence of water in the ear can cause a sensation of hearing impairment, localized discomfort, or a sensation of fullness. Heat and humidity can lead to swelling within the ear canal, skin maceration, itching, and possible infection.[32,33] Patients experiencing pain or other symptoms suggestive of otitis externa, infection, or inflammation with the ear canal should be referred to an HCP.

Treatment of Water-Clogged Ears

Treatment Goals

The goals of treating a water-clogged ear are to dry it using a safe and effective agent and to prevent recurrences in persons who are prone to retaining moisture in the ears.

General Treatment Approach

Before recommending an agent to treat water-clogged ears, the HCP should determine whether the patient has a ruptured tympanic membrane or has a tympanostomy tube in place. Ear-drying agents are very painful if instilled in either of these situations. Figure 30–3 includes a list of additional exclusions for self-treatment. The algorithm presented in Figure 30–3 outlines the appropriate self-treatment approach for water-clogged ears.

Nonpharmacologic Therapy

Nonpharmacologic measures include tactics to prevent exposure to and accumulation of moisture within the ear canal. The use of ear plugs or a bathing cap can be recommended for swimming.[32,33] A variety of products intended to protect the ears from exposure to water, or to absorb water when present, are available, including AquaEars, BioEars, and ClearEars. The ClearEars water-absorbing ear plugs are inserted into the ear canal to absorb trapped water; adult supervision is required for use in children younger than 11 years of age. The ear plugs are left within the canal for 5 to 10 minutes to absorb any trapped water and then gently removed and discarded.[34] Patients may attempt to dispel excessive moisture from the ear canal by tilting the head downward while pulling the ear to straighten the EAC, which promotes gravity drainage. Another method is to use the lowest heat setting on a blow dryer to help dry the ear canal.[32] A nonpharmacologic measure for use *before* exposure to moisture is to block the ear canal entrance with cotton swabs that have been "waterproofed" with petroleum jelly.[28,32] In one study, insertion of cotton wool coated with petrolatum was ranked the most effective means for preventing water from entering the ears and the easiest to implement.[32]

Pharmacologic Therapy

FDA has approved only isopropyl alcohol 95% in anhydrous glycerin 5% as a safe and effective "ear-drying aid."[19] No minimum age is listed on the ear-drying products generally accepted for use when the ears are exposed to moisture. Patients are instructed to apply 4 to 5 drops into the affected ear. The active ingredient contains a warning to keep the product away from fire, because it is flammable. It should also not be used within the eye. Medical referral is indicated if pain, burning, or irritation occurs with application or if symptoms persist after several days of use.[35] (See Table 30–3 for examples of products containing these agents.)

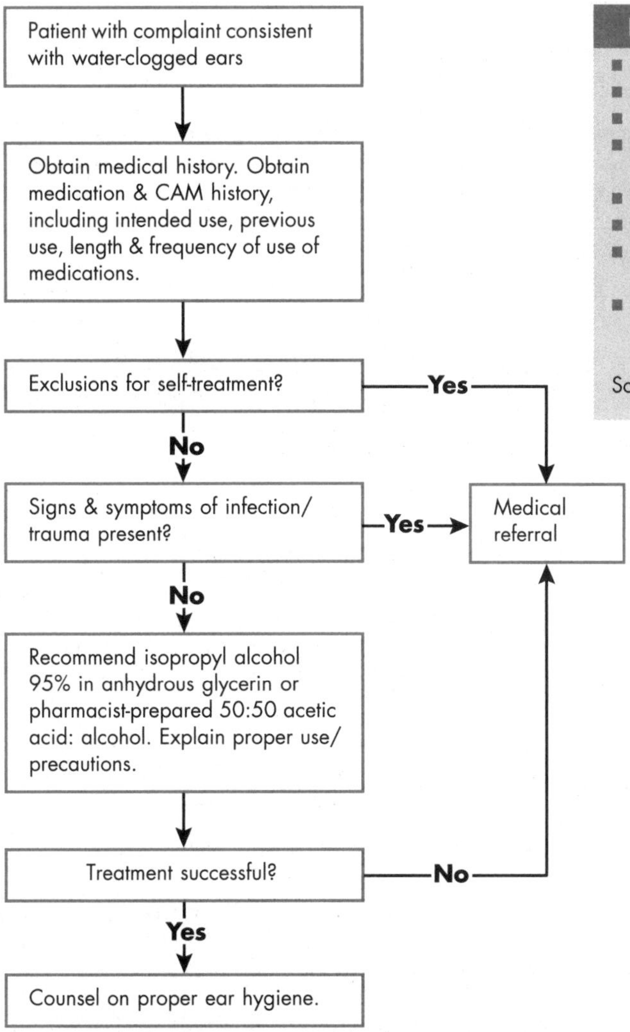

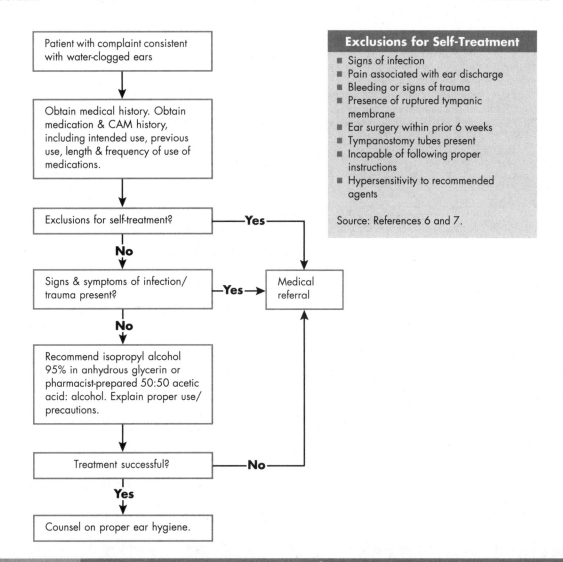

Exclusions for Self-Treatment

- Signs of infection
- Pain associated with ear discharge
- Bleeding or signs of trauma
- Presence of ruptured tympanic membrane
- Ear surgery within prior 6 weeks
- Tympanostomy tubes present
- Incapable of following proper instructions
- Hypersensitivity to recommended agents

Source: References 6 and 7.

FIGURE **30–3** Self-care for water-clogged ears. Key: CAM, complementary and alternative medicine.

Isopropyl Alcohol in Anhydrous Glycerin

Alcohol is highly miscible with water and acts as a drying agent. In concentrations greater than 70%, alcohol is also an effective skin disinfectant.[36] Glycerin has been used in pharmaceutical preparations for its solvent, emollient, or hygroscopic properties. It is safe but stings when applied to open wounds or abraded skin. Repeated use of alcohol alone can cause overdrying of tissue in the canal. The combination of alcohol and glycerin, however, provides a product that reduces moisture in the ear without overdrying.

Acetic Acid

A combination of acetic acid and water or isopropyl alcohol has been used as a preventive antiseptic, to be used after swimming or bathing. The acetic acid solution is made by creating a 50:50 concentrated mixture of acetic acid 5% and isopropyl alcohol 95%.[35,37] *Pseudomonas*, *Candida*, and *Aspergillus* organisms are particularly susceptible to this agent. A 50:50 mixture of white vinegar 5% and isopropyl alcohol 95% provides an acetic acid 2.5% solution. Concentrations of acetic acid between 2% and 3% may lower the pH of the ear canal below the optimal pH of 6.5–7.5 needed for bacterial growth.[36]

The solution is well tolerated and nonsensitizing and does not induce resistant organisms. It may sting or burn slightly, especially if the EAC skin is abraded. The provider should direct the patient in how to properly compound this solution by ensuring use of ingredients that are not expired, and to discard any remainder after use. An additional point is to use white vinegar only, rather than cider or other types of vinegar. Cider and wine vinegars, for example, are produced from fruit and contain impurities that could hinder antibacterial activity.

Product Selection Guidelines

Table 30–3 lists examples of ear-drying and other otic products. No special consideration is necessary for use of these preparations in pregnant, lactating, or geriatric patients.

Assessment of Otic Disorders: A Case-Based Approach

The most common complaints in ear disorders are otalgia, pruritus (itching), and hearing loss. Evaluating the characteristics of particular symptoms, such as pain and hearing loss, as well as the specific combination of symptoms, is key to assessing otic disorders. Cases 30–1 and 30–2 provide examples of the assessment of two different patients with otic disorders; common otic symptoms and possible causes are highlighted. Table 30–4 compares the signs and symptoms and other features of common otic disorders.[38–40] and Table 30–5 summarizes common causative disorders and their treatment for primary presenting complaints related to the ear: otalgia, otic pruritus, hearing loss, dizziness, tinnitus, and foreign body.[30–33,41–46] A verbal 5-minute hearing loss test for use in adults is available at the American Academy of Otolaryngology–Head and Neck Surgery website (www.entnet.org/healthinformation/hearing-loss.cfm) and will quickly assess how often the patient experiences hearing loss, along with the attendant circumstances.[37]

CASE 30-1

Relevant Evaluation Criteria	Scenario/Model Outcome
Collect	
1. Gather essential information about the patient's symptoms and medical history, including	
a. Description of symptom(s) (i.e., nature, onset, duration, severity, associated symptoms)	Three days ago, the patient started to experience a sense of fullness in her ears.
b. Description of any factors that seem to precipitate, exacerbate, and/or relieve the patient's symptom(s)	She experienced slight hearing loss in her ears. She tried to dry her ears with a cotton swab after exposure to moisture. She denies experiencing pain in her ear. She is on the school swim team, which practices 4 times a week.
c. Description of the patient's efforts to relieve the symptoms	She has used cotton swabs and towel drying.
d. Patient's identity	Kimberly Smithson
e. Patient's age, gender, height, and weight	10 years old, female, 4 ft 7 in., 34 kg (75 lb)
f. Patient's occupation	Student
g. Patient's dietary habits	She is a vegetarian and tries to eat a healthy diet. She eats low-carbohydrate foods when possible and eats three meals a day. Has two high protein snacks on swim practice days.
h. Patient's sleep habits	She sleeps 7 hours each night on weekdays and ~9 hours a night on weekends.
i. Concurrent medical conditions, prescription and nonprescription medications, and dietary supplements	Children's multivitamin supplement 1 tablet daily; Stress B complex vitamin supplement 1 tablet daily; calcium citrate 600 mg 1 caplet daily.
j. Allergies	Seasonal allergies in the spring and fall
k. History of other adverse reactions to medications	Sulfa antibiotics
l. Other (describe) ______	The patient swims 4 afternoons a week; swim competitions can occur up to twice on weekends. She wears a swim cap during competitions but does not always wear it during practice. She has a hot tub at home and uses it a couple of times per week to ease sore muscles. The patient is easily distracted and wears ear plugs during exams at school.
Assess	
2. Differentiate patient's signs/symptoms, and correctly identify the patient's primary problem(s) (Table 30–4).	Patient is experiencing cerumen impaction that is likely to be the result of improper attempts to remove water from the ear, and of the use of ear plugs during exams.
3. Identify exclusions for self-treatment (Figure 30–2).	None
4. Formulate a comprehensive list of therapeutic alternatives for the primary problem to determine whether triage to a health care provider is required, and share this information with the patient or caregiver.	Options include (1) Refer the patient to an appropriate HCP. (2) Recommend a nonprescription cerumen-softening agent with proper ear hygiene (Table 30–3). (3) Recommend use of a nonprescription ear-drying agent (Table 30–3). (4) Recommend self-care until the patient can see an appropriate HCP. (5) Take no action.

CASE 30-1 *continued*

Relevant Evaluation Criteria	Scenario/Model Outcome
Plan	
5. Select an optimal therapeutic alternative to address the patient's problem, taking into account patient preferences.	The patient should be referred to a HCP because of her young age. She can continue with nonpharmacologic recommendations but needs further medical evaluation.
6. Describe the recommended therapeutic approach to the patient or caregiver.	Refer to HCP.
7. Explain to the patient or caregiver the rationale for selecting the recommended therapeutic approach from the considered therapeutic alternatives.	"Attempting to use cotton swabs to dry the water in your ears can lead to cerumen impaction. Use of ear plugs can also exacerbate cerumen impaction. Because of your age, it is recommended that you be evaluated by a health care provider before use of a nonprescription product to relieve the impaction."
Implement	
8. When recommending self-care with nonprescription medications and/or nondrug therapy, convey accurate information to the patient or caregiver.	"You should use proper ear hygiene and avoid placing objects such as cotton-tipped swabs into the ear." See the box "Patient Education for Self-Treatable Otic Disorders."
Solicit follow-up questions from the patient or caregiver.	"Should I stop using ear plugs?"
Answer the patient's or caregiver's questions.	"If you can compete without using them, it would be advised to discontinue their use. If you still need to use ear plugs, carefully follow the package insert for directions. In addition, daily safe ear hygiene techniques will help reduce risk."
Follow-up: Monitor and Evaluate	
9. Assess patient outcome.	Contact the patient's caregiver in 2 days to determine whether the symptoms have resolved.

Key: HCP = Health care provider.

CASE 30-2

Relevant Evaluation Criteria	Scenario/Model Outcome
Collect	
1. Gather essential information about the patient's symptoms and medical history, including	
a. Description of symptom(s) (i.e., nature, onset, duration, severity, associated symptoms)	Two days ago, the patient started to experience "itching" within the ear canal, slight difficulty in hearing, and a feeling of excess moisture in her ears.
b. Description of any factors that seem to precipitate, exacerbate, and/or relieve the patient's symptom(s)	The patient denies experiencing pain, even on attempts to dry her ears with a cotton swab after exposure to moisture. She has recently joined a gym and works out 5 days a week. She ends each workout session with 20 minutes in the steam room followed by a shower.
c. Description of the patient's efforts to relieve the symptoms	She has used cotton swabs and towel drying. She states that she has also used a hairpin and the cap of an ink pen to try to "scratch" within the ear canal to relieve the itching.
d. Patient's identity	Susan McKindley
e. Patient's age, gender, height, and weight	26 years old, female, 5 ft 4 in., 185 lb
f. Patient's occupation	Patient is a kindergarten teacher.

CASE 30-2 *continued*

Relevant Evaluation Criteria	Scenario/Model Outcome
g. Patient's dietary habits	Patient is attempting to lose weight and has recently joined a gym. She is on a strict diet of 1100 calories/day in an attempt to lose weight. She is skipping breakfast and eating only lunch and dinner in an attempt to cut her caloric intake.
h. Patient's sleep habits	She sleeps ~7 hours a day. Some nights it is only 5 hours.
i. Concurrent medical conditions, prescription and nonprescription medications, and dietary supplements	Multivitamin supplement for women 1 tablet daily. Alli weight loss aid 1 60-mg capsule with each meal (3 times daily).
j. Allergies	NKA
k. History of other adverse reactions to medications	Iodine
l. Other (describe) ______	The patient participates in a high-intensity "cardio" exercise class 5 days a week in an attempt to lose weight quickly. Patient states that she has been sweating profusely during the workouts and that she enters the sauna (steam room) after each session to "cleanse my pores" and allow more sweating to occur.
Assess	
2. Differentiate patient's signs/symptoms, and correctly identify the patient's primary problem(s) (Table 30–4).	Patient is experiencing water-clogged ears. Her complaints are likely to be the result of improper attempts to remove any water from the ear and of excessive exposure to moisture from sweating, sitting in a sauna, and showering.
3. Identify exclusions for self-treatment (Figure 30–3).	None
4. Formulate a comprehensive list of therapeutic alternatives for the primary problem to determine whether triage to a health care provider is required, and share this information with the patient or caregiver.	Options include (1) Refer the patient to an appropriate HCP. (2) Recommend a nonprescription ear-drying agent with proper ear hygiene (Table 30–3). (3) Recommend self-care until the patient can see an appropriate HCP. (4) Take no action.
Plan	
5. Select an optimal therapeutic alternative to address the patient's problem, taking into account patient preferences.	The patient would like to use a self-care product.
6. Describe the recommended therapeutic approach to the patient or caregiver.	"Auro-Dri drops contain isopropyl alcohol and anhydrous glycerin, which will help to remove the excessive moisture in your ears without overdrying."
7. Explain to the patient or caregiver the rationale for selecting the recommended therapeutic approach from the considered therapeutic alternatives.	"Attempting to use cotton swabs to dry the ear may be ineffective and is not recommended. The use of ear-drying products can help in removing excessive moisture from within the ear."
Implement	
8. When recommending self-care with nonprescription medications and/or nondrug therapy, convey accurate information to the patient or caregiver.	"You should use proper ear hygiene and avoid placing objects like cotton-tipped swabs in your ears. You should also avoid placing other objects such as hairpins within the ear canal, as this can lead to tissue damage to the ear canal or tympanic membrane." See the box "Patient Education for Self-Treatable Otic Disorders."
a. Appropriate dose and frequency of administration	"Ensure that there is no damage to the ear canal before using an ear-drying product containing isopropyl alcohol in anhydrous glycerin." "Apply 4 or 5 drops into affected ear(s)." "Use nonpharmacologic ear-drying techniques to prevent recurrence of symptoms."
b. Maximum number of days the therapy should be employed	"The Auri-Dri drops can be used for up to 4 days."
c. Product administration procedures	See Table 30–1.

CASE 30-2 *continued*

Relevant Evaluation Criteria	Scenario/Model Outcome
d. Expected time to onset of relief	"Symptoms of water-clogged ears should diminish after first use. However, it may take additional treatments to obtain full symptom relief."
e. Degree of relief that can be reasonably expected	"Full resolution of symptoms can be expected within a few days."
f. Most common adverse effects	"The medication may cause stinging or burning if the ear canal has sustained injury."
g. Adverse effects that warrant medical intervention should they occur	"You may experience pain, rash, irritation, tenderness, redness, discharge, or dizziness from the medication. If you have a perforated tympanic membrane, do not use this product."
h. Patient options in the event that condition worsens or persists	"Stop using the product and see your primary care provider."
i. Product storage requirements	Keep cap on bottle when not in use. Store drops in original carton at room temperature. Store product in a dry place and in its original container.
j. Specific nondrug measures	See the box "Patient Education for Self-Treatable Otic Disorders."
Solicit follow-up questions from the patient or caregiver.	"Should I stop exercising?"
Answer the patient's or caregiver's questions.	"You can continue to exercise if you would like to continue as part of a healthy lifestyle. You should use nonpharmacologic measures to help remove moisture from the ear canal, such as towel-drying the outer ear area or using a blow dryer set on a cool setting."
Follow-up: Monitor and Evaluate	
9. Assess patient outcome.	Contact the patient in 2 days to evaluate her response to treatment and resolution of symptoms.

Key: HCP = Health care provider; NKA = no known allergies.

TABLE **30–4** **Differentiation of Common Otic Disorders**

Disorder	Etiology	Pain	Itching	Loss of Hearing	Discharge	Other Features
Ruptured tympanic membrane	Otitis media or trauma to ear such as a sharp blow, diving into water, forceful irrigation of ear	Brief, severe	No	Abrupt	If associated with otitis media	May be associated with otitis media (see that entry)
External otitis (swimmer's ear)	Local trauma to EAC caused by excessive moisture or abrasions; subsequent fungal/bacterial infections	Acute onset, ranges from mild to severe, increases with movement of tragus or auricle	Yes	Occasional	Occasionally, clear discharge changing to seropurulent	Swollen ear canal, stuffiness, discharge, swollen lymph nodes, fever; usually occurs in summer or in warm, humid climates
Otitis media	Bacterial infection of middle ear, usually following an upper respiratory tract infection	Sharp, steady, frequently unilateral; does not increase with movement of tragus or auricle	No	Is sometimes decreased	Possible exudate through perforated eardrum	Perforated or bulging eardrum, lymph nodes sometimes swollen, fever, dizziness; usually occurs in winter
Foreign object in ear	Insects, insertion of objects by children, hearing aids, sound attenuators	Dull-severe, with sense of fullness or pressure during chewing	Yes	Yes	Possible exudate from secondary bacterial infection	If obstruction not removed promptly, acute otitis externa and tinnitus may develop.

(continued)

TABLE 30–4 Differentiation of Common Otic Disorders *(continued)*

Disorder	Etiology	Pain	Itching	Loss of Hearing	Discharge	Other Features
Trauma to ear	Burns from curling iron, frostbite, hematomas/injuries from contact sports or ill-fitting helmets, ear piercing, improper cerumen removal techniques, abrasions of EAC, rapid changes in air pressure	Ranges from sharp and steady to brief and severe	Rare	Varies, can be abrupt to seldom	Seldom	Untreated hematomas may cause swelling/scarring; ear piercing may cause metal sensitivities, keloids, perichondritis, toxic shock syndrome, hepatitis B.
Tinnitus	Hearing disorders, blockage of EAC, exposure to high noise levels, acoustic trauma, systemic diseases, drug toxicity (from salicylate, quinidine, aminoglycosides and other antibiotics)	Possible	No	Sometimes	None	Continuous or intermittent alien noises in ear such as ringing, roaring, or humming
Excessive/impacted cerumen	Overactive ceruminous glands, obstructed migration of cerumen	Rare, dull pain if present	No	Often	None	Sense of fullness or pressure in the ears
Water-clogged ears	Excessive moisture in EAC	None	No	Often	None	Sense of fullness or wetness

Key: EAC = External auditory canal.
Source: References 4, 6, 8, and 38–40.

TABLE 30–5 Etiology and Treatment of Common Otic Complaints

Complaint	Etiology	Treatment
Otalgia	*Intrinsic:* infection, trauma, foreign objects, perichondritis *Extrinsic:* dental or jaw problems, nasopharyngeal infections, tumors, cysts, migraine headaches, neuralgias, cervical arthritis	Medical referral unless cause is clearly obvious, self-limiting, and self-treatable; always refer patients with suspected infection; self-care may delay seeking proper treatment.
Otic pruritus	Seborrhea, psoriasis, contact dermatitis; infection (external otitis); excessive dryness related to decreased sebum production	See Chapters 34 and 35; medical referral is indicated for suspected infection; excessive dryness: administer 1–2 drops of mineral oil.
Hearing loss	Foreign objects or water trapped in EAC; infection, congestion, neoplasms, tympanic membrane perforation, medication effects; excessive pressure or cerumen in EAC, or exposure to high noise levels	Medical referral is indicated unless hearing loss is related to excessive water or impacted cerumen in EAC.
Dizziness	Inner ear lesions, otitis media, rapid change in pressure on the tympanic membrane, migraine headache, ototoxic drugs, postural hypotension, cardiac disease, neoplasms, irrigation of ear canal with very hot or cold water, motion sickness	Medical referral is indicated unless complaint is related to motion sickness.
Tinnitus	See Table 30–4	Check for impacted cerumen; otherwise, medical referral is indicated.
Foreign body	Insects, beads, seeds, small batteries, or other objects in ear canal	Medical referral; mineral oil can be used to quickly suffocate an insect, with relief of distressing symptoms, until it can be removed by an HCP; moisture causes seeds to swell, making removal more difficult.

Key: EAC = External auditory canal; HCP = health care provider.
Source: References 4, 6–8,38, and 40–43.

Patient Counseling for Otic Disorders

For patients attempting to self-treat otic disorders, it is crucial to recognize how easily the EAC can be injured. The HCP should discourage common harmful practices of relieving itching of the ear using cotton swabs, fingernails, or other devices, and provide instruction on the proper methods of removing excessive cerumen and moisture from the ears. Patients who are susceptible to these disorders should be advised to incorporate proper removal methods in their "aural hygiene" regimen. The provider should explain the proper use and possible adverse effects of all recommended medications. The box "Patient Education for Self-Treatable Otic Disorders" lists specific information to provide in patient counseling.

Evaluation of Patient Outcomes for Otic Disorders

The recommended self-treatment measures for impacted or excessive cerumen and water-clogged ears have been proved to be effective in most uncomplicated cases. If symptoms related to these conditions persist or worsen after 4 days of appropriate self-treatment, the patient should consult a primary care provider. Another important indication for referral to a primary

PATIENT EDUCATION FOR Self-Treatable Otic Disorders

Excessive or Impacted Cerumen

Cerumen is necessary to lubricate the canal, trap dust and foreign materials, and provide a waxy, waterproof barrier to the entry of pathogens. The objective of self-treatment is to soften and remove any waxy accumulation or to prevent the disorder from recurring in susceptible individuals. For most patients, carefully following product instructions and the self-care measures listed here will help ensure optimal therapeutic outcomes.

Nondrug Measures

- Use a washcloth draped over a finger to remove earwax from the outer canal.
- Do not insert objects into the ear to remove earwax. Such attempts may injure the ear canal or push the wax farther into the canal.
- Never use the hollow candle method to remove earwax. This practice can cause serious ear injury or burns to other areas of the body.

Nonprescription Medications

- A combination of carbamide peroxide and anhydrous glycerin is recommended to soften and mechanically break down excessive or impacted cerumen.
- See Tables 30–1 and 30–2 for guidelines on using carbamide peroxide to remove excessive or impacted earwax.
- Do not let the medication come into contact with the eyes.
- Do not use this medication if you have a fever, ear drainage, pain more severe than a dull pain, dizziness, or a ruptured eardrum, or if you had ear surgery within the past 6 weeks.
- Do not use this medication to treat inflamed ear tissue, swimmer's ear, or itching of the ear canal.
- Prolonged contact between carbamide peroxide solution and the skin of the ear canal can cause dermatitis. Discontinue treatment if irritation or a rash appears.
- Store product in a cool, dry area, and check expiration date before using.

When to Seek Medical Attention

- Monitor for changes in your hearing and symptoms of infection such as pain and itching.
- If severe pain occurs or your hearing worsens, see a primary care provider immediately. Severe pain may indicate a ruptured eardrum.

Water-Clogged Ears

Water can become trapped in the ear, causing a sense of fullness or wetness. The objective of self-treatment is to remove excess moisture from the ear canal or to prevent the disorder in persons who are susceptible to retention of water in the ears. For most patients, carefully following product instructions and the self-care measures listed here will help ensure optimal therapeutic outcomes.

Nondrug Measures

- Tilt the head with the affected ear down, and gently manipulate the outer ear to help drain water from the ear. Gently towel dry the outer ear area.
- Immediately after swimming or bathing, use a blow dryer on low-heat and low-speed settings to help dry the ear canal. Do not blow air directly into the ear.

Nonprescription Medications

- Use a product that reduces moisture content in the ear without overdrying. Isopropyl alcohol 95% in anhydrous glycerin 5% is the only formula approved by the Food and Drug Administration.
- Do not use the medication if you have a ruptured eardrum or have a tympanostomy tube in place.
- Place 5–10 drops of the solution in the ear canal, and allow the solution to remain for 1–2 minutes.
- See Table 30–1 for further instructions on instilling the medication.
- Do not let the medication come into contact with the eyes.
- Discontinue use of the medication if stinging or burning occurs.
- Store product in a cool, dry area, and check expiration date before using.

When to Seek Medical Attention

- If pain, fever, or discharge develops, see a primary care provider immediately.

Dermatologic Disorders of the Ear

The objective of self-treatment for dermatologic disorders of the ear is to relieve the symptoms. For most patients, carefully following product instructions and the self-care measures described in Chapters 34 and 35 will help ensure optimal therapeutic outcomes.

care provider is the development of ear pain or discharge during treatment.

The provider can follow up by telephone in 4 days to determine whether the therapy is successful.

Key Points for Otic Disorders

- Limit self-treatment of otic disorders to relief of minor symptoms such as a sense of fullness, pressure, or wetness in the ears.
- Refer for further evaluation patients younger than 12 years of age with impacted cerumen, as well as patients with signs and symptoms of ear infection, bleeding or signs of trauma, tympanostomy tubes, or ruptured tympanic membrane and those who have had ear surgery within the past 6 weeks.
- Instruct patients on how to use specific otic products that have been proved safe and effective (Tables 30–1 and 30–2).
- Advise patients with self-treatable symptoms to contact a primary care provider if symptoms worsen or no improvement occurs after 4 days.
- Educate patients about proper ear hygiene, along with the role of cerumen in the healthy ear canal, to prevent further problems.

REFERENCES

1. CDC/National Center for Health Statistics. *National Ambulatory Medical Care Survey: 2010 Summary Tables.* Atlanta, GA: Centers for Disease Control and Prevention; 2010. Available at: http://www.cdc.gov/nchs/data/ahcd/namcs_summary/2010_namcs_web_tables.pdf. Accessed June 20, 2017.
2. CDC/National Center of Health Statistics. *National Health and Nutrition Examination Survey: 2009–2010.* Atlanta, GA: Centers for Disease Control and Prevention; 2012. Available at: https://wwwn.cdc.gov/nchs/nhanes/continuousnhanes/default.aspx?BeginYear=2009. Accessed June 20, 2017.
3. Tueh B, Shapiro N, MacLean CH, et al. Screening and management of adult hearing loss in primary care. *JAMA.* 2003;289(15):1976–85. doi: 10.1001/jama.289.15.1976
4. McCarter DF, Courtney AU, Pollart SM. Cerumen impaction. *Am Fam Physician.* 2007;75(10):1523–8. PMID: 17555144.
5. Schwartz SR, Magit AE, Rosenfeld RM, Ballachanda BB, et al. Clinical practice guideline (update): earwax (cerumen impaction). *Otolaryngol Head Neck Surg.* 2017 Jan;156(1 Suppl):S1–S29. doi: 10.1177/0194599816671491.
6. Beatrice F, Bucolo S, Cavallo R. Earwax, clinical practice. *Acta Otorhinolaryngol Ital.* 2009;29(Suppl 1):1–20.
7. Brown K, Banuchi V, Selesnick S. Diseases of the external ear. In: Lalwani AK, ed. *Current Diagnosis and Treatment: Otolaryngology Head and Neck Surgery.* 3rd ed. New York, NY: Lange Medical Books/McGraw-Hill; 2012:645–60.
8. National Institute on Deafness and Other Communication Disorders. *Ear Infections in Children.* Rockville, MD: National Institutes of Health; 2010. NIH Publication No. 10-4799. Available at: https://www.nidcd.nih.gov/health/ear-infections-children. Accessed June 20, 2017.
9. Oghalai JS, Brownell WE. Anatomy and physiology of the ear. In: Lalwani AK, ed. *Current Diagnosis and Treatment: Otolaryngology Head and Neck Surgery.* 3rd ed. New York, NY: Lange Medical Books/McGraw-Hill; 2012:599–616.
10. Hersh SP. Cerumen: insights and management. *Ann Longterm Care.* 2010;18(7):39–42.
11. Poulton S, Yau S, Anderson D, Bennett D. Ear wax management. *Aust Fam Physician.* 2015;44(10):731–4. PMID: 26484488.
12. Meador JA. Cerumen impaction in the elderly. *J Gerontol Nurs.* 1995; 21(12):43–5. PMID: 8537620.
13. Manchaiah V, Arthur J, Williams H. Does hearing aid use increase the likelihood of cerumen impaction? *J Audiol Otol.* 2015;19(3):168–71. doi: 10.7874/jao.2015.19.3.168.
14. Macknin ML, Talo H, Medendrop SV. Effect of cotton-tipped swab use on ear-wax occlusion. *Clin Pediatr.* 1994; 33(1):14–8. doi: 10.1177/000992289403300103.
15. Guest JF, Greener MJ, Robinson AC, Smith AF. Impacted cerumen: composition, production, epidemiology and management. *QJM.* 2004;97(8):477–88. doi: 10.1093/qjmed/hch082.
16. Subha, ST, Raman R. Role of impacted cerumen in hearing loss. *ENT J.* 2006;85(10):650–3. PMID: 17124935.
17. Moore AM, Voytas J, Kowalski D, et al. Cerumen, hearing and cognition in the elderly. *J Am Med Dir Assoc.* 2002;3(3):136–9.
18. Mayo Clinic Staff. Earwax blockage: lifestyle and home remedies. Available at: http://www.mayoclinic.org/diseases-conditions/earwax-blockage/basics/lifestyle-home-remedies/con-20018904. Accessed June 20, 2017.
19. U.S. Food and Drug Administration. OTC ingredient list. Updated August 2006. Available at: http://www.fda.gov/downloads/aboutfda/centersoffices/officeofmedicalproductsandtobacco/cder/ucm106426.pdf. Accessed June 20, 2017.
20. Burton MK, Doree C. Ear drops for the removal of ear wax. *Cochrane Database Syst Rev.* 2009;1:CD004326. doi: 10.1002/14651858.CD004326.pub2.
21. Miscellaneous otic preparations. *Facts & Comparisons eAnswers.* St. Louis, MO: Wolters Kluwer Health. Available at: http://online.factsandcomparisons.com/index.aspx. Accessed April 1, 2016.
22. Coppin R, Wicke D, Little P. Managing earwax in primary care: efficacy of self-treatment using a bulb syringe. *Br J Gen Pract.* 2008;58(546):44–9. doi: 10.3399/bjgp08X263811.
23. McEvoy GK, ed. *AHFS Drug Information.* 58th ed. Bethesda, MD: American Society of Health-System Pharmacists; 2016.
24. Coppin R, Wicke D, Mehta R, Little P. Management of ear wax in primary care—postal survey of UK GPs and practice nurses. *Fam Pract.* 2004;21(4):413–4. doi: 10.1093/fampra/cmh410.
25. Ototekloop [product information]. Earest Inc., Columbia, MO, 2015. Available at: https://www.ototekloop.com/instructions.aspx. Accessed June 20, 2017.
26. Clinere [product information]. Clinere Products Inc. Mudelein, IL; 2015. Available at: http://www.clinere.com/ear-cleaning.html. Accessed June 20, 2017.
27. Rafferty J, Tsikoudas A, Davis BC. Ear candling: should general practitioners recommend it? *Can Fam Physician.* 2007;53(12):2121–2. PMCID: PMC2231549.
28. Ernst E. Ear candles: a triumph of ignorance over science. *J Laryngol Otol.* 2004;118(1):1–2. doi: 10.1258/002221504322731529.
29. U.S. Food and Drug Administration. Ear candling: ineffective and risky [consumer video]. Available at: http://www.fda.gov/forconsumers/protectyourself/healthfraud/ucm267550.htm. Accessed June 20, 2017.
30. U.S. Food and Drug Administration. Electronic Code of Federal Regulations. Title 21, Food and Drugs Chapter 1, Subchapter D, Part 344. Updated April 1, 2015. U.S. Government Publishing Office. Available at: http://www.accessdata.fda.gov/scripts/cdrh/cfdocs/cfcfr/CFRSearch.cfm?CFRPart=344. Accessed June 20, 2017.
31. *Stedman's Medical Dictionary.* 28th ed. Baltimore, MD: Lippincott Williams & Wilkins; 2006.
32. Wang M, Liu C, Shiao A, Wang T. Ear problems in swimmers. *J Chin Med Assoc.* 2005;68(8):347–52. doi: 10.1016/S1726-4901(09)70174-1.
33. Kaushilk V, Malik T, Saeed R. Interventions for acute otitis externa. *Cochrane Database Syst Rev.* 2010;1:CD004740. doi: 10.1002/14651858.CD004740.pub2.
34. Clear Ears [product information]. Cirrus Healthcare Products, LLC, Cold Spring Harbor, NY. Available at: https://cirrushealthcare.com/products/clearearsa-water-removing-earplugs-10-count. Accessed June 20, 2017.

35. Schaefer P, Baugh RF. Acute otitis externa: an update. *Am Fam Physician.* 2012;86(11):1055–61. PMID: 23198673.
36. Allen LV, ed. *Remington: The Science and Practice of Pharmacy.* 22nd ed. Philadelphia, PA: Pharmaceutical Press and University of the Sciences, Philadelphia College of Pharmacy; 2013:1081–2, 1631.
37. Domino F. *The 5-Minute Clinical Consult.* Philadelphia, PA: Wolters Kluwer Health; 2015.
38. U.S. Food and Drug Administration. Topical OTC drug products for over-the-counter human use; final monopgraph; final rule. *Fed Regist.* August 8, 1986;51:28656–61.
39. Eye, ear, nose and throat (EENT) preparations: carbamide peroxide. *AHFS Drug Information.* Bethesda, MD: American Society of Health System Pharmacists; 2007:2807.
40. Johnson J, Lalwani AK. Vestibular disorders. In: Lalwani AK, ed. *Diagnosis and Treatment: Otolaryngology Head and Neck Surgery.* 3rd ed. New York, NY: Lang Medical Books/McGraw-Hill; 2012:729–38.
41. Pai S, Parikh, SR. Otitis media. In: Lalwani AK, ed. *Current Diagnosis and Treatment: Otolaryngology Head and Neck Surgery.* 3rd ed. New York, NY: Lang Medical Books/McGraw-Hill; 2012:674–81.
42. Dekelboum AM. Driving machine. In: Lalwani AK, ed. *Current Diagnosis and Treatment: Otolaryngology Head and Neck Surgery.* 3rd ed. New York, NY: Lang Medical Books/McGraw-Hill; 2012:739–46.
43. Gates GA, Clark WW. Occupational hearing loss. In: Lalwani AK, ed. *Current Diagnosis and Treatment: Otolaryngology Head and Neck Surgery.* 3rd ed. New York, NY: Lang Medical Books/McGraw-Hill; 2012: 747–59.

CHAPTER 31

PREVENTION OF HYGIENE-RELATED ORAL DISORDERS

KARLEEN MELODY

Dental diseases and disorders are recognized to affect the health and well-being of Americans throughout their lifespan. Dental caries (tooth decay) is the most common pathologic condition of childhood, being five times more prevalent than asthma and seven times more prevalent than hay fever.

Professional dental care is essential to maintain oral health. The most commonly recommended interval of examination is every 6 months; however, this frequency should be individualized according to historical, clinical, and radiographic findings. Patients at high risk for periodontal disease need more frequent visits, and low-risk patients are recommended to return for follow-up assessments at a minimum of once a year. Children should have their first visit to a dental care provider at the time of the first tooth eruption, at no later than 12 months of age. Despite these recommendations for optimal oral health, more than 30% of people have not visited the dentist in the past year.[1] In the United States, 21% of children 6 to 11 years of age and 15% of those 12 to 19 years of age have at least one untreated dental caries.[2] Furthermore, rates of dental caries in Hispanic children and non-Hispanic black children are above the national average at 46% and 44%, respectively.[2] The overall frequency increases to 60%–90% for school-age children.[3] Poor oral health is particularly detrimental for children in that it affects nutrition, growth, and development.

Improper oral hygiene is a direct cause of dental caries, periodontal disease (gingivitis and periodontitis), halitosis, and some cases of denture-related discomfort. Nonprescription products for prevention of oral disease are widely available in pharmacies, food stores, and other retail venues; educating the public about proper use of these products is key to preventing dental diseases.

The teeth and supporting structures are necessary for normal mastication and articulation, as well as for normal appearance. The primary (deciduous or baby) dentition first appears at the age of approximately 6 months, when the mandibular (lower jaw) central incisors erupt; the process is usually complete with the eruption of the upper second molars at approximately 24 months of age. Each of the upper and lower arches holds 10 deciduous teeth, 20 in all. Generally, emergence of the permanent dentition (adult teeth) begins when the mandibular first molar erupts behind the deciduous second molar at the age of approximately 6 years, and the process continues in a regular pattern, usually with replacement of deciduous teeth as they are shed. Of the 32 total permanent teeth, 28 usually are present by the age of 14 years; third molars (wisdom teeth) may appear between the ages of 17 and 21 years.

Anatomically, the teeth are viewed grossly as having two parts, the roots and the crown (Figure 31–1). Normally, the roots are located below the gingival (gum) line or margin; roots are essential in supporting and attaching the tooth to the surrounding tissues. The crown is the part of the tooth visible above the gingival margin and provides appropriate surfaces for effective mastication. Each tooth has four major components: enamel, dentin, pulp, and cementum.

Enamel is composed of very hard, crystalline calcium phosphate salts (hydroxyapatite). It is 1.5–2 mm thick at its thickest part and protects the underlying tooth structure. It covers the crown of the tooth, ending around the gum line at the cementoenamel junction. Enamel's hardness enables the crown to withstand the wear of mastication. *Dentin,* which is softer, lies beneath the enamel and makes up the largest part of the tooth structure. It contains a network of microscopic tubules that transport nutrients from the dental pulp. Dentin protects the dental pulp from mechanical, thermal, and chemical irritation. The bone-like *cementum* is softer than dentin and covers the root of the tooth, extending apically from the cementoenamel junction.

The *pulp* occupies the pulp chamber and canal. It is continuous with the tissues surrounding the tooth by an opening at the apex of the root (apical foramen). The pulp consists primarily of vascular and neural tissues. The only nerve endings in the pulp are free nerve endings; therefore, any type of stimulus to the pulp is interpreted as pain.

The *periodontium* comprises the hard and soft tissues that surround the teeth, including the periodontal ligament, the encompassing alveolar bone, and the gingiva. The tooth is suspended hammock-like in bone by the *periodontal ligament.* The cementum's major function is to attach the tooth to the periodontal ligament by periodontal fibers. The periodontal ligament is connective tissue that attaches the tooth to the surrounding alveolar bone and gingival tissue. The periodontal ligament performs supportive, formative, sensory, and nutritive functions. The *alveolar bone* forms the sockets of the teeth. The *gingiva* is the soft tissue surrounding the teeth. Gingiva is categorized as either attached gingiva or unattached gingiva. Attached gingiva normally is pink and stippled (like an orange peel), and is attached to the cementum by periodontal ligament fibers. Unattached gingiva appears light pink or coral in color, is not bound to the underlying tissue of the tooth, and is the first tissue to respond to inflammation.

The major salivary glands—parotid, submandibular, and sublingual—are responsible for secreting *saliva,* an alkaline,

Editor's Note: This chapter is based on the 18th edition chapter of the same title, written by Daniel Forrister.

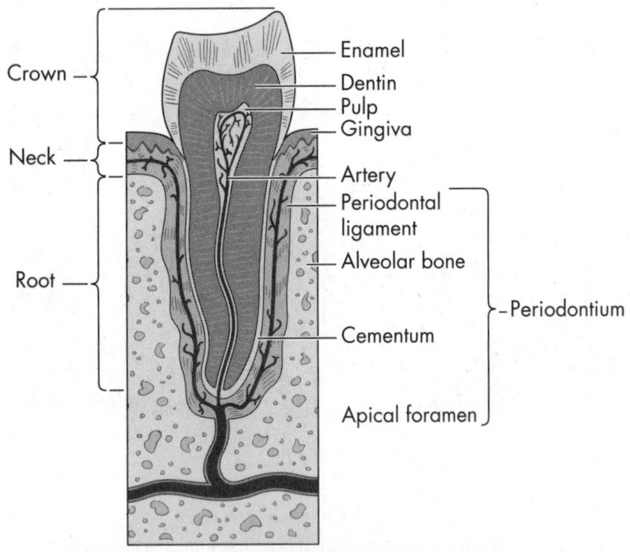

FIGURE 31–1 Anatomy of the tooth.

slightly viscous, clear secretion that contains enzymes (lysozymes and ptyalin), albumin, epithelial mucin (a mucopolysaccharide), immunoglobulin, leukocytes, and minerals. Normal salivary gland function promotes good oral health in several ways. First, saliva lubricates and facilitates the removal of carbohydrates and microorganisms from the oral cavity. Second, saliva also buffers the decline in pH caused by the acid formed by carbohydrate fermentation. Third, the mineral components of saliva have a protective role in the demineralization and remineralization of tooth enamel.

CARIES

The increase in dental caries globally among both children and adults is a great public health concern. Although no consensus has emerged regarding the cause of this increase, health care providers (HCPs) should focus attention on public health strategies that have been successful in reducing caries in the past (e.g., fluoridation of the municipal water supply, topical fluoride treatments, education on proper tooth brushing with a fluoride dentifrice, daily flossing, a proper diet, regular dental office visits).[4]

Patients with poor oral hygiene are at greatest risk for developing caries. Other risk factors for the development of caries include presence of orthodontic appliances, xerostomia (dry mouth), and gum tissue recession that exposes root surfaces. Certain medications may cause xerostomia (see Chapter 32); this condition also is more likely to manifest in patients who have undergone head and neck radiation therapy.

Increased dental caries also is associated with the use of tobacco products, which may be attributable to changes in salivary function, buffering capacity, or composition, including bacterial flora.[5] Because alcohol consumption can cause xerostomia, people who consume alcohol may also be at higher risk for the development of caries.

Access to dental care remains a major issue for one-third of the U.S. population (most notably among racial and ethnic minorities and people with chronic diseases); access often is limited owing to financial barriers, with prioritization of health crises and basic living needs. Access may also be influenced by government legislation pertaining to health insurance coverage. The Affordable Care Act specified that dental care for children is an Essential Health Benefit; however, purchasing a dental plan was not mandatory under federal law, and ultimately the decision was left up to the family, with cost often remaining a frequent deterrent.[6] The American Health Care Act (AHCA) allows states to choose which Essential Health Benefits to cover; this coverage would begin in 2020. The impact of the AHCA on dental care is unknown: although uninsured rates could potentially increase if Medicaid is converted to a block grant program, the use of health savings accounts to cover dental care may become more widespread.[7] Delayed access to dental care for children adversely affects not only their oral health but also their general health, well-being, and readiness to start school.

Pathophysiology of Caries

Dental caries is now considered an infectious disease that affects the calcified tissues of the teeth. Certain plaque bacteria generate acid from dietary carbohydrates; the acid demineralizes tooth enamel and dentin, leading to the formation of soft carious lesions (pits or fissures of smooth surface that, if left untreated, will eventually destroy the tooth). Formation of dental caries requires growth and attachment of cariogenic microorganisms of various species (e.g., *Streptococcus mutans, Lactobacillus casei, Actinomyces viscosus*) to exposed tooth surfaces. If oral hygiene is neglected, dental plaque (the biofilm containing these organisms) remains on the tooth surfaces and over time attracts more bacteria, thereby promoting decay.

The carious process is characterized by alternating periods of destruction (demineralization) and repair (remineralization). Demineralization is caused by organic acids (e.g., lactic and formic acids), which are produced (usually anaerobically) by microbial metabolism of low-molecular-weight carbohydrates (sugars) that readily diffuse into plaque. The resulting reduction in pH on the tooth surface leads to demineralization of dental enamel. Saliva, which is rich in calcium and phosphate ions, is crucial in remineralizing early carious lesions. The presence of fluoride ions in the mouth also promotes remineralization and slows demineralization, thereby retarding enamel dissolution.

A carious lesion starts slowly on the enamel surface and initially produces no clinical symptoms. Once demineralization progresses through the enamel to the softer dentin, the destruction proceeds much more rapidly, becoming clinically or radiographically evident as a carious lesion. At this point, the patient can become aware of the lesion either by observing it or by experiencing symptoms of sensitivity to stimuli (e.g., heat, cold, sweet foods) or chewing. If untreated, the carious lesion can progress to involve the dental pulp (with continuous pain as a common symptom), with eventual necrosis of vital pulp tissue. In addition to pain and difficulty chewing, untreated caries can lead to abscess formation, tooth loss, and serious infections.

Clinical Presentation of Caries

Plaque is commonly recognized as the source of microbes that cause caries and periodontal disease. After meals, food residue may be incorporated into plaque by bacterial degradation. Left undisturbed, plaque thickens, and bacteria proliferate. Plaque growth begins in protected cracks and fissures and along the gingival margin. If not removed within 24 hours, dental plaque (especially in areas opposite the salivary glands) begins to calcify by calcium salt precipitation from the saliva, forming calculus, or tartar. This hardened, adherent deposit is removable only by professional dental cleaning.

Calculus is generally considered to be a substrate on which additional plaque can develop and is not considered the primary cause in periodontal disease. However, most periodontists agree that supragingival and subgingival calculus (located above and below the gingival margins, respectively) can promote the progression of periodontal disease by accumulating new bacterial plaque in contact with sensitive tissue sites and by interfering locally with dental self-hygiene efforts to remove plaque.

Prevention of Caries

General Approach

The key to preventing caries is controlling dental plaque. Because a combination of diet (providing carbohydrate substrate), oral bacteria, and host resistance is involved in developing caries, prevention should be aimed at modifying these factors. The amount and frequency of refined carbohydrate intake should be reduced; plaque should be regularly removed, usually by mechanical means (e.g., brushing; flossing); and host resistance should be increased through appropriate exposure to fluoride ion.

Efforts to reduce childhood caries can begin in infancy. Parents should avoid putting the child to bed with a bottle, and cleaning the teeth before placing the child in bed can help reduce future caries. For toddlers, filling training cups with water instead of milk or juice between meals can reduce the exposure to cavity-causing bacteria.[8]

The declining prevalence of dental caries in permanent teeth among youths, adolescents, and most adults in the United States may be attributed to a combination of these interventions (e.g., increased exposure to fluoride in drinking water, dentifrices, and mouth rinses; changed patterns of diet; overall improved oral hygiene).

Mechanical removal (brushing with a dentifrice and flossing) and chemical management (e.g., using specific products to prevent plaque accumulation or aid its removal) are two methods used to manage plaque. Plaque found on interproximal (between the teeth) surfaces can be removed efficiently only with dental floss and other interdental cleaning aids (e.g., interproximal brush, dental tape, tapered picks).

Nonpharmacologic Therapy

Dietary Measures

Cariogenic foods and beverages, which predispose the tooth enamel to deleterious effects (i.e., erosion), should be avoided in favor of those that are less cariogenic. A food is considered highly cariogenic if it contains more than 15% sugar, clings to the teeth, and remains in the mouth after it is chewed. Conversely, foods are less cariogenic if they have a high water content (e.g., fresh fruit), stimulate the flow of saliva (e.g., carrots, other fibrous foods that require a lot of chewing), or are high in protein (e.g., dairy products). Both the water content of fresh fruit and the resulting flow of saliva tend to wash away the fruit's sugar and neutralize the acid it creates. Milk protein also raises pH and tends to inhibit binding of bacteria. Chewing sugarless gum for 20 minutes after meals helps reduce tooth decay as an adjunct to brushing and flossing.[9] The associated increase in salivary flow helps wash out food debris, and saliva neutralizes acid produced by plaque bacteria.

Plaque Removal Devices

Toothbrushes, dental floss, oral irrigating devices, and specialty aids (e.g., interproximal dental brushes) are the primary devices used in facilitating plaque removal. To ensure the health of teeth and gingival tissues, it is recommended to brush at least twice daily and to floss at least once daily.

Toothbrushes

The toothbrush is the most universally accepted device available for removing dental plaque and maintaining good oral hygiene. Toothbrushing removes plaque from the lingual (tongue side), buccal (cheek side), and occlusal (biting) surfaces of the teeth.

The proper frequency and method of brushing will vary from patient to patient. Thoroughness of plaque removal without gingival trauma is more important than the method used. Table 31–1 describes the proper method of brushing teeth.

Manual toothbrushes vary in size, shape, texture, and design, with new product designs proliferating rapidly. These toothbrushes have either nylon or natural bristles that usually are rated as soft, medium, or firm.

Powered toothbrushes, which are widely available on the market, either are battery-operated or have a rechargeable battery system. Battery-operated devices (e.g., Arm & Hammer Spinbrush, Colgate 360 Sonic Power Toothbrush) use a rotary and/or vibratory motion and are less expensive, but their effectiveness deteriorates over time as the disposable battery loses power. Rechargeable battery toothbrushes may also use a rotary and/or vibrating motion (e.g., Oral B) or ultrasonic vibration (e.g., Sonicare, Oral B) to remove plaque. These powered brushes tend to be more expensive, but they maintain constant efficiency because of their rechargeability. Powered toothbrushes may be of benefit for certain patients, such as those who are disabled or who have dexterity issues.

No definite guideline specifies how often a patient should buy a new toothbrush, although 3 months has been suggested as the average toothbrush life expectancy. Children's toothbrushes often need to be replaced more frequently than adult brushes. Two compelling reasons are recognized for replacing toothbrushes

TABLE 31-1 Guidelines for Brushing Teeth

- Brush teeth after each meal or at least twice a day.
- If using toothpaste, apply a small amount of paste to the toothbrush.
- Use a gentle scrubbing motion with the bristle tips at a 45-degree angle against the gum line so that the tips of the brush do the cleaning.
- Do not use excessive force because it may result in bristle damage, cervical abrasion, irritation of delicate gingival tissue, and gingival recession with associated hypersensitivity.
- Brush for at least 2 minutes, cleaning all tooth surfaces systematically.
- Gently brush the upper surface of the tongue to reduce debris, plaque, and bacteria that can cause oral hygiene problems.
- Rinse the mouth, and spit out all of the water (do not swallow).

frequently: bristle wear and bacterial accumulation. Different brushing methods cause bristles to wear differently. Worn, bent, or matted bristles do not remove plaque effectively. Accordingly, toothbrushes should be replaced at the first sign of bristle wear, rather than after a defined period of use. Ideally, the toothbrushing regimen should rotate among 2 or 3 toothbrushes to allow each to dry completely between uses, thereby decreasing bristle wear and matting. Some brands of toothbrushes have color-impregnated bristles that indicate the need for replacement when the color disappears halfway down the bristles.

PRODUCT SELECTION GUIDELINES. HCPs should recommend toothbrushes that carry the American Dental Association's (ADA) Seal of Acceptance, as described in the box "American Dental Association (ADA) Seal of Acceptance."[10] ADA criteria for acceptance are based on safety and efficacy concerns. Currently, no powered toothbrushes have the ADA Seal of Acceptance, which may reflect previously limited research. A recent Cochrane review, however, found that powered toothbrushes do provide a statistically significant reduction in the occurrence of plaque and gingivitis from that for manual brushes.[11]

Dental professionals recommend toothbrushes according to the individual patient's manual dexterity, oral anatomy, and periodontal health. The toothbrush should be of a size and shape to allow the user to reach every tooth in the mouth. Innovations in head shapes and bristle configurations continue to be introduced in an attempt to improve cleaning contact with tooth and gum line surfaces. Toothbrush firmness is not standardized; toothbrushes designated as soft, medium, or hard may not be comparable across manufacturers. Use of medium- or hard-bristle toothbrushes may result in damage to the tooth enamel and gingival tissue. Softer bristles are more effective at working themselves into crevices and spaces between the teeth, and they are less abrasive on teeth with exposed recession, as well as gentler on soft tissue. Many dental providers and dental hygienists prefer soft, rounded, multitufted, nylon bristle brushes, both because nylon bristles are more durable and easier to clean than natural bristles and because soft, rounded bristle tips are more effective in removing plaque below the gingival margin and on proximal tooth surfaces.

The handle size and shape of a toothbrush should allow the user to maneuver the brush easily while maintaining a firm grasp. Many modifications (e.g., angle bends or flexible areas in the handle) that may improve contact between the bristles and some less-accessible tooth surfaces have been introduced. Dental providers can fabricate customized handles for physically impaired individuals by adding moldable acrylic to the handles.

Children's toothbrushes are smaller than adult toothbrushes and typically are sized by age. Toothbrush size and shape should be individualized according to the size of the child's mouth. Soft bristles are recommended for children's toothbrushes. Children usually can remove plaque more easily with a brush that has short and narrow bristles.

Dental Floss

Plaque accumulation in the interdental spaces contributes to proximal caries and periodontal pocketing. Interdental plaque removal has been reported to reduce gingival inflammation and prevent periodontal disease and dental caries. Dental flossing is the most widely recommended method of removing dental plaque from proximal tooth surfaces that are not adequately cleaned by toothbrushing alone. By removing plaque and debris interproximally, proper flossing also polishes the tooth surfaces and reduces gingival inflammation. Proper flossing technique requires some finger dexterity and practice. If performed improperly, flossing can injure gingival tissue and cause cervical wear on proximal root surfaces. Table 31–2 describes the proper use of dental floss.

Floss is a multifilament nylon yarn that is available in waxed or unwaxed form and in various widths, ranging from thin thread to thick tape. Many brands feature product lines of flosses that are coated with additives, such as flavoring, baking soda, and fluoride. In addition, several manufacturers are marketing floss made of materials with superior antishredding properties (e.g., Glide, Oral B Essential).

PRODUCT SELECTION GUIDELINES. The HCP should recommend a dental floss product with the ADA Seal of Acceptance.[10] Clinical studies have not shown any differences among various floss types in terms of removing plaque and preventing gingivitis, so patient factors (e.g., tightness of tooth contacts, tooth roughness, manual dexterity, personal preference) should be considered in product selection.[12]

Waxed or antishredding floss may be passed between tight-fitting teeth with less shredding and resistance than unwaxed floss. If contacts at the crowns of teeth are too tight to permit interdental flossing, floss threaders can be used to pass floss between the teeth and under the replacement teeth (pontics) of fixed

AMERICAN DENTAL ASSOCIATION (ADA) Seal of Acceptance

ADA evaluates the safety and efficacy of dental products used by dental professionals and the public through the Council on Scientific Affairs' Seal of Acceptance evaluation program. Manufacturers of dentifrices or mouth rinses with therapeutic potential for gingivitis and supragingival dental plaque control may voluntarily submit data to ADA for evaluation. Product labels and promotional material must also comply with ADA standards.

The ADA Council on Scientific Affairs allows only products that demonstrate a significant effect against gingivitis to make plaque-control or plaque-modification claims. A product for which significant plaque reduction but no concomitant significant reduction in gingivitis has been demonstrated will not be eligible for acceptance.[18] ADA has approved the following statements to be used for products classified under these guidelines—the first for both gingivitis and plaque reduction, and the second for gingivitis reduction only:

- "The ADA Council on Scientific Affairs' Acceptance of (product name) is based on its finding that the product is effective in helping to prevent and reduce gingivitis and plaque above the gumline, when used as directed."
- "The ADA Council on Scientific Affairs' Acceptance of (product name) is based on its finding that the product is effective in helping to prevent and reduce gingivitis, when used as directed."[18]

Once a product has earned the ADA seal, it may display that seal for 5 years, provided that it continues to meet all of the requirements.[9] The ADA online home page (www.ada.org) provides searchable access to a current listing of dental consumer products that have been awarded the ADA Seal of Acceptance.

TABLE 31-2 **Guidelines for Using Dental Floss**

- Pull out approximately 18 inches of floss from the dispenser, and wrap most of it around the middle finger.
- Wrap the remaining floss around the same finger of the opposite hand. Approximately an inch of floss should be held between the thumbs and forefingers.
- Do not "snap" the floss down between the teeth; instead, use a gentle, sawing motion to guide the floss to the gum line.
- When the gum line is reached, curve the floss into a C shape against one tooth, and gently slide the floss into the space between the gum and the tooth until you feel resistance.
- Hold the floss tightly against the tooth, and gently scrape the side of the tooth with an up-and-down motion.
- Curve the floss around the adjoining tooth, and repeat the procedure.
- Use a new section of floss for each tooth surface, to avoid the transfer of plaque and bacteria to other teeth.

bridges. Floss threaders, available in reusable and disposable forms, usually are thin plastic loops or soft plastic, needle-like appliances. Patients who wear braces may find that the use of threaders aids in the flossing process. Floss holders have one or two forks that are rigid enough to keep floss taut and a mounting mechanism that allows quick rethreading of floss. These products are recommended for patients who lack manual dexterity and for caregivers who assist disabled or hospitalized patients. Electrically powered interdental cleaning devices may be used to remove interproximal debris. Such devices, including floss threaders, should be used cautiously to avoid physical trauma to the gingiva.

Specialty Aids

Cleaning devices that adapt to irregular tooth surfaces better than dental floss are recommended for interproximal cleaning of teeth with large interdental spaces. Increased interdental spacing often is characteristic of periodontal disease. The G-U-M Flossbrush is such a device; it features woven dental floss that contains a timed-release fluoride system and is molded into a plastic handle for interdental cleaning. The most commonly used aids are tapered triangular wooden toothpicks (Stim-U-Dent), holders for round toothpicks (Perio-Aid), interdental brushes (Proxabrush), rubber stimulator tips, denture brushes, and denture clasp brushes.

Oral Irrigating Devices

Oral irrigators work by directing a high-pressure stream of water through a nozzle to the tooth surfaces. These devices can remove only a minimal amount of plaque from tooth surfaces. Therefore, oral irrigators cannot be viewed as substitutes for a toothbrush, dental floss, or other plaque-removal devices, but they should be considered as adjuncts in maintaining good oral hygiene. These devices are useful for removing loose debris from those areas that cannot be cleaned with a toothbrush (e.g., around orthodontic bands or fixed bridges). Several brands on the market carry the ADA Seal of Acceptance.[10]

Oral irrigators are also valuable as vehicles for administering chemotherapeutic agents that inhibit microbial growth in inaccessible regions of the mouth. Patients with advanced periodontal disease should use these devices only under professional supervision, because transient bacteremia may occur after manipulative procedures with the oral irrigator. Oral irrigation devices are also contraindicated in patients who are at risk for the development of bacterial endocarditis.

Pharmacologic Therapy

Chemical Management of Plaque

Chemical management of plaque and calculus can enhance mechanical removal either by acting directly on the plaque bacteria or by disrupting components of plaque to aid in its removal during routine oral hygiene. The use of chemical agents in plaque control may be particularly appropriate for selected patients who may be unable to brush and floss effectively. Physically or mentally disabled individuals (who may not be able to master the manual techniques necessary to brush and floss effectively) and patients with orthodontic appliances (i.e., fixed prostheses) may benefit from adding antiplaque agents to their oral hygiene regimen.

Desirable characteristics for antiplaque agents include the following:

- selective antibacterial activity; interference with the rate of accumulation or metabolism of supragingival plaque
- substantivity (sustained retention of the agent in the mouth)
- compatibility with dentifrice ingredients
- lack of undesirable adverse effects for the user
- noninterference with the natural ecology of the normal oral microflora

Use of Fluoride

Fluoride is believed to help prevent dental caries through a combination of effects. When it is incorporated into developing teeth, fluoride acts systemically to reduce the solubility of dental enamel by enhancing the development of a fluoridated hydroxyapatite, which is more resistant to demineralizing acids, at the enamel surface. When applied topically, fluoride facilitates remineralization of early carious lesions during repeated cycles of demineralization and remineralization. Some evidence suggests that fluoride interferes with the bacterial cariogenic process. Fluoride that is chemically bound to organic constituents of plaque may interfere with plaque adherence and may inhibit glycolysis (the process by which sugar is metabolized to produce acid).[13]

Fluoridation of the public water supply is an effective and economically sound public health measure that has played a major role in decreasing the incidence of caries.[13] According to the Centers for Disease Control and Prevention, more than 75% of the U.S. population resides in communities in which the public water supply contains either naturally occurring or added fluoride at optimal levels for decay prevention (1 ppm or 1 mg/L).[14] In addition to reducing dental caries in children, fluoridation has benefits that extend through adulthood, resulting in (1) fewer decayed, missing, or filled teeth; (2) better tooth retention; and (3) a lower incidence of root caries. Current concepts of the action of fluoride relative to its presence in saliva and plaque provide a rationale for its topical application to prevent caries in all age groups. Most bottled water does not contain fluoride. If manufacturers choose to add fluoride, the U.S. Food and Drug Administration (FDA) recommends limiting the concentration to no more than 0.7 mg/L.[15] This recommendation replaces the previously recommended level of 0.7–1.2 mg/L and aims to promote balance between protection from dental caries, which lead to tooth decay, and the risk of dental fluorosis. The FDA recommendation is specific only to fluoride added to bottled water. Mouth rinses and gels that contain sodium fluoride are therapeutic topical applications of fluoride for prevention of dental caries (Table 31–3). Fluoride mouth rinsing enables patients to apply fluoride interproximally.

Patients who may benefit from fluoride rinsing include those with fixed orthodontic appliances, those with decreased salivary flow, those at risk for developing root caries, and anyone with difficulty maintaining good oral hygiene. Orthodontic appliance–wearing patients are at risk for the development of decalcified areas during treatment, because the ability to thoroughly clean interdental spaces may be inhibited by presence of the appliance or its attachments.

Package directions of fluoride rinses and gels should be followed closely to maximize the safe and effective use of these products. Table 31–4 describes the proper method of applying fluoride treatments. When recommending a nonprescription fluoride mouth rinse, the HCP should emphasize the need for parents and caregivers to supervise children younger than 12 years as necessary until they are capable of using the product correctly. Furthermore, children younger than 6 years should use these products only as directed by a dental care or primary care provider.

Dental fluorosis—evident as a mottled appearance of the surface enamel of the tooth—may develop in children who receive excess fluoride intake during the time of tooth formation. Although a mild degree of fluorosis is an aesthetic concern, more severe cases can result in pitting and surface defects (see Color Plates, photograph 10).

In response to the aesthetic concerns related to fluorosis, FDA considered issuing comments regarding formulation of a reduced-strength fluoride dentifrice during the anticaries final rule process. FDA determined that unlike dental caries, mild dental fluorosis does not compromise oral health or tooth function; therefore, the risk of dental caries from inadequate fluoride protection is a greater health hazard than the cosmetic detriment of fluorosis.

Dentifrices

Dentifrices (e.g., toothpastes) are used with a toothbrush for cleaning accessible tooth surfaces. Use of a dentifrice enhances removal of dental plaque and stains, resulting in a decreased incidence of dental caries and gum disease, reduced mouth odors, and enhanced personal appearance.

Dentifrices are available as pastes or gels (Table 31–5). The gels and pastes commonly contain an abrasive, a surfactant, a humectant (moistening agent), a binder or thickener, a sweetener, flavoring agents, and one or more therapeutic agents (e.g., fluoride) for anticaries activity.

Dentifrice abrasives are pharmacologically inactive and insoluble compounds. Common abrasives include silicates, dicalcium phosphate, alumina trihydrate, calcium pyrophosphate, calcium carbonate, and sodium metaphosphate. Dentifrices vary in their degree of abrasiveness; factors such as the size and shape of the abrasive particle, individual brushing technique, and individual salivary characteristics affect the abrasive's potential effectiveness. The ideal abrasive would provide maximal cleaning while causing minimal damage to tooth surfaces. Unfortunately, because of the variability in patients' brushing techniques and oral health status, the ideal dentifrice abrasive does not exist. Low-abrasive dentifrices (including most dentifrice formulations currently marketed in the United States) usually have a low concentration of silica abrasives (10%–25%), whereas high-abrasive dentifrices typically have higher concentrations of the inorganic calcium or aluminum salts previously mentioned (40%–50%). Baking soda, a mild abrasive, is found in a number of dentifrices. Recent studies have demonstrated that toothpastes with baking soda are more effective at removing plaque than toothpastes without it.[16,17] Sodium lauryl sulfate, a chemical used to create a foaming action, is present in nearly all toothpastes and has been implicated as a cause of irritative lesions of the oral mucosa such as aphthous ulcers (i.e., canker sores; see Chapter 32).[18] Some dentifrices that do not contain sodium lauryl sulfate are listed in Table 31–5.

Fluoride Dentifrices

Fluoride dentifrices are indicated for both preventing and treating carious lesions. In all countries that show a reduction in caries, use of fluoride-containing dentifrices for caries prevention is the norm. ADA accepts fluoride-containing toothpaste and fluoride-containing gel dentifrice formulations with compatible abrasives as safe and effective. The most commonly used fluoride sources are sodium fluoride, sodium monofluorophosphate, and stannous fluoride. The first two forms remineralize and strengthen weakened enamel in addition to reducing gingivitis and sensitivity. In addition to these beneficial effects, stannous fluoride also creates a protective mineral layer over the teeth to prevent plaque.

Patients may experience slight (but noticeable) tooth discoloration after using stannous fluoride dentifrices continuously for 2–3 months. The staining is not permanent and is readily removed

TABLE 31-3 Selected Nonprescription Topical Fluoride Products

Trade Name	Primary Ingredient
ACT Anticavity Fluoride Rinse	Sodium fluoride 0.05%
Crest Pro-Health For Me Anti-Cavity Fluoride Rinse	Sodium fluoride 0.022%
Colgate Phos-Flur Fluoride Rinse	Sodium fluoride 0.044%
Alpha-Dent Home Care Fluoride Gel	Stannous fluoride 0.4%

TABLE 31-4 Guidelines for Using Topical Fluoride Treatments

- Use topical fluoride treatments no more than once a day.
- Brush teeth with a fluoride dentifrice before using a fluoride treatment.
- If using a fluoride rinse, measure the recommended dose (most commonly 10 mL), and vigorously swish it between the teeth for 1 minute.
- If using a fluoride gel, brush the gel on the teeth. Allow the gel to remain for 1 minute.
- After 1 minute, spit out the fluoride product. Do not swallow it.
- Do not eat or drink for 30 minutes after the treatment.
- Supervise children receiving fluoride treatments as necessary until they can use the product without supervision.
- Instruct children younger than 12 years in good rinsing habits to minimize swallowing of the product.

TABLE 31-5 Selected Nonprescription Dentifrices

Trade Name	Primary Ingredients
Fluoride Toothpastes	
Arm & Hammer Dental Care Toothpaste	Sodium fluoride (fluoride 0.24%)
Colgate Cavity Protection Toothpaste	Sodium monofluorophosphate (fluoride 0.15%)
Crest Cavity Protection Gel	Sodium fluoride (fluoride 0.15%)
Tartar-Control Toothpastes	
Colgate Total Toothpaste	Sodium fluoride (fluoride 0.24%); triclosan 0.3%
Crest Tartar Protection Gel/Toothpaste	Sodium fluoride (0.15%)
Antiplaque/Antigingivitis Toothpastes	
Colgate Total Toothpaste	Sodium fluoride (fluoride 0.24%); triclosan 0.3%
Crest Pro-Health Toothpaste	Stannous fluoride (fluoride 0.16%)
Whitening Toothpastes	
Colgate Total Whitening Gel/Toothpaste	Sodium fluoride (fluoride 0.24%); triclosan 0.3%
Crest Pro-Health Extra Whitening Power Toothpaste	Stannous fluoride (fluoride 0.16%)
Sodium Lauryl Sulfate–Free Toothpastes[a]	
Toms of Maine Clean & Gentle	Sodium monofluorophosphate (fluoride 0.13%)
Sensodyne Pronamel Toothpaste	Sodium fluoride (fluoride 0.15%)
Botanical-Based Toothpastes[a]	
Tom's of Maine Botanically Bright	Peppermint or spearmint; xylitol; carrageenan; stevia; propolis
Jason Powersmile Whitening Toothpaste	Calcium carbonate; carrageenan; bamboo powder; parsley extract; grapefruit seed extract; peppermint; sodium bicarbonate

[a] These products do not have the ADA Seal of Acceptance.

at the next professional dental cleaning. Stannous fluoride is indicated for use by adults and children 12 years of age and older.

Tartar-Control Dentifrices

A number of fluoride dentifrices contain anticalculus compounds for tartar control. Although plaque—not supragingival calculus—is the primary etiologic factor in marginal periodontal disease, reducing calculus formation remains a goal of good oral hygiene. The ingredients of tartar-control dentifrices that prevent or retard new calculus formation are zinc chloride, zinc citrate, and soluble pyrophosphates, which act to inhibit crystal growth. ADA regards the inhibition of supragingival calculus as a nontherapeutic use and therefore does not evaluate anticalculus claims. However, all advertising claims made for accepted products are reviewed for accuracy as described in the box "American Dental Association (ADA) Seal of Acceptance."[19]

The use of tartar-control toothpastes has been associated with a type of contact dermatitis in the perioral region. The addition of pyrophosphate compounds to these products to increase alkalinity requires increased concentrations of other components for solubilizing (e.g., flavorings, surfactants); presence of such ingredients at high levels is hypothesized to be the cause of irritant contact dermatitis. Patients experiencing such a reaction should be advised to discontinue the tartar-control dentifrice and to switch to a non–tartar-control fluoride product.

Antiplaque and Antigingivitis Dentifrices

Two toothpastes that are currently accepted by ADA for both antiplaque and antigingivitis indications include Colgate Total, containing triclosan, and Crest Pro-Health, containing stannous fluoride. These dentifrices are not intended for use in children younger than 6 and 12 years respectively.[10]

Whitening/Antistain Dentifrices

Cosmetic dentifrices make no therapeutic claims and are usually chosen by patients for whitening ability or antistain properties, as well as taste. Some dentifrices that claim to remove coffee or tobacco stains may contain higher concentrations of abrasives. High-abrasive formulations are not advised for long-term use or for use by patients with exposed root surfaces. Plain baking soda (a water-soluble, mild abrasive) and toothpastes containing baking soda (e.g., Arm & Hammer Truly Radiant) have been shown to be effective at stain removal.[20] Other products may contain a pigment (e.g., titanium dioxide) that produces a temporary brightening effect. Rembrandt Whitening Toothpaste contains a chemical complex of aluminum oxide, a citrate salt, and papain. Whitening dentifrices that incorporate oxygenating agents rely on a debriding action to remove stained pellicle. Numerous products offer a combination of baking soda and peroxide with fluoride. Whitening dentifrices should not be confused with tooth-bleaching products, as described in the box "A Word About Tooth-Bleaching Products."

A WORD ABOUT
Tooth-Bleaching Products

The popularity of tooth bleaching has increased in the United States in recent years. Three methods are currently in use: (1) in-office dental bleaching, (2) dental office–supported home bleaching, and (3) nonprescription home bleaching. All three methods use basically the same chemical agents: carbamide peroxide or hydrogen peroxide in various strengths. The in-office method has the advantage of a one-time treatment, but the stronger bleach and the accelerator light are not necessary to obtain the same result with the dental office–supported home-bleaching process. The latter method involves the use of custom trays. With this process, patients can fine-tune the extent of lightening to their own preferences.

The following two nonprescription products (from among many) may aid in lightening teeth:

- Rembrandt Intense Stain Dissolving Strips contain hydrogen peroxide. The kit contains 56 whitening strips that are applied to upper and lower teeth. Strips dissolve in 5–10 minutes with nothing to remove. The kit is designed for use over a 2-week period.
- Crest 3D WhiteStrips Vivid are translucent film strips impregnated with hydrogen peroxide and other ingredients. The strips are peeled away from a protective backing and then applied by folding them over the 6 upper or lower front teeth (different strips are provided for upper and lower teeth). The teeth will look as though they are covered with small pieces of transparent food wrap. The strips are applied once a day and left in place for 30 minutes. A kit contains enough strips for 10 days.

Botanical-Based Dentifrices

Some evidence indicates that nonbotanical-based and botanical-based dentifrices are equally effective at reducing plaque. Reported studies, however, have small sample sizes and were conducted outside of the United States.[21]

Administration Guidelines

Table 31–1 describes the proper method for brushing teeth using a fluoride dentifrice. Children usually are unable to brush by themselves until they are 4–5 years of age; to clean their teeth effectively, children may require supervision until 8–9 years of age. FDA recommends that caregivers instruct children 6–12 years of age about good brushing and rinsing habits to minimize swallowing of fluoride. ADA recommends that caregivers use a smear (approximately the size of a grain of rice) of fluoride toothpaste for children younger than 3 years and no more than a pea-sized amount of toothpaste for children 3 to 6 years of age.[22] Non-fluoridated pediatric toothpastes can be recommended for young children, who may ingest toothpaste instead of rinsing and expectorating.

All fluoride dentifrice products must contain the following warning on the labeling: "Warning: Keep out of the reach of children under 6 years of age. If you accidentally swallow more than used for brushing, seek professional assistance or contact a poison control center immediately."

Product Selection Guidelines

Unless otherwise advised by their dental providers, patients (especially those with periodontal disease, significant gum recession, and/or exposed root surfaces) should choose the least abrasive dentifrice that effectively removes stained pellicle. Although dentifrice abrasives do not pose a risk to dental enamel, toothbrushing action and excessive abrasiveness (which may lead to tooth hypersensitivity) can damage the cementum (the softer material of exposed root surfaces) and dentin.

ADA now recommends fluoride dentifrices for all children regardless of age, because the benefit of reducing dental caries outweighs any associated risks. Extra-strength fluoride dentifrices may be beneficial to patients who have a greater tendency to develop cavities or who reside in an area with non-fluoridated water. HCPs should recommend a dentifrice that is sodium lauryl sulfate–free for patients with a history of canker sores.

Flavored gel dentifrices disperse rapidly in the mouth and are popular with children. Manufacturers of gel dentifrices have advertised that children brush longer and more thoroughly because of the preferable consistency, translucence, dispersibility, and flavor of these products. This claim has not been substantiated, but many dentifrices marketed for children are of the gel type. Children's products usually have fruit flavors rather than "breath-freshening" minty or cinnamon flavors, which adults prefer.

Mouth Rinses

Regular use of a mouth rinse with plaque- or calculus-control properties is indicated as an adjunct to proper flossing and toothbrushing with fluoride toothpaste. Further research is necessary to determine the efficacy of the antiplaque activity of these products. Mouth rinse and dentifrice formulations are very similar. As with dentifrices, mouth rinses may be cosmetic or therapeutic (Table 31–6). Both may contain surfactants, humectants, flavor, coloring, water, and therapeutic ingredients.

TABLE 31-6 Selected Nonprescription Mouth Rinses

Trade Name	Primary Ingredients
Cosmetic Mouth Rinses[a]	
Bioténe	Glycerin; xylitol; sorbitol; propylene glycol
Lavoris	Cinnamon and clove oil; zinc oxide; sodium hydroxide; citric acid
Therapeutic Mouth Rinses[a]	
Crest Pro-Health Rinse	Cetylpyridinium chloride 0.07%
Crest Pro-Health Clinical Rinse	Cetylpyridinium chloride 0.1%
Gly-Oxide	Carbamide peroxide 10%
Scope	Cetylpyridinium chloride
Plaque/Gingivitis Control Rinse	
Listerine Antiseptic	Thymol; eucalyptol; methyl salicylate; menthol

[a] These products do not have the ADA Seal of Acceptance.

A mouth rinse approximates a diluted liquid dentifrice that contains alcohol but no abrasive. Alcohol adds bite and freshness, enhances flavor, solubilizes other ingredients, and contributes to the mouth rinse's cleansing action and antibacterial activity. Flavor contributes pleasant taste and breath-freshening action. Surfactants are foaming agents that aid in the removal of debris. Other active ingredients may include astringents (alum or zinc chloride), demulcents (sorbitol or glycerin), antibacterial agents (cetylpyridinium chloride or thymol), and fluoride.

Cosmetic mouth rinses freshen the breath and clean some debris from the mouth. Mouth rinses can be classified by appearance, flavor, alcohol content, and active ingredients. In general, mouth rinses contain various ingredients such as (1) glycerin, a topical protectant that tastes sweet and is soothing to oral mucosa; (2) benzoic acid, an antimicrobial agent; or (3) zinc chloride or zinc citrate, both astringents that neutralize odoriferous sulfur compounds produced in the oral cavity. The most popular cosmetic mouth rinses are medicinal and mint-flavored. Healthy individuals normally have some degree of oral malodor, typically on awakening (i.e., "morning breath"). This malodor results from reduced nighttime activity of tongue and cheek muscles and of salivary flow, contributing to enhanced bacterial activity and production of odoriferous sulfur compounds. (Other causes of oral malodor in healthy persons are noted later in the "Halitosis" section.) The FDA Advisory Review Panel on Over-the-Counter Oral Health Care Products considers products that are intended to eliminate or suppress mouth odor of local origin in healthy people with healthy mouths to be cosmetics unless they contain antimicrobial or other therapeutic agents. ADA does not evaluate mouth rinses labeled and advertised as only cosmetic agents.

One important consideration is the potential for breath-freshening mouth rinses to disguise or delay treatment of pathologic conditions that may contribute to lingering oral malodor (e.g., periodontal disease, purulent oral infections, respiratory infections). If marked breath odor persists after proper toothbrushing, investigation for an underlying cause is warranted; masking the odor with mouth rinse will not address the issue.

Since the 1990s, nonprescription mouth rinses promoted for antiplaque or tartar-control activity have proliferated. Plaque control ingredients include (1) aromatic oils (thymol, eucalyptol, menthol, and methyl salicylate), which are antibacterial and have some local anesthetic activity, and (2) agents with antimicrobial activity (e.g., quaternary ammonium compounds). Listerine, containing the active ingredients thymol, eucalyptol, methyl salicylate, and menthol, was the first mouth rinse to be accepted by ADA as a nonprescription antiplaque/antigingivitis mouth rinse. The phenol oils control plaque by destroying bacterial cell walls, inhibiting bacterial enzymes, and extracting bacterial lipopolysaccharides.

Many dental providers have found anecdotally that use of rinses containing phenol oils, methyl salicylate, and alcohol may bring about a sloughing of the oral epithelium, which subsides when the rinse is discontinued. A similar effect has been observed with the use of lozenges or candies containing cinnamon or other common flavoring substances.

Mouth rinses and gels are generally safe when used as directed, but occasional adverse reactions (e.g., burning sensation, irritation) have been reported. Overuse should be discouraged. Consultation with a health professional is indicated if irritation persists after the patient discontinues use of the product.

Unsupervised use of mouth rinses is contraindicated in patients with mouth irritation or ulceration. These products should be kept out of children's reach. In case of accidental ingestion, the caregiver should seek professional assistance or contact a poison control center.

The alcohol content in mouth rinses ranges from 0% to 27%; the most popular adult mouth rinses contain between 14% and 27%. Ingestion of alcohol-containing rinses poses a danger for children, who may be attracted by the bright colors and pleasant flavors of these products. Toxicity data concerning children's ingestion of alcohol-containing mouth rinses demonstrate that the amount of alcohol in available mouth rinse preparations is sufficient to cause serious illness and injury. The generally accepted lethal dose of ethanol in children is 3 g/kg; however, toxic reactions have been reported from doses as small as 0.6 g/kg. Responding to concern over the potential danger to children, the Consumer Products Safety Commission issued a final rule that required child-resistant packaging for mouth rinses containing 3 g or more of absolute alcohol per package—the amount that is present in a small quantity (approximately 2.6 ounces) of a mouth rinse with alcohol 5%. For the purposes of this final rule, the term *mouthwash* includes liquid products that are variously called mouthwashes, mouth rinses, oral antiseptics, gargles, fluoride rinses, antiplaque rinses, and breath fresheners. The rule does not include throat sprays or aerosol breath fresheners. These products should be kept out of children's reach and should not be administered to children younger than 12 years. Labeling includes a warning not to swallow the product but to seek professional assistance or contact a poison control center immediately in case of accidental ingestion.

Special Population Considerations for Plaque Removal

At birth, the 20 primary teeth that will erupt are present but not visible. Oral hygiene must be started early in life. Accordingly, HCPs should recommend that caregivers remove plaque and milk residue from the baby's mouth after each feeding by wiping the gums with a wet gauze pad. The deciduous teeth usually start to erupt at the age of approximately 6 months and without proper oral care can begin to decay at any time. "Baby bottle caries" results when an infant is allowed to nurse continuously from a bottle of juice, milk, or sugar water. The prolonged contact of teeth with the cariogenic liquid promotes conditions conducive to decay.

When the teeth have erupted, a soft, child-sized toothbrush can be used for cleaning. Parents must do the brushing and should take care to use a smear of fluoride toothpaste. Children at this age will swallow the toothpaste, which will contribute to overall systemic fluoride ingestion. Therefore, younger children need to be taught the proper brushing technique and should be supervised while brushing.

In patients with fixed orthodontic appliances, very careful attention to oral hygiene to prevent gingivitis and caries is required because of the ease with which plaque accumulates along the orthodontic brackets. Patients with these appliances require a combination of toothbrush types to clean all surfaces effectively. Use of power toothbrushes or oral irrigating devices may help remove plaque and debris around orthodontic bands. Orthodontic patients may want to use a nonprescription fluoride mouth rinse while undergoing treatment.

Patients with removable orthodontic appliances should consult their orthodontist about using a denture cleanser. In addition to brushing orthodontic appliances, some dental providers recommend a denture cleanser to remove plaque, tartar, odor-causing bacteria, and stain that accumulate on orthodontic appliances.

In patients of advanced age who have natural dentition, topical fluoride application in the form of a dentifrice, rinse, or gel is indicated to prevent coronal and root caries. HCPs should continue to recommend fluoride anticaries products to older adult patients. For counseling on oral health care in this age group, review and update of the medication history are essential. Because senior patients are more likely to be taking multiple medications, the incidence of drug-induced or disease-related changes in oral physiology is increased.

No special considerations related to plaque removal have been identified for pregnant or lactating women or for males and females of reproductive age.

Assessment of Caries

When asked to recommend plaque-control products, the HCP should determine what dental care measures the patient is taking, whether these measures meet recommended oral hygiene standards, and how often the patient sees a dental care provider. It also is important to ascertain whether the patient has a history of caries or if the patient suspects that a new carious lesion has developed. Presence of dental caries symptoms—toothache, tooth sensitivity with chewing, or tooth pain with exposure to hot, cold, or sweet foods or beverages—warrants referral to a dental care provider for evaluation and treatment.

Patient Counseling for Caries Prevention

In patient counseling for caries prevention, all explanations of the purposes of various oral hygiene products and the methods for using them should be tailored to the patient's level of knowledge. Patients with a history of caries should be encouraged to brush after meals and to consult with a dental provider about the use of topical fluoride products. The HCP may recommend products with anticaries agents (e.g., chlorhexidine, xylitol). If caries recurs or is widespread, the patient should be encouraged to visit a dental care provider for treatment. The HCP should explain the precautions for these products as well as the possible adverse effects of certain therapeutic ingredients in other products. The box "Patient Education for Prevention of Caries, Gingivitis, and Halitosis" lists specific information for patient counseling on plaque-induced oral disorders.

PATIENT EDUCATION FOR Prevention of Caries, Gingivitis, and Halitosis

The primary objective of self-care for oral hygiene is the removal of plaque to prevent caries, gingivitis, and halitosis. For most patients, carefully following product instructions and the self-care measures listed here will help ensure good oral hygiene.

Nondrug Measures and Other Considerations

- Avoid cariogenic foods, such as foods that contain more than 15% sugar, cling to the teeth, and remain in the mouth after they are chewed.
- Eat low-cariogenic-index foods, such as foods that have a high water content (e.g., fresh fruit), stimulate the flow of saliva (e.g., fibrous foods that take longer to chew), or are high in protein (e.g., dairy products).
- To help prevent mouth odor, maintain proper oral hygiene and limit or avoid foods and products that may cause oral malodor. Also, if you wear dentures, do not wear them while sleeping.
- Note that use of alcohol and tobacco are associated with caries, gingivitis, and halitosis.
- Note that hormonal changes during pregnancy increase the risk of gingivitis.
- Chewing sugarless gum for 20 minutes after meals helps reduce tooth decay as an adjunct to brushing and flossing.

Plaque Removal

Brushing Teeth

- Mechanically remove plaque buildup by brushing teeth at least twice daily with a fluoride dentifrice. (See Table 31–1 for proper brushing technique.)
- Use a brush with soft nylon bristles.
- Replace the brush when the bristles show signs of wear.
- For children younger than 3 years, use a smear (a grain of rice size) of fluoride gel once teeth erupt.
- For children 3–6 years of age, apply a pea-sized amount of toothpaste to a child-sized toothbrush, and brush the child's teeth until the child can brush properly.
- Teach children how to rinse the mouth and spit out the toothpaste to avoid swallowing fluoride.
- Note that tartar-control toothpastes have been related to a type of contact dermatitis in the perioral region. If you experience itching or irritation of the mouth after brushing, discontinue the tartar-control toothpaste, and switch to a non–tartar-control fluoride toothpaste.
- If you are prone to developing caries or gingivitis, consider using a toothpaste with antiplaque or antigingivitis activity. Such toothpastes contain stannous fluoride.
- If you are prone to developing aphthous ulcers, consider using a toothpaste that does not contain sodium lauryl sulfate.

Flossing Teeth

- Floss your teeth at least once a day. (See Table 31–2 for proper flossing technique.)
- Use waxed or Teflon-coated floss for teeth with tight contacts.

Using Mouth Rinses and Gels

- To freshen breath, use a mouth rinse that contains zinc chloride and zinc citrate to eliminate odoriferous volatile sulfur compounds.
- If you are prone to developing caries or gingivitis, consider using a mouth rinse classified as having antiplaque/antigingivitis activity. Such mouth rinses contain cetylpyridinium chloride or a combination of thymol, eucalyptol, methyl salicylate, and menthol.
- Note that overuse of mouth rinses containing cetylpyridinium can stain teeth.

Using Topical Fluoride Treatments

- If your drinking water is not fluoridated (including bottled water), or if you are prone to developing caries, consider using topical fluoride treatments. (See Table 31–4 for proper use of these products.)
- Supervise children younger than 12 years of age until they are capable of using the product correctly.

When to Seek Medical Attention

- See a dental provider if any of the following occurs:
  - You experience symptoms of a toothache.
  - Your teeth develop a mottled appearance.
  - Your gums bleed, swell, or become red.
  - Mouth odor persists despite regular use of fluoride toothpaste, or the cause of the mouth odor cannot be identified.

GINGIVITIS

Periodontal disease (which may result in tooth loss) affects an estimated 46% of U.S. adults 30 years of age and older.[22] Curtailing buildup of plaque can prevent or control this common and significant public health problem. All forms of periodontal disease are associated with oral hygiene status, not with age. However, as life spans increase and people retain more teeth later in life, both the number of teeth at risk and the susceptible period for development of periodontal disease increase.

Gingivitis, the mildest form of periodontal disease, is common and reversible. Gingivitis may progress to more severe periodontal diseases (specifically, acute necrotizing ulcerative gingivitis and periodontitis, the latter of which can cause significant, irreversible alveolar bone loss).

Gingivitis is inflammation of the gingiva without loss or migration of epithelial attachment to the tooth, but periodontitis occurs when the periodontal ligament attachment and alveolar bone support of the tooth have been compromised or lost. This process involves apical migration of the epithelial attachment. (See Color Plates, photographs 11 and 12.)

Pregnant patients are more susceptible to the development of dental caries and gingivitis. *Pregnancy gingivitis* is characterized by red, swollen gingival tissue that bleeds easily. Local factors are the cause, as with any form of gingivitis, but the varying hormone levels in pregnancy may make gingival tissue more sensitive to bacterial dental plaque. These changes in the connective tissues that compose the periodontium appear to be the primary pathogenic mechanism. Pregnancy gingivitis can be prevented or resolved with thorough plaque control. The severity of the inflammatory response and the resulting gingivitis decrease postpartum, returning to pre-pregnancy levels after about 1 year.[24]

Pathophysiology of Gingivitis

Gingivitis results from the accumulation of supragingival bacterial plaque. If this accumulation is not controlled, the plaque proliferates and invades subgingival spaces. Although not all gingivitis progresses to periodontitis, the progression from supragingival plaque to gingivitis to periodontitis is well documented, so controlling gingivitis is a reasonable approach to limiting periodontitis.

Other possible etiologic factors include effects of medications such as calcium channel blockers, cyclosporine, and phenytoin. Anticholinergics and antidepressants may cause gingivitis by reducing the flow of saliva. The use of tobacco (both smokeless and smoked) has also been linked to periodontal disease.

Clinical Presentation of Gingivitis

The marginal gingiva (the border of the gingiva surrounding the neck of the tooth) is held firmly to the tooth by a network of collagen fibers. Microorganisms present in the plaque in the gingival sulcus (the space between the gingiva and the tooth) are capable of producing harmful products (e.g., acids, toxins, enzymes) that damage cellular and intercellular tissue. Early-stage gingivitis signs and symptoms include dilation and proliferation of gingival capillaries, increased flow of gingival fluid, and increased blood flow with resulting erythema of the gingiva. The gingivae may also enlarge, change contour, and appear puffy or swollen as a result of the inflammation (see Color Plates, photograph 11). The inflammatory process of early-stage gingivitis is reversible with effective oral hygiene.

Some common indications that early-stage gingivitis has become chronic gingivitis include changes in gingival color, size, and shape, as well as changes in the ease with which gingival bleeding occurs. Both the patient and the dental care provider can recognize these symptoms. Additionally, the flat, knife-edge appearance of healthy gingiva is replaced by a ragged or rounded edge. Progression of these conditions usually is slow and insidious—and often painless.

Left untreated, chronic gingivitis may advance to the inflammatory condition of chronic destructive periodontal disease, or periodontitis (see Color Plates, photograph 12). Progression of gingivitis may parallel an increase in the proportion of bacterial species implicated in the genesis of periodontitis.

Prevention of Gingivitis

Because prevention of gingivitis and caries depends on calculus prevention and plaque control, the same measures described for prevention of caries pertain to gingivitis. Active ingredients that prevent gingivitis and are commonly found in dentifrices, mouth rinses, and other antiplaque products include triclosan, cetylpyridinium chloride, and stabilized stannous fluoride. Brushing and flossing can cure early gingivitis that arises from irritating food debris and plaque. The most important factors in reversing gingivitis and in preventing and controlling periodontal disease are adequate removal and control of supragingival plaque. Patients who notice signs of early gingivitis such as bleeding gums during tooth brushing should be referred to a dental provider.

Special Population Considerations for Gingivitis

In general, self-care for prevention of gingivitis requires no specific considerations for the following patient populations: children, pregnant or lactating women, males and females of reproductive age, and older adults.

Assessment of Gingivitis: A Case-Based Approach

Before recommending oral hygiene products, the HCP should evaluate the patient's oral hygiene regimen. An important issue is whether the patient has a history of gingivitis or current signs and symptoms of gingivitis, as well as what preventive measures the patient has tried or is using. Checking the medical and medication histories will identify asymptomatic patients who are at risk for gingivitis. Any signs or symptoms of gingivitis—swollen gums, gums that bleed with brushing or flossing, receding gums, or gums that appear darker red than usual—warrant referral to a dental provider for evaluation and treatment.

The HCP should be cognizant of the association between pregnancy and gingivitis and should address this potential issue during counseling on prescription prenatal vitamins. Besides monitoring the pregnant patient's medications for safety, the provider has an opportunity to encourage the patient to have a dental checkup and to stress the importance of careful attention to brushing and flossing to avoid oral health problems.

Patient Counseling for Gingivitis

Because gingivitis is not usually associated with pain, patients are unlikely to seek dental care for this problem alone. A more likely scenario is patient-initiated contact with an HCP to request oral hygiene information and product recommendations. In such encounters, it may be appropriate to suggest specific oral hygiene methods and emphasize possible adverse effects of certain products.

Case 31–1 provides an example of assessment of a patient with gingivitis. The box "Patient Education for Prevention of Caries, Gingivitis, and Halitosis" lists specific information for patient counseling.

The HCP should also use such clinical encounters as an opportunity to warn patients with suspected gingivitis that the disease is a serious problem warranting professional attention. Counseling should emphasize that adherence to an oral hygiene program is vital to preventing gingivitis.

CASE 31-1

Relevant Evaluation Criteria	Scenario/Model Outcome
Collect	
1. Gather essential information about the patient's symptoms, including	
a. Description of symptom(s) (i.e., nature, onset, duration, severity, associated symptoms)	Patient has had red, bleeding, swollen gums for the past 2 weeks.
b. Description of any factors that seem to precipitate, exacerbate, and/or relieve the patient's symptom(s)	Patient notices blood when she rinses her mouth after toothbrushing.
c. Description of the patient's efforts to relieve the symptoms	Patient continues to brush her teeth twice daily.
d. Patient's identity	Laura James
e. Patient's age, sex, height, and weight	32 years old, female, 5 ft 6 in., 165 lb
f. Patient's occupation	Accountant
g. Patient's dietary habits	Normal, healthy diet
h. Patient's sleep habits	6–8 hours of sleep each night
i. Concurrent medical conditions, prescription and nonprescription medications, and dietary supplements	Patient is pregnant with her first child. Just started her second trimester. Takes prenatal vitamins.
j. Allergies	Sulfa
k. History of other adverse reactions to medications	None
l. Other (describe) ______	n/a
Assess	
2. Differentiate patient's signs/symptoms, and correctly identify the patient's primary problem(s).	The patient appears to have pregnancy gingivitis.
3. Identify exclusions for self-treatment.	Bleeding, swollen gums (see the box "Patient Education for Prevention of Caries, Gingivitis, and Halitosis")
4. Formulate a comprehensive list of therapeutic alternatives for the primary problem to determine whether triage to a medical provider is required, and share this information with the patient or caregiver.	Options include (1) Refer Laura to a dental care provider. (2) Recommend appropriate nonprescription products along with education about proper oral care and referral to a dental care provider. (3) Take no action.
Plan	
5. Select an optimal therapeutic alternative to address the patient's problem, taking into account patient preferences.	Refer the patient to a dental care provider.
6. Describe the recommended therapeutic approach to the patient or caregiver.	"You need to see a dental care provider because you have signs of gingivitis."
7. Explain to the patient or caregiver the rationale for selecting the recommended therapeutic approach from the considered therapeutic alternatives.	"Although there are steps you can take to improve your oral hygiene, pregnant women are at increased risk of developing gingivitis. Therefore, a dental care provider will need to evaluate your condition and develop a treatment plan. You should get a thorough checkup and cleaning from your dental health care provider to ensure that you and your teeth and gums stay healthy."

CASE 31-1 *continued*

Relevant Evaluation Criteria	Scenario/Model Outcome
Implement	
8. When recommending self-care with nonprescription medications and/or nondrug therapy, convey accurate information to the patient or caregiver.	Criterion does not apply in this case.
Solicit follow-up questions from the patient or caregiver.	"Is there a nonprescription medication that might work?"
Answer the patient's or caregiver's questions.	"Nonprescription medications do not treat gingivitis. They may reduce the symptoms, but ultimately your dental care provider will need to develop a treatment strategy. Once your condition has been diagnosed, there are nonprescription products you may use as part of your oral care regimen. Gingivitis and periodontal disease, if left untreated, may result in tooth loss and other complications."
Follow-up: Monitor and Evaluate	
9. Assess patient outcome.	Contact Laura in 1–2 days to ensure that she made an appointment and sought dental care.

Key: n/a = Not applicable.

HALITOSIS

Halitosis, or oral malodor (usually known as bad breath), affects greater than 40% of U.S. adults older than 60 years of age.[25]

Pathophysiology of Halitosis

Causes of halitosis may be related to both systemic and oral conditions. Approximately 85% of cases are related to oral causes, including dental caries, periodontal disease, oral infections, mucosal ulcerations, tongue coating, and impacted food or debris.[25]

Medications that have anticholinergic properties often cause xerostomia, which also can lead to mouth odor. Many foods and products such as garlic, tobacco, onions, alcohol, and other substances may contribute to mouth odor as well.

Most foul breath odors arise from volatile sulfur compounds (VSCs), which can be produced by breakdown of food debris left in the mouth or by systemic conditions that eliminate VSCs in exhaled air.[25]

Prevention of Halitosis

Prevention of halitosis relies on the removal of plaque and the prevention of calculus formation as described for prevention of caries. One of the primary sites for the formation of VSCs is the back of the tongue. Plaque and VSCs in this area of the mouth can seed the tonsillar crypts with malodorous debris. Brushing both the teeth and tongue is helpful, but some dental care providers have found that the use of a tongue-cleaning device (e.g., a tongue blade) may be the best way to clean the circumvallate papillae area of the tongue. Cleaning this posterior dorsal area not only will remove the fetid VSCs but also will prevent them from spreading to the tonsils.

Zinc salts and chlorine dioxide are most effective in the chemical prevention of oral malodor. These two agents are combined in two-part rinses such as SmartMouth or as single ingredients in CloSYS (chlorine dioxide) or Listerine Tartar Control (zinc chloride). Zinc salts reduce the receptor binding necessary for VSC production and kill gram-negative bacteria. Chlorine dioxide breaks disulfide bonds and oxidizes the precursors of VSCs.

Any patient who complains of severe or lingering halitosis without a readily identifiable cause (e.g., smoking) should be advised to see a dental provider for a thorough evaluation. Masking foul taste and odor with cosmetic mouth rinses may delay necessary dental or medical assessment and any needed treatment.

Special Population Considerations for Halitosis

No self-care considerations related to prevention of halitosis have been identified for the following patient populations: children, pregnant or lactating women, males and females of reproductive age, and older adults.

Assessment of Halitosis: A Case-Based Approach

When assessing a patient for halitosis, the HCP should evaluate the patient's dental hygiene. Ideally, both medication and medical histories are obtained to help identify the cause of the halitosis, as discussed in the "Pathophysiology of Halitosis" section (see also "Xerostomia" in Chapter 32). Patients with medical conditions associated with halitosis and those with halitosis that persists despite proper dental hygiene should be referred to their dental care provider for evaluation and treatment.

Patient Counseling for Halitosis

For patients with mouth odor related to poor dental hygiene, the HCP should reinforce proper techniques for maintaining dental hygiene to prevent tooth and gum problems, including brushing and flossing, and should recommend appropriate products, with explanations of their use. The box "Patient Education for Prevention of Caries, Gingivitis, and Halitosis" lists specific information for patient counseling on prevention of halitosis.

HYGIENE-RELATED DENTURE PROBLEMS

Pain along the gingival ridge under a denture prosthesis suggests conditions such as *denture stomatitis* (an inflammation of the oral tissue in contact with a removable denture), inflammatory papillary hyperplasia, and chronic candidiasis. Denture stomatitis, which results from poor cleaning of dentures, can lead to chronic candidiasis.[26]

Pathophysiology of Hygiene-Related Denture Problems

Dentures accumulate plaque, stain, and calculus by a process very similar to that occurring on natural teeth. Contact of the denture plaque mass with oral tissues leads to predictable toxic results. Poor denture hygiene contributes to fungal and bacterial growth that not only affects the patient aesthetically (with unpleasant odors and staining) but also seriously compromises the patient's oral health (from inflammation and mucosal disease) and ability to wear the dentures successfully.

Chronic atrophic candidiasis is common in patients with full or partial dentures. This condition may be attributed to infection with *Candida* organisms, which is more prevalent in denture wearers.[26] Symptomatically, the inflamed denture-bearing area may appear granular or erythematous and edematous, associated with soreness or a burning sensation (see Color Plates, photograph 13). Inflammation secondary to *Candida* infection is generalized, involving the entire denture-bearing tissue area, whereas inflammation secondary to the trauma of ill-fitting dentures usually is localized to the specific area of the trauma. Failure to remove the denture at bedtime and to clean it regularly worsens this condition. Angular cheilitis (soreness and cracking at the corners of the mouth) is commonly associated with chronic atrophic candidiasis, other forms of oral candidiasis, and poor denture fit. The cheilitis lesions often can be treated effectively with terbinafine cream. If a staphylococcal organism also is involved, a prescription from the patient's HCP will be needed.

Prevention of Hygiene-Related Denture Problems

Removing plaque from dentures helps prevent gum infections, staining of dentures, and mouth odor. Specialty brushes and aids are available to remove plaque from hard-to-clean areas on fixed orthodontic appliances (e.g., spaces around a bridge, implant, or orthodontic band) and dentures. Dentures should be cleaned thoroughly at least once daily to remove unsightly stains, debris, and plaque. Abrasive and chemical cleansers formulated specifically for dentures are available (Table 31–7).

TABLE 31–7 Selected Nonprescription Denture Products

Trade Name	Primary Ingredient
Efferdent Denture Cleanser Tabs	Sodium bicarbonate
Fresh 'N Brite Denture Cleaning Paste	n/a

Key: n/a = Not applicable.

A combination regimen of brushing dentures with an abrasive cleaner and soaking them in a commercial cleaning solution is recommended.

Denture cleansers for brushing, in either a paste or powder formulation, contain mild abrasives (e.g., calcium carbonate) and must be applied properly with specialty brushes adapted to the denture's contour to remove stains, plaque, and calculus. Overly vigorous scrubbing can abrade the denture's acrylic materials and bend the metal clasps. To prevent irritation of oral tissues, the patient should thoroughly rinse the abrasive cleaner from the denture. After initial brushing, the denture should be soaked in a cleansing solution (alkaline peroxide, hypochlorite, or dilute acids) to help remove remaining plaque and bacteria. Brushing the denture after it has soaked further enhances plaque removal; instructions for this procedure are included with some products.

Alkaline peroxide products are the most commonly used chemical denture soaking cleansers. These powders or tablets are dissolved in water to become alkaline solutions of hydrogen peroxide, causing oxygen to be released for a mechanical cleaning effect. These products are most effective on new plaque and stains when the denture is soaked for 4–8 hours. The alkaline peroxides have few serious disadvantages and do not damage the surface of acrylic resins.

Hypochlorite (bleach) removes stains, dissolves mucin, and is both bactericidal and fungicidal. *Denture plaque* consists of cells embedded in a matrix that serves as a surface on which calculus may develop. Hypochlorite cleansers act directly on the organic plaque matrix to dissolve its structure, but they cannot dissolve calculus once it has formed. The most serious disadvantage of hypochlorite is that it corrodes metal denture components (e.g., the framework and clasps of removable partial dentures, solder joints, and possibly the pins holding the teeth). The addition of anticorrosive phosphate compounds has greatly reduced this problem, but these products should be used for only 10-minute soaks (to limit exposure) and not more often than once a week.

Acid-containing soaking solutions can also be corrosive to metals, and short soaking times are recommended with use of these solutions. A sonic or ultrasonic cleaning device, when used with a commercially prepared solution, is easy to use and cleans more effectively than soaking alone. However, some hand brushing may still be required.

All denture-cleansing products should be rinsed off the denture completely before it is inserted into the mouth, to reduce tissue irritation. All denture cleansers should be kept out of children's reach because of the potential for eye or skin irritation, and because they are toxic if accidentally ingested. Stains that are resistant to proper denture brushing and soaking in available solutions should be evaluated by a dental care provider.

Only products that are specifically formulated for denture cleansing should be used. Household cleansers (sometimes used by patients for soaking dentures) are not appropriate and may be ineffective or may damage the denture material. The use of whitening toothpastes (which are formulated for use with natural dentition) should be discouraged as well, because they are too abrasive to be used safely on denture material.

Patients should not soak or clean dentures in hot water or hot soaking solutions, because distortion or warping may occur.

Patients of advanced age or disabled persons may prefer an alkaline peroxide soak solution for daily, overnight cleaning. Unlike alkaline hypochlorite and acid cleansers, alkaline peroxide cleansers do not corrode metal components of dentures.

Assessment of Hygiene-Related Denture Problems

Before recommending any type of oral hygiene product, the HCP should identify what denture care measures the patient is taking and assess whether those measures are adequate for oral health and successful wear of dentures or other appliance. Another important aspect of the HCP's assessment is to determine whether the patient suffers from denture stomatitis or inflammation secondary to ill-fitting dentures, necessitating referral to a dental care provider for evaluation and treatment. Case 31–2 illustrates assessment of a patient with a hygiene-related denture problem.

Patient Counseling for Hygiene-Related Denture Problems

Denture wearers may tend to blame the appliances for any oral discomfort, rather than their hygiene regimen. The HCP should emphasize that diligent plaque removal from dentures is the key to preventing denture stomatitis. The methods of cleaning dentures, including their advantages and disadvantages, should be explained. The HCP should recommend a denture cleanser that

CASE 31-2

Relevant Evaluation Criteria	Scenario/Model Outcome
Collect	
1. Gather essential information about the patient's symptoms, including	
a. Description of symptom(s) (i.e., nature, onset, duration, severity, associated symptoms)	The patient feels that he is unable to get his dentures as clean as he would like.
b. Description of any factors that seem to precipitate, exacerbate, and/or relieve the patient's symptom(s)	n/a
c. Description of the patient's efforts to relieve the symptoms	He started brushing his dentures with toothbrush and whitening toothpaste last week, which has not helped. Previously just soaked then overnight in a dental cleanser.
d. Patient's identity	Stewart Johnson
e. Patient's age, sex, height, and weight	68 years old, male, 5 ft 11 in., 210 lb
f. Patient's occupation	Retired school bus driver
g. Patient's dietary habits	Normal healthy diet; enjoys his nightly ice cream.
h. Patient's sleep habits	Averages 6 hours per night and takes a 1-hour nap every afternoon.
i. Concurrent medical conditions, prescription and nonprescription medications, and dietary supplements	High blood pressure: lisinopril 20 mg, 1 tablet daily, and hydrochlorothiazide 25 mg, 1 tablet daily; high cholesterol: atorvastatin 20 mg, 1 tablet daily.
j. Allergies	NKA
k. History of other adverse reactions to medications	Amoxicillin: upset stomach
l. Other (describe) ______	n/a
Assess	
2. Differentiate patient's signs/symptoms, and correctly identify the patient's primary problem(s).	Patient seems to have residual plaque on dentures and is inappropriately using a tooth dentifrice on dentures.
3. Identify exclusions for self-treatment.	None
4. Formulate a comprehensive list of therapeutic alternatives for the primary problem to determine whether triage to a medical provider is required, and share this information with the patient or caregiver.	Options include (1) Refer Mr. Johnson to a dental care provider. (2) Recommend appropriate nonprescription products along with education about proper oral care and a referral to a dental care provider. (3) Take no action.

CASE 31-2 *continued*

Relevant Evaluation Criteria	Scenario/Model Outcome
Plan	
5. Select an optimal therapeutic alternative to address the patient's problem, taking into account patient preferences.	Mr. Johnson should stop using the whitening toothpaste and brush the dentures using a denture brush and denture paste daily. After this, he should also soak the dentures in a dental cleanser.
6. Describe the recommended therapeutic approach to the patient or caregiver.	"Only products that are specifically formulated for denture cleansing should be used. Whitening toothpastes are too abrasive to use on dentures. Denture brushes and pastes are specially designed to remove deposits from dentures. Resume daily soaking of dentures in a dental cleanser."
7. Explain to the patient or caregiver the rationale for selecting the recommended therapeutic approach from the considered therapeutic alternatives.	"Effective manual brushing removes more plaque and biofilm from dentures than soaking alone. Soaking the dentures after brushing can help remove any residual plaque."
Implement	
8. When recommending self-care with nonprescription medications and/or nondrug therapy, convey accurate information to the patient or caregiver.	
a. Appropriate dose and frequency of administration	"Dentures should be brushed daily and then soaked in a dental cleanser."
b. Maximum number of days the therapy should be employed	n/a
c. Product administration procedures	"All surfaces of the denture should be brushed. To avoid breaking the denture, brush it over a folded towel or a sink filled with water. Thoroughly rinse the denture after brushing. Then soak it in a denture cleanser solution after brushing. After soaking, the denture can be brushed again for further removal of plaque."
d. Degree of relief that can be reasonably expected	"Daily brushing may help remove plaque and stains."
e. Most common adverse effects	"Only denture paste should be used, because dentures are easily scratched by regular toothpastes. The resulting damage may include changes in surface or contour that lead to poorly fitting dentures and irritation or infection."
f. Adverse effects that warrant medical intervention should they occur	n/a
g. Patient options in the event that condition worsens or persists	"A dental care provider should evaluate stains that are resistant to proper brushing and soaking in available solutions."
h. Product storage requirements	n/a
i. Specific nondrug measures	"Continue regular denture hygiene and maintenance."
Solicit follow-up questions from the patient or caregiver.	"Can I increase the frequency of brushing to provide additional cleaning?"
Answer the patient's or caregiver's questions.	"No. Brushing too often may scratch and damage dentures."
Follow-up: Monitor and Evaluate	
9. Assess patient outcome.	Ask the patient to call to update you on his response to your recommendations, or follow up with a telephone call in 1 week to evaluate his response.

n/a = Not applicable; NKA = no known allergies.

PATIENT EDUCATION FOR Hygiene-Related Denture Problems

The objective of self-care is to prevent bacterial or fungal infections of the mouth by removing plaque from the dentures. For most patients, carefully following product instructions and the self-care measures listed here will help ensure good denture hygiene.

- Thoroughly clean dentures at least once daily to remove unsightly stain, debris, and potentially harmful plaque.
- Preferably, brush dentures with an abrasive cleaner, and then soak them in a chemical cleanser. This combination regimen is more effective in removing plaque and bacteria.
- Apply the abrasive cleaner to the denture, using a brush designed to adapt to the denture's contour.
- Do not scrub the denture surface vigorously; this action can abrade the acrylic materials and bend the metal clasps.
- To prevent irritation of oral tissues, thoroughly rinse the abrasive cleaner from the denture.
- After brushing the dentures, soak them in an alkaline peroxide or sodium hypochlorite cleansing solution for 10 minutes to avoid corrosion of metal denture components. Rinse the dentures thoroughly to avoid chemical burns of the mouth.
- If possible, brush the dentures again, and rinse them thoroughly.
- Keep all denture cleansers out of children's reach. These agents can cause eye or skin irritation or toxicity if accidentally ingested.
- Do not use household cleansers or whitening toothpastes to clean dentures. These agents may damage denture material.
- Do not soak or clean dentures in hot water or hot soaking solutions. Distortion or warping of the denture may occur.
- Do not sleep while wearing your dentures. Decreased levels of saliva during sleep may contribute to plaque buildup on the denture.

When to Seek Medical Attention

- If your mouth becomes sore or shows sign of infection, see a dental provider.

accommodates the patient's preferences and should reinforce the methods of use. The box "Patient Education for Hygiene-Related Denture Problems" lists specific information for patient counseling.

Key Points for Prevention of Hygiene-Related Oral Disorders

- Removing plaque and modifying the diet are the main goals of self-care to prevent caries, gingivitis, and halitosis.
- Mechanical removal of plaque by brushing and flossing is essential for good oral health.
- Mouth rinses may augment the benefits of brushing and flossing procedures and may be used to freshen breath or as antiplaque or antigingivitis adjuncts.
- Topical fluorides may be used in patients with high caries activity.
- Parents must supervise oral hygiene measures in children younger than 12 years as necessary until they can use the products without supervision.
- Denture cleaners may be used to remove debris physically and to prevent bacterial and/or fungal infections.
- If a patient has specific problems related to the purpose or use of these products, consultation with a dental care provider should be recommended.

REFERENCES

1. Soderlund K. Gallup: One-third of Americans had no dental visit in past year. *ADA News.* May 5, 2014. Available at: http://www.ada.org/en/publications/ada-news/2014-archive/may/gallup-one-third-of-americans-had-no-dental-visit-in-past-year. Accessed June 5, 2017.
2. Dye BA, Thornton-Evans G, Li X, Iafolla TJ. Dental caries and sealant prevalence in children and adolescents in the United States, 2011–2012. NCHS data brief, no 191. Hyattsville, MD: National Center for Health Statistics. 2015. Available at: http://www.cdc.gov/nchs/products/databriefs/db191.htm. Accessed June 5, 2017.
3. World Health Organization. Oral Health. Fact sheet no. 318. April 2012. Available at: http://www.who.int/mediacentre/factsheets/fs318/en/. Accessed June 5, 2017.
4. Bagramian RA, Garcia-Godoy F, Volpe AR. The global increase in dental caries. A pending public health crisis. *Am J Dent.* 2009;22(1):3–8. PMID: 19281105.
5. Warnakulasuriya S. Oral health risks of tobacco use and effects of cessation. *Int Dent J.* 2010;60(1):7–30. doi: 10.1922/IDJ_2532 Warnakulasuriya24.
6. Wall T, Nasseh K, Vujicic M. Most important barriers to dental care are financial, not supply related. Health Policy Institute Research Brief. American Dental Association, October 2014. Available at: http://www.ada.org/~/media/ADA/Science%20and%20Research/HPI/Files/HPI Brief_1014_2.ashx. Accessed June 5, 2017.
7. Vujicic M. Obamacare, Trumpcare, and Your Mouth. Health Affairs Blog. Available at http://healthaffairs.org/blog/2017/01/13/obamacare-trump care-and-your-mouth. Accessed May 21, 2017.
8. American Academy of Pediatric Dentistry. Guideline on periodicity of examination, preventative dental services, anticipatory guidance/counseling, and oral treatment for infants, children, and adolescents. *Pediatr Dent.* 2013;35(5):148–56. PMID:19216408.
9. American Dental Association. Chewing Gum: Key Points. Available at: http://www.ada.org/en/science-research/ada-seal-of-acceptance/product-category-information/chewing-gum. Accessed June 5, 2017.
10. American Dental Association. ADA Seal of Acceptance FAQ. Available at: http://www.ada.org/en/science-research/ada-seal-of-acceptance/ada-seal-faq. Accessed June 5, 2017.
11. Yaacob M, Worthington HV, Deacon SA, et al. Powered versus manual toothbrushing for oral health. *Cochrane Database Syst Rev.* 2014;6: CD002281. doi: 10.1002/14651858.CD002281.pub3.
12. Terzhalmy GT, Bartizek RD, Biesbrock AR. Plaque-removal efficacy of four types of dental floss. *J Periodontol.* 2008;79(2):245–51. doi: 10.1902/jop.2008.070345.
13. Ran T, Chattopadhyay SK. Economic evaluation of community water fluoridation: a community guide systematic review. *Am J Prev Med.* 2016; 50(6):790–6. doi: 10.1016/j.amepre.2015.10.014.
14. Centers for Disease Control and Prevention. 2012 Water Fluoridation Data & Statistics. Available at: http://www.cdc.gov/fluoridation/statistics/. Accessed March 27, 2016.
15. U.S. Public Health Service. U.S. Public Health Service recommendations for fluoride concentration in drinking water for the prevention of dental caries. *Public Health Rep.* 2015;130(4):14. Available at: http://www.ada.

org/~/media/EBD/Files/PHS_2015_Fluoride_Guidelines.pdf?la=en. Accessed June 5, 2017.
16. Putt MS, Milleman KR, Ghassemi A, et al. Enhancement of plaque removal efficacy by tooth brushing with baking soda dentifrices: results of five clinical studies. *J Clin Dent.* 2008;19(4):111–9. PMID:19278079.
17. Thong S, Hooper W, Xu Y, et al. Enhancement of plaque removal by baking soda toothpastes from less accessible areas in the dentition. *J Clin Dent.* 2011;22(5):171–8. PMID: 22403983.
18. Moore C, Addy M, Moran J. Toothpaste detergents: a potential source of oral soft tissue damage? *Int J Dent Hyg.* 2008;6(3):193–8. doi: 10.1111/j.1601-5037.2008.00307.x.
19. American Dental Association Council on Scientific Affairs. *Acceptance Program Guidelines: Chemotherapeutic Products for the Control of Gingivitis.* Chicago, IL: American Dental Association; November 2011. Available at: http://www.ada.org/en/science-research/ada-seal-of-acceptance/how-to-earn-the-ada-seal/general-criteria-for-acceptance. Accessed June 5, 2017.
20. Ghassemi A, Vorwerk L, Hooper W, et al. Extrinsic stain removal effectiveness of a new whitening dentifrice. *J Clin Dent.* 2015;26(3):72–5. PMID: 26665289.
21. Tatikonda A, Debnath S, Chauhan VS, et al. Effects of herbal and non-herbal toothpastes on plaque and gingivitis: a clinical comparative study. *J Int Soc Prev Community Dent.* 2014;4(Suppl 2):S126–9. doi: 10.4103/2231-0762.146220.
22. American Dental Association Council on Scientific Affairs. Fluoride toothpaste use for young children. *J Am Dent Assoc.* 2014;145(2):190–1. doi: 10.14219/jada.2013.47.
23. Eke PI, Dye BA, Wei L, et al. Update on prevalence of periodontitis in adults in the United States: NHANES 2009 to 2012. *J Periodontol.* 2015;86(5):611–22. doi: 10.1902/jop.2015.140520.
24. Wu M, Chen S, Jiang S. Relationship between gingival inflammation and pregnancy. *Mediators Inflamm.* 2015;(2015):1–11. doi:10.1155/2015/623427.
25. Bollen CM, Beikler T. Halitosis: the multidisciplinary approach. *Int J Oral Sci.* 2012;4(2):55–63. doi: 10.1038/ijos.2012.39.
26. Gonsalves WC, Chi AC, Neville BW. Common oral lesions: Part I. Superficial mucosal lesions. *Am Fam Physician.* 2007;75(4):501–7. PMID: 17323710.
27. Marcos-Arias C, Vicente JL, Sahand IH, et al. Isolation of Candida dubliniensis in denture stomatitis. *Arch Oral Biol.* 2009;54(2):127–31. doi: 10.1016/j.archoralbio.2008.09.005.

CHAPTER 32

OROFACIAL PAIN AND DISCOMFORT

NICOLE PAOLINI ALBANESE AND MARK DONALDSON

Orofacial pain and discomfort are common ailments throughout the lifespan.[1] Many children experience irritation and soreness during the teething process. Both before and after eruption of the teeth, various etiopathogenic factors and conditions may be responsible for pain and discomfort. In adulthood, orofacial pain may be associated with sudden exposure of, or damage to, nerves in a tooth; unexpected cracking or breaking of teeth necessitating fillings or crowns (caps) may also occur. Similarly, pain in the mucosa of the oral cavity and lips can be generated by traumatic injury to the mouth or may accompany recurrent aphthous stomatitis (i.e., "canker sores") or herpes simplex labialis (i.e., "cold sores"). Another common problem is xerostomia (dry mouth), which may be significant enough to require treatment with nonprescription medications. Orofacial pain and discomfort can interfere with daily activities such as drinking, eating, and speaking; cause mental anxiety and distress, affecting school and work performance and quality of life; and result in costly visits to health care providers (HCPs).[2,3] Distinguishing the patient's self-treatable problems from those potentially requiring professional dental or medical care is an important advisory role for all HCPs.

TOOTH HYPERSENSITIVITY

Tooth hypersensitivity, or *dentin hypersensitivity*, is characterized by a short, sharp pain arising from exposed dentin (i.e., mineralized tissue of teeth internal to crown enamel and root cementum) in response to a stimulus—thermal, chemical, or physical—that cannot be ascribed to any other form of dental defect or disease.[4–8] Tooth hypersensitivity affects 15%–20% of the adult population, with peak incidence between the ages of 30 and 39 years.[5]

Pathophysiology of Tooth Hypersensitivity

Two processes are required for the development of dentin hypersensitivity: (1) dentin must become exposed (lesion localization) through loss of enamel or gingival recession, and (2) the dentin tubules must be open to both the oral cavity and the pulp (lesion initiation).[4–8] The roots of teeth are usually covered by gum tissues (gingiva), but infection (e.g., periodontal disease) or injury (e.g., aggressive or improper brushing) can cause the gums to recede. The cementum covering affected root surfaces may be reduced by further injury (attrition, abrasion, or erosion), eventually exposing the underlying porous dentin. When stimuli such as heat, cold, pressure, or acid touch exposed dentin or reach an open tubule, fluid flow in the dentin tubule is increased, and the underlying nerves are stimulated, resulting in pain.[4–8]

Enamel, which covers the anatomic crowns of the teeth and is the most densely mineralized body tissue, is resistant to abrasion by normal toothbrushing, but aggressive or improper brushing with an abrasive dentifrice (toothpaste) or a medium- or hard-bristle toothbrush can be problematic. The primary contributing or etiologic factor in dental erosion is the presence of extrinsic or intrinsic acid.[6,7] Extrinsic sources of acid include acidic medications, foods, and drinks, especially with frequent consumption. Persons who regularly consume citrus juices and fruits, carbonated drinks, wines, and ciders may be at risk for tooth hypersensitivity. The most common source of intrinsic acid is regurgitation of gastric contents into the mouth, which occurs with disorders such as gastroesophageal reflux disease or bulimia nervosa.[6,7]

Tooth hypersensitivity is more common in individuals with periodontitis or after procedures such as deep scaling, root planing, orthodontic tooth movement, or periodontal (gum) surgery.[4–8] Sensitivity to hot and cold for several weeks after dental therapy is normal. Hypersensitivity can also occur as a result of clenching or grinding teeth and from gumline grooves formed by aggressive or inappropriate toothbrushing technique.[6] Tooth whitening procedures, whether done at home or by a trained clinician, can also cause dentin sensitivity. Tooth sensitivity is the most common reason why patients fail to complete or adhere to a tooth whitening regimen.[7] Tooth whitening products are discussed in more detail in Chapter 31.

Clinical Presentation of Tooth Hypersensitivity

The patient with tooth hypersensitivity experiences pain from hot, cold, sweet, or sour solutions, as well as when hot or cold air touches the teeth. As individual pain thresholds vary, so does the pain experienced from tooth hypersensitivity. Pain varies in intensity, ranging from mild discomfort to sharp, excruciating pain. Although tooth hypersensitivity is self-treatable, toothache is not; therefore, it is critical to differentiate between these two conditions (Table 32–1).

TABLE 32–1 **Differentiation of Tooth Hypersensitivity and Toothache**

Feature	Tooth Hypersensitivity	Toothache
Etiology	Exposed and open dentin tubules	Bacterial invasion extending to the pulp
Pathophysiology	Stimuli (heat, cold, pressure, acid) cause fluid in the dentinal tubules to expand and shrink, stimulating pulp nerve fibers and resulting in pain	Inflammatory response to invading bacteria stimulates free nerve endings in the pulp.
Causes	Attrition, abrasion, erosion, tooth/restoration fracture, faulty restoration, or gingival recession	Cavitation/decay present in tooth/teeth under existing restoration, tooth/restoration fracture, or trauma to the dentition
Symptoms	A quick, fleeting, sharp, or stabbing pain on stimulation by thermal, chemical, or physical stimuli, which stops after stimuli are no longer present	Pain that remains even in the absence of stimulus; intermittent, short, and sharp pain on stimulation may indicate reversible damage; continuous, dull, and throbbing pain without stimulation usually indicates irreversible damage.
Assessment	Hypersensitivity due to attrition, abrasion, or erosion is not serious and is self-treatable; sensitivity due to fracture, faulty restoration, or gingival recession warrants referral to a dentist.	Requires dental care for resolution

Source: References 4, 6, and 7.

Resolution of pain associated with toothache, fractured dentition, ill-fitting dentures, or suspected infection (abscess) requires professional dental care. Only a dentist can adequately evaluate and treat these conditions; therefore, the patient should see a dentist without delay.

Treatment of Tooth Hypersensitivity

Treatment Goals

The goals of self-treating tooth hypersensitivity are (1) to repair the damaged tooth surface using an appropriate toothpaste and (2) to replace aggressive or improper toothbrushing practices with optimal technique. When these goals have been achieved, tooth hypersensitivity may be eliminated.

General Treatment Approach

Pain related to tooth hypersensitivity can be challenging. Acute pain may cause anxiety, and the patient may not seek care from a dentist but rather will try to self-treat with the aid of a pharmacist.[5,6] Before recommending self-treatment for tooth pain, the provider should determine if the patient is a candidate for self-care. Figure 32–1 outlines the self-treatment of tooth hypersensitivity and lists exclusions for self-care.[4–9]

Nonpharmacologic Therapy

Treatment plans for tooth hypersensitivity should include identification and elimination of predisposing factors, such as extrinsic and intrinsic acid exposure and improper or aggressive toothbrushing technique. Tooth hypersensitivity often can be limited or reversed by less vigorous brushing using a standard fluoride dentifrice and a soft-bristle toothbrush. Brushing teeth within 30–60 minutes of consuming acidic foods or drinks should be avoided, to reduce the effects of acids and abrasions. If correct brushing techniques with a fluoride toothpaste do not effect improvement, a desensitizing dentifrice should be used. For this purpose, a 1-inch strip of a desensitizing toothpaste is applied to a soft-bristle toothbrush, followed by brushing as usual. Dentin permeability can be increased after ingesting acidic foods or beverages.[6] Fluoride is discussed in further detail in Chapter 31.

Pharmacologic Therapy

In general, two pharmacologic mechanisms have been recruited for the treatment of tooth hypersensitivity. The first mechanism involves depolarizing the excited nerves in the tubules and pulp to disrupt the pain stimuli neuronal response.[8] A potassium salt, usually potassium nitrate, diffuses along the dentin tubules to decrease the excitability of intradental nerves and alter its membrane potential. The potassium nitrate acts on the dentin to block the perception of stimuli that patients with healthy teeth usually do not experience. The second mechanism involves minimizing the flow of fluid by sealing the exposed dentin.[8] A new technology using 8% arginine, an amino acid naturally found in saliva, combined with calcium carbonate, works by occluding the exposed dentinal tubules.[8] This treatment prevents the fluid from moving into the tubules, which is the cause of hypersensitivity. Both of these mechanisms have been implemented in the design and manufacture of desensitizing dentifrices. Table 32–2 lists selected desensitizing toothpastes and their active ingredients.

Potassium nitrate 5% is the most widely used and generally accepted ingredient used for treatment of teeth sensitivity. Most commercially available desensitizing dentifrices are combination products containing potassium nitrate and sodium fluoride, in various concentrations. Studies have shown these products to be efficacious for the treatment of tooth sensitivity, but debate continues regarding the efficacy of potassium nitrate.[9,10] The Pro-Argin technology, which combines 8% arginine and calcium carbonate, although highly efficacious,[8,11] is not currently available to consumers for home use.

Exclusions for Self-Treatment

- Toothache (Table 32–1)
- Mouth soreness associated with poor-fitting dentures
- Presence of fever or swelling
- Loose teeth
- Bleeding gums in the absence of trauma
- Broken or knocked-out teeth
- Severe tooth pain triggered or worsened by hot, cold, or chewing
- Trauma to the mouth with bleeding, swelling, and soreness

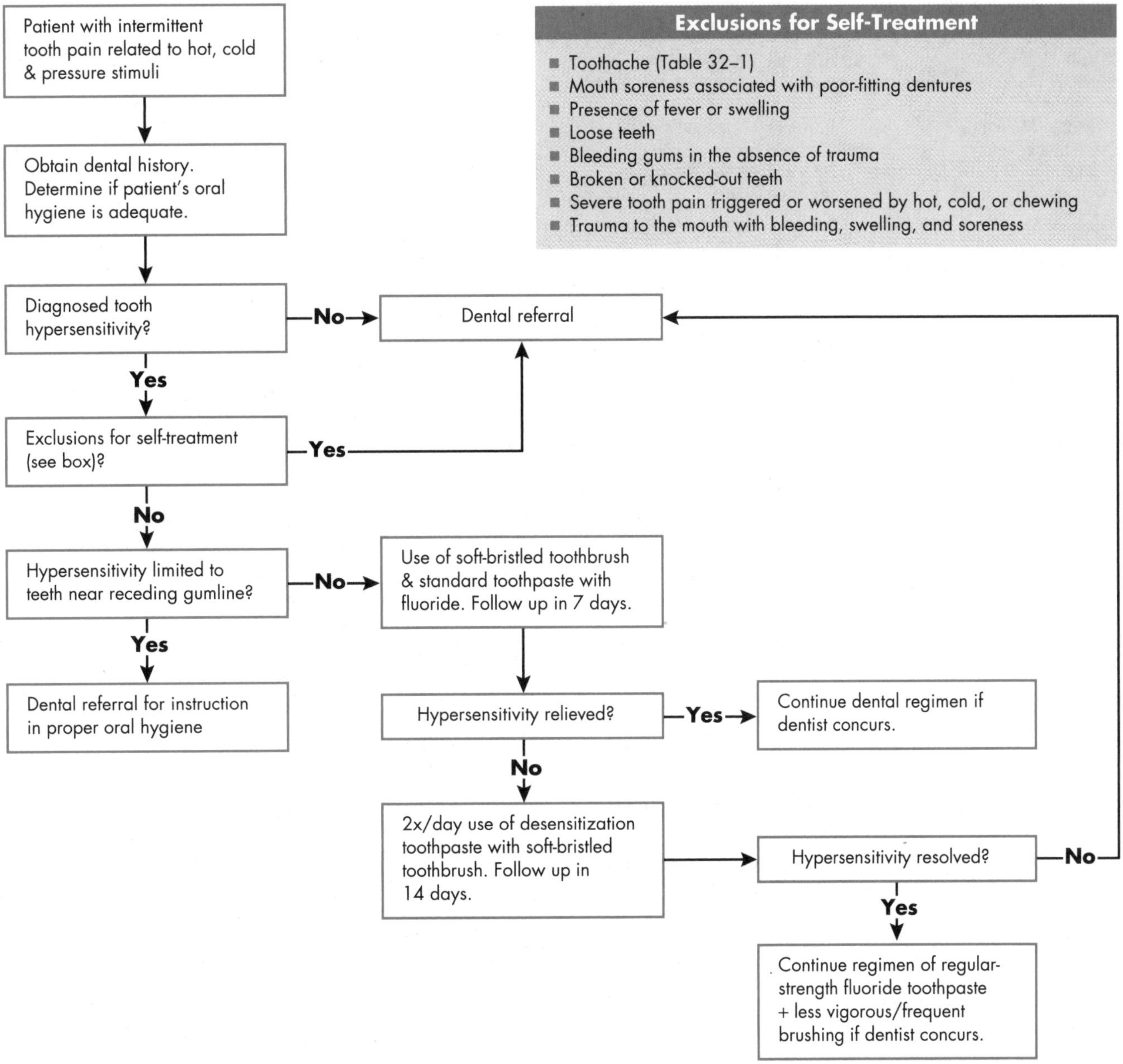

FIGURE 32–1 Self-care for tooth hypersensitivity. (Source: References 5–9.)

Clinically important drug interactions for desensitizing toothpastes are listed in Table 32–3. Patients consuming calcium-containing products need to be aware that the excess calcium can affect the bioavailability of fluoride. This potential adverse interaction should be emphasized by the HCP during counseling before initiation of fluoride-containing products.

Guidelines for brushing teeth can be found in the previous chapter (Table 31–1) and can be applied to brushing with desensitizing dentifrices.[9,10] A single application typically has no effect; for some patients, long-term use (2–4 weeks) may be necessary to relieve the symptoms. The desensitizing dentifrice should be used until the sensitivity subsides or for as long as the dentist recommends. In approximately 25% of adults, tooth hypersensitivity is a chronic problem and necessitates long-term treatment provided by a dentist.[5,6] If the hypersensitivity is not relieved within 14–21 days of using a desensitizing dentifrice, the patient should see a dentist for an in-office method of treatment or an appropriate HCP for further evaluation.[5,6]

Product Selection Guidelines

Patients with hypersensitive teeth should be cautioned against using high-abrasion toothpastes such as cosmetic pastes that whiten teeth or remove stains.

Special Populations

Dentifrices containing potassium nitrate 5% are not recommended for children younger than 12 years. Toothpastes containing potassium nitrate have earned the American Dental Association (ADA) Seal of Acceptance, which means they have been shown to not

TABLE 32-2 Selected Nonprescription Desensitizing Toothpastes

Trade Name	Primary Ingredients
Colgate Sensitive Multiprotection	Potassium nitrate 5%; sodium fluoride 0.24%
Colgate Sensitive Pro-Relief Original	Potassium nitrate 5%; sodium fluoride 0.24%
Colgate Sensitive Pro-Relief Enamel Repair	Potassium nitrate 5%; sodium monofluorophosphate 1.14%
Colgate Sensitive Pro-Relief Whitening	Potassium nitrate 5%; sodium fluoride 0.24%
Colgate Total Zx Pro-Shield Plus Sensitivity	Potassium nitrate 0.24%; sodium monofluoride 0.055%; zinc citrate trihydrate 0.096%
Crest Pro-Health[a]	Potassium nitrate 5%; stannous fluoride 0.454%
Crest Pro-Health Whitening[a]	Potassium nitrate 5%; stannous fluoride 0.454%
Crest Sensitivity: Clinical Sensitivity Relief Extra Whitening	Potassium nitrate 5%; sodium fluoride 0.243%
Crest Sensitivity Whitening Plus Scope	Potassium nitrate 5%; sodium fluoride 0.243%
Sensodyne Fresh Impact[a]	Potassium nitrate 5%; sodium fluoride 0.15%
Sensodyne Maximum Strength with Fluoride	Potassium nitrate 5%; sodium fluoride 0.15%
Sensodyne ProNamel	Potassium nitrate 5%; sodium fluoride 0.15%
Tom's Sensitive	Potassium nitrate 5%; sodium fluoride 0.24%

[a] Carries the American Dental Association (ADA) Seal of Acceptance.

only be efficacious but also safe. Therefore, no special considerations are necessary in choosing products for pregnant or lactating women or for geriatric patients.

Assessment of Toothache and Tooth Hypersensitivity: A Case-Based Approach

The primary objectives of the assessment are to determine whether the patient has a history of dental problems, whether the patient's oral self-care regimen is adequate, and whether the patient receives regular professional dental care. This information will help determine the patient's level of care and risk for a toothache versus tooth hypersensitivity (Table 32–1).

Patient Counseling for Tooth Hypersensitivity

Subsequent to a definite diagnosis of tooth hypersensitivity, patients should be counseled on the proper use of desensitizing toothpastes and safe methods of toothbrushing, as outlined in the box "Patient Education for Tooth Hypersensitivity." Use of the desensitizing toothpaste should continue for as long as the dentist recommends, and then switching to a low-abrasion (nonwhitening) fluoride dentifrice is appropriate.

Evaluation of Patient Outcomes for Tooth Hypersensitivity

The patient with tooth hypersensitivity should use a desensitizing dentifrice for a maximum of 4 weeks. If the pain is resolved, the patient should continue treatment as recommended by a dentist. The patient should be advised to continue the recommended dental hygiene measures (i.e., regular flossing, brushing teeth twice daily, and visiting the dentist twice a year). If the pain persists or worsens, or if new symptoms develop after 14–21 days, the patient should see the dentist for further evaluation.[5,6,8]

TEETHING DISCOMFORT

Not all babies suffer discomfort during teething. For those who do, nonprescription products can provide symptomatic relief.

Pathophysiology of Teething Discomfort

Teething is the eruption of the deciduous (primary or baby) teeth through the gingival tissues. Usually, this normal physiologic process is essentially uneventful. In some children, however, it can cause pain, sleep disturbances, or irritability.

Clinical Presentation of Teething Discomfort

Mild pain, irritation, reddening, excessive drooling, mouth biting, gum rubbing, low-grade fever, or slight swelling of the gums while teething may precede or accompany sleep disturbances or irritability.[12] Teething is not associated with vomiting, diarrhea, nasal congestion, malaise, fever, or rashes; these signs and symptoms may indicate presence of an ear or stomach infection. Bluish, soft, round swellings (called eruption cysts) sometimes form over emerging incisors and molars. Eruption cysts are not the result of infection and will disappear if left alone. In addition, three bumps, called mamelons, may be present on the biting surfaces (*incisal edges*) of emerging incisors. The mamelons will wear away as the teeth begin to occlude against the opposing dentition. If the underside of the tongue becomes irritated, a dentist may try to smooth the edges of the mamelons to prevent further irritation. Teeth eruption can begin as early as the age of 6 months, and for each tooth that erupts, the teething period usually extends over an 8-day window.[12]

Treatment of Teething Discomfort

Treatment Goals

The goal of self-care for teething discomfort is to relieve gum pain and irritation, thereby reducing the child's distress and sleep disturbances.[12]

TABLE 32–3 Clinically Important Drug–Drug Interactions With Nonprescription Orofacial Pain and Discomfort Agents

Active Ingredient	Interacting Drug	Potential Interaction	Management/ Preventive Measures
Desensitizing Toothpastes			
Potassium nitrate	ACEIs, ARBs, potassium-sparing diuretics	These agents increase the risk of hyperkalemia.	Be cautious with this combination.
Sodium fluoride	Calcium-rich foods	Foods rich in calcium can decrease the bioavailability of fluoride by up to 25%.	Avoid concurrent use if possible.
Stannous fluoride	Calcium	Calcium can form insoluble compounds with fluoride and reduce absorption by 10%–25%.	Avoid concurrent use if possible.
Oral Debriding and Wound-Cleansing Agents			
Carbamide peroxide	No drug interactions with topical carbamide peroxide have been reported.		
Hydrogen peroxide	No drug interactions with topical hydrogen peroxide have been reported.		
Topical Oral Anesthetics			
Benzocaine	Concurrent use of other drugs that can cause methemoglobin formation, such as prilocaine, nitrates, or sulfonamides	Rare and sometimes fatal cases of methemoglobinemia have been reported with the use of topical or oromucosal benzocaine products.	Avoid concurrent use.
Camphor	Hepatotoxic herbs and supplements	Theoretically, concomitant use of camphor with other potentially hepatotoxic herbs and supplements might increase the risk of developing liver damage.	Avoid concurrent use with androstenedione, chaparral, comfrey, DHEA, germander, kava, niacin, pennyroyal oil, red yeast, and others if possible.
Herpicin-L Lip Balm	No drug or herbal interactions with any of the individual ingredients comprising topical Herpicin-L Lip Balm have been reported.		
Topical Oral Protectants			
Menthol	No drug interactions with topical menthol have been reported.		
Glycyrrhiza (licorice) extract	Antihypertensive medications	Theoretically, licorice might reduce the effect of antihypertensive drug therapy as licorice increases blood pressure in a dose-dependent manner.	Avoid concurrent use if possible.
	Warfarin	Licorice seems to increase metabolism and decrease levels of warfarin, likely by induction of CYP2C9 metabolism.	Avoid concurrent use.
	CYP3A4 substrates (lovastatin, clarithromycin, cyclosporine, diltiazem, estrogens, indinavir, triazolam, numerous others)	Licorice appears to induce CYP3A4 metabolism.	Avoid concurrent use if possible.
Oral Rinses			
Eucalyptol	Antidiabetic medications	Preliminary research suggests eucalyptus might have hypoglycemic activity and might have additive effects when used with antidiabetes medications.	Avoid concurrent use if possible and monitor blood glucose levels closely.
Bee Propolis	Anticoagulant and antiplatelet medications	In vitro evidence suggests that the propolis constituent caffeic acid phenethyl ester can inhibit platelet aggregation.	Avoid concurrent use if possible.

(continued)

TABLE 32-3 **Clinically Important Drug–Drug Interactions With Nonprescription Orofacial Pain and Discomfort Agents** *(continued)*

Active Ingredient	Interacting Drug	Potential Interaction	Management/ Preventive Measures
Topical Treatments			
Docosanol	No drug or herbal interactions with topical docosanol have been reported.		
Saliva Substitutes and Other Xerostomia Products			
Isomalt	No drug or herbal interactions with isomalt have been reported.		
Xylitol	No drug or herbal interactions with xylitol have been reported.		
Glucose oxidase	No drug or herbal interactions with glucose oxidase have been reported.		
Sodium carboxymethylcellulose	No drug or herbal interactions with sodium carboxymethylcellulose have been reported.		
Sorbitol	Sodium polystyrene sulfonate	Concomitant use has been implicated in cases of colonic necrosis.	Avoid concurrent use.
	Dichlorphenamide	Metabolic acidosis is associated with the use of dichlorphenamide and large volumes of sorbitol.	Avoid concurrent use.
Sodium monofluorophosphate	Calcium	Calcium can form insoluble compounds with fluoride, with consequent reduction in its absorption by 10%–25%.	Avoid concurrent use if possible.

Key: ACEIs = Angiotensin-converting enzyme inhibitors; ARBs angiotensin receptor blockers; CYP = cytochrome P450; DHEA = dehydroepiandrosterone.

Source: References 25, 26, 29, and 44.

General Treatment Approach

Parents and caregivers should be cautioned to exercise restraint in treating a child's teething discomfort. Eruption cysts are a part of the normal physiologic process and should be left alone to resolve spontaneously. If cut or punctured, the cysts will form scars that may delay the tooth's eruption. Parents should try all nonpharmacologic measures to determine which ones are helpful. If additional treatment is needed, pediatric doses of systemic analgesics can be used. Furthermore, the use of teething necklaces should be discouraged, in view of the potential risk of strangulation versus accessorizing the child with a product that has never been proven to be effective.[12]

Nonpharmacologic Therapy

If the baby cooperates, massaging the gum around the erupting tooth may provide relief. Babies may be made more comfortable

PATIENT EDUCATION FOR

Tooth Hypersensitivity

The objectives of self-treatment of tooth hypersensitivity are (1) to repair the damaged tooth surface using the appropriate toothpaste and (2) to replace abrasive toothbrushing practices with preferred technique. For most patients, carefully following product instructions, the dentist's recommendations, and the self-care measures listed here will help ensure optimal therapeutic outcomes.

- If adherence to correct brushing techniques with a fluoride toothpaste fails to effect improvement, a desensitizing toothpaste should be used.
- If a desensitizing toothpaste is needed, apply a 1-inch strip of toothpaste to a soft-bristle toothbrush. Brush at least twice daily.
- Note that relief of the sensitivity may take several days to several weeks. The better the patient is at removing bacterial plaque, the quicker the sensitivity will resolve.
- Use the toothpaste for as long as the dentist recommends, and then switch to a low-abrasion (nonwhitening) fluoride dentifrice.
- Note that some cases of tooth hypersensitivity require long-term treatment or several repeated treatments.
- Do not use desensitizing toothpastes in children younger than 12 years.
- Do not use high-abrasion toothpastes, such as cosmetic pastes that whiten or remove stains.

When to Seek Medical Attention

- See a dentist if the pain worsens during treatment or if new symptoms develop.

Source: References 5–9.

by giving them a cold teething ring. Teething products made of plastic and filled with fluid should not be subjected to extreme temperatures, as with boiling to sanitize or freezing, because such exposure can weaken the plastic with subsequent leakage of the fluid.[12] The cold temperature causes local vasoconstriction in addition to the pressure on the gums that the child feels on biting down on the object. If the child is at an age to tolerate food such as dry toast or teething biscuits, such foods may be offered to chew on. Foods high in sucrose should be avoided.[12]

Pharmacologic Therapy

Pharmacologic management of infant teething discomfort is limited to pediatric doses of systemic analgesics. Topical oral anesthetics carry strict FDA warnings against their use. Clinically important drug interactions for topical oral anesthetics are listed in Table 32–3.

Topical Oral Anesthetics

Benzocaine is available in concentrations ranging from 5% to 20% and is generally not accepted as a safe topical anesthetic for teething pain. In addition, the safety of benzocaine use during pregnancy has not been established.[13] Table 32–4 provides additional information regarding use of benzocaine in pregnancy.[13] (See the Preface for a detailed explanation of the pregnancy data.)

In the highest concentration approved for nonprescription use (20%), benzocaine is too potent for infants and can even cause death from drug overdose.[12] In April 2011, the U.S. Food and Drug Administration (FDA) released a MedWatch safety alert that warned HCPs of the reports linking benzocaine use and methemoglobinemias.[14] FDA recommends that benzocaine products not be used by children younger than 2 years, except under the advice and supervision of a health care professional.[12,14] Patients

TABLE 32–4 Selected Nonprescription Medications for RAS and HSL

Trade Name	Primary Ingredients	Pregnancy Data[a]
Oral Debriding and Wound-Cleansing Agents[b]		
Cankaid Liquid Oral Antiseptic	Carbamide peroxide 10%	Information is not available about the use of carbamide peroxide in pregnancy, but it is unlikely that any significant concentration reaches the fetus. Pregnant patients should consult a dentist along with their health care provider before considering use of these products. No adequate and well-controlled studies have been conducted in pregnant women.
Gly-Oxide Antiseptic Oral Cleanser	Carbamide peroxide 10%	
Orajel Antiseptic Rinse for Mouth Sores	Hydrogen peroxide 1.5%	Pregnant patients should consult a dentist along with their health care provider before considering use of these products. No adequate and well-controlled studies have been conducted in pregnant women.
Colgate Peroxyl Mouth Sore Rinse	Hydrogen peroxide 1.5%	
Topical Oral Anesthetics		
Anbesol Regular Strength Gel/Liquid	Benzocaine 10%	Pregnant patients should consult a dentist along with their health care provider before considering use of these products. No adequate and well-controlled studies have been conducted in pregnant women.
Zilactin-B Gel	Benzocaine 10%	
Anbesol Maximum Strength Gel	Benzocaine 20%	
Kank-A Liquid	Benzocaine 20%	
Orabase Paste	Benzocaine 20%	
Benzodent	Benzocaine 20%	
Orajel Mouth Sore Gel	Benzocaine 20%; benzalkonium chloride 0.02%; zinc chloride 0.1%	
Campho-Phenique Gel/Liquid	Camphor 10.8%; phenol 4.7%	Pregnant patients should consult a dentist along with their health care provider before considering use of these products. No adequate and well-controlled studies have been conducted in pregnant women.

(continued)

TABLE 32-4 **Selected Nonprescription Medications for RAS and HSL** *(continued)*

Trade Name	Primary Ingredients	Pregnancy Data[a]
Blistex Lip Medex Ointment	Camphor 1%; menthol 1%; phenol 0.54%; petrolatum 59.14%	
Carmex Lip Balm Ointment	Menthol 0.7%; camphor 1.7%; phenol 0.4%	
Herpicin-L Lip Balm	Dimethicone 1%; meradimate 5%; octinoxate 7.5%; octisalate 5%; oxybenzone 5%	
Topical Oral Protectants[b]		
Canker Cover	Menthol 2.5 mg	Pregnant patients should consult a dentist along with their health care provider before considering use of these products. No adequate and well-controlled studies have been conducted in pregnant women.
Cankermelts	Glycyrrhiza extract (GX) 30 mg (includes 1.4 mg glycyrrhizin) per disc	
Oral Rinses		
Original Listerine Antiseptic	Eucalyptol 0.092%; menthol 0.042%; methyl salicylate 0.060%; thymol 0.064%	Pregnant patients should consult a dentist along with their health care provider before considering use of these products. No adequate and well-controlled studies have been conducted in pregnant women.
Canker-Rid	Bee propolis	
Topical Treatments[c]		
Abreva cream	Docosanol 10%	Pregnant patients should consult a dentist along with their health care provider before considering use of these products. No adequate and well-controlled studies have been conducted in pregnant women.

Key: FDA = U.S. Food and Drug Administration; HSL = herpes simplex labialis; ID = insufficient data to determine pregnancy category; RAS = recurrent aphthous stomatitis.

[a] See the Preface for a detailed explanation of the pregnancy data.

[b] Use limited to RAS.

[c] Use limited to HSL.

Source: References 13, 23, 28, 29, and 44.

with known hypersensitivity to common local anesthetics should not use products containing benzocaine. Benzocaine is a known sensitizer (allergen), and its use in these patients can cause a hypersensitivity reaction.

In June 2014, FDA released a Drug Safety Communication regarding the use of topical agents for infant and child teething discomfort.[15] The communication warned that prescription oral viscous lidocaine 2% solution should not be used to treat infants and children with teething pain. Furthermore, the agency requires the following boxed warning to appear on the product packaging: "Oral viscous lidocaine solution is not approved to treat teething pain, and use in infants and young children can cause serious harm, including death." In addition, this safety communication recommends against use of nonprescription topical medications for teething pain, which would include benzocaine-containing products. These products are sold under different brand names, such as Anbesol, Hurricaine, Orajel, Baby Orajel, Orabase, and various store brands. FDA supports following the American Academy of Pediatrics' recommendations to help lessen teething pain. These modalities are discussed in detail earlier in the "Nonpharmacologic Therapy" section.

A warning released by FDA in September 2016 warns of the risk that homeopathic teething tablets and gels can pose to children, including those distributed by CVS, Hyland's, and possibly other companies, although other manufacturers were not named specifically.[16] FDA recommends that consumers stop using these products immediately and seek medical attention if their child experiences symptoms consistent with belladonna toxicity after using any of these products.[16] Teething should be managed using nonpharmacologic modalities, which are described in detail above.

Systemic Analgesics

Pediatric doses of systemic nonprescription analgesics (e.g., acetaminophen) may be used to relieve teething discomfort. (See Chapter 5 for discussion of these agents, recommended dosages, clinically important drug interactions, and pregnancy safety data.)

Product Selection Guidelines

Topical teething products labeled for the temporary relief of sore gums due to teething in infants and children are no longer recommended by FDA as safe and effective.[13–16] Nonpharmacologic management and systemic analgesics, given at the appropriate pediatric doses, should be used for symptom management.

Special Populations

The pediatric population should avoid topical teething products.[13–16] No special considerations are necessary in choosing products for older adults.[13] It is unknown how topical teething products may affect pregnant or lactating women.[13]

Assessment of Teething Discomfort: A Case-Based Approach

In most cases, teething discomfort must be assessed on the basis of the parent's description of the child's symptoms. If the child cooperates, visual inspection of the gums may confirm that the child is teething. Nonetheless, the signs and symptoms of teething must be distinguished from those of an infection. Case 32–1 provides an example of the assessment of a patient with teething discomfort.

Patient Counseling for Teething Discomfort

Patient counseling for parents should include both nonpharmacologic and pharmacologic remedies for teething discomfort, as outlined in the box "Patient Education for Teething Discomfort." Parents should be urged to contact a primary care

CASE 32-1

Relevant Evaluation Criteria	Scenario/Model Outcome
Collect	
1. Gather essential information about the patient's symptoms and medical history, including	
a. Description of symptom(s) (i.e., nature, onset, duration, severity, associated symptoms)	The father of an infant reports that his baby has been crying all night for the past few nights and he doesn't know why. He reports that the pediatrician did say teething is common at this age, but he doesn't see any teeth, so he is unsure if that is causing the baby's pain and subsequent crying.
b. Description of any factors that seem to precipitate, exacerbate, and/or relieve the patient's symptom(s)	During the day teething rings seem to help, but at night the baby won't use them.
c. Description of the patient's efforts to relieve the symptoms	Chewing on teething rings
d. Patient's identity	Grace T. Savarino
e. Patient's age, gender, height, and weight	9 months old, female, 28 in., 17 lb
f. Patient's occupation	n/a
g. Patient's dietary habits	Breast milk and some cereal
h. Patient's sleep habits	10 hours at night and two 2-hour naps during the day
i. Concurrent medical conditions, prescription and nonprescription medications, and dietary supplements	None
j. Allergies	NKDA
k. History of other adverse reactions to medications	None
l. Other (describe) ______	n/a
Assess	
2. Differentiate patient's signs/symptoms, and correctly identify the patient's primary problem(s).	Patient's symptoms seem to be consistent with teething, even though the teeth have not broken through the gums yet.
3. Identify exclusions for self-treatment.	None
4. Formulate a comprehensive list of therapeutic alternatives for the primary problem to determine whether triage to a health care provider is required, and share this information with the patient or caregiver.	Options include (1) Refer Grace to her pediatrician. (2) Recommend an OTC product to relieve the teething pain. (3) Recommend nondrug measures. (4) Take no action.

CASE 32-1 *continued*

Relevant Evaluation Criteria	Scenario/Model Outcome
Plan	
5. Select an optimal therapeutic alternative to address the patient's problem, taking into account patient preferences.	Grace is a candidate for self-care provided by the parent or caregiver.
6. Describe the recommended therapeutic approach to the patient or caregiver.	"A systemic analgesic at appropriate pediatric doses can be used." (See Chapter 5.)
7. Explain to the patient or caregiver the rationale for selecting the recommended therapeutic approach from the considered therapeutic alternatives.	"Topical oral anesthetics are not recommended for use in infants and children, so a systemic analgesic at an appropriate pediatric dose is the recommended pharmacologic agent, in addition to nondrug measures." (See Chapter 5 and the box "Patient Education for Teething Discomfort.")
Implement	
8. When recommending self-care with nonprescription medications and/or nondrug therapy, convey accurate information to the patient or caregiver.	See the box "Patient Education for Teething Discomfort."
Solicit follow-up questions from the patient or caregiver.	"Can we put the teething rings in the freezer to get them cold fast?"
Answer the patient's or caregiver's questions.	"You should avoid putting the teething rings in the freezer to get them cold because doing so can weaken the plastic and lead to leakage of the fluid inside."
Follow-up: Monitor and Evaluate	
9. Assess patient outcome	Ask the father to call to update you on Grace's response to your recommendations, or you could call him in 2 days to evaluate her response.

Key: OTC = Over-the-counter; n/a = not applicable; NKDA = no known drug allergy.

PATIENT EDUCATION FOR Teething Discomfort

The objective of parent or caregiver self-treatment for teething discomfort is to relieve gum pain and irritation, thereby reducing the affected child's distress and sleep disturbances. For most patients, the parent's or caregiver's careful following of product instructions and the self-care measures listed here will help ensure optimal therapeutic outcomes.

Nondrug Measures

- If possible, massage the gum around the erupting tooth to provide relief.
- Give the baby a cold teething ring or cold wet cloth or an appropriate food (e.g., dry toast or teething cookies) to chew on.
- The American Dental Association recommends regular dental checkups, which includes a dental visit within 6 months of eruption of the child's first tooth but no later than the child's first birthday.

Nonprescription Medications

Topical Analgesics

- Do not use teething preparations containing benzocaine in infants and young children.
- Do not use prescription viscous lidocaine 2% solution in infants and young children.

Systemic Analgesics

- If desired, use pediatric formulations of oral nonprescription analgesics such as acetaminophen to relieve teething discomfort.
- Read the label carefully, and do not exceed recommended doses or frequency of use.

When to Seek Medical Attention

- If the baby is vomiting or has diarrhea, fever, nasal congestion, malaise, pain, or other symptoms not typical of teething discomfort, take the baby to a health care provider.

Source: References 12, 14, and 15.

provider (PCP) when uncharacteristic symptoms of teething discomfort are present.

Evaluation of Patient Outcomes for Teething Discomfort

The parent should be asked to call back after 2 days of treatment. If neither nonpharmacologic therapy nor nonprescription medications are relieving the symptoms, the parent should be advised to take the baby to a PCP, pediatrician, or pediatric dentist. Furthermore, if symptoms uncharacteristic of teething discomfort have developed, the baby should be evaluated by a PCP or pediatrician.

RECURRENT APHTHOUS STOMATITIS

Recurrent aphthous stomatitis (RAS), in which the lesions are also known as canker sores or aphthous ulcers, affects approximately 2.5 billion people worldwide.[17] The onset of RAS appears to peak between the ages of 10 and 19 years.[18] Eighty percent of patients with RAS are considered to have a mild form of the disease. The lesions affect only nonkeratinized mucosa (e.g., labial, buccal) and will spontaneously heal in 10–14 days.[19,20]

Pathophysiology of Recurrent Aphthous Stomatitis

The cause of RAS is unknown in most patients. Precipitating factors such as local, systemic, immunologic, genetic, allergic, and nutritional factors have been proposed. Local trauma (e.g., smoking, chemical irritation, biting the inside of cheeks or lips, injury caused by toothbrushing or braces) has been implicated as a leading cause of lesions.[18–20] Streptococci and varicella-zoster virus have been implicated as infectious agents.[18–20] Systemic conditions associated with RAS include Behçet disease, systemic lupus erythematosus, neutrophil dysfunction, inflammatory bowel disease, and human immunodeficiency virus infection/acquired immunodeficiency syndrome (HIV/AIDS). Nutritional conditions associated with RAS include gluten-sensitive enteropathy and deficiencies of iron, B vitamins (B_1, B_2, B_6, B_{12}), and folic acid. A genetic component to the disease is possible: 40% of patients with RAS have a familial history, and children with parents who have RAS have a 90% chance of developing RAS themselves, compared with a 20% chance in children whose parents do not have RAS.[17] Additional precipitating or contributing factors may include food allergy (e.g., preservatives) and hormonal changes (e.g., menstrual cycle).[19,20]

Clinical Presentation of Recurrent Aphthous Stomatitis

RAS manifests as an epithelial ulceration on nonkeratinized mucosal surfaces of movable mouth parts, such as the tongue, floor of the mouth, soft palate, or inside lining of the lips and cheeks. Rarely, ulcerations affect keratinized tissue such as the gingiva or the external lips (vermilion). Individual ulcers are usually: (1) round or oval, (2) flat or *crateriform* (having a depressed, crater-like center), and (3) gray to grayish yellow, with an erythematous halo of inflamed tissue surrounding the ulcer (see Color Plates, photograph 14).

RAS occurs in three clinical forms: minor, major, and herpetiform. The RAS form can be distinguished primarily by the number of lesions, the size of the ulcer, and the number of days that the lesion persists. Table 32–5 compares the features of the three forms of RAS and cold sores.[18,20–23] Some patients may experience a pricking or burning sensation (prodrome) approximately 2–48 hours before the lesion actually appears.[18] The lesions can be very painful, with the pain increasing with eating and drinking, and may inhibit normal eating, drinking, swallowing, talking, and routine oral hygiene. Usually, fever or lymphadenopathy does not accompany RAS; however, such symptoms may arise if a secondary bacterial infection is present.

Treatment of Recurrent Aphthous Stomatitis

RAS cannot be cured; however, nonprescription medications can provide symptomatic relief.

Treatment Goals

The primary objective of self-treatment for RAS is to relieve pain and irritation so that the lesions can heal and the patient can eat, drink, and perform routine oral hygiene. The secondary objective is to prevent complications, such as secondary infection.[24]

General Treatment Approach

If possible, the lesions should be inspected to determine whether their appearance and location are characteristic of RAS. If possible, factors that may have led to development of the ulcer should be identified, and precipitating or contributing factors should be removed. For example, if local trauma is suspected, perhaps a softer toothbrush and gentler brushing technique could be suggested. It is also helpful to determine whether the patient has a history of RAS. If the treatments used are appropriate and previously have been successful for the patient, they should be continued. Figure 32–2 outlines the self-treatment of RAS and lists exclusions for self-care.[13,18–20,24,25]

Nonpharmacologic Therapy

If a nutritional deficiency (e.g., iron, folate, vitamins) is diagnosed as a contributing factor, the patient should increase consumption of foods high in the deficient nutrients or take appropriate nutritional supplements. For patients in whom a food allergy is thought to be a contributing factor, elimination of the offending agent from the diet may help to improve or resolve RAS. Because stress may play a role in the development of RAS, relaxation and stress removal may be useful and have shown reductions in ulcer frequency.[18] The box "Patient Education for Recurrent Aphthous Stomatitis" lists additional nonpharmacologic measures.

Pharmacologic Therapy

Several types of nonprescription medications (oral debriding and wound-cleansing agents, topical oral anesthetics, topical oral

TABLE 32-5 **Differentiation of RAS and HSL**

Feature	RAS (canker sores) Minor	RAS (canker sores) Major	RAS (canker sores) Herpetiform	HSL (cold sores)
Clinical manifestation	Oval, flat ulcer; erythematous tissue around ulcer	Oval, ragged, gray/yellow ulcers; crateriform	Small, oval ulcers in crops, similar to minor RAS	Red, fluid-filled vesicles; lesions may coalesce; crusted when mature
Location	All areas except gingiva, hard palate, vermilion border (at junction of oral mucosa and external skin)	Any intraoral area, but predilection for lips, soft palate, and throat	Any intraoral area	Junction of oral mucosa and skin of lip and nose
Incidence	13%–26%	1.5%–3%	0.5%–1%	20%–30%
Incidence among RAS sufferers	80%	10%	5%–10%	n/a
Number of lesions	1–5	Several (1–10)	10–100 (in crops)	Several
Size of lesion	<0.5 cm	>0.5 cm	<0.5 cm	1–3 mm
Duration	10–14 days	≥6 weeks	7–10 days	10–14 days
Pain	None–moderate	None–moderate	Moderate–severe	None–moderate
Scarring	None	Common	None	Rare
Comments	Immunologic defect	Immunologic defect	Immunologic defect	Induced by HSV-1

Key: HSL = Herpes simplex labialis; HSV-1 = herpes simplex virus type 1; n/a = not applicable; RAS = recurrent aphthous stomatitis.
Source: References 18 and 21–23.

protectants, oral rinses, systemic analgesics) provide symptomatic relief of RAS, but they do not prevent its recurrence. Table 32–4 lists a variety of the commercially available products for relief of orofacial pain and discomfort and their pregnancy category rating, if known.

Clinically important drug interactions with these agents—oral debriding and wound-cleansing agents, topical oral anesthetics, topical oral protectants, and oral rinses—are discussed in Table 32–3.

Oral Debriding and Wound-Cleansing Agents

Oral debriding agents and wound cleansers may be used (1) to aid in the removal of debris, phlegm, mucus, or other secretions associated with a sore mouth; (2) to cleanse minor wounds or areas of minor gum inflammation; and (3) to cleanse recurrent aphthous ulcers. Products that release nascent oxygen can be used as debriding and cleansing agents to provide temporary relief of RAS discomfort. Hydrogen peroxide and carbamide peroxide release oxygen immediately on contact with tissue enzymes (catalase and peroxidase), but tissue and bacterial exposure to the oxygen is very brief.[25,26]

For direct application, a few drops of carbamide peroxide (10%–15%) or hydrogen peroxide (1.5%) are applied to the affected area and allowed to remain in place for 1 minute before expectorating. This can be done up to four times a day. As a rinse, carbamide peroxide drops are placed on the tongue, mixed with saliva, and swished in the mouth for 1 minute. An aqueous solution of hydrogen peroxide 3% should be mixed with an equal amount of water before rinsing the mouth. Some products (e.g., Colgate Peroxyl Rinse) are provided as a solution of hydrogen peroxide 1.5% and should be used without dilution. Prolonged rinsing with oxidizing products can lead to soft-tissue irritation, transient tooth sensitivity from decalcification of enamel, cellular changes, and overgrowth of undesirable organisms that could possibly result in development of a black hairy tongue.[25] Self-medication with any of these products should not be continued for longer than 7 days, and patients should contact an HCP if symptoms (i.e., irritation or inflammation of the mouth or throat) worsen or persist beyond that time. If at any time a rash develops during the self-treatment regimen, the patient should discontinue use of the product and contact an HCP.

Topical Oral Anesthetics

Topical oral anesthetic/analgesic products, including benzocaine 5%–20%, benzyl alcohol 0.05%–0.1%, butacaine sulfate 0.05%–0.1%, dyclonine 0.05%–0.1%, hexylresorcinol 0.05%–0.1%, and salicylic alcohol 1%–6%, are generally recognized as effective for temporary relief of pain associated with RAS.[18] To reduce the incidence of RAS, patients should also avoid the use of dentifrices containing sodium lauryl sulfate.[18–20]

Topical Oral Protectants

Oral mucosal protectants are pharmacologically inert substances that coat and protect the ulcerated area. Coating the ulcer with a topical oral protectant can be effective in protecting ulcerations, decreasing friction, and giving temporary symptomatic relief. These products create a barrier by using a paste, an adhering film, or a dissolvable patch to cover the lesion. Some products

Exclusions for Self-Treatment

- Lesions associated with underlying pathology
- Lesions present ≥14 days
- Frequently recurring lesions
- Symptoms of systemic illness
- Failure of prior appropriate self-treatment

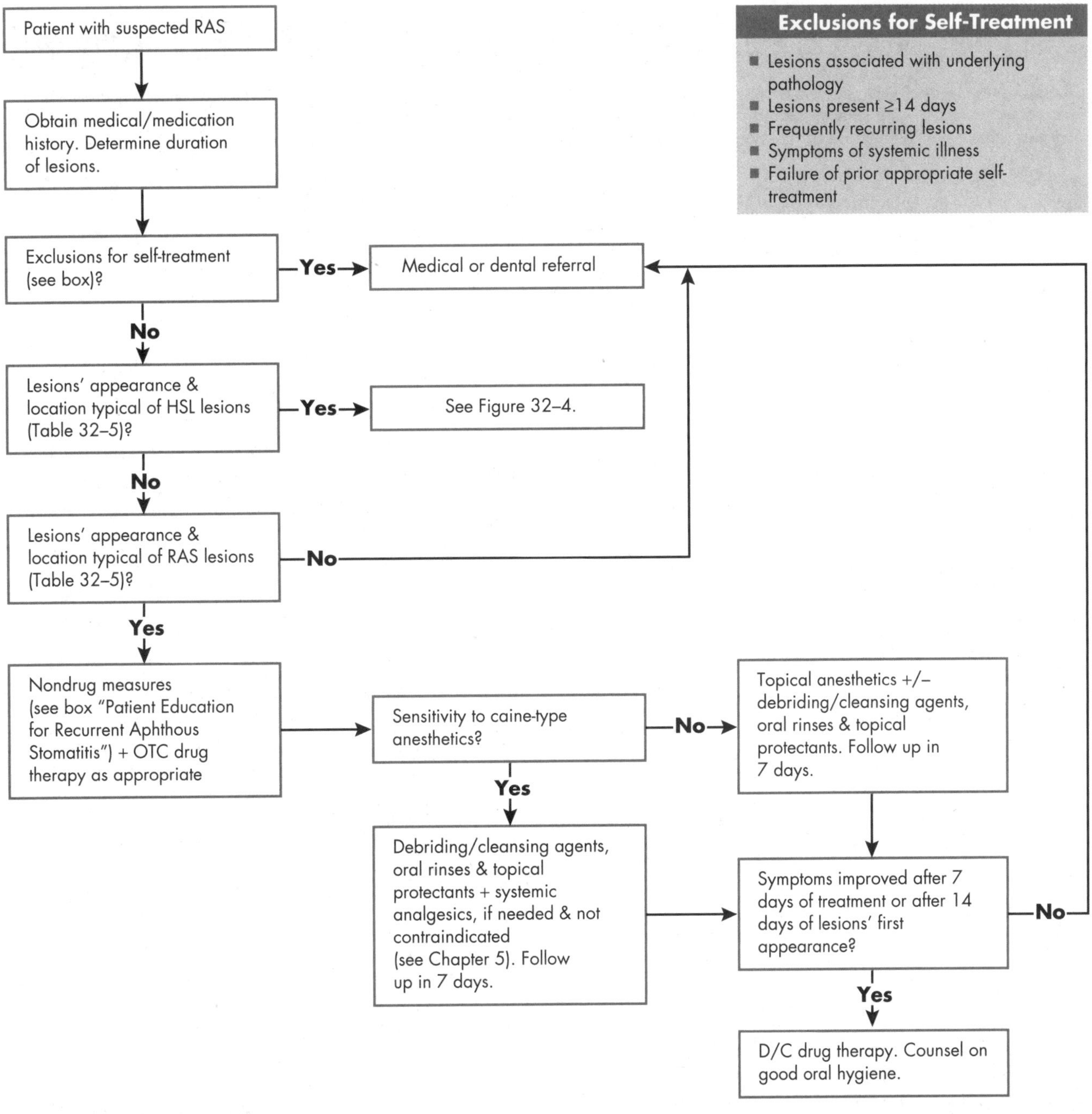

FIGURE **32–2** Self-care for recurrent aphthous stomatitis (RAS). Key: D/C = Discontinue; HSL = herpes simplex labialis; OTC = over-the-counter. (Source: References 13, 18–20, 24–26, and 44.)

are available in combination with an oral anesthetic. Products available as a patch or dissolving disc must be placed against the sore for 10–20 seconds. Once the disc adheres to the lesion, the barrier is formed and the disc will stay in place until dissolved, approximately 8–12 hours.[27]

Oral Rinses

Rinsing the mouth with an antiseptic rinse will hasten the healing of the lesions. Saline rinses (1–3 teaspoons of salt in 4–8 ounces of warm tap water) may soothe ulcers and can be used before topical application of a medication. Similarly, a paste of baking soda applied to the lesions for a few minutes may soothe irritation.

Systemic Analgesics

Systemic nonprescription analgesics (e.g., aspirin, nonsteroidal anti-inflammatory drugs, acetaminophen) give additional relief of mouth discomfort. (See Chapter 5 for discussion of these agents, recommended dosages, clinically important drug interactions,

PATIENT EDUCATION FOR Recurrent Aphthous Stomatitis

The primary objective of self-treatment of recurrent aphthous stomatitis is to relieve pain and irritation so that the lesions can heal and the patient can eat, drink, and perform routine oral hygiene. The secondary objective is to prevent complications, such as secondary infection. For most patients, carefully following product instructions and the self-care measures listed here will help ensure optimal therapeutic outcomes.

Nondrug Measures

- If a deficiency of iron, folate, or vitamin B_{12} is diagnosed as a contributing factor, increase consumption of foods high in the deficient nutrient, or take appropriate nutritional supplements.
- Avoid spicy or acidic foods until the lesions heal.
- Avoid sharp-textured foods that may cause increased trauma to the lesion.
- If desired, apply ice directly to the lesions in 10-minute increments but for no longer than 20 minutes in a given hour.
- Do not use heat. If an infection is present, heat may spread the infection.

Nonprescription Medications

- If longer-lasting relief is desired, nonprescription medications such as oral debriding and cleansing agents, topical oral anesthetics, topical oral protectants, oral rinses, and systemic analgesics can be used.

Oral Debriding and Wound-Cleansing Agents

- Use a product containing one of the following ingredients: carbamide peroxide 10%–15% or hydrogen peroxide 1.5%. Apply after meals up to 4 times daily.
- Do not use these medications longer than 7 days. Chronic use can cause tissue irritation, decalcification of enamel, and black hairy tongue.
- Do not swallow these medications.

Topical Oral Anesthetics

- Use products containing one of the following medications: benzocaine 5%–20%, benzyl alcohol 0.05%–0.1%, butacaine sulfate 0.05%–0.1%, dyclonine 0.05%–0.1%, hexylresorcinol 0.05%–0.1%, or salicylic alcohol 1%–6%.
- Do not use benzocaine if you have a history of hypersensitivity to other benzocaine-containing products.

Topical Oral Protectants

- Use topical oral protectants or denture adhesives to coat and protect the lesions. These agents also will provide temporary relief of discomfort.
- Apply these products as needed.

Oral Rinses

- Rinse the mouth with Original Listerine Antiseptic to hasten healing of the lesions.
- Rinse the mouth with a saline solution to soothe discomfort or to prepare the lesion for application of a topical medication. For saline solution, add 1–3 teaspoons of salt to 4–8 ounces of warm tap water.

Systemic Analgesics

- Oral analgesics (e.g., aspirin or other NSAID, acetaminophen) can be used for additional relief of mouth discomfort.
- Do not hold aspirin in the mouth or place it on oral lesions. The acid can cause a chemical burn and tissue damage.

When to Seek Medical Attention

- See a primary care provider if any of the following occur:
  - Symptoms do not abate after 7 days of treatment with oral debriding or wound-cleansing agents.
  - The lesions do not heal in 14 days.
  - Symptoms worsen during self-treatment.
  - Manifestations of systemic infection, such as fever, rash, or swelling, develop.

Key: NSAID = Nonsteroidal anti-inflammatory drug.
Source: References 13, 17–20, 24–26, and 44.

and pregnancy safety data.) Aspirin should not be retained in the mouth before swallowing, nor placed in the area of the oral lesions. The acetylsalicylic acid can cause a chemical burn with subsequent tissue damage (see Color Plates, photograph 15).

Product Selection Guidelines

Patients with known hypersensitivity to common local anesthetics should not use a product containing a local anesthetic. Benzocaine is a known sensitizer (allergen), and its use in these patients can cause a hypersensitivity reaction. Patients with known sensitivity to aspirin should also avoid salicylic acid. Various dosage forms are available (e.g., liquid, gel, rinse, dissolvable patch); drug delivery is a major concern, however, because topical applications can be easily washed away by saliva. Gels are the preferred drug delivery application because they are easy to apply and are not as easily washed away.[18–20,24] A topical anesthetic will provide short-term relief of the pain and discomfort associated with RAS, and the oral debriding agents will help to keep the ulcer clean. Using both of these agents should help alleviate immediate discomfort and heal the ulcer quickly.

Special Populations

The safety of these agents (oral debriding and wound-cleansing agents, topical oral anesthetics, topical oral protectants, and oral rinses) with use during pregnancy is mostly unknown. Table 32–4 provides additional information regarding use of these agents. (See the Preface for detailed explanation of the pregnancy data.) No special considerations are necessary in choosing products for older adults. It is unknown how these products affect lactating women. These products should not be used or are not approved for use in pediatric patients.[13,25,26,28–30]

Assessment of Recurrent Aphthous Stomatitis: A Case-Based Approach

Controlling the pain and preventing infection are the primary concerns when RAS is suspected. If possible, factors that may have precipitated or contributed to the development of the ulcer should be identified and then removed. The patient should be asked about previous self-treatments and their effectiveness. If the treatments used are appropriate and have been successful for the patient, they should be continued.

Patient Counseling for Recurrent Aphthous Stomatitis

All nonpharmacologic and pharmacologic measures for treating RAS, as outlined in the box "Patient Education for Recurrent Aphthous Stomatitis," should be explained to the patient. The patient should also be cautioned about using ineffective or harmful therapies. Possible adverse effects, drug interactions, contraindications, and precautions should then be explained for all nonprescription agents. In addition, patients must be alerted to the conditions that warrant dental or medical evaluation.

Evaluation of Patient Outcomes for Recurrent Aphthous Stomatitis

Minor RAS lesions are typically self-limiting and resolve within 14 days. Oral debriding and wound-cleansing agents are labeled for use for up to 7 days. If the symptoms have improved, the patient should discontinue treatment but continue other dental hygienic measures (e.g., regular flossing and twice-daily toothbrushing). Symptoms that are unimproved or that have worsened during treatment require medical evaluation.

MINOR ORAL MUCOSAL INJURY OR IRRITATION

Pathophysiology of Minor Oral Mucosal Injury or Irritation

Minor wounds or inflammation resulting from minor dental procedures; accidental injury (e.g., biting of the tongue, cheek or abrasion from sharp, crisp foods); or other irritations of the mouth, gums, or palate may be treated with various nonprescription medications.

Treatment of Minor Oral Mucosal Injury or Irritation

Treatment of mouth injury (traumatic laceration or ulcer) and irritation is similar to that for RAS. Mouth injury and irritation differ from RAS with regard to etiology and certain treatment considerations.

Treatment Goals

The goals of treating minor mucosal injury and irritation are (1) to control discomfort and pain, (2) to aid healing with the appropriate use of nonpharmacologic and pharmacologic measures, and (3) to prevent secondary bacterial infection.

General Treatment Approach

Treatment should focus first on relieving discomfort. Application of ice can accomplish this. Local anesthetics, oral analgesics, and saline rinses are also safe and effective.[18–20,24] Once the discomfort has resolved, patients should focus on healing the affected area. Homemade sodium bicarbonate rinses and oral debriding and wound-cleansing agents can help achieve this objective. Finally, concomitant use of oral protectants can relieve discomfort and aid healing by protecting the area from further irritation. Figure 32–3 outlines this approach and lists exclusions for self-care.[21–23]

Nonpharmacologic Therapy

When tissues of the lips, tongue, cheeks, or palate are bruised, direct application of ice may reduce the swelling. Ice should be applied in 10-minute increments but not longer than 20 minutes in a given hour. Longer application times may cause local tissue damage. Sodium bicarbonate solutions (½–1 teaspoon of household baking soda in 4 ounces of water) can act as an oral debriding agent and wound cleanser.[23] The solution is swished in the mouth over the affected area for at least 1 minute and then expectorated. Sodium bicarbonate's mucolytic action is related to its alkalinity. Saline rinses (1–3 teaspoons of salt in 4–8 ounces of warm tap water) can cleanse and soothe the affected area.

Pharmacologic Therapy

As with RAS, topical analgesics/anesthetics, oral protectants, and oral debriding and wound-cleansing agents are the mainstay of pharmacologic therapy. The "Pharmacologic Therapy" section for treatment of RAS discusses these agents in further detail. In addition to these agents, astringents may be used. Astringents cause tissues to contract or arrest secretions by causing proteins to coagulate on the cell surface.[31] Dentists may suggest that their patients use oxidizing mouth rinses or topically applied steroids (which are available only by prescription) as an adjunctive treatment for specific conditions or as a postoperative aid in cleaning the affected area, relieving discomfort, and assisting the healing process.

Assessment of Minor Oral Mucosal Injury or Irritation: A Case-Based Approach

The cause and nature of the injury or irritation are the primary considerations in patient assessment. If the disorder is self-treatable, the HCP should ascertain whether the injury or irritation has occurred previously, how it was treated, and whether the patient has known contraindications to the nonprescription medications used to treat the disorder.

Patient Counseling for Minor Oral Mucosal Injury or Irritation

Once the problem is determined to be a minor irritation or injury of the mouth, the patient should be counseled on (1) the steps in

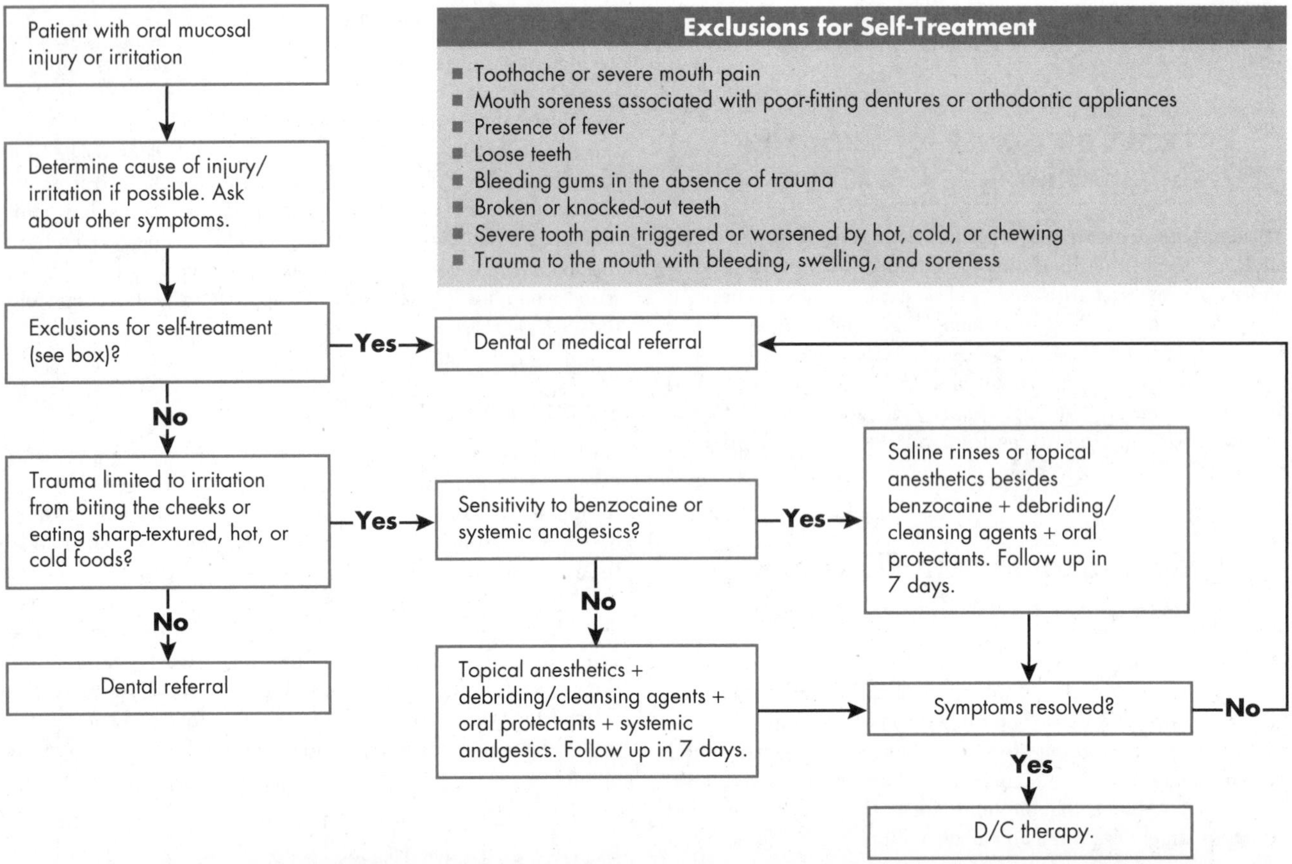

FIGURE 32-3 Self-care for minor oral mucosal injury or irritation. Key: D/C = Discontinue. (Source: References 21, 22, 25, 26, and 44.)

the treatment regimen, (2) the purpose of each agent, and (3) the length of time the products can be used safely. Signs and symptoms that indicate infection should also be explained. See the box "Patient Education for Minor Oral Mucosal Injury or Irritation."

Evaluation of Patient Outcomes for Minor Oral Mucosal Injury or Irritation

Minor injury or irritation should resolve within 7 days of treatment and within 10 days of the initial insult or injury.[31] If the symptoms resolve, no further treatment is necessary. If symptoms persist or worsen, or swelling, rash, or fever develops, the patient should be evaluated by a PCP.

HERPES SIMPLEX LABIALIS

Herpes simplex labialis (HSL), manifesting as cold sores or fever blisters, is a disorder caused by a virus of the family Herpesviridae. Herpes simplex virus type 1 (HSV-1) is primarily associated with oral and labial lesions, whereas herpes simplex virus 2 (HSV-2) usually produces genital sores. However, predilection of a specific HSV infection for an anatomic site is changing, in part because of variable sexual practices.[23] Any of the human herpesviruses (e.g., cytomegalovirus, Epstein–Barr virus), not just HSV-1 and HSV-2, can cause oral lesions. Anyone who comes in contact with the herpesvirus can potentially become infected. After the primary infection, HSV infection can be latent and reactivate at a later date as the more commonly known herpes labialis, or cold sores.[21]

Pathophysiology of Herpes Simplex Labialis

HSV infection is contagious and believed to be transmitted by direct contact. Fluid from herpes vesicles contains live virus, which can be transmitted from patient to patient. Because the virus remains viable on surfaces for several hours, contaminated objects may also be a source of infection. Transmission commonly occurs through kissing or sharing utensils or drinking vessels.[21] HSV enters the host through a break in the skin or intact mucous membranes. Once the virus has infected a host, it remains in a latent state in the trigeminal ganglia. The virus can be reactivated on exposure to a triggering stimulus, such as ultraviolet radiation, stress, fatigue, cold, and windburn. Other possible triggers include

PATIENT EDUCATION FOR

Minor Oral Mucosal Injury or Irritation

The objectives of self-treatment of minor oral mucosal injury or irritation are (1) to control discomfort and pain, (2) to aid healing with the appropriate use of drug and nondrug measures, and (3) to prevent secondary bacterial infection. For most patients, carefully following product instructions and the self-care measures listed here will help ensure optimal therapeutic outcomes.

Nondrug Measures

- Rinse with a sodium bicarbonate solution to remove injured tissue and cleanse the affected area. Add ½–1 teaspoon of sodium bicarbonate to 4 ounces of water. Swish the solution in the mouth over the affected area for at least 1 minute, then spit out the solution. This can be done up to four times a day.
- Use saline rinses to cleanse and soothe the affected area. Add 1–3 teaspoons of salt to 4–8 ounces of warm tap water. This can be done up to 4 times a day.
- For bruised lips or cheeks, apply ice in 10-minute increments to reduce swelling. Do not apply ice for longer than 20 minutes in a given hour.

Nonprescription Medications

- If longer-lasting relief is desired, use the following types of nonprescription medications: oral debriding and wound-cleansing agents, topical oral anesthetics, topical oral protectants, and systemic analgesics.

Debriding and Cleansing Agents

- Use a product containing carbamide peroxide 10%–15% or hydrogen peroxide 1.5%.
- Do not use these medications for longer than 7 days. Chronic use can cause tissue irritation, decalcification of enamel, and black hairy tongue.
- Do not swallow these medications.
- These products should be used after meals (3–4 times a day), and the patient should avoid eating or drinking for at least 30 minutes after application. Swish the liquid around the mouth for 10–15 minutes (or as long as the patient can tolerate, but no longer than 15 minutes).

Topical Oral Anesthetics

- Use a product containing one of the following medications: benzocaine 5%–20%, benzyl alcohol 0.05%–0.1%, butacaine sulfate 0.05%–0.1%, dyclonine 0.05%–0.1%, hexylresorcinol 0.05%–0.1%, or salicylic alcohol 1%–6%.
- Do not use benzocaine if you have a history of hypersensitivity to other benzocaine-containing products.
- Avoid potentially inflammatory products containing substantial amounts of menthol, phenol, or camphor. These agents may cause tissue irritation and damage or systemic toxicity.
- These products should be used after meals (3–4 times a day), and the patient should avoid eating or drinking for at least 30 minutes after application.

Topical Oral Protectants

- Use topical oral protectants or denture adhesives to coat and protect the lesions.
- These products should be used after meals (3–4 times a day), and the patient should avoid eating or drinking for at least 30 minutes after application.

Systemic Analgesics

- If desired, take an oral analgesic (e.g., aspirin or other NSAID, acetaminophen) for additional relief of mouth discomfort.
- Do not hold aspirin in the mouth or place it on oral lesions. The acid can cause a chemical burn and tissue damage.

When to Seek Medical Attention

- See a primary care provider if any of the following occur:
  - Symptoms persist after 7 days of treatment.
  - Symptoms worsen during self-treatment.
  - Manifestations of systemic infection such as fever, redness, or swelling develop.

Key: NSAID = Nonsteroidal anti-inflammatory drug.
Source: References 21, 22, 25, 26, and 44.

fever, injury, menstruation, dental work, infectious diseases, and factors that suppress the immune system (e.g., chemotherapy, radiation therapy).[21] Although the virus can go through periods of dormancy and reactivation, the person is infected for life. On reactivation, the lesions often arise repeatedly in the same location.

Clinical Presentation of Herpes Simplex Labialis

HSL is so named because it commonly affects the lip or areas bordering the lips; the usual site is at the junction of mucous membrane and skin of the lips or nose. HSL lesions may also occur intraorally (primarily involving keratinized mucosa such as the hard palate or gingiva). The lesions are recurrent, painful, and cosmetically objectionable. Onset of HSL often is preceded by a prodrome in which the patient notices burning, *pruritus* (itching), tingling, or numbness in the area of the forthcoming lesion. Other signs and symptoms include pain, fever, localized bleeding, swollen lymph nodes, and malaise.

The initial lesion in an episode of HSL is a collection of small red papules of fluid-containing vesicles 1–3 mm in diameter. Often, many lesions coalesce to form a larger area of involvement. An erythematous, inflamed border around the fluid-filled vesicles may be present. In mature lesions, a crust often forms over the top of many coalesced, burst vesicles; its base is erythematous (see Color Plates, photograph 16). Pustules or pus present under the crust of a herpesvirus lesion may indicate a secondary bacterial infection; prompt evaluation and treatment with a targeted antibiotic, if indicated, are appropriate. Table 32–5 further describes the clinical presentation of HSL and compares its features with those of RAS.

A related disease, acute (primary) herpetic gingivostomatitis, is seen mainly in children but can occur in adults, especially those who are immunocompromised. Although the oral lesions of this disease can develop anywhere on the oral mucosal surface, they commonly occur on the lips, areas bordering the lips, or the gums. Herpetic gingivostomatitis is distinguished from RAS gingivostomatitis by infected gums, which are very red and covered by a pseudomembrane or studded with ulcerations.

Other symptoms of herpetic gingivostomatitis may include submandibular lymphadenitis, swallowing difficulties, and halitosis. Referral to a health care professional is warranted if this disorder is suspected.

On the basis of clinical appearance, HSL and RAS should be easy to distinguish from oral candidiasis, which develops as part of yeast infections. In the mouth, candidiasis is often referred to as thrush and is characterized by white plaques with a milk curd appearance. These plaques, which are attached to the oral mucosa, can usually be detached easily, revealing erythematous, bleeding, sore areas beneath (see Color Plates, photograph 13).

Treatment of Herpes Simplex Labialis

Although HSL and RAS differ in etiology, global treatment for these disorders is similar. The patient should be instructed to avoid circumstances that induce more lesions (e.g., stress), to keep the lesions free of counterirritants, and to keep existing lesions as clean as possible, thereby avoiding secondary infections. Table 32–4 lists common classes of nonprescription medications used to treat RAS and HSL. (Note: Of the products listed in Table 32–4, oral debriding and wound-cleansing agents and oral mucosal protectants are *not* used to treat HSL.)

Treatment Goals

The objectives of self-treatment for HSL (cold sores) are (1) to relieve pain and irritation while the sores are healing, (2) to prevent secondary infection, and (3) to curtail spread of the lesions.

General Treatment Approach

The lesions should be inspected to determine whether their appearance and location are characteristic of HSL. If possible, factors that may have led to development of lesions should be identified; then precipitating or contributing factors should be removed. For example, if trauma is suspected, perhaps a gentler toothbrush and gentler brushing technique could be suggested. It is also helpful to determine whether the patient has a history of HSL. The medical history should be reviewed to determine whether an underlying pathologic process predisposes the patient to recurrent HSL or could complicate treatment. The interviewing provider should inquire about previous self-treatments and their effectiveness. If the treatments used are appropriate and have been successful for the patient, they should be implemented and continued. Treatment should focus on cleansing the affected area, protecting the lesions from infection, and relieving the discomfort of burning, itching, and pain. Figure 32–4 outlines the self-treatment of HSL and lists exclusions for self-care.[21,22,28–33]

Nonpharmacologic Therapy

Lesions should be kept clean by gently washing with mild soap solutions. Handwashing is important in preventing lesion contamination and minimizing autoinoculation of herpesvirus. The involved skin should be kept moist to prevent drying and *fissuring* (cracking). Cracking may render lesions more susceptible to secondary bacterial infection, may delay healing, and usually increases discomfort. Factors that delay healing (e.g., stress, local trauma, wind, excessive sun exposure, fatigue) should be avoided. Patients who identify sun exposure as a precipitating event should be advised to routinely use a lip and face sunscreen product. (See Chapter 39 for more detail about sunscreens and sun protection factor (SPF) requirements.)

Pharmacologic Therapy

Topical skin protectants help to protect the lesions from infection, relieve dryness, and keep the involved tissue soft, but they do not reduce the duration of symptoms. These products should be used after meals (3–4 times a day), and the patient should avoid eating or drinking for at least 30 minutes after application.[24]

Externally applied analgesics or anesthetics, in bland, emollient vehicles, also relieve the discomfort of burning, itching, and pain, but they do not reduce the duration of symptoms. Ingredients that are generally used include benzocaine 5%–20%, dibucaine 0.25%–1%, dyclonine hydrochloride 0.5%–1%, benzyl alcohol 10%–33%, camphor 1%–20%, and menthol 0.1%–1%. Menthol in concentrations greater than 1% can stimulate cutaneous sensory receptors and produce a counterirritant effect; such preparations are therefore contraindicated.[29]

Docosanol 10% (Abreva Cream) is the only FDA-approved nonprescription product proven to reduce the duration and severity of symptoms. The agent inhibits direct fusion between the herpes virus and the human cell plasma membrane, thereby preventing viral replication.[33] Docosanol should be applied at the first sign of an outbreak (prodromal stage), 5 times a day, until the lesion is healed, but for no more than 10 days. Treatment with docosanol reduces the median healing time to healing by approximately 1 day (18 hours) compared with placebo. Docosanol-treated patients also note a significant reduction in the duration of symptoms, including pain and/or burning, itching, or tingling, compared with placebo (20% reduction in the median time to complete cessation of these symptoms).[33] The safety of docosanol with use during pregnancy is unknown. Table 32–4 provides additional information regarding use of docosanol. (See the Preface for detailed explanation of the pregnancy data.) Clinically important drug interactions with docosanol are discussed in Table 32–3.

Abreva Cream, which contains docosanol 10%, should not be mistaken for Abreva Conceal, which is a nonmedicated patch.[28]

If evidence of secondary bacterial infection is seen (e.g., failure of crusting to occur, persistence of an erythematous border), topical application of a thin layer of triple-antibiotic ointment 3–4 times daily is recommended. (See Chapter 41 for more information about these agents.) Systemic nonprescription analgesics may provide additional pain relief.

Studies suggest that patients suffering from sideropenia, a condition resulting from a deficiency of iron in the body, and those who have recurrent HSL may experience fewer episodes after treatment with iron replacement therapy.[34]

HSL is not considered a steroid-responsive dermatosis; therefore, the use of topical steroids is contraindicated. Products that are highly astringent should also be avoided. Zinc sulfate should be avoided as well, because oral mucosal absorption and toxicity could occur with frequent application of these agents to the lip and oral cavity.[30]

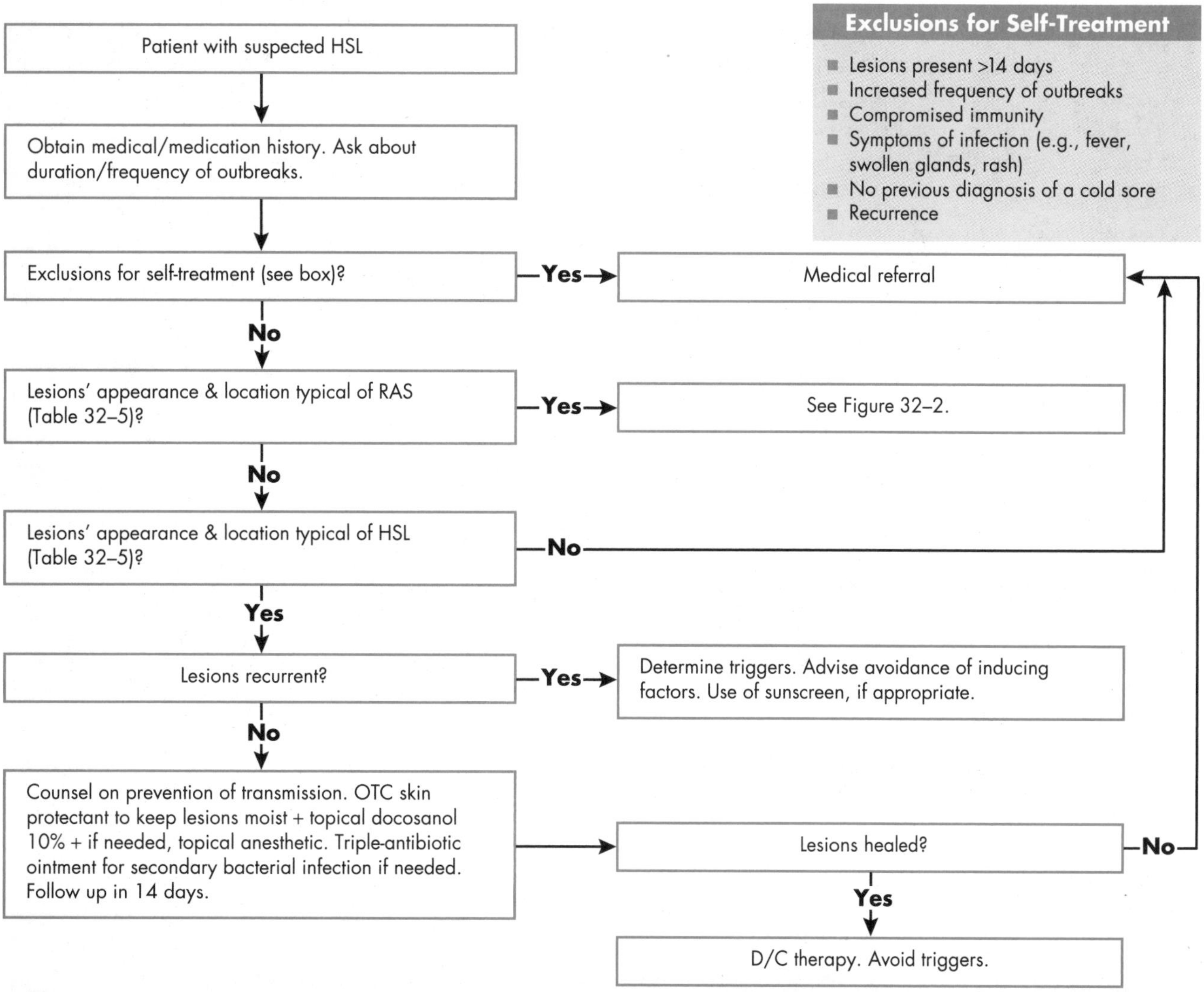

FIGURE 32–4 Self-care for herpes simplex labialis (HSL). Key: D/C = Discontinue; OTC = over-the-counter; RAS = recurrent aphthous stomatitis. (Source: References 21, 22, 28–30, and 32–34.)

Complementary Therapies

The essential oil of *Melaleuca alternifolia*, or tea tree oil, has activity against HSV in vitro. Studies have shown that, compared with placebo, the healing time is reduced with use of tea tree oil and is similar to that of topical acyclovir 5%.[35] Lysine has preventive effects and has been shown to decrease the frequency of outbreaks when taken daily.[31,36] Extract of the leaves of *Melissa officinalis*, or lemon balm, has also been used in patients with HSL. Studies comparing lemon balm with placebo have shown a reduction in symptoms, shortened healing time, prevention of infection spread, and patient preference for lemon balm.[36]

Assessment of Herpes Simplex Labialis: A Case-Based Approach

Although many of the same nonprescription medications are indicated for RAS and HSL, the disorders still need to be differentiated. Because herpes simplex lesions are contagious, additional measures are necessary to prevent transmission of the virus. The medical history will help determine the presence of an underlying pathologic process that predisposes the patient to recurrent HSL or could complicate treatment.

Patient Counseling for Herpes Simplex Labialis

Patient counseling should emphasize that HSL lesions are contagious and should include appropriate measures to prevent transmission of the virus, as outlined in the box "Patient Education for Herpes Simplex Labialis." Patients should be advised that the disorder is self-limiting, and that pharmacologic therapy with appropriate agents can keep the affected tissue moist and supple, decrease the itching and pain, protect involved skin from secondary bacterial infection, and help reduce the duration of active infection. The action of each recommended

PATIENT EDUCATION FOR Herpes Simplex Labialis

The objectives of self-treatment of herpes simplex labialis (cold sores) are (1) to relieve pain and irritation while the sores are healing, (2) to prevent secondary infection, and (3) to prevent spread of the lesions. For most patients, carefully following product instructions and the self-care measures listed here will help ensure optimal therapeutic outcomes.

Nondrug Measures

- Keep labial or extraoral lesions clean by gently washing them with mild soap solutions.
- Wash hands frequently to prevent contaminating the lesions and to avoid spreading the virus.
- Avoid factors believed to delay healing such as stress, local injury, wind exposure, excessive sun exposure, and fatigue.
- If outbreaks are related to sun exposure, always use a lip and face sunscreen with appropriate SPF protection. (See Chapter 39, "Prevention of Sun-Induced Skin Disorders," for further discussion related to SPF.)

Nonprescription Medications

- Use topical anesthetics such as benzocaine or dibucaine to relieve burning, itching, and pain. Do not use benzocaine if you have a history of hypersensitivity to other benzocaine-containing products.
- If using products containing camphor and menthol, make sure that the concentration of camphor does not exceed 3% and the concentration of menthol does not exceed 1%.
- Do not apply hydrocortisone to the lesions.
- If evidence of secondary bacterial infection is seen, apply a thin layer of triple-antibiotic ointment 3–4 times daily.
- Apply the topical agent docosanol 10% (Abreva Cream) to limit the burning, tingling, and itching sensations. Docosanol 10% can also speed up the healing process, thereby reducing the duration of the symptoms.
- If desired, take an oral nonprescription analgesic (e.g., aspirin or other NSAID, acetaminophen) for additional pain relief.
- Do not hold aspirin in the mouth or place it on oral lesions. The acid can cause a chemical burn and tissue damage.
- These products should be used after meals (3–4 times a day), and the patient should avoid eating or drinking for at least 30 minutes after application.

When to Seek Medical Attention

- See a primary care provider if any of the following occurs:
  - The lesions do not heal in 14 days.
  - The lesions recur despite appropriate self-care.
  - The self-treatment measures do not relieve discomfort.
  - Signs or symptoms of systemic illness such as fever, malaise, rash, or swollen lymph glands emerge.
  - Symptoms change or worsen.

Key: NSAID = Nonsteroidal anti-inflammatory drug; SPF = sun protection factor.
Source: References 21, 22, 28–30, and 32–34.

product, its proper use, and possible adverse effects should also be explained.

Evaluation of Patient Outcomes for Herpes Simplex Labialis

In immunocompetent patients, HSL is typically mild and self-limiting, with healing of lesions within 10–14 days.[24,25,33] If the symptoms have resolved, no further treatment is necessary. However, if the condition worsens (pain and itching persist, redness increases, or signs of secondary infection are apparent), referral to the patient's PCP is warranted.

XEROSTOMIA

Xerostomia, commonly referred to as *dry mouth,* is a syndrome in which salivary flow is limited or completely arrested. A person with normal salivary flow produces up to 1.5 L of saliva every 24 hours. Between 10% and 50% of the population is said to be afflicted with persistent dry mouth.[37]

Pathophysiology of Xerostomia

Patients with certain disease states, including *Sjögren syndrome* (an autoimmune condition in which the salivary glands become partly or completely dysfunctional and the presenting manifestations typically include dry mouth and/or dry eyes), diabetes mellitus, depression, and Crohn's disease, are prone to xerostomia.[37,38] In addition, radiation therapy of the head and neck can cause atrophy of the salivary glands; in the vast majority of treated patients, irreversible compromise of salivary gland function results. Medications that have anticholinergic activity or cause depletion of salivary flow volume (e.g., antihistamines, decongestants, antihypertensives, diuretics, antidepressants, antipsychotics, sedatives) can also cause xerostomia.[39,40] Older patients, who are more likely to be taking multiple medications for chronic diseases, typically are more commonly affected. However, if the xerostomia is drug-induced and the causative medication can be discontinued, normal salivary flow may resume in some cases.[41] Nonpharmacologic causes of xerostomia include the use or consumption of alcohol, tobacco, caffeine, or hot spicy food; blockage of ducts by salivary gland stones (*sialolithiasis*); and mouth breathing.

Clinical Presentation of Xerostomia

Xerostomia can result in difficulty talking and swallowing, stomatitis, burning tongue, and halitosis. Unmoistened food cannot be tasted; therefore, xerostomia can cause loss of appetite with eventual decline in nutritional status.[37–40] As a consequence of the decrease in salivary flow and the lack of buffering capacity that saliva provides, the teeth can become hypersensitive.[39,40] Xerostomia can also result in an increased incidence of *cervical caries* (decay around the root surfaces of teeth) despite excellent oral hygiene. The inadequacy of salivary flow, which normally washes away food and debris from the teeth, is responsible for this increase in tooth decay.[39,40] Depending on the status of the patient's dentition, xerostomia can increase the incidence of caries, gingivitis, and more severe periodontal disease or can reduce denture-wearing time. Furthermore, reduced flow of saliva can disturb the balance of microflora species in the oral cavity and predispose affected patients to the development of candidiasis.

Treatment of Xerostomia

Dry mouth should never be discounted as inconsequential. Failure to treat it can result in serious complications for some patients.

Treatment Goals

The objectives of self-treatment of xerostomia are (1) to relieve the discomfort of dry mouth, (2) to reduce the risk of dental decay, and (3) to prevent and treat infections and periodontal disease.

General Treatment Approach

The patient should stop using substances that dry the mouth or erode tooth enamel. If possible, medications that are known to cause xerostomia should be discontinued. To reduce the risk of caries, the patient must maintain good oral hygiene. In mild cases, using sugarless sweets and chewing gums or sucking on ice chips can help to stimulate residual salivary flow.

Commercial artificial saliva products can be used as needed to relieve soft tissue discomfort. Figure 32–5 outlines the self-treatment of xerostomia and lists exclusions for self-care.[37–42]

Nonpharmacologic Therapy

The patient should avoid exposure to substances that reduce salivation, including tobacco (smoked and smokeless), caffeine, hot spicy foods, and alcohol (including mouth rinses). Medication schedules should be modified in consultation with the treating HCP to coincide with periods of natural stimulation. For example, patients could take medications that cause dry mouth 1 hour before meals, because eating naturally stimulates an increase in salivary flow. Consequently, the duration of dry mouth would be reduced.

To prevent tooth decay, the xerostomic patient should limit their intake of sugary (e.g., candy), starchy (e.g., cookies, potato chips), and acidic foods (e.g., orange juice) that may have been tolerated before but now pose significant danger to the patient's oral health.[42,43] Sugar promotes the bacterial production of acid, which causes tooth decay. Acidic foods may also decrease the pH of saliva, resulting in caries and tooth erosion. Chewing gum sweetened with sugar alcohols (e.g., xylitol), however, may be beneficial. Chewing gum increases salivary flow, and xylitol has not been shown to be cariogenic.[37–40,43] Increasing water intake, especially if it is fluoridated, will also be of benefit. Using a humidifier at home can help to add moisture in the air, which may provide some level of relief.[42] Finally, the use of very soft-bristle toothbrushes will help prevent decay by minimizing tissue abrasion.

Pharmacologic Therapy

Artificial saliva products are the primary agents for relieving the discomfort of dry mouth. They are designed to mimic natural saliva both chemically and physically. However, they do not contain the many

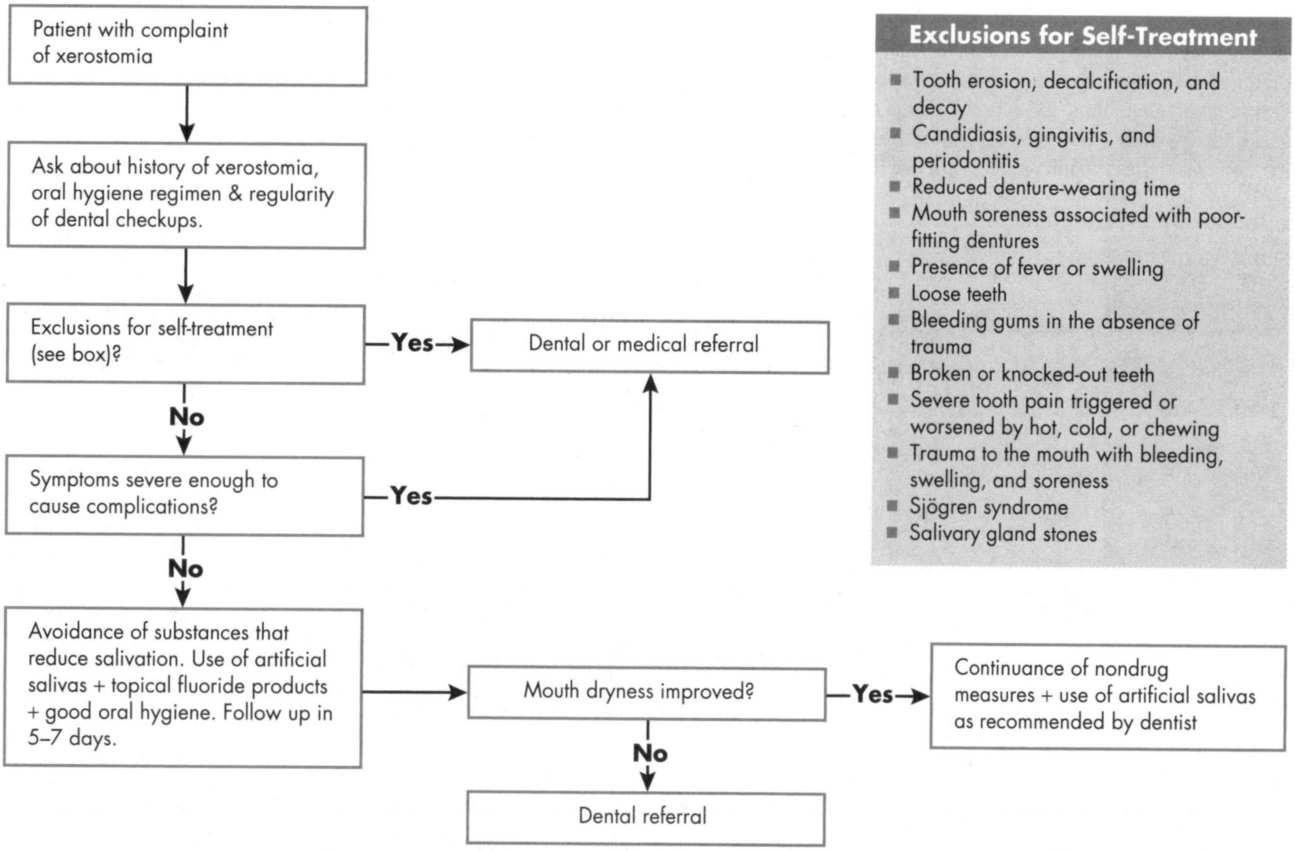

FIGURE 32–5 Self-care for xerostomia. (Source: References 37–42.)

TABLE 32–6 Selected Nonprescription Saliva Substitutes and Other Xerostomia Products

Trade Name	Primary Ingredients
ACT Total Care Dry Mouth Lozenges	Isomalt, Xylitol, Glycerin
Biotene Oral Balance Gel/Liquid Biotene Moisturizing Mouth Spray	Glucose oxidase 10,000 units; lactoferrin 16 mg; Lactoperoxidase 15,000 units; lysozyme 16 mg; sodium monofluorophosphate 0.14% (w/v fluoride ion)
Entertainer's Secret Spray	Sodium carboxymethylcellulose; dibasic sodium phosphate; potassium chloride; parabens; aloe vera gel; glycerin
Biotene Dry Mouth Gum	Sorbitol; gum base; xylitol; maltitol syrup
Biotene Dry Mouth Toothpaste	Sodium monofluorophosphate 0.14%

Key: w/v = Weight per volume.
Source: Reference 44.

naturally occurring protective components that are present in innate saliva. Because these products do not stimulate salivary glands to increase natural saliva production, they must be considered to provide replacement therapy, not a cure for xerostomia. However, such products can be used on an as-needed basis in patients with little or no salivary flow. Table 32–6 lists selected nonprescription saliva substitutes and other xerostomia products. Clinically important drug interactions for xerostomia products are listed in Table 32–3.

Product Selection Guidelines

A majority of artificial saliva products are available as sprays and gels; however, gums and toothpastes are also available. Proper use of a gel involves placing approximately a ½-inch length of extruded product onto the tongue and spreading it thoroughly in the mouth. These products can be used at any time; a minimum suggested regimen is after all meals and before going to bed. Products that contain preservatives, such as methyl- or propylparaben, may cause hypersensitivity reactions in certain patients. Patients on low-sodium diets should avoid artificial salivas that contain sodium.

Special Populations

No special considerations are required with use of these products in children, pregnant or lactating women, or older adults.[44]

Assessment of Xerostomia: A Case-Based Approach

The patient should be asked about any history of xerostomia, oral hygiene practices, and regularity of dental visits. The patient's symptoms should be evaluated to determine whether the condition has progressed to the point that complications are likely. A review of the patient's medical and medication history can identify medical conditions and/or medications known to reduce salivation. Furthermore, the provider should determine whether lifestyle or other practices could be contributing to the condition. Asking the patient about concurrent dry eyes or joint symptoms will assess the risk for Sjögren syndrome. Similarly, the assessment should establish whether any salivary gland pain or swelling occurs with meals to determine the risk for salivary gland stones. Case 32–2 provides an example of the assessment of a patient with xerostomia.

CASE 32–2

Relevant Evaluation Criteria	Scenario/Model Outcome
Collect	
1. Gather essential information about the patient's symptoms and medical history, including	
a. Description of symptom(s) (i.e., nature, onset, duration, severity, associated symptoms)	Patient is concerned about developing dry mouth, because she just completed the first round of radiation therapy for thyroid cancer. Her oncologist told her that dry mouth would be a likely side effect of the radiation, and she has already noticed the classic "cotton mouth" sensation. This adverse effect has made eating and chewing an issue, because her dentures are not fitting quite right and her mouth is now sore because of these changes.
b. Description of any factors that seem to precipitate, exacerbate, and/or relieve the patient's symptom(s)	The radiation therapy has left the patient with oral discomfort.
c. Description of the patient's efforts to relieve the symptoms	Drinking water
d. Patient's identity	Ginger Moutheski
e. Patient's age, gender, height, and weight	72 years old, female, 5 ft 2 in., 110 lb
f. Patient's occupation	Retired schoolteacher

CASE 32-2 *continued*

Relevant Evaluation Criteria	Scenario/Model Outcome
g. Patient's dietary habits	Usually a "good eater," but recently she finds it difficult to eat.
h. Patient's sleep habits	The patient sleeps only approximately 5–6 hours a night, but she takes a nap at mid-day.
i. Concurrent medical conditions, prescription and nonprescription medications, and dietary supplements	Thyroid cancer: atorvastatin 20 mg PO once daily; hypertension: lisinopril/HCTZ 10/25 PO once daily; migraines: sumatriptan 50 mg prn; also takes multivitamin PO daily.
j. Allergies	NKDA
k. History of other adverse reactions to medications	None
l. Other (describe) ______	n/a
Assess	
2. Differentiate patient's signs/symptoms, and correctly identify the patient's primary problem(s).	It is highly likely that the patient has xerostomia. This is a known consequence of radiation therapy, and her description of "cotton mouth" indicates dry mouth.
3. Identify exclusions for self-treatment (Figure 32–5).	■ Reduced denture-wearing time ■ Mouth soreness associated with poor-fitting dentures
4. Formulate a comprehensive list of therapeutic alternatives for the primary problem to determine whether triage to a health care provider is required, and share this information with the patient or caregiver.	Options include (1) Refer patient to an appropriate HCP (2) Recommend self-care with a nonprescription product for xerostomia. (3) Recommend self-care until patient can see an appropriate HCP. (4) Take no action.
Plan	
5. Select an optimal therapeutic alternative to address the patient's problem, taking into account patient preferences.	Patient should consult an HCP for treatment.
6. Describe the recommended therapeutic approach to the patient or caregiver.	"You should consult a health care provider for treatment."
7. Explain to the patient or caregiver the rationale for selecting the recommended therapeutic approach from the considered therapeutic alternatives.	"This option is best because you have additional conditions that can be contributing to your dry mouth."
Implement	
8. When recommending self-care with nonprescription medications and/or nondrug therapy, convey accurate information to the patient or caregiver.	Criterion does not apply in this case.
Solicit follow-up questions from the patient or caregiver.	"Is there anything I can do in the meantime?"
Answer the patient's or caregiver's questions.	"Yes, see the box 'Patient Education for Xerostomia.'"
Follow up: Monitor and Evaluate	
9. Assess patient outcome.	Contact the patient in a day or two to ensure she has called or made an appointment with her health care provider.

Key: HCP = Health care provider; HCTZ = hydrochlorothiazide; n/a = not applicable; NKDA = No known drug allergy.

PATIENT EDUCATION FOR Xerostomia

The objectives of self-treatment of xerostomia (dry mouth) are (1) to relieve the discomfort of dry mouth, (2) to reduce the risk of dental decay, and (3) to prevent and treat infections and periodontal disease. For most patients, carefully following product instructions and the self-care measures listed here will help ensure optimal therapeutic outcomes.

Nondrug Measures

- To help prevent reduction in salivary flow, avoid use of cigarettes and smokeless tobacco.
- Do not drink or use products that contain alcohol (including mouth rinses) or medications that cause depletion of salivary flow.
- Avoid food or drinks that contain caffeine.
- Avoid hot spicy foods.
- To prevent tooth decay, limit consumption of sugary (e.g., candy), starchy (e.g., cookies, potato chips), and acidic foods (e.g., orange juice). Do not suck on hard candy or lozenges sweetened with sugar.
- If desired, chew gum sweetened with sugar alcohols, such as xylitol, to help increase flow of saliva.
- If possible, take medications 1 hour before meals so that the natural saliva flow caused by food can counteract any mouth dryness.
- To help prevent tooth decay, use a very soft toothbrush to reduce abrasion of the teeth.
- Drink plenty of water.
- Use a humidifier at home to help moisten the air.

Nonprescription Medications

- Use artificial saliva products that contain fluoride to relieve the discomfort of dry mouth and to prevent tooth decay.
- If you are on a low-sodium diet, avoid artificial salivas that contain sodium.
- Brush and floss your teeth at least twice daily using a regular toothpaste with fluoride, and see your dentist regularly.

When to Seek Medical Attention

- If your symptoms do not improve or if they worsen, see a dentist.

Source: References 37–42.

Patient Counseling for Xerostomia

In general, patients with xerostomia require professional dental management of the condition, in addition to the self-care methods discussed previously and outlined in the box "Patient Education for Xerostomia." Patients should be encouraged to practice good oral hygiene measures and to see their dentist regularly. In addition, patient counseling should include appropriate information about nonpharmacologic and pharmacologic measures for keeping the oral cavity moist and treating dry mouth, to minimize the increased risk for tooth decay associated with xerostomia. Finally, patient education should highlight signs and symptoms that indicate complications from dry mouth.

Evaluation of Patient Outcomes for Xerostomia

The patient with xerostomia should return for evaluation after 5–7 days of self-treatment. If the mouth dryness is lessened, the patient should continue using artificial saliva and fluoride products as recommended by an HCP. The patient should also be advised to continue with nonpharmacologic measures. If the dryness becomes worse or symptoms of complications develop, the patient should return to a dental HCP for further evaluation.

Key Points for Orofacial Pain and Discomfort

- ➤ Tooth hypersensitivity and teething discomfort are not serious and are self-treatable problems.
- ➤ Self-treatment of toothache should be limited to the temporary relief of pain, because professional treatment is required for complete resolution of the underlying condition.
- ➤ RAS is amenable to self-treatment for the relief of pain and irritation so that the lesions can heal, thereby allowing the patient to eat, drink, and perform routine oral hygiene while preventing further complications.
- ➤ Minor oral mucosal injury or irritation may be self-treated by controlling discomfort and pain, by using appropriate drug and nondrug measures to aid healing, and by preventing secondary bacterial infection.
- ➤ The goals of self-treatment of HSL (cold sores) are to relieve pain and irritation while the sores are healing, to prevent secondary infection, and to prevent spread of the lesions to other areas of the body and to other individuals.
- ➤ Self-treatment of xerostomia (dry mouth) can relieve discomfort from dry mouth, thereby reducing the risk of dental decay as well as preventing and, at times, treating infections.
- ➤ If the pain or discomfort worsens or persists after appropriate self-treatment and nondrug measures, medical referral for further treatment is imperative.

REFERENCES

1. Jin LJ, Lamster IB, Greenspan JS, et al. Global burden of oral diseases: emerging concepts, management and interplay with systemic health. *Oral Dis.* 2016;22(7):609–19. doi: 10.1111/odi.12428.
2. Benjamin RM. *Oral Health: The Silent Epidemic.* Rockville, MD: Department of Health and Human Services, Office of the Surgeon General; 2010. Public Health Rep No. 125:158–9.
3. Bress LE. Improving oral health literacy—the new standard in dental hygiene practice. *J Dent Hyg.* 2013;87(6):322–9. PMID: 24357560.
4. Gillam D, Chesters R, Attrill D, et al. Dentine hypersensitivity—guidelines for the management of a common oral health problem. *Dent Update.* 2013;40(7):514–6, 518–20, 523–4. PMID: 24147382.
5. Cummins D. Advances in the clinical management of dentin hypersensitivity: a review of recent evidence for the efficacy of dentifrices in providing instant and lasting relief. *J Clin Dent.* 2011;22:100–7. PMID: 22403985.
6. Jones JA. Dentin hypersensitivity: etiology, risk factors, and prevention strategies. *Dent Today.* 2011;30(11):108, 110, 112–3. PMID: 22187808.
7. da Rosa WL, Lund RG, Piva E, da Silva AF. The effectiveness of current dentin desensitizing agents used to treat dental hypersensitivity: a systematic review. *Quintessence Int.* 2013;44(7):535–6. doi: 10.3290/j.qi.a29610.
8. Li Y. Innovations for combating dentin hypersensitivity: current state of the art. *Compend Contin Educ Dent.* 2012;33(Spec no. 2):10–6. PMID: 22774324.

9. Schmidlin PR, Sahrmann P. Current management of dentin hypersensitivity. *Clin Oral Invest.* 2013;17(Suppl 1):S55–9. doi: 10.1007/s00784-012-0912-0.
10. Poulsen S, Errboe M, Lescay-Mevil Y, et al. Potassium containing toothpastes for dentine hypersensitivity. *Cochrane Database Syst Rev.* 2012;4: CD001476. doi:10.1002/14651858.CD001476.pub2.
11. Magno MB, Nascimento GC, Da Penha NK, et al. Difference in effectiveness between strontium acetate and arginine-based toothpastes to relieve dentin hypersensitivity. A systematic review. *Am J Dent.* 2015;28(1):40–4. PMID: 25864241.
12. Sood S, Sood M. Teething: myths and facts. *J Clin Pediatr Dent.* 2010; 35(1):9–13. PMID: 21189758.
13. Benzocaine. Lexi-Drugs™ Online. Hudson, OH: Lexi-Comp. Available at: http://www.crlonline.com. Accessed January 25, 2016.
14. U.S. Food and Drug Administration. MedWatch safety alert. Benzocaine topical products: sprays, gels and liquids—risk of methemoglobinemia. Available at: http://www.fda.gov/drugs/drugsafety/postmarketdrugsafetyinformationforpatientsandproviders/ucm273111.htm. Accessed June 20, 2017.
15. U.S. Food and Drug Administration. Drug Safety Communications. FDA recommends not using lidocaine to treat teething pain and requires new Boxed Warning. June 24, 2014. Available at: http://www.fda.gov/downloads/Drugs/DrugSafety/UCM402241.pdf. Accessed June 20, 2017.
16. U.S. Food and Drug Administration. Consumer Safety Alert. Homeopathic Teething Tablets and Gels: FDA Warning—Risk to Infants and Children. September 30, 2016. Available at: http://www.fda.gov/Safety/MedWatch/SafetyInformation/SafetyAlertsforHumanMedicalProducts/ucm523435.htm. Accessed June 20, 2017.
17. Lalla RV, Choquette LE, Feinn RS, et al. Multivitamin therapy for recurrent aphthous stomatitis: a randomized, double-masked, placebo-controlled trial. *J Am Dent Assoc.* 2012;143(4):370–6. PMCID: PMC3880249.
18. Chavan M, Jain H, Diwan N, et al. Recurrent aphthous stomatitis: a review. *J Oral Pathol Med.* 2012;41(8):577–83. doi: 10.1111/j.1600-0714.2012.01134.x. Available at: https://www.researchgate.net/publication/221891773_Recurrent_aphthous_stomatitis_A_review. Accessed June 20, 2017.
19. Tarakji B, Gazal G, Al-Maweri SA, et al. Guideline for the diagnosis and treatment of recurrent aphthous stomatitis for dental practitioners. *J Int Oral Health.* 2015;7(5):74–80. PMCID: PMC4441245. Available at: https://www.ncbi.nlm.nih.gov/pmc/articles/PMC4441245/. Accessed June 20, 2017.
20. Altenburg A, El-Haj N, Micheli C, et al. The treatment of chronic recurrent oral aphthous ulcers. *Dtsch Arztebl Int.* 2014;111(40):665–73. doi: 10.3238/arztebl.2014.0665.
21. Bascones-Martínez A, García-García V, Meurman JH, Requena-Caballero L. Immune-mediated diseases: what can be found in the oral cavity? *Int J Dermatol.* 2015;54(3):258–70. doi: 10.1111/ijd.12681.
22. Sardana K, Bansal S. Palatal ulceration. *Clin Dermatol.* 2014;32(6): 827–38. doi: 10.1016/j.clindermatol.2014.02.023.
23. Klein RS, Hirsch MS, Mitty J. Treatment of herpes simplex virus type 1 infection in immunocompetent patients. UpToDate; 2015. Available at: http://www.uptodate.com. Accessed January 25, 2016.
24. Stoopler ET, Sollecito TP. Oral mucosal diseases: evaluation and management. *Med Clin North Am.* 2014;98(6):1323–52. doi: 10.1016/j.mcna.2014.08.006.
25. Carbamide peroxide. *Lexi-Drugs Online.* Hudson, OH: Lexi-Comp. Available at: http://www.crlonline.com. Accessed January 25, 2016.
26. Hydrogen peroxide. *Lexi-Drugs Online.* Hudson, OH: Lexi-Comp. Available at: http://www.crlonline.com. Accessed June 21, 2017
27. Shemer A, Amichai B, Trau H, et al. Efficacy of a mucoadhesive patch compared with an oral solution for treatment of aphthous stomatitis. *Drugs R D.* 2008;9(1):29–35. PMID: 18095751.
28. Docosanol. *Lexi-Drugs Online.* Hudson, OH: Lexi-Comp. Available at: http://www.crlonline.com. Accessed January 25, 2016.
29. Menthol. *Lexi-Drugs Online.* Hudson, OH: Lexi-Comp. Available at: http://www.crlonline.com. Accessed January 25, 2016.
30. Zinc sulfate. *Lexi-Drugs Online.* Hudson, OH: Lexi-Comp. Available at: http://www.crlonline.com. Accessed January 25, 2016.
31. Messier C, Epifano F, Genovese S, Grenier D. Licorice and its potential beneficial effects in common oro-dental diseases. *Oral Dis.* 2012; 18(1):32–9. doi: 10.1111/j.1601-0825.2011.01842.x.
32. Chi CC, Wang SH, Delamere FM, et al. Interventions for prevention of herpes simplex labialis (cold sores on the lips). *Cochrane Database Syst Rev.* 2015;8:CD010095. doi: 10.1002/14651858.CD010095.pub2.
33. McCarthy JP, Browning WD, Teerlink C, et al. Treatment of herpes labialis: comparison of two OTC drugs and untreated controls. *J Esthet Restor Dent.* 2012;24(2):103–9. doi: 10.1111/j.1708-8240.2011.00417.x.
34. Willis A, Hyland P, Lamey PJ. Response to replacement iron therapy in sideropenic individuals with recrudescent herpes labialis. *Eur J Clin Microbiol Infect Dis.* 2000;19(5):355–7.
35. Carson CF, Ashton L, Dry L, et al. Melaleuca alternifolia (tea tree) oil gel (6%) for the treatment of recurrent herpes labialis. *J Antimicrob Chemother.* 2001;48(3):450–1. PMID: 11533019.
36. Ciuman RR. Phytotherapeutic and naturopathic adjuvant therapies in otorhinolaryngology. *Eur Arch Otorhinolaryngol.* 2012;269(2):389–97. doi: 10.1007/s00405-011-1755-z.
37. Furness S, Worthington HV, Bryan G, et al. Interventions for the management of dry mouth: topical therapies. *Cochrane Database Syst Rev.* 2011;12:CD008934. doi:10.1002/14651858. CD008934.pub2.
38. Donaldson M, Epstein J, Villines D. Managing patients with Sjögren syndrome and dry mouth: comorbidities, medication use and dental care considerations. *J Am Dent Assoc.* 2014;145(12):1240–7. doi: 10.14219/jada.2014.83.
39. Kramer JM. Current concepts in Sjögren's syndrome and considerations for the dental practitioner. *N Y State Dent J.* 2015;81(1):24–9. PMID: 25707165.
40. Villa A, Connell CL, Abati S. Diagnosis and management of xerostomia and hyposalivation. *Ther Clin Risk Manag.* 2014;11:45–51. doi: 10.2147/tcrm.s76282.
41. Yellowitz JA, Schneiderman MT. Elder's oral health crisis. *J Evid Based Dent Pract.* 2014;14(Suppl):191–200. doi: 10.1016/j.jebdp.2014.04.011.
42. Singh M, Tonk RS. Xerostomia: etiology, diagnosis, and management. *Dent Today.* 2012;31(10):80, 82–3. PMID: 23156632.
43. Donaldson M, Goodchild JH, Epstein JB. Sugar content, cariogenicity, and dental concerns with commonly used medications. *J Am Dent Assoc.* 2015;146(2):129–33. doi: 10.1016/j.adaj.2014.10.009.
44. Lexicomp Online Clinical Database 2016. Alphen aan den Rijn, Netherlands: Wolters Kluwer; 2016. Available at: http://www.crlonline.com. Accessed February 24, 2016.

section

VIII

DERMATOLOGIC DISORDERS

CHAPTER 33

ATOPIC DERMATITIS AND DRY SKIN

KIMBERLEY W. BENNER

An estimated 5% of the U.S. population suffers from a chronic skin, hair, or nail disorder, and many other Americans experience acute or seasonal skin disorders.[1] In the United States, 15%–20% of children ages 0–17 years and 1%–3% of adults are estimated to have atopic dermatitis (AD).[2] Furthermore, most patients with this disorder are believed either to be undertreated or to be self-treating with primarily nonprescription medications.[3] Therefore, it is essential for health care providers to be able to recognize and differentiate common skin disorders, suggest appropriate treatment, and know when to refer patients to a primary care provider or a dermatologist.

Dermatitis is a nonspecific term describing numerous dermatologic disorders that are generally characterized by erythema and inflammation. The terms *eczema* and *dermatitis* are used interchangeably to describe a group of inflammatory skin disorders that are often of unknown etiology. *AD* (or *atopic eczema*) is a form of eczema that describes inflammatory skin conditions that are typically erythematous, edematous, papular, and crusty.[4] This chapter focuses on AD and dry skin, because dry skin is a common complaint in many dermatoses and its incidence increases with age.[5] Dry skin may be associated with decreased quality of life for patients with mild–moderate dryness because of the accompanying pruritus and, in some cases, the infection, pain, and inflammation that may occur.

Role of Skin in Drug Absorption

The most important function of skin and its appendages (hair and nails) is to protect the body from external harmful agents such as pathogenic organisms and chemicals. The skin's ability to exert this function depends on an individual's age, immunologic status, underlying disease states, medication use, and preservation of his or her intact stratum corneum. Skin is also important in hydroregulation, controlling moisture loss from the body and moisture penetration into the body. If the stratum corneum becomes dehydrated, it loses elasticity and its permeation characteristics are altered. Although skin is exposed to a variety of chemical and environmental insults, it demonstrates remarkable resiliency and recuperative ability.[6]

Human skin has three functionally distinct regions: epidermis, dermis, and hypodermis (Figure 33–1). The epidermis, the outermost thin layer of the skin, regulates the water content of the skin and controls drug transport into the lower layers and systemic circulation. The middle layer, the dermis, is 40 times thicker than the epidermis and contains nerve endings, vasculature, and hair follicles. The hypodermis primarily provides nourishment and cushioning for the upper two layers.

The skin is involved in numerous physical and biochemical processes. Skin thickness is variable but averages about 1–2 mm. The thickest skin is on the palms and soles, and the thinnest skin is on the genitalia. Thinner skin areas are more permeable, allowing substances to be absorbed more easily than through thicker skin. As individuals age, their skin becomes more fragile, requiring a longer recovery time after injury.[7]

A drug applied topically must be released from its vehicle if it is to exert an effect at the desired site of activity (skin surface, epidermis, or dermis). Release occurs at the area of contact between the skin surface and the applied layer of product. The physical–chemical relationship between the drug and the vehicle determines the rate and amount of drug released. A drug's solubility in the vehicle, its diffusion coefficient in the vehicle, and its partition coefficient into the sebum and stratum corneum are significant considerations for its efficacy.[8] The major mechanism of drug absorption is passive diffusion through the stratum corneum, followed by transport through the deeper epidermal regions and then the dermis. The stratum corneum is often a rate-limiting barrier to percutaneous absorption and its hydration status can thus affect drug diffusion. Occlusion (blocking or covering) increases hydration of the stratum corneum, which enhances the transfer of most drugs.[8] Wounds, burns, chafed areas, and dermatitis can alter the integrity of the stratum corneum and can result in increased absorption. Inflammation can also enhance percutaneous absorption of topically applied medications, which may result in higher systemic drug levels. Therefore, caution should be used in applying topical medication to compromised skin, particularly if large surface areas are involved.

ATOPIC DERMATITIS

AD is a common, pervasive inflammatory condition of the epidermis and dermis that is characterized by episodic flares and periods of remission. Fifty percent of patients are diagnosed within the first year of life, with as many as 85% presenting before the age of 5 years.[2] Prevalence of AD worldwide is increasing, possibly because of environmental influences such as climate, urbanization, diet, and pollution/tobacco smoke, but microbial exposure may also be an influence.[2]

Asthma and allergic rhinitis can occur in up to 80% of patients with AD, either in childhood or as individuals age[9]; this phenomenon has been referred to as the "atopic march."

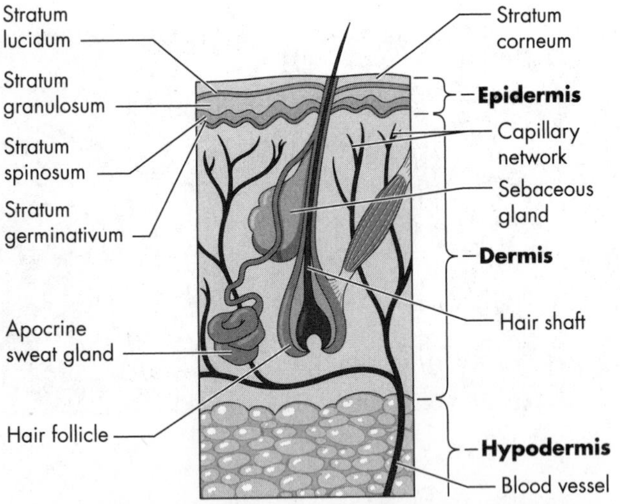

FIGURE 33-1 Cross section of human skin.

However, *atopic triad* describes the simultaneous occurrence of asthma, allergic rhinitis, and atopic dermatitis.[10] Eighty percent of AD is classified as mild and can be safely treated with nonprescription products in patients older than 2 years of age.[11] In addition, many patients with AD do not seek medical care and therefore are likely to look for advice regarding self-care of this disorder.[12]

Pathophysiology of Atopic Dermatitis

AD has a genetic basis, but its expression is modified by a broad spectrum of exogenous manifestations.[12] Atopic skin is inflamed with an expression of cytokines and chemokines; inflammatory cytokines such as interleukin-4 and 13 and tumor necrosis factor are produced.[10,13] A protein in the epidermal differentiation complex, filaggrin (FLG), is related to the development of AD. Even one mutation in FLG increases one's risk of AD, and 35 mutations are known to exist in the FLG gene.[4] The filaggrin mutation can lead to the deficient skin barrier characteristic of AD, including an increased penetration of allergens, a decrease in skin barrier proteins, higher peptidase activity, and lack of protease inhibitors.[14,15] In addition, because of a decreased concentration of lipid and ceramides, atopic skin has a decreased ability to retain moisture.[16] Seventy percent of AD cases have an atopic family history; if one parent is atopic, the rate of similar symptoms in their children is approximately 50%, whereas if both parents are atopic, this risk rises to 79%.[4]

AD is diagnosed according to clinical criteria (Table 33–1).[17] No established confirmatory laboratory tests exist, although many patients have shown an elevated immunoglobulin (Ig) E level and peripheral blood eosinophilia. This elevated IgE level typically does not appear early on, and may never occur in some children.[18] There are currently three validated assessments for AD, the SCORAD (SCORing Atopic Dermatitis), EASI (Eczema Area and Severity Index), and POEM (Patient-Oriented Eczema Measure).[19,20]

TABLE 33-1 **Diagnostic Criteria for Atopic Dermatitis**

Essential features include
- Pruritus
- Eczema

Important features include
- Early age of onset
- Atopy
- Xerosis

Note: There are other associated features and exclusionary conditions to consider.
Source: Reference 17.

Clinical Presentation of Atopic Dermatitis

AD is often first manifested within the first year of life, often beginning at 2–3 months of age. Infantile or childhood AD initially appears as erythema and scaling of the infant's cheeks, which may progress to affect the face, neck, forehead, and extremities (see Color Plates, photographs 17A, B, and C). Crusts and pustules can form from the effects of scratching and rubbing. Remission can occur by the end of the second year; however, AD or xerosis (dry skin) can continue into adulthood in up to 30% of patients.[21] AD presents quite differently in adults and children and may be less severe in adults.[13,21] Plaques appear erythematous, scaly, exudative, or lichenified. Areas affected include antecubital and popliteal fossae, neck, forehead, eyes, and hands.[21] The trigger in adults is often environmental, attributed to chemicals or skin trauma.[15] Pruritus, the hallmark symptom of AD, causes morbidity and is sometimes referred to as the "itch that rashes." Patients with AD are more susceptible to pruritic-inducing stimuli. Scratching and lichenification can produce a vicious cycle and lead to excoriation.[4,15] It is important to note that patients can present atypically, and any undiagnosed skin lesions that do not improve over time or that get worse with self-treatment should be evaluated by a primary care provider.

AD has three clinical forms: acute AD, subacute AD, and chronic AD. *Acute AD*, which is characterized by intensely pruritic, erythematous *papules* (small, firm, elevated lesions) or *vesicles* (fluid or air-filled sacs) over erythematous skin, is often associated with excoriation and *serous exudates* (secretions). *Subacute AD* is characterized by erythematous, excoriated papules and *plaques* (large, slightly elevated lesions with a flat surface) that can be scaly. *Chronic AD* is characterized by thickened plaques of skin and accentuated skin markings.[22]

Secondary or associated cutaneous infections, especially bacterial, can be common and difficult to prevent, and typically aggravate AD. More than 90% of the skin lesions in patients with AD (in contrast to 5% of unaffected individuals) harbor *Staphylococcus aureus*.[10,12] Although *S. aureus* is the most common cause of infection, streptococci may also be found alone or in association with *S. aureus*. Infections present as yellowish crusting of the eczematous lesions.

Patients with AD may also develop viral infections such as herpes simplex or *Molluscum contagiosum*.[10,22] Although true infection of the skin is more common in children with AD, colonization is higher in adult patients.[13] Patients should be counseled to seek medical attention promptly when signs of bacterial or viral skin infections, such as *pustules* (circumscribed, elevated lesions, 1 cm in diameter containing pus), vesicles (especially those filled with exudate or pus), and crusting are noticed.[12]

Treatment of Atopic Dermatitis

Treatment Goals

The goals of self-treatment of AD are (1) to stop the itch–scratch cycle, (2) to maintain skin hydration and barrier function, (3) to avoid or minimize factors that trigger or aggravate the disorder, and (4) to prevent secondary infections.

General Treatment Approach

Health care providers should stress to patients that AD cannot be cured but that most patients' symptoms can be managed. The disorder should be explained as being multifactorial, and just as there is no cure, there is no single cause. Often no explanation can be found for a particular flare-up of the disorder, and many factors can contribute simultaneously.

Enhancing hydration and achieving barrier repair in atopic skin can be achieved through nonpharmacologic measures, including the use of emollients and moisturizers. Hydrocortisone can relieve itching and inflammation. An effective preventive measure is to minimize exposure to factors known to trigger AD. The algorithm in Figure 33–2 outlines the self-treatment of this disorder and lists exclusions for self-treatment.[10,22]

Nonpharmacologic Therapy

Treatment should be tailored to a patient's needs and preferences, bearing in mind the patient's age, gender, and social conditions, along with the site(s) and severity of the lesions. Successful treatment of AD includes (1) the identification and elimination of triggers; (2) skin hydration/barrier protection; and (3) the use of topical therapy and possibly systemic therapy for refractory cases.

Education on trigger avoidance and hydration of the skin are of utmost importance in the prevention as well as treatment of AD. Common triggers that patients should avoid are listed in Table 33–2.[10,14,23] Compared with nonaffected individuals, skin in a patient with AD may be more reactive to irritants. Therefore, patients with AD can take additional preventive measures and make lifestyle changes. Suggestions include using cotton sheets, laundering them in gentle detergents, and using two rinse cycles. Laundering and thoroughly rinsing new clothing with unscented laundry detergent is recommended, as is avoiding fabric softeners. If used, liquid fabric softeners are preferred over dryer sheets. Bathing can provide hydration and remove bacteria.[24] Recent guidelines state that baths should be of limited duration and taken in lukewarm water without additives; moisturizers should be applied immediately after bathing to rehydrate the skin.[25,26] However, there is no standard for frequency or duration of bathing.[26] Because some soaps can be irritating and cause dry skin, mild nonsoap cleansers that are hypoallergenic and fragrance free (e.g., Cetaphil) are preferred.[25]

Although allergens such as plant or animal proteins from food, pollens, or pets can aggravate AD, the role of food allergies in exacerbating AD is unclear. It has been previously reported that in about one-third of children, food allergies may exacerbate moderate-severe AD.[27] These allergies often include egg, milk, peanut, soy, and wheat. Patients with food allergies often have more severe AD, with an earlier onset.[26] Children who present with food allergies and AD should be evaluated by a primary care provider, particularly if they are younger than 5 years of age with severe AD.[11,26] Dietary restriction, especially in children, is difficult to maintain, and although it may produce some improvement in AD symptoms initially, complete resolution is unlikely. Experts have maintained that patients with moderate–severe AD eliminate known food allergens.[10,14,23] However, recent guidelines state that restriction of offending foods does not alter the risk of developing AD[17] and that although food allergies are prevalent in patients with AD, they are not always the cause. Other preventive measures, such as breastfeeding and delaying introduction of solid food, remain controversial. There are limited studies that investigate these interventions and their role in the prevention of AD; guidelines state that no definite evidence indicates that breastfeeding and solid food introduction will significantly affect AD.[17,26]

Patients with AD are often intolerant of extreme temperatures as well as sudden and drastic changes in temperature and humidity. High temperature may enhance perspiration, leading to increased itching, whereas low humidity can dry the skin and increase itching. Use of humidifiers in dry environments can provide some benefit.

Pruritus is often bothersome for many patients. Recommending that patients keep their fingernails short, smooth, and clean is important to avoid introduction of bacteria through microfissures; patients can consider the use of cotton gloves at night to prevent constant scratching of the itchy skin. Moisturization using an emollient is standard of care for AD, because maintaining skin hydration and patency is important. Emollient use at least twice daily is recommended for preventive and maintenance therapy to keep skin soft and pliable. Furthermore, the use of natural moisturizing factors (NMFs), ceramides or pseudoceramides in emollients, can aid in preventing epidermal water loss via "barrier repair therapy."[28] Patient preference should direct specific emollient choice; however, the higher water content in lotions can have a drying effect and their use should be avoided. Ointments may have more effective dermal penetration, but some patients find them greasy.[23,25] Little evidence exists to support one product over the other; therefore, choosing a product that the patient is satisfied with is paramount.[10]

Pharmacologic Therapy

Corticosteroids are the standard of care for AD when nonprescription anti-inflammatory therapy is warranted during acute flare-ups.[25] Although their exact mechanism is unknown, corticosteroids most likely suppress cytokines associated with the development of inflammation and itching, symptoms that are associated with various dermatoses. Hydrocortisone, a low-potency corticosteroid, is the primary nonprescription active ingredient available for self-care. This corticosteroid is safe to use short term on virtually any area of the body (including the face, neck, axillae, and groin) and safe to use in children older than 2 years.[13,25] Compared with high-potency topical corticosteroid products, hydrocortisone 0.5% and 1% products, when used properly, are associated with a very low risk of local and systemic adverse effects.[22,24] Hydrocortisone cream is often the preferred dosage form. Ointment formulations, while often greasy, are preferred on areas of thick skin or if a patient's skin is dry, lichenified, or scaly.[22,24,29] Hydrocortisone should be applied sparingly twice daily during AD flare-ups, usually before application of any moisturizers.[8,10,25] Ointments should be avoided if the AD lesions are weeping, and all hydrocortisone products should be avoided if the skin is infected, open, or cracked.[30]

Topical hydrocortisone rarely produces systemic complications, because its systemic absorption in adults is relatively minimal (approximately 1%). Therefore, the risk of adrenal suppression,

Exclusions for Self-Treatment

- Moderate–severe condition with intense pruritis
- Involvement of large area of body
- <1 years of age
- Skin appears to be infected
- Involvement of face or intertriginous areas

Source: References 11 and 12.

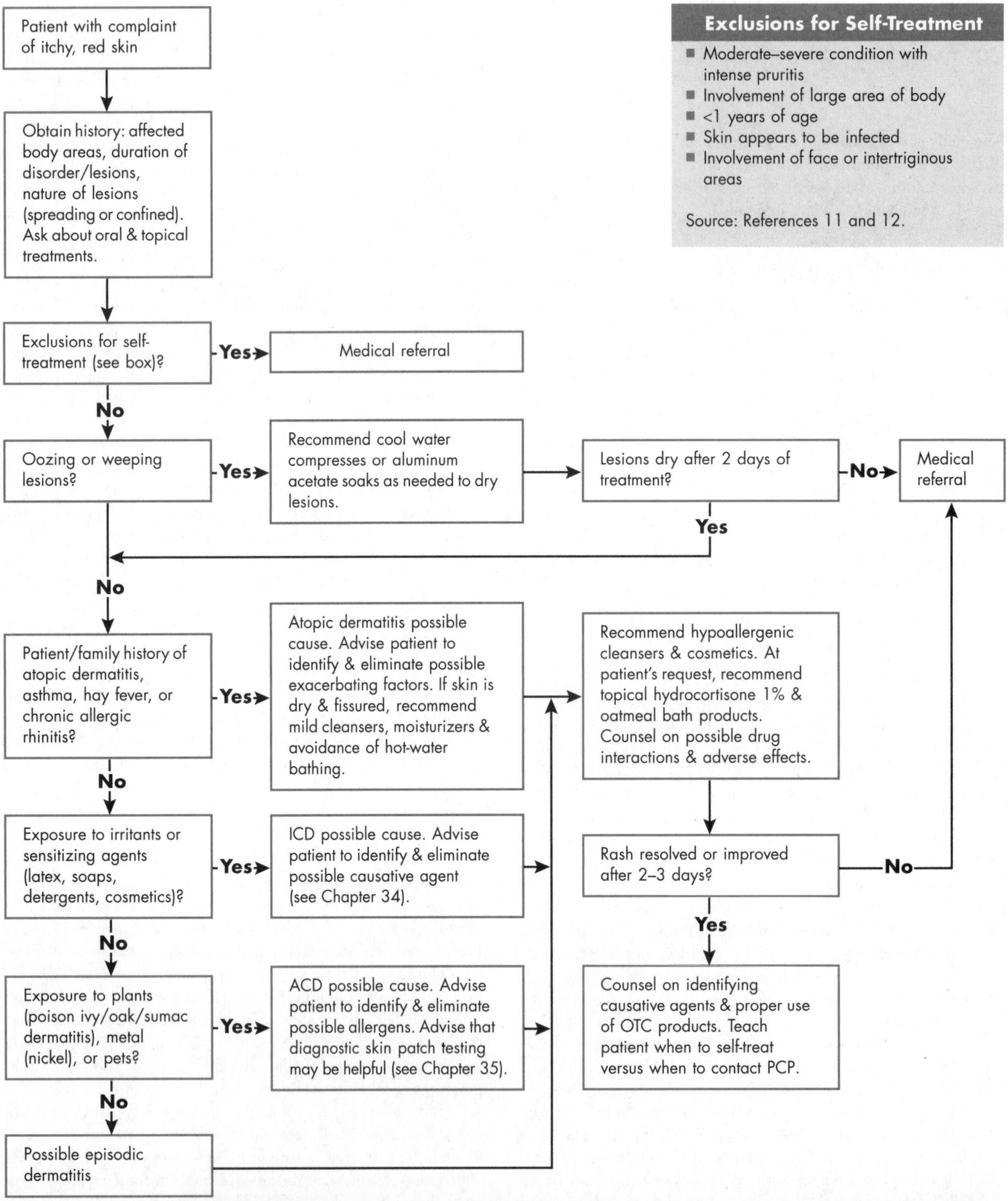

FIGURE 33-2 Self-care of dermatitis. Key: ACD = Allergic contact dermatitis; ICD = irritant contact dermatitis; OTC = over-the-counter; PCP = primary care provider.

TABLE 33-2 Triggers Associated With Atopic Dermatitis

Food allergens (e.g., egg, milk, peanut, soy, wheat, nuts)
Aeroallergens (e.g., dust mites, cat dander, molds, grass, ragweed, pollen)
Stress
Airborne irritants (tobacco smoke, air pollution, traffic exhaust)
Cosmetics, fragrances, and astringents
Exposure to temperature extremes (heat or cold)
Electric blankets
Excessive hand or skin washing
Use of irritating soaps, detergents, and scrubs
Tight-fitting or irritating clothes (wool or synthetics)
Dyes and preservatives

Source: References 10, 14, and 23.

growth suppression, osteoporosis, and other metabolic complications is slight when low-potency hydrocortisone is used on a short-term basis or rotated with other agents. Certain local adverse effects such as skin atrophy rarely occur with nonprescription concentrations; they are more common with the more-potent prescription products. Intermittent courses of therapy are advised when possible, because response to topical hydrocortisone may decrease with continued use owing to tachyphylaxis. These intermittent courses can include daily use of hydrocortisone only during periods of flare-ups and once weekly dosing, or no hydrocortisone at all, during remission phases, accompanied by continued maintenance strategies such as emollient use.[24]

Refractory cases of AD should be referred to a primary care provider for prescribed therapy with a higher-potency topical corticosteroid; a topical calcineurin inhibitor (e.g., tacrolimus, pimecrolimus); or a systemic immunomodulator (e.g., cyclosporine, azathioprine, methotrexate).[31]

Preventing and managing infections is important in AD patients, because their altered skin barrier predisposes them to infection. Guidelines state the use of topical antibiotics may reduce skin colonization; however, this effect does not appear to improve patient outcomes and these products are not routinely recommended.[25] Twice daily diluted bleach baths and intranasal mupirocin have been associated with decreased disease severity and is recommended in moderate–severe AD.[25,32] Patients should be instructed to prepare a diluted bleach bath by adding one-half cup of bleach per 40 gallons of water (a full bathtub).[14,23,24]

Although time consuming for patients and caregivers, the use of "wet wraps" can increase skin hydration and help decrease scratching. Wet wraps entail applying a steroid or emollient to affected lesions, wrapping the lesions in a wet then dry layer, and retaining the wraps for an overnight period.[10] A growing body of literature is available on the use and efficacy of wet wraps[33,34]; recent guidelines recommend their use to decrease disease severity.[25]

Antipruritics

The pruritus associated with dermatitis may be mediated through several mechanisms, which may explain how local anesthetics, antihistamines, and hydrocortisone are all useful as antipruritics. Older guidelines do not recommend routine use of these local anesthetics (e.g., lidocaine, benzocaine),[14] and newer guidelines do not even mention their potential use.[25] Itching may also be mediated by various endogenous substances, including histamine. Therefore, it is thought that topical antihistamines (e.g., diphenhydramine) can be effective in alleviating pruritus and can exert a topical anesthetic effect. Although topical antihistamines may provide some short-term relief from itching, their use is not recommended and, furthermore, may be associated with sensitization.[14,25] Oral antihistamines are not recommended for the routine treatment for pruritus in AD because of the lack of demonstrated efficacy and the hypothesis that the pruritus in AD often is not histamine related.[14,25] However, an oral antihistamine may help with sleep in the patient who has been staying up all night scratching, and if concurrent depression is a problem, an antidepressant with anticholinergic properties may help further with itching. In either case, sedation may be a problem as may the anticholinergic adverse effects in patients with disorders such as benign prostatic hypertrophy or closed-angle glaucoma.[35]

Complementary Therapies

Few complementary therapies exist to manage atopic dermatitis. Some researchers thought that the use of probiotics in infants, such as *Lactobacillus*, may delay the presentation of AD; however, a review of 12 trials revealed no significant difference in AD symptoms.[36,37] The use of phototherapy in patients with AD has documented benefit and is recommended in the guidelines as second-line therapy for acute and chronic AD.[31] The use of certain Chinese herbal mixtures has shown benefit in AD,[38] but recent guidelines state insufficient evidence exists to support their use. Although not specifically mentioned in the guidelines, some evidence exists to support the use of topical coconut oil in mild–moderate AD.[39] Other botanicals used in skin disorders are discussed in Chapter 51.

DRY SKIN

Xerosis, or *dry skin*, is the result of decreased water content of the skin with resultant abnormal loss of cells from the stratum corneum. Dry skin is a common problem and affects more than 50% of older adults. It is also the most common cause of pruritus.[40] Dry skin is a frequent cause of pruritus in cooler climates during the winter season (i.e., "winter itch"). Individuals who live or work in arid, windy, or cold environments also have an increased risk for dry skin. Environmental dry skin often is associated with long, hot showers or not consuming enough water. The prevention and care of dry skin may become a major focus for health care providers as the population of older adults continues to increase. Among those caring for these older adults, a heightened awareness exists that prophylactic dry skin care can reduce morbidity by minimizing the risk of skin breakdown and, therefore, can ultimately reduce the cost of dermatologic health care.[5]

Pathophysiology of Dry Skin

Dry skin can result from various etiologies. It can be caused by disruption of keratinization and desquamation.[40] Dry skin may also occur secondary to prolonged detergent use, malnutrition, or physical damage to the stratum corneum. Furthermore, dry skin may signal a systemic disorder such as hypothyroidism or dehydration.

Dry skin is related to a decreased amount of ceramides—not to a lack of natural skin oils; the loss of ceramides leads to water loss in the stratum corneum.[28] Dry air allows the outer skin layer to lose moisture, become less flexible, and crack when flexed, leading to an increased rate of moisture loss. Exposure of skin to high wind velocity will result in moisture loss.

With advancing age, the epidermis changes because of abnormal maturation or adhesion of the keratinocytes, resulting in a superficial, irregular layer of corneocytes. This disorder may be described as a thinning of the entire epidermis, which produces a roughened skin surface. The skin's hygroscopic substances also decrease in quantity with advancing age. Hormonal changes that accompany aging result in lowered sebum output.[5,6]

Clinical Presentation of Dry Skin

Dry skin is characterized by one or more of the following signs and symptoms: roughness, scaling, loss of flexibility, fissures, inflammation, and pruritus. Common clinical findings include fine plate-like scaling, particularly on the arms and legs, that may be associated with a "cracked" appearance (eczema craquelé) or fish-scaling (ichthyosis) appearance of the skin.[40]

Treatment of Dry Skin

Treatment Goals

The goals of self-treatment of dry skin are (1) to restore skin hydration, (2) to restore the skin's barrier function, and (3) to educate the patient about prevention and treatment of this chronic disorder.

General Treatment Approach

Treatment involves recognizing the problem as well as modifying the environment and bathing habits to maintain skin hydration. Nonprescription products such as bath oils, emollients, and moisturizers containing humectants, keratolytic agents, or both, aid in restoring and maintaining barrier function. If needed, topical hydrocortisone can be used to reduce pruritus and erythema.

Nonpharmacologic Therapy

The most important aspects of care are the proper use of emollients that soften the skin, and modifications to bathing practices. The patient should apply oil-based emollients immediately after bathing while the skin is damp and should reapply them frequently. The room humidity can be increased with a portable cool-mist humidifier, or a humidification unit can be added to the home heating system. The patient should be encouraged to stay well hydrated by drinking ample water daily unless contraindicated by any medical disorders. Table 33–3 reviews nonpharmacologic therapy of dry skin.

TABLE 33-3 Nonpharmacologic Therapy of Dry Skin

- Take tub baths with addition of bath oil 2–3 times per week for brief periods (3–5 minutes). Take sponge baths on other days.
- Bathe in tepid water, not more than 3°F above body temperature.
- Within 3 minutes of getting out of the tub, pat the body dry, leaving beads of moisture, and generously apply body moisturizer to trap the moisture.
- Apply the body moisturizer at least 3 more times during the day to the whole body (preferably) or at least to the most affected areas.
- Additional measures include
  - Use corticosteroid ointments rather than creams if short-term use is indicated.
  - Keep room humidity high.

Pharmacologic Therapy

Dry skin is more prone to itching, inflammation, and development of secondary infections. Most moisturizers are mixtures of oils and water, but more severe cases of dry skin may require a product containing a humectant (e.g., glycerin, urea, lactic acid) to enhance hydration. Other agents that can be added to these emollients or moisturizers include alpha hydroxy acids and lipid moisturizers such as phospholipids and ceramides.[41] Dry skin responds minimally to topical corticosteroid therapy, although short-term (≤7 days) use of topical corticosteroids may reduce symptoms of erythema and pruritus.[40] If resolution does not occur within 1 week, a primary care provider should be consulted because other options may be required to improve the dry skin.

Nonprescription Medications Used to Treat Atopic Dermatitis and Dry Skin

Nonprescription products for dermatitis and dry skin that restore skin hydration include bath products and emollients, which can contain hydrating, keratolytic, and keratin-softening agents. Often these products are combined in commonly available nonprescription products (Table 33–4). Many ingredients are available for use on AD lesions or dry skin. These products are reviewed below and can be recommended according to patient preference and therapeutic response.

Bath Products

Bath Oils

Bath oils generally consist of a mineral or vegetable oil plus a surfactant. Some commercially available bath oil products are combined with colloidal oatmeal in an attempt to provide better relief of itching. Bath oils are minimally effective in improving a dry skin disorder, because they are greatly diluted in water. When applied as wet compresses, bath oils (1 teaspoon in one-fourth cup of warm water) help lubricate dry skin and may allow a decrease in the frequency of full-body bathing. Bath oils make the tub and floor slippery, creating a safety hazard, especially for older adults or children.

Cleansers

Typical bath soaps generally contain salts of long-chain fatty acids (commonly oleic, palmitic, or stearic acid) and alkali metals (e.g., sodium, potassium). Combined with water, these products act as

TABLE 33-4 **Selected Nonprescription Dry Skin Products**

Trade Name	Primary Ingredients
Petrolatum-Containing Products	
Absorbase Ointment[a]	Petrolatum; mineral oil; ceresin wax; wool wax alcohol; potassium sorbate
AmLactin Cream/Lotion	Ammonium lactate 12%
Aquaphor Ointment	Petrolatum 41%; water
Cetaphil Cream[a]	Petrolatum; glycerin
Cetaphil Gentle Cleansing Bar[a]	Sodium cocoyl isethionate; stearic acid; sodium tallousate; PEG-20; petrolatum
Eucerin Cream[a]	Petrolatum; mineral oil; mineral wax; wool wax alcohol
Jergens Ultra Healing Lotion	Petrolatum; mineral oil; dimethicone; cetearyl alcohol; cetyl alcohol; glycerin
Moisturel Cream/Lotion[a]	Petrolatum; dimethicone; cetyl alcohol; glycerin
Vaseline Intensive Care Lotion	White petrolatum; mineral oil; dimethicone; glyceryl stearate; cetyl alcohol; glycerin
Ceramide Containing Products	
CeraVe Moisturizing Lotion	Glycerin; ceramide 1, 3, 6, and 11; hyaluronic acid; dimethicone; petrolatum, potassium phosphate
Eucerin Professional Repair Concentrated Lotion	Ceramide 3; glycerin; urea
Urea-Containing Products	
Carmol 10 Lotion	Urea 10%
Carmol 20 Cream	Urea 20%
Lac-Hydrin Five Lotion	Urea 5%
Counterirritants	
Sarna Anti-Itch Lotion	Camphor 0.5%; menthol 0.5%; carbomer 940; cetyl alcohol; DMDM hydantoin; glyceryl stearate; petrolatum
Miscellaneous Emollients	
Cetaphil Gentle Skin Cleanser Liquid[a]	Cetyl alcohol; stearyl alcohol; PEG
Gold Bond Ultimate Healing Lotion	Glycerin; petrolatum; cetyl alcohol; aloe; cetearyl alcohol; propylene glycol; glyceryl stearate
Keri Original Dry Skin Lotion	Mineral oil; lanolin oil; glyceryl stearate; propylene glycol
Lubriderm Advanced Therapy Lotion	Cetyl alcohol; glycerin; mineral oil; PEG-40; emulsifying wax; vitamin E
Lubriderm Daily Moisturizing Lotion	Mineral oil; petrolatum; sorbitol; lanolin; lanolin alcohol; triethanolamine
Neutrogena Body Oil	Isopropyl myristate; sesame oil
Neutrogena Soap	TEA-stearate; triethanolamine; glycerin
Nivea Body Lotion	Glycerin; mineral oil; isopropyl palmitate; vitamin E; lanolin alcohol
Purpose Gentle Cleansing Bar	Sodium tallowate; sodium cocoate; glycerin; BHT

Key: BHT = Butylhydroxytoluene; DMDM = dimethylol dimethyl; PEG = polyethylene glycol; TEA = triethanolamine.
[a] Fragrance-free formulation.

surfactants that remove many substances from the skin, including the lipids that normally keep the skin soft and pliable. Health care providers often recommend special soaps, such as those including glycerin, that contain extra oils to minimize the drying effect of washing. However, these soaps usually lather and clean poorly. Glycerin soaps, which are transparent and more water soluble, have a higher oil content than standard soaps because of the addition of castor oil. They are closer to a neutral pH and are regarded as less drying than traditional soaps, which are alkaline. Although little objective proof exists to prove their superiority, glycerin soaps are advertised for, and well accepted by, people with skin disorders. Mild cleansers such as Cetaphil or pHisoDerm can be recommended if soap is to be avoided.

Emollients and Moisturizers

Emollients function to soften the skin by filling the space between the desquamating skin scales with oil droplets through which moisture cannot readily escape, but their effect is only temporary. Cosmetically, emollients make the skin feel soft and smooth by helping reestablish the integrity of the stratum corneum. Lipid components make the scales on the skin translucent and flatten them against the underlying skin. This flattening eliminates air between the scales and the skin surface, which is partly responsible for a white, scaly appearance.[41]

Moisturizers impart moisture to the skin, thereby increasing skin flexibility. Most moisturizers consist of water (60%–80%), which functions as a diluent and evaporates, leaving behind active agents. Moisturizers can contain several components, some of which include emulsifiers, which keep water and lipids in one continuous phase; humectants, such as glycerin, propylene glycol, alpha hydroxy acids, and urea, which help skin retain water; preservatives; fragrance (or may be fragrance free); and color (dyes). Specialty additives, such as vitamins (vitamins A, C, D, B complex), which have no known clinical effect, and natural moisturizing factors (e.g., lactate, urea, ammonia, uric acid, glucosamine) can also be added and are reported to regulate the moisture content of the stratum corneum. Lipid additives such as ceramides or pseudoceramides, are being added to some products for added skin barrier protection.[24,28] The differences between moisturizer products are often due to the addition of fragrances, exotic oils, vitamins, protein or amino acid products, and other minor moisturizing aids. Moisturizers come in lotions, creams, ointments, gels, oils, and butters. Creams, ointments, and butters are more difficult to spread, especially in hairy areas. Butters are stiffer moisturizing formulations sold in jars and often contain shea butter, which is extracted from the nut of the African shea tree. Patients with tree nut allergies appear to be able to use these products without fear of an allergic reaction. The simplest and most economical hand ointment is petroleum jelly. Although it is greasy, petroleum jelly is effective when applied at bedtime and covered with wraps or clothing. Because sebum and skin surface lipids contain a relatively high concentration of fatty acid glycerides, vegetable and animal oils derived from avocado, cucumber, mink, peanut, safflower, sesame, turtle, and shark liver are included in dry skin products, presumably because of their unsaturated fatty acid content. Although use of these oils contributes to skin flexibility and lubricity, they are less occlusive than white petrolatum. Use of these products should be avoided in individuals with an allergy to any component.

Ointments are typically water-in-oil emulsions. Often containing petrolatum, they are typically greasy and generally lack consumer appeal because of their texture, difficulty of spreading and removing, and staining properties. To avoid a greasy feel, patients can gently warm the product in the hands, apply a very thin layer, and massage it into the skin. Ointments are inappropriate for oozing AD, because they do not allow the lesions to dry and ultimately heal. Additionally, petrolatum should not be applied over puncture wounds, infections, or lacerations, because its high-occlusive property may lead to maceration and further inflammation. Application of petrolatum to intertriginous areas (e.g., armpits, groin, perianal region), mucous membranes, and acne-prone areas should be minimized; only a preparation with a low concentration of petrolatum is tolerated in these areas. In addition, ointments may be too occlusive in very warm weather, making creams a better choice.[24]

Lotions and creams are typically oil-in-water emulsions that are less greasy. These agents help alleviate the pruritus associated with dry skin by virtue of their cooling effect as water evaporates from the skin surface. Lotions may be preferred in milder cases of dryness or in warm weather when the occlusive properties of ointments are an issue.[24]

Frequency of application depends on the severity of the dry skin disorder and the hydration efficiency of the occlusive agent. Generally, moisturizers should be applied liberally and frequently, or a minimum of 3 times daily, to achieve maximum benefit.[25] For dry hands, the patient may need to apply the moisturizing agent after each hand washing, as well as at numerous other times during the day.

Topical Hydrocortisone

Hydrocortisone (0.5% or 1%) is currently the only corticosteroid available without a prescription for the topical treatment of dermatitis. Although its exact mechanism is unknown, hydrocortisone most likely suppresses cytokines associated with the development of inflammation and itching, which is associated with various dermatoses. Food and Drug Administration monograph indications for use of hydrocortisone in patients older than 2 years include temporary relief of itching associated with minor skin irritations, inflammation, and rashes caused by dermatitis, seborrheic dermatitis, insect bites, poison ivy/oak/sumac dermatitis, soaps, detergents, cosmetics, and jewelry.[42] Concentrations of 0.5% or 1% are considered appropriate for treating localized dermatitis. Many commercially available nonprescription hydrocortisone products now also contain aloe. (The "Pharmacologic Therapy" section under "Atopic Dermatitis" provides more information on hydrocortisone.) Aloe may serve as a potential irritant to some patients with dermatitis, so this population should avoid use of products containing this agent. (See Chapter 51 for more information on aloe.)

For mild dry skin, a cream is acceptable; however, an ointment formulation generally provides the best results for chronic, nonoozing dermatoses. Maximizing the application of moisturizers (lotions, creams, ointments) to dry, itchy skin disorders may lessen the frequency that medicated products, such as hydrocortisone, have to be applied.[22,32]

Product Selection Guidelines

Special Populations

Topical medications are used to treat many common skin disorders in infants and children. Infants have a reduced capability to biotransform drugs absorbed by the cutaneous route, because they have immature hepatic enzyme systems. In addition, because the ratio of surface area to body weight in a neonate is approximately two to three times that of an adult, the proportion of drug absorbed per kilogram of body weight is greater in a newborn.[43] Therefore, patients younger than 1 year should be referred to a primary care provider for the care of skin disorders.

Patient Factors and Preferences

When deciding which product to recommend for dermatitis or dry skin, the health care provider must evaluate the active ingredients and the vehicle. Primary active ingredients contained in nonprescription skin products are water and oil. However, a variety of secondary ingredients is added to enhance product elegance and stability, and many of these ingredients, such as preservatives like parabens or benzyl alcohol, have the potential to produce contact dermatitis through either an irritant or a sensitizing effect.[29]

The type of vehicle (e.g., ointment, cream, lotion, gel, solution, aerosol) may significantly affect treatment of dermatitis, so product selection should be based on patient preference and location of lesions. Ointments provide lubrication and may be useful if occlusion is desired or if the lesion is dry, thick, or scaly. However, use of ointments in intertriginous areas (e.g., groin, axillae) should be avoided because of the potential for maceration. Alternatively, creams may be less potent than ointments and contain preservatives previously mentioned as potential irritants. Lotions and gels are not as greasy, and both dry quickly. Lotions can be useful in hairy areas, as can foams and mousses.[29] Gels, foams, and mousses can feel good on patients' skin, because the alcohol component produces a "cooling" effect. This component also has a drying effect and can cause hypersensitivity in some patients. In addition, some novel formulations (foams and mousses) can be more expensive than traditional creams and ointments.

Cases 33–1 and 33–2 are examples of the assessment of patients with AD or dry skin, respectively.

Patient Counseling for Atopic Dermatitis and Dry Skin

Patients with AD should be counseled about achieving control of their disease, the chronic nature of the condition, exacerbating factors, and appropriate treatment options. The health care provider should also explain factors that cause dry skin and the appropriate measures for restoring barrier function. Finally, health care providers should ensure that patients are aware of potential duplicate drug therapy; that is, they should be advised to stop using a nonprescription hydrocortisone product if a prescription corticosteroid is prescribed but to continue using emollients. The box "Patient Education for Atopic Dermatitis and Dry Skin" lists specific information to provide patients.

CASE 33-1

Relevant Evaluation Criteria	Scenario/Model Outcome
Collect	
1. Gather essential information about the patient's symptoms and medical history, including	
a. Description of symptom(s) (i.e., nature, onset, duration, severity, associated symptoms)	The patient presents with pruritic, scaly skin on both forearms and lower legs. He claims the soles of his feet and palms of his hands are very rough, with some fissures but no open wounds. Significant flaking of the affected areas is observed, especially in the morning.
b. Description of any factors that seem to precipitate, exacerbate, and/or relieve the patient's symptom(s)	He states the skin symptoms are more bothersome in the winter months and have worsened as he has aged.
c. Description of the patient's efforts to relieve the symptoms	He has tried a store-brand lotion on "most" mornings with minimal improvement.
d. Patient's identity	Tyler Brown
e. Age, gender, height, and weight	79 years old, male, 5 ft 7 in., 230 lb
f. Patient's occupation	Retired engineer
g. Patient's dietary habits	MNT diet for patients with diabetes
h. Patient's sleep habits	6–7 hours of sleep per night
i. Concurrent medical conditions, prescription and nonprescription medications, and dietary supplements	Hypertension: lisinopril 20 mg once daily; prophylaxis for CVD: ASA 81 mg once daily; type 2 diabetes: metformin 500 mg twice daily
j. Allergies	None
k. History of other adverse reactions to medications	None
l. Other (describe) ______	Tyler bathes 5–6 times per week in a tub for 30 minutes at a time. He lives in Madison, Wisconsin. He keeps the temperature in his home at 75 degrees and says that he uses a humidifier in his bedroom during the winter months.
Assess	
2. Differentiate patient's signs/symptoms, and correctly identify the patient's primary problem(s).	Tyler has dry skin that is most likely caused by environmental factors in combination with his advancing age.
3. Identify exclusions for self-treatment (Figure 33–2).	None
4. Formulate a comprehensive list of therapeutic alternatives for the primary problem to determine whether triage to a health care provider is required, and share this information with the patient or caregiver.	Options include (1) Refer Tyler to his PCP or a dermatologist. (2) Recommend self-care with nonprescription product(s) and nondrug measures. (3) Recommend appropriate self-care until Tyler can see an appropriate provider. (4) Take no action.

CASE 33-1 *continued*

Relevant Evaluation Criteria	Scenario/Model Outcome
Implement	
5. Select an optimal therapeutic alternative to address the patient's problem, taking into account patient preferences.	A nonprescription emollient will be appropriate for Tyler. Applying white petrolatum at bedtime on his arms, legs, and feet and then covering them with sleeves or stockings, as appropriate, will provide the fastest results. A moisturizing cream could be used 2–3 times daily in place of the petrolatum. Hand lotion should be applied liberally and frequently, at least 3–4 times daily. If intense itching is troublesome, nonprescription hydrocortisone 1% cream or ointment may be applied to the affected area 2 times daily followed by an emollient. (Table 33–3 provides other information on dry skin therapy.)
6. Describe the recommended therapeutic approach to the patient or caregiver.	"Take brief (3- to 5-minute) full-body baths 2–3 times per week using warm (tepid) water. (Bath oils should be avoided because of the risk of falling). Pat dry after bathing; apply moisturizer generously. Drink plenty of water daily. Increase the humidity in your house to minimize evaporation from the skin."
7. Explain to the patient or caregiver the rationale for selecting the recommended therapeutic approach from the considered therapeutic alternatives.	"Dry skin can be managed but not cured with nonprescription topical therapy plus changes in your bathing habits."
Implement	
8. When recommending self-care with nonprescription medications and/or nondrug therapy, convey accurate information to the patient or caregiver.	
a. Appropriate dose and frequency of administration	See the box "Patient Education for Atopic Dermatitis and Dry Skin."
b. Maximum number of days the therapy should be employed	"It is likely the emollient will need to be used chronically. Avoid daily prolonged use (>7 days) of topical hydrocortisone, if possible." (See the box "Patient Education for Atopic Dermatitis and Dry Skin.")
c. Product administration procedures	See the box "Patient Education for Atopic Dermatitis and Dry Skin."
d. Expected time to onset of relief	See the box "Patient Education for Atopic Dermatitis and Dry Skin."
e. Degree of relief that can be reasonably expected	See the box "Patient Education for Atopic Dermatitis and Dry Skin."
f. Most common adverse	See the box "Patient Education for Atopic Dermatitis and Dry Skin."
g. Adverse effects that warrant medical intervention should they occur	See the box "Patient Education for Atopic Dermatitis and Dry Skin."
h. Patient options in the event that condition worsens or persists	If the symptoms progress or if your lesions, particularly those on the feet, become open, seek assistance from a primary care provider.
i. Product storage requirements	Store in a cool, dry place out of children's reach.
j. Specific nondrug measures	See the box "Patient Education for Atopic Dermatitis and Dry Skin."
Solicit follow-up questions from the patient or caregiver.	"Can I just use my Jergen's Lotion rather than using the Vaseline on my feet and legs?"
Answer the patient's or caregiver's questions.	"Ointments such as Vaseline hold moisture in the skin better than creams or lotions do. Although you may be able to use only your lotion after your disorder improves, you would have to apply it 4–5 times daily to achieve the same results that Vaseline will provide."
Follow-up: Monitor and Evaluate	
9. Assess patient outcome.	Ask the patient to call you to report how he responded to the recommended therapy, or call the patient in a week to evaluate his response.

Key: ASA = Acetyl salicylic acid; CVD = cardiovascular disease; MNT = medical nutrition therapy.

CASE 33-2

Relevant Evaluation Criteria	Scenario/Model Outcome
Collect	
1. Gather essential information about the patient's symptoms and medical history, including	
a. Description of symptom(s) (i.e., nature, onset, duration, severity, associated symptoms)	The patient presents with persistent itching on her wrist and elbow areas, which has intensified during the past 2–3 months. The skin is dry and thickened, and within the past week, yellowish exudates and crusting appeared in both areas.
b. Description of any factors that seem to precipitate, exacerbate, and/or relieve the patient's symptom(s)	The patient states that the symptoms seem to have worsened after the move into a new house. The itching is much worse and has caused the patient to frequently scratch the affected areas.
c. Description of the patient's efforts to relieve the symptoms	The patient has tried hydrocortisone 1% cream applied twice daily over the past 2 months, but this regiment has not helped to date.
d. Patient's identity	Cathy Smith
e. Patient's age, gender, height, and weight	28 years old, female, 5 ft, 4 in., 135 lb
f. Patient's occupation	Salesperson
g. Patient's dietary habits	Normal diet
h. Patient's sleep habits	Sleeps 6–7 hours per night.
i. Concurrent medical conditions, prescription and nonprescription medications, and dietary supplements	Allergic rhinitis: loratadine 10 mg once daily
j. Allergies	House dust
k. History of other adverse reactions to medications	None
l. Other (describe) ______	Cathy was diagnosed with atopic dermatitis at 12 years of age. It has been controlled fairly well with topical corticosteroids used on an as-needed basis.
Assess	
2. Differentiate patient's signs/symptoms, and correctly identify the patient's primary problem(s).	Patient has lesions associated with atopic dermatitis that vary with time and are likely to worsen with continued irritation from scratching.
3. Identify exclusions for self-treatment (Figure 33–2).	The recent development of yellow exudates may indicate a secondary infection; thus, any form of self-treatment should be avoided. The patient should undergo further evaluation prior to using any pharmacologic agent on a chronic basis.
4. Formulate a comprehensive list of therapeutic alternatives for the primary problem to determine whether triage to a health care provider is required, and share this information with the patient or caregiver.	Options include (1) Refer Cathy to her primary care provider or a dermatologist for a differential diagnosis. (2) Recommend an appropriate nonprescription product. (3) Recommend an appropriate nonprescription product until Cathy can be seen by primary care provider or a dermatologist. (4) Take no action.
Plan	
5. Select an optimal therapeutic alternative to address the patient's problem, taking into account patient preferences.	Cathy should apply a topical emollient cream or lotion to the lesions 3–4 times daily with clean hands. She should try to keep the lesions and surrounding skin as clean as possible. In addition, she should be seen by her primary care provider or a dermatologist. Hydrocortisone should be avoided, because it could delay the healing of a skin infection.
6. Describe the recommended therapeutic approach to the patient or caregiver.	"Until you can see your primary care provider or a dermatologist, you may apply a topical emollient cream or lotion 3–4 times daily to the lesions. You may have a skin infection, so you should stop using the hydrocortisone. It could delay the healing of the infection."
7. Explain to the patient or caregiver the rationale for selecting the recommended therapeutic approach from the considered therapeutic alternatives.	"Because of the likelihood of a skin infection, it is important to be sure what the lesions are prior to recommending any long-term treatment with any pharmacologic agent, such as hydrocortisone."

Relevant Evaluation Criteria	Scenario/Model Outcome
Implement	
8. When recommending self-care with nonprescription medications and/or nondrug therapy, convey accurate information to the patient or caregiver.	"Try not to scratch the lesions; wearing cotton gloves at night may help with this." See the box "Patient Education for Atopic Dermatitis and Dry Skin" for additional information that can be discussed with the primary care provider or a dermatologist.
Solicit follow-up questions from the patient or caregiver.	"Is there a nonprescription medication that might help?"
Answer the patient's or caregiver's questions.	"Use of a nonprescription topical antibiotic ointment may not be adequate therapy to eradicate the skin infection. Nonprescription medications are not appropriate to recommend without a definite diagnosis from a health care provider or dermatologist."
Follow-up: Monitor and Evaluate	
9. Assess patient outcome.	Contact the patient in a day or two to ensure that she sought further medical care.

PATIENT EDUCATION FOR Atopic Dermatitis and Dry Skin

The primary objectives of self-treating atopic dermatitis are (1) to stop the itch–scratch cycle, (2) to maintain skin hydration, (3) to avoid or minimize factors that trigger or aggravate the disorder, and (4) to prevent secondary infections. The primary objective in self-treating dry skin—restoring skin moisture and the skin's barrier function—can also help relieve the discomfort of atopic dermatitis. For most patients, carefully following product instructions and the self-care measures listed here will help ensure optimal therapeutic outcomes. Understanding that implementing a treatment plan for AD requires patience is key to a successful outcome, because some therapeutic measures can be time consuming to implement and often a delay occurs in the time to maximal benefit.

Atopic Dermatitis

Nondrug Measures

- Avoid factors that trigger allergic reactions. Do not wear tight clothing. Remain in areas that have a moderate temperature and low humidity.
- Take short showers or baths, using warm (tepid) water and a nonsoap cleanser.
- If possible, substitute sponge baths (with tepid water) for full-body bathing.
- Pat dry after bath or shower.
- To dry weeping lesions, apply cool tap water compresses for 5–20 minutes, 4–6 times daily.
- To prevent injury to the affected area caused by scratching, keep your fingernails short, smooth, and clean. At night, wear cotton gloves or socks on your hands to lessen scratching.

Nonprescription Medications

- Gently wash the affected areas with a nonsoap cleanser before applying any emollient or medication. Gently pat skin dry, and apply an emollient within 3 minutes after washing while skin is still damp.
- Wash hands before and after applying any medication.
- Apply a thin layer of medication over the affected areas.
- Apply hydrocortisone 1–2 times daily to dry lesions to relieve itching. Do not use this medication longer than 7 days.
- With proper use of medications and nondrug measures, noticeable improvement can be observed in 24–48 hours.
- Although completely eliminating the rash and itch is possible, the lesions likely could get worse, especially during the winter and summer months.

When to Seek Medical Attention

- If the atopic dermatitis does not improve or worsens after 2–3 days of treatment, consult your primary care provider.

Dry Skin

Nondrug Measures

- Avoid excessive bathing; take brief full-body baths 2–3 times per week, using bath oil and warm (tepid) water.
- If possible, take sponge baths on other days using warm water to maintain skin hydration.
- Pat dry after bathing or showering.
- Drink plenty of water daily.
- Moisturizer should be generously applied 3–4 times daily and continued as long as dry skin persists.
- Moisturizers should be applied within 3 minutes after bathing, plus an additional 3 times per day.
- Although getting rid of the dry skin completely may be difficult, initial improvement should be seen within 24 hours.
- Avoid caffeine, spices, and alcohol, because they can contribute to dehydration.
- Keep the room humidity higher than normal to minimize evaporation from the skin.

Nonprescription Medications

- Add products such as oilated oatmeal or bath oil near the end of your bath to improve skin hydration. Colloidal oatmeal products, if used on a regular basis, may clog plumbing pipes and can leave the tub slick.
- Apply an oil-based emollient immediately after bathing while your skin is damp. Reapply the emollient frequently.
- For more severe cases of dry skin, use a product that contains urea or lactic acid.
- Apply nonprescription topical hydrocortisone ointment to reduce inflammation and itching. Do not use this medication longer than 7 days.

When to Seek Medical Attention

- If skin dryness worsens after 7 days of treatment, consult a primary care provider.

Evaluation of Patient Outcomes for Atopic Dermatitis and Dry Skin

A patient with dry skin should be reevaluated 7 days after initiation of therapy. Visual assessment is the best method of determining treatment response. Therefore, a scheduled visit is the preferred follow-up method. If the symptoms have not improved or have worsened (continued or additional itching, redness, scaling, lesions, or tissue breakdown), medical referral is appropriate.

Key Points for Atopic Dermatitis and Dry Skin

- Most patients with mild–moderate AD or dry skin are candidates for self-treatment with a combination of nonprescription and nonpharmacologic therapies.
- Refer patients with yellow, crusting, eczematous AD lesions and all children younger than 1 year of age with AD to a primary care provider or a dermatologist for evaluation and treatment.
- Question patients presenting with dry or eczematous skin lesions about new or changes in exposure to soaps, detergents, fragrances, chemicals, irritants, temperature extremes, allergens, and other triggers; then provide information about avoidance of such triggers.
- Counsel patients with dry skin disorders to take brief baths, use tepid water, pat dry, and apply moisturizers within 3 minutes of completing the bath or shower.
- Advise patients to use mild skin cleansers and to apply copious quantities of moisturizers 3–4 times daily.
- Educate the patient with chronic dry skin disorders about the importance of stopping the itch–scratch cycle and maintaining adequate hydration.
- Advise patients to use ointment-based products, whenever possible, to maximize the hydrating properties of the product. Cream-based products can be recommended for patients who will not comply with use of ointments or for patients with weeping lesions.
- Instruct patients how to properly apply topical emollients, anti-inflammatory agents, and antipruritic agents, using the smallest amount possible and thoroughly rubbing in the product.
- Advise patients with self-treatable symptoms to contact their primary care provider if symptoms worsen or do not improve within 7 days.

REFERENCES

1. Weller R, Hunter JAA, Savin J, et al. *Clinical Dermatology.* 6th ed. Hoboken, NJ: Wiley-Blackwell; 2015:1–14.
2. Nutten S. Atopic Dermatitis: Global epidemiology and risk factors. *Ann Nutr Metab.* 2015;66(Suppl 1):8–16. doi: 10.1159/000370220.
3. Hanifin JM, Reed ML. A population-based survey of eczema prevalence in the United States. *Dermatitis.* 2007;18(2):82–91. PMID: 17498413.
4. Atopic dermatitis, eczema, and noninfectious immunodeficiency disorders. In: James WD, Berger TG, Elston DM, eds. *Andrews' Diseases of the Skin: Clinical Dermatology.* 11th ed. London: Saunders Elsevier; 2011: 62–70.
5. House AA. Issues in geriatric dermatology. In: Olsen CG, Tindall WN, Clasen ME, eds. *Geriatric Pharmacotherapy: A Guide for the Helping Professional.* Washington, DC: American Pharmacists Association; 2007:137–61.
6. Micali G, Lacarrubba F, Bongu A, et al. The skin barrier. In: Freinkel R, Woodely D, eds. *The Biology of the Skin.* New York, NY: Parthenon; 2001:227.
7. Law RM, Law DTS. eChapter 23. Dermatologic drug reactions and common skin conditions. In: DiPiro JT, Talbert RL, Yee GC, et al., eds. *Pharmacotherapy: A Pathophysiologic Approach.* 9th ed. New York, NY: McGraw-Hill. 2014.
8. Burkhart C, Morrell D, Goldsmith L. Dermatological pharmacology. In: Brunton L, ed. *Goodman and Gilman's the Pharmacological Basis of Therapeutics.* 12th ed. New York, NY: McGraw-Hill; 2011:1803–32.
9. Bieber T, Cork M, Reitamo S. Atopic dermatitis: a candidate for disease-modifying strategy. *Allergy.* 2012;67(8):969–75. doi: 10.1111/j.1398-9995.2012.02845.x.
10. Krakowski AC, Eichenfield LF, Dohil MA. Management of atopic dermatitis in the pediatric population. *Pediatrics.* 2008;122(4):812–24. doi: 10.1542/peds.2007-2232.
11. Sabin BR, Peters N, Peters AT. Atopic dermatitis. *Allergy Asthma Proc.* 2012;33(Suppl 1):S67–9. doi: 10.2500/aap.2012.33.3553.
12. Thompson J, Avery M, Honeywell M, et al. Atopic dermatitis: a review of clinical management. *US Pharm.* 2006;31:89–96.
13. Eichenfield LR, Ellis CN, Mancini AJ, et al. Atopic dermatitis: epidemiology and pathogenesis update. *Semin Cutan Med Surg.* 2012;31 (3 Suppl):S3–5. doi: 10.1016/j.sder.2012.07.002.
14. Ring J, Alomar A, Bieber T, et al. Guidelines for treatment of atopic eczema (atopic dermatitis) part I. *J Eur Acad Dermatol Venereol.* 2012; 26(8):1045–60. doi: 10.1111/j.1468-3083.2012.04635.x.
15. Law RM, Kwa P. Atopic dermatitis. In: DiPiro JT, Talbert RL, Yee GC, et al, eds. *Pharmacotherapy: A Pathophysiologic Approach.* 9th ed. New York, NY: McGraw-Hill; 2014:1595–604.
16. Condren M, Miller JL. Pediatric dermatology. In: Benevades S, Nahata MC. *Pediatric Pharmacotherapy.* Lenexa, KS: American College of Clinical Pharmacy; 2013:92–107.
17. Eichenfield LF, Tom WL, Chamlin SL, et al. Guidelines of care for the management of atopic dermatitis. Section 1. Diagnosis and assessment of atopic dermatitis. *J Am Acad Dermatol.* 2014;70:338-51. doi: 10.1016/j.jaad.2013.10.010.
18. Beiber T. Mechanisms of disease: Atopic dermatitis. *N Engl J Med.* 2008; 358(14):1483–94. doi: 10.1056/NEJMra074081.
19. Schram ME, Spuls PI, Leeflang MM, et al. EASI, (objective) SCORAD and POEM for atopic eczema: responsiveness and minimal clinically important difference. *Allergy.* 2012;67(1):99–106. doi: 10.1111/j.1398-9995.2011.02719.x.
20. Ricci G, Dondi A, Patrizi A. Useful tools for the management of atopic dermatitis. *Am J Clin Dermatol.* 2009;10(5):287–300. doi: 10.2165/11310760-000000000-00000.
21. Ellis CN, Mancini AJ, Paller AS, et al. Understanding and managing atopic dermatitis in adult patients. *Semin Cutan Med Surg.* 2012;31(3 Suppl): S18–22. doi: 10.1016/j.sder.2012.07.006.
22. Berke R, Singh A, Guralnick M. Atopic dermatitis: an overview. *Am Fam Physician.* 2012:86 (1):35–42. PMID: 22962911.
23. Eichenfield LF, Boguniewicz M, Simpson EL, et al. Translating atopic dermatitis management guidelines into practice for primary care providers. *Pediatrics.* 2015;136(3):554–65. doi:10.1542/peds.2014-3678.
24. Paller AS, Simpson EL, Eichenfield LF, et al. Treatment strategies for atopic dermatitis: optimizing the available therapeutic options. *Semin Cutan Med Surg.* 2012;31(3 Suppl):S10–7. doi: 10.1016/j.sder.2012.07.004.
25. Eichenfield LF, Tom WL, Berger TG, et al. Guidelines of care for the management of atopic dermatitis. Section 2. Management and treatment of atopic dermatitis with topical therapies. *J Am Acad Dermatol.* 2014; 71:116–132. doi:10.1016/j.jaad.2014.03.023.
26. Tollefson MM, Bruckner AL. Atopic dermatitis: skin-directed management. *Pediatrics.* 2014;124(6): e1735–44. doi: 10.1542/peds.2014-2812.
27. Lieberman JA, Sicherer SH. The diagnosis of food allergy. *Am J Rhinol Allergy.* 2010;24(6):439–43. doi: 10.2500/ajra.2010.24.3515.
28. Hon KL, Leung AKC, Barankin B. Barrier repair therapy in atopic dermatitis: an overview. *Am J Clin Dermatol.* 2013;14:389–99. doi: 10.1007/s40257-013-0033-9.
29. Ference JD, Last AR. Choosing topical corticosteroids. *Am Fam Physician.* 2009;79(2):135–40. PMID: 19178066.
30. Buys LM. Treatment options for atopic dermatitis. *Am Fam Physician.* 2007;75(4):523–8. PMID: 17323714.

31. Sidbury R, Davis DM, Cohen DE, et al. Guidelines of care for the management of atopic dermatitis. *J Am Acad Dermatol.* 2014;71:327–49. doi:10.1016/j.jaad.2014.03.030
32. Huang JT, Abrams M, Tlougan B, et al. Treatment of *Staphylococcus aureus* colonization in atopic dermatitis decreases disease severity. *Pediatrics.* 2009;123:e808–14. doi: 10.1542/peds.2008-2217.
33. Devillers AC, Oranje AP. Wet-wraps treatment in children with atopic dermatitis: a practical guide. *Pediatr Dermatol.* 2012;29(1):24–7. doi: 10.1111/j.1525-1470.2011.01691.x.
34. Song T. The efficacy of wet wrap treatment in children with atopic dermatitis. *J Allergy Clin Immunol.* 2011;127(2):AB36. doi: https://doi.org/10.1016/j.jaci.2010.12.155.
35. Sidbury R, Tom WL, Bergman JN, et al. Guidelines of care for the management of atopic dermatitis. Section 4. Prevention of disease flares and use of adjunctive therapies and approaches. *J Am Acad Dermatol.* 2014;71(6):1218–33.doi:10.1016/j.jaad.2014.08.038.
36. Wickens K Black PN, Stanley TV, et al. A differential effect of 2 probiotics in the prevention of eczema and atopy: a double-blind, randomized, placebo-controlled trial. *J Allergy Clin Immunol.* 2008;122(4):788–94. doi: 10.1016/j.jaci.2008.07.011.
37. Boyle RJ, Bath-Hextall FL, Leonardi-Bee J, et al. Probiotics for the treatment of eczema: a systemic review. *Clin Exp Allergy.* 2009;39:1117–27. doi: 10.1111/j.1365-2222.2009.03305.x.
38. Armstrong N, Ernst E. The treatment of eczema with Chinese herbs: a systematic review of randomized clinical trials. *Br J Clin Pharm.* 1999; 48:262–4. PMID: 10417508.
39. Evangelista MT, Abad-Casintahan F, Lopez-Villafuerte L. The effect of topical virgin coconut oil on SCORAD index, transepidermal water loss, and skin capacitance in mild to moderate pediatric atopic dermatitis: a randomized, double-blind, clinical trial. *Int J Dermatol.* 2014;53(1):100–8. Available at: http://www.druglib.com/abstract/ev/evangelista-mt1_int-j-dermatol_20140000.html. Accessed June 1, 2017.
40. Zagaria MAE. Xerosis: treating clinically dry skin. *US Pharm.* 2006;31:28–32.
41. Lazar AP, Lazar P. Dry skin, water, and lubrication. *Dermatol Clin.* 1991;9(1):45–51. PMID: 2022097.
42. U.S. Food and Drug Administration. Hydrocortisone monograph. Available at http://www.fda.gov/Drugs/default.htm. Accessed March 31, 2016.
43. Buck ML. Pediatric pharmacotherapy. In: Alldredge BK, Corelli RL, Ernst ME, et al., eds. *Applied Therapeutics: The Clinical Use of Drugs.* 10th ed. Philadelphia, PA: Lippincott Williams and Wilkins; 2013:2265–76.

CHAPTER 34

SCALY DERMATOSES

RUPAL PATEL MANSUKHANI AND LUCIO VOLINO

Chronic scaly dermatoses include dandruff, seborrheic dermatitis, and psoriasis. These disorders involve the uppermost layer of skin, the epidermis. Their primary manifestation is scaling of the skin with varying degrees of inflammation, erythema, and appearance. *Dandruff* is a less inflammatory form of seborrhea manifested as dermatitis with relatively fine scaling confined to the scalp and, occasionally, mild erythema or inflammation.[1–3] *Seborrheic dermatitis,* which affects the scalp, face, and chest (usually the sternum), typically involves significant inflammation and erythema; their degree and extent are based on severity of the disorder.[2] *Psoriasis* is a highly inflammatory skin disorder with raised plaques and adherent thick silvery white scales.[1,4]

Nonprescription products are appropriate treatment for most cases of dandruff and seborrheic dermatitis. Mild psoriasis may be responsive to nonprescription treatment, but the initial diagnosis of psoriasis and the management of acute flares require the attention of a primary care provider or dermatologist.

DANDRUFF

Dandruff is a mildly inflammatory scalp disorder that results in excessive scalp scaling.[2,4] It can be a substantial cosmetic concern and associated with social stigma and distress.[3,4] Previously thought to be a separate entity, this disorder represents the milder side of the seborrheic dermatitis spectrum.[2,5]

Dandruff generally appears around the onset of puberty as sebaceous gland and hormonal activity increase.[6,7] Dandruff shows no gender preference and bald spots are typically dandruff free. Sebaceous secretions and individual factors such as skin permeability and fatty acid penetration may also play a role in both disorders.[7,8] Finally, intrinsic (e.g., psychological stress) and extrinsic (e.g., cold temperatures) factors may affect hormone levels and skin moisture, respectively, to exacerbate dandruff symptoms.[6]

Pathophysiology of Dandruff

Dandruff is a hyperproliferative epidermal disorder, characterized by an accelerated epidermal cell turnover and an abnormal keratinization, resulting in inflammation, flaking, and pruritus.[2,6] This process involves the presence of *Malassezia* yeast, inflammation, and disruption in skin proliferation, differentiation, and barrier function.[2] The accelerated cell turnover rate is thought to be caused by the irritant inflammatory effects of fatty acids and cytokines produced by *Malassezia* species.[2,6,7] With dandruff, crevices occur deep in the stratum corneum, which cause cracking and the development of large flakes.[9] If the large scales are broken down to smaller units, dandruff becomes less visible.

Clinical Presentation of Dandruff

Scalp scaling, the sloughing of small white or gray loosely bound flakes, is the only visible manifestation of dandruff. The scaling may occur in small patches or may be distributed across the scalp surface. Patients may experience additional, less common symptoms such as scalp pruritus, dryness, tightness, and irritation. Unlike seborrheic dermatitis and psoriasis, dandruff involves minimal to no inflammation or erythema.[2,10]

Treatment for Dandruff

Treatment Goals

The goals of self-treatment for dandruff are (1) to reduce the epidermal turnover rate of the scalp skin by reducing the number of *Malassezia* species in the scalp, (2) to minimize the cosmetic embarrassment of visible scaling, and (3) to minimize itch.

General Treatment Approach

Routine shampooing with a general-purpose nonmedicated shampoo daily to every other day is often sufficient to control mild–moderate dandruff. If this approach is not effective, the health care provider may recommend nonprescription medicated antidandruff products. Shampoos with harsh surfactants containing sodium lauryl sulfate or sodium laureth sulfate should be avoided because of their damaging effects on the stratum corneum.[6]

Editor's Note: This chapter is based on the 18th edition chapter of the same title, written by Richard N. Herrier.

A cytostatic agent (e.g., pyrithione zinc, selenium sulfide) is generally recommended initially. Contact time is the key to effectiveness of cytostatic medicated shampoos that contain pyrithione zinc or selenium sulfide to suppress the replication of *Malassezia* species.[11,12] The patient should massage the medicated shampoo into the scalp and leave on the hair for 3–5 minutes before rinsing. Repeated (2–3 times) rinsing of the hair after the desired contact time is suggested with medicated shampoos that contain selenium sulfide to ensure that a residue is not left on the hair and possibly cause discoloration. The patient should be instructed to use the medicated shampoo daily for 1 week, then 2–3 times weekly for 2–3 weeks, and thereafter once weekly or every other week to control the disorder.[13] Scalp scrubbers are useful in all patients, especially those with longer hair, to help ensure adequate contact of the medicated shampoo with the scalp.

Alternatively, nonprescription ketoconazole shampoo, an antifungal shampoo that also has anti-*Malassezia* activity, can be used. Shampoos containing coal tar are usually of limited use and reserved for second-line therapy, because they may discolor light hair, clothing, and jewelry. These agents reduce scaling by decreasing the turnover rate of scalp cells.[14,15]

A keratolytic shampoo containing salicylic acid or sulfur may also be used but requires far longer treatment periods and is of limited efficacy.

The section "Nonprescription Medications for Scaly Dermatoses" provides more information on these agents. If dandruff proves resistant to these agents, the patient should be referred to a primary care provider or dermatologist for further evaluation.

SEBORRHEIC DERMATITIS

Seborrheic dermatitis is a chronic inflammatory disorder that occurs predominantly in the areas of greatest sebaceous gland activity (e.g., scalp, face, chest).[3,11,16] It commonly presents as a red, scaly, itchy rash affecting infants (up to 30 months old), adolescents/young adults, and 1%–3% of adults (more commonly men).[5,16,17] Typically more severe during the winter and in low-humidity environments, seborrheic dermatitis may also be aggravated by emotional stress.[16,18] The risk for experiencing seborrheic dermatitis is increased in patients with immunosuppressive disorders (e.g., human immunodeficiency virus [HIV], acquired immunodeficiency syndrome [AIDS], organ transplants) and those with chronic neurologic disorders (e.g., Parkinson disease).[19–21]

Pathophysiology of Seborrheic Dermatitis

Similar to dandruff, seborrheic dermatitis involves *Malassezia* species and accelerated epidermal proliferation. Areas with dense distribution of sebaceous glands are predominantly affected and exhibit more inflammation compared with dandruff.[5,7,19] The characteristic accelerated cell turnover and enhanced sebaceous gland activity give rise to prominent yellow, greasy scales with erythema.[4,5]

Clinical Presentation of Seborrheic Dermatitis

Seborrheic dermatitis can present in a variety of forms based on its severity and affected body area. It can affect the scalp, eyebrows, glabella, eyelid margins, cheeks, paranasal areas, nasolabial folds, beard area, presternal area, central back, retroauricular creases, and in and about the external ear canal. The disorder typically presents as fairly well-demarcated, dull, yellowish, oily, scaly areas on red skin. Pruritus is common.[1,4]

The infantile form of seborrheic dermatitis, also known as *cradle cap,* is common in the first 3 months of life. The prevalence diminishes significantly by 1 year of age and then gradually over the next few years.[22] In the infant population, thick, white to yellow-brown greasy scales tend to concentrate on the scalp, but the scales can extend across the entire scalp and into the face, neck, trunk, and extremity regions with subsequent redness and inflammation.[16,18]

The most common presentation of seborrheic dermatitis in adults is characterized by yellow, greasy scales on the scalp that often extend to the middle third of the face with subsequent eyebrow involvement (see Color Plates, photograph 18). Typically, seborrheic dermatitis manifests as greasy, scaling patches or plaques, exudation, and thick crusting. On the face, flaky scales or yellowish scaling patches on red, itchy skin are seen in the eyebrows and glabella.[3,18] Red scaling, fissures, and swelling may be present in the ear canals, around the auditory meatus, in the postauricular region, or under the earlobe. V-shaped areas of the chest and back intertriginous areas, such as the side of the neck, axillae, submammary region, umbilicus, groin, and gluteal crease, may also be involved.[1,18] In adults, the disease is chronic, lasting for years to decades, with periods of improvement in warmer seasons and periods of exacerbation in the colder months.[18]

Treatment for Seborrheic Dermatitis

Treatment Goals

The goals of self-treatment for seborrheic dermatitis are (1) to reduce inflammation and the epidermal turnover rate of the scalp skin by reducing the level of *Malassezia* species, (2) to minimize or eliminate visible erythema and scaling, and (3) to minimize itch.[16]

General Treatment Approach

Because of the inflammatory nature of seborrheic dermatitis, its treatment is similar to but more aggressive than that of dandruff. Patients should be educated that therapy works by controlling the disease rather than by curing it. Therapy is directed toward loosening and removal of scales and crusts, inhibiting yeast colonization, controlling secondary infection, and reducing erythema and itching. The scales and crust loosen with the use of topical antifungal agents, which are first-line treatment for seborrheic dermatitis.[13] Because seborrheic dermatitis is a chronic disorder, other medicated shampoos such as pyrithione zinc and selenium sulfide may be used. Patients should work the shampoo into the scalp and then leave the lather on the hair and affected areas for 3–5 minutes. Initially, the shampoo should be used daily for the first week or 2, then 2–3 times per week for the next 4 weeks. When the disorder is controlled, the shampoo is applied once a week to prevent relapse.

In infants, seborrheic dermatitis is usually self-limited and treated primarily by gently massaging the scalp with baby oil, followed by the use of a nonmedicated shampoo (e.g., Johnson's baby shampoo, Mustela Foam Shampoo) to remove scales.[1] For cases that do not respond to this treatment, the patient should be referred to a pediatrician. Shampooing is the foundation of treatment in adults, regardless of skin lesion location. Once the disorder is controlled, at least weekly use of shampoos containing pyrithione zinc, selenium sulfide, or ketoconazole should be used to prevent relapse. If the odor of a medicated shampoo is objectionable, its use can be followed by a more cosmetically acceptable shampoo or conditioner. A regular nonmedicated shampoo or liquid dishwashing soap can be used to soften and remove crusts or scales.[12] Topical corticosteroids are not useful in treating dandruff; however, these agents are needed more frequently to treat the greater levels of inflammation in seborrheic dermatitis.[16] These products may be used to manage seborrheic dermatitis whenever erythema persists after therapy with medicated shampoos. Hydrocortisone ointment should be applied no more than twice daily because of the reservoir effect of the stratum corneum that slowly releases the corticosteroid over time. Treatment should continue until symptoms subside but for no more than 7 consecutive days. If the disorder worsens or symptoms persist longer than 7 days, a primary care provider or dermatologist should be consulted, because a more potent topical corticosteroid may be indicated.[12]

PSORIASIS

Psoriasis is a chronic inflammatory disease estimated to affect approximately 7.5 million Americans.[23] Lesions are often localized, but they may become generalized over much of the body surface. Remissions and exacerbations are unpredictable.[1,24] Approximately 50% of people with psoriasis find that lesions may clear spontaneously and remain clear for varying periods of time.[18] Unrelenting generalized psoriasis may cause enough psychological and physical distress to adversely affect a patient's quality of life.[24,25]

The incidence of psoriasis is distributed almost equally among men and women. Psoriasis is seen in all races and geographic regions, but the incidence is lower among people living in countries close to the equator and among people of African American, West African, Native American, and Asian descent.[1,18]

Although the cause of psoriasis is unknown, exacerbations can be triggered by the following[1,18,24,25]:

- Environmental factors such as physical, ultraviolet, and chemical injury
- Various infections (streptococcal infection, HIV infections)
- Prescription drug use (e.g., antimalarials, beta blockers, interferons, lithium, nonsteroidal anti-inflammatory drugs) and withdrawal of systemic corticosteroids
- Emotional and psychological stress
- Obesity
- Use of alcohol and tobacco

Pathophysiology of Psoriasis

Immunologic mechanisms such as T-cell induction, cytokine production, and keratinocyte and epidermal proliferation are believed to contribute to the development and exacerbation of psoriasis. A genetic predisposition is also associated with early-onset disease and first-degree familial history.[25] Epidermal cell turnover rate is approximately 8 times shorter in psoriatic skin than in normal skin.[26] The duration of psoriasis is variable with spontaneous exacerbations and remissions possible. Lesions may last a lifetime or disappear quickly.[18,24]

Clinical Presentation of Psoriasis

Regardless of the clinical form, psoriasis is typically symmetrical. Approximately 90% of patients experiencing psoriasis present with plaque psoriasis. Lesions start as small papules that grow and unite to form plaques. Plaques are typically well marked with a silvery-white scale covering them. Plaques may also be painful or itchy.[18,24,25] (see Color Plates, photographs 19A, B, C). Common sites for psoriasis plaques include the extensor surfaces of the elbows and knees, lumbar region of the back, scalp, trunk, and genital area. When the scale is lifted from the base of the plaque, punctate bleeding points sometimes occur at the plaque site (Auspitz sign).[18,24]

Treatment of Psoriasis

Treatment Goals

The goals of self-treatment for psoriasis are (1) to control or eliminate the signs and symptoms (inflammation, scaling, itching) and (2) to prevent or minimize the likelihood of flare-ups.

General Treatment Approach

Mild cases of psoriasis, characterized by a few localized lesions no larger than a quarter, can be self-treated with topical agents such as hydrocortisone or emollients. Areas of involvement greater than 5%, involvement of the face, or the presence of joint pain dictate that the patient be treated by a primary care provider with more effective prescription medications and phototherapy.[27] Cases not responding to emollients and nonprescription strengths of hydrocortisone or cases in children younger than 2 years should also be referred to a primary care provider or dermatologist.

Numerous nondrug measures can be used by patients in the treatment of psoriasis for both mild and moderate-severe cases. Although these treatments can help symptoms and enhance the local effectiveness of nonprescription and prescription products, these measures alone are unlikely to control the signs and symptoms of the disorder. Patients should avoid physical, chemical, or ultraviolet (UV) trauma to the skin because of the likelihood of lesions developing at the site of skin trauma. Scale removal is an important treatment modality, because scales facilitate the continuation of psoriatic plaques and interfere with the penetration of topical agents.[28] Patients with psoriasis should be encouraged to bathe with lubricating bath products (see Chapter 33) 2–3 times per week using tepid water.[29]

Daily lubrication of the skin after a bath or shower is an essential part of therapy. Emollients moisturize, lubricate, and soothe dry and flaky skin, as well as reduce fissure formation within plaques and help maintain flexibility of the surrounding skin. Emollients (e.g., Lubriderm Lotion, Nivea Cream) should be applied to the lesions within minutes of bathing. Pruritic dry skin is common in psoriasis, and emollients and lubricating bath products often provide some relief for this symptom.[30] To be effective, these products need to be applied liberally with gentle rubbing, up to 4 times daily. Loose scales can be removed by gently rubbing with a soft cloth.

Hydrocortisone ointment 1% is the nonprescription treatment of choice for individuals with bright red lesions. Typically, soothing local therapy with emollients and hydrocortisone ointment 1% can be beneficial. In some patients, nonprescription treatment may be ineffective and more aggressive treatments may be needed.[25]

In most cases, psoriasis will not be controlled by nonprescription treatment, and referral to a primary care provider or dermatologist will be necessary. For patients who are not candidates for nonprescription treatment, the selection of therapy must be individualized based on the site, severity, duration, and previous treatment of the disorder, and the patient's age. Treatment may be topical, systemic, or a combination of both. Factors in determining appropriate therapy include body surface area affected by psoriasis, patient's age, treatment cost, and ability of the patient to adhere to the regimen. For moderate–severe or recalcitrant psoriasis, more aggressive treatment is necessary. Dermatologists can help treat this type of psoriasis.

Psoriasis can be controlled but not cured, and remissions do occur. Patients should be educated on controlling the disorder to increase compliance with burdensome and prolonged treatment regimens. In addition, education on understanding and acceptance of the disorder may help reduce the patient's emotional stress and psychogenic exacerbations. Prevention of flare-ups should be emphasized. During flare-ups, however, signs and symptoms can usually be controlled adequately with appropriate patient education and treatment. Flare-ups can be prevented by minimizing identified precipitating factors, such as emotional stress, skin irritation, and physical trauma.

Nonprescription Medications Used to Treat Scaly Dermatoses

A variety of products are used to treat or reduce scaly dermatoses. In addition, hydrocortisone is used to control the inflammation associated with seborrheic dermatitis and psoriasis. Table 34–1 summarizes the concentrations and indications of currently approved agents,[18,31] and the algorithm in Figure 34–1 outlines self-treatment with these agents.

Patients should shampoo with a nonmedicated, nonresidue regular shampoo to remove dirt, oil, and scales from scalp and hair before they use a medicated shampoo. Many shampoos leave a residue on the hair shaft and scalp that may aggravate scaly dermatoses of the scalp. Nonresidue shampoos do not interfere with these scalp disorders; rather they leave the scalp clean and receptive to optimal effects from medicated shampoos. After the nonresidue shampoo is rinsed, a medicated shampoo can be left on the scalp for up to 5 minutes. The patient can use this treatment daily, if needed, until symptoms are relieved and then 2–3 times weekly.[12]

TABLE 34–1 Concentrations of Approved Nonprescription Ingredients for Products Used to Treat Scaly Dermatoses

	Concentration (%)		
Ingredient	Dandruff	Seborrheic Dermatitis	Psoriasis
Coal tar	0.5–5	0.5–5	0.5–5
Hydrocortisone	—	0.5–1	0.5–1
Ketoconazole	1	1	1
Pyrithione zinc (brief exposure)	0.3–2	0.95–2	2
Pyrithione zinc (residual)	0.1–0.25	0.1–0.25	0.25
Salicylic acid	1.8–3	1.8–3	1.8–3
Selenium sulfide	1	1	1
Sulfur	2–5	2–5	—

Source: References 18 and 31.

Cytostatic Agents

Topical cytostatic agents are known to decrease the rate of epidermal cell replication. This action increases the time required for epidermal cell turnover, which in turn allows the possibility of normalizing epidermal differentiation, resulting in a slow decline in visible scales. However, these products have limited efficacy and multiple other issues that make them poor alternatives to anti-*Malassezia* products.[3]

Pyrithione Zinc

Pyrithione zinc's mechanism of action is its anti-*Malassezia* activity, which reduces the yeast count in the scalp and skin. Product effectiveness is influenced by several factors. Pyrithione zinc binds strongly to both hair and the external skin layers of the scalp, and the extent of binding correlates with clinical performance. The Food and Drug Administration (FDA) recommends concentrations of 0.3%–2.0% for treating dandruff and 0.95%–2.0% for treating seborrheic dermatitis.[32] Nonprescription shampoos and soaps are currently available in 1% and 2% concentrations. Pyrithione zinc shampoo is well tolerated when used as directed and is not associated with any major adverse effects. Contact with the eyes should be avoided to prevent stinging.

Selenium Sulfide

Selenium sulfide and pyrithione zinc have a similar mechanism of action.[19] As with pyrithione zinc, selenium sulfide is more effective with longer contact time and therefore should be applied in a similar manner.[11,12] Selenium sulfide must be rinsed from the hair thoroughly or discoloration may result, especially in light or dyed hair. Frequent use may leave a residual odor and an oily scalp.

Selenium sulfide is approved in a 1% concentration in nonprescription products to treat dandruff and seborrheic

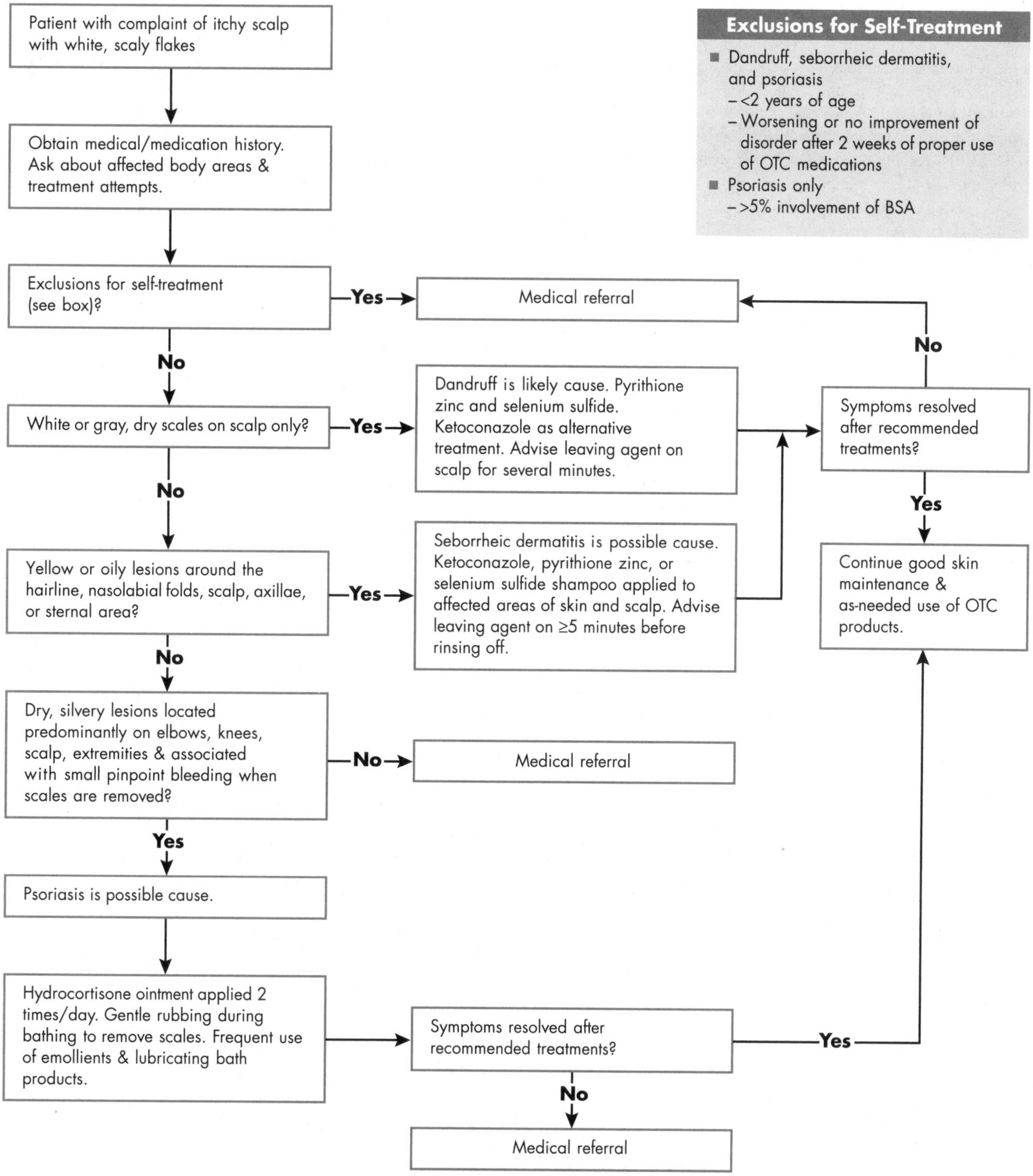

FIGURE 34–1 Self-care for scaly dermatoses. Key: BSA = Body surface area; OTC = over-the-counter

dermatitis.[32] A 2.5% lotion formulation is available by prescription for use in resistant cases and other topical fungal infections. The risk of irritation of the mucous membranes and scalp from selenium sulfide is minimal, and no adverse effects are associated with routine use of the 1% shampoo. Contact with the eyelids should be avoided because of the potential for eye irritation.

Coal Tar

For many years, the therapeutic response to coal tar products was believed to be caused solely by its phototoxicity. Now it is believed that coal tar may work by its ability to cross-link with DNA and arrest excessive skin cell proliferation. Coal tar products have long been popular for treating dandruff, seborrheic dermatitis, and psoriasis. Although many nonprescription products are available, their usefulness is limited because of their potentially unacceptable cosmetic properties and limited clinical efficacy.[15]

Coal tar is available in concentrations of 0.5%–5% as creams, ointments, pastes, lotions, bath oils, shampoos, soaps, and gels to self-treat dermatologic disorders.[32] This variety of dosage forms is partly a result of an attempt to develop a cosmetically acceptable product: one that masks the odor, color, and staining properties of crude coal tar, which most patients find esthetically unappealing.

Adverse effects associated with the use of coal tar include folliculitis (particularly of the axilla and groin), stains to the skin and hair (particularly blond, gray, and dyed hair), photosensitization, and irritant contact dermatitis.[33] Rarely, the disorder may worsen on exposure to coal tar products. This situation is of particular concern in the acute phase of psoriasis, when topical corticosteroids are recommended to reduce inflammation before coal tar preparations are used.

Coal tar products may be applied to the body, arms, and legs, preferably at bedtime. Because coal tar stains most materials, the patient should use bed linen and clothing for which staining would not present a problem. Overnight application is followed by a bath in the morning to remove residual coal tar and loosen psoriatic scales. Patients using coal tar preparations should avoid sun exposure for 24 hours after application.

Antifungal Agent

Ketoconazole

Ketoconazole, a synthetic azole antifungal agent, is available as a nonprescription shampoo formulation. Ketoconazole 1% is active against most pathogenic fungi but is indicated specifically for *Malassezia.* Patients should use ketoconazole shampoo twice a week for 4 weeks, with at least 3 days between each treatment. Once the disorder is controlled, the shampoo can be applied once weekly to prevent relapse. Adverse effects associated with 1% ketoconazole shampoo are minimal, but hair loss, skin irritation, abnormal hair texture, and dry skin have been reported. Patients should be advised to avoid contact of ketoconazole shampoo with the eyes, because irritation may occur.

Keratolytic Agents

The keratolytic agents, salicylic acid and sulfur, can be used in dandruff and seborrheic dermatitis to loosen and lyse keratin aggregates, thereby facilitating their removal from the scalp in smaller particles. These agents act by dissolving the "cement" that holds epidermal cells together. Vehicle composition, contact time, and concentration are important factors in the success of a keratolytic agent. Keratolytic concentrations in nonprescription scalp products (Table 34–2) are not sufficient to impair the normal skin barrier, but they do affect the abnormal, incompletely keratinized stratum corneum.

Keratolytic agents have a primary, concentration-dependent irritant effect, particularly on mucous membranes and the conjunctiva of the eye. The directions and precautions for the use of keratolytic shampoos are similar to those for shampoos containing other therapeutic agents, with the exception that prolonged use is usually necessary to obtain a therapeutic response.

Salicylic Acid

Salicylic acid decreases skin pH, which causes increased hydration of keratin and therefore facilitates its loosening and removal. Topical salicylic acid is useful for psoriasis when thick scales are present. However, application over extensive areas should be avoided because of the potential for percutaneous absorption. Salicylic acid has been approved in concentrations of 1.8%–3% to self-treat dandruff, seborrheic dermatitis, and psoriasis.[32] One study showed shampoo containing 1.5% ciclopirox olamine and 3% salicylic acid had efficacy similar to that of 2.0% ketoconazole shampoo for dandruff.[34] The combination product with ciclopirox is not available in the United States. At these concentrations, the keratolytic effect typically takes 7–10 days.

Sulfur

Sulfur is believed to cause increased sloughing of cells and to reduce corneocyte counts. Sulfur has been approved in concentrations of 2%–5% to self-treat dandruff only.[32] Although it is approved as a single-entity active ingredient, sulfur is often combined with salicylic acid. Although not an FDA-approved indication, this combination has been commonly used to self-treat seborrheic dermatitis.[24] The use of nonprescription topical preparations containing sulfur has not been associated with any significant adverse effects.

Topical Hydrocortisone

Topical hydrocortisone 0.5% and 1% is available without a prescription and is FDA approved for inflammatory skin disorders such as allergic contact dermatitis, insect bites, eczema, and psoriasis. It may be useful for seborrheic dermatitis accompanied by inflammation that is unresponsive to medicated shampoos and is the nonprescription treatment of choice for mild psoriasis.[11,12,18,19]

Nonprescription hydrocortisone products can play a role in managing mild psoriasis. Topical corticosteroids have several effects (e.g., anti-inflammatory, vasoconstrictive, immunosuppressive) on cellular activity, which can result in decreased redness and itching. Hydrocortisone ointment is the most potent and effective dosage form. Ointment can be enhanced in psoriasis by waiting 30 minutes after its application and then covering the area of the psoriatic plaque with a greasy emollient such as petrolatum, which acts as an occlusive dressing.

Adverse effects associated with the use of topical corticosteroids include local atrophy after prolonged use and aggravation of certain cutaneous infections. The possibility of systemic sequelae exists and is enhanced by the use of the more potent compounds, use of occlusive dressings, or application to large areas of the body.

Assessment of Scaly Dermatoses: A Case-Based Approach

Differentiation of the scaly dermatoses involves several factors. The appearance of the scales in the early stages of a disorder is not always definitive. In these cases, the presence and nature of other symptoms or the location of the dermatitis provides additional important clues to its assessment. Factors that precipitate or exacerbate the disorder are also helpful in defining the disorder. Table 34–3 describes the distinguishing features of these three dermatoses. Cases 34–1 and 34–2 illustrate the assessment of patients with scaly dermatoses.

TABLE 34–2 Selected Nonprescription Products to Treat Dandruff and Scaly Dermatoses

Trade Name	Primary Ingredients
Cytostatic Products	
DHS Zinc Shampoo	Pyrithione zinc 2%
DHS Tar Shampoo	Coal tar 0.5%
DHS Tar Gel Shampoo	Coal tar 0.5%
Head & Shoulders Dandruff Shampoo	Pyrithione zinc 1%
Head & Shoulders Clinical Strength Shampoo	Selenium sulfide 1%
Neutrogena T/Derm Body Oil	Tar 5% (equivalent to coal tar 1.2%)
Neutrogena T/Gel Extra Strength Therapeutic Shampoo	Tar 4% (equivalent to coal tar 1%)
Neutrogena T/Gel Shampoo	Tar 2% (equivalent to coal tar 0.5%)
Pentrax Shampoo	Coal tar extract 5%
Sebulon Shampoo	Pyrithione zinc 2%
Selsun Blue Medicated Treatment Shampoo	Selenium sulfide 1%
Zincon Shampoo	Pyrithione zinc 1%
ZNP Cleansing Bar	Pyrithione zinc 2%
Keratolytic Products	
Denorex Extra Strength	Salicylic acid 3%
MG217 Medicated Tar-Free Shampoo	Salicylic acid 3%; sulfur 5%
Sebucare Lotion	Salicylic acid 1.8%
Sebulex Conditioning Shampoo with Protein	Salicylic acid 2%; sulfur 2%
Sulfoam Medicated Antidandruff Shampoo	Sulfur 2%
Sul-Ray Cleansing Bar	Sulfur 5%
Sul-Ray Dandruff Shampoo	Sulfur 2%
X-Seb Shampoo	Salicylic acid 4%
Antifungal Products	
Nizoral A-D Shampoo	Ketoconazole 1%
Combination Products	
Neutrogena T/Sal Maximum Strength Therapeutic Shampoo	Salicylic acid 3%; coal tar extract 2%
P&S Plus Gel	Coal tar solution 8%; salicylic acid 2%
Scalpicin Maximum Strength Foam/Solution	Salicylic acid 3%; menthol
Sebutone Shampoo	Coal tar 0.5%; sulfur 2%; salicylic acid 2%
X-Seb Plus Shampoo	Pyrithione zinc 1%; salicylic acid 2%
X-Seb T Shampoo	Coal tar solution 10%; salicylic acid 4%
X-Seb T Plus Shampoo	Coal tar solution 10%; salicylic acid 3%; menthol 1%

TABLE 34-3 **Distinguishing Features of Scaly Dermatoses**

	Dandruff	Seborrheic Dermatitis	Psoriasis
Location	Scalp	Scalp, face, trunk	Scalp, elbows, knees, trunk, lower extremities
Exacerbating factors	Generally a stable condition, but may be exacerbated by psychological stress, cold temperatures, dry climate	Immunosuppression, neurologic conditions, environmental factors, stress	Environmental factors, infection, medications, stress, obesity, alcohol, tobacco
Appearance	Thin, white, or grayish flakes; even distribution on scalp	Macules, patches, and thin plaques of discrete yellow, oily scales on red skin	Discrete symmetrical, red plaques with sharp borders; silvery white scales; small bleeding points when scale is removed; difficult to distinguish from seborrhea in early stages or in intertriginous zones
Inflammation	Absent	Present	Present
Epidermal hyperplasia	Absent	Present	Present
Epidermal kinetics	Turnover rate 2 times faster than normal	Turnover rate about 3 times faster than normal	Turnover rate about 8 times faster than normal

Source: References 1, 4, 6, 16, 18, 19, 24, and 25.

CASE 34-1

Relevant Evaluation Criteria	Scenario/Model Outcome
Collect	
1. Gather essential information about the patient's symptoms, including	
a. Description of symptom(s) (i.e., nature, onset, duration, severity, associated symptoms)	Patient complains of yellow, oily scales along his hairline and around his nose. Some minor erythema is also present in these areas.
b. Description of any factors that seem to precipitate, exacerbate, and/or relieve the patient's symptom(s)	The condition has grown worse since the onset of cold weather.
c. Description of the patient's efforts to relieve the symptoms	Washing the face twice daily with hand soap has not proven beneficial.
d. Patient's identity	Robert Plant
e. Patient's age, gender, height, and weight	57 years old, male, 5 ft 9 in., 185 lb
f. Patient's occupation	Sales manager
g. Patient's dietary habits	Normal healthy diet
h. Patient's sleep habits	6–7 hours per night
i. Concurrent medical conditions, prescription and nonprescription medications, and dietary supplements	Depression: sertraline 50 mg daily; hypertension: hydrochlorothiazide 25 mg daily
j. Allergies	NKA
k. History of other adverse reactions to medications	None
l. Other (describe) ______	n/a
Assess	
2. Differentiate patient's signs/symptoms, and correctly identify the patient's primary problem(s) (Table 34–3).	Robert appears to have seborrheic dermatitis on his face. His scalp should be examined closely for involvement as well.
3. Identify exclusions for self-treatment (Figure 34–1).	None

CASE 34-1 *continued*

Relevant Evaluation Criteria	Scenario/Model Outcome
4. Formulate a comprehensive list of therapeutic alternatives for the primary problem to determine whether triage to a medical provider is required, and share this information with the patient or caregiver.	Options include (1) Recommend self-care with an appropriate OTC product and nondrug measures. (2) Recommend self-care with an appropriate OTC product and nondrug measures until a PCP or dermatologist can be consulted. (3) Refer Robert to a PCP or dermatologist. (4) Take no action.
Plan	
5. Select an optimal therapeutic alternative to address the patient's problem, taking into account patient preferences.	OTC treatment with pyrithione zinc shampoo can be used initially. Ketoconazole or selenium sulfide shampoo is a good alternative agent to recommend if the patient prefers to use an alternative product. Hydrocortisone 1% ointment can be added to red areas if 1 week of treatment with medicated shampoo does not resolve redness.
6. Describe the recommended therapeutic approach to the patient or caregiver.	"For the first week, shampoo the hair with the medicated shampoo and apply it to the affected areas of the face daily. Leave on for 5 minutes; then rinse off. For the next 4 weeks, repeat the preceding procedure only 2–3 times per week. Regardless of the location of the lesions, the hair needs to be shampooed to prevent relapse. Once the condition is controlled, the hair should be shampooed at least once a week to prevent relapse."
7. Explain to the patient or caregiver the rationale for selecting the recommended therapeutic approach from the considered therapeutic alternatives.	"You may use the pyrithione zinc, selenium sulfide, or ketoconazole shampoo according to personal preference and cost."
Implement	
8. When recommending self-care with nonprescription medications and/or nondrug therapy, convey accurate information to the patient or caregiver.	See the box "Patient Education for Dandruff and Seborrheic Dermatitis."
Solicit follow-up questions from the patient or caregiver.	"What should I use on my hair on the days I do not use the medicated shampoo?"
Answer the patient's or caregiver's questions.	"Any type of nonmedicated shampoo is fine to use. One that does not leave a residue is preferred. Once your condition is controlled, daily use of a shampoo is not necessary unless your scalp is especially oily."
Follow-up: Monitor and Evaluate	
9. Assess patient outcome.	Contact the patient in a week to assess his progress in resolving his seborrheic dermatitis.

Key: n/a = Not applicable; NKA = no known allergies; OTC = over-the-counter; PCP = primary care provider.

Patient Counseling for Scaly Dermatoses

Patients need to know that scaly dermatoses are rarely cured by pharmacotherapy; rather, nonprescription agents help control the signs and symptoms of the disorders. Patients should also be advised that fluctuation in severity of seborrheic dermatitis and psoriasis may be related to emotional, physical, or environmental factors.

Explanations of the proper use of antifungal, cytostatic, and keratolytic agents should include information about the contact time of the agent on the affected area(s), possible adverse effects, and signs and symptoms that may indicate a need for medical attention. The box "Patient Education for Dandruff and Seborrheic Dermatitis" and the box "Patient Education for Psoriasis" list specific information to provide patients.

Evaluation of Patient Outcomes for Scaly Dermatoses

Follow-up on the patient's progress should occur after 1 week of self-treatment. If the symptoms have worsened after this period, the patient should consult a primary care provider or dermatologist. If

CASE 34-2

Relevant Evaluation Criteria	Scenario/Model Outcome
Collect	
1. Gather essential information about the patient's symptoms, including	
a. Description of symptom(s) (i.e., nature, onset, duration, severity, associated symptoms)	The patient has had shiny scales bilaterally on her elbows for longer than 6 months. Some minor bleeding occurs when the scales are removed. She now complains of the development of lesions on both of her knees.
b. Description of any factors that seem to precipitate, exacerbate, and/or relieve the patient's symptom(s)	The lesions appeared to worsen after her recent divorce from her husband.
c. Description of the patient's efforts to relieve the symptoms	Use of hydrocortisone 1% cream once daily has been marginally effective. Use of lotion on the lesions is soothing.
d. Patient's identity	Elaine Abel
e. Patient's age, gender, height, and weight	43 years old, female, 5 ft 6 in., 195 lb
f. Patient's occupation	Factory line worker
g. Patient's dietary habits	Normal diet
h. Patient's sleep habits	Averages 6–8 hours per night.
i. Concurrent medical conditions, prescription and nonprescription medications, and dietary supplements	Diabetes × 2 years: fairly well controlled with metformin 500 mg twice daily; hypothyroidism × 15 years: well controlled with levothyroxine 100 mcg once daily; allergic rhinitis × 20+ years: controlled with loratadine 10 mg once daily
j. Allergies	Penicillin: rash
k. History of other adverse reactions to medications	None
l. Other (describe) ______	Elaine showers once or twice daily.
Assess	
2. Differentiate patient's signs/symptoms, and correctly identify the patient's primary problem(s) (Table 34–3).	Elaine possibly has a flare of psoriasis. The type of lesions and bilateral appearance support this assessment.
3. Identify exclusions for self-treatment (Figure 34–1).	The worsening symptoms and appearance of the lesions on the patient's knees indicate a worsening condition that requires more than self-care.
4. Formulate a comprehensive list of therapeutic alternatives for the primary problem to determine whether triage to a medical provider is required, and share this information with the patient or caregiver.	Options include (1) Refer Elaine to a PCP or dermatologist for a differential diagnosis. (2) Recommend an OTC product (hydrocortisone ointment 1% and emollient therapy) to use until the PCP appointment. (3) Take no action.
Plan	
5. Select an optimal therapeutic alternative to address the patient's problem, taking into account patient preferences.	Refer the patient to a PCP or dermatologist for a differential diagnosis and treatment.
6. Describe the recommended therapeutic approach to the patient or caregiver.	"Contact your primary care provider or dermatologist to accurately diagnose your condition. Until the time of your appointment, you could switch to applying hydrocortisone ointment 1% to the affected areas 2 times daily. Wait 30 minutes and then liberally apply an emollient."
7. Explain to the patient or caregiver the rationale for selecting the recommended therapeutic approach from the considered therapeutic alternatives.	"You need to see a primary care provider or dermatologist, because nonprescription therapy won't be as effective as prescription medications for disease as extensive as yours."

CASE 34-2 *continued*

Relevant Evaluation Criteria	Scenario/Model Outcome
Implement	
8. When recommending self-care with nonprescription medications and/or nondrug therapy, convey accurate information to the patient or caregiver.	See the box "Patient Education for Psoriasis" for nondrug measures to treat psoriasis.
Solicit follow-up questions from the patient or caregiver.	"I saw on the internet that treatment with coal tar products is an option for psoriasis. Should I use one of these products?"
Answer the patient's or caregiver's questions.	"Although coal tar products have been used for a long time, topical corticosteroid therapy is now considered the first-line topical therapy for most patients. The smell and mess associated with using coal tar products are major drawbacks, plus they have limited efficacy."
Follow-up: Monitor and Evaluate	
9. Assess patient outcome.	Call patient in 2 days to ensure that she made an appointment with her PCP or a dermatologist.

Key: OTC = Over-the-counter; PCP = primary care provider.

PATIENT EDUCATION FOR

Dandruff and Seborrheic Dermatitis

The primary objective of self-treating dandruff and seborrheic dermatitis is to reduce the turnover rate of skin cells, which is responsible for the scaly lesions. Controlling inflammation and itching of the affected areas is another treatment objective. Although these disorders are chronic and incurable, carefully following product instructions and the self-care measures can help ensure optimal therapeutic outcomes for many patients.

General Measures

- Shampoo the hair with the medicated shampoo. Leave the shampoo on the hair for 5 minutes. Then rinse the scalp and face thoroughly.
- Use the shampoo for a minimum of 2 weeks to determine effectiveness; after 4 weeks of use, apply the shampoo once a week to control the condition.
- If you are experiencing persistent itching and inflammation, apply a thin layer of hydrocortisone cream no more than 2 times a day. Wash the affected area(s) before use.
- With use of medication and proper nondrug therapy, noticeable improvement could be observed within 7–14 days. Complete control of the disorder is possible with weekly use of the medicated shampoo. It is likely that exacerbations may occasionally appear, especially during the winter months.
- Stinging or burning may occur if a medicated shampoo enters the eyes.

Dandruff

- Use a medicated shampoo containing pyrithione zinc or selenium sulfide. If these agents are ineffective, consult your primary care provider or a dermatologist. Massage the medicated shampoo and leave on the hair for 3–5 minutes before rinsing. Repeated rinsing (2–3 times) after the desired contact time is suggested. Use the shampoo daily for 1 week; then use it 2–3 times weekly for 2–3 weeks, and thereafter once weekly or every other week to control the disorder.
- Coal tar products can be used; however, they have limited efficacy. Coal tar shampoos can stain light hair and cause *folliculitis* (inflammation of hair follicles), dermatitis, and *photosensitization* (sensitivity of the skin to sunlight).

Seborrheic Dermatitis

- More aggressive doses of the anti-*Malassezia* shampoos are used for seborrheic dermatitis than for dandruff. Regardless of the location of the lesions, the hair needs to be shampooed. The scalp always has the highest concentration of *Malassezia* yeast and is the source of the yeast that causes skin lesions. Apply the shampoo to hair, scalp, and to any lesions on face, hairline, or body; then massage these areas thoroughly. Use product once daily for the first week; then reduce use to 2–3 times a week thereafter. Use a medicated shampoo containing ketoconazole, pyrithione zinc, or selenium sulfide. Shampoo the hair and scalp, and apply shampoo directly to any lesions on the face and hairline. Daily use for seborrheic dermatitis is appropriate for the first week; after that reduce use to 2–3 times a week. Washing the hair at least weekly with a cytostatic agent is absolutely essential to prevent relapses, even when lesions appear only on the face.
- If redness persists after therapy with medicated shampoos, apply hydrocortisone ointment 2 times a day until symptoms subside, and then apply the ointment intermittently to control acute exacerbations. Do not use this agent longer than 7 days. Prolonged use can cause rebound flare-ups when the hydrocortisone is discontinued.

When to Seek Medical Attention

- Consult a primary care provider or dermatologist if the condition does not improve or if it worsens after 2 weeks of treatment with nonprescription medications.

PATIENT EDUCATION FOR Psoriasis

The primary objective of self-treating psoriasis is to reduce the turnover rate of skin cells, which is responsible for the scaly lesions. Controlling inflammation and itching of the affected areas and hydrating the skin are other treatment objectives. Although psoriasis is chronic and incurable, carefully following product instructions and self-care measures can help ensure optimal therapeutic outcomes for many patients.

- For itchy, dry skin, use emollients and lubricating bath products (see Chapter 33). Remove scales by gently rubbing them with a soft cloth after the bath. Do not rub vigorously.
- For psoriasis involving more than one or two coin-sized lesions, consult a primary care provider or dermatologist.
- Prevent flare-ups by minimizing factors that you know will exacerbate the disorder, such as emotional stress, skin irritation, and physical trauma.

When to Seek Medical Attention

- If you have psoriasis lesions plus joint pain, consult a primary care provider or dermatologist for treatment.
- If hydrocortisone ointment and emollients are not effective, or if the affected area has more than a few less-than-quarter-size lesions, consult a primary care provider or dermatologist for treatment with prescription products.
- Consult a primary care provider or dermatologist if the condition does not improve or if it worsens after 2 weeks of treatment with nonprescription medications.

the disorder has not worsened, the provider should ask the patient to return after a second week of treatment. If the symptoms persist or have worsened after this period, the patient should consult a primary care provider.

Key Points for Scaly Dermatoses

- Mild–moderate scaly dermatoses can often be effectively managed with topical nonprescription products.
- Product selection should be based on an evaluation of the patient's history and prior response to treatment, as well as a careful evaluation of the risks and benefits of using the nonprescription products.
- The provider should be sure to educate patients about the proper application of topical therapy, which greatly impacts the efficacy of therapy.

REFERENCES

1. James WD, Berger TG, Elston DM. *Andrews' Diseases of the Skin: Clinical Dermatology.* 11th ed. Philadelphia, PA: Saunders Elsevier; 2011.
2. Schwartz JR, Messenger AG, Tosti A, et al. A comprehensive pathophysiology of dandruff and seborrheic dermatitis—towards a more precise definition of scalp health. *Acta Derm Venereol.* 2013;93(2):131–7. doi: 10.2340/00015555-1382.
3. Hay RJ, Graham-Brown RA. Dandruff and seborrhoeic dermatitis: causes and management. *Clin Exp Dermatol.* 1997;22(1):3–6. doi: 10.1046/j.1365-2230.1997.d01-231.x.
4. Naldi L, Rebora A. Seborrheic dermatitis. *N Engl J Med.* 2009;360(4):387–96. doi: 10.1056/NEJMcp0806464.
5. Dessinioti C, Katsambas A. Seborrheic dermatitis: etiology, risk factors, and treatments: facts and controversies. *Clin Dermatol.* 2013;31(4):343–51. doi: 10.1016/j.clindermatol.2013.01.001.
6. Turner GA, Hoptroff M, Harding CR. Stratum corneum dysfunction in dandruff. *Int J Cosmet Sci.* 2012;34(4):298–306. doi: 10.1111/j.1468-2494.2012.00723.x.
7. Ro BI, Dawson TL. The role of sebaceous gland activity and scalp microfloral metabolism in the etiology of seborrheic dermatitis and dandruff. *J Investig Dermatol Symp Proc.* 2005;10(3):194–7. doi: 10.1111/j.1087-0024.2005.10104.x.
8. DeAngelis YM, Gemmer CM, Kaczvinsky JR, et al. Three etiologic facets of dandruff and seborrheic dermatitis: Malassezia fungi, sebaceous lipids, and individual sensitivity. *J Investig Dermatol Symp Proc.* 2005;10(3):295–7. doi: 10.1111/j.1087-0024.2005.10119.x.
9. Ackerman AB, Kligman AM. Some observations on dandruff. *J Soc Cosmet Chem.* 1969;20:81–101.
10. Grimalt R. A practical guide to scalp disorders. *J Investig Dermatol Symp Proc.* 2007;12(2):10–4. doi: 10.1038/sj.jidsymp.5650048.
11. Shin H, Kwon OS, Won CH, et al. Clinical efficacies of topical agents for the treatment of seborrheic dermatitis of the scalp: a comparative study. *J Dermatol.* 2009;36(3):131–7. doi: 10.1111/j.1346-8138.2009.00607.x.
12. Stefanaki I, Katsambas A. Therapeutic update on seborrheic dermatitis. *Skin Therapy Lett.* 2010;15(5):1–4. PMID: 20505895.
13. Johnson BA, Nunley JR. Treatment of seborrheic dermatitis. *Am Fam Physician.* 2000;61(9):2703–10. PMID: 10821151.
14. PC-TAR (coal tar shampoo) [package insert]. Mt Vernon, NY: Geritrex LLC; 2016.
15. Piérard-Franchimont C, Piérard GE, Vroome V, et al. Comparative anti-dandruff efficacy between a tar and a non-tar shampoo. *Dermatology.* 2000;200(2):181–4. doi: 10.1159/000018362.
16. Clark GW, Pope SM, Jaboori KA. Diagnosis and treatment of seborrheic dermatitis. *Am Fam Physician.* 2015;91(3):185–90. PMID: 25822272.
17. Gupta AK, Bluhm R. Seborrheic dermatitis. *J Eur Acad Dermatol Venereol.* 2004;18(1):13–26. doi: 10.1111/j.1468-3083.2004.00693.x.
18. Goldsmith LA, Katz SI, Gilchrest BA, et al., eds. *Fitzpatrick's Dermatology in General Medicine.* 8th ed. New York, NY: McGraw-Hill; 2012.
19. Hay RJ. Malassezia, dandruff and seborrheic dermatitis: an overview. *Brit J Derm.* 2011:165(Suppl 2):2–8. doi: 10.1111/j.1365-2133.2011.10570.x.
20. Lally A, Casabonne D, Imko-Walczuk B, et al. Prevalence of benign cutaneous disease among Oxford renal transplant recipients. *J Eur Acad Dermatol Venereol.* 2011;25(4):462–70. doi: 10.1111/j.1468-3083.2010.03814.x.
21. Blanes M, Belinchón I, Merino E, et al. Current prevalence and characteristics of dermatoses associated with human immunodeficiency virus infection. *Actas Dermosifiliogr.* 2010;101(8):702–9. doi: 10.1016/s1578-2190(10)70700-9.
22. Foley P, Zuo Y, Plunkett A, et al. The frequency of common skin conditions in preschool-aged children in Australia: seborrheic dermatitis and pityriasis capitis (cradle cap). *Arch Dermatol.* 2003;139(3):318–22. doi: 10.1001/archderm.139.3.318.
23. National Psoriasis Foundation. Fact sheet. Available at: https://www.psoriasis.org/sites/default/files/psoriasis_fact_sheet.pdf. Accessed June 2, 2017.
24. Menter A, Gottleib A, Feldman S, et al. Guidelines of care for the management of psoriasis and psoriatic arthritis. *J Am Acad Dermatol.* 2008;58(5):826–50. doi: 10.1016/j.jaad.2008.02.039.
25. Luba KM, Stulberg DL. Chronic plaque psoriasis. *Am Fam Physician.* 2006;73(4):636–44. PMID: 16506705.

26. Weinstein GD, McCullough JL, Ross P. Cell proliferation in normal epidermis. *J Invest Dermatol.* 1984;82(6):623–8. PMID: 6725985.
27. Patrizi A, Raone B, Ravaioli GM. Management of atopic dermatitis: safety and efficacy of phototherapy. *Clin Cosmet Investig Dermatol.* 2015;8:511–20. doi: 10.2147/CCID.S87987.
28. Stern, RS. Psoralen and ultraviolet A light therapy for psoriasis. *N Engl J Med.* 2007;357(4):682–90. doi: 10.1056/nejmct072317.
29. Schiener R, Brockow T, Franke A, et al. Bath PUVA and saltwater baths followed by UV-B phototherapy as treatments for psoriasis: a randomized controlled trial. *Arch Dermatol.* 2007; 143(5):586-96. doi: 10.1001/archderm.143.5.586.
30. Eichenfield LF, Totri C. Optimizing outcomes for paediatric atopic dermatitis. *Br J Dermatol.* 2014;170:31–7. doi: 10.1111/bjd.12976.
31. U.S. Food and Drug Administration. Final rule: dandruff, seborrheic dermatitis and psoriasis drug products for over-the-counter human use. *Fed Regist.* December 4, 1991;56:63554–69.
32. U.S. Food and Drug Administration. *CFR: Code of Federal Regulations.* Title 21. Available at: http://www.accessdata.fda.gov/scripts/cdrh/cfdocs/cfcfr/CFRSearch.cfm?fr=358.710. Accessed June 2, 2017.
33. Schwartz RA, Janusz CA, Janniger CK. Seborrheic dermatitis: an overview. *Am Fam Physician.* 2006;74(1):125–30. PMID: 16848386.
34. Squire RA, Goode K. A randomised, single-blind, single-centre clinical trial to evaluate comparative clinical efficacy of shampoos containing ciclopirox olamine (1.5%) and salicylic ac-id (3%), or ketoconazole (2%, Nizoral) for the treatment of dandruff/seborrhoeic dermatitis. *J Dermatolog Treat.* 2002 Jun;13(2):51–60. doi: 10.1080/095466302317584395.

CHAPTER 35

CONTACT DERMATITIS

PATRICIA L. DARBISHIRE AND KIMBERLY S. PLAKE

Contact dermatitis is a condition characterized by inflammation, redness, itching, burning, stinging, and vesicle and pustule formation on dermal areas exposed to irritant or antigenic agents.[1,2] The two primary types of contact dermatitis, classified by etiology and presentation, are discussed in this chapter. *Irritant contact dermatitis* (ICD) is an inflammatory reaction of the skin caused by exposure to an irritant substance. *Allergic contact dermatitis* (ACD) is an immunologic reaction of the skin caused by exposure to an antigen.[2]

According to the U.S. Bureau of Labor Statistics, work-related skin disorders comprised 14.9% of total workplace injuries in 2014.[3] Individuals employed in forestry, agriculture, and hunting and fishing industries have the greatest incidence of work-related skin diseases or disorders at 9.7 per 10,000 workers.[3] Educational and health services sectors have an incidence of 4 per 10,000 workers. This sector is followed by manufacturing with an incidence of 3.6 per 10,000, and leisure, entertainment, and hospitality with an incidence of 3.2 per 10,000.[3] Of the reported 2014 U.S. occupational dermatitis cases, 32.5% were identified as ACD, 15.5% as ICD, and 45.2% as unspecified.[4] The estimated cost for managing contact dermatitis, which includes treatment and workdays lost, is $1 billion annually.[5,6]

IRRITANT CONTACT DERMATITIS

Individuals who frequently wash their hands, handle food, and/or have repeated contact with irritants, for example, hairstylists and restaurant dishwashers are at increased risk for ICD.[1,7–9] Substances associated with ICD are listed in Table 35–1. The majority of ICD cases are related to occupation, particularly jobs that involve work with water or exposure to irritant substances. ICD also occurs in the home; however, the only available statistics are those associated with employment.

Pathophysiology of Irritant Contact Dermatitis

Most instances of ICD occur on exposed skin surfaces, such as the face and dorsal surfaces of the hands and forearms. ICD may appear after a single exposure or after multiple exposures to an irritant. Mechanisms responsible for causing ICD include disruption of the skin barrier, changes in the cells of the epidermis, and release of proinflammatory cytokines.[7] The irritant may be absorbed through the cell membrane, thus destroying cell systems. Destruction to epidermal cells may also occur as a result of the release of cytokines from chemical exposure.[1,5,7]

Several factors may affect the magnitude of the skin response. The presence of existing skin conditions, such as atopic dermatitis, can result in a more profound dermatitis because of the increased or enhanced permeability of the dermis. The quantity and concentration of substance exposure also affects the severity of the response. Chemical irritants, acids, and alkalis are likely to produce immediate and severe inflammatory reactions. Mild irritants, such as detergents, soaps, and solvents, often require repeated exposures before the dermatitis appears. Occlusive clothing and diapers can prolong skin contact with the irritant, allowing greater skin penetrability of the irritant and leading to a more severe reaction. In addition, environmental factors, such as warmer ambient temperature and higher humidity, may contribute to more severe ICD.[5]

Clinical Presentation of Irritant Contact Dermatitis

Following exposure to an irritant, the skin becomes inflamed, swells, and turns erythematous. Symptoms often are delayed and generally do not occur immediately after exposure. ICD presents primarily as dry or macerated, painful, cracked, and inflamed skin. Itching, stinging, and burning commonly occur with the rash. The inflammatory reaction varies, ranging from these initial symptoms to ulcer formation and localized necrosis. Within days, the dermatitis may crust. If the patient avoids further contact with the irritant, the dermatitis generally resolves in several days. In patients chronically exposed to an irritant, the affected areas of skin will remain inflamed, may develop fissures and scales, and may become hyper- or hypopigmented.[10] Some patients who are chronically exposed to irritants recover completely, whereas others improve but continue to have recurrences. In some patients who are chronically exposed to an irritant, necrosis, inflammation, and crusting comparable to or worse than the original insult may be observed. Chronic forms of ICD can present with *lichenification*, or leathery thickening of the skin.[1]

TABLE 35–1 Selected Substances Commonly Associated With Irritant Contact Dermatitis

- Acids, strong (e.g., hydrochloric, nitric, sulfuric, hydrofluoric)
- Alkalis, strong (e.g., sodium, potassium, calcium hydroxides)
- Detergents, soaps, and hand sanitizers
- Epoxy resins
- Ethylene oxide
- Fiberglass
- Flour
- Oils (e.g., cutting, lubricating)
- Oxidants, plasticizers, and activators in athletic shoes
- Oxidizing agents
- Reducing agents
- Solvents
- Urine and feces
- Water
- Wood dust and products

Source: References 7 and 11.

Treatment of Irritant Contact Dermatitis

Treatment Goals

The goals in self-treating ICD are (1) to remove the offending agent and to prevent future exposure to the irritant; (2) to relieve the inflammation, dermal tenderness, and irritation; and (3) to educate the patient on self-management to prevent or treat recurrences.

General Treatment Approach

The primary treatment advice is institution of preventive measures to avoid further irritant exposure and appropriate selection and use of therapy.

Nonpharmacologic Therapy

Patients should wash the exposed area with copious amounts of tepid water and cleanse with a mild or hypoallergenic soap, such as Cetaphil or Dove, to reduce contact time with the irritant and minimize local symptoms.[2,7]

Pharmacologic Therapy

Liberal application of emollients to the affected area can restore moisture to the stratum corneum and protect the area from further exposure. Colloidal oatmeal baths may help relieve itching.[7] Corticosteroids have questionable efficacy as they do not address the process directly; however, they may reduce inflammation and relieve itching. Topical caine-type anesthetics and agents commonly found in therapeutic products, including propylene glycol, lactic acid, urea, and salicylic acid, should be avoided because of their ability to cause further skin irritation and potential ACD.[7,11]

Preventive Measures

Irritant exposure can be reduced by using protective clothing, gloves, or other equipment. Frequent changes in coverings can limit the time skin areas are occluded. Emollients, moisturizers, and barrier creams can be recommended to assist in repairing the epidermis and to prevent future exposures.[7,8]

ALLERGIC CONTACT DERMATITIS

Three thousand chemicals have been cited as causes of ACD.[12] The most common causes of ACD in the United States are poison ivy, poison oak, and poison sumac, as well as nickel used in jewelry, clothing, and electronics. Nickel is found in some food items, but dermatitis related to nickel is generally localized to areas of contact.[12,13] Approximately 19% of patients patch-tested for allergies are allergic to nickel, including 11 million children in the United States.[13,14] Latex allergies are commonly seen in health care workers, and latex found in waistbands and socks can also cause ACD. Fragrances, cosmetics, and skin care products may cause ACD.[12] Table 35–2 lists select allergenic substances.

TABLE 35–2 Selected Substances Commonly Associated With Allergic Contact Dermatitis

Allergen	Sources of Allergen
Balsam of Peru	Cough syrups, flavors
Benzocaine	The caine-type anesthetics have crossover allergy to other caine-type local anesthetics, topical medications (for skin, eye, ear), other oral medications.
Chromium salts	Potassium dichromate electroplating, cement, leather-tanning agents, detergents, dyes
Cobalt chloride	Cement, metal plating, pigments in paints
Colophony (rosin)	Rosin cake for string instrument bows, sport rosin bags, cosmetics, adhesives
Epoxy resins	Constituents prior to mixing and hardening
Formaldehyde	Germicides, plastics, clothing, glue, adhesives
Fragrances	Cosmetics, household products, eugenol, cinnamic acid, geraniol, oak moss absolute
Lanolin	Lotions, moisturizers, cosmetics, soaps
Latex	Gloves, syringes, vial closures, elastic waistbands, socks, condoms
Nickel sulfate	In jewelry, blue jean studs, utensils, pigments, coins, tools, many metal alloys encountered daily
Neomycin sulfate	Medications, antibiotic ointments, other aminoglycosides
Plants	*Toxicodendron* species (poison ivy, oak, sumac), primrose (*Primula obconica*), tulips, others
Rubber (carba mix)	Added ingredients, accelerators, activators, other processing chemicals
Thimerosal	Preservative in many medications, injectables, cosmetics

Source: References 1, 11, 12, and 24.

Pathophysiology of Allergic Contact Dermatitis

ACD is an inflammatory dermal reaction related to allergen exposure. Sensitized T cells are activated and migrate to the site of contact to release inflammatory mediators. ACD ordinarily does not appear on first contact. Several steps occur before dermatitis is manifested. During the induction phase, initial exposure to the antigen sensitizes the immune system. Subsequent contact with the antigen induces a cell-mediated, type IV delayed hypersensitivity reaction, within 24 hours to 21 days. This reaction results in dermatitis and symptoms associated with ACD. In people previously sensitized, the rash and related symptoms typically appear within 24–48 hours after exposure.[1,2,11,12]

Urushiol-Induced ACD

In the United States, four species of *Toxicodendron* plants belonging to the family Anacardiaceae (Northern or Western poison ivy, Eastern and Western poison oak, and poison sumac) cause dermatoses on exposure (Table 35–3). Many of these plants previously belonged to the genus *Rhus*, but *Toxicodendron* is now the accepted genus and is used throughout this chapter.[15,16]

As much as 80% of the U.S. population is estimated to be sensitive to urushiol, the antigenic oleoresin in these plants. On exposure, urushiol enters the skin within 10 minutes, starting the sensitivity process. Poison ivy/oak/sumac dermatitis has been reported in toddlers, but sensitivity increases into adulthood; sensitivity appears to be reduced in older individuals, but their dermatitis tends to take longer to heal.[10,17]

If patients have sensitivity to any one *Toxicodendron* species, they are generally allergic to all. These species are most easily identified as having three leaves emanating from a central stem, with the middle leaflet appearing at the terminal end of the stem. The plants flower in the spring and produce small, waxy, white, five-petaled flowers. In the late fall, the leaves turn brilliant red or orange, and the plants develop berries that are greenish white, pale yellow, or tan. Although "Leaves of three; let it be!" is a helpful, common warning, some members of the genus differ in the number of leaflets attached to the central stalk, and in berry and leaf morphology.[15,16]

Urushiol is contained and carried within resin canals of the plant. The release of urushiol occurs only through damage to the plant, either directly by an individual or by damage from natural causes (e.g., wind, rain, insects, animals).[15,16]

Urushiol is not a volatile substance, but when the plant is burned, urushiol particulates in the smoke may affect the lungs or other protected areas.[16] Unwashed, contaminated hands, feet, or shoes may transfer urushiol to other areas of the body and to other individuals. Dermatitis can occur on any skin surface, including the eyes, lips, underarms, buttocks, anus, and genitalia, on contact with or transfer of urushiol.

Poison Ivy

The most common *Toxicodendron* plant found throughout central and northeastern United States and Canada is poison ivy (*Toxicodendron radicans* and *Toxicodendron rydbergii*). The leaves are reddish in the spring, green in the summer, and yellow, orange, or red in the fall. The plant may have greenish-white flowers and whitish-yellow berries. It commonly grows up poles, trees, and buildings, along roads, hiking trails, streams, dry rocky canyons, and embankment slopes (see Color Plates, photograph 20A). *Toxicodendron radicans* is composed of nine subspecies of small shrubs or climbing vines with aerial rootlets. Each leaf has three glossy leaflets with smooth or toothed edges. *Toxicodendron rydbergii* is a dwarf shrub with large, broad, spoon-shaped leaves that have a hairy underside; *T. rydbergii* is the principal variety of poison ivy growing in the northern United States and southern Canada.[15,16]

Poison Oak

Poison oak has two species indigenous to the United States: *Toxicodendron diversilobum*, which grows in tall clumps or as long vines along the West Coast, and *Toxicodendron toxicarium*, a low-growing shrub found in the eastern and southern areas of the United States. Both species possess leaves similar to those of oak trees, with three fuzzy leaflets per stem. Leaflets edges may be unlobed, lobed, or deeply toothed with rounded tips. The plant may have yellow-white berries. (See Color Plates, photograph 20B.) It is found along streams, in thickets, on wooded slopes, and in dry woodlands. Western poison oak (*T. diversilobum*) may have 3–11 leaflets per stem with leaves similar to those of California live oak.[15,18,19]

TABLE 35–3 Toxicodendron Plants Indigenous to North America

Plant	Other Common Names	Common Geographic Location
Poison ivy (*Toxicodendron radicans*)	Poison vine, mark weed, three-leaved ivy, poor man's liquid amber	Exists throughout North America, ranging throughout the United States (central plains, Midwest, south central, southeastern, lower Mississippi Valley regions); Canada (Ontario, Nova Scotia); and Mexico
Poison oak, Eastern (*Toxicodendron toxicarium*)	—	Exists widely in the southeastern United States
Poison oak, Western (*Toxicodendron diversilobum*)	—	Exists throughout the Pacific Coast
Poison sumac (*Toxicodendron vernix*)	Poison elder, poison ash	Exists from Quebec to Florida, primarily in the eastern third of the U.S. coast

Source: References 18–20.

Poison Sumac

Poison sumac (*Toxicodendron vernix*) grows in remote areas of the eastern third and Midwest areas of the United States in bogs and swampy areas. It appears as a tall shrub or small tree, attains a height of roughly 9.8 ft (3 m), and may resemble an elder or ash tree. Hence, it is also known as "poison elder" and "poison ash." Its leaves are odd numbered and pinnate and may be 16 in. (40 cm) long, with 7–13 smooth-edged leaflets that come to a tip. The leaves are orange in the spring, green in the summer, and yellow, orange, or red in the fall. The plant may have greenish-yellow flowers and whitish-green fruits that hang in clusters. (See Color Plates, photograph 20C.) [15,19,20]

Clinical Presentation of Allergic Contact Dermatitis

General Presentation

ACD is initially distinguished from ICD by the distribution and presentation of the rash, although differentiation is difficult in chronic cases. Both ICD and ACD can occur anywhere on the body that is exposed to an irritant, but ICD is often limited to the hands and forearms as a result of occupational exposure. The rash in ACD is limited to the area of antigen contact and the area immediately surrounding the antigen contact. For example, reactions to latex gloves involve only the areas covered by the glove. Sensitivity to latex in undergarments occurs in areas touched by the latex, such as the waist (by waistbands) or calves (from socks). Urushiol-induced ACD, however, is often linear and/or occurs over a broad area, because urushiol may be transferred to other parts of the body from the hands or inanimate objects, for up to 5 years in the latter case. ACD generally presents with papules, small vesicles, and/or bullae over inflamed, swollen skin. Significant itching is a prominent feature of ACD. Chronic forms of ACD can present with lichenification.[1,7,11,12]

Presentation of Urushiol-Induced Dermatitis

Symptoms occur only where contact was made with urushiol and begin within a few hours to several days (generally within 24–48 hours). The rash does not spread but may appear to do so, because urushiol is absorbed at different rates on different areas of the body. The individual may also incur inadvertent repeated exposure from contaminated objects, clothing, or bed linens or from transfer of urushiol under the fingernails during scratching. Intense itching of exposed skin surfaces is followed by erythema and formation of vesicles or bullae. Presentation depends on patient sensitivity and extent of exposure. The vesicles or bullae may break open, releasing vesicular fluid. This fluid does not contain antigenic material and cannot be transferred to other areas of the body or to others. Oozing and weeping of vesicular fluid generally occur for several days. It is a common patient misconception that poison ivy spreads through the oozing; the patient should be educated that the development of the rash over time in different areas is caused by the response time, skin thickness, and severity of exposure. Papules and plaques may develop in addition to or instead of vesicles and bullae (see Color Plates, photograph 21A). Streaks of vesicles that correspond to the points of urushiol contact from the damaged plant suggest *Toxicodendron* exposure (see Color Plates, photograph 21B). In the last stage of the dermatitis, the affected area develops crusts and begins to dry (see Color Plates, photograph 21C).

Severity of Poison Ivy/Oak/Sumac Dermatitis

Mild dermatitis is localized to the unprotected areas of the body exposed to the urushiol oil. Linear streaks may be seen and itching may be minimal. Signs of moderate dermatitis include the appearance of erythema, bullae, papules, vesicles, and inflammation of the exposed skin, in addition to pruritus. Severe dermatitis is distinguished by extensive involvement and edema of the extremities and/or face. Marked swelling or closure of the eyelids, caused by rubbing the eyelids with urushiol-contaminated hands, may occur. Extreme itching, irritation, and formation of numerous vesicles and bullae may be present, affecting daily activities.[21] Medical referral for systemic therapy is warranted for dermatitis or edema affecting the eyes, genitalia, face, or large surface areas, as well as secondary infections from scratching.[22]

Treatment of Allergic Contact Dermatitis

Treatment Goals

The goals of self-treating ACD are (1) to remove and avoid further contact with the offending agent; (2) to treat the inflammation; (3) to relieve itching and prevent excessive scratching; (4) to relieve the accumulation of debris from oozing, crusting, and scaling of the vesicle fluids; and (5) to prevent secondary skin infections.

General Treatment Approach

Because of intense itching and discomfort, the widespread nature of the dermatitis, and/or the magnitude of other symptoms, patients will seek advice on treatment. Treated or untreated dermatitis will naturally resolve in approximately 10–21 days as a result of the patient's own immune system. Topical nonprescription products may be used for symptomatic relief.[1,23,24] Removing the antigen from the skin as soon as possible may reduce the chance and severity of the immune response (e.g., avoiding jewelry or leather watch bands; switching to latex-free underwear and socks; washing urushiol-contaminated clothes, such as dog leashes or boots; washing affected areas of the body with mild soap and tepid water).

Customarily, the first several days after the initial appearance of ACD are the most uncomfortable. Treatment depends on the severity of the symptoms from the antigenic reaction (Figure 35–1). Hydrocortisone 1% cream may be applied to localized areas to reduce inflammation and relieve itching. The cream allows weeping lesions to dry and is preferred over the occlusive ointment for weeping areas. The patient also may use astringent compresses and tepid baths to dry oozing vesicles.

Other symptomatic treatment options for non-weeping lesions include products containing calamine to assist in drying and colloidal oatmeal to relieve itching. Patients should be advised that calamine leaves a visible pink film on the skin, and that colloidal oatmeal makes the bathtub slippery and can clog the drain if oatmeal clumps are not removed.

Medical referral is appropriate for children younger than 2 years; for patients with involvement of the eyes, eyelids, mouth, and genitals; and for patients with dermatitis that involves more than 20% of the skin's surface. Medical referral is also appropriate when

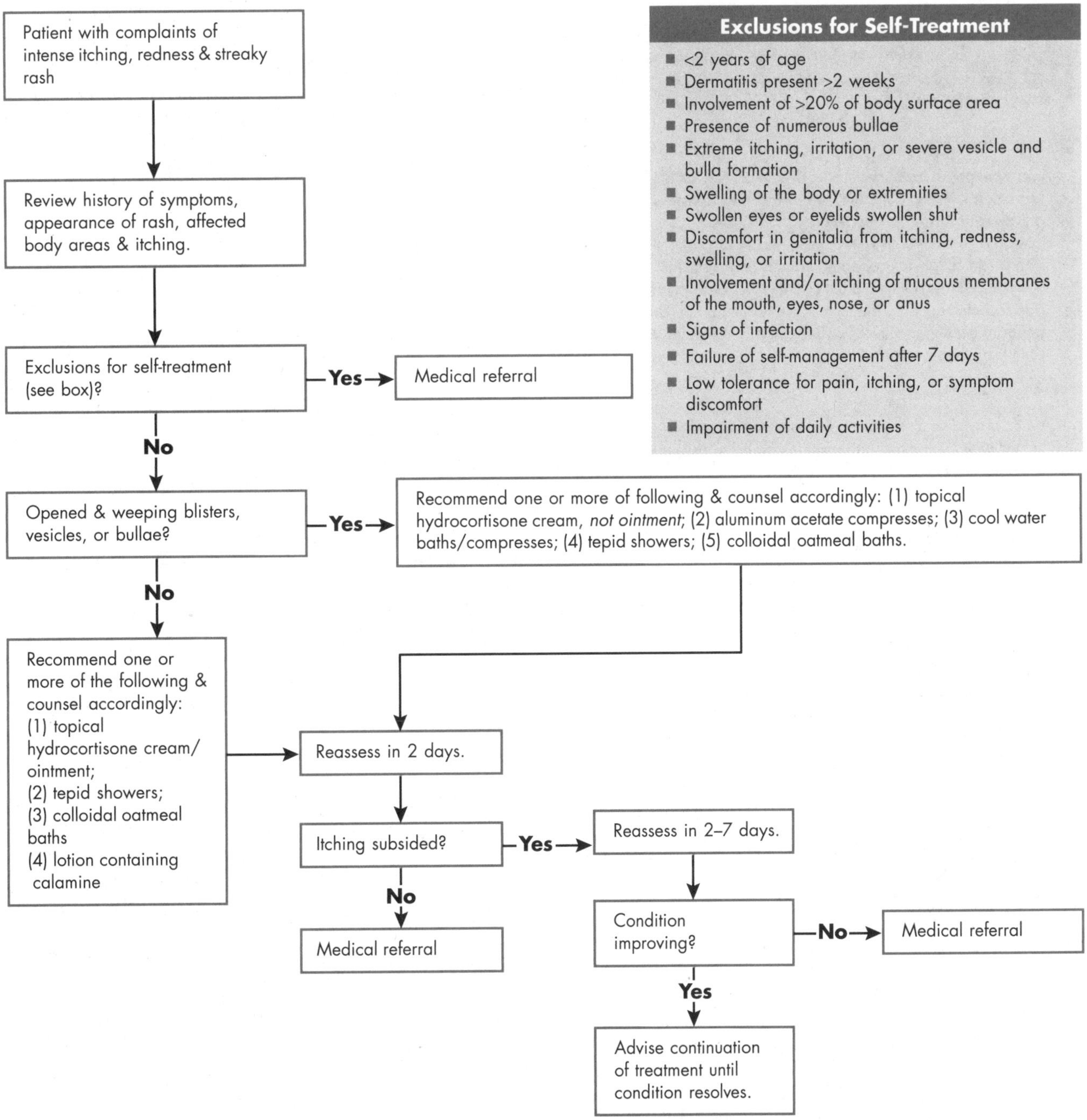

FIGURE 35–1 Self-care for allergic contact dermatitis.

(1) signs and symptoms of infection occur (a temperature >100.0°F [37.8°C] or pus or tenderness on the rash); (2) numerous large bullae are present; or (3) the rash has not improved within 1–2 weeks.

Nonpharmacologic Therapy

Prevention of Urushiol-Induced Allergic Contact Dermatitis

Patients presenting with ACD should be provided descriptions and/or photographs of *Toxicodendron* plants. Patients involved in outdoor work or activities should survey the surrounding vegetation to determine the potential risk of exposure and, if needed, take preventive measures. Table 35–4 provides preventive and protective measures, such as how to clean contaminated clothing and items. Urushiol may linger on almost any surface for years until it is washed off with soap and water or rubbing alcohol.[21]

Use of Barrier Products

In a double-blind study, the ability of a topical organoclay preparation to provide protection from urushiol was compared with that of

TABLE 35-4 Preventive and Protective Measures for Poison Ivy/Oak/Sumac Dermatitis

Preventive Measures

- Learn the physical characteristics and usual habitat of *Toxicodendron* plants. When outdoors, survey the area to assess potential risk for exposure to *Toxicodendron* plants.
- Cover nose and mouth with a mask and wear protective clothing when eradicating *Toxicodendron* plants near your residence. Mechanically remove the plant and its roots or apply an herbicide recommended by the State Farm Bureau or the United States Department of Agriculture (USDA) extension services. Do not burn the leaves of plants.

Protective Measures

- Wear protective clothing to cover exposed areas.
- Immediately after exposure, remove and wash clothes with ordinary laundry detergent.
- Wash contaminated clothing separately from non-contaminated clothing.
- Wash bed linens to prevent the transfer of urushiol to other parts of the body.
- Take a shower or wash suspected areas of exposure with soap as soon as possible. Avoid tub baths after initial exposure, because oleoresin may remain in the tub and contaminate body areas that were not originally exposed.
- Clip and meticulously clean fingernails to avoid transferring trapped urushiol to other skin surfaces.
- If dry cleaning clothes, put contaminated clothing in a plastic bag for transport, and warn personnel of possible contamination.
- As soon as possible, thoroughly wash shoes, gloves, jackets, or other protective garments, sports equipment, garden and work tools, and equipment suspected of carrying urushiol.
- Wear vinyl gloves when washing contaminated objects.
- Wash pets after known or suspected exposures to *Toxicodendron* plants.

Source: References 18–20.

bentonite, kaolin, and silicone products. The organoclay preparation gave 95.3% protection against topical urushiol applications. Bentonite, kaolin, and silicone gave 29.6%, 37.9%, and 32.9% protection, respectively. The author concluded that organoclay is significantly more effective than other agents.[25] However, no currently available barrier product contains organoclay.

Eradication of Toxicodendron *Plants*

The eradication of *Toxicodendron* plants may be required when extremely sensitive individuals live in close proximity to the plant and its oleoresin. The plant may be mechanically removed by hand grubbing the plants and the root system using protective equipment, such as gloves and long sleeves and pants, or by applying an appropriate herbicide. Individuals also should cover their noses and mouths with a mask when eradicating the plants. Patients should contact the U.S. Department of Agriculture (USDA) or contact the appropriate state or county agency to determine the recommended herbicide and its prescribed methods of application.

Patients presenting with *Toxicodendron* ACD in midwinter or during off-season periods may have come in contact with urushiol-contaminated objects. Urushiol remains active within dead and dried parts of plants and on inanimate objects for long periods of time, sometimes years. It is not unusual for objects to become contaminated with urushiol in one growing season and retain its antigenicity throughout the winter, causing rashes with each use of the object in succeeding seasons. This is commonly seen with shoes, boots, and clothing; upholstery and carpets; garden and work tools; and recreational equipment, such as golf clubs, baseball bats, fishing rods, and tents and other camping equipment. Urushiol is often carried into the home or transferred to people via the fur of pets.[19,26]

Removal of Antigen at Time of Exposure

Urushiol quickly binds to skin, but it is readily degraded in the presence of water. Washing exposed areas with mild soap and water reduces the risk of transfer and the severity of the rash. Immediate washing is preferred, although washing within 30 minutes of urushiol contact may still remove urushiol that has not yet entered the dermal layers. Once urushiol has entered the skin and attached to tissue proteins, the antigenic process and reaction begins.[27,28] Good handwashing, including meticulous cleansing under or clipping of the fingernails, is necessary to avoid contaminating additional skin surfaces. Anitgen removal methods such as vigorous scrubbing of contaminated skin with a harsh soap or household bleach, or the use of isopropyl alcohol, hand sanitizers, and other cleansers and organic solvents are not recommended, because they may cause further damage to the skin.

Several products are marketed to wash or cleanse the skin following urushiol exposure. Product prices range considerably and cost should be a consideration in selecting a product. One such product, Zanfel, a poison ivy, oak, and sumac wash (a mixture of alcohol solubles and anionic surfactants), is a nonprescription topical soap scrub that can be used at any time following urushiol exposure, even after rash develops, to provide relief from pain and itching. It is intended to prevent or relieve the rash by bonding with urushiol within the dermal layer of the skin to create an aggregate that can be washed away with water.[29] Small studies suggest that Zanfel ameliorates or prevents *Toxicodendron*-induced ACD and reduces the redness and blistering after urushiol exposure, but larger-scale studies are needed to confirm Zanfel's efficacy.[30–32] Anecdotally, it also has been used to clean equipment such as garden tools that have been exposed to urushiol. The product has a 10-year shelf life. Tecnu Original Outdoor Skin Cleanser is another agent intended to remove urushiol from the skin to prevent rash and itching. The product contains deodorized mineral spirits, water, propylene glycol, octylphenoxypolyethoxyethanol, mixed fatty acid soap, and fragrance. TEC Labs also markets Tecnu Extreme Medicated Poison Ivy Scrub, which contains the anti-itch ingredient Grindelia robusta 3X.[33] Table 35–5 provides usage guidelines for these three products.

A study evaluated the efficacy of three different modes of post-contact rash prevention versus no treatment: a chemical inactivator (Tecnu), a surfactant (Dial Ultra dishwashing soap), and an oil-removing compound (Goop). All three products provided good protection against poison ivy rash when used to cleanse skin exposed to urushiol. The difference in protective ability among the products was not significant, but Tecnu had a substantially higher cost.[34]

Relief of Itching

Cold or tepid soapless showers temporarily relieve the itching associated with ACD. Hot showers typically intensify itching and may cause scalding or thermal skin injuries to affected areas. Patients may use hypoallergenic soap to maintain cleanliness.

TABLE 35-5 Usage Guidelines for Products That Remove Urushiol

Zanfel

1. Wet the affected area.
2. Measure 1½ inches of the product into one palm.
3. Wet both hands and rub the product into a paste.
4. Rub both hands on the affected area until there is no sign of itching (up to 3 minutes).
5. Rinse the affected area thoroughly.
6. If itching returns after several hours, the product may be used again.

Tecnu Original Outdoor Skin Cleanser

1. Rub product into dry, contaminated areas as soon after exposure as possible.
2. Cleanse the area by rubbing vigorously for 2 minutes.
3. Wipe away product using a cloth, or rinse the area with cool water.
4. Product can be used up to 8 hours after exposure to remove any free oil from the skin.
5. Product may also be used to remove urushiol from objects and pet fur.

Tecnu Extreme Medicated Poison Ivy Scrub

1. Squeeze product into one hand.
2. Add an equal amount of water to the product and mix.
3. Apply the product to affected skin, and gently rub the skin for 15 seconds.
4. Rinse with cool water and gently towel dry.
5. Repeat as needed.

Source: References 29 and 33.

Patients should trim fingernails to reduce the risk of secondary bacterial skin infections from scratching.

Pharmacologic Therapy

Itching

Topical ointments and creams containing anesthetics (e.g., benzocaine), antihistamines (e.g., diphenhydramine), or antibiotics (e.g., neomycin) should not be used for itching related to ACD. These agents are known sensitizers and can cause a drug-induced ACD superimposed on the existing ACD.[35] If the patient requires nighttime sedation because of itching, then first-generation oral antihistamines can be used.[35] If itching is not alleviated, patients can be referred to a primary care provider (PCP) for further care.

Weeping

Astringents applied to unhealthy serous skin or mucous membranes decrease weeping, oozing, discharge, or bleeding from dermatitis. They decrease edema, exudation, and inflammation by reducing cell membrane permeability and by hardening the intercellular cement of the capillary epithelium. When applied as a wet dressing or compress, astringents cool and dry the skin through evaporation. They cause vasoconstriction and reduce blood flow in inflamed tissue. They also cleanse the skin of exudates, crust, and debris. Because astringents generally have low cell penetrability, their activity is limited to the cell surface and interstitial spaces. The protein precipitate that forms may serve as a protective coat, allowing new tissues to grow underneath.

Aluminum acetate solution USP, or Burow's solution, contains approximately 5% aluminum acetate. Its drying ability likely involves complexing of the astringent agent with proteins, thereby altering the proteins' ability to swell and hold water. Table 35–6 provides guidelines for preparing and applying Burow's solution to affected areas. In addition to softening and removing crusting, Burow's solution has a mild antipruritic effect.[12,36,37] Less expensive alternatives to aluminum acetate include isotonic saline solution (1 teaspoon of salt in 2 cups of tap or unchlorinated water), diluted white vinegar (¼ cup per 1 pint of water), or baking soda mixed with water to make a solution for a wet compress, or mixed with water to make a paste and applied to the rash.[38]

Inflammation

Hydrocortisone (0.5% and 1%) is the most effective nonprescription topical therapy for treating symptoms of mild–moderate ACD that do not involve edema or extensive areas of the skin. Hydrocortisone is a low-potency corticosteroid capable of vasoconstriction, thereby reducing inflammation and pruritus. It is approved for use in minor skin irritations, itching, and rashes caused by eczema, insect bites, poison ivy, poison oak, poison sumac, soaps, detergents, cosmetics, and jewelry.[39,40] However, urushiol ACD may require a prescription corticosteroid, because the nonprescription strength may be too weak to treat the rash effectively. Hydrocortisone is recognized as safe to apply to all parts of the body except the eyes and eyelids. Although systemic absorption is minimal when used on intact skin, use of topical hydrocortisone over large surface areas, prolonged use, use with an occlusive dressing, or use when skin integrity is compromised can lead to systemic absorption. Hydrocortisone cream can be applied as frequently as 3–4 times per day.[39–41]

Generally, topical hydrocortisone is well tolerated, with limited adverse reactions such as burning and irritation. Pharmacists should be aware that, rarely, topical hydrocortisone causes contact dermatitis.[39,42]

No dressing or bandages should be applied when hydrocortisone is used as a self-care treatment. Topical hydrocortisone should not be used on children younger than 2 years of age, except on a PCP's advice. Hydrocortisone should not be used if the dermatitis persists longer than 7 days, or if symptoms clear and then reappear in a few days, unless patients have consulted with a PCP. When greater than 20% of the body is affected, systemic therapy is recommended and patients should be referred to a PCP.[39]

TABLE 35-6 Usage Guidelines for Burow's Solution

- Prepare a 1:40 solution using prepackaged tablets or powder, or add 1–3 tablets or powder packets to 1 pint of cool tap water.
- Stir or shake until fully dissolved.
- Soak affected area 15–30 minutes 3–4 times daily.
- Alternatively, loosely apply a compress to the affected area:
  - Prepare compress by soaking a washcloth, cheesecloth, or small towel in the Burow's solution.
  - Gently wring the compress and apply it to the affected area.
  - Rewet and reapply the compress for 20–30 minutes, 4–6 times daily.
- Prepare a fresh solution for each soak or application of a compress.

Source: References 12, 36, and 37.

Product Selection Guidelines

Special Populations

Treatment of contact dermatitis in pediatric patients is similar to the approach used in adults. Emollients, barrier creams, and topical corticosteroids can be used in pediatric patients as described for adults (refer to product label instructions). Use of pharmacologic products in pediatric patients younger than 2 years without the advice of a PCP is discouraged.[21]

Topical preparations are generally considered safe for use during pregnancy, as long as they are not used for long periods of time or over extensive areas of the body. The risk in pregnancy is considered limited with low-potency, topical nonprescription formulations.[43,44] Other topical preparations (e.g., calamine, colloidal oatmeal, aluminum acetate) have an "undetermined" pregnancy category. The same precautions described for self-treatment in adults apply to pregnant women. For other treatments, pregnant patients should be referred for medical evaluation. (See the Preface for a detailed explanation of the pregnancy data.)

In geriatric patients, avoid first-generation antihistamines (e.g., diphenhydramine) because of sedation and anticholinergic effects. Itching should be addressed in geriatric patients because of increased risk for skin damage and accompanying infections from scratching. If used on a small area, oatmeal baths, creams, and topical hydrocortisone can be used to address itching in these patients.

Patient Preferences

Nonprescription medications for ACD are available in numerous dosage forms. Creams allow vesicle fluid to flow freely from blisters and do not trap bacteria, because the medication is quickly absorbed into the skin. Because a cream is an oil-in-water emulsion, it tends to be drying and is best for open weeping lesions. In addition, creams are more cosmetically appealing to patients.[45] Gels offer ease of application and rapid absorption of active ingredients into the skin. Some gels may contain alcohol or similar organic solvents that may cause irritation or burning when applied to open lesions. The use of ointments is not recommended in plant-based ACD and when weeping lesions are present. Ointments also should not be applied to open lesions, because their removal from the skin is difficult, and they may trap bacteria beneath the oleaginous film, leading to secondary infections. Spray products are convenient and easily applied to large areas of skin. The use of a spray does not require touching the dermatitis, which could trigger itching. However, aerosol sprays may contain propellants that cause inflammation and/or alcohol that causes drying and irritation. Table 35–7 lists specific products to treat poison ivy/oak/sumac dermatitis.

TABLE 35–7 Select Topical Products for Treatment of Poison Ivy/Oak/Sumac Dermatitis

Trade Name	Primary Ingredients
Aveeno Soothing Bath Treatment	Colloidal oatmeal 100%
Burow Solution	Aluminum acetate 5%
Caladryal Lotion	Calamine 8%; pramoxine hydrochloride 1%
Cortaid Cream	Hydrocortisone cream 1% or 0.5%
Domeboro Astringent Solution Powder Packets	Aluminum sulfate 1347 mg; calcium acetate 952 mg

Assessment of Contact Dermatitis: A Case-Based Approach

Circumstances surrounding the occurrence of the dermatitis can help determine the type of dermatitis (Table 35–8). The factors that help to distinguish ICD from ACD include (1) history of irritant or allergen exposure, (2) history of known sensitivity on previous exposure, (3) time from exposure (at home, at work, during recreation) to appearance of rash, (4) distribution and appearance of the lesions, (5) severity of symptoms, and (6) improvement of the dermatitis with avoidance of irritants.[1,7,11,12,27] Much of the information that distinguishes between ICD and ACD is obtained by taking the patient's history; the distribution and appearance of lesions will be the only factor directly observable at the time of the patient visit. Determining the type and success of previous treatments of similar rashes will aid in selecting the appropriate nonprescription medications.

Cases 35–1 and 35–2 illustrate the assessment of patients with contact dermatitis.

Patient Counseling for Contact Dermatitis

Counseling of a patient who presents with possible ICD or ACD but cannot identify contact with irritant chemicals, allergens, or *Toxicodendron* plants should begin with a review of chemicals or allergens likely to cause dermatitis. Then preventive and protective measures, as well as nonprescription pharmacologic treatment options, should be explained. Counseling for nonprescription agents should include information about their purpose and appropriate use, their possible adverse effects, expected time to experience relief, and signs and symptoms that indicate the need for medical referral for further evaluation. The box "Patient Education for Contact Dermatitis" lists specific information to provide patients.

Evaluation of Patient Outcomes for Contact Dermatitis

The patient should be encouraged to call for additional advice if the itching has not subsided significantly within 5–7 days. If, at follow-up, the rash has significantly increased in size, displays signs of infection, affects the eyes or genitals, or covers extensive areas of the face, the patient must be referred to his or her PCP. Overall, complete remission of the dermatitis may take up to 3 weeks. However, the patient should see slow but steady reduction in itching, weeping, and dermatitis after 5–7 days of therapy.

Key Points for Contact Dermatitis

- The leading cause of ICD is frequent, unprotected exposure to wet environments that may contain irritant substances, such as detergents and cleaning solutions.
- ACD is produced through sensitization to an antigenic substance.

TABLE 35–8 Differentiation of Irritant and Allergic Contact Dermatitis

Symptom or Characteristic	Irritant Contact Dermatitis	Allergic Contact Dermatitis
Itching	Yes, later	Yes, early
Stinging, burning	Early	Late or not at all
Erythema	Yes	Yes
Vesicles, bullae	Rarely or no	Yes
Papules	Rarely or no	Yes
Dermal edema	Yes	Yes
Time to reaction (rash) after exposure	Dependent on irritant	Dependent on antigen
Appearance of symptoms in relation to exposures	Initial or repetitive exposures	Delayed for first exposure; in subsequent exposures, varies based on antigen and sensitivity
Causative substances	Water, urine, flour, detergents, hand sanitizers, soap, alkalis, acids, solvents, salts, surfactants, oxidizers	*Toxicodendron* plants, fragrances, nickel, latex, benzocaine, neomycin, leather
Substance concentration at exposure	Important	Less important
Mechanism of reaction	Direct tissue damage	Immunologic reaction
Common location	Hands, wrist, forearms, diaper area	Anywhere on body that comes in contact with antigen
Presentation	No clear margins	Clear margins based on contact of offending substance

Source: References 1, 7, and 11–13.

CASE 35–1

Relevant Evaluation Criteria	Scenario/Model Outcome
Collect	
1. Gather essential information about the patient's symptoms and medical history, including	
a. Description of symptom(s) (i.e., nature, onset, duration, severity, associated symptoms)	Patient has a rash on both hands and is seeking treatment. She has been working as a waitress for the past 2 months and noticed the problem shortly after beginning her new job. She notes that she regularly cleans tables with the solution that the restaurant provides. She also washes her hands frequently. The rash is becoming increasingly more diffuse, and the affected area is substantially larger than a month ago. The patient also complains of minor itching and dryness in the area of the rash. Upon examination, there are no vesicles, bullae, open lesions, or signs of infection. Irritation is confined to the upper arms.
b. Description of any factors that seem to precipitate, exacerbate, and/or relieve the patient's symptom(s)	Symptoms worsened as the weather became colder and as she started working more shifts. Dryness and itching progressively increased over the last month.
c. Description of the patient's efforts to relieve the symptoms	She tried a "generic lotion" she had on hand, and although it felt soothing upon application, there was no improvement in the rash.
d. Patient's identity	Joanna Dinkins
e. Patient's age, gender, height, and weight	24 years old, female, 5 ft 3 in., 110 lb
f. Patient's occupation	Waitress
g. Patient's dietary habits	Normal diet with weekend use of alcohol
h. Patient's sleep habits	Averages 6–8 hours per night.
i. Concurrent medical conditions, prescription and nonprescription medications, and dietary supplements	The patient has taken the same oral contraceptive (ethinyl estradiol/levonorgestrel) for the past 4 years. She occasionally uses ibuprofen 600 mg by mouth every 6 hours as needed for headache.
j. Allergies	Sulfa
k. History of other adverse reactions to medications	None
l. Other (describe) ______	n/a

CASE 35-1 *continued*

Relevant Evaluation Criteria	Scenario/Model Outcome
Assess	
2. Differentiate patient's signs/symptoms, and correctly identify the patient's primary problem(s).	Joanna is likely suffering from irritant contact dermatitis. The likely source is the chemical(s) used to clean tables and excessive hand washing while on the job.
3. Identify exclusions for self-treatment (Figure 35–1).	None
4. Formulate a comprehensive list of therapeutic alternatives for the primary problem to determine whether triage to a medical provider is required, and share this information with the patient or caregiver.	Options include (1) Refer Joanna to the appropriate HCP. (2) Recommend self-care with a nonprescription product and/or nondrug measures. (3) Recommend self-care until she can be seen by an appropriate HCP. (4) Take no action.
Plan	
5. Select an optimal therapeutic alternative to address the patient's problem, taking into account patient preferences.	Joanna should take protective measures when at work to prevent irritant exposure to cleaning products. When necessary, she should use a mild cleanser, such as Cetaphil. She should apply hand cream or ointment such as Aquaphor. She can wear gloves if they are not an additional source of irritation.
6. Describe the recommended therapeutic approach to the patient or caregiver.	"Completely dry your hands after washing with a mild cleanser such as Cetaphil; then use a hypoallergenic hand cream or ointment. Also, apply cream or ointment to your hands, and cover them with cotton gloves overnight."
7. Explain to the patient or caregiver the rationale for selecting the recommended therapeutic approach from the considered therapeutic alternatives.	"Drying your hands will cleanse them of irritants. The hypoallergenic hand cream or ointment will relieve dryness. The addition of cotton gloves will increase the amount of moisture retained in your skin."
Implement	
8. When recommending self-care with nonprescription medications and/or nondrug therapy, convey accurate information to the patient or caregiver.	
a. Appropriate dose and frequency of administration	See the box "Patient Education for Contact Dermatitis."
b. Maximum number of days the therapy should be employed	See the box "Patient Education for Contact Dermatitis."
c. Product administration procedures	See the box "Patient Education for Contact Dermatitis."
d. Expected time to onset of relief	See the box "Patient Education for Contact Dermatitis."
e. Degree of relief that can be reasonably expected	"Complete symptomatic relief is likely."
f. Most common adverse effects	See the box "Patient Education for Contact Dermatitis."
g. Adverse effects that warrant medical intervention should they occur	See the box "Patient Education for Contact Dermatitis."
h. Patient options in the event that condition worsens or persists	"You should consult a primary care provider if the condition does not improve or if irritation is intolerable."
i. Product storage requirements	See the box "Patient Education for Contact Dermatitis."
j. Specific nondrug measures	See the box "Patient Education for Contact Dermatitis."
Solicit follow-up questions from the patient or caregiver.	"When should the irritation get better?"
Answer the patient's or caregiver's questions.	"You should see a difference in 1 week. If you do not see improvement, contact your primary care provider."
Follow-up: Monitor and Evaluate	
9. Assess patient outcome.	Ask the patient to contact you and report how she responded to the recommended therapy, or call her in a week to evaluate her treatment outcome.

Key: HCP = Health care provider; n/a = not applicable.

CASE 35-2

Relevant Evaluation Criteria	Scenario/Model Outcome
Collect	
1. Gather essential information about the patient's symptoms and medical history, including	
a. Description of symptom(s) (i.e., nature, onset, duration, severity, associated symptoms)	Patient complains of redness, swelling, and intense itching around her eyes and eyelids. She is having difficulty with vision because of swelling, and symptoms have worsened over the past week. She states that she recently started wearing a new brand of eye shadow.
b. Description of any factors that seem to precipitate, exacerbate, and/or relieve the patient's symptom(s)	After washing her face at night, she notices some relief.
c. Description of the patient's efforts to relieve the symptoms	Patient reports that no treatment has been used.
d. Patient's identity	Anna Drake
e. Patient's age, gender, height, and weight	15 years old, female, 5 ft 5 in., 120 lb
f. Patient's occupation	High school student
g. Patient's dietary habits	Normal diet with junk food
h. Patient's sleep habits	5–6 hours a night
i. Concurrent medical conditions, prescription and nonprescription medications, and dietary supplements	Drospirenone/ethinyl estradiol, 1 tablet by mouth daily for painful menses; leflunomide 10 mg daily for arthritis
j. Allergies	Nickel
k. History of other adverse reactions to medications	Upset stomach with codeine
l. Other (describe) ______	n/a
Assess	
2. Differentiate patient's signs/symptoms, and correctly identify the patient's primary problem(s).	Anna is suffering from an allergic reaction to her new eye shadow. Her symptomatology (e.g., redness, swelling, mild itching) has worsened over time as a result of continued use.
3. Identify exclusions for self-treatment (Figure 35–1).	None
4. Formulate a comprehensive list of therapeutic alternatives for the primary problem to determine whether triage to a medical provider is required, and share this information with the patient or caregiver.	Options include (1) Refer Anna to the appropriate HCP. (2) Recommend self-care with an OTC product and/or nondrug measures. (3) Recommend self-care until Anna can see an appropriate HCP. (4) Take no action.
Plan	
5. Select an optimal therapeutic alternative to address the patient's problem, taking into account patient preferences.	Recommend self-care until Anna can see an appropriate HCP.
6. Describe the recommended therapeutic approach to the patient or caregiver.	"Discontinue use of the eye makeup. Keep areas around your eyes clean, and avoid using additional eye care products until your condition is resolved."
7. Explain to the patient or caregiver the rationale for selecting the recommended therapeutic approach from the considered therapeutic alternatives.	"Allergic contact dermatitis involving the eyes should not be treated with self-care products."
Implement	
8. When recommending self-care with nonprescription medications and/or nondrug therapy, convey accurate information to the patient or caregiver.	"Expect some relief within 2 or 3 days of discontinuation of the eye makeup. Complete relief of your symptoms is likely. If, after removing the source of the allergy, your condition does not improve or the irritation is intolerable, contact your primary care provider."

Relevant Evaluation Criteria	Scenario/Model Outcome
Solicit follow-up questions from the patient or caregiver.	"Can I wear any eye makeup?"
Answer the patient's or caregiver's questions.	"Once the condition is resolved, you might consider trying a hypo-allergenic brand of eye makeup. If symptoms return, stop using the product."
Follow-up: Monitor and Evaluate	
9. Assess patient outcome.	Ask the patient to contact you and report whether the recommendation resolved the rash, or call the patient in a week to evaluate her condition.

Key: HCP = Health care provider; n/a = not applicable; OTC = over-the-counter.

PATIENT EDUCATION FOR Contact Dermatitis

Irritant Contact Dermatitis

The goals in self-treating irritant contact dermatitis (ICD) are (1) to remove the offending agent and prevent future exposure to the irritant; (2) to relieve the inflammation, dermal tenderness, and irritation; and (3) to educate the patient on self-management to prevent and treat recurrences. For most patients, carefully following product instructions and the self-care measures listed here will help ensure optimal therapeutic outcomes.

Nondrug Measures

- Avoid or limit contact with common skin irritants, such as detergents, soaps, and solvents.
- Change clothing and gloves used for cleaning more frequently.
- Wash the affected area gently to remove the skin irritant.

Nonprescription Medications

- Use emollients liberally to restore moisture to skin.
- Use colloidal oatmeal baths or soaks to soothe and cleanse areas of the rash and to reduce itching:
  - Sprinkle a 30-g packet or a cup full of milled oatmeal into fast-running bath water, and mix the water to avoid lumping of the oatmeal.
  - Soak for 15–20 minutes in the oatmeal bath at least twice a day.
  - Pat skin dry rather than wiping it.
  - Oatmeal baths can leave the tub slippery and can clog the drain.
- Store nonprescription medications in a cool, dry place out of children's reach.
- Rash and itching should improve within 5–7 days. If either the rash or the itching worsens, consult your primary care provider.
- Using nonprescription medications longer than 7 days for dermatitis without consulting a primary care provider is not recommended.

Allergic Contact Dermatitis

The goals of self-treating allergic contact dermatitis (ACD) are (1) to remove and/or avoid further contact with the offending agent; (2) to treat the inflammation; (3) to relieve itching and excessive scratching; (4) to relieve the accumulation of debris that arises from oozing, crusting, and scaling of the vesicle fluids; and (5) to prevent secondary skin infections. For most patients, carefully following product instructions and the self-care measures listed here will help ensure optimal therapeutic outcomes.

Nondrug Measures

- Use the measures outlined in Table 35–4 to prevent poison ivy/oak/sumac dermatitis.
- Take cold or tepid, soapless showers to relieve itching.
- When cleansing the affected areas, do not use harsh cleansers or scrub vigorously.
- Use clean white cloths to apply cool water compresses; apply for 20–30 minutes as often as needed or desired.
- To avoid potential allergic reactions, use hypoallergenic cosmetics and soapless cleansers.

Nonprescription Medications

- If desired, to reduce inflammation and the itching and redness, apply topical hydrocortisone cream *only* as follows:
  - Apply a small amount to affected areas up to 3–4 times a day.
  - Avoid applying the cream around the eyes or eyelids.
- To avoid infection, do not apply ointments to open lesions.
- Apply aluminum acetate (Burow solution) compresses to areas with vesicles, bullae, and/or weeping lesions as follows:
  - Mix a prepackaged tablet or packet of aluminum acetate with a pint of cool tap water, wet a cloth with the solution, and apply the compress to rash areas.
  - Apply compresses for 20–30 minutes at least 4–6 times a day or as needed.
  - Prepare fresh Burow solution for each application.
- Use colloidal oatmeal baths or soaks to soothe and cleanse areas of the rash and to reduce itching:
  - Sprinkle a 30-g packet or a cup full of milled oatmeal into fast-running bath water, and mix the water to avoid lumping of the oatmeal.
  - Soak for 15–20 minutes in the oatmeal bath at least twice a day.
  - Pat skin dry rather than wiping it.
  - Oatmeal baths can leave the tub slippery and can clog the drain.
- Use a sedating oral antihistamine, such as diphenhydramine or doxylamine, for nighttime sedation, and follow the label instructions. These medications can cause drowsiness that might extend to the next morning.
- Store nonprescription medications in a cool, dry place out of children's reach.
- Using nonprescription medications for dermatitis longer than 7 days without consulting a primary care provider is not recommended.

When to Seek Medical Attention

- Contact a primary care provider for the following situations:
  - The rash does not begin to improve in 7 days.
  - The symptoms from the rash worsen.
  - The rash continues to develop for several weeks after initial exposure.
  - Joints are swelling or evidence of other systemic involvement exists.
  - The rash covers large areas of the face or causes swelling of the eyelids.
  - The rash involves the genitals.

- Many substances are antigenic. Common antigens include fragrances, metals, medications, plants, and chemicals. Urushiol from poison ivy/oak/sumac is one of the most common allergens.
- Patients who are sensitive to irritants, allergens, or urushiol should take precautions to eliminate exposure by avoiding these agents, limiting exposure time, and wearing protective clothing and equipment.
- Patients should be advised to avoid geographic areas with endemic *Toxicodendron* plants and wear clothing (e.g., gloves, long sleeves, long pants) that limits exposure of the skin to the environment.
- Once exposed to an irritant or antigen, the patient should shower with mild soap and water or apply large volumes of cool water to the area immediately after exposure to reduce the risk of dermatitis.
- ACD may begin as localized streaks or patches of highly pruritic rash that, with time, may become more numerous or coalesce into larger plaques on exposed dermal areas. The rash may affect the eyelids or face and, in some cases, areas ordinarily considered to be protected.
- Patients should be referred for further evaluation if there is involvement of the face, genitalia, or anus; signs of infection; considerable edema anywhere on the body (including eyelids); or extensive lesions covering a large portion of the body.
- Treatment of localized, pruritic rash consists of a topical application of hydrocortisone cream, compresses, or baths. Zanfel is also recommended to treat localized rash, because it may be used for relief anytime a rash develops. Weeping vesicles or bullae may be treated with aluminum acetate compresses.
- Irritant and allergic contact dermatitis will resolve in approximately 10–21 days with or without topical therapy. Nonprescription medications primarily relieve symptoms.

REFERENCES

1. Usatine RP, Riojas M. Diagnosis and management of contact dermatitis. *Am Fam Physician.* 2010;82(3):249–55. Available at: http://www.aafp.org/afp/2010/0801/p249.html. Accessed June 2, 2017.
2. Wolff K, Johnson RA, Saavedra AP. Contact dermatitis. In: *Color Atlas and Synopsis of Clinical Dermatology.* 7th ed. New York, NY: McGraw-Hill; 2013:18–30.
3. Bureau of Labor Statistics. Incidence rates of nonfatal occupational illness by industry and category of illness, 2014. Available at: http://www.bls.gov/iif/oshwc/osh/os/ostb4354.pdf. Accessed June 2, 2017.
4. Bureau of Labor Statistics. Occupational injuries/illnesses and fatal injuries profile, 2014. Available at: http://data.bls.gov/gqt/InitialPage. Accessed June 2, 2017.
5. Cashman MW, Reutemann PA, Erhlich A. Contact dermatitis in the United States: epidemiology, economic impact, and workplace prevention. *Dermatol Clin.* 2012;30(1):87–98. doi: 10.1016/j.det.2011.08.004.
6. Developing dermal policy based on laboratory and field studies: a new National Institute for Occupational Safety and Health (NIOSH) research program in response to the National Occupational Research Agenda (NORA). Cincinnati, OH: National Institute for Occupational Safety and Health. Publication No. 2000142. Available at: http://www.cdc.gov/niosh/docs/2000-142/pdfs/2000-142.pdf. Accessed June 2, 2017.
7. Hogan DJ. Irritant contact dermatitis. Available at: http://emedicine.medscape.com/article/1049353-overview. Updated September 26, 2016. Accessed June 2, 2017.
8. Mostosi C, Simonart T. Effectiveness of barrier creams against irritant contact dermatitis. *Dermatology.* 2016;232:353–62. doi: 10.1159/000444219.
9. Corazza M, Minghetti S, Bianchi A, et al. Barrier creams: facts and controversies. *Dermatitis.* 2014;25(6):327–33. doi: 10.1097/DER.0000000000000078.
10. Honari G, Talor JS, Sood A. Occupational skin diseases due to irritants and allergens. In: Goldsmith LA, Katz SI, Gilchrest BA, et al., eds. *Fitzpatrick's Dermatology in General Medicine.* 8th ed. New York, NY: McGraw-Hill; 2012.
11. Cher-Han T, Rasool S, Johnston GA. Contact dermatitis: allergic and irritant. *Clin Dermatol.* 2014;32(1):116–24. doi: 10.1016/j.clindermatol.2013.05.033.
12. Hogan DJ. Allergic contact dermatitis. Available at: http://emedicine.medscape.com/article/1049216-overview. Accessed June 2, 2017.
13. American Academy of Dermatology and AAD Association. Position statement on nickel sensitivity. August 22, 2015. Available at: https://www.aad.org/forms/policies/uploads/ps/ps-nickel%20sensitivity.pdf. Accessed June 2, 2017.
14. Warshaw EM, Maibach HI, Taylor JS, et al. North American contact dermatitis group patch test results: 2011–2012. *Dermatitis.* 2015;26:49–59. doi: 10.1097/DER.0000000000000097.
15. Botanical Dermatology Database. Anacardiaceae. Available at: http://www.botanical-dermatology-database.info/BotDermFolder/ANAC-6.html. Accessed June 2, 2017.
16. Innes RJ. Toxicodendron radicans, T. rydbergii. In: Fire Effects Information System, U.S. Department of Agriculture, Forest Service, Rocky Mountain Research Station, Fire Sciences Laboratory [producer]. Available at: https://www.fs.fed.us/database/feis/plants/shrub/toxspp/all.html. Accessed June 2, 2017.
17. Prakash AV, Davis MDP. Contact dermatitis in older adults: a review of the literature. *Am J Clin Dermatol.* 2010;11(6):373–81. doi: 10.2165/11319290-000000000-00000.
18. U.S. Department of Agriculture, Forest Service Pacific Southwest Region. Poison oak. Available at: http://www.fs.usda.gov/Internet/FSE_DOCUMENTS/stelprdb5110489.pdf. Accessed June 2, 2017.
19. Park Brown S, Grace P. Identification of poison ivy, poison oak, poison sumac, and poisonwood. Gainesville, FL: University of Florida IFAS Extension, document ENH866. Available at: https://edis.ifas.ufl.edu/pdffiles/EP/EP22000.pdf. Accessed June 2, 2017.
20. U.S. Department of Agriculture, Natural Resources Conservation Service. *Toxicodendron vernix* (L.) Kuntze poison sumac. Available at: http://plants.usda.gov/core/profile?symbol=TOVE. Accessed June 2, 2017.
21. Jacob SH, Herro EM, Taylor JS. Contact dermatitis: diagnosis and therapy. In: Elzouki AY, Harfi HA, Nazer HM, et al., eds. *Textbook of Clinical Pediatrics.* 2nd ed. Verlag Berlin Heidelberg: Springer; 2012.
22. Stephanides SL. Toxicodendron poisoning. Updated January 3, 2017. Available at: http://emedicine.medscape.com/article/817671-overview#a5. Accessed June 2, 2017.
23. Svedman C, Bruze M. Allergic contact dermatitis. In: Krieg T, Bickers DR, Miyachi Y, eds. *Therapy of Skin Diseases.* Verlag Berlin Heidelberg: Springer; 2010.
24. Flohr C, English JSC. Allergic contact dermatitis. In: Irvine AD, Hoeger PH, Yan AC., eds. *Harper's Textbook of Pediatric Dermatology.* 3rd ed. Oxford, UK: Wiley-Blackwell; 2011.
25. Epstein WL. Topical prevention of poison ivy/oak dermatitis. *Arch Dermatol.* 1989;125(4):499–501. Available at: https://www.ncbi.nlm.nih.gov/pubmed/2522756. Accessed June 2, 2017. doi:10.1001/archderm.1989.01670160047005.
26. American Academy of Dermatology. Poison ivy, oak, and sumac. Available at: https://www.aad.org/public/diseases/itchy-skin/poison-ivy-oak-and-sumac#.UWBrKRlU9Ok. Accessed June 2, 2017.
27. Fonacier L, Bernstein DI, Pachecok, et al. Contact dermatitis: a practice parameter update 2015. *J Allergy Clin Immunol Pract.* 2015;3:S1–39. doi.org/10.1016/j.jaip.2015.02.009.
28. Fisher AA. Poison ivy/oak dermatitis, part 1: prevention soap and water, topical barriers, and hyposensitization. *Cutis.* 1996;57(6):384–6. Available at: http://www.conovers.org/ftp/Poison-Ivy-Guin.pdf. Accessed June 2, 2017.
29. Zanfel [package insert]. Peoria, IL: Zanfel Laboratories; 2016. Available at: http://www.zanfel.com/help/productfaq.html. Accessed June 2, 2017.
30. Boelman DJ. Emergency: Treating poison ivy, oak, and sumac. *Am J Nurs.* 2010;210(6):49–52. doi: 10.1097/01.NAJ.0000377690.87350.36.
31. Davila A, Lucas J, Laurora M, et al. A new topical agent, Zanfel, ameliorates urushiol-induced toxicodendron allergic contact dermatitis. *Ann Emerg Med.* 2003;42(Suppl):601.

32. Stankewicz H, Cancel G, Eberhardt M, et al. Effective topical treatment and post-exposure prophylaxis of poison ivy: objective confirmation [Research Gate abstract 81]. *Ann Emerg Med.* 2007;50(3):S26–7.
33. Tec Labs. Products: poison oak and poison ivy solutions. Available at: http://www.teclabsinc.com/products/poison-oak-ivy/. Accessed June 2, 2017.
34. Stibich AS, Yagan M, Sharma V, et al. Cost-effective post-exposure prevention of poison ivy dermatitis. *Int J Dermatol.* 2000 Jul;39(7):515–8. doi: 10.1046/j.1365-4362.2000.00003.x.
35. Boelman DJ. Treating poison ivy, oak, and sumac. *Am J Nurs.* 2010; 210(6):49–52. doi: 10.1097/01.NAJ.0000377690.87350.36.
36. Goodman R, Hollimon D. Allergic contact dermatitis: poison ivy. *Dermatol Nurs.* 2010;22(4):26–8.
37. Aluminum acetate topical. Facts & Comparisons eAnswers. Available at: http://online.factsandcomparisons.com/index.aspx. Accessed June 2, 2017.
38. Emedicinehealth. Poison ivy, oak, or sumac: relieving the itch. Last revised August 30, 2011. Available at: http://www.emedicinehealth.com/poison_ivy_oak_or_sumac_relieving_the_itch-health/article_em.htm. Accessed June 2, 2017.
39. Hydrocortisone topical. Facts & Comparisons eAnswers. Available at: http://online.factsandcomparisons.com/index.aspx. Accessed June 2, 2017.
40. U.S. National Library of Medicine, MedlinePlus. Hydrocortisone topical. Available at: https://www.nlm.nih.gov/medlineplus/druginfo/meds/a682793.html. Accessed June 2, 2017.
41. Hydrocortisone topical [monograph]. Facts & Comparisons. Available at: http://online.factsandcomparisons.com/index.aspx. Accessed June 2, 2017.
42. D'Erme AM, Gola M. Allergic contact dermatitis induced by topical hydrocortisone-17-butyrate mimicking papular rosacea. *Dermatitis.* March/April 2012;23(2):95–6. doi: 10.1097/DER.0b013e31824a609f.
43. Chi CC, Mayon-White RT, Wojnarowska FT. Safety of topical corticosteroids in pregnancy: a population-based cohort study. *J Invest Derm.* 2011; 131(4):884–91. doi: 10.1038/jid.2010.392.
44. Cortaid Maximum Strength Hydrocortisone Cream [package insert]. Bridgewater, NJ: Valeant Pharmaceuticals North America; 2013.
45. Silverberg NB. Pediatric contact dermatitis medication. Updated August 22, 2016. Available at: http://emedicine.medscape.com/article/911711-medication#3. Accessed June 2, 2017.

CHAPTER 36

DIAPER DERMATITIS AND PRICKLY HEAT

KATELYN ALEXANDER AND CORTNEY MOSPAN

Irritant contact diaper dermatitis (commonly referred to as diaper rash) and prickly heat (also known as miliaria, miliaria rubra, or heat rash) are acute dermatologic conditions that primarily affect infants. This chapter will review presentation of these conditions and appropriate use of nonprescription products to treat symptoms related to these conditions. In most circumstances, neither diaper dermatitis nor prickly heat causes serious illness. These conditions typically produce discomfort, irritation, and itching. They may lead to fussiness, agitation, and irritability, especially in the infant population.

DIAPER DERMATITIS

Diaper dermatitis is an acute inflammation of the skin occurring in the region of the perineum, buttocks, lower abdomen, and inner thighs. Despite the perception that this condition is limited to infancy, it can and does occur in any population in which incontinence presents.[1] This chapter focuses primarily on infant diaper dermatitis. Information presented in this chapter may be generalized to the adult population. Readers are referred to Chapter 49 for specific information regarding treatment of adult incontinence. Both irritant contact and allergic contact diaper dermatitis can present in the diaper area.[2] The primary focus of this chapter is irritant contact diaper dermatitis. Irritant contact diaper dermatitis is referred to simply as *diaper dermatitis* or *diaper rash* throughout. Allergic contact dermatitis will be discussed briefly.

Diaper dermatitis is the most common dermatologic disorder of infancy, resulting in more than 1 million primary care provider office visits per year.[3] The majority of diaper dermatitis cases appear in infants 2 years of age and younger.[3,4] Diaper dermatitis can present as early as 7 days after birth.[4] Given the common nature of diaper dermatitis, the actual incidence of the condition is likely underreported. Literature has suggested a prevalence rate of 4%–35% in the first 2 years of life.[3] However, a majority of children experience diaper dermatitis at least once by the time they are out of diapers. The steady decline in the number of cases of diaper dermatitis in infants since the 1970s is attributed to the increased use of disposable diapers. The decline was accelerated in the 1980s and 1990s with improvements in diaper technology and the rise of superabsorbent core materials and breathable diaper coverings.[5–7]

Pathophysiology of Diaper Dermatitis

Diaper dermatitis can be caused by multiple factors. Occlusion, moisture, microbes, gastrointestinal tract proteolytic enzymes and bile salts, a shift from the normal acidic skin pH (pH 4.0–5.5) to a more alkaline pH, mechanical chafing, and friction can cause skin compromise and, in additive or synergistic ways, present as diaper dermatitis.[1,4,8–15]

The skin of the infant perineal region is about one-half to one-third the thickness of adult skin. Because the perineal region is typically occluded by a diaper, this area tends to hold moisture and wetness, predisposing it to irritation and infection.[16] Frequent urination and defecation, combined with infrequent changing of the diaper, contributes to increased skin moisture. The development of diaper dermatitis is closely related to the exposure to urine and feces from occlusion caused by a diaper. Younger infants will urinate and defecate more frequently. Newborns will typically require a diaper change every 2 hours because of a high wetting frequency, but frequency of diaper changes in older infants can be decreased to every 3–4 hours.[17] Skin left in contact with wetness for long periods becomes waterlogged or hyperhydrated, which plugs sweat glands, increases susceptibility to abrasion and frictional harm, and diminishes the barrier function of the stratum corneum in the diaper area. Diminished barrier capabilities, in turn, make the skin more susceptible to irritation, absorption of chemicals, and opportunistic microbes.

Urine and fecal bacteria can contribute to skin breakdown. Urea-splitting bacteria from the colon are believed to convert urine contents into ammonia. Ammonia raises the pH of the skin, making it more susceptible to damage or infection. This etiologic factor has been lessened by the use of absorbent disposable diapers, which minimize mixing of urine and feces in the diaper area.[5,18] Mechanical irritation can also lead to epidermal breakdown, allowing other irritants (e.g., fecal bacteria) to harm the skin. Tight-fitting, stiff, or rough diapers and the use of occlusive plastic or rubberized covers or pants over cloth diapers can contribute to occlusion and mechanical friction of the skin.

Medications and foods that affect the motility or microbial flora of the gastrointestinal tract, or that hinder autonomic control

Editor's Note: This chapter is based on the 18th edition chapter of the same title, written by Nicholas E. Hagemeier.

of urination and defecation may contribute to diaper dermatitis. Foods high in hexitols, sorbitol, sucrose, and fructose may induce diarrhea and predispose to diaper dermatitis. Dairy products can induce diarrhea, especially if the child is lactose intolerant. Compared with infants fed bottle formula, breastfed infants have decreased incidences of diaper dermatitis.[19] The feces of breastfed infants are less copious, less alkaline, and less caustic to the skin. Transitions in the type of food consumed (e.g., from breast milk to solid foods) can also contribute to diaper dermatitis.

Some products (e.g., detergent or soap residues, household cleaning products, lotions, sunscreens, insect repellents), plant materials (e.g., ragweed, thistle), and diaper product ingredients can produce an allergic contact dermatitis that resembles diaper dermatitis.[20] Although many of these agents may not be purposefully or intentionally used in the diaper region, if present, they may have an unexpected effect on skin under a diaper. Chemicals used to launder reusable cloth diapers, for example, can contribute to diaper dermatitis and skin irritation if the diapers are not adequately washed and rinsed. Harsh chemicals used to clean and sanitize the diapers may leave chemical residues that exacerbate diaper dermatitis. Allergic contact dermatitis in the diaper region routinely presents only in areas of contact with the allergen, often sparing the inguinal skin folds. Allergic contact dermatitis should be considered when standards of care do not lead to healing in the diaper area.[2] (See Chapter 35 for discussion of allergic contact dermatitis.)

Clinical Presentation of Diaper Dermatitis

Diaper dermatitis usually presents as red to bright red (erythematous), sometimes shiny, wet-looking patches and lesions on the skin (see Color Plates, photograph 22). Lesions may appear dusky maroon or purplish on darker skin. Generally, diaper dermatitis occurs on the skin spaces covered by the diaper, but severe cases can spread outside the diaper area. If an infant, for example, lies primarily on his or her abdomen, the rash may appear more anterior to the perineum. In the same manner, if the infant lies primarily on his or her back, the rash may appear more posterior to the perineum.

A disconcerting feature of diaper dermatitis is that it can perceivably present in a matter of hours, yet it can often take days to completely resolve. Most likely, the process of skin breakdown is not pronounced or visible initially but quickly transitions from unobservable to observable. The entire process from normal to noticeably erythematous skin takes longer than the time between normal diaper changes.

Although uncommon, severe diaper dermatitis can progress to maceration, papule formation, the presence of vesicles or bullae, oozing, erosion of the skin, or ulceration. Diaper dermatitis can also predispose infants to secondary infections and genital damage. As skin pH changes, it can foster the growth of opportunistic infections that can be bacterial (e.g., streptococci or staphylococci), fungal (e.g., yeasts), and viral (e.g., herpes simplex) in nature. If infection is a concern, visual inspection of the diaper area is beneficial for proper diagnosis. *Candida* infections, for example, can present in the diaper area secondary to diaper dermatitis. The presentation of a *Candida* infection is distinct from that of uncomplicated diaper dermatitis. The typical *Candida* superinfection presents as papular or pustular lesions around the margins of the diaper dermatitis. Additionally, *Candida* infections in the diaper area often present in the skin folds or creases. Untreated or infected diaper dermatitis can progress to skin ulceration, infections of the penis or vulva, and urinary tract infections, all requiring medical referral.

Diaper dermatitis can also be a manifestation of other diseases, such as Kawasaki syndrome, granuloma gluteale infantum, cytomegalovirus infection, and nutritional deficiencies. Infants born to immunocompromised mothers (e.g., those with human immunodeficiency virus [HIV]; genital herpes) should be considered at increased risk for unusual manifestations of diaper dermatitis or diaper dermatitis–like presentations. Primary infections of the skin can resemble diaper dermatitis and be misdiagnosed. Inguinal swelling, fever, chills, tachycardia, blisters, vesicles, and irregular borders bounded by bumps are indicators of infections that require medical referral.[4,21] Diaper dermatitis can exist concurrently with other skin conditions such as psoriasis and seborrhea[10]; therefore, these skin conditions may be misdiagnosed as diaper dermatitis.

Treatment of Diaper Dermatitis

Treatment Goals

The goals of diaper dermatitis treatment are (1) to relieve symptoms, (2) to rid the patient of the rash, (3) to prevent secondary infection, and (4) to prevent recurrences.

General Treatment Approach

The general treatment approach for diaper dermatitis is the use of nonpharmacologic therapy or a combination of pharmacologic and nonpharmacologic therapy as outlined in Figure 36–1. The ideal, yet often impractical, preventive therapy would be to change the diaper immediately after the infant defecates or urinates. Self-treatment will often involve increased vigilance in keeping the infant dry and use of skin protectants in the diaper area. Self-treatment should be limited to diaper dermatitis that is uncomplicated (e.g., absence of comorbid conditions or constitutional symptoms) and mild-moderate (e.g., absence of oozing or blood at lesion sites, or lesions present less than 7 days) in presentation. Figure 36–1 presents a thorough list of characteristics of complicated and severe diaper dermatitis. Medical referral should occur when diaper dermatitis manifests one or more of the exclusions listed.

Nonpharmacologic Therapy

Nonpharmacologic therapy plays an integral role in the treatment of diaper dermatitis. These nonpharmacologic approaches can be remembered through the mnemonic ABCDE: air, barrier, cleansing, diaper, and education.[22] The goals of nonpharmacologic therapy are (1) to reduce occlusion, (2) to reduce contact time of urine and feces with skin, (3) to reduce mechanical irritation and trauma, (4) to protect the skin from further irritation, (5) to encourage healing, and (6) to discourage the onset of secondary infection.

Treatment of uncomplicated diaper dermatitis should be initiated with nonpharmacologic therapy. Increasing the frequency of diaper changes to a minimum of six per day is advisable. Although challenging to implement, an effective strategy to prevent diaper dermatitis, known as a *diaper holiday*, is to expose the buttocks to air as long as possible to reduce contact of the skin with wet fabric, in an attempt to reduce friction.[17]

Exclusions for Self-Treatment of Diaper Dermatitis and Prickly Heat

- Lesions present >7 days
- Lesions have not improved in 7 days despite appropriate care
- Therapy complicated by secondary infection (viral, bacterial, fungal)
- Lesions part of or caused by another disease state
- Presence of *diaper dermatitis* outside diaper region
- *Diaper dermatitis* possibly associated with urinary tract infection (painful urination) or disfigurement of penis or vulva
- Presence of broken skin (ulceration, blistering, or peeling of skin) due to disease progression or patient action (e.g., scratching)
- Onion-skin–like appearance or bulla formation in affected area
- Oozing, blood, vesicles, or pus at lesion sites
- Chronic or frequently recurrent lesions
- Presence of constitutional symptoms (e.g., fever, diarrhea, nausea, vomiting, swollen inguinal lymph nodes, rapid pulse, rash or skin lesions on other parts of body)
- Significant behavioral changes in patient (e.g., lethargy, incessant crying) associated with the rash
- Comorbid conditions (e.g., HIV, organ transplantation, immune suppressive therapy, a history of dermal hepatic infections)

Source: References 4, 10, 20, and 28.

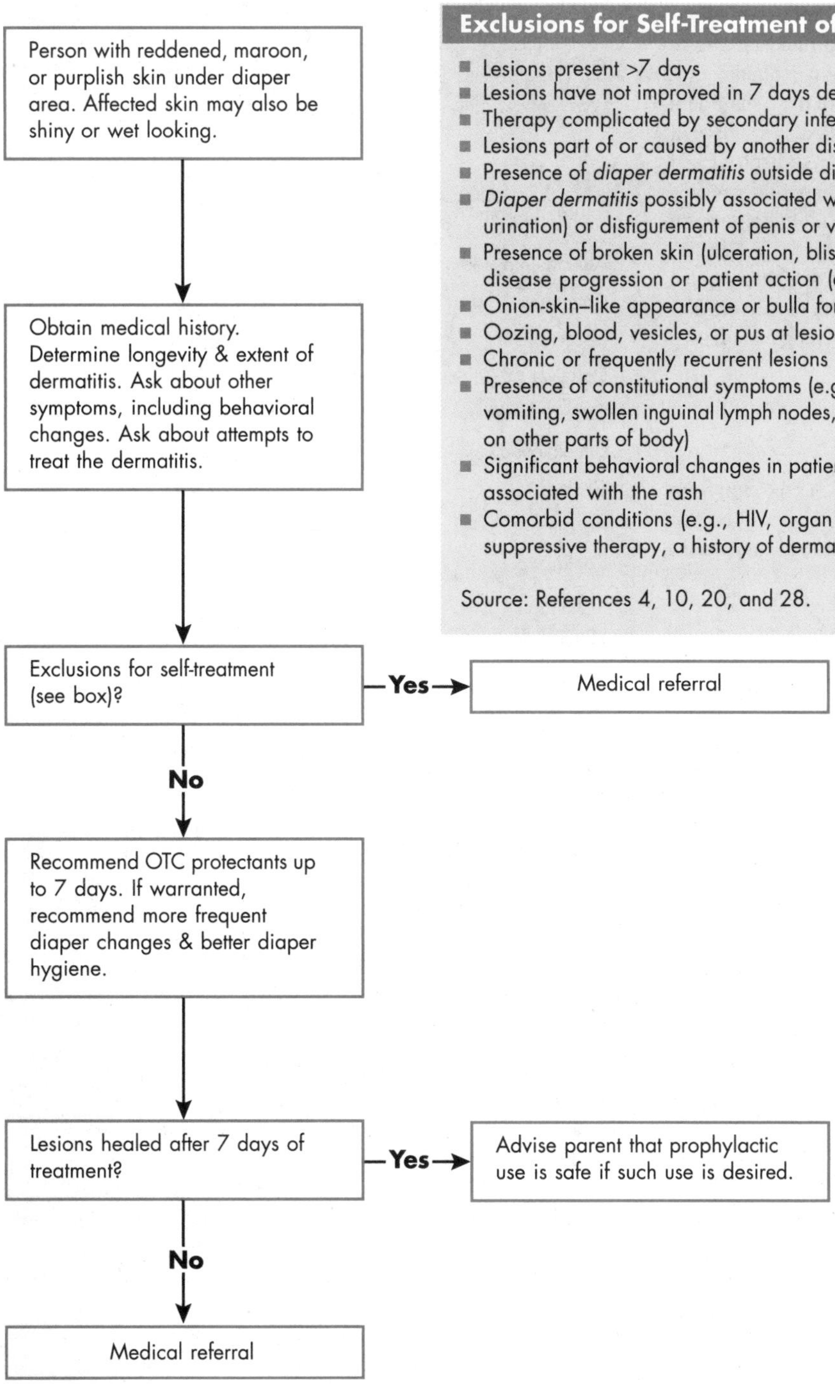

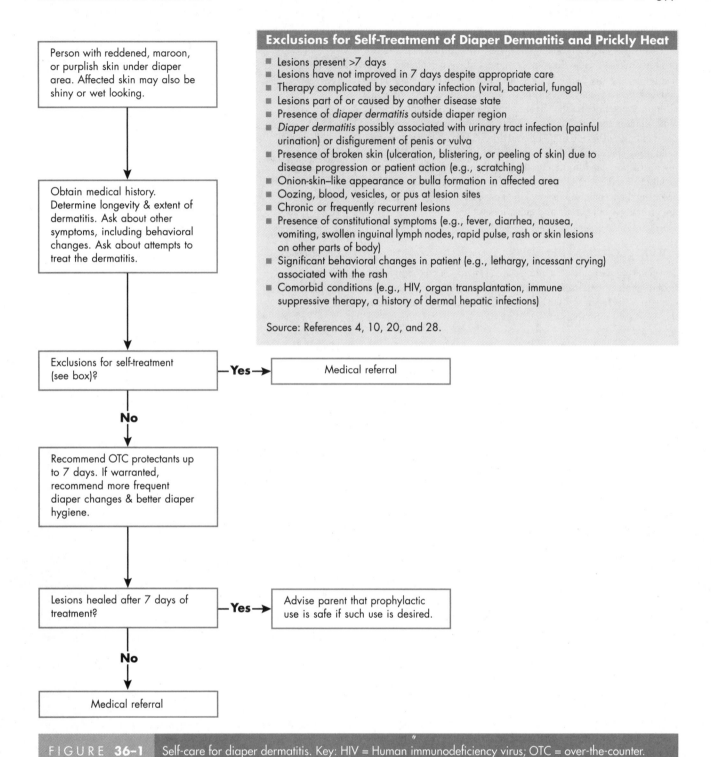

FIGURE 36–1 Self-care for diaper dermatitis. Key: HIV = Human immunodeficiency virus; OTC = over-the-counter.

When the perianal area requires cleansing (C of the ABCDE mnemonic), gentle patting with a chemically bland, soft cloth or low-abrasive baby wipe is appropriate. Sensitive-skin baby wipe products are readily available. Used with finesse and gentle wiping, baby wipes are as mild as or milder than washcloths.[23] Few baby wipes still contain alcohol, perfumes, soap, or other ingredients that can cause contact dermatitis or actually burn or sting the infant. Products that list such ingredients on the label should be avoided. Importantly, the unsoiled part of a diaper should not be used to clean or wipe the infant, because it may harbor bacteria. An alternative to wipes can be careful rinsing of the skin with warm water followed by gentle nonfriction drying. The infant's diaper area should be allowed to thoroughly air dry prior to rediapering. Cleansing should be limited to occasions when stool is present to minimize irritation from excessive cleansing.[24]

With improving technology, the disposable diaper has become a critical component of nonpharmacologic therapy for diaper dermatitis.[5,7] Caregivers should consider the following about diapers (D of the ABCDE mnemonic). Some disposable diapers have absorptive materials that pull moisture away from direct contact with the skin to reduce skin hyperhydration and mixing of urine with feces. Some disposable diapers already contain a protectant (e.g., petrolatum). Disposable diapers with dyes should be avoided, because they recently have been identified as a source of allergic contact dermatitis. Research that compared disposal and cloth diapers indicates that use of disposable diapers decreases the incidence of severe diaper dermatitis.[6,25–27] If cloth diapers are used, they should be laundered with a mild detergent; if sanitizing agents are used in the laundering process, extra rinse cycles should be used. Discussing the treatment plan with caregivers and ensuring their comprehension of the nonpharmacologic measures are critical for adherence and quick resolution.[24]

Pharmacologic Therapy

The goals of pharmacologic therapy are (1) to protect the skin from further contact with urine and feces, (2) to soothe any discomfort caused by the lesions, (3) to encourage healing, and (4) to prevent the onset of secondary infection.

Skin Protectants

Overall, skin protectants serve as physical barriers (B of the ABCDE mnemonic) between the skin and external irritants. Protectants also serve as lubricants in areas in which skin-to-skin or skin-to-diaper friction could aggravate diaper dermatitis or predispose the area to development of diaper dermatitis. Protectants absorb moisture or prevent moisture from coming into direct contact with skin. Protective effects of these products allow the body's normal healing processes to work. Because skin protectants are remarkably safe, their use as both treatment and prevention is acceptable. A skin protectant should be applied with each diaper change to aid in preventing diaper dermatitis.[17]

Protectants are the only products considered safe and effective for use in diaper dermatitis without medical referral. The Food and Drug Administration (FDA) has approved 17 ingredients, all skin protectants, for treatment of infant diaper dermatitis (Table 36–1).[28] Two or more of the approved ingredients are commonly combined in commercial products for treating diaper dermatitis. Importantly, some products contain an approved ingredient in combination with other ingredients that are unsafe or of dubious value for treating diaper dermatitis. The other ingredients may be unsuitable or even toxic when applied to skin compromised by diaper dermatitis. Therefore, a general rule of thumb is to suggest the simplest possible products that contain FDA-approved ingredients. By law, products that contain antimicrobials, topical analgesics, and antifungals cannot claim they are for treatment of diaper dermatitis. Ingredients routinely included in skin protectant formulations but not approved for treatment of diaper dermatitis are listed in Table 36–2.

Of the skin protectants listed in Table 36–1, a select few are commonly incorporated into trade-name skin protectant products. Useful comparative studies of the skin protectants are lacking. Zinc oxide is one of the most commonly used semisolid skin protectants in products that treat diaper dermatitis. A major drawback of many zinc oxide ointment preparations and other hydrophobic diaper dermatitis preparations is the necessity of soap to remove the product from the skin. However, the hydrophobic nature of the preparations is beneficial in forming a protective barrier for the compromised skin. Some zinc oxide preparations are formulated to be more washable and creamlike and therefore are easier to apply and remove. However, one must weigh the ease of use with the ability of the preparation to adequately protect the skin.

Petrolatum and white petrolatum are commonly used oleaginous ingredients that serve as excellent skin protectants. These products are ubiquitous ointment bases. Petrolatum may be listed as an active or inactive ingredient in skin protectant formulations. Lanolin is a bacteriostatic product obtained from a fatty substance found in wool and is also commonly used alone or in combination with other skin protectants. Although approved for use in diaper dermatitis, lanolin also is a common contact sensitizer. The risk for sensitization should be noted if lanolin is applied in the diaper

TABLE 36–1 FDA-Approved Skin Protectants to Treat Diaper Rash[a]

Agent	Concentration (%)
Allantoin	0.5–2
Aluminum hydroxide[b]	0.15–5
Calamine	1–25
Cocoa butter	50–100
Cod liver oil (in combination)	5.0–13.56
Colloidal oatmeal	≤0.007
Dimethicone	1–30
Glycerin[b]	20–45
Hard fat	50–100
Kaolin	4–20
Lanolin	12.5–50
Mineral oil	50–100
Petrolatum	30–100
Topical cornstarch	10–98
White petrolatum	30–100
Zinc carbonate	0.2–2
Zinc oxide	1–25

[a] Due to safety concerns, products containing sodium bicarbonate and zinc acetate are not appropriate for use in children younger than 2 years of age and have been excluded from this list.

[b] Consultation with a primary care provider is suggested prior to use in infants.

Source: Reference 28.

TABLE 36–2 Selected Nonmonograph Ingredients in Diaper Dermatitis Products

Aloe	Flower extract	Sweet clover
Beeswax	Honey	Tea tree oil
Calendula	Goldenseal	Vitamin A
Castor oil	Jojoba	Vitamin D
Chamomile	Lavender	Vitamin E
Comfrey	Peruvian balsam	

area where the skin is inflamed and more likely vulnerable to contact allergens.

Calamine is a mixture of zinc and ferrous oxides. It has absorptive, antiseptic, and antipruritic properties and is available in numerous dosage forms. Mineral oil coats the skin with a water-impenetrable film that must be washed off with each diaper change to avoid buildup in pores and subsequent folliculitis. Mineral oil often is used in small quantities in skin protectant products. It is often listed as an inactive ingredient in formulations despite FDA approval for use as an active ingredient. Dimethicone is a silicone-based oil that repels water and soothes and counteracts inflammation. It is used in combination with other skin protectants such as petrolatum.

Topical cornstarch and talc are used as loose powders. They provide benefit by reducing moisture and friction.[24] Topical cornstarch is an absorbent material, whereas talc functions as a lubricant. Both products carry warnings against inhalation of the powder because of an associated risk of severe respiratory disease. The warning states, "Keep powder away from child's face to avoid inhalation, which can cause breathing problems."[28] Some health care providers (HCPs) suggest pouring the powder into the hands away from the infant and gently rubbing it onto the perineal area; however, because of the inhalation risk, these products should likely be avoided.[24] Talc specifically should not be applied to broken or oozing skin; it can cake on the edges of wounds and precipitate infection or retard healing.

Although it has not been studied for safety and efficacy, Maalox (aluminum hydroxide and magnesium hydroxide) oral antacid suspension has become a popular topical therapy for diaper dermatitis when mixed with Aquaphor.[24] Burow's solution (aluminum acetate in water) has been compounded with petrolatum and zinc oxide to form 1-2-3 Paste, which has also been used in irritant contact dermatitis in the diaper area despite the lack of clinical evidence. Table 36–3 lists selected widely available trade-name products and their active ingredients.

Skin protectant dosing and application are straightforward. The protectant is applied liberally to the skin in the diaper area. Any remaining protectant from the previous diaper change should not be removed to minimize additional irritation that may result from the rubbing. Special attention should be paid to completely cover erythematous areas with the protectant if diaper dermatitis is already present. Overapplication (overdosage) of approved skin protectants is not a concern. Underapplication, however, can reduce the protective effectiveness of the product. The protectant should be reapplied as needed and with every diaper change. Research suggests that applying a skin protectant regularly with each diaper change is one element of preventing diaper dermatitis.[12] Skin protectants do not interact with other agents; however, the use of ointment preparations will occlude other topically applied products. Diaper dermatitis that does not necessitate medical referral commonly improves dramatically within 24 hours of initiating pharmacologic and nonpharmacologic treatment.

Contraindicated Agents

Topical nonprescription antibiotic and antifungal agents are not appropriate to use in the self-treatment of diaper dermatitis. If an infection is suspected, medical referral is advised. Topical

TABLE 36–3 Selected Nonprescription Products for Diaper Dermatitis

Trade Name	Primary Ingredients (and selected additional ingredients)
A + D Original Ointment	Petrolatum 53.4%; lanolin 15.5% (cod liver oil; mineral oil; beeswax[a])
A + D Diaper Rash Cream	Zinc oxide 10%; dimethicone 1% (aloe vera[a]; coconut oil[a]; cod liver oil; mineral oil; beeswax[a])
Aquaphor Healing Ointment	Petrolatum 41% (lanolin; mineral oil)
Aveeno Baby Soothing Relief Diaper Rash Cream	Zinc oxide 13% (oat kernel extract[a]; beeswax[a]; dimethicone; willowherb extract[a]; glycerin; mineral oil; evening primrose[a])
Baby Anti Monkey Butt Diaper Rash Powder	Calamine powder 8% (cornstarch)
Balmex Diaper Rash Cream	Zinc oxide 11.3% (beeswax[a]; dimethicone; mineral oil; soybean oil[a]; evening primrose[a]; olive leaf extract[a])
Boudreaux's Butt Paste	Zinc oxide 16% (castor oil[a]; mineral oil; Peruvian balsam[a]; petrolatum)
Burt's Bees Baby Diaper Rash Ointment	Zinc oxide 40% (sweet almond oil[a]; beeswax[a]; lanolin; castor oil[a]; jojoba oil[a]; shea butter[a]; olive oil[a]; chamomile[a]; lavender oil[a]; calendula[a]; rosemary[a]; soybean oil[a]; canola oil[a])
CeraVe Baby Diaper Rash Cream	Dimethicone 1%; zinc oxide 1% (mineral oil)
Desitin Maximum Strength Original Paste	Zinc oxide 40% (cod liver oil; lanolin; petrolatum; talc[a])
Desitin Multi-Purpose Skin Protectant and Diaper Rash Ointment	Petrolatum 70.3% (mineral oil; paraffin[a]; cocoa butter; retinyl palmitate [vitamin A palmitate][a]; cholecalciferol [vitamin D][a])
Desitin Rapid Relief Cream	Zinc oxide 13% (mineral oil; petrolatum; beeswax[a]; dimethicone; aloe[a]; glycerin)
Flanders Buttocks Ointment	White petrolatum 66.2%; zinc oxide 13.4% (beeswax[a]; castor oil[a]; mineral oil; Peruvian balsam[a])
Palmer's Cocoa Butter Formula Bottom Butter Diaper Rash Cream	Zinc oxide 10% (petrolatum; mineral oil; cocoa butter; beeswax[a]; dimethicone; corn oil[a]; soybean oil[a])
Triple Paste Medicated Ointment	Zinc oxide 12.8% (cornstarch; lanolin; white petrolatum; beeswax[a])

[a] Nonmonograph ingredients.

analgesics are not recommended, because they can alter sensory perception in a population that often cannot communicate perceptual changes. These agents may also excoriate macerated skin, cause pain, retard healing, and further complicate diaper dermatitis.

Hydrocortisone is indicated for minor skin irritation, but it should not be used in diaper dermatitis without supervision by an HCP. Hydrocortisone can increase the risk of secondary infection via immune response suppression. Additionally, the diaper area is a significant portion of the infant's body surface area. Hydrocortisone absorption into the skin is enhanced under occlusive conditions. When applied to macerated skin or a large surface area, absorption of hydrocortisone may lead to serum levels that interfere with the infant's pituitary–adrenal axis. Nonprescription hydrocortisone is labeled to be avoided in patients younger than 2 years. (See Chapter 35 for additional information on the use of hydrocortisone.)

Product Selection Guidelines

Whereas no particular product among the approved products possesses evidence-based advantages, personal preferences for particular product characteristics will likely determine which product caregivers use to treat diaper dermatitis. As previously mentioned, some commonly used products contain nonapproved (i.e., nonmonograph) ingredients. These products may be used for formulation purposes, or they may be unregulated nutraceuticals listed as inactive or active ingredients. Unapproved ingredients could also be included in preparations to support marketing claims. For example, camphor may be present to provide a "medicated" fragrance; aloe may be present to appeal to the public perception that aloe is a wound-healing agent; or vitamins may be present to convey "natural" characteristics. To make the claim to treat diaper dermatitis, the product, however, must meet FDA-published guidelines for active ingredients. Because diaper dermatitis is a condition primarily of special populations (infants and geriatrics), there are no additional concerns related to product selection in those populations.

Complementary Therapies

Complementary therapies are not recommended for use in newborns and infants because of insufficient evidence regarding their safety and effectiveness in these populations. Rates of systemic absorption are unknown. Although some of these agents have been used without incident in adults, no credible data exist on their safety or efficacy in infants. Recently, honey has received attention as a treatment for diaper dermatitis; it has been used for several years in wound care. Manuka honey in particular has been shown to provide hygroscopic, fungicidal, and antibacterial properties and helps to regulate the mildly acidic pH of the skin. Initial studies have shown honey, beeswax, and olive oil to be effective in management of diaper dermatitis.[29] Although these agents should not be recommended at this time, with more robust studies, they may become acceptable recommendations in the future.

Assessment of Diaper Dermatitis: A Case-Based Approach

When a caregiver or patient consults an HCP about a suspected diaper dermatitis, the provider should evaluate the presentation of the diaper rash itself and determine the extent to which factors conducive to exacerbation of diaper dermatitis are present. If appropriate, the provider should visually inspect the diaper dermatitis. If such inspection is inappropriate, the provider should use open-ended questioning techniques to gain a description of the dermatitis. Case 36–1 illustrates assessment of patients with diaper dermatitis. If the dermatitis is deemed to be uncomplicated diaper dermatitis warranting self-care, nonpharmacologic and pharmacologic suggestions can be made by the HCP. From a nonpharmacologic perspective, the caregiver should be asked what type of diaper is being used and how frequently diapers are changed. Drawing on that response, the provider must consider whether increasing the frequency of diaper changes and other nonpharmacologic measures are likely sufficient to heal the diaper dermatitis or whether pharmacologic treatment is warranted. Given the minimal risk associated with pharmacologic treatment, many available options are often appropriate to suggest to the caregiver.

Patient Counseling for Diaper Dermatitis

The HCP should educate (E of the ABCDE mnemonic) the caregiver on proper cleaning of the diaper area. Additionally, the provider should advise the caregiver to avoid occlusion of the area, when feasible, and to avoid prolonged contact of urine or feces with the infant's skin. The provider should explain the proper methods of applying nonprescription skin protectants and should describe to the caregiver signs and symptoms that indicate the dermatitis has worsened and warrants medical attention. The box "Patient Education for Diaper Dermatitis" lists specific information to provide caregivers.

Evaluation of Patient Outcomes for Diaper Dermatitis

Treatment of diaper dermatitis should be relatively short. If 7 days of treatment have elapsed and the condition is not showing signs of healing, medical referral should occur. At the conclusion of therapy, the skin should return to its pre-diaper dermatitis condition. If diaper dermatitis presents routinely or has a severe presentation, prophylactic use of skin protectants is suggested, given the safety of preparations presented in Table 36–1.

PRICKLY HEAT

Prickly heat, also known as heat rash, is a transient inflammation of the skin that appears as a very fine, pinpoint, and usually red raised rash. It can appear on any part of the body that has sweat glands (e.g., groin, chest, axillae). This condition occurs in any aged patient with active sweat glands.[30] It affects up to 40% of infants, with the greatest incidence during the first month of life.[30] It is likely underreported, because it is less troublesome than diaper dermatitis and generally clears up rapidly. Prickly heat often presents in hot working conditions and with activities associated with sweating (e.g., manual labor, exercise, athletics).[31,32]

CASE 36-1

Relevant Evaluation Criteria	Scenario/Model Outcome
Collect	
1. Gather essential information about the patient's symptoms and medical history, including	
a. Description of symptom(s) (i.e., nature, onset, duration, severity, associated symptoms)	Mrs. Tate has noticed her daughter Brooklyn has been very fussy lately. While changing Brooklyn's diapers over the past few days, she noticed that her baby's bottom has been getting progressively redder and is now bright red. It also appears shiny and is sensitive to touch. Brooklyn cries with each diaper change, especially when her mother uses wipes to clean her.
b. Description of any factors that seem to precipitate, exacerbate, and/or relieve the patient's symptom(s)	Similar rashes have occurred before, but Mrs. Tate mentions that this rash seems to be much worse. In the past, symptoms have resolved before she has needed to see the pediatrician. Mrs. Tate does mention that they have been introducing some solid foods into her daughter's diet within the past few weeks, which coincides with worsening symptoms.
c. Description of the patent's efforts to relieve the symptoms	Mrs. Tate has been trying to change Brooklyn's diaper more often at home, but she is not sure if this is continuing while her daughter is at daycare. She also purchased disposable diapers that were specially formulated for infants with sensitive skin, but she has not seen much difference so far.
d. Patient's identity	Brooklyn Tate
e. Patient's age, gender, height, and weight	5 months old, female, 24 in., 15 lb
f. Patient's occupation	n/a
g. Patient's dietary habits	Breastfed, 5–6 feedings per day; beginning to introduce dry rice cereal
h. Patient's sleep habits	Normal for age
i. Concurrent medical conditions, prescription and nonprescription medications, and dietary supplements	None
j. Allergies	NKA
k. History of other adverse reactions to medications	None noted
l. Other (describe) ______	n/a
Assess	
2. Differentiate patient's signs/symptoms, and correctly identify the patient's primary problem(s).	Symptoms are consistent with mild–moderate diaper dermatitis in the groin area. The description of the rash, along with the quick onset and the child's irritability and sensitivity, support this diagnosis.
3. Identify exclusions for self-treatment (Figure 36–1).	None noted.
4. Formulate a comprehensive list of therapeutic alternatives for the primary problem to determine whether triage to a health care provider is required, and share this information with the patient or caregiver.	Options include (1) Refer Brooklyn immediately to her pediatrician or other PCP. (2) Recommend self-care until an appropriate PCP can be consulted. (3) Recommend self-care with nonprescription product(s). (4) Recommend self-care with nonpharmacologic methods. (5) Recommend both nonprescription self-care product(s) and non-pharmacologic treatment. (6) Take no action.
Plan	
5. Select an optimal therapeutic alternative to address the patient's problem, taking into account patient preferences.	The best recommendation would be to use both nonprescription and nonpharmacologic methods to treat Brooklyn's rash. Suggest Mrs. Tate continue with increased diaper changes and allow the area to completely air dry between diaper changes. She may also try cleansing the skin gently with warm water when stool is present and then thoroughly drying. Recommend liberal application of a skin protectant with every diaper change, as needed. (See Table 36–3 for a listing of available products.) Mrs. Tate can be encouraged to continue use of the product even after the current rash heals to prevent future diaper rash.

CASE 36-1 *continued*

Relevant Evaluation Criteria	Scenario/Model Outcome
6. Describe the recommended therapeutic approach to the patient or caregiver.	"A skin protectant will help protect Brooklyn's skin from further irritation and will allow the diaper rash to heal. Changing her diaper more often and allowing the skin to air dry will quicken healing time and reduce the likelihood of the rash coming back. You should also use plain, warm water or sensitive wipes to clean the area prior to air drying."
7. Explain to the patient or caregiver the rationale for selecting the recommended therapeutic approach from the considered therapeutic alternatives.	"Based on the appearance of Brooklyn's diaper rash, you should be able to use nonprescription products. She currently does not need to see her pediatrician, but one should be contacted if her rash has not improved within 7 days, if the skin under her diaper becomes broken, or if she develops any symptoms not limited to the diapering area."
Implement	
8. When recommending self-care with nonprescription medications and/or nondrug therapy, convey accurate information to the patient or caregiver.	
a. Appropriate dose and frequency of administration	"Apply Boudreaux's Butt Paste liberally to the affected area with every diaper change and as needed."
b. Maximum number of days the therapy should be employed	"Skin protectants can be applied to both treat and prevent diaper rash. There is no maximum length of therapy for this medication. However, if symptoms do not improve within 7 days, seek medical attention."
c. Product administration procedures	"Wash your hands and clean the diaper region with a sensitive baby wipe or plain warm water. Allow the area to thoroughly air dry. Once dry, apply the paste to the diaper region liberally. Change diapers at least 6 times a day, every 3–4 hours as a minimum."
d. Expected time to onset of relief	"You should see noticeable improvement in the rash within 24 hours."
e. Degree of relief that can be reasonably expected	"The rash will become less tender with continued application. Skin should return to normal within 7 days—quicker if diapering technique is adjusted."
f. Most common adverse effects	"There are no common adverse effects reported with this product."
g. Adverse effects that warrant medical intervention should they occur	n/a
h. Patient options in the event that condition worsens or persists	See the box "Patient Education for Diaper Dermatitis" and Figure 36–1.
i. Product storage requirements	"Store this product out of reach of children and away from heat and moisture."
j. Specific nondrug measures	See the box "Patient Education for Diaper Dermatitis."
Solicit follow-up questions from the patient or caregiver.	"What are the differences between the various diaper rash products?"
Answer the patient's or caregiver's questions.	"Ointments, pastes, and creams are usually preferred over powders that can be dangerous if inhaled. Most all of the agents provide similar benefit and lack any major adverse effects. Children may be sensitive to products containing lanolin, especially if they suffer from other allergies. Products containing mineral oil must be washed off with each diaper change to avoid occurrence of folliculitis. Zinc oxide and other greasy products require soap to be removed from the skin. It is probably best to avoid products containing any extra 'natural' ingredients, which usually lack evidence of benefit."
Follow-up: Monitor and Evaluate	
9. Assess patient outcome.	Ask Mrs. Tate to call you in 2 days to discuss how Brooklyn's rash is resolving with the suggested treatment plan.

Key: n/a = Not applicable; NKA = no known allergies; PCP = primary care provider.

PATIENT EDUCATION FOR
Diaper Dermatitis

The goals of diaper rash treatment are (1) to relieve the symptoms, (2) to rid the patient of the rash, (3) to prevent secondary infection, and (4) to prevent recurrences. For most patients, carefully following product instructions and the self-care measures listed here will help ensure optimal therapeutic outcomes.

Nondrug Measures

- Use the mnemonic ABCDE (air, barrier, cleansing, diaper, education) in managing diaper dermatitis.
- Change diapers frequently, at least six times a day, to prevent exposure of the infant's skin to moisture and feces.
- Do not use rubber or plastic pants over cloth diapers. Tightly covering the skin encourages skin breakdown.
- During every diaper change, use plain water to clean the diaper area. Gently dry area or allow it to air dry.
- Do not wipe the infant with any part of the diaper. Even areas that appear clean may be contaminated with fecal bacteria.
- Avoid commercial baby wipes that contain alcohol, perfumes, and soap, which may burn or sting the skin.
- If feasible, allow the infant to go without a diaper, even for short instances, in an effort to dry the rash.

Nonprescription Medications

- To treat diaper rash, use a product containing one or more of the skin protectants listed in Table 36–1. The product can be used even after the rash clears to prevent recurrences.
- Do not use products that contain ingredients listed in Table 36–1 if they are combined with benzocaine or an antibacterial such as benzethonium chloride. Benzocaine can cause an allergic reaction; antibacterials are not suitable for use on diaper rash.
- Do not use hydrocortisone.
- Do not use topical (external) analgesics such as phenol, menthol, methyl salicylate, or capsaicin to treat diaper rash. These medications are inappropriate for use on infant skin and may cause harm.
- Powders for children or infants should ideally be avoided; if used, they should be gently poured into the caregiver's hands away from the infant's face and then rubbed onto the skin, using a sufficient amount to cover the affected area. Do not vigorously shake powders near infants. Avoid infant inhalation of powders.
- Apply cream or ointment liberally to cover the affected area.
- If mineral oil has been applied, wash it off at every diaper change to avoid clogging skin pores.
- Throw away products that are discolored or whose expiration dates have passed. (The health care provider should point out expiration dates on the products.)

When to Seek Medical Attention

- Consult a primary care provider if any of the exclusions in Figure 36–1 apply.

Pathophysiology of Prickly Heat

Prickly heat results from partially clogged sweat glands. (See Chapter 38 for a review of the anatomy of the sweat gland.) The trapped sweat causes dilation and rupture of epidermal sweat pores, resulting in acute inflammation of the dermis that may manifest as stinging, burning, or itching.[33]

Prickly heat can arise from normal skin with little or no anatomic prodrome. The condition is most often associated with very hot, humid weather or during illnesses that cause significant or profuse sweating. It is commonly associated with the inability of the skin to "breathe" because of excessive tight, flame-resistant, or occlusive clothing such as leather, polyester, athletic clothing materials (i.e. neoprene), or athletic protective or safety garments and devices.[34] Chemicals added during the laundering process can also be a cause of prickly heat.[35]

Clinical Presentation of Prickly Heat

The hallmark presentation of prickly heat is pinpoint-sized lesions that are raised and red or maroon, forming erythematous papules (see Color Plates, photograph 23). The lesions may appear in small numbers clustered together or spread over the occluded area on a pink to red field (miliaria rubra). Common sites for prickly heat dermatitis include the axillae, chest, upper back, back of the neck, abdomen, and inguinal area. The lesions often trace the pattern of the occlusion and, in uncomplicated cases, do not extend beyond the occluded area. If lesions are not resolved in a reasonable length of time (approximately 3–10 days), they can evolve into the same kinds of complications seen in diaper dermatitis (e.g., infection, pustule formation, generalized dermatitis). Complications, however, are extremely rare.

Treatment of Prickly Heat

Treatment Goals

The primary goal of treatment in prickly heat is removal of the causative agent or agents. Lesions associated with prickly heat usually resolve without pharmacologic treatment if the cause is removed. A secondary goal in the treatment of prickly heat is alleviation of symptoms associated with the condition.

General Treatment Approach

The nonpharmacologic treatment goals for prickly heat include (1) eliminating occlusion of skin, (2) protecting skin from further irritation, (3) promoting healing of skin, and (4) discouraging onset of secondary infection.

Pharmacologic therapy and nonpharmacologic therapy have the same goals. Pharmacologic products help (1) keep skin dry, (2) promote healing, (3) soothe any discomfort caused by lesion(s), and (4) discourage onset of secondary infection. The algorithm in Figure 36–2 outlines the self-treatment of prickly heat.

Nonpharmacologic Therapy

Nondrug therapy for prickly heat includes measures to decrease sweating and increase air flow to the affected area. If the sweating

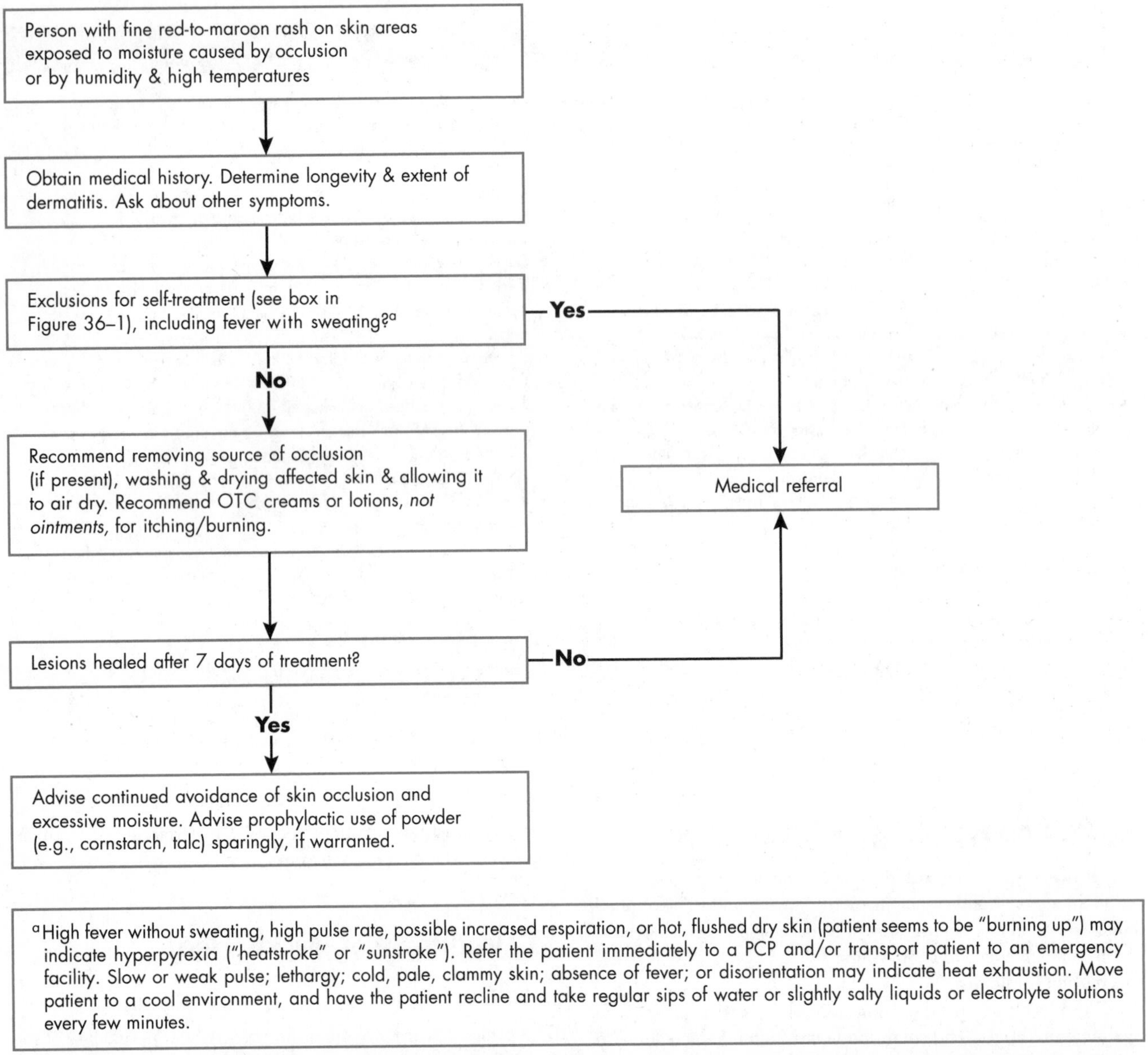
Person with fine red-to-maroon rash on skin areas exposed to moisture caused by occlusion or by humidity & high temperatures
Obtain medical history. Determine longevity & extent of dermatitis. Ask about other symptoms.
Exclusions for self-treatment (see box in Figure 36–1), including fever with sweating?[a]
Yes
No
Recommend removing source of occlusion (if present), washing & drying affected skin & allowing it to air dry. Recommend OTC creams or lotions, *not ointments*, for itching/burning.
Medical referral
Lesions healed after 7 days of treatment?
No
Yes
Advise continued avoidance of skin occlusion and excessive moisture. Advise prophylactic use of powder (e.g., cornstarch, talc) sparingly, if warranted.
[a]High fever without sweating, high pulse rate, possible increased respiration, or hot, flushed dry skin (patient seems to be "burning up") may indicate hyperpyrexia ("heatstroke" or "sunstroke"). Refer the patient immediately to a PCP and/or transport patient to an emergency facility. Slow or weak pulse; lethargy; cold, pale, clammy skin; absence of fever; or disorientation may indicate heat exhaustion. Move patient to a cool environment, and have the patient recline and take regular sips of water or slightly salty liquids or electrolyte solutions every few minutes.

FIGURE 36–2 Self-care for prickly heat. Key: OTC = Over-the-counter; PCP = primary care provider.

is caused by a fever, use of systemic antipyretics may be appropriate, unless contraindicated. Wearing loose, light-colored, and lightweight clothing is palliative in prickly heat, allowing airflow to the skin. Cooling baths and use of air conditioning will also be helpful in symptoms management. Keeping that in mind, all excessive clothing should be removed. HCPs should warn patients not to apply oleaginous substances to prickly heat lesions, because these substances plug pores that need to be patent.

Pharmacologic Therapy

Nonprescription treatment of prickly heat should be limited to mild–moderate, uncomplicated cases. Affected areas should not be occluded during therapy. Cooling baths and use of air conditioning will be helpful in symptom management. Overall, this disorder can be ameliorated in less time and with less total drug exposure than are required for diaper dermatitis.

Emollients, Skin Protectants, and Antipruritics

A drug product that relieves burning and itching and does not block exposure of skin to air should be used. Water-washable antipruritic products, as well as bland emollients and protectants that soothe the skin and maintain skin moisture and texture, can be used to treat the symptoms of prickly heat. Colloidal oatmeal bath products and lotions are useful because of their antipruritic and soothing properties. Powders should be used only prophylactically to absorb moisture and keep skin dry. (See Table 36–4 for selected trade-name products and Chapter 33 for a discussion of skin emollients.)

TABLE 36–4 **Selected Nonprescription Products for Prickly Heat**

Trade Name	Primary Ingredients (and selected additional ingredients)
Aveeno Daily Moisturizing Lotion	Dimethicone 1.2% (glycerin; colloidal oatmeal)
Extra Strength Benadryl Itch Stopping Cream	Diphenhydramine HCl 2%; zinc acetate 0.1%
Cortizone-10 Maximum Strength Anti-Itch Cream	Hydrocortisone 1% (aloe; beeswax; glycerin; mineral oil; petrolatum)
Eucerin Calming Itch Relief Treatment	Menthol 0.1% (glycerin; colloidal oatmeal; dimethicone; evening primrose oil; castor oil)
Lubriderm Daily Moisture Lotion	Water; glycerin; mineral oil; petrolatum; dimethicone

Other Pharmacologic Agents

As with diaper dermatitis, hydrocortisone is contraindicated in infants. In adults, hydrocortisone may be useful if the body surface area involved is 10% or less. (See Figure 41–4 for information on calculating body surface area.) Because prickly heat rapidly clears without drug therapy, hydrocortisone should be used only when relief of itching is required. Topical antihistamines and local anesthetics (see Chapter 37) carry the risk of sensitization, but they can be used as antipruritic agents. Patients who have a fever and the associated sweating may be causing prickly heat can use standard systemic analgesics to manage the fever (see Chapter 5).

Product Selection Guidelines

When treating prickly heat, the skin needs to dry and dissipate moisture. Therefore, only water-washable, cream-based products should be used. For moisture absorption and prevention of wetness, powders are reasonable; however, prolonged use or overuse can lead to clogged pores, precipitating prickly heat. When applied to the chest or neck, cornstarch or talc powder should be placed in the hand and applied manually to the skin with light friction. Any product that has a potentially toxic ingredient (e.g., phenols, boric acid) if absorbed through thin, compromised skin should not be recommended for infants. Bathing children and infants who have prickly heat in colloidal oatmeal or lukewarm water may be recommended as a first option.

Assessment of Prickly Heat: A Case-Based Approach

Patient assessment for prickly heat involves identifying the site(s) of the lesions and potential causes. If the patient is an infant, the HCP should gather information regarding potential environmental characteristics (e.g., sleeping conditions, presence/absence of air conditioning) that could be exacerbating the condition.

Case 36–2 provides an example of assessment of a patient with prickly heat.

Patient Counseling for Prickly Heat

The HCP should stress to the patient that prickly heat is usually easily treated by removing factors that clog skin pores, while also explaining appropriate nonpharmacologic and pharmacologic measures for healing or alleviating symptoms. The provider should explain that excessive use of skin protectants could exacerbate the disorder. The box "Patient Education for Prickly Heat" lists specific information to provide patients.

Evaluation of Patient Outcomes for Prickly Heat

Treatment of prickly heat should be relatively short. Considerable improvement is commonly noted in as little as 24 hours after initiation of nonpharmacologic and pharmacologic treatment. If the condition is not completely resolved or has worsened after 7 days of treatment, the patient should be referred for further evaluation. Monitoring of treatment success involves simple observation of lesions. At the end of therapy, the affected skin should have returned to its precondition state.

Key Points for Diaper Dermatitis and Prickly Heat

Diaper Dermatitis

- Diaper dermatitis is exacerbated by moisture and occlusion.
- Increasing the frequency of diaper changes (i.e., decreasing contact time between skin and excrement) plays a major role in the nonpharmacologic treatment of diaper dermatitis.
- Pharmacologic treatment should be limited to products containing FDA-approved ingredients indicated for the treatment of diaper dermatitis (Table 36–1); exotic additives and complementary therapies should be avoided.
- Apply hydrophobic skin protectants liberally to diaper dermatitis areas; overapplication should not be a concern.
- Do not use hydrocortisone in the self-treatment of diaper dermatitis.
- The majority of diaper dermatitis cases will resolve when occlusion and wetness are adequately suppressed.
- Cases of diaper dermatitis that are still present after 7 days of treatment should be referred for further evaluation.

Prickly Heat

- Prickly heat is exacerbated by heat, humidity, and occlusion.
- Generally, prickly heat will resolve when occlusion and wetness are adequately suppressed.

CASE 36-2

Relevant Evaluation Criteria	Scenario/Model Outcome
Collect	
1. Gather essential information about the patient's symptoms and medical history, including	
a. Description of symptom(s) (i.e., nature, onset, duration, severity, associated symptoms)	Patient states he has a "red, itchy rash in tiny dots" on his upper arms, back, and shoulders. He has had the rash for 2 days. He states that the rash is not painful.
b. Description of any factors that seem to precipitate, exacerbate, and/or relieve the patient's symptom(s)	Patient seems to get this rash every few months, but notices that it happens more often in warm weather. He is a firefighter and notices the rash when he has to wear his gear a lot. He still gets the rash occasionally in the winter when he plays in his intramural basketball league.
c. Description of the patent's efforts to relieve the symptoms	Patient tries to prevent rash through good personal hygiene techniques (e.g., taking showers more frequently) and applying a thick cream to problem areas to keep them moist; however, these measures do not always prevent the rash.
d. Patient's identity	D.R. Myers
e. Patient's age, gender, height, and weight	28 years old, male, 6 ft 1 in., 200 lb
f. Patient's occupation	Firefighter
g. Patient's dietary habits	Normal diet; minimal vegetables; social drinker
h. Patient's sleep habits	Averages 7 hours of sleep nightly.
i. Concurrent medical conditions, prescription and nonprescription medications, and dietary supplements	None
j. Allergies	Allergy to penicillin (hives)
k. History of other adverse reactions to medications	None
l. Other (describe) ______	D.R. is a very fit individual who plays several intramural sports and coaches high school football. He often joins his students during drills at practice.
Assess	
2. Differentiate patient's signs/symptoms, and correctly identify the patient's primary problem(s).	Prickly heat secondary to sweating, exercise, heat, and athletic clothing and equipment
3. Identify exclusions for self-treatment (Figure 36–1).	None
4. Formulate a comprehensive list of therapeutic alternatives for the primary problem to determine whether triage to a health care provider is required, and share this information with the patient or caregiver.	Options include (1) Refer D.R. to a dermatologist or his PCP. (2) Recommend self-care until an appropriate HCP can be consulted. (3) Recommend self-care with nonprescription product(s). (4) Recommend self-care with nonpharmacologic methods. (5) Recommend both nonprescription self-care products and nonpharmacologic treatment. (6) Take no action.
Plan	
5. Select an optimal therapeutic alternative to address the patient's problem, taking into account patient preferences.	Patient education about the cause of prickly heat is important in prevention of future occurrences. Colloidal oatmeal lotions should provide relief from itching and also provide soothing benefits. Powders may be used prophylactically to absorb moisture. Cooling baths and air conditioning should also be used.
6. Describe the recommended therapeutic approach to the patient or caregiver.	"Discontinue the thick cream, because it can block pores, worsening your prickly heat. Topical hydrocortisone will help with the itching, but do not apply it to more than 10% of your body."
7. Explain to the patient or caregiver the rationale for selecting the recommended therapeutic approach from the considered therapeutic alternatives.	"Prickly heat often heals with time and can be effectively managed with nonprescription products and hygiene practices. Keeping the area dry and minimizing clogged pores are key measures. If relief of itching is needed, hydrocortisone is preferred, because topical antihistamines and local anesthetics carry the risk of sensitization."

Relevant Evaluation Criteria	Scenario/Model Outcome
Implement	
8. When recommending self-care with nonprescription medications and/or nondrug therapy, convey accurate information to the patient or caregiver.	
a. Appropriate dose and frequency of administration	"Cortizone 10 Maximum Strength: apply to affected area(s) not more than 3–4 times daily as needed. Johnson's Baby Powder: apply 1 time daily after showering. Do not inhale powder."
b. Maximum number of days the therapy should be employed	"Nonprescription protectants and self-treatment of prickly heat are limited to 7 days."
c. Product administration procedures	See the box "Patient Education for Prickly Heat."
d. Expected time to onset of relief	"Twenty-four hours or less if nonpharmacologic measures are employed as directed"
e. Degree of relief that can be reasonably expected	"Skin should return to normal within 7–10 days; protectants may not provide sufficient itch relief." Prickly heat is likely to return if nonpharmacologic strategies not implemented.
f. Most common adverse effects	Powders used in excess may clog pores, exacerbating the condition.
g. Adverse effects that warrant medical intervention should they occur	Respiratory inhalation of powders
h. Patient options in the event that condition worsens or persists	See "Exclusions for Self-Treatment" in Figure 36–1.
i. Product storage requirements	"Keep product out of reach of children."
j. Specific nondrug measures	See "Nondrug Measures" in the box "Patient Education for Prickly Heat."
Solicit follow-up questions from the patient or caregiver.	"Are there specific athletic clothing items that make this better or worse?"
Answer the patient's or caregiver's questions.	"Any type of tight or occlusive clothing will worsen or make prickly heat more likely. Neoprene materials in athletic clothing have been found to make prickly heat more likely. Wearing loose athletic clothing and removal of clothing immediately after working out and then showering will minimize your risk."
Follow-up: Monitor and Evaluate	
9. Assess patient outcome.	Ask Mr. Myers to call you in 3 days to update you on his response to your treatment plan.

Key: HCP = Health care provider; PCP = primary care provider.

PATIENT EDUCATION FOR

Prickly Heat

The objectives of self-treatment are (1) to relieve the discomfort of prickly heat and (2) to eliminate its cause. For most patients, following product instructions and the self-care measures listed here will help ensure optimal therapeutic outcomes.

Nondrug Measures

- To prevent clogging skin pores, avoid excessive sweating by resting, cooling off, or going to a cool environment.
- Wear loose, light-colored, porous, and lightweight clothing to allow airflow to the skin.
- Shower, bathe, or change clothes immediately after heavy sweating, and wear loose-fitting clothes when such activity is anticipated. Remember to drink plenty of fluids, and allow the body to cool down after any strenuous activity.

Nonprescription Medications

- Unless a health care provider advises otherwise, use systemic analgesics, such as, aspirin, acetaminophen, or ibuprofen, to reduce a fever and the sweating it can cause. (See Chapter 5 for dosing information.)
- Do not apply oily substances to prickly heat lesions, because they clog skin pores.
- Use powdered skin protectants to absorb moisture and help prevent wetness (Table 36–3). Place cornstarch or talc powder in the hand, and apply to the skin with light friction. Note that prolonged use or overuse of powders can lead to clogged pores and can precipitate prickly heat in adults.
- Do not use hydrocortisone on infants. However, it may be used to relieve itching in adult cases of prickly heat if no more than 10% of the body surface area is involved.
- Water-washable emollients applied in a thin film twice a day can help the skin return to normal (see Chapter 33).
- If redness, burning, itching, peeling, or swelling develops after a product is applied, rinse any remaining product off the skin and avoid further use.
- To soothe discomfort in adults or infants, wash the affected skin with bland soap or soak the skin in a colloidal oatmeal solution.
- The condition should show observable improvement in 24 hours.

When to Seek Medical Attention

- If the condition persists after 7 days of treatment, consult a primary care provider.

- Products containing emollients or anti-itch ingredients in water-washable dosage forms are favored in the treatment of prickly heat. Powders may be used to help dry the skin, but they must be used judiciously to prevent clogged pores.
- Pharmacologic treatment of prickly heat should be targeted at providing relief from itching or burning.
- Cases of prickly heat that persist after 7 days of treatment should be referred for further evaluation.

REFERENCES

1. Foureur N, Vanzo B, Meaume S, et al. Prospective aetiological study of diaper dermatitis in the elderly. *Br J Dermatol.* 2006;155(5):941–6. doi:10.1111/j.1365-2133.206.07423.x.
2. Ravanfar P, Wallace JS, Pace NC. Diaper dermatitis: a review and update. *Curr Opin Pediatr.* 2012;24(4):472–9. doi: 10.1097/MOP.0b013e32835585f2.
3. Ward DB, Fleischer Jr AB, Feldman SR, et al. Characterization of diaper dermatitis in the United States. *Arch Pediatr Adolesc Med.* 2000;154(9): 943–6. PMID: 10980800.
4. Nield LS, Kamat D. Prevention, diagnosis, and management of diaper dermatitis. *Clin Pediatr (Phila).* 2007;46(6):480–6. doi: 10.1177/0009922806292409.
5. Erasala GN, Romain C, Merlay I. Diaper area and disposable diapers. *Curr Probl Dermatol.* 2011;40:83–9. doi: 10.1159/000321057.
6. Akin F, Spraker M, Aly R, et al. Effects of breathable disposable diapers: reduced prevalence of Candida and common diaper dermatitis. *Pediatr Dermatol.* 2001;18(4):282–90. PMID: 11576399.
7. Odio M, Friedlander SF. Diaper dermatitis and advances in diaper technology. *Curr Opin Pediatr.* 2000;12(4):342–6. PMID: 10943814.
8. Shin HT. Diaper dermatitis that does not quit. *Dermatol Therapy.* 2005;18(2):124–35. doi: 10.1016/j.pcl.2013.11.009.
9. Adam R. Skin care of the diaper area. *Pediatr Dermatol.* 2008;25(4): 427–33. doi: 10.1111/j.1525-1470.2008.00725.x.
10. Scheinfeld N. Diaper dermatitis: a review and brief survey of eruptions of the diaper area. *Am J Clin Dermatol.* 2005;6(5):273–81. PMID: 16252927.
11. Borkowski S. Diaper rash care and management. *Pediatr Nurs.* 2004;30(6): 467–70. PMID: 15704594.
12. Atherton DJ. A review of the pathophysiology, prevention and treatment of irritant diaper dermatitis. *Curr Med Res Opin.* 2004;20(5):645–9. doi: 10.1185/030079904125003575.
13. Adalat S, Wall D, Goodyear H. Diaper dermatitis—frequency and contributory factors in hospital attending children. *Pediatr Dermatol.* 2007;24(5): 483–8. doi: 10.1111/j.1525-1470.2007.00499.x.
14. Berg RW. Etiologic factors in diaper dermatitis: a model for development of improved diapers. *Pediatrician.* 1986;14(Suppl 1):27–33. PMID: 3601827.
15. Stamatas GN, Zerweck C, Grove G, et al. Documentation of impaired epidermal barrier in mild and moderate diaper dermatitis in vivo using noninvasive methods. *Pediatr Dermatol.* 2011;28(2):99–107. doi: 10.1111/j.1525-1470.2011.01308.x.
16. Wolf R, Wolf D, Tuzun B, et al. Diaper dermatitis. *Clin Dermatol.* 2000; 18(6):657–60. PMID: 11173200.
17. Stamatas GN, Tierney NK. Diaper dermatitis: etiology, manifestations, prevention, and management. *Pediatr Dermatol.* 2014;31(1):1–7. doi: 10.1111/pde.12245.
18. Beguin AM, Malaquin-Pavan E, Guihaire C, et al. Improving diaper design to address incontinence associated dermatitis. *BMC Geriatr.* 2010;10(86): 1–10. doi: 10.1186/1471-2318-10-86.
19. Benjamin L. Clinical correlates with diaper dermatitis. *Pediatrician.* 1987; 14(suppl 1):21–6. PMID: 3299331.
20. Smith WJ, Jacob SE. The role of allergic contact dermatitis in diaper dermatitis. *Pediatr Dermatol.* 2009;26(3):369–70. doi: 10.1111/j.1525-1470.2009.00934.x.
21. Gupta AK, Skinner AR. Management of diaper dermatitis. *Int J Dermatol.* 2004;43(11):830–4. doi: 10.1111/j.1365-4632.2004.02405.x.
22. Boiko S. Treatment of diaper dermatitis. *Dermatol Clin.* 1999;17:235–40. PMID: 9987005.
23. Odio M, Streicher-Scott J, Hansen RC. Disposable baby wipes: efficacy and skin mildness. *Dermatol Nurs.* 2001;13(2):107–13. PMID: 11917305.
24. Klunk C, Domingues E, Wiss K. An update on diaper dermatitis. *Clin Dermatol.* 2014;32:477–87. doi: 10.1016/j.clindermatol.2014.02.003.
25. Visscher MO, Chatterjee R, Munson KA, et al. Development of diaper rash in the newborn. *Pediatr Dermatol.* 2000;17(1):52–7. PMID: 10720989.
26. Liu N, Wang X, Odio M. Frequency and severity of diaper dermatitis with use of traditional Chinese cloth diapers: observations in 3- to 9-month-old children. *Pediatr Dermatol.* 2011;28(4):380–6. doi: 10.1111/j.1525-1470.2011.01494.x.
27. Lavender T, Furber C, Campbell M, et al. Effect on skin hydration of using baby wipes to clean the napkin area of newborn babies: assessor-blinded randomised controlled equivalence trial. *BMC Pediatr.* 2012;12(59):1–9. doi: 10.1186/1471-2431-12-59.
28. U.S. Food and Drug Administration. Skin protectant drug products for over-the-counter human use; final monograph. Final rule. *Fed Regist.* June 4, 2003;68(107):33362–81.
29. Burlando B, Cornara L. Honey in dermatology and skin care: a review. *J Cosmet Dermatol.* 2013;12(4):306–13. doi: 10.1111/jocd.12058.
30. Feng E, Janniger CK. Miliaria. *Cutis.* 1995;55(4):213–6. PMID: 7796612.
31. Howe AS, Boden BP. Heat-related illness in athletes. *Am J Sports Med.* 2007;35(8):1384–95. doi: 10.1177/0363546507305013.
32. Bray P, Sokas R, Ahluwalia J. Heat-related illnesses: opportunities for prevention. *J Occup Environ Med.* 2010;52(8):844–5. doi: 10.1097/JOM.0b013e3181ed4c36.
33. Zaidi Z, Lanigan SW. Diseases of the sebaceous, sweat, and apocrine glands. In: *Dermatology in Clinical Practice.* 1st ed. London: Springer; 2010:337–57.
34. Schulmerich SC. When nature turns up the heat. *RN.* 1999;62(8):35–8. PMID: 10481729.
35. Carter III R, Garcia AM, Souhan BE. Patients presenting with miliaria while wearing flame resistant clothing in high ambient temperatures: a case series. *J Med Case Rep.* 2011;5:474. doi: 10.1186/1752-1947-5-474.

CHAPTER 37

INSECT BITES AND STINGS AND PEDICULOSIS

PATRICIA H. FABEL AND ELIZABETH W. BLAKE

Insect bites and stings are common, and anyone who spends time outdoors is at risk. These injuries usually cause only a local reaction, but they can produce a mild allergic reaction or life-threatening anaphylaxis in patients who are sensitive to compounds in the insect's saliva. Approximately 0.5% of the population may show signs of systemic allergic reactions to insect stings, and simultaneous multiple insect stings of 500 or more may cause death from toxicity. In the United States, more people die of insect stings than of bites from all poisonous animals combined. The exact number of people who experience systemic allergic reactions to insect bites is unknown.

Despite the potentially fatal consequences, encounters with biting and stinging insects are typically brief. Pediculosis (lice infestation) and scabies, by contrast, are parasitic infections, and the arachnids remain on the host until eradicated. Approximately 10–12 million people in the United States are affected by pediculosis each year, most of them children ages 3–12 years.

This chapter covers the stings of insects only but discusses the bites of both insects and arachnids (e.g., ticks, mites, spiders, lice). The term *insect* is used to cover general statements about these invertebrates.

INSECT BITES

Pathophysiology and Clinical Presentation of Insect Bites

Bites from insects (e.g., mosquitoes, fleas, bedbugs) and from arachnids (e.g., ticks, chiggers) are nonvenomous. Each insect has distinctive biting organs and salivary secretions that contribute to the characteristic signs and symptoms for each type of bite.

Mosquitoes

Mosquitoes are found in abundance worldwide, particularly in humid, warm climates. After landing on the skin, mosquitoes inject an anticoagulant saliva into the victim, which causes the characteristic welt and itching.

Mosquitoes serve as vectors for spreading serious systemic infections including malaria and West Nile, Chikungunya, and Zika viruses.[1] Although most infected patients do not experience symptoms, about 20% of infected patients experience influenza-like symptoms with fever, fatigue, and possible joint pain. Few patients experience severe symptoms, and the illnesses are rarely fatal. New outbreaks of Zika virus in 2016 prompted the World Health Organization to issue a public health emergency of international concern.[2] At the time of this publication, most cases reported in the United States have been associated only with travel to areas of outbreaks rather than from local transmission of the virus. Although most of those infected will have generalized symptoms, there is a small risk of microcephaly in fetuses of infected mothers and Guillain-Barré syndrome in children and adults.[3] Controlling mosquito populations is particularly important in preventing the spread of these diseases.

Fleas

Fleas are tiny bloodsucking insects that can be found worldwide but breed best in a humid climate. Humans are often bitten after moving into a vacant flea-infested habitat or when living with infested pets. Flea bites are usually multiple and grouped and, in humans, occur primarily on legs and ankles. Each lesion is characterized by an erythematous region around the puncture and intense itching. In addition to being annoying, fleas can transmit diseases such as bubonic plague and endemic typhus.

Sarcoptes scabiei

Scabies is a contagious parasitic skin infection caused by *Sarcoptes scabiei*, a very small and rarely seen arachnid mite. The mites burrow up to 0.4 in. (1 cm) into the stratum corneum, and the females deposit eggs in their "tunnels." Common infestation sites are interdigital spaces of fingers, flexor surfaces of the wrists, external male genitalia, buttocks, and anterior axillary folds (see Color Plates, photograph 24). Scabies infection is characterized by inflammation and intense itching. Mites are transmitted from an infected individual to others through physical contact. A scabies infection requires prescription therapy rather than nonprescription treatment.

Bedbugs

Bedbugs usually hide and deposit their eggs in crevices of walls, floors, picture frames, bedding, folds of linens, corners of suitcases, and furniture during the day; they bite their victims at night. The increased mobility of society worldwide has heightened concern for an increased incidence of bedbug infestations in the United States in places frequented by travelers, such as hotels.[4] Additionally, bedbugs have developed resistance to commonly used pesticides that contain pyrethroids.[5] Bedbug bites typically appear along exposed areas of skin, such as the head, neck, and arms. Bites occur in clusters of twos and threes and usually in a straight line. The reaction to a bedbug bite can range from irritation at the site to a small dermal hemorrhage, depending on the sensitivity of the individual, but most involve intense itching.

Ticks

Ticks feed on the blood of humans and animals. During feeding, the tick's mouthparts are introduced into the skin, enabling it to hold firmly (see Color Plates, photograph 25). If the tick is removed, but the mouthparts are left behind, intense itching and nodules requiring surgical excision may develop. If left attached, the tick becomes fully engorged with blood and remains for up to 10 days before dropping off. Ticks should be removed intact within 36 hours of attachment using fine tweezers. Tick removal by heating methods, such as a match or hot nail, or by painting substances onto the tick, such as nail polish or petrolatum, is not recommended, because these methods can irritate the tick, causing it to secrete more saliva or even regurgitate gut contents, thereby increasing the likelihood of transmission of a tick-borne illness.[6]

The local reaction to tick bites consists of itching papules that disappear within 1 week. Certain species of ticks, however, can transmit systemic diseases such as Rocky Mountain spotted fever and Lyme disease. Rocky Mountain spotted fever, transmitted by wood ticks or dog ticks, is characterized by severe headache, rash, high fever, and extreme exhaustion.[7] Lyme disease is caused by a spirochete found in deer ticks that is transmitted into the victim after the tick is attached for 36 hours.[7] About 300,000 cases of Lyme disease are diagnosed annually, with a greater incidence in the northeast and upper Midwest.[8] Most acute stages of Lyme disease are heralded by skin rash and influenza-like symptoms. The rash appears first as a papule at the bite site and may become an enlarged circle with a clear center called a "bull's-eye rash" or erythema migrans. Tender urticarial lesions appear 3–32 days after the bite and disappear spontaneously within 3–4 weeks. If left untreated, complications such as neurologic symptoms, cardiac disturbances, musculoskeletal symptoms, and arthritis may occur. Early diagnosis and prompt treatment by a health care provider are essential to prevent development of these serious manifestations.

Chiggers

Chiggers, or red bugs, live in shrubbery, trees, and grass. A common myth is that chiggers burrow into the skin and stay there. After attaching to the skin, the larvae secrete a digestive fluid that causes cellular disintegration of the affected area, a red papule, and intense itching. This fluid also causes the skin to harden and form a tiny tube in which the chigger remains to feed until engorged. It then drops off and changes into an adult.

Spiders

Although all species of spiders are venomous, most are unable to penetrate the skin, because their fangs are too short or too fragile. The black widow, brown recluse, and hobo spiders are three major exceptions. Deaths from spider bites are rare, but symptoms can be serious. Reaction to black widow bites includes delayed intense pain, stiffness and joint pain, abdominal disturbances, fever, chills, and dyspnea. Brown recluse bites can cause these symptoms as well as a spreading ulcerated wound at the bite site. Hobo spider bites typically present with a moderate–severe, slow-healing wound.[9] If a spider bite is suspected but cannot be confirmed, the wound area should be monitored for these symptoms.

Complications of Insect Bites

Secondary bacterial infection of insect bites can occur if skin of the affected area is abraded from scratching. Skin infections, such as impetigo, may be a complication of insect bites; these infections may appear as yellow crusting, purulent drainage, and/or significant redness and swelling of the skin around the bite.

Treatment of Insect Bites

Specific nonprescription external analgesics are labeled for use in treating minor insect bites.

Treatment Goals

The goals of self-treating insect bites are to relieve symptoms and prevent secondary bacterial infections.

General Treatment Approach

Application of an ice pack wrapped in a washcloth may provide sufficient relief of the pain and irritation of bites from mosquitoes, chiggers, bedbugs, or fleas: apply the ice pack to the affected area for up to 10 minutes with at least 10 minutes between applications. If this treatment does not work, applying an external analgesic to the site should relieve symptoms. Patients should be advised to avoid scratching the bite. Prevention of future insect bites is also important.

Self-treatment of insect bites with a nonprescription product is appropriate if the reaction is confined to the site of the bite and the patient is older than 2 years. No effective nonprescription product is available to treat scabies. Patients with bites from ticks and spiders require medical referral because of possible systemic effects. Figure 37–1 outlines treatment of insect bites and lists exclusions for self-treatment.

Nonpharmacologic Therapy

Nondrug measures include the two methods of preventing insect bites: avoiding insects and using repellents. Specific measures are discussed in the box "Patient Education for Insect Bites."

Avoidance of Insects

Recommendations for avoiding insects are included in the box Patient Education for Insect Bites.

Use of Insect Repellents

Insect repellents are useful in preventing bites from insects such as mosquitoes, fleas, and ticks, but these products are not effective in repelling stinging insects. Selection of an insect repellent

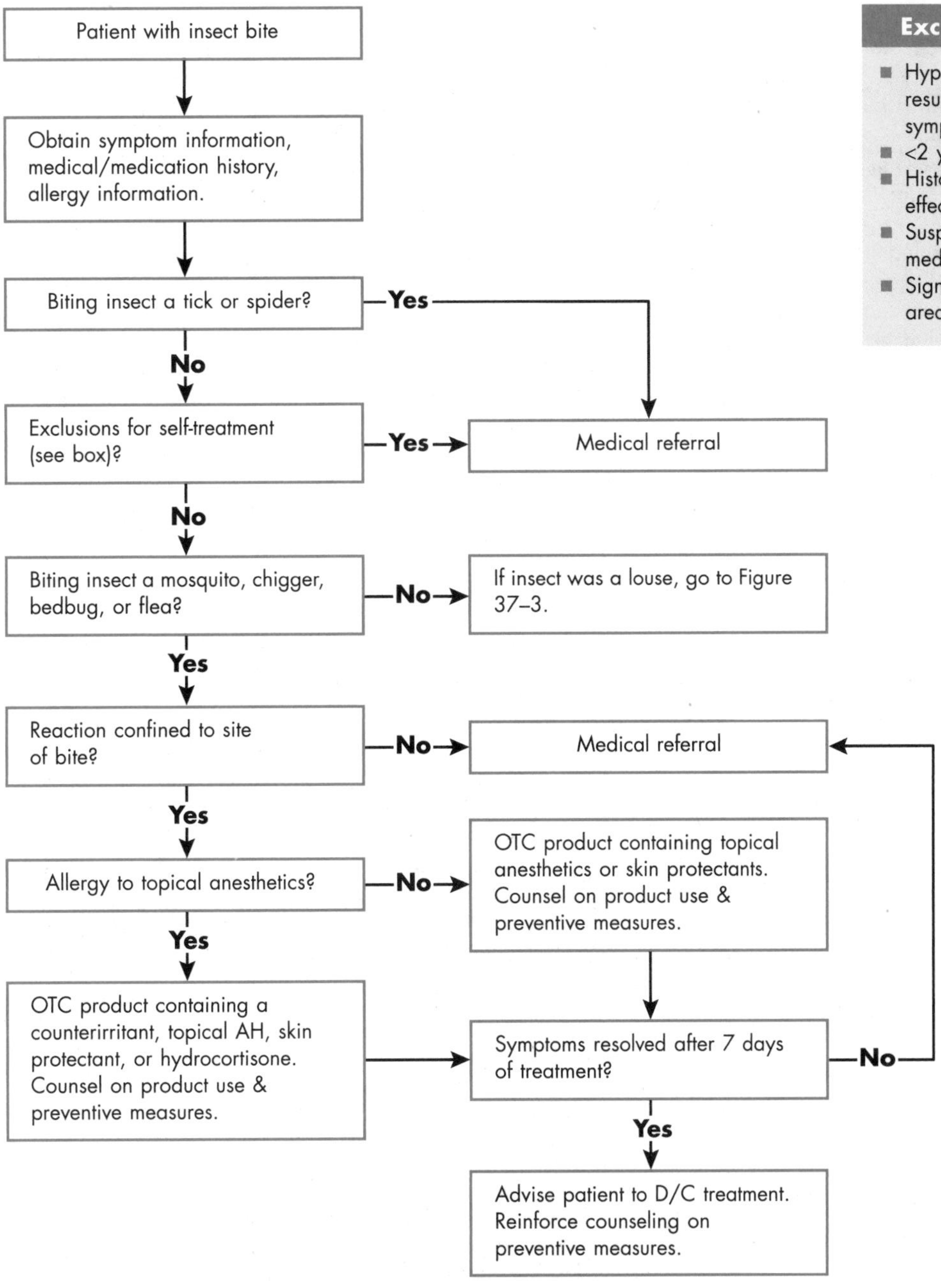

Exclusions for Self-Treatment

- Hypersensitivity to insect bites, resulting in systemic symptoms or symptoms away from bite area
- <2 years of age
- History of tick bite and systemic effects indicating possible infection
- Suspected spider bite requiring medical attention
- Signs of secondary infection of bite area

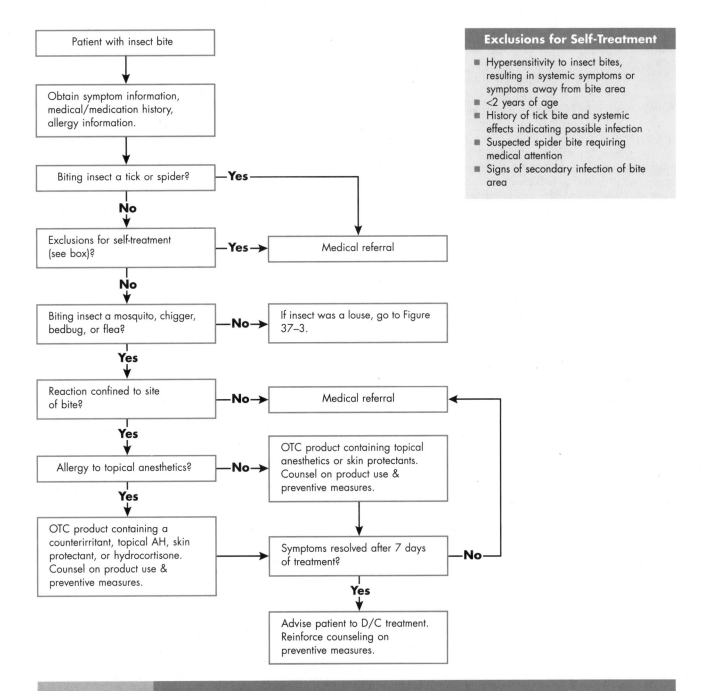

FIGURE **37–1** Self-care for insect bites. Key: AH = Antihistamine; D/C = discontinue; OTC = over-the-counter.

should be based on product ingredients, concentration, and the anticipated type and length of exposure. Most commercial products contain *N,N*-diethyl-*m*-toluamide, commonly called DEET, in concentrations ranging from 4% to 100%. Other ingredients that may be combined with DEET include ethyl butylacetylaminopropionate (IR3535) and dimethyl phthalate (Table 37–1).

N,N-Diethyl-m-Toluamide

The best all-purpose repellent is *N,N*-diethyl-*m*-toluamide, or DEET.

Repellents protect the skin against insect bites. The exact mechanism of action is not fully known, but DEET, like other repellents, does not kill insects. When applied to skin or clothing, the volatile repellent releases vapors that tend to discourage the approach of insects.

Repellents, available in sprays, solutions, creams, wipes, and other forms, are applied as needed to skin or clothing according to package directions, which usually is no more frequently than every 4–8 hours. Concentrations below 30% are preferable for children, but use of DEET insect repellents on children younger than 2 months should be discouraged.[10] Products with DEET concentrations ranging from 10% to 35% provide adequate effect and sufficient protection for adults in routine situations, with concentrations at 20% or higher recommended to prevent tick bites. Concentrations greater than 50% do not offer any additional protection, but they may have a longer repellent effect. Unfortunately, products with such concentrations may also be associated with a higher incidence of skin reactions.[11] Table 37–2 provides a summary from the Environmental Protection Agency, as well as other sources, regarding the application and safe use of DEET products.[11–14]

Though rare, skin irritation is the most frequent DEET-related problem, with occlusion of the application area possibly contributing to skin rashes or eruptions.[13] Central nervous system reactions, including seizures, ataxia, hypotension, encephalopathy, and angioedema, have been reported in association with improper use or ingestion.[14–16] The Food and Drug Administration (FDA) advises against the use of products that combine insect repellents and sunscreen. Sunscreen products require more frequent applications than insect repellents; therefore, use of combination products can increase the risk of too much DEET absorption.[11,14] These products are considered safe if used appropriately, even in women who are pregnant or breastfeeding.[14–16] Table 37–2 lists warnings and precautions for use of DEET.

Other Insect Repellents

Alternative products include citronella, lemon eucalyptus oil, soybean oil, cedar oil, lavender oil, tea tree oil, garlic, and scented moisturizers in mineral oil (e.g., Skin-So-Soft). These products generally have been found to be less effective than DEET as repellents against mosquitoes, particularly with regard to length of action. Picaridin, an alternative to DEET, is being promoted as being less odorous and less irritating to skin.[11] Insect repellents containing permethrin 0.5% are designed for use only on clothing and camping equipment.

Pharmacologic Therapy

External analgesics, such as local anesthetics, topical antihistamines, hydrocortisone, and some counterirritants, are approved for treating pain and itching associated with insect bites. These agents are not approved for use in children younger than 2 years.

TABLE 37–1 Selected Nonprescription Insect Repellents

Trade Name	Primary Ingredients
Cutter Skinsations Insect Repellent Pump Spray	DEET 7%; aloe vera; vitamin E
Cutter Sport Insect Repellent	DEET 15%
OFF! Deep Woods Sportsmen Insect Repellent I Pump Spray	DEET 98.25%
OFF! EXPLORE Insect Repellent I	DEET 25%
OFF! FamilyCare Pump	DEET 7%
OFF! Deep Woods Insect Repellent Towelettes	DEET 25%
Skin So Soft Bug Guard Plus IR3535 Gentle Breeze SPF 30 Lotion	IR3535 7.5%; SPF 30 sunscreen
Skin So Soft Bug Guard Plus Picaridin Aerosol Spray	Picaridin 10%
Repel Plant-Based Lemon Eucalyptus Insect Repellent Pump Spray	Lemon eucalyptus oil 30%
Repel Insect Repellent Sportsmen Max Formula Aerosol	DEET 40%
Repel Insect Repellent Mosquito Wipes	DEET 30%
Coleman Insect Treatment Gear & Clothing Aerosol Spray	Permethrin 0.5%
Sawyer Fisherman's Formula	Picaridin 20%

Key: DEET = *N,N*-Diethyl-*m*-toluamide.

TABLE 37–2 EPA Guidelines for Safe Use of DEET

- Read and follow all directions and precautions on the product label.
- Do not apply product over cuts, wounds, or irritated skin.
- Do not apply product to hands or near eyes and mouth of young children.
- Do not allow young children to apply this product.
- Use just enough repellent to cover exposed skin and/or clothing.
- Apply the sunscreen first, followed by the repellent, when sunscreen needs to be used in conjunction with a repellent.
- Do not use product under clothing.
- Avoid overapplication of this product.
- After returning indoors, wash treated skin with soap and water.
- Wash treated clothing before wearing it again.
- Product may damage synthetic fibers and plastics.
- Use of this product may cause skin reactions in rare cases.
- Do not spray product in enclosed areas.
- To apply to face, spray product on hands first, and then rub on face.
- Do not spray product directly onto face.

Key: DEET = *N,N*-Diethyl-*m*-toluamide; EPA = Environmental Protection Agency.
Source: References 11–14.

Topical skin protectant agents may be used to reduce inflammation and promote healing. First-aid antiseptics and antibiotics can help prevent secondary infections (see Chapter 41).

Systemic antihistamines often are used in treating itching related to insect bites, but this use is not a label indication. Chapter 11 discusses systemic antihistamines in detail.

Local Anesthetics

Local anesthetics such as benzocaine, pramoxine, benzyl alcohol, lidocaine, dibucaine, and phenol are approved in topical preparations for relief of itching and irritation caused by insect bites.

Local anesthetics cause a reversible blockade of conduction of nerve impulses at the site of application, thereby producing loss of sensation. Phenol exerts topical anesthetic action by depressing cutaneous sensory receptors.

Topical preparations containing local anesthetics are applied in the form of creams, ointments, aerosols, or lotions. These products are generally applied to the bite area up to 3–4 times daily for no longer than 7 days.

Local anesthetics are relatively nontoxic when applied topically as directed, and systemic absorption does not typically occur with these topical products. However, allergic contact dermatitis may occur. Compared with other local anesthetics, pramoxine and benzyl alcohol do not commonly cause adverse effects and exhibit less cross-sensitivity. Dibucaine, a common allergen, may cause systemic toxicity if excessive absorption occurs. Convulsions, myocardial depression, and death have been reported from systemic absorption.[17] Phenol solutions of greater than 2% are irritating and may cause sloughing and necrosis of skin, but the concentration of phenol in nonprescription products ranges from 0.5% to 1.5%. Nonprescription products containing phenol should not be applied to extensive areas of the body, especially under compresses or bandages because of the risk of skin damage and systemic absorption.[17] Products containing phenol should be avoided in pregnant patients and children.

Topical Antihistamines

Diphenhydramine hydrochloride in concentrations of 0.5%–2% is the agent used in most products that contain a topical antihistamine.

Topical antihistamines exert an anesthetic effect by depressing cutaneous receptors and are approved for temporary relief of pain and itching related to minor insect bites.[18] Products are available in several topical dosage forms; they are generally applied to the bite area up to 3–4 times daily for no longer than 7 days.

Although absorption occurs through skin, topical antihistamines generally are not absorbed in sufficient quantities to cause systemic adverse effects, even when applied to damaged skin. Systemic absorption is of more concern when these products are used over large body areas, especially in young children. Topical antihistamines can cause photosensitivity and hypersensitivity reactions; continued use of these agents for 3–4 weeks increases the possibility of contact dermatitis.

Counterirritants

Low concentrations of the counterirritants camphor and menthol are used in some topical analgesic products. Chapter 7 discusses these agents in more detail. These products generally are applied to the bite area 3–4 times daily for up to 7 days.

Camphor

At concentrations of 0.1%–3%, camphor depresses cutaneous receptors, thereby relieving itching and irritation by exerting an anesthetic effect. However, camphor-containing products can be very dangerous if ingested. Patients should be warned to keep these products out of children's reach.

Menthol

In concentrations of less than 1%, menthol depresses cutaneous receptors and exerts an analgesic effect. Menthol is considered a safe and effective antipruritic when applied to the affected area in concentrations of 0.1%–1%.

Hydrocortisone

Hydrocortisone 1% topical preparations are indicated for temporary relief of minor insect bites.

A wide variety of topical hydrocortisone dosage forms are available and should be applied as directed to the bite area 3 or 4 times daily for up to 7 days. Chapter 35 provides more information about topical hydrocortisone.

Skin Protectants

Medications such as zinc oxide, calamine, and titanium dioxide are applied to insect bites mainly in the form of lotions, ointments, and creams. These agents act as protectants and tend to reduce inflammation and irritation. Zinc oxide works as a mild astringent with weak antiseptic properties.[18] Zinc oxide and calamine also absorb fluids from weeping lesions.

FDA considers nonprescription drugs containing zinc oxide and calamine to be safe and effective in concentrations of 1%–25%. Although its mechanism of action is similar to that of zinc oxide, titanium dioxide's safety and effectiveness have not been determined by FDA. These preparations should be applied to the affected area as needed. They have minimal adverse effects and are recommended for adults, children, and infants.

Product Selection Guidelines

Sensitization, specifically contact dermatitis, can occur with use and overuse of local anesthetics. If these agents are preferred, pramoxine and benzyl alcohol have a low incidence of adverse effects. Dibucaine and phenol have the most potential for adverse effects, especially if systemic absorption occurs from improper application.

Adverse effects and systemic absorption generally are not a concern with short-term use of the topical antihistamine diphenhydramine hydrochloride. Its prolonged use, however, can cause allergic or photoallergic contact dermatitis. Similarly, short-term use of hydrocortisone usually does not cause adverse effects or clinically significant systemic absorption. Patients with scabies, bacterial infections, or fungal infections should not use hydrocortisone without medical supervision, because it can worsen or mask these disorders. Camphor-containing products can be very dangerous if ingested, making them an inappropriate choice for use in children. Patients must understand that topical antipruritics and anesthetics should not be used for longer than 7 days.

The patient's preference of dosage forms should also guide product recommendations. Table 37–3 lists selected trade-name products in various dosage forms.

TABLE 37-3 Selected Nonprescription External Analgesic Products for Insect Bites and Stings

Trade Name	Primary Ingredients
Local Anesthetics	
Itch-X Gel/Pump Spray	Pramoxine HCl 1%; benzyl alcohol 10%
Lanacane First Aid Aerosol Spray 2-in-1 Fast Acting Pain Relief	Benzocaine 20%; benzethonium chloride 0.2%
Solarcaine Pain Relieving Aerosol Spray	Lidocaine 0.5%; aloe
Topical Antihistamines	
Benadryl Itch Relief Spray	Diphenhydramine HCl 1%; zinc acetate 0.1%
Benadryl Extra Strength Topical Analgesic Itch Stopping Gel	Diphenhydramine HCl 2%
Counterirritants	
Blue Star Ointment	Camphor 1.24%
Sarna Anti-itch Lotion Original	Camphor 0.5%; menthol 0.5%
Corticosteroids	
Aveeno Maximum Strength Anti-itch Cream	Hydrocortisone 1%; aloe vera
Cortaid Intense Therapy Cooling Spray	Hydrocortisone 1%
Cortizone-10 Easy Relief Liquid	Hydrocortisone 1%; aloe vera
Combination Products	
Aveeno Anti-Itch Concentrated Lotion	Pramoxine HCl 1%; calamine 3%; dimethicone
Caladryl Clear Lotion	Pramoxine HCl 1%; acetate 0.1%; camphor
Campho-Phenique Gel	Camphor 10.8%; phenol 4.7%; eucalyptus oil
Chigarid External Analgesic	Camphor 2.8%; phenol 1.5%; menthol 0.1%; eucalyptus oil 0.5% in collodion
StingEze Insect Bite Relief	Benzocaine 5%; phenol 1.35%
Sting-Kill Swabs	Benzocaine 20%; menthol 1%

Assessment of Insect Bites: A Case-Based Approach

The type of insect that inflicted the patient's injury should be determined first. Patients with suspected spider or tick bites require a medical referral because of the risk of complications. For other insect bites, the seriousness of the reaction should be evaluated before a nonprescription product or nondrug measure is recommended. If a nonallergic reaction is present, the appropriate external analgesic for symptomatic relief should be recommended. Recommending a skin protectant to reduce irritation and inflammation or to prevent secondary bacterial infection is appropriate.

Patient Counseling for Insect Bites

Counseling for insect bites includes an explanation of how to treat the injury and how to prevent recurrences. Nondrug measures and proper use of recommended nonprescription products should be explained. The explanation should include potential adverse effects of these agents, plus signs and symptoms that indicate the injury needs medical attention. Appropriate use of insect repellents to prevent further bites should also be discussed. The box "Patient Education for Insect Bites" lists specific information to provide patients.

Evaluation of Patient Outcomes for Insect Bites

Follow-up should occur after 7 days of self-treatment. The patient should be advised to seek medical attention if symptoms such as redness, itching, and localized swelling worsen during treatment, or if the patient develops secondary infection, fever, joint pain, or lymph node enlargement. Medical attention is also necessary if symptoms persist after 7 days of treatment.

INSECT STINGS

Pathophysiology and Clinical Presentation of Insect Stings

Venomous insects such as bees, wasps, hornets, yellow jackets, and fire ants belong to the order Hymenoptera. They attack their victims to defend themselves or to kill other insects. The injected venom contains allergenic proteins and pharmacologically active molecules. Because venom contents vary within the Hymenoptera order, venom is discussed here in general terms.

Most people will complain of pain, itching, and irritation at the site following an insect sting, but they generally will have no systemic symptoms. Individuals who are allergic to insect stings may experience hives, itching, swelling, and burning sensations of the skin. Although anaphylaxis is rare, those with severe allergies may experience a fall in blood pressure, light-headedness, chest tightness, dyspnea, and even loss of consciousness.

Wild Honeybees, Wasps, Hornets, and Yellow Jackets

Wild honeybees are most commonly found in the western and midwestern United States; they usually nest in hollow tree trunks. Because the honeybee stinger is barbed, it remains embedded in the skin, even after the bee pulls away or is brushed off, and continues to inject venom. Paper wasps, hornets, and yellow jackets are found more commonly in the southern, central, and southwestern United States. Paper wasps tend to nest in high places, under eaves of houses or on branches of high trees, whereas hornets prefer to nest in hollow spaces, especially hollow trees. Yellow jackets, considered the most common stinging culprits, usually nest in low places, such as burrows in the ground, cracks in sidewalks,

PATIENT EDUCATION FOR Insect Bites

The objectives of self-treatment for insect bites are (1) to relieve swelling, pain, and itching; (2) to prevent scratching that may lead to secondary bacterial infection; (3) to monitor for infections transmitted by ticks; and (4) to prevent future insect bites. For most patients, carefully following product instructions and the self-care measures listed here will help ensure optimal therapeutic outcomes.

Nondrug Measures

- Apply ice pack promptly to bite area to reduce swelling, itching, and pain.
- Avoid scratching the affected area; keep fingernails trimmed.
- Remove ticks with tweezers by grasping the tick's head and gently pulling; the head should be removed. Keep the removed tick in a sealed container for future identification in case of systemic symptoms. After removal of the tick, clean the affected area with rubbing alcohol to disinfect the skin.
- Do not wear rough, irritating clothing over bite area.

Preventive Measures

- To prevent exposure, cover skin as much as possible with clothing and socks, and cuff clothing around ankles, wrists, and neck.
- Avoid swamps, dense woods, and dense brush that harbor mosquitoes, ticks, and chiggers.
- Keep pets free of pests.
- Remove standing water from around the home to reduce breeding areas for mosquitoes.
- Limit the amount of time spent outside at dawn and dusk.
- Use barriers such as window screens and netting.
- Apply insect repellent according to package recommendations to repel biting insects (see Table 37–2); these repellents do not deter stinging insects.
- To prevent transmission of scabies, avoid close, physical contact with infected individuals.

Nonprescription Medications

Topical Analgesics

- Use an external analgesic to relieve pain and itching of insect bites. Choice of medications includes local anesthetics, topical antihistamines, counterirritants, and hydrocortisone.
- These products can be applied to the bite area 3–4 times daily. Do not use on children younger than 2 years. Do not use longer than 7 days.
- Note that local anesthetics can cause sensitization. If these agents are preferred, pramoxine and benzyl alcohol are less likely to cause adverse effects.
- Do not use dibucaine in large quantities, particularly over raw surfaces or blistered areas. Such use could cause myocardial depression, convulsions, or death.
- Do not apply phenol to extensive areas of the body or under compresses and bandages. Such application increases the possibility of skin damage or systemic absorption.
- Do not use topical diphenhydramine longer than the recommended 7 days. Prolonged use can cause hypersensitivity reactions or systemic effects.
- Do not use hydrocortisone on scabies, bacterial infections, or fungal infections without a medical recommendation. Hydrocortisone can mask or worsen these disorders.
- Do not allow children to ingest camphor-containing products. Camphor is toxic when ingested.

Skin Protectants

- If a medication is needed to reduce irritation or inflammation, or if bacterial infection is a concern, use a skin protectant such as zinc oxide or calamine.
- Apply protectant to affected area as needed up to 4 times daily.
- Protectants can be applied to skin of children younger than 2 years.
- Some insect bite products contain external analgesics and skin protectants.

When to Seek Medical Attention

- Seek medical attention if the condition worsens during treatment or if symptoms persist after 7 days of topical treatment.

or small shrubs. The stinging mechanism of wasps, hornets, and yellow jackets resembles that of the honeybee, except their stingers are not barbed. Their stingers can be withdrawn easily after venom is injected, enabling them to sting repeatedly.

Fire Ants

Fire ants, imported from South America early in the 20th century, are now found in the southern and western United States, live in underground colonies, and form large raised mounds. Some ants only bite, whereas others bite and sting simultaneously; however, the bite is believed to cause the reactions. Fire ant bites cause intense itching, burning, vesiculation, tissue necrosis, and anaphylactic reactions in hypersensitive individuals.

Treatment of Insect Stings

Although labeling of nonprescription products for insect-related injuries mentions only "insect bites" as an indication, it is generally accepted that FDA had intended the term to also cover insect stings.

Treatment Goals

The goal of self-treating insect stings is to relieve the itching and pain of cutaneous nonallergic reactions. Allergic reactions require medical referral.

General Treatment Approach

Removal of the stinger followed by application of an ice pack in 10-minute intervals is the first step in treating insect stings. Application of a local anesthetic, skin protectant, antiseptic, or counterirritant to the sting site is appropriate if the reaction is confined to the site and if no exclusions for self-treatment apply. Figure 37–2 lists exclusions for self-treatment and outlines the treatment of insect stings.

Avoiding future insect stings can prevent an individual from developing allergic reactions to stings. If symptoms of an allergic reaction develop, emergency treatment should be administered, and the patient should seek medical attention. Patients with severe allergic reactions should be advised to wear a bracelet or carry a card identifying the nature of the allergy. They should also contact their primary care provider about carrying an injectable form of epinephrine.

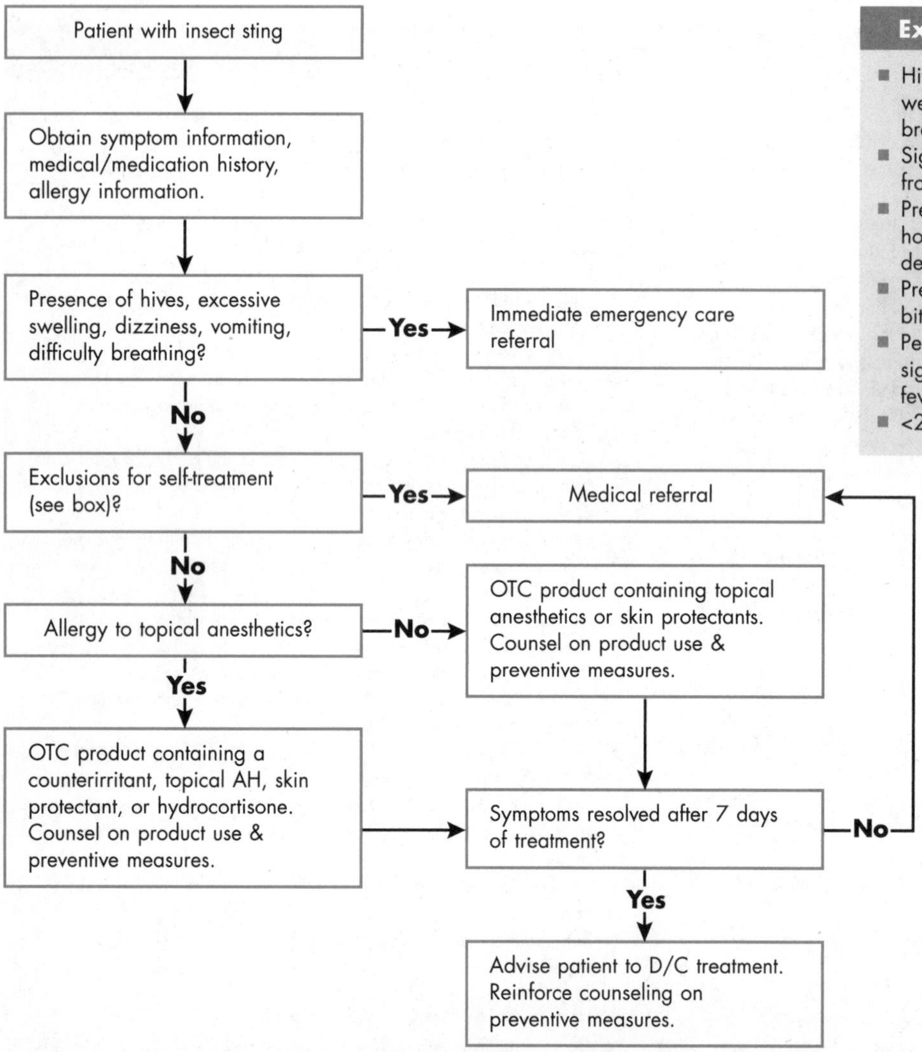

Exclusions for Self-Treatment

- Hives, excessive swelling, dizziness, weakness, nausea, vomiting, difficulty breathing
- Significant allergic response away from site of sting
- Previous sting by honeybee, wasp, or hornet (need to evaluate possible development of hypersensitivity)
- Previous severe reaction to insect bites
- Personal or family history of significant allergic reactions (e.g., hay fever)
- <2 years of age

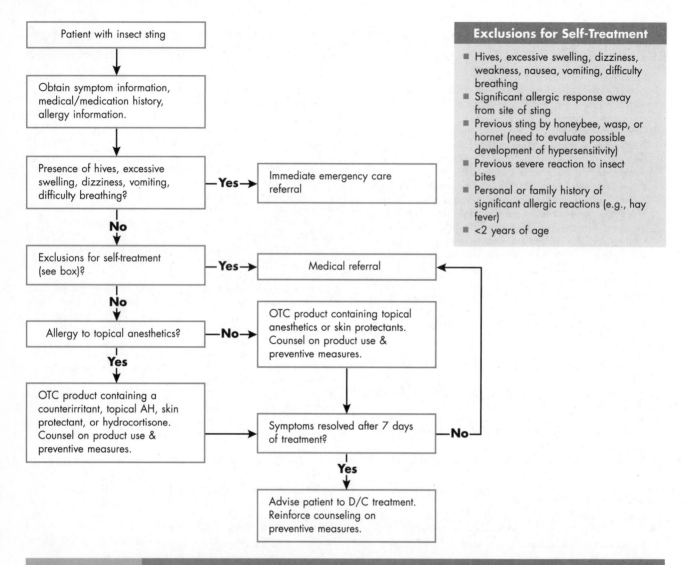

FIGURE 37-2 Self-care for insect stings. Key: AH = Antihistamine; D/C = discontinue; OTC = over-the-counter.

Nonpharmacologic Therapy

Prompt application of cold packs to the sting site in 10-minute intervals helps slow absorption and reduce itching, swelling, and pain. Removal of the honeybee's stinger and venom sac, which are usually left in the skin, is important. The patient should remove the stinger before all venom is injected; approximately 2–3 minutes are needed to empty all contents from the honeybee's venom sac. The patient should not use tweezers or squeeze the sac, because rubbing, scratching, or grasping it releases more venom. Scraping away the stinger with a fingernail or the edge of a credit card minimizes the venom flow. After the stinger is removed, an antiseptic, such as hydrogen peroxide or alcohol, should be applied.

Measures to avoid attracting stinging insects are included in the box "Patient Education for Insect Stings."

Pharmacologic Therapy

The section Treatment of Insect Bites discusses the following external analgesics approved for treatment of insect bites and, by inference, insect stings: local anesthetics, topical antihistamines, counterirritants, hydrocortisone, and skin protectants.

Product labels for systemic antihistamines do not include treatment of itching associated with insect stings as an indication, even though these products are often used for this purpose.

Complementary Therapies

Meat tenderizer has been used on insect stings to "break down" proteins in venom. Ammonia and baking soda have been used to "neutralize" venom in insect bites. These products may affect itching. Most reports of their success are anecdotal, however, and to date their effectiveness has not been determined.

Assessment of Insect Stings

The critical determination in assessing a patient with an insect sting is whether the patient is allergic to the venom. Patients experiencing allergic reactions should be referred immediately for emergency medical attention.

PATIENT EDUCATION FOR Insect Stings

The objectives of self-treatment for insect stings are (1) to relieve the swelling, pain, and itching of insect stings; (2) to monitor any reaction to the sting to determine whether an allergic reaction is developing; and (3) to prevent future insect stings. For most patients, carefully following product instructions and the self-care measures listed here will help ensure optimal therapeutic outcomes.

Nondrug Measures

- For honeybee stings, removing the honeybee stinger immediately is important. Scraping the stinger away with the edge of a credit card is effective. Try not to squeeze or rub the stinger; these actions will actually release more venom.
- Apply an ice pack or a cold compress promptly to the sting site to help slow absorption of the venom. This action will reduce itching, swelling, and pain.
- Avoid scratching the affected area; keep fingernails trimmed. Gloves or mittens may be used on small children during sleep to avoid unconscious scratching.
- To avoid attracting stinging insects, avoid wearing perfume, scented lotions, and brightly colored clothes; control odors in picnic and garbage areas; change children's clothing if it becomes contaminated with summer foods such as fruits; wear shoes when outdoors; and destroy nests of stinging insects near homes.
- If you are hypersensitive to stings, wear a bracelet or carry a card showing the nature of the allergy.

Nonprescription Medications

- For nonallergic stings, apply a topical nonprescription external analgesic such as a local anesthetic, topical antihistamine, counterirritant, or hydrocortisone to the affected site to relieve pain and itching. A skin protectant can also be recommended to prevent irritation and inflammation as well as prevent secondary bacterial infection.
- These products can be applied 3–4 times daily for up to 7 days.

When to Seek Medical Attention

- If you have experienced previous severe reactions to insect stings, seek emergency medical care immediately. If a primary care provider has prescribed epinephrine or an oral antihistamine and you have it on your person, administer it according to the provider's instructions.
- Seek medical attention if you develop symptoms of an allergic reaction, such as hives, excessive swelling, dizziness, vomiting, or difficulty breathing.
- Seek medical attention if the pain and itching worsen during treatment or if they do not improve after 7 days of topical treatment.

Patient Counseling for Insect Stings

The health care provider should advise the patient that local reactions to insect stings usually are transient, but that severe reactions to insect stings can occur if sensitization to the insect venom develops with repeated exposure. The symptoms of allergic reactions should be explained. Patients who have a known hypersensitivity to insect stings should have epinephrine injection available at all times for emergency self-treatment.

For nonallergic reactions to stings, the provider should recommend one or more topical medications to manage immediate symptoms. The patient should be advised about adverse effects and any contraindications. The box "Patient Education for Insect Stings" lists specific information that should be provided.

Evaluation of Patient Outcomes for Insect Stings

Follow-up for nonallergic reactions to insect stings should occur within 7 days. The patient should be advised to seek medical attention if symptoms of pain, itching, and localized swelling worsen during the treatment period or persist after 7 days of treatment. Symptoms of secondary infection or fever also warrant medical attention. Follow-up for patients who have allergic reactions should occur the same day, if possible.

Case 37–1 illustrates assessment of a patient who has an insect sting.

CASE 37-1

Relevant Evaluation Criteria	Scenario/Model Outcome
Collect	
1. Gather essential information about the patient's symptoms and medical history, including	
a. Description of symptom(s) (i.e., nature, onset, duration, severity, associated symptoms)	A mother brings her 7-year-old son to the pharmacy stating that he was playing near the neighborhood creek when he ran to her screaming that something had stung him. He said that other kids were also running from the creek and were worried about the flying yellow and black bugs there. The boy complains that his arm really hurts and itches. He has a swollen, bright red patch on his right upper arm.
b. Description of any factors that seem to precipitate, exacerbate, and/or relieve the patient's symptom(s)	The mother says that she used her credit card to remove the stinger from his arm and then applied an ice pack to his arm. This helped initially, but she thinks that his arm looks like it continued to swell. Development of hives distal to the bite site is noted.

Relevant Evaluation Criteria	Scenario/Model Outcome
c. Description of the patient's efforts to relieve the symptoms	The mother used an ice pack to help with swelling and pain.
d. Patient's identity	George Hill
e. Patient's age, gender, height, and weight	7 years old, male, 45 in., 53 lb
f. Patient's occupation	First-grade student
g. Patient's dietary habits	George is thin but well-nourished. His mother says that he eats a varied diet.
h. Patient's sleep habits	Sleeps 9–10 hours a night.
i. Concurrent medical conditions, prescription and nonprescription medications, and dietary supplements	Asthma and seasonal allergies; nonprescription loratadine 10 mg daily and prescription montelukast 5 mg once daily
j. Allergies	Amoxicillin (rash)
k. History of other adverse reactions to medications	None
l. Other (describe) ______	n/a
Assess	
2. Differentiate patient's signs/symptoms, and correctly identify the patient's primary problem(s).	George appears to have been stung by a yellow jacket (based on the mother's description) on his upper right arm. The swelling in his arm appears to be worsening, and hives have begun to appear down his arm.
3. Identify exclusions for self-treatment (Figure 37–2).	Hives, excessive swelling of affected area
4. Formulate a comprehensive list of therapeutic alternatives for the primary problem to determine whether triage to a health care provider is required, and share this information with the patient or caregiver.	Options include (1) Application of local anesthetic, topical antihistamine, counterirritant, antiseptic, or hydrocortisone, including the following: a. anesthetic: Lanacane First Aid 2-in-1 Aerosol Spray (benzocaine 20%; benzethonium chloride 0.2%) b. antihistamine: Maximum Strength Benadryl Cream/Spray (diphenhydramine 2%) c. counterirritant: Blue Star Ointment (camphor 1.24%) d. antiseptic: hydrogen peroxide or alcohol e. hydrocortisone: Cortizone-10 Cream (hydrocortisone 1%) (2) Refer George for immediate medical referral. (3) Recommend self-care until the PCP can be consulted. (4) Take no action.
Plan	
5. Select an optimal therapeutic alternative to address the patient's problem, taking into account patient preferences.	Refer George for immediate medical attention, because he is developing signs of anaphylaxis (hives and excessive swelling) to the insect sting.
6. Describe the recommended therapeutic approach to the patient or caregiver.	Call 911 for immediate care.
7. Explain to the patient or caregiver the rationale for selecting the recommended therapeutic approach from the considered therapeutic alternatives.	"George needs immediate treatment, because it appears he is having an allergic reaction to the insect sting. I have called 911."
Implement	
8. When recommending self-care with nonprescription medications and/or nondrug therapy, convey accurate information to the patient or caregiver.	Criterion does not apply in this case.
Solicit follow-up questions from the patient or caregiver.	"What do I do if my son is stung again?"
Answer the patient's or caregiver's questions.	"If symptoms of an allergic reaction develop, emergency treatment should be administered, and you should seek immediate medical attention for your son. Patients with severe allergic reactions might be advised to carry a bracelet or card identifying the allergy and to carry an injectable form of epinephrine. Your son's primary care provider can prescribe the injectable epinephrine if it is needed."
Follow-up: Monitor and Evaluate	
9. Assess patient outcome.	Call the patient's mother in 1–2 days to assess his outcome.

Key: n/a = Not applicable; PCP = primary care provider.

PEDICULOSIS

Pathophysiology and Clinical Presentation of Pediculosis

Lice are irritating pests, and lice infestations in the United States are common. Three types of lice that infest humans are head lice (*Pediculus humanus capitis*), body lice (*Pediculus humanus corporis*), and pubic lice (*Phthirus pubis*).

Head Lice

Head lice are the most common cause of lice infestation; outbreaks of lice infestation are common in places such as schools and day-care centers. Infestations are most commonly spread through direct head-to-head contact with an infected person. Sharing personal items such as caps, hairbrushes, and combs is unlikely to cause spreading.[19] Outbreaks usually peak after the opening of schools each year, between August and November. All socioeconomic groups are affected. Head lice create problematic infestations, but they generally do not contribute to the spread of other diseases in the United States.[20]

Head lice usually infest the head and live on the scalp (see Color Plates, photographs 26A and B). A lice egg or nit is about 0.04 in. (1 mm) in diameter and is typically found within 0.16 in. (4 mm) of the scalp. Once hatched, the louse must begin feeding within 24 hours or it dies. The nymph, or newly hatched, immature louse, resembles an adult and matures within 8–9 days. Without treatment, this cycle may repeat every 3 weeks.[20] The bite of a louse causes an immediate wheal to develop around the bite, with a local papule appearing within 24 hours. Itching and subsequent scratching may result in secondary infection. Adult lice, which are about the size of a sesame seed, often are difficult to locate, because they move when the hair is moved during inspection of the scalp. However, nits and nit casings generally can be spotted at the base of hair shafts when hair is parted for physical inspection. Hair inspections should focus on the crown of the head, near ears, and at the base of the neck. The grayish nits blend in well with the hair, but nit casings (hatched nits) are a lighter color and are more easily located. Nits and nit casings may be differentiated from dandruff, dirt, and so forth because of their firm attachment to the hair shaft. The presence of black powdery specks, lice feces, is also evidence of an infestation.

Body Lice

Body lice (or "cooties") live, hide, and lay their eggs in clothing, particularly in the seams and folds of underclothes. They periodically attack body areas for blood feedings and can transmit infections such as typhus and trench fever.[21] Body lice infestations generally occur in individuals who do not shower or change clothing frequently, such as the homeless.[21]

Pubic Lice

Pubic lice or "crabs," referring to their crab-like appearance, are generally transmitted through high-risk sexual contact, but they may also spread by way of toilet seats, shared undergarments, or bedding. The lice usually are found in the pubic area but may infest armpits, eyelashes, mustaches, beards, and eyebrows.[22]

Treatment of Pediculosis

Nonprescription pediculicide agents, appropriate hair combing for nit removal, and home vacuuming and cleaning of personal items are primary treatments for lice infestation.[20]

Treatment Goals

The goal of treating pediculosis is to rid the infested patient of lice by killing adult and nymph lice and by removing nits from the patient's hair.

General Treatment Approach

A pediculicide is applied to the infested body area for the designated amount of time to rid the patient of lice. The hair is then combed with a lice or nit comb to remove nits from the hair shaft; combing will also remove dead lice. Once rid of lice, patients should be instructed on how to avoid future infestations. Figure 37–3 outlines treatment of lice infestations and lists exclusions for self-treatment.

Nonpharmacologic Therapy

Because none of the pediculicides kills 100% of lice eggs, the National Pediculosis Association recommends careful visual inspection of the hair for nits and combing with an FDA-approved nit comb, such as the LiceMeister comb; removal of nits is helpful in treating and controlling head lice.[20] The AirAllé (formerly called the LouseBuster) is a machine that applies heat to the hair and scalp to dehydrate and kill lice and nits. Preliminary evidence suggests this procedure kills more than 90% of nits.[23] Unfortunately, it is expensive and requires a certified technician to operate the machine.

Direct physical contact with an infested individual should be avoided, and articles such as combs, brushes, towels, caps, and hats should not be shared; however protective head gear should not be avoided due to fear of transmission. Clothing and bedding should be washed in hot water and dried in a clothes dryer to kill lice and their nits; an alternative to washing would be to seal contaminated items in a plastic bag for 2 weeks. Hairbrushes and combs should be washed in very hot water. Carpets, rugs, and furniture should be vacuumed thoroughly and regularly.[20] Use of insecticidal sprays on these items is not generally recommended, because lice usually survive for less than 48 hours when not in contact with a host.[20] Given the increasing resistance to pediculicides, some patients are choosing to use nondrug therapy exclusively; these nondrug methods, specifically combing and vacuuming, can be effective, but they are labor intensive and tedious.[24] Complete head shaving has also been used as a lice treatment, but the social stigma involved makes this a distasteful option. Body lice are controlled by appropriate body hygiene and frequent changing and appropriate laundering of clothing and bed linens.[22]

Pharmacologic Therapy

Two nonprescription pediculicide agents are available for treating pediculosis: permethrins and synergized pyrethrins. Health care providers should be concerned about increasing resistance to the nonprescription pediculicides. Research conducted in 2015 found that 25 states in the United States had lice with genetic mutations

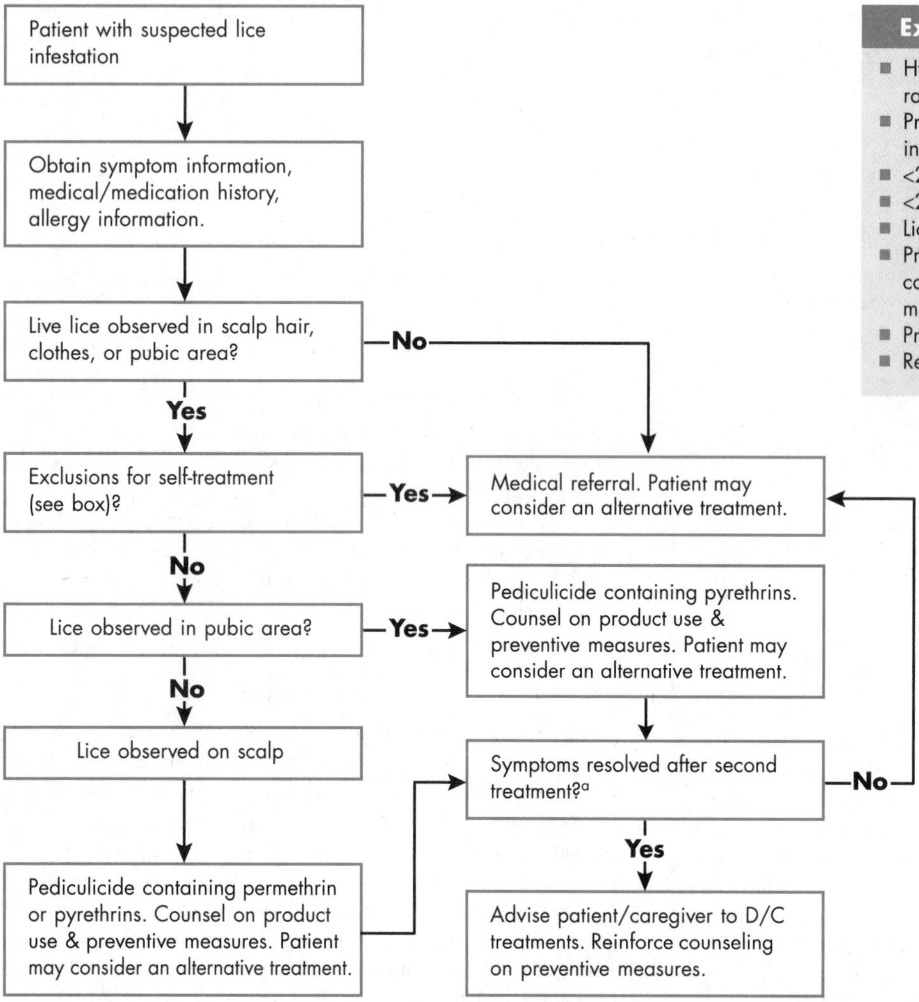

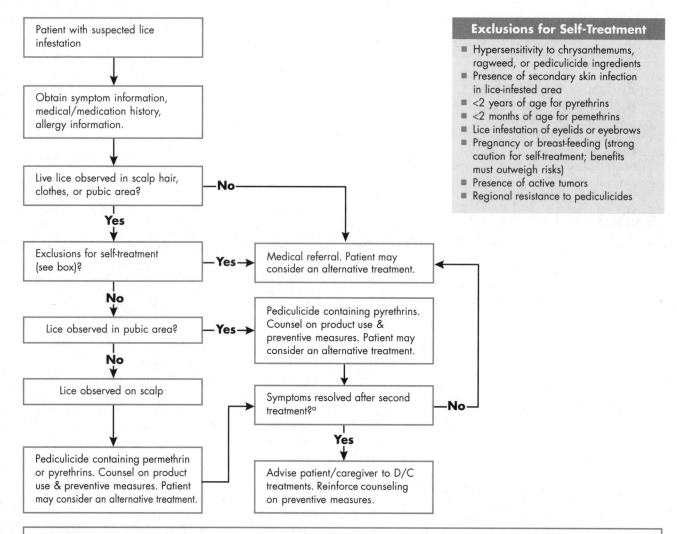

Exclusions for Self-Treatment

- Hypersensitivity to chrysanthemums, ragweed, or pediculicide ingredients
- Presence of secondary skin infection in lice-infested area
- <2 years of age for pyrethrins
- <2 months of age for pemethrins
- Lice infestation of eyelids or eyebrows
- Pregnancy or breast-feeding (strong caution for self-treatment; benefits must outweigh risks)
- Presence of active tumors
- Regional resistance to pediculicides

[a] Permethrin rinse has residual effects for up to 10 days; therefore, retreatment in 7–10 days is not required unless active lice are detected.

FIGURE 37–3 Self-care for pediculosis. Key: D/C = Discontinue.

indicating resistance to nonprescription pediculicides; with lice in California, Texas, Florida, and Maine being the most resistant.[25]

Synergized Pyrethrins

Synergized pyrethrins are approved for the treatment of head and pubic lice. Pyrethrins are synergized by addition of piperonyl butoxide. This agent limits the ability of lice to break down pyrethrins. As a result, higher, more toxic concentrations of pyrethrins are achieved.

Pyrethrins block nerve impulse transmission, causing the insect's paralysis and death. Addition of piperonyl butoxide to pyrethrins synergizes their insecticidal effect through inhibition of pyrethrin breakdown, increasing insecticide levels within the louse.[20,26] Excessive contact time or occlusion of the scalp after product application may increase skin absorption of topical pyrethrins.

Pyrethrins, in concentrations ranging from 0.17 to .33%, generally are used in combination with 2%–4% piperonyl butoxide. This combination is considered an effective pediculicide when applied topically as shampoos, foams, solutions, or gels. The medication is applied to the affected area for 10 minutes; then the treated area is rinsed or shampooed as recommended. Combing with a lice comb should follow the treatment. The treatment is repeated in 7–10 days to kill any remaining nits that have since hatched. The drug should not be applied more than twice in 24 hours.

When applied according to directions, pyrethrins have a low order of toxicity. Most adverse reactions are cutaneous and include irritation, erythema, itching, and swelling.[19,27] Contact with eyes and mucous membranes should be avoided.

Individuals allergic to pyrethrins or chrysanthemums should not use this agent; ragweed-sensitive individuals risk cross-sensitivity.

Permethrin

Permethrin, a synthetic pyrethroid, is available as a nonprescription cream rinse for treating head lice only. Permethrin acts on the nerve cell membrane of lice. It disrupts the sodium channel, delaying repolarization and causing paralysis and death of the parasite.

When permethrin is applied, an estimated less than 2% is absorbed, after which the agent is metabolized.

The 1% cream rinse is applied in sufficient quantities to cover or saturate washed hair and scalp. It is left on the hair for 10 minutes before rinsing; the hair is then combed with a lice comb. The rinse has residual effects for up to 10 days; therefore, retreatment in 7–10 days is not required unless active lice are detected.

Primary adverse effects, which can occur in up to 10% of the patient population, include transient pruritus, burning, stinging, and irritation of the scalp. Contact with eyes and mucous membranes should be avoided.

Permethrin is contraindicated in patients who are sensitive to pyrethrins or chrysanthemums. Permethrin should not be used on infants younger than 2 months.

Pharmacotherapeutic Comparison

When treatment involves a single application of a pediculicide, permethrin is more effective than the pyrethrin and piperonyl butoxide combination. However, to date, no significant difference exists in effectiveness of these agents when treatment consists of two applications. A comprehensive meta-analysis is ongoing.[20]

Product Selection Guidelines

Preparations that contain synergized pyrethrins may be used on children ages 2 years and older, but they should be used in pregnancy and lactation only if prescribed by a health care provider.

Synergized pyrethrins may be recommended for treating pubic lice. For treatment of head lice, synergized pyrethrins or permethrin may be selected on the basis of preferred dosage form, desire for single application, or patient allergies and sensitivities. Table 37–4 lists selected trade-name products containing available nonprescription pediculicides agents.

TABLE 37–4 Selected Nonprescription Pediculicides and Alternative Therapies

Trade Name	Primary Ingredients
A-200 Lice Killing Shampoo	Pyrethrins 0.33%; piperonyl butoxide 3%
RID Lice Killing Shampoo, Maximum Strength	Pyrethrins 0.33%; piperonyl butoxide 4%
Nix Lice Killing Cream Rinse	Permethrin 1%
Pronto Lice Killing Shampoo	Pyrethrins 0.33%; piperonyl butoxide 4%
LiceMD	Dimethicone 100%
Vamousse Lice Treatment	Natrum muriaticum 2X (HPUS)
Licefreee Spray	Natrum muriaticum 2X (HPUS)
Clearlice Shampoo	Proprietary blend: enzyme proteins, neem oils, *Wrightia tinctoria*, tea tree oil, *Acorus calamus*, peppermint oil, *Cocos nucifera*, Natrum muriaticum

Alternative Therapies

A variety of alternative therapies have been used to eliminate lice infestations. However, none of them are FDA approved. Lice enzyme shampoos, which claim to break down the lice exoskeleton, are being promoted as an alternative to traditional pediculicides. A product containing 10% tea tree oil and 1% lavender oil applied weekly for 3 weeks was more effective at eradicating lice than a pyrethrin/piperonyl butoxide product applied twice (1 week apart).[28] Tea tree oil must be used with caution because of potential significant allergic reactions and possible liver toxicity.[29] Other oil-based products such as petroleum jelly and mayonnaise also are being used on the basis of the theory that they impair lice respiration; however, these products are not very effective and most likely only slow the movement of lice.[19,27] Dangerous alternative treatments such as gasoline and kerosene should always be avoided because of their flammability and potential for toxicity.[20,24]

A homeopathic remedy containing *Natrum muriaticum*, also known as sodium chloride, works by drying out lice and their eggs. In a randomized trail including 42 pediatric patients with head lice, the sodium chloride spray demonstrated efficacy superior to that of permethrin.[30] These products are applied to sections of dry hair for 15 minutes followed by combing with a nit comb. Table 37–4 lists specific sodium chloride products available in the United States.

Battery-operated louse combs with oscillating teeth (MagiComb and RobiComb) are also available; although they claim to kill lice, there are no published studies that evaluate their effectiveness. The electronic combs should be avoided in patients with pacemakers or histories of seizures.[20]

Emerging Therapies

A new potential treatment under study uses dry-on, suffocation-based pediculicide (DSP) lotions. The Nuvo method, which uses Cetaphil Gentle Skin Cleanser, the first DSP product to be tested, is a nontoxic lotion that "shrink-wraps" lice. It is applied to hair and dried with a hairdryer to form a shrink-wrap film over hair and lice. The lotion covers breathing holes, suffocating the louse. One study suggests suffocation products may be more effective than pyrethrins/piperonyl butoxide; however, additional research is needed.[28]

Dimethicone 100% gel also has been shown to cure pediculosis while causing less irritation than traditional therapy. Furthermore, dimethicone works by coating the lice and irreversibly immobilizing them within 5 minutes of application.[31]

Assessment of Pediculosis: A Case-Based Approach

In many cases of pediculosis, visual inspection of the scalp will verify the presence or absence of head lice or nits. Similarly, presence of body lice can be determined by identifying adult lice and nits in seams of clothing. If a patient does not want such an inspection or if lice/nits have not been confirmed by another health care provider, a pediculicide should not be recommended. When the disorder is confirmed, the appropriate pediculicide should be recommended. If resistance to pyrethrins or permethrin has been reported in the region, patients should be referred to a health care provider for a prescription pediculicide. However, because of the cost of prescription products for head lice, an alternative therapy can be recommended.[20]

Case 37–2 illustrates assessment of a patient who has a head lice infestation.

CASE 37-2

Relevant Evaluation Criteria	
Collect	
1. Gather essential information about the patient's symptoms and medical history, including	
a. Description of symptom(s) (i.e., nature, onset, duration, severity, associated symptoms)	A mother comes to the pharmacy concerned that her daughter is constantly scratching her head. She also reports that seeing little white specks in her daughter's hair. It is the start of the school year, and her daughter attends kindergarten with many other children. The mother is concerned that her daughter has head lice, because the school has notified all the parents of a potential lice outbreak.
b. Description of any factors that seem to precipitate, exacerbate, and/or relieve the patient's symptom(s)	Nothing has seemed to relieve the symptoms.
c. Description of the patient's efforts to relieve the symptoms	The child keeps scratching her head to relieve the itching.
d. Patient's identity	Sally Joseph
e. Patient's age, gender, height, and weight	5 years old, female, 41 in., 44 lb
f. Patient's occupation	Kindergartener
g. Patient's dietary habits	Sally appears well-nourished and has a normal appetite.
h. Patient's sleep habits	Sally sleeps in her own room with many stuffed animals.
i. Concurrent medical conditions, prescription and nonprescription medications, and dietary supplements	No significant past medical history
j. Allergies	None
k. History of other adverse reactions to medications	None
l. Other (describe) ______	n/a
Assess	
2. Differentiate patient's signs/symptoms and correctly identify the patient's primary problem(s).	Patient appears to have multiple grayish-colored specks in her hair, and she is scratching her head constantly. Resistance to pyrethrins or permethrin has not been reported in the region.
3. Identify exclusions for self-treatment (Figure 37–3).	
4. Formulate a comprehensive list of therapeutic alternatives for the primary problem to determine whether triage to a health care provider is required, and share this information with the patient or caregiver.	Options include 1. Use permethrin 1% cream rinse products or pyrethrins 33% with piperonyl butoxide 4% shampoo products. 2. Refer patient to an HCP. 3. Advise self-care until an HCP is consulted. 4. Take no action.
Plan	
5. Select an optimal therapeutic alternative to address the patient's problem, taking into account patient preferences.	■ Permethrin 1% cream rinse products or ■ Pyrethrins 33% with piperonyl butoxide 4% shampoo products
6. Describe the recommended therapeutic approach to the patient or caregiver.	■ "Your daughter appears to have head lice and is eligible for self-treatment. I recommend a nonprescription product to kill the head lice." ■ "Use a pyrethrin shampoo first: – Apply enough to wet the dry hair and scalp. – Allow the treatment to stay for 10 minutes. – Lather the shampoo throughout the hair and then rinse. – Use a nit comb to remove dead lice and eggs. – Repeat this in 7–10 days if lice or nits are detected." ■ "After shampooing her hair, apply a permethrin cream rinse: – Wash hair with regular shampoo and then towel dry hair. – Apply enough cream rinse to wet hair and scalp.

CASE 37-2 *continued*

Relevant Evaluation Criteria	Scenario/Model Outcome
	– Allow treatment to remain for 10 minutes and then rinse and towel dry. – Use nit comb to remove dead lice and eggs." ■ "When using the nit comb, part the hair into segments, and comb each segment to ensure thoroughness."
7. Explain to the patient or caregiver the rationale for selecting the recommended therapeutic approach from the considered therapeutic alternatives.	"This product should kill the head lice."
Implement	
8. When recommending self-care with nonprescription medications and/or nondrug therapy, convey accurate information to the patient or caregiver.	"To prevent the lice from spreading, make sure to follow all directions on the product labeling and wash or seal items that the patient may have come in contact with."
Solicit follow-up questions from the patient or caregiver.	"What else should I do to help prevent the spread of lice?"
Answer the patient's or caregiver's questions.	■ "Wash hairbrushes, combs, and toys that have come in contact with the patient in water that is 130°F (39.4°C) or higher for 10 minutes." ■ "Clothes, bedding, and towels used by the patient should be washed in water that is 130°F (39.4°C) or higher. They should be dried on the hottest dryer setting possible." ■ "Items that cannot be washed should be sealed in plastic bags for 2 weeks" ■ "Vacuum living areas regularly." ■ "Visually inspect hair and scalp before, during, and after treatment for lice or nits."
Follow-up: Monitor and Evaluate	
9. Assess patient outcome.	■ "If there are still head lice after 2 treatment rounds, we will need to contact your primary care provider to see if we can try a prescription product." ■ Advise patient and caregiver that significant skin irritation or exposure of eyes to pediculicides require medical attention.

Patient Counseling for Pediculosis

Control of pediculosis requires both pharmacologic and nonpharmacologic intervention. The health care provider should reassure parents of children with head lice that the condition is not the result of poor hygiene. Patients with confirmed head or pubic lice infestations should be counseled on which product is best for the situation and how to use the product properly; preventive measures should also be discussed. Additional information regarding patient counseling for pediculosis can be found in the box "Patient Education for Pediculosis."

Evaluation of Patient Outcomes for Pediculosis

Follow-up of lice infestations should occur within 10 days. If signs of lice infestation persist after a second application of a pediculicide, the patient should be advised to seek medical attention. Overuse of these products should be discouraged, and use of nonpharmacologic control measures should be emphasized.[24]

Key Points for Insect Bites and Stings and Pediculosis

- Insect stings and bites cause local irritation, inflammation, swelling, and itching; a cold pack may be applied to reduce local symptoms.
- For relief of the itching and pain resulting from insect bites, topical nonprescription preparations that contain local anesthetics, antihistamines, hydrocortisone, or counterirritants can be used in patients ages 2 years and older.
- In hypersensitive people, anaphylactic reactions may pose serious emergency problems; these patients require immediate medical attention.
- Suspected spider bites should be referred; nonprescription treatments are not appropriate. If possible, the spider should be sealed in a container for identification.

PATIENT EDUCATION FOR Pediculosis

The objectives for self-treatment of pediculosis are (1) to rid the body of lice and nits and (2) to implement measures to prevent future infestations. For most patients, carefully following product instructions and the self-care measures listed here will help ensure optimal therapeutic outcomes.

Nondrug Measures

- Wash hairbrushes, combs, and toys of infested patients in water at a temperature of 130°F (39.4°C) or higher for 10 minutes.[20]
- Use water at a temperature of 130°F (39.4°C) or higher to wash the clothes, bedding, and towels of infested patients. Dry the items on the hottest dryer setting that the fabric permits.[20]
- Objects or clothing that cannot be washed should be sealed in plastic bags for the length of the louse's life cycle (2 weeks) so that it is unable to feed on a host.
- Avoid close physical contact with an infested patient; do not share articles such as combs, brushes, towels, caps, and hats.
- Vacuum living areas thoroughly and regularly during treatment period.
- Visually inspect the hair and scalp before, during, and after treatment for evidence of lice or nits.
  - Use a nit comb diligently to remove nits.
  - Part hair into segments and comb the hair in each segment. (Individual hairs can be trimmed if nit removal proves difficult.)

Nonprescription Medications

- Treatment of other family members should be determined on the basis of presence of lice or nits and the family members' level of contact with the infested individual; unnecessary treatment should be avoided.
- Application steps for a pyrethrin shampoo include the following:
  - Apply sufficient quantity to wet the dry hair and scalp. (Foams should also be applied to dry hair.)
  - Allow the treatment to remain for 10 minutes.
  - Work the shampoo into a lather and then rinse thoroughly. (Remove foams with shampoo or soap and water.)
  - Use a nit comb to remove dead lice and eggs as described previously.
- Application steps for a permethrin cream rinse include the following.
  - Shampoo with regular shampoo, rinse, and towel dry hair.
  - Apply sufficient cream rinse to wet hair and scalp.
  - Allow the treatment to remain for 10 minutes; then rinse and towel dry.
  - Use a nit comb as described previously.
- Avoid contact of the pediculicide with eyes and mucous membranes.
- The pediculicide can cause temporary irritation, erythema, itching, swelling, and numbness of the scalp; itching should be relieved in a few days.
- For pyrethrin products, repeat entire process in 7–10 days; permethrin products can be used again in 7–10 days if lice or nits are detected. Because of treatment resistance, proper use of these products is required and overuse must be avoided.
- If desired, contact the National Pediculosis Association at www.headlice.org or 1-617-905-0176 for information about treatment of lice infestations.
- If pediculicides are ruled out as a treatment option, alternative products such as citronella, lemon eucalyptus oil, soybean oil, cedar oil, lavender oil, tea tree oil, garlic, and scented moisturizers in mineral oil (e.g., Skin-So-Soft) may be tried.

When to Seek Medical Attention

- Significant skin irritation or excessive exposure of eyes or mucous membranes to pediculicides warrants medical intervention.
- Seek medical attention if symptoms of lice infestation persist after the second treatment.
- Seek medical attention if resistance to pyrethrins or permethrin has been reported in the region.

➤ A tick should be removed by grasping it near the head with tweezers and gently pulling to cause the tick to release from the skin. The patient should be monitored for systemic effects such as Lyme disease and Rocky Mountain spotted fever.

➤ Appropriate use of insect repellents containing DEET will help prevent insect bites from mosquitoes, ticks, and chiggers.

➤ Exposure to mosquito bites warrants monitoring the patient for symptoms of mosquito-borne viruses.

➤ Nondrug measures are an important component in treatment of lice infestation.

➤ Available nonprescription pediculicides contain either synergized pyrethrins or permethrin.

➤ Pediculicides are designed for initial treatment and retreatment in 7–10 days; hair should be combed with a nit comb after treatment.

➤ If resistance to pyrethrins and permethrin has been reported in the region, patients should be referred to a medical provider for a prescription pediculicide or an alternative therapy should be recommended.

REFERENCES

1. Centers for Disease Control and Prevention. Avoid mosquito bites. Updated March 18, 2016. Available at: http://www.cdc.gov/features/stopmosquitoes/. Accessed June 26, 2017.
2. Centers for Disease Control and Prevention. About Zika virus disease. Updated February 22, 2016. Available at: http://www.cdc.gov/zika/about/index.html. Accessed June 26, 2017.
3. Centers for Disease Control and Prevention. Zika virus: clinical evaluation and disease. Updated February 5, 2016. Available at: http://www.cdc.gov/zika/hc-providers/clinicalevaluation.html. Accessed June 26, 2017.
4. Kolb A, Needham GR, Neyman KM, et al. Bedbugs. *Dermatol Ther.* 2009;22(4):347–52. doi: 10.1111/j.1529-8019.2009.01246.x.
5. Doggett SL, Dwyer DR, Peñas PF, et al. Bed bugs: Clinical relevance and control options. *Clin Microbiol Rev.* 2012;25(1):164–92. doi: 10.1128/CMR.05015-11.
6. Due C, Fox W, Medlock JM, et al. Tick bite prevention and tick removal. *BMJ.* 2013;347:f7123. doi: 10.1136/bmj.f7123.
7. Bratton RL, Corey GR. Tick-borne disease. *Am Fam Physician.* 2005; 71(12):2323–30.
8. Centers for Disease Control and Prevention. Lyme disease data and statistics. Updated September 24, 2015. Available at: http://www.cdc.gov/lyme/stats/index.html. Accessed June 26, 2017.

9. Centers for Disease Control and Prevention. National Institute for Occupational Safety and Health (NIOSH) workplace safety and health topics: venomous spiders. Updated July 30, 2015. Available at: http://www.cdc.gov/niosh/topics/spiders/default.html. Accessed June 26, 2017.
10. Katz TM, Miller JH, Hebert AA. Insect repellents: historical perspective and new developments. *J Am Acad Dermatol.* 2008;58:865–71. doi: 10.1016/j.jaad.2007.10.005.
11. Diaz JH. Chemical and plant-based insect repellents: efficacy, safety, and toxicity. *Wilderness Environ Med.* 2016;27(1):153–63. doi: 10.1016/j.wem.2015.11.007.
12. Centers for Disease Control and Prevention. West Nile virus: frequently asked questions: insect repellent use and safety. Updated March 31, 2015. Available at: http://www.cdc.gov/westnile/faq/repellent.html. Accessed June 26, 2017.
13. U.S. Environmental Protection Agency. Insect repellents: skin-applied repellent ingredients. Updated March 11, 2016. Available at: https://www.epa.gov/insect-repellents/skin-applied-repellent-ingredients. Accessed June 26, 2017.
14. Alpern JD, Dunlop SJ, Dolan BJ, et al. Personal protection measures against mosquitoes, ticks, and other arthropods. *Med Clin North Am.* 2016;100:303–16. doi: 10.1016/j.mcna.2015.08.019.
15. Koren G, Matsui D, Bailey B. DEET-based insect repellants: safety implications for children and pregnant and lactating women. *CMAJ.* 2003; 169(3):209–12. PMCID: PMC167123.
16. Sudakin D, Trevathan W. DEET: a review and update of safety and risk in the general population. *J Toxicol.* 2003;42(6):831–9. doi: 10.1081/CLT-120025348.
17. Dibucaine. Wolters Kluwer Clinical Drug Information (Lexi-Drugs). Available at: http://www.crlonline.com. Accessed April 20, 2013.
18. Zinc oxide. Wolters Kluwer Clinical Drug Information (Lexi-Drugs). Available at: http://www.crlonline.com. Accessed April 20, 2013.
19. Center for Disease Control and Prevention. Head lice: epidemiology and risk factors. Updated September 24, 2013. Available at: https://www.cdc.gov/parasites/lice/head/epi.html. Accessed June 26, 2017.
20. Devore CD, Schutze GE. Head lice. *Pediatrics.* 2015;135(5):1355–65. doi: 10.1542/peds.2015-0746.
21. Raoult D, Roux V. The body louse as a vector of reemerging human diseases. *Clin Infect Dis.* 1999;29(4):888–911. doi: 10.1086/520454.
22. Leone PA. Scabies and pediculosis pubis: an update of treatment regimens and general review. *Clin Infect Dis.* 2007;44(Suppl 3):S153–9. doi: 10.1086/511428.
23. Goates BM, Atkin JS, Wilding KG, et al. An effective nonchemical treatment for head lice: a lot of hot air. *Pediatrics.* 2006;118(5):1962–70. doi: 10.1542/peds.2005-1847.
24. Pray S. Pediculicide resistance in head lice: a survey. *Hosp Pharm.* 2003;38:241–6. doi: 10.1111/j.1365-2583.2011.01097.x.
25. Lice in at least 25 states show resistance to common treatment [press release]. Boston, MA: American Chemical Society; August 18, 2015.
26. Burkhart C. Relationship of treatment-resistant head lice to the safety and efficacy of pediculicides. *Mayo Clin Proc.* 2004;79(5):661–6. doi: 10.1016/S0025-6196(11)62289-1.
27. Pearlman D. Nuvo lotion and the future of head-lice treatment. *Pediatrics.* 2005;115(5):1452-3. doi: 10.1542/peds.2005-0396.
28. Barker SC, Altman PH. A randomized assessor blind, parallel group comparative efficacy trial of three products for the treatment of head lice in children—melaleuca oil and lavender oil, pyrethrins and piperonyl butoxide, and a suffocation product. *BMC Dermatol.* 2010;10:1–7. doi: 10.1186/1471-5945-10-6.
29. HeadLice.org. Alternative treatments: what the NPA is saying about mayonnaise, Vaseline, and tea tree oil. Available at: http://www.headlice.org/faq/treatments/alternatives.htm. Accessed June 26, 2017.
30. Serrano L, Decesar L, Pham L. Evaluation of the efficacy and safety of sodium chloride (LiceFreee Spray) against 1% permethrin crème rinse on head lice infested individuals. *Pharmacology & Pharmacy.* 2013:4(2); 266–73. doi: 10.4236/pp.2013.42038.
31. Ihde ES, Boscamp JR, Loh JM, et al. Safety and efficacy of a 100% dimethicone pediculicide in school-age children. *BMC Pediatrics.* 2015; 15(70):1–6. doi: 10.1186/s12887-015-0381-0.

CHAPTER 38

ACNE

KARLA T. FOSTER

Acne, also known as *acne vulgaris* (AV), is an inflammatory skin disease that affects 40–50 million people in the United States.[1] *Vulgaris* is a Latin term that means common or affecting the masses. The 2010 Global Burden of Disease study ranks acne as the eighth most prevalent disease worldwide.[2] AV affects the pilosebaceous glands, resulting in lesions most commonly found on the face. Extrafacial lesions are also found on the back (52%), chest (30%), lower back (22%), shoulders and arms (16%), and neck 8%.[3]

Acne is most prevalent during adolescence. Cordain et al. describes acne as a universal disease that affects 79%–95% of adolescents in Westernized societies.[4] One study conducted from 1971 to 1989 showed a prevalence of acne in nearly 100% of boys ages 16–17 years and more than 85% of 16-year-old girls.[5] AV peaks between the ages of 14 and 17 years in girls and 16 and 19 years in boys. Acne begins to improve between the ages of 20 and 25 years but may persist in 7%–17% of individuals, with a prevalence of nearly 24% in women in this age group. Late-onset acne, defined as acne symptoms in persons older than 25 years, occurs in 8% of patients.[5] Acne persists in 1% of men and 5% of women after the age of 40.[5]

Acne was once considered a disease of teenagers.[6] The onset of acne correlates with the onset of puberty; however, acne is occurring in adolescents younger than 12 years.[6] Recently, reports of acne in children have increased, with acne reported in children ages 10–12 years at a rate of 28%–61%.[4] Eichenfield et al. reports that acne is common in preadolescents (ages 7–12 years).[6] Additionally, acne has also been observed in children ages 4–7 years.[4]

The effect of acne on patients should not be overlooked. Associations have been shown between acne and lower self-esteem.[7] Acne also has a negative impact on quality of life similar to that in patients with asthma or epilepsy.[7] In 2014, the manufacturing industry for nonprescription acne treatments reported revenue of $621.3 million.[8] Manufacturers expected a slight decrease in revenue related to the younger age of buyers (adolescents are the most common buyers of nonprescription drugs) and the recession.[8] Revenue from nonprescription products is also expected to fall by 0.6% a year due to competition with prescription acne products and a decreased adolescent population.[8] In 2016, sales of nonprescription acne products totaled $607 million.[9] In the United States, the direct and indirect costs related to acne was reported at $3 billion.[10]

Pathophysiology of Acne

Acne is the result of several pathologic processes that occur within the pilosebaceous unit located in the *dermis,* or middle layer of the skin (Figure 38–1A). These units consist of a hair follicle and associated sebaceous glands and are connected to the skin surface by a duct (*infundibulum*) lined with epithelial cells through which the hair shaft passes. The sebaceous glands produce sebum. Sebum normally functions to protect the skin from light and to retain moisture. It possesses an antibacterial property that is both pro- and anti-inflammatory and is involved in the wound-healing process.[11] A greater understanding of the molecular function of the sebaceous glands has helped to explain the role of these glands in skin function. The sebaceous gland acts as an endocrine organ and responds to changes in androgens and hormones similar to the action of the hypothalamic–pituitary–adrenal axis; hence, the sebaceous gland has been called "the brain of the skin." Corticotrophin-releasing hormone (CRH) influences the sebaceous glands' endocrine function.[12] CRH is the primary hormone involved in neuroendocrine and behavioral responses to stress. In acne-prone skin, CRH is found throughout the sebaceous glands and has been associated with the immune and inflammatory processes that lead to stress-induced acne.[11]

The etiology of acne is multifactorial. In addition to its intricate pathophysiology, diet, as well as genetics and gender, play an important role in acne. In one study of 200 patients with post-adolescent acne, Ebede et al. found that 50% of patients reported at least one first-degree family relative with acne.[13]

Genetic factors have long been discussed as a possible factor in the susceptibility to acne. However, more research is needed to explore the role of genetics in acne.[3] Recent literature has increasingly discussed the role of environmental factors, such as diet, in the etiology of acne. Cordain et al. observed acne prevalence in adolescents from non-Westernized countries.[4] Scientists observed 1200 Kitavan subjects (including 300 subjects ages 15–25 years) in whom no case of acne was observed. Cordain et al. also observed 115 Aché subjects (including 15 subjects ages 15–25 years) for more than 843 days and observed no cases of active acne.[4] The authors of this study noted differences between the Westernized population and the non-Westernized population who had little to no acne. They concluded that environmental factors such as diets that consist of a high glycemic load, found in the Westernized population, and the resulting increase in insulin may play a more important role in the correlation in the incidence of acne.[4] Researchers noted that clinicians should look toward these differences to treat acne.[4] Several more epidemiologic studies have correlated acne with the Western diet.[14] The non-Western diets had low-glycemic loads. These diets consisted of lower consumption of dairy products, alcohol, cereals, oil, sugar, and salt.[14] Foods with a high-glycemic load elevate plasma concentrations of insulin, which regulates insulinlike growth factor-1 (IGF-1) and IGF-binding protein, promotes unregulated tissue

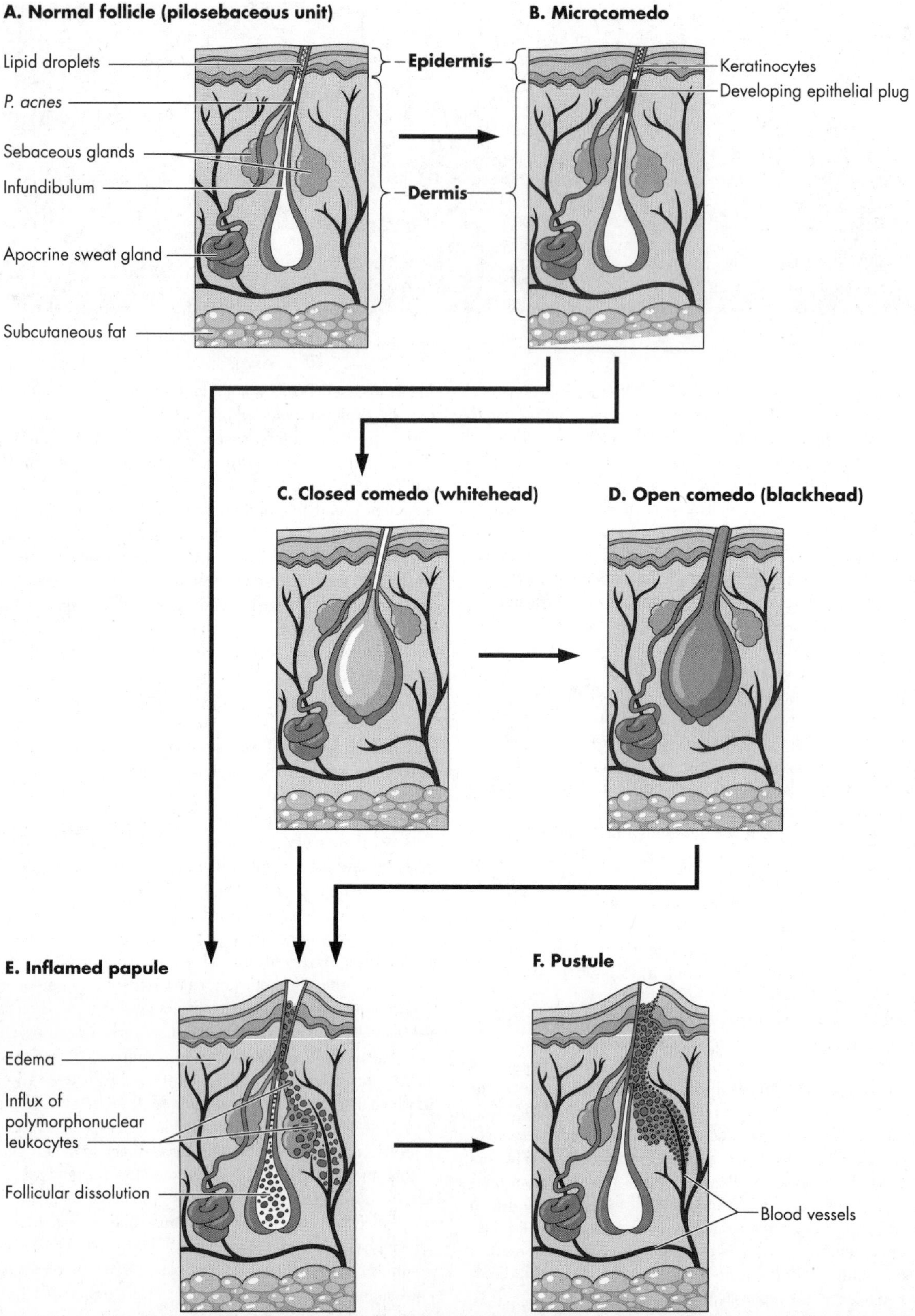

FIGURE **38–1** Pathogenesis of acne. Key: *P. acnes* = *Propionibacterium acnes*. (Source: Adapted with permission from Fulton JE, Bradley S. The choice of vitamin A acid, erythromycin, or benzoyl peroxide for the topical treatment of acne. *Cutis*.1976;17(3):560.)

growth, and enhances androgen synthesis.[15] Hormones, such as androgens and IGF-1, act on sebaceous glands and keratinocytes.[15] Dietary milk also causes a rise in the serum level of IGF-1 through a high rise in blood glucose and serum insulin levels.[14] Melnik discusses the role of mammalian target of rapamycin complex 1 (mTORC1) as a nutrient-derived signal involved in the exacerbation of acne through diet.[16] The mTORC1 signal is activated in the presence of foods with a high-glycemic load, high fat intake, high dairy intake, and high meat consumption. These foods are characteristic of those found in the Western diet.[16] The mTORC1 kinase integrates signals of cellular energy, growth factors (insulin, IGF-1), and protein-derived signals, predominantly leucine, which is provided in high amounts by milk proteins and meat, with resultant increases in androgen and sebum production, respectively, which further perpetuates the pathogenesis of acne.[16] Melnik goes on to explain that the role of diet in acne pathogenesis is still controversial. However, the discovery of nutrient signaling pathways, such as mTORC1, helps explain the link between diet and acne exacerbation.[16] Currently no specific dietary changes are recommended in the management of acne, although emerging data show evidence that diets consisting of high-glycemic-index foods may be associated with acne.[17]

Pathologic factors involved in the development of acne are (1) sebum production by the sebaceous gland, (2) *Propionibacterium acnes (P. acnes)* follicular colonization, (3) alteration in the keratinization process, and (4) release of inflammatory mediators in the skin.[12]

The rise in androgenic hormones coincides with the start of puberty and the appearance of acne. The conversion of testosterone to dihydrotestosterone stimulates an increase in the size and metabolic activity of sebaceous glands. The excessive sebum serves as a breeding ground for *P. acnes* as the comedo develops. Increases in androgen levels are also partly responsible for abnormal follicular desquamation within the infundibulum. Sebum includes several matrix metalloproteinases.[12] This enzyme has a prominent role in inflammatory matrix remodeling and proliferative skin disorders.[13] Prescription medications are being aimed at these enzymes to target acne. Examples of these prescription medications include adapalene and antibiotics such as tetracyclines and macrolides.[18] Evidence also exists that follicular keratinocytes release interleukin-1, which may stimulate comedone formation. Recent studies show that the skin of people without acne have inflammatory responses that occur before the hyperproliferation of keratinocytes in acne.[12] The understanding of the pathophysiology of acne is still evolving. Kircik discusses a "new paradigm shift" in the way that we think of the pathogenesis of acne.[19] Kircik reevaluated a 2003 landmark study that showed the pathogenesis of acne begins with an inflammatory process, rather than with hyperkeratinization and comedogenesis.[19] Further, the study authors found that inflammatory responses are a key component in the early stages of acne lesion formation.[19]

Figures 38–1 and 38–2 illustrate the complex interplay of the pathophysiology of acne. Hyperproliferation of keratinocytes results in cell cohesion and formation of a plug that blocks the follicular

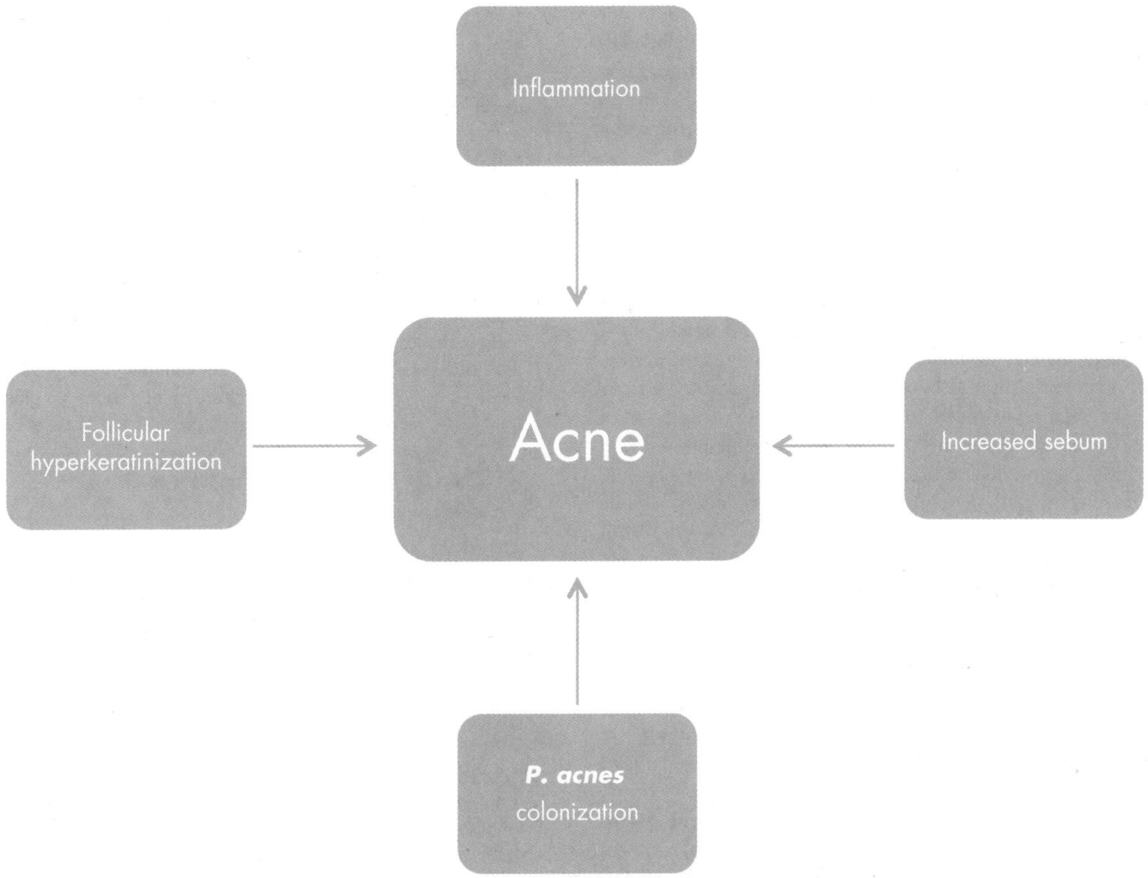

FIGURE 38-2 Pathophysiology of acne. (Source: References 5 and 20.)

orifice. This plug distends the follicle to form a *microcomedo*, the initial pathologic lesion of acne (Figure 38–1B).[20] As more cells and sebum accumulate, the microcomedo enlarges and becomes visible as a *closed comedo*, or *whitehead*, that is, a small, pale nodule just beneath the skin surface (Figure 38–1C). If the contents of the plug cause distention of the pore's orifice, the plug will protrude from the pore, causing an *open comedo*, or *blackhead*. The lesion is named a blackhead because of the presence of melanin and oxidation of lipids upon exposure to air.

Currently, there is no exact and clear explanation behind the pathogenesis of acne.[21] The authors believe the factors involved in acne are more intricately related than previously thought. New factors involved may include T-helper cells, *P. acnes* subtypes, and nutritional factors.[21] Research has led to the discovery that several types of *P. acnes* exist. Information on the types of acne may one day help health care providers (HCPs) develop specific treatment plans for acne.[22,23]

Clinical Presentation of Acne

More information continues to evolve around the presentation of acne. Through production of lipases, *P. acnes* breaks down sebum into highly irritating free fatty acids. As a result of the irritation and inflammation, localized tissue destruction occurs. Toll-like receptors (TLRs) are mammalian proteins that have emerged as a vital regulator of host responses to infection.[12] Research shows that cytokine induction by *P. acnes* occurs through TLR-2, which stimulates inflammatory lesions. In acne, TLR-2 invokes a significant inflammatory response as well as cellular apoptosis and tissue injury.[24] Redness and inflammation in and around the follicular canal constitute a *papule* (Figure 38–1E). A *pustule* (Figure 38–1F) possesses the same qualities as a papule but has visible purulence in the center of the lesion. *Nodules* result from disruption of the follicular wall and release of its contents into the surrounding dermis.[20]

Several factors contribute to the exacerbation of existing acne and cause periodic flare-ups of acne in some patients (Table 38–1).[25–27]

Until recently acne was categorized as noninflammatory or inflammatory (see the Color Plates, Photographs 27 and 28). Noninflammatory lesions included open or closed comedones. Inflammatory lesions included papules, pustules, or nodules. Do et al. discovered that although 54% of inflammatory lesions were preceded by comedones, 28% of inflammatory lesions were preceded by normal skin. Furthermore, it was demonstrated that cellular inflammatory lesions could occur at every stage of acne. In this update, the authors explain that noninflammatory lesions should be considered comedones with probable new evidence of the inflammatory process occurring at every stage of acne.[28] Acne lesions are commonly found on the face, chest, upper back, and upper arms.[20] Women in their 30s and 40s not uncommonly have acne that is concentrated on the chin and along the jaw line.[29] On presentation to an HCP, the patient may exhibit one or more types of lesions. Acne severity is defined by the number and type of acne lesions[30]; however, there is no consensus on the type of grading system to use.[17,31] Table 38–2 describes a commonly used acne grading system used to assess the severity of acne.[30]

If acne lesions persist beyond an individual's mid-20s or develop in the mid-20s or later, the symptoms may signal rosacea, rather than AV. A differential diagnosis is necessary, because the treatment of rosacea, although similar to that for acne, has unique elements. Erythema and telangiectasias or facial flushing present on the cheeks, but no comedones are present.[31]

TABLE 38-1 Exacerbating Factors in Acne

Factor	Description of Factor
Acne cosmetica	Noninflammatory comedones on the face, chin, and cheek caused by occlusion of the pilosebaceous unit by oil-based cosmetics, moisturizers, pomades, or other health and beauty products
Acne excoriee (excoriated)	A form of acne caused by constant picking, squeezing, or scratching at the skin, which causes the acne to look worse
Acne mechanica	Local irritation or friction from occlusive clothing, headbands, helmets, or other friction-producing devices
	Excessive contact between face and hands, such as resting the chin or cheek on the hand
Chloracne	An acneiform eruption caused by exposure to chlorine compounds
Drug-induced acne	*More common:* Anabolic steroids, bromides, corticosteroids, corticotrophin, isoniazid, lithium, phenytoin
	Less common: Azathioprine; cyclosporine; disulfiram; phenobarbital; quinidine; tetracycline; vitamins B_1, B_6, B_{12}, and D_2
Hormone-induced acne	Hormonal alterations, specifically increased androgen levels induced by medical conditions, pregnancy, or medications
Hydration-induced acne	Hydration-induced decrease in size of pilosebaceous duct orifice and prevention of loosening of comedone caused by high-humidity environments and prolonged sweating
Occupational acne	Exposure to dirt, vaporized cooking oils, or certain industrial chemicals, such as coal tar and petroleum derivatives
Stress- and extreme emotion–induced acne	May induce expression of neuroendocrine modulators and release of CRH, which play a role in centrally and topically induced stress of the sebaceous glands and possibly progression of acne

Key: CRH = Corticotrophin-releasing hormone.
Source: References 25–27

TABLE 38-2 Grading and Classification of Acne

Mild	Moderate	Severe
Few erythematous papules and occasional pustules mixed with comedones	Many erythematous papules and pustules and prominent scarring	Extensive pustules, erythematous papules, and multiple nodules in an inflamed background

Source: Reference 31.

In addition to the negative psychosocial impact of acne, physical scarring is also a complication of acne.[32] Scarring presents as (1) hypertrophic scars and keloids caused by increased tissue formation and (2) a loss of skin resulting in ice picks or boxcar scars.[32] Kircik explains that scientists observed patients with and without scarring. It was concluded that patients with scarring had an initial cellular response to AV that was weaker and less effective throughout the resolution of acne. Patients with scarring also experienced a later influx of macrophages and increased inflammatory responses that resulted in persistent inflammatory hyperpigmentation.[19]

Treatment of Acne

In most cases, acne is self-limiting and can be controlled to varying degrees. Adherence to therapeutic regimens will reduce symptoms and minimize scarring. Because acne persists for long periods, treatment must be long term, continuous, and consistent.

Treatment Goals

Patients and HCPs should identify any exacerbating factors of acne (Table 38–1). It is also imperative that patients and providers classify the acne (Table 38–2) to allow selection of the most appropriate therapeutic options.[31] Once the classification has been determined, treatment should be initiated and adherence to medication therapy should be encouraged.[12] A major global problem with acne treatment is adherence.[33]

General Treatment Approach

Gollnick describes a general treatment approach that involves three categories in which acne treatment should fall: (1) eliminate the visual lesions of acne that occur during the acute phase of acne, (2) maintain treatments that prevent relapse, and (3) implement adjunctive procedures that treat scarring or other complications that result from acne.[33]

Nonpharmacologic Therapy

Patients with acne should eliminate exacerbating factors of acne (Table 38–1). This measure should promote understanding and prevention of the disease as well as adherence to therapy. Patients seeking self-care options should cleanse the skin with a mild soap or nonsoap cleanser twice daily. The use of abrasive products and excessive cleansing may worsen the acne. Self-care options should also include staying well hydrated. Dehydration may increase the inflammatory chemicals in the cell and may cause dysfunction in the natural desquamation process of the stratum corneum. Decker and Graber explain that the normal skin has a pH of 5.3–5.9. Washing the face with harsh soaps that can increase the pH by at least 2 units can cause skin dryness and create an environment that supports growth of *P. acnes*.[34] Facial toners may decrease oily skin. They may also help remove makeup and traces of dirt. However, patients should not overuse toners, because they could cause increased skin irritation.[6] Patients could also consider dietary changes by eliminating or cutting back on foods with a high glycemic index to determine whether the acne improves or remains the same.[35]

Physical Treatments

Physical treatments include light therapies and mechanical therapies such as scrubs, cleansing clothes, brushes, and heating devices (Table 38–3).[34] Comedo extraction is also an example of a physical treatment.[17] A wide range of self-applied, acrylate glue–based material strips can aid in the extraction of impacted comedones.[34] The working group for the guidelines of care and management of AV note that professional comedo extraction is a useful adjunct to the overall acne regimen and often results in immediate improvement; however, there is limited evidence to recommend physical therapies.[17]

The U.S. Food and Drug Administration (FDA) has approved several light-based therapies for the treatment of acne. These treatments target reduction of *P. acnes* and disruption of sebaceous gland function. *P. acnes* produce porphyrin compounds during normal metabolism. Porphyrins absorb visible light at a variety of wavelengths, which excites the porphyrin compound, causing the formation of oxygen and free radicals.[36] The oxygen radicals are thought to destroy *P. acnes* by damaging lipids in the cell wall of the organism.[12] For now, light therapy is considered a device to be used in conjunction with traditional pharmacologic therapy for acne. More well-designed trials that include light therapy as a standard of treatment are needed.[17]

Pharmacologic Therapy

Researchers advise that nonprescription therapy offers benefits to and should have a role in the treatment of acne.[34] Topical therapy is the standard of care in acne treatment.[37] HCPs should be familiar with the nonprescription products available for treatment of acne.

Adapalene

On July 8, 2016, FDA approved adapalene gel 0.1% (Differin Gel) for nonprescription treatment of acne. It is the first new ingredient

TABLE 38-3 Description of Physical Treatments

Implement	Treatment
Brushes	The oscillating motion of the brush is used to deeply cleanse the skin while removing makeup. The impact of this treatment has not been clinically evaluated.
Cleansing cloth	Cloths are less abrasive than scrubs while providing conditioning and exfoliation of the skin.
Cosmetic adhesive pads	Pads were developed to remove adherent corneocytes, dirt, oil, or to loosen open comedones from the skin.
Heating devices	Heating devices are marketed to directly treat acne vulgaris by contacting the lesion. The device is thought to treat acne through heat and phototherapy.
Light therapy	Examples include visible light, pulsed dye laser, and photodynamic therapies. The most evidence exists for photodynamic therapy in treating acne. A photosensitizer is applied to the affected skin for 15 minutes to 3 hours.
Scrubs	Abrasion opens closed comedones and prevents their progression; however, the abrasive nature of this action could damage the integrity of the skin.

Source: Reference 34

approved for acne treatment since the 1980s and the first full prescription-strength retinoid to become available without a prescription.[38] Adapalene is a first-line topical drug for acne treatment.[20,38] Its mechanism of action differs from that of other available nonprescription acne agents and offers patients another option to manage acne. Adapalene appears to modulate epithelial cell differentiation, keratinization, and inflammation.[39]

Patients should follow all label directions for this product. A thin layer of the product should be applied to affected, intact skin areas once daily. The affected areas should be protected from sun exposure, because adapalene increases susceptibility to sunburn.[39]

Redness, scaling, dryness, itching, and burning are the most common adverse effects of adapalene, but they often diminish after the first month of therapy. Acne may worsen during the first weeks of therapy, because this medication affects lesions that are not yet visible on the skin. The full therapeutic effect of adapalene will become apparent after 8–12 weeks of treatment.[39]

If symptoms worsen or fail to improve in 3 months with proper use of the agent, patients should consult their primary care providers. In addition, product users who experience allergic reactions, become pregnant, or are planning to become pregnant should discontinue use of this product and consult their primary care providers for other treatment options.[39]

Benzoyl Peroxide

Benzoyl peroxide (BP) is the most common topical acne product available both with and without a prescription. BP has keratolytic and antibacterial properties against skin *P. acnes*.[17] BP kills bacteria by introducing oxygen into the environment, thereby killing *P. acnes*, which can thrive only in an oxygen-free environment.[20]

BP has been the mainstay of treatment for acne since the 1930s.[34] In March 2010, FDA issued a final rule for topical acne drug products that included BP as a generally recognized as safe and effective (GRASE) active ingredient in nonprescription topical acne products.[40] BP had been classified as a non-GRASE ingredient since 1995 because of concern about benzoyl's weak mutagenic effect in vitro and BP's tumor promotion potential.[40] FDA later concluded that BP in concentrations of 2.5%–10% is a GRASE ingredient for acne based on animal studies that suggest BP is not carcinogenic or photocarcinogenic.[40]

One of the main benefits of BP is its ability to prevent or eliminate the development of treatment resistance by *P. acnes*, which has increased with the use of conventional antibiotics (macrolides, tetracyclines) over the last 3 decades.[12] Resistant strains have been found in 50% of acne patients who had close contact with a resistant organism.[12] *Close contact* is defined as those individuals living in the same household with family members with acne. The use of BP in combination with antibiotics is recommended to minimize *P. acnes* resistance.[12] BP is often used in combination with other oral or topical antibiotics. In a recent literature review, BP was more effective than topical antibiotics such as clindamycin and erythromycin. In addition, BP in combination with either of these antibiotics was more effective and better tolerated than either of the antibiotics alone.[12]

Nonprescription formulations of BP are available in concentrations of 2.5%–10% as a gel, wash, or cream. Higher strengths of BP have the same antibacterial effects as the lower strengths,[34] but may cause more skin irritation.[41] All new users of nonprescription acne products should test the product by applying it sparingly to 1–2 small affected areas over the first 3 days. If discomfort does not occur, the product should be used according to label directions.[40] Avoidance of contact with clothes or hair is advised, because this product may cause bleaching. In addition, BP can cause photosensitivity, so avoidance of excessive sun exposure and use of a broad-spectrum sunscreen product with a sun protection factor (SPF) of 15 or higher are recommended. Minor improvement may occur with daily application of BP. The number of applications can be increased or decreased until a mild peeling occurs. Results have been seen in as few as 5 days or by week 3 of treatment. Maximum lesion reduction may occur after 8–12 weeks of use. Some patients may experience only mild erythema and scaling during the first few days, which usually subside within 1–2 weeks. BP is recommended for mild acne in adults and pediatric populations (preadolescents and adolescents).[6] Allergic contact dermatitis reactions, characterized by a sudden onset of erythema and vesiculation, are considered rare and occur in a minority of the population (1 in 500). A 2014 FDA Drug Safety Communication reported rare but serious allergic reactions to BP and salicylic acid that ranged from symptoms of local irritation to local and systemic hypersensitivity, including anaphylaxis.[41] FDA has not determined if the products' active ingredients, inactive ingredients, or both are responsible for these reactions. Use of BP products should be discontinued when an allergic reaction such as itching or hives occurs. Medical attention should be sought for hypersensitivity reactions such as throat tightness; difficulty breathing; feeling faint; or swelling of the eyes, face, lips, or tongue.[34] The box "Patient Education for Acne" presented at the end of the chapter lists other precautions for use of BP.

Other Nonprescription Acne Agents

Other FDA-approved nonprescription topical anti-acne ingredients include hydroxy acids in various strengths, sulfur 3%–10% (in single-ingredient products), and a combination of sulfur 3%–8% with either resorcinol 2% or resorcinol monoacetate 3%.[42]

Hydroxy Acids

Keratolytic agents such as alpha hydroxy acids (AHAs) and beta hydroxy acids (BHAs) are also common nonprescription acne products. Hydroxy acids are considered less potent and are often used when patients cannot tolerate other topical acne products.[42] Some hydroxy acids have comedolytic properties and are moderately effective in the treatment of acne.[42]

AHAs are natural exfoliating acids that occur in sugar cane, milk products, and fruits; the most common AHAs are glycolic, lactic, and citric acids, respectively.[33] AHAs are not able to penetrate the pilosebaceous unit to cause a comedolytic effect. AHAs are available in several nonprescription formulations in concentrations of 4%–10% or through dermatologists at higher concentrations. In a study comparing BP with AHAs, BP demonstrated a superior effect at 8 weeks. However, once acne is controlled, a light chemical peel with AHAs may be useful to help correct scarring and hyperpigmentation.[12] However, several treatments are needed and the results are not long lasting. The duration of dosing is once every 15 days for 4–6 months.[17] Table 38–4 lists contraindications to glycolic acid peels that HCPs should be aware of.

Polyhydroxy acids comprise a category of AHAs that has fewer adverse effects, such as irritation and stinging. They are marketed for patients with more clinical sensitivity. They are also said to have moisturizing and humectant properties.[32] Lactobionic acid, a type of polyhydroxy acid, has been said to inhibit the breakdown of matrix metalloproteinase enzymes that occurs from sun exposure. This reduces the appearance of photoaging on the skin.[32]

Salicylic acid, often described as a BHA, is a comedolytic agent available in various nonprescription acne products in concentrations of 0.5%–2%.[32,42] The comedolytic effect is concentration

TABLE 38-4 **Glycolic Acid Peel Contraindications**

Glycolic Acid Peel Contraindications
Active infection or open wounds (herpes simplex, excoriations, open acne cysts)
For medium and deep peels: medium-depth or deep resurfacing procedure within the last 3–12 months
For medium and deep peels: recent facial surgery involving extensive undermining
History of abnormal scar formation or delayed wound healing
History of rosacea, seborrheic dermatitis, atopic dermatitis, psoriasis, vitiligo, active retinoid dermatitis
History of therapeutic radiation exposure
Isotretinoin therapy within the last 6 months
Lack of psychological stability and mental preparedness
Poor general health and nutritional status
Unrealistic expectations

Source: Reference 17.

dependent. Higher concentrations are used in prescription products and chemical peels.[32] Salicylic acid provides a milder, less effective alternative to prescription agents, such as topical retinoids.[15] In cleansing preparations, salicylic acid is considered adjunctive treatment. It should be applied 1–3 times daily, working up to 3 times daily if needed. If dryness or peeling occurs, reduce application to once daily or every other day.[35] Salicylic acid is a phytohormone and is chemically similar to the active component of aspirin. Salicylic acid has the potential drug–drug interactions listed in Table 38–5. Salicylic acid is lipid soluble and able to penetrate the pilosebaceous unit to produce a comedolytic effect.[42] A 2% topical application of salicylic acid can be absorbed up to 20% in the skin. The amount of absorption depends on several factors including the vehicle used, the pH of the drug, skin structure, the frequency of application, and whether or not it is occluded on the skin. Therefore, a patient may be susceptible to salicylism or salicylic acid toxicity with topical application to extensive areas of the skin, especially in children who metabolize drugs differently. A patient would need additional monitoring and possible dose adjustments of their maintenance medications with chronic use of salicylic acid or with application to extensive areas of the body.[17] It is important for HCPs to be aware of potential drug–drug interactions that could occur with the use of salicylic acid.

Salicylic acid products also offer protection from the sun by inhibiting ultraviolet B (UVB) radiation-induced formation of sunburn cells that occurs after the cell has been exposed to UVB rays that cause an irreversible damage to the cell's DNA and by increasing the removal of UVB-induced *dimers* (premutagenic lesions) in skin.[42] However, patients using these products should continue to wear a broad-spectrum sunscreen with an SPF of 15 or higher to protect their skin from further skin damage. BHA products are contraindicated in diabetic patients or patients with poor blood circulation. Use of these products should be limited to the affected area. Use of the products over a large area for prolonged periods could result in toxicity. Signs of salicylate toxicity include nausea, vomiting, dizziness, loss of hearing, tinnitus, lethargy, hyperpnea, diarrhea, psychic disturbances, toxic inner ear damage, hypoglycemia, and hypersensitivity.[42] In 2014, FDA warned of potentially life-threatening hypersensitivity reactions for nonprescription acne products containing salicylic acid or BP (see the section "Benzoyl Peroxide").

Sulfur

Sulfur, precipitated or colloidal, is included in acne products as a keratolytic and antibacterial in concentrations of 3%–10%.[42] Sulfur is generally accepted as effective in promoting the resolution of existing comedones, but with continued use it may have a comedogenic effect. Alternative forms of sulfur such as sodium thiosulfate, zinc sulfate, and zinc sulfide are not recognized as safe and effective.

TABLE 38-5 **Drug–Drug Interactions With Nonprescription Acne Agents**

Acne Agent	Drug	Potential Interaction	Management
Salicylic acid	Anticoagulants	Increased anticoagulation	Use with caution and monitor closely.
Salicylic acid	Antidiabetic agents	Increased activity of glyburide; hypoglycemia	Monitor closely; use alternative acne agent, if possible.
Salicylic acid	Aspirin	Increased anticoagulation; increased serum level of potassium	Monitor closely; consider alternative agent.
Salicylic acid	Corticosteroids	Prednisone may increase renal clearance; increased risk of GI ulceration	Monitor closely.
Salicylic acid	Diuretics	Increased serum level or effect of salicylates	Monitor closely.
Salicylic acid	Methotrexate	Increased serum level of methotrexate	Monitor closely.
Salicylic acid	Heparin	Salicylate decreases platelet adhesiveness and interferes with hemostasis in heparin-treated patients.	Monitor closely.
Salicylic acid	Uricosuric	Effect of probenemide, sulfinpyrazone, and phenylbutazone inhibited	Monitor closely.
Salicylic acid	Pyrazinamide	Pyrazinamide-induced hyperuricemia inhibited	Monitor closely; may consider alternative acne agent.

Source: Reference 17.

Adverse effects with these products are rare but include noticeable odor and dry skin, depending on the formulation used.[34] Sulfur is often combined with sodium sulfacetamide to mask the odor of sulfur in prescription drugs, and sulfur is combined with resorcinol in nonprescription medications for treatment of acne.[42]

Sulfur/Resorcinol

Combinations of sulfur 3%–8% with resorcinol 2% or resorcinol monoacetate 3%, which enhances the effect of sulfur, are available in nonprescription acne products.[34,42] The products function primarily as keratolytics, fostering cell turnover and desquamation. Resorcinol is not effective when used as a monotherapy. However, it is believed to have antibacterial, antifungal, and keratolytic effects when used with other anti-acne products such as sulfur.[34] Resorcinol produces a reversible, dark brown scale on some darker-skinned individuals.[34]

Pharmacotherapeutic Comparison

Table 38–6 provides a comparison of the therapeutic properties of the major acne products.

Product Selection Guidelines

Product selection should be based on individual patient needs, skin type, and severity of acne. Nonprescription acne medications are indicated for mild acne. Skin cleansers and topical acne products are available in a variety of vehicles and strengths. Medicated cleansing products (bars and liquids) are of small value; they leave little active ingredient residue on the skin. Generally, gels are the most effective formulations, because they are astringents and remain on the skin the longest. Gels and solutions have a drying effect that may sometimes cause contact dermatitis. However, these dosage forms are not greasy and may be more beneficial in patients with oily skin. Creams and lotions are generally less irritating to the skin compared with gels and solutions.[43] They are acceptable alternatives to the more effective gels and are recommended for dry or sensitive skin and for use during dry winter weather. Ointment vehicles are not used, because they are occlusive and tend to worsen acne. Patients should start with the lowest strength available and gradually increase the concentration to minimize the irritating effects of the product. They should apply the product only once daily; as they are able to tolerate the applications with no redness or skin irritation, they may increase to twice daily applications. Table 38–7 lists selected nonprescription trade-name acne products in these and other formulations.

Many patients will use nonprescription medications in combination with prescription products to manage acne. Patients should be aware of current medications that may cause acne as well as potential drug interactions that may occur with nonprescription products. Product selection is important for the successful treatment and management of acne. It is important that patients seek medical referral for proper diagnosis and grading of acne. For example, women who experience acne related to hormonal imbalance may benefit more from correction of the imbalance with hormone therapy, such as oral contraceptives, whereas a peripubertal teenager or young adult may benefit more from consultation on avoidance of comedogenic products and adherence with nonprescription products such as BP.[43]

Special Populations

Pregnant patients may have problems with acne because of hormonal imbalances. In most cases, if pregnancy occurs during treatment with any acne medication, the medication should be discontinued and the obstetrician should be advised of current or previous product use because of the potential for teratogenic effects. Little, if any, human data are available to describe the use of topical BP, sulfur, hydroxyl acids, and photodynamic therapy during pregnancy.[44] (See the Preface for a detailed explanation of the pregnancy data.) Glycolic acid peels have not been rated for use in pregnancy.

Acne occurs in all age groups, including the pediatric population. This population comprises neonates, infants, and young children. Most infantile and neonatal acne is self-limiting; however, differential diagnoses by appropriate HCPs, which may include a pediatric endocrinologist, are needed for treatment recommendations.[6] Use of aspirin and aspirin-containing products, such as salicylic acid, in children or teenagers who have or are recovering from chicken pox or flu-like symptoms should be avoided because of the risk of Reye's syndrome. (See Chapter 5 for further discussion of Reye's syndrome.)

Complementary Medicine, Vitamins, and Vitamin Analogs

Tea tree oil is widely known for its antibacterial and antifungal properties. *Staphylococcus aureus,* a common pathogen found on the skin, is sensitive to tea tree oil. Tea tree oil also has anti-inflammatory properties.[45] Terpinen-4-ol, the active ingredient in tea tree oil, has been thought to suppress production of inflammatory mediators and inflammation.[34] Studies have shown that tea tree oil was effective at reducing lesion counts, but there have not

TABLE 38–6 Comparison of Properties for Nonprescription Topical Acne Agents

	Property			
Agent	**Antibacterial**	**Comedolytic**	**Anti-inflammatory**	**Keratolytic**
Adapalene 0.1%	No	Yes	Yes	Yes
Benzoyl peroxide 2.5%–10%	Yes	Yes	No	Yes
Salicylic acid 0.5%–2%	No	Yes	Yes	No
Sulfur 3%–10%	Yes	No	No	Yes
Resorcinol 2% with sulfur 3%–8%	Yes	No	No	Yes
Resorcinol monoacetate 3% with sulfur 3%–8%	Yes	No	No	Yes

Note: Limited data exist to support the recommendation of nicotinamide and zinc for the treatment of acne.[17]
Source: References 6, 17, 33, 34, and 41.

TABLE 38-7 Selected Nonprescription Acne Products

Trade Name	Primary Ingredients
Retinoid Product	
Differin Gel, 15 g	Adapalene 0.1%
Benzoyl Peroxide Products	
Proactiv Repairing Treatment, 2 oz	Benzoyl peroxide 2.5%
Neutrogena Rapid Clear Stubborn Acne Cleanser, 5 oz	Benzoyl peroxide 10%
Clearasil Ultra Rapid Action Vanishing Treatment Cream, 1 oz	Benzoyl peroxide 10%
Salicylic Acid Products	
Neutrogena Oil-Free Acne Stress Control Power Cream Wash, 6 oz	Salicylic acid 2%
Clean & Clear Advantage Acne Spot Treatment, 0.75 oz	Salicylic acid 2%
Alpha Hydroxy Acid Products	
Alpha Hydrox AHA Soufflé 12% Glycolic AHA, 1.6 oz	Glycolic acid 12%
Gly Derm Face Lotion Lite Plus 10, 4 oz	Glycolic acid 10%
Alpha/Beta Hydroxy Acid Products	
M.D. Forté Skin Rejuvenation Hydra-Masque, 4 oz	Glycolic acid; salicylic acid
Polyhydroxy Acid Products	
NeoStrata Bionic Face Cream, 1.4 oz	Gluconolactone 8%; lactobionic acid 4%
Sulfur Product	
De La Cruz Sulfur Ointment 10% Acne Medication, 2.6 oz	Sulfur 10%
Sulfur/Resorcinol Product	
Adult Acnomel Tinted Cream, 1.3 oz	Resorcinol 2%; sulfur 8%
Physical Treatments	
Bioré Deep Cleansing Pore Strips	Comedone extraction strip
BlueMD Blue Light Therapy	Light therapy
Garnier SkinActive Clean+ Refreshing Remover Cleansing Towelettes	Cleansing cloth
Olay Pro-X Advanced Cleansing System	Acne brush
Tanda Zap Acne Spot Treatment Device	Heat therapy

been any robust conclusive studies on the efficacy of tea tree oil use in acne.[34]

Oral zinc may be considered an alternative to tetracyclines.[12,34] Zinc is bacteriostatic against *P. acnes*, inhibits chemotaxis, and has shown effectiveness against severe acne. One study found that zinc was 17% less effective than minocycline but that zinc could be used as an alternative to tetracycline therapy, especially in the summer, because it does not cause phototoxicity. However, zinc's adverse effects of nausea, vomiting, and diarrhea have made it a less attractive therapy.[34,42] Poor patient compliance as a result of these adverse effects has limited its use.

Vitamin A is naturally occurring and is a retinol.[42] Vitamin A is transformed into several metabolites. One metabolite, retinoic acid, is used in cosmetics to help eliminate wrinkles and fine lines. Theoretically, retinol should also work against acne. However, few studies exist to validate this claim. Oral vitamin A or retinol may be beneficial in acne in doses up to 300,000 units daily for women and 500,000 daily for men.[42] Common adverse effects include xerosis and chelitis.

Nicotinamide, a water-soluble derivative of vitamin B_3 is also used for AV.[34] Nicotinamide is an active form of niacin and has been postulated to have several roles in the treatment of acne. It is an anti-inflammatory that improves the texture of photoaged skin and decreases sebum production.[21,46] Data on nicotinamide's role in acne are still limited, and more research needs to be facilitated to assess the role of nicotinamide in acne.

Limited data exist regarding the safety and efficacy of other complementary and alternative therapies for their use in acne.[17]

Assessment of Acne: A Case-Based Approach

Patient assessment begins with asking questions to define the condition. Physical assessment, which involves observing the affected area and questioning the patient further, is the next step in evaluating the disorder. This evaluation helps determine whether the

Exclusions for Self-Treatment

- Moderate–severe acne (Table 38–2)
- Exacerbating factors (e.g., comedogenic drugs, mechanical irritation)
- Possible rosacea

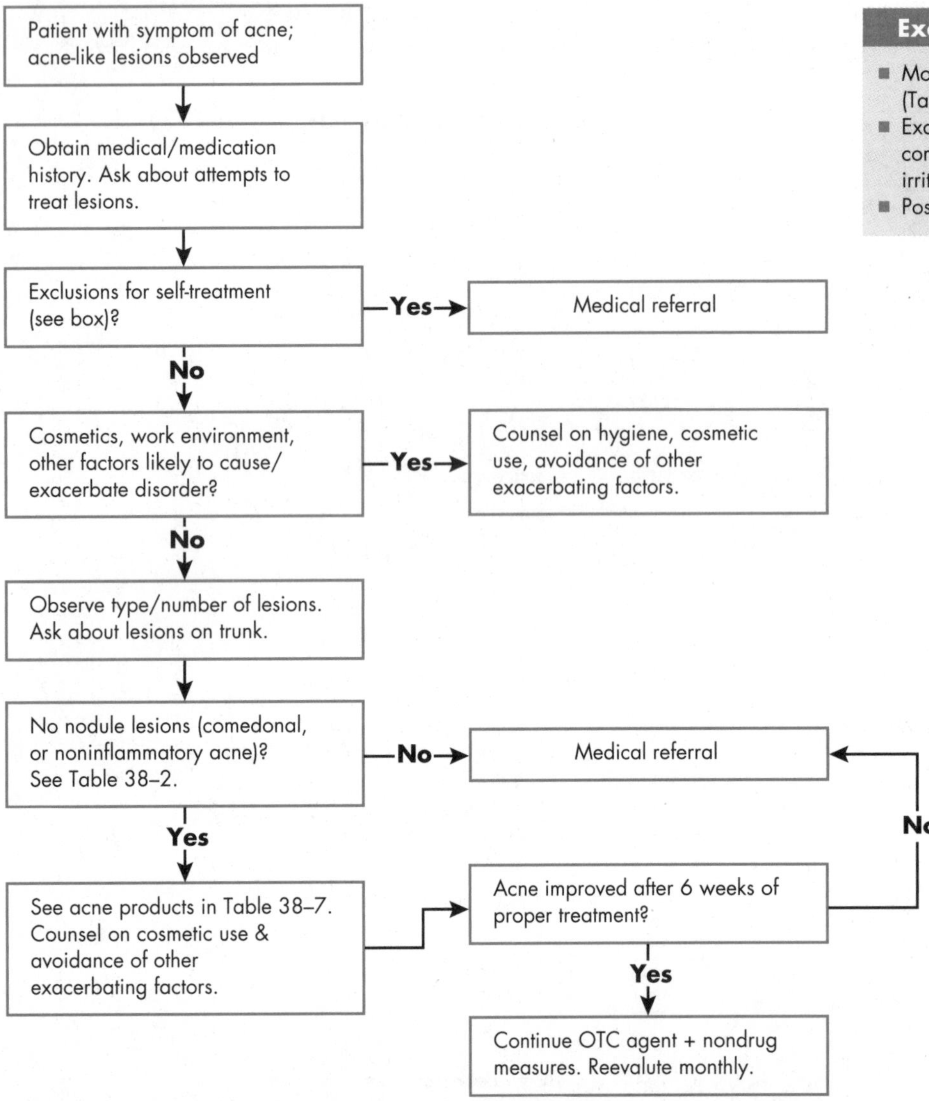

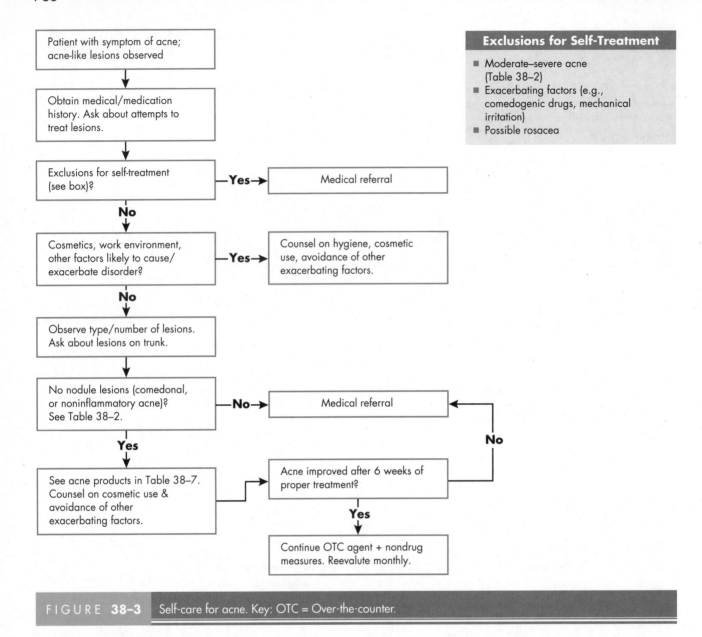

FIGURE 38–3 Self-care for acne. Key: OTC = Over-the-counter.

condition is AV or another dermatologic condition with similar signs and symptoms. Physical assessment also determines whether the severity of the condition precludes self-treatment (Figure 38–3). Before self-care is recommended, an assessment of current medication use, prescription and nonprescription, is necessary to reveal prescribed treatments for the disorder or use of medications known to cause acne (Table 38–1).

Cases 38–1 and 38–2 are examples of assessment of patients presenting with acne.

Patient Counseling for Acne

The success of the treatment regimen depends largely on the patient. Therefore, it is crucial that the HCP communicates with the patient on the causes of acne, corrects any misconceptions, and clearly explains the rationale for treatment. Patient buy-in will facilitate adherence and increase the likelihood of a successful outcome. The HCP must also evaluate the patient's maturity and willingness to adhere to a skin care program that involves a continued daily regimen of washing affected areas and applying medication. Reassurance and emotional support are often necessary to reduce patient concern, because acne cannot be cured—only controlled. The box "Patient Education for Acne" lists specific information to provide patients.

The internet lists supplemental information about acne in lay language, including discussions of acne, nonprescription drugs used to treat it, and treatment expectations. Selected sites that appear to provide accurate information are listed in Table 38–8. If not copyrighted, these materials can be printed and given to the patient during the consultation. If the material is copyrighted, the HCP should instead give the patient the website address.

Evaluation of Patient Outcomes for Acne

Although the patient may expect complete resolution of the acne, an improvement in the disorder, as defined by a decrease in both the number and severity of lesions, is a more realistic expectation

CASE 38-1

Relevant Evaluation Criteria	Scenario/Model Outcome
Collect	
1. Gather essential information about the patient's symptoms and medical history, including	
a. Description of symptom(s) (i.e., nature, onset, duration, severity, associated symptoms)	A mother presents to the pharmacy with her 11-year-old daughter and asks a pharmacist for advice on selecting an acne medication for her daughter. "She has had bumps along her forehead and cheeks for a month or two. The bumps are small and round and the same color as her skin."
b. Description of any factors that seem to precipitate, exacerbate, and/or relieve the patient's symptom(s)	The mother reports that nothing her daughter is doing makes the bumps better or worse.
c. Description of the patient's efforts to relieve the symptoms	She washes her face more frequently with soap.
d. Patient's identity	Leslie Phillips
e. Patient's age, gender, height, and weight	11 years old, female, 4 ft 5 in., 70 lb
f. Patient's occupation	None
g. Patient's dietary habits	Eats three meals a day and dessert every night.
h. Patient's sleep habits	Bedtime is 8:00 PM.
i. Concurrent medical conditions, prescription and nonprescription medications, and dietary supplements	n/a
j. Allergies	NKDA
Assess	
2. Differentiate patient's signs/symptoms, and correctly identify the patient's primary problem(s).	Exacerbation of acne could be due to onset of puberty during preadolescence
3. Identify exclusions for self-treatment (Figure 38–3).	None
4. Formulate a comprehensive list of therapeutic alternatives for the primary problem to determine whether triage to a medical provider is required, and share this information with the patient or caregiver.	Options include (1) Refer Leslie to an appropriate HCP. (2) Recommend self-care with an OTC product and nondrug measures. (3) Recommend self-care until Leslie can see an appropriate HCP. (4) Take no action.
Plan	
5. Select an optimal therapeutic alternative to address the patient's problem, taking into account patient preferences.	Recommend self-care options until Leslie can see an appropriate HCP.
6. Describe the recommended therapeutic approach to the patient or caregiver.	"Try a self-care option that includes nondrug measures."
7. Explain to the patient or caregiver the rationale for selecting the recommended therapeutic approach from the considered therapeutic alternatives.	"Acne is very common in preadolescence and occurs in more than 60% of 10- to 12-year-olds. It is appropriate to be aware of nondrug treatments. If these self-care treatments do not improve the acne in 6 weeks, take your daughter to her pediatrician." See the box "Patient Education for Acne."
Implement	
8. When recommending self-care with nonprescription medications and/or nondrug therapy, convey accurate information to the patient or caregiver.	
a. Appropriate dose and frequency of administration	See the box "Patient Education for Acne."
b. Maximum number of days the therapy should be employed	See the box "Patient Education for Acne."
c. Product administration procedures	See the box "Patient Education for Acne."
d. Expected time to onset of relief	See the box "Patient Education for Acne."

CASE 38-1 *continued*

Relevant Evaluation Criteria	Scenario/Model Outcome
e. Degree of relief that can be reasonably expected	"Acne varies and may be self-limiting. It may take up to 6 weeks to see improvement with the nondrug therapy."
f. Most common side effects	See the box "Patient Education for Acne."
g. Adverse effects that warrant medical intervention should they occur	None
h. Patient options in the event that condition worsens or persists	"If the acne worsens, take your daughter to her pediatrician."
i. Product storage requirements	See the box "Patient Education for Acne."
j. Specific nondrug measures	See the box "Patient Education for Acne."
Solicit follow-up questions from the patient or caregiver.	"Can I just use benzoyl peroxide on her bumps?"
Answer the patient's or caregiver's questions.	"Recommendations and guidelines on the care of acne in pre-adolescents do state that benzoyl peroxide is safe for use in this age group. However, the product guidelines are recommended for ages 12 years and older. You should see your daughter's pediatrician to obtain guidance on product selection in this age group and a plan for appropriate follow-up."
Follow-up: Monitor and Evaluate	
9. Assess patient outcome.	Contact the parent in 3 weeks to see whether she has noticed any improvement in her daughter's acne symptoms. Ask her to call her daughter's pediatrician in 6 weeks if the symptoms have not improved.

Key: BP = Benzoyl peroxide; HCP = health care provider; n/a = not applicable; NKDA = no known drug allergies; OTC = over-the-counter.

CASE 38-2

Relevant Evaluation Criteria	Scenario/Model Outcome
Collect	
1. Gather essential information about the patient's symptoms and medical history, including	
a. Description of symptom(s) (i.e., nature, onset, duration, severity, associated symptoms)	Patient has come into the pharmacy for advice on options for acne. She occasionally gets a few pimples on her forehead and cheeks. The acne is not too bad, but she believes she gets acne because her skin is very oily.
b. Description of any factors that seem to precipitate, exacerbate, and/or relieve the patient's symptom(s)	She started seeing more pimples on her face within the last 2 months.
c. Description of the patient's efforts to relieve the symptoms	She has not tried anything yet. She wanted some recommendations first, because she does not want to spend a lot of money trying a lot of different products.
d. Patient's identity	Lela Watkins
e. Patient's age, gender, height, and weight	17 years old, female, 5 ft 8 in., 170 lb
f. Patient's occupation	High school student
g. Patient's dietary habits	Normal vegetarian diet
h. Patient's sleep habits	Sleeps well. Her bedtime is 10:00 PM.
i. Concurrent medical conditions, prescription and nonprescription medications, and dietary supplements	None
j. Allergies	None

CASE 38–2 *continued*

Relevant Evaluation Criteria	Scenario/Model Outcome
Assess	
2. Differentiate patient's signs/symptoms, and correctly identify the patient's primary problem(s).	Patient's acne symptoms are normal for her age. Acne may also be exacerbated by oily skin.
3. Identify exclusions for self-treatment (Figure 38–3).	Moderate–severe acne
4. Formulate a comprehensive list of therapeutic alternatives for the primary problem to determine whether triage to a medical provider is required, and share this information with the patient or caregiver.	Options include (1) Refer Lela to an appropriate HCP. (2) Recommend self-care with an OTC product and nondrug measures. (3) Recommend self-care until patient can see an appropriate HCP. (4) Take no action.
Plan	
5. Select an optimal therapeutic alternative to address the patient's problem, taking into account patient preferences.	Recommend self-care with an OTC product and nondrug measures.
6. Describe the recommended therapeutic approach to the patient or caregiver.	"I would recommend BP and nondrug measures, because you have mild acne." See the box "Patient Education for Acne."
7. Explain to the patient or caregiver the rationale for selecting the recommended therapeutic approach from the considered therapeutic alternatives.	"BP is a safe and effective nonprescription product for mild acne. It is also important to incorporate nondrug self-care treatments."
Implement	
8. When recommending self-care with nonprescription medications and/or nondrug therapy, convey accurate information to the patient or caregiver.	See the box "Patient Education for Acne."
Solicit follow-up questions from the patient or caregiver.	"Is there anything else that I can do about my oily skin? Sometimes I look shiny by midday."
Answer the patient's or caregiver's questions.	"Everyone produces sebum at different rates. You could use towelettes or a skin toner occasionally to remove excess oil from the skin. This will also decrease the shine that you mentioned throughout the day. You should not wash your face too often though. Sometimes excessive cleaning of your face can make your acne worse."
Follow-up: Monitor and Evaluate	
9. Assess patient outcome.	Contact the patient in 6 weeks to see if her acne hast improved or gotten worse.

Key: HCP = Health care provider; n/a = not applicable; OTC = over-the-counter.

PATIENT EDUCATION FOR Acne

The goal of self-treatment is to control mild acne, thereby preventing more serious forms from developing. Symptoms can usually be managed with diligent and long-term treatment. The best approaches to controlling acne are using cleansers and medications to keep the pores open and avoiding situations that worsen acne. For most patients, carefully following product instructions and the self-care measures listed here will help ensure optimal therapeutic outcomes.

Disease Information

- Acne is the result of several factors that occur within the pilosebaceous unit located in the dermis, or middle layer of the skin.
- Acne can be controlled by using certain medications, but it cannot be cured.

Nondrug and Preventive Measures

- Cleanse skin thoroughly but gently twice daily to produce a mild drying effect that loosens comedones. Use a mild, oil-free cleanser and warm water.
- To prevent or minimize acne flare-ups, consider using a skin toner to remove excess dirt and oil. Also avoid or reduce exposure

PATIENT EDUCATION FOR Acne *(continued)*

to environmental factors such as dirt, dust, petroleum products, cooking oils, or chemical irritants.

- To prevent friction or irritation that may cause acne flare-ups, do not wear tight-fitting clothes, headbands, or helmets; avoid resting the chin on the hand.
- To minimize acne related to cosmetic use, use noncomedogenic, oil-free makeup
- To prevent excessive hydration of the skin, which can cause flare-ups, avoid areas of high humidity. In addition, do not wear tight-fitting clothes that restrict air movement.
- Avoid stressful situations when possible and practice stress-management techniques. Stress can worsen existing acne.
- Do not pick or squeeze pimples, which can further irritate skin and possibly lead to infection, worsening of acne, and scarring.
- Note that sexual activity plays no role in the occurrence or worsening of acne, although the onset of sexual activity and occurrence of acne may take place within the same time span.

Nonprescription Medications

- Most commonly available nonprescription products contain adapalene, benzoyl peroxide, salicylic acid, or sulfur, and these products come in a variety of formulations (e.g., cleansers, creams, gels, astringents).
- Benzoyl peroxide is the most effective and widely used non-prescription medication for treating acne.

Adapalene

- Adapalene is believed to normalize the development of skin cells, resulting in decreased acne symptoms.
- Do not use adapalene if you have very sensitive skin or are sensitive to benzoyl peroxide.
- When using this product, avoid unnecessary sun exposure, and use a broad-spectrum sunscreen with an SPF of 15 or higher.
- To avoid possible excessive irritation, avoid contact of adapalene with eyes, lips, mouth, and nose, as well as cuts, scrapes, and other abrasions.
- Note that use of other acne medications with adapalene may cause excessive dryness and peeling. Such combination therapy should be directed by a health care provider.
- Redness, itching, dryness, scaling, and burning are common adverse effects that tend to diminish after the first month of treatment.
- Acne symptoms may worsen temporarily after beginning treatment with adapalene.
- It will take 8–12 weeks of treatment with adapalene before acne symptoms noticeably improve. Adapalene appears to work by modulating epithelial cell differentiation, keratinization, and inflammation.
- Avoid unnecessary sun exposure and use a broad-spectrum sunscreen with an SPF of 15 or higher, because adapalene increases susceptibility to sunburn.
- The redness, scaling, dryness, itching, and burning that commonly occur with use of adapalene often diminish after the first month of therapy.
- If symptoms worsen or fail to improve in 3 months with proper use of the agent, consult your primary care provider.
- The full therapeutic effect of adapalene usually becomes apparent after 8–12 weeks of treatment.
- If you experience allergic reactions, become pregnant, or are planning to become pregnant, discontinue use of adapalene and consult your primary care provider for other treatment options.

Benzoyl Peroxide

- Benzoyl peroxide inhibits the growth of *Propionibacterium acnes,* the bacteria involved in acne development; it also helps unclog pores by causing a mild peeling effect.
- Do not use benzoyl peroxide if you have very sensitive skin or are sensitive to it.
- When using this product, avoid unnecessary sun exposure and use a broad-spectrum sunscreen with an SPF of 15 or higher.
- To prevent possible excessive irritation, avoid contact of benzoyl peroxide with eyes, lips, mouth, and nose, as well as cuts, scrapes, and other abrasions. Avoid contact of benzoyl peroxide with hair and dyed fabrics, which may be bleached by this product.
- Skin irritation, characterized by redness, burning, itching, peeling, or possibly swelling, may occur with the recommended treatment regimen. Irritation may be reduced by using the product less frequently or in a lower concentration.
- Note that use of other acne medications with this product may cause excessive dryness and peeling. Do this only as directed by a health care provider.
- After the initial 1–2 weeks of treatment, applications can be increased up to 2–3 times per day over a period of 2–3 days, as tolerated.
- Slight improvement may be noticed in as little as a few days, but maximum effectiveness may take up to 3–6 weeks of continued use.
- If treatment is tolerated, but the problem persists, the strength may be increased to 5% after 1 week and to 10% after 2 weeks, if necessary.
- Continue the treatment regimen even after lesions have cleared to prevent the formation of new ones.

Salicylic Acid

- Salicylic acid helps unclog pores by causing slight peeling.
- This medication is less effective than benzoyl peroxide.
- Salicylic acid can be used 1–3 times daily as a cleanser or as a topical gel.
- Gel formulations should be applied to only the affected area.
- If excessive peeling occurs, limit use to once daily or every other day.
- Salicylic acid may cause sun sensitivity, so use a broad-spectrum sunscreen with an SPF of 15 or higher (see the previous section "Benzoyl Peroxide").
- Maximum effectiveness and duration of use are similar to those of benzoyl peroxide.
- Lack of response after 6 weeks is an indication of need for medical referral.

Sulfur

- Sulfur is believed to work by inhibiting the growth of *P. acnes*.
- This medication can be applied 1–3 times daily, but its use is limited by its chalky yellow color and characteristic unpleasant odor.
- Use of sulfur is mostly adjunctive; it is not as effective as benzoyl peroxide.
- Patients who are allergic to sulfa drugs should not use sulfur-containing acne products.

When to Seek Medical Attention

- If severe skin irritation or sensitivity develops, stop use of benzoyl peroxide and sunscreen, and see a health care provider.
- If improvement has not occurred after 6 weeks of treatment with benzoyl peroxide, seek medical evaluation.
- If you experience tightness in the throat; breathing problems; feeling faint; or swelling of the eyes, face, tongue, or lips with use of an acne product, seek emergency medical attention.

TABLE 38-8 Selected websites for Acne Information

Organization	Website
Acne.com	www.acne.com
Acne.org	www.acne.org
U.S. Food and Drug Administration	www.fda.gov

for effective self-treatment. The HCP should determine whether patients whose acne shows no improvement after 6 weeks of self-treatment or 6 months with diet change are following the recommended regimen. If they have been adherent, medical referral is appropriate. Patients who have not diligently followed the regimen should be encouraged to do so. The provider should again explain the expected results and the rigor with which treatment must be pursued. If some improvement is evident, the provider may suggest monthly follow-up to check for improvement in the condition and potential adjustment of the maintenance regimen.

Key Points for Acne

- Acne cannot be cured, but it may be controlled enough to improve cosmetic appearance and prevent development of severe acne with resultant scarring.
- Adherence to any regimen to treat acne is a crucial factor in achieving a successful outcome.
- Minimizing environmental and physical factors that exacerbate acne can help limit the extent of the condition.
- Pharmacologic and nonpharmacologic therapies should be tailored to the patient.
- Medical referral should be considered for grading acne lesions and diagnosing the severity of acne.
- Some people have chronic acne into adulthood and must care for their skin for a long time before improvement will occur.
- If given proper counseling, including empathy and reassurance, patients with acne may understand that the condition may not exist forever.

REFERENCES

1. Basra M, Shahrukh M. Burden of skin diseases. *Expert Rev Pharmacoecon Outcome Res.* 2009;9(3):271–83. doi: 10.1586/erp.09.23.
2. Hay RJ, Johns NE, Williams HC, et al. The global burden of skin disease in 2010: an analysis of the prevalence and impact of skin conditions. *J Invest Dermatol.* 2014;134(6):1527–34. doi: 10.1038/jid.2013.446.
3. Tan JK, Bhate K. A global perspective on the epidemiology of acne. *Br J Dermatol.* 2015;172(Suppl 1):3–12. doi: 10.1111/bjd.13462.
4. Cordain L, Lindeberg S, Hurtado M, et al. Acne vulgaris: a disease of Western civilization. *Ach Dermatol.* 2002;138(12):1584–90. doi:10.1001/archderm.138.12.1584.
5. Archer CB, Cohen SN, Baron SE, et al. Guidance on the diagnosis and clinical management of acne. *Clin Exp Dermatol.* 2012;37(1):1–6. doi: 10.1111/j.1365-2230.2012.04335.x.
6. Eichenfield LF, Krakowski AC, Piggott C et al. Evidence-based recommendations for the diagnosis and treatment of pediatric acne. *Pediatrics.* 2013;131(3):S163–86. doi: 10.1542/peds.2013-0490B.
7. Keri J, Shiman M. An update on the management of acne vulgaris. *Clin Cosmet Investig Dermatol.* 2009;2:105–10.
8. Acne treatment manufacturing OTC in the US industry market research report from IBISWorld has been updated [news release]. Insurancenews net.com; August 3, 2014. Available at: http://insurancenewsnet.com/article/acne-treatment-manufacturing-OTC-in-the-US-industry-market-research-report-from-a-539286. Accessed June 9, 2017.
9. Consumer Healthcare Products Association OTC sales by category. Available at: https://www.chpa.org/OTCsCategory.aspx. Accessed June 9, 2017.
10. Tuchayi SM, Makrantonaki E, Ganceviciene R, et al. Acne vulgaris. *Nat Rev Dis Primers.* 2015;1:15029. doi: 10.1038/nrdp.2015.29.
11. Makrantonaki E, Ganceviciene R, Zouboulis C. An update on the role of the sebaceous gland in the pathogenesis of acne. *Dermatoendocrinol.* 2011;3(1):41–9. doi: 10.4161/derm.3.1.13900.
12. Thiboutot D, Gollnick H, Bettoli V, et al. New insights into the management of acne: an update from the Global Alliance to Improve Outcomes in Acne group. *J Am Acad Dermatol.* 2009;60(5):S1–50. doi: 10.1016/j.jaad.2009.01.019.
13. Ebede TL, Arch EL, Berson D. Hormonal treatment of acne in women. *J Clin Aesthet Dermatol.* 2009;2(12):16–22. PMID:20725580.
14. Spencer EH, Ferdowsian HR, Barnard ND. Diet and acne: a review of evidence. *Int J Dermatol.* 2009;48(4):339-47. doi: 10.1111/j.1365-4632.2009.04002.x.
15. Lolis MS, Bowe WP, Shalita AR. Acne and systemic disease. *Med Clin North Am.* 2009;93(6):1161–81. doi: 10.1016/j.mcna.2009.08.008.
16. Melnik B. Dietary intervention in acne. *Dermatoendocrinol.* 2012;4(1):20–32. doi: 10.4161/derm.19828.
17. Zaenglein AL, Pathy AL, Schlosser BJ, et al. Guidance of care for the management of acne vulgaris. *J Am Acad Dermatol.* 2016;74(5):945–73.e33. doi: 10.1016/j.jaad.2015.12.037.
18. Das S, Reynolds RV. Recent advances in acne pathogenesis: implications for therapy. *Am J Clin Dermatol.* 2014;15(6):479–88. doi: 10.1007/s40257-014-0099-z.
19. Kircik LH. Advantages in the understanding of the pathogenesis of inflammatory acne. *J Drugs Dermatol.* 2016;15(1 Suppl):S7–10. PMID:26741393.
20. Suh DH, Kwon HH. What's new in the pathophysiology of acne? *Br Journal Dermatol.* 2015;172:13–9. PMID: 25645151.
21. Fox L, Csongradi C, Auscamp M, et al. Treatment modalities for acne. *Molecules.* 2016;21(8). pii: E1063. doi: 10.3390/molecules21081063.
22. Barnard E, Liu J, Yankova E, et al. Strains of the *Propionibacterium acnes* type III lineage are associated with the skin condition progressive macular hypomelanosis. *Sci Rep.* 2016;6:31968. doi: 10.1038/srep31968.
23. Gibbon SF, Tomida S, Chiu BH, et al. *Propionibacterium acnes* strain population in the human skin microbiome associated with acne. *J Invest Dermatol.* 2013;133(9):2152–60. doi: 10.1038/jid.2013.21.
24. Hari A, Flach TL, Shi Y, et al. Toll-like receptors: role in dermatological disease. *Mediators Inflamm.* 2010;2010:437246. doi: 10.1155/2010/437246.
25. Clark C. Acne treatment. *Clin Pharm.* 2009;1:168–9. Available at: http://www.pharmaceutical-journal.com/files/rps-pjonline/pdf/cp200904_168.pdf. Accessed June 9, 2017.
26. Knutsen-Larson S, Dawson AL, Dunnick CA, et al. Acne vulgaris: pathogenesis, treatment, and needs assessment. *Dermatol Clin.* 2012;30(1):99–106, viii-ix. doi: 10.1016/j.det.2011.09.001.
27. Feldman S. Careccia RE, Barham KL. Diagnosis and treatment of acne. *Am Fam Physician.* 2004;69(9):2123–30. PMID:15152959.
28. Do TT, Zarkhin S, Orringer JS, et al. Computer assisted alignment and tracking of acne lesions indicate that most inflammatory lesions arise from comedones and de novo. *J Am Acad Dermatol.* 2008;58(4):603–8. doi: 10.1016/j.jaad.2007.12.024.
29. Dreno B, Layton A, Zouboulis CC, et al. Adult female acne: a new paradigm. J *Eur Acad Dermatol Venereol.* 2013;27(9):1063–70. doi: 10.111/jdv.12061.
30. Kraft J, Freiman A. Management of acne. *CMAJ.* 2011;183(7):E430–5. doi: 1.1503/cmaj.090374.
31. Titus S, Hodge J. Diagnosis and treatment of acne. *Am Fam Physician.* 2012;86(8):734–40. PMID:23062156.

32. Rivera AE. Acne scarring: a review and current treatment modalities. *J Am Acad Dermatol.* 2008;59(4):659–76. doi: 10.1016/j.jaad.2008.05.029.
33. Gollnick HP. From new findings in acne pathogenesis, to new approaches in treatment. *J Eur Acad Dermatol Venereol.* 2015;29(Suppl 5):1–7. doi: 10.1111/jdv.13186.
34. Decker A, Graber EM. Over-the-counter acne treatments. *J Clin Aesthetic Dermatol.* 2012;5(5):32–40. PMCID: PMC3366450.
35. Kurokawa L, Danby FW, Ju Q, et al. New developments in our understanding of acne pathogenesis and treatment. *Exp Dermatol.* 2009;18(10): 821–32. doi: 10.1111/j.1600-0625.2009.00890.x.
36. Rathi SK. Acne vulgaris treatment: the current scenario. *Indian J Dermatol.* 2011;56(1):7–13. doi:10.4103/0019-5154.77543.
37. Strauss JS, Krowchuk DP, Leyden JJ, et al. Guidelines of care for acne vulgaris management. *J Am Acad Dermatol.* 2007;56(4):651–63. doi: 10.1016/j.jaad.2006.08.048.
38. FDA approves Differin Gel 0.1% for over-the-counter use to treat acne [news release]. July 8, 2016. Available at: http://www.fda.gov/newsevents/newsroom/pressannouncements/ucm510362.htm. Accessed June 21, 2017.
39. Adapalene. Updated March 2, 2017. Available at: https://www.drugs.com/pro/adapalene.html. Accessed June 21, 2017.
40. U.S. Food and Drug Administration. Classification of benzoyl peroxide as safe and effective and revision of labeling to drug facts format; topical acne drug products for over-the-counter human use; final rule. *Fed Regist.* 2010;75(42):9767–77.
41. U.S. Food and Drug Administration. FDA Drug Safety Communication: FDA warns of rare but serious hypersensitivity reactions with certain over-the-counter topical acne products. June 25, 2014. Updated January 15, 2016. Available at: https://www.fda.gov/Drugs/DrugSafety/ucm400923.htm. Accessed June 9, 2017.
42. Bowe WP, Shalita AR. Effective over-the-counter acne treatments. *Semin Cutan Med Surg.* 2008;27(3):170–6. doi: 10.1016/j.sder.2008.07.004.
43. Federman DG, Kirsner RS. Acne vulgaris: pathogenesis and therapeutic approach. *Am J Manag Care.* 2000;6(1):78–87. PMID: 11009749.
44. Whitney KM, Ditre CM. Management strategies for acne vulgaris. *Clin Cosmet Investig Dermatol.* 2011;4:41–53. doi: 10.2147/CCID.S10817.
45. Cao H, Wang Y, Liu JP, et al. Complementary therapies for acne vulgaris. *Cochrane Database Syst Rev.* 2015;1:CD009436. doi: 10.1002/14651858.CD009436.pub2.
46. Ebanks JP, Wickett RR, Boissy RE. Mechanisms regulating skin pigmentation: the rise and fall of complexion coloration. *Int J Mol Sci.* 2009; 10(9):4066–87. doi: 10.3390//ijms10094066.

CHAPTER 39

PREVENTION OF SUN-INDUCED SKIN DISORDERS

KIMBERLY M. CROSBY AND KATHERINE S. O'NEAL

Exposure to ultraviolet radiation (UVR) is cumulative and can produce serious, long-term problems. The most common skin problem caused by excessive UVR exposure is sunburn. However, other conditions that are either directly caused or exacerbated by exposure to UVR include a group of photoaggravated skin disorders: premature aging, skin cancers, cataracts, and photodermatoses (Table 39–1).[1–3]

In addition to the idiopathic photodermatoses, UVR can precipitate or exacerbate many photoaggravated dermatologic conditions, including herpes simplex labialis (cold sores), systemic lupus erythematosus (SLE), and associated skin lesions. The common factor in the development of a photodermatosis is the onset or exacerbation of signs and symptoms after exposure to UVR.[1–3]

The most serious skin disorder caused by UVR is skin cancer. Cumulative exposure from childhood to adulthood, even without serious sunburn, may predispose a person to develop precancerous and cancerous skin conditions. Epidemiologic studies conducted since the 1950s demonstrate a strong relationship between chronic, excessive, and unprotected sun exposure and human skin cancer. Nonmelanoma skin cancers are the most common type of cancer malignancy in the United States. According to the American Cancer Society, 3.5 million basal and squamous cell carcinomas (nonmelanoma skin cancers [NMSCs]) are diagnosed in the United States annually. An estimated 73,000 cases of malignant melanoma were diagnosed in 2015.[4–6]

Avoiding excessive exposure to UVR through the use of sunscreens and other sun protection measures will reduce the incidence of the sun-induced skin disorders: sunburn, premature aging of the skin, photodermatoses, skin cancer, and other long-term dermatologic effects. Education about the safe and effective use of sunscreen and suntan products is a public health need. To perform this function, health care providers should be aware of the hazards of UVR and the criteria for selecting and properly using sunscreen products. Providers are encouraged to become involved in educational efforts to help minimize the morbidity and mortality associated with UVR exposure.[4,5]

Pathophysiology of Sun-Induced Skin Disorders

Ultraviolet Radiation

The UV spectrum is divided into 3 major bands: ultraviolet C (UVC), ultraviolet B (UVB), and ultraviolet A (UVA), all of which can cause or exacerbate sun-induced skin disorders.

UVA radiation (wavelength between 320 and 400 nm) is involved in suppressing the immune system and damaging DNA, which result in premature photoaging and skin cancers.[5–7] In addition, UVA can produce photosensitivity reactions in patients who have ingested or applied photosensitizing agents.[2,3]

UVB (wavelength between 290 and 320 nm) is the most active UVR wavelength for producing erythema, which is why it is called *sunburn radiation.* The intensity of UVB radiation reaching the Earth is the highest from 10:00 AM to 4:00 PM. UVB is considered the primary inducer of skin cancer, however, its carcinogenic effects are believed to be augmented by UVA. UVB is also primarily responsible for photoaging changes. The only true therapeutic effect of UVB exposure is synthesis of vitamin D_3 in the skin.[5–8] However, with the wide availability of vitamin D–rich foods and the availability of vitamin D supplements, the need for UVB exposure to increase vitamin D production is not necessary. In fact, the American Academy of Dermatology position statement on vitamin D states that UVR exposure should not be used as a source of vitamin D because of the risks associated with sun exposure.[8–10]

Most UVC radiation (wavelength between 200 and 290 nm) is screened out by the ozone layer of the upper atmosphere and little of it reaches Earth. However, UVC is emitted by some artificial sources of UVR. Most of the UVC that strikes the skin is absorbed by the dead cell layer of the stratum corneum.[11–13]

Many factors contribute to the amount of UVR exposure received. Cloud cover filters very little UVR. Seventy-ninety percent of UVR will penetrate through cloud cover. However, clouds tend to filter out the infrared radiation that contributes to the sensation of heat, creating a false sense of security against a burn. White or light-colored surfaces (e.g., snow, sand) reflect the UVR that strikes them. Also, the irradiance of UVB increases by 4% for every 1000-foot increase in altitude. These factors all contribute to the overall radiation received, and severe sunburn may result even if the individual is sitting in the shade or if there is cloud cover.[11–15] Water reflects no more than 5% of UVR, allowing the remaining 95% to penetrate and burn the swimmer. Therefore, time in the water, even if the swimmer is completely submerged, should be considered part of the total time spent in the sun. Dry clothes reflect almost all UVR. If light passes through dry clothing when held up to the sun, however, UVR will also penetrate the clothing. Tightly woven material offers the greatest protection. Wet clothes allow transmission of approximately 50% of UVR.[13,15]

Although UVB does not penetrate window glass, UVA does. Most automobile windshields are made from laminated glass that filters most of the UVA. However, side windows are not made from laminated glass; therefore, a significant amount of UVA may pass

TABLE 39–1 Common Photodermatoses

Idiopathic Disorders
Actinic prurigo
Chronic actinic dermatitis
Hydroa vacciniforme
Polymorphous light eruption
Solar urticaria
Photoaggravated Dermatoses
Atopic dermatitis
Chronic actinic dermatitis
Cutaneous T-cell lymphoma
Dermatomyositis
Disseminated superficial actinic porokeratosis
Drug-induced photosensitivity
Erythema multiforme
Herpes simplex labialis
Lichen planus actinicus
Pellagra
Pemphigus
Porphyrias
Psoriasis
Reticular erythematous mucinosis
Rosacea
Systemic lupus erythematosus
Transient acantholytic dermatosis

Source: References 1–3.

through to riders in the vehicle. Therefore, patients sensitive to UVA (e.g., those with photodermatoses, those taking photosensitizing drugs) should use appropriate sunscreens even when driving with the windows closed.[16]

The Environmental Protection Agency has developed a UV index that uses a scale to rate the amount of skin-damaging UVR that reaches the earth's surface at any instance in time (Table 39–2). As the rating increases, the risk of exposure increases. When a UV index is given in the United States, it typically is given for noon; however, the UV index changes throughout the day. Factors that influence the UV index are time of day (UVR exposure is greater at midday than in the early morning or late afternoon); ozone (limited amounts of ozone increase the amount of UVR exposure); altitude; season (UVR exposure is greater in spring and summer); surface reflectivity; latitude (UVR exposure is increased in areas closer to the equator); and land cover (less tree cover increases UVR exposure).[17]

TABLE 39–2 Global Solar UV Index

Rating Number	Interpretation of UVR Exposure Risk
1–2	Low
3–5	Moderate
6–7	High
8–10	Very high
11+	Extreme

Key: UV = Ultraviolet; UVR = ultraviolet radiation.
Source: Reference 17.

Sunburn and Suntan

Sunburn and suntan present as reactions to UVR exposure. The degree to which a person will develop a sunburn or a tan depends on several factors, including type and amount of radiation received, thickness of the epidermis and stratum corneum, skin pigmentation, skin hydration, and distribution and concentration of peripheral blood vessels. Most UVR that strikes the skin is absorbed by the epidermis.

A sunburn is an acute reaction to excessive UVR exposure, resulting in inflammation of the exposed skin. Both UVA and UVB exposure can result in sunburn. The cellular mechanism for this response is complex, involving skin cells and numerous inflammatory mediators. Erythema, swelling, and pain occur usually 3–5 hours after the UVR exposure, reaching a maximum response at 12–24 hours. A sunburn usually resolves in 72 hours. However, the sunburn may occur sooner and last longer if the time of exposure to UVR is greater.[12,18]

A suntan is produced when UVR stimulates the melanocytes in the skin layers to generate and redistribute melanin in the skin. Tanning can be described as immediate or delayed. Delayed tanning serves as a protective mechanism for the skin to diffuse and absorb additional UVR. However, tanning does not protect an individual from developing skin cancer, photodermatoses, premature photoaging, or other UVR-related negative health risks. Tanning also does not protect against future sunburns. UVA and UVB both contribute to the development of a suntan. *Immediate tanning*, which is caused by a redistribution of melanosomes, begins to be visible rapidly after exposure and may last for 3–4 days after UVR exposure. The pigment darkening may not be visible on lighter skin types. *Delayed tanning* occurs as a result of the increase in number and activity of melanocytes after UVR exposure. Delayed tanning of the skin becomes visible 3–4 days after exposure to UVR and will last from 10 to 30 days depending on skin type and amount of UVR exposure.[12,18]

Photodermatoses

The exact pathologic mechanism for the development of photodermatoses is unknown. UVB most often is responsible for these reactions; however, UVA and some visible light may also cause photodermatoses.

Photosensitivity encompasses two types of conditions: photoallergy and phototoxicity. *Drug photoallergy* involves an increased, chemically induced reactivity of the skin to UVR and/or visible light. UVR (primarily UVA) triggers an antigenic reaction in the skin. This reaction, which is not dose related, is usually seen after at least one prior exposure to the involved chemical agent or drug.

Similar to photoallergy, *phototoxicity* is an increased, chemically induced reactivity of the skin to UVR and/or visible light. However, phototoxicity is not immunologic. It is often seen on first exposure to a chemical agent or drug, is dose related, and usually exhibits no drug cross-sensitivity. Some drugs associated with phototoxicity are listed in Table 39–3. This type of reaction is not limited to drugs: it is also associated with plants, cosmetics, and soaps.[1-3]

Skin Cancer

The majority of NMSCs occur on the most exposed areas of the body (face, head, neck, backs of the hands). The two most common types of NMSC are basal cell carcinoma (BCC) and squamous cell carcinoma (SCC). BCC is often an aggressive, invasive disorder of the epidermis and dermis that can cause serious damage to the skin and underlying tissue. However, it rarely metastasizes. SCC is found in epithelial keratinocytes and grows very slowly.

The pathophysiology of melanoma differs from that of the NMSCs. Although most melanomas come from normal skin, about 30% arise from existing nevi (moles). Some of the risk factors for skin cancer include a family or personal history of melanoma; sun sensitivity (e.g., difficulty tanning, burning easily); large numbers of atypical nevi; a previous history of SCC or BCC; tanning bed use; and a history of excessive sun exposure and sunburns. Regardless of risk factors, skin cancer may develop in all individuals with increased exposure to UVR.[5] A growing amount of evidence supports the supposition that sun exposure plays a role in the development of all types of skin cancers.[6,19–21]

TABLE 39-3 Selected Medications (by Drug Category) Associated With Photosensitivity Reactions

Anticancer Drugs
- Dacarbazine
- Daunorubicin
- Fluorouracil
- Methotrexate
- Vinblastine

Anticonvulsants
- Carbamazepine
- Gabapentin
- Lamotrigine
- Phenytoin

Antidepressants
- Bupropion
- Selective serotonin reuptake inhibitors
- Trazodone
- Venlafaxine

Antihistamines
- Cetirizine
- Diphenhydramine

Antihypertensives
- Angiotensin-converting enzyme inhibitors
- Calcium channel blockers
- Hydralazine
- Labetalol
- Methyldopa
- Minoxidil
- Sotalol

Anti-infectives
- Azithromycin
- Ceftazidime
- Dapsone
- Gentamicin
- Griseofulvin
- Itraconazole
- Ketoconazole
- Metronidazole
- Pyrazinamide
- Quinolones
- Ritonavir
- Saquinavir
- Sulfonamides
- Tetracyclines
- Trimethoprim
- Trovafloxacin
- Zalcitabine

Antimalarials
- Chloroquine
- Quinine

Antipsychotics/Phenothiazines
- Haloperidol
- Olanzapine
- Ziprasidone

Coal Tar and Derivatives
- DHS Tar Gel Shampoo
- Ionil T Plus Shampoo
- Neutrogena T/Derm Body Oil
- Neutrogena T/Gel Extra Strength

Diuretics
- Acetazolamide
- Amiloride
- Furosemide
- Metolazone
- Triamterene
- Thiazide diuretics

Nonsteroidal Anti-inflammatory Drugs
- Celecoxib
- Ibuprofen
- Indomethacin
- Methoxsalen
- Naproxen

Sunscreens
- Aminobenzoic acid
- Aminobenzoic acid derivatives
- Benzophenones
- Cinnamates
- Homosalate
- Menthyl anthranilate
- Oxybenzone

Miscellaneous
- Amiodarone (antiarrhythmic)
- Benzoyl peroxide
- Gold salts (antiarthritic)
- Isotretinoin (antiacne)
- Quinidine sulfate (antiarrhythmic)
- Retinoids
- Statins

Source: References 1–3 and Stein KR, Scheinfeld NS. Drug-induced photoallergic and phototoxic reactions. *Expert Opin Drug Saf.* 2007;6(4):431–43.

Clinical Presentation of Sun-Induced Skin Disorders

Sunburn

Sunburn is usually seen as a superficial burn with a reaction that ranges from mild erythema to tenderness, pain, and edema (see Color Plates, photograph 29). Severe reactions to excessive UVR exposure can sometimes produce burns that range in severity from superficial partial thickness to full thickness with the development of *vesicles* (blisters) or *bullae* (many large blisters), as well as fever, chills, weakness, and shock. Shock caused by heat prostration or hyperpyrexia can lead to death.[12] (See Chapter 41 for treatment of sunburn.)

Drug Photosensitivity

Drug photoallergy presents similar to allergic contact dermatitis (e.g., poison ivy) and is characterized by pruritus with erythematous papules, vesicles, bullae, and/or urticaria (see Color Plates, photograph 30). *Phototoxicity* is most likely to appear as exaggerated sunburn with pruritis,[1–3] but urticaria may also occur (see Color Plates, photograph 31).

Photodermatoses

Each photodermatosis has a unique morphology. *Polymorphous light eruption* alone can have multiple morphologic presentations of pruritus with papules, vesicles, plaques, and/or urticaria.[1–3]

Premature Aging

Premature aging is characterized by wrinkling and yellowing of the skin. Conclusive evidence reveals that prolonged exposure to UVR results in *elastosis* (degeneration of the skin caused by a breakdown of the skin's elastic fibers). Pronounced drying, thickening, and wrinkling of the skin may also result. Other physical changes include cracking, *telangiectasia* (spider vessels), *solar keratoses* (growths), and *ecchymoses* (subcutaneous hemorrhagic lesions).[2,5,14] (See Chapter 40 for measures to reverse photoaging.)

Skin Cancer

BCC is a translucent nodule with a smooth surface. It is usually firm to the touch and may be ulcerated or crusted. It is generally found as an isolated lesion on the nose or other parts of the face, although multiple lesions are sometimes found. Conversely, *SCC*, is a slow-growing, isolated papule or plaque on sun-exposed areas of the body.

Self-examination for melanoma uses four factors (A-B-C-D-E) for evaluation: Asymmetric shape; Border irregularity or poorly defined border; Color variation within the same mole or a change in color; Diameter larger than 6 mm; and Evolving or changing mole. A mole with these characteristics and any new growth or change in appearance of the skin (including the lips) should be evaluated by a dermatologist.[22,23]

Prevention of Sun-Induced Skin Disorders

The short-term goals in preventing sun-induced skin disorders are relatively simple: avoid or minimize sunburn, photosensitivity reactions, and photodermatoses induced or exacerbated by UVR. The expected long-term outcomes are prevention of skin cancer and avoidance of premature aging of the skin.

UVR-induced skin disorders can be prevented by minimizing exposure to UVR and by using sunscreen agents. The sunscreen product selected and the degree of protection will vary, depending on the patient's intended use for the product and the conditions under which the product will be used (Figure 39–1).

The greater the risk a patient has of developing a UVR-induced skin disorder, the greater the need to avoid sun exposure. However, most people neither spend warm, sunny afternoons sitting inside, nor do they go to the beach or pool wearing lots of clothing. Providers can assist the patient in striking a balance between completely avoiding sun exposure, wearing protective clothing, and using sunscreen

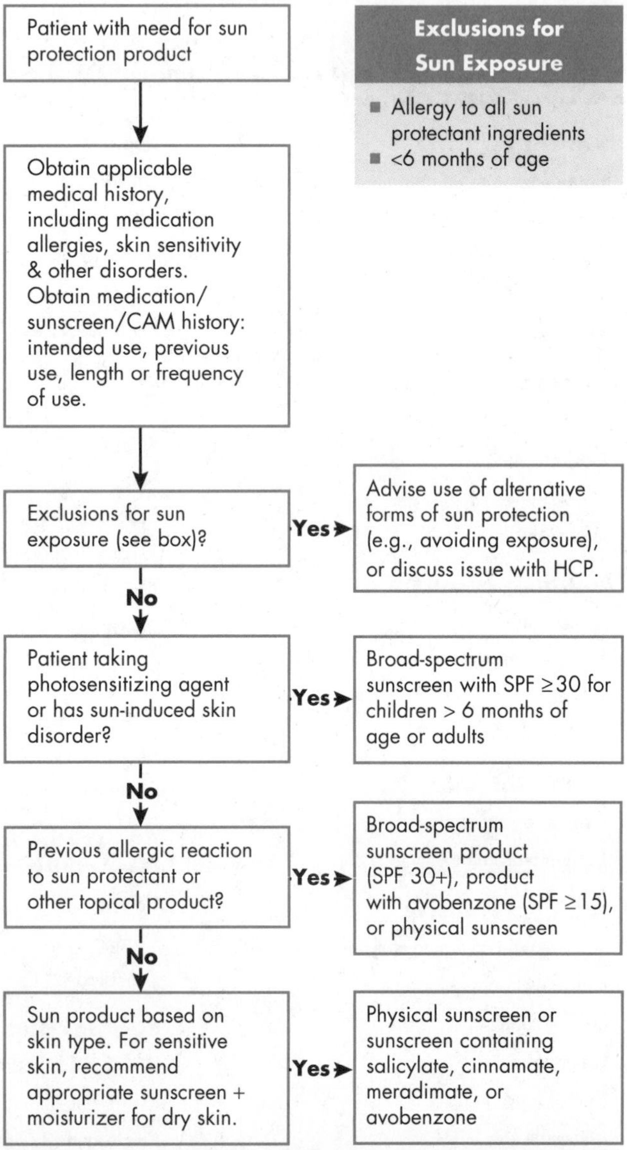

FIGURE 39–1 Self-care for sun protection. Key: CAM = Complementary and alternative medicine; HCP = health care provider; SPF = sun protection factor. Source: References 2, 3, 19–21, and 38.

products. If, however, the patient suffers from a UVR-induced skin disorder (e.g., SLE), few options are available other than complete avoidance. With regard to preventing sunburn, the patient's natural skin type will be the primary factor in determining the sun protection factor (SPF) of the sunscreen product to be used. The lighter the natural skin color a patient has and the more *quickly* the patient develops a burn, the higher the SPF required for the sunscreen product to prevent sunburn. However, all skin colors, including darker skin, can suffer UVR damage, so patients of all skin types should be advised about protection from UVR.

Avoidance of Sun Exposure

Although unrealistic, complete avoidance of UVR is often the best approach for patients who have the physical characteristics or history listed in Table 39–4. People who refuse to stay indoors or who must be outdoors for extended periods should wear protective clothing. (e.g., a hat with a 4-inch brim, long pants, a long-sleeved shirt or special sun protective clothing embedded with agents that absorb UVR). Many clothing items now list an *ultraviolet protection factor* (UPF) rating on their label, which identifies how much UVR is filtered out with wearing of the clothing. Clothing items that are darker in color, have a tighter weave, or contain UVR-absorbing agent tend to block out more UVR. In situations in which the patient is unwilling or unable to avoid the sun or to wear protective clothing, the next best choice is to use a sunscreen product.[24]

Measures of UVR Protection

SPF

Purchasers of sunscreens are usually familiar with SPF, which is one parameter for determining a sunscreen's effectiveness for UV protection. Another parameter, minimal erythema dose (MED), is used to calculate a sunscreen's SPF. The *MED* is defined as the "minimum UVR dose that produces clearly marginated erythema in the irradiated site, given as a single exposure."[24] It is a dose of radiation, not a grade of erythema. Generally, 2 MEDs will produce a bright erythema; 4 MEDs, a painful sunburn; and 8 MEDs, a blistering burn. However, because of variations in thickness of the stratum corneum, different parts of the body may respond differently to the same MED. Furthermore, the MED for individuals with heavily pigmented skin is estimated to be 33 times higher than that for individuals with lightly pigmented skin.

The important measure for sunscreens is the SPF, which is derived by dividing the MED on protected skin by the MED on unprotected skin. For example, if a person requires 25 mJ/cm^2 of UVB radiation to experience 1 MED on unprotected skin and requires 250 mJ/cm^2 of radiation to produce 1 MED after applying a given sunscreen, the product would be given an SPF rating of 10. The higher the SPF, the more effective the agent is in preventing sunburn. If 60 minutes of sun exposure is usually required for someone to experience 2 MEDs (a bright erythematous sunburn), a sunscreen with an SPF of 6 will allow that person to stay in the sun 6 times longer (or 6 hours) before receiving the same degree of sunburn (assuming the sunscreen is reapplied in sufficient amounts at the recommended intervals). The SPF is product specific, because it is calculated on the basis of the final formulation of the product and cannot be determined on the basis of the active ingredient alone.[17,20,21] A product with an SPF of 15 blocks 93% of UVB. Raising the SPF to 30 increases UVB protection to only 96.7%, and an SPF of 40 blocks 97.5%.[19] A hypothetical SPF of 70 would increase UVB protection to only 98.6%.[24,25]

With concern growing about the long-term adverse effects of UVA, the utility of the SPF value in measuring photoprotection from UVA has been questioned. The Food and Drug Administration (FDA) has concluded that the SPF test in combination with a new broad-spectrum in vitro test can effectively assess both UVA and UVB radiation protection. Products that pass the new test will offer higher protection against both UVA and UVB, and they will be labeled as broad-spectrum sunscreens.[26]

On June 17, 2011, FDA announced new requirements for nonprescription sunscreens. These changes are outlined in four regulatory documents: a final rule, a proposed rule, an advanced notice of proposed rulemaking, and a draft guidance for industry.[27–29] These regulations became effective in June 2012.

The final rule mandates that all sunscreens labeled as "broad spectrum" must pass FDA's new, standardized broad-spectrum procedure that measures a product's UVA protection relative to its UVB protection. This procedure is in addition to the SPF test mandated previously. Only broad-spectrum sunscreens with an SPF value of 15 or higher will be able to claim to reduce the risk of skin cancer and early skin aging if they are used as directed along with other skin protection measures. Broad-spectrum sunscreens with an SPF value between 2 and 14 and products that protect against only UVB (not broad spectrum) can claim only to help prevent sunburn. Products that are not broad spectrum must carry a label warning: "Skin Cancer/Skin Aging Alert: Spending time in the sun increases your risk of skin cancer and early skin aging. This product has been shown only to help prevent sunburn, not skin cancer or early skin aging."[26]

A sunscreen's efficacy is also related to its *substantivity*—that is, its ability to remain effective during prolonged exercising, sweating, and swimming. This property can be a function of the active sunscreen, the vehicle, or both. Generally speaking, products with cream-based (water-in-oil) vehicles appear more resistant to removal by water than those with alcohol bases. The final rule prohibits "waterproof," "sweatproof," and "sunblock" claims, because these terms overstate product effectiveness. Further, water-resistance claims on the front label must indicate whether the sunscreen remains effective for either 40 or 80 minutes during swimming or sweating. These times are based on the standard testing procedure. Products that are not water resistant must instruct users to wear a water-resistant product while swimming

TABLE 39–4 Patient Risk Factors for the Development of UVR-Induced Problems

- Fair skin that always burns and never tans
- A history of one or more serious or blistering sunburns
- Blonde or red hair
- Blue, green, or gray eyes
- A history of freckling
- A previous growth on the skin or lips caused by UV exposure
- The existence of a UV-induced disorder
- A family history of melanoma
- Current use of an immunosuppressive drug
- Current use of a photosensitizing drug
- Excessive lifetime exposure to UVR, including tanning beds and booths
- History of an autoimmune disease

Key: UV = Ultraviolet; UVR = ultraviolet radiation.
Source: References 6, 15, 22, and 23.

or sweating. Finally, all sunscreen products must include standard "Drug Facts" labeling on the back or side of the container.[26]

The final rule limited the maximum SPF value on sunscreen levels to "50+." This rule is based on the lack of sufficient evidence that products with SPF values higher than 50 provide more protection than products with SPF values of 50.[27,30]

The application dosage forms eligible for review and inclusion in the final monograph (FM) are oils, lotions, creams, gels, butters, pastes, ointments, sticks, and sprays. Other application dosage forms (e.g., towelettes and wipes) are not included in the FM.[28,29,31]

The draft guidance for industry is an enforcement guide for manufacturers of sunscreens. It provides information to help manufacturers understand how to label and test their products in light of the new final rule, proposed rule, and advance notice of proposed rulemaking.[29]

Types of Sunscreens

According to the therapeutic definitions, topical sunscreens can be divided into two major subgroups: chemical sunscreens and physical sunscreens. *Chemical sunscreens* absorb and thus block the transmission of UVR to the epidermis. An active ingredient absorbs at least 85% of the radiation in the UV range at wavelengths from 290 to 320 nm, but the agent may or may not allow transmission of radiation to the skin at wavelengths longer than 320 nm. *Physical sunscreens* are generally opaque; instead of absorbing UVR, they reflect and scatter it. An opaque sunscreen active ingredient reflects or scatters all light in the UV and visible ranges at wavelengths from 290 to 777 nm. The sunscreen thereby minimizes suntan and sunburn.

The FM for sunscreens includes 15 chemical agents and 2 physical agents as safe and effective for use as sunscreens. Table 39–5 lists these agents, their UVR absorbance range, and their maximum concentrations. Because the SPF is product specific and does not depend on the sunscreen's active agent alone, the FM has eliminated a required minimum strength for sunscreens that contain a single active ingredient.[31–33]

TABLE 39–5 Sunscreens Considered Safe and Effective

Sunscreen Agent	UV Spectrum Activity	Approved Maximum Concentration (%)
ABA and Derivatives		
Aminobenzoic acid (PABA)	UVB	15
Padimate O	UVB	8
Anthranilates		
Meradimate	UVA II	5
Benzophenones		
Dioxybenzone	UVB, UVA II	3
Oxybenzone	UVB, UVA II	6
Sulisobenzone	UVB, UVA II	10
Cinnamates		
Cinoxate	UVB	3
Octocrylene	UVB, UVA II	10
Octinoxate	UVB	7.5
Dibenzoylmethane Derivatives		
Avobenzone[b]	UVA I	3
Salicylates		
Homosalate	UVB	15
Octisalate	UVB	5
Trolamine salicylate	UVB	12
Miscellaneous		
Ensulizole	UVB	4
Ecamsule (terephthalylidene dicamphor sulfonic acid)	UVB, UBA	2
Titanium dioxide[c]	290–770	25
Zinc oxide[c]	290–770	24

Key: ABA = Aminobenzoic acid; UV = ultraviolet; UVA = ultraviolet A; UVB = ultraviolet B.

[a] Values are achieved when used in combination with other sunscreen agents.

[b] Agent is currently marketed through a new drug application.

[c] Agent scatters (rather than absorbs) radiation in the 290–770 nm range.

Source: References 11, 20, 24, 25, 27, and 33–35.

Chemical Sunscreens

Aminobenzoic Acid and Derivatives

Aminobenzoic acid (formerly para-aminobenzoic acid [PABA]), once was the most widely used sunscreen agent; however, it has been replaced by other agents because it is a major sensitizer. Because of the continuing confusion about the name of this common sunscreen agent, the FM requires that product labels list it as "aminobenzoic acid"; in addition, each time this name appears on product labeling, it must be followed by "(PABA)" so patients know which chemical entity they are using.

Aminobenzoic acid is an effective UVB sunscreen, especially when formulated in a hydroalcoholic base (maximum of 50%–60% alcohol). The SPF of such formulations increases proportionally as the concentration of aminobenzoic acid increases from 2% to 5%. One advantage of this agent is its ability to penetrate into the horny layer of the skin and provide lasting protection. Its substantivity on sweating skin is significant but is reduced on skin that is immersed in water. The only derivative of aminobenzoic acid approved for use in sunscreens is padimate O.

The disadvantages of alcoholic solutions of aminobenzoic acid include contact dermatitis, photosensitivity, stinging and drying of the skin, and yellow staining of clothes on exposure to the sun. Products containing padimate O will not cause staining of the clothing, which may offer an advantage over aminobenzoic acid–containing products. Patients who have experienced a photosensitivity reaction to a sunscreen product containing aminobenzoic acid or any of its derivatives should avoid using these products.[11,20,24,25,33]

Anthranilates

The anthranilates are ortho-aminobenzoic acid derivatives. Meradimate, the menthyl ester of anthranilic acid, is a weak UV sunscreen with maximal absorbance in the UVA range. It is usually found in combination with other sunscreen agents to provide broader UV coverage.[11,24,20,25,33]

Benzophenones

The benzophenone group comprises three agents: dioxybenzone, oxybenzone (benzophenone-3), and sulisobenzone (benzophenone-4). As a group, these agents are primarily UVB absorbers, with maximum absorbance between 282 and 290 nm. However, their absorbance extends well into the UVA range (up to 350 nm with oxybenzone, and up to 380 nm with dioxybenzone). Many sunscreen formulations now contain benzophenones, because these agents have a broad spectrum of action and are less likely to cause allergic reactions than some of the other sunscreen classes. Oxybenzone, also found in some cosmetic formulations, is a significant sensitizing agent among sunscreens. As the use of these agents has increased, reports of sensitivity to the benzophenones have also increased.[11,20,24,25,33]

Cinnamates

Cinnamates include cinoxate, octinoxate, and octocrylene. As shown in Table 39–5, cinoxate and octinoxate have similar absorbance ranges and maximum absorbances. Octocrylene, however, has an absorbance range of 250–360 nm, well into the UVA range. Octocrylene is currently found in more commercial sunscreen preparations than it was in the past, possibly reflecting its broader spectrum of absorbance. It is also an effective photostabilizer. *Photostablizers* are compounds often used with sunscreens to prevent the sunscreen agent from losing effectiveness upon exposure to sunlight.[31] Octocrylene can decrease the rate at which other sunscreens degrade upon sun exposure. It often is combined with other sunscreens to improve their stability.

Unfortunately, cinnamates do not adhere well to the skin and must rely on the vehicle in a given formulation for their substantivity.[11,20,24,25,32–34]

Dibenzoylmethane Derivatives

Avobenzone (butyl methoxydibenzoylmethane, originally known as Parsol 1789) is the first of a new class of sunscreen agents effective throughout the entire UVA range (320–400 nm; full spectrum). It has maximum absorbance at approximately 360 nm. Although avobenzone absorbs UVR throughout the UVA spectrum, its absorption capacity falls off sharply at 370 nm. Therefore, reactions from photosensitive drugs and chemicals that are highly reactive in the 370–400 nm range still could occur. Compared with the other chemical sunscreens on the market, avobenzone, offers the best protection in the UVA range. It is commonly included in sunscreen products to increase UVA coverage. Avobenzone is easily degraded by exposure to sunlight; it is found in newer sunscreen products combined with octocrylene, salicylates, 4-methylbenzylidene camphor, and micronized zinc oxide and/or titanium dioxide to enhance stability of the product and to extend the product's spectrum of coverage through the UVA and UVB spectrum.[11,20,24,25,33]

Salicylates

Salicylic acid derivatives are weak sunscreens and must be used in high concentrations. They do not adhere well to the skin and are easily removed by perspiration or swimming.[11,20,33,34]

Other Chemical Sunscreens

Ensulizole does not fit into any of the preceding classes. It is a pure UVB sunscreen with an absorbance range of 290–320 nm. Ecamsule (terephthalylidene dicamphor sulfonic acid) is a new molecule that FDA approved in 2006. It is a water-resistant broad-spectrum sunscreen. Ecamsule is often combined with octocrylene to increase its stability to light.[11,20,34]

Physical Sunscreens

Physical sunscreens (zinc oxide and titanium dioxide) are considered broad-spectrum UV protectants. They are used most often on small and prominently exposed areas by patients who cannot limit or control their exposure to the sun (e.g., lifeguards). Earlier formulations of these agents were opaque and had an undesirable sticky or gritty sensation. Current formulations contain micro- or nano-sized particles of the agent. These formulations are transparent, which improves their cosmetic appeal. Because titanium dioxide increases the effective SPF of a product and extends the spectrum of protection well into the UVA range, the number of commercial products containing this agent has increased. The FM allows zinc oxide to be used alone or in combination with any of the other sunscreen agents except avobenzone; this exception results from a lack of data on effectiveness.[11,20,24,25,33]

Combination Products

FDA has not recommended limits on the number of sunscreen agents that may be used together. However, each sunscreen agent must contribute to the efficacy of a product and must not be included merely for marketing promotion purposes. Therefore, the FM requires that each active ingredient contribute a minimum SPF of not less than 2; in addition, the finished product must have a minimum SPF of not less than the number of sunscreen active ingredients used in the combination multiplied by 2.[25]

Dosage and Administration Guidelines

The two major causes of poor sun protection with sunscreen use are application of inadequate amounts and infrequent reapplication. Although many sunscreen products that prevent burning of the lips (or nose) are available, the lips often are neglected. Products for the lips differ in ingredients and in the UVA and UVB spectrum, but they carry most of the same labeling used on sunscreen lotions (including the SPF). The SPF of these products is usually at least 15. Studies have shown that lip protection not only helps prevent drying and burning of the lips, but that it also helps prevent the development of cold sores or fever blisters caused by the herpes simplex virus in patients who are susceptible to recurrent outbreaks.

For maximum effectiveness, sunscreens must be applied liberally to all exposed areas of the body and reapplied at least as often as the label recommends. FDA-approved labeling recommends that sunscreens be applied 15–30 minutes before UV exposure and at least every 2 hours thereafter. Reapplication after every episode of swimming, towel drying, or excessive sweating is also recommended.[35]

The FDA standard for application of sunscreens is 2 mg/cm^2 of body surface area. This standard means that, for sufficient protection, the average adult in a bathing suit should apply 9 portions of sunscreen of approximately ½ teaspoon each, or approximately 4 and ½ teaspoons (22.5 mL) total. The sunscreen should be distributed as follows:

- Face and neck: ½ teaspoon.
- Arms and shoulders: ½ teaspoon to each side of body.
- Torso: ½ teaspoon each to front and back.
- Legs and tops of feet: 1 teaspoon to each side of body.

Because of the cost of sunscreen products and the need to apply them often and in sufficient amounts, users may apply substantially less sunscreen than is necessary to provide adequate protection. Exposure to UVR should be within the limits of the SPF value of the sunscreen for the individual using the sunscreen. A higher SPF may be needed for longer or more intense exposure to UVR. The final rule requires that the sunscreen label recommend the following with regard to sunscreen application: Regardless of the water resistance of the product, it should be applied 15 minutes before sun exposure. Non–water-resistant products should be reapplied at least every 2 hours. Water-resistant products should be reapplied every 2 hours, after 40 or 80 minutes of swimming or sweating (as designated on the label), and immediately after towel drying.[26]

Safety Considerations

The development of a rash, vesicles, hives, or exaggerated sunburn after use of the sunscreen product is most likely a sign of either a photosensitivity or allergic reaction.[1–3] Product labels must state the following: "Stop use if skin rash occurs."[25] The patient should be referred for medical evaluation of the situation. The degree of the reaction will determine what type of medical intervention (if any) is necessary.

If a patient has experienced a prior reaction to a sunscreen product, the product's name and ingredients should be identified, if possible. This action may be difficult, because product formulations change frequently. Photosensitivity and contact dermatitis have been reported with aminobenzoic acid and its derivatives, benzophenones, cinnamates, homosalate, avobenzone, and meradimate. Although no evidence exists of significant effects from eye contact, FDA requires the label warning "Keep out of eyes."[27,36,37]

The FM also addresses a gray area that has allowed the proliferation of cosmetics claiming to offer sun protection. It stipulates that sunscreen products will be classified as drugs rather than cosmetics, because users expect that sunscreens will protect them from some of the sun's damaging effects. However, cosmetics that contain sunscreen agents will be classified as cosmetics as long as no therapeutic claims are made and the sunscreen is intended for a nontherapeutic, nonphysiologic purpose. If the cosmetic makes a claim for use as a sunscreen product, it will have to include the appropriate labeling. Under the directions for use, the optional statement "for sunscreen use" may be added.[22,23,25,26]

Product Selection Guidelines

Two primary factors will determine the best product for a given patient: the intended use of the product and specific patient characteristics. The decision of which sunscreen product to use must be based on the information obtained from both categories.

Intended Use

Some patients may want to use sunscreens to prevent sunburn or the photoaging effects of UVR or to protect themselves from skin cancer. Others may need protection from sun exposure, because they are taking photosensitive drugs or they suffer from a photodermatosis.

The higher the SPF of the sunscreen product, the greater the protection it provides against sunburn and tanning. Studies have shown that sunscreens can protect against the long-term hazards of skin cancer.[11,20,24] Considerable research is currently being conducted on all aspects of UVR and its effects. However, experts are debating whether low-SPF products protect individuals from UV skin damage or allow them to receive dangerously high levels of UVR over extended periods of time. Because of the known hazards associated with UVR, FDA and other organizations such as the American Academy of Dermatology recommend the use of sunscreen products of at least SPF 15. Generally, if a product is to be used to prevent skin cancer, reduce the chances of a photosensitivity reaction, or reduce the risk of triggering a skin disorder induced or aggravated by UVR, a broad-spectrum SPF value of 15 or higher is recommended.

Patient Factors

For patients not concerned with photosensitivity or photodermatoses, product selection is much simpler. The following factors can serve as a guide in selecting products with the appropriate properties for a patient's particular situation.

The most important factors in product selection are the individual's natural skin type and tanning history. An SPF product of 30+ should be used by people who burn easily and tan minimally at best. If the individual plans to swim, participate in vigorous activity (e.g., sand volleyball), or work outdoors, the sunscreen product must be able to adhere to the skin more substantially than if the individual just lies on the beach. The expected duration of the physical activity can also help to determine which sunscreen to use. Water-resistant products are usually effective for at least 40 or 80 minutes when used during the preceding activities.[26]

At least one-third of the current commercial products are labeled "noncomedogenic," "fragrance-free," and "hypoallergenic." Noncomedogenic products do not plug the pores and, therefore, do not exacerbate acne. This property is especially important for teenagers, who usually spend more time outdoors than other age groups and generally would prefer not to use comedogenic sunscreens. Many patients are sensitive to various ingredients (e.g., fragrances, emulsifiers, preservatives). These patients should try to choose fragrance-free formulations or those that are hypoallergenic. The prevalence of a true allergy to sunscreen products has been reported as low as 1% in North Americans. However, adverse reactions to sunscreens are more common. Patients may develop phototoxic or photoallergic reactions to any sunscreen or other inactive ingredient in the product. Although it may not be possible to figure out which specific ingredient a patient is sensitive to, patients who have a history of sensitivity to sunscreens would do well to use a fragrance-free, hypoallergenic product and to try to avoid using a product containing a sunscreen with which they have had a previous reaction.[36,37]

Some patients have normally dry skin; sunbathing can further exacerbate this problem. These patients should avoid ethyl and isopropyl alcohols, which are included in a number of commercial sunscreen products and can further dry the skin.

Use in Special Populations

Absorptive characteristics of human skin in children younger than 6 months differ from those of adult skin. The metabolic and excretory systems of infants are not fully developed to handle any sunscreen agent absorbed through the skin. Therefore, only patients older than 6 months are considered to have skin with adult characteristics. FDA requires that sunscreen products be labeled with the statement "children under 6 months of age: ask a doctor." Caregivers should be extremely wary regarding sun exposure in children, especially infants. Although the evidence is not yet conclusive, researchers and providers agree that use of an SPF-15 product starting after 6 months of age and continuing throughout an individual's lifetime can reduce the incidence of long-term skin damage related to UVR. A product with an SPF of 30+ may result in even higher reductions in sunburn, premature skin aging, skin cancer, and other skin problems. No special consideration is needed for other special populations such as pregnant or lactating women or geriatric patients.[26–31,38]

Assessment of Sun-Induced Skin Disorders

The approach to UVR-induced skin disorders differs from that used in most self-care situations. These disorders are addressed from a preventive, rather than a treatment, standpoint.

Consequently, assessment of the patient should focus on *the individual patient characteristics and intended use* of the product. Clinical providers' interventions with patients occur in two primary situations. The first situation occurs when a patient requests a recommendation for a sunscreen product to prevent a burn and/or to allow development of a tan. The second situation is initiated by the provider when a patient is placed on a drug that can produce a photosensitivity reaction. In this second scenario, no real patient assessment is needed, because prevention of exposure to UVR is the standard approach. Cases 39–1 and 39–2 are examples of assessment of patients with sun-induced skin disorders.

Patient Counseling for Sun-Induced Skin Disorders

Health care providers can provide a great service by counseling patients about the suntanning process and about properly selecting and using sunscreens.

One simple way to find out whether a patient is using a sunscreen properly is to ask how long the product currently being

CASE 39-1

Relevant Evaluation Criteria	Scenario/Model Outcome
Collect	
1. Gather essential information about the patient's symptoms and medical history, including	
a. Description of symptom(s) (i.e., nature, onset, duration, severity, associated symptoms)	The patient would like help choosing a sunscreen to use while on spring break in Mexico. She has a history of getting sunburned and would like to avoid this.
b. Description of any factors that seem to precipitate, exacerbate, and/or relieve the patient's symptom(s)	Staying completely out of the sun has been the only thing she has found that keeps her from getting burned, but she doesn't want to have to spend this vacation indoors. She likes to spend a lot of time in the water so she would like a sunscreen that protects her in the water.
c. Description of the patient's efforts to relieve the symptoms	She has tried using sunscreens in the past before she went out in the sun. She usually did not reapply her sunscreen.
d. Patient's identity	Katie Grant
e. Patient's age, gender, height, and weight	21 years old, female, 5 ft 2 in., 115 lb
f. Patient's occupation	College student
g. Patient's dietary habits	n/a
h. Patient's sleep habits	n/a
i. Concurrent medical conditions, prescription and nonprescription medications, and dietary supplements	Contraception: norgestimate and ethinyl estradiol (Sprintec) 1 tablet by mouth daily
j. Allergies	None
k. History of other adverse reactions to medications	Katie reacted to sunscreen products in the past. She developed a rash when using the sunscreen. She is not sure which product it was.
l. Other (describe) ______	n/a

CASE 39-1 *continued*

Relevant Evaluation Criteria	Scenario/Model Outcome
Assess	
2. Differentiate patient's signs/symptoms, and correctly identify the patient's primary problem(s).	The patient desires a sunscreen product that will allow her to spend time in the sun while on vacation.
3. Identify exclusions for sun exposure (Figure 39–1).	None
4. Formulate a comprehensive list of therapeutic alternatives for the primary problem to determine whether triage to a health care provider is required, and share this information with the patient or caregiver.	Options include (1) Use an OTC sunscreen product regularly while in the sun. (2) Avoid sun exposure by staying in the shade or indoors. (3) Take no action.
Plan	
5. Select an optimal therapeutic alternative to address the patient's problem, taking into account patient preferences.	Regularly using a sunscreen product while outdoors will allow the patient to enjoy the outdoor activities she would like to do on vacation. Because the patient has a history of rash when using sunscreen, it will be important to consider this during product selection and avoid agents that are more likely to cause skin reactions (e.g., agents that have caused previous reactions or agents commonly causing reactions, such as PABA, padimate O, benzophenones).
6. Describe the recommended therapeutic approach to the patient or caregiver.	"Use a sunscreen product of SPF 15 or greater that provides both UVA and UVB coverage. A product that is water resistant will be a better choice if you plan to be in the water during the day. Because you have a history of a reaction to sunscreens in the past, I would recommend a sunscreen containing ecamsule, with octocrylene and zinc or titanium dioxide. Apply the product liberally to all sun-exposed areas of the body."
7. Explain to the patient or caregiver the rationale for selecting the recommended therapeutic approach from the considered therapeutic alternatives.	"Correct use of a sunscreen product will allow you to enjoy time outdoors without getting a sunburn. With past burns, you may not have applied an appropriate amount of sunscreen or the right type: a broad-spectrum sunscreen that provides both UVA and UVB coverage. Additionally, using a sunscreen like ecamsule, which is water resistant, will be preferred because you like to spend time in the water. Finally, choosing products that do not commonly cause skin reactions will be important since you have a history of a skin reaction in the past."
Implement	
8. When recommending self-care with nonprescription medications and/or nondrug therapy, convey accurate information to the patient or caregiver.	"Apply the sunscreen product every day 15 or 30 minutes prior to going out into the sun. Reapply the sunscreen at least every 2 hours and every 40 or 80 minutes as directed on the product label if sweating or in the water. You will need to apply the sunscreen as follows: ■ Face and neck: ½ teaspoon. ■ Arms and shoulders: ½ teaspoon to each side of body. ■ Torso: ½ teaspoon each to front and back. ■ Legs and tops of feet: 1 teaspoon to each side of body."
Solicit follow-up questions from the patient or caregiver.	"What should I do if I have a reaction to sunscreen again?"
Answer the patient's or caregiver's questions.	"If you develop a rash or other skin reaction to the sunscreen, stop using it and see your provider."
Follow-up: Monitor and Evaluate	
9. Assess patient outcome.	n/a

Key: n/a = Not applicable; PABA = aminobenzoic acid; OTC = over-the-counter; SPF = sun protection factor; UVA = ultraviolet A; UVB = ultraviolet B.

CASE 39-2

Relevant Evaluation Criteria	Scenario/Model Outcome
Collect	
1. Gather essential information about the patient's symptoms and medical history, including	
a. Description of symptom(s) (i.e., nature, onset, duration, severity, associated symptoms)	The patient has a history of acne, and she has noticed that her skin becomes much more sensitive after she spends any time in the sun. She would like something to help limit this sun sensitivity. She has noticed that the skin on her face has become red and she is having some skin peeling.
b. Description of any factors that seem to precipitate, exacerbate, and/or relieve the patient's symptom(s)	Sun exacerbates the adverse effects from her acne medication.
c. Description of the patient's efforts to relieve the symptoms	She used sunscreen prior to being in the sun, but she failed to reapply it throughout the day.
d. Patient's identity	Alex Jones
e. Patient's age, gender, height, and weight	22 years old, female, 5 ft 10 in., 145 lb
f. Patient's occupation	College student
g. Patient's dietary habits	She eats at home for most meals and tries to eat a healthy diet. Occasionally (1–2 meals per week), she eats out or picks up fast food.
h. Patient's sleep habits	She gets between 7 and 8 hours of sleep a night.
i. Concurrent medical conditions, prescription and nonprescription medications, and dietary supplements	Acne: topical tretinoin applied at bedtime to face.
j. Allergies	Penicillins
k. History of other adverse reactions to medications	None
Assess	
2. Differentiate patient's signs/symptoms, and correctly identify the patient's primary problem(s).	Patient with history of acne. Adverse effects to topical tretinoin are exacerbated by sun exposure.
3. Identify exclusions for sun exposure (Figure 39–1).	None
4. Formulate a comprehensive list of therapeutic alternatives for the primary problem to determine whether triage to a health care provider is required, and share this information with the patient or caregiver.	Options include (1) Avoidance of additional sun exposure until her symptoms improve. (2) Use of a sunscreen product in future sun exposures. (3) Referral to her dermatologist to treat current adverse effects and consider changing acne medication.
Plan	
5. Select an optimal therapeutic alternative to address the patient's problem, taking into account patient preferences.	The patient is experiencing significant adverse effects from her tretinoin, which have been worsened by sun exposure. Recommend that Alex follow up with her dermatologist to treat current symptoms and discuss options for treatment of acne, which she may tolerate better.
6. Describe the recommended therapeutic approach to the patient or caregiver.	"You should see your dermatologist for treatment of your skin sensitivity reaction. In the future, apply a sunscreen at least 15 minutes prior to sun exposure, and reapply it every 2 hours during sun exposure for non–water-resistant products. Also, you should consider wearing a long-sleeved shirt and a hat with a 4-inch brim prior to sun exposure, and you should avoid sunburns."
7. Explain to the patient or caregiver the rationale for selecting the recommended therapeutic approach from the considered therapeutic alternatives.	"The adverse effects of skin sensitivity, burning, redness, and peeling skin to tretinoin are worsened by exposure to the sun."

CASE 39-2 *continued*

Relevant Evaluation Criteria	Scenario/Model Outcome
Implement	
8. When recommending self-care with nonprescription medications and/or nondrug therapy, convey accurate information to the patient or caregiver.	Criterion does not apply in this case.
Solicit follow-up questions from the patient or caregiver.	"Is there any sunscreen that only needs to be used once a day?"
Answer the patient's or caregiver's questions.	"No, all sunscreens, even water-resistant ones, must be reapplied."
Follow-up: Monitor and Evaluate	
9. Assess patient outcome.	n/a

Key: n/a = Not applicable.

used has lasted. When applied properly, according to the suggested dosing guidelines and in accordance with the appropriate substantivity of the product, a sunbather could easily use about 1 ounce every 80–90 minutes. This use would amount to several ounces a day and several product containers per week. Incredibly, many frequent sunbathers use only one container in an entire season. This diminished usage demonstrates the importance of individuals' receiving adequate counseling to get the protection they desire. The box "Patient Education for Protection from Sun Exposure" lists specific information to provide patients.

Patients should also be advised to wear sunglasses to protect their eyes from sun-induced damage. The box "A Word about Sun-Induced Ocular Damage" describes the categories of available sunglasses and their UVR filtration properties.[39]

PATIENT EDUCATION FOR Protection From Sun Exposure

The objectives of self-treatment depend on a patient's specific goal or health status. Protection from sun exposure can prevent sunburn or tanning, photosensitivity reactions in susceptible persons, or exacerbation of sun-induced photodermatoses. The primary long-term benefits are to prevent skin cancer and premature aging of the skin. For most patients, carefully following product instructions and the self-care measures listed here will help ensure optimal therapeutic outcomes.

Avoiding/Minimizing Sun Exposure

- Avoid exposure to the sun and other sources of ultraviolet radiation (UVR), such as tanning beds/booths and sunlamps.
- The sun's rays are the most direct and damaging between 10:00 AM and 4:00 PM. Avoid sun exposure as much as possible during this time of day.
- Sunburn can occur on a cloudy or overcast day; 70%–90% of UVR penetrates clouds.
- Wear protective clothing (e.g., long pants, a long-sleeved shirt, and a hat with a brim). Tightly woven fabrics that do not allow light to pass through will provide the most protection.
- Use a beach umbrella or other protection to reduce UVR.
- Water and wet clothing allow significant transmission of UVR. Even if the body is completely submerged, consider time in the water as part of the total time spent in the sun.

Use of Sunscreens

- An SPF of 15 or greater provides the greatest protection against sunburn and other UVB-induced skin problems.
- A broad-spectrum sunscreen product (e.g., avobenzone used in combination with padimate O and/or octocrylene, meradimate, titanium dioxide, or one of the benzophenones) provides optimal protection against UVA and UVB sun exposure. This type of sunscreen is especially recommended if you have a sun-induced disorder, if you are taking photosensitizing drugs, or if you just want to reduce sun exposure as much as possible to prevent long-term effects.
- Apply first dose 15 minutes before exposure.
- Apply approximately 1 ounce of sunscreen over the exposed areas of the body, avoiding contact with the eyes. The sunscreen should be distributed as follows: ½ teaspoon to the face and neck area, ½ teaspoon to the arms and shoulders, ½ teaspoon to the front and back each, and 1 teaspoon to each side on the leg and top of the foot.
- Use the most substantive sunscreen available; water-resistant sunscreens are recommended if you will be in water or perspiring excessively.
- Reapply the sunscreen according to the label instructions, usually every 40 minutes or 80 minutes (as directed on the label) for water-resistant sunscreens while swimming or sweating or after towel drying. Apply every 2 hours for non–water-resistant products or for water-resistant products if you are not swimming or sweating.
- Always check the expiration date on the sunscreen product. Sunscreens can lose their effectiveness.
- Higher altitudes and lower latitudes increase the amount of UVR to which an individual is exposed. Take proper precautions (e.g., use a sunscreen with a high SPF) to protect skin from UVR.
- Snow and sand reflect UVR. Take proper precautions to protect exposed skin (e.g., wear sunglasses and use high-SPF sunscreens).
- Keep sunscreen out of direct sun, which can reduce its potency.
- Continue to use a sunscreen as long you are taking a photosensitizing drug or exhibiting signs and symptoms of photodermatitis.
- Avoid sunscreens containing aminobenzoic acid derivatives, benzophenones, cinnamates, or meradimate if you have had a prior allergic reaction to a sunscreen product.
- Stop using the sunscreen if redness, itching, rash, or exaggerated sunburn occurs.

Key: SPF = Sun protection factor; UVA = ultraviolet A; UVB = ultraviolet B.

A WORD ABOUT
Sun-Induced Ocular Damage

Recent studies have demonstrated a relationship between both UVA and UVB in cataract formation. UVR has been shown to cause temporary injuries such as photokeratitis (a painful type of snow blindness associated with highly reflective surfaces). Another concern involves an increase in the incidence of uveal (iris plus ciliary body) melanoma. These concerns are even more serious because of the erroneous belief that all sunglasses screen out UVR. In response, the Sunglass Association of America, working with FDA, has developed a voluntary labeling program. Abbreviated information concerning sunglasses' UVR-screening properties is directly attached to each pair, and brochures describing the appropriate use of each type of lens are available at outlets selling the sunglasses.[39]

According to its UVR filtration properties, each pair of sunglasses is placed in one of the following three categories:

1. Cosmetic sunglasses block at least 70% UVB and 20% UVA. They are recommended for activities in nonharsh sunlight (e.g., shopping).
2. General-purpose sunglasses block at least 95% UVB and 60% UVA. With shades that range from medium to dark, they are recommended for most activities in sunny environments (e.g., boating, driving, flying, or hiking).
3. Special-purpose sunglasses block at least 99% UVB and 60% UVA. They are recommended for activities in very bright environments (e.g., ski slopes and tropical beaches).[39]

Key: FDA = Food and Drug Administration; UVA = ultraviolet A; UVB = ultraviolet B; UVR = ultraviolet radiation.

Evaluation of Patient Outcomes for Sun-Induced Skin Disorders

The short-term outcomes for sunscreen use are readily apparent. Twenty-four hours after use, there will be no obvious sunburn, photosensitivity reaction, or eruption of photodermatosis. This success indicates that the appropriate sunscreen agents and/or SPF were used. However, the long-term effects of UVR (e.g., skin cancer, premature aging of the skin) may take up to 20–30 years to become evident.

Key Points for Sun-Induced Skin Disorders

- UVR (UVA and UVB) triggers a variety of photodermatoses and causes sunburn, photosensitivity, skin cancer, premature aging of the skin, cataracts, and a variety of other medical problems.
- There is no safe form of UVR exposure. Tanning and use of tanning beds can result in negative health effects.
- The effects of UVR are cumulative over an individual's lifetime.
- The best protection against UVR is avoidance. The next best approach is to wear a hat, long sleeves, pants, and UV-protective sunglasses.
- Maximum protection is provided by using a broad-spectrum sunscreen of SPF 15+.
- Because broad-spectrum sunscreens provide added UVA protection, they are the best sunscreen for preventing long-term effects, regardless of the patient's history.

Providers need to appreciate sunscreen products as therapeutic agents rather than cosmetics. Unfortunately, most patients have the latter view. This perception makes good patient counseling even more important. Reinforcing the need for proper selection of the appropriate sunscreen product and correct use of these products are key to educating the public and reducing the risks of UVR exposure.

REFERENCES

1. O'Gorman SM, Murphy GM. Photoaggravated disorders. *Dermatol Clin.* 2014;32(3):385–98. doi: 10.1016/j.det.2014.03.008.
2. Vandergriff TW, Bergstresser PR. Abnormal responses to ultraviolet radiation: idiopathic, probably immunologic, and photoexacerbated. In: Goldsmith LA, Katz SI, Gilchrest BA, et al., eds. *Fitzpatrick's Dermatology in General Medicine.* 8th ed. New York: McGraw-Hill; 2012:chp 91. Available at: http://www.accessmedicine.com/content.aspx?aID=56051339. Accessed April 2, 2016.
3. Lim HW. Abnormal responses to ultraviolet radiation: photosensitivity induced by exogenous agents. In: Goldsmith LA, Katz SI, Gilchrest BA, et al., eds. *Fitzpatrick's Dermatology in General Medicine.* 8th ed. New York: McGraw-Hill; 2012:chp 92. Available at: http://www.accessmedicine.com/content.aspx?aID=56051779. Accessed April 2, 2016.
4. American Cancer Society. Skin cancer. Atlanta, GA: American Cancer Society; 2016. Available at: http://www.cancer.org/cancer/cancercauses/sunanduvexposure/skin-cancer-facts. Accessed June 22, 2017.
5. Gonzaga ER. Role of UV light in photodamage, skin aging, and skin cancer. *Am J Clin Dermatol.* 2009;10(Suppl 1):19–24. doi: 10.2165/0128071-200910001-00004.
6. Kennedy C, Bajdik CD, Willemze R, et al. The influence of painful sunburns and lifetime sun exposure on the risk of actinic keratosis, seborrheic wards, melanocytic nevi, atypical nevi and skin cancer. *J Invest Dermatol.* 2003;120(6):1087–93. doi: 10.1046/j.1523-1747.2003.12246.x.
7. El Ghissassi F, Baan R, Straif K, et al. A review of human carcinogens—Part D: radiation. *Lancet Oncol.* 2009;10(8):294–304. PMID: 19655431.
8. Reichrath J. Skin cancer prevention and UV-protection: how to avoid vitamin D-deficiency? *Br J Dermatol.* 2009;161(Suppl 3):54–60. doi: 10.1111/j.1365-2133.2009.09450.x.
9. Diehl JW, Chiu MW. Effects of ambient sunlight and photoprotection on vitamin D status. *Dermatol Ther.* 2010;23(1):48–60. doi: 10.1111/j.1529-8019.2009.01290.x.
10. American Academy of Dermatology. Position statement on vitamin D. Amended December 22, 2010. Available at: http://www.aad.org/forms/policies/uploads/ps/ps-vitamin%20d%20postition%20statement.pdf. Accessed June 22, 2017.
11. Palm MD, O'Donoghue MN. Update on photoprotection. *Dermatol Ther.* 2007;20(5):360–76. doi: 10.1111/j.1529-8019.2007.00150.x.
12. Kochevar IE, Taylor CR, Krutmann J. Fundamentals of cutaneous photobiology and photoimmunology. In: Goldsmith LA, Katz SI, Gilchrest BA, et al., eds. *Fitzpatrick's Dermatology in General Medicine.* 8th ed. New York, NY: McGraw-Hill; 2012:ch. 90. Available at: http://accessmedicine.mhmedical.com/content.aspx?bookid=392&Sectionid=41138799. Accessed April 1, 2016.
13. U.S. Environmental Protection Agency. *The Burning Facts.* Washington, DC: U.S. Environmental Protection Agency; September 2006. Publication No. EPA430-F-060-013.
14. Auerbach H. Geographic variation in incidence of skin cancer in the United States. *Public Health Rep.* 1961;76:345–8. PMID: 13685076.
15. American Cancer Society. Skin cancer prevention and early detection. Atlanta, GA: American Cancer Society; July 6, 2010. Available at: http://www.cancer.org/cancer/cancercauses/sunanduvexposure/skincancerpreventionandearlydetection/skin-cancer-prevention-and-early-detection-intro. Accessed June 22, 2017.

16. Tuchinda C, Srivannaboon S, Lim HW. Photoprotection by window glass, automobile glass, and sunglasses. *J Am Acad Dermatol.* 2006;54(5):845–54. doi: 10.1016/j.jaad.2005.11.1082.
17. U.S. Environmental Protection Agency. *A Guide to the UV Index.* Washington, DC: U.S. Environmental Protection Agency; May 2004. Publication No. EPA30-F-04-020. Available at: http://www.epa.gov/sunwise/publications.html. Accessed June 22, 2017.
18. Park H, Yaar M. Biology of melanocytes. In: Goldsmith LA, Katz SI, Gilchrest BA, et al., eds. *Fitzpatrick's Dermatology in General Medicine.* 8e. New York, NY: McGraw-Hill; 2012:Chp 72. Available at: http://accessmedicine.mhmedical.com/content.aspx?bookid=392&Sectionid=41138774. Accessed April 03, 2016.
19. Skotarczak K, Osmola-Man'Kowska A, Lodyga M. Photoprotection: facts and controversies. *Eur Rev Med Pharmacol Sci.* 2015;19(1):98–112. PMID: 25635982.
20. Mancebo SE, Hu JY, Wang SQ. Sunscreens a review of health benefits, regulations and controversies. *Dermatol Clin.* 2014;32(3):427–38. doi: 10.1016/j.det.2014.03.011.
21. Kaur A, Thatai P, Sapra B. Need of UV protection and evaluation of efficacy of sunscreens. *J Cosmet Sci.* 2014;65(5):315–45. PMID: 25682622.
22. Melanoma Research Foundation. The ABCDEs of melanoma. Washington, DC: Melanoma Research Foundation; 2016. Available at: https://www.melanoma.org/understand-melanoma/diagnosing-melanoma/detection-screening/abcdes-melanoma. Accessed June 22, 2017.
23. Wolff K, Johnson R, Saavedra AP. Precancerous lesions and cutaneous carcinomas. In: Wolff K, Johnson R, Saavedra AP, eds. *Fitzpatrick's Color Atlas and Synopsis of Clinical Dermatology.* 7th edition. New York, NY: McGraw-Hill; 2013:sect. 11. Available at : http://accessmedicine.mhmedical.com/content.aspx?bookid=1700&Sectionid=113783499. Accessed April 03, 2016.
24. Kullavanijaya P, Lim HW. Photoprotection. *J Am Acad Dermatol.* 2005; 52(6):937–58. doi: 10.1016/j.jaad.2004.07.063.
25. U.S. Food and Drug Administration. Over-the-counter human drugs; labeling requirements; delay of implementation date. Final rule: delay of implementation date of certain provisions. *Fed Regist.* 2004;69(171): 53801–4. Available at: https://www.gpo.gov/fdsys/pkg/FR-2004-09-03/pdf/04-18842.pdf. Accessed June 22, 2017.
26. U.S. Food and Drug Administration. Labeling and effectiveness testing: sunscreen drug products for over-the-counter human use. Final rule. *Fed Regist.* 2011;76(117):35620–65. Available at: http://www.regulations.gov/#!documentDetail;D=FDA-1978-N-0018-0698. Accessed June June 22, 2017.
27. U.S. Food and Drug Administration. Agency information collection activities; proposals, submissions, and approvals: SPF labeling and testing requirements and drug facts labeling for over-the-counter sunscreen drug products. *Fed Regist.* 2011;76(117):35678–81. Available at: http://www.regulations.gov/#!documentDetail;D=FDA-2011-N-0449-0001. Accessed June 22, 2017.
28. U.S. Food and Drug Administration. Sunscreen drug products for over-the-counter human use; request for data and information regarding dosage forms. *Fed Regist.* 2011;76(117):35669–72. Available at: http://www.regulations.gov/#!documentDetail;D=FDA-1978-N-0018-0697. Accessed June 22, 2017.
29. U.S. Department of Health and Humans Services, Food and Drug Administration, Center for Drug Evaluation and Research (CDER). Guidance for industry: enforcement policy—OTC sunscreen drug products marketed without an approved application: draft guidance. Silver Spring, MD: Office of Communications, Division of Drug Information; June 2011. Available at: http://www.fda.gov/downloads/Drugs/GuidanceComplianceRegulatoryInformation/Guidances/UCM259001.pdf. Accessed June 22, 2017.
30. U.S. Food and Drug Administration. Revised effectiveness determination; sunscreen drug products for over-the-counter human use. *Fed Regist.* 2011; 76(117):35672–8. Available at: http://www.regulations.gov/#!documentDetail;D=FDA-1978-N-0018-0699. Accessed June 22, 2017.
31. U.S. Food and Drug Administration. Sunscreen drug products for over-the-counter human use. Final monograph. *Fed Regist.* 1999;64(98):27666–93. PMID: 10558542.
32. Wang SQ, Balagula Y, Osterwalder U. Photoprotection: a review of the current and future technologies. *Dermatol Ther.* 2010;23(1):31–47. doi: 10.1111/j.1529-8019.2009.01289.x.
33. Tuchinda C, Lim HW, Osterwalder U, et al. Novel emerging sunscreen technologies. *Dermatol Clin.* 2006;24(1):105–17. doi: 10.1016/j.det.2005.09.003.
34. U.S. Food and Drug Administration. Sunscreen drug products for over-the-counter human use. Final monograph; technical amendment. *Fed. Regist.* 2002;67(119):41821–3. Available at: https://www.gpo.gov/fdsys/pkg/FR-2002-06-20/pdf/01-15632.pdf. Accessed June 22, 2017.
35. Burnett ME, Hu JY, Wang SQ. Sunscreens: obtaining adequate photo protection. *Dermatol Ther.* 2012;25(3):244–51. doi: 10.1111/j.1529-8019.2012.01503.x.
36. Herung AR, Raju SI, Warshaw EM. Adverse reactions to sunscreen agents: epidemiology, responsible irritants and allergens, clinical characteristics, and management. *Dermatitis.* 2014;25(6):289–326. doi: 10.1097/DER.0000000000000079.
37. Scheuer E, Warshaw E. Sunscreen allergy: a review of epidemiology, clinical characteristics, and responsible allergens. *Dermatitis.* 2006;17(1):3–11. PMID: 16800271.
38. U.S. Food and Drug Administration. Consumer updates: should you put sunscreen on infants? Not usually. June 25, 2013. Updated July 7, 2016. Available at: http://www.fda.gov/forconsumers/consumerupdates/ucm309136.htm. Accessed June 22, 2017.
39. Sunglass Association of America (SAA). SAA UV labeling program. Norwalk, CT: SAA; 1997.

CHAPTER 40

SKIN HYPERPIGMENTATION AND PHOTOAGING

KATHERINE S. O'NEAL AND KIMBERLY M. CROSBY

Skin hyperpigmentation may result from serious or benign medical conditions. Photoaging of the skin is directly related to exposure to ultraviolet radiation (UVR). This chapter focuses on the nonprescription product treatment of hyperpigmentation and photoaging once they have occurred. Nonprescription products used to minimize sun exposure are discussed in Chapter 39.

SKIN HYPERPIGMENTATION

Hyperpigmentation, manifested as an area of skin darker than the surrounding skin, is usually a benign phenomenon that is challenging to treat. Hyperpigmentation may be perceived by the patient as a disfigurement, especially when the altered pigmentation occurs on the face and neck and is in noticeable contrast to the surrounding normal skin color. Although products used to treat hyperpigmentation serve a cosmetic function, it is important to emphasize that they are drugs with potential toxicity and adverse effects.[1]

Pathophysiology of Skin Hyperpigmentation

Systemic illnesses as well as localized skin diseases may cause pigment cells to become overactive (resulting in skin darkening) or underactive (resulting in skin lightening).[2] Endocrine imbalances caused by Addison disease, Cushing disease, or hyperthyroidism and conditions such as pregnancy are capable of altering skin pigmentation. Metabolic alterations affecting the liver, as well as certain nutritional deficiencies, can be associated with diffuse melanosis. Inflammatory dermatoses (e.g., contact dermatitis from poison ivy or acne lesions) or physical trauma to the skin (e.g., thermal burn) may cause prolonged postinflammatory hyperpigmentation. In addition, certain drugs (Table 40–1) have an affinity for melanin and may cause hyperpigmentation. Skin hyperpigmentation resulting from these conditions may occur as a result of increased melanin and melanocyte production accompanied by increased activity of melanocytes or deposits of other darkening chemicals in the skin.[3–5] *Melanocytes* (pigment cells) produce *melanosomes,* pigment granules that contain the protein melanin, a brown-black pigment. These cells can be viewed as tiny single-celled glands with long projections used to pass pigment particles into the keratinocytes, from which the particles migrate upward to the skin surface. The melanocyte is believed to provide protection from UVR. Dark skin usually has a greater number of melanocytes than light skin, which explains why UVR-induced skin cancers of all types are less common in dark skin than in light skin.[6–8] This may be why individuals with dark hair or darker complexions (Fitzpatrick skin types IV–VI; Table 40–2) and individuals who are Hispanic, African American, African, or Asian have been found to be more susceptible to hyperpigmentation.[9]

The three types of hyperpigmentation that may be self-treated with topical nonprescription agents include ephelides, solar lentigines, and melasma.[10] *Ephelides,* or *freckles,* are spots of uneven skin pigmentation that first appear in childhood, are exacerbated by the sun, and tend to fade with reduced sun exposure. *Solar* or "*senile*" *lentigines* (age spots or liver spots) appear on exposed skin surfaces, particularly in fair-skinned people, and are induced by UVR. *Melasma* (also called *chloasma*), a condition in which macular hyperpigmentation appears, usually on the face or neck, is often associated with pregnancy ("the mask of pregnancy"), the use of oral contraceptives, and sun exposure.

Clinical Presentation of Skin Hyperpigmentation

Melasma is a common form of hyperpigmentation that occurs more often in women than in men.[2] Depending on the etiology of hyperpigmentation, patients can present with varying signs and symptoms.[1,11] Most notably, patients complain of persistent macular discoloration on the face or other sun-exposed areas. The centrofacial pattern (forehead, cheeks, upper lip, nose, chin) is the most common pattern.[1,2] Discoloration typically consists of a more intense brown coloration than that of surrounding normal skin and may range from dark to faint in appearance. Clinical evidence of hyperpigmentation and photoaging, and their response to treatment, are not easily quantifiable by standard light photography or by routine clinical evaluation. Fluorescence photography is used to detect subtle but significant decreases in diffuse and mottled hyperpigmentation after topical treatment, which helps to clinically evaluate and effectively assess the efficacy of topical products.[11]

TABLE 40-1 Medications That May Cause Hyperpigmentation

Amiodarone
Anticonvulsants (e.g., carbamazepine, phenobarbital, phenytoin)
Antimalarial agents (e.g., chloroquine, hydroxychloroquine)
Antineoplastic agents (e.g., busulfan, cyclophosphamide, daunorubicin, doxorubicin, fluorouracil)
Clofazimine
Heavy metals (e.g., arsenic, bismuth, gold compounds, mercury, silver)
Hormone replacement therapy
Minocycline
Oral contraceptives
Phenothiazines (e.g., chlorpromazine, clomipramine, imipramine, thioridazine)
Tricyclic antidepressants (e.g., amitriptyline, desipramine, imipramine)
Zidovudine

Source: Adapted from references 1, 2, and Law RM, Law DT. Dermatologic drug reactions and common skin conditions. In: DiPiro JT, Talbert RL, Yee GC, et al., eds. *Pharmacotherapy: A Pathophysiologic Approach.* 10th ed. New York, NY: McGraw-Hill Professional; 2017:e99.

TABLE 40-2 Fitzpatrick Skin Types

Fitzpatrick Skin Type	Characteristics	Response to UV
I	Unexposed skin is bright white Blue/green eyes typical Freckling frequent	Always burns Peels Never tans
II	Unexposed skin is white Blue, hazel, or brown eyes Red, blonde, or brown hair European/Scandinavian	Burns easily Peels Tans minimally
III	Unexposed skin is fair Brown eyes Southern or Central European	Burns moderately Average tanning ability
IV	Unexposed skin is light brown Dark eyes Dark hair Mediterranean, Asian, or Latino	Burns minimally Tans easily
V	Unexposed skin is brown Dark eyes Dark hair East Indian, Native American, Latino, or African	Rarely burns Tans easily
VI	Unexposed skin is black Dark eyes Dark hair African or Aboriginal ancestry	Almost never burns Tans readily

Key: UV = Ultraviolet light.
Source: Adapted from reference 50.

Treatment of Skin Hyperpigmentation

Treatment Goals

The goal of treating skin hyperpigmentation is to diminish the degree of pigmentation of affected areas so the skin tone of these areas is consistent with surrounding normal skin.

General Treatment Approach

The treatment approach for hyperpigmentation focuses on the melanin production pathway and falls into two broad categories: (1) stopping the skin cells from overproducing melanin and inhibiting melanosome formation and melanin synthesis, and (2) chemically or mechanically removing the top few layers of the skin's surface.[11] Although good results can be achieved by using either approach, the best results are accomplished through a combination of approaches.

Exfoliation used to treat hyperpigmentation involves physically buffing away surface-layer skin (*microdermabrasion*) and applying chemical agents (e.g., alpha hydroxy acids [AHAs]). Chemical peels, used as adjunct therapy, may enhance the efficacy of topical products.[11] Because of the risk of hyperpigmentation and other adverse events, microdermabrasion is not considered standard therapy. Abrading skin may also cause irritation and burning.

To prevent negation of the effects of treatment with either bleaching agents or pharmacologic therapy, patients must avoid even minimal exposure to UVR. On an ongoing basis, they must also use broad-spectrum sunscreen agents with a sun protection factor (SPF) of at least 30 in combination with a physical blocker, such as titanium dioxide, and wear protective clothing and broad-brimmed hats, even after discontinuing the bleaching agent.[1]

The algorithm in Figure 40–1 outlines the self-treatment of skin hyperpigmentation.[1,12–20]

Pharmacologic Therapy

Management of hyperpigmentation as directed by a primary care provider may include topical prescription agents composed of ingredients known to cause lightening of the skin primarily through inhibition of tyrosinase, the rate-limiting step in melanin biosynthesis. These products include tretinoin (retinoic acid), azelaic acid, hydroquinone, and corticosteroids. The disorder may also be treated with laser therapy alone. Combination products or laser therapy sometimes may be effective for postinflammatory hyperpigmentation that is resistant to treatment with a single agent nonprescription product.[14]

A number of nonprescription agents have been used in skin-bleaching preparations. These agents have included hydroquinone 2%, ascorbic acid, *N*-acetyl glucosamine, arbutin, glycolic

Exclusions for Self-Treatment

- <12 years of age
- Hyperpigmentation of large BSA
- Disease-induced or drug-induced hyperpigmentation
- Lesions that are changing in size, shape, or color

Source: References 9 and 12–20.

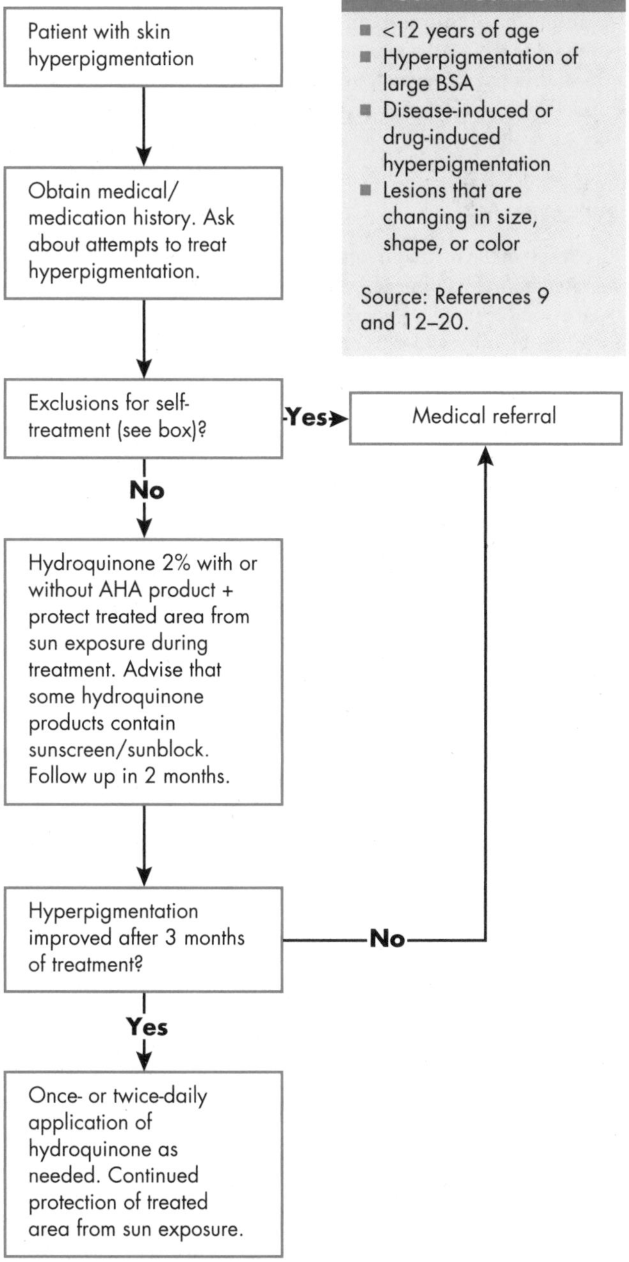

FIGURE 40–1 Self-care of skin hyperpigmentation. Key: AHA = Alpha hydroxy acid; BSA = body surface area.

acid, vitamin C, licorice extract, niacinamide, and kojic acid. Newer products are being formulated with synthetic oligopeptide, rucinol, tranexamic acid, deoxyarbutin, dioic acid, and aloesin.[5,15] However, only preparations containing hydroquinone were submitted to the Food and Drug Administration (FDA) Advisory Review Panel on Over-the-Counter Miscellaneous External Drug Products, and products containing this agent remain the most effective nonprescription skin-bleaching products available. AHAs, promoted as nonprescription treatments for photoaging, are used to treat both disorders. Table 40–3 lists selected trade-name products.

TABLE 40–3 Selected Nonprescription Skin Bleaching/Fading Products

Trade Name	Primary Ingredients
Alpha Hydrox Spot Light Targeted Skin Lightener	Hydroquinone 2%; glycolic acid 10%; vitamin E
Civant Meladerm	Niacinamide; kojic acid; bear-berry extract; licorice extract; alpha arbutin; lactic acid
Clinicians Complex 6% Skin Bleaching Cream	Hydroquinone 2%; kojic acid 2%
DDF Fade Gel 4	Hydroquinone 2%; kojic acid; azelaic acid; salicylic acid
Exuviance Brighten Up Kit	Hydroquinone 2%; glycolic acid; PHA/kojic acid complex
La Roche-Posay Mela-D Pigment Control Concentrated Serum	Glycolic acid; lipo-hydroxy acid
Lumixyl	Synthetic oligopeptide 0.1%
Murad Rapid Age Spot and Pigment Lightening Serum	Hydroquinone 2%; glycolic acid
Noreva IKLEN Depigmenting Serum	Rucinol
Philosophy Miracle Worker Dark Spot Corrector	Niacinamide
Shiseido White Lucent Intensive Spot Targeting Serum	Tranexamic acid
SkinCeuticals Pigment Regulator	Kojic acid 2%; emblica extract 2%; glycolic acid
Verso Skincare Dark Spot Fix	Retinol 8 with retinyl retinoate, niacinamide

Key: PHA = Polyhydroxy acid.

Hydroquinone

Skin-bleaching agents diminish hyperpigmentation by inhibiting melanin production within the skin.[1] Hydroquinone (*p*-dihydroxybenzene), a skin-bleaching agent, in concentrations of 1.5%–2% is currently available for self-treatment of skin hyperpigmentation.[10] Hydroquinone is considered the mainstay and gold standard of hyperpigmentation therapy.[5,12,15] However, the safety of bleaching creams that contain hydroquinone continues to be reviewed in the literature.[16,17] In 2006, FDA proposed withdrawing the tentative final monograph that approved skin-bleaching creams to replace it with a final rule stating that all drug products (including hydroquinone) used in nonprescription products to lighten skin are no longer generally recognized as safe and effective owing to the potential increased risk of cancer and *ochronosis,* a bluish-black discoloration of skin that occurs where hydroquinone has been applied. If this final monograph is published, hydroquinone products will be removed from the nonprescription marketplace. In December 2009, FDA nominated hydroquinone to undergo additional studies to determine whether its use poses a risk to humans.[19] The National Toxicology Program's review of the agent is ongoing.[19] In the interim, FDA believes that hydroquinone should remain available as a nonprescription drug product.

Hydroquinone and its derivatives act by reducing conversion of tyrosine to dopa and, subsequently, to melanin by inhibiting the enzyme tyrosinase. Other possible mechanisms of action include destruction of the melanocyte or melanosomes.[1,12] Hydroquinone is available in concentrations of 2%, 3%, and 4%.[21] The 2% concentration is safer and produces results equivalent to those of higher concentrations.[17] The combination of hydroquinone with an antioxidant and exfoliant is considered efficacious, giving patients acceptable outcomes with minimal adverse effects.[1,5,13] Combining hydroquinone with an exfoliant, such as topical glycolic acid (an AHA), topical tretinoin, or a corticosteroid, has shown increased efficacy compared with hydroquinone monotherapy.[11,20]

Hydroquinone 2% should be rubbed gently but thoroughly into affected areas twice daily. The agent should be applied to clean skin before application of moisturizers or other skin care products. It should not be applied to damaged skin or near the eyes. If no improvement is seen within 2 months, its use should be discontinued and a primary care provider should be consulted.[1,21] Once the desired benefit is achieved, hydroquinone can be applied as often as needed in a once- or twice-daily regimen to maintain lightening of the skin. Because of the lack of safety data, hydroquinone is not recommended for children younger than 12 years. Contraindications to the use of hydroquinone include hypersensitivity to the product. Although not directly contraindicated, hydroquinone should be used during pregnancy only if absolutely needed as it is currently labeled as Pregnancy Category C. It is not known if topical hydroquinone can cause fetal harm.[21,22] (See the Preface for a detailed explanation of the pregnancy data.)

Alternative Agents

Synthetic Oligopeptide

Synthetic oligopeptide 0.01% (decapeptide-12) is a newer agent that has been shown in clinical trials to produce improvement in hyperpigmentation of various severities.[23–25] Oligopeptide's mechanism of action, inhibiting tyrosinase thereby reducing melanin synthesis, is similar to that of hydroquinone.[11,23–25] The studies concluded that the decapeptide-12 was efficacious, well tolerated, and less toxic than hydroquinone. This oligopeptide is currently available only in the nonprescription product Lumixyl, which also contains 20% glycolic acid, licorice root extract, phenylethyl resorcinol, and a broad-spectrum sunscreen with an SPF of at least 30. It is not an FDA-approved skin-bleaching product. A pea-size amount should be applied twice daily, with results expected in 8–16 weeks.[23–25]

Kojic Acid

Kojic acid, a product derived from certain species of fungus (e.g., *Acetobacter, Aspergillus, Penicillium*), can be found in cosmetic products promoted to treat hyperpigmentation in concentrations ranging from 1% to 4%.[11] This product is usually found in combination with AHAs, with or without hydroquinone. It is dosed and applied according to the product type (e.g., cream, soap, lotion, drops). Kojic acid works primarily by inhibiting the production of tyrosinase through chelation of its copper, which reduces melanin synthesis. It also, however, can help reduce melanin proliferation.[11] Adverse effects associated with this product include contact dermatitis, stinging, and erythema. One study comparing the combination of 2% kojic acid and 10% glycolic acid with that of 2% hydroquinone and 10% glycolic acid demonstrated similar results for the two therapies.[5,12–14]

Rucinol

Rucinol is a resorcinol derivative that has a unique mechanism of action that inhibits both tyrosinase and tyrosinase-related protein-1 (TRP-1), the enzyme used in melanin synthesis.[12,15] Several studies have demonstrated that rucinol 0.3% serum or cream, applied twice daily, improved pigmentation within 8–12 weeks and was well tolerated.[12,15,25]

Tranexamic Acid

As a result of the hydroquinone controversy, tranexamic acid (trans-4-aminomethylcyclohexanecarboxylic acid), an agent that has been available for many years, is receiving more attention. It works by inhibiting ultraviolet (UV)-induced plasmin activity, which, in turn, reduces inflammatory mediators and tyrosinase activity in melanocytes.[1,15,25] Although some studies have shown no benefit, a few have shown improvement within 12 weeks of inception of use.[26] Studies have evaluated topical, intravenous, and oral dosage forms.[27] The oral dose most commonly being studied is 250 mg twice daily, and the currently available topical application is twice daily. The most common adverse effect of the topical form was irritation to the applied area. Currently, tranexamic acid can be found as an adjunct ingredient in some nonprescription serums.

Mandelic Acid

Mandelic acid is a type of AHA that penetrates the epidermis more slowly and uniformly.[28] It is used in the treatment of several skin conditions, including hyperpigmentation. When combined with salicylic acid and administered as a peel, it has fewer adverse effects than a glycolic acid peel and has demonstrated better efficacy. The adverse effects most commonly seen were dryness and burning.

Niacinamide

Niacinamide is a form of vitamin B_3 and acts as an anti-inflammatory agent. Although most pharmacologic treatments of hyperpigmentation disrupt tyrosinase activity, niacinamide instead works by preventing the transfer of melanin to keratinocytes, improving appearance of not only hyperpigmentation but also photoaged skin (redness and wrinkles).[29–33] Topical niacinamide 2% has been shown to reduce hyperpigmentation after 4 weeks of treatment.[29] The most common adverse effects are redness, burning, and itching.[31] Niacinamide has also demonstrated efficacy when used topically in combination with other agents, such as desonide 0.05%, 2% tranexamic acid, or 2% *N*-acetyl glucosamine.[30–32]

Arbutin

Arbutin is a beta-D-glucopyranoside derivative of hydroquinone and is derived from the extract of the bearberry plant.[1,12] It works by inhibiting tyrosinase and melanosome maturation.[1] Studies have used concentrations ranging from 1% to 3%, applied twice daily to the affected areas, with beneficial effects seen in about 6 months. Although the effect is dose dependent, higher concentrations have been found to induce hyperpigmentation.

Product Selection Guidelines

Product selection should be based on a suitable dosage form (e.g., cream, lotion, gel) for the patient's skin type (dry, normal, oily) and anatomic site (face, neck). For example, an emollient cream-based product may be more suitable for dry skin, whereas a gel-based preparation may be preferable for an oily skin type.

Assessment of Skin Hyperpigmentation: A Case-Based Approach

Assessment should involve evaluating the affected areas to determine whether they are characteristic of freckles, melasma, or lentigines. The patient's medication history and health status are important factors in pinpointing possible causes of the hyperpigmentation.

Case 40–1 is an example of the assessment of a patient with skin hyperpigmentation.

Patient Counseling for Skin Hyperpigmentation

The types of hyperpigmentation that are self-treatable should be explained to the patient, and the importance of avoiding sun exposure during and after treatment should be stressed. The product instructions should be reviewed with the patient to ensure a successful therapeutic outcome. The box "Patient Education for Skin Hyperpigmentation" lists specific information to provide patients. In addition, the Melasma Quality of Life Scale has shown that

CASE 40–1

Relevant Evaluation Criteria	Scenario/Model Outcome
Collect	
1. Gather essential information about the patient's symptoms and medical history, including	
a. Description of symptom(s) (i.e., nature, onset, duration, severity, associated symptoms)	The patient has been experiencing darkening areas of skin on her forehead, cheeks, and upper lip, which first appeared last summer.
b. Description of any factors that seem to precipitate, exacerbate, and/or relieve the patient's symptom(s)	Patient says that she had been on an oral contraceptive for 10 years but stopped taking it at the beginning of the summer last year. The affected skin areas appear darker when the patient spends more time in sunlight. The darkened areas faded slightly over the winter but now, with the onset of summer, the patient has noticed the spots are darkening again.
c. Description of the patient's efforts to relieve the symptoms	The patient tried topical moisturizing lotions and hydroquinone 2% per her pharmacist's recommendation for 2 months last summer.
d. Patient's identity	Jane Doe
e. Patient's age, gender, height, and weight	36 years old, female, 5 ft 6 in., 160 lb
f. Patient's occupation	Full-time daycare worker
g. Patient's dietary habits	Diet is well balanced. She drinks wine and beer occasionally.
h. Patient's sleep habits	She averages 5 hours per night during the week and 10 hours on the weekend.
i. Concurrent medical conditions, prescription and nonprescription medications, and dietary supplements	Diabetes: metformin (Glucophage XR) 500 mg daily; hypertension: lisinopril 20 mg once daily
j. Allergies	None
k. History of other adverse reactions to medications	None
l. Other (describe) ______	n/a
Assess	
2. Differentiate patient's signs/symptoms, and correctly identify the patient's primary problem(s).	The patient has hyperpigmentation of the centrofacial region, which appeared last summer when she discontinued her oral contraceptive and seems to be aggravated by sun exposure.
3. Identify exclusions for self-treatment (Figure 40–1).	The patient has tried OTC products, including hydroquinone, for 2 months without benefit.
4. Formulate a comprehensive list of therapeutic alternatives for the primary problem to determine whether triage to a medical provider is required, and share this information with the patient or caregiver.	Options include (1) Refer Jane to an HCP or dermatologist for further evaluation. (2) Try a different skin-lightening agent. (3) Take no action.

CASE 40-1 *continued*

Relevant Evaluation Criteria	Scenario/Model Outcome
Plan	
5. Select an optimal therapeutic alternative to address the patient's problem, taking into account patient preferences.	Patient should be referred to an HCP or dermatologist, because the OTC treatment has been unsuccessful.
6. Describe the recommended therapeutic approach to the patient or caregiver.	"Because you have tried self-treatment unsuccessfully for 2 months, you should see a health care provider or dermatologist for further evaluation."
7. Explain to the patient or caregiver the rationale for selecting the recommended therapeutic approach from the considered therapeutic alternatives.	"Continuing treatment with the current product will most likely not provide any benefit. A health care provider or dermatologist can evaluate your condition and suggest alternative treatments."
Implement	
8. When recommending self-care with nonprescription medications and/or nondrug therapy, convey accurate information to the patient or caregiver.	Criterion does not apply in this case.
Solicit follow-up questions from the patient or caregiver.	"A friend told me about Shiseido White Lucent Intensive Spot Targeting Serum. Do you think I should try this first?"
Answer the patient's or caregiver's questions.	"Hydroquinone is currently the nonprescription product with the most evidence supporting its effectiveness. Because you tried it for 2 months with no improvement, I would recommend further evaluation of your condition to see if a combination of medications would be more efficacious."
Follow-up: Evaluate and Monitor	
9. Assess patient outcome.	Contact the patient in a couple of days to ensure that she made an appointment for further evaluation.

Key: HCP = Health care provider; n/a = not applicable; OTC = over-the-counter.

PATIENT EDUCATION FOR

Skin Hyperpigmentation

The objective of self-treatment with skin-bleaching products is to diminish the degree of pigmentation in affected areas. For most patients, carefully following product instructions and the self-care measures listed here will help ensure optimal therapeutic outcomes.

Hydroquinone

- Use hydroquinone to lighten only limited areas of hyperpigmented skin that show brownish discoloration.
- Do not use these products on nevi (moles) or reddish or bluish areas, such as port wine discoloration.
- Time to initial response averages 6–8 weeks, but it may take up to 3 months to see noticeable results.
- Test for possible irritant reactions to the product by applying it to a small test area and checking the area for redness, itching, or swelling after 24 hours.
- Do not apply the product near the eyes or to damaged skin.
- Apply a thin layer of the product to clean, dry skin in the affected area only. Rub product into the skin gently but thoroughly.
- If moisturizers or other topical agents are being used at the same time, apply the hydroquinone first.
- When outdoors for even a short time, apply an opaque sunblock or broad-spectrum sunscreen (see Chapter 39) to the affected area after applying the hydroquinone, unless the product already contains a sunscreen in the formulation.
- Once the desired lightening of skin is reached, apply the hydroquinone once or twice daily to prevent hyperpigmentation from recurring. Continue to protect the treated area from sun exposure.

When to Seek Medical Attention

- Consult a primary care provider if
  - No improvement is seen after 2 months of using hydroquinone.
  - Skin pigmentation becomes darker during treatment with hydroquinone.

melasma, at any level, negatively affects a patient's quality of life, especially social life, recreation, and emotional well-being.[12] Pharmacists, therefore, can potentially make a significant impact when they counsel patients about hyperpigmentation.

Evaluation of Patient Outcomes for Skin Hyperpigmentation

Follow-up on the patient's progress should occur after 2 months of therapy. If the pigmented area shows no improvement, the patient should consult a primary care provider or a dermatologist. If the desired outcome has been achieved, the patient should continue applying the agent once or twice daily, as needed, and using a sunscreen to maintain lightening of the skin.

PHOTOAGING

Photoaging, also referred to as premature aging or dermatoheliosis, is the pattern of characteristic skin changes associated with sun exposure. Individuals with Fitzpatrick skin types I–III (Table 40–2) are more susceptible to photoaging. Most fair-skinned Americans will have some signs of photodamaged skin by 50 years of age. A variety of therapies are available to treat photodamaged skin; these therapies range from use of topical products and cosmetics to more invasive procedures such as facelifts, botulinum toxin A injections, and laser resurfacing. Although some products are available by prescription only, many others are nonprescription, with AHAs being widely used to combat photoaged skin.[34]

Pathophysiology of Photoaging

Aging skin results from a combination of intrinsic and extrinsic factors. Clinical and histologic changes that occur intrinsically include genetically controlled skin and muscle changes, expression lines, sleep lines, and hormonal changes. The second component, extrinsic factors, pertains to environmental influences such as UVR, smoking, wind, and chemical exposure.[35–37] Medications known to induce photosensitivity can contribute to photoaging by making the skin sensitive to UVR (see Chapter 39).

Prematurely aged facial skin, with creases and wrinkles, dry texture, and blotchy hyperpigmentation, is largely attributed to cumulative UVR, or photoaging. Exposure to ultraviolet B (UVB) (290–320 nm) is primarily responsible for photoaging, although the longer ultraviolet A (UVA) wavelengths (320–400 nm) contribute to damage as well.[34] The amount of UVA present in sunlight is 10 times that of UVB, which allows greater amounts of skin exposure. UVA can also penetrate into the deeper dermal layer and can work synergistically with UVB to cause photodamage and skin cancers.

Microscopically, sun-damaged skin shows *dysplasia* (abnormal tissue development), atypical keratinocytes, and occasional cell necrosis. Irregularity of epidermal cell alignment is also common. Loss of collagen and elastin is seen deeper in the dermal layer.[35–37]

Clinical Presentation of Photoaging

Clinical signs of photoaging include changes in color, surface texture, and functional capacity (Table 40–4). Photoaged skin may have a sallow yellow color with discoloration and may show telangiectasias (visible distended capillaries). Textural changes include loss of smoothness, loss of subcutaneous tissue around the mouth, and epidermal thinning around the lips. As sebaceous glands hypertrophy, the skin begins to show coarse texture with increased pore size. In addition, fine vellus hairs can develop into unwanted terminal hairs. Other manifestations of photoaged skin may include development of precancerous (actinic keratosis) and cancerous (basal cell, squamous cell, melanoma) tumor development.[34–37] Cosmetically, patients may notice freckling, discolorations, or *crow's feet* (small parallel lines around the eyes). Postmenopausal skin is susceptible to reduced estrogen receptor stimulation of dermal metabolism and undergoes significant changes in collagen and moisture content. These changes lead to signs of skin aging, as evidenced by diminished elasticity and wrinkles.[38]

Treatment of Photoaging

Treatment Goals

The first goal is to prevent or minimize the likelihood of skin photoaging by using appropriate sun protection.[39] The goals of treating photoaging are (1) to reverse cumulative skin damage with prescription and nonprescription products and (2) to maintain the skin and protect it from further extrinsic damage by making lifestyle changes and, most importantly, protecting the skin from further and prolonged sun exposure.

General Treatment Approach

The first step in preventing and treating photoaged skin is for the patient to commit to minimizing sun exposure by wearing sun-protective clothing, using large-brimmed hats, avoiding the sun during peak UVR times, and wearing sunscreen daily. Broad-spectrum sunscreens (UVA and UVB coverage) with an SPF

TABLE 40–4 Glogau Classification of Photoaging

Type I (mild)	No wrinkles, early photoaging, mild pigment changes
	20–30 years of age
Type II (moderate)	Wrinkles in motion, early–moderate photoaging, keratoses palpable
	30–40 years of age
Type III (advanced)	Wrinkles at rest, advanced photoaging, obvious dyschromia and keratoses
	≥50 years of age
Type IV (severe)	Only wrinkles, severe photoaging, yellow-gray skin
	≥60 years of age

Source: Glogau RG. Aesthetic and anatomic analysis of the aging skin. *Semin Cutan Med Surg.* 1996;15(3):134–8.

of 30 or greater can minimize further photodamage during UVR exposure[35,36,40] (see Chapter 39).

Proper cleansing of the skin removes bacteria, dirt, desquamated keratinocytes, cosmetics, sebum, and perspiration. However, excessive use of soap can lead to xerosis, eczematous dermatitis, and other skin conditions.[41]

Pharmacologic Therapy

Various topical products are being used to treat aging skin. These products include coenzyme Q10, *N*-furfuryladenine (Kinerase), AHAs, and beta hydroxy acids (BHAs). Many cosmeceutical ingredients, such as AHAs, function as active pharmaceuticals that are known to have a sustained effect on the skin.[42] Of the vitamins, A, C, B_3, and E have the most evidence supporting their use in treatment and/or prevention of photoaging.[43]

Hydroxy Acids

Current labeling on hydroxy acid (HA) cosmetic products includes recommendations for melasma, acne, solar lentigines, and fine wrinkling of photoaging.[12] The AHAs are used in various concentrations and in a wide array of available products. Most AHAs are sold as cosmeceuticals, some are sold as cosmetics, and yet others are sold as pharmaceuticals through a primary care provider. These products range in concentration from 2% to 20% (as nonpeeling AHAs). As peeling agents (as used by estheticians or dermatologists), they are available in concentrations greater than 20%.

Of the available nonprescription products, AHAs currently play a major role in reliably reversing and cosmetically improving aging skin.[12,44] Many types of AHAs are available, with the most common being lactic and glycolic acids (Table 40–5). The Cosmetic Ingredient Review Expert Panel, the cosmetic industry's self-regulatory body, concluded that use of AHAs in cosmetic products is safe if (1) concentrations are less than or equal to 10%, (2) the final pH is greater than or equal to 3.5, and (3) the product is formulated with a sunscreen or includes directions to use a sunscreen.[45]

Of the BHAs, salicylic acid is used widely, even as a chemical peel.[46,47] Compared with AHA products, BHAs are more lipophilic and demonstrate keratolytic effects. Products containing BHAs as the active ingredients may be beneficial to acne-prone skin.

Polyhydroxy acids are the new generation of AHAs that appear to have results similar to those of the alpha and beta hydroxy products, but with less irritation.[40]

Used appropriately, HA products act as exfoliants by causing detachment of keratinocytes, resulting in a smoother, nonscaly skin surface with eventual normalization of keratinization. The effect of the AHA product depends on the concentration and pH.[40] The lower the pH, the more effective the product is, and the higher the AHA concentration, the more deeply it affects the stratum corneum. By improving skin elasticity, HAs have been shown to make skin more flexible and less vulnerable to cracking and flaking. Long-term use has led to an increase in skin collagen and elastin.[39,43] Regular application of HAs results in smoother skin texture, lessening of fine lines, and normalization of pigmentation.[43]

Guidelines for treatment with HAs include identification of patient factors such as medications, prior procedures, and medical history, all of which may affect treatment outcome and realistic patient expectations.[48] Care should be taken to apply HAs to dry skin, with an estimated wait time of 10–15 minutes after cleansing the face. It is also prudent to begin application gradually, starting every other night for approximately 1 week and then increasing the frequency, as tolerated, to a maximum of twice-daily application.[22] HA products may make the skin more sensitive to sun exposure. Patients should be advised to use daily sunscreen or sunblock with an SPF of 30 or greater during use of AHAs and after discontinuation of their use.[35]

Common adverse effects of AHA and BHA products include mild transient stinging, burning, pruritus, skin lightening, and dryness. BHA products may be less irritating. Many of these effects can be ameliorated if products are used with caution and proper counseling. Patients should also note that other topically applied products, both medications and cosmetics, may contain active ingredients capable of exacerbating irritation (e.g., AHA, BHA, hydroquinone). Information regarding use during pregnancy and lactation is lacking; therefore, such use is not recommended.[22]

TABLE 40–5 Selected Nonprescription Products for Photoaged Skin

Trade Name	Active Ingredients
Glycolic Acid–Containing Products	
Aqua Glycolic Hand and Body Lotion	Glycolic acid 14%
Alpha Hydrox AHA Enhanced Anti-Wrinkle Crème	Glycolic acid 10%
Alpha Hydrox AHA Souffle	Glycolic acid 12%
DDF Glycolic Exfoliating Oil Control Gel	Glycolic acid 10%
DermaQuest Skin Therapy	Glycolic acid 5%; azelaic acid 2.5%; salicylic acid 2%
Dr. Michelle Copeland AHA Face Cream	Glycolic acid 10%
M.D. Forte Facial Cleanser III	Glycolic acid 30%
Peter Thomas Roth Glycolic Acid Hydrating Gel	Glycolic acid 10%
Peter Thomas Roth Glycolic Acid Moisturizer	Glycolic acid 10%
Reviva Labs Glycolic Acid Cream Exfoliation and Cell Renewal	Glycolic acid 10%
Retinol-Containing Products	
GlyMed Plus Retinol Restart Rejuvenation Serum	Retinol 5%
Paula's Choice Clinical 1% Retinol Treatment	Retinol 1%; vitamin C
Proactiv+ Skin Revitalizing Pads	Retinol
Salicylic Acid–Containing Products	
Paula's Choice Skin Perfecting 2% BHA Lotion Exfoliant	Salicylic acid 2%
Peter Thomas Roth Beta Hydroxy 2% Acne Wash	Salicylic acid 2%

Retinol and Retinaldehyde (Vitamin A Derivative)

Topical retinoids (tretinoin, isotretinoin, tazarotene, adapalene, retinol, alitretinoin) are the mainstay of treatment of photoaging.[34,40] Retinol and its derivatives have been incorporated into many skin care products and are available in both prescription and nonprescription products. Retinoids increase collagen production and induce epidermal hyperplasia, which helps reduce the appearance of fine lines, improves skin texture, and corrects tone and skin elasticity. Retinol is very unstable and, with light exposure, easily degrades to biologically inactive forms.[40] Thus, higher concentrations may be needed for efficacy. Retinol is transformed into retinaldehyde and then into retinoic acid with a two-step enzymatic process that involves dehydrogenase in human keratinocytes. Topical retinaldehyde is not only well tolerated by human skin but has also been shown to have several effects identical to that of tretinoin. Common adverse effects of topical retinoids include scaling, redness, burning, and dermatitis. Retinoids may have to be used for at least 4 months before benefit can be seen. The use of vitamin A in excess of recommended amounts is contraindicated in women who are pregnant or may become pregnant.[21]

Ascorbic Acid (Vitamin C)

Ascorbic acid (vitamin C) is a plentiful antioxidant in the skin.[40] It neutralizes reactive oxygen species caused by UV irradiation and functions as a scavenger of free radicals. Several studies have demonstrated reduced skin roughness and wrinkles with application of topical ascorbic acid 3%–5% for 12 weeks.[1,49] Ascorbic acid has also been reported to have at least some photoprotective properties. Compared with hydroquinone 4%, ascorbic acid 5% was better tolerated and had fewer adverse effects.[1] Ascorbic acid is a vitamin and is currently labeled as Pregnancy Category C.[21] (See the Preface for a detailed explanation of the pregnancy data.)

Coenzyme Q10

Ubiquinone (coenzyme Q10) is a lipophilic antioxidant that is synthesized by all mammalian cells and is critical for the protection of mitochondrial membranes.[40] Idebenone, a synthetic derivative of ubiquinone, is more soluble and has potent antioxidant properties. It has been suggested that idebenone exerts a beneficial effect on preventing and/or reversing photoaging by quenching free radicals in the epidermis. These products often are found in concentrations ranging from 0.3% to 1% in cosmetic creams and lotions promoted as anti-aging and/or antioxidant products.[49] Information regarding its use during pregnancy and lactation is lacking; therefore, such use is not recommended.[21]

Product Selection Guidelines

Skin type should determine the selection of product type. Creams are appropriate for drier skin types, lotions are best for combination or normal skin, and gels or solutions are useful for oilier skin. Use of products with higher concentrations and a lower pH may produce faster results. However, the patient should be warned that these products may also cause greater skin irritation.

Assessment of Photoaging: A Case-Based Approach

If visual inspection of the patient's skin indicates photoaging, the patient should be questioned about his or her history of UVR (sunlight as well as artificial light) exposure. Knowing whether the patient's current occupational or recreational habits require excessive exposure is useful not only in determining the cause of the skin disorder but also in developing a treatment plan. It is important to assess for a history of diseases or medications that may predispose the patient to premature photodamage or photosensitivity. The patient's health status, lifestyle practices, and daily skin maintenance regimen are other pertinent assessment criteria.[34]

Case 40–2 is an example of assessment of a patient with photoaging.

CASE 40-2

Relevant Evaluation Criteria	Scenario/Model Outcome
Collect	
1. Gather essential information about the patient's symptoms and medical history, including	
a. Description of symptom(s) (i.e., nature, onset, duration, severity, associated symptoms)	Patient complains of wrinkles, dry skin, crow's feet around her eyes, and dark skin pigmentation.
b. Description of any factors that seem to precipitate, exacerbate, and/or relieve the patient's symptom(s)	These skin changes have occurred over the past several years and are progressively becoming more noticeable. She retired 2 years ago and is spending a lot more time outside gardening and enjoying her pool.
c. Description of the patient's efforts to relieve the symptoms	She uses daily moisturizer but wants to "have less wrinkles."
d. Patient's identity	Ginger Smith
e. Patient's age, gender, height, and weight	65 years old, female, 5 ft 4 in., 145 lb
f. Patient's occupation	Retired
g. Patient's dietary habits	Patient eats fast food often while running errands and babysitting her grandkids. She denies drinking alcohol. She quit smoking 15 years ago.
h. Patient's sleep habits	Normal sleep schedule; she averages 7 hours per night.
i. Concurrent medical conditions, prescription and nonprescription medications, and dietary supplements	Osteoporosis prevention: calcium 600 mg + vitamin D 400 international units

CASE 40-2 *continued*

Relevant Evaluation Criteria	Scenario/Model Outcome
j. Allergies	None
k. History of other adverse reactions to medications	None
l. Other (describe) ______	n/a
Assess	
2. Differentiate patient's signs/symptoms, and correctly identify the patient's primary problem(s).	The patient has noticeable wrinkles, crow's feet, dry skin, and hyper-pigmented areas on her face caused by photoaging.
3. Identify exclusions for self-treatment.	The patient has no exclusions for self-treatment.
4. Formulate a comprehensive list of therapeutic alternatives for the primary problem to determine whether triage to a medical provider is required, and share this information with the patient or caregiver.	Options include (1) Refer Ginger to an HCP or dermatologist for further evaluation. (2) Recommend a 2-month trial of a topical retinoid product and use of daily sunscreen. (3) Take no action.
Plan	
5. Select an optimal therapeutic alternative to address the patient's problem, taking into account patient preferences.	The patient would like to try an OTC product.
6. Describe the recommended therapeutic approach to the patient or caregiver.	"Apply the chosen product, such as GlyMed Retinol Restart Rejuvenation Serum, to your clean, dry face once or twice a day in the morning and/or evening. Smooth the serum over your face and neck, allowing the product to absorb completely. Then apply a broad-spectrum sunscreen with an SPF of at least 30. Use this sunscreen daily."
7. Explain to the patient or caregiver the rationale for selecting the recommended therapeutic approach from the considered therapeutic alternatives.	"Seeing a dermatologist may not be necessary with proper use of this product. Wrinkles will not be completely removed, because they are part of the natural aging process."
Implement	
8. When recommending self-care with nonprescription medications and/or nondrug therapy, convey accurate information to the patient or caregiver.	
a. Appropriate dose and frequency of administration	"Apply once or twice a day in the morning and/or evening. Smooth the serum over the face and neck, allowing the product to absorb completely. Apply a broad-spectrum sunscreen with an SPF of at least 30 after applying the product. Use this sunscreen daily."
b. Maximum number of days the therapy should be employed	"Improvement may be seen in as little as 4 weeks but may take as long as 6 months."
c. Product administration procedures	"The product should be applied after cleansing the face."
d. Expected time to onset of relief	"Improvement may be seen in as little as 4 weeks."
e. Degree of relief that can be reasonably expected	"Fine lines may be reduced, pore size may decrease, dark spots may improve, and dryness should be improved. All signs of wrinkles, however, may not disappear completely."
f. Most common adverse effects	"Mild irritation may occur. In addition, the areas being treated may appear to be lighter than surrounding skin."
g. Adverse effects that warrant medical intervention should they occur	"If the treated areas of the skin become severely irritated or darken significantly, you should see your health care provider or a dermatologist."
h. Patient options in the event that condition worsens or persists	"If no improvement is seen within 2 months, you should see your health care provider or a dermatologist."
i. Product storage requirements	"When not in use, the product should be stored at normal room temperature and tightly closed."
j. Specific nondrug measures	"This product may make the skin more sensitive to sun exposure. A sunscreen with an SPF of at least 30 should be applied daily while using this product and for up to a week afterward."

CASE 40-2 *continued*

Relevant Evaluation Criteria	Scenario/Model Outcome
Solicit follow-up questions from the patient or caregiver.	(1) "May I use this product more than twice a day?" (2) "Should I always wear sunscreen or only when I am using this product?"
Answer the patient's or caregiver's questions.	(1) "No, this product should be used a maximum of twice daily." (2) "This product will increase the overall sensitivity of your skin to the sun. In addition, because you often are outside, it is advisable to use a moisturizer or foundation with an SPF of at least 30 every day."
Follow-up: Evaluate and Monitor	
9. Assess patient outcome.	Ask the patient to call and update you on her response to your recommendation. Or you could call her in a month to evaluate response.

Key: HCP = Health care provider; n/a = not applicable; OTC = over-the-counter; SPF = sun protection factor.

Patient Counseling for Photoaging

Patients should be advised that premature wrinkling, creases, dry texture, and blotchy hyperpigmentation are not inevitable, and that proper R protection from UVR can limit the effects of photoaging.[37] The provider should be proactive in identifying and recommending products that are appropriate for a specific patient. The box "Patient Education for Photoaging" lists specific information to provide patients.

Evaluation of Patient Outcomes for Photoaging

Patients using nonprescription products for photoaging should set a reasonable goal. Obviously, these preparations cannot "erase wrinkles." The provider should monitor the progress of the treatment and be sensitive to issues that may require medical referral (e.g., reactive hyperpigmentation, bacterial or fungal infections, epidermal cysts, acneiform eruption, scarring).[48]

Key Points for Skin Hyperpigmentation and Photoaging

- Photoaging and hyperpigmentation are cosmetically unacceptable skin conditions. Patients who have reasonable expectations should be able to achieve even skin tone and to minimize appearance and occurrence of fine wrinkling with the use of nonprescription products.
- Hydroquinone is the only FDA-approved nonprescription skin-bleaching product. Patients should apply a 2% concentration to skin up to twice daily, as tolerated.
- Patients younger than 12 years; those with large areas of hyperpigmentation or disease- or drug-induced hyperpigmentation; or those with lesions that have changed in size, shape, or color should consult their primary care provider.[21]
- Patients should be referred to a primary care provider if no improvement occurs within 2 months or if skin darkens during treatment of hyperpigmentation.[13]

PATIENT EDUCATION FOR Photoaging

The objectives of self-treatment are (1) to reverse skin damage by using available nonprescription products and (2) to protect the skin from further damage by making lifestyle changes and protecting skin from sun exposure. For most patients, carefully following product instructions and the self-care measures listed here will help ensure optimal therapeutic outcomes.

Alpha Hydroxy Acids

- Protect the skin from sun exposure by covering it with clothing. The Food and Drug Administration (FDA) recommends advising patients to wear long-sleeved clothing and hats with brims of at least 4 inches. Patients should also use a sunblock or sunscreen product with an SPF of 30 or greater during use of alpha hydroxy acids (AHAs) and regularly in the future to prevent further damage.
- To prevent dry skin, cleanse the skin with a mild soap or a soap-free liquid cleanser. Do not cleanse skin more often than twice daily. Apply a pea-sized amount of an AHA product to clean, dry skin.
- To minimize transient mild tingling and stinging, wait 10–15 minutes after cleansing the face to apply an AHA product.
- Excessive skin dryness or irritation warrants decreased application.
- Note that AHA products contain an active ingredient and that the use of other products, including cosmetics, could result in skin irritation, including mild stinging, burning, or erythema.
- Do not apply the product too close to the eyes or mucous membranes.
- Begin applying this product once at bedtime every other day for approximately 1 week. Gradually increase application to twice a day.
- Use a daily moisturizer with sunscreen after applying the AHA product to minimize dry skin and maintain the antiphotoaging effect.
- Store this product in a cool dry place out of children's reach.
- Discontinue the AHA product if severe irritation, such as redness or excessive dryness, or a rash occurs.

- Patients should avoid applying hydroquinone-containing products near the eye area or on damaged skin areas.
- Patients using HAs to reduce photoaging should be advised to apply the products to dry skin up to twice daily. Patients should be counseled that it may take up to 6 months to see the effect.
- Patients who use products to prevent photoaging or hyperpigmentation should be instructed to protect their skin from daily sun exposure by using a sunscreen with an SPF of 30 or greater to maintain results.[36]

REFERENCES

1. Sheth VM, Pandya AG. Melasma: a comprehensive update: part II. *J Am Acad Dermatol.* 2011;65(4):699–714. doi: 10.1016/j.jaad.2011.06.001.
2. Nicolaidou E, Katsambas A. Pigmentation disorders: Hyperpigmentation and hypopigmentation. *Dermatol Clin.* 2014;32(1):66–72. doi: 10.1016/j.clindermatol.2013.05.026.
3. Nicolaidou E, Antoniou C, Katsambas A. Origin, clinical presentation and diagnosis of facial hypermelanoses. *Dermatol Clin.* 2007;25(3):321–6. doi: 10.1016/j.det.2007.05.002.
4. Plensdorf S, Martinez J. Common pigmentation disorders. *Am Fam Physician.* 2009;79(2):109–16. PMID: 19178061.
5. Callender VD, St. Surin-Lord S, Davis EC, et al. Postinflammatory hyperpigmentation. *Am J Clin Dermatol.* 2011;12(2):87–99. doi: 10.2165/11536930-000000000-00000.
6. Park H, Yaar M, Lee J, et al. Biology of melanocytes. In: Goldsmith LA, Katz SI, Gilchrest BA, eds. *Fitzpatrick's Dermatology in General Medicine.* 8th ed. New York: McGraw-Hill; 2012. Available at: http://accessmedicine.mhmedical.com/book.aspx?bookID=392. Accessed March 18, 2016.
7. Parvez S, Kang M, Chung H, et al. Survey and mechanism of skin depigmenting and lightening agents. *Phytother Res.* 2006;20(11):921–34. doi: 10.1002/ptr.1954.
8. Fisher JM, Fisher DE. From suntan to skin cancers: molecular pathways and prevention strategies. *Targ Oncol.* 2008;3(1):41–4. doi:10.1007/s11523-007-0066-1.
9. Shankar K, Godse K, Aurangabadkar S, et al. Evidence-based treatment for melasma: expert opinion and review. *Dermatol Ther (Heidelb).* 2014;4(2)165–86. doi: 10.1007/s13555-014-0064-z.
10. U.S. Food and Drug Administration. Skin bleaching drug products for over-the-counter human use; proposed rule. *Fed Regist.* 2006;71(167): 51146–55.
11. Rigopoulos D, Gregoriou S, Katsambas A. Hyperpigmentation and melasma. *J Cosmet Dermatol.* 2007;6(3):195–202. doi: 10.1111/j.1473-2165.2007.00321.x.
12. Arefiev KL, Hantash BM. Advances in the treatment of melasma: a review of the recent literature. *Dermatol Surg.* 2012;38(7 Pt 1):971–84. doi: 10.1111/j.1524-4725.2012.02435.x.
13. Gupta AK, Gover MD, Nouri K, et al. The treatment of melasma: a review of clinical trials. *J Am Acad Dermatol.* 2006;55(6):1048–65. doi: 10.1016/j.jaad.2006.02.009.
14. Davis E, Callender V. Postinflammatory hyperpigmentation: a review of the epidemiology, clinical features, and treatment options in skin of color. *J Clin Aesthetic Dermatol.* 2010;3(7):20–31. PMC2921758.
15. Konda S, Geria AN, Halder RM. New horizons in treating disorders of hyperpigmentation in skin of color. *Semin Cutan Med Surg.* 2012;31(2):133–9. doi: 10.1016/j.sder.2012.03.001.
16. Rajatanavin N, Suwanachote S, Kulkollakarn S. Dihydroxyacetone: a safe camouflaging option in vitiligo. *Int J Dermatol.* 2008;47(4):402–6. doi: 10.1111/j.1365-4632.2008.03356.x.
17. Nordlund JJ, Grimes PE, Ortonne JP. The safety of hydroquinone. *J Eur Acad Dermatol Venereol.* 2006;20(7):781–7. doi: 10.1111/j.1468-3083.2006.01670.x.
18. Draelos Z. Skin lightening preparations and the hydroquinone controversy. *Dermatol Ther.* 2007;20(5):308–13. doi: 10.1111/j.1529-8019.2007.00144.x.
19. U.S. Food and Drug Administration. Hydroquinone studies under the National Toxicology Program (NTP). Available at: http://www.fda.gov/AboutFDA/CentersOffices/OfficeofMedicalProductsandTobacco/CDER/ucm203112.htm. Accessed June 26, 2017.
20. Azzam OA, Leheta TM, Nagui NA, et al. Different therapeutic modalities for treatment of melasma. *J Cosmet Dermatol.* 2009;8(4):275–81. doi: 10.1111/j.1473-2165.2009.00471.x.
21. McEvoy GK, ed. Hydroquinone. In: *AHFS Drug Information 2007.* Bethesda, MD: American Society of Health-System Pharmacists; 2007: 3551–2.
22. Hydroquinone. Lexicomp Online. Hudson, OH: Lexi-Comp. Available at http://www.crlonline.com. Accessed May 8, 2017.
23. Hantash BM, Jimenez F. A split-face, double-blind, randomized and placebo-controlled pilot evaluation of a novel oligopeptide for the treatment of recalcitrant melasma. *J Drugs Dermatol.* 2009;8(8):732–5. doi: 10.1111/j.1365-4632.2009.04105.x.
24. Kassim AT, Hussain M, Goldberg DJ. Open-label evaluation of the skin-brightening efficacy of a skin-brightening system using decapeptide-12. *J Cosmet Laser Ther.* 2012;14(2):117–21. doi: 10.3109/14764172.2012.672745.
25. Woolery-Lloyd H, Kammer JN. Treatment of hyperpigmentation. *Semin Cutan Med Surg.* 2011;30(3):171–5. doi: 10.1016/j.sder.2011.06.004.
26. Tse TW, Hui E. Tranexamic acid: an important adjuvant in the treatment of melasma. *J Cosmet Dermatol.* 2012;12(1):57–66. doi: 10.1111/jocd.12026.
27. Ayuthaya P, Niumphradit N, Manosrol A, et al. Topical 5% tranexamic acid for the treatment of melasma in Asians: A double-blind randomized controlled clinical trial. *J Cosmet Laser Ther.* 2012;14(3):150–4. doi: 10.3109/14764172.2012.685478.
28. Garg VK, Sinha S, Sarkar R. Glycolic acid peels versus salicylic-mandelic acid peels in active acne vulgaris and post-acne scarring and hyperpigmentation: a comparative study. *Dermatol Surg.* 2009;35(1):59–65. doi: 10.1111/j.1524-4725.2008.34383.x.
29. Vashi NA, Kundu RV. Facial hyperpigmentation: causes and treatment. *Br J Dermatol.* 2013;169(3):41–56. doi: 10.1111/bjd.12536.
30. Navarrete-Solis J, Castandeo-Cazares JP, Torres-Alvarez B, et al. A double-blind, randomized clinical trial of niacinamide 4% versus hydroquinone 4% in the treatment of melasma. *Dermatol Res Pract.* 2011;2011:379173. doi: 10.1155/2011/379173.
31. Castenado-Cazares J, Larraga-Pinones G, Ehnis-Perez A, et al. Topical niacinamide 4% and desonide 0.05% for treatment of axillary hyperpigmentation: A randomized, double-blind, placebo-controlled study. *Clin Cosmet Investig Dermatol.* 2013;6:29–36. doi: 10.2147/CCID.
32. Lee D, Oh I, Koo K, et al. Reduction in facial hyperpigmentation after treatment with a combination of topical niacinamide and tranexamic acid: a randomized, double-blind, vehicle-controlled trial. *Skin Res Technol.* 2014;20(2):208–12. doi: 10.1111/srt.12107.
33. Kimball A, Kaczvinsky J, Li J, et al. Reduction in the appearance of facial hyperpigmentation after use of moisturizers with a combination of topical niacinamide and N-acetyl glucosamine: results of a randomized, double-blind, vehicle-controlled trial. *Br J Dermatol.* 2010;162(2):435–41. doi: 10.1111/j.1365-2133.2009.09477.x.
34. Han A, Chien A, Kang S. Photoaging. *Dermatol Clin.* 2014;32(3):291–9. doi: 10.1016/j.det.2014.03.015.
35. Rabe JH, Mamelak AJ, McElgunn PJ, et al. Photoaging: mechanisms and repair. *J Am Acad Dermatol.* 2006;55(1):1–19. doi: 10.1016/j.jaad.2005.05.010.
36. Rodriques M, Pandya AG. Melasma: clinical diagnosis and management options. *Australas J Dermatol.* 2015;56(3):151–63. doi: 10.1111/ajd.12290.
37. Yarr M, Gilchrest B. Aging of skin. In: Goldsmith LA, Katz SI, Gilchrest BA, eds. *Fitzpatrick's Dermatology in General Medicine.* 8th ed. New York, NY: McGraw-Hill; 2012. Available at: http://accessmedicine.mhmedical.com/book.aspx?bookID=392. Accessed March 18, 2016.
38. Yaar M, Gilchrest BA. Photoaging: mechanism, prevention and therapy. *Br J Dermatol.* 2007;157(5):874–87. doi: 10.1111/j.1365-2133.2007.08108.x.
39. Archer DF. Postmenopausal skin and estrogen. *Gynecol Endocrinol.* 2012;28(Suppl 2):2–6. doi: 10.3109/09513590.2012.705392.
40. Antoniou C, Kosmadaki MG, Stratigos AJ, et al. Photoaging: prevention and topical treatments. *Am J Clin Dermatol.* 2010;11(2):95–102. doi: 10.2165/11530210-000000000-00000.

41. Baumann L. Cosmetics and skin care in dermatology. In: Goldsmith LA, Katz S, Gilchrest BA, eds. *Fitzpatrick's Dermatology in General Medicine.* 8th ed. New York, NY: McGraw-Hill; 2012. Available at: http://accessmedicine.mhmedical.com/book.aspx?bookID=392. Accessed March 18, 2016.
42. Newburger AE. Cosmeceuticals: myths and misconceptions. *Clin Dermatol.* 2009;27(5):446–52. doi: 10.1016/j.clindermatol.2009.05.008.
43. Zussman J, Ahdout J, Kim J. Vitamins and photoaging: do scientific data support their use? *J Am Acad Dermatol.* 2010;63(3):507–25. doi: 10.1016/j.jaad.2009.07.037.
44. Huang CK, Miller TA. The truth about over-the-counter topical anti-aging products: a comprehensive review. *Aesthetic Surg J.* 2007;27(4): 402–12. doi: 10.1016/j.asj.2007.05.005.
45. U.S. Food and Drug Administration. Guidance for industry: labeling for cosmetics containing alpha hydroxy acids. January 10, 2005. Last updated June 30, 2016. Available at: http://www.fda.gov/Cosmetics/GuidanceRegulation/GuidanceDocuments/ucm090816.htm. Accessed June 22, 2017.
46. Fabbrocini G, De Padova MP, Tosti A. Chemical peels: what's new and what isn't new but still works well. *Facial Plast Surg.* 2009;25(5): 329–36. doi: 10.1055/s-0029-1243082.
47. Kessler E, Flanagan K, Chia C, et al. Comparison of a- and b-hydroxy acid chemical peels in the treatment of mild to moderately severe facial acne vulgaris. *Dermatol Surg.* 2008;34(1):45–51. doi: 10.1111/j.1524-4725.2007.34007.x.
48. Landau M. Chemical peels. *Clin Dermatol.* 2008;26(2):200–8. doi: 10.1016/j.clindermatol.2007.09.012.
49. Bradley EJ, Griffiths C, Sherratt MJ, et al. Over-the-counter anti-ageing topical agents and their ability to protect and repair photoaged skin. *Maturitas.* 2015;80:265–72. doi: 10.1016/j.maturitas.2014.12.019.
50. D'Orazio J, Jarrett S, Amaro-Ortiz A, Scott T. UV radiation and the skin. *Int J Mol Sci.* 2013;14(6):12222–48. doi: 10.3390/ijms140612222.

CHAPTER 41

MINOR BURNS, SUNBURN, AND WOUNDS

DAPHNE B. BERNARD

Pharmacists often provide guidance to patients needing treatment for minor burns and wounds. A quick assessment helps to identify appropriate products and procedures to manage cuts, burns, and scrapes and to speed the healing process. Burn and wound care management can be quite resource intensive, with much of the cost related to fees for emergency department visits and the expense of the medications and supplies used for wound healing. Thousands of people seek medical treatment for skin injuries each year. For example, approximately 450,000 patients per year are estimated to receive burn injuries that require medical treatment.[1]

Because patients commonly use self-care in burn and wound management, a thorough knowledge of skin injuries and how they heal is essential for health care providers likely to be consulted regarding treatment of such injuries. Although healthy skin is well equipped for effective and efficient repair of minor burns and wounds, selection of the proper dressing and appropriate use of antiseptics and antibiotics will facilitate healing, minimize scar formation, and prevent secondary bacterial skin infections. At the initial patient–provider encounter, an accurate assessment of the injury is essential to determine whether self-care or referral for further evaluation is appropriate.

Pathophysiology of Minor Burns, Sunburn, and Wounds

Skin injuries are described according to cause and depth of damage. *Acute* wounds include burns, abrasions, punctures, and lacerations—in this chapter, those designated as minor. These types of wounds typically are caused by trauma of lesser degree and, with proper care, tend to heal within 1 month in healthy adults. By contrast, any wound that does not heal properly through the normal stages of tissue repair is considered a *chronic* wound and requires referral for more intensive medical care. Chronic wounds are not discussed in this chapter.

Burns are wounds caused by thermal, electrical, chemical, or ultraviolet radiation (UVR) exposure.

Thermal burns result from skin contact with flames, scalding liquids, or hot objects (e.g., irons, oven broiler elements, hot pans, curling irons, radiators) or from the inhalation of smoke or hot vapors. Figure 41–1 shows a cross section of the anatomy of the skin and the depth of injury with thermal burns of increasing severity. (See Chapter 33 for further discussion of skin anatomy and physiology.)

Chemical burns occur secondary to exposure to corrosive or reactive chemicals that cause tissue damage, ulceration, and sloughing. The necrotic tissue often acts as a reservoir of the harmful chemical, allowing its continued absorption and prolonging exposure of adjacent skin, with increased cutaneous damage and tissue injury.[2] If not adherent to the skin, clothing that has been exposed to chemicals should be removed to prevent continued burn insult to the affected area. The provider should refer all patients with chemical burns to a hospital emergency department for evaluation.

Sunburn is caused by too much exposure to ultraviolet A (UVA) and ultraviolet B (UVB) light in natural sunlight, and from use of commercial tanning beds and tanning lamps (see Color Plates, photograph 29). UVA radiation accounts for approximately 95% of the radiation that reaches the surface of the earth. It penetrates the skin more deeply than UVB radiation and is responsible for tanning and photoaging of the skin. It also plays a role in the development of skin cancers and drug-induced photoallergy and photosensitivity reactions that can resemble sunburn (see Color Plates, photographs 30 and 31). UVB radiation is the primary cause of the erythema associated with sunburn. It also contributes to tanning and photoaging, but to a much more restricted extent than for UVA radiation.[3] (See Chapter 39 for a discussion of UVR bands.)

Abrasions usually result from rubbing or friction and affect the epidermal layer of the skin, extending to the uppermost portion of the dermis. *Punctures* usually result from piercing of the epidermis by a sharp-pointed object and may reach into the dermis or deeper tissues. *Lacerations* result from cutting through the various layers of the skin by a sharp-edged object.[4]

Self-treatment of acute wounds such as abrasions, cuts (lacerations), punctures, and burn wounds that do not extend beyond the dermis is generally deemed appropriate.

For providers to identify the appropriate course of action, including patient counseling, understanding the physiology of wound healing is just as important as understanding the pathology of the wound itself. Skin integrity depends on a delicate balance between structure and function. When a burn or other wound disturbs this balance, prompt restoration is required to ensure body homeostasis and proper wound healing.

The process of wound healing begins immediately after injury and consists of three overlapping phases: inflammatory, proliferative, and maturation (remodeling).[5]

The *inflammatory phase* is the body's immediate response to injury. This phase, which lasts approximately 3–4 days, is responsible for preparing the wound for subsequent tissue development

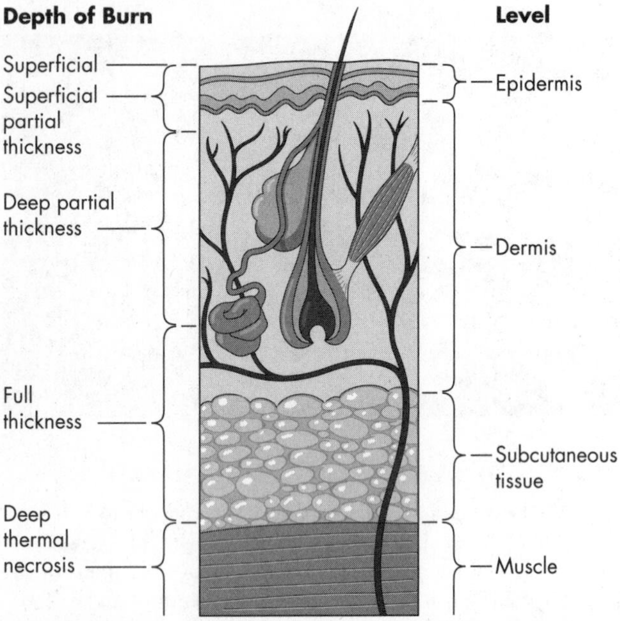

FIGURE 41-1 Cross section of skin showing depth of injury in burns of increasing severity.

and consists of two primary parts: hemostasis and inflammation. Hemostasis is initiated by the release of thromboplastin from injured cells to form a clot, the main event in the physiologic process that stops bleeding, so that tissue repair can begin. Later in the inflammatory phase, debris and bacteria are removed from the wound area. Collagen is formed to stimulate wound healing, and epithelial cells migrate to cover the wound bed and provide the initial layer (just one cell thick) of new skin that will cover the wound.[5]

In the next phase of healing, the *proliferative phase,* the wound is filled with new connective tissue and covered with new epithelium. This phase starts on day 3 or 4 and continues for approximately 3 weeks. It involves the formation of granulation tissue, which is a collection of new connective tissue (fibroblasts and newly synthesized collagen), new capillaries, and inflammatory cells.[5]

The final phase of healing is known as the *maturation* or *remodeling phase.* This is the longest phase, beginning at approximately week 3, when the wound is completely closed by connective tissue and resurfaced by epithelial cells. It involves a continual process of collagen synthesis and breakdown, with replacement of earlier-constituted, weak collagen by high-tensile-strength collagen; this process peaks approximately 60 days after the injury occurred.[5]

Several local and systemic factors can affect how efficiently and to what extent a wound will heal. *Local* factors associated with delayed or otherwise poor healing include inadequate tissue perfusion and oxygenation, infection, and unfavorable wound characteristics. The most important *systemic* factors that can impair the healing process are poor vascularization, bacterial contamination, inadequate nutrition, coexisting medical conditions, and medication effects.

Poor vascularization delays wound healing. The resulting poor oxygenation leads to impaired leukocyte activity, decreased production of collagen, decreased epithelialization, and reduced resistance to infection. Common disorders that may cause decreased perfusion include diabetes, severe anemia, hypotension, peripheral vascular disease, and congestive heart failure.[6]

Wound infection occurs as a consequence of deposition and multiplication of organisms in tissue with an associated host reaction. Some fungi and protozoa have been implicated as pathogens in this setting, but most minor wound infections are caused by bacteria, especially *Streptococcus pyogenes, Enterococcus faecalis,* and *Staphylococcus aureus.* Of these, *S. aureus* is the most common. When the number of bacteria is excessive, wounds can become infected. Localized infection in the wound delays collagen synthesis and epithelialization, prolongs the inflammatory phase, and causes additional tissue destruction.[7]

Adequate nutrition provides the building blocks for wound repair. Protein, carbohydrates, vitamins, and trace elements are needed for collagen production and cellular energy.[8] Vitamin supplements are commonly used to manage wound healing. Vitamin C has many roles in wound healing, so a deficiency of this vitamin has multiple adverse effects on tissue repair. A well-recognized result of such deficiency is impaired healing, with links to decreased collagen synthesis and fibroblast proliferation, decreased angiogenesis, and increased capillary fragility. In addition, deficiency of vitamin C is associated with an impaired immune response and increased susceptibility to wound infection. Vitamin E also has anti-inflammatory properties and has been suggested to have a role in decreasing excess scar formation in chronic wounds. Animal experiments have indicated that vitamin E supplementation is beneficial to wound healing, and topical vitamin E has been widely promoted as an antiscarring agent.[9]

It is commonly recognized that even in healthy older adults, the effects of aging include a temporal delay in wound healing, but not an actual impairment in terms of the quality of healing.[10] Patients who are obese have problems with poor perfusion (adipose tissue lacks blood flow) and tend to have delayed wound healing.[11]

Poorly controlled diabetes usually is associated with reduced collagen synthesis, impaired wound contraction, delayed epidermal migration, and reduced polymorphonuclear leukocyte chemotaxis and phagocytosis. Because of these inherent difficulties, strict professional attention is warranted for wounds in patients with diabetes.[12] Some medications have the capacity to affect wound healing, such as those that interfere with clot formation or platelet function or with inflammatory responses and cell proliferation. Glucocorticosteroids inhibit wound repair through global anti-inflammatory effects and suppression of cellular wound responses, including fibroblast proliferation and collagen synthesis. Systemic steroids cause wounds to heal with incomplete granulation tissue and reduced wound contraction. In addition, chemotherapeutic drugs delay cell migration into the wound, decrease early wound matrix formation, lower collagen production, impair proliferation of fibroblasts, and inhibit contraction of wounds.[11] In patients with wounds who are taking these medications, careful follow-up by a wound care specialist is indicated to ensure that proper healing occurs.

Local features that may impair wound closure include poor oxygenation resulting from inadequate perfusion, with chronic hypoxia and inflammation largely secondary to infection; the presence of necrotic tissue, eschar (i.e., scab), or foreign bodies (e.g., glass, dirt); inadequate moisture; and infection.[13] Providers who are aware of and can recognize problems associated with these local factors can provide more effective wound care management instructions to ensure faster wound healing.

Clinical Presentation of Minor Burns, Sunburn, and Wounds

The clinical presentation of burns, sunburn, and wounds is largely determined by the depth of skin damage. For simplification, this depth classification (Figure 41–2) has been divided into four descriptive stages of injury.

Stage I skin injuries (i.e., minor sunburn and superficial burns) involve only the epidermis, with no loss of any skin layers, and consist primarily of reddened, nonblanching, unbroken, nonblistering skin. Minor sunburn causes a superficial burn injury characterized by erythema and slight dermal edema that results from increased blood flow to the affected skin. The increase in blood flow begins approximately 4 hours after exposure, peaking between 12 and 24 hours. Other superficial burns usually result from a brief exposure to low heat, causing a painful area of erythema similar to sunburn but without significant damage to epithelial cells. Avoidance of additional injury and symptomatic relief of pain and fever are usually the only treatment measures required. A majority of superficial burns can be managed with self-care or through ambulatory care centers and will heal within 3–6 days.[14]

Stage II skin injuries (i.e., severe sunburn, abrasions, superficial lacerations and punctures, superficial partial-thickness burns, and deep partial-thickness burns) include blistering or partial-thickness skin loss that involves all of the epidermis and part of the dermis. Because the injury involves a break in the skin, drainage from the wound area may occur, in addition to pain, edema, and erythema. Severe sunburns fall into this category and result in blisters that subsequently desquamate or "peel" over a period of several days. There is a slight chance of bacterial infection because of the loss of the outer skin barrier (see Color Plates, photograph 29). Pain, edema, and skin tenderness accompany the erythema. Systemic signs and symptoms such as vomiting, low-grade fever, chills, weakness, and shock are not uncommon in patients in whom a large portion of the skin surface has been affected. After exfoliation and for several weeks thereafter, the skin will be more susceptible than normal to sunburn.[14]

In addition to sun exposure, stage II burns may result from higher levels of heat or longer exposures than in superficial burns. Damage to the epidermis and dermis layers produces painful blistering, and these lesions can be superficial partial-thickness or deep partial-thickness injuries. The burns often occur from a splash or spill of hot liquid, brief contact with a hot object, flash ignition, chemical contact, or exposure to a flame. Stage II burns are painful and sensitive to temperature and air. A specific feature of such burns is blanching, indicating loss of blood vessels to the area. The burned area may be patchy white to red in appearance, often with large blisters. Pain may be more intense than with superficial burns because of the irritation to nerve endings, although some affected areas may lack sensation. Wound resurfacing can occur because nests of epithelial cells that line the hair follicles and sweat glands that survive in the burned area will initiate the healing process. In such cases, however, healing may be slow, and scarring is likely.

Stage II burns are prone to infection because of the loss of barrier function and vasculature. Infection will increase the severity of a burn injury or its depth, or both. If the damage does not involve the deeper proliferating area of the epidermis (as in superficial partial-thickness burns), rapid regeneration of a normal epidermis usually results within 2–3 weeks, with minimal or no scarring. If more of the dermis is involved (as in deep partial-thickness burns), the wound will take longer to heal (up to 6 weeks), with the potential for thick scar formation (hypertrophic scarring or cheloid), as well as contractures of the skin and underlying tissues that can affect use of the involved areas.

Small stage II burns restricted to 1%–2% of body surface area (BSA) usually can be managed with self-care measures. However, superficial partial-thickness burns in a child or a patient with multiple medical problems or those involving more than 10% of BSA necessitate hospitalization with fluid restoration. All stage II burns that fail to heal within 2–3 weeks or those associated with pain, redness, exudate formation, fever, odor, or malaise that persists days or weeks after the initial injury warrant referral for medical evaluation. Finally, patients with deep partial-thickness burns should be evaluated in a hospital emergency department. These burn injuries can convert to full-thickness injuries if not properly and promptly managed.[14]

Stage III skin injuries (i.e., full-thickness burns and deep lacerations and punctures) include those with full-thickness skin loss associated with damage to the entire epidermis, dermis, and dermal appendages and may involve subcutaneous tissue. Heat exposure that is more intense than that causing deep partial-thickness burns will cause death of the entire skin layer (i.e., full-thickness injury) in the affected area, resulting in dry, leathery tissue that is painless and insensate. Deep punctures and lacerations can be quite painful. Deep lacerations bleed profusely, and underlying tissue layers may be visible in the wound bed. The body attempts to heal such wounds by sloughing off the dead layer and contracting the

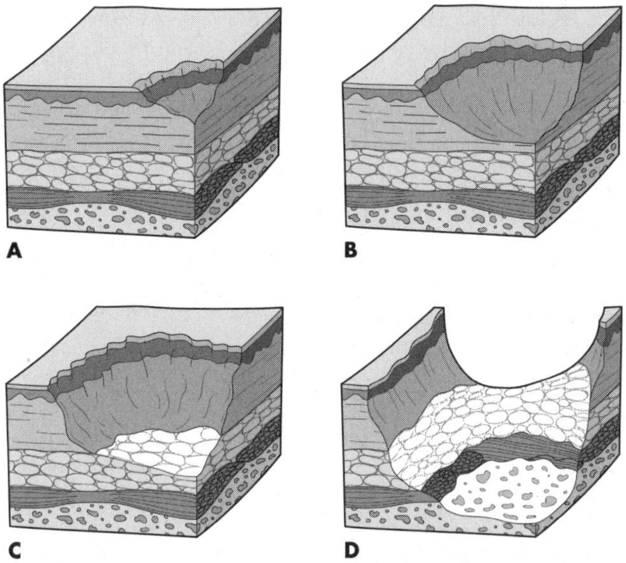

FIGURE **41–2** Stages of wounds. **A**, Stage I: Nonblanchable erythema of intact skin with warmth and redness. **B**, Stage II: Superficial lesions with partial-thickness skin loss involving the epidermis with or without extension into the dermis. **C**, Stage III: Full-thickness skin loss with damage to subcutaneous tissue. **D**, Stage IV: Full-thickness skin loss with extensive tissue necrosis and damage to underlying muscle, tendon, and bone.

wound edges. Hospitalization is normally required for treatment of full-thickness burns.[14] Patients suffering from deep lacerations or punctures should seek emergency care as soon as possible.

Stage IV skin injury is an extension of Stage III injury and involves the subcutaneous tissue and underlying muscle, tendon, and bone.[4]

For both providers and patients, an understanding of these skin injury stages will help in selecting appropriate dressings for optimal wound closure.

Figures 41–1 and 41–2 illustrate the depth and associated stages of skin injury.

Treatment of Minor Burns, Sunburn, and Wounds

Treatment Goals

The goals in treating acute, minor skin injury are (1) to relieve symptoms, (2) to promote healing by protecting the burn or wound from infection and further trauma, and (3) to minimize scarring. Treatment should include a stepwise approach that involves careful cleansing of the damaged area, selective use of antiseptics and antibiotics, and closing or covering the wound with an appropriate dressing.

General Treatment Approach

The extent and depth of stage I and stage II burns should be assessed for self-treatment, both initially and again in 24–48 hours. The inflammatory response to a burn injury evolves over the first 24–48 hours, so the initial appearance of the injury often leads to an underestimation of its actual severity. If the patient has none of the exclusions for self-treatment listed in Figure 41–3, the provider should recommend appropriate measures using the treatment approach outlined in the algorithm. If the burned area is 2% of BSA or larger and consists of superficial partial-thickness or deeper injury, medical attention is needed. Figure 41–4 illustrates the rule-of-nines method for estimating the percentage of affected BSA. Stage III and Stage IV skin injuries (e.g., animal or human bites, puncture wounds, severe burns) require immediate medical evaluation. Specifically, these injuries necessitate primary care provider consultation to assess the need for systemic or topical prescription antibiotics and a tetanus booster to prevent infection from the tetanus toxin occasionally found in dust, soil, and animal waste.

Treatment of uncontaminated acute skin injuries rated as stages I and II (Figure 41–2), such as minor cuts, scrapes, and burns, requires only basic supportive measures, including irrigation with saline or water for removal of debris from the damaged area and use of a wound dressing to keep the area moist and to prevent entry of bacteria into the affected area. Topical nonprescription antibiotic and antiseptic preparations can also be useful in preventing secondary infection, especially when debris or other foreign particulate matter that increases the risk of infection is present. Figure 41–5 outlines the triage and treatment of acute skin injuries.

Nonpharmacologic Therapy

Nonpharmacologic therapy used in the treatment of stage I and stage II skin injuries primarily involves first aid measures to relieve pain, prevent contamination, and promote healing. The approach involves steps to remove exposure to the offending agent, stop bleeding and weeping from exudates, cool burned skin, provide pain relief, decrease infection risk, and protect the area from further trauma.

Wound irrigation is often necessary to clean the wound surface by removing dirt and debris. Flushing with normal saline or tap water usually is sufficient for irrigation; however, mechanical removal of debris with clean gauze is sometimes appropriate. Minor abrasions and lacerations should be cleansed with water or sterile saline to remove any debris. They should then be covered with an appropriate wound dressing.

The patient or the provider should inspect puncture wounds to ensure that no foreign bodies are retained, and tetanus prophylaxis should be updated if necessary. If no debris is present, the wound should then be cleansed with either water or sterile saline. The wound should be left open and soaked with soapy water for 30 minutes, at least 4 times a day initially, to allow for proper healing.[10] The wound should then be covered with an appropriate wound dressing.

Specific first aid measures for the care of burns are described in Figure 41–3. Reducing further trauma to the site of skin injury caused by burns is done by immediately removing the source of heat and actively cooling the burn wound with cool tap water (by means of lavage, soaks, application of compresses, or immersion). Continuous cooling for the first 10 minutes dissipates heat, reduces pain, and delays onset and minimizes the extent of burn edema by decreasing histamine release from skin mast cells. Cooling beyond 10 minutes may provide pain relief to the patient. It is best to avoid the application of ice or ice-cold water because this may cause numbness and intense vasoconstriction, resulting in further tissue damage. Chemical burns should be irrigated with copious amounts of water to reduce the size and extent of the injury.[15]

A nonadherent, hypoallergenic dressing may be applied to the wound to protect the damaged area and speed wound healing (Table 41–1). Minor skin injuries usually heal without additional treatment. Patients should be advised not to pull at loose skin or peel off burned skin because viable skin may be removed in the process, thereby delaying healing.

In the case of chemical burns, the patient should immediately remove any clothing on or near the affected area. The affected area should then be washed with tap water for at least 15 minutes or longer until the offending agent has been removed. This treatment, however, should not delay transport to a hospital emergency department.

If the eye is involved, the eyelid should be pulled back and the eye irrigated with tap water for at least 15–30 minutes. The irrigation fluid should flow from the nasal side of the eye to the outside corner, to prevent washing the contaminant into the other eye. The area poison control center should be contacted immediately at 800-222-1222 for treatment recommendations. Referral for further evaluation is frequently encouraged for eye injuries, and medical attention should be sought as soon as possible.

Wound Dressing

Traditional wound management involves leaving the wound open to air or covering it with a nonocclusive textile dressing (gauze). However, this type of management leads to eschar (i.e., scab) formation, which impedes reepithelialization of wounds and creates

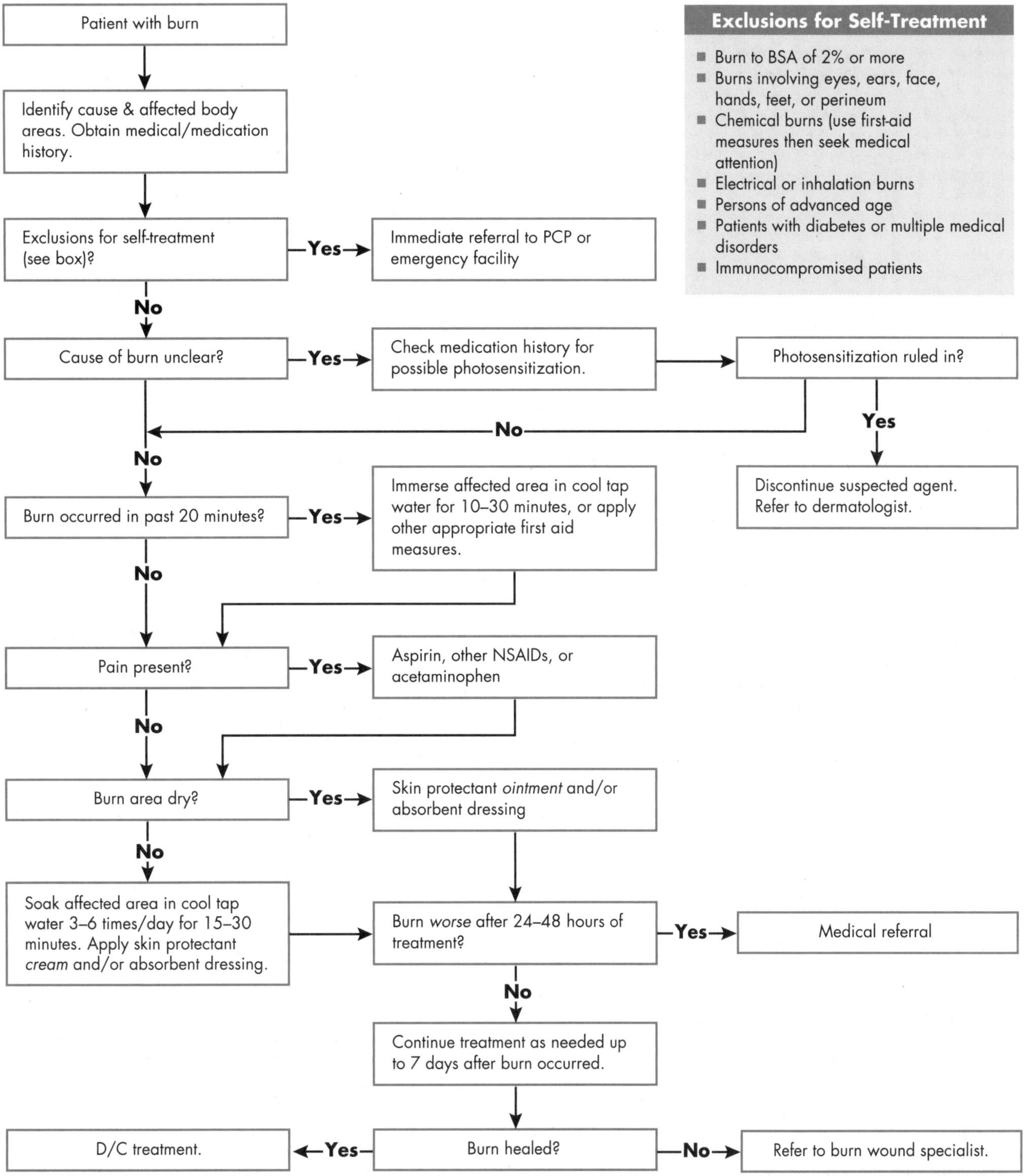

FIGURE 41–3 Self-care for minor burns and sunburn. Key: BSA = Body surface area; D/C = discontinue; NSAID = nonsteroidal anti-inflammatory drug; PCP = primary care provider.

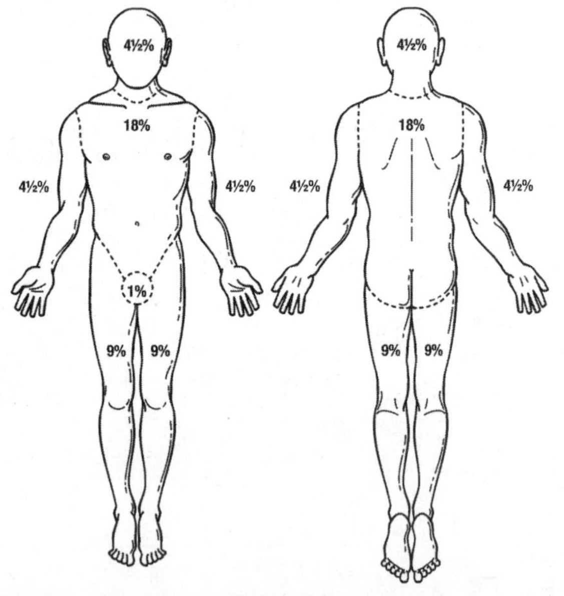

FIGURE 41–4 Rule-of-nines method for quickly establishing the percentage of adult body surface burned. (Source: Adapted with permission from *The Guide to Fluid Therapy*. Deerfield, IL: Baxter Laboratories; 1969:111.)

unwanted scar tissue (Figure 41–6A). Wound dehydration with delayed healing and increased risk of bacterial entry into the wound also may occur. Removal of gauze dressings often tears away not only the eschar but also the new tissue under the eschar. These cumulative problems have led primary care providers and nurses to develop new treatment strategies that are based on creating a moist wound environment (Figure 41–6B). The moist environment reduces the loss of protein, electrolytes, and fluid from the wound to help minimize pain and reduce the risk of infection.[16] Providers should still recommend the use of gauze and gauze-type adhesive dressings under certain circumstances; for example, gauze pads may be used with more advanced semiocclusive dressings such as foams for better exudate absorption. Gauze dressings also assist with the removal of eschar and necrotic tissue when wound debridement is necessary. In addition, gauze-type adhesive bandages may be used for stage I skin injuries for which the possible removal of excess granulation tissue is not a concern.

Selection Criteria for Wound Dressings

Choosing the right dressing depends on proper assessment of skin injury and of characteristics of the wound bed. Healing requires the appropriate type and amount of moisture in the wound bed to enhance healing. The role of a wound dressing is to provide the right environment to enhance and promote wound healing. A moist healing environment stimulates cell proliferation and encourages epithelial cells to migrate. Moisture-retentive dressings also act as a barrier against bacteria and absorb excess wound fluid, creating opportune conditions for healing. Today's wound dressings can also help decrease or eliminate pain, reduce the need for dressing changes, and provide autolytic debridement. Used appropriately, they are also cost-effective.[17]

An understanding of the potential use and function of specific wound dressings should guide the provider in proper product selection. Also, wound dressing requirements may change with each healing phase. In terms of promoting moist wound healing, the wound dressing may be used to absorb excess moisture, maintain optimal moisture, or provide moisture when it is lacking. Table 41–1 and Figure 41–7 describe the major categories of available wound care products and give an overview of their indications, advantages, and disadvantages.[17,18]

Types of Wound Dressings

Gauze

Gauze is available in a variety of forms and is generally used in the care of minor burns and wounds that are draining or those requiring debridement. It is available in woven and nonwoven forms and can be impregnated with nonadherent products such as petrolatum, as well as with antiseptics and antimicrobials. Some advantages of gauze are that it is readily available in many sizes and forms, it is affordable, and it can be combined with other topical products. Disadvantages of gauze are that it must be held in place by a second agent, its fibers may adhere to the wound bed, and it must be changed often (preferably several times a day) to prevent the wound from drying out. In addition, gauze alone is not recommended for moist wound treatment. Examples of gauze products are Kerlix, Kling, and Conform.[17]

Antimicrobial

Antimicrobial dressings contain products like silver and iodine and are often used in the management of wounds that are colonized or infected. As exudates from the wound bed are slowly absorbed, silver and iodine are gradually released to decrease the bacterial load within the wound bed. Examples are Acticoat, Actisorb, and Iodoflex.[19]

Specialty Wound Dressings

Often the practitioner must maintain a delicate balance of moisture and wound healing.[17] Specialty dressings are available that absorb excess moisture (e.g., foams, alginates), maintain moisture (e.g., hydrocolloid and transparent film dressings), or provide moisture when it is lacking (e.g., hydrogels).

Dressings that absorb moisture are beneficial early in the inflammatory phase of healing. The wound tissue may be overly moist as a result of the accumulation of fluid evaporated by exposed damaged tissue and from blood and serous drainage. With a wound that is "too wet," maceration of the surrounding tissue may result.[20] A wound that exudes moderate–high levels of drainage requires use of absorbent dressings (e.g., foam, alginates, carbon-impregnated, composite dressings). Such dressings offer the benefit of requiring fewer changes than are needed with the nonabsorbent type, enabling undisturbed wound healing. Examples are Kaltostat, Repel, Mepilex, and Actisorb.

Dressings that maintain moisture are preferred as healing moves to the proliferative phase, with the formation of new connective tissue. Dressings that maintain natural moisture, such as hydrocolloid and transparent film dressings, are preferred in this phase.[17,18] Examples are Exuderm and Suresite.

Dressings that provide moisture are preferred when a dry wound that is covered with dead tissue needs to be rehydrated before optimal healing can occur. Providing moisture will soften the dead tissue for easier removal while promoting autolytic debridement, which facilitates the migration of newly formed epithelial tissue to

Exclusions for Self-Treatment

- Wound containing foreign matter after irrigation
- Chronic wound
- Wound secondary to an animal or human bite
- Signs of infection
- Involvement of face, mucous membrane, or genitalia
- Deep, acute wound
- Patients with diabetes

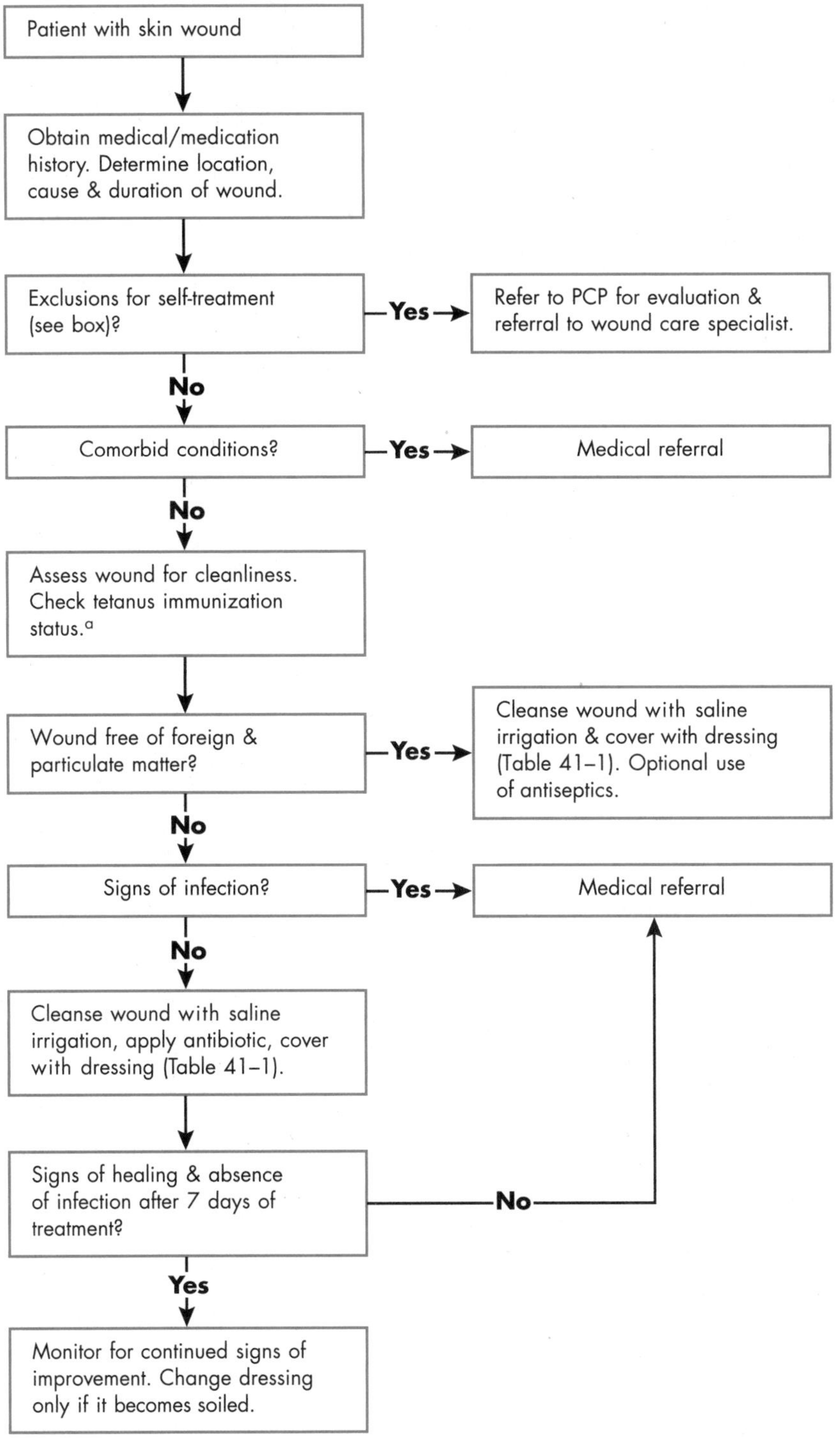
Patient with skin wound
Obtain medical/medication history. Determine location, cause & duration of wound.
Exclusions for self-treatment (see box)?
Yes
Refer to PCP for evaluation & referral to wound care specialist.
No
Comorbid conditions?
Yes
Medical referral
No
Assess wound for cleanliness. Check tetanus immunization status.[a]
Wound free of foreign & particulate matter?
Yes
Cleanse wound with saline irrigation & cover with dressing (Table 41–1). Optional use of antiseptics.
No
Signs of infection?
Yes
Medical referral
No
Cleanse wound with saline irrigation, apply antibiotic, cover with dressing (Table 41–1).
Signs of healing & absence of infection after 7 days of treatment?
No
Yes
Monitor for continued signs of improvement. Change dressing only if it becomes soiled.

[a] If basic series has been completed, one dose is required every 10 years.

FIGURE 41-5 Self-care for acute skin wounds. Key: PCP = Primary care provider.

TABLE 41–1 Options in Wound Dressings

Description (With Trade Names for Product Type)[a]	Uses/Indications	Advantages	Disadvantages
Gauze Dressings			
Nonocclusive fiber dressing with loose, open weave (Sterilux Bulky Gauge Bandage, Conform, Kerlix Rolls and Sponges, Kling Rolls)	Stages II–IV Minimal–heavy exudate/topicals Debridement Wound rehydration May use with semiocclusive dressings	Readily available in many sizes Deep wound packing May use with infected wounds/topicals Nonocclusive Conformable	Wound bed may desiccate if dressing is dry. Nonselective debridement May cause bleeding/pain on removal Need secondary dressing Frequent dressing changes
Nonadherent (Gauze-Type) Dressings			
Nonadherent, porous dressings lightly coated (Adaptic, Nexcare Non-Stick Pads, Telfa, Vaseline Gauze)	Skin donor sites Stage II, shallow Stage III Staple/suture lines Abrasions Lacerations Punctures May use with semiocclusive dressings	Readily available Less adherent than plain gauze Lightly coated dressings allow exudate to flow through.	Need secondary dressing May cause bleeding/pain on removal Some impregnated dressings may delay healing. Frequent dressing changes may be required. Some may cause exudate pooling.
Foams			
Semipermeable, nonwoven, absorptive, inert polyurethane foam dressings (Allevyn, Hydrasorb, Lyofoam) (Figure 41–6C)	Stage II, shallow stage III Minimal–moderate drainage	Most are nonadhesive. Some can be used with infected wounds/topicals. Thermal insulation Reduce pain Nonocclusive Moist environment Conformable Less frequent dressing changes Trauma-free removal Absorbent	Most require secondary dressing. May require cutting May cause wound desiccation May be difficult to determine wound contact surface
Alginates			
Hydrophilic, nonwoven dressings composed of calcium-sodium (percentages vary) alginate fibers (Algosteril, Nu-Derm, Kaltostat, Sorbsan) Alginates are processed from brown seaweed into pad or twisted fiber form; exudate transforms fibers to gel at wound interface.	Light–heavy exudate Stages II, III, IV Skin donor sites	Absorptive Reduce pain Nonocclusive Moist environment Conformable Easy, trauma-free removal Can use on infected wounds Accelerate healing time Less frequent dressing changes Potential to aid in control of minor bleeding	Secondary dressing required Characteristic odor May need wound irrigation May desiccate May promote hypergranulation

TABLE 41–1 Options in Wound Dressings *(continued)*

Description (With Trade Names for Product Type)[a]	Uses/Indications	Advantages	Disadvantages
Carbon-Impregnated (Odor Control) Dressings			
Dressings with an outer layer of carbon for odor control (Carboflex, Actisorb)	Malodorous wounds	Control odor	Appropriate seal required to prevent odor escaping Carbon is inactivated when it becomes wet.
Composite/Island Dressings			
Nonadherent, absorptive center barrier with adhesive at perimeter (Allevyn Island, Lyofoam A, Viasorb)	Stages II, III Moderate–heavy exudate	Nonadherent over wound Semiocclusive Autolysis Suture/staple lines Protective and reduce pain No secondary dressing required Impermeable to fluids/bacteria	May cause periwound trauma on removal
Hydrocolloids			
Wafer dressings composed of hydrophilic particles in an adhesive form covered by a water-resistant film or foam (Band-Aid Brand Advanced Healing Strips, Comfeel Plus, Cutinova, DuoDERM CGF Dressing, Exuderm, Tega-sorb, ULTEC Pro, Nu-Derm) (Figure 41–6D)	Stages I, II, shallow stage III Clean, granular wounds Autolysis Minimal–moderate exudate Can use with absorption products and alginates	Occlusive Manage exudate by particle swelling Autolysis Long wear time Self-adherent Impermeable to fluids/bacteria Conformable Protective Thermal insulation Reduce pain Moist environment	For uninfected wounds only May cause periwound trauma on removal Difficult wound assessment Characteristic odor Impermeable to gases Some may leave residue on skin or in wound.
Transparent Adhesive Films			
Semiocclusive, translucent dressings with partial or continuous adhesive composed of polyurethane or copolyester thin film (BIOCLUSIVE, Blisterfilm, OpSite, Suresite, Tegaderm) (Figure 41–6E)	Stages I, II, shallow stage III Clean granular wounds Minimal exudate Autolysis Can use with absorption products and alginates Can be used in conjunction with some enzymatic debriders	Semiocclusive Gas-permeable Easy inspection Autolysis Protective Impermeable to fluids/bacteria Comfortable Self-adherent Reduce pain Moist environment Shear-resistant	For uninfected wounds only Not absorptive May cause periwound trauma on removal With continuous adhesive, may reinjure wound on removal With large amounts of exudate, maceration may occur.

(continued)

TABLE 41-1 **Options in Wound Dressings** *(continued)*

Description (With Trade Names for Product Type)[a]	Uses/Indications	Advantages	Disadvantages
Hydrogels/Gels			
Nonadherent, nonocclusive dressings with high moisture content that come in the form of sheets and gels (Aquasite, FlexiGel, Burn Free, MoistBurn, 2nd Skin Moist Burn Pads, Vigilon Primary Wound Dressing) (Figure 41–6F)	Stages II, III, some approved for stage IV Granular or necrotic wound beds Autolysis Some used on partial- and full-thickness burns Punctures	Nonadherent Most are nonocclusive. Trauma-free removal Varying absorption capabilities Conformable Some can be used in conjunction with topicals. Thermal insulation Reduce pain Moist environment	Most require secondary dressings. May macerate periwound skin Some products may dehydrate. Slow to minimal absorption rate in most Most require frequent/daily dressing changes.
Antimicrobial			
Dressings that contain an antimicrobial agent to reduce bacterial contamination (Acticoat, Actisorb Silver 220, Aquacel Hydrofiber Dressing, Iodoflex Pad)	Stages II, III, and IV All locally infected wounds	Nonadherent Absorbent Reduce infection	Use caution in patients with thyroid disease because of increased iodine absorption. Skin allergy

[a] The trade names that appear with each type of wound dressing are given as examples of available products; these examples do not constitute an all-inclusive list of such products.

Source: Adapted with permission from an unpublished document prepared by McIntosh A, Raher E. Silver Cross Hospital, Joliet, IL; 1991.

the wound bed. A wound dressing must contain water to effectively add moisture to a wound and promote healing. Hydrogel dressings can consist of 80%–99% water on a nonadherent, cross-linked polymer, and the different products have various absorptive properties.[18,21,22] Examples are AquaSite and FlexiGel.

Adhesive Bandages

Most superficial wounds (minor abrasions and lacerations) may simply require the application of adhesive gauze-type bandages such as regular Band-Aid brand bandages. Recognition of the importance of the moist wound healing method has led to the development and marketing of more moisture-retaining hydrocolloid-based bandages that promote wound healing (e.g., Band-Aid Brand Advanced Healing Strips, New Skin). Another alternative to conventional bandages is the cyanoacrylate tissue adhesives, also known as liquid adhesive bandages (e.g., Liquiderm), which are used on small cuts and abrasions. These bandages are preferred either for cosmetic considerations (as when a wound is located on the face) or when a more flexible dressing product is needed (as when a wound is located on the finger or elbow). They are easy and rapid to apply, and the adhesives have a high bonding strength.

Surgical Tape

As the name implies, surgical tape is primarily used to hold in place bandages that cover a wound or surgical incision. The tape should be chosen on the basis of its adhesive properties, but it should be easy to remove. To minimize skin irritation, paper and cloth tapes should not contain latex and should be hypoallergenic. The most adherent, but potentially irritating, tape is clear surgical tape, so it should be reserved for wounds that do not require frequent dressing changes (e.g., to secure IV lines or surgical drains). Examples are Blenderm, Medipore, and Micropore.

Pharmacologic Therapy

Various products are useful in treating minor burns, sunburn, and wounds. Some agents cleanse the area and/or relieve pain, swelling, and/or inflammation. Others either protect the damaged area from infection or otherwise aid in healing the skin.

Systemic Analgesics

An initial step in treating the patient with a minor skin injury is to recommend short-term administration of a systemic analgesic, preferably one with anti-inflammatory activity, such as the nonsteroidal anti-inflammatory drugs (NSAIDs) (e.g., aspirin, naproxen, ibuprofen). As prostaglandin inhibitors, NSAIDs may decrease erythema and edema in the injured area. NSAIDs may be especially beneficial in the patient with mild sunburn, especially in the first 24 hours after overexposure to UVR. Use of these agents has been shown to decrease inflammation caused by exposure to UVR. However, this effect has been found to last only approximately

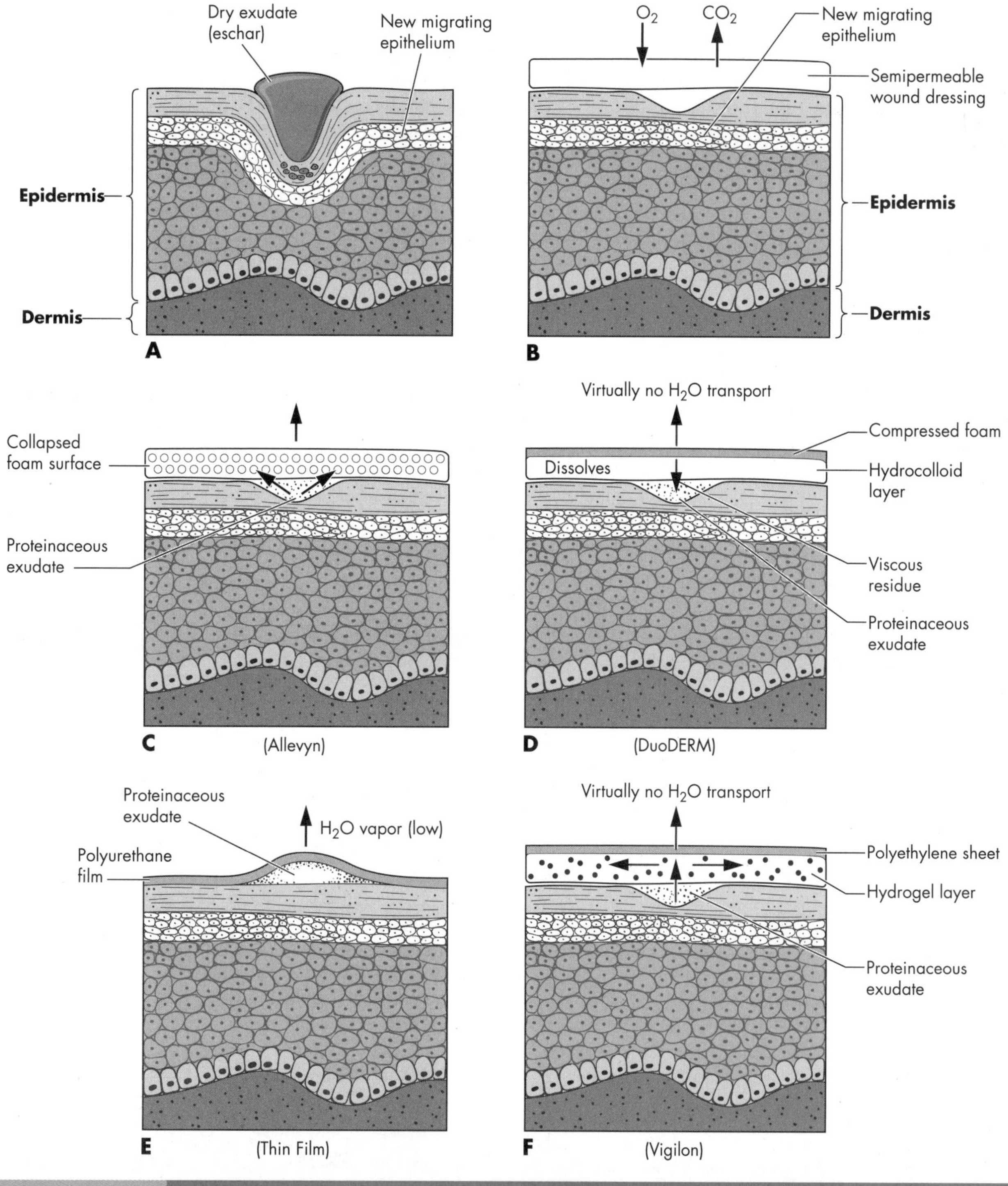

FIGURE **41–6** Mechanisms by which semipermeable wound dressings create a moist environment for wound healing. **A**, Regenerating epidermal cells are forced to "tunnel" below the dry wound eschar to attain wound closure. This tunneling delays wound closure. **B**, Semipermeable wound dressings prevent formation of eschar by maintaining optimal moisture level at the wound bed. Unhindered by the presence of a dry eschar, migrating epithelial cells are able to migrate and close the wound. **C**, Mechanism of action of a hydrophilic polyurethane foam dressing (Allevyn). **D**, Mechanisms of action of a hydrocolloid wound dressing (DuoDERM). **E**, Mechanism of water vapor transmission in thin films. **F**, Mechanism of action of a hydrogel wound dressing (Vigilon). (Source: Adapted with permission from Syzcher M, Lee SJ. Modern wound dressings: a systemic approach to wounds. *J Biomater Appl.* 1992;7:142–213.)

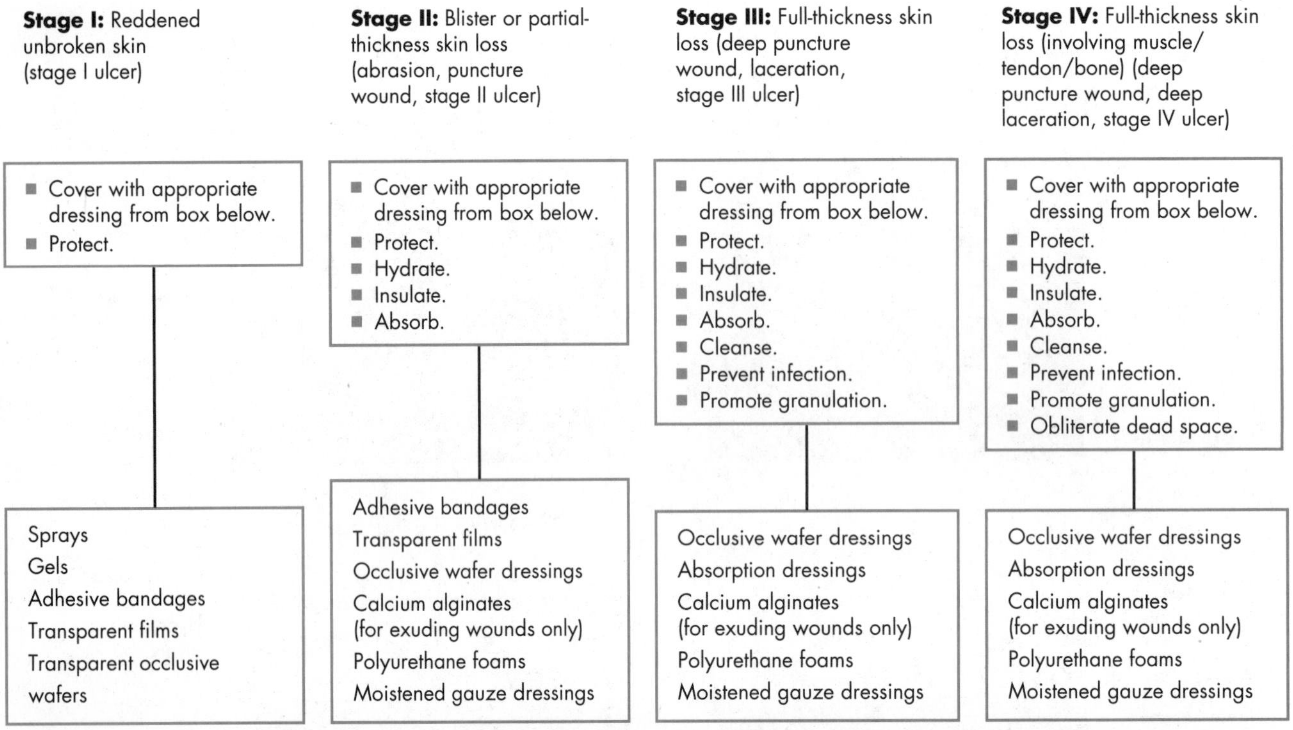
Stage I: Reddened unbroken skin (stage I ulcer)
Stage II: Blister or partial-thickness skin loss (abrasion, puncture wound, stage II ulcer)
Stage III: Full-thickness skin loss (deep puncture wound, laceration, stage III ulcer)
Stage IV: Full-thickness skin loss (involving muscle/tendon/bone) (deep puncture wound, deep laceration, stage IV ulcer)
■ Cover with appropriate dressing from box below.
■ Protect.
■ Cover with appropriate dressing from box below.
■ Protect.
■ Hydrate.
■ Insulate.
■ Absorb.
■ Cover with appropriate dressing from box below.
■ Protect.
■ Hydrate.
■ Insulate.
■ Absorb.
■ Cleanse.
■ Prevent infection.
■ Promote granulation.
■ Cover with appropriate dressing from box below.
■ Protect.
■ Hydrate.
■ Insulate.
■ Absorb.
■ Cleanse.
■ Prevent infection.
■ Promote granulation.
■ Obliterate dead space.
Sprays
Gels
Adhesive bandages
Transparent films
Transparent occlusive wafers
Adhesive bandages
Transparent films
Occlusive wafer dressings
Calcium alginates (for exuding wounds only)
Polyurethane foams
Moistened gauze dressings
Occlusive wafer dressings
Absorption dressings
Calcium alginates (for exuding wounds only)
Polyurethane foams
Moistened gauze dressings
Occlusive wafer dressings
Absorption dressings
Calcium alginates (for exuding wounds only)
Polyurethane foams
Moistened gauze dressings

FIGURE **41–7** Guidelines for product selection on the basis of wound severity. (Source: Adapted with permission from Jeter KF, Tintle TE. Wound dressings of the nineties: indications and contraindications. *Clin Podiatr Med Surg.* 1991;8:799–816.)

24 hours,[23] possibly because the initial inflammation of sunburn is mediated by prostaglandins, whereas the later inflammation is associated primarily with leukocytes. For patients who cannot tolerate NSAIDs, acetaminophen can provide pain relief, although it is a weak prostaglandin inhibitor and does not have any anti-inflammatory effect. (See Chapter 5 for discussion of dosages and safety considerations for systemic analgesics.)

Skin Protectants

The U.S. Food and Drug Administration (FDA) has recognized the skin protectants listed in Table 41–2 as safe and effective for the temporary protection of minor burns and abrasions.

Skin protectants benefit patients with minor skin injuries by making the damaged area less painful. They protect the area from mechanical irritation caused by friction and rubbing, and they prevent drying of the stratum corneum. Products that prevent dryness and provide lubrication should be selected. Generally, the patient may apply a skin protectant as often as needed. However, skin protectants are recommended for use on dry wound beds, as opposed to those that have exudates, to prevent maceration and impaired wound healing. If improvement is not seen in 7 days or if the injury worsens during or after treatment, the patient should seek medical attention promptly.

Topical Anesthetics

The pain of minor burns, wounds, and sunburn can be attenuated by the judicious use of topical anesthetics. Agents proposed as safe and effective in providing temporary relief of pain specifically associated with minor burns are listed in Table 41–3.

Topical anesthetics relieve pain by inhibiting the transmission of pain signals from pain receptors. Relief is short-lived, lasting only 15–45 minutes.[24]

Benzocaine (0.5%–20%) and lidocaine (2%–5%) are the two anesthetics most often used in nonprescription drug preparations. Dibucaine (0.25%–1%), tetracaine (0.5%–2%), butamben (1%), and pramoxine (0.5%–1%) are also found in external anesthetic

TABLE **41–2** **Skin Protectant Ingredients Used in Treatment of Minor Burns and Sunburn**

Ingredient	Proposed Concentration (%)
Allantoin	0.5–2
Cocoa butter	50–100
Petrolatum	30–100
Shark liver oil	3
White petrolatum	30–100

Source: U.S. Food and Drug Administration. Skin protectant drug products for over-the-counter human use. Final rule. *Fed Regist.* 2003;68:33377.

TABLE 41-3 Nonprescription Topical Analgesic Ingredients for Treatment of Minor Burns and Sunburn

Agent	FDA-Approved Concentration (%)
Amine and Caine-Type Local Anesthetics	
Benzocaine	5
Dibucaine	1
Lidocaine	2–4
Pramoxine hydrochloride	1
Antihistamines	
Diphenhydramine hydrochloride	1–2
Tripelennamine hydrochloride	0.5–2

Source: Wolters Kluwer Drug Facts and Comparisons eFacts. Local anesthetics, topical. Available at: http://online.factsandcomparisons.com/index.aspx. Accessed April 24, 2016.

preparations. The higher concentrations of the topical anesthetics are appropriate for skin injuries in which the skin is intact. Lower concentrations are preferred when the skin surface is not intact because drug absorption is enhanced under such conditions. These agents should be applied only to small areas of no more than 1%–2% of BSA to avoid systemic toxicity.[24,25]

Topical anesthetics should be applied no more often than 3–4 times daily. Because their duration of action is short, continuous pain relief cannot be obtained with these agents. Increasing the number of applications increases the risk of a hypersensitivity reaction and, more important, the chance for systemic toxicity.

Benzocaine produces a hypersensitivity reaction in approximately 1% of patients, a higher incidence than that seen with lidocaine. By contrast, benzocaine is essentially free of systemic toxicity, whereas the systemic absorption of lidocaine can lead to a number of adverse effects. However, systemic toxicities caused by lidocaine are rare if the product is used on intact skin, on localized areas, and for short periods.[24]

First Aid Antiseptics

Antiseptics are chemical substances designed for application to intact skin up to the edges of a damaged skin area for disinfection purposes. When effective antisepsis is combined with proper skin injury care technique, including gentle handling of tissue, the infection rate is low. Ideally, antiseptics should exert a sustained effect against all microorganisms, without causing tissue damage. However, even therapeutic concentrations of antiseptics can harm tissue. For example, alcohol-containing preparations should not be used within the wound bed because they dehydrate the area and also cause pain and cell damage. Therefore, antiseptics should be used to disinfect only intact skin surrounding the wound after the removal of all organic matter.

Antiseptic active ingredients recognized as safe and effective for clinical use include hydrogen peroxide topical solution USP, ethyl alcohol (48%–95%), isopropyl alcohol (50%–91.3%), iodine topical solution USP, iodine tincture USP, povidone/iodine complex (5%–10%), and camphorated phenol[25] (Tables 41–4 and 41–5).

TABLE 41-4 Nonprescription First Aid Antiseptic Ingredients

Antiseptic Agent	Concentration (%)
Chlorhexidine gluconate	2–4
Isopropyl alcohol	70

Source: Wolters Kluwer Drug Facts and Comparisons eFacts. Anti-infectives, topical. Available at: http://online.factsandcomparisons.com/index.aspx. Accessed April 24, 2016.

Hydrogen Peroxide

Hydrogen peroxide 3% topical solution USP is a widely used antiseptic. Enzymatic release of oxygen occurs when the hydrogen peroxide comes in contact with the skin, causing an effervescent, mechanical cleansing action. Hydrogen peroxide should be used only when released gas can escape; therefore, it should not be used in abscesses, nor should bandages be applied before the compound dries. Because of the limited bactericidal effect and the risk of tissue toxicity, hydrogen peroxide is of little benefit over soapy water for antisepsis.

Ethyl Alcohol

Alcohol has good bactericidal activity in 20%–70% concentrations. Caution is essential, however, with application of alcohol to the intact skin surrounding the injured area, because inadvertent, direct contact with the wound bed can cause tissue irritation.

TABLE 41-5 Selected Nonprescription Wound Irrigant and Antiseptic Products

Trade Name	Primary Ingredients
Wound Irrigants	
Wound Wash Saline Aerosol	
Saline Wound Flush	Sodium chloride 0.9%
Antiseptics	
Betadine Skin Cleanser Liquid	Povidone/iodine 7.5%
Campho-Phenique Gel/Liquid	Camphor 10.8%; phenol 4.7%
Hibiclens	Chlorhexidine gluconate 4%
Neosporin Wound Cleanser	Benzalkonium chloride 0.013%

Source: Wolters Kluwer Drug Facts and Comparisons eFacts. Genitourinary irrigants; Antiseptics and germicides. Available at: http://online.factsandcomparisons.com/index.asp. Accessed July 28, 2014.

Ethyl alcohol may be used 1–3 times daily, and the wound may be covered with a sterile bandage only after the washed area has dried.[25]

Isopropyl Alcohol

Compared with ethyl alcohol, isopropyl alcohol 70% aqueous solution has somewhat stronger bactericidal activity and lower surface tension. Isopropyl alcohol is generally used for its cleansing and antiseptic effects on intact skin. It should not be used to clean open wound beds because of possible cytotoxic effects and higher reported infection rates. Isopropyl alcohol also has a greater potential for drying the skin (astringent action) because its lipid solvent effects are stronger than those of ethyl alcohol. Similar to ethyl alcohol, isopropyl alcohol is flammable and must be kept away from a flame.[25]

Iodine

An iodine solution USP of iodine 2% and sodium iodide 2.5% is used as an antiseptic for superficial skin injuries. An iodine tincture USP of iodine 2%, sodium iodide 2.5%, and alcohol (approximately 50%) is less preferable than the aqueous solution because the tincture is irritating to the tissue. Strong iodine solution (Lugol's solution) must not be used as an antiseptic. In general, bandaging should be discouraged after iodine application, to avoid tissue irritation. Iodine solutions stain skin, may be irritating to tissue, and may cause allergic sensitization in some people. Iodine products are recommended, however, if patients have chlorhexidine allergy.[26]

Povidone/Iodine

Povidone/iodine is a water-soluble complex of iodine with povidone. It contains 9%–12% available iodine, which accounts for its rapid bactericidal activity. Povidone/iodine is nonirritating to skin and mucous membranes. Of note, however, when used as a wound irrigant, povidone/iodine is absorbed systemically; the extent of iodine absorption is related to the concentration used and the frequency of application. The final serum level also depends on the patient's intrinsic renal function. When severe burns and large wounds are treated with povidone/iodine, iodine absorption through the skin and mucous membranes can result in excess systemic iodine concentrations, possibly leading to transient thyroid dysfunction, clinical hyperthyroidism, or thyroid hyperplasia.[26]

Camphorated Phenol

Oily solutions of phenol and camphor are often used as nonprescription first aid antiseptics. These products contain relatively high concentrations of phenol (4%) and must be used with caution. If oleaginous phenolic solutions are applied to moist areas, the phenol is partitioned out of the vehicle into water, resulting in caustic concentrations of phenol on the skin. These damaging effects can be avoided by applying these products only to dry, intact skin. Wounds treated with camphorated phenol should not be bandaged, because the trapped moisture would result in tissue damage.[27]

First Aid Antibiotics

Nonprescription first aid antibiotics available in the United States consist of the active ingredients bacitracin, neomycin, and polymyxin B sulfate[28] (Table 41–6). These topical agents help prevent infection in minor cuts, wounds, scrapes, and burns. They are not indicated for the treatment of wounds that are already infected. They are especially beneficial if the wound contains debris or foreign matter. Topical and, in some cases, oral antibiotics are indicated in contaminated wounds that carry a moderately high risk of infection. However, clean wounds free of contamination have a low infection rate and do not warrant the use of prophylactic antibiotics. If questions arise concerning the degree of contamination and the need for oral antibiotics, the patient should seek medical attention.

Topical antibiotic preparations should be applied to the wound bed after cleansing and before applying a sterile dressing. Special caution should be taken with use of these preparations on large areas of denuded skin, however, because the potential for systemic toxicity can increase. Prolonged use of these agents may result in the development of resistant bacteria and secondary fungal infection. If significant signs of improvement are not seen within 7 days, the patient should seek medical attention.

TABLE 41-6 Selected Nonprescription Antibiotic Products

Trade Name	Primary Ingredients
Lanabiotic Ointment	Polymyxin B sulfate 10,000 U/g; bacitracin zinc 500 U/g; neomycin base 3.5 mg/g
Neosporin Ointment	Polymyxin B sulfate 5000 U/g; bacitracin zinc 400 U/g; neomycin base 3.5 mg/g
Neosporin Plus Pain Relief Ointment	Bacitracin zinc 500 U/g; polymyxin B sulfate 10,000 U/g; neomycin base 3.5 mg/g; pramoxine HCl 10 mg
Neosporin Plus Pain Relief Cream	Polymyxin B sulfate 10,000 U/g; neomycin base 3.5 mg/g; pramoxine HCl 10 mg
Polysporin Ointment/Powder	Polymyxin B sulfate 10,000 U/g; bacitracin zinc 500 U/g

Source: Wolters Kluwer Drug Facts and Comparisons eFacts. Anti-infectives, topical; antibiotic agents. Available at: http://online.factsandcomparisons.com/index.asp. Accessed April 24, 2016.

Bacitracin

Bacitracin is a polypeptide bactericidal antibiotic that inhibits cell wall synthesis in several gram-positive organisms. The development of resistance in previously sensitive organisms is rare. Minimal absorption occurs with topical administration. The frequency of allergic contact dermatitis (erythema, infiltration of macrophages, papules, or edematous or vesicular reaction) is approximately 2%. Topical nonprescription preparations usually contain 400–500 U/g of ointment and are applied 1–3 times a day.[28]

Neomycin

Neomycin is an aminoglycoside antibiotic; it exerts its bactericidal activity by irreversibly binding to the 30S ribosomal subunit to inhibit protein synthesis in gram-negative organisms and some species of *Staphylococcus.* Neomycin has been demonstrated to decrease the severity of clinical infection 48 hours after treatment of tape-stripped wounds. Resistant organisms may develop. Neomycin applied topically is associated with a relatively high rate of hypersensitivity; reactions occur in 3.5%–6% of patients. Although neomycin is not absorbed when applied to intact skin, application to large areas of denuded skin may cause systemic toxicity (specifically, ototoxicity and nephrotoxicity). It is most frequently used in combination with polymyxin and bacitracin in a concentration of 3.5 mg/g to prevent the development of neomycin-resistant organisms. Applications are made 1–3 times a day.[28]

Polymyxin B Sulfate

Polymyxin B sulfate is a polypeptide antibiotic that is effective against several gram-negative organisms because it alters the bacterial cell wall permeability. Topical preparations may be compounded in either a solution or ointment base, and numerous prepackaged antibiotic combinations containing polymyxin B are available. Applications are usually made 1–3 times a day.[28]

Antibacterial Soaps

In September 2016, FDA concluded that the available scientific evidence was not sufficient to demonstrate that nonprescription antibacterial soaps are better at preventing infections than washing with plain soap and water. An additional concern is that long-term exposure to antibacterial ingredients in these products may contribute to microbial resistance. As a result, FDA has banned 19 antibacterial ingredients from wash products including liquid, foam, gel hand soaps, bar soaps, and body washes. The most commonly used of the banned ingredients include triclosan and triclocarban.[29]

Product Selection Guidelines

If a topical anesthetic is to be used, the provider should recommend the most appropriate product formulation. These products are available as ointments, creams, solutions (lotions), and sprays (aerosols).

Ointments are oleaginous-based preparations. They provide a protective film to impede the evaporation of water from the wound area, which helps keep the skin from drying. If the skin is broken, however, an ointment may not be appropriate because of its impermeability. The presence of excessive moisture trapped beneath the ointment may promote bacterial growth or maceration of the skin, thereby delaying healing. Ointments are more appropriate for minor burns and wounds in which the skin is intact. Creams are emulsions that allow some fluid to pass through the film and are best for broken skin. Generally, it is easier to apply and remove creams than ointments. To prevent contamination of the preparation, the patient should not apply ointments and creams directly from the container onto the burn or wound. A preferred technique is to apply the topical product to a clean or gloved hand or gauze and then apply it directly to the injury site.

Lotions spread easily and are easier to apply when the burn or wound area is large. However, lotions that produce a powdery cover should not be used on a wound bed because they tend to dry out the area, are difficult (and possibly painful) to remove, and provide a medium for bacterial growth under the caked particles.

Generally, aerosol and pump sprays are more costly than other topical dosage forms. Sprays offer the advantage of precluding the need to physically touch the injured area, so the application process is associated with less pain. Proper application requires holding the container approximately 6 inches from the wound and spraying for 1–3 seconds. This method decreases the chances of chilling the area (from the aerosol). However, sprays are not usually protective in that the aerosol is typically water- or alcohol-based and will evaporate. In addition, alcohol-based sprays can irritate or dehydrate the wound bed.

Table 41–7 lists selected trade name topical products appropriate for treating minor burns, sunburn, and wounds.

Normal saline is the preferred choice for effective wound irrigation. The issue of which is the best antiseptic solution to use remains unresolved. In choosing an antiseptic product, important considerations include the potential for tissue toxicity and the cost of the different ingredients.

A topical antibiotic applied 1–3 times a day to a contaminated wound is effective in eradicating bacteria and producing faster wound healing when the agent is combined with appropriate cleansing of the wound and the use of proper dressings.

Special Populations

The approach to treating minor burns, sunburn, and wounds in special populations (e.g., pediatric patients, pregnant and lactating women, older adults) is the same as that in the general population.

Complementary Therapies

Natural products such as honey, *Calendula officinalis*, *Aloe vera*, *Garcinia morella*, and *Datura metel* are said to have healing

TABLE 41–7 Selected Nonprescription Topical Products for Minor Burns, Sunburn, and Wounds

Trade Name	Primary Ingredients
Skin Protectants	
A + D Prevent	Petrolatum 53.4%; lanolin 15.5%; cod liver oil (contains vitamins A and D)
Zinc Oxide Ointment	Zinc oxide 20%; petrolatum, mineral oil, lanolin, and olive oil
Local Anesthetics	
Solarcaine Aerosol	Benzocaine 20%
Xolido Cream	Lidocaine 2%
Dermoplast Spray	Benzocaine 8%; menthol 0.5%
Dibucaine Topical Ointment	Dibucaine 1%
Itch-X Spray/Gel	Pramoxine HCl 1%; benzyl alcohol 10%
Solarcaine Lotion	Benzocaine
Local Anesthetics/Antiseptics	
Dermoplast Lotion	Benzocaine 8%; menthol 0.5%
Lanacane Maximum Strength Anti-Itch Cream	Benzocaine 20%; benzethonium chloride 0.2%
Bicozene Cream	Benzocaine 6%; resorcinol 1.67%

Source: Wolters Kluwer Drug Facts and Comparisons eFacts. Protectants; Local anesthetics, topical. Available at: http://online.factsandcomparisons.com/index.asp. Accessed April 24, 2016.

properties.[30,31] (See Chapter 51 for a more in-depth review of natural products for skin care.)

Aloe vera gel is obtained from the mucilaginous center of the leaf of the aloe vera plant. It has been used for many centuries and is the major ingredient in various commercial skin and wound care products. The aloe vera gel contains vitamins A, B, C, and E, as well as enzymes, polysaccharides, amino acids, sugars, and minerals. In the management of acute and chronic wounds, several studies using aloe vera have reported variable results.[30]

Calendula (as *C. officinalis*) has been widely used in homeopathic medicine for the treatment of many diseases. It is thought to promote wound healing by its reported anti-inflammatory and antibacterial properties. Results of one study indicate the effectiveness of *C. officinalis* extract for enhancing the antioxidant defense mechanism, thereby decreasing healing time in a group of rats exposed to burn injury.[31]

The use of honey in wound management dates back many centuries. Honey consists of approximately 40% fructose, 30% glucose, 5% sucrose, and 20% water. It also contains several amino acids, antioxidants, vitamins, minerals, glucose oxidase (which produces hydrogen peroxide), and gluconic acid. Honey is highly viscous and delivers a moist wound healing environment. Also, because of the hyperosmolarity of honey, it is able to absorb the exudates from the wound and allow healing in a moist environment. Honey also has antibacterial, anti-inflammatory, and antifungal properties.[32]

One prospective randomized trial of honey versus silver sulfadiazine (SSD) for superficial burns demonstrated that honey dressings showed greater efficacy over SSD cream for treating superficial and partial-thickness burns; however, honey dressings are not advocated by burn centers.[33]

Assessment of Minor Burns, Sunburn, and Wounds: A Case-Based Approach

The assessment approach for burns differs slightly from the approach for wounds. When a patient presents with a burn, the severity of the burn should be immediately assessed by determining the depth of the injury and the percentage of BSA involved. The percentage of the adult body that has been burned can be estimated by the *rule-of-nines method* (Figure 41–4). The total BSA is divided into 11 areas, each accounting for 9% or a multiple of 9. An easy way to estimate the percentage of burned BSA is to use the back of the hand as 1% of BSA. The rule of nines is reliable for adults but inaccurate for children and smaller-sized patients.

Case 41–1 is an example of the assessment of a patient with a minor burn.

When a patient presents with a minor wound, the type, depth, location, and degree of contamination should be assessed. Visual inspection of the affected area usually provides an accurate evaluation of these factors. The wound should also be assessed for signs of infection, including whether drainage of yellow or greenish fluid (pus) is present or whether the skin around the wound has become increasingly erythematous, swollen, and painful. Because noninfectious processes such as drug-induced eruptions could be involved, the patient's health status and current medication use should also be determined. A nonprescription antibiotic ointment should generally be recommended when secondary infection is present or might occur.

Case 41–2 is an example of the assessment of a patient with a minor wound.

CASE 41-1

Relevant Evaluation Criteria	Scenario/Model Outcome
Collect	
1. Gather essential information about the patient's symptoms and medical history, including	
a. Description of symptom(s) (i.e., nature, onset, duration, severity, associated symptoms)	The patient complains of pain and extreme tenderness on her right shoulder due to a "spot" sunburn that she incurred despite sitting under an umbrella while at the beach for most of the previous day. She has a lesion approximately 6 inches in diameter on her right shoulder.
b. Description of any factors that seem to precipitate, exacerbate, and/or relieve the patient's symptom(s)	The patient reports that the pain is constant but gets a bit more intense when she moves.
c. Description of the patient's efforts to relieve the symptoms	The patient has applied Vaseline to the area twice, with little relief.
d. Patient's identity	Michelle Lauer
e. Patient's age, gender, height, and weight	35 years old, female, 5 ft 8 in., 160 lb
f. Patient's occupation	School teacher
g. Patient's dietary habits	Eats a regular diet with limited carbohydrates.
h. Patient's sleep habits	At least 7 hours nightly
i. Concurrent medical conditions, prescription and nonprescription medications, and dietary supplements	None
j. Allergies	None
k. History of other adverse reactions to medications	None
l. Other (describe) ______	None

CASE 41–1 *continued*

Relevant Evaluation Criteria	Scenario/Model Outcome
Assess	
2. Differentiate patient's signs/symptoms, and correctly identify the patient's primary problem(s).	Mrs. Lauer is suffering from a common sunburn secondary to prolonged sun exposure.
3. Identify exclusions for self-treatment (Figure 41–3).	None
4. Formulate a comprehensive list of therapeutic alternatives for the primary problem to determine whether triage to a health care provider is required, and share this information with the patient or caregiver.	Options include (1) Refer the patient to an appropriate HCP. (2) Recommend self-care with a nonprescription skin protectant and OTC analgesics. (3) Recommend self-care until the patient can see an appropriate HCP. (4) Take no action.
Plan	
5. Select an optimal therapeutic alternative to address the patient's problem, taking into account patient preferences.	Mrs. Lauer should use self-care measures to treat her sunburn using topical and systemic OTC products.
6. Describe the recommended therapeutic approach to the patient or caregiver.	"Take frequent showers to provide cool relief to the area. The sunburned area should be gently patted dry, and then a skin protectant should be applied to help to hold in moisture. If the pain is significant, take a nonprescription analgesic for relief. Leave the area uncovered unless blistering occurs. If blisters form, gently cover the area with a nonadherent gauze or a transparent film dressing to protect the area. Protective clothing to cover the area is also advised."
7. Explain to the patient or caregiver the rationale for selecting the recommended therapeutic approach from the considered therapeutic alternatives.	"Minor burns can be properly managed with nonprescription skin protectants and nonprescription analgesics as long as there are no exclusions for self-treatment, as in your case."
Implement	
8. When recommending self-care with nonprescription medications and/or nondrug therapy, convey accurate information to the patient or caregiver.	
a. Appropriate dose and frequency of administration	See the box "Patient Education for Minor Burns and Sunburn."
b. Maximum number of days the therapy should be employed	See the box "Patient Education for Minor Burns and Sunburn."
c. Product administration procedures	See the box "Patient Education for Minor Burns and Sunburn."
d. Expected time to onset of relief	"You should experience significant healing in about 7 days."
e. Degree of relief that can be reasonably expected	"The burn should heal well with proper use of a skin protectant and recommended nonprescription analgesics."
f. Most common adverse effects	See the box "Patient Education for Minor Burns and Sunburn."
g. Adverse effects that warrant medical intervention should they occur	See the box "Patient Education for Minor Burns and Sunburn."
h. Patient options in the event that condition worsens or persists	See the box "Patient Education for Minor Burns and Sunburn."
i. Product storage requirements	"Store in a cool, dry place out of children's reach."
j. Specific nondrug measures	See the box "Patient Education for Minor Burns and Sunburn."
Solicit follow-up questions from the patient or caregiver.	"Should I exfoliate the peeling skin for faster healing?"
Answer the patient's or caregiver's questions.	"No, applying harsh products that contain an exfoliant will further damage the sensitive skin and prolong healing and is likely to cause pain."
Follow-up: Monitor and Evaluate	
9. Assess patient outcome.	"If you provide me with your phone number, I will give you a call in 7–10 days to see how you are healing."

Key: HCP = Health care provider; OTC = over-the-counter.

CASE 41-2

Relevant Evaluation Criteria	Scenario/Model Outcome
Collect	
1. Gather essential information about the patient's symptoms and medical history, including	
a. Description of symptom(s) (i.e., nature, onset, duration, severity, associated symptoms)	The patient's wife calls to report that he stepped on a nail while working in their garage about 10 minutes ago. She says he is not complaining of much pain, but there is lots of bleeding. The affected area is the heel of his right foot. He removed the nail and is currently applying pressure to the area with a shop towel that he was using when changing the oil in his car.
b. Description of any factors that seem to precipitate, exacerbate, and/or relieve the patient's symptom(s)	Her husband reports mild pain at the site of the wound. It does not seem to be getting any worse since the injury occurred.
c. Description of the patient's efforts to relieve the symptoms	He is applying pressure to the area with a towel.
d. Patient's identity	Ronnie Coulter
e. Patient's age, gender, height, and weight	46 years old, male, 6 ft 2 in., 180 lb
f. Patient's occupation	Computer programmer
g. Patient's dietary habits	Vegetarian
h. Patient's sleep habits	6–8 hours a night
i. Concurrent medical conditions, prescription and nonprescription medications, and dietary supplements	Amlodipine 10 mg daily for high blood pressure
j. Allergies	NKA
k. History of other adverse reactions to medications	None
l. Other (describe) ______	None
Assess	
2. Differentiate patient's signs/symptoms, and correctly identify the patient's primary problem(s).	The patient has mild pain and bleeding at the site of injury, a puncture wound from a nail.
3. Identify exclusions for self-treatment (Figure 41–5).	Deep acute wound
4. Formulate a comprehensive list of therapeutic alternatives for the primary problem to determine whether triage to a health care provider is required, and share this information with the patient or caregiver.	Options include (1) Refer the patient to an appropriate HCP. (2) Recommend self-care with a nonprescription analgesic and nondrug measures. (3) Recommend self-care until the patient can see an appropriate HCP. (4) Take no action.
Plan	
5. Select an optimal therapeutic alternative to address the patient's problem, taking into account patient preferences.	Mr. Coulter should consult an HCP.
6. Describe the recommended therapeutic approach to the patient or caregiver.	"You should consult a health care provider for treatment because self-treatment is not recommended."
7. Explain to the patient or caregiver the rationale for selecting the recommended therapeutic approach from the considered therapeutic alternatives.	"Puncture wounds require immediate medical attention to assess the need for systemic or topical antibiotics and possibly a tetanus booster to prevent infection. Provide your husband with a clean towel to use to apply pressure to the injured site and seek medical help immediately."

CASE 41–2 *continued*

Relevant Evaluation Criteria	Scenario/Model Outcome
Implement	
8. When recommending self-care with nonprescription medications and/or nondrug therapy, convey accurate information to the patient or caregiver.	Criterion does not apply in this case.
Solicit follow-up questions from the patient or caregiver.	"Should I flush the wound with hydrogen peroxide to sterilize the area?"
Answer the patient's or caregiver's questions.	"No, agents such as hydrogen peroxide cause damage to injured skin and should be avoided. You may use warm soapy water to clean the area and help remove dirt and oil caused by contact from the towel that was used initially."
Follow-up: Monitor and Evaluate	
9. Assess patient outcome.	Contact Mr. Coulter in 1–2 days to ensure that he sought proper medical care.

Key: HCP = Health care provider; NKA = no known allergies; OTC = over-the-counter.

Patient Counseling for Minor Burns, Sunburn, and Wounds

Once a burn is assessed as self-treatable, the patient's immediate concern, relieving the pain and swelling, should be addressed. Some patients may not realize the potential complications associated with even minor burns; therefore, advice on how to protect the injury is vital in preventing possible infection and minimizing scarring.

After a 24- to 48-hour follow-up evaluation of the burn, either continuation of self-treatment or referral for further evaluation should be recommended. If self-treatment continues, the patient needs to know how long healing of the burn will take, as well as the signs and symptoms that indicate worsening of the injury. Burned skin is more susceptible to sunburn for several weeks after initial injury, so avoiding sun exposure and using sunscreen agents during this period are recommended. The box "Patient Education for Minor Burns and Sunburn" lists specific measures for successful self-treatment of these injuries.

When assessing a wound, the provider should remember that minor cuts and abrasions may be self-treated, whereas chronic and more severe acute wounds or those that appear infected should first be evaluated by a primary care provider (Figure 41–5). Irrigation with soapy water or normal saline is generally recommended if the wound is dirty. Patients should be instructed to change the dressing only when it is soiled or not intact. The provider should ensure that the patient understands the basic steps in wound care, especially the selection of appropriate wound dressings.

PATIENT EDUCATION FOR Minor Burns and Sunburn

The objectives of self-treatment are (1) to relieve the pain and swelling, (2) to protect the burned area from further physical injury, and (3) to avoid infection and scarring of the burned area. For most patients, carefully following product instructions and the self-care measures listed here will help ensure optimal therapeutic outcomes.

Nondrug Measures

- Treat superficial burns with no blistering as follows:
  - Immerse the affected area in cool tap water for 10–30 minutes.
  - Cleanse the area with water and a mild soap.
  - Apply a nonadherent dressing or skin protectant to the burn.
- For small burns with minor blistering, follow the first two steps above, but use a hydrocolloid dressing to protect the burn.
- If possible, avoid rupturing blisters.
- For sunburns, avoid further sun exposure and follow the previous procedures according to whether blistering is present.

Nonprescription Medications

- For superficial burns (including sunburn) with unbroken skin, treat the affected area with thin applications of a skin protectant or topical anesthetic, using a tissue to reduce the risk of infection from the fingertips.
- If the skin is broken, use topical antibiotics to prevent infection.
- If nutritional status is poor, take supplements for vitamins A, B, and C.
- Do not apply products containing camphor, menthol, or ichthammol (also called "drawing salve") to the burn.
- For temporary relief of pain, take aspirin, acetaminophen, ibuprofen, or naproxen. (See Chapter 5 for dosage guidelines and safety considerations.)

When to Seek Medical Attention

- If a skin rash, weight gain, local swelling, or blood in the stool occurs with use of a pain reliever, report these adverse effects to a primary care provider.
- Report immediately to a primary care provider any redness, pain, or swelling that extends beyond the boundaries of the original injury.
- If the burn seems to worsen or is not healed significantly in 7 days, see a primary care provider for further treatment.

PATIENT EDUCATION FOR Acute Wounds

The objective of self-treatment is to promote healing by protecting the wound from infection or further trauma. For most patients, carefully following product instructions and the self-care measures listed here will help ensure optimal therapeutic outcomes.

- Position the affected area with the wound above the level of the heart, to slow bleeding and to help relieve throbbing pain.
- If the wound is dirty, irrigate it with tepid tap water or normal saline solution, which is not toxic to cells. Use antiseptic solutions selectively and cautiously. Any inflammation should subside within 12–24 hours.
- When cleansing with soapy water, first wash hands. Then apply mild liquid soap (e.g., Dove soap) to a wet cotton ball and gently wash the wound area; rinse the wound under running warm water and gently pat the area dry.
- Cover the wound with a dressing that will keep the wound site moist. Make sure the dressing is the appropriate size and contour for the affected body part.
- Continue using a wound dressing until the wound bed has firmly closed and signs of inflammation in surrounding tissue have subsided. This process usually takes 2–3 weeks. Failure to keep the wound covered may delay healing.
- Avoid disrupting the dressing unnecessarily; change it only if it becomes soiled or is not intact. Most dressings should be changed every 3–5 days. More frequent changes may remove resurfacing layers of epithelium and slow the healing process. Change the dressing if excessive fluid is released.
- Use a mild analgesic to control pain.
- All wound dressings should be kept in their original packaging and stored away from moisture.
- Observe the wound for signs of infection. Redness, swelling, and exudate are normal during healing; foul odor is not.

When to Seek Medical Attention

- Consult a primary care provider if infection is suspected or if the wound does not show signs of healing after 7 days of self-treatment.

An explanation of basic skin physiology and the wound healing process will enhance patient adherence to the wound care regimen. The box "Patient Education for Acute Wounds" lists specific information to include in patient counseling. Medical referral for further evaluation is warranted if the wound does not show signs of healing after 7 days of self-treatment.

Evaluation of Patient Outcomes for Minor Burns, Sunburn, and Wounds

Burn should be reassessed after 24–48 hours because the full extent of skin damage may not be initially apparent. If the burn extent or severity has progressed or worsened, the patient should be referred to an appropriate health care provider for further evaluation.

Minor wounds should exhibit decreased redness during healing. Signs that indicate the need for further evaluation by a primary care provider include evidence of cellulitis or tissue infection, such as increasing redness, pain, and swelling that extend beyond the boundaries of the original wound. Patients in whom contact dermatitis develops with topical treatments should also be evaluated further.

The patient's progress should be checked after 7 days to assess the healing process; therefore, a scheduled visit to see the provider is preferable. If the wound shows no signs of healing or has worsened in nature or degree (as indicated by a foul odor or increasing inflammation), the patient should be referred for more aggressive therapy.

Key Points for Minor Burns, Sunburn, and Wounds

- Minor burns and sunburn can often be treated with self-care measures. However, deeper burn injuries or burns affecting more than 1%–2% of BSA require medical attention.
- Burn injuries may increase in severity over the first 24–48 hours, so frequent reassessment is always necessary.
- Patient complaints usually focus on pain. Skin protectants and dressings should be recommended, and aspirin or other NSAIDs are often helpful if not contraindicated. The type of dressing or skin protectant used depends on whether the wound is dry or weeping. Blisters should not be ruptured. Topical hydrocortisone or anesthetics may provide additional relief in some patients but should be used sparingly on broken skin. Counterirritants such as camphor, menthol, and ichthammol ("drawing salve") should be avoided.
- Vitamins, whether systemic or topical, are generally of no value unless the patient is malnourished.
- Photosensitization reactions can often be assessed by reviewing the patient's history and must be distinguished from ordinary sunburns.
- Self-treatment of minor acute wounds is appropriate.
- First aid antibiotics are used to prevent infection.
- Moist wound healing is now considered the standard of care.
- Proper selection of first aid products, including appropriate wound dressing, is essential.

REFERENCES

1. American Burn Association. Burn incidence and treatment in the United States: 2011 fact sheet. Available at: http://www.ameriburn.org/resources_factsheet.php. Accessed June 26, 2017.
2. Rice RH, Mauro TM. Toxic responses of the skin. In: Rice RH, Mauro TM, eds. *Casarett & Doull's Essentials of Toxicology*. 2nd ed. New York, NY: McGraw-Hill; 2010. Available at: http://www.accesspharmacy.com/content.aspx?aID=6484631. Accessed June 8, 2013.
3. Skin Cancer Foundation. UVA & UVB. May 24, 2013. Available at: http://www.skincancer.org/prevention/uva-and-uvb. Accessed June 26, 2017.
4. Internal Medicine and Pediatric Clinic of New Albany. Skin wounds (lacerations, punctures, and abrasions). 2007. Available at: http://www.impcna.com/intranet/Nelson%20Pediatric/Emergency/SkinWounds%5B1%5D.pdf. Accessed June 26, 2017.
5. Barrett KE, Barman SM, Boitano S, Brooks HL. Immunity, Infection, & Inflammation. In: Barrett KE, Barman SM, Boitano S, Brooks HL, eds. *Ganong's Review of Medical Physiology*. 25th ed. New York, NY: McGraw-

Hill; 2016. Available at: http://accesspharmacy.mhmedical.com/content.aspx?bookid=1587&Sectionid=97162342. Accessed April 24, 2016.

6. Guo S, Dipietro LA. Factors affecting wound healing. *J Dent Res.* 2010; 89(3):219–29.
7. Wolff K, Johnson R, Saavedra AP. Bacterial colonizations and infections of skin and soft tissues. In: Wolff K, Johnson R, Saavedra AP, eds. *Fitzpatrick's Color Atlas and Synopsis of Clinical Dermatology.* 7th ed. New York, NY: McGraw-Hill; 2013. Available at: http://accessmedicine.mhmedical.com/content.aspx?bookid=1700&Sectionid=113786500. Accessed April 24, 2016.
8. Demling RH. Nutrition, anabolism, and the wound healing process: an overview. *Eplasty.* 2009;9:e9-65–94.
9. Arnold M, Barbul A. Nutrition and wound healing. *Plast Reconstr Surg.* 2006;117(7 Suppl):42S–58S.
10. Keylock KT, Vieira VJ, Wallig MA, et al. Exercise accelerates cutaneous wound healing and decreases wound inflammation in aged mice. *Am J Physiol Regul Integr Comp Physiol.* 2008;294(1):R179–84.
11. Franz MG, Steed DL, Robson MC. Optimizing healing of the acute wound by minimizing complications. *Curr Probl Surg.* 2007;44(11):691–763.
12. Velander P, Theopod C, Hirsch T, et al. Impaired wound healing in an acute diabetic pig model and the effects of hyperglycemia. *Wound Repair Regen.* 2008;16(2):288–93.
13. Menke NB, Ward KR, Witten TM, et al. Impaired wound healing. *Clin Dermatol.* 2007;25(1):19–25.
14. Alsbjorn B, Gilbert P, Hartmann B, et al. Guidelines for the management of partial-thickness burns in a general hospital or community setting—recommendations of a European working party. *Burns.* 2007;33(2):155–60.
15. Shrivastava P, Goel A. Pre-hospital care in burn injury. *Indian J Plast Surg.* 2010;43(Suppl):S15–22.
16. Sarabahi S. Recent advances in topical wound care. *Indian J Plast Surg.* 2012;45(2):379–87.
17. Baranoski S. Choosing a wound dressing, part 1. *Nursing.* 2008;38(1): 60–1.
18. Baranoski S. Choosing a wound dressing, part 2. *Nursing.* 2008;38(2): 14–5.
19. Jones V, Grey J, Harding K. ABC of wound healing: wound dressing. *BMJ.* 2006;332(7554):777–80.
20. Thompson G, Stephen-Hayes J. An overview of wound healing and exudates management. *Br J Community Nurs.* 2007;12(12):S22, S24–6, S28–30.
21. Lee K, Mooney DJ. Alginate: properties and biomedical implications. *Prog Polym Sci.* 2012;37(1):106–26.
22. Okan D, Woo K, Ayello E. The role of moisture balance in wound healing. *Adv Skin Wound Care.* 2007;20(1):39–53.
23. Young AR, Walker SL. Acute and chronic effects of ultraviolet radiation on the skin. In: Wolff K, Goldsmith LA, Katz SI, et al., eds. *Fitzpatrick's Dermatology in General Medicine.* 7th ed. New York, NY: McGraw-Hill; 2007.
24. McEvoy GK, Miller J, eds. Antipruritics and local anesthetics. In: *AHFS Drug Information.* Bethesda, MD: American Society of Health-System Pharmacists; 2007:2844–5.
25. Wolters Kluwer Health, Inc. Antiseptics and germicides. Drug Facts and Comparisons eFacts. Available at: http://online.factsandcomparisons.com/MonoDisp.aspx?monoid=fandc-hcp10207&book=DFC. Accessed July 28, 2014.
26. Eloot S, Dhondt A, Hoste E, et al. How to remove accumulated iodine in burn-injured patients. *Nephrol Dial Transplant.* 2010;25(5):1614–20.
27. Wolters Kluwer Health, Inc. Topical combinations: miscellaneous. Drug Facts and Comparisons eFacts. Available at: http://online.factsandcomparisons.com/index.asp. Accessed July 28, 2014.
28. Robertson DB, Maibach HI. Chapter 61. Dermatologic pharmacology. In: Katzung BG, Masters SB, Trevor AJ, eds. *Basic & Clinical Pharmacology.* 12th ed. New York, NY: McGraw-Hill; 2012. Available at: http://www.access pharmacy.com/content.aspx?aID=55832444. Accessed June 9, 2013.
29. U.S. Food and Drug Administration. FDA Consumer Update. Antibacterial Soap? You Can Skip It—Use Plain Soap and Water. September 2016. Available at: http://www.fda.gov/downloads/ForConsumers/ConsumerUpdates/UCM378615.pdf. Accessed October 21, 2016.
30. Khorasani G, Hosseinimehr SH, Azadbakht M, et al. Aloe vs silver sulfadiazine creams for second degree burns: a randomized controlled study. *Surg Today.* 2009;39(7):587–91.
31. Chandran O, Kuttan R. Effect of *Calendula officinalis* flower extract on acute phase proteins, antioxidant defense mechanism and granuloma formation during thermal burns. *J Clin Biochem Nutr.* 2008;43(2):58–64.
32. Bittmann S, Luchter E, Thiel M, et al. Does honey have a role in paediatric wound management? *Br J Nurs.* 2010;19(15):19–24.
33. Malik KI, Malik MA, Aslam A. Honey compared with silver sulphadiazine in the treatment of superficial partial-thickness burns. *Int Wound J.* 2010; 7(5):413–7.

CHAPTER 42

FUNGAL SKIN INFECTIONS

APRIL GARDNER AND NATALIE WALKUP

Approximately 20%–25% of the world's population suffers from fungal skin infections, including dermatophyte, non-dermatophyte, and candidal infections, with dermatophyte fungi being responsible for the majority of fungal infections.[1,2] Most fungal infections are a result of a barrier breakdown in either the skin or nail or an associated comorbidity affecting the host's defense, including diabetes, obesity, or an immunocompromised state.[1,3]

Fungal infections are usually superficial and can involve the hair, nails, and skin. The term *tinea* refers exclusively to dermatophyte infections. Most often, tinea infections are named according to the area of the body that is affected (e.g., scalp [tinea capitis]; groin [tinea cruris]; body [tinea corporis]; feet [tinea pedis]; nails [tinea unguium]). These infections are generally caused by three genera of fungi including *Microsporum, Trichophyton,* and *Epidermophyton.*[3–5]

Dermatomycoses are often referred to as ringworm, because their characteristic lesions are ring shaped with clear centers and red, scaly borders. However, these lesions can vary from the ring form and may present as single or multiple lesions that range from mild scaling to deep *granulomas* (inflamed, nodular lesions). The most common causative agents of dermatomycoses are *Trichophyton rubrum, Trichophyton tonsurans,* and *Trichophyton mentagrophytes. Trichophyton rubrum* is the most commonly isolated dermatophyte in the United States.[1,6] Non-dermatophytes and species of *Candida* and other yeasts may also be involved in fungal skin infections; however, currently, no nonprescription antifungals are available for self-management of cutaneous infections secondary to yeasts.[7]

Although many pathogenic fungi exist, the overall prevalence of actual superficial fungal infections is remarkably low. An estimated 10%–20% of the U.S. population suffers from a tinea infection at any one time.[8,9] Many degrees of susceptibility, from instantaneous "takes" by a single spore to severe trauma with massive exposure, produce a clinical infection. Trauma to the skin, especially trauma that produces blisters (e.g., from wearing ill-fitting footwear), appears to be significantly more important than simple exposure to the offending pathogens.[9] Other predisposing factors for the development of tinea infections include diabetes and other diseases associated with immunodeficiency, use of immunosuppressive drugs, impaired circulation, poor nutrition and hygiene, occlusion of the skin, and warm, humid climates.[9,10]

The most prevalent cutaneous fungal infection in humans is *tinea pedis* (dermatophytosis of the foot, or athlete's foot). Tinea pedis afflicts approximately 26.5 million people in the United States every year; 7 of every 10 sufferers are male. Approximately 45% will suffer with tinea pedis episodically for more than 10 years. When exposure to infectious environments is equal, the incidence of tinea pedis infections in women approaches that in men.[8,9,11,12] Tinea pedis is rare among blacks but common in whites, particularly whites who live in urban tropical areas.[13] An estimated 70% of people will be afflicted with tinea pedis in their lifetime. Although tinea pedis may occur at all ages, it is more common in adults, presumably because of their increased opportunities for exposure to pathogens.[9]

The risk for development of tinea pedis is greater in individuals who use public pools or bathing facilities than in the general population. However, tinea pedis may be acquired in the home if one or more members of the household are already infected. High-impact sports that cause chronic trauma to the feet (e.g., long-distance running) also predispose athletes to tinea pedis.[6,9] The trauma affords infecting fungi the opportunity to invade the outer layers of the skin. In addition, wearing socks and shoes exacerbates the problem by impeding the dispersion of heat and the evaporation of moisture, both of which facilitate fungal growth. In contrast, individuals who most often use footwear that allows the feet to remain cool and dry (e.g., sandals) are less likely to develop tinea pedis.

Tinea unguium (ringworm of the nails or onychomycosis) causes about half of all nail disorders and is sometimes associated with tinea pedis. The estimated prevalence of tinea unguium is between 2% and 8%, depending on the population.[14] The Food and Drug Administration (FDA) has not approved self-treatment of onychomycosis with topical nonprescription antifungals. Rather, the affected nail must be treated with systemic prescription drug therapy (e.g., terbinafine, itraconazole), prescription combination topical (e.g., ciclopirox olamine 8% or efinaconazole 10% nail solutions) and systemic oral therapy, or surgical removal to rid the area of the offending fungus.[4]

The next two most common infections are tinea corporis and tinea cruris. *Tinea corporis,* also called ringworm of the body, is most common in prepubescent individuals. It is frequently transmitted among children in daycare centers and among child participants in contact sports, such as wrestling. However, it is also more prevalent in adults and children who live in hot, humid climates. Individuals who are under stress or overweight are also at increased risk to develop tinea corporis.[1,15]

Tinea cruris, or jock itch, often presents as a pruritic, red rash and is most common during warm weather; however, it can occur at any time of the year if the skin in the groin area stays warm and moist for long periods. For example, sweating or prolonged contact with wet clothing provides an ideal environment for the growth of

Editor's Note: This chapter is based on the 18th edition chapter of the same title, written by Gail D. Newton.

fungi. Tinea cruris occurs more often in men than in women and rarely affects children.[9] Close indirect or direct physical contact between infected males and noninfected females does not mitigate the higher prevalence of tinea cruris in males. For example, females who live in the same household with infected males do not develop infections at the same rate as noninfected males in the same household.[9]

Although its true incidence is unknown, *tinea capitis*, or ringworm of the scalp, occurs most often in children, because their likelihood of having contact with infected individuals is higher and because they are less attentive than adults to personal hygiene. Tinea capitis is the most common dermatophyte infection in children 3–14 years of age.[6,9] Compared with black males and white children, black female children are infected more often, possibly because of the hair care products and practices (e.g., occlusive hair dressings, tight braiding) that are unique to this population.[9,15]

Tinea capitis can be spread by direct contact with an infected person, but it is often spread by contact with infected fomites (e.g., using infected combs, hats, toys, or telephones; wearing infected clothing; using infected towels; sleeping on infected linens). In some instances, tinea capitis is spread through contact with other infected individuals or with infected cats or dogs.[16] As with onychomycosis, tinea capitis cannot be managed with topical nonprescription antifungals.

Pathophysiology of Fungal Skin Infections

Tinea infections are caused by three genera of pathogenic fungi: *Trichophyton*, *Microsporum*, and *Epidermophyton*.[3–5] Tinea pedis and tinea cruris are caused by species of *Epidermophyton* and *Trichophyton*. Species of *Trichophyton* and *Microsporum* cause ringworm of the scalp. *Trichophyton* species also cause onychomycosis. All species of the three genera can cause tinea corporis.[9] Fungal transmission can occur through contact with infected people, animals, soil, or fomites. Dermatophytes are classified according to their habitat: anthropophilic (humans), zoophilic (animals), and geophilic (soil). Most tinea infections are caused by person-to-person contact with individuals infected with anthropophilic dermatophytes.[15]

In addition to specific fungi, other environmental factors, such as climate and social customs, contribute to dermatophytosis development. Footwear is a key variable, as illustrated by the incidence of tinea pedis in any population that wears occlusive footwear, especially in the summer and in tropical or subtropical climates. Nonporous shoe material increases temperature and hydration of the skin, which interferes with the barrier function of the stratum corneum. Similarly, sweating or wearing wet clothing for long periods of time can predispose individuals to the development of tinea corporis and tinea cruris.

Chronic health problems and medications that weaken or suppress the immune system can also increase the risk for development of tinea infections. For example, patients with diabetes or human immunodeficiency virus and older persons taking medications such as glucocorticoids should be instructed to monitor themselves for signs and symptoms of tinea infections. They should also be instructed about the importance of proper hygiene and diet to prevent tinea infections and other health problems.

After a dermatophyte is inoculated into the skin under suitable conditions, a tinea infection progresses through several stages. The stages include periods of incubation and then enlargement, followed by a refractory period and a stage of involution. During the incubation period, the dermatophyte grows in the stratum corneum, sometimes with minimal signs of infection. After the incubation period and once the infection is established, two factors appear to play a role in determining the size and duration of the lesions: the growth rate of the organism and the epidermal turnover rate.[17] The fungal growth rate must equal or exceed the epidermal turnover rate, or the organism will be quickly shed.

Dermatophytid infestations remain within the stratum corneum. Resistance to the spread of infection seems to involve both immunologic and nonimmunologic mechanisms. For example, the presence of a serum inhibitory factor (SIF) appears to limit the growth of dermatophytes beyond the stratum corneum. SIF is not an antibody but a dialyzable, heat-labile component of fresh sera. It appears that SIF chelates the iron that dermatophytes need for continued growth.[17] Once in the stratum corneum, dermatophytes produce keratinases and other proteolytic enzymes that cause allergic reactions when they reach living epidermis.[9]

The major immunologic defense against fungal skin infections is the type IV delayed-hypersensitivity response. The refractory period precedes complete development of this cell-mediated immunity. The fungal growth rate typically exceeds epidermal turnover, and inflammation and pruritus are at their peak. After development of an adequate immune response, symptoms of superficial fungal infections diminish, and the infection may clear spontaneously during the involution period. Patients with chronic infections typically present with much less inflammation. This presentation may be caused by a suppressed hypersensitivity response, which in turn reduces the inflammatory response.[18]

Clinical Presentation of Fungal Skin Infections

The clinical spectrum of tinea infections ranges from mild itching and scaling to a severe, exudative inflammatory process characterized by denudation, fissuring, crusting, and/or discoloration of the affected skin. Individuals experiencing their first tinea infection and patients with infections secondary to zoophilic fungi tend to present with greater inflammation.[15] Table 42–1 summarizes key differences between fungal skin infections, contact dermatitis, and bacterial skin infections to distinguish the underlying cause of a patient's symptoms from other conditions that may have a similar clinical presentation.

Tinea Pedis

Clinically, tinea pedis has four accepted variants; two or more of these types may overlap. The most common is the chronic intertriginous type,[9] characterized by fissuring, scaling, or maceration in the interdigital spaces; malodor; pruritus; and/or a stinging sensation on the feet (see Color Plates, photograph 32). Typically, the infection involves the lateral toe webs, usually between either the fourth and fifth or the third and fourth toes. From these sites, the infection may spread to the sole or instep of the foot but rarely to the dorsum. Warmth and humidity aggravate this condition; consequently, *hyperhidrosis* (excessive sweating) becomes an underlying problem and must be treated along with the dermatophyte infestation.[9]

After initial invasion of the stratum corneum by dermatophytes, enough moisture may accumulate to trigger a bacterial overgrowth. Increased moisture and temperature then lead to the release of

TABLE 42-1 **Differentiation of Fungal Skin Infections and Skin Disorders With Similar Presentation**

Criterion	Fungal Skin Infections	Contact Dermatitis	Bacterial Skin Infection
Location	On areas of the body where excess moisture accumulates, such as the feet, groin area, scalp, and under the arms	Any area of the body exposed to the allergen/irritant; hands, face, legs, ears, eyes, and anogenital area most often involved	Anywhere on the body
Signs	Presents either as soggy malodorous, thickened skin; acute vesicular rash; or fine scaling of affected area with varying degrees of inflammation; cracks and fissures may also be present	Presents as a variety of lesions: raised wheals, fluid-filled vesicles, or both	Presents as a variety of lesions from macules to pustules to ulcers with redness surrounding the lesion; lesions are often warmer than surrounding, unaffected skin
Symptoms	Itching and pain	Itching and pain	Irritation and pain
Quantity/severity	Usually localized to a single region of the body but can spread	Affects all areas of exposed skin but does not spread	Usually localized to a single region of the body but can spread
Timing	Variable onset	Variable onset from immediately after exposure to 3 weeks after contact	Variable onset
Cause	Superficial fungal infection	Exposure to skin irritants or allergens	Superficial bacterial infection
Modifying factors	Treated with nonprescription astringents, antifungals, and nondrug measures to keep the area clean and dry	Treated with topical antipruritics, skin protectants, astringents, and non-drug measures to avoid reexposure	Treated with prescription antibiotics

metabolic products that diffuse easily through the underlying horny layer already damaged by fungal invasion. In more severe cases, gram-negative organisms intrude and may exacerbate the condition, causing skin maceration, white hyperkeratosis, or erosions with increased patient symptomatology.[9]

The second variant of tinea pedis is known as the chronic papulosquamous pattern.[9] It is usually found on both feet and is characterized by mild inflammation and diffuse, moccasin-like scaling on the soles of the feet. Tinea unguium of one or more toenails may also be present and may continue to fuel the infection.

The third variant of tinea pedis is the vesicular type, usually caused by *T. mentagrophytes* var. *interdigitale.*[5] Small vesicles or vesicopustules are observed near the instep and on the mid-anterior plantar surface. Skin scaling is seen on these areas as well as on the toe webs. This variant is symptomatic in the summer and is clinically quiescent during the cooler months.

The acute ulcerative type is the fourth and least common variant of tinea pedis. It is often associated with macerated, denuded, weeping ulcerations on the sole of the foot. Typically, white hyperkeratosis and a pungent odor are present. The term *dermatophytosis complex* has been used to describe this type of infection, which is complicated by an overgrowth of opportunistic, gram-negative bacteria such as *Proteus* and *Pseudomonas;* the infection may produce an extremely painful, erosive, purulent interdigital space that can impede the patient's ability to walk.[9]

Tinea Unguium

Nails affected by tinea unguium gradually lose their normal shiny luster and become opaque. If left untreated, the nails become thick, rough, yellow, opaque, and friable. The nail may separate from the nail bed if the infection progresses secondarily to subungual hyperkeratosis. Ultimately, the nail may be lost altogether. Subungual debris also provides an excellent medium for the growth of opportunistic bacteria and other microorganisms, which can lead to further infectious complications.[9]

Tinea Corporis

Tinea corporis may have a diverse clinical presentation. Most often, the lesions, which involve *glabrous* (smooth and bare) skin, begin as small, circular, erythematous, scaly areas. The lesions spread peripherally, and the borders may contain vesicles or pustules. Infected individuals may also complain of pruritus.[19]

Tinea corporis can occur on any part of the body. However, the location of the infection can provide clues to the type of infecting dermatophyte. For example, zoophilic dermatophytes often infect areas of exposed skin such as the neck, face, and arms. In contrast, infections secondary to anthropophilic dermatophytes often occur in occluded areas or in areas of trauma.[9]

Tinea Cruris

Tinea cruris is more common in males and occurs on the medial and upper parts of the thighs and the pubic area. The lesions have well-demarcated margins that are elevated slightly and are more erythematous than the central area; small vesicles may be seen, especially at the margins. Acute lesions are bright red, and chronic cases tend to have more of a hyperpigmented appearance; fine scaling is usually present. This condition is generally bilateral with significant pruritus; however, the lesions usually spare the penis and scrotum. This characteristic can help to distinguish tinea cruris from candidiasis, which also causes lesions in these areas.[20] Pain may also be present during periods of sweating or when the skin becomes macerated or infected by a secondary microorganism.[8,9]

Tinea Capitis

Clinically, tinea capitis may present as one of four variant patterns, depending on the causative dermatophyte. In noninflammatory tinea capitis, lesions begin as small papules surrounding individual hair shafts. Subsequently, the lesions spread centrifugally to involve all hairs in their path. Although there is some scaling of the scalp, little inflammation is present (see Color Plates, photograph 33). Hairs in the lesions are a dull gray color and usually break off above the scalp level.[9]

The inflammatory type of tinea capitis produces a spectrum of inflammation, ranging from pustules to kerion formation. *Kerions* are weeping lesions whose exudate forms thick crusts on the scalp.[12] In addition to fever and pain, individuals with this type of tinea capitis may experience a higher degree of pruritus. Regional lymph nodes may also be enlarged.[9]

The black dot variety of tinea capitis was named for the appearance of infected areas of the scalp. The location of arthrospores on the hair shaft causes hairs to break off at the level of the scalp, leaving black dots on the scalp surface. Hair loss, inflammation, and scaling with this type of tinea capitis range from minimal to extensive. Therefore, this variant is especially challenging to diagnose.[9,21,22]

The favus variant of tinea capitis typically presents as patchy areas of hair loss and *scutula* (yellowish crusts and scales). Ultimately, these lesions can coalesce to involve a major portion of the scalp. If left untreated, this condition can lead to secondary bacterial infections, scalp atrophy, scarring, and permanent hair loss.[9]

Treatment of Fungal Skin Infections

Overall, fungal skin infections do not have a significant impact on mortality; however, they can be difficult to treat, leading to chronic lesions and a decrease in quality of life.[5]

Treatment Goals

The goals of treating fungal skin infections are (1) to provide symptomatic relief, (2) to eradicate existing infection, and (3) to prevent future infections.

General Treatment Approach

In many instances, patients can effectively self-treat tinea pedis, tinea corporis, and tinea cruris with nonprescription topical antifungals and nonpharmacologic measures. However, individuals with tinea unguium or tinea capitis should be referred to a primary care provider (PCP) for treatment.

Before recommending therapy, the provider must be reasonably sure that the lesions are consistent with a tinea infection. Their appearance should conform to the descriptions provided in Clinical Presentation of Fungal Skin Infections, and photographs 32 and 33 of tinea lesions (see Color Plates) should be consulted for comparison. Furthermore, the lesions should not resemble any other skin conditions. When in doubt about the true cause of a condition, the patient should be advised to consult a PCP or dermatologist. Figure 42–1 outlines the appropriate self-treatment options for fungal skin infections.

A number of topical antifungals are available in a variety of dosage forms for self-treatment of fungal skin infections. The selection of a particular product depends on the type of infection and on individual patient characteristics and preferences. For example, in acute, inflammatory tinea pedis, characterized by reddened, oozing, and vesicular eruptions, the inflammation must be counteracted with solutions of astringent aluminum salts before antifungal therapy can be instituted.

A critical determinant of the outcome of therapy is the patient's ability to adhere to the recommended therapy for the appropriate length of time. Adherence may be difficult, because these conditions may take between 2 and 4 weeks or up to 6 weeks to resolve (Table 42–2). Patients may be tempted to terminate therapy when their symptoms subside but before the infection has been eradicated.

Nonpharmacologic Therapy

Another determinant of therapeutic outcome relates to the patient's adherence to the nonpharmacologic measures intended to complement the effects of nonprescription antifungals and to prevent future infections. These measures include keeping the skin clean and dry, avoiding the sharing of personal articles, and avoiding contact with infected fomites or persons who have a fungal infection.

The box "Patient Education for Fungal Skin Infections" describes nonpharmacologic measures intended to complement the effects of nonprescription antifungals and to prevent future infections. The patient should follow these measures during and after treatment of the infection.

Pharmacologic Therapy

An antifungal ingredient must have at least one well-designed clinical trial that demonstrates its effectiveness in treating tinea infections before FDA will classify it as a monograph antifungal.[23] Clotrimazole, miconazole nitrate, terbinafine hydrochlorate, butenafine hydrochloride, tolnaftate, clioquinol, undecylenic acid, and imidazoles are considered safe and effective for nonprescription use in the treatment of fungal skin infections.[7] Rare cases of mild skin irritation, burning, and stinging have occurred with use of nonprescription topical antifungals. These agents are labeled for treatment of athlete's foot, jock itch, and body ringworm.

Clotrimazole and Miconazole Nitrate

Topical clotrimazole and miconazole nitrate are imidazole derivatives that demonstrate fungistatic/fungicidal activity (depending on concentration) against *T. mentagrophytes, T. rubrum, Epidermophyton floccosum,* and *Candida albicans.*

These agents act by inhibiting the biosynthesis of ergosterol and other sterols and by damaging the fungal cell wall membrane, thereby altering its permeability and resulting in the loss of essential intracellular elements. These drugs have also been shown to inhibit the oxidative and peroxidative enzyme activity that results in intracellular buildup of toxic concentrations of hydrogen peroxide; this toxicity may then contribute to the degradation of subcellular organelles and to cellular necrosis. In *C. albicans* infections, these drugs have been shown to inhibit the transformation of blastospores into the invasive mycelial form that causes infection.

FDA classifies clotrimazole 1% and miconazole nitrate 2% as safe and effective for topical nonprescription use in treating tinea pedis, tinea cruris, and tinea corporis. Clotrimazole and miconazole nitrate are applied twice daily. For athlete's foot and ringworm, these drugs should be applied twice daily for 4 weeks; for jock itch they should be applied twice daily for 2 weeks.

A drug–drug interaction between warfarin and topical miconazole cream is possible: coadministration of the drugs may increase the effects of warfarin.[24] No other drug–drug interactions have been reported with topical use of clotrimazole and miconazole nitrate for up to 4 weeks.[7]

Terbinafine Hydrochloride

Topical terbinafine hydrochloride 1% is an antifungal agent that inhibits squalene epoxidase, a key enzyme in fungi sterol

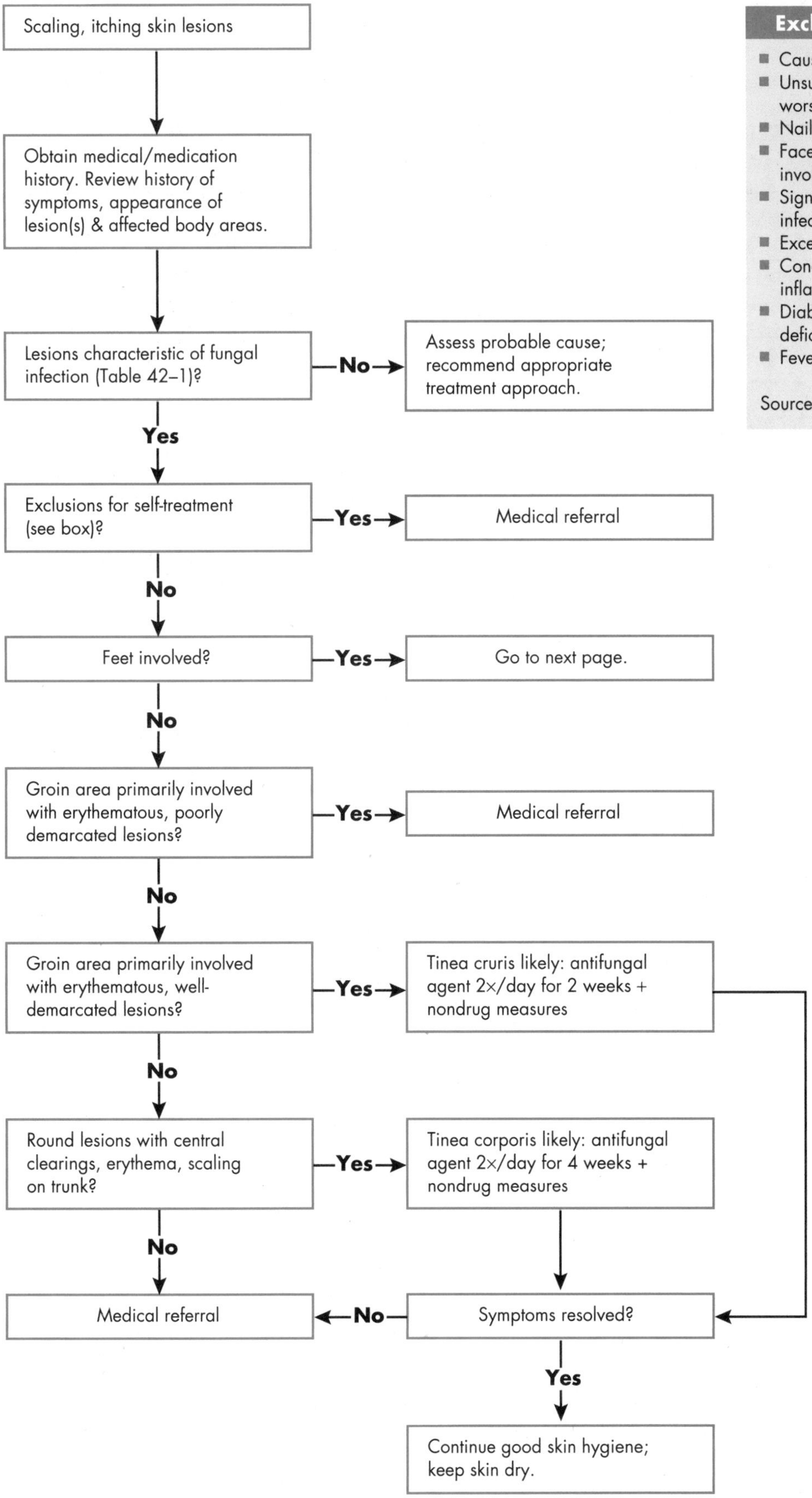

Exclusions for Self-Treatment

- Causative factor unclear
- Unsuccessful initial treatment, or worsening of condition
- Nails or scalp involved
- Face, mucous membranes, or genitalia involved
- Signs of possible secondary bacterial infection (oozing purulent material)
- Excessive and continuous exudation
- Condition extensive, seriously inflamed, or debilitating
- Diabetes, systemic infection, immune deficiency
- Fever, malaise, or both

Source: Reference 38.

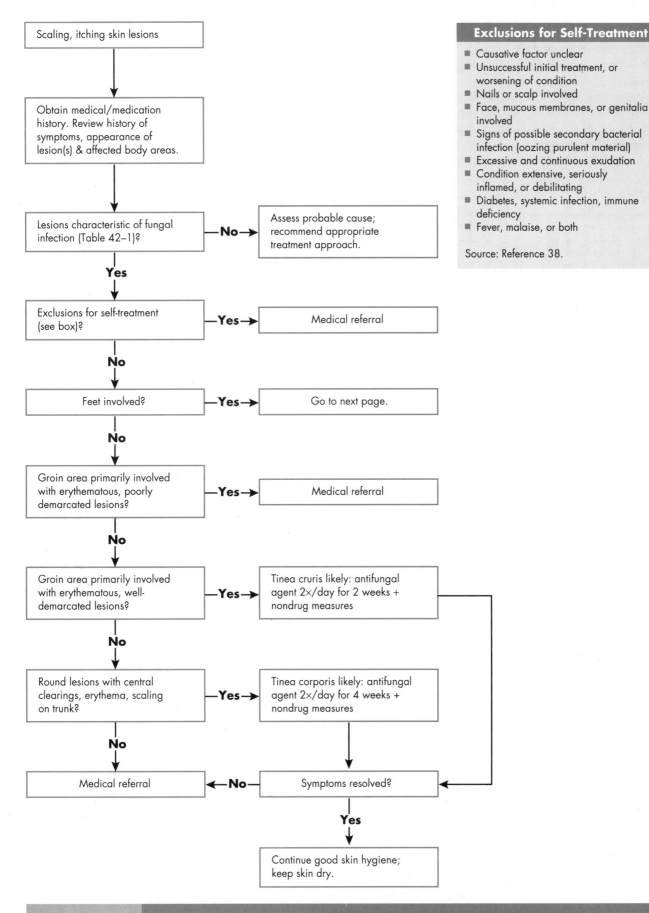

FIGURE **42–1** Self-care for fungal skin infections. (*continued on next page*)

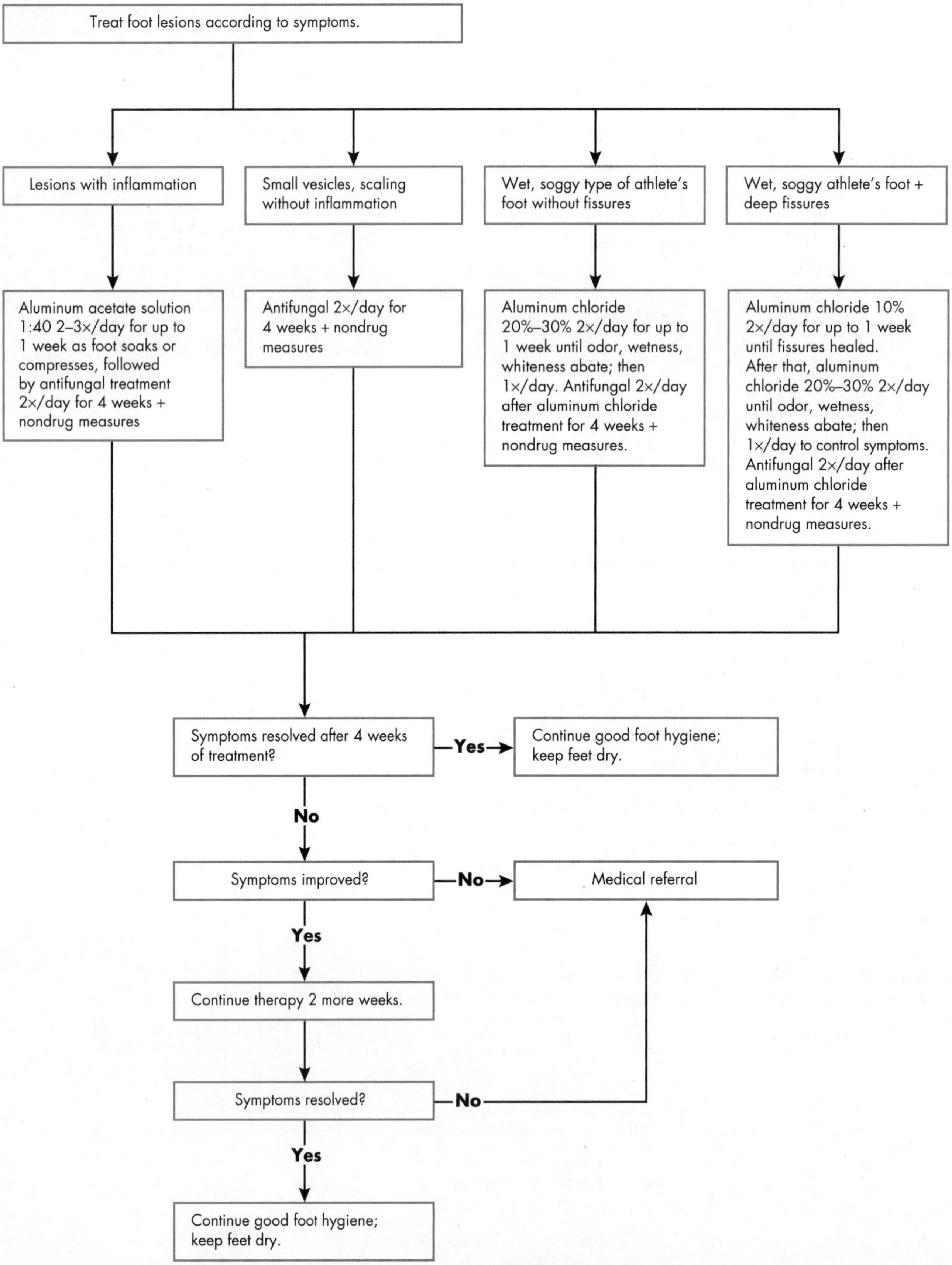

FIGURE 42-1 Self-care for fungal skin infections. (*continued*)

TABLE 42–2 Selected Nonprescription Topical Antifungal Products

Trade Name	Active Ingredient	Indications for Use	Directions for Use
Cruex Antifungal Spray Powder	Miconazole 2%	For adults and children older than 2 years of age	Clean skin, shake well, and apply 4–6 inches from site. For treatment of tinea cruris, apply twice daily for 2 weeks. For treatment of tinea corporis and pedis, apply twice daily for 4 weeks.
Desenex Antifungal Liquid Spray Powder	Miconazole 2%	For adults and children older than 2 years of age	For tinea cruris and corporis, apply twice daily for 2 weeks. For tinea pedis, apply twice daily for 4 weeks.
Lotrimin AF Jock Itch Antifungal Powder Spray	Miconazole 2%	For adults and children 12 years of age and older	For athlete's foot and ringworm, use twice daily for 4 weeks. For jock itch, use twice daily for 2 weeks.
Micatin Antifungal Cream	Miconazole 2%	For adults and children 2 years of age and older	For athlete's foot and ringworm, use twice daily for 4 weeks. For jock itch, use twice daily for 2 weeks.
Lotrimin AF Clotrimazole Jock Itch Cream	Clotrimazole 1%	For adults and children 3 years of age and older	For athlete's foot and ringworm, use twice daily for 4 weeks. For jock itch, use daily for 2 weeks.
Lotrimin Ultra Jock Itch Cream	Butenafine 1%	For adults 18 years of age and older	For athlete's foot between the toes, apply to affected skin between and around the toes twice a day for 1 week (morning and night), or once a day for 4 weeks. For jock itch and ringworm, apply once a day to affected skin for 2 weeks.
Tinactin Athlete's Foot Cream	Tolnaftate 1%	For adults and children 2 years of age and older	For athlete's foot and ringworm, use daily for 4 weeks. For jock itch, use daily for 2 weeks.
Tinactin Powder Spray	Tolnaftate 1%	For adults and children 2 years of age and older	For athlete's foot and ringworm, spray twice daily for 4 weeks. For prevention, spray 1–2 times daily.
Fungicure (solution, cream)	Undecylenic acid 10%, 22%, 25%	For adults 18 years of age and older	For tinea corporis and pedis, apply twice daily for 4 weeks

biosynthesis. This action results in a deficiency in ergosterol and a corresponding accumulation of squalene within the fungal cell, causing fungal cell death. Terbinafine hydrochloride is indicated for interdigital tinea pedis, tinea cruris, and tinea corporis caused by *E. floccosum*, *T. mentagrophytes*, and *T. rubrum*. Similar to miconazole and clotrimazole, terbinafine hydrochloride should be applied sparingly to the affected area twice daily.

In clinical trials, this drug demonstrated that it could cure tinea pedis with 1 week of treatment. However, complete resolution of symptoms may require up to 4 weeks of treatment. For athlete's foot between the toes, patients should apply terbinafine twice a day for 1 week. For athlete's foot on the bottom or sides of the foot, it should be applied twice a day for 2 weeks. For jock itch and ringworm, patients should apply terbinafine once a day for 1 week or as directed by a PCP.

Clinical trials to date have demonstrated a low incidence of adverse effects for terbinafine hydrochloride. These adverse effects include irritation (1%), burning (0.8%), and itching/dryness (0.2%).[25,26] No drug–drug interactions have been reported with topical use of this agent.

Butenafine Hydrochloride

Topical butenafine hydrochloride 1% is also an antifungal squalene epoxidase inhibitor. This action results in a deficiency in ergosterol, a corresponding accumulation of squalene within the fungal cell, and eventually cell death.

Butenafine hydrochloride is indicated as a cure for tinea pedis between the toes, tinea cruris, and tinea corporis caused by *E. floccosum*, *T. mentagrophytes*, and *T. rubrum*. Similar to other nonprescription topical antifungals, butenafine hydrochloride also relieves the itching, burning, cracking, and scaling that can accompany these conditions. This agent's effectiveness on infection of the bottom or sides of the foot is unknown.

Patients suffering from tinea pedis should be advised to apply a thin film to affected skin between and around toes twice daily for 1 week, once a day for 4 weeks, or as directed by a PCP. Patients with tinea cruris or tinea corporis should apply a thin film to the affected area once daily for 2 weeks or as directed by a PCP.

Effective treatment rates of butenafine for interdigital tinea pedis with 1-week and 4-week application durations are reported to be approximately 38% and 74%, respectively. In clinical trials, butenafine kept users free of tinea pedis for up to 3 months.[27] To date, clinical trials demonstrate a low incidence of adverse effects for this agent. Further, no drug–drug interactions have been reported with its topical use.

Tolnaftate

Topical tolnaftate has demonstrated clinical efficacy since its commercial introduction in the United States in 1965. In addition, for many years, it was the standard against which the efficacy of other topical antifungals was compared. Tolnaftate is approved for treatment of tinea pedis, tinea cruris, and tinea corporis.

Although tolnaftate's exact mechanism of action has not been reported, tolnaftate is thought to distort the hyphae and stunt the mycelial growth of the fungi species. Tolnaftate is the only nonprescription drug approved for both preventing and treating tinea infections.[7] It acts on fungi that are typically responsible for tinea infections, including *T. mentagrophytes, T. rubrum,* and *E. floccosum.*

Tolnaftate is valuable primarily in treating the dry, scaly lesions. Relapse of superficial fungal infections has occurred after discontinuation of tolnaftate therapy. Relapse may be caused by inadequate duration of treatment, patient nonadherence with the medication, or use of tolnaftate when an oral antifungal should have been used.

As a cream, tolnaftate is formulated in a polyethylene glycol 400/propylene glycol vehicle. The 1% solution is formulated in polyethylene glycol 400 and may be more effective than the cream. The solution solidifies when exposed to cold but liquefies with no loss in potency if allowed to warm. These vehicles are particularly advantageous in superficial antifungal therapy, because they are nonocclusive, nontoxic, nonsensitizing, water miscible, anhydrous, easy to apply, and efficient in delivering the drug to the affected area.

The topical powder formulation of tolnaftate uses cornstarch/talc as the vehicle. The two agents combined absorb excess moisture in the affected area that allows fungus to thrive. The topical aerosol formulation of tolnaftate includes talc, alcohol, and the propellant vehicle.

Tolnaftate (1% solution, cream, gel, powder, spray powder, or spray liquid) is applied sparingly twice daily. Effective therapy usually takes 2–4 weeks, depending on the type of infection. For example, a patient should experience improvement of symptoms with tinea cruris within 2 weeks, but treatment for tinea pedis and tinea corpus may take 4-6 weeks. Tolnaftate is well tolerated when applied to intact or broken skin, although it usually stings slightly when applied. Delayed hypersensitivity reactions to tolnaftate are extremely rare. No drug–drug interactions have been reported with topical use of tolnaftate.

Clioquinol/Undecylenic Acid

FDA has approved clioquinol 3%, and undecylenic acid for nonprescription use. Two nonprescription products are commercially available that contain undecylenic acid 25% that can be applied twice daily for 4 weeks. These products are approved for treatment of tinea pedis and tinea cruris. Both products work by preventing fungal growth. Undecylenic acid is a fatty acid and clioquinol has antibiotic effects. However, these products are less effective on the scalp or nails, despite commercial advertisement. Common adverse effects include local skin irritation and burning sensations.

Salts of Aluminum

Because aluminum salts do not have any direct antifungal activity, these drugs were not included in the FDA final monograph for topical antifungal drug products. Rather, they are approved for the relief of inflammatory conditions of the skin, such as tinea pedis. However, their effectiveness as astringents and their possible use in treating tinea pedis merit their inclusion in this chapter. Historically, aluminum acetate has been the foremost astringent used for both the acute, inflammatory type and the wet, soggy type of tinea pedis. Aluminum chloride is also used to treat the wet, soggy type of infection.

Aluminum salts do not cure athlete's foot entirely but are useful when combined with other topical antifungal drugs. Application of aluminum salts merely shifts the disease process back to the simple dry type of athlete's foot, which can then be controlled with other agents, such as tolnaftate or an imidazole.

The action and efficacy of aluminum salts appear to be double-pronged. First, these compounds act as astringents. Their drying ability probably involves complexing of the astringent agent with proteins, thereby altering the proteins' ability to swell and hold water. Astringents decrease edema, exudation, and inflammation by reducing cell membrane permeability and by hardening the intercellular cement of the capillary epithelium. Second, aluminum salts in concentrations greater than 20% possess antibacterial activity, which may help to prevent the development of secondary bacterial infections. Aluminum chloride solution (20%) may exhibit that activity in two ways: by directly killing bacteria and by drying the interdigital spaces. Solutions of 20% aluminum acetate and 20% aluminum chloride demonstrate equal in vitro antibacterial efficacy.

Aluminum acetate for use in tinea pedis is generally diluted with about 10–40 parts of water. Depending on the situation, the whole foot may be immersed in the solution for 20 minutes up to 3 times a day (every 6–8 hours), or the solution may be applied to the affected area in the form of a wet dressing.

For patient convenience, aluminum acetate solution (Burow solution) or modified Burow solution (which includes dextrin, polyethylene glycol, and sodium bicarbonate as inactive ingredients) is available for immediate use in solution or in forms to be dissolved in water (powder packets, powder, effervescent tablets) (see Chapter 35).

Aqueous solutions of 20%–30% aluminum chloride have been the most beneficial for the wet, soggy type of athlete's foot.[11] Twice-daily applications are generally used until the signs and symptoms (odor, wetness, whiteness) abate. After that, once-daily applications may control the symptoms. In hot, humid weather, the original condition may return within 7–10 days after the application is stopped.

Because aluminum salts penetrate the skin poorly, their toxicity is low. However, a few cases of irritation have been reported in patients with deep fissures. Therefore, the use of concentrated aluminum salt solutions on severely eroded or deeply fissured skin is contraindicated. In this case, the salts must be diluted to a lower concentration (10% aluminum chloride) for initial treatment.

Solutions of aluminum acetate or aluminum chloride have the potential for misuse (e.g., accidental childhood poisoning by ingestion of the solutions or the solid tablets), so precautions must be taken to prevent this misuse. Products containing these ingredients are intended for external use only and should not be applied near the eyes. Prolonged or continuous use of aluminum acetate solution may produce tissue necrosis. In the acute inflammatory stage of tinea pedis, this solution should be used less than 1 week. The provider should instruct the patient to discontinue its use if inflammatory lesions appear or worsen.

Pharmacotherapeutic Comparison

All the topical antifungals approved for treating cutaneous fungal infections have demonstrated effectiveness. The allure of butenafine hydrochloride and terbinafine hydrochloride is their ability to cure athlete's foot in some patients after 1 week. However, a close analysis of the data demonstrates that the number of patients achieving complete resolution of the problem is low, and that the effectiveness of these agents parallels that of other antifungals previously approved for nonprescription use (e.g., clotrimazole, miconazole nitrate).[28]

Controlled studies have demonstrated the efficacy of clotrimazole and miconazole nitrate for tinea pedis. Both agents would be expected to demonstrate efficacy comparable to that of tolnaftate for tinea infections. If patient factors (e.g., nonadherence, improper foot hygiene) can be ruled out as a cause of treatment failure, both can be suggested as alternative treatment modalities.

Product Selection Guidelines

Cutaneous antifungals are available as ointments, creams, powders, and aerosols (Table 42–2). Creams or solutions are the most efficient and effective dosage forms for delivery of the active ingredient to the epidermis. Sprays and powders are less effective, because they often are not rubbed into the skin. They are probably more useful as adjuncts to a cream or a solution or as prophylactic agents in preventing new or recurrent infections.

Patient adherence is influenced by product selection. Therefore, the provider should recommend a drug and dosage form that are likely to cause the least interference with daily habits and activities, without sacrificing efficacy. For example, older patients may require a preparation that is easy to use. Obese patients, in whom excessive sweating may contribute to the disease, should sprinkle talcum powder on the feet and in the shoes as adjunctive therapy to keep the feet dry. Under certain circumstances, the provider may need to instruct the caregiver instead of the patient in the proper use of foot products.

Before recommending a nonprescription product, the provider should review the patient's medical history. For example, patients with diabetes should have their blood glucose levels under control, because increased glucose in perspiration may promote fungal growth. Patients with allergic dermatitis often have a history of asthma, hay fever, or atopic dermatitis; therefore, they are extremely sensitive to many oral and topical agents. Acquiring a good medical history may aid in distinguishing a tinea infection from atopic dermatitis and may avoid the recommendation of a product that might cause further skin irritation.

In addition, product line extensions that carry the same brand name do not necessarily have the same active ingredient(s). For example, the cream and solution formulations of Lotrimin AF contain clotrimazole 1%, whereas the topical spray and powder formulations contain miconazole nitrate 2%. Indeed, Lotrimin Ultra, the newest line extension, contains butenafine hydrochloride. Similarly, Desenex spray liquid, spray powder, and spray powder formulations contain miconazole nitrate 2%, whereas these products formerly contained undecylenic acid.

Complementary Therapies

Bitter orange, tea tree oil, and garlic have been used with some success in the management of fungal skin infections, with few or no adverse effects. None of the studies that examined these ingredients included more than 60 patients, but the results suggest that further investigation of each complementary therapy is warranted.

Bitter orange has the least evidence of safety and efficacy. However, in one controlled trial, topical application of oil of bitter orange 3 times daily demonstrated benefit in most patients with tinea corporis, tinea cruris, or tinea pedis in 1–4 weeks. The only reported side effect was mild, local irritation.[29]

Investigations into the efficacy of tea tree oil for tinea pedis have yielded mixed results. In one study that compared tolnaftate 1% cream with tea tree oil 10% cream, both agents were equally effective in relieving the scaling, inflammation, itching, and burning, but neither agent was more effective than placebo in achieving mycologic cure.[30] Results of two other studies suggest that tea tree oil 25% and 50% appear to result in both symptomatic and mycologic cure of tinea pedis. However, the mycologic cure rates were inferior to those for butenafine and clotrimazole.[31,32]

Research relative to the efficacy of topical garlic for the management of tinea infections has been positive. For example, application of a garlic gel containing 0.6% ajoene (a constituent of garlic believed to have antifungal activity) was demonstrated to be as effective as terbinafine 1% cream in a study of subjects with either tinea corporis or cruris.[33] In another study ($n = 34$), the use of ajoene 0.4% as a cream resulted in clinical and mycologic cure of all research subjects after 2 weeks of use.[34] In the most recent study published in 2000, researchers reported evidence that ajoene 1% cream produces a higher mycologic cure rate than that of ajoene 0.6% and terbinafine 1% creams.[35]

Assessment of Fungal Skin Infections: A Case-Based Approach

Fungal skin infections must be differentiated from bacterial skin infections and noninfectious dermatitis. If possible, the provider should examine the affected area to determine whether the disorder's manifestation is typical of a fungal infection (Table 42–1).[36] The only true determinant of a fungal infection is a clinical laboratory evaluation of tissue scrapings from the affected area.

The provider should question the patient thoroughly regarding the condition and its characteristics to determine symptoms, extent of disease, previous patient adherence with medications, and any compounding disorders (e.g., diabetes, obesity) that might render the patient susceptible. Patients with diabetes, for example, may present with a mixed dermatophytid and monilial infection. In general, it is appropriate to inspect the affected area if privacy and sanitary conditions allow. Inspection is especially appropriate for patients with diabetes.

Cases 42–1 and 42–2 are examples of the assessment of patients with a fungal skin infection.

The most common symptom of patients with a cutaneous fungal infection is pruritus. However, if fissures are present, particularly between the toes, painful burning and stinging may also occur. If the area is abraded, denuded, or inflamed, weeping or oozing may be present in addition to pain. Some patients may merely remark on the bothersome scaling of dry skin, particularly if the infection involves the soles of the feet. In other instances, small vesicular lesions may combine to form a larger bullous eruption marked by pain and irritation, or the only symptoms may be brittleness and discoloration of a hypertrophied nail.

The provider should seek to distinguish a tinea infection from diseases with similar symptoms, such as bacterial infection, irritant contact dermatitis, allergic contact dermatitis, and atopic

CASE 42-1

Relevant Evaluation Criteria	Scenario/Model Outcome
Collect	
1. Gather essential information about the patient's symptoms and medical history, including	
a. Description of symptom(s) (i.e., nature, onset, duration, severity, associated symptoms)	The patient presents to the pharmacy with redness in the shape of eyeglasses on her nose and around both eyes. Scaling and weeping vesicles on both eyelids extend into both eyebrows. The patient has an open sore on the bridge of her nose that she admits she caused by scratching the area. She also complains of intense itching. Her symptoms began about a month ago, right after she started to swim competitively at school. She denies changes in swimming equipment, including goggles.
b. Description of any factors that seem to precipitate, exacerbate, and/or relieve the patient's symptom(s)	She says that the itching is worse after she removes her swim goggles.
c. Description of the patient's efforts to relieve the symptoms	She has tried hydrocortisone ointment with no relief.
d. Patient's identity	Sara Lansbury
e. Patient's age, gender, height, and weight	21 years old, female, 5 ft 6 in, 128 lb
f. Patient's occupation	College student
g. Patient's dietary habits	Patient is a vegetarian.
h. Patient's sleep habits	Number of hours that patient sleeps each night varies.
i. Concurrent medical conditions, prescription and nonprescription medications, and dietary supplements	Seasonal allergies: Claritin D (loratadine/pseudoephedrine) in the spring and fall
j. Allergies	Ragweed and maple trees
k. History of other adverse reactions to medications	None
l. Other (describe) _______	Patient has a history of ringworm during swim season.
Assess	
2. Differentiate patient's signs/symptoms, and correctly identify the patient's primary problem(s) (Table 42–1).	Patient is suffering from inflammation, weeping, denudation, and intense itching on her face, secondary to ringworm.
3. Identify exclusions for self-treatment (Figure 42–1).	Severe symptoms, eye involvement, eyebrow involvement
4. Formulate a comprehensive list of therapeutic alternatives for the primary problem to determine whether triage to a medical provider is required, and share this information with the patient or caregiver.	Options include (1) Refer patient to an appropriate HCP (2) Recommend self-care with a nonprescription antifungal and nondrug measures. (3) Recommend self-care until patient can see an appropriate HCP. (4) Take no action.
Plan	
5. Select an optimal therapeutic alternative to address the patient's problem, taking into account patient preferences.	Patient should consult an HCP.
6. Describe the recommended therapeutic approach to the patient or caregiver.	"You should consult a health care provider for treatment."
7. Explain to the patient or caregiver the rationale for selecting the recommended therapeutic approach from the considered therapeutic alternatives.	"This option is best, because your problem is severe and is affecting skin near your eyes. You will need oral medication that is available only by prescription to treat your condition."
Implement	
8. When recommending self-care with nonprescription medications and/or nondrug therapy, convey accurate information to the patient or caregiver.	"Make sure you dry off well after swimming, and allow your face to air dry completely. Do not share towels or other sports equipment."

CASE 42-1 *continued*

Relevant Evaluation Criteria	Scenario/Model Outcome
Solicit follow-up questions from the patient or caregiver.	"One of my teammates said that I should suffocate the ringworms by applying clear nail polish on the itchy spots. Does this really work?"
Answer the patient's or caregiver's questions.	"Ringworm is not actually caused by worms. It is caused by a fungus that lives in the superficial skin layers. Nail polish will have no effect on your symptoms. It can, however, cause severe irritation if you get it in your eyes."
Follow-up: Monitor and Evaluate	
9. Assess patient outcome.	Contact the patient in a day or two to ensure that she made an appointment and sought medical care.

Key: HCP = Health care provider.

CASE 42-2

Relevant Evaluation Criteria	Scenario/Model Outcome
Collect	
1. Gather essential information about the patient's symptoms and medical history, including	
a. Description of symptom(s) (i.e., nature, onset, duration, severity, associated symptoms)	The patient describes intense itching and a red, scaly rash on and between the third, fourth, and fifth toes of each foot. He says that the symptoms began a week ago, soon after he began his summer job at a lawn maintenance service.
b. Description of any factors that seem to precipitate, exacerbate, and/or relieve the patient's symptom(s)	The patient says that the itching is worse after he gets home from work in the evening.
c. Description of the patient's efforts to relieve the symptoms	The patient has not tried anything other than scratching the affected area when the itching becomes unbearable.
d. Patient's identity	Robert Grees
e. Patient's age, gender, height, and weight	17 years old, male, 5 ft 11 in., 175 lb
f. Patient's occupation	Lawn maintenance worker
g. Patient's dietary habits	Eats fast food for breakfast and lunch.
h. Patient's sleep habits	6–7 hours nightly
i. Concurrent medical conditions, prescription and nonprescription medications, and dietary supplements	None
j. Allergies	None
k. History of other adverse reactions to medications	None
l. Other (describe) _______	n/a
Assess	
2. Differentiate patient's signs/symptoms, and correctly identify the patient's primary problem(s) (Table 42–1).	Robert is suffering from a scaling red rash and itching secondary to athlete's foot. He likely contracted this problem from mowing lawns.
3. Identify exclusions for self-treatment (Figure 42–1).	None
4. Formulate a comprehensive list of therapeutic alternatives for the primary problem to determine whether triage to a medical provider is required, and share this information with the patient or caregiver.	Options include (1) Refer Robert to an appropriate HCP. (2) Recommend self-care with a nonprescription antifungal and nondrug measures. (3) Recommend self-care until Robert can see an appropriate HCP. (4) Take no action.

CASE 42-2 *continued*

Relevant Evaluation Criteria	Scenario/Model Outcome
Plan	
5. Select an optimal therapeutic alternative to address the patient's problem, taking into account patient preferences.	Robert should use a nonprescription antifungal and nondrug measures to treat his problem.
6. Describe the recommended therapeutic approach to the patient or caregiver.	"Regular use of any of the commercially available nonprescription antifungals in any dosage form except a spray or powder should alleviate the problem. However, for the medication to be optimally effective, you will have to take several measures to keep the affected area clean and dry."
7. Explain to the patient or caregiver the rationale for selecting the recommended therapeutic approach from the considered therapeutic alternatives.	"Athlete's foot can be effectively managed with nonprescription antifungals and nondrug measures (if the area is kept clean and dry) as long as there is no evidence of secondary infection or preexisting medical conditions that would preclude self-treatment, as in your case. Sprays and powders are less effective, because they often are not rubbed into the skin."
Implement	
8. When recommending self-care with nonprescription medications and/or nondrug therapy, convey accurate information to the patient or caregiver.	
a. Appropriate dose and frequency of administration	See the box "Patient Education for Fungal Skin Infections."
b. Maximum number of days the therapy should be employed	See the box "Patient Education for Fungal Skin Infections."
c. Product administration procedures	See the box "Patient Education for Fungal Skin Infections."
d. Expected time to onset of relief	"Itching may be relieved somewhat within a few days, but eradication of the causative microorganism may take up to 4–6 weeks, depending on the agent used."
e. Degree of relief that can be reasonably expected	"Athlete's foot can be cured if you use the antifungal and nondrug measures properly."
f. Most common adverse effects	See the box "Patient Education for Fungal Skin Infections."
g. Adverse effects that warrant medical intervention should they occur	See the box "Patient Education for Fungal Skin Infections."
h. Patient options in the event that condition worsens or persists	See the box "Patient Education for Fungal Skin Infections."
i. Product storage requirements	"Store in a cool, dry place out of children's reach."
j. Specific nondrug measures	See the box "Patient Education for Fungal Skin Infections."
Solicit follow-up questions from the patient or caregiver.	"Why do I have this? I am not an athlete."
Answer the patient's or caregiver's questions.	"Your feet are sweating more than usual now, because you are working outside. As a result, the skin on your feet remains damp until you remove your shoes and socks after work. Moisture helps the fungus that causes ringworm to thrive."
Follow-up: Monitor and Evaluate	
9. Assess patient outcome.	Ask the patient to call to update you on his response to your recommendations 1 week after initiating treatment. Or you could call him in a week to evaluate the outcome.

Key: HCP = Health care provider; n/a = not applicable.

dermatitis. For this reason, the manifestation of these disorders is briefly discussed here. In children, peridigital dermatitis or atopic dermatitis is more common than tinea pedis. Shoe dermatitis is perhaps the most common form of allergic contact dermatitis from clothing. Therefore, the provider should inquire about the type of footwear worn by the patient and about recent footwear changes. The increased use of rubber and adhesives in footwear has paralleled the increase in reports of shoe dermatitis in the dermatologic and podiatric literature. Contact allergy to accelerators (the chemical compounds used to speed the processing of rubber used in sponge-rubber insoles for tennis shoes) has also been reported.[37] In addition to accelerators, antioxidants have been implicated as major chemical allergens, and various phenolic resins used in adhesives are also troublesome. The patient is usually unaware that his or her footwear may be causing the problem.

Hyperhidrosis of interdigital spaces and of the sole of the foot is common, as is infection of the toe interspaces by gram-negative bacteria. In hyperhidrosis, tender vesicles cover the sole of the foot and toes, and these areas may be quite painful. The skin generally turns white, erodes, and becomes macerated. This condition is accompanied by a foul foot odor. A soggy wetness of the toe webs and the immediately adjacent skin characterizes infection by gram-negative bacteria; the affected tissue is damp and softened. The last toe web (adjacent to the little toe) is the most common area of primary or initial involvement, because it is deeper and extends more proximally than the web between the other toes. Furthermore, abundant exocrine sweat glands, a semiocclusive anatomic setting, and the added occlusion provided by footwear enhance development of the disease at this site. The provider must be careful not to confuse this condition with soft corns, which also appear between the fourth and fifth toes.

Patient Counseling for Fungal Skin Infections

The proper application technique for topical antifungals and required duration of therapy should be described to the patient to prevent over- or undermedication. The patient should be told to apply the medication regularly throughout a complete course of therapy. Information that will help to control or eradicate the infection and that will minimize the likelihood of recurrent infections may also be provided. This information should address proper care of the infected skin site, appropriate laundry techniques and products, minimal use of occlusive clothing, and avoidance of habits or behavior that may lead to recurring infections. The patient should also be told which conditions indicate the need to consult a PCP (e.g., the development of a secondary bacterial infection). The box "Patient Education for Fungal Skin Infections" lists information to provide patients.

PATIENT EDUCATION FOR Fungal Skin Infections

The objectives of self-treatment are (1) to relieve itching, burning, and other discomfort; (2) to inhibit the growth of fungi and cure the disorder; and (3) to prevent recurrent infections. For most patients, carefully following product instructions and the self-care measures listed here will help ensure optimal therapeutic outcomes.

Nondrug Measures

- To prevent spreading the infection to other parts of the body, either use a separate towel to dry the affected area or dry the affected area last.
- Do not share towels, clothing, or other personal articles with household members, especially when an infection is present.
- Launder contaminated towels and clothing in hot water, and dry them on a hot dryer setting to prevent spreading the infection.
- Cleanse skin daily with soap and water, and thoroughly pat dry to remove oils and other substances that promote growth of fungi.
- If possible, do not wear clothing or shoes that cause the skin to stay wet. Wool and synthetic fabrics prevent optimal air circulation.
- If needed, allow shoes to dry thoroughly before wearing them again. Dust shoes with medicated or nonmedicated foot powder to help keep them dry.
- If needed, place odor-controlling insoles in casual or athletic shoes. These insoles also provide some support and cushioning for the feet. Change insoles routinely every 3–4 months or more often if their condition warrants. Take care that the shoe fit is not compromised by the insoles.
- As with all topical medications, discontinue the use of an antifungal if irritation, sensitization, or worsening of the skin condition occurs.
- Avoid contact with people who have fungal infections. Wear protective footwear (e.g., rubber or wooden sandals) in areas of family or public use, such as home bathrooms or community showers.

Nonprescription Medications

- Ask a health care provider for assistance in picking the appropriate antifungal agent and dosage form for your infection.
- Available agents include butenafine, clotrimazole, miconazole nitrate, terbinafine, and tolnaftate.
- It usually takes 2–4 weeks to cure tinea infections. Some cases may require 4–6 weeks of treatment.
- Apply the antifungal to the clean, dry affected area as directed (in the morning or evening if once daily, or both times if twice daily). Massage the medication into the area. Note that creams and solutions are easier to work into the skin; therefore, they are probably more effective treatment forms.
- Avoid getting the product in your eyes.
- Wash hands thoroughly with soap and water before and after applying the product.
- Topical antifungals themselves may cause itching, redness, and irritation.
- Tolnaftate may sting slightly upon application.
- When the medication is to be applied to pressure areas of the foot, where the horny skin layer is thicker, apply a keratolytic agent (e.g., Whitfield ointment) to the affected area first to help the antifungal penetrate the skin.
- If oozing lesions are present, apply aluminum acetate solution (1:40) to the area before applying the antifungal:
  - Soak the area in an aluminum acetate solution for 20 minutes up to 3 times a day (every 6–8 hours), or apply the solution to the affected area in the form of a wet dressing.
  - Note that aluminum acetate solution (Burow solution) or modified Burow solution is available for immediate use as a solution or as forms to be dissolved in water (powder packets, powder, and effervescent tablets).
  - Avoid getting the product in your eyes.
  - To avoid skin damage, use the solution for no more than 1 week. Discontinue use of the solution if inflammatory lesions appear or worsen.

PATIENT EDUCATION FOR Fungal Skin Infections *(continued)*

- For the wet, soggy type of athlete's foot, apply to or soak foot in aluminum acetate solution (1:40) before applying the antifungal:
  - Soak feet with aluminum acetate solution (1:40) twice daily until the odor, wetness, and whiteness are gone. After that, soak once daily to control the symptoms.
  - If deep fissures are present in the skin, use a more dilute solution of aluminum acetate for initial treatment.
  - A solution of 30% aluminum chloride twice daily can be applied for treating athlete's foot.

When to Seek Medical Attention

- Discontinue use of the product and contact a primary care provider if itching or swelling occurs, or if the infection worsens.
- Consult a primary care provider if the infection worsens or persists beyond the recommended length of therapy.
- Consult a primary care provider if the infection worsens, does not improve within a week or persists beyond the recommended length of therapy.

Evaluation of Patient Outcomes for Fungal Skin Infections

In general, the patient should begin to see some relief of the itching, scaling, and/or inflammation within 1 week. If the disorder shows improvement within this time frame, continuing treatment for 1–3 weeks (depending on the type of tinea infection and medication being used) should be recommended. If the disorder has not improved or has worsened, referring the patient to a PCP for more aggressive therapy is appropriate. Recurrent skin infections may be a sign of undiagnosed diabetes, immunodeficiency, or another organic problem that requires medical evaluation.

Key Points for Fungal Skin Infections

- Tinea corporis, tinea cruris, and tinea pedis can be treated with nonprescription drugs. Clotrimazole, miconazole nitrate, terbinafine hydrochloride, butenafine hydrochloride, tolnaftate, and undecylenic acid are efficacious for this purpose.
- The effectiveness of topical antifungals will be limited unless the patient eliminates other predisposing factors to tinea infections.
- These drugs are effective in all their delivery vehicles, but the powder forms should be reserved only for extremely mild conditions or as adjunctive therapy.
- Because solutions and creams can spread beyond the affected area, they should be used sparingly.
- When recommended for suspected or actual dermatophytosis, these topical antifungals should be used once or twice daily (morning and night), depending on the indication. Treatment should be continued for 1–4 weeks, depending on the symptoms and the type of fungal infection. After that time, the patient and/or provider should evaluate the effectiveness of the therapy.
- To minimize nonadherence, the provider should advise patients that alleviation of symptoms will not occur overnight. Patients should also be cautioned that frequent recurrence of any of these problems is an indication that they should consult a PCP.
- Immunocompromised patients and those with diabetes or circulatory problems should be treated by a PCP.
- Pregnant patients should be treated by a PCP or obstetrician.
- The only antifungal currently approved for prevention of athlete's foot is tolnaftate.

REFERENCES

1. Havlickova B, Czaika VA, Friedrich M. Epidemiological trends in skin mycoses worldwide. *Mycoses.* 2008;51(4):2–15, doi: 10.1111/j.1439-0507.2008.01606.x.
2. Sahoo AK, Mahajan R. Management of tinea corporus, tinea cruris, and tinea pedis: a comprehensive review. *Indian Dermatol Online J.* 2016;7(2): 77–86, doi: 10.4103/2229-5178.178099.
3. Pathangani AP, Tidman MJ. Diagnosis directs treatment in fungal infections of the skin. *Practitioner.* 2015;259(1786):25–9. PMID: 26738249.
4. Jaulim Z, Salmon N, Fuller C. Fungal skin infections: current approaches to management. *Prescriber.* 2015;5(10):31–5, doi: 10.1002.
5. Pires CA, Santos da Cruz NF, Lobato AM, et al. Clinical, epidemiological, and therapeutic profile of dermatophytosis. *An Bras Dermatol.* 2014; 89(2):259–64. PMID: 24770502.
6. Nenoff P, Krüger C, Schaller J, et al. Mycology: an update part 2: dermatomycoses: clinical picture and diagnostics. *J Dtsch Dermatol Ges.* 2014; 12(9):749–77, doi: 10.1111/ddg.12420.
7. U.S. Department of Food and Drug Administration. Topical antifungal drug products for over-the-counter human use; proposed amendment of final monograph. *Fed Regist.* 2001;66(103)46744–5. Available at: https://www.federalregister.gov/documents/2001/05/29/01-13299/topical-antifungal-drug-products-for-over-the-counter-human-use-proposed-amendment-of-final. Accessed July 24, 2017.
8. Drake LA, Dinehart SM, Farmer ER, et al. Guidelines for care of superficial mycotic infections of the skin: tinea corporis, tinea cruris, tinea faciei, tinea manuum and tinea pedis. *J Am Acad Dermatol.* 1996;34(2 Pt 1): 282–6. PMID: 8642096.
9. Schieke SM, Garg A. Chapter 188. Superficial fungal infection. In: Goldsmith LA, Katz SI, Gilchrest BA, et al., eds. *Fitzpatrick's Dermatology in General Medicine.* 8th ed. New York, NY: McGraw-Hill; 2012. Available at: http://accessmedicine.mhmedical.com/content.aspx?bookid=392&sectionid=41138916. Accessed March 09, 2016.
10. Lesher J, Levine N, Treadwell P. Fungal skin infections. *Patient Care.* 1994;28:16–44.
11. Shrum JP, Millikan LE, Bataineh O. Superficial fungal infections in the tropics. *Dermatol Clin.* 1994;12(4):687–93. PMID: 7805297.
12. Bergus GR, Johnson JS. Superficial tinea infections. *Am Fam Physician.* 1993;48(2):259. PMID: 8342479.
13. Evans EG. Tinea pedis: clinical experience and efficacy of short treatment. *Dermatology.* 1997;194(Suppl 1):3–6. PMID: 9154392.
14. Szepietowski JC, Reich A, Carlowska E, et al. Factors influencing co-existence of toenail onychomycosis with tinea pedis and other dermatomycoses. *Arch Dermatol.* 2006;142(10):1279–84, doi: 10.1001/archderm.142.10.1279.
15. Hasan MA, Fitzgerald SM, Saoudin M, et al. Dermatology for the practicing allergist: tinea pedis and its complications. *Clinical and Molecular Allergy.* 2004; (2):5-11, doi: 10.1186/1476-7961-2-5.
16. Pray SW. *Nonprescription Product Therapeutics.* 2nd ed. Philadelphia, PA: Lippincott Williams & Wilkins; 2006:591. PMCID: PMC1636993.
17. Dahl MV. Dermatophytosis and the immune response. *J Am Acad Dermatol.* 1994;31(3 Pt 2):S34–41. PMID: 8077506.
18. Schieke SM, Garg A. Superficial fungal infection. In: Goldsmith LA, Katz SI, Gilchrest BA, et al *Fitzpatrick's Dermatology in General Medicine.*

8th ed. Eds. New York, NY: McGraw-Hill; 2012. Available at: http://accessmedicine.mhmedical.com/content.aspx?bookid=392&sectionid=41138916. Accessed July 30, 2017.
19. Pray SW. Recognizing and eradicating tinea pedis (athlete's foot). *US Pharm.* 2010;35(8):10–5.
20. Watkins J. Fungal infection of the skin, part 2: cutaneous candida. *Br J Sch Nurse.* 2013;8(6):284–6, doi: 10.12968/bjsn.2013.8.6.294.
21. Elewski BE, Silverman RA. Clinical pearl: diagnostic procedures for tinea capitis. *J Am Acad Dermatol.* 1996;34(3):498–9. PMID: 8609265.
22. Drake LA, Dinehart SM, Farmer ER, et al. Guidelines for care of superficial mycotic infections of the skin: tinea capitis and tinea barbae. *J Am Acad Dermatol.* 1996;34(2 Pt 1):290. PMID: 8642096.
23. U.S. Food and Drug Administration. History and overview of OTC monograph for topical antifungal drug products [memo]. 2004. Available at: https://www.fda.gov/ohrms/dockets/ac/04/briefing/4036B1_06_OTC%20Monograph%20Topical.htm. Accessed July 24, 2017.
24. Devaraj A, O'Beirne J, Veasey R, et al. Interaction between warfarin and topical miconazole cream. *BMJ.* 2002;325(7355):77. PMID: 12114237.
25. Savin RC. Treatment of chronic tinea pedis (athlete's foot type) with topical terbinafine. *J Am Acad Dermatol.* 1990;23(4 Pt 2):786–9. PMID: 2229524.
26. Savin RC, Zaias N. Treatment of chronic moccasin-type tinea pedis with terbinafine: a double-blind, placebo-controlled trial. *J Am Acad Dermatol.* 1990;23(4 Pt 2):804–7. PMID: 2229528.
27. Mentax (butenafine HCl cream) Cream, 1% [package insert]. Morgantown, WV: Bertek Pharmaceuticals; Available at: http://www.accessdata.fda.gov/drugsatfda_docs/label/2001/20524s5lbl.pdf. Accessed.
28. Gupta AK, Einarson TR, Summerbell RC, et al. An overview of topical antifungal therapy in dermatomycoses: a North American perspective. *Drugs.* 1998;55(5);645–74. PMID: 9585862.
29. Ramadan W, Ibrahim S, Sonbol F. Oil of bitter orange: new topical antifungal agent. *Int J Dermatol.* 1996;35(6):448–9. PMID: 8737885.
30. Tong MM, Altman PM, Barneston RS. Tea tree oil in the treatment of tinea pedis. *Australas J Dermatol.* 1992;33(3):145–9. PMID: 1303075.
31. Buck, DS, Nidor DM, Addino JD. Comparison of two topical preparations for the treatment of onychomycosis: *Melaleuca alternifolia* (tea tree) oil and clotrimazole. *J Fam Pract.* 1994;38(6):601–5. PMID: 8195735.
32. Syed TA, Qureshi ZA, Ali SM, et al. Treatment of toenail onychomycosis with 2% butenafine and 5% *Melaleuca alternifolia* (tea tree) oil in cream. *Trop Med Int Health.* 1999;4(4):284–7. PMID: 10357864.
33. Ledezma E, Lopez JC, Marin P, et al. Ajoene in the topical short term treatment of tinea cruris and tinea corporis in humans. Randomized comparative study with terbinafine. *Arzneimittelforschung.* 1999;49(6):554–7. doi: 10.1055/s-0031-1300459.
34. Ledezma E, DeSousa L, Jorquera A, et al. Efficacy of ajoene, an organosulphur derived from garlic, in the short-term efficacy of tinea pedis. *Mycoses.* 1996;39(9–10):393–5. PMID: 9009665.
35. Ledezma E, Marcano K, Jorquera A, et al. Efficacy of ajoene in the treatment of tinea pedis: a double-blind comparative study with terbinafine. *J Am Acad Dermatol.* 2000;43(5 Pt 1):829–32. PMID: 11050588.
36. Bruinsma W, ed. *A Guide to Drug Eruptions.* 6th ed. Amsterdam, The Netherlands: Free University Press; 1995.
37. Jung JH, McLaughlin JL, Stannard J, et al. Isolation, via activity-directed fractionation, of mercaptobenzothiazole and dibenzothiazyl disulfide as 2 allergens responsible for tennis shoe dermatitis. *Contact Dermat.* 1988; 19:254–9. PMID: 3219832.
38. U.S. Food and Drug Administration. Topical anti-microbial drug products for over-the-counter human use. *CFR: Code of Federal Regulations.* Title 21, Part 333, Section 333.150. Updated April 1, 2016. Available at: https://www.accessdata.fda.gov/scripts/cdrh/cfdocs/cfcfr/CFRSearch.cfm?CFRPart=333. Accessed August 5, 2017.

CHAPTER 43

WARTS

DONNA M. ADKINS

Warts, or verrucae, are a common skin disorder caused by human papillomaviruses (HPVs).[1–12] Approximately 7%–10% of the general population has warts, with approximately 70% of the cases being attributed to common warts.[1–4] Warts occur more frequently in children and adolescents than in infants and adults, with the peak incidence among 12- to 16-year-olds.[1,2,5] Warts are a benign condition and often go away without treatment. Approximately 23% of warts regress within 2 months and 65%–78% within 2 years.[1,6,11] This chapter discusses treatments for common warts and plantar warts that are found on areas of the body and are amenable to self-treatment.

Pathophysiology of Warts

HPVs are double-stranded DNA viruses.[1–6,8] More than 150 related viruses and more than 200 subgroups have been identified through DNA sequencing.[2] HPV infection occurs via person-to-person contact, autoinoculation, or fomites found on contaminated surfaces.[1,3,7] Warts may affect skin and mucous membranes anywhere on the body. HPV infection is limited to the epidermal tissues and does not spread systemically. When minor skin abrasions are present, HPV may enter the epidermal layer and infect the basal keratinocytes.[1] The incubation period may be long (i.e., months).[2,11] The manifestation of warts may depend on the immune response of the infected individual. How quickly warts are cleared is influenced by factors such as viral type, patient immune status, and the extent and duration of time the warts have been present.[1] Several risk factors exist for the development of warts, such as having previous or existing warts; having a depressed immune system; going barefoot, especially on wet surfaces; using swimming pools and public showers; working in a meat-handling occupation; and biting one's fingernails.[1–3,5,9]

Clinical Presentation

The appearance, size, shape, and response to treatment of individual warts vary by HPV type and the specific location of the warts on the body.[1,3,9] Although different types of HPV are not found exclusively in specific areas of the body, HPV-2, HPV-4, HPV-27, and HPV-57 are the most common cause of warts on the hands, and HPV-1 is the most common cause of warts on the feet.[1,7,12]

Table 43–1 describes the categories of warts.

Common warts are skin-colored or brown, hyperkeratotic, dome-shaped papules with a rough cauliflower-like appearance; they frequently occur on the hands (see Color Plates, photograph 34).[1,2] Common warts often are painless.[2] Plantar warts are skin-colored callous-like lesions that occur on the feet (see Color Plates, photograph 35).[2] Because of their deeply penetrating sloping sides and central depressions, plantar warts may be painful, especially if they occur in a weight-bearing location.[1] When tightly clustered, multiple plantar warts may appear as one large wart. In this presentation, the warts are called a mosaic wart.[1,2]

Plantar warts can be confused with corns or calluses.[1] If there is any question about whether the lesion is a wart, the patient should be referred to a medical provider for evaluation and treatment. To distinguish plantar warts from calluses, the medical provider may remove the outer keratinous layer of the lesion. When the surface layer is removed, the warts exhibit pinpoint bleeding, which looks like small black dots. The bleeding is from thrombosed capillaries in the warts.[1]

Plantar warts can also be confused with malignant growths.[6] The latter are usually very painful and discolored, and they bleed and grow quickly.[7] Patients with lesions displaying these characteristics should be referred for medical evaluation and treatment.

Treatment of Warts

No single regimen is universally effective in the treatment of warts.[1,4,9] Although several treatment options are available for relief of symptoms associated with warts and for their removal, none cure the HPV infection.[1,4,9] Limited high-quality evidence exists for the efficacy of most wart treatments, and a placebo effect cannot be ruled out.[1,4,7]

Because many warts will resolve without treatment, one treatment option is a wait-and-see approach. However, many patients seek treatment because of the pain, cosmetic appearance, and social stigma associated with warts or because of concern about transmitting warts to others. The decision to treat a wart is based on the patient's desire for treatment; the presence of pain or bleeding, disabling and/or disfiguring lesions, or large or multiple lesions; the desire to prevent transmission of the warts; and the presence of an immunocompromising condition.[4,8] Warts often recur after treatment. Some warts, especially recurrent or persistent warts, will require a combination of treatments.[1]

Treatment Goals

The goals for treatment of warts are (1) to eliminate signs and symptoms associated with the warts, (2) to remove the wart without

TABLE 43–1 Types of Nongenital Warts

Type	Common Location	Populations Commonly Affected	Characteristics
Common (verruca vulgaris)	Hands	Children and adolescents	Skin-colored or brown, dome-shaped, hyperkeratotic papules with a rough surface
Flat (verruca plana)	Face	Children	Smooth, flat topped, yellow-brown papules; common in children but rare in adults
Plantar (verruca vulgaris)	Feet	Adolescents and young adults	Skin-colored, flat, callous-like, hyperkeratotic lesions with disruption of normal skin markings; located on the feet
Mosaic	Feet	Adolescents and young adults	Multiple, closely grouped plantar warts
Periungual	Nails	Persons who bite their nails	Thickened, fissured, cauliflower-like skin around the nail plate
Filiform	Face		Flesh-colored, rapidly growing with thread-like projections

Source: References 1, 2, 5, and 9.

scarring, (3) to prevent recurrence of the warts, and (4) to prevent spread of HPV through autoinoculation of one's self or transmission to others.[8]

General Treatment Approach

Determining the optimal treatment for a patient with warts depends on a number of factors, including the patient's age; the type, number, size, location, and duration of the lesions; the patient's immune status; the cost of therapy; access to therapies; adverse effects; and treatment preference.[1,4]

Although approximately 70% of warts will resolve after 2 years, even without treatment, only 46% of affected individuals will remain wart free.[6] Warts are less likely to resolve spontaneously in adults, immunocompromised patients, and patients with other warts that persist despite treatment.[1] A wait-and-see approach allows the continued spread of warts through autoinoculation and transmission to others.[4,6,7] Patient education regarding the cause of warts and ways to prevent their transmission to others is a key part of the treatment plan for any patient with warts.

Figure 43–1 outlines the treatment of warts and lists exclusions for self-treatment. A medical provider should evaluate patients with multiple warts, warts in any area other than the hands and feet, warts on the fingernails, large warts, and/or painful warts to determine whether the warts may be caused by a more serious condition. Patients with poor circulation or decreased sensitivity (e.g., patients with diabetes or peripheral vascular disease) should not self-treat warts because of the potential for injury.

Nonpharmacologic Therapy

Nonpharmacologic therapies focus mainly on preventing the spread of the HPV virus. To prevent spreading warts through autoinoculation, patients should be instructed to avoid cutting, shaving or picking at warts; to wash hands before and after treating or touching warts; to use a designated towel to dry warts; and to avoid using the designated towel to dry other body areas. To prevent transmission of the virus to others, patients should be instructed to avoid sharing towels, razors, socks, shoes, and so forth; to keep the wart covered; and to not walk barefoot, especially in bathrooms or in public places. For patients experiencing discomfort from plantar warts, padding such as lamb's wool or moleskin may be used over the pressure points to help relieve the discomfort.

Pharmacologic Therapy

Salicylic Acid

Salicylic acid is a keratolytic agent available in several formulations for use in self-treatment of common and plantar warts: salicylic acid 17% liquid and gel, and salicylic 40% plaster, pads, strips, and stick.[2,13] Table 43–2 lists selected products that contain salicyclic acid products. Salicylic acid concentrations of 17% or less are generally used for common warts, and higher concentrations (i.e., 40%) are used for plantar warts.[9]

Salicylic acid slowly destroys the virus-infected cells. It may also induce an immune response secondary to mild irritation.[1,3–5,9] The Food and Drug Administration (FDA) recommends that use of salicyclic acid for self-treatment of warts be restricted to common and plantar warts.[13] Self-treatment is not recommended for other types of warts because of the difficulty in accurately recognizing and treating warts without medical oversight. A medical provider should evaluate patients with painful plantar warts and lesions that are not easily recognizable as common or plantar warts.

The advantages of topical nonprescription products that contain salicyclic acid include low cost, ease of access, few adverse effects if used as directed, and reasonable effectiveness.[1,3,5] Compared with placebo, salicyclic acid is more effective in treating warts at all locations, but it may be more effective for warts on the hands than those on the feet.[5] Disadvantages include the need for consistent, frequent application; the potential for damage to healthy skin surrounding the wart; and the duration of treatment needed to see a therapeutic response.[1,3,5,9] Adverse effects include skin irritation and the potential for systemic toxicity.[1,3,9]

In most instances, warts will begin to improve within a couple of weeks of treatment with salicylic acid. Self-treatment of common and plantar warts should not continue past 12 weeks. A medical provider should evaluate patients who have warts that do not completely resolve after 12 weeks.

Table 43–3 provides guidelines for using salicylic acid products.[14–16]

Cryotherapy

Medical providers have used cryotherapy with liquid nitrogen and other agents for many years to treat warts in their offices.[6] Cryotherapy destroys the wart by freezing the wart tissue.[6,9] Liquid nitrogen can freeze tissue to temperatures of approximately −196°C

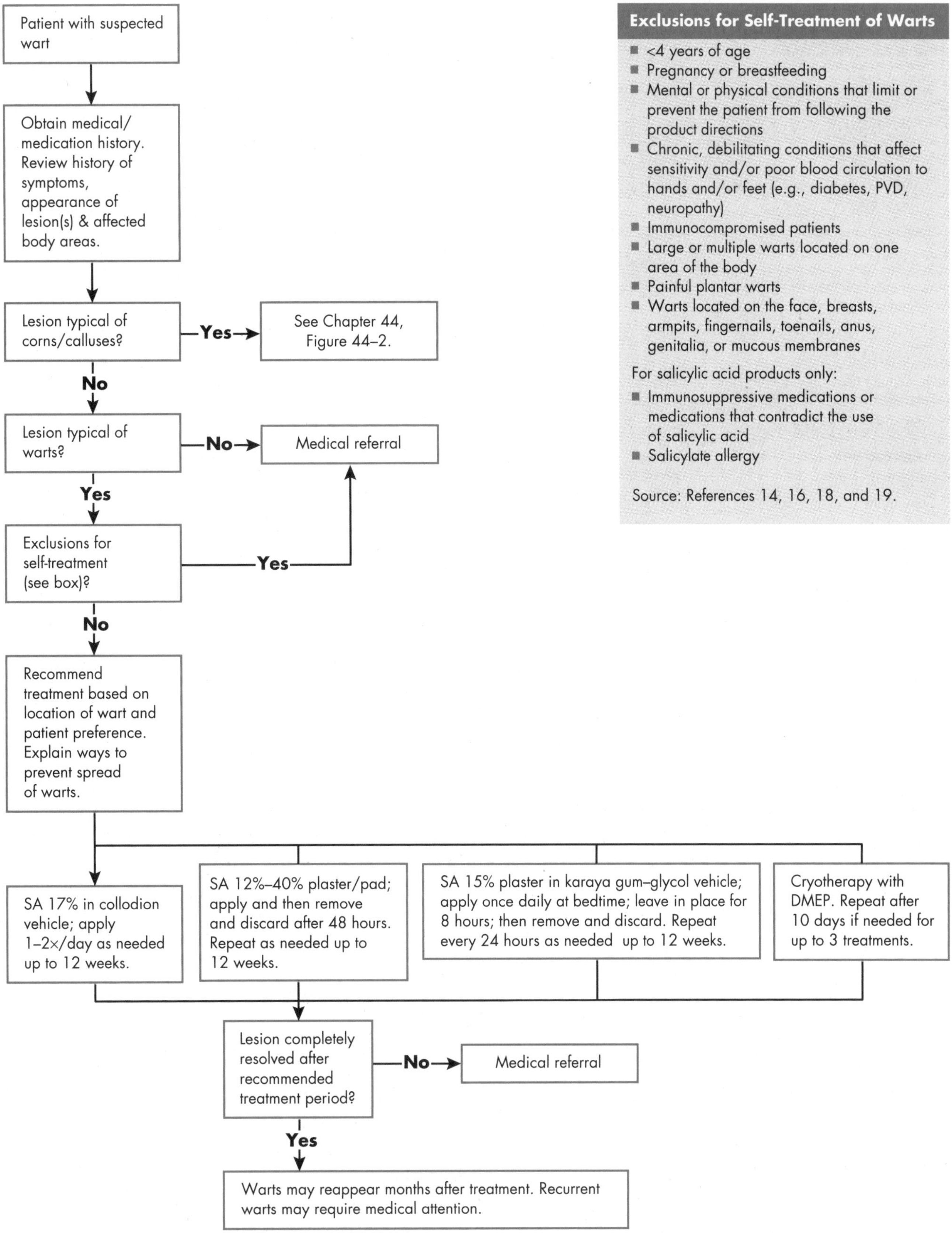
Patient with suspected wart
Obtain medical/ medication history. Review history of symptoms, appearance of lesion(s) & affected body areas.
Lesion typical of corns/calluses?
Yes
See Chapter 44, Figure 44–2.
No
Lesion typical of warts?
No
Medical referral
Yes
Exclusions for self-treatment (see box)?
Yes
No
Recommend treatment based on location of wart and patient preference. Explain ways to prevent spread of warts.
SA 17% in collodion vehicle; apply 1–2×/day as needed up to 12 weeks.
SA 12%–40% plaster/pad; apply and then remove and discard after 48 hours. Repeat as needed up to 12 weeks.
SA 15% plaster in karaya gum–glycol vehicle; apply once daily at bedtime; leave in place for 8 hours; then remove and discard. Repeat every 24 hours as needed up to 12 weeks.
Cryotherapy with DMEP. Repeat after 10 days if needed for up to 3 treatments.
Lesion completely resolved after recommended treatment period?
No
Medical referral
Yes
Warts may reappear months after treatment. Recurrent warts may require medical attention.

Exclusions for Self-Treatment of Warts

- <4 years of age
- Pregnancy or breastfeeding
- Mental or physical conditions that limit or prevent the patient from following the product directions
- Chronic, debilitating conditions that affect sensitivity and/or poor blood circulation to hands and/or feet (e.g., diabetes, PVD, neuropathy)
- Immunocompromised patients
- Large or multiple warts located on one area of the body
- Painful plantar warts
- Warts located on the face, breasts, armpits, fingernails, toenails, anus, genitalia, or mucous membranes

For salicylic acid products only:

- Immunosuppressive medications or medications that contradict the use of salicylic acid
- Salicylate allergy

Source: References 14, 16, 18, and 19.

FIGURE 43–1 Self-care of warts. Key: DMEP = Dimethyl ether and propane; PVD = peripheral vascular disease; SA = salicylic acid.

TABLE 43-2 Selected Self-Care Products for Warts

Trade Name	Primary Ingredients
Compound W One Step Pads	Salicylic acid 40%
Curad Mediplast Pads	Salicylic acid 40%
Dr. Scholl's Clear Away One Step Clear Strips	Salicylic acid 40%
DuoFilm Wart Remover Patch	Salicylic acid 40%
WartStick	Salicylic acid 40%
Compound W Fast Acting Wart Removal Gel	Salicylic acid 17%
Compound W Fast Acting Wart Removal Liquid	Salicylic acid 17%
Dr. Scholl's Clear Away Fast-Acting Liquid	Salicylic acid 17%
DuoFilm Liquid Wart Remover	Salicylic acid 17%
Compound W Freeze Off Wart Removal System	Cryotherapy (dimethyl ether; propane)
Compound W Freeze Off Advanced	Cryotherapy (dimethyl ether; propane)
Dr. Scholl's Freeze Away Wart Remover	Cryotherapy (dimethyl ether; propane)
Wartner Cryogenic Wart Removal System	Cryotherapy (dimethyl ether; propane)

Source: Reference 25.

TABLE 43-3 Guidelines for Treating Warts With Selected Salicylic Acid Products

General Guidelines

- Wash hands before and after use.
- Soak the affected area in warm water for 5 minutes.
- Wash and dry the affected area thoroughly.

Salicylic Acid 40% Plasters/Pads/Strips/Stick[14]

- Apply disc of appropriate size to wart and cover with pad. Or trim a plaster to fit the wart, apply plaster, and cover with an occlusive tape. Or, apply stick to wart or bandage and cover.
- Remove plasters/pads/strips/stick after 48 hours.
- Repeat procedure every 48 hours as needed until the wart is removed. These products may be used for up to 12 weeks.

Salicylic Acid 17% Liquid/Gel[15,16]

- Apply 1 drop at a time to cover the wart. Protect adjacent healthy skin from coming into contact with the drug.
- Let solution dry completely.
- Cover wart with self-adhesive discs or an occlusive tape.
- Repeat procedure 1–2 times a day until the wart is removed. This product may be used for up to 12 weeks.

(−385°F).[3,7] As temperatures decrease to −5°C to −15°C (−41°F to −59°F), extracellular ice crystals form.[6] At −40°C (−104°F) and below, intracellular ice crystals form.[6] As tissue freezes, microthrombi form, leading to ischemic necrosis and destruction of the HPV-infected keratinocytes.[6] The freezing also causes local inflammation that may clear the wart through a cell-mediated response.[1,4]

FDA has approved a mixture of dimethyl ether and propane (DMEP) for the self-treatment of common and plantar warts. Compared with liquid nitrogen used in medical providers' offices, nonprescription products containing dimethyl ether reach only temperatures around −70°C (−158°F).[1,3]

Nonprescription cryotherapy products have similar, but product-specific, directions for preparing the applicator. Table 43–4 provides guidelines for using cryotherapy products and illustrates the procedural differences between two selected nonprescription cryotherapy products.[17–19] The cryotherapy is applied directly to the wart. Patients must follow the directions carefully to avoid damaging the healthy skin surrounding the wart. A blister will form under the wart and, after about 10 days, the wart will fall off. Applicators must not be used more than once to avoid reinfecting the tissue or spreading the virus to others.

With regard to evaluating the effectiveness of cryotherapy in the treatment of both common and plantar warts, cryotherapy is no more effective than salicyclic acid or placebo.[3,5,9] One study found that cryotherapy may be more effective than salicyclic acid for warts on the hands but not on the feet.[20] The use of two freeze–thaw cycles, instead of one, during a treatment may improve the clearance of plantar warts, but this approach has not been shown to improve clearance of common warts on the hands.[1,3,11] However, nonprescription cryotherapy products are not approved to be used with two freeze-thaw cycles during a treatment. Aggressive cryotherapy treatments are more effective (52%) than gentle treatments (31%) but have an increased incidence of adverse effects.[1,3,5,9] Treating the wart every 2–3 weeks with cryotherapy yields the best results.[5,11]

The advantages of nonprescription cryotherapy products include their easy access and lower cost, compared with the liquid nitrogen used in the medical provider's office, and a single treatment may be sufficient to clear the wart. Disadvantages of cryotherapy include pain and the potential for damage to healthy skin surrounding the wart, and self-treatments may not be as effective as the liquid nitrogen used in the medical provider's office. Potential adverse effects include blistering, scarring, hypo- or hyperpigmentation, and tendon damage or nerve damage with aggressive therapy.[1,3,9]

In some cases, warts will resolve after a single treatment with cryotherapy. Self-treatment of common and plantar warts may be repeated every 2 weeks, if the wart does not resolve after the first treatment. However treatments should not continue beyond a maximum of 4 treatments or for more than 12 weeks duration. If this regimen does not completely resolve the wart, the patient should be referred to a medical provider for evaluation and treatment.

Other Pharmacologic Therapies

Numerous prescription products, laser treatments, immunotherapies, and combinations of treatments are used to treat warts. Discussion of prescription products and procedures is outside the scope of this chapter. Limited or inconsistent data exist for the effectiveness of using products other than salicyclic acid and cryotherapy for self-treatment of common and plantar warts

TABLE 43-4 Guidelines for Treating Warts With Selected Cryotherapy Products

General Guidelines

- Wash hands before and after use.
- Soak the affected area in warm water for 5 minutes.
- Wash and dry the affected area thoroughly.
- May use a file or pumice stone to lightly remove the surface of plantar warts.
- Do not hold the canister close to the face, body, or clothing.
- Products are flammable. Do not use near heat sources.
- Discard the foam applicator after a single use.
- Repeat after 2 weeks, if needed.
- Do not use product if
  - You cannot follow the instructions exactly as written.
  - You are not sure if the condition is a wart.
  - The wart is on children younger than 4 years.
  - You are pregnant or breastfeeding.
  - You have diabetes or poor circulation.
  - The wart is on thin, sensitive, or irritated skin such as the face, breasts, genitals, or armpits.

Compound W Freeze Off[17,18]

- Keep the protective cap on the canister. Hold the Compound W Freeze Off applicator by the plastic stick. Attach the applicator to the canister by firmly inserting the applicator stick into the opening.
- Place the canister on a sturdy surface.
- Remove the protective cap from the canister. Keeping the can upright, press the dispensing valve all the way down for 3–5 seconds to saturate the applicator. Release finger from the dispensing valve when droplets start to fall from the applicator tip.
- Turn the canister so that the applicator is pointing straight down and wait 15 seconds.
- Position the wart so that it faces upward.
- While keeping the applicator pointing straight down, lightly place the tip of the applicator on the center of the wart. Do not press the valve while the applicator is in contact with the skin. The applicator should be applied to the skin for no more than 40 seconds. Do not dab applicator onto the wart.
- Replace the protective cap after use.
- This product may be used for up to 3 treatments.

Wartner Wart Removal System[17,19]

- Holding the end of the foam applicator between the thumb and index finger, squeeze until a small opening appears.
- Slide the opening of the foam applicator over the stick of the holder until the stick is no longer visible. You will find the holder in the bag containing the foam applicators.
- Insert the holder with the applicator in the opening on the top of the cap so that the foam applicator is no longer visible.
- Place the aerosol spray can on a sturdy surface.
- Holding the can firmly at the bottom, press down the valve for 2–3 seconds.
- Leave the foam applicator on the holder and wait 20 seconds.
- Lightly place the tip of the foam applicator to the wart.
  - Apply 20 seconds for common warts.
  - Apply 40 seconds for plantar warts.
- This product may be used for up to 4 treatments.

Product Selection Guidelines in Special Populations

Several factors should be considered when selecting a wart remover product, including the patient's age, whether the patient is pregnant or lactating, and whether the patient has certain comorbid conditions. The specific product chosen must also be compatible with the patient's lifestyle and personal preference.

Pregnancy

The effects of topical salicylic acid on an unborn child are not known. Therefore, because of the risk for systemic absorption from topical application, products containing salicylic acid should not be used for self-treatment by patients who are pregnant. Cryotherapy products should also not be used for self-treatment by patients who are pregnant, because it is uncertain how cryotherapy will affect the patient or unborn child. Patients who are pregnant should be referred to a medical provider for treatment of warts.

Lactation

It is not known if topical salicylic acid passes into breast milk in sufficient amounts to harm a nursing child. Products containing salicylic acid should not be used for self-treatment by patients who are lactating. However, if patients who are lactating wish to self-treat warts with these products, they should be instructed to discontinue nursing for the duration of use. Cryotherapy products should not be used for self-treatment of warts in patients who are lactating as it is uncertain how cryotherapy will affect the patient or child. Patients who are lactating should be referred to a medical provider for treatment of warts.

Children

Topical salicylic acid products should not be used for self-treatment of warts in children younger than 4 years, because of the potential for systemic absorption and the potential for damage to the young child's skin. Further, salicylic acid–containing products should not be used in children or teenagers who have or are recovering from chickenpox or influenza-like symptoms because of the risk of Reye's syndrome (see Chapter 5 for further information). In addition, cryotherapy products should not be used for self-treatment of warts in children younger than 4 years. It is uncertain how these products may affect the skin of young children. Because of the nature of the skin in young children, these products have the potential to cause significant damage.

Patients of Advanced Age

Both cryotherapy products and products containing salicylic acid may be used in patients of advanced age in a manner similar to that in younger adults. Care should be taken not to damage the normal skin tissue around the wart when using these products, because these patients often have thinner, more friable skin.

Comorbid Conditions

Patients with diabetes or poor circulation should not use cryotherapy or salicylic acid–containing products because of the risk for delayed healing.

Dosage Form Considerations

The salicylic acid–containing products come in a variety of dosage forms that may appeal to specific patient preferences, such as colored pads for children to cover the wart or strips or pads that may be easier for some patients to apply than the liquid. Cryotherapy products may appeal more to patients who are looking for a product that requires minimal applications.

Complementary Therapies

Folklore

There are numerous folk remedies for warts. Most of these are based on anecdotal success and highlight the probability that many warts resolve spontaneously without treatment.[1]

Vitamin A

Retinoids such as vitamin A regulate epithelial cell differentiation and keratin expression. Vitamin A may interfere with HPV replication. One case report of a 30-year-old woman found topical vitamin A to be effective in clearing recalcitrant warts. The woman's warts had been present for a 9-year period despite various treatments. The treatment required 6 months to clear the largest wart. The report noted that untreated warts on the opposite hand cleared without application of vitamin A, which may illustrate either a placebo effect or an unknown mechanism of action.[12]

Dietary Zinc

Deficiencies of zinc lead to decreased immunity.[1,10] Dietary zinc is postulated to improve immune response and inhibit HPV replication.[10] One placebo-controlled trial evaluated 10 mg/kg/day of zinc to treat recalcitrant warts. Complete clearance was reported in 35 of the 40 patients, 87%, in the treatment group versus no clearance in the placebo group.[1,10]

*Garlic (*Allium sativum*)*

Garlic is thought to inhibit cellular proliferation of virus-infected cells.[1,21] One placebo-controlled trial reported that application of chloroform extracts of garlic resulted in complete resolution of warts for all 23 patients after 1–2 weeks, with no recurrence after 3–4 months.[1,21]

Occlusion With Duct Tape

Duct tape is an inexpensive, potentially less painful self-treatment for warts. The mechanism by which duct tape clears warts is still unclear, but local irritation may cause stimulation of the patient's immune response.[5]

One randomized controlled study[22] compared duct tape occlusion with cryotherapy for the treatment of common warts. In one treatment group, liquid nitrogen was applied to warts every 2–3 weeks, for a maximum of 6 treatments or until the warts resolved. In the other treatment group, duct tape was applied to the wart, left in place for 6 days, removed in the evening of the sixth day, and replaced with a new piece of duct tape the next morning; this procedure was repeated for up to 2 months or until the wart resolved. The treated warts were completely resolved in 84.6% of the patients in the duct tape group and 60% of the patients in the cryotherapy group.[1,5]

Another randomized controlled trial[23] yielded conflicting results. This trial compared occlusion of warts with either duct tape or moleskin. In each group, the wart was shaved and the pad applied for 1 week. The wart was then debrided with an emery board, and the pad was reapplied for an additional week. This procedure was repeated for up to 2 months or until the wart resolved. Six months later, patients were asked if the wart had recurred. The treatment groups demonstrated no difference in resolution or recurrence of the warts.[5,24]

More evidence on the effectiveness of therapy with duct tape is needed. Duct tape may have a place in therapy for small children with warts or in combination with other treatments.[1]

Assessment of Warts: A Case-Based Approach

When a patient presents with a wartlike lesion, the health care provider should gather information from multiple sources to determine whether the lesion is suitable for self-treatment and whether available treatments are appropriate for that individual. Before a treatment plan is recommended, the provider should inspect the wart to accurately identify the lesion as a wart and to determine whether self-treatment is appropriate. The provider should then question the patient about medication use and the existence of medical conditions that would preclude self-treatment. The patient should also be asked about previous attempts to treat the lesion and whether the lesion showed improvement with those attempts Patient preferences for type of treatment may be used to help guide product selection.

Table 43–5 compares characteristics of warts, corns, calluses, and malignant growths. Cases 43–1 and 43–2 illustrate the assessment of patients with warts.

Patient Counseling for Warts

Patients must understand that warts are caused by the HPV virus and are contagious. Health care providers should discuss with patients measures to prevent the spread of warts (see Nonpharmacologic Therapy) to other parts of the body or to other individuals. Health care providers should also point out the differences between available products, including their indications, contraindications, warnings, and precautions. The box Patient Education for Warts lists specific information for patients who are using either salicylic acid products or cryotherapy products. If warts persist despite self-treatment for a maximum of 12 weeks of therapy, patients should be referred to a medical provider for evaluation and treatment.

Evaluation of Patient Outcomes for Warts

Salicyclic acid may require up to 12 weeks of treatment to completely resolve the wart. Patients should see some improvement in 1–2 weeks. Follow-up with the health care provider should occur after 4–6 weeks to evaluate the wart. If the wart does not appear to be resolved, the patient should be encouraged to continue treatment. If the wart has not cleared after 12 weeks, prescription therapies may be warranted. The patient should be referred to a medical provider for further evaluation and treatment.

Cryotherapy may be repeated after 2 weeks for up to 12 weeks or 4 treatments. If the wart is not cleared after 12 weeks or 4 treatments, the patient should be referred to a medical provider for evaluation and treatment.

TABLE 43–5 **Differentiation of Warts and Skin Disorders With Similar Presentation**

Criterion	Warts	Corns	Calluses	Malignant Growth
Location	Any area of skin susceptible to the virus	Over bony prominences in the feet	Weight-bearing areas of the feet	Any area of the skin
Signs	Rough cauliflower-like appearance; plantar warts disrupt normal skin ridges	Raised, sharply demarcated, hyperkeratotic lesions with a central core	Raised, yellowish thickening of the skin; broad based with diffuse borders; normal pattern of skin ridges	Bleeding; swelling; red, discolored, or multicolored and swollen
Symptoms	Usually not painful but pain may occur if the wart is located in areas undergoing repeated pressure (i.e., soles of the feet)	Pain	Usually not painful but pain may occur if the callus is located in an area where significant pressure may occur (i.e., soles of the feet)	Pain
Quantity/severity	Varies; may grow to approximately 1 inch in diameter	Varies; a few millimeters to 1 cm	Varies; a few millimeters to several centimeters	Varies; grows rapidly
Timing	Incubation period may be several months in length; may progressively enlarge	Variable onset; may progressively enlarge	Variable onset; may progressively enlarge	Variable onset; grows rapidly
Cause	HPV infection of the epidermal layer	Friction	Friction, walking barefoot, structural foot problems	Mutations related to damaged DNA cause skin cells to grow unchecked
Modifying factors	Prevention of spread; treatment with salicylic acid or cryotherapy	Alleviation of causative factors; treatment with salicylic acid	Alleviation of causative factors; treatment with salicylic acid	Surgical removal; prescription medications

Key: HPV = Human papillomavirus.

CASE 43–1

Relevant Evaluation Criteria	Scenario/Model Outcome
Collect	
1. Gather essential information about the patient's symptoms and medical history, including	
a. Description of symptom(s) (i.e., nature, onset, duration, severity, associated symptoms)	A male middle school student, accompanied by his mother, is in the self-care section of the pharmacy. The mother tells you that her son has a rough callus-like spot on the bottom of his foot. She asks if you can suggest anything to help her get rid of it. He noticed it about a month ago but did not tell his mother about it until it started getting bigger. He says it is not painful, but he does not like it being on his foot and he is afraid it will keep getting bigger. There is no inflammation, bleeding, significant discoloration, or discharge from the lesion.
b. Description of any factors that seem to precipitate, exacerbate, and/or relieve the patient's symptom(s)	The student is on the wrestling team, which practices 4–5 days a week and has matches most weekends. After practice and matches, he showers barefoot in the communal showers.
c. Description of the patient's efforts to relieve the symptoms	He has used no previous treatments on the lesion.
d. Patient's identity	Luke Harrison
e. Patient's age, gender, height, and weight	12 years old, male, 4 ft 10 in., 80 lb
f. Patient's occupation	Middle school student

CASE 43-1 *continued*

Relevant Evaluation Criteria	Scenario/Model Outcome
g. Patient's dietary habits	Luke follows a generally healthy diet avoiding excess carbohydrates and concentrated sweets.
h. Patient's sleep habits	8–10 hours a night
i. Concurrent medical conditions, prescription and nonprescription medications, and dietary supplements	No medical conditions; medication(s): children's chewable multivitamin daily
j. Allergies	Penicillin
k. History of other adverse reactions to medications	None
l. Other (describe) _______	Luke lives at home and shares a bedroom and bathroom with his twin brother.
Assess	
2. Differentiate patient's signs/symptoms, and correctly identify the patient's primary problem(s).	Luke most likely has a plantar wart.
3. Identify exclusions for self-treatment (Figure 43–1).	None
4. Formulate a comprehensive list of therapeutic alternatives for the primary problem to determine whether triage to a medical provider is required, and share this information with the patient or caregiver.	Options include (1) Recommend self-care with an OTC wart removal product and nondrug measures. (2) Recommend self-care until Luke can consult a medical provider for evaluation and treatment. (3) Refer Luke for medical evaluation and treatment (4) Take no action.
Plan	
5. Select an optimal therapeutic alternative to address the patient's problem, taking into account patient preferences.	Because Luke is concerned about the possibility that the wart will continue to enlarge and because there is significant possibility of transmitting the virus to others, pharmacologic treatment of the wart should be considered. Because the wart is a single, small, painless lesion confined to a single area, and the patient has no identifiable exclusions for self-treatment, he can be treated with a nonprescription wart removal product. He can prevent transmitting the wart to others by wearing shoes or covering the wart, especially when showering or when using his bathroom. He should not share towels with his teammates or family members.
6. Describe the recommended therapeutic approach to the patient or caregiver.	See Figure 43–1 and the box Patient Education for Warts. "Salicylic acid in a pad or strip would be a good choice in this situation. Salicylic acid pads/strip products have to be applied, removed after 48 hours, and a new pad applied. The pad should be covered with occlusive tape. Salicyclic acid therapy might take up to 12 weeks for the wart to resolve."
7. Explain to the patient or caregiver the rationale for selecting the recommended therapeutic approach from the considered therapeutic alternatives.	"Salicylic acid in a strip or pad form is an appropriate recommendation for your son, because salicylic acid is effective for this type of wart, easy to use, and less painful than some other treatment options. Cryotherapy is another self-care option for the treatment of warts. However, cryotherapy is more painful than salicyclic acid, and small warts may be adequately treated with salicylic acid." "The wart is not severe enough to warrant a referral to a health care provider at this time. Self-treatment is more cost-effective and should provide acceptable results in resolving your son's wart."

CASE 43-1 *continued*

Relevant Evaluation Criteria	Scenario/Model Outcome
Implement	
8. When recommending self-care with nonprescription medications and/or nondrug therapy, convey accurate information to the patient or caregiver.	Table 43–3 and the box Patient Education for Warts provide information on removing warts safely. Also, be sure to read and follow the directions that come with the product. "The wart may be soaked in warm water for 5 minutes to soften the outer surface. The pad or strip should be applied directly over the wart. Remove the pad or strip every 48 hours and replace it with a new one. Treatment with salicylic acid may be continued for up to 12 weeks." "If there is any irritation to the healthy tissue surrounding the wart, wash the area immediately with soap and water."
Solicit follow-up questions from patient or caregiver.	(1) "Can his teammates or family members get warts from him?" (2) "What should he do if the wart is not gone after 12 weeks?"
Answer patient or caregiver's questions.	(1) "Yes, warts are caused by a virus that is spread from person to person or by touching surfaces that have come in contact with the wart. See the box Patient Education for Warts for preventive measures." (2) "If after 12 weeks of treatment, the wart is still present, you should consult a medical provider."
Follow-up: Monitor and Evaluate	
9. Assess patient outcome.	Follow up in 4–6 weeks to assess the patient's progress in clearing the wart with the recommended therapy.

Key: OTC = Over-the-counter.

CASE 43-2

Relevant Evaluation Criteria	Scenario/Model Outcome
Collect	
1. Gather essential information about the patient's symptoms and medical history, including	
a. Description of symptom(s) (i.e., nature, onset, duration, severity, associated symptoms)	A middle-aged male asks for something to get rid of a lesion at the base of his fingernail on his right index finger. The lesion has a rough cauliflower-like surface. He has had similar lesions on this and other fingers in the past. It is currently about the size of a pea and is not painful. There is no inflammation, bleeding, significant discoloration, or discharge from the growth.
b. Description of any factors that seem to precipitate, exacerbate, and/or relieve the patient's symptom(s)	None
c. Description of the patient's efforts to relieve the symptoms	He has treated the wart with both salicylic acid liquid and OTC cryotherapy products over the past 6 months. The wart would go away for a while then return.
d. Patient's identity	Simon Bridges
e. Patient's age, gender, height, and weight	52 years old, male, 5 ft 10 in., 185 lb
f. Patient's occupation	High school math teacher and football coach
g. Patient's dietary habits	Simon follows a healthy diet most of the time.

CASE 43-2 *continued*

Relevant Evaluation Criteria	Scenario/Model Outcome
h. Patient's sleep habits	Averages 6 hours a night.
i. Concurrent medical conditions, prescription and nonprescription medications, and dietary supplements	Hypertension: lisinopril 10 mg daily; dyslipidemia: atorvastatin 20 mg daily
j. Allergies	None
k. History of other adverse reactions to medications	None
l. Other (describe) _______	Smoker: 30 pack years (30-year history × 1 ppd)
Assess	
2. Differentiate patient's signs/symptoms, and correctly identify the patient's primary problem(s).	Simon most likely has a common wart on his finger.
3. Identify exclusions for self-treatment (Figure 43–1).	Recurrent common wart on the fingernail
4. Formulate a comprehensive list of therapeutic alternatives for the primary problem to determine whether triage to a medical provider is required, and share this information with the patient or caregiver.	Options include (1) Recommend self-care with a nonprescription wart removal product and nondrug measures. (2) Recommend self-care until Simon can consult a medical provider for evaluation and treatment. (3) Refer Simon for medical evaluation and treatment. (4) Take no action.
Plan	
5. Select an optimal therapeutic alternative to address the patient's problem, taking into account patient preferences.	Simon should be referred to a medical provider for evaluation and treatment, because the wart is located on the fingernail and it has recurred despite treatment with both OTC salicylic acid and cryotherapy.
6. Describe the recommended therapeutic approach to the patient or caregiver.	"You should consult a medical provider to evaluate and treat the wart."
7. Explain to the patient or caregiver the rationale for selecting the recommended therapeutic approach from the considered therapeutic alternatives.	"Self-treatment is not recommended, because the wart is on the fingernail and because you have already used two different types of nonprescription wart removal products without success."
Implement	
8. When recommending self-care with nonprescription medications and/or nondrug therapy, convey accurate information to the patient or caregiver.	Criterion does not apply in this case.
Solicit follow-up questions from patient or caregiver.	(1) "Is there anything I can do to keep this wart from coming back again after it is treated?" (2) "Will the wart spread to other people or other areas of my body?"
Answer patient or caregiver's questions.	(1) "It is common for warts to recur even after treatment. The box Patient Education for Warts lists things you can do to reduce the risk of reinfection." (2) "Warts are spread through person-to-person contact or by contact with contaminated surfaces such as towels or exercise equipment. The box Patient Education for Warts provides information on how to prevent spreading warts to other areas of your body or to other persons."
Follow-up: Monitor and Evaluate	
9. Assess patient outcome.	The patient should follow-up with the medical care provider as directed.

Key: OTC = Over-the-counter; ppd = pack per day.

PATIENT EDUCATION FOR Warts

When treating warts, the goals are (1) to eliminate signs and symptoms associated with the warts, (2) to remove the wart without causing scars, (3) to prevent the wart from recurring, and (4) to prevent spreading of warts to self or others. To ensure the best possible treatment outcomes, patients must follow product instructions carefully and must consistently use measures to prevent the spread of warts.

Nondrug Measures

- To decrease the chance of getting warts, avoid nail-biting; do not go barefoot; and keep feet clean and dry.
- To avoid spreading warts from one part of your body to another, do not cut, shave, or pick at warts; wash hands before and after treating or touching warts; use a single specific towel to dry warts; and do not use the same towel to dry other areas of the body.
- To avoid spreading warts to others, do not share towels, razors, socks, shoes, and so forth; keep the wart covered; and do not walk barefoot, especially in bathrooms or in public places.

Nonprescription Medications

- Select only nonprescription salicylic acid or cryotherapy products approved for self-treatment of warts. Follow the instructions on the label closely.
- Use these products only on common or plantar warts. Do not use on moles, birthmarks, warts with hairs growing from them, irritated or inflamed skin, or infected skin.
- If you are not certain that the condition is a wart, consult a health care provider before using these products.
- Do not use these products to treat warts on the face, mucous membranes, armpits, breasts, genitals, or around fingernails.
- Do not use these products on children who are younger than 4 years, women who are pregnant or breastfeeding, or patients who have diabetes or poor circulation.
- Some of these products are flammable or contain collodions that are poisonous if ingested. Keep away from heat and out of children's reach.
- Warts may recur after treatment.

Salicylic Acid Products

- Keep these products away from the eyes. If they come into contact with the eyes, seek medical help immediately.
- Do not apply these products to healthy skin. If they come into contact with healthy skin, wash the area with soap and water immediately.
- Improvement should be seen within a week or two of beginning treatment. The wart should completely clear within 6–12 weeks. Self-treatment should not continue longer than 12 weeks.

Cryotherapy Products

- You will feel an aching, stinging sensation when the product is applied.
- A blister will form and the wart should fall off after about 10 days.
- If the wart does not completely clear after the first treatment, the procedure may be repeated in 2 weeks. The product should not be used for more than 12 weeks or repeated more than 4 times.

When to Seek Medical Attention

- Stop using the products and consult a medical provider if severe irritation or pain occurs immediately after application.
- If the wart has not cleared after 12 weeks of treatment, consult a medical provider for evaluation and treatment.

Source: References 7, 8, 14–16, 18–19, and 25.

Key Points for Warts

- Because many warts will resolve without treatment, a wait-and-see approach may be an appropriate treatment option in some patients. However, this approach allows the continued transmission of the highly contagious HPV virus.
- Patients with multiple warts, warts in any area other than the hands and feet, warts on the fingernails, or large warts should be evaluated by a medical provider.
- Plantar warts should be treated with higher concentrations of salicylic acid (≤40%). Warts on the hands or areas with thinner epidermis should be treated with lower concentrations of salicylic acid (<17%).
- DMEP products are available for home cryotherapy treatments, but cryotherapy is no more effective than salicylic acid.
- The directions for use of nonprescription salicylic acid and cryotherapy products should be followed to prevent injury to healthy tissue surrounding the wart.
- Patients with diabetes, poor circulation, or immunodeficiencies should not self-treat with salicylic acid or cryotherapy without first consulting a medical provider.
- Patients who experience adverse effects from nonprescription wart removal products or have warts that recur frequently should be evaluated by a medical provider.

REFERENCES

1. Lipke MM. An armamentarium of wart treatments. *Clin Med Res.* 2006; 4(4):273–93. PMCID: PMC1764803.
2. Pray WS, Pray GE, Pray M. Removing warts with nonprescription treatments. *US Pharm.* 2011;36(8):15–23.
3. Mulhem E, Pinelis S. Treatment of non-genital cutaneous warts. *Am Fam Physician.* 2011;84(3):288–93.
4. Micali G, Dall'Oglio F, Nasca MR, et al. Management of cutaneous warts. *Am J Clin Dermatol.* 2004;5(5):311–7. doi: 10.2165/00128071-200405050-0004.
5. Kwok CS, Gibbs S, Bennett C, et al. Topical treatments for cutaneous warts. *Cochrane Database Syst Rev.* 2012;9:CD001781. doi: 10.1002/14651858.CD004976.pub3.
6. Nguyen NV, Burkhart CG. Cryotherapy treatment of warts: dimethyl ether and propane versus liquid nitrogen—case report and review of the literature. *J Drugs Dermatol.* 2011;10(10):1174–6. PMID: 21968668.
7. Watkins P. Identifying and treating plantar warts. *Nurs Stand.* 2006; 20(42):50–4. doi: 10.7748/ns2006.06.20.42.50.c6554.
8. Drake LA, Celley RI, Cornelison R. Guidelines of care: guidelines of care for warts: human papillomavirus. *J Am Acad Dermatol.* 1995;32:98–103.
9. Dall'Oglio F, D'Amico V, Nasca MR, et al. Treatment of cutaneous warts: an evidence-based review. *Am J Clin Dermatol.* 2012;13(2):72–96. doi: 10.2165/11594610-000000000-0000.
10. Al-Gurairi FT, Al-Waiz M, Sharquie KE. Oral zinc sulphate in the treatment of recalcitrant viral warts: randomized placebo controlled clinical trial. *Br J Dermatol.* 2002;146:423–31. doi: 10.1046/j1365-2133.2002.04617x.
11. Kuykendall-IVY TD, Johnson SM. Evidence based review of management of non-genital cutaneous warts. *Cutis.* 2003;71:213–22.
12. Gaston A, Garry R. Topical vitamin A treatment of recalcitrant common warts. *Virol J.* 2012;9:21. doi: 10.1186/1743-422x-9-21
13. U.S. Food and Drug Administration. Wart remover products for over-the-counter human use; Final monograph. *Fed Regist.* 1990;55:33246. Available at http://loc.heinonline.org/loc/page?handle=hein.fedreg/055157&co. Accessed June 16, 2017.
14. Compound W [product information]. Lynchburg, VA and Tarrytown, NY: Prestige Brands. Available at: http://compoundw.com/compound-w-one-strp-pads. Accessed June 16, 2017.
15. Compound W [product information]. Lynchburg, VA and Tarrytown, NY: Prestige Brands. Available at: http://www.compoundw.com/compound-w-fast-acting-wart-removal-liquid. Accessed June 16, 2017.

16. Compound W [product information]. Lynchburg, VA and Tarrytown, NY: Prestige Brands. Available at: http://www.compoundw.com/compound-w-fast-acting-wart-removal-gel. Accessed June 16, 2017.
17. Newton GD, Pray WS, Popovich NG. New OTC drugs and devices 2003: a selective review. *J Am Pharm Assoc.* 2004;44:211–25.
18. Compound W Freeze Off [patient instruction leaflet]. Lynchburg, VA and Tarrytown, NY: Prestige Brands. Available at: http://www.compoundw.com/compound-w-freeze-advanced. Accessed: June 16, 2017.
19. Wart and Verruca Remover [instruction leaflet]. Dublin, Ireland: Wartner/Omega Pharma. Available at: http://wartner.eu/wp-content/uploads/Wartner-Corporate-Leaflet-Unilingual.pdf. Accessed June 22, 2017.
20. Bruggink SC, Gussekloo J, Berger MY, et al. Cryotherapy with liquid nitrogen versus topical salicylic acid application for cutaneous warts in primary care: randomized controlled trial. *CMAJ.* 2010;182(15):1624–30. doi: 10.1503/cmaj.092194.
21. Dehghani F, Merat A, Panjehshahin MR, et al. Healing effect of garlic extract on warts and corns. *Int J Dermatol.* 2005;44:612–5. doi:10.1111/j.1365-4632.2004.02348.x.
22. Christakis DA, Lehmann HP. Is duct tape occlusion therapy as effective as cryotherapy for the treatment of the common wart? *Arch Pediatr Adolesc Med.* 2002;156:975–7. PMID: 12361440.
23. U.S. Food and Drug Administration. For consumers: some wart removers are flammable. January 16, 2014. Available at: https://www.fda.gov/ForConsumers/ConsumerUpdates/ucm381429.htm. Accessed June 8, 2017.
24. Wenner R, Askari SK, Cham PM, et al. Duct tape for the treatment of common warts in adults: a double-blind randomized controlled trial. *Arch Dermatol.* 2007;143:309–13. doi:10.1001/archderm.143.3.309.
25. U.S. News & World Report and Pharmacy Times. Health: wart removers. Available at http://health.usnews.com/health-products/top-rec-wart-removers-146. Accessed June 8, 2017.

CHAPTER 44

MINOR FOOT DISORDERS

CYNTHIA W. COFFEY AND SNEHA BAXI SRIVASTAVA

Containing one-quarter of the bones in the body, the feet are designed to absorb shock from pressure and to assist in movement. On average, a person walks 115,000 miles in a lifetime, which is equivalent to circling the world nearly four times. Up to 75% of Americans will experience foot health problems of variable degree at one time or another in their lives.[1] Many minor foot disorders and injuries can be prevented with adequate precautions.[1] Among the most common such disorders are corns, calluses, and ingrown toenails.[1,2] Accordingly, for today's health care providers (HCPs), the clinical encounter should include recognizing these and other minor foot health problems from the patient's symptoms and recommending appropriate measures for their prevention and treatment.

In some instances, self-care for foot disorders is inappropriate. For instance, children with a congenital malformation, a deformity, or a specific disease that affects the foot (e.g., juvenile arthritis) require medical care by an orthopedic surgeon or a podiatrist. Rapid growth in adolescents can result in foot irritation from changes in growth plates, which is a condition excluded from use of self-care measures. Patients may also encounter foot problems related to aging (e.g., arthritis) or disease (e.g., peripheral vascular disease). Common foot disorders can potentially have severe consequences in patients with comorbid disorders (e.g., diabetes) and may also indicate other serious underlying conditions.[3] In some instances, inappropriate foot care practices may be life-threatening in patients with diabetes, severe arthritis, or impaired circulation[3–7] (see the box "A Word about Chronic Diseases and Foot Disorders"). For most patients, however, such problems cause nominal measures of discomfort and impaired mobility, which can be treated with self-care measures.

Pathophysiology of the Foot

At birth, an infant's foot has 33 joints, 19 muscles, 107 ligaments, and cartilage that will develop into 26 bones. The feet continue to develop and mature until the ages of 14–16 years for females and 15–21 years for males. Women and men generally will begin to notice changes in their feet in their 40s and 50s, respectively.[8] After years of bearing the body's weight, feet tend to broaden and flatten, thereby stretching ligaments and causing bones to shift positions. These changes subject feet to stress, which is compounded by prolonged standing. An estimated 40% of U.S. workers spend approximately 75% of the day on their feet, increasing the potential for painful foot conditions.[1,2]

CORNS AND CALLUSES

Although corns and calluses are common foot disorders, they should not be ignored. These lesions may indicate a biomechanical problem and lead to serious complications if left untreated.

Pathophysiology of Corns and Calluses

Under normal conditions, the cells in the skin's basal cell layer (*stratum basale*) undergo mitotic division at a rate equal to the continual surface cellular desquamation, eventuating in complete replacement of the epidermis in approximately 1 month. During corn or callus development, however, friction and pressure increase mitotic activity of the basal cell layer, leading to the migration of maturing cells through the prickle cell (*stratum spinosum*) and granular (*stratum granulosum*) skin layers (see Chapter 33, Figure 33–1). As more cells reach the outer skin surface, they produce a thicker horny layer (*stratum corneum*). This process is a natural protective mechanism of the skin surface and may signal biomechanical problems that result in abnormal weight distribution on the foot. When friction or pressure is relieved, mitotic activity returns to normal, with consequent remission and disappearance of the lesion.[8–10]

Clinical Presentation of Corns and Calluses

Corns and calluses are similar in that both produce a marked hyperkeratosis of the stratum corneum, but they have marked differences.

Corns

A *corn* (*clavus*) is a small, raised, sharply demarcated, hyperkeratotic lesion with a central core; the lesion is caused by pressure from underlying bony prominences or joints. The central core of the corn differentiates it from a wart (see Chapter 43, Table 43–5). Misidentification of warts and corns is common. Differentiation can be made by shaving the central core. A corn has a hard center, whereas a wart will bleed because of the multiple capillary loops in its center.[9] Corns are yellowish gray and well circumscribed,

A WORD ABOUT

Chronic Diseases and Foot Disorders

Some chronic diseases can predispose affected patients to foot complications. Patients with diabetes often have poor circulation and diminished limb sensitivity, making them especially vulnerable to infectious foot problems. Other susceptible patients include those with peripheral vascular disease or arthritis. The HCP can identify these patients by asking about daily medication use or reviewing the patient's drug profile. Typical drug use patterns for high-risk patients include regimens of insulin; oral antidiabetic drugs (e.g., glipizide, glyburide, metformin); drugs for circulation disorders (e.g., clopidogrel, pentoxifylline); drugs for neuropathic pain (e.g., gabapentin, duloxetine); and drugs for arthritic disorders (e.g., aspirin, other NSAIDs).

If not properly supervised in patients with impaired circulation, self-treatment with nonprescription products may induce more inflammation, ulceration, or even gangrene, particularly in cases of vascular insufficiency in the foot. Affected tissues in patients with diabetes and those with peripheral circulatory impairments are particularly susceptible to gangrene. In addition, simple lesions may mask more serious abscesses or ulcerations. If left medically unattended, these lesions may lead to conditions such as osteomyelitis, which may necessitate hospitalization and aggressive intravenous antibiotic therapy.

Diabetes Mellitus

Patients who have poorly controlled diabetes are at greater risk for lower extremity complications, associated with increased health care costs, decreased quality of life, and increased morbidity. Two major causes of foot ulcerations are peripheral neuropathy, which results in loss of injury perception and subsequently excessive plantar pressure, which contributes to decreased mobility and foot deformities. Other factors contributing to foot complications in patients with diabetes are poor foot hygiene such as extremely hot water soaks, wearing inappropriate footwear, and lack of daily foot self-examinations. Patients with diabetes need to be educated on proper foot care, such as trimming toenails appropriately, not applying creams/lotions between the toes, keeping socks clean and dry, performing foot examinations at home, and scheduling regular foot examinations in the HCP's office. The following self-care and other preventative measures can help reduce the risks diabetes complications.

Foot Care

- Perform annual foot examination.
  - Have patient remove shoes at each visit with the primary care provider for visual inspection.
  - Evaluate for any changes in foot appearance or tactile sensation.
  - Advise patients known to be at high risk for skin ulcers (e.g., neuropathy) to see a podiatrist regularly.
- Teach patient to clean and inspect feet daily for any changes (e.g., corn, callus, open wound, fungal infection).
- Instruct patient to trim nails carefully (straight across) and file them with an emery board to the contour of the toe.
- Instruct patient to avoid walking barefoot.
- Recommend use of soft cotton, synthetic blend, or wool socks to absorb moisture.
- Recommend that patient wear properly fitting, comfortable shoes and use caution when "breaking in" new shoes.
- Recommend that patient inspect shoes for foreign objects before inserting feet.
- Recommend that patient (1) use moisturizing lotion sparingly for the tops and bottoms of dry feet, (2) allow feet to completely dry before wearing shoes to prevent excess moisture buildup, and (3) avoid use of moisturizers between the toes.

Peripheral Vascular Disease

Patients with peripheral vascular disease often have poor circulation in the feet and legs. Because of decreased blood flow and low oxygen perfusion, skin ulcerations and decreased wound healing may be problematic in these patients. They may complain of persistent and unusual feelings of cold, numbness, tingling, burning, or fatigue. Other manifestations of this disease may include discolored skin, dry skin, absence of hair on the feet or legs, or a cramping or tightness in the leg muscles. The provider should palpate for pedal pulses. The most discriminating questions that a provider can ask this type of patient are as follows: (1) Do you experience aching in your calves when you walk? (2) Do you have to hang your feet over the edge of the bed during sleep to relieve the soreness in your calves? A yes response to either question warrants referral to an HCP.

Localized redness or unilateral coldness may indicate a possible blockage (a clot) of circulation to the foot. The involved foot or lower leg may appear physically larger than the other, may be red or waxy in appearance, may have no hair growth on the toes, and will exhibit thickened nails. If the medication history of the patient with suspected circulatory problems does not list medications intended to relieve such symptoms, the patient should be referred immediately for further evaluation.

A daily footbath is a simple measure for peripheral vascular disease. After the foot is patted dry, an emollient foot cream can be applied to aid the skin in retaining moisture and pliability. The footbath will also soften brittle toenails for clipping and filing. The feet should be kept warm and moderately exercised every day.

Arthritis

Osteoarthritis is a noninflammatory, degenerative joint disease that occurs primarily in older people. Degeneration of the articular cartilage and changes in the bone result in a loss of resilience and a decrease in the skeleton's shock absorption capability. This condition, however, is also experienced by young individuals in their late teens and early 20s as a secondary complication of a previous athletic injury. This condition can be evidenced by the development of hallux limitus or *rigidus* of the big toe (e.g., a painful flexion or extension of the big toe related to stiffness and spur formation in the metatarsophalangeal joint or a stiff toe, respectively). Subsequently, these patients have a lot of difficulty with their shoes not fitting properly. Development of an osteoarthritic condition in the ankle joint is another possible complication. Referral for further evaluation is appropriate.

Most patients with rheumatoid arthritis eventually have foot involvement. The major forefoot deformities in these patients are painful metatarsal heads, hallux valgus, and clawfoot. Corrective surgical procedures are often indicated to reduce pain and improve function and mobility. Little evidence exists that conventional nonsurgical therapy (e.g., orthopedic shoes, metatarsal inserts, conventional arch supports, metatarsal bars) is effective.

Proper palliative foot care is especially important for arthritic patients. They should wear properly fitted shoes, pad their shoes with insoles to protect their feet from the shock of hard surfaces, and undergo regular podiatric or medical examinations. (See Chapters 5 and 7, respectively, for use of systemic or topical nonprescription analgesics for osteoarthritis.)

Key: HCP = Health care provider; NSAID = nonsteroidal anti-inflammatory drug.

Source: American Diabetes Association. Standards of medical care in diabetes—2013. *Diabetes Care.* 2013;36(Suppl 1):S11–66; Centers for Disease Control and Prevention. *National Diabetes Facts Sheet: National Estimates and General Information on Diabetes and Prediabetes in the United States, 2011.* Atlanta, GA: U.S. Department of Health and Human Services, Centers for Disease Control and Prevention; 2011; Evert AB, Boucher JL, Cypress M, et al. Nutrition therapy recommendations for the management of adults with diabetes. *Diabetes Care.* 2013;36(11):3821–42; and Mullooly CA. Physical activity. In: Mensing C, ed. *The Art and Science of Diabetes Self-Management Education.* 1st ed. Chicago, IL: American Association of Diabetes Educators; 2006:297–330.

with a diameter of 1 cm or less. The base of the corn is on the skin surface; its apex points inward and presses on the nerve endings in the dermis, causing pain.[7,11]

Polished, shiny, dry *hard corns* (*heloma durum*) are the most prevalent and usually occur on the bulb of the great toe, the dorsum of the fourth or fifth toe, or tips of the middle toes. *Soft corns* (*heloma molle*) are whitish thickenings of the skin and may be extremely painful. Accumulated perspiration macerates the epidermis, giving this corn a soft appearance. Soft corns may occur between any adjacent toes but are most frequently found between the fourth and fifth toes[8,9] (Figure 44–1).

Pressure from inappropriate, tight-fitting shoes is the most frequent cause of pain from corns. As narrow-toed or high-heeled shoes crowd toes into a narrow toe box, the most lateral toe, the fifth, sustains the most pressure and friction and is the usual site of a corn. The resulting pain may be severe and sharp (on application of downward pressure) or dull and discomforting. Consumer research approximates that 82% of women 35–54 years of age suffer moderate–severe pain from corns and that 35% are consequently limited or restricted in their activities.[7,10,11]

Calluses

A *callus* has a broad base, with relatively even thickening of skin, and is generally found on the bottom of the foot in areas such as the heel, ball of the foot, and toes, and on the sides of the foot (Figure 44–1). A callus has indefinite borders and ranges in diameter from a few millimeters to several centimeters. The indefinite borders help in differentiating calluses from corns, which have well-circumscribed margins. A callus is usually raised and yellow, with a normal pattern of skin ridges on its surface. Calluses form over joints and on weight-bearing areas of the hands and feet[7,9–11] (see Color Plates, photograph 36).

Friction (caused by loose-fitting shoes or tight-fitting hosiery), walking barefoot, and structural biomechanical problems contribute to the development of calluses. Calluses can be symptomatic and protective.

Two most common calluses found on the feet are discrete-nucleated and diffuse-shearing calluses. The *discrete-nucleated callus* is smaller and has a localized translucent center; this type of callus is painful with applied pressure because of its central keratin plug. The *diffuse-shearing callus* covers a larger surface area and does not have a central core; therefore, this callus is not associated with pain.[9–11]

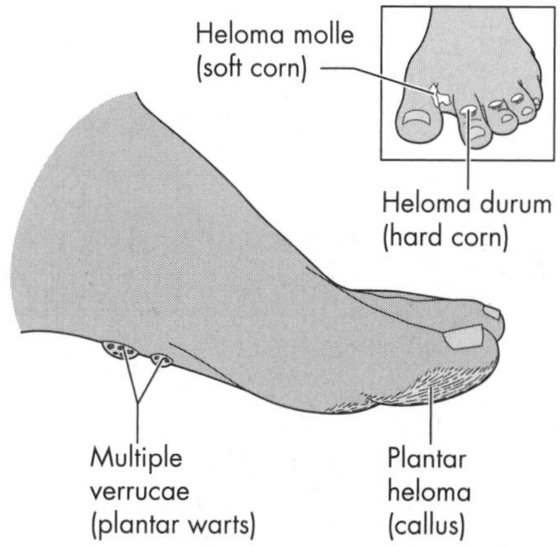

FIGURE 44–1 Disorders affecting top and sole of foot: corns, callus, and plantar warts.

Treatment of Corns and Calluses

Treatment Goals

The goals of self-treatment are (1) to provide symptomatic relief, (2) to remove corns and calluses, and (3) to prevent their recurrence by correcting underlying causes.

General Treatment Approach

Although effective nonprescription products are available for removing corns and calluses, ultimate success depends on eliminating the causes. The algorithm in Figure 44–2 outlines self-treatment of corns and calluses and lists potential exclusions for self-care.

Nonpharmacologic Therapy

Daily soaking of the affected skin area (for at least 5 minutes in warm, not hot, water) throughout the treatment period aids in softening dead tissue for removal. After normal washing of the foot, dead tissue should be removed gently, rather than forcibly, to avoid further damage. A callus file or pumice stone effectively accomplishes this purpose. Power-operated foot files may be too aggressive. Sharp knives or razor blades should not be used, because these instruments may lacerate the skin, which could allow bacteria to enter the wound, potentially resulting in localized infection.[9]

Cushioning pads are another option. Correct placement of circular foam cushioning pads may aid in relieving painful pressure from inflamed tissue. Some podiatrists recommend that the pads be changed every day because of concerns that the pad adhesive may degrade the skin, leading to infection. Disadvantages associated with older pads have been overcome with polymer gel pads, which provide a protective cushion without leaving a sticky residue. Another advantage of gel pads is that the smooth outer surface does not cause snags and runs in socks and hosiery.[9,12] A silicone toe sleeve impregnated with mineral oil, such as the Pedifix Visco-Gel Toe Protector, is an option for toes affected by corns. The mineral oil is slowly released to soften the skin. The sleeve also protects and cushions the corn area. A foam spacer or lamb's wool may be used to provide relief in areas with soft corns. Placement of a metatarsal pad or lamb's wool may help relieve pain and pressure from a callus.[8,13]

Eliminating the pressure and friction that induce corns and calluses entails using well-fitting, nonbinding footwear that evenly distributes body weight[13] (Table 44–1). The stratum corneum will normalize after topical keratolytics are applied and total desquamation of the hyperkeratotic tissue occurs. For anatomic foot deformities, orthopedic corrections must be made. Orthotics (i.e., arch supports) may be needed to help compensate for deformities by redistributing the mechanical forces. These measures relieve pressure and friction, which allow normal mitosis of the basal cell layer to resume. Ultimately, surgical correction of toe deformities and resection of the underlying bone may be necessary.

Pharmacologic Therapy

Salicylic Acid

Salicylic acid, the oldest of the keratolytic agents, is formulated in various strengths (0.5%–40%). For the treatment of corns and

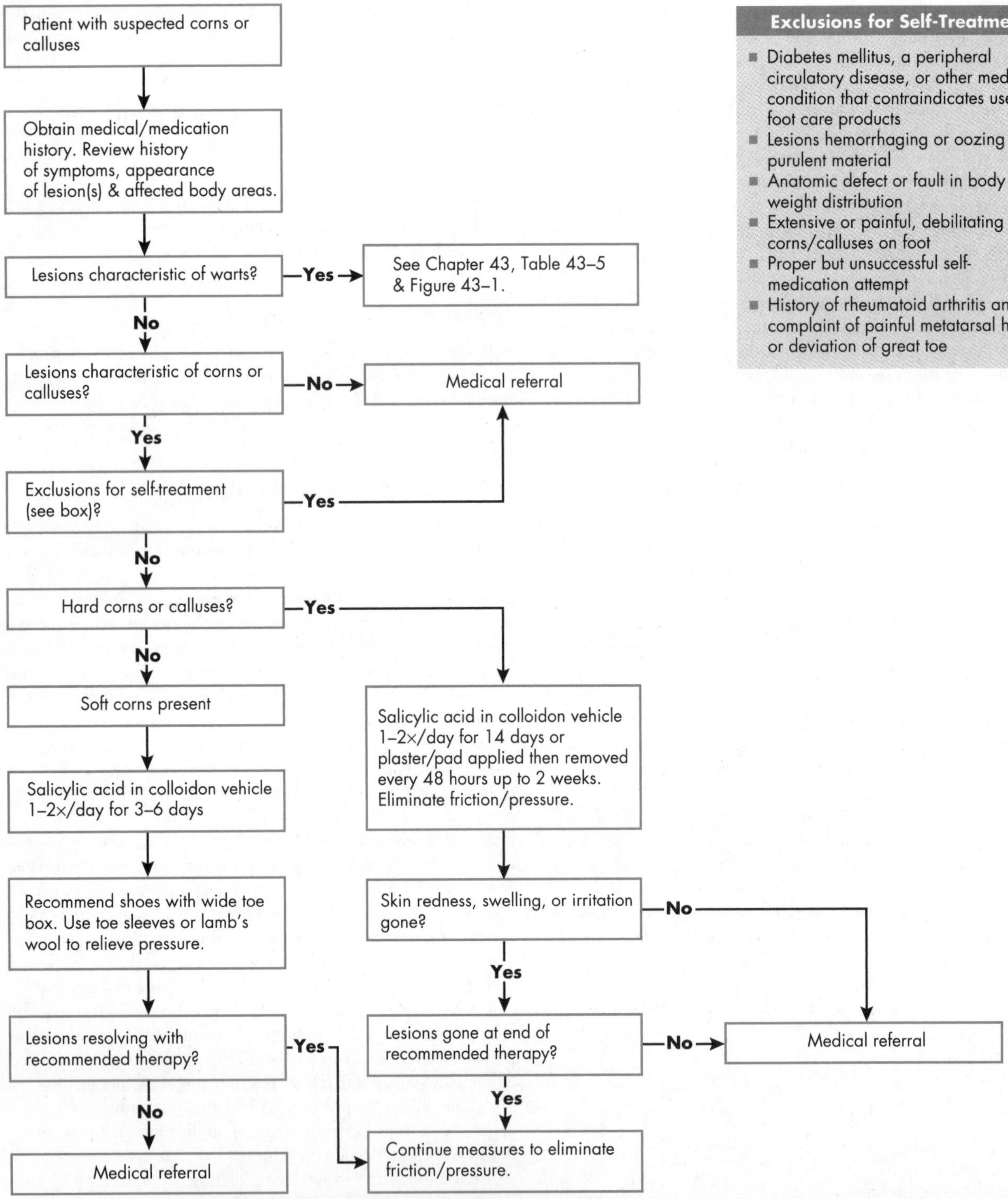

Exclusions for Self-Treatment

- Diabetes mellitus, a peripheral circulatory disease, or other medical condition that contraindicates use of foot care products
- Lesions hemorrhaging or oozing purulent material
- Anatomic defect or fault in body weight distribution
- Extensive or painful, debilitating corns/calluses on foot
- Proper but unsuccessful self-medication attempt
- History of rheumatoid arthritis and complaint of painful metatarsal heads or deviation of great toe

FIGURE **44–2** Self-care for corns and calluses.

calluses, the approved concentration ranges are 6%–17% in a topical gel (i.e., Hydrisalic gel), 12%–40% in a plaster vehicle, and 12%–27.5% in a collodion-like vehicle.[14–16]

Salicylic acid is believed to act on hyperplastic keratin, without affecting viable epidermis. Product application will cause the area to swell, soften, macerate, and then desquamate the affected epithelium. The U.S. Food and Drug Administration (FDA) has stated that presoaking the affected area before application of salicylic acid produced no significant positive effects. In its final rule, FDA proposed allowing manufacturers of these products to use the following statement as an optional direction to the consumer: "May soak corn/callus (or wart) in warm water for 5 minutes to assist in removal."[14–16]

The FDA advisory review panel evaluated more than 20 agents for the treatment of corns and calluses. Of these agents, only salicylic acid in a plaster, pad, disk, gel, or collodion vehicle dosage form

TABLE 44–1 Selection of Properly Fitted Footwear

- Buy shoes in the proper size (width and length). To obtain an accurate measurement, ask a trained salesperson to measure your feet. Recheck shoe size every 2 years.
- Base shoe length on the longest toe of your longest foot. The optimum distance between the tip of the shoe and the longest toe is approximately ½ inch. In an athletic shoe, 1 inch is needed.
- For proper arch length, choose a shoe in which the first metatarsal head of the foot fits the metatarsal break of the shoe.
- For proper shoe width, choose a shoe that feels comfortable at the first metatarsal joint (i.e., toes do not feel cramped in the toe box).
- Once the shoe size is determined, choose a shoe shaped to match the shape of your foot.
- If you have abnormalities of the toes (e.g., hammer toes) or use orthotics or padding in your shoes, select a shoe with a toe box of adequate depth (vertical height) to prevent friction on the tops of the toes. A wide toe box will help relieve pressure between toes.
- Make sure the heel area fits snugly and helps hold the foot straight.
- If you are physically active, make sure the shoe's midsole provides adequate cushioning and support.
- Try on both shoes at the time of purchase, preferably wearing a pair of socks or stockings of the type that will usually be worn with the new pair of shoes.
- If your feet tend to swell, select shoes at the end of the day.

Source: References 1, 8, 10, 13, and 18.

is approved as safe and effective as a nonprescription preparation marketed for the removal of corns and calluses (Table 44–2). FDA recognizes that the term *plaster* includes disks and pads, because these dosage forms are similar.[15,16]

Salicylic acid is usually applied to a corn, callus, or common wart in a collodion or collodion-like vehicle. These vehicles contain pyroxylin and various combinations of volatile solvents (e.g., ether, acetone, alcohol) or a plasticizer, which is usually castor oil. Pyroxylin is a nitrocellulose derivative that remains on the skin as a water-repellent film after the volatile solvents have evaporated.[14–16]

The advantages of collodions and liquid dosage forms are that they form an adherent flexible or rigid film and prevent moisture evaporation. These qualities aid penetration of the active ingredient into the affected tissue, resulting in sustained local action of the drug. The delivery systems are largely water-insoluble, as are most of their active ingredients, such as salicylic acid. They are also less prone than other aqueous solutions to run onto surrounding skin.[14–16]

A disadvantage of collodions is that they are extremely flammable and volatile. Some patients may inhale and abuse these vehicles. Another disadvantage is the occlusion of normal water transport through the skin, which allows systemic absorption of some drugs (e.g., salicylic acid). Percutaneous absorption may be problematic with prolonged use on large surface areas in children and patients with renal or hepatic impairment, because salicylic acid is largely metabolized in the liver and excreted in the urine. Although occlusive vehicles can enhance the percutaneous absorption of salicylic acid, it is highly unlikely that salicylate toxicity will result during corn, callus, or wart therapy at recommended dosages. However, if signs and symptoms of possible salicylism (nausea, vomiting, dizziness, hearing loss, tinnitus, lethargy, hyperpnea, diarrhea, or psychiatric disturbances) occur, use of these products should be discontinued immediately.[14–16]

Salicylic acid may also be delivered to the skin through the use of a plaster, disk, or pad. This delivery system provides direct and prolonged contact of the drug with the affected area, resulting in quicker resolution of the condition. Salicylic acid plaster is a uniform solid or semisolid adhesive mixture of salicylic acid in a suitable base that is spread on appropriate backing material (e.g., felt, moleskin, cotton, plastic). The usual concentration of salicylic acid in the base is 40%; these dosage forms may be applied directly to the corn or callus.[9,14–16] Table 44–3 provides instructions for applying salicylic acid products.

Caution should be used in applying topical salicylic acid because misapplication may lead to inflammation or ulcer formation (see the box "A Word about Chronic Diseases and Foot Disorders"). Use of these products may be hazardous in pregnancy, and they should also not be used in patients who are breastfeeding because of systemic absorption and the potential for Reye syndrome. Salicylic acid may be used in pediatric patients older than 2 years at concentrations of 1.8%–6%. FDA requires the following warning on salicylic acid product labels:

> Do not use this product on irritated skin, any area that is infected or reddened, moles, birthmarks, warts with hair growing from them, genital warts, warts on the face, or warts on the mucous membranes, such as inside the mouth, nose, anus, genitals, or lips. Do not use if you are diabetic, or if you have poor blood circulation.[14–16]

TABLE 44–2 Selected Corn and Callus Products

Trade Name	Primary Ingredients
Curad Mediplast Corn, Callus & Wart Remover	Salicylic acid 40%
Dr. Scholl's Corn/Callus Remover Liquid	Salicylic acid 12.6%
Hydrisalic Gel	Salicylic acid 6%
Dr. Scholl's Cushlin Gel Corn/ Callus Remover Disk	Salicylic acid 40%
Freezone One Step Corn/ Callus Remover Pads	Salicylic acid 40%

Source: Reference 14.

Assessment of Corns and Calluses: A Case-Based Approach

The clinical encounter should be in a private area where the patient can be comfortable removing the shoe(s) to allow direct inspection of the feet and enable accurate assessment of the nature and extent of the problem and its underlying cause. The patient should be asked about any self-care attempts and their outcome. The patient's health status and current medication regimen should also be assessed. Lifestyle factors (e.g., occupation, daily exercise, footwear), underlying pathology (e.g., circulatory or neurologic disorders), the possibility of an aggravating event, and the walking/working surface must also be evaluated. This information should be recorded and regularly updated in the patient's medication profile.

Case 44–1 illustrates the assessment of a patient with corns.

TABLE 44-3 Guidelines for Treating Corns and Calluses With Salicylic Acid Products

- Wash and dry the affected area thoroughly before applying any product.
- May soak the affected foot in warm water for 5 minutes. Then remove the macerated, soft white skin of the corn or callus by scrubbing gently with a rough towel, pumice stone, or callus file. Do not debride the healthy skin.

Salicylic Acid 12%–17.6% in Collodion-Like Vehicle

- Apply product no more than twice daily. Morning and evening are usually the most convenient times.
- Do not let adjacent areas of normal healthy skin come in contact with the drug. If this happens, immediately wash off the solution with soap and water.
  - A coating of petroleum jelly on the healthy skin will serve as protection if delivery of the medication accidentally extends beyond the intended treatment area.
- Apply 1 drop at a time directly to the corn or callus until the affected area is well covered. Do not overuse the product.
- Allow the drops to dry and harden so that the solution does not run.
- The solution is applied once or twice daily for up to 14 days.
- After use, cap the container tightly to prevent evaporation, which would result in a greater, potentially harmful concentration of the active ingredients.
- Store the product in an amber or otherwise light-resistant container away from direct sunlight or heat.

Salicylic Acid 12%–40% Plasters/Pads

- If using a plaster, trim it to follow the contours of the corn or callus. Apply the plaster to the affected skin, and cover it with adhesive occlusive tape.
- If using medicated disks with pads, apply the appropriately sized disk directly on the affected area, and then cover the disk with the pad.
- Remove the plaster/pad and occlusive tape within 48 hours.
- After removing the softened skin, reapply the plaster every 48 hours as needed to remove the corn/callus, but do not treat for longer than 14 days.
  - Seek medical attention if redness or irritation of the skin occurs or if corn or callus is not removed after 14 days of treatment.

Source: References 8 and 14–16.

CASE 44-1

Relevant Evaluation Criteria	Scenario/Model Outcome
Collect	
1. Gather essential information about the patient's symptoms and medical history, including	
a. Description of symptom(s) (i.e., nature, onset, duration, severity, associated symptoms)	The patient describes a large raised thick dry area of thick skin on the ball of his foot that has been present for approximately 2 months.
b. Description of any factors that seem to precipitate, exacerbate, and/or relieve the patient's symptom(s)	The patient says the thickened area bothers him when he stands for long periods of time. He tried using his wife's pumice stone on the affected area, but the thick skin comes back.
c. Description of the patient's efforts to relieve the symptoms	The patient has not tried anything other than "sanding down" the area of irritation.
d. Patient's identity	Lincoln James
e. Patient's age, gender, height, and weight	41 years old, male, 6 ft 2 in., 226 lb
f. Patient's occupation	Construction worker
g. Patient's dietary habits	Gas station breakfast (pastry, or sandwich), peanut butter and jelly sandwich, chips, banana, and water. Typical family dinner (e.g., hamburgers, spaghetti, pork chops)
h. Patient's sleep habits	8 hours nightly
i. Concurrent medical conditions, prescription and nonprescription medications, and dietary supplements	Lisinopril 10 mg every day for hypertension
j. Allergies	No allergies
k. History of other adverse reactions to medications	None
l. Other (describe) ______	None

CASE 44-1 *continued*

Relevant Evaluation Criteria	Scenario/Model Outcome
Assess	
2. Differentiate patient's signs/symptoms, and correctly identify the patient's primary problem(s).	Mr. James has developed diffuse shearing calluses (Figures 44–1 and 44–2).
3. Identify exclusions for self-treatment (Figure 44–2).	None
4. Formulate a comprehensive list of therapeutic alternatives for the primary problem to determine whether triage to a health care provider is required, and share this information with the patient or caregiver.	Options include (1) Refer Mr. James to an appropriate HCP. (2) Recommend self-care with a nonprescription callus remover and nondrug measures. (3) Recommend self-care until Mr. James can see an appropriate provider. (4) Take no action.
Plan	
5. Select an optimal therapeutic alternative to address the patient's problem, taking into account patient preferences.	Mr. James should use a nonprescription callus remover, callus cushioning pads, and nondrug measures to treat his condition.
6. Describe the recommended therapeutic approach to the patient or caregiver.	"Daily foot soaks and a pumice stone or foot file may be used to reduce roughness of your calluses. Completely dry the feet before applying the callus remover. Use of cushioning pads will help to protect pressure point areas on your feet, allowing the affected skin to improve. You should also consider selection of appropriate shoes as outlined in Table 44–1."
7. Explain to the patient or caregiver the rationale for selecting the recommended therapeutic approach from the considered therapeutic alternatives.	"Calluses can be removed by nonprescription products and the use of foot files. However, it is important to assess the cause of the callus formation and to correct the cause with appropriate measures including selection of well-fitting footwear."
Implement	
8. When recommending self-care with nonprescription medications and/or nondrug therapy, convey accurate information to the patient or caregiver.	See Table 44–3 for instructions for applying salicylic acid products. Also see the box "Patient Education for Corn and Calluses." Mr. James should see a response to treatment recommendations within 14 days.
Solicit follow-up questions from the patient or caregiver.	(1) "Will a couple of days be long enough to treat my foot? I really don't have the time to deal with this." (2) "Can I speed up the process by cutting the callus down with a razor blade before applying the nonprescription medication?"
Answer the patient's or caregiver's questions.	(1) "You should follow the appropriate treatment duration to receive the maximum benefit. You should see resolve in symptoms within 14 days." (2) "It is best to soak the feet and use foot files to pare down the callus. Do not cut on your feet because of the risk of injury and infection."
Follow-up: Monitor and Evaluate	
9. Assess patient outcome.	Ask Mr. James to call in 14 days to update you on the response to your treatment recommendations. Or you could call him into the pharmacy to evaluate the response.

Key: HCP = Health care provider.

Patient Counseling for Corns and Calluses

Remission of corns and calluses can take several days to several months. Patients suffering from corns and calluses should understand that effective treatment and maintenance depend on eliminating predisposing factors that contributed to the foot problem. It is important to emphasize the need for wearing footwear of adequate width and length. Pads and cushions also help to reduce the pressure and shearing associated with corn and callus development.

The patient or caregiver should be counseled on how to use nonprescription medications that remove corns and calluses. Because many products contain corrosive materials, they must be applied to only the corn or callus. Patients should be alerted that products containing collodions are poisonous when ingested and that these products, as well as all other medications, should be stored out of children's reach. The box "Patient Education for Corns and Calluses" lists specific information to provide in patient counseling.

Evaluation of Patient Outcomes for Corns and Calluses

The progress of the patient's self-treatment regimen for corns or calluses should be checked after 14 days. The affected area should be visually inspected to determine whether the corns or calluses have decreased in size or resolved. The methods used to eliminate the corns or calluses should also be evaluated. If these conditions are still present, the patient should seek further medical evaluation.

TIRED, ACHING FEET AND EXERCISE-INDUCED FOOT INJURIES

With every step taken (8000–10,000 steps each day), gravity-induced pressure of up to twice the body's weight bears down on each foot, releasing powerful shocks of energy that the foot's natural padding must struggle to absorb.[1,17,18] In an unpadded shoe, the shock as the foot strikes the ground is absorbed throughout the foot, ankle, leg, and back. This shock can fatigue muscles, resulting in tired, aching feet and/or back pain.[17–19]

An estimated two-thirds of Americans complain of tired, aching feet (the most common foot problem). In addition, 2 million adults are estimated to suffer from heel pain. People simply do not realize the daily abuse their feet endure.[20] In addition to recognizing the foot disorders due to daily impact, HCPs should be familiar with possible exercise-induced foot injuries, particularly those caused by running, jogging, or other high-impact physical activities (Figure 44–3). Often, individuals seeking to increase their daily activity level are unaware of certain important precautions and may plunge head first into a strenuous exercise program. To minimize potential injuries and dangers, individuals who are typically sedentary, are older than 35 years of age, suffer from hypertension, or have a history of heart disease or diabetes should seek medical evaluation before beginning a high-level exercise regimen. Patients with potential orthopedic problems may benefit from walking instead of engaging in more demanding activities.[21]

PATIENT EDUCATION FOR Corns and Calluses

The objectives of self-treatment are (1) to provide symptomatic relief, (2) to remove corns or calluses, and (3) to prevent their recurrence by correcting underlying causes. For most patients, carefully following product instructions and the self-care measures listed here will help ensure optimal therapeutic outcomes.

Nondrug Measures

- After use, carefully clean instruments used to remove dead skin to avoid subsequent bacterial contamination and infection when used again.
- Do not use sharp knives or razor blades to remove dead skin from corns and calluses. These instruments may cause bacterial infections.
- If you have trouble applying the product only to the affected area, use petroleum jelly to coat healthy skin surrounding the treatment area before applying the corn and callus remover.
- For temporary relief of painful pressure in the area under a corn or callus, cover the affected area with a pad.
- Consult a health care provider if the symptoms described recur.

Preventive Measures

- To eliminate the pressure and friction that cause corns and calluses, wear well-fitting shoes that evenly distribute body weight (Table 44–1).
- Consult a podiatrist about foot deformity corrections.

Nonprescription Medications

- To remove corns and calluses, use a salicylic acid product labeled for use on these types of lesions (Tables 44–2 and 44–3).
- Do not use this product on irritated, infected, or reddened skin.
- Do not use this product if you are diabetic or have poor blood circulation.
- Salicylic acid is poisonous. Do not allow it to come in contact with the mouth, and keep it out of children's reach.
- Note that the medication sloughs off skin, which may leave an unsightly pinkish tinge to the affected area.

When to Seek Medical Attention

- Stop treatment and consult a health care provider if swelling, reddening, or irritation of the skin develops, or if pain occurs immediately with product application.

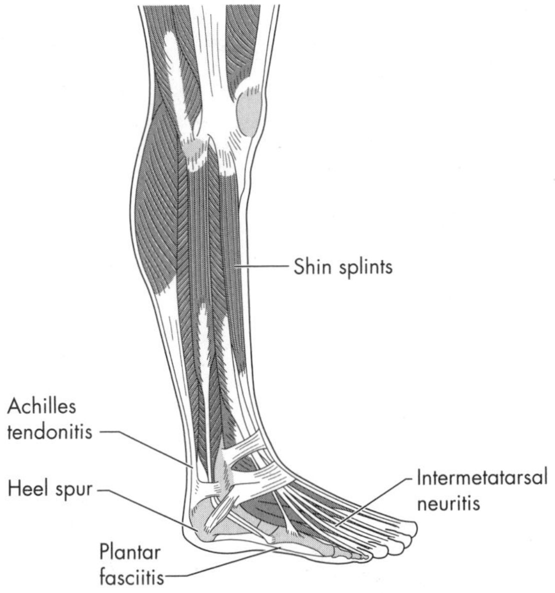

FIGURE 44–3 Selected foot and leg injuries associated with excessive impact shock.

Pathophysiology of Tired, Aching Feet and Exercise-Induced Foot Injuries

Aching feet can be caused by increased frequency of standing and/or walking (especially on hard surfaces), age-related erosion of the fat padding on the bottom of the foot, circulatory or neurologic disorders, and poor-fitting or inappropriate footwear.[17,18,20]

Because the cause of heel pain is difficult to determine, treatment often can be prolonged and expensive. The three most common types of heel pain are heel spurs, plantar fasciitis, and Sever's disease. Exercise-induced injuries include shin splints, stress fractures, Achilles tendonitis, blisters, ankle sprains, intermetatarsal neuritis, and toenail loss. The common causes, pathophysiology, clinical presentation, and therapeutic recommendations are discussed in Table 44–4 for each of these conditions.

Assessment of Tired, Aching Feet and Exercise-Induced Foot Injuries

Treatment of tired, aching feet requires evaluation of lifestyle factors (e.g., occupation, daily exercise, footwear); the possibility of underlying pathology (e.g., circulatory or neurologic disorders);

TABLE 44–4 Differentiation and Management of Exercise-Induced Foot Injuries

Type of Injury	Common Causes	Pathophysiology	Clinical Presentation	Recommendations
Shin splints	Overzealous workout; inappropriate stretching; running/walking on sloped or hard surfaces; wearing ill-fitting footwear; over striding	Excessive pronation weakens/strains posterior tibialis; anterior tibia muscle stretches away from periosteum that lines shinbone.	Pain in medial lower third of shin, or below knee and above ankle; pain worsens with exercise; cramping, burning, and tightness on anterior lateral section of shin	PRICE or RICE therapy; acetaminophen or ibuprofen; shoe orthotic; medical referral
Stress fracture	Running on hard, rigid surfaces; rapid increase in physical activity; jumping; estrogen deficiency; nutritional deficiencies; obesity; ill-fitting footwear	Outer cortex of long bones of leg or foot cracks from tensile forces sent by ligaments, tendons, and muscles.	Deep pain in lower leg; tender to the touch; swelling; pain worsens with exercise.	Medical referral; complete rest; NSAID therapy
Achilles tendonitis	Running on hills or in sand; ill-fitting footwear; excessive pronation; arthritis	Inflammation of Achilles tendon; rupture of tendon	Posterior heel pain; tenderness; swelling	Medical referral
Blisters	Repetitive movement; ill-fitting footwear; tight hosiery	Continual friction on small surface of foot separates stratum corneum and stratum lucidum skin layers, causing space between layers to fill with fluid	Accumulation of fluid beneath stratum corneum; may be painful	Do not remove blister; protect with topical bandage; medical referral for drainage, if needed.
Ankle sprains	Ankle rotating outside acceptable range	Lateral ligament damage	Pain; bruising; tenderness; difficulty walking	PRICE or RICE therapy; compression bandage
Intermetatarsal neuritis	Small toe box space	Inflammation of nerves from compression of or entanglement between metatarsal heads and digital bases	Pain and numbness between toes	Proper footwear

(continued)

TABLE 44-4 **Differentiation and Management of Exercise-Induced Foot Injuries** *(continued)*

Type of Injury	Common Causes	Pathophysiology	Clinical Presentation	Recommendations
Toenail loss	Long, thick toenails in small toe box space; friction and pressure from running in "stop and go" sports, such as tennis	Fluid beneath nail plate pushes toenail from nail bed.	Dark discoloration from blood underneath nail plate; pain at toe; nail loss	Referral to podiatrist or PCP
Plantar fasciitis	High arches, flat feet, repetitive stress during athletic activity, pronated feet, prolonged standing	Strain on the connective tissue that attaches the arch to the front of the heel	Manifests with pain upon rising from bed in the morning or standing up after sitting; the pain results from tissue contraction. The sensation on the bottom of the heel is quite painful, and the patient may complain of a burning sensation.	
Heel spurs	Incorrect walking or running technique, excessive running, poor-fitting shoes, obesity, aging	Bony growth on the underside of the heel bone Calcium deposits may form on the calcaneous bone detected via X-ray; they cause pain of increasing intensity after prolonged periods of rest.	Strained foot muscles, deterioration of fat tissue surrounding heel bone	
Sever's disease	Seen in children (predominantly occurs in males between ages 8 and 15 years) that is precipitated by running, jumping, and excessive walking; usually resolves once the bone has completed growth or activity is lessened	Calcaneal apophysitis	Manifests with no swelling, skin changes, erythema, or visible abnormalities. The *squeeze test* aids in the diagnosis of Sever's disease: pressure is applied at the point of attachment of the calcaneal apophysis to the main body of the os calcis to determine if the patient experiences pain.	

Key: NSAID = Nonsteroidal anti-inflammatory drug; PCP = primary care provider; PRICE = protection, rest, ice, compression, elevation; RICE = rest, ice, compression, elevation.

Source: References 8, 9, 11, 13, 15, 19, and 21–29.

the possibility of an aggravating event; and the walking/working surface. If underlying pathology is suspected, the patient should be referred to a primary care provider or podiatrist for initial evaluation. The provider may be called on to play a triage role in treating an exercise-induced injury to the foot (Figure 44–4). Identifying the location of the pain will help determine the type and extent of the injury. Establishing the nature and duration of the pain will help in determining whether the injury is self-treatable.

Treatment of Tired, Aching Feet and Exercise-Induced Foot Injuries

Treatment Goals

The primary goal in self-treatment is to provide additional support and shock absorbance for the feet in order to reduce foot pain and fatigue. Stretching muscles to prevent limitations on daily activities is also desired. The goals in self-treating exercise-induced foot problems are (1) to relieve any pain, (2) to prevent secondary bacterial infection if the skin is broken, and (3) to institute measures to prevent further injury.

General Treatment Approach

The first measure to avoid tired, aching feet is to choose well-fitted footwear that has sufficient padding and cushioning (Table 44–1). The second is to identify appropriate measures personalized to individual patient needs. For athletes, wearing sport-specific shoes with good arch support (e.g., running shoes) is an excellent measure for preventing heel pain. Individuals who are physically active or stand for prolonged periods during the day may need to take additional measures, such as replacing worn shoes or heel pads, using a night splint, strapping or taping the arch, decreasing the amount of weight-bearing activity, and, if necessary, entering a weight reduction program.[21] Oral nonprescription anti-inflammatory agents

Exclusions for Self-Treatment

- Patients with inappropriate gait
- Patients with malformations of the foot
- Diabetes mellitus or peripheral circulatory diseases

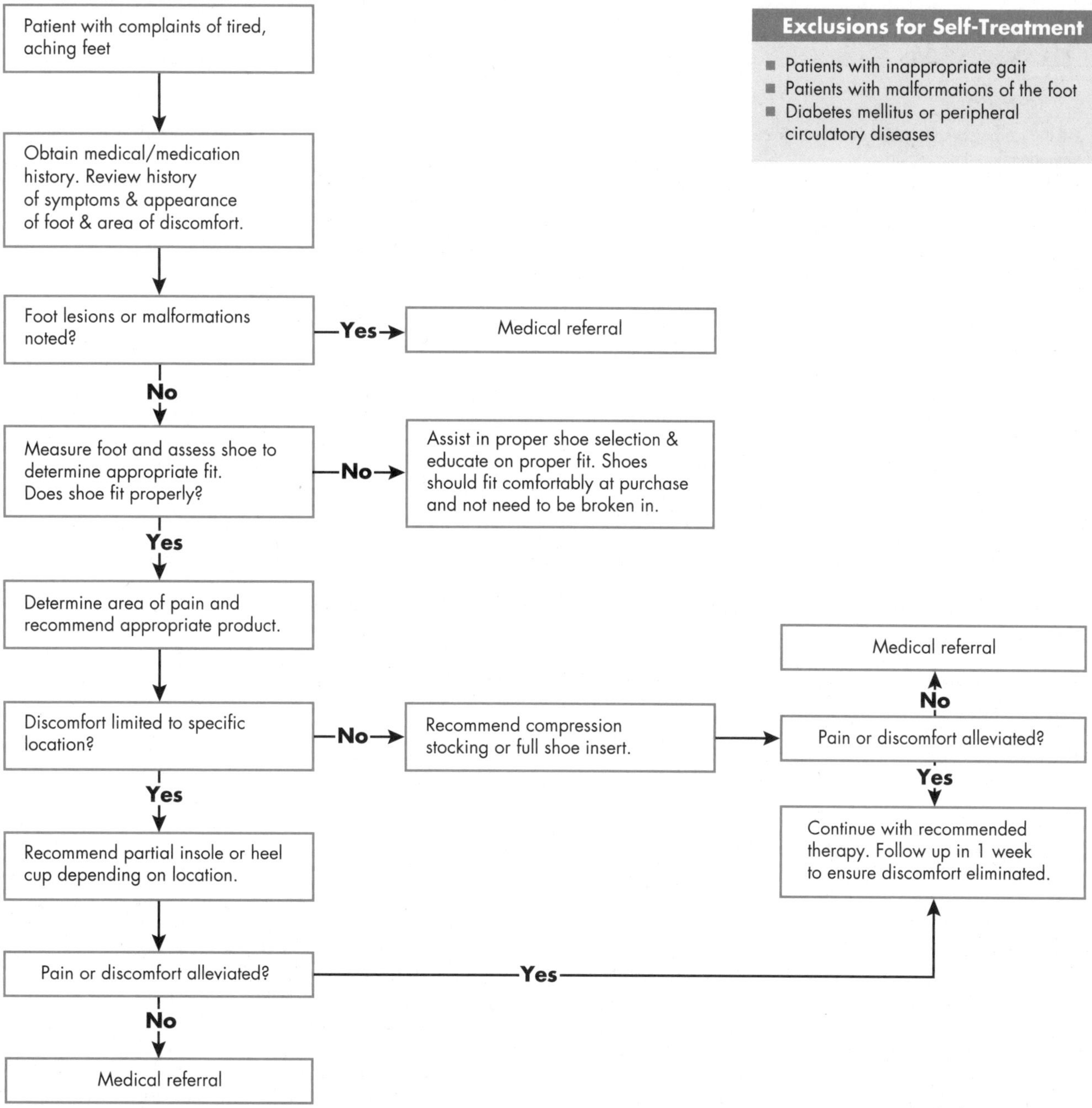

Patient with complaints of tired, aching feet
Obtain medical/medication history. Review history of symptoms & appearance of foot & area of discomfort.
Foot lesions or malformations noted?
Yes
Medical referral
No
Measure foot and assess shoe to determine appropriate fit. Does shoe fit properly?
No
Assist in proper shoe selection & educate on proper fit. Shoes should fit comfortably at purchase and not need to be broken in.
Yes
Determine area of pain and recommend appropriate product.
Discomfort limited to specific location?
No
Recommend compression stocking or full shoe insert.
Pain or discomfort alleviated?
No
Medical referral
Yes
Continue with recommended therapy. Follow up in 1 week to ensure discomfort eliminated.
Yes
Recommend partial insole or heel cup depending on location.
Pain or discomfort alleviated?
Yes
No
Medical referral

FIGURE 44–4 Self-care for exercise-induced injuries. Key: PRICE = Protection, rest, ice, compression, and elevation; RICE = rest, ice, compression, and elevation.

and topical anti-inflammatory treatments such as ice applications (Table 44–5) are also appropriate. Magnesium sulfate (Epsom salts) baths have historically been used for soothing tired aching muscles, sprains, and bruising, but no scientific evidence supports these claims. When self-treatment fails, patients should be referred to an appropriate HCP for evaluation for any bone malalignments and possible orthotic therapy. Figure 44–5 outlines self-treatment for tired, aching feet.

Measures to prevent exercise-induced injuries entail using suitable footwear that fits properly (Table 44–1); running on the proper surface; using correct posture (i.e., running erect); and stretching muscles before exercising. Most running injuries can be successfully treated with measures such as shoe modifications, shoe inserts, and in-shoe supports.

If an injury to the leg or foot occurs, activity must usually be interrupted to allow the injured leg or foot to rest and heal. Relative rest (i.e., avoiding activities that produce the symptoms) is often indicated. Alternative exercise such as swimming, rowing, and/or bicycling (stationary or outdoor) should be encouraged. If the injury warrants, the patient can be instructed on selecting and using nonprescription accessories (e.g., compression bandages, arch supports, heel cushions) and related modalities (e.g., cryotherapy, PRICE [protection, rest, ice, compression, and elevation]) that will alleviate injuries or other underlying problems. Systemic

TABLE 44-5 Table 44-5 Guidelines for Applying Cold Compresses

Ice Bag Method

- Fill the ice bag with crushed or shaved ice to one-half to two-thirds of its capacity, if possible. These forms of ice will promote greater contact with the injured body part.
- If necessary, break ice into walnut-sized pieces with no jagged edges. An overfilled bag will be difficult to apply because it will not rest on the contour of the body area.
- After filling the bag, squeeze out trapped air. Then dry the outside of the bag and check for leaks.
- Bind the injured body part with a wet elastic wrap. The wet wrap aids transfer of cold to the injured area.
- If the ankle is being treated, keep it in a dorsiflexed position (foot tipped toward the nose) when it is wrapped in the elastic bandage.
- Apply the ice bag to the specific body part.
- To avoid tissue damage, apply the ice bag for 10 minutes and then remove it for 10 minutes. If the bag is not cloth-covered, wrap the injured area or the ice bag in a thin towel to prevent tissue damage.
- Follow this procedure 3–4 times a day.
- For most injuries, continue the cryotherapy until swelling decreases or for a maximum of 12–24 hours. Application of ice may be necessary for up to 48–72 hours, depending on the severity of the injury. (For example, the maximum swelling of ankle injuries may occur up to 48 hours after the injury.)
- Before storing the ice bag, drain it and allow it to air dry. If possible, turn it inside out for more efficient drying. Cap the bag and store it in a cool, dry place.

Cold Wraps

- To activate a single-use cold pack, squeeze the middle of the pack to burst the bubble. This action initiates an endothermic reaction of ammonium nitrate, water, and special additives.
- For a reusable cold wrap (cold pack or gel pack), store it in the freezer for 2 hours. Do not put the cloth cover in the freezer.
- Remove the cold wrap from the freezer, insert it in the cloth cover, and apply it to the injured body part.
- If the cold wrap is uncomfortable, remove it for 1–2 minutes and then reapply it.
- Alternate application of the cold wrap (10 minutes on, 10 minutes off) 3–4 times a day for 24–48 hours.
- After use, store the cold wrap in the freezer.
- Although some gel packs are nontoxic, keep all cold wraps out of children's reach.

Source: References 20 and 26.

analgesics can also relieve the pain and inflammation associated with minor foot injuries (see Chapter 5).

Nonpharmacologic Therapy

Shoe Inserts, Partial Insoles, and Heel Cups/Cushions

Full-shoe inserts, which can provide cushioning and absorb shock, are available in various sizes and thicknesses to accommodate most individuals with exercise-related foot problems. These inserts help decrease the incidence of lower back pain associated with the impact from walking. The patient must select an insert that conforms to the type of shoe worn.[8,9]

Partial insoles are preferred when a patient needs cushioning or support in a certain portion of the shoe. For example, metatarsal arch supports, which fit into the ball-of-foot region of the shoe, help lift the arch behind the toes to alleviate pain associated with the spreading of the foot, a condition that occurs with increasing age in women. Inserts specifically designed to fit in high heels (e.g., Dr. Scholl's for Her High Heel Insoles) are also available. Finally, the arch support insert is intended to cushion and support painful longitudinal arches.[9,13]

A heel cup or heel cushion may be indicated, depending on the location and extent of the pain. For example, a heel cushion might be appropriate when the pain is confined to the bottom of the heel. A heel cushion supports the entire heel as it elevates the sensitive area to prevent further irritation. Alternatively, when the pain is widespread and diffuse, a heel cup might be more appropriate. Heel cups help relieve the pain caused by the breakdown of the heel's natural padding or by intense athletic activity.

Caution should be used in selecting shoe inserts. If an added insole affects the gait, the patient should be referred to a podiatrist or pedorthist; the latter specializes in the designing, manufacturing, modifying, and fitting of footwear and orthotics. Insoles should be used only to cushion the foot, not to correct malformation, which requires a specialist's attention.

Athletic Footwear

Appropriate footwear can be a powerful tool for manipulating human movement and can greatly influence the healing of injured tissues, both positively and negatively. The importance of neutral shoes or motion controlled footwear has been reported.[22] A study demonstrated that the type of footwear chosen by recreational runners is important to prevent injury. Consequently, inappropriate or worn-out shoes can result in foot injuries and pain. Athletic shoes should be replaced after 200–400 miles of use.[23]

Compression Stockings

Compression stockings are also an option to enhance support for individuals who spend many hours on their feet. Compression stockings may be purchased without a prescription in compressions ranging from 8 to 30 mm Hg. These stockings will decrease inflammation by improving circulation, thereby reducing fatigue of the feet, legs, and back.[24,25]

Compression Bandages

Typically, a compression bandage (e.g., Ace Bandage) is used for an ankle or knee sprain. If a compression bandage is to be used,

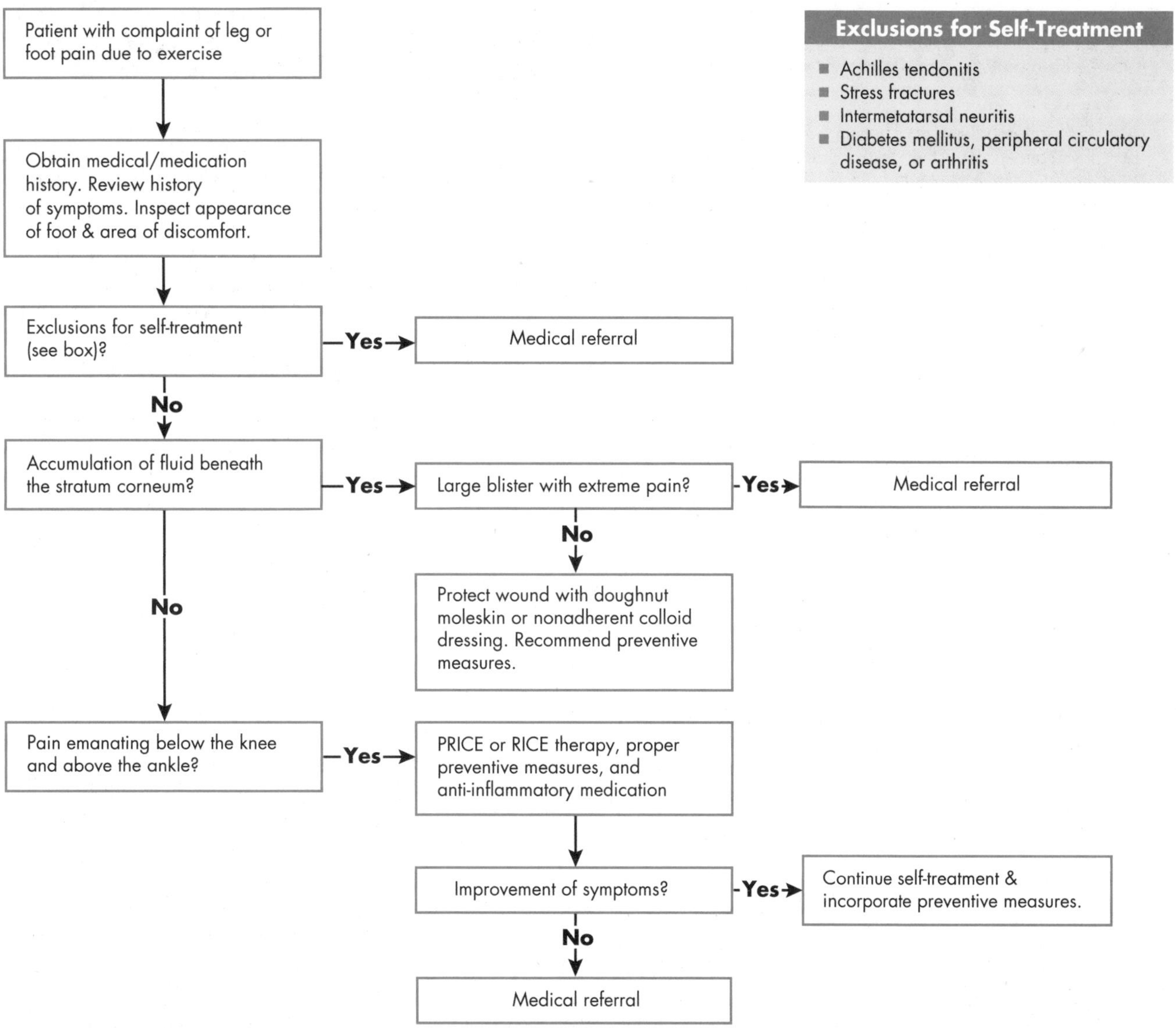

FIGURE 44–5 Self-care for tired, aching feet.

the width of the bandage depends on the injury site. For example, a foot or an ankle requires a 2- to 3-inch bandage.[26] Table 44–6 describes the proper method of applying this type of bandage.

Cryotherapy

Applying cold compresses to an injury such as a muscle sprain anesthetizes the area and decreases pain and inflammation. Ice bags or cold wraps are useful for cold application in 10-minute increments. Table 44–5 describes the proper method of cold application to injuries.

Contrast Bath Soaks

For acute injury, cold application is beneficial during the first 48 hours to decrease ensuing inflammation. After the acute injury, some podiatrists advocate the use of alternating applications of cold therapy and warm therapy for chronic, nagging pain. Specifically, the cold therapy is intended to decrease inflammation. The warm therapy attempts to bring increased blood flow to the affected area and to effect smooth muscle relaxation.

Patient Education and Evaluation of Patient Outcomes for Tired, Aching Feet and Exercise-Induced Injuries

Recommendations to resolve pain in the soles or heels of the feet depends on whether the patient has exclusions for self-treatment and how long the foot problem has persisted. Follow-up evaluation is indicated after 1 week, to determine whether the treatment recommendations such as the use of new shoes and/or in-shoe supports, compression bandages, cryotherapy, or other anti-inflammatory therapy has reduced or eliminated the discomfort. If the initial swelling and/or pain persist, medical referral is appropriate, and

TABLE 44-6 Application Guidelines for Compression Bandages

- Choose the appropriate size of bandage for the injured body part. If you are unsure of the size, purchase a product designed for the appropriate body part.
- Recommended elastic bandage width for coverage area:
  - 2 inches: foot, wrist, ankle
  - 3 inches: elbow, knee, ankle
  - 4 inches: knee, lower leg, shoulder
  - 6 inches: shoulder, upper leg, chest
- Unwind approximately 12–18 inches of bandage at a time, and allow the bandage to relax.
- If ice is also being applied to the injured area, soak the bandage in water to aid the transfer of cold (Table 44–5).
- Wrap the injured area by overlapping the previous layer of bandage by approximately one-third to one-half of its width.
- Snugly wrap the point most distal from the injury. For example, if the ankle is injured, begin wrapping just above the toes.
- Decrease the tightness of the bandage as you continue to wrap. (Follow package directions on how far to extend the bandage past the injury.) If the bandage feels tight or uncomfortable or if circulation is impaired, remove the compression bandage and rewrap it. Cold or swollen toes and fingers indicate that the bandage is too tight.
- After using the bandage, wash it in lukewarm, soapy water; do not scrub it. Rinse the bandage thoroughly, and allow it to air-dry on a flat surface. Roll up the bandage to prevent wrinkles, and store it in a cool, dry place. Do not iron the bandage to remove wrinkles.

Source: Reference 27.

depending on the acuity of the symptoms, patient should consult their primary care provider (for exercise-induced injuries) or podiatrist for appropriate evaluation. The boxes "Patient Education for Tired, Aching Feet" and "Patient Education for Exercise-Induced Injuries" detail the patient counseling that should be provided as well as when to seek medical attention.

INGROWN TOENAILS

The most frequent cause of ingrown toenail, or *onychocryptosis*, is incorrect trimming of the nails. The correct method is to cut the nail straight across, without tapering the corners. Wearing pointed-toe or tight shoes or too-tight hosiery has also been implicated. Other causes are hyperhidrosis, trauma, obesity, and excessive pressure on the toes. Direct pressure on a toe can force the lateral or medial edge of the nail into the soft tissue. The embedded nail may then continue to grow, resulting in swelling and inflammation of the nail fold.[8,10,23,27]

Bedridden patients may develop ingrown toenails if tight or heavy bedcovers press the soft skin tissue against the nails. Nail curling, which can be hereditary or secondary to incorrect nail trimming; onychomycosis; or a systemic, metabolic disease, can also result in ingrown toenails.

Pathophysiology of Ingrown Toenails

An ingrown toenail occurs when the nail curves and becomes embedded into the flesh at the corner(s) of a toe, causing pain (Figure 44–6). Puncture of the skin that is accompanied by soft tissue hypertrophy and subsequent invasion by opportunistic resident foot bacteria can cause a superficial infection. Swelling, inflammation, and ulceration are secondary complications that can accompany an ingrown toenail.[23]

Treatment of Ingrown Toenails

Treatment Goals

The goals of self-treating ingrown toenails are (1) to relieve pressure on the toenails, (2) to relieve pain, (3) to prevent recurrence of the disorder, and (4) to prevent infection.

PATIENT EDUCATION FOR Tired, Aching Feet

The objectives of self-treatment are (1) to reduce impact on the feet by providing additional support and shock absorbance and (2) to relieve foot discomfort. For most patients, carefully following product instructions and the self-care measures listed here will help ensure optimal therapeutic outcomes.

- To reduce friction of the feet and impact on weight-bearing parts of the feet, wear well-fitted footwear that has sufficient padding and cushioning (Table 44–1).
- Consider other measures to further decrease impact on the feet, such as decreasing the length of time you stand or exercise, switching to exercises that have less impact on the feet, and, if necessary, losing weight.
- To relieve swelling or discomfort, apply an ice bag or cold wrap to the affected area (Table 44–5).
- For acute pain relief, NSAID medications such as ibuprofen or naproxen may be used.
- To improve circulation, select a compression stocking with mild–moderate compression (<20 mm Hg).
- Choose a full-shoe insert when the entire foot aches. Make sure the insert conforms to the shoe. For example, choose a thin insole for a woman's pump and a thicker insole for a sneaker.
- Use partial insoles to cushion or support a certain portion of the foot, such as the ball of the foot, the arch, or the toes.
- Use a heel cushion for pain confined to the bottom of the heel.
- Use a heel cup when the pain is widespread and diffuse.

When to Seek Medical Attention

- If discomfort or swelling continues after 1 week of implementing appropriate self-care measures, consult a health care provider.

Key: NSAID = Nonsteroidal anti-inflammatory drug.

PATIENT EDUCATION FOR Exercise-Induced Injuries

The objectives of self-treatment are (1) to rest the injured foot or limb to allow healing, (2) to relieve discomfort, and (3) to implement measures to prevent further injury. For most patients, carefully following product instructions and the self-care measures listed here will help ensure optimal therapeutic outcomes.

General Measures

- When a leg or foot injury occurs, rest the injured limb. If desired, perform other types of exercise that do not put a great deal of force on the feet, such as swimming or bicycling (stationary or outdoor).
- Take the following actions to prevent exercise-induced injuries:
  - Stretch muscles before exercising.
  - Choose sport-specific shoes with good arch support for athletic activities.
  - Run or walk on a relatively smooth, level, and resilient surface.
  - Keep the back straight when running.

Shin Splints

- Rest the feet and apply an ice bag or a cold wrap to the painful area (Table 44–5).
- If desired, take aspirin or another NSAID to relieve pain and reduce tissue inflammation.
- Do not use analgesics before a workout to suppress pain or to increase your endurance.

When to Seek Medical Attention

- Seek medical attention if the discomfort becomes a cramping, burning tightness that repeatedly occurs at the same distance or time during a run.

Blisters

- To prevent blisters during running, wear moisture-wicking socks (e.g., wool or acrylic). If desired, wear two pairs of socks with ordinary talcum powder sprinkled between them. Using an acrylic sock next to the foot will assist in drawing moisture from the foot.
- Apply compound tincture of benzoin or a flexible collodion product (e.g., New Skin) to the blister before exercise to decrease pain and accelerate healing by promoting reepithelialization.
- Apply an antiperspirant that contains aluminum chloride 20% to the feet, to decrease incidence of blisters.
- If blisters break, apply a first aid antibiotic to the broken skin to prevent secondary bacterial infection.
- Cover blistered area with moleskin to protect the surface.

Ankle Sprains

- Although maximum swelling will not occur for 48 hours, begin treatment as soon as possible.
- Stay off the injured foot, wrap a compression bandage around the ankle, apply ice, and elevate the ankle. (Tables 44–5 and 44–6 provide guidelines on applying ice and compression bandages, respectively.)

When to Seek Medical Attention

- Seek medical attention if swelling persists more than 72 hours.

Toenail Blisters/Loss

- To prevent blisters under the toenail, keep toenails trimmed and run in properly fitted shoes.
- Should a blister develop, do not disturb or puncture the blister roof.

When to Seek Medical Attention

- If the toenail separates from the skin or is lost, consult a primary care provider or podiatrist for proper treatment.

Key: NSAID = Nonsteroidal anti-inflammatory drug

General Treatment Approach

Patient education is the best means of preventing the development of ingrown toenails. In the early stages of development, therapy is directed at providing adequate room for the nail to resume its normal position adjacent to soft tissue. This therapy is accomplished by relieving the external source of pressure. Warm water soaks for 10–20 minutes several times a day until resolution will help soften the area. Topical antiseptics prescribed by a primary care provider can be applied to prevent possible opportunistic infections. Insertion of small cotton wisps or dental floss under the impinged nail edge is associated with a 79% rate of symptomatic improvement. No evidence is linked to secondary infection from the cotton wisps or dental floss.[27] Medical referral is necessary if the condition is recurrent or gives rise to an oozing discharge, pain, or severe inflammation. Sometimes surgery is warranted; with subsequent systemic antibiotic therapy, the toe may take up to 3–4 weeks to heal. The most common surgical procedure is removal of the lateral edge of the nail followed by chemical matricectomy achieved by phenolization. This process destroys the exposed nail-forming matrix.[23,27] Figure 44–7 outlines self-treatment options for ingrown toenails.[22]

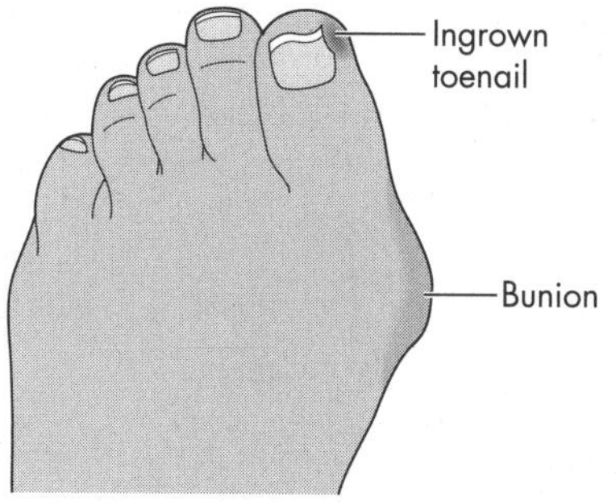

FIGURE 44–6 Bunion and ingrown toenail.

Pharmacologic Therapy

Sodium Sulfide Gel

Sodium sulfide 1% gel is applied topically and a retainer ring is then placed around the affected area to help maintain the product at the site of action. The mechanism of action of sodium sulfide

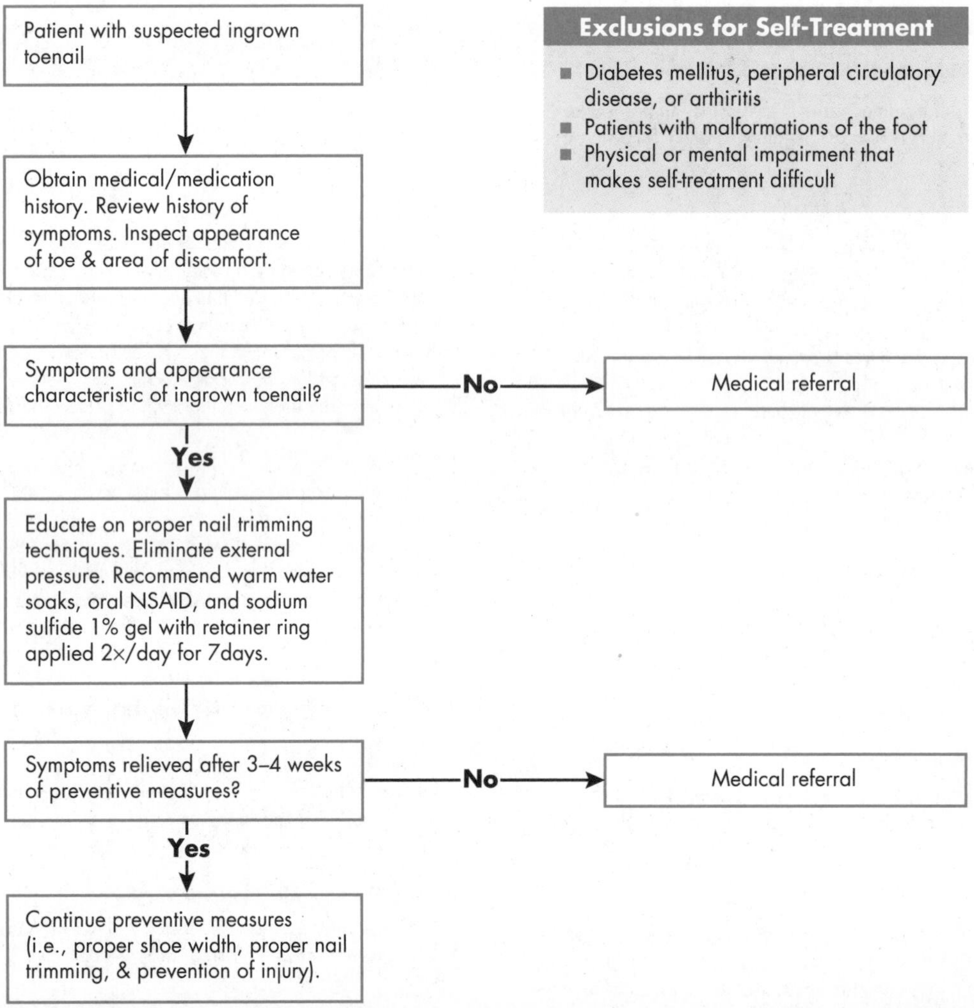
Patient with suspected ingrown toenail
Exclusions for Self-Treatment
■ Diabetes mellitus, peripheral circulatory disease, or arthiritis
■ Patients with malformations of the foot
■ Physical or mental impairment that makes self-treatment difficult
Obtain medical/medication history. Review history of symptoms. Inspect appearance of toe & area of discomfort.
Symptoms and appearance characteristic of ingrown toenail?
No
Medical referral
Yes
Educate on proper nail trimming techniques. Eliminate external pressure. Recommend warm water soaks, oral NSAID, and sodium sulfide 1% gel with retainer ring applied 2×/day for 7days.
Symptoms relieved after 3–4 weeks of preventive measures?
No
Medical referral
Yes
Continue preventive measures (i.e., proper shoe width, proper nail trimming, & prevention of injury).

FIGURE **44-7** Self-care for ingrown toenail. Key: NSAID = Nonsteroidal anti-inflammatory drug.

1% is relief of pain by softening the nail or by hardening the nail bed. It may be applied twice daily for up to 7 days for relief of the discomfort of ingrown toenails.[28,29] HCPs must be aware of misleading trade-name products marketed for ingrown toenails. Products containing benzocaine 20% relieve pain associated with ingrown toenails, but this agent does not treat the underlying problem.[29–31]

Patients with ingrown toenails often fail to realize that oral medications to alleviate pain and inflammation may help their condition. In the absence of any contraindications to their use, oral aspirin, ibuprofen, or naproxen may be recommended; all are proven analgesics with anti-inflammatory activity (see Chapter 5).

Assessment of Ingrown Toenail: A Case-Based Approach

The HCP can play a vital role in recommending measures for relieving acute pain from ingrown toenails and in preventing their recurrence. For relief of ingrown toenail, initial recommendations include warm bath soaks to soften the skin and oral anti-inflammatory therapy for temporary pain relief. If the toenail or nail bed is infected, immediate referral for medical care is warranted.

Case 44–2 illustrates the assessment of a patient with an ingrown toenail.

Patient Counseling for Ingrown Toenails

The box "Patient Education for Ingrown Toenails" lists specific information to include in patient counseling.

Evaluation of Patient Outcomes for Ingrown Toenails

Patient reevaluations should be made after 3–4 weeks to determine whether pressure relief and preventive measures have been successful. Medical referral is appropriate if the condition shows no improvement or worsens or if a discharge from the site of irritation is noted.

CASE 44-2

Relevant Evaluation Criteria	Scenario/Model Outcome
Collect	
1. Gather essential information about the patient's symptoms and medical history, including	
a. Description of symptom(s) (i.e., nature, onset, duration, severity, associated symptoms)	Patient presents with a swollen great toe that she states is causing her extreme pain.
b. Description of any factors that seem to precipitate, exacerbate, and/or relieve the patient's symptom(s)	Wearing dress shoes with a narrow toe box makes the pain unbearable. Relieving pressure from the toes relieves discomfort.
c. Description of the patient's efforts to relieve the symptoms	The patient has tried to dig her embedded toenail out of the skin. It just continues to hurt.
d. Patient's identity	Jennifer Clark
e. Patient's age, gender, height, and weight	21 years old, female, 5 ft 8 in., 138 lb
f. Patient's occupation	Baker
g. Patient's dietary habits	Eats a relatively healthy diet, 2 to 3 meals a day.
h. Patient's sleep habits	Typically sleeps 6 hours per night.
i. Concurrent medical conditions, prescription and nonprescription medications, and dietary supplements	No medical conditions
j. Allergies	NKDA
k. History of other adverse reactions to medications	None
l. Other (describe) ______	Ms. Clark is experiencing a lot of pain.
Assess	
2. Differentiate patient's signs/symptoms, and correctly identify the patient's primary problem(s).	The patient has an ingrown toenail. Upon closer inspection you note that it is oozing a yellow discharge, indicating infection.
3. Identify exclusions for self-treatment (Figure 44–7).	Infection
4. Formulate a comprehensive list of therapeutic alternatives for the primary problem to determine whether triage to a health care provider is required, and share this information with the patient or caregiver.	Options include (1) Recommend OTC products for treating ingrown toenail. (2) Refer patient for medical care of ingrown toenail with secondary infection. (3) Take no action.
Plan	
5. Select an optimal therapeutic alternative to address the patient's problem, taking into account patient preferences.	Ms. Clark should consult an HCP because of the presence of an infection seen on assessment. Appropriate footwear to prevent pressure will assist to prevent pressure. She can also take an anti-inflammatory such as naproxen or ibuprofen to help relieve some discomfort until she is seen.
6. Describe the recommended therapeutic approach to the patient or caregiver.	"You should consult a health care provider about your ingrown toenail. In the interim you can take ibuprofen to help alleviate some of the discomfort. Wear shoes with a large toe box to prevent pressure on your toe."
7. Explain to the patient or caregiver the rationale for selecting the recommended therapeutic approach from the considered therapeutic alternatives.	"This option is best for you since there is an appearance of infection present. You may need antibiotics to treat the infection."

CASE 44-2 *continued*

Relevant Evaluation Criteria	Scenario/Model Outcome
Implement	
8. When recommending self-care with nonprescription medications and/or nondrug therapy, convey accurate information to the patient or caregiver.	"Take ibuprofen 200 mg: 2 tablets by mouth every 6 to 8 hours as needed for pain."
Solicit follow-up questions from the patient or caregiver.	"What can I do to prevent this from happening in the future?"
Answer the patient's or caregiver's questions.	"Ensure that your shoes fit properly to eliminate pressure on toes. Cut your toenails straight across, rather than at an angle."
Follow-up: Monitor and Evaluate	
9. Assess patient outcome.	Contact Ms. Clark in a day or two to ensure she made an appointment and sought medical care.

Key: HCP = Health care provider; NDKA = no known drug allergies; OTC = over-the-counter.

PATIENT EDUCATION FOR Ingrown Toenails

The ultimate goals for self-treatment of ingrown toenails are (1) to relieve the pain and pressure associated with the condition and (2) to prevent recurrence.

- Ensure that shoes fit properly to eliminate pressure on the toenails (Table 44–1).
- Prevent recurrence of ingrown toenails by cutting toenails straight across, rather than at an angle.
- Decrease pain and swelling of the ingrown toenail by taking an NSAID medication such as ibuprofen or naproxen.
- Relieve impingement of the nail by soaking your feet in warm water to soften the nail and the skin around it.
- Place cotton wisps or dental floss under the edge of the ingrown nail for almost immediate pain relief.

Key: NSAID = Nonsteroidal anti-inflammatory drug.

Key Points for Minor Foot Disorders

- The nonprescription drug of choice to treat corns and calluses is salicylic acid in a collodion-like vehicle or plaster form.
- Predisposing factors responsible for corns and calluses must be corrected.
- Patients should also be cautioned that frequent recurrence of any of these foot disorders is an indication to consult a podiatrist or an HCP.
- Patients with diabetes, circulatory problems, and/or arthritis should be counseled to avoid self-medicating with any topical or oral nonprescription drug without first checking with their HCP.
- Nonprescription products are powerful drugs and may exacerbate certain conditions; the HCP must monitor patient progress carefully and be attuned to patient comments that might indicate the occurrence of drug-related problems.
- HCPs should be prepared to educate and assist patients who develop exercise-induced injuries.
- Most exercise-induced injuries can be treated with shoe modifications, in-shoe supports, modified training methods, ice applications, and stretching exercises.
- Counseling on proper foot hygiene is an important aspect of caring for the patient as a whole.

REFERENCES

1. Foot health facts. Available at: https://www.foothealthfacts.org/foot-ankle-conditions/browse-foot-ankle-conditions. Accessed July 20, 2017.
2. Khan M. Podiatric management in epidermolysis bullosa. *Dermatol Clin.* 2010;28(2):325–33. doi:10.1016/j.det.2010.02.006.
3. Singh N, Armstrong DG, Lipsky BA. Preventing foot ulcers in patients with diabetes. *JAMA.* 2005;293(2):217–28. doi:10.1001/jama.293.2.217.
4. Stolt M, Suhonen R, Puukka P, et al. Foot health and self-care activities of older people in home care. *J Clin Nurs.* 2012;21(21–22):3082–95. doi: 10.1111/j.1365-2702.2012.04223.x.
5. Smith RG. Common foot disorders in patients with diabetes. *Drug Top.* 2005;149(9):57–66.
6. Schroeder SM, Blume P. Foot infections. Available at: http://www.emedicine.com/orthoped/topic601.htm. Accessed July 20, 2017.
7. Corns and calluses—baby your feet. *Mayo Clin Health Lett.* 2008;26(4):7. Available at: http://healthletter.mayoclinic.com/health/pdf/88/200804.PDF. Accessed July 20, 2017.
8. Auerbach. *Wilderness Medicine.* 6th ed. Maryland Heights, MO: Mosby; 2011:580–93.
9. Lyman TP, Vlahovac TC. Foot care from A to Z. *Dermatol Nurs.* 2010; 22(5):2–7.
10. Menz HB, Morris ME. Footwear characteristics and foot problems in older people. *Gerontology.* 2005;51(5):346–51. doi: 10.1159/000086373.
11. DeLee D. *Orthopaedic Sports Medicine.* 3rd ed. Philadelphia, PA: Saunders; 2010:chap 25.
12. Mayo Clinic Store: Healthy Living. 2013–2014 Medical Supplies Catalog. Available at: http://www.mayoclinic.org/mcitems/mc1200-mc1299/mc1234-20.pdf. Accessed July 20, 2017.

13. How your feet work—and three steps for keeping them healthy. *Harvard Health Lett.* 2009;34(10):3–5. PMID: 20821859.
14. Salicylic acid topical. Facts and Comparisons eAnswers [subscription database]. Available at: http://online.factsandcomparisons.com. Accessed July 20, 2017.
15. U.S. Food and Drug Administration. Wart remover drug products for over-the-counter human use. Final monograph. *Fed Regist.* 1990;55(358): 33258–62.
16. U.S. Food and Drug Administration. Wart remover drug products for over-the-counter human use. Correction. *Fed Regist.* 1990;55:33246–56.
17. California Podiatric Medical Association. Top 10 foot problems. Available at: https://www.podiatrists.org/visitors/foothealth/other/common. Accessed July 20, 2017.
18. Cushing M. You *Can Cope with Peripheral Neuropathy: 365 Tips for Living A Better Life.* New York, NY: Demos Medical Publishing; 2009:chap 2.
19. Kennedy JG, Knowles B, Dolan M, et al. Foot and ankle injuries in the adolescent runner. *Curr Opin Pediatr.* 2005;17(1):34–42. PMID: 15659961.
20. The New York Times Health. Foot pain in-depth report. Available at: http://www.nytimes.com/health/guides/symptoms/foot-pain/print.html?module=Search&mabReward=relbias%3Ar. Accessed July 20, 2017.
21. McDermott AY, Mernitz H. Exercise and older patients: prescribing guidelines. *Am Fam Physician.* 2006;74:437–44. PMID: 15659961.
22. Cheung RT, Ng G. Influence of different footwear on force of landing during running. *Phys Ther.* 2008;88(5):620–8. doi: 10.2522/ptj.20060323.
23. Meadows M. Taking care of your feet. *FDA Consum.* 2006;40(2):16–24. PMID: 16671196.
24. Bope ET, Kellerman RD. *Conn's Current Therapy.* 1st ed. Philadelphia, PA: Saunders; 2013.
25. Flore R, Gerardino L, Santoliquido A, et al. Reduction of oxidative stress by compression stockings in standing workers. *Occup Med (Oxford).* 2007;57:337–41. doi: 10.1093/occmed/kqm021.
26. Nicola TL. Rehabilitation of running injuries. *Clin Sports Med.* 2012; 31(2):351–72. doi: 10.1016/j.csm.2011.10.002.
27. Heidelbaugh JJ, Lee H. Management of the ingrown toenail. *Am Fam Physician.* 2009;79(4):303–8. PMID: 19235497.
28. U.S. Food and Drug Administration. Ingrown toenail relief drug products for over-the-counter human use. Final rule. *Fed Regist.* 2003;68(88): 24347–9.
29. U.S. Food and Drug Administration. Ingrown toenail relief drug products for over-the-counter human use. Final rule. *Fed Regist.* 1993;58(88): 47602–6.
30. U.S. Food and Drug Administration. Ingrown toenail relief drug products for over-the-counter human use. Tentative final monograph. *Fed Regist.* 1982;47:39120–5.
31. Benzocaine. Lexi-Drugs Online [subscription database]. Hudson, OH: Lexi-Comp, Inc.; 2010. Available at: http://online.lexicomp. Accessed July 20, 2017.

CHAPTER 45

HAIR LOSS

TRICIA M. BERRY

A significant number of men and women experience hair loss, with up to 50% of men and women affected at some point in their life.[1] Hair loss has many potential contributing factors (Table 45–1).[1–9] Regardless of the cause, hair loss can have a significant psychological and social impact. Individuals affected by hair loss often experience low self-esteem; personal, social, and work-related challenges; and psychiatric disorders, such as depression and anxiety.[10] The economic impact is also substantial, with patients spending approximately $3.5 billion each year on products and procedures to treat hair loss.[11]

Hair loss is broadly categorized as nonscarring or scarring alopecia. Forms of nonscarring alopecia include *androgenetic alopecia* (AGA, or pattern hereditary hair loss); *alopecia areata* (rapid onset, patchy hair loss); *anagen effluvium* (rapid shedding of growing hairs); *telogen effluvium* (rapid shedding of resting hairs); cosmetic hair damage; *trichotillomania* (a compulsive pulling out of one's hair); and tinea capitis. Types of hair loss secondary to medication use, acute or chronic illness, or dietary changes typically are also nonscarring. Table 45–2 provides information on common types of nonscarring alopecia.[1,3,7,12] Scarring alopecia may be related to conditions such as discoid lupus erythematosus, syphilis, sarcoidosis, or lichen planus. Severe forms of tinea capitis and chronic hair care practices that significantly damage the hair and scalp may also lead to scarring alopecia.

AGA is the most common form of hair loss and the only type of alopecia for which Food and Drug Administration (FDA)–approved nonprescription medications are available. AGA is characterized by progressive, patterned hair loss from the scalp. Caucasian men are more likely than Asian, American Indian, or African American men to experience baldness.[12] Caucasian men often experience more extensive hair loss than men of the aforementioned ethnicities.[12]

Pathophysiology of Hair Loss

Hair follicle activity is cyclic (Figure 45–1). A variety of triggers can alter the hair follicle cycle, resulting in hair loss. A brief discussion of the proposed pathophysiologic mechanisms for several common types of nonscarring alopecia, with a focus on AGA, follows.

In AGA, the hair follicle undergoes a stepwise miniaturization and change in growth dynamics. With each successive cycle, the anagen phase becomes shorter and the telogen phase becomes longer. Consequently over time, the anagen–telogen ratio decreases from 12:1 to 5:1. Because telogen hairs are more loosely anchored to follicles, their presence in increased numbers eventually manifests as increased shedding. In addition, the catagen phase lengthens, reducing the number of hairs. As telogen hairs are shed, they are gradually replaced by *vellus-like* (short and fine) hairs or by anagen hairs that are too short to reach the surface.

Hair follicles and their sebaceous glands produce enzymes that convert weak androgens to estrogens, testosterone, and dihydrotestosterone (DHT) (Figure 45–2). These enzymes are believed to maintain androgen balance in the follicle, thereby regulating the hair cycle. Although the mechanisms are not completely understood, estrogen is proposed to affect androgen metabolism in the hair follicle and prolong the anagen phase. Testosterone and DHT stimulate production of growth factors and proteases, affect vascularization of the follicle and the composition of basement membrane proteins, and alter the amounts of cofactors required for follicle metabolism.

DHT is believed to be a primary repressor of hair growth. It binds five times more readily than testosterone to androgen receptors. Increased 5-alpha-reductase–mediated conversion of testosterone to DHT in the balding areas of women with AGA also supports the contention that DHT is important in this process. In contrast to men, women with AGA rarely lose all their hair, not only because they have less 5-alpha-reductase but also because they have more aromatase that converts testosterone into estradiol, thereby reducing the level of androgen and increasing the estrogen level.[13] In addition, women are more likely to have follicles with fewer localized androgen receptors and, therefore, are more likely to retain actively growing hair.[14]

Although not fully understood, alopecia areata is thought to have an autoimmune etiology and genetic influences (e.g., HLA-DRB1*0401 and DQB1).[7]

Chemotherapeutic agents (e.g., antimitotic drugs) are identified as a potential cause of anagen effluvium. They cause narrowing of the hair shaft, which may fracture the hair or stop hair growth. Current nonprescription drug therapies are not FDA approved for the treatment of alopecia that is related to anagen effluvium.

Certain triggers (e.g., severe illness, injury, stress, metabolic changes, autoimmune disorders) may precipitate telogen effluvium, which occurs when an increased number of hairs shift from the anagen phase to telogen phase.

Hair care products and hair-grooming methods associated with scarring or burns on the scalp may result in scarring alopecia. *Traction alopecia* is seen primarily in individuals who braid their hair tightly every day. Braiding traumatizes the hair follicles, causing hairs to loosen and break. Patients who use oily moisturizers to

TABLE 45-1 Causes of Hair Loss

General Causes	Specific Examples
Hormonal changes	Hyperandrogenic conditions (e.g., polycystic ovary syndrome)
	Menopause
	Postpartum
	Pregnancy
Physiologic stress	Fever, infections
	Hemorrhage
	Surgery
	Trauma
Chronic illnesses	Autoimmune diseases (e.g., rheumatoid arthritis, lupus)
	Eating disorders (e.g., anorexia, bulimia)
	Endocrine disorders (e.g., hypo/hyperthyroidism, hypopituitarism, diabetes mellitus, growth hormone deficiency, hyperprolactinemia)
	Hepatic or renal failure
	Infections (e.g., HIV, syphilis)
Medications	ACE inhibitors (e.g., enalapril, captopril)
	Allopurinol
	Androgenic action (e.g., oral contraceptives, danazol, testosterone, anabolic steroids)
	Anticonvulsants (e.g., phenytoin, carbamazepine, valproate)
	Anticoagulants (e.g., warfarin, heparin)
	Antidepressants (e.g., SSRIs, tricyclic antidepressants)
	Beta-blockers (e.g., propranolol, metoprolol)
	Cholesterol-lowering drugs (e.g., clofibrate, gemfibrozil)
	Chemotherapeutic agents
Dietary changes or deficiencies	Protein restriction/deficiency
	Rapid weight loss including weight loss associated with bariatric surgery
	Strict vegetarian diet
	Zinc, biotin, or iron deficiencies
Local trauma	Hair care practices
	Tinea capitis
	Trichotillomania (compulsive hair pulling)
Genetics	Chromosome 3q26 and 20p11 in AGA[9]
	HLA genes, such as HLA-DRB1*0401 and DQB1*0301, in alopecia areata[7]
	Polymorphisms in the androgen-receptor gene in AGA[8,9]

Key: ACE = Angiotensin-converting enzyme; AGA = androgenetic alopecia; HIV = human immunodeficiency virus; HLA = human leukocyte antigen; SSRI = selective serotonin reuptake inhibitor.
Source: References 1–9.

make hair more manageable and to stop the scalp from flaking may develop folliculitis and hair loss.

Psychological stress may potentiate several types of hair loss, although the literature on this subject is conflicting. Trichotillomania, a compulsive psychiatric disorder most common in children, involves an individual repetitively pulling or plucking hairs, leading to patchy hair loss.

Untreated or improperly treated tinea capitis may lead to hair loss. This disease must be treated with prescription systemic antifungals; hair regrowth occurs after eradication of the dermatophyte.

Scaly dermatoses (e.g., psoriasis, seborrheic dermatitis) may also lead to scarring alopecia. Nonprescription agents marketed for the treatment of psoriasis and seborrheic dermatitis are not effective in treating alopecia. Chapter 34 provides additional information on self-care for scaly dermatoses.

Clinical Presentation of Hair Loss

The scalp of a patient with AGA shows no signs of inflammation or scarring. Hair loss is gradual; in contrast to other types of alopecia, the number of hairs that come out during brushing or shampooing does not suddenly increase. Typically, male pattern hair loss (MPHL) is insidious in onset and usually does not start until after puberty. Progression fluctuates considerably, with 3–6 months of accelerated loss followed by 6–18 months of no loss. Most men take 15–25 years to lose their hair. The loss begins with a recession of the frontal hairline and continues with thinning at the vertex until only a fringe of hair at the occipital and temporal margins remains. The pattern and extent of MPHL are often characterized using the Norwood Scale; images are viewable at the referenced website.[15]

In women with alopecia, hair loss is typically more diffuse. Female pattern hair loss (FPHL) manifests as gradual hair thinning over the crown and mid-frontal portion of the scalp. Several scales (e.g., Ludwig, Sinclair, Savin) have been used to classify the extent of FPHL.[4,16] The Ludwig and Savin scales use similar images for degrees of hair loss; these images can be viewed at the referenced website.[16] In contrast, the Sinclair Scale uses 5 ratings for severity of hair loss.[4] These scales are helpful in visualizing the typical progression of hair loss in MPHL and FPHL, and in assessing the patient's pattern of hair loss as MPHL or FPHL and whether self-care is appropriate.

FPHL is often classified as AGA; genetic components along with hormonal factors contribute to the hair loss.[3,8,17] Women with AGA may present with symptoms of *hyperandrogenism* (an excess of androgen), such as significant acne; *hirsutism* (hairiness in other parts of the body); menstrual irregularities; and infertility. It is conceivable that a patient with FPHL may be using a hair regrowth treatment agent on the scalp while using an antihirsute agent (e.g., topical eflornithine, oral spironolactone [off label]) to remove excess hair on the face. Androgen excess may indicate serious metabolic disturbances, such as cardiovascular disease, diabetes mellitus, polycystic ovarian syndrome, and endometrial cancer.[17] Women with multiple symptoms should be referred for medical evaluation and treatment.[1,8,17]

Alopecia areata has three stages: sudden loss of hair in patches, enlargement of the patches, and regrowth. The cycle may take months or sometimes years and can occur in any hair-bearing area. Up to 5% of patients lose all their scalp hair (*alopecia totalis*), and 1% of patients lose all their body and scalp hair, including eyebrows and eyelashes (*alopecia universalis*).[3] Hair loss may accompany or be preceded by nail pitting or other nail

TABLE 45-2 **Characteristics of Common Types of Nonscarring Alopecia**

Type of Hair Loss	Etiology	Epidemiology	Clinical Presentation
Androgenetic alopecia/ pattern hereditary hair loss	Hormonal, hereditary	Female: 40%–50% by age 70 years[1,3] Male: 80% by age 70 years[12] Affects white men more often than men of other ethnicities[12]	Gradual onset with progression of patterned hair loss Female: Central portion of scalp, sparing frontal hairline; wide midline part on the crown with progression to diffuse thinning over crown Male: Top rear of the head (vertex), frontal hairline, and occipital regions
Alopecia areata	Autoimmune	2% of U.S. population; affects men and women of all races equally; most cases (70%) occur in children and young adults[1,7]	Abrupt onset (may wax and wane with relapses); usually patchy but can be generalized; can occur in any hair-bearing area; can progress to complete loss of scalp hair (alopecia totalis) or total loss of body hair (alopecia universalis)[1,3]
Anagen effluvium	Chemotherapy, radiation, heavy metal poisoning	Data not available	Abrupt loss of 80%–90% of body hair[1]
Telogen effluvium	Metabolic or hormonal disturbances, stress; severe illness or injury; medications[1]	Exact prevalence unknown; can occur in either gender at any age, but not common in childhood[3]	Generalized, abrupt onset (often with trigger factor); rapid hair thinning without bare patches
Cosmetic hair damage[a]	Hair care practices (e.g., braiding, permanents, bleaching)	Any age; associated with specific social, cultural, and cosmetic practices[1]	Gradual or abrupt loss on any area of the scalp depending on cause; broken hairs with blunt rather than tapered tips
Trichotillomania	Psychiatric compulsive disorder	More common in children but may persist into adulthood[1]	Twisted and broken-off hairs are visible in patchy areas across the scalp[1]
Tinea capitis[a]	*Trichophyton tonsurans*	Any age; common in childhood[1]	Any area of the scalp; usually round patch(es) of hair loss

[a] In rare circumstances, chronic and/or severe cases can lead to scarring alopecia.

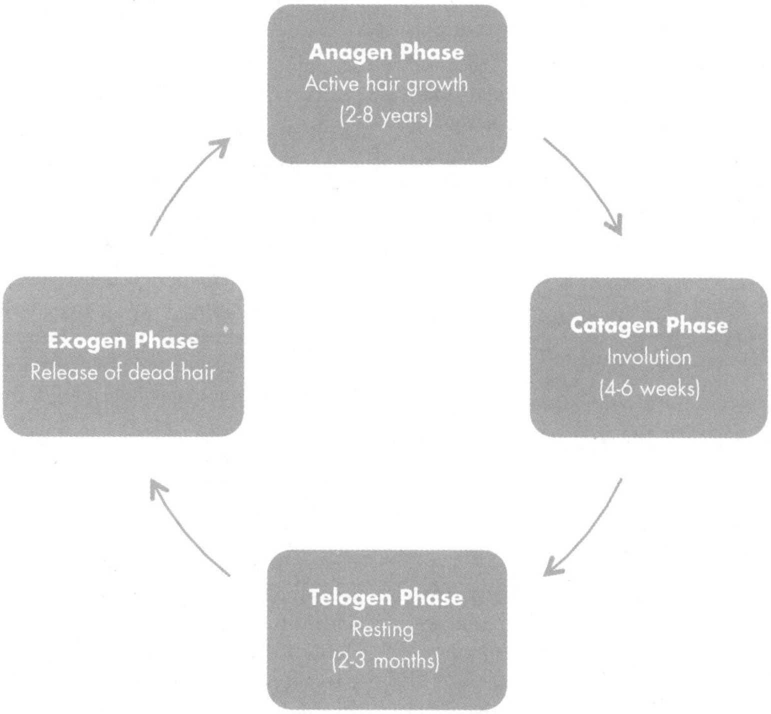

FIGURE 45-1 Normal hair follicle cycle.

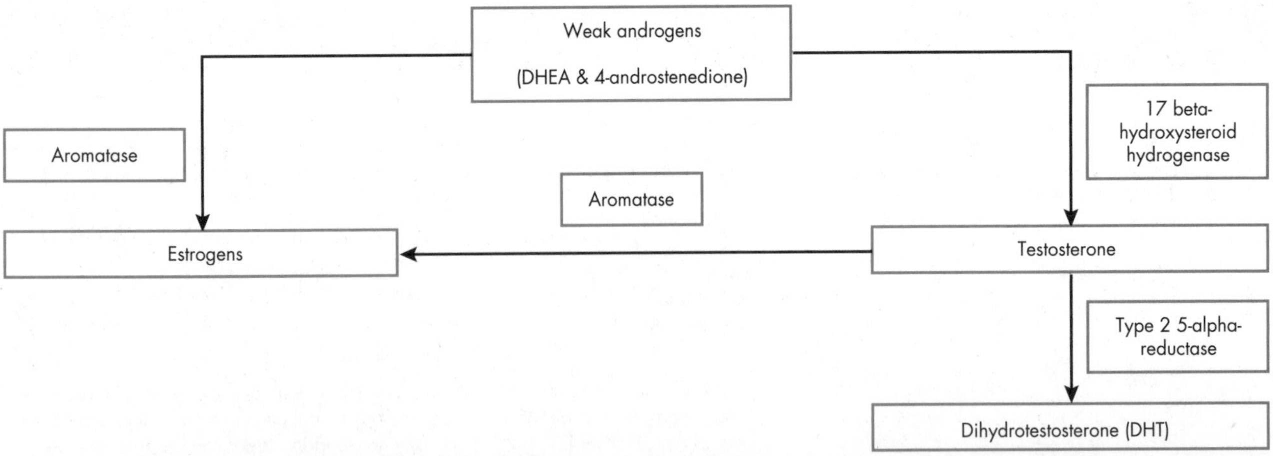

FIGURE 45–2 Androgen metabolism within the hair follicle. Key: DHEA = Dehydroepiandrosterone.

abnormalities. Itching, tingling, burning, or other painful sensations may also be experienced in the patch of hair loss.

Telogen effluvium (also known as diffuse alopecia) can be acute (lasting <6 months) or chronic (lasting >6 months). The precipitating factor usually precedes shedding by 1–6 months, but identifying a specific causal event is often difficult, if not impossible. This point is especially important to note with medication use, because hair loss will often occur one to several months after the patient has begun a particular drug therapy. Health care providers should assess the start date of all medications as a part of the clinical workup of patients with telogen effluvium. This type of hair loss is usually reversible.[1]

Hair loss may be assessed by using a variety of tests (e.g., biopsy of the scalp, daily hair loss count, hair-pull test).[2,18] A *hair-pull test* is done by holding 40–60 hairs between the thumb and forefinger and firmly (but not forcefully) pulling the hairs away from the scalp. A positive test, noted when more than 10% of the hairs are removed, suggests types of alopecia other than AGA (e.g., effluvium, alopecia areata).[2,3] All patients presenting with hair loss that is not considered androgenetic should be referred to a primary care provider (PCP) for complete medical evaluation.

Treatment of Hair Loss

Treatment Goals

The goal in self-treating hair loss is to achieve an appearance the patient considers acceptable.

General Treatment Approach

Treatment goals for hair loss can be accomplished through the following nonprescription measures: (1) nonpharmacologic therapy such as cosmetic camouflage and/or (2) the use of topical minoxidil to stimulate hair growth, if applicable. With the exception of AGA, all other types of hair loss should be referred to a PCP to determine the cause and proper treatment. The algorithm in Figure 45–3 outlines the self-treatment of hair loss and lists specific exclusions for self-treatment.

Nonpharmacologic Therapy

Hair loss that is dramatic and extensive can be emotionally distressing. Camouflaging thinning hair with wigs and hair weaves may help relieve the distress of hair loss. Technological advances have made production of custom wigs that match the wearer's original hair a standard practice. Approaches to treating less severe hair loss include hair sprays, gels, colorants, permanents, and scalp camouflaging products (e.g., topical hair fibers, powder cakes, scalp lotions, scalp sprays, hair crayons); these products can create an illusion of fullness without decreasing hair loss.[19]

Scalp massage, frequent shampooing, and electrical stimulation have been proposed as treatments for hair loss; however, these remedies are considered ineffective.[20] Although its efficacy remains unknown, low-level light therapy is a safe therapy marketed for hair growth.[21]

Both acute and chronic telogen effluvium should be referred to a PCP for further evaluation. Acute telogen effluvium usually resolves spontaneously, and treatment is limited to comforting and reassuring the patient. Chronic telogen effluvium is slower to resolve, but the patient will still need comfort and reassurance. If a patient's hair loss is caused by poor diet or iron deficiency, the patient may benefit from consulting a dietitian. In deficiency states, increasing protein intake or taking iron supplements may be simple solutions to reversing hair loss.

Surgical transplantation of terminal hair follicles from another anatomic site is an alternative nonpharmacologic approach to hair loss. This method may be useful in frontal and vertex hair loss.

Pharmacologic Therapy

Minoxidil

Minoxidil, the only FDA-approved self-treatment option for AGA, is available as a 2% and 5% hydroalcoholic solution and a 5% solvent-free foam. Minoxidil can be applied by various methods (Table 45–3), depending on the applicator (spray, dropper, rub-on assembly).[22] This treatment is indicated for AGA of the scalp.[22] Specifically, nonprescription topical minoxidil is labeled for baldness at the crown of the head in men and for hair thinning in the frontoparietal area in women. The 2% and 5% solutions and 5% foam are approved for use in men, whereas only the 2%

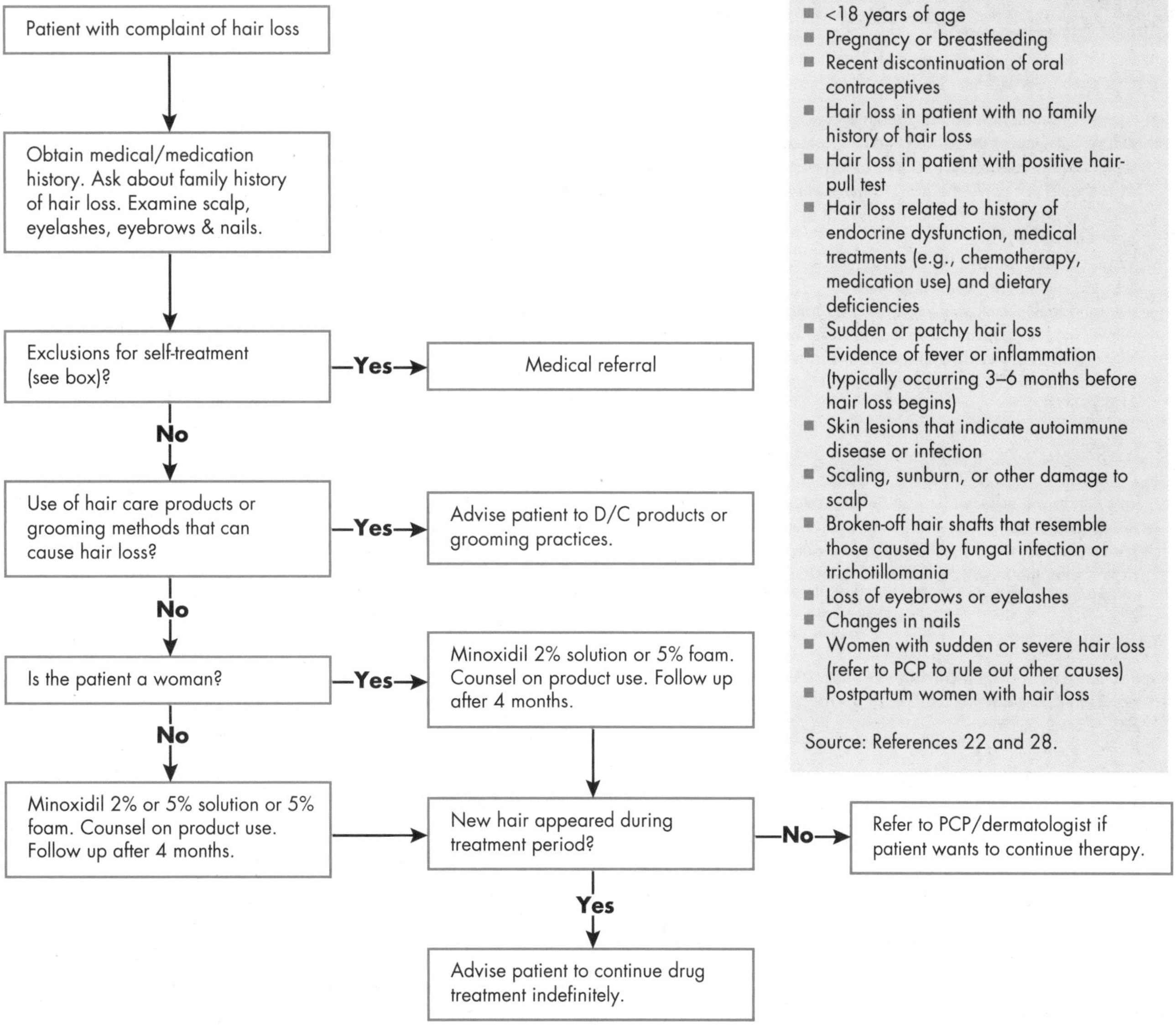

Exclusions for Self-Treatment

- <18 years of age
- Pregnancy or breastfeeding
- Recent discontinuation of oral contraceptives
- Hair loss in patient with no family history of hair loss
- Hair loss in patient with positive hair-pull test
- Hair loss related to history of endocrine dysfunction, medical treatments (e.g., chemotherapy, medication use) and dietary deficiencies
- Sudden or patchy hair loss
- Evidence of fever or inflammation (typically occurring 3–6 months before hair loss begins)
- Skin lesions that indicate autoimmune disease or infection
- Scaling, sunburn, or other damage to scalp
- Broken-off hair shafts that resemble those caused by fungal infection or trichotillomania
- Loss of eyebrows or eyelashes
- Changes in nails
- Women with sudden or severe hair loss (refer to PCP to rule out other causes)
- Postpartum women with hair loss

Source: References 22 and 28.

FIGURE **45–3** Self-care for hair loss. Key: D/C = Discontinue; PCP = primary care provider.

solution and 5% foam products are approved for use in women.[22] When used orally to control hypertension, minoxidil is a potassium channel opener and vasodilator. When used topically for hair loss, the drug appears to increase cutaneous blood flow, promote and maintain vascularization of hair follicles, directly stimulate follicular hypertrophy, and prolong the anagen phase. Minoxidil may also transform resting (*telogen phase*) hair follicles into active (*anagen phase*) hair follicles, resulting in a lower percentage of hairs in the telogen phase, which are shed more easily.[23–25] It is also proposed that minoxidil enhances hair growth by stimulating prostaglandin endoperoxide synthase-1, leading to increased production of prostaglandin E2.[25,26]

For men undergoing hair transplantation whose hair follicles may be viable but not functioning optimally in the area to be transplanted, topical minoxidil can increase hair density, speed regrowth in transplanted follicles, and complement the surgical outcome by minimizing the likelihood of progression of hair loss.[27]

After initiation of minoxidil treatment, an increase in hair loss may occur within the first few weeks of product usage.[28] Several months may elapse before hair growth is apparent. If increased hair density fails to appear after 4–6 months of using minoxidil, the patient should consider ending treatment and discussing other options with his or her PCP.[22,28] For many patients, increased hair density is minimal and treatment response is difficult to assess. Once the drug is discontinued, hair density returns to pretreatment levels in a matter of months; therefore, the patient must continue to use the product indefinitely to maintain new growth.[22]

Several studies have evaluated the effectiveness and safety of topical minoxidil 2% and 5% preparations. In a 48-week study, men using 5% minoxidil had an earlier response and greater hair regrowth (45% more hair regrowth) than did men using 2% minoxidil.[29] Increased frequency in itching and local irritation was also noted in the 5% minoxidil treatment group compared with the 2% minoxidil group.[29] A randomized, double-blind, placebo-controlled

TABLE 45-3 Administration Guidelines for Nonprescription Minoxidil

Minoxidil Solution

- Apply minoxidil to clean, dry scalp and hair.
- Rub about 1 mL of the product into the affected area of the scalp. Some products have a measuring cap with a 1 mL fill line. Men should not apply the product more often than twice daily (morning and night). Women should not apply the product more often than once daily.
- Wash and dry hands after applying the medication. If it gets into the eyes, mouth, or nose, rinse these areas thoroughly.
- Do not double the dose if you miss an application.
- Allow 2–4 hours for the drug to penetrate the scalp. Do not participate in any activity that might wash away or dilute the drug (e.g., bathing or swimming without a cap) for 2–4 hours after application.
- At night, apply the drug 2–4 hours before bedtime; if minoxidil is not fully dry, it can stain clothing and bed linen.
- Do not dry the scalp with a hair dryer after applying the drug. This action will reduce the drug's effectiveness.
- If applicable, apply hair grooming and styling products (e.g., sprays, mousses, gels), coloring agents, permanents, or relaxing agents after the minoxidil has dried. These products usually do not affect the efficacy of topical minoxidil.

Minoxidil Foam

- The foam may melt on contact with warm skin. Therefore, wash hands in cold water before applying. Dry hands thoroughly before applying foam.
- Within the thinning hair area, part the hair into one or more rows to maximize contact of the foam with the scalp. The hair should be completely dry before application.
- Holding the can upside down, apply one-half capful of the foam to the fingertips. The 5% product for men should be applied twice daily, in the morning and at night. The 5% product for women should be applied once daily.
- Using the fingertips, spread the foam over the thinning scalp area, and then massage gently into the scalp. Wash hands thoroughly after application.
- Allow the product to dry completely before lying down or applying grooming, styling, or coloring products.

Source: References 22 and 28.

trial compared the efficacy and safety of 5% topical minoxidil with 2% topical minoxidil and placebo in the treatment of FPHL.[30] Both 5% and 2% minoxidil were superior to placebo, and the 5% topical minoxidil group showed statistically significant benefits over the 2% topical minoxidil group.[30] The incidence of itching, local irritation, and *hypertrichosis* (excessive hair growth) in the group receiving 5% minoxidil was greater than that of the 2% minoxidil and placebo groups; however, both concentrations were considered well tolerated with no evidence of systemic side effects.[30] In a randomized, single-blind trial studying 113 women with androgenetic alopecia, once-daily 5% minoxidil foam was found to be as effective as twice-daily 2% minoxidil solution; the 5% concentration was also associated with several aesthetic and practical advantages (e.g., once-daily administration; lower rates of side effects, such as itching and dandruff; less interference with hair styling).[31]

Some patients who require prescription treatment with finasteride may still use topical minoxidil as an adjunct therapy. Topical minoxidil solution 2% has been investigated in combination with oral finasteride 1 mg in male patients. The outcomes of this study indicate a higher percentage of responders with the combination treatment than with either agent alone. It is inferred that efficacy may be enhanced by the two-drug regimen, which acts on multiple AGA etiologies.[32]

The most common side effect associated with minoxidil—local itching, irritation, and dryness or scaling at the site of application—may be related to the hydroalcoholic/propylene glycol vehicle. The 5% minoxidil topical formulation in a propylene glycol-free foam vehicle reduces the risk of local side effects.

Transient hypertrichosis, usually on the forehead and cheeks, is a possible side effect with long-term use. Occasionally, patients may notice hypertrichosis on the chest, back, forearms, and ear rims, which could indicate that the product has been applied excessively.[33] Rare side effects include acne at the site of application, increased hair loss, inflammation (soreness) of the hair roots, reddened skin, swelling of the face, and allergic contact dermatitis.[22,28]

Minoxidil is absorbed through the skin in relatively low concentrations; documented systemic side effects are rare. In the unlikely event of an accidental ingestion, the patient should seek emergency medical attention. Symptoms may include the following[28]:

- Low blood pressure (dizziness, confusion, fainting, lightheadedness)
- Blurred vision or other changes in vision
- Headache or chest pain
- Irregular heart rate
- Swollen hands or feet
- Flushing of the skin
- Numbness or tingling of the face, hands, or feet

Although minoxidil-induced hemodynamic changes have not been detected in most controlled clinical studies, patients with cardiovascular disorders may have an increased risk of cardiotoxicity.[34]

Researchers have found little evidence of a potential effect of minoxidil on systemic endocrine functions.[35] Their measurement of plasma testosterone and excretion of urinary hydroxysteroids and ketosteroids in hypertensive patients who had been treated with oral minoxidil did not reveal any effects. In a study of topical minoxidil, serum cortisol, testosterone, and thyroid indexes were unchanged, but modification of follicular testosterone metabolism did occur.[36]

The use of topical minoxidil is not associated with any known drug–drug interactions. Topical application of corticosteroids, petrolatum, or retinoids (e.g., adapalene, tretinoin) to the scalp in combination with minoxidil should be avoided because of possible increased absorption of minoxidil and increased risk of side effects. In addition, minoxidil should not be used for 24 hours before or after application of a hair permanent, hair color, or hair relaxant.[22,28]

Patients who are allergic to minoxidil or to any component of the preparation should avoid this medication. Patients with scalp damage from psoriasis, severe sunburn, or abrasions should also avoid topical minoxidil; these conditions may increase minoxidil absorption.

The solution formulation has an alcohol base and will burn or irritate eyes, mucous membranes, and abraded skin. If the product gets into the eyes, mouth, or nose, the patient should thoroughly rinse these areas. Patients should wash and dry their hands after using the product. These precautions are also intended to prevent the systemic entry of minoxidil by alternative routes. Products containing minoxidil should not be used on any other part of the body.[28]

Product Selection Guidelines

Safety and efficacy of the product in children younger than 18 years have not been established, so the use of minoxidil in this population is contraindicated.[22]

The limited human and animal data available for topical minoxidil suggest moderate fetal risk.[37] (See the Preface for a detailed explanation of the pregnancy data.) Pregnant women should be advised to consult their PCP before using minoxidil. Minoxidil is excreted in breast milk. Even though the American Academy of Pediatrics considers minoxidil compatible with breastfeeding, patients should consult their PCP rather than initiate self-treatment with topical minoxidil.[37]

Either the 2% solution or 5% foam formulations can be recommended for use by women; however, men are usually advised to use the 5% concentration. One study demonstrated a lower incidence of contact dermatitis with propylene glycol–free foam products than with topical solutions.[3,21] Accordingly, the foam formulation *may* be more desirable in patients with a history of sensitive skin or dermatitis. Patient preference for method of application is a critical factor in product selection. Patients with impaired vision or physical dexterity may find the rub-on method of application preferable to using sprays or droppers. Table 45–4 lists examples of commercially available products.

Complementary Therapies

In the past, FDA advisory panels have proposed removing from the market a number of ingredients that were known to be safe for external use but lacked scientific data to support their purported efficacy in preventing hair loss or promoting hair growth.[38] The false claims generally are no longer made, but many of these ingredients are still available today in nonprescription lotions and shampoos. In addition, oral and topical dietary supplements marketed to improve the structure and function of hair growth have become more popular. Despite the lack of sufficient evidence to document effectiveness, shampoos, topical solutions, and dietary supplements for hair loss include ingredients such as amino acids, aminobenzoic acid, B vitamins, jojoba oil, lanolin, maidenhair fern (*Adiantum capillis-verneris*), polysorbates 20 and 660, royal jelly (white secretion of *Apis melliferis* worker bees), tetracaine hydrochloride, urea, and wheat germ oil.[20,38,39] Saw palmetto administered orally demonstrated increased hair growth in 6 of 10 men with AGA in one randomized, double-blind, placebo-controlled study.[40]

TABLE 45–4 Selected Nonprescription Hair Regrowth Products

Trade Name	Primary Ingredient
Hair Regrowth Treatment Men Topical Solution	Minoxidil 5%
Minoxidil for Men 2% Topical Solution	Minoxidil 2%
Minoxidil for Men 5% Topical Solution	Minoxidil 5%
Rogaine Extra Strength for Men Topical Solution	Minoxidil 5%
Rogaine Men's Extra Strength Topical Foam	Minoxidil 5%
Rogaine Men's Topical Foam	Minoxidil 5%
Rogaine Women's Topical Foam	Minoxidil 5%
Rogaine Topical Solution	Minoxidil 2%

Source: Reference 22.

Assessment of Hair Loss: A Case-Based Approach

Before recommending a treatment for hair loss, the health care provider should first identify any possible underlying medical cause. To assess alopecia areata or telogen effluvium, the provider can direct the patient to perform a gentle hair-pull test. The patient should be referred to a dermatologist if a hair-pull test is positive. However, the test may be falsely negative if the patient's hair has been recently combed, brushed, or shampooed.[6] If pathology-induced hair loss and active hair loss are ruled out, the provider should determine whether the balding fits the criteria for AGA.

Cases 45–1 and 45–2 illustrate the assessment of patients with hair loss.

Patient Counseling for Hair Loss

Patients who want to use nonprescription minoxidil should be advised that most treatment regimens for hair loss do not alter its progression and that the longer the hair thinning or loss has continued, the less likely it is that the agent will elicit a regrowth response. If the patient still wants to use minoxidil, the provider should review product instructions with the patient, making sure that the patient understands the possible adverse effects and the signs and symptoms that indicate the need for medical attention. In addition, the patient should be counseled that if hair regrowth is achieved, indefinite use of minoxidil will be necessary to maintain the regrowth. If the patient is concerned about long-term use of minoxidil or a desired endpoint is not achieved with minoxidil, cosmetic products, camouflaging options, and hair transplants/surgical interventions may be acceptable alternatives. The box "Patient Education for Hair Loss" lists specific information to provide patients.

Evaluation of Patient Outcomes for Hair Loss

Patients should use minoxidil for the minimum recommended period. If new hair growth does not occur after using minoxidil 2% or 5% for 4–6 months, the patient should consider ending treatment and consulting his or her PCP.[22,28] If new hair does appear within the recommended period, the patient should be advised to continue the drug treatment indefinitely.

Key Points for Hair Loss

- Minoxidil is not effective for everyone.
- Positive treatment results may take several weeks to be noticed. Additional hair loss may occur during the first few weeks of therapy.
- Adherence is critically important for pharmacologic treatment. Hair loss will recur if therapy is stopped.

CASE 45-1

Relevant Evaluation Criteria	Scenario/Model Outcome
Collect	
1. Gather essential information about the patient's symptoms and medical history, including	
a. Description of symptom(s) (i.e., nature, onset, duration, severity, associated symptoms)	Patient has had gradual hair loss with thinning in the crown and a "widening part" on top of her head but no signs of inflammation or scarring on scalp.
b. Description of any factors that seem to precipitate, exacerbate, and/or relieve the patient's symptom(s)	None
c. Description of the patient's efforts to relieve the symptoms	Has tried OTC "vitamins" and switched shampoos.
d. Patient's identity	Lisa Loomis
e. Patient's age, gender, height, and weight	62 years old, female, 5 ft 4 in., 190 lb
f. Patient's occupation	Restaurant manager
g. Patient's dietary habits	Has toast or oatmeal for breakfast; often eats at the restaurant (at least one meal a day).
h. Patient's sleep habits	Sleeps ~7–8 hours nightly.
i. Concurrent medical conditions, prescription and nonprescription medications, and dietary supplements	GERD: omeprazole 20 mg daily; osteoarthritis: piroxicam 20 mg daily; hypertension: hydrochlorothiazide 25 mg daily
j. Allergies	None
k. History of other adverse reactions to medications	ACE inhibitor (angioedema)
l. Other (describe) _______	She remembers that her grandmother had thinning hair. She prefers to use a topical treatment, because she does not want to add any new medications.
Assess	
2. Differentiate patient's signs/symptoms, and correctly identify the patient's primary problem(s) (Table 45–2).	The patient has androgenetic alopecia, as evidenced by gradual hair loss at crown and mid-frontal areas. She has no signs of inflammation or scarring on scalp. Eyebrows and eyelashes are normal.
3. Identify exclusions for self-treatment (Figure 45–3).	None
4. Formulate a comprehensive list of therapeutic alternatives for the primary problem to determine whether triage to a medical provider is required, and share this information with the patient or caregiver.	Options include (1) Recommend self-care using OTC minoxidil topical treatment and/or camouflage measures. (2) Refer Lisa to her PCP for treatment. (3) Recommend self-care until a PCP can be consulted. (4) Take no action.
Plan	
5. Select an optimal therapeutic alternative to address the patient's problem, taking into account patient preferences.	Only topical minoxidil 2% solution or 5% foam are approved for use in women. Lisa can use either formulation along with nondrug measures to treat the alopecia. The foam formulation may be preferred: it may cause less irritation.
6. Describe the recommended therapeutic approach to the patient or caregiver.	"Apply approximately ½ capful of 5% topical foam once daily to a clean, dry scalp."
7. Explain to the patient or caregiver the rationale for selecting the recommended therapeutic approach from the considered therapeutic alternatives.	"Minoxidil 2% solution and 5% foam are available and FDA-approved for use in females with androgenetic alopecia. The foam formulation may cause less irritation."
Implement	
8. When recommending self-care with nonprescription medications and/or nondrug therapy, convey accurate information to the patient or caregiver.	See the box "Patient Education for Hair Loss" for specific nondrug measures.
a. Appropriate dose and frequency of administration	"Apply approximately ½ capful of 5% topical foam once daily to a clean, dry scalp."

CASE 45-1 *continued*

Relevant Evaluation Criteria	Scenario/Model Outcome
b. Maximum number of days the therapy should be employed	"If no new hair growth is noted within 4–6 months, discuss continued use of the product with your primary care provider."
c. Product administration procedures	See Table 45–3.
d. Expected time to onset of relief	"It may take 4–6 months to experience increased hair growth."
e. Degree of relief that can be reasonably expected	"Progressive hair loss will be slowed."
f. Most common adverse effects	"Local itching, irritation, and dryness or scaling at the site of application may occur."
g. Adverse effects that warrant medical intervention should they occur	"Contact your primary care provider if you experience increased hair growth in areas beyond the scalp, acne, reddened skin/scalp, or swelling of the face."
h. Patient options in the event that condition worsens or persists	"If increased hair growth is not experienced within 4–6 months, contact your primary care provider. Also contact your primary care provider, if side effects are noted."
i. Product storage requirements	"Store product in a cool, dry place out of children's reach."
j. Specific nondrug measures	"Minimize exposure to factors that may trigger hair loss (e.g., certain medications, stress, illness, injury)."
Solicit follow-up questions from the patient or caregiver.	"How can I tell if I am responding to the treatment?"
Answer the patient's or caregiver's questions.	"Hair density will increase if the treated area involves early thinning. Look for fine, short hairs as a first response. Additional hair loss may occur during the first few weeks of therapy."
Follow-up: Monitor and Evaluate	
9. Assess patient outcome.	Ask the patient to call you right away with significant concerns of side effects (skin irritation, redness). Ask the patient to monitor and report any hair regrowth in 1–4 months.

Key: ACE = Angiotensin converting enzyme; FDA = Food and Drug Administration; GERD = gastroesophageal reflux disease; OTC = over-the-counter; PCP = primary care provider.

CASE 45-2

Relevant Evaluation Criteria	Scenario/Model Outcome
Collect	
1. Gather essential information about the patient's symptoms and medical history, including	
a. Description of symptom(s) (i.e., nature, onset, duration, severity, associated symptoms)	Patient has noticed a sudden increase in hair loss. He sees a large amount of hair in the shower, in the bathroom sink and on his pillow. The hair loss has resulted in noticeable patchy hair loss over the past week. No signs of inflammation or scarring of scalp are present. Hair-pull test is positive.
b. Description of any factors that seem to precipitate, exacerbate, and/or relieve the patient's symptom(s)	None
c. Description of the patient's efforts to relieve the symptoms	Patient has not tried anything for the hair loss.
d. Patient's identity	George Tuhl
e. Patient's age, gender, height, and weight	19 years old, male, 5 ft 7 in., 165 lb
f. Patient's occupation	Freshman in college, electrical engineering major
g. Patient's dietary habits	Eats in the college residence hall cafeteria 3 meals per day. Has had a lot of past education about diabetes diet and follows it for the most part. Late night snacks are his weakness.

CASE 45-2 *continued*

Relevant Evaluation Criteria	Scenario/Model Outcome
h. Patient's sleep habits	Sleeps ~6 hours a night.
i. Concurrent medical conditions, prescription and nonprescription medications, and dietary supplements	Type 1 diabetes treated with regular insulin pump and glucose tablets as needed for hypoglycemia; daily multivitamin.
j. Allergies	None
k. History of other adverse reactions to medications	None
l. Other (describe) ______	"I think I had a problem like this when I was in elementary school. It seemed to eventually go away. I have had type 1 diabetes since I was 6. I have learned to manage it pretty well; my A1c is 6%."
Assess	
2. Differentiate patient's signs/symptoms, and correctly identify the patient's primary problem(s) (Table 45–2).	The patient likely has alopecia areata, as evidenced by rapid, patchy hair loss and a positive hair-pull test. He has no signs of inflammation or scarring on the scalp. Alopecia areata is often associated with autoimmune disorders; this patient has type 1 diabetes.
3. Identify exclusions for self-treatment (Figure 45–3).	Hair loss with positive hair-pull test
4. Formulate a comprehensive list of therapeutic alternatives for the primary problem to determine whether triage to a medical provider is required, and share this information with the patient or caregiver.	Options include (1) Refer George to his PCP for evaluation and treatment. (2) Recommend self-care until he can see his PCP. (3) Take no action.
Plan	
5. Select an optimal therapeutic alternative to address the patient's problem, taking into account patient preferences.	Refer George to his PCP for evaluation and treatment.
6. Describe the recommended therapeutic approach to the patient or caregiver.	"You should consult a primary care provider for evaluation and treatment."
7. Explain to the patient or caregiver the rationale for selecting the recommended therapeutic approach from the considered therapeutic alternatives.	"The hair loss may spontaneously stop with a return of hair growth. Nonprescription therapy available for hair loss is not recommended for this type of hair loss. It is best to see your primary care provider for evaluation and subsequent treatment."
Implement	
8. When recommending self-care with nonprescription medications and/or nondrug therapy, convey accurate information to the patient or caregiver.	See the box "Patient Education for Hair Loss" for specific nondrug measures.
Solicit follow-up questions from the patient or caregiver.	"Will this happen again? Is it possible it will continue to get worse?"
Answer the patient's or caregiver's questions.	"It is possible that you will experience hair loss again. In some patients with this type of hair loss, it does recur periodically. Sometimes you will have only small patches of hair loss, but it is possible that it may progress to complete loss of hair on the scalp or the whole body. It is important to see your primary care provider to be evaluated and to determine appropriate treatment."
Follow-up: Monitor and Evaluate	
9. Assess patient outcome.	Ask the patient to report to you the outcome of the PCP evaluation and recommendations.

Key: PCP = primary care provider.

PATIENT EDUCATION FOR Hair Loss

The goal in self-treating hair loss is to achieve an appearance the patient considers acceptable. This objective can be accomplished through nonprescription means by recommending (1) cosmetic camouflage and/or (2) the use of topical minoxidil to stimulate hair growth, when appropriate. To ensure optimal therapeutic outcomes, it is essential that patients carefully follow product packaging information and consider the following measures.

Nondrug Measures

- If desired, use wigs to cover severe hair loss until hair is regrown.
- For less severe hair loss, use hair sprays, gels, colorants, permanents, or hair-building products in moderation to create the illusion of full hair. These cosmetics will not affect the rate of hair loss.
- Avoid the use of oily hair products that can cause folliculitis.
- Avoid hairstyles that pull on the hair, such as tight braids.
- Avoid heat from hair dryers and curling/flat irons, because their use can make the hair more brittle.

Nonprescription Medications

- During the first few weeks of minoxidil use, continued hair loss may occur. Note that use of minoxidil must be continuous and indefinite to maintain regrowth. It may take up to 4–6 months to see any results. If treatment is interrupted, regrowth will typically be lost within 4 months or less, and progression of hair loss will begin again.
- Minoxidil is not recommended in patients who are pregnant, breastfeeding, or planning to become pregnant while using this product. Consult a primary care provider before you use this product.
- See Table 45–3 for instructions on how to use this product.
- Do not apply the product more often than directed. More frequent applications will not achieve better regrowth or a faster response but may increase side effects.
- Do not apply the product to damaged or inflamed areas of the scalp, including areas with active scalp psoriasis or eczema lesions and open scalp wounds of any kind.
- Note that local itching or irritation at the site of application may occur. More rarely, allergic contact dermatitis or transient hypertrichosis (unwanted facial hair growth) may occur.
- Keep product container in a cool, dry place, but do not put it in the refrigerator.
- Keep the product out of children's reach. Ingestion of minoxidil is potentially hazardous, and a poison control center should be contacted immediately.
- The solution is flammable. Keep away from fire or flame.
- Do not use on infants or children ages 18 years or younger.
- Do not use if you have heart disease except under the supervision of a primary care provider.
- If hair fails to appear within the time specified on the product (generally 4–6 months) despite consistent use of the product, consider stopping the treatment and seeing your primary care provider for further evaluation.

Source: References 22 and 28.

- Offering cosmetic solutions may also be helpful.
- Patients, particularly women, are seeking treatment not only for hair loss but also for lost self-esteem resulting from the association of hair loss with illness and advanced age.
- Providers should dispense medication with a dose of emotional support and should describe the limitations of the existing treatment.

REFERENCES

1. Mounsey AL, Reed SW. Diagnosing and treating hair loss. *Am Fam Physician.* 2009;80(4):356–62, 373–4. PMID: 19678603.
2. Harrison S, Bergfield W. Diffuse hair loss: its triggers and management. *Cleve Clin J Med.* 2009;76(6):361–7. doi: 10.3949/ccjm.76a.08080.
3. Shapiro J. Hair loss in women. *N Eng J Med.* 2007:357(16);1620–30. doi: 10.1056/NEJMcp072110.
4. Dinh QQ, Sinclair R. Female pattern hair loss: current treatment concepts. *Clin Inter Aging.* 2007;2(2):189–99. PMID: 18044135.
5. Shinkai K, Stern RS, Wintroub BU. Cutaneous drug reactions. In: Kasper D, Fauci A, Hauser S, et al., eds. *Harrison's Principles of Internal Medicine.* 19th ed. New York, NY: McGraw-Hill; 2015. Available at: http://accesspharmacy.mhmedical.com/content.aspx?bookid=1130&Sectionid=79727466. Accessed July 11, 2016.
6. American Hair Loss Association. Drug induced hair loss. Available at: http://www.americanhairloss.org/drug_induced_hair_loss/. Accessed June 12, 2017.
7. Alzolibani AA. Epidemiologic and genetic characteristics of alopecia areata (part 1). *Acta Dermatoven APA.* 2011;20(4):191–8. PMID: 22367375.
8. Mesinkovska NA, Bergfeld WF. Hair: what is new in diagnosis and management? Female pattern hair loss update: diagnosis and treatment. *Dermatol Clin.* 2013;31(1):119–27. doi: 10.1016/j.det.2012.08.005.
9. Rathnayake D, Sinclair R. Male androgenetic alopecia. *Expert Opin Pharamcother.* 2010;11(8):1295–304. doi: 10.1517/14656561003752730.
10. Hunt N, McHale S. The psychological impact of alopecia. *BMJ.* 2005; 331(7522):951–3. doi: 10.1136/bmj.331.7522.951.
11. Hume AL. Viviscal: an answer for hair loss in women? *Pharm Today.* 2013;9:22.
12. Stough D, Stenn K, Haber R, et al. Psychological effect, pathophysiology, and management of androgenetic alopecia in men. *Mayo Clin Proc.* 2005;80(10):1316–22. doi: 10.4065/80.10.1316.
13. Sawaya ME, Price VH. Different levels of 5 alpha-reductase type I and II, aromatase, and androgen receptor in hair follicles of women and men with androgenetic alopecia. *J Invest Dermatol.* 1997;109(3):296–300. PMID: 9284093.
14. Randall VA, Hibberts NA, Thornton MJ, et al. The hair follicle: a paradoxical androgen target organ. *Horm Res.* 2000;54(5–6):243–50. doi: 53266.
15. American Hair Loss Association. The Norwood Scale. Available at: http://www.americanhairloss.org/men_hair_loss/the_norwood_scale.asp. Accessed June 12, 2017.
16. American Hair Loss Association. Degree of hair loss. Available at: http://www.americanhairloss.org/women_hair_loss/degree_of_hair_loss.asp. Accessed June 12, 2017.
17. van Zuuren EJ, Fedorowicz Z, Carter B, et al. Interventions for female pattern hair loss. *Cochrane Database System Rev.* 2012;5:CD007628. doi: 10.1002/14651858.CD007628.pub3.
18. Sinclair R, Patel M, Dawson TL, et al. Hair loss in women: medical and cosmetic approaches to increase scalp hair fullness. *Br J Derm.* 2011; 165(Suppl 3):12–8. doi: 10.1111/j.1365-2133.2011.10630.x.
19. Donovan JC, Shapiro RL, Shapiro P, et al. A review of scalp camouflaging agents and prostheses for individuals with hair loss. *Dermatol Online J.* 2012;18(8):1. PMID: 22948051.
20. Ross E, Shapiro J. Management of hair loss. *Dermatol Clin.* 2005:23;227–43. doi: 10.1016/j.det.2004.09.008.
21. Rogers NE, Avram MR. Medical treatments for male and female pattern hair loss. *J Am Acad Dermatol.* 2008;59(4):547–66. doi: 10.1016/j.jaad.2008.07.001.

22. Minoxidil topical. Facts and Comparisons eAnswers. Wolters Kluwer Health, Inc., St. Louis, MO. Available at: http://online.factsandcomparisons.com. Accessed November 27, 2016.
23. Otomo S. Hair growth effect of minoxidil. *Nippon Yakurigaku Zasshi.* 2002;119(3):167–74. PMID: 11915519.
24. Tosti A, Duque-Estrada B. Treatment strategies for alopecia. *Expert Opin Pharmacother.* 2009;10(6):1017–26. doi: 10.1517/14656560902876368.
25. Varothai S, Bergfeld WF. Androgenetic alopecia: An evidence-based treatment update. *Am J Clin Dermatol* 2014;15:217–30. doi: 10.1007/s40257-014-0077-5.
26. Iorizzo M, Tosti A. Treatment options for alopecia. *Expert Opin Pharmacother* 2015;16(15):2343–54. doi: 10.1517/14656566.2015.1084501.
27. Avram MR, Cole JP, Gandelman M, et al. The potential role of minoxidil in the hair transplantation setting. *Dermatol Surg.* 2002;28(10):894–900. PMID: 12410672.
28. McNeill-PPC, Inc. Rogaine. Available at: http://www.rogaine.com. Accessed June 12, 2017.
29. Olsen EA, Dunlap FE, Funicella T, et al. A randomized clinical trial of 5% topical minoxidil versus 2% topical minoxidil and placebo in the treatment of androgenetic alopecia in men. *J Am Acad Dermatol.* 2002;47(3):377–85. PMID: 12196747.
30. Lucky AW, Piacquadio DJ, Ditre CM, et al. A randomized, placebo-controlled trial of 5% and 2% topical minoxidil solutions in the treatment of female pattern hair loss. *J Am Acad Dermatol.* 2004;50(4):541–53. doi: 10.1016/j.jaad.2003.06.014.
31. Blume-Peytavi U, Hillmann K, Dietz E, et al. A randomized, single-blind trials of 5% minoxidil foam once daily versus 2% minoxidil solution twice daily in the treatment of androgenetic alopecia in women. *J Am Acad Dermatol.* 2011;65(6):1126–34. doi: 10.1016/j.jaad.2010.09.724.
32. Khandpur S, Suman M, Reddy BS. Comparative efficacy of various treatment regimens for androgenetic alopecia in men. *J Dermatol.* 2002;29(8):489–98. PMID: 12227482.
33. Peluso AM, Misciali C, Vincenzi C, et al. Diffuse hypertrichosis during treatment with 5% topical minoxidil. *Br J Dermatol.* 1997;136(1):118–20. PMID: 9039309.
34. Satoh H, Morikaw S, Fujiwara C, et al. A case of acute myocardial infarction associated with topical use of minoxidil (RiUP) for treatment of baldness. *Jpn Heart J.* 2000;41(4):519–23. PMID: 11041102.
35. Nguyen KH, Marks JG Jr. Pseudoacromegaly induced by the long-term use of minoxidil. *J Am Acad Dermatol.* 2003;48(6):962–5. doi: 10.1067/mjd.2003.325.
36. Sato T, Tadokoro T, Sonoda T, et al. Minoxidil increases 17 beta-hydroxysteroid dehydrogenase and 5 alpha-reductase activity of cultured human dermal papilla cells from balding scalp. *J Dermatol Sci.* 1999;19(2):123–5. PMID: 10098703.
37. Topical minoxidil. *Briggs' Drugs in Pregnancy and Lactation.* Facts & Comparisons eAnswers. Wolters Kluwer Health, Inc., St. Louis, MO. Available at: http://online.factsandcomparisons.com. Accessed December 3, 2016.
38. Hanover L. Hair replacement. *FDA Consum.* 1997;31:7–10.
39. Maidenhair fern and royal jelly monographs. In: Fetrow CW, Avila JR, eds. *Professional's Handbook of Complementary & Alternative Medicines.* Philadelphia, PA: Lippincott Williams & Wilkins; 2004:530, 718.
40. Prager N, Bickett K, French N, Marcovici G. A randomized, double-blind, placebo-controlled trial to determine the effectiveness of botanically derived inhibitors of 5-alpha-reductase in the treatment of androgenetic alopecia. *J Altern Complement Med* 2002;8(2): 143–52. doi: 10.1089/acm.2002.8.143.

section

IX

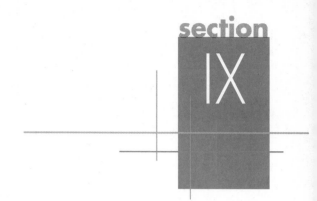

OTHER MEDICAL DISORDERS

CHAPTER 46

INSOMNIA, DROWSINESS, AND FATIGUE

SARAH T. MELTON AND CYNTHIA K. KIRKWOOD

INSOMNIA

Insomnia is one of the most common patient complaints, ranking second behind the common cold. Insomnia is a symptom with diverse etiologies, and it can progress to a disorder.[1] Insomnia occurs when a person has trouble falling or staying asleep, wakes up too early and cannot return to sleep, or does not feel refreshed after sleeping. Patients with other sleep disorders, such as sleep apnea, narcolepsy, and restless legs syndrome, may also seek nonprescription sleep aids. Because of potentially significant adverse clinical effects, patients with these disorders require referral to a sleep specialist.

Although the average adult requires 8 or more hours of sleep nightly, the typical American gets 6.7 hours.[2] An estimated 64% of the U.S. population experiences sleep problems at least a few nights a week, with 7% of adults reporting the use of alcohol, 7% a nonprescription sleep aid, and 8% a prescription hypnotic to manage their insomnia.[2] Patients with insomnia are more likely to report being unable to work efficiently, exercise, eat healthfully, and engage in leisure activities because they are too sleepy.[2]

Total annual cost estimates for insomnia in the United States range from $30 billion to $107.5 billion, depending on the prevalence rates assumed.[3] Compared with patients without insomnia, this disorder is associated with a significant economic burden for younger (ages 18–64 years) and older (>65 years) patients in terms of the average and indirect costs.[4] More than half of adults older than 65 report at least one sleep complaint, with 3%–21% of men and 7%–29% of women reporting the use of hypnotics.[5] Approximately 20% of American adults use a medication for insomnia in a given month, with nearly 60% of medications used being nonprescription sleep aids, primarily antihistamines, which are associated with adverse effects in older adults.[6] This group also has an increased incidence of sleep apnea and restless legs syndrome. Significant morbidity is associated with obstructive sleep apnea, including increased mortality from cardiovascular death.[7] As a result, complaints of insomnia in older patients should be carefully evaluated.

Despite these data, only a small percentage of patients with symptoms of insomnia actually consult their health care provider (HCP).[6] The combination of frequent misuse of hypnotics and availability of nonprescription agents makes insomnia a disorder of significant concern.

Pathophysiology of Insomnia

Sleep can be categorized into different stages by using the sleeping electroencephalogram (EEG) in conjunction with electro-oculography and electromyography. *Stage 1 sleep* is a transitional stage, occurring as the patient falls asleep; the EEG resembles the waking state more than sleep. *Stage 2 sleep* constitutes about 50% of sleep time and is light sleep. *Stages 3 and 4 of sleep,* collectively known as deep sleep or delta sleep, are characterized by the patterns of delta waves, or slow-frequency waves, on the EEG. *Rapid eye movement (REM) sleep* is neither light nor deep, and the EEG manifests an increase in high-frequency waves. REM sleep is characterized by physiologic activity such as changes in blood pressure not found in other sleep stages; skeletal muscle movement is inhibited. The eyes move rapidly from side to side, whereas blood pressure, heart rate, temperature, respiration, and metabolism are increased.[7,8]

Upon falling asleep, an individual progresses through four stages. The first REM period, usually 5–7 minutes in length, starts in about 70–90 minutes. The time from falling asleep to the first REM period is referred to as *REM latency.* The sleep cycle then repeats about every 70–120 minutes, with each progressive REM period becoming longer and the time spent in deep sleep becoming shorter. Prolonged suppression of REM sleep can result in psychological and behavioral changes, including anxiety, irritability, and difficulty concentrating.[7,8]

Sleep physiology changes with increasing age. Among older adults, the total duration of sleep is shorter, the number of nocturnal awakenings increases, and less time is spent in stage 4 and REM sleep. *Sleep latency* (time to fall asleep) usually remains normal with increasing age. Despite these changes, older adults cannot be assumed to require less sleep.[7]

Insomnia can be classified as transient, short term, or chronic according to the duration of sleep disturbance. *Transient insomnia* is often self-limiting, lasting less than 1 week. *Short-term insomnia* usually lasts from 1–3 weeks.[3] *Chronic, or long-term, insomnia* persists for more than 3 weeks to years and is often the result of medical problems, psychiatric disorders, or substance abuse.[1,3]

Insomnia can also be classified on the basis of an identifiable cause. *Primary insomnia* is the term used to describe patients who have sleep difficulty that lasts at least 1 month; that affects psychosocial functioning; and that is not caused by another sleep disorder, general medical disorder, psychiatric disorder, or medication (i.e., *secondary insomnia*).[9] All underlying causes of insomnia must be identified and managed to relieve the sleep disturbance.[1,3,9]

Difficulty falling asleep often is associated with acute life stresses or medical illness, anxiety, and poor sleep habits. The severity of stressful situations can affect the length of insomnia. Travel, hospitalization, or anticipation of an important or stressful event can cause transient insomnia. If more severe stressors such as the death of a loved one, recovery from surgery, or divorce are present, transient insomnia can become short-term insomnia. Unless managed appropriately, short-term insomnia can progress to chronic insomnia.

Shift workers often complain of sleep disturbances, excessive sleepiness, or both. Sleep problems occur more frequently in individuals who must rotate shifts. Some nighttime workers adjust to a change in their sleep schedule, whereas others never do. Some individuals are extremely sensitive to the stimulant effects of caffeine and nicotine. Drinking caffeinated beverages in the late afternoon or evening hours can cause insomnia. Late-night exercise and late-evening meals as well as environmental distractions such as noise, lighting, uncomfortable temperatures, or new surroundings can also interfere with sleep.[7,8]

Several medical disorders, in addition to psychiatric disorders, are associated with chronic insomnia (Table 46–1). Chronic insomnia is a key complaint of patients experiencing pain syndromes. Chronic insomnia can also be secondary to use of medications or other substances or to *circadian rhythm sleep disorders* (i.e., abnormalities in length, timing, and/or rigidity of the sleep–wake cycle relative to the day–night cycle).[1,6,9] Early morning awakening is often associated with depression. Nonprescription hypnotics are generally not helpful in patients with chronic insomnia, and medical referral is indicated.

Medications, including both prescription and nonprescription drugs, can produce either insomnia or withdrawal insomnia (Table 46–2).[1,6–8] Antidepressants, antihypertensive agents, and sympathomimetic amines such as pseudoephedrine and phenylephrine are commonly associated with causing insomnia. Alcohol can cause insomnia after acute use and as a withdrawal effect after chronic use.

TABLE 46–1 Medical Disorders Associated With Insomnia

General Medical Disorders
Allergies
Arthritis
Benign prostatic hyperplasia
Chronic pain syndromes
Diabetes mellitus
Gastroesophageal reflux disease
Heart failure
Peptic ulcer disease

Respiratory Disorders
Asthma
Chronic obstructive pulmonary disease

Psychiatric Disorders
Anxiety disorders
Depression

Sleep Disorders
Obstructive sleep apnea
Psychophysiologic insomnia
Restless legs syndrome
Shift-work sleep disorder

Other Conditions
Menopause
Pregnancy

Source: References 1, 3, 5, and 7.

TABLE 46–2 Drugs That Can Exacerbate Insomnia

Drugs That Can Cause Insomnia	Drugs That Can Produce Withdrawal Insomnia
Alcohol	Alcohol
Anabolic steroids	Amphetamines
Antidepressants (e.g., bupropion, fluoxetine, venlafaxine)	Antihistamines (first generation)
Anticonvulsants (e.g., lamotrigine)	Barbiturate
Antihypertensives (e.g., clonidine)	Benzodiazepines
Antineoplastics	Illicit drugs (e.g., cocaine, marijuana, phencyclidine)
Amphetamines	Monoamine oxidase inhibitors
Anorexiants (e.g., phentermine)	Opiates
Beta-adrenergic agonists (e.g., albuterol)	Tricyclic antidepressants
Beta-blockers (especially propranolol)	
Caffeine	
Corticosteroids	
Decongestants	
Diuretics (at bedtime)	
Levodopa	
Nicotine	
Oral contraceptives	
Thyroid preparations	

Source: References 1 and 6–8.

Clinical Presentation of Insomnia

Patients with insomnia may have varying complaints, such as difficulty falling asleep, frequent awakening, early morning awakening and inability to fall back to sleep, disturbed quality of sleep with unusual or troublesome dreams, or just poor sleep in general. Their actual duration of sleep, as determined by sleep laboratory studies, may or may not differ from that of individuals who report normal sleep. However, these patients usually report they need more than 30 minutes to fall asleep and/or their duration of sleep is less than 6–7 hours nightly. The National Sleep

Foundation recommends an average sleep requirement of 8 hours for adults older than 18 years.[2] Patients who complain of insomnia characterized by frequent nighttime awakenings or early morning awakenings with difficulty going back to sleep or those whose symptoms have lasted 4 weeks or longer should be referred to their HCP for further evaluation.

Sleep-deprived individuals are highly symptomatic, and their quality of life is negatively affected. Some impairment in daytime functioning is typical, and most untreated patients with insomnia report symptoms of fatigue, drowsiness, anxiety, irritability, depression, decreased concentration, and memory impairment. If untreated, insomnia is associated with an increase in motor vehicle and occupational accidents as well as a rise in morbidity and mortality rates from general medical and psychiatric disorders, such as cardiovascular disease, pain syndromes, depression, anxiety, and substance abuse.[1,6]

Treatment of Insomnia

Treatment Goals

Treatment goals are to improve the patient's presenting symptoms, quality of life, and functioning.[1]

General Treatment Approach

For patients with transient or short-term insomnia but no underlying medical or psychiatric conditions that cause insomnia, reestablishing the normal sleep cycle with good sleep hygiene practices, with or without a nonprescription sleep aid, should help to normalize sleep patterns. The algorithm in Figure 46–1 outlines the assessment and self-treatment of transient and short-term insomnia, and lists exclusions for self-treatment.

Nonpharmacologic Therapy

Cognitive behavioral therapy for insomnia (CBI) addresses dysfunctional behaviors and beliefs that contribute to insomnia and is considered first-line therapy for all patients.[6,10] CBI is multimodal and consists of a combination of cognitive therapy, behavioral interventions such as sleep restriction and stimulus control, and educational interventions such as sleep hygiene. The sleep hygiene measures in Table 46–3 are recommended for all patients with insomnia.[7–10] In most patients with sleep disturbances, these measures should be tried before starting drug therapy. Patients should be encouraged to try one or two measures at a time.

Pharmacologic Therapy

When the Food and Drug Administration (FDA) issued its final monograph on nonprescription sleep aids in 1989, diphenhydramine, as either the hydrochloride or citrate salt, was the only sleep aid deemed to be safe and effective for self-administration.[11]

Antihistamines

Diphenhydramine and doxylamine belong to the ethanolamine group of antihistamines. Ethanolamines affect sleep through their affinity for blocking histamine-1 and muscarinic receptors.[12] Although the safety and efficacy of doxylamine have not been fully established, FDA has allowed the drug to remain on the market.[13] Few studies supporting the efficacy of doxylamine as a hypnotic are available.[13,14]

Both diphenhydramine and doxylamine are well absorbed from the gastrointestinal tract, with similar times to maximum plasma concentrations (1–4 hours and 2–3 hours, respectively). The elimination half-life of diphenhydramine is 2.4–9.3 hours, whereas that of doxylamine is 10 hours.[11,13] Diphenhydramine is metabolized in the liver through two successive N-demethylations, and its apparent half-life can be prolonged in patients with hepatic cirrhosis.[11] Studies have shown a positive relationship between diphenhydramine plasma concentrations and drowsiness and cognitive impairment. Maximum sedation with diphenhydramine occurs between 3 and 6 hours after a dose.[11]

The primary indication for diphenhydramine is the symptomatic management of transient and short-term sleep difficulty, particularly in individuals who complain of occasional problems falling asleep. The efficacy of diphenhydramine in patients with chronic insomnia is poor.[14] Tolerance to the sedative effect of diphenhydramine develops in healthy volunteers within days of repeated use.[14]

Although the usual diphenhydramine dosage is 50 mg nightly, some individuals benefit from a 25 mg dosage. Intermittent use for 3 days with an "off" night to assess sleep quality without medication may reduce tolerance to the hypnotic effect. Diphenhydramine should be used for no more than 7–10 consecutive nights, because insomnia may be a symptom of an undiagnosed medical or psychiatric illness that requires further evaluation.[11]

Additive sedation or anticholinergic effects occur when diphenhydramine is used in combination with other medications that have these properties.[12] Diphenhydramine, an inhibitor of the hepatic enzyme CYP2D6, causes more than a twofold decrease in the clearance of metoprolol, especially in women.[15] Table 46–4 describes clinically significant drug–drug interactions that can occur with diphenhydramine.[16] These potential interactions should be carefully monitored and alterations made to pharmacotherapy if indicated.

The primary adverse effects of diphenhydramine and doxylamine are anticholinergic.[11,13] Dry mouth and throat, constipation, blurred vision, urinary retention, and tinnitus commonly occur. Older patients, patients with comorbid medical disorders, and patients taking multiple medications are particularly susceptible to developing adverse effects.

Anticholinergic toxicity can result from excessive antihistamine dosages. Factors such as drug–drug interactions, intentional overdosage, or individual sensitivity can also lead to toxicity.[12,17] Central nervous system (CNS) anticholinergic toxicity is one of the primary presenting features of antihistamine excess. Patients exhibiting excessive anticholinergic effects can be anxious, excited, delirious, hallucinating, or stuporous. In more severe cases, coma or seizures may occur. Other physical signs of anticholinergic toxicity include dilated pupils, flushed skin, hot and dry mucous membranes, and elevated body temperature. Tachycardia and moderate QTc prolongation on the electrocardiogram are common. In severe cases, rhabdomyolysis, dysrhythmias, cardiovascular collapse, and death can occur.[11,12,17] In the case of diphenhydramine overdose, patients should be referred for emergency treatment, which includes gastric lavage and activated charcoal via gastric tube, and further symptomatic treatment.

Diphenhydramine is contraindicated in several situations. Older men with prostatic hyperplasia and difficulty urinating should not use diphenhydramine, because urinary retention can occur. Because anticholinergic agents can increase intraocular pressure, angle-closure glaucoma is another contraindication. Patients with

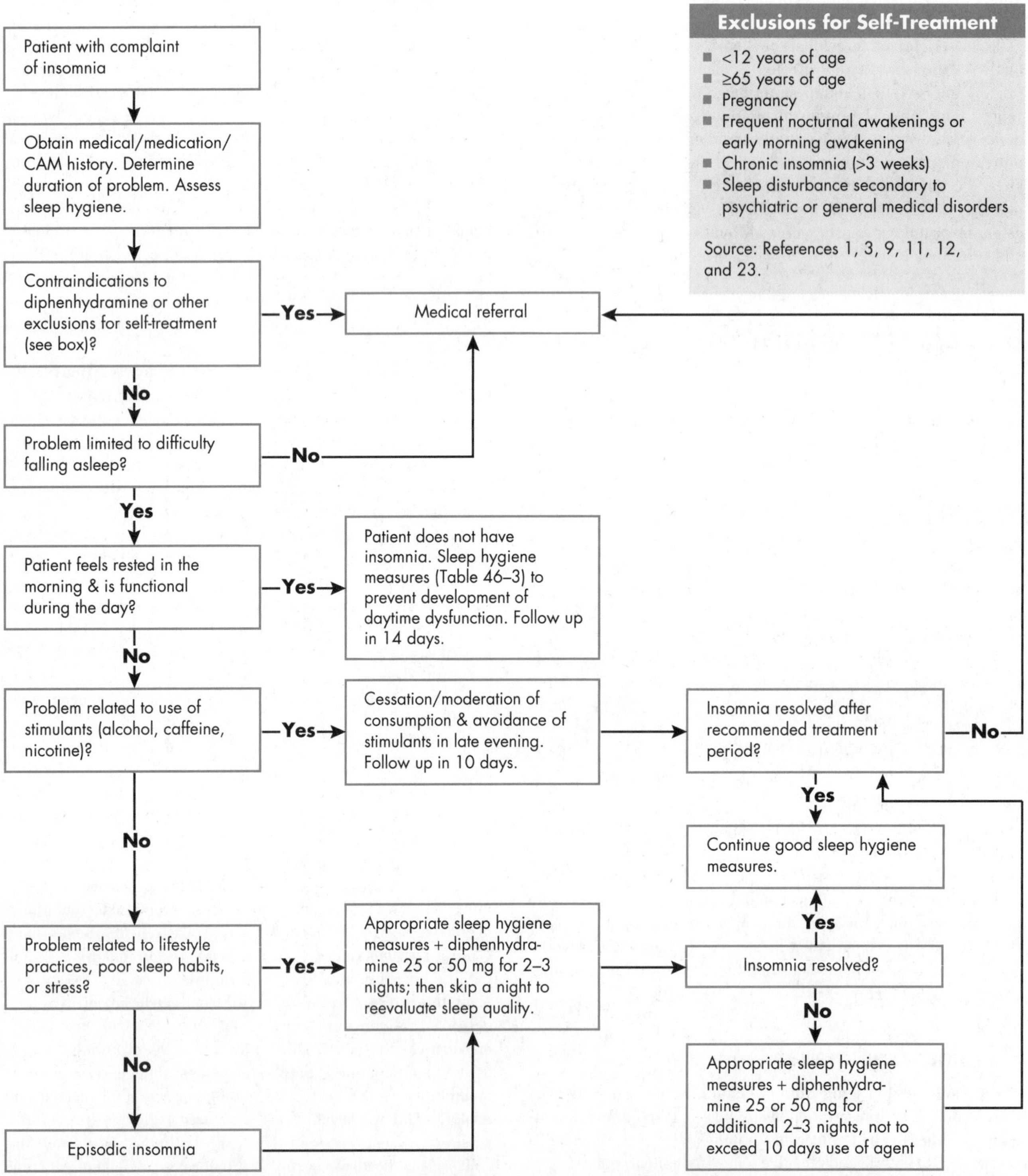

FIGURE 46–1 Self-care of transient and short-term insomnia. Key: CAM = Complementary and alternative medication.

TABLE 46–3 Principles of Good Sleep Hygiene

- Use bed for sleeping or intimacy only.
- Establish a regular sleep pattern. Go to bed and arise at about the same time daily, even on the weekends.
- Make the bedroom comfortable for sleeping. Avoid temperature extremes, noise, and light.
- Engage in relaxing activities before bedtime.
- Avoid using electronic devices (particularly videos, television, and tablets) around bedtime.
- Exercise regularly but not within 2–4 hours of bedtime.
- If hungry eat a light snack, but avoid eating meals within 2 hours before bedtime.
- Avoid daytime napping.
- Avoid using caffeine, alcohol, or nicotine for at least 4–6 hours before bedtime.
- If unable to fall asleep, do not continue to try to sleep; get out of bed and perform a relaxing activity until you feel tired.
- Do not watch the clock at night.

Source: References 7–10.

cardiovascular disease, such as angina or arrhythmias, may be particularly susceptible to the anticholinergic adverse effects and should not use these agents.[12] Anticholinergic agents decrease cognition and increase confusion in patients with dementia; diphenhydramine should be avoided in these patients. In addition, higher cumulative anticholinergic use is associated with an increased risk for dementia. Efforts to increase awareness among HCPs and older adults about this potential medication-related risk are important to minimize anticholinergic use of medications such as diphenhydramine over time.[18]

Patients should be cautioned to avoid performing tasks that require their full attention or coordination, such as driving, cooking, or operating machinery, until their response is known. They should be discouraged from drinking alcoholic beverages while taking diphenhydramine. Some patients can develop excitation from diphenhydramine and other highly anticholinergic antihistamines.[12] This paradoxical effect occurs more often in children, older patients, and patients with organic mental disorders. Symptoms include nervousness, restlessness, agitation, tremors, insomnia, delirium, and, in rare cases, seizures.

Combination products containing diphenhydramine and acetaminophen, ibuprofen, or aspirin are available,[12] although no published studies establish whether these products are of benefit in inducing sleep in patients who complain of insomnia caused by pain. Gastrointestinal adverse effects are of concern with frequent use of combination products containing ibuprofen and aspirin.

Several case reports of diphenhydramine abuse in patients taking antipsychotic medications have been published.[19] Animal studies indicate that selected antagonists of the histamine-1 receptors enhance dopamine release in the mesolimbic areas similar to that produced by cocaine.[20] HCPs should carefully assess for abuse in individuals making repeated purchases of diphenhydramine, especially in patients being treated for psychosis.[19]

Ethanol

Use of alcohol to induce sleep is common in patients with chronic insomnia and is associated with hazardous drinking behavior.[21] Alcohol, in both small and large quantities, initially improves sleep in people who do not abuse alcohol, but sleep disturbances occur in the second half of the night at high doses. Tolerance quickly develops after the initial beneficial effects, often leading to the use of higher doses. Individuals whose alcohol use is heavy or continuous usually experience restless sleep, often awaken within 2–4 hours, and have reduced total sleep duration. People who chronically drink alcohol usually have a marked disorganization of the sleep cycle. A worsening of sleep or rebound insomnia can occur when alcohol use ceases.[22]

Alcohol is present in some liquid nonprescription combination cold products, which can contain up to 10% alcohol by volume. Products of this type are marketed to induce sleep. However, data regarding the efficacy and safety of these products as hypnotics are limited. The multiple ingredients increase the risk of adverse effects and interactions with other drugs.

Pharmacotherapeutic Comparisons

Most clinical trials indicate that diphenhydramine is effective in decreasing sleep latency and in improving the reported quality of sleep for individuals with occasional insomnia.[11,14] Compared with placebo, diphenhydramine improved sleep efficiency for 2 weeks in patients with mild insomnia.[22] In general, diphenhydramine should not be recommended for a chronic sleep disturbance.[1,6,10]

Product Selection Guidelines

Because the value of doxylamine as a hypnotic is not well established, only diphenhydramine should be recommended to patients for such use. Nonprescription diphenhydramine is available as capsules, gelcaps, tablets, chewable tablets, solutions, and elixirs (Table 46–5) to meet different patient preferences.[12]

Special Population Considerations

The safety of antihistamines during pregnancy has not been established.[12] Therefore, the benefit–risk ratio of using these drugs to manage insomnia during pregnancy should be carefully evaluated. In April 2013, FDA approved the combination of doxylamine succinate and pyridoxine HCl for treatment of pregnant women experiencing nausea and vomiting. Most epidemiologic studies have not demonstrated increased risk of teratogenicity with the use of diphenhydramine during the first trimester, but one trial reported cleft palate alone and other fetal abnormalities.[11] Nevertheless, rather than recommending a nonprescription product, pregnant women should be referred for further evaluation.

An increased risk of CNS adverse effects can occur in breastfed neonates after maternal intake of a sedating antihistamine. The intermittent use of low dosages of diphenhydramine by the mother after the last daytime feeding would lessen potential drug effects in the infant. Use of large dosages for sustained periods of time may inhibit lactation and cause drowsiness in breastfed infants.[24] Continued use of sedating antihistamines for insomnia are not recommended for use in nursing mothers.[11–13]

Children and adolescents may present with insomnia caused by a circadian rhythm disorder. Teenagers should be asked about their use of nonprescription remedies and intake of caffeine, nicotine, alcohol, or illicit substances. Behavioral interventions and good sleep hygiene are first-line treatment for insomnia in children and adolescents. Diphenhydramine and doxylamine are not indicated to treat insomnia in children younger than 12 years. Diphenhydramine may cause paradoxical excitation in younger children and is not recommended to induce sleep in infants.[11]

TABLE 46–4 Clinically Significant Drug Interactions With Diphenhydramine

Interacting Drugs or Drug Classes	Description	Monitoring Recommendation
Acetylcholinesterase inhibitors	Acetylcholinesterase inhibitors may diminish the therapeutic effect of diphenhydramine.	Monitor therapy.
Alcohol (ethyl)	Diphenhydramine may enhance the CNS depressant effect of ethanol.	Monitor therapy.
Aripiprazole, brexpiprazole	Diphenhydramine may increase serum concentrations of aripiprazole and brexpiprazole.	Monitor for increased pharmacologic effects. Dose adjustments may be required based on concomitant therapy and/or indication.
Buprenorphine	Diphenhydramine may enhance the CNS depressant effect of buprenorphine.	Consider reduced doses of other CNS depressants, and avoiding such drugs in patients at high risk of buprenorphine overuse/self-injection.
Cannabis	Cannabis may enhance the CNS depressant effect of diphenhydramine.	Monitor therapy.
Gastrointestinal Agents (prokinetic)	Diphenhydramine may diminish the therapeutic effect of prokinetic gastrointestinal agents.	Monitor therapy.
Glucagon	Diphenhydramine may enhance the adverse and toxic GI effects of glucagon.	Avoid combination.
Kava	Kava may enhance the adverse/toxic effect of diphenhydramine.	Monitor therapy.
Metoprolol	Diphenhydramine may increase the serum concentration of metoprolol and cause decreased heart rate and blood pressure.	Consider an alternative for one of the interacting drugs in order to avoid metoprolol toxicity. If the combination must be used, monitor response to metoprolol closely. Metoprolol dose reductions may be necessary.
Minocycline	Minocycline may enhance the CNS depressant effect of diphenhydramine.	Monitor therapy.
Mirtazapine	Diphenhydramine may enhance the CNS depressant effect of mirtazapine.	Monitor therapy.
Opioid analgesics (codeine, hydrocodone, oxycodone, tapentadol, etc)	Diphenhydramine may enhance the CNS depressant effect of opioid analgesics. Diphenhydramine may diminish the therapeutic effect of codeine by preventing the metabolic conversion of codeine to its active metabolite morphine.	When opioid analgesics are combined with diphenhydramine, a dose reduction of one or both agents should be considered. Consider therapy modification and monitor for pain relief if codeine is used.
Potassium chloride	Diphenhydramine may enhance the ulcerogenic effect of potassium chloride.	Patients on diphenhydramine should avoid using any solid oral dosage form of potassium chloride because of anticholinergic effects. Avoid combining use of these drugs.
Selective serotonin reuptake inhibitors (SSRIs)	Diphenhydramine may enhance the adverse effects of SSRIs. Risk of psychomotor impairment may be enhanced.	Monitor therapy.
Tamoxifen	Diphenhydramine may decrease serum concentrations of the active metabolite(s) of tamoxifen.	When possible, consider alternatives that have less of an inhibitory effect on CYP2D6 activity. Consider therapy modification.
Topiramate	Diphenhydramine may enhance the adverse and toxic effects of topiramate.	Monitor therapy.
Tramadol	Diphenhydramine may diminish the therapeutic effect of tramadol by preventing the metabolic conversion of tramadol to its active metabolite.	Monitor therapy.

Source: Reference 16.

TABLE 46–5 **Selected Nonprescription Sleep Aid Products**

Trade Name	Primary Ingredients
Single-Entity Antihistamine Products	
Unisom SleepGels Capsules, liquid filled	Diphenhydramine HCl 50 mg
Sominex Nighttime Sleep-Aid Tablets	Diphenhydramine HCl 25 mg
ZzzQuil Nighttime Sleep-Aid Liquid	Diphenhydramine HCL 50 mg/300 ml
Antihistamine/Analgesic Combination Products	
Advil PM Caplets	Diphenhydramine citrate 38 mg; ibuprofen 200 mg
Excedrin PM Headache Caplets	Diphenhydramine citrate 38 mg; acetaminophen 250 mg; aspirin 250 mg
Tylenol PM Extra Strength Caplets	Diphenhydramine HCl 25 mg; acetaminophen 500 mg

Note: Information is not all inclusive. Product formulations may have changed since time of publication.

Anticholinergic toxicity is common in children, and their symptoms may be more severe than those of adults. Diphenhydramine toxicity was reported in children using the topical application over large areas of their bodies, as well as in those using the topical and oral preparations simultaneously.[11] FDA requires a warning statement advising consumers not to use oral nonprescription diphenhydramine with other products containing the drug, including topical agents.[11]

Treatment of insomnia in older adults consists of behavioral therapy and pharmacotherapy with approved agents. The Beers criteria recommend avoiding the use of anticholinergic drugs in older adults.[25] Concerns about diphenhydramine and doxylamine include falls and cognitive and memory impairment in older patients.[1,26] Therefore, nonprescription antihistamines should not be recommended to treat insomnia in this age group, and the patients should be referred to their HCP for further evaluation.

Complementary Therapies

Complementary therapies such as melatonin and valerian are commonly used for insomnia. (See Chapter 51 for a thorough discussion of these two supplements). Overall, evidence of the efficacy of melatonin is conflicting and likely depends on many factors.

Valerian (*Valeriana officinalis*) has limited benefit in insomnia compared with placebo.[27] Clinical trials have used 400–900 mg of the valerian root extract. Continuous nightly use for several days or weeks is required for an effect, so valerian is not useful for acute insomnia. Patients using large dosages of valerian may experience severe benzodiazepine-like withdrawal symptoms and cardiac complications.[27] Valerian should be slowly tapered after extended use.

Kava (*Piper methysticum*) has been used in insomnia and has been associated with severe hepatotoxicity.[28] Therefore, kava should not be recommended as a sleep aid.

The American Academy of Sleep Medicine recommends that dietary supplements not be used to treat insomnia or any other sleep problem, unless their use is approved by an HCP.[29] Complementary therapies such as acupuncture, tai chi, and light therapy may be useful in the treatment of insomnia.[1,28] However, these treatments have not been adequately evaluated.

Assessment of Insomnia: A Case-Based Approach

In assessing whether to recommend a nonprescription sleep aid, the HCP should determine whether use of such products is appropriate, what nondrug interventions should be recommended, and whether referral to another HCP is indicated. Identifying acute causes of insomnia, poor sleep hygiene practices, or underlying medical disorders can assist the provider in making a recommendation.

Case 46–1 illustrates the assessment of a patient with insomnia.

Patient Counseling for Insomnia

Patients with sleep disorders should be encouraged to practice good sleep hygiene measures. For some patients, these measures alone will resolve insomnia. If use of a nonprescription sleep aid is appropriate, the dosage guidelines and recommended duration of therapy should be reviewed with the patient. Potential adverse effects, drug–drug interactions, and any precautions or warnings should be carefully explained. In addition, patient education should include the signs and symptoms that indicate the need for further visits to the HCP. Taking a combination of products (i.e., prescription and nonprescription drugs, and dietary supplements) concomitantly to treat insomnia should be discouraged; this approach increases the risk of adverse effects. The box "Patient Education for Insomnia" lists specific information to provide patients.

Evaluation of Patient Outcomes for Insomnia

Successful outcomes include decreased time to fall asleep, improved sleep quality, and decreased daytime fatigue and drowsiness. The patient should be advised to seek medical evaluation if sleep has not improved in 10 days.[12]

Key Points for Insomnia

- Refer patients with chronic insomnia or sleep disturbance caused by an underlying disorder for medical evaluation.
- Advise patients with self-treatable symptoms that if symptoms worsen or do not improve after 10 days, they should contact their HCP.
- Counsel patients with insomnia on nondrug measures such as good sleep hygiene (Table 46–3).
- Refer children younger than 12 years, pregnant women, and adults older than 65 years with insomnia to their HCP.
- Advise patients about the different dosage forms of sleep aids so they can select a product that is best suited for them.

CASE 46–1

Relevant Evaluation Criteria	Scenario/Model Outcome
Collect	
1. Gather essential information about the patient's symptoms and medical history, including	
a. Description of symptom(s) (i.e., nature, onset, duration, severity, associated symptoms)	Patient complains of difficulty sleeping for the past 2 weeks. She feels tired and irritable during the day and a need for a nap every afternoon.
b. Description of any factors that seem to precipitate, exacerbate, and/or relieve the patient's symptom(s)	Difficulty falling asleep began after the patient was promoted to a new job with added responsibilities. Previously, she typically slept well.
c. Description of the patient's/caregiver's efforts to relieve the symptoms	She tries to stay up until she is sleepy at night. She says that she usually lies in bed and begins worrying when she cannot fall asleep. She becomes frustrated watching the alarm clock, knowing that she has to get up in a few hours to get ready for work. When she cannot fall asleep, she will get up and do housework (i.e., washing clothes, ironing). She is concerned about being sleepy during the daytime, because the drowsiness interferes with her work and interaction with the public.
d. Patient's identity	Kayla Johnson
e. Patient's age, gender, height, and weight	39 years old, female, 5 ft 5 in., 120 lb
f. Patient's occupation	Vice President at National American Bank
g. Patient's dietary habits	Patient is fairly conscientious about eating a healthy diet, low in fat and sodium. She drinks 1 large mug of coffee in the morning, a 12-ounce Mountain Dew at lunch, and a 5-hour ENERGY Extra Strength in the afternoon when she feels drowsy.
h. Patient's sleep habits	Stays up late working, especially when a financial project is due; sleeps in on the weekends often until noon. She has been napping 30 minutes or more when she gets home from work on a nearly daily basis.
i. Concurrent medical conditions, prescription and nonprescription medications, and dietary supplements	Allergic rhinitis: Claritin D 24-hour Extended Release tablets (loratadine 10 mg/pseudoephedrine 240 mg) daily; nasal saline as needed
j. Allergies	Sulfa (rash)
k. History of other adverse reactions to medications	None
l. Other (describe) _______	Drinks 2 glasses of wine nightly to help her relax and go to sleep. Denies use of tobacco.
Assess	
2. Differentiate patient's signs/symptoms, and correctly identify the patient's primary problem(s).	Poor sleep, likely secondary to the stress of promotion and poor sleep hygiene. Possible use of alcohol on a daily basis, use of a decongestant, and excessive caffeine are disrupting sleep.
3. Identify exclusions for self-treatment (Figure 46–1).	None
4. Formulate a comprehensive list of therapeutic alternatives for the primary problem to determine whether triage to a health care provider is required, and share this information with the patient or caregiver.	Options include (1) Refer Kayla to her HCP. (2) Recommend diphenhydramine until Kayla can make an appointment with her HCP. (3) Recommend diphenhydramine and good sleep hygiene, including limiting daily alcohol and caffeine use and engaging in regular physical activity. (4) Take no action.
Plan	
5. Select an optimal therapeutic alternative to address the patient's problem, taking into account patient preferences.	Diphenhydramine 50 mg tablets and good sleep hygiene measures, as well as limited alcohol and caffeine consumption
6. Describe the recommended therapeutic approach to the patient or caregiver.	"Take 1 diphenhydramine 50 mg tablet ½–1 hour before your anticipated bedtime every night for 3 nights. Skip 1 night and evaluate your ability to sleep. If not improved, continue diphenhydramine for 3 more nights, and reevaluate your ability to sleep without taking it. If symptoms persist for 10 days, seek medical evaluation."

CASE 46-1 *continued*

Relevant Evaluation Criteria	Scenario/Model Outcome
	"Follow measures for positive sleep hygiene." (See Table 46–3.) "Limit alcohol consumption to 1–2 glasses of wine or less, consumed no later than 2 hours before bedtime. Limit overall intake of caffeine, and at a minimum, avoid caffeine 6 hours before bedtime."
7. Explain to the patient or caregiver the rationale for selecting the recommended therapeutic approach from the considered therapeutic alternatives.	"A consistent sleep pattern will help resolve your insomnia. Seeing your health care provider may not be necessary if you take the diphenhydramine and follow good sleep hygiene measures. Poor sleep practices are a common cause of insomnia. If these practices are continued, they can create a chronic sleep disturbance. A medicine such as diphenhydramine can facilitate falling asleep, but it must be combined with measures of good sleep hygiene." "Alcohol in more than modest quantities can disrupt sleep and make insomnia worse. Therefore, alcohol consumption should be limited and avoided before bedtime. In addition, caffeine is a stimulant that promotes wakefulness. Caffeine intake should be limited and not occur within 6 hours of bedtime. Reduce intake of sodas and stop the 5-hour ENERGY Extra Strength drinks. The Mountain Dew contains 54 mg of caffeine in each 12-ounce drink. The 5-hour ENERGY Extra Strength contains 242 mg of caffeine, which is equivalent to 2.5 cups of coffee. All dietary sources of caffeine, for example, coffee, sodas, and energy drinks, as well as hidden sources of caffeine, such as chocolate, should be identified." "The pseudoephedrine in the Claritin-D Extended Release tablets may also contribute to insomnia. You may take loratadine tablets without the decongestant for your allergies."
Implement	
8. When recommending self-care with nonprescription medications and/or nondrug therapy, convey accurate information to the patient or caregiver.	"Take diphenhydramine 50 mg nightly for 3 nights; then reevaluate sleep for 1 night without the medication. Do not exceed this nightly dose. Always use sleep aids in combination with good sleep hygiene measures." (See Table 46–3). "Do not take sleep aids nightly longer than 10 days without seeing your health care provider." "Avoid drinking alcohol with the diphenhydramine because of the risk of increased sedation and negative effects of alcohol on sleep patterns." "Adverse effects may include sedation, next-morning hangover, and anticholinergic effects, for example, dry mouth, urinary retention, blurry vision, and constipation."
Solicit follow-up questions from the patient or caregiver.	(1) "May I repeat the dose of diphenhydramine if I do not fall asleep within 2 hours?" (2) "May I take diphenhydramine with my Claritin-D allergy medication?"
Answer the patient's or caregiver's questions.	(1) "No, repeating the dose increases the risk of side effects and will likely not improve sleep." (2) "You should continue the saline nasal spray while using the diphenhydramine. Do not take the Claritin-D on the days you take diphenhydramine, because both are antihistamines."
Follow-up: Monitor and Evaluate	
9. Assess patient outcome.	Contact the patient in 2–3 days to assess the efficacy of diphenhydramine and improved sleep hygiene measures. Remind the patient that if the insomnia continues for longer than 10 days, she should make an appointment with her HCP for evaluation.

Key: HCP = Health care provider.

PATIENT EDUCATION FOR Insomnia

The objectives of self-treatment are (1) to improve the duration and quality of sleep, (2) to reduce fatigue and drowsiness during the day, (3) to improve daytime functioning, and (4) to minimize adverse effects of treatment. Carefully following product instructions and the self-care measures listed here will help ensure optimal therapeutic outcomes for most patients.

Disease Information

- Insomnia is difficulty getting enough sleep or trouble sleeping without interruption. Insomnia may be described as difficulty falling asleep, waking up too early, or waking up periodically during the night and not feeling rested during the day. Insomnia can cause fatigue and drowsiness during the day. Insomnia is *chronic* when it happens almost nightly for at least 1 month. Insomnia can be caused by medical or psychiatric conditions, mental stress or excitement, or certain daytime and bedtime habits. If prescribed a medication that can exacerbate insomnia, talk with your health care provider about taking the medication in the morning (e.g., corticosteroids).

Nondrug Measures

- See Table 46–3 for nondrug measures to prevent insomnia.
- Using principles of good sleep hygiene can help improve bad sleep habits and enhance quality sleep.
- If insomnia worsens or continues beyond 2 weeks, seek medical attention.

Nonprescription Medications

- Do not drive or operate machinery after taking sleep aids, including melatonin and valerian.
- Diphenhydramine is not expected to harm an unborn baby; however, you should not use diphenhydramine for sleep during pregnancy unless your health care provider recommends its use. It is important to tell your health care provider if you are pregnant or plan to become pregnant during treatment.
- Diphenhydramine may pass into breast milk and may harm a nursing baby. Antihistamines may also slow breast milk production. Do not use this medication without medical advice if you are breastfeeding a baby.

Diphenhydramine

- Establish a regular bedtime and take diphenhydramine 30–60 minutes before you want to go to sleep. Do not take more than 50 mg of diphenhydramine each night.
- After 2–3 nights of improved sleep, skip taking the medication for 1 night to see if the insomnia is relieved.
- Do not take the medication longer than 10 days. Longer use will cause tolerance to the medication's sleep-inducing effects but not necessarily to its side effects, and you may have an underlying disorder that is causing insomnia.
- Note that diphenhydramine can cause morning grogginess or excessive sedation, dry mouth, blurred vision, constipation, and difficulty urinating (particularly in older men).
- Do not take diphenhydramine with alcohol; alcohol can increase the effects of the medication on the central nervous system. Alcohol also disrupts the sleep cycle.
- Do not take diphenhydramine with prescription sleep aids to improve sleep further.
- Consult your health care provider before taking diphenhydramine with other medications.

- ➤ Advise patients that diphenhydramine is the only antihistamine recommended as a sleep aid for occasional insomnia.
- ➤ Counsel patients that nonprescription sleep aids can cause next-day sedation.
- ➤ Counsel patients on the adverse effects of diphenhydramine and other sleep aids, particularly drowsiness and the additive CNS depressant effects of alcohol and other sedating drugs.
- ➤ Advise patients not to take other oral medications that contain diphenhydramine with a nonprescription sleep aid that also contains diphenhydramine.
- ➤ Advise patients not to apply topical products that contain diphenhydramine if they are also taking a nonprescription sleep aid that contains diphenhydramine.
- ➤ Advise patients to discuss the potential risks and benefits of complementary therapies with their HCP before selecting an agent.

DROWSINESS AND FATIGUE

Drowsiness or fatigue may be acute in onset or chronic and can increase the risk of workplace or transport-related accidents, as well as adversely impact productivity, mood, and overall health.[30] Evidence indicates an increased incidence of sleep-related crashes in young drivers who report an average of less than 6 hours of sleep per night.[31]

Caffeine is the most frequently used CNS stimulant in the world. Men and women consume an average of 196 mg daily and 151 mg daily, respectively, through ingestion of coffee, tea, and soft drinks. Youths consume less caffeine than adults daily; caffeine consumption averaged 61 mg in those ages 14–19 years, 26 mg in those ages 9–13 years, and 15 mg in those ages 4–8 years.[32] Energy drinks are popular with adolescents and young adults. Table 46–6 lists the caffeine content of commonly consumed beverages. Caffeine is in many nonprescription, prescription, and dietary supplements. Total daily caffeine intake leads to adverse effects, withdrawal reactions, or, rarely, interactions with drugs.

Pathophysiology of Drowsiness and Fatigue

Daytime drowsiness and fatigue are most often caused by *inadequate sleep,* that is, sleep of both insufficient duration and quality. The degree of sleepiness is determined by two factors that regulate sleep and wakefulness: (1) a homeostatic process involving an increase in sleepiness as time since the most recent period of sleep increases and (2) a circadian process by which the master biological clock in the suprachiasmatic nucleus varies alertness over the course of the 24-hour day.[33] Other possible contributing factors include the use of CNS depressants, such as antihistamines, antipsychotics, anticonvulsants, and opioids.

TABLE 46-6 **Caffeine Content in Common Beverages**

Coffees, Teas, and Soft Drinks	Ounces	Caffeine Content (mg)
Coffee	8	108
Coffee, decaffeinated	8	6
Starbucks coffee, tall	12	260
Starbucks coffee, grande	16	330
Espresso	2	100
Instant coffee	8	57
Brewed tea, U.S. brands	8	40
Snapple Iced Tea	8	21
Mountain Dew	12	54
Diet Coke	12	46.5
Coca-Cola	12	34.5
Dr. Pepper	12	41

Note: The listed caffeine content for the brewed coffees and teas may vary according to brewing methods.

Dopamine agonists, antibiotics, and antihypertensive agents may also increase the risk of drowsiness. Increased susceptibility to the sedating effects of these agents can be particularly troublesome in older patients. Other etiologies include depression, cancer, anemia, hypothyroidism, chronic pain, overexertion, or imbalances in diet and exercise.[30]

Clinical Presentation of Drowsiness and Fatigue

The subjective experience of sleepiness includes yawning, eye rubbing, a tendency to fall asleep, and decreased ability to focus and concentrate. Self-reported measures of sleepiness include the Stanford Sleepiness Scale and the Epworth Sleepiness Scale.[34]

Treatment of Drowsiness and Fatigue

Treatment Goals

The goal in treating daytime drowsiness and fatigue is to identify and eliminate the underlying cause to improve mental alertness and productivity. The algorithm in Figure 46–2 outlines the approach to self-treatment.

General Treatment Approach

Many consumers use dietary sources of caffeine to self-treat occasional symptoms of fatigue and drowsiness. Nonprescription caffeine-containing products may also be used. Caffeine as a supplement, or in dietary form, is not a substitute for adequate sleep. Before recommending any caffeine-containing nonprescription product, the HCP should rule out any drug-induced cause of daytime drowsiness and fatigue. If symptoms are chronic, especially with 7–8 hours of sleep, referral is indicated.

Nonpharmacologic Therapy

Good sleep hygiene principles should be emphasized (Table 46–3).

Pharmacologic Therapy

Caffeine is a nonselective adenosine antagonist at the A_1 and A_{2A} receptors. Adenosine acts centrally to promote sleep. Secondary effects on other neurotransmitters such as dopamine and acetylcholine may also increase alertness.[35]

Low–moderate caffeine doses increase arousal, decrease fatigue, and elevate mood; higher doses are associated with anxiety, nausea, jitteriness, and nervousness.[36] Caffeine possesses weak bronchodilatory action and stimulates the sympathetic nervous system. Moderate caffeine doses (250 mg) can cause a transient increase in heart rate and blood pressure.[37]

Caffeine is completely absorbed, reaching a peak concentration within 30–75 minutes. It is rapidly and widely distributed, with an almost immediate effect on alertness. Caffeine is metabolized in the liver by the CYP1A2 isoenzyme; the primary demethylated metabolite is paraxanthine, which predominantly exerts a sympathomimetic effect. Other active metabolites are theobromine and theophylline. Paraxanthine can accumulate with higher dosages and reduce the clearance of caffeine. The elimination half-life is 3–6 hours.[37]

Caffeine is the only FDA-approved nonprescription stimulant, and Table 46–7 lists selected trade-name products that contain caffeine. The labeled dosages of approved nonprescription supplements for adults and children 12 years of age and older is 100–200 mg every 3–4 hours as needed. Caffeine is marketed for occasional use to help restore mental alertness or wakefulness.[38]

Rapid tolerance to the effects of caffeine on the respiratory and cardiovascular systems is common. Habitual caffeine drinkers who routinely consume as little as 1–2 cups of coffee and abruptly

TABLE 46-7 **Selected Caffeine-Containing Products**

Trade Name	Caffeine Content (mg)
Nonprescription Caffeine-Only Products	
NoDoz Maximum Strength	200
Vivarin	200
Nonprescription Combination Products	
Excedrin Migraine Caplets	65
Midol Complete Caplets	60
Prescription Combination Products	
Cafergot	100
Fioricet	40
Fiorinal	40

Note: Information is not all inclusive. Products may have changed formulations or caffeine content since time of publication.

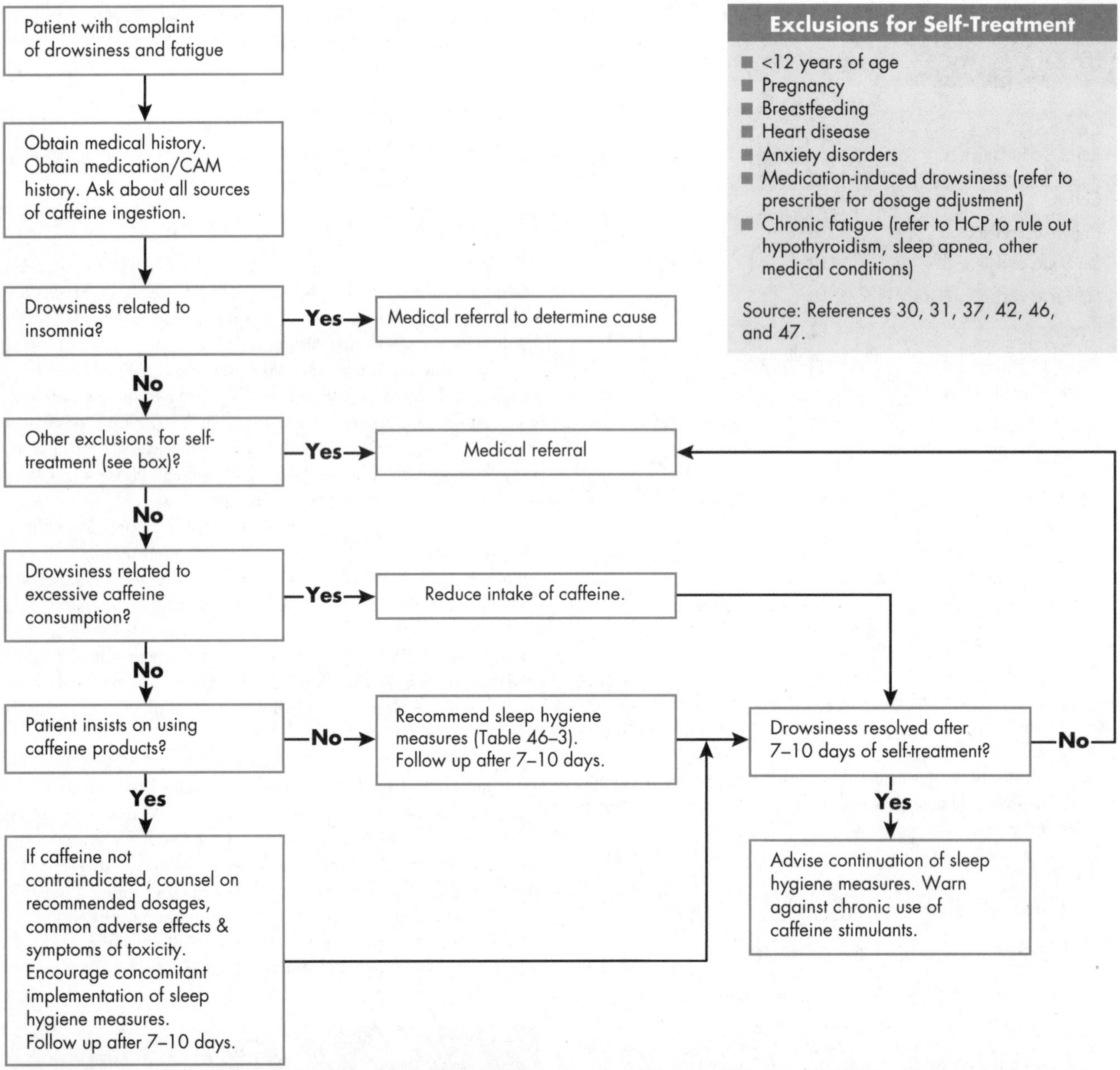

FIGURE 46–2 Self-care of drowsiness and fatigue. Key: CAM = Complementary and alternative medication; HCP = health care provider.

discontinue caffeine may experience mild signs and symptoms of withdrawal. Symptoms include headache, fatigue, decreased concentration, and irritability, starting within 12–24 hours after cessation and persisting for 1–5 days.[39]

An exaggerated pharmacologic effect can occur when nonprescription caffeine is combined with dietary sources, or with prescription or nonprescription medications that contain caffeine. Caffeine may increase the absorption of aspirin or reduce the clearance of theophylline to cause additive sympathetic effects such as an increased heart rate.

The CYP1A2 isoenzyme can be induced or inhibited by other drugs. The routine use of high dosages of caffeine (400 mg/day) could theoretically saturate the binding sites and increase the risk of interactions with drugs that share this metabolic pathway. Cigarette smoking increases the clearance of caffeine by 56%.[40] Individuals who are quitting smoking should be counseled to reduce their caffeine intake by half.[41] Conversely, hormonal contraceptives and ciprofloxacin can inhibit the CYP1A2 isoenzyme. The clinical significance of these interactions is unknown, but at-risk patients should be cautioned to moderate their use of caffeine. They should also be monitored for signs of such interactions.[36] Clinically significant drug interactions with caffeine are listed in Table 46–8.[42] Genetic polymorphisms at CYP1A2 and adenosine receptors may also influence response to caffeine.

Patients who take monoamine oxidase inhibitors or have existing coronary heart disease, uncontrolled hypertension, or preexisting arrhythmias should be counseled to avoid nonprescription caffeine-containing preparations and to moderate their intake of

TABLE 46–8 Clinically Significant Drug Interactions With Caffeine

Interacting Drugs or Drug Classes	Description	Monitoring Recommendation
Adenosine	Caffeine may diminish the therapeutic effect.	Monitor for decreased effect of adenosine if patient is receiving caffeine. Discontinue caffeine in advance of scheduled diagnostic use of adenosine whenever possible.
Atomoxetine	Atomoxetine may increase the hypertensive or tachycardic effect of caffeine.	Monitor therapy.
Cannabinoid-containing products	These products may increase the tachycardic effect of caffeine.	Monitor therapy.
Ciprofloxacin	Ciprofloxacin (oral) may increase serum concentration of caffeine.	Monitor therapy.
Linezolid	Linezolid may enhance the hypertensive effect of caffeine.	Reduce initial doses of caffeine, and closely monitor blood pressure.
Lithium	Caffeine may decrease the serum concentration of lithium.	Monitor therapy.
Norfloxacin	Norfloxacin may increase the serum concentration of caffeine.	Monitor therapy.
Tizanidine	Caffeine may increase the serum concentration of tizanidine.	Avoid combinations when possible. If combined use cannot be avoided, initiate tizanidine at 2 mg and increase in 2–4 mg increments based on patient response. Monitor for adverse reactions. Consider therapy modification.

Source: Reference 42.

dietary caffeine. The consumption of coffee increases blood pressure. An increase in systolic blood pressure by 2 mm Hg occurred after acute administration of caffeinated coffee for 1–12 weeks.[43] A small increase in blood pressure was demonstrated in healthy individuals and in patients with hypertension after chronic consumption of caffeine (4.2 mm Hg systolic; 2.4 mm Hg diastolic, respectively).[43]

When taken before sleep, caffeine delays sleep onset, reduces deep sleep, and increases nocturnal awakenings. After sleep deprivation, caffeine improved psychomotor performance, maintained alertness, and reduced fatigue.[39] In driving simulation tests, caffeine 200 mg was compared with placebo on driving performance and sleepiness during early morning hours.[44] After "restricted sleep," caffeine reduced early morning sleepiness for 2 hours; after "no sleep," caffeine delayed sleep by only 30 minutes. Patients should be counseled that caffeine cannot compensate for an inadequate amount of sleep.

The use of caffeinated coffee to counter the effects of excessive alcohol ingestion is a common practice. While the combination of energy drinks or caffeine with alcohol increased alertness and reduced alcohol-related fatigue, it failed to reverse alcohol-induced deficits on simple psychomotor tasks.[45] In 2010, FDA banned production of caffeinated alcoholic beverages secondary to safety concerns.[46]

Patients should be cautioned about excessive consumption of caffeine in weight-loss supplements and energy sports drinks. Natural caffeine, other methylxanthines, and caffeine-containing herbs such as guarana, green tea, yerba mate, and cola nut are common ingredients in products that are marketed to young consumers for energy or weight loss. The caffeine content often is not listed on the label of energy drinks.[47] Table 46–9 lists the amount of caffeine that is contained in both selected weight-loss dietary supplements and sports energy drinks.

TABLE 46–9 Caffeine Content in Selected Dietary Supplements and Energy Drinks

Trade Name	Caffeine Content per Serving (mg)
Dietary Supplements	
Dexatrim Max Daytime Appetite Control	200
Pro Clinical Hydroxycut[a]	200
Energy Drinks[b]	
Monster Energy	80[c]
Red Bull	80[d]
Rockstar Juiced	80[e]

Note: Information is not all inclusive. Products may have changed formulations or caffeine content since time of publication.

[a] Also contains calcium 145 mg, Hydroxycut Blend™ 441 mg (robusta coffee extract, papaya, blackberry, saffron extract, maqui, and amla extract).

[b] Caffeine content based on serving size sold.

[c] Also contains 1000 mg taurine, 200 mg Panax ginseng, and guarana seed extract.

[d] Also contains 1000 mg taurine.

[e] Also contains 1000 mg taurine, 25 mg Panax ginseng, and 25 mg guarana seed extract.

Product Selection Guidelines

Special Populations

Caffeine freely crosses the placenta.[47] The American College of Obstetricians and Gynecologists has concluded that moderate caffeine consumption (≤200 mg/day) does not contribute to miscarriages or preterm births.[48] Total daily caffeine intake should be limited to less than 200 mg during pregnancy. The American Academy of Pediatrics considers usual dietary amounts of caffeine compatible with breastfeeding.[49] Infants unable to metabolize caffeine or those who receive large quantities of caffeine through breast milk may have symptoms of nervousness, increased heart rate, sleeplessness, poor feeding, and irritability. Nursing women should consume caffeine only in small–moderate amounts (2–3 cups daily), preferably after breastfeeding to minimize effects on the infant.

Children are more susceptible to the cardiovascular and CNS adverse effects of caffeine because of their lower body weight. In one study of adolescents (ages 12–17 years), dosages of 50 mg, 100 mg, and 200 mg of caffeine per day significantly increased diastolic blood pressure.[50] Nonprescription caffeine products are not indicated in children younger than 12 years.

The elimination half-life of caffeine is prolonged in older adults, increasing their susceptibility to an exaggerated pharmacologic effect and interference with sleep.[42] Older adults should avoid consuming caffeine in the diet or as an ingredient in a medication after dinner.

Complementary Therapies

Ginseng is frequently used to boost physical and mental energy and a sense of well-being. A review of randomized controlled trials reveals contradictory scientific evidence to support these claims (see Chapter 51). Caffeine-containing dietary supplements that patients may be using include cola nut, guarana, and yerba mate. Ingredients purported to counteract fatigue that are often found in sports energy drinks include taurine and guarana, although the amounts are unlikely to produce either therapeutic or adverse effects.

Assessment of Drowsiness and Fatigue: A Case-Based Approach

When assessing a patient with a complaint of daytime drowsiness, the HCP should determine the cause of the patient's fatigue. Evaluating the patient's medical or psychiatric problems, current medication use, dietary caffeine consumption, sleep patterns, and lifestyle will help in determining the underlying cause. In light of the lack of data supporting the efficacy of caffeine and the adverse effects associated with recommended and excessive dosages, HCPs should recommend improved sleep hygiene and lifestyle modifications or medical referral before recommending the use of a caffeine-containing product.

Case 46–2 provides an example of the assessment of a patient with drowsiness and fatigue.

CASE 46-2

Relevant Evaluation Criteria	Scenario/Model Outcome
Collect	
1. Gather essential information about the patient's symptoms and medical history, including	
a. Description of symptom(s) (i.e., nature, onset, duration, severity, associated symptoms)	Patient requests advice on choosing an OTC product to improve her energy levels. She is tired upon awakening in the mornings, and the fatigue becomes progressively worse as the day goes on. Her roommate often has to wake her up during class and at night when she falls asleep on the couch.
b. Description of any factors that seem to precipitate, exacerbate, and/or relieve the patient's symptom(s)	She started graduate school a month ago and is extremely worried about her move to a new city and about passing graduate courses. Over the past 2 weeks she noticed a decrease in her ability to concentrate and having to re-read her notes several times to study and complete assignments. This has never happened before. Her muscles have also been tense. She was late for her part-time job as an interpreter last weekend, because she was so exhausted. The symptoms tend to worsen when she drinks wine.
c. Description of the patient's/caregiver's efforts to relieve the symptoms	The patient usually drinks 2 Starbucks Tall coffees daily and started purchasing 1–2 Red Bulls daily this past week.
d. Patient's identity	Amanda Mays
e. Patient's age, gender, height, and weight	25 years old, female, 5 ft 5 in., 136 lb
f. Patient's occupation	Graduate student
g. Patient's dietary habits	Normal diet. Usually drinks 2 medium cups of coffee daily and recently started drinking energy drinks.
h. Patient's sleep habits	Stays up late studying each evening; has trouble falling asleep and waking up in the mornings because she is tired.

CASE 46-2 *continued*

Relevant Evaluation Criteria	Scenario/Model Outcome
i. Concurrent medical conditions, prescription and nonprescription medications, and dietary supplements	Migraines: frovatriptan 2.5 mg as needed, may repeat in 2 hours (takes once every other month); generalized anxiety disorder: escitalopram 5 mg daily; no dietary supplements
j. Allergies	Tree nuts: hives, skin rash
k. History of other adverse reactions to medications	None
l. Other (describe) _______	n/a
Assess	
2. Differentiate patient's signs/symptoms, and correctly identify the patient's primary problem(s).	Daytime fatigue
3. Identify exclusions for self-treatment (Figure 46–2).	OTC stimulants should not be used in patients with anxiety disorders.
4. Formulate a comprehensive list of therapeutic alternatives for the primary problem to determine whether triage to a health care provider is required, and share this information with the patient or caregiver.	Options include (1) Refer Amanda to an appropriate HCP. (2) Recommend self-care with a nonprescription stimulant and nondrug measures. (3) Recommend self-care until Amanda can see an appropriate provider. (4) Take no action.
Plan	
5. Select an optimal therapeutic alternative to address the patient's problem, taking into account patient preferences.	Amanda should be referred to her HCP for evaluation of generalized anxiety disorder. Patient findings that suggest that the anxiety disorder is not optimally controlled include her daily worries, fatigue, inability to fall asleep and feeling tired upon awakening, muscle tension, and decreased concentration. Sleep hygiene education (Table 46-3) should be offered.
6. Describe the recommended therapeutic approach to the patient or caregiver.	"You should make an appointment to see your health care provider."
7. Explain to the patient or caregiver the rationale for selecting the recommended therapeutic approach from the considered therapeutic alternatives.	"Because this problem of fatigue may be caused by anxiety, you should make an appointment with your health care provider for a physical examination. Stimulant medication is not indicated at this time, because your provider will have to decide on the best method of treatment. Even before you see your health care provider, you should reduce your intake of energy drinks and coffee, and begin sleep hygiene measures."
Implement	
8. When recommending self-care with nonprescription medications and/or nondrug therapy, convey accurate information to the patient or caregiver.	Criterion does not apply to this case.
Solicit follow-up questions from the patient or caregiver.	"Can I use my roommate's Fioricet instead of the frovatriptan when I have a headache?"
Answer the patient's or caregiver's questions.	"It is never advisable to use medications prescribed for other people. Fioricet contains caffeine that may contribute to your symptoms of anxiety."
Follow-up: Monitor and Evaluate	
9. Assess patient outcome.	Contact the patient in 1–2 days to be sure that she made an appointment for medical care.

Key: HCP = Health care provider; n/a = not applicable; OTC = over-the-counter.

PATIENT EDUCATION FOR Drowsiness and Fatigue

The objective of self-treatment is to maintain wakefulness. For most patients, improved sleep hygiene will help ensure optimal therapeutic outcomes. If the patient insists on taking a caffeine-containing product, carefully following product instructions and the self-care measures listed here will help ensure optimal therapeutic outcomes for most patients.

Disease Information

- Symptoms of drowsiness and fatigue often include yawning, a tendency to fall asleep, and decreased ability to focus and concentrate.

Nondrug Measures

- Practice principles of good sleep hygiene (Table 46–3.)
- If drowsiness or fatigue persists or recurs, consult your health care provider.

Nonprescription Medications

- Do not exceed the recommended dose of 200 mg every 3–4 hours. Note that higher doses of caffeine may cause side effects and that chronic use may result in tolerance as well as withdrawal symptoms upon abrupt discontinuation.
- Do not use caffeine tablets in combination with coffee or other caffeinated products, including dietary supplements.
- Do not use if you are pregnant or breastfeeding.
- Do not use in children younger than 12 years.
- If you are taking atomoxetine or ciprofloxacin, consult your health care provider before using caffeine-containing products.
- If you have a history of peptic ulcer disease, psychiatric disorders, symptomatic heart disease, or uncontrolled hypertension, consult your health care provider before using caffeine products.

When to Seek Medical Attention

- Seek medical attention immediately if the following symptoms of caffeine toxicity occur at the same time:
  - Increases in heart rate and blood pressure
  - Headache
  - Symptoms of anxiety and insomnia
  - Increase in hand tremor

Patient Counseling for Drowsiness and Fatigue

Counseling on the treatment of drowsiness and fatigue should focus on practicing good sleep hygiene and eliminating factors that may interfere with normal sleep. If a caffeine product is indicated, the HCP should review dosage guidelines with the patient and emphasize the potential adverse effects and drug interactions. The patient should be counseled on symptoms of excessive caffeine ingestion, such as irritability, tremor, rapid pulse, dizziness, or heart palpitations. Regular users of caffeine should also be counseled on withdrawal symptoms such as headache and anxiety, which can occur if caffeine from any source is stopped abruptly. The box "Patient Education for Drowsiness and Fatigue" lists information to provide patients.

Evaluation of Patient Outcomes for Drowsiness and Fatigue

Successful outcomes include daytime alertness, increased productivity, and peak performance with respect to psychomotor tasks and cognitive function, including attention and concentration. An individual should seek medical evaluation if, after 7–10 days, drowsiness and fatigue persist despite the limited use of caffeine and the establishment of good sleep hygiene.

Key Points for Drowsiness and Fatigue

- ➤ Advise patients that caffeine appears to be safe and effective in low–moderate doses in the diet, as well as for occasional use as a nonprescription supplement during completion of tasks of short duration when enhanced alertness is desired.
- ➤ Instruct patients that caffeine is most effective when taken intermittently at dosages of 100 or 200 mg every 3–4 hours as needed.
- ➤ Pregnant or nursing women, children younger than 12 years, patients with heart disease, and patients with anxiety disorders should avoid caffeine.
- ➤ HCPs should be aware of the prescription and nonprescription medications and diet supplements that contain caffeine, as well as the patient's dietary consumption of caffeine.
- ➤ Adverse effects of caffeine are more likely to occur in occasional users and patients of advanced age.
- ➤ Advise patients taking higher daily dosages of caffeine that drug interactions can occur with some medications.
- ➤ Counsel patients that dietary supplements should not be used to increase energy or decrease fatigue.

REFERENCES

1. Schutte-Rodin S, Broch L, Buysse D, et al. Clinical guideline for the evaluation and management of chronic insomnia in adults. *J Clin Sleep Med.* 2008;4(5):487–504. PMID: 18853708.
2. National Sleep Foundation. 2009 Sleep in America Poll. Available at: http://www.sleepfoundation.org/article/sleep-america-polls/2009-health-and-safety. Accessed June 27, 2017.
3. Rosekind MR, Gregory KB. Insomnia risks and costs: health, safety, and quality of life. *Am J Manag Care.* 2010;16(8):617–26. PMID: 20712395.
4. Ozminkowski RJ, Wang S, Walsh JK. The direct and indirect costs of untreated insomnia in adults in the United States. *Sleep.* 2007;30(3): 263–73. PMID: 17425222.
5. Tariq SH, Pulisetty S. Pharmacotherapy for insomnia. *Clin Geriatr Med.* 2008;24:93–105.
6. Winkelman JW. Insomnia disorder. *N Engl J Med.* 2015;373(15):1437–44. doi: 10.1056/NEJMcp1412740.
7. Bloom HG, Ahmed I, Alessi CA, et al. Evidence-based recommendations for the assessment and management of sleep disorders in older persons. *J Am Geriatr Soc.* 2009;57(5):761–89. PMID: 19484833.
8. Morin AK, Jarvis CI, Lynch AM. Therapeutic options for sleep maintenance and sleep-onset insomnia. *Pharmacotherapy.* 2007;27(1):89–110. doi: 10.1592/phco.27.1.89.

9. Kraus SS, Rabin LA. Sleep America: managing the crisis of adult chronic insomnia and associated conditions. *J Affect Disord.* 2012;138(3):192–212. doi: 10.1016/j.jad.2011.05.014.
10. Qaseem A, Kansagara D, Forciea MA, et al. Management of chronic insomnia disorder in adults: a clinical practice guideline from the American College of Physicians. *Ann Intern Med.* 2016;165(2):125–33. doi: 10.7326/M15-2175.
11. Diphenhydramine. In: Gerald K. McEvoy, Pharm.D., ed. 2017. AHFS Drug Information. 59th ed. Bethesda, MD. American Society of Health-System Pharmacists. STAT!Ref Online Electronic Medical Library. Available at: http://online.statref.com/publictitleinfo/titleinfo.aspx?fxid=1. Accessed July 10, 2017.
12. Antihistamine drugs. In: Gerald K. McEvoy, PharmD, ed. AHFS Drug Information. 59th ed. STAT!Ref Online Electronic Medical Library. Bethesda, MD: American Society of Health-System Pharmacists: 2017. Available at: http://online.statref.com/publictitleinfo/titleinfo.aspx?fxid=1. Accessed July 10, 2017.
13. Doxylamine. In: Gerald K. McEvoy, PharmD, ed. AHFS Drug Information. 59th ed. STAT!Ref Online Electronic Medical Library. Bethesda, MD: American Society of Health-System Pharmacists; 2017. Available at: http://online.statref.com/publictitleinfo/titleinfo.aspx?fxid=1. Accessed July 10, 2017.
14. Culpepper L, Wingertzahn MA. Over-the-counter agents for the treatment of occasional disturbed sleep or transient insomnia: a systematic review of efficacy and safety. *Prim Care Companion CNS Disord.* 2015; 17(6). doi: 10.4088/PCC.
15. Sharma A, Pibarot P, Pilote S, et al. Toward optimal treatment in women: the effect of sex on metoprolol-diphenhydramine interaction. *J Clin Pharmacol.* 2010;50(2):214–25. doi: 10.1177/0091270009340417.
16. Diphenhydramine. Drug Facts and Comparisons. Facts & Comparisons [database online]. St. Louis, MO: Wolters Kluwer Health, Inc; May 2015. Available at: http://online.factsandcomparisons.com/. Accessed May 24, 2016.
17. Church MK, Maurer M, Simons FER, et al. Risk of first-generation H_1-antihistamines: a GA²LEN position paper. *Allergy.* 2010;65(4):459–66. doi: 10.1111/j.1398-9995.2009.02325.x.
18. Gray SL, Anderson ML, Dublin S, et al. Cumulative use of strong anticholinergics and incident dementia: a prospective cohort study. *JAMA Intern Med.* 2015;175(3):401–7. doi: 10.1001/jamainternmed.2014.7663.
19. Thomas A, Nallur DG, Jones N, et al. Diphenhydramine abuse and detoxification: a brief review and report. *J Psychopharmacol.* 2009;23(1): 101–5. doi: 10.1177/0269881107083809.
20. Tanda G, Kopajtic TA, Katz JL. Cocaine-like neurochemical effects of antihistaminic medications. *J Neurochem.* 2008;106(1):147–57. doi: 10.1111/j.1471-4159.2008.05361.x.
21. Vinson DC, Manning BK, Galligher JM, et al. Alcohol and sleep problems in primary care patients: a report from the AAFP National Research Network. *Ann Fam Med.* 2010;8(6):484–92. doi: 10.1370/afm.1175.
22. Roth T. Does effective management of sleep disorders reduce substance dependence? *Drugs.* 2009;69(Suppl 2):65–75. doi: 10.2165/11531120-000000000-00000.
23. Morin CM, Koetter U, Bastien C, et al. Valerian-hops combination and diphenhydramine for treating insomnia. *Sleep.* 2005;28(11):1465–71. PMID: 16335333.
24. Diphenhydramine. U.S. National Library of Medicine, Toxicology Data Network, LactMed database. Available at: http://toxnet.nlm.nih.gov. Accessed July 10, 2017.
25. The American Geriatrics Society. American Geriatrics Society 2015 Updated Beers Criteria for potentially inappropriate medication use in older adults. *J Am Geriatr Soc.* 2015;63(11):2227–46. doi: 10.1111/jgs.13702.
26. Zisapel N. Drugs for insomnia. *Expert Opin Emerg Drugs.* 2012;17(3): 299–317. doi: 10.1517/14728214.2012.690735.
27. Taibi DM, Landis CA, Petry H, et al. A systematic review of valerian as a sleep aid: safe but not effective. *Sleep Med Rev.* 2007;11(3):209–30. doi: 10.1016/j.smrv.2007.03.002.
28. Kava. National Center for Complementary and Integrative Health. Available at: https://nccih.nih.gov/. Accessed July 10, 2017.
29. American Academy of Sleep Medicine. AASM position statement: treating insomnia with herbal supplements. Available at: http://www.aasmnet.org/Articles.aspx?id=254. Accessed June 27, 2017.
30. Schwartz JRL, Roth T, Hirshkowitz M, et al. Recognition and management of excessive sleepiness in the primary care setting. *Prim Care Companion J Clin Psychiatry.* 2009;11(5):197–204. doi: 10.4088/PCC.07r00545.
31. Martiniuk AL, Senserrick T, Lo S, et al. Sleep-deprived young drivers and the risk for crash: the DRIVE Prospective Cohort Study. *JAMA Pediatr.* 2013;167(7):647–55. doi: 10.1001/jamapediatrics.2013.1429.
32. Drewnowski A, Rehm CD. Sources of caffeine in diets of US children and adults: trends by beverage type and purchase location. *Nutrients.* 2016 Mar 10;8(3):E154. doi:10.3390/nu8030154.
33. Silver R, LeSauter J. Circadian and homeostatic factors in arousal. *Ann NY Acad Sci.* 2008;1129:263–74. doi: 10.1196/annals.1417.032.
34. Task Force for the Handbook of Psychiatric Measures. *Handbook of Psychiatric Measures.* Washington, DC: American Psychiatric Association; 2000:682–5.
35. Ferré S. An update on the mechanisms of the psychostimulant effects of caffeine. *J Neurochem.* 2008;105(4):1067–79. doi: 10.1111/j.1471-4159.2007.05196.x.
36. Yang A, Palmer AA, de Wit H. Genetics of caffeine consumption and responses to caffeine. *Psychopharmacol.* 2010;211(3):245–57. doi: 10.1007/s00213-010-1900-1.
37. Roehrs T, Roth T. Caffeine: sleep and daytime sleepiness. *Sleep Med Rev.* 2008;12(2):153–62. doi: 10.1016/j.smrv.2007.07.004.
38. U.S. Food and Drug Administration. Stimulant drug products for over-the-counter human use. CFR: Code of Federal Regulations. Title 21, Part 340, Section 340.50. Revised April 1, 2010. Available at: http://www.accessdata.fda.gov/scripts/cdrh/cfdocs/cfcfr/cfrsearch.cfm?fr=340.50. Accessed June 27, 2017.
39. Snel J, Lorist MM. Effects of caffeine on sleep and cognition. In: Van Dongen HPA, Kerkhof GA, eds. *Progress in Brain Research.* Vo.l 190. London: Elsevier; 2011;105–17.
40. Drug interactions with tobacco smoke. Rx For Change. Available at: https://smokingcessationleadership.ucsf.edu/sites/smokingcessation leadership.ucsf.edu/files/Drug-Interactions-with-Tobacco-Smoke.pdf. Accessed June 27, 2017.
41. Kroon LA. Drug interactions with smoking. *Am J Health-System Pharm.* 2007;64(18):1917–21. doi: 10.2146/ajhp060414
42. Caffeine. Drug Facts and Comparisons. Facts & Comparisons [database online]. St. Louis, MO: Wolters Kluwer Health, Inc; May 2015. Available at: http://fco.factsandcomparisons.com/action/home. Accessed May 24, 2016.
43. Higdon JV, Frei B. Coffee and health: a review of recent human research. *Crit Rev Food Sci Nutr.* 2006;46(2):101–23. doi: 10.1080/104083905 00400009.
44. Reyner LA, Horne JA. Early morning driver sleepiness: effectiveness of 200 mg caffeine. *Psychophysiology.* 2000;37(2):251–6. PMID:10731775.
45. McKetin R, Coen A, Kaye S. A comprehensive review of the effects of mixing caffeinated energy drinks with alcohol. *Drug Alcohol Depend.* 2015;151:15–30. doi: 10.1016/j.drugalcdep.2015.01.047.
46. U.S. Food and Drug Administration. Update on caffeinated alcoholic beverages. FDA announces progress on removal of certain caffeinated alcoholic beverages from the market. November 24, 2010. Available at: http://www.fda.gov/NewsEvents/PublicHealthFocus/ucm234900.htm. Accessed June 27, 2017.
47. Caffeine. Drug Monograph. ClinicalKey. Available at: https://www.clinical key.com. Accessed May 18, 2017.
48. American College of Obstetricians and Gynecologists Committee on Obstetric Care. Moderate caffeine consumption during pregnancy. *Obstet Gynecol.* 2010;116(2 Pt 1):467–8. doi: 10.1097/AOG.0b013e3181eeb2a1.
49. American Academy of Pediatrics Committee on Drugs. The transfer of drugs and other chemicals into human milk. *Pediatrics.* 2001;108:776–89. PMID: 11533352.
50. Temple JL, Dewey AM, Briatico LN. Effects of acute caffeine administration on adolescents. *Exp Clin Psychopharmacol.* 2010;18(6):510–20. doi: 10.1037/a0021651.

CHAPTER 47

TOBACCO CESSATION

BETH A. MARTIN AND MARIA C. WOPAT

In 1982, the U.S. Surgeon General C. Everett Koop stated that cigarette smoking was the "chief, single, avoidable cause of death in our society and the most important public health issue of our time."[1] This statement remains true more than 3 decades later. In the United States, cigarette smoking is the leading known cause of preventable death,[2] responsible for an estimated 480,000 deaths each year.[3] In addition to lives lost, the economic impact of smoking is enormous, costing society approximately $300 billion annually for smoking-attributable health expenditures and lost productivity.[3]

The negative effects of smoking are both well established and well publicized, yet according to recent data reported over the period 2009–2014, an estimated 40.0 million adult Americans (16.8% of the overall population in 2014—18.8% of males and 14.8% of females) smoked either every day (76.8%) or some days (23.2%).[4] The prevalence of smoking varies in accordance with sociodemographic factors including gender, race/ethnicity, education level, age, and socioeconomic status. The prevalence of smoking in the United States was highest among non-Hispanic American Indians/Alaska Natives (29.2%) and lowest among non-Hispanic Asians (9.5%). Smoking is more common among people ages 25–44 years (20.0%) and those living below the federal poverty level (26.3%).[4] Smoking is also more prevalent for those with less than a post-secondary education, ranging from high school graduates (21.7%) to those who have completed a General Educational Development test (43.0%).[4] The median prevalence of smoking varies by state, with Utah exhibiting the lowest prevalence at 10.3% and West Virginia exhibiting the highest at 27.3%.[5] The concurrent use of cigarettes and smokeless tobacco is lowest in Vermont at 3.1% and as high as 13.5% in Idaho.[5] Smoking prevalence differs in patients with various medical conditions, with the highest rates among patients with mental illness. Thirty-six percent of patients with mental health conditions smoke cigarettes, and this group consumed approximately one-third of all cigarettes sold in the United States during 2009–2011.[6]

Despite tobacco control efforts at the state and national levels and a rate decline in the United States since 2010 to a national average below 20%,[4] tobacco use is a public health issue of great importance, and only Utah has met the *Healthy People 2020* target goal of a 12% or lower prevalence of smoking.[7] Worldwide, nearly 6 million deaths attributable to tobacco occur annually; unless tobacco control efforts are able to reverse this trend, the number of annual deaths is likely to exceed 8 million by 2030.[8]

Pathophysiology of Tobacco Use and Dependence

In 1988, the U.S. Surgeon General released a landmark report concluding that tobacco products are effective nicotine delivery systems capable of inducing and sustaining chemical dependence.[9] The primary criteria used to categorize nicotine as an addictive substance were its (1) psychoactive effects, (2) use in a highly controlled or compulsive manner, and (3) reinforcement of behavioral patterns of tobacco use. The underlying pharmacologic and behavioral processes associated with tobacco dependence are considered to be similar to those that determine addiction to drugs such as heroin and cocaine.[9]

As with other addictive substances (e.g., opiates, cocaine, amphetamines), nicotine stimulates the mesolimbic dopaminergic system in the midbrain, inducing pleasant or rewarding effects that promote continued use.[10] This effect is also known as the dopamine reward pathway. Nicotine binds to the alpha$_4$beta$_2$ nicotinic cholinergic receptors in the ventral tegmental area of the brain, triggering the release of dopamine in the nucleus accumbens. Psychosocial, behavioral, genetic, and environmental factors also play an important role in establishing and maintaining dependence.[10,11] For example, smoking commonly is associated with specific activities such as driving, talking on the telephone, eating, drinking coffee or alcohol, and being around others who smoke. Over time, the habitual use of cigarettes under these circumstances can lead to the development of smoking routines that can be difficult to break. Indeed, specific environmental situations can become powerful conditioned stimuli or cues associated with smoking and are capable of triggering "automatic" smoking patterns.[10]

Tobacco use dramatically increases one's odds of dependence, disease, disability, and death. Cigarettes are carefully engineered and heavily marketed products. For example, although the design of cigarettes and other tobacco products has evolved over the past five decades (e.g., filtered, menthol, low-tar, "light" cigarettes; e-cigarettes; dissolvable tobacco), overall disease risk has not been reduced among smokers.[11] The tobacco industry spends nearly $20 to market its products for every $1 that states spend on tobacco control.[12] Cigarettes are the *only* marketed consumable product that, when used persistently, will kill half or more of its users.[13]

Cigarette smoke, which is classified by the Environmental Protection Agency (EPA) as a Class A carcinogen (i.e., a carcinogen with no safe level of exposure for humans), is a complex mixture of thousands of compounds—including nitrogen, carbon monoxide, ammonia, hydrogen cyanide, benzene, and nicotine—in gaseous and particulate phases. The particulate fraction, excluding the nicotine and water components, is collectively referred to as tar. Numerous carcinogens, including polycyclic aromatic hydrocarbons (PAHs) and nitrosamines, have been identified in the tar fraction of tobacco smoke.[11,14]

Nicotine, the addictive component of tobacco, is distilled from burning tobacco and carried in tar droplets to the small airways of the lung, where it is absorbed rapidly into the arterial circulation and distributed throughout the body. Nicotine readily penetrates the central nervous system and is estimated to reach the brain within seconds after inhalation.[15] Nicotine binds to receptors in the brain and other organs, inducing a variety of predominantly stimulatory effects on the cardiovascular, endocrine, nervous, and metabolic systems.[10,16] Pharmacodynamic effects associated with nicotine administration include arousal and increases in the heart rate and blood pressure. In the brain, smoking leads to the activation of nicotinic cholinergic receptors and release of numerous neurotransmitters, which induce a range of effects such as pleasure (dopamine), arousal (acetylcholine and norepinephrine), cognitive enhancement (acetylcholine), appetite suppression (dopamine, norepinephrine, and serotonin), learning and memory enhancement (glutamate), mood modulation (serotonin), and reduction of anxiety and tension (beta-endorphin and gamma-aminobutyric acid).[10,11,15]

Clinical Presentation of Tobacco Use and Dependence

Most chronic tobacco users develop tolerance to the effects of nicotine, and abrupt cessation precipitates symptoms of nicotine withdrawal.[10] The symptoms and their severity vary from person to person but generally include irritability, frustration, anger, anxiety, depression, difficulty concentrating, impatience, insomnia, and restlessness.[17,18] Other symptoms that patients may report include cravings, impaired performance, constipation, cough, dizziness, and increased dreaming. Typically, the physiologic nicotine withdrawal symptoms manifest within the first 1–2 days, peak within the first week, and gradually dissipate over 2–4 weeks.[18] Increased appetite and weight gain may persist for 6 or more months after quitting.[17]

According to reports issued by the U.S. Surgeon General in 2004,[2] 2010,[11] and 2014,[3] smoking adversely affects nearly every organ system in the body and plays a causal role in the development of numerous diseases, including many cancers (Table 47–1). Furthermore, smoking cigarettes with lower machine-measured yields of tar and nicotine provides no clear benefit to health. Involuntary exposure to secondhand smoke, which includes the smoke emanating from a cigarette and that exhaled by the smoker, is associated with adverse health effects in nonsmokers, including cardiovascular disease, respiratory disease, and lung cancer.[19] Even low levels of exposure, such as secondhand smoke exposure, are associated with rapid increases in endothelial dysfunction and inflammation, which lead to acute cardiovascular events and thrombosis.[11] In children, secondhand smoke exposure can increase the risk of ear infections, precipitate more frequent and severe asthma attacks, worsen respiratory symptoms (e.g., coughing, sneezing, shortness of breath), increase the risk of respiratory infections, and increase the risk for sudden infant death syndrome (SIDS).[19] There is no risk-free level of exposure to tobacco smoke.[11,20]

Tobacco smoke interacts with medications through pharmacokinetic or pharmacodynamic mechanisms that can lead to reduced therapeutic efficacy or, less commonly, increased toxicity. Most of the pharmacokinetic interactions are the result of induction of hepatic cytochrome P450 (CYP) enzymes (primarily the CYP1A2 isoenzyme) by PAHs present in tobacco smoke.[21] Induction of the CYP1A2 isoenzyme can increase the hepatic metabolism of certain drugs (Table 47–2), potentially resulting in a reduced therapeutic response or a need for higher dosages in smokers; conversely, the dosages of some drugs might need to be reduced in patients who quit smoking.[21] Similarly, the clearance of caffeine is significantly increased (by 56%) in smokers. After cessation, ex-smokers who drink caffeinated beverages should be advised to decrease their usual caffeine intake, to avoid higher levels of caffeine, which may induce symptoms similar to nicotine withdrawal.

A significant pharmacodynamic drug interaction occurs with tobacco smoke and combination hormonal contraceptives (pills, patch, ring). Data indicate that cigarette smoking substantially increases the risk of serious adverse cardiovascular events (e.g., stroke, myocardial infarction, thromboembolism) in women using oral contraceptives.[22–26] This risk is markedly increased in women 35 years of age or older who smoke 15 or more cigarettes per day.[22] Accordingly, most experts consider use of hormonal contraceptives to be a contraindication in smokers and recommend use of an alternative form of contraception.[23,26] Additional interactions, with their corresponding underlying mechanisms, are provided in Table 47–2.[21,27] During the course of routine patient care, it is important to assess for potential drug and smoking interactions and to make appropriate adjustments to the medication regimen.

Smoking Cessation Treatment

The 1990 Surgeon General's Report on the health benefits of smoking cessation outlined the numerous and substantial health benefits realized when patients quit smoking.[28] Some health benefits are incurred shortly after quitting (e.g., within 2 weeks–3 months), and others are incurred over time (Figure 47–1). On average, cigarette smokers die approximately 10 years earlier than nonsmokers; among those who continue smoking, at least half will eventually die of a tobacco-related disease. Quitting at the ages of 30, 40, 50, and 60 years results in a gain of 10, 9, 6, and 3 years of life, respectively.[3,13] Consequently, although it is important to educate tobacco users that it is never too late to quit to achieve many of the associated health benefits, significant benefits to quitting earlier in life should be emphasized as well.

Treatment Goals

Tobacco dependence is a chronic disease typically characterized by multiple failed attempts to quit before long-term cessation is achieved. Because tobacco use is a complex, addictive behavior, helping patients quit and preventing relapse are best achieved by combining appropriate pharmacotherapy with counseling.[29] For any patient who uses tobacco, the primary goal is complete, long-term abstinence from all nicotine-containing products.

General Treatment Approach

Most smokers use no cessation treatments for their quit attempts, an approach known as quitting "cold turkey,"[30] and approximately 95% of all attempts to quit using this method end in relapse.[29] Yet decades of research clearly show that patients who receive assistance have increased odds of quitting. In 2008, the U.S. Public Health Service published an updated clinical practice guideline for treating tobacco use and dependence[29] that presents evidence-based recommendations and effective strategies for HCPs who provide tobacco cessation counseling. Although even brief advice from a provider is associated with increased odds of quitting,[29,31] more

TABLE 47-1 Health Consequences of Smoking

Cancer

Acute myeloid leukemia
Bladder
Breast
Cervical
Colorectal
Esophageal
Gastric
Kidney
Laryngeal
Liver
Lung
Oral cavity and pharyngeal
Pancreatic
Prostate

Cardiovascular Diseases

Abdominal aortic aneurysm
Coronary heart disease—e.g., angina pectoris, ischemic heart disease, myocardial infarction
Cerebrovascular disease—e.g., transient ischemic attacks, stroke
Peripheral arterial disease

Pulmonary Diseases

Acute respiratory illnesses
- Upper respiratory tract disease—e.g., rhinitis, sinusitis, laryngitis, pharyngitis
- Lower respiratory tract disease—e.g., bronchitis, pneumonia

Chronic respiratory illnesses
- Chronic obstructive pulmonary disease
- Respiratory symptoms
- Exacerbation of asthma
- Reduced lung function
- Tuberculosis

Reproductive Effects

Reduced fertility in women
Pregnancy and pregnancy outcomes
- Premature rupture of membranes
- Placenta previa
- Placental abruption
- Preterm delivery
- Low infant birth weight
- Ectopic pregnancy
- Infant mortality
- Sudden infant death syndrome (SIDS)
- Erectile dysfunction

Ophthalmic Effects

Cataract
Neovascular and atrophic forms of age-related macular degeneration

Other Effects

Diabetes (30%–40% higher risk for active smokers, with a dose-response relationship between the number of cigarettes smoked and this risk)
Osteoporosis (reduced bone density in postmenopausal women, with increased risk of hip fracture)
Periodontitis
Peptic ulcer disease (in patients infected with *Helicobacter pylori*)
Rheumatoid arthritis
Surgical outcomes—suboptimal
- Poor wound healing
- Respiratory complications

Source: References 2, 3, and 11.

intensive counseling (longer and more frequent counseling sessions, or greater overall contact time) and use of pharmacotherapy (except in patients with exclusions for self-treatment with medications, as listed in Figure 47–2) result in increased quit rates. Two particularly effective types of counseling are practical counseling (behavior change counseling, including problem-solving and skills training) and social support delivered as part of treatment.[29]

Patients who receive a tobacco cessation intervention from a provider, either nonphysician or physician, are 1.7 or 2.2 times, respectively, more likely to quit (and remain tobacco free at >5 months after cessation), respectively, than are patients who do not receive a provider's intervention.[29] Self-help materials are only slightly better than no provider intervention. Although the length of an intervention increases effectiveness, even minimal interventions (<3 minutes) increase cessation rates.[29] In a meta-analysis of 46 studies, four or more intervention sessions were found to approximately double cessation rates.[29]

Although the use of pharmacotherapy substantially increases patients' chances of quitting, the addition of counseling further increases cessation rates (by a factor of 1.4).[29] Similarly, adding pharmacotherapy to counseling increases cessation rates. Cessation interventions should therefore consist of pharmacotherapy (one or a combination of medications) and counseling, when medications are not contraindicated (see later under "Special Populations").[29] Figure 47–2 outlines a self-treatment approach for tobacco cessation.

Nonpharmacologic Therapy

Helping Patients Quit: The 5 A's Approach (Comprehensive Counseling)

As delineated in the U.S. Public Health Service Clinical Practice Guideline for Treating Tobacco Use and Dependence,[29] the five

TABLE 47-2 **Drug Interactions With Tobacco Smoke**

Drug/Class (Trade Name)	Mechanism of Interaction and Effects
Pharmacokinetic Interactions	
Alprazolam (Xanax)	Conflicting data on significance, but possible decreased plasma concentrations (up to 50%); decreased half-life (35%).
Bendamustine (Treanda)[a]	Metabolized by CYP1A2. Manufacturer recommends using with caution in smokers owing to likely decreased bendamustine concentrations, with increased concentrations of its two active metabolites.
Caffeine[a]	Increased metabolism (induction of CYP1A2); increased clearance (56%). Caffeine levels are likely increased after cessation.
Chlorpromazine (Thorazine)	Decreased AUC (36%) and serum concentrations (24%).
	Decreased sedation and hypotension possible in smokers; smokers may require increased dosages.
Clopidogrel (Plavix)[a]	Increased metabolism (induction of CYP1A2) of clopidogrel to its active metabolite.
	Clopidogrel's effects are enhanced in smokers (≥10 cigarettes/day): significant increased platelet inhibition, decreased platelet aggregation. Although improved clinical outcomes have been shown, risk of bleeding may also be increased.
Clozapine (Clozaril)[a]	Increased metabolism (induction of CYP1A2); decreased plasma concentrations (18%).
	Increased levels may occur upon cessation; closely monitor drug levels and reduce dose as required to avoid toxicity.
Erlotinib (Tarceva)[a]	Increased clearance (24%); decreased trough serum concentrations (twofold).
Flecainide (Tambocor)	Increased clearance (61%); decreased trough serum concentrations (25%). Smokers may need increased dosages.
Fluvoxamine (Luvox)[a]	Increased metabolism (induction of CYP1A2); increased clearance (24%); decreased AUC (31%); decreased plasma concentrations (32%).
	Dosage modifications are not routinely recommended, but smokers may need increased dosages.
Haloperidol (Haldol)[a]	Increased clearance (44%); decreased serum concentrations (70%).
Heparin	Mechanism unknown but increased clearance and decreased half-life are observed. Smoking has prothrombotic effects.
	Smokers may need increased dosages owing to PK and PD interactions.
Insulin, subcutaneous	Possible decreased insulin absorption secondary to peripheral vasoconstriction; smoking may cause release of endogenous substances that cause insulin resistance.
	PK and PD interactions are likely not clinically significant; smokers may need increased dosages and should monitor blood sugar closely.
Irinotecan (Camptosar)[a]	Increased clearance (18%); decreased serum concentrations of active metabolite, SN-38 (~40%), via induction of glucuronidation; decreased systemic exposure resulting in lower hematologic toxicity; may reduce efficacy.
	Smokers may need increased dosages.
Methadone	Possible increased metabolism (induction of CYP1A2, a minor pathway for methadone).
	Carefully monitor response upon cessation.
Mexiletine (Mexitil)	Increased clearance (25%; via oxidation and glucuronidation); decreased half-life (36%).
Olanzapine (Zyprexa)[a]	Increased metabolism (induction of CYP1A2); increased clearance (98%).
	Dosage modifications are not routinely recommended, but smokers may need increased dosages.
Propranolol (Inderal)	Increased clearance (77%), via side chain oxidation and glucuronidation.
Riociguat (Adempas)[a]	Increased metabolism (induction of CYP1A1, a major pathway for riociguat); decreased plasma concentrations (by 50%–60%)
	Smokers may require dosages higher than 2.5 mg 3 times a day; consider dose reduction upon cessation.
Ropinirole (Requip)[a]	Decreased maximum concentration (30%) and AUC (38%) in study with patients with restless legs syndrome.
	Smokers may need increased dosages.

TABLE 47-2 Drug Interactions With Tobacco Smoke *(continued)*

Drug/Class (Trade Name)	Mechanism of Interaction and Effects
Tacrine (Cognex)[a]	Increased metabolism (induction of CYP1A2); decreased half-life (50%); serum concentrations threefold lower.
	Smokers may need increased dosages.
Tasimelteon (Hetlioz)[a]	Increased metabolism (induction of CYP1A2); drug exposure decreased by 40%.
	Smokers may need increased dosages.
Theophylline[a]	Increased metabolism (induction of CYP1A2); increased clearance (58%–100%); decreased half-life (63%).
	Levels should be monitored if smoking is initiated, discontinued, or changed. Maintenance doses are considerably higher in smokers.
	Increased clearance with secondhand smoke exposure.
Tizanidine (Zanaflex)	Decreased AUC (30%–40%) and decreased half-life (10%) observed in male smokers.
Tricyclic antidepressants (e.g., imipramine, nortriptyline)	Possible interaction with tricyclic antidepressants in the direction of decreased blood levels, but the clinical significance is not established.
Warfarin	Increased metabolism (induction of CYP1A2) of R-enantiomer; however, S-enantiomer is more potent, and the effect on the international normalized ratio (INR) is inconclusive. Consider monitoring INR more closely upon smoking cessation.
Pharmacodynamic Interactions	
Benzodiazepines (diazepam, chlordiazepoxide)	Decreased sedation and drowsiness, possibly caused by nicotine stimulation of central nervous system.
Beta blockers	Less effective antihypertensive and heart rate control effects, possibly caused by nicotine-mediated sympathetic activation.
	Smokers may need increased dosages.
Corticosteroids, inhaled[a]	Smokers with asthma may have less of a response to inhaled corticosteroids.
Hormonal contraceptives[a]	Increased risk of cardiovascular adverse effects (e.g., stroke, myocardial infarction, thromboembolism) in women who smoke and use oral contraceptives. Ortho Evra patch users have twofold increased risk of venous thromboembolism compared with oral contraceptive users, likely owing to increased estrogen exposure (60% higher levels).
	Increased risk with age and with heavy smoking (≥15 cigarettes per day) that is quite marked in women ≥35 years of age
Serotonin 5-HT_1 receptor agonists (triptans)	This class of drugs may cause coronary vasospasm; caution is indicated for use in smokers owing to possible unrecognized CAD.

Key: AUC = Area under the curve; CAD = coronary artery disease; HT_1 = hydroxytryptamine (receptor) class 1; PD = pharmacodynamic; PK = pharmacokinetic.

Note: Many interactions between tobacco smoke and medications have been identified. In most cases, the tobacco smoke—not the nicotine—causes these drug interactions. Tobacco smoke interacts with medications through PK and PD mechanisms. PK interactions affect the absorption, distribution, metabolism, or elimination of other drugs, potentially causing an altered pharmacologic response. A majority of PK interactions with smoking are the result of induction of hepatic cytochrome P450 enzymes (primarily CYP1A2). PD interactions alter the expected response or actions of other drugs. The amount of tobacco smoking necessary to have an effect has not been established, and the assumption is that any smoker is susceptible to the same degree of interaction. Those exposed regularly to secondhand smoke may also be at risk.

[a] Clinically significant interaction.

Source: Reproduced with permission from Rx for Change: Clinician-Assisted Tobacco Cessation program. The Regents of the University of California. Copyright © 1999–2015.

key components of comprehensive counseling for tobacco cessation are (1) asking patients whether they use tobacco, (2) advising tobacco users to quit, (3) assessing patients' readiness to quit, (4) assisting patients with quitting, and (5) arranging follow-up care. These steps are referred to as the "5 A's."[29]

Ask About Tobacco Use

A key first step in the cessation process, and in all patient interactions, is asking about tobacco use. Because tobacco use is the primary known preventable cause of mortality in the United States, and because tobacco smoke interacts with multiple medications, screening for tobacco use is crucial and should be a routine component of care. The following question can be used to identify all types of tobacco use, even for infrequent users: "Do you ever smoke or use any type of tobacco?" In clinic or hospital settings, tobacco use status should be considered a component of vital sign assessment and collected routinely, along with blood pressure, pulse, weight, temperature, and respiratory rate.[29] In community pharmacies, tobacco use status should be assessed, documented

TIME ELAPSED

- **20 minutes after quitting:** Blood pressure drops to a level close to that before the last cigarette. Temperature of hands and feet increases to normal.
- **8 hours after quitting:** Blood levels of carbon monoxide drop to normal.
- **24 hours after quitting:** Chance of having a heart attack decreases.
- **2 weeks to 3 months after quitting:** Circulation improves, and lung function improves by up to 30%.
- **1 to 9 months after quitting:** Coughing, sinus congestion, fatigue, and shortness of breath decrease, and cilia regain normal function in the lungs, increasing the ability to handle mucus, clear the lungs, and reduce infection.
- **1 year after quitting:** Excessive risk of coronary heart disease is half that of a smoker's.
- **5 years after quitting:** Risk of stroke is reduced to that of a nonsmoker 5 to 15 years after quitting.
- **10 years after quitting:** Lung cancer death rate is about half that of continuing smokers. Risk of cancer of the mouth, throat, esophagus, bladder, kidney, and pancreas are also lower than that of continuing smokers.
- **15 years after quitting:** Risk of coronary heart disease is similar to that of a nonsmoker.

FIGURE **47-1** Health benefits of smoking cessation. (Source: References 2, 3, and 11.)

in the patient profile, and reassessed periodically. Asking about exposure to secondhand smoke should also be considered.

Advise to Quit

All tobacco users should be advised to quit. The advice should be clear, strong, and personalized, yet delivered with sensitivity and in a tone of voice that communicates concern for the patient and a willingness to provide appropriate assistance with quitting when the patient is ready. When possible, primary care providers should individualize the message by linking their advice to the patient's health status, current medication regimen, personal reasons for wanting to quit, or the effect of tobacco on others. The following example highlights this approach: "Ms. Bettis, I see that you now are on two different inhalers for your emphysema. Quitting smoking is the single most important treatment for your emphysema and can improve how well your inhalers work. I strongly encourage you to quit, and I would like to help you."

Assess Readiness to Quit

Because many patients will not be ready to quit when they are first approached, it is important for providers to gauge each patient's readiness to quit before recommending a treatment regimen. Patients should be categorized as (1) not ready to quit in the next month; (2) ready to quit in the next month; (3) a recent quitter, having quit in the past 6 months; or (4) a former user, having quit more than 6 months ago.[29] This classification defines the provider's next course of action, which is to provide counseling that is tailored to the patient's readiness to quit. The following approach is an example for a current smoker: "Mr. Crosby, what are your thoughts about quitting? Is this something that you might consider doing in the next month?" Counseling a patient who is ready to quit in the next month should differ from counseling a patient who is not considering quitting in the near future.

Assist With Quitting

Important elements of the assisting component of treatment include (1) helping patients to make the decision to quit and (2) setting a quit date. Providers should be empathetic and acknowledge that quitting is a challenge for most patients. Accordingly, the goal is to help maximize each patient's chances of success by designing an individualized treatment plan.

All patients attempting to quit should be encouraged to use pharmacotherapy combined with counseling. This combination will yield higher quit rates than either approach alone, except in special circumstances or in specific populations for which adequate evidence of the combined method's effectiveness is lacking (pregnant women, smokeless tobacco users, people who smoke fewer than 10 cigarettes per day, and adolescents).[29] Counseling interventions, which focus on promoting behavior change and enhancing adherence with medication regimens, may include individualized counseling (e.g., in person or by telephone), a group cessation program, an internet-based program, or a combination of these approaches.

Arrange Follow-up Counseling

Because the patient's ability to quit increases substantially when multiple counseling interactions are provided, arranging follow-up counseling is an important, yet typically neglected, element of treatment for tobacco dependence. Follow-up contact should occur soon after the quit date, preferably during the first week. Follow-up does not have to be done in person and could be performed by telephone or e-mail. A second follow-up contact is recommended within the first month after quitting.[29] Additional follow-up contacts should occur periodically to monitor patient progress (including adherence to pharmacotherapy regimens) and to provide ongoing support. Quit rates at 5 or more months after cessation are positively associated with the total number of person-to-person encounters (both individual and group): 12.4% for 0–1 contact, 16.3% for 2–3 contacts, 20.9% for 4–8 contacts, and 24.7% for more than 8 contacts.[29] A dose-response relationship has also been seen for length of contact.[29]

Counseling Interventions for Quitting

In providing counseling for quitting smoking, the goal is to facilitate the process of change by helping to ready the patient for permanent cessation. It is important to convey the view of quitting as a learning process that might take months or even years to achieve, rather than as a now-or-never event.

Counseling Patients Who Are Not Ready to Quit: Ongoing Assessment and the 5 R's

In counseling patients who are not ready to quit, an important first step is to encourage the patient to start thinking about quitting and to consider making a commitment to quit sometime in the foreseeable future. Sometimes patients who are not ready truly do not understand the need to quit. In general, most smokers will recognize the need to quit but are not yet ready to make the commitment to quit. Many patients will have tried to quit multiple times and relapsed; thus, they might feel too discouraged to try again.

Strategies for working with patients who are not ready to quit include increasing patient awareness of the available treatment options, having patients identify their reasons for smoking and

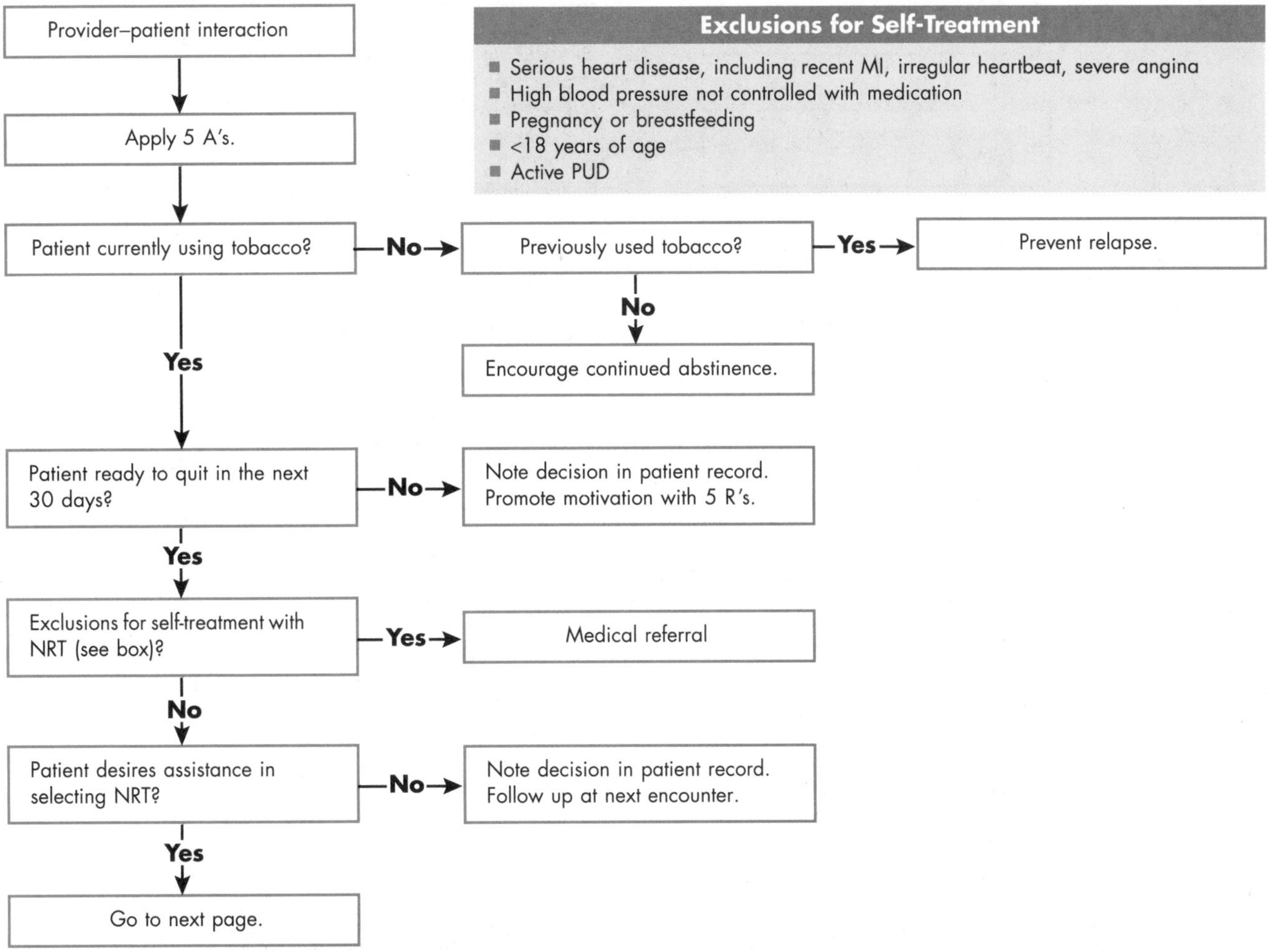

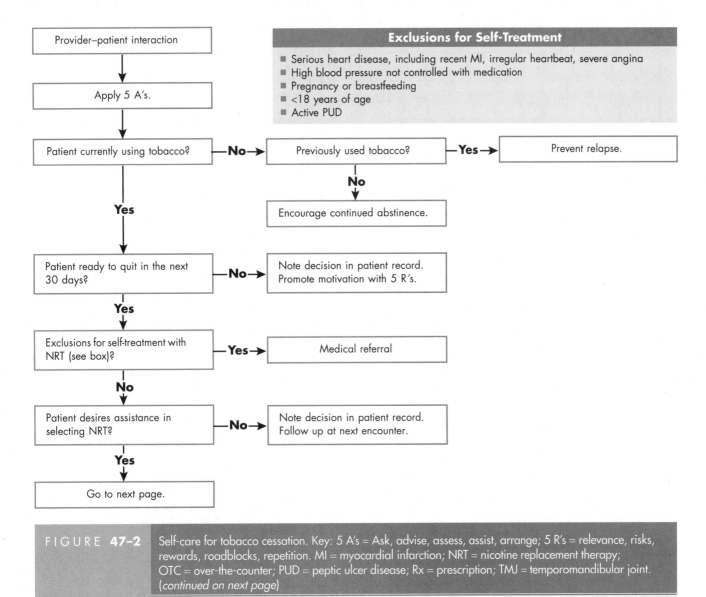

FIGURE 47–2 Self-care for tobacco cessation. Key: 5 A's = Ask, advise, assess, assist, arrange; 5 R's = relevance, risks, rewards, roadblocks, repetition. MI = myocardial infarction; NRT = nicotine replacement therapy; OTC = over-the-counter; PUD = peptic ulcer disease; Rx = prescription; TMJ = temporomandibular joint. (*continued on next page*)

for wanting to quit, and identifying barriers to quitting. Providers can also engage patients in thinking about quitting by raising awareness of specific drug interactions between medications and tobacco smoke (Table 47–2) and how tobacco use can induce or exacerbate medical conditions (e.g., chronic obstructive pulmonary disease, coronary heart disease). Providers should also discuss the importance of preventive health, such as the recommendation for all adult smokers, 19–64 years of age, to receive the pneumococcal vaccine to aid in the prevention of invasive pneumococcal disease.[32]

Although it may be useful to provide patients with information about the medications available for quitting, it is not appropriate to recommend a treatment regimen until the patient is ready to quit in the near future (e.g., within the next month). A treatment goal at this stage should be to promote motivation to quit. Providers can encourage patients to seriously consider quitting by asking the following series of three questions:

1. "Do you ever plan to quit?"
   If the patient responds "no," the provider should inquire, "What would have to change for you to decide to quit?" If the patient indicates that nothing would change his or her opinion about quitting, then the provider should offer to assist if or when the patient changes his or her mind. If the patient responds "yes," the provider should continue to question 2.
2. "How would it benefit you to quit now, instead of later?"
   Quitting generally becomes more difficult the longer a patient smokes. Most patients will agree that there is never an ideal time to quit, and that postponing quitting has more negative effects than positive.
3. "What would have to change for you to decide to quit sooner?"
   This question probes patients' perceptions about quitting and can reveal specific barriers to quitting that can be discussed and addressed.

Motivation can also be enhanced by applying the "5 R's": relevance, risks, rewards, roadblocks, and repetition.[29]

RELEVANCE. The intervention begins by encouraging patients to think about why quitting is important to them. Because information has a greater effect if it takes on a personal meaning, counseling should be framed to relate to the patient's risk of disease or exacerbation of disease, other health concerns, family or social situation

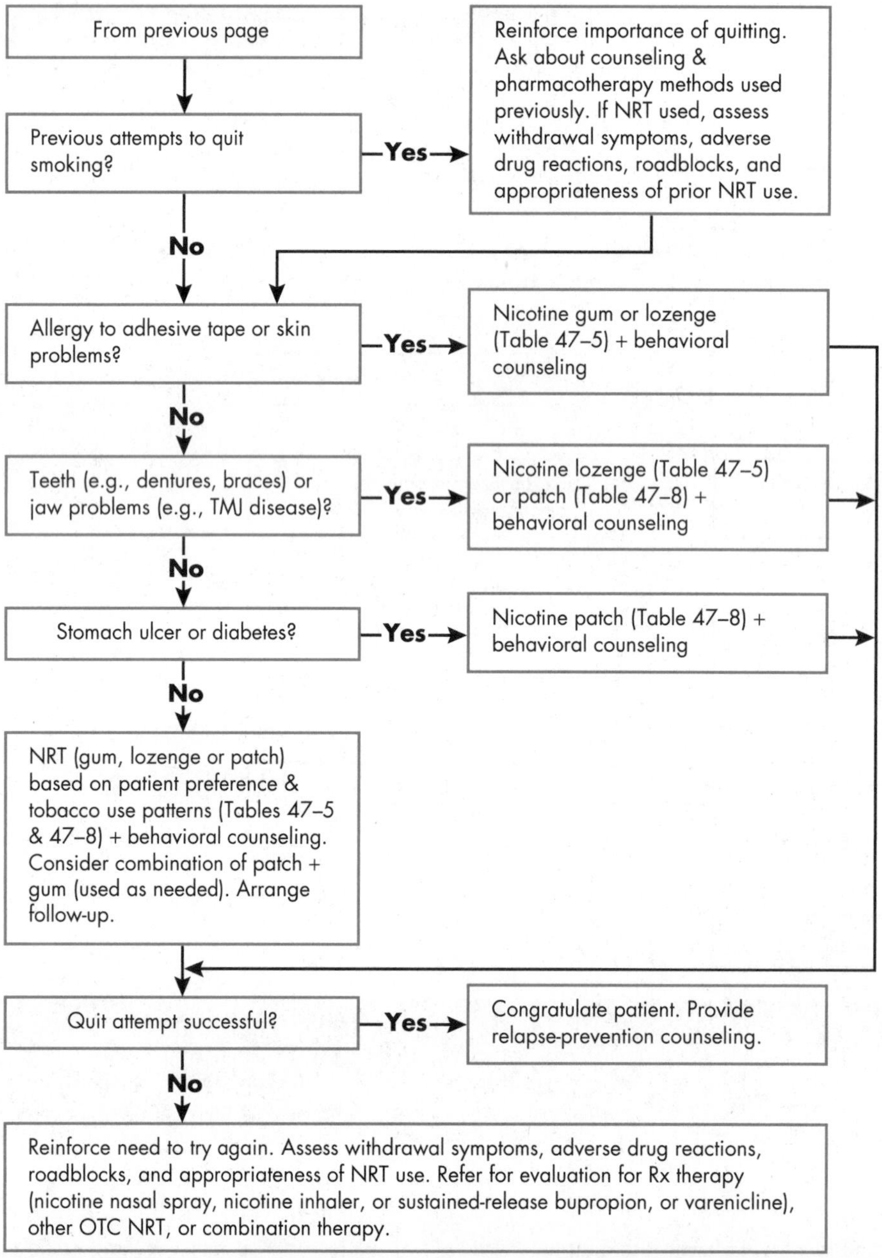

FIGURE **47–2** Self-care for tobacco cessation. Key: 5 As = Ask, advise, assess, assist, arrange; 5 Rs = relevance, risks, rewards, roadblocks, repetition. MI = myocardial infarction; NRT = nicotine replacement therapy; OTC = over-the-counter; PUD = peptic ulcer disease; Rx = prescription; TMJ = temporomandibular joint. (*continued*)

(e.g., having children with asthma), age, and other patient factors such as previous experience with quitting.

RISKS. This intervention entails asking patients to identify negative health consequences of smoking, such as acute risks (e.g., shortness of breath, exacerbation of asthma, pregnancy complications, infertility); long-term risks (e.g., cancer, cardiac and pulmonary disease); and environmental risks (e.g., effects of secondhand smoke on others, including children and pets). The risks also include patients demonstrating unhealthy behaviors around children and adolescents such as smoking near them.

REWARDS. Patients can be asked to identify specific benefits of quitting, such as improved health, enhanced physical performance, acuity of taste and smell, reduced expenditures for tobacco, less time wasted or work missed, reduced health risks to others (e.g., fetus, children, housemates), and reduced aging of the skin.

ROADBLOCKS. This step entails helping patients identify significant barriers to quitting and helping them develop coping skills to address or circumvent each such barrier. Common barriers include nicotine withdrawal symptoms, fear of failure, a need for social support while quitting, depression, concern about weight gain, and a sense of deprivation or loss.

REPETITION. The provider continues to work with patients who are either not motivated to quit or who have been unsuccessful in quitting. Discussing circumstances in which smoking occurs will help identify triggers for relapse and should be viewed as part of the learning process. It is also beneficial to repeat the intervention steps whenever possible.

Counseling Patients Who Are Ready to Quit

The goal for patients who are ready to quit in the next month is to achieve cessation by providing an individualized treatment plan that addresses the key issues listed in Table 47–3. The first step is to discuss the patient's tobacco use history by inquiring about levels of smoking (cigarettes/day), number of years smoked, methods used previously for quitting (if any), and reasons for previous failed quit attempts. Providers should fully understand the basis for personal preferences for the different pharmacotherapies for quitting and work with each patient in selecting the quitting methods (e.g., medications or behavioral counseling programs). It is important to recognize that pharmacotherapy might not be desirable or affordable for all patients. However, providers should educate patients that medications, when taken correctly, can substantially increase the likelihood of quitting successfully,[29] and that the costs of continuing smoking far outweigh the costs of the medications.

Ideally, patients will select a quit date that is within the next 2 weeks, allowing ample time to prepare themselves and their environment before the actual quit date. This preparation includes removing all tobacco products and ashtrays from the home, car, and workplace. Patients should be advised to discuss their desire to quit with their family, friends, and coworkers and to request their support and assistance. Having patients think about when and why they smoke can help them anticipate situations that might trigger a desire to smoke and contribute to relapse. Additional counseling strategies to address with patients during a quit attempt are listed in Table 47–4. Patients should be counseled on proper medication use (including administration), adverse effects,

TABLE 47–3 Key Topics for Individualized Tobacco Cessation Plans

Topic	Description
Assess tobacco use history	■ Current use: – Type(s) and amount of tobacco used ■ Past use: – Duration of smoking – Recent changes in levels of use ■ Past quit attempts: – Number of attempts, date of most recent attempt, duration of abstinence – Previous methods: What did or did not work? Why or why not? – Previous experience with cessation pharmacotherapy: agent used, adequacy of dose, adherence, duration of treatment – Reasons for relapse ■ Reasons or motivation for wanting to quit (or stay quit) ■ Confidence in ability to quit (or stay quit) ■ Triggers for smoking ■ Routines and situations associated with smoking ■ Stress-related smoking ■ Social support for quitting ■ Concerns about weight gain ■ Concerns about withdrawal symptoms
Facilitate the quitting process	■ Discuss methods for quitting: pros and cons of the different methods ■ Set a quit date, ideally within the next 2 weeks ■ Discuss coping strategies ■ Discuss withdrawal symptoms ■ Discuss concept of a slip (occasional smoking) versus full relapse ■ Provide medication counseling: adherence and proper use ■ Offer to assist throughout the quit attempt
Arrange and provide follow-up counseling	■ Monitor the patient's progress throughout the quit attempt ■ Evaluate the current quit attempt – Status of attempt – Slips (occasional smoking) and relapses – Medication use: ■ Adherence with regimen ■ Plans for discontinuation – Address temptations and triggers; discuss relapse prevention strategies – Provide encouragement throughout the quit attempt ■ Follow-up contacts (face-to-face, by telephone, or by e-mail): first contact during first week after quitting, second contact within the first month, additional contacts scheduled as needed

Source: Reproduced with permission from Rx for Change: Clinician-Assisted Tobacco Cessation program. The Regents of the University of California. Copyright © 1999–2015.

TABLE 47–4 Cognitive and Behavioral Strategies for Smoking Cessation

Cognitive Strategies	
Cognitive strategies focus on retraining of the way a patient thinks. Often, patients mentally deliberate on the fact that they are thinking about a cigarette, and this leads to relapse. Patients must recognize that thinking about a cigarette does not mean they need to have one.	
Review of the commitment to quit, with focus on the downside of tobacco	Remind oneself that cravings and temptations are temporary and will pass. Announcing, either silently or aloud, "I want to be a nonsmoker," may make overcoming the temptation easier.
Distractive thinking	Practice deliberate, immediate refocusing of thinking when cued by thoughts about tobacco use.
Positive self-talk, pep talks	Say: "I can do this," and remember difficult situations in which tobacco use was avoided with success.
Relaxation through imagery	Mentally focus on a scene, place, or situation that is peaceful, relaxing, and positive.
Mental rehearsal, visualization	Prepare for situations that might arise by envisioning how best to handle them. For example, envision what would happen if offered a cigarette by a friend, mentally craft and rehearse a response, and perhaps even practice it by saying it aloud.
Behavioral Strategies	
Behavioral strategies involve specific actions to reduce the risk of relapse. For maximal effectiveness, patient-specific triggers for smoking should first be identified; then these behavioral strategies should be considered before quitting. Below are some strategies for responding to several common cues or triggers for relapse.	
Stress	Anticipate upcoming challenges at work, at school, or in personal life. Develop a substitute plan for smoking during times of stress (e.g., practice deep breathing, take a break or leave the situation, call a supportive friend or family member, perform self-massage, use nicotine replacement therapy).
Alcohol	Drinking alcohol can lead to relapse. Consider limiting or abstaining from alcohol during the early stages of quitting.
Other smokers	Quitting is more difficult when other smokers are around. This is especially difficult if there is another smoker in the household. During the early stages of quitting, limit prolonged contact with people who are smoking. Ask coworkers, friends, and housemates not to smoke in your presence.
Oral gratification needs	Have nontobacco oral substitutes (e.g., gum, sugarless candy, straws, toothpicks, lip balm, toothbrush, nicotine replacement therapy, bottled water) readily available.
Automatic smoking routines	Anticipate routines that are associated with tobacco use and develop an alternative plan. *Examples:* ■ Smoking with morning coffee: Change morning routine; drink tea instead of coffee; take shower before drinking coffee; take a brisk walk shortly after awakening. ■ Smoking while driving: Remove all tobacco from car; have car interior detailed; listen to an audiobook or talk radio; use oral substitute. ■ Smoking while on the phone: Stand while talking; limit call duration; change phone location; keep hands occupied by doodling or sketching. ■ Smoking after meals: Get up and immediately do dishes or take a brisk walk after eating; call a supportive friend.
Postcessation weight gain	Most tobacco users gain weight after quitting. Most quitters will gain less than 10 pounds, but a broad range of weight gain is reported, with up to 10% of quitters gaining as much as 30 pounds.[29] In general, attempting to modify multiple behaviors at one time is not recommended. If the prospect of weight gain is a barrier to quitting, engage in regular physical activity and adhere to a healthy diet (as opposed to strict dieting). Carefully plan and prepare meals; increase fruit, vegetable, and water intake to create a feeling of fullness; and chew sugarless gum or eat sugarless candy. Consider use of pharmacotherapy shown to delay weight gain (e.g., 4 mg nicotine gum, 4 mg nicotine lozenge, bupropion).
Cravings for tobacco	Cravings for tobacco are temporary and usually pass within 5–10 minutes. Handle cravings by using distractive thinking, taking a break, changing activities or tasks, taking deep breaths, or performing self-massage.

Source: Reproduced with permission from Rx for Change: Clinician-Assisted Tobacco Cessation program. The Regents of the University of California. Copyright © 1999–2015.

and adherence, and it is crucial to emphasize the importance of receiving behavioral counseling throughout the quit attempt. Additionally, patients should be advised to adhere to the entire course of pharmacotherapy, even though most withdrawal symptoms subside within 2–4 weeks.[18]

Counseling Patients Who Recently Quit

Patients who recently quit will face frequent, difficult challenges in countering withdrawal symptoms and cravings or temptations to use tobacco. An important step is to help them identify situations that might trigger relapse and to suggest appropriate coping strategies. Because smoking is also a habitual behavior, patients should be advised to alter daily routines that were previously associated with tobacco use. These changes will help to disassociate the behaviors from the tobacco.

Many people who quit using tobacco will experience cravings for years and even decades after quitting. Thus, relapse prevention counseling should be part of every follow-up contact with patients who have recently or ever quit smoking. Patients who slip and smoke a cigarette (or use any form of tobacco) or experience a full relapse back to smoking should be encouraged to think through the scenario in which smoking first recurred and identify the trigger for relapse. Identifying triggers will provide valuable information for future quit attempts.

Counseling Patients Who Are Former Smokers

The strategies to be applied for former tobacco users are similar but typically less intensive than those to be applied for recent quitters. The goal for former tobacco users is to remain tobacco-free for life. Providers should evaluate the patient's resolve for staying tobacco-free and ongoing coping strategies; in this context, it is appropriate to ascertain whether the patient has had any strong temptations to use tobacco or has occasionally used any tobacco product. Also, it is important to ensure that patients are appropriately terminating or tapering pharmacotherapy products. Patients who have been tobacco-free should be congratulated for their success. For patients who have intermittently used tobacco, situations in which tobacco use occurred should be reviewed, and additional coping strategies should be discussed.

Helping Patients Quit: The Ask-Advise-Refer Approach (Brief Intervention)

Providers should familiarize themselves with local resources for tobacco cessation, including group programs and telephone quit lines. When time or lack of expertise limits the ability to provide comprehensive cessation counseling, providers are encouraged to apply an "abbreviated 5 A's" model whereby they *ask* about tobacco use, *advise* tobacco users to quit, and *refer* patients to other resources, including local services and group counseling programs, for additional assistance. Telephone-based counseling is available throughout the United States. These services provide low-cost interventions that can reach patients who might otherwise have limited access to medical treatment because of remoteness of geographic location or lack of financial resources. In clinical trials, telephone counseling services for which at least some of the contacts are initiated by the quit line counselor were shown to be effective in promoting abstinence.[29] Combining medication with quit line counseling significantly improves abstinence rates compared with medication alone.[29] The national telephone number for the toll-free tobacco quit line is 1-800-Quit-Now.

Pharmacologic Therapy

Although in some situations pharmacotherapy should be used with caution or only under the supervision of a primary care provider (see later under Special Populations), most patients who are attempting to quit should be advised to incorporate pharmacotherapy in their treatment plan. Currently, seven first-line agents are approved by the U.S. Food and Drug Administration (FDA) for smoking cessation[29]: five formulations of nicotine replacement therapy (NRT), sustained-release bupropion, and varenicline. Three of the NRT formulations—gum, lozenge, and transdermal patch—are nonprescription, but the nicotine inhaler and nicotine nasal spray, as well as bupropion and varenicline, require a prescription.

Nicotine Replacement Therapy

NRT is the most commonly used pharmacotherapy for smoking cessation.[30] NRT products are often used to help noncigarette tobacco users to quit, but these products are FDA labeled only to help cigarette smokers quit. Similar to the nicotine present in tobacco, the active agents in NRT stimulate the release of dopamine in the central nervous system.[10] The rationale underlying the use of NRT for smoking cessation is twofold. First, NRT provides smokers with a nontobacco source of nicotine to reduce the physiologic symptoms of nicotine withdrawal that typically occur after abstinence from tobacco. Second, by attenuating the symptoms of withdrawal, NRT assists quitters by allowing them to focus on the behavioral and psychological aspects of smoking cessation. A key advantage of NRT is that patients, as well as those in the smoker's environment, are not exposed to the carcinogens and other toxic constituents present in tobacco and tobacco smoke. Furthermore, compared with cigarettes, NRT formulations provide lower, slower, and less-variable plasma nicotine concentrations,[15] thereby eliminating the almost immediate reinforcing effects of nicotine obtained through smoking.

Nicotine is well absorbed (Figure 47–3) from many sites, including the lungs, skin, and nasal and buccal (oral) mucosa. Nicotine absorption is pH-dependent, and lower systemic concentrations are achieved under acidic conditions. Nicotine is also well absorbed from the gastrointestinal tract (small intestine) but undergoes extensive first-pass hepatic metabolism, resulting in negligible systemic levels of nicotine.[15]

The main difference between the various NRT formulations is the site and rate of nicotine absorption (Figure 47–3). Compared with cigarettes, all of the NRT formulations deliver nicotine less rapidly and achieve lower serum nicotine levels, thereby lowering the likelihood of developing physical dependence. Peak serum concentrations are achieved most rapidly with the nasal spray (11–18 minutes), followed by the gum, lozenge, and inhaler (30–60 minutes) and then by the transdermal patch (3–12 hours). In contrast, significantly higher peak nicotine levels are attained within 10 minutes of smoking a cigarette.[15]

Patients should begin NRT on their quit date and discontinue use of all forms of tobacco on initiation of the NRT regimen. Use of tobacco in combination with NRT may result in serum nicotine concentrations that are higher than those achieved from tobacco products alone, increasing the likelihood of nicotine-related adverse effects, including nausea, vomiting, hypersalivation, perspiring, abdominal pain, dizziness, weakness, and palpitations.

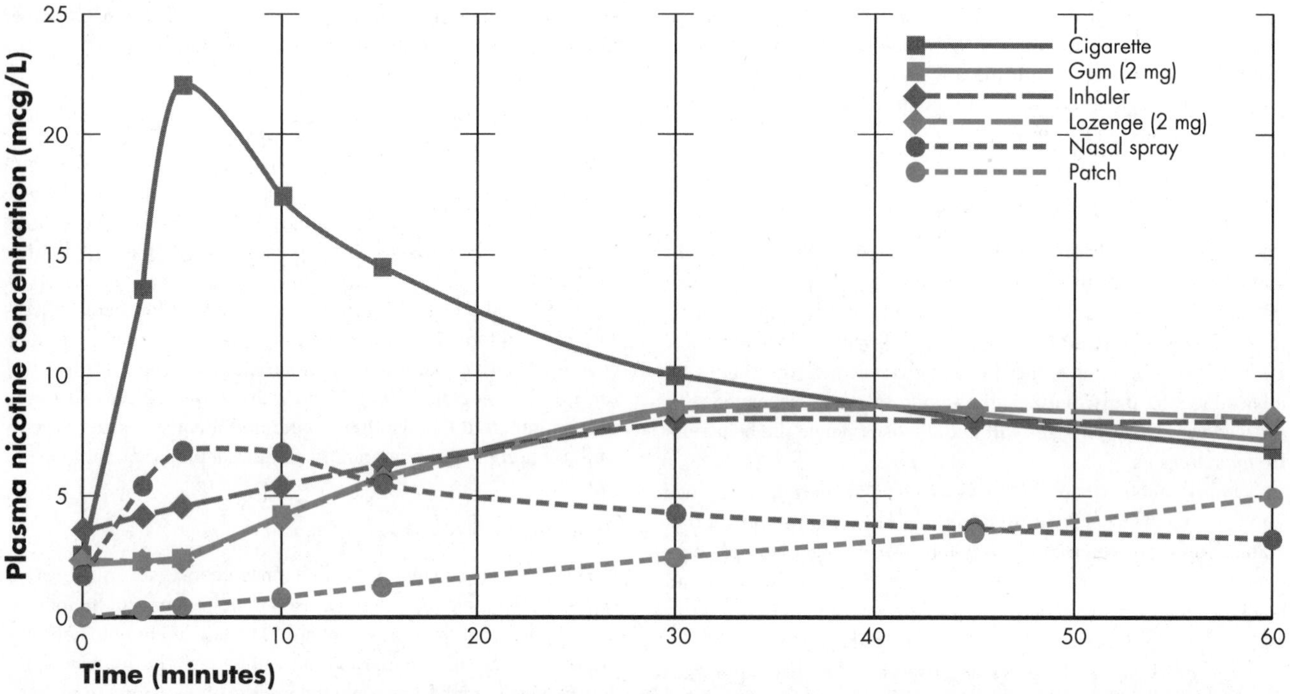

FIGURE 47–3 Plasma nicotine concentrations over time for various nicotine delivery systems. (Source: Reproduced with permission from Rx for Change: Clinician-Assisted Tobacco Cessation program. The Regents of the University of California. Copyright © 1999–2015.)

Nicotine Polacrilex Gum

Nicotine polacrilex gum is a resin complex of nicotine and polacrilin in a sugar-free (<3 calories/piece) chewing gum base. The product is available as 2 mg and 4 mg strengths, in original (tobacco-like, peppery), cinnamon, fruit, and mint flavors (Table 47–5). All gum formulations contain buffering agents (sodium carbonate and sodium bicarbonate) to increase salivary pH, thereby enhancing absorption of nicotine across the buccal mucosa. When the 2 mg and 4 mg gums are used properly, approximately 1.6 mg and 2.2 mg of nicotine is absorbed from each dose, respectively. Peak serum concentrations of nicotine are achieved approximately 30 minutes after chewing a single piece of gum and then slowly decline over 2–3 hours.[15]

The recommended dosage of nicotine gum is based on the "time to first cigarette" (TTFC) of the day. Having a strong desire or need to smoke soon after waking is viewed as a key indicator of nicotine dependence. Therefore, patients who smoke their first cigarette of the day within 30 minutes of waking are likely to be more highly dependent on nicotine and require higher dosages than those who delay smoking for more than 30 minutes after waking. Specifically, if the TTFC is 30 minutes or less, therapy should be initiated with the 4 mg gum. If the TTFC is more than 30 minutes, therapy should be initiated with the 2 mg gum. Table 47–5 provides the manufacturer's recommended dosing schedule. During the initial 6 weeks of therapy, patients should use one piece of gum every 1–2 hours while awake. In general, this amounts to at

TABLE 47–5 **Dosages for Nonprescription Nicotine Polacrilex Gum and Lozenge**

	Gum	Lozenge
Product strength	Nicorette: 2 mg, 4 mg; original, cinnamon, fruit, mint Generic: 2 mg, 4 mg; original, fruit, mint	Nicorette (standard): 2 mg, 4 mg; mint Nicorette (mini): 2 mg, 4 mg; mint Generic (standard): 2 mg, 4 mg; mint, cherry
Dose	First cigarette ≤30 minutes after waking: 4 mg First cigarette >30 minutes after waking: 2 mg *Weeks 1–6:* 1 piece every 1–2 hours *Weeks 7–9:* 1 piece every 2–4 hours *Weeks 10–12:* 1 piece every 4–8 hours	First cigarette ≤30 minutes after waking: 4 mg First cigarette >30 minutes after waking: 2 mg *Weeks 1–6:* 1 lozenge every 1–2 hours *Weeks 7–9:* 1 lozenge every 2–4 hours *Weeks 10–12:* 1 lozenge every 4–8 hours

least 9 pieces of gum daily which improves the overall chances of quitting. Table 47–6 provides specific instructions for proper use of the nicotine gum. The "chew and park" method described in the table allows for the slow, consistent release of nicotine from the polacrilin resin. Patients can use additional pieces of gum (up to the maximum of 24 pieces per day) if cravings occur between the scheduled doses. In general, individuals who smoke heavily will need more pieces to alleviate their cravings.

An important point to note is that patients often do not use enough of the gum to derive its full benefit or they use it incorrectly (e.g., incorrect chewing technique or concurrent consumption of beverages or foods that alter the pH of the mouth). Commonly, patients chew too few pieces per day or shorten the duration of treatment. For this reason, recommending a fixed schedule of administration, tapering over 1–3 months, is preferable to having the patient use the gum as needed to control cravings.[29]

The most common adverse effects associated with the use of the nicotine gum include unpleasant taste, mouth irritation, jaw muscle soreness or fatigue, hypersalivation, hiccups, and dyspepsia. Many of these effects can be minimized or prevented by using proper chewing technique.[29] The nicotine polacrilin resin is more viscous than ordinary chewing gum and more likely to adhere to fillings, bridges, dentures, crowns, and braces. Patients should be warned that chewing the gum too rapidly may result in excessive release of nicotine, leading to lightheadedness, nausea, vomiting, irritation of the throat and mouth, hiccups, and indigestion.

Patients with active temporomandibular joint (TMJ) disease should not use the nicotine gum because the highly viscous consistency of the formulation and the need for frequent chewing may exacerbate the jaw condition. In addition, the manufacturer recommends that patients with stomach ulcers or diabetes contact their HCP before use of the product because these more serious conditions may potentially necessitate further monitoring.

TABLE 47–6 Usage Guidelines for Nicotine Polacrilex Gum

- Begin NRT on quit date and discontinue all forms of tobacco upon initiation of NRT regimen.
- Note that nicotine gum is a nicotine delivery system, not a chewing gum.
- Proper administration technique is necessary when using this product. Nicotine from the gum is released using the "chew and park" method:
  - Chew each piece of gum *slowly* several times.
  - Stop chewing at the first sign of a peppery, minty, fruity, or citrus taste, or after experiencing a slight tingling sensation in the mouth. This usually occurs after approximately 15 chews, but the time to effect onset varies.
  - Park the gum between the cheek and gum to allow absorption of nicotine across the lining of the mouth.
  - When the taste or tingling dissipates (generally after 1–2 minutes), slowly resume chewing.
  - When the taste or tingle returns, stop chewing and park the gum in a different place in the mouth. This will decrease the incidence of mouth irritation.
  - The chew-and-park steps should be repeated until most of the nicotine is gone, which is when the taste or tingle does not return after continued chewing. On average, each piece of gum lasts 30 minutes.
- To minimize withdrawal symptoms, use the nicotine gum on a scheduled basis rather than as needed.
- Follow the dosage regimen carefully; reduce the dosage at the recommended intervals; if needed for longer than 12 weeks of treatment to keep from smoking, talk to your HCP.
- Do not chew more than 24 pieces per day.
- Acidic beverages such as coffee, juices, wine, or soft drinks may transiently reduce the salivary pH, resulting in decreased absorption of nicotine across the buccal mucosa. Do not eat or drink anything (except water) 15 minutes before or while using the nicotine gum.
- Note that chewing the gum too quickly will result in an unpleasant taste caused by too much nicotine in the saliva, and that if the nicotine is swallowed, it may cause effects similar to those produced by excessive smoking (e.g., nausea, throat irritation, light-headedness, hiccups).
- Have nicotine gum readily available at all times. Keep the nicotine gum in the same place you previously kept your cigarettes (e.g., shirt pocket, purse, desk).
- Keep this product, including used pieces, out of the reach of children and pets.

Key: HCP = Health care provider; NRT = nicotine replacement therapy.

Nicotine Polacrilex Lozenge

The nicotine polacrilex lozenge is a resin complex of nicotine and polacrilin in a sugar-free mint- or cherry-flavored lozenge (Table 47–5). The lozenges are available in 2 mg and 4 mg strengths with two different physical sizes (regular and mini) and should be used similarly to other medicinal lozenges or troches (i.e., suck and rotate it within the mouth until it dissolves). Because the mini-lozenge is smaller, it is more easily concealed and dissolves more quickly. The pharmacokinetics of the nicotine lozenge and gum formulations are comparable, but a nicotine lozenge delivers approximately 25% more nicotine than an equivalent dose of nicotine gum because of complete dissolution of the dosage form.[33] The lozenge form contains buffering agents (sodium carbonate and potassium bicarbonate) to increase salivary pH, enhancing the buccal absorption of nicotine.

As with nicotine gum, dosing for the lozenge is based on the TTFC. If the TTFC is 30 minutes or less, therapy should be initiated with the 4 mg lozenge. If the TTFC is more than 30 minutes, therapy should be initiated with the 2 mg lozenge. During the initial 6 weeks of therapy, patients should use 1 lozenge every 1–2 hours while awake. In general, this amounts to at least 9 lozenges daily. Table 47–7 provides further instructions for proper use of the nicotine lozenge. Patients can use additional lozenges (up to 5 lozenges in 6 hours or a maximum of 20 lozenges per day) if cravings occur between the scheduled doses. The manufacturer recommends that patients with stomach ulcers or diabetes contact their HCP before using the lozenges because these more serious conditions may necessitate further monitoring.

Adverse effects associated with the nicotine lozenge include mouth irritation, nausea, hiccups, cough, heartburn, headache, flatulence, and insomnia. Patients who use more than 1 lozenge at a time, continuously use 1 lozenge after another, or chew or swallow the lozenge are more likely to experience heartburn or indigestion.

Nicotine Transdermal Systems (Nicotine Patch)

Nicotine transdermal systems deliver continuous, low levels of nicotine through the skin over 24 hours. The patch consists of a waterproof surface layer, a nicotine reservoir, an adhesive layer, and a disposable protective liner.

The dosing schedules for the nicotine patches vary slightly (Table 47–8). Before recommending a specific product and a dosing

TABLE 47-7 Usage Guidelines for Nicotine Polacrilex Lozenge

- Begin NRT on quit date and discontinue use of all forms of tobacco on initiation of NRT regimen.
- Proper administration technique is necessary when using the nicotine lozenge:
  - Place the lozenge in the mouth and allow it to dissolve slowly (20–30 minutes for standard lozenge; 10 minutes for mini-lozenge). As the nicotine is released from the lozenge, you may experience a warm, tingling sensation.
  - To reduce the risk of side effects (e.g., nausea, hiccups, and heartburn), do not chew or swallow the lozenge.
  - Occasionally rotate the lozenge to different areas of the mouth to decrease mouth irritation.
- To minimize withdrawal symptoms, use the nicotine lozenge on a scheduled basis rather than as needed.
- Follow the dosage regimen carefully; reduce the dosage at the recommended intervals; if needed for longer than 12 weeks of treatment to keep from smoking, talk to your HCP.
- Do not use more than 5 lozenges in 6 hours or more than 20 lozenges per day.
- Acidic beverages such as coffee, juices, wine, or soft drinks may transiently reduce the salivary pH, resulting in decreased absorption of nicotine across the buccal mucosa. Do not eat or drink anything (except water) 15 minutes before or while using the nicotine lozenge.
- Patients who use more than 1 lozenge at a time, continuously use 1 lozenge after another, or chew or swallow the lozenge are more likely to experience heartburn or indigestion.
- Have nicotine lozenges readily available at all times. Keep the nicotine lozenges in the same place you previously kept your cigarettes (e.g., shirt pocket, purse, desk).
- Keep this product out of the reach of children and pets.

Key: HCP = Health care provider; NRT = nicotine replacement therapy.

schedule, the provider should know how many cigarettes the patient smokes per day. In general, heavier smokers will require higher-strength formulations for a longer duration of therapy. Patients who experience adverse effects such as dizziness, perspiration, nausea, vomiting, diarrhea, or headache, should consider a lower-strength patch. Additional instructions for proper use of the nicotine patch are listed in Table 47–9.

TABLE 47-8 Dosages for Nonprescription Nicotine Transdermal Systems (Patch)

Dosage Feature	NicoDerm CQ and Generic Patch
Product strength	7, 14, 21 mg (24 hour)
Dose	*>10 cigarettes/day*
	21 mg/day × 4–6 weeks
	14 mg/day × 2 weeks
	7 mg/day × 2 weeks
	≤10 cigarettes/day
	14 mg/day × 6 weeks
	7 mg/day × 2 weeks

TABLE 47-9 Usage Guidelines for Nicotine Transdermal Systems (Nicotine Patch)

- Begin NRT on quit date and discontinue use of all forms of tobacco on initiation of NRT regimen.
- Apply the patch to a clean, dry, hairless area of the skin on the upper body or the upper outer part of the arm at approximately the same time each day.
- The patch should be applied to a different area of skin each day. To minimize the potential for local skin reactions, the same area should not be used again for at least 1 week.
- During application, apply firm pressure to the patch with the palm of the hand for 10 seconds. Be sure that the patch adheres well to the skin, especially around the edges; this is necessary for a good seal.
- Wash your hands after applying or removing the patch.
- The patch should not be left on the skin for more than 24 hours because prolonged use may lead to skin irritation.
- Any adhesive remaining on the skin after patch removal can be removed with rubbing alcohol.
- Water will not reduce the effectiveness of the nicotine patch if it is applied correctly. You may bathe, swim, shower, or exercise while wearing the patch.
- Do not cut patches in half or into smaller pieces to adjust or reduce the nicotine dosage. Nicotine in the patch may evaporate from the cut edges and the patch may be less effective.
- Local skin reactions (e.g., itching, burning, redness) are common with the nicotine patch. These reactions are generally caused by adhesives; they can be minimized by rotating patch application sites and, if they occur, treated with nonprescription hydrocortisone cream.
- Remove the nicotine patch before having a magnetic resonance imaging (MRI) procedure. Burns from nicotine patches worn during MRI scanning have been reported and probably are caused by the metallic component in the backing of some patches.
- Users experiencing troublesome dreams or other sleep disruptions should remove the patch before bedtime.
- Discard the removed nicotine patch by folding it onto itself, completely covering the adhesive area.
- Keep new and used patches out of the reach of children and pets.

Key: NRT = Nicotine replacement therapy.

The most common adverse effects associated with the nicotine patch are local skin reactions (erythema, burning, pruritus) at the application site, which generally are caused by skin occlusion or sensitivity to the patch adhesives. If the skin reaction is bothersome, the patient can apply nonprescription hydrocortisone cream to the site or try another manufacturer's product that uses a different adhesive. Other, less common adverse effects include vivid or abnormal dreams, insomnia, and headache. Sleep disturbances might be caused by nocturnal nicotine absorption. If this effect becomes troublesome, patients should be instructed to remove the patch at bedtime; of note, a new patch should be applied as soon as possible after waking the following morning because the lack of nicotine coverage throughout the night may lead to an increased urge to smoke.[29]

Prescription Medications for Smoking Cessation

Detailed information about prescription products for tobacco cessation is outside the scope of this discussion. The following information is a summary of key information; for further details, the reader is encouraged to consult another reference that specializes in this content.

Nicotine Inhaler

The nicotine inhaler consists of a plastic mouthpiece and a nicotine-containing cartridge that delivers 4 mg of nicotine as an inhaled vapor, 2 mg of which is absorbed across the oropharyngeal mucosa. The inhaler reduces nicotine withdrawal symptoms and may give some degree of comfort by providing a hand-to-mouth ritual that emulates the act of smoking. However, reinforcing the hand-to-mouth ritual can make quitting more difficult. The inhaler has not been evaluated for use in patients with bronchospastic diseases, such as asthma, so it should be used with caution in these patients because of the risk of exacerbation.[34] Adverse effects of the inhaler include mild mouth and throat irritation, cough, and rhinitis.

Nicotine Nasal Spray

The nicotine nasal spray is an aqueous solution of nicotine for administration to the nasal mucosa. Each actuation delivers a 0.5 mg bolus of nicotine that is absorbed across the nasal mucosa. Because of its rapid onset of action (relative to other NRT formulations), the spray is a potential option for patients who prefer a medication to manage withdrawal symptoms rapidly; however, in 15%–20% of patients, use of the nasal spray can result in dependence. Some patients with asthma have reported bronchospasm after using the nasal spray, so use of this medication in patients with bronchospastic disease should be avoided.[34] Initially, most patients will experience nose and throat irritation (peppery sensation), watery eyes, sneezing, or coughing when using this product. This product is to be administered without sniffing (i.e., not administered using the same technique as for standard allergy nasal sprays). After the first week, most patients have minimal difficulty with the product, and tolerance generally develops with regular use.

Sustained-Release Bupropion

Sustained-release bupropion was the first non-nicotine medication approved for smoking cessation. This agent is a prescription antidepressant medication that is believed to promote smoking cessation by blocking the reuptake of dopamine and norepinephrine in the brain, thereby decreasing the cravings for cigarettes and symptoms of nicotine withdrawal.[29]

Therapy is started with a dose of 150 mg orally every morning for 3 days, followed by 150 mg twice daily for 7–12 weeks. Because steady-state blood levels are reached after approximately 7 days of therapy, patients set their quit date for 1–2 weeks after starting therapy. Insomnia and dry mouth are the most common adverse effects reported with bupropion. Because seizures have been reported in approximately 0.1% of patients, bupropion is contraindicated in patients who (1) have a seizure disorder, (2) have a current or previous diagnosis of anorexia or bulimia nervosa, (3) are undergoing abrupt discontinuation of alcohol or sedatives (including benzodiazepines), (4) are currently using or have used a monoamine oxidase inhibitor within the past 14 days, or (5) are currently being treated with any other medications that contain bupropion. Other factors that may potentially increase the odds of seizure and are classified as warnings for use of this medication include history of head trauma or previous seizure, central nervous system tumor, severe hepatic cirrhosis, and concomitant use of medications that lower the seizure threshold. In July 2009, FDA mandated that the prescribing information for all bupropion-containing products include a black-box warning that highlights the risk of serious neuropsychiatric symptoms, including changes in behavior, hostility, agitation, depressed mood, suicidal thoughts and behavior, and attempted suicide.[35] Advise patients to stop taking bupropion SR and contact an HCP immediately if they experience any of these symptoms that are not typical of nicotine withdrawal, or if they experience suicidal thoughts or behavior. If treatment is stopped due to neuropsychiatric symptoms, patients should be monitored until the symptoms resolve. These additional warnings were based on postmarketing adverse event surveillance reports received by FDA.

Varenicline

Varenicline (Chantix) is a partial agonist and is highly selective for the alpha-4 beta-2 nicotinic receptor. The efficacy of varenicline in smoking cessation is believed to be the result of sustained, low-level agonist activity at the receptor site that is combined with competitive inhibition of nicotine binding. The partial agonist activity induces modest receptor stimulation, leading to increased dopamine levels that attenuate the symptoms of nicotine withdrawal. In addition, by competitively blocking the binding of nicotine to nicotinic acetylcholine receptors in the central nervous system, varenicline inhibits the surges of dopamine release that occur immediately after inhalation of tobacco smoke. The latter mechanism may be effective in preventing relapse by reducing the pleasure associated with smoking.[36]

As with sustained-release bupropion, treatment with varenicline should be started 1 week before the patient stops smoking. This regimen allows for gradual escalation of the dose to minimize treatment-related nausea and insomnia. Therapy is generally started at 0.5 mg daily on days 1–3; 0.5 mg twice daily on days 4–7; and 1 mg twice daily for weeks 2–12. Nausea, insomnia, abnormal dreams, and headache are the most commonly reported adverse effects. Some people have experienced increased drunkenness (intoxication), unusual or sometimes aggressive behavior, and/or having no memory of things that have happened while drinking alcohol and using this medication.[37] In July 2009, FDA mandated that the prescribing information for varenicline contain a black-box warning that highlights the risk of serious neuropsychiatric symptoms, including changes in behavior, hostility, agitation, depressed mood, and suicidal events including ideation, behavior changes, and attempted suicide.[38] Advise patients to stop taking varenicline and contact an HCP immediately if they experience any of these symptoms, which are not typical of nicotine withdrawal, or if they experience suicidal thoughts or behavior. If emergence of neuropsychiatric symptoms necessitates stopping treatment, patients should be monitored until the symptoms resolve. These additional warnings were based on continued postmarketing adverse event surveillance reports received by FDA. Although these reports are rare in comparison with the total number of patients exposed to varenicline, providers and patients should monitor for changes in mood and behavior during treatment with varenicline.[38]

A small increased risk of cardiac events has been reported in some patients with existing cardiovascular disease.[39] In December 2012, FDA shared results of a meta-analysis conducted by the manufacturer of varenicline, reporting that a higher occurrence of major adverse cardiovascular events was observed in patients using varenicline than in persons taking a placebo (although the increased risk was not statistically significant).[39] The warnings and precautions labeling was updated to include the results of the meta-analysis and included instructions to patients to notify their HCPs of new or worsening cardiovascular symptoms and to seek immediate medical attention if they experience signs and symptoms of myocardial infarction or stroke.[38]

Pharmacotherapeutic Comparison

Few trials have directly compared the various agents for smoking cessation. In general, compared with placebo, regimens with the first-line agents approximately double the long-term quit rates[29] (Table 47–10).

Product Selection Guidelines

Because all first-line, FDA-approved cessation medications enhance quit rates, the choice of therapy is based largely on contraindications or precautions, patient preference, tolerability of the available dosage forms, use during previous quit attempts (i.e., what worked well and what did not, regardless of whether or not the medication was being used correctly), and cost. For whatever regimen selected, the cost of treatment will be insignificant compared with the costs of continued smoking and the costs of managing the resultant complications.

The number of smokeless tobacco products available on the market is on the rise, including dissolvable tobacco and electronic cigarettes. Currently no guidelines exist for the treatment of tobacco cessation for people using these products. A randomized, clinical trial comparing varenicline and placebo showed positive results for smokeless tobacco users; however, more studies are needed.[40]

In May 2016, the FDA announced it would begin regulating the sales of all tobacco products, including cigars, electronic cigarettes, and hookah and pipe tobacco. This change also includes restricting these products to purchasers older than 18 years of age. Finally, manufacturers now have to comply with all FDA requirements, including reporting all ingredients and listing health warnings on packaging and advertising. Two states, California and Hawaii, have also raised the age at which people can purchase tobacco products to 21.

Special Populations

NRT should be used with caution in patients with serious underlying cardiovascular disease, including those who have had a recent myocardial infarction (i.e., within the preceding 2 weeks), those with serious arrhythmias, and those with serious or worsening angina pectoris.[29] Nicotine may increase the myocardial workload by increasing the heart rate and blood pressure and may constrict coronary arteries, leading to cardiac ischemia.[41] Although most experts believe that the risks of NRT in patients with cardiovascular disease are small relative to the risks of continued smoking,[42–44] patients with serious underlying cardiovascular disease are advised to use NRT only while under the supervision of an HCP.

Evidence exists for risk to the human fetus when prescription formulations of nicotine are used during pregnancy.[45] (See the

TABLE 47–10 Methods for Smoking Cessation: Estimates of Treatment Efficacy for First-Line Agents Compared With Placebo at 6 Months After Quitting

Pharmacotherapy	Estimated Odds Ratio[a] (95% CI)	Estimated Abstinence Rate[b] (95% CI)
Placebo	1.0	13.8
Monotherapy (first-line agents)		
Sustained-release bupropion	2.0 (1.8–2.2)	24.2 (22.2–26.4)
Nicotine gum (6–14 weeks)	1.5 (1.2–1.7)	19.0 (16.5–21.9)
Nicotine inhaler	2.1 (1.5–2.9)	24.8 (19.1–31.6)
Nicotine lozenge (2 mg)	2.0 (1.4–2.8)	24.2[c]
Nicotine patch (6–14 weeks)	1.9 (1.7–2.2)	23.4 (21.3–25.8)
Nicotine nasal spray	2.3 (1.7–3.0)	26.7 (21.5–32.7)
Varenicline (2 mg/day)	3.1 (2.5–3.8)	33.2 (28.9–37.8)
Combination Therapy (first-line agents)		
Nicotine patch (>14 weeks) + as-needed NRT (gum, nasal spray, or lozenge[d])	3.6 (2.5–5.2)	36.5 (28.6–45.3)
Nicotine patch + bupropion SR	2.5 (1.9–3.4)	28.9 (23.5–35.1)
Nicotine patch + nicotine inhaler	2.2 (1.3–3.6)	25.8 (17.4–36.5)

Key: CI = Confidence interval; NRT = nicotine replacement therapy; SR = sustained release.

[a] Estimated relative to placebo.

[b] Abstinence percentages for specified treatment.

[c] One qualifying randomized trial; 95% CI not reported in the 2008 clinical practice guideline.

[d] A recent trial, not included in the clinical practice guideline, supports the combination of the nicotine patch and nicotine lozenge.[45]

Source: Reproduced with permission from Rx for Change: Clinician-Assisted Tobacco Cessation program. The Regents of the University of California. Copyright © 1999–2015.

Preface for a detailed explanation of the pregnancy data.) Although NRT may pose a risk to the developing fetus, some experts have argued that NRT use during pregnancy is safer than continued smoking.[44,45] However, because data showing effectiveness of NRT in pregnancy are inconclusive and because nicotine has the potential to cause fetal harm, the 2008 clinical practice guideline states that pregnant women should be encouraged to quit without the use of medication. Instead, providers are advised to offer interventions of person-to-person behavioral counseling for their pregnant patients who smoke.[29]

The efficacy of NRT, sustained-release bupropion, and varenicline has not been established in pediatric or adolescent smokers, and no NRT product is currently indicated for use in these populations.[29] Accordingly, counseling is the recommended treatment method for smokers younger than 18 years.

People older than 65 years can benefit greatly from quitting smoking. Pharmacologic therapy and counseling are recommended. If mobility is an issue, referral to a quit line may be useful.[13,29]

The manufacturers of nicotine gum, lozenge, and patch products recommend that patients taking a prescription medicine for asthma or depression speak with their HCP before using nonprescription NRT. Fluvoxamine and theophylline (both now used infrequently) and inhaled corticosteroids have known clinically significant interactions with tobacco smoke (Table 47–2).

For light smokers (those who smoke fewer than 10 cigarettes per day and those who do not smoke every day), counseling is the recommended treatment method for this population.[29] However, the nicotine patch is approved for use in light smokers, and the nicotine lozenge was shown to be effective in individuals who smoke 15 or fewer cigarettes daily.[46] Use of smokeless tobacco (e.g., snuff, moist snuff, chewing tobacco, dissolvable tobacco), cigars, and pipes can produce nicotine addiction and lead to serious health consequences. Behavioral counseling is the recommended treatment method for these tobacco users.[29]

Patient Factors

When recommending a nonprescription agent for smoking cessation, HCPs should determine the patient's smoking patterns, lifestyle habits, and coexisting medical conditions. In general, higher levels of smoking will require higher dosages of NRT and longer durations of treatment.

Some patients might need to use their smoking cessation medication longer than the usual recommended treatment duration. Although the general goal is complete, long-term abstinence from all nicotine-containing products, some smokers may benefit from long-term medication use.[29] If continued use helps prevent relapse, this approach is considered preferable to the patient returning to smoking.[29]

Patients who smoke continuously throughout the day may have better success with a nicotine patch because it provides a sustained, steady release of nicotine. Conversely, patients who smoke intermittently throughout the day or who smoke intensely for short periods of time, followed by long periods of abstinence, might prefer a relatively short-acting formulation, such as a nicotine gum or lozenge, to more closely mimic their tobacco use patterns. For some quitters, frequent gum chewing may not be feasible or socially acceptable. The nicotine patch, which can be concealed under clothing, might be a reasonable choice for these patients. Others may find nicotine lozenges, which can be used more discreetly, to be an acceptable alternative. Patients with underlying dermatologic conditions (e.g., psoriasis, eczema, atopic dermatitis) or allergy to adhesive tape are more likely to experience skin irritation and should not use the nicotine patch. The nicotine lozenge or patch is more appropriate than the nicotine gum for patients with TMJ disease or dentures. Finally, patients with serious cardiovascular disease, women who are pregnant or nursing, light smokers, and adolescents should be referred for further evaluation by their primary provider before starting treatment with NRT.

Patient Preferences

Identifying the patient's perceptions and expectations about pharmacotherapy is particularly important, including the ability to adhere to the regimen, previous experience with smoking cessation medications, and concern about weight gain. Because NRT formulations require frequent dosing or nontraditional routes of administration, patient education about proper use of these products is essential. Patients who have difficulty taking multiple doses of medications throughout the day or those who want a simplified regimen might achieve greater success with the nicotine patch. By contrast, the gum or lozenge may be preferable for patients who want to titrate nicotine levels to manage withdrawal symptoms. Some people may find that they need an oral substitute for tobacco; the oral gratification given by the nicotine gum, lozenge, or inhaler might be beneficial in these patients. Others may prefer the idea of using a combination of medications, such as the nicotine patch plus gum or lozenge, on an as-needed basis, as discussed later in this section.

All smokers making a repeat quit attempt should be queried about their previous use of pharmacotherapy and their perceptions of available treatment options. For patients reporting a favorable past experience with a given product, repeated treatment with the same agent may be appropriate, with consideration given to increasing the dose, frequency of dosing, or duration of therapy. For patients who report a negative experience with a particular medication (e.g., poor adherence, adverse effects, palatability issues, cost), a different regimen should be considered. For example, for a quitter who had short-term success with the patch but discontinued therapy because of intolerable nightmares, a second trial of the patch that is removed at bedtime is more likely to be successful. A patient who is unable to tolerate nicotine gum because of jaw muscle ache could be advised to switch to the nicotine lozenge or patch. For a patient who expresses concern about postcessation weight gain, use of the 4 mg nicotine gum or lozenge or sustained-release bupropion may be particularly helpful in that that these products were shown to delay weight gain after quitting.[29] Among patients for whom the out-of-pocket expense poses a potential barrier to pharmacologic treatment, use of the generic formulations is preferable.

Combination therapy should be considered a first-line treatment and might be particularly appropriate in patients who have experienced numerous failed attempts using monotherapy. Combination therapy generally involves the use of a long-acting medication (nicotine patch or sustained-release bupropion) in combination with a short-acting nicotine formulation (nicotine gum, lozenge, inhaler, or nasal spray). The long-acting nicotine formulation, which delivers relatively constant concentrations of drug, is used to prevent the onset of severe withdrawal symptoms, whereas the short-acting nicotine formulation, which delivers nicotine more rapidly, is used as needed to control withdrawal symptoms that may emerge during potential relapse situations (e.g., after meals, during episodes of stress, being around other smokers). Research suggests that combination therapy may be somewhat more efficacious than monotherapy.[29,47] Disadvantages of combination therapy are the possibility of additional adverse effects (e.g., nicotine toxicity), difficulty with adherence, and increased cost. For other combination regimens, patients should be referred to their primary care provider to determine the most appropriate option.

Complementary Therapies

Although a variety of herbal and homeopathic products are available to aid cessation, data supporting their safety and efficacy are lacking. Many herbal preparations for cessation contain lobeline (derived from *Lobelia inflata*), an herbal alkaloid with partial nicotinic agonist properties. A meta-analysis[48] and a multicenter trial[49] found no evidence to support the role of lobeline as an aid for smoking cessation. Similarly, controlled trials did not find hypnosis or acupuncture to be an effective treatment for smoking cessation.[29,50]

Electronic Cigarettes

More recently, electronic cigarettes (e-cigarettes) have become available in the United States. These devices are being marketed as a substitute for cigarettes in situations that do not allow smoking. The National Youth Tobacco Survey, which focuses on middle and high school students, showed that between 2011 and 2013, the number of youth who had never smoked a conventional cigarette but had used an e-cigarette increased three-fold (from 79,000 in 2011 to 263,000 in 2013).[51] These youth were also nearly twice as likely to have an intention to smoke conventional cigarettes compared with those who had never smoked conventional or e-cigarettes: of those who had used e-cigarettes but not conventional cigarettes, 43.9% had an intention to smoke conventional cigarettes, and 21.5% of those who had never used either type of cigarette had an intention to smoke conventional cigarettes. It was concluded that enhanced prevention efforts for youth are important for use of all forms of tobacco, including e-cigarettes.

A common misperception is that e-cigarettes are safe alternatives to conventional cigarettes. However, data are currently insufficient to support their safety or efficacy in reducing or stopping smoking.[52] E-cigarettes have been found to contain carcinogens such as nitrosamines and diethylene glycol, which are toxic to humans.[53] Continued vigilance and research in this area are needed.

Assessment of Tobacco Cessation: A Case-Based Approach

To help patients succeed at tobacco cessation, the provider must assist them in evaluating their patterns of smoking, identify medications and quitting methods they have or have not tried in the past, and determine appropriate cessation therapies. Analysis of smoking patterns and triggers for smoking will help the provider work with the patient to develop an appropriate treatment plan.

Cases 47–1 and 47–2 illustrate the assessment of two patients in different phases of quitting smoking.

CASE 47–1

Relevant Evaluation Criteria	Scenario/Model Outcome
Collect	
1. Gather essential information about the patient's symptoms, including	
a. Description of symptom(s) (i.e., nature, onset, duration, severity, associated symptoms)	Patient would like information about the various nonprescription medications for tobacco cessation. He is noticing that he gets more "winded" when he walks, and he is concerned about the effects of smoking on his health. He has smoked one pack per day (or 20 cigarettes) for 21 years. He smokes 2 cigarettes with his morning coffee and smokes in social situations such as when having a few drinks with coworkers. He has not received cessation counseling from a provider. He has tried the nicotine patch and gum in the past and wants to try Chantix (varenicline).
b. Description of any factors that seem to precipitate, exacerbate, and/or relieve the patient's symptom(s)	He is in a rush because he has to get back to work. He smokes mostly on work breaks and at home in the morning and in the evenings after dinner.
c. Description of the patient's efforts to relieve the symptoms	He has tried to quit smoking approximately 5 times to date, 3 times using NRT.
d. Patient's identity	Kevin Stills
e. Patient's age, gender, height, and weight	61 years old, male, 5 ft 8 in., 170 lb
f. Patient's occupation	Accountant
g. Patient's dietary habits	Reasonably healthy diet; walks 30 minutes daily during his lunch break.
h. Patient's sleep habits	Sleeps 7 hours/night during the workweek; does not have trouble sleeping.
i. Concurrent medical conditions, prescription and nonprescription medications, and dietary supplements	Hypertension: controlled on lisinopril 10 mg daily
j. Allergies	NKA
k. History of other adverse reactions to medications	None
l. Other (describe)	Mr. Stills is married, with no children. His wife is supportive of his attempt to quit. Some close friends and coworkers also smoke.

CASE 47–1 *continued*

Relevant Evaluation Criteria	Scenario/Model Outcome
Assess	
2. Differentiate patient's signs/symptoms, and correctly identify the patient's primary problem(s).	Patient is a middle-aged man who would like to quit smoking to improve his breathing and overall health.
3. Identify exclusions for self-treatment (Figure 47–2).	None
4. Formulate a comprehensive list of therapeutic alternatives for the primary problem to determine whether triage to a medical provider is required, and share this information with the patient or caregiver.	Options include (1) Recommend pharmacotherapy and counseling. Pharmacotherapy options include ■ Nicotine patch ■ Nicotine gum ■ Nicotine lozenge ■ Combination therapy with the nicotine patch plus a short-acting NRT formulation ■ Referral to PCP for prescription pharmacotherapy (nicotine inhaler, nicotine nasal spray, bupropion SR, varenicline) (2) Refer Mr. Stills to telephone counseling (1-800-Quit-Now) because he is in a hurry. (3) Recommend that he set a quit date in 1–2 weeks. (4) Take no action.
Plan	
5. Select an optimal therapeutic alternative to address the patient's problem, taking into account patient preferences.	Mr. Stills expressed interest in taking varenicline. Refer him to his PCP for a prescription. For behavioral counseling, refer him to the quit line. (See Tables 47–3 and 47–4.)
6. Describe the recommended therapeutic approach to the patient or caregiver.	"Medication is recommended. Although you have no contraindications or precautions for medication use as part of a self-care quit program, varenicline is available only by prescription."
7. Explain to the patient or caregiver the rationale for selecting the recommended therapeutic approach from the considered therapeutic alternatives.	"Use of Chantix, or varenicline, is considered a first-line treatment for smoking cessation. Because you would like to take this medication and it is available by prescription only, you will need to contact your primary care provider to obtain a prescription. I can also call your provider for you now if you would like. Receiving counseling, in addition to taking Chantix as directed, will increase your chances of success with quitting."
Implement	
8. When recommending self-care with nonprescription medications and/or nondrug therapy, convey accurate information to the patient or caregiver.	Criterion does not apply in this case.
Solicit follow-up questions from the patient or caregiver.	"What should I do if I am tempted to smoke when I am around my friends?"
Answer the patient's or caregiver's questions.	"The quit line counselor will be able to talk to you about problem-solving and coping skills for your smoking triggers. It is important that your friends and wife support you when you quit. To minimize relapse, reduce or avoid use of alcohol during the first 2 weeks of your quit attempt. The counselor will arrange follow-up contacts after your quit date."
Follow-up: Monitor and Evaluate	
9. Assess patient outcome.	Mr. Stills plans to contact his PCP and will return to the pharmacy to fill his prescription. He also set a quit date in 2 weeks with plans to follow up with the quit line.

Key: NKA = No known allergies; NRT = nicotine replacement therapy; PCP = primary care provider; SR = sustained release.

CASE 47-2

Relevant Evaluation Criteria	Scenario/Model Outcome
Collect	
1. Gather essential information about the patient's symptoms, including	
a. Description of symptom(s) (i.e., nature, onset, duration, severity, associated symptoms)	Patient quit smoking 7 days ago and is using the generic 21 mg nicotine patch. She complains of trouble sleeping and is experiencing disturbing dreams since starting to use the patch. She had been smoking approximately 1.5 packs per day (approximately 30 cigarettes daily) for 10 years before quitting.
b. Description of any factors that seem to precipitate, exacerbate, and/or relieve the patient's symptom(s)	Before quitting, patient used to have a cigarette before even getting out of bed, because she had such intense cravings.
c. Description of the patient's efforts to relieve the symptoms	Patient has been using the 21 mg nicotine patch for 7 days. She had not previously tried pharmacotherapy for quitting. She purchased the patch after speaking to an HCP. She has not received any formal counseling from a provider. She feels a bit agitated and irritable from time to time during the day; she is very tempted to smoke in the morning when she wakes up. Overall, she likes the patch and is not experiencing any significant skin reactions.
d. Patient's identity	Kristen Brady
e. Patient's age, gender, height, and weight	28 years old, female, 5 ft 6 in., 140 lb
f. Patient's occupation	Web designer
g. Patient's dietary habits	Tries to "eat healthy"; drinks approximately 8 cups of caffeinated coffee per day.
h. Patient's sleep habits	Sleeps 7–8 hours a night. Since using the patch, she has experienced trouble sleeping and disturbing dreams.
i. Concurrent medical conditions, prescription and nonprescription medications, and dietary supplements	Ms. Brady is not pregnant or lactating. She has temporomandibular joint (TMJ) disease, for which she takes acetaminophen 325 mg every 6 hours as needed for pain, but uses rarely.
j. Allergies	NKA
k. History of other adverse reactions to medications	None
l. Other (describe)	Patient is single. Her boyfriend and her roommate are supportive of her desire to quit.
Assess	
2. Differentiate patient's signs/symptoms, and correctly identify the patient's primary problem(s).	Patient quit smoking 1 week ago and is experiencing "intolerable" adverse effects from the nicotine patch (i.e., sleep disturbances), daily withdrawal symptoms (i.e., agitation and irritability), and morning cravings.
3. Identify exclusions for self-treatment (Figure 47–2).	None
4. Formulate a comprehensive list of therapeutic alternatives for the primary problem to determine whether triage to a medical provider is required, and share this information with the patient or caregiver.	Options include (1) Recommend continued pharmacotherapy and counseling. Pharmacotherapy options include: ■ Removal of nicotine patch at night and addition of a lozenge as needed (particularly in the morning upon waking). ■ Alternative NRT agent, such as lozenge alone. ■ Referral to PCP for prescription pharmacotherapy (nicotine inhaler, nicotine nasal spray, bupropion SR, varenicline). (2) Take no action.

CASE 47-2 *continued*

Relevant Evaluation Criteria	Scenario/Model Outcome
Plan	
5. Select an optimal therapeutic alternative to address the patient's problem, taking into account patient preferences.	Because Ms. Brady has expressed that she thinks the patch is working well to manage her withdrawal symptoms, continue the nicotine patch, but advise her to take the patch off before bedtime. This change should help reduce the sleep disturbances and disturbing dreams. She can use combination therapy with a nicotine lozenge, as needed. The nicotine gum would not be a good choice because she has TMJ disease. A 2 mg lozenge dose to be used on an as-needed basis is reasonable.
6. Describe the recommended therapeutic approach to the patient or caregiver.	"It's great that the patch is working for you so far. You have no contraindications or precautions for use of the nicotine patch and as-needed 2 mg lozenge. I have some ideas that should help you with your sleep problems and some other information for you, including how to manage morning cravings."
7. Explain to the patient or caregiver the rationale for selecting the recommended therapeutic approach from the considered therapeutic alternatives.	"You do not have any medical conditions for which nicotine replacement medications should be used with caution (e.g., recent heart attack, serious arrhythmias, angina). The nicotine patch provides a low, constant level of nicotine to help reduce nicotine withdrawal symptoms. By taking it off at night, you should no longer experience sleep disturbances. The nicotine lozenge should be used only when you experience situations in which you are craving a cigarette, such as when you wake up. Receiving counseling, in addition to taking your medications as directed, will increase your chances of quitting."
Implement	
8. When recommending self-care with nonprescription medications and/or nondrug therapy, convey accurate information to the patient or caregiver.	
a. Appropriate dose and frequency of administration	"Use the 2 mg nicotine lozenge if you experience situations in which you are craving a cigarette, such as when you wake up." (See Tables 47–5 and 47–8.)
b. Maximum number of days the therapy should be employed	See Table 47–8.
c. Product administration procedures	See Tables 47–7 and 47–9.
d. Expected time to onset of relief	"With the lozenge, nicotine levels will peak 30–60 minutes after you start using it. You are already using the nicotine patch, which provides a steady amount of nicotine throughout the day. The blood nicotine levels from the patch and lozenge are lower than those from smoking but should be sufficient to help control your nicotine withdrawal. Most patients find that nicotine withdrawal symptoms peak in the first few days after the last cigarette; withdrawal symptoms then gradually diminish over the next 2–4 weeks."
e. Degree of relief that can be reasonably expected	"Over time, you may find you need to use the lozenge less often. Be sure to stick with the recommended daily dosing schedule for the patch and the duration of use needed for the best chance of success. This will help you to be more comfortable while you are quitting."
f. Most common adverse effects	"The most common adverse effects of the nicotine patch are skin reactions (redness, burning, itching) at the application site and headaches. The sleep disturbances (vivid dreams, insomnia) that you are currently experiencing from the patch should resolve when you remove it before bedtime. The most common adverse effects of the nicotine lozenge are nausea, hiccups, and heartburn."
g. Adverse effects that warrant medical intervention should they occur	"If you find that reducing your caffeine intake and using the nicotine lozenge do not help relieve your morning cravings and irritability during the day, contact your PCP. If you experience symptoms of nicotine excess (e.g., nausea, vomiting, dizziness, weakness, rapid heartbeat), also contact your PCP."

CASE 47-2 *continued*

Relevant Evaluation Criteria	Scenario/Model Outcome
h. Patient options in the event that condition worsens or persists	"Contact your PCP for the following reasons: ■ If you experience withdrawal symptoms or severe cigarette cravings, you may need a higher dosage of nicotine. ■ If you have adverse effects related to nicotine excess." (see outcome in 8g.)
i. Product storage requirements	"Store the patches and lozenges at room temperature. Keep unused patches in the closed, protective pouch. Keep all new and used patches and lozenges out of the reach of children and pets."
j. Specific nondrug measures	"Reduce caffeine use by half to minimize agitation and trouble sleeping. In addition to the counseling I can provide, other counseling programs are available, including the telephone quit line (1-800-QUIT NOW), group classes, and internet-based programs. We can discuss which options you feel might be useful to you."
Solicit follow-up questions from the patient or caregiver.	"How often can I use the lozenge?"
Answer the patient's or caregiver's questions.	"You should use the lozenge when you feel a strong craving to smoke, such as when you wake up in the morning. The patch will provide a consistent low level of nicotine to help reduce withdrawal symptoms. You should use the nicotine lozenge only when you feel a need, or urge, to smoke. Even though the box says you can use up to 20 lozenges a day, you should not need this many when you use them with the patch. Also remember to switch to the lower-strength 14 mg patch after 6 weeks; use this for 2 weeks, and then use the 7 mg patch for 2 weeks."
Follow-up: Monitor and Evaluate	
9. Assess patient outcome.	Confirm that Ms. Brady will reduce caffeine use, remove patch before bedtime, and use lozenge as needed for cravings. Will call patient in 1 week to assess quit plan.

Key: NKA = No known allergies; NRT = nicotine replacement therapy; PCP = primary care provider; SR = sustained release.

Patient Counseling for Tobacco Cessation

Substantial benefits of quitting can be realized at any age. Although approximately 70% of adult smokers would like to quit,[4] few are able to do so on their own. Research has shown that tobacco cessation rates can be substantially improved with treatment that includes counseling and pharmacotherapy.[29] (See Nonpharmacologic Therapy for a detailed discussion of counseling.) HCPs are in an ideal position to identify tobacco users and to either provide assistance throughout the cessation attempt or refer the patient to a tobacco cessation resource. The box Patient Education for Tobacco Cessation describes specific information to include in patient counseling.

Evaluation of Patient Outcomes for Tobacco Cessation

Follow-up contact is an essential component of treatment for tobacco use and dependence.[29] At each follow-up encounter, the provider should do the following:

- Assess a patient's tobacco use status and, if appropriate, evaluate and monitor pharmacotherapy use.
- Congratulate abstinent patients and encourage them to remain tobacco free.
- In cases of relapse, review the specific circumstances; reassess the commitment to abstinence; encourage the patient to learn from identified mistakes; and identify strategies to prevent future lapses.
- Determine whether the patient is experiencing nicotine withdrawal symptoms or adverse effects from the pharmacotherapy.
- Offer ongoing support. If providing that level of support is not possible, refer the patient to a specialist for more intensive treatment.

Key Points for Tobacco Cessation

- ➤ Apply the 5 As approach in providing tobacco cessation counseling: ask, advise, assess, assist, and arrange.
- ➤ For a patient who is not ready to quit, provide brief counseling by addressing the 5 Rs: relevance, risks, rewards, roadblocks, and repetition.
- ➤ For a patient who is ready to quit, offer counseling and pharmacotherapy. If time is limited, ask about tobacco use, advise the patient to quit, and refer the patient to the toll-free quit line (1-800-Quit-Now), web-based resources, and mobile apps.

PATIENT EDUCATION FOR
Tobacco Cessation

Tobacco dependence is a chronic disease optimally treated with a combination of counseling and medications. The primary goal of tobacco cessation treatment is to attain complete, long-term abstinence from all nicotine-containing products. For most people, carefully following product instructions and the self-care measures listed here will help ensure optimal treatment outcomes.

Nondrug Methods

- Receiving counseling from a HCP will increase the success of tobacco cessation. A provider can help develop a tailored tobacco cessation treatment plan.
- Telephone quit lines (e.g., 1-800-Quit-Now) are also available to provide comprehensive counseling services at no cost.
- Internet-based resources and mobile apps are also available, many at no cost.

Nonprescription Medications

Nicotine Replacement Therapy (NRT)

- NRT helps relieve and prevent symptoms of nicotine withdrawal by partially replacing the high levels of nicotine that your body is used to obtaining from cigarettes. Use of NRT helps you to focus on changing your smoking routines and to practice new coping skills while decreasing your withdrawal symptoms.
- NRT does not contain any of the harmful tars and other toxins present in tobacco smoke.
- Symptoms of nicotine withdrawal are common and should subside over 2–4 weeks.
- Recommended daily dosages for NRT are shown in Tables 47–5 and 47–8.
- See Table 47–6 for usage guidelines for nicotine gum, Table 47–7 for the nicotine lozenge, and Table 47–9 for the nicotine patch.
- Carefully follow the dosage regimen for the selected product. Failure to do so will increase the chance of having withdrawal symptoms. Discontinuing therapy early might lead to relapse.
- Signs and symptoms of nicotine excess include nausea, vomiting, dizziness, diarrhea, weakness, and rapid heartbeat.
- Do not eat or drink (except water) 15 minutes before or while using the nicotine gum or lozenge.
- Store NRT products at room temperature and protect from light.
- Keep new and used products out of the reach of children and pets.
- For all forms of NRT, consult your primary care provider before use if you have had a recent (in the past 2 weeks) heart attack, experience frequent pain caused by severe angina, have an irregular heartbeat, are pregnant or lactating, are younger than 18 years, or smoke fewer than 10 cigarettes a day.
- You may consider use of nicotine gum with the patch (gum used only on as-needed basis). For other possible medication combinations, speak to your primary care provider first.

When to Seek Medical Attention

- For all forms of NRT, stop use and seek medical attention if irregular heartbeat or palpitations occur, or if you have symptoms of nicotine overdose, such as nausea, vomiting, dizziness, diarrhea, or weakness.
- For nicotine gum: Stop use if mouth, teeth, or jaw problems develop.
- For nicotine lozenge: Stop use if mouth problems, persistent indigestion, or severe sore throat develops.
- For nicotine patch: Stop use if the skin swells, a rash develops, or skin redness caused by the patch does not subside with use of nonprescription hydrocortisone cream or does not go away after 4 days.

➤ Numerous effective medications are available for tobacco dependence; encourage their use by all patients attempting to quit smoking—except when medically contraindicated or in specific populations for which evidence of effectiveness is insufficient (i.e., pregnant women, smokeless tobacco users, light smokers, and adolescents). For patients with exclusions for self-treatment with NRT, referral to a primary care provider for further assessment is warranted.

➤ Advise patients that it is never too late for them to quit, but that quitting earlier in life is clearly advantageous. Quitting smoking at any age has immediate as well as long-term benefits by reducing the risk for smoking-related diseases and improving health in general.

REFERENCES

1. U.S. Department of Health and Human Services. *The Health Consequences of Smoking: Cancer. A Report of the Surgeon General.* Rockville, MD: Public Health Service, Office on Smoking and Health; 1982. DHHS Publication No. (PHS) 82-50179.
2. U.S. Department of Health and Human Services. *Adult Cigarette Smoking in the United States: Current Estimate.* Atlanta, GA: U.S. Department of Health and Human Services, Centers for Disease Control and Prevention, National Center for Chronic Disease Prevention and Health Promotion, Office on Smoking and Health; 2012.
3. U.S. Department of Health and Human Services. *The Health Consequences of Smoking—50 Years of Progress: A Report of the Surgeon General.* Atlanta, GA: U.S. Department of Health and Human Services, Centers for Disease Control and Prevention; 2014.
4. Centers for Disease Control and Prevention. Current cigarette smoking among adults—United States, 2005–2014. *MMWR Morb Mortal Wkly Rep.* 2015;64(44):1233–40. doi: 10.15585/mmwr.mm6444a2.
5. Centers for Disease Control and Prevention. State-specific prevalence of current cigarette smoking and smokeless tobacco use among adults aged ≥18 years—United States, 2011–2013. *MMWR Morb Mortal Wkly Rep.* 2015;64(19):532–6. PMID: 25996096.
6. Centers for Disease Control and Prevention. Vital signs: current cigarette smoking among adults aged ≥18 years with mental illness—United States, 2009–2011. *MMWR Morb Mortal Wkly Rep.* 2013;62(05):81–7. PMID: 23388551.
7. U.S. Department of Health and Human Services. *Healthy People 2020.* Washington, DC: U.S. Department of Health and Human Services; 2010. Available at: https://www.healthypeople.gov/. Accessed August 5, 2017.
8. World Health Organization. *Report on the Global Tobacco Epidemic, 2008.* Geneva, Switzerland: World Health Organization; 2008.
9. U.S. Department of Health and Human Services. *The Health Consequences of Smoking: Nicotine Addiction: A Report of the Surgeon General.* Washington, DC: U.S. Government Printing Office; 1988.
10. Benowitz NL. Nicotine addiction. *N Engl J Med.* 2010;362(24):2295–303. doi: 10.1056/NEJMra0809890.
11. U.S. Department of Health and Human Services. *How Tobacco Smoke Causes Disease: The Biology and Behavioral Basis for Smoking-Attributable Disease: A Report of the Surgeon General.* Atlanta, GA: U.S. Department of Health and Human Services, Centers for Disease Control and Prevention, National Center for Chronic Disease Prevention and Health Promotion, Office on Smoking and Health; 2010.
12. Campaign for Tobacco-Free Kids. Broken Promises to Our Children. Available at: http://www.tobaccofreekids.org/microsites/statereport2016/. Accessed August 5, 2017.

13. Doll R, Peto R, Boreham J, et al. Mortality in relation to smoking: 50 years' observations on male British doctors. *BMJ.* 2004;328(7455):1519. doi: 10.1136/bmj.38142.554479.AE.
14. National Cancer Institute. *Risks Associated with Smoking Cigarettes with Low Machine-Measured Yields of Tar and Nicotine.* Smoking and Tobacco Control Monograph No. 13. Bethesda, MD: U.S. Department of Health and Human Services, National Institutes of Health, National Cancer Institute; 2001. NIH Publication No. 02-5074.
15. Benowitz NL, Hukkanen J, Jacob P 3rd. Nicotine chemistry, metabolism, kinetics and biomarkers. *Handb Exp Pharmacol.* 2009;192:29–60. doi: 10.1007/978-3-540-69248-5_2.
16. Benowitz NL. Clinical pharmacology of nicotine: implications for understanding, preventing, and treating tobacco addiction. *Clin Pharmacol Ther.* 2008;83(4):531–41. doi: 10.1038/clpt.2008.3.
17. American Psychiatric Association. *Diagnostic and Statistical Manual of Mental Disorders.* 5th ed. Washington, DC: American Psychiatric Association; 2013.
18. Hughes JR. Effects of abstinence from tobacco: valid symptoms and time course. *Nicotine Tob Res.* 2007;9(3):315–27. PMID: 17365764
19. U.S. Department of Health and Human Services. *Secondhand Smoke (SHS) Facts.* Atlanta, GA: U.S. Department of Health and Human Services, Centers for Disease Control and Prevention, Coordinating Center for Health Promotion, National Center for Chronic Disease Prevention and Health Promotion, Office on Smoking and Health; 2013.
20. U.S. Department of Health and Human Services. *The Health Consequences of Involuntary Exposure to Tobacco Smoke: A Report of the Surgeon General.* Bethesda, MD: U.S. Department of Health and Human Services, Centers for Disease Control and Prevention, Coordinating Center for Health Promotion, National Center for Chronic Disease Prevention and Health Promotion, Office on Smoking and Health; 2006.
21. Zevin S, Benowitz NL. Drug interactions with tobacco smoking. *Clin Pharmacokinet.* 1999;36(6):425–38. PMID: 10427467.
22. Kroon LA. Drug interactions with smoking. *Am J Health Syst Pharm.* 2007; 64(18):1917–21. PMID: 17823102.
23. World Health Organization. *Medical Eligibility Criteria for Contraceptive Use.* 5th ed. Geneva, Switzerland: World Health Organization; 2015: 1–1267. Available at: http://apps.who.int/iris/bitstream/10665/181468/1/9789241549158_eng.pdf/. Accesssed July 1, 2011.
24. Pomp ER, Rosendaal FR, Doggen CJ. Smoking increases the risk of venous thrombosis and acts synergistically with oral contraceptive use. *Am J Hematol.* 2008;83(2):97–102. PMID: 17726684.
25. Tanis BC. Oral contraceptives and the risk of myocardial infarction. *Eur Heart J.* 2003;24(5):377–80. PMID: 12633537.
26. American College of Obstetricians and Gynecologists. ACOG practice bulletin no. 73: use of hormonal contraception in women with coexisting medical conditions. *Obstet Gynecol.* 2006;107(6):1453–72. PMID: 16738183.
27. University of California San Francisco. Rx for Change: Clinician-Assisted Tobacco Cessation. San Francisco, CA: University of California San Francisco; 2004–2014. Available at: http://rxforchange.ucsf.edu. Accessed August 5, 2017.
28. U.S. Department of Health and Human Services. *The Health Benefits of Smoking Cessation. A Report of the Surgeon General.* Rockville, MD: U.S. Department of Health and Human Services, Public Health Service, Office on Smoking and Health; 1990. DHHS Publication No. (CDC) 90-8416.
29. Fiore MC, Jaén CR, Baker TB, et al. *Treating Tobacco Use and Dependence: 2008 Update.* Clinical Practice Guideline. Rockville, MD: U.S. Department of Health and Human Services, Public Health Service; 2008.
30. Shiffman S, Brockwell SE, Pillitteri JL, et al. Use of smoking-cessation treatments in the United States. *Am J Prev Med.* 2008;34(2):102–11. doi: 10.1016/j.amepre.2007.09.033.
31. Stead LF, Bergson G, Lancaster T. Physician advice for smoking cessation. *Cochrane Database Syst Rev.* 2008;2:CD000165. doi:10.1002/14651858.CD000165.pub3.
32. Centers for Disease Control and Prevention. Updated recommendations for prevention of invasive pneumococcal disease among adults using the 23-valent pneumococcal polysaccharide vaccine (PPSV23). *MMWR Morb Mortal Wkly Rep.* 2010;59(34):1102–6. PMID: 20814406.
33. Shiffman S, Dresler CM, Hajek P, et al. Efficacy of a nicotine lozenge for smoking cessation. *Arch Intern Med.* 2002;162(11):1267–76. PMID: 12038945.
34. Stead LF, Perera R, Bullen C, et al. Nicotine replacement therapy for smoking cessation. *Cochrane Database Syst Rev.* 2012;11:CD000146. doi:10.1002/14651858.CD000146.pub4.
35. GlaxoSmithKline Inc. Zyban [package insert]. Research Triangle Park, NC: GlaxoSmithKline Inc.; September 2010.
36. Foulds J. The neurobiological basis for partial agonist treatment of nicotine dependence: varenicline. *Int J Clin Pract.* 2006;60(5):571–6. PMID: 16700857.
37. U.S. Food and Drug Administration. FDA Drug Safety Communication: FDA updates label for stop smoking drug Chantix (varenicline) to include potential alcohol interaction, rare risk of seizures, and studies of side effects on mood, behavior, or thinking. March 9, 2015. Available at: www.fda.gov/downloads/Drugs/DrugSafety/UCM436960.pdf. Accessed August.5, 2017.
38. Pfizer, Inc. Chantix [package insert]. New York, NY: Pfizer, Inc.; December 2012.
39. U.S. Food and Drug Administration. FDA Drug Safety Communication: Chantix (varenicline) may increase the risk of certain cardiovascular adverse events in patients with cardiovascular disease. July 22, 2011. Available at: http://www.fda.gov/Drugs/DrugSafety/ucm259161.htm#data. Accessed August 5, 2017.
40. Fagerstrom K, Gilljam H, Metcalfe M, et al. Stopping smokeless tobacco use with varenicline: randomized double-blind placebo-controlled trial. *BMJ.* 2010;341:c6549. doi: 10.1136/bmj.c6549.
41. U.S. Food and Drug Administration. FDA Drug Safety Communication: safety review update of Chantix (varenicline) and risk of cardiovascular adverse events. December 12, 2012. Available at: http://www.fda.gov/Drugs/DrugSafety/ucm330367.htm. Accessed August 5, 2017.
42. Benowitz NL. Cigarette smoking and cardiovascular disease: pathophysiology and implications for treatment. *Prog Cardiovasc Dis.* 2003;46(1): 91–111. PMID: 12920702.
43. Joseph AM, Fu SS. Safety issues in pharmacotherapy for smoking in patients with cardiovascular disease. *Prog Cardiovasc Dis.* 2003;45(6):429–41. PMID: 12800126.
44. Henningfield JE, Shiffman S, Ferguson SG, et al. Tobacco dependence and withdrawal: science base, challenges and opportunities for pharmacotherapy. *Pharmacol Ther.* 2009;123(1):1–16. doi: 10.1016/j.pharmthera.2009.03.011.
45. Benowitz N, Dempsey D. Pharmacotherapy for smoking cessation during pregnancy. *Nicotine Tob Res.* 2004;6(Suppl 2):S189–202. PMID: 15203821.
46. Shiffman S. Nicotine lozenge efficacy in light smokers. *Drug Alcohol Depend.* 2005;77(3):311–4. PMID: 15734231.
47. Cahill K, Stevens S, Perera R, et al. Pharmacological interventions for smoking cessation: an overview and network meta-analysis. *Cochrane Database Syst Rev.* 2013;5:CD009329. doi:10.1002/14651858. CD009329.pub2.
48. Stead LF, Hughes JR. Lobeline for smoking cessation. *Cochrane Database Syst Rev.* 2000;2:CD000124. doi:10.1002/14651858.CD000124.
49. Glover ED, Rath JM, Sharma E, et al. A multicenter phase 3 trial of lobeline sulfate for smoking cessation. *Am J Health Behav.* 2010;34(1):101–9. PMID:19663757.
50. White AR, Rampes H, Campbell JL. Acupuncture and related interventions for smoking cessation. *Cochrane Database Syst Rev.* 2006;1:CD000009. doi:10.1002/14651858.CD000009.
51. US Department of Health and Human Services. E-Cigarette Use Among Youth and Young Adults. A Report of the Surgeon General. Atlanta, GA: U.S. Department of Health and Human Services, CDC; 2016. Available at: https://www.cdc.gov/tobacco/data_statistics/sgr/e-cigarettes/pdfs/2016_sgr_entire_report_508.pdf. Accessed August 5, 2017.
52. Cobb NK, Abrams DB. E-cigarette or drug-delivery device? Regulating novel nicotine products. *N Engl J Med.* 2011;365(3):193–5. doi: 10.1056/NEJMp1105249.
53. U.S. Food and Drug Administration. Summary of results: laboratory analysis of electronic cigarettes conducted by FDA. April 22, 2014. Available at: https://www.fda.gov/newsevents/publichealthfocus/ucm173146.htm. Accessed August 5, 2017.

section

X

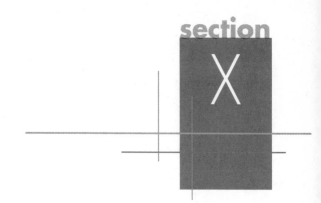

HOME MEDICAL EQUIPMENT

CHAPTER 48

HOME TESTING AND MONITORING DEVICES

GENEVA CLARK BRIGGS

Warner-Lambert's introduction of the first home pregnancy test kit in 1977 led to the current home testing market. Annual sales of just three home pregnancy test brands, First Response, ept, and Clearblue, totaled $162.7 million in 2013.[1] The home testing market continues to grow, offering an expanded array of products that are also more user friendly. Forces driving the growth in home diagnostics include (1) increased public interest in health and preventive medicine; (2) reduced health care costs, because patients can avoid unnecessary visits to health care providers (HCPs) and can seek earlier treatment of a medical condition; (3) reduced access and availability of health care resources; (4) increased number of available tests; and (5) important advances in technology that have led to simplified, accurate tests that can be easily performed at home.

Home testing and monitoring kits are designed to detect the presence or absence of a medical or physiologic condition and to monitor disease therapy. The Food and Drug Administration (FDA) requires home tests to perform as well as the professional-use equivalent. However, these products must be used properly to achieve accurate results.

This chapter discusses home test kits that aid in detecting the following conditions: pregnancy, female fertility, male fertility, colorectal cancer (fecal occult blood tests), high cholesterol, urinary tract infections (UTIs), human immunodeficiency virus (HIV), hepatitis C, and drug abuse. This chapter also covers proper selection and use of blood pressure monitors. In addition, a table of miscellaneous tests is included at the end of the chapter. For other products used in self-monitoring of disorders, see Chapter 8 for discussion of self-treatment for vaginal fungal infections.

Selection Criteria

With the variety of diagnostic and monitoring products available, deciding which test to recommend to a given patient can be challenging. The major product variables to consider include test complexity, ease of reading results, presence of a control, and cost. Table 48–1 addresses these variables as well as the major patient assessment variables, which fall within three general areas:

1. Appropriateness of testing
2. Ability to accurately conduct the test and interpret the results
3. Potential interference with test results

PREGNANCY DETECTION TESTS

Women are now able to detect pregnancy earlier, including before the day of the missed period, because of the heightened sensitivity of at-home pregnancy tests. Early detection of pregnancy is desirable for many reasons, including allowing the woman to make decisions regarding prenatal care and lifestyle changes to avoid potential harm to the fetus.

Physiology of the Female Reproductive Cycle

The female reproductive cycle is approximately 28 days and is hormonally controlled. At the beginning of the cycle (day 1 through approximately day 12), low levels of circulating estrogen and progesterone cause the hypothalamus to secrete gonadotropin-releasing hormone (GnRH). In turn, GnRH stimulates release of follicle-stimulating hormone (FSH) and low levels of luteinizing hormone (LH) from the anterior pituitary gland. This combination of hormones promotes development of several follicles within an ovary during each cycle. One follicle continues to mature while the others regress. At midcycle (approximately day 14 or 15), circulating and urinary LH levels significantly increase and cause final maturation of the follicle. *Ovulation* (rupturing of the follicle and release of the ovum) occurs approximately 20–48 hours after the LH surge. Cells in the ruptured follicle form the corpus luteum, which begins to secrete progesterone and estrogen. For approximately 7–8 days after ovulation, the corpus luteum continues to develop and secrete estrogen and progesterone, inhibiting further secretion of FSH and LH.

Once ovulation occurs, the ovum remains viable for fertilization for only 12–24 hours. Because sperm may live up to 72 hours, optimal days for fertilization to occur include the 2 days before ovulation, the day of ovulation, and the day after ovulation. For the greatest chance of achieving pregnancy, intercourse should take place within 24 hours after the LH surge.

If fertilization occurs, trophoblastic cells produce human chorionic gonadotropin (hCG) hormone. This hormone causes the corpus luteum to continue to produce progesterone and estrogen, forestalling the onset of menses while the placenta develops and

TABLE 48–1 Selection and Use of Home Tests and Devices

- Not all available tests are FDA-approved for home use. Check the status of a particular test at www.accessdata.fda.gov/scripts/cdrh/cfdocs/cfIVD/Search.cfm.
- Always check the expiration date before purchasing a product to ensure that reagents are not outdated. For example, a test that has an expiration date of 07/19 expires at the end of July 2019.
- Follow the manufacturer's instructions for storing the tests to ensure that reagents remain stable.
- When selecting a test, consider simplicity of use. Single-step tests are usually desirable, because each step is a potential source of error.
- When considering cost, determine the cost per test unit and whether kits with multiple tests are needed. Generic or store-brand kits may cost significantly less.
- When possible, select a test that includes a control to ensure that the test is functioning correctly.
- Read all instructions carefully and completely before attempting to perform a test.
- Note the time of day that the test is to be conducted, the length of time required, and any necessary supplies or equipment; then schedule the best time and place to conduct the test.
- Follow instructions exactly as described and in the order described. If you have questions about the testing procedure or interpretation of the results, consult a health care provider, or call the test manufacturer's toll-free number, if provided, for customer assistance.
- Use an accurate timing device that measures seconds to ensure that you wait the specified length of time between steps. In addition, waiting longer than the specified time to read test results could affect test reliability.
- If the selected test requires observation of a color change, read the test in good lighting. If you have color-defective vision or other visual impairment, ask someone without vision problems to observe the color change and/or read the test results.
- If you have physical limitations that could interfere with performing the test, ask someone to help you perform the test.
- If the test requires a fingerstick and you have a medical condition or take medications that may cause excessive bleeding, consult your health care provider before performing the test.
- Food, medications, and certain diseases or conditions can sometimes interfere with test results.

Key: FDA = Food and Drug Administration.

becomes functional. As early as day 7 after conception, the placenta produces hCG, some of which is excreted in the urine. The concentration of hCG continues to increase during early pregnancy, reaching maximum levels 6 weeks after conception. The levels of hCG decline over the following 4–6 weeks and then stabilize for the remainder of the pregnancy.

If fertilization does not occur during a cycle, the corpus luteum degenerates, circulating levels of progesterone and estrogen diminish, and menstruation occurs (days 1–5). Resulting low levels of progesterone and estrogen cause release of GnRH from the hypothalamus, and the hormonal cycle begins again.

Usage Considerations

Numerous pregnancy tests with different reaction times and hCG sensitivity are available for home use. Table 48–2 lists some available products that have been tested for accuracy.[2–5] Because it has the lowest detection level, First Response Early Result may be the best test for detecting pregnancy at the time of missed menses or a few days before, when hCG levels are low. After that point, most of the tests are equivalent.

Mechanism of Action

Home pregnancy tests detect hCG in the urine by using monoclonal or polyclonal antibodies in an enzyme immunoassay. The antibodies are bound to a solid surface of the stick. If urinary hCG is present, it will form a complex with the antibodies. Another antibody is added, one that is linked to an enzyme and that will react with a chromogen to produce a distinctive color. The hCG is sandwiched between the antibody linked to the enzyme and the antibodies bound to the solid surface. Filtering within the testing device removes unbound substances; a chromogen then reacts with the enzyme, causing a color change. Digital devices contain optical readers that provide results in words or icons.

Accuracy Rate

A pregnancy cannot be detected before implantation. Because of natural variability in the timing of ovulation, implantation does not necessarily occur before the expected onset of the next menses. One study found that the highest possible screening sensitivity for an hCG-based pregnancy test conducted on the first day of a missed period is 90%, because 10% of women may not have an implanted embryo at that point. Although most pregnancy tests are advertised as 99% accurate on the day of expected period, studies estimate that the highest possible screening sensitivity of a home pregnancy test by 1 week after the first day of the missed period is 97%.[5] A test sensitivity for hCG of 12.4 mIU/mL is needed to detect 95% of pregnancies on the expected day of a missed period.[6] Many tests now include a table in the package insert that details the accuracy rates based on the number of days before the expected period. The actual accuracy rate of these tests is lower, because users do not carefully follow the directions; digital readouts appear to improve the patient's ability to use home pregnancy tests and to accurately interpret results and are rated highly by users.[4,7]

Interferences

A false-positive result may occur if the woman has had a miscarriage or given birth within the previous 8 weeks, because hCG may still be present in the body. Medications such as Pergonal (menotropins for injection) and Profasi (chorionic gonadotropin for injection) can produce false-positive results. Unreliable results may occur in women who have ovarian cysts, women who have ectopic pregnancy, or women who are perimenopausal. Oral contraceptive use does not affect test results.

Because hCG levels are very low in early pregnancy and may be below the sensitivity of a particular test, false-negative results may occur with home pregnancy tests if they are performed on or before the first day of a missed period.

Usage Guidelines

See the box "Patient Education for Pregnancy Tests."

Product Selection Guidelines

Product labeling for most tests states that women may use the test as early as the first day of a missed menstrual period. Some tests

TABLE 48-2 Selected Nonprescription Pregnancy Tests

Trade Name	hCG Sensitivity[a]	Product Features
First Response Early Result	<6.3 mIU/mL	Test stick; best combination of sensitivity and reliability; can test up to 6 days before missed period; digital display test also available. First Response Rapid Result produces a result in 1 minute.
Clearblue Plus/ Advanced/Digital	25 mIU/mL	Test stick; can test up to 4 days before missed period; color-change tip so user knows urine has been absorbed; digital display test is also available (50 mIU/mL). Clearblue Advanced also gives estimate of weeks since ovulation (1–2 weeks, 2–3 weeks, 3+ weeks). >95% agreement between consumer and laboratory technician conducting test for Clearblue Plus/Digital.[3]
Store brands	25–50 mIU/mL	Test sticks; some CVS samples failed to work.[2]
E.P.T.	25–50 mIU/mL	Test sticks; some samples failed to work[2]; digital display test also available.
Accu-Clear	50 mIU/mL	Test sticks; 1% of samples failed to work.[2]
Fact Plus	25–40 mIU/mL	Test sticks

Key: hCG = Human chorionic gonadotropin [hormone].
[a] Manufacturer's claimed sensitivity.
Source: References 2–5.

that can detect hCG levels at 25 mIU/mL or less can be used 3 days before the missed period. The earlier a pregnancy test is used, the greater is the likelihood of a false-negative result. Most pregnancy tests are one-step procedures. Some tests have clear test sticks or a color change indicator that allows the woman to see the reaction occurring; this feature serves as a check that the stick absorbed sufficient urine. Other tests include two devices, which can be helpful if the first test is negative. The newest tests are digital and display the results as "pregnant" or "not pregnant," or "yes" or "no," instead of showing colored lines, which eliminates the need to interpret the results. Test results are generally obtained in 3 minutes.

A study of seven nonprescription pregnancy tests found that First Response Early Result was the most sensitive and most reliable test. It detected hCG at concentrations as low as 6.5 mIU/mL. In addition, this product was expected to detect more than 95% of pregnancies on the first day of a missed period.[3]

Assessment of Pregnancy Test Use

Whether a pregnancy test is appropriate for the patient should be determined first by asking questions about her menstrual cycle and the number of days since intercourse. If product use is appropriate, the patient should be asked about previous use of pregnancy tests and any difficulties the patient had with the tests. Questions about medical disorders and medication use should also be asked to determine whether inaccurate test results are possible or whether special measures may be required to protect the unborn child.

Patient Counseling for Pregnancy Tests

During counseling on the use of pregnancy tests, the HCP should emphasize the importance of following package instructions carefully, especially the instruction for when to begin testing. Pregnancy tests are very sensitive; therefore, the patient should be advised of medical and environmental factors that can cause inaccurate test results. The box "Patient Education for Pregnancy Tests" lists specific information to provide patients.

Evaluation of Patient Outcomes With Pregnancy Tests

If the pregnancy test result is positive, the woman should assume that she is pregnant and contact her HCP as soon as possible. In addition, if the patient is taking a medication that has teratogenic potential (e.g., Accutane, methotrexate) or any medications for chronic conditions, she should be advised to discuss with her HCP any possible effects the drugs may have on the fetus. If the test result is negative, the woman should review the procedure and make sure she performed the test correctly. She should test again in 1 week if menses has not begun. If the results of the second test are negative and menses still has not begun, the woman should seek the advice of an HCP.

FEMALE FERTILITY TESTS

Women use basal thermometers and ovulation prediction test kits and devices to time sexual intercourse to coincide with optimal fertility. These tests and devices are also useful for women who want to be more aware of their time of ovulation. However, they are not a reliable means of birth control.

It may take several months of attempting pregnancy for a fertile woman to be successful. *Infertility,* however, is defined as the medical inability to conceive after 1 year of unsuccessful attempts. Infertility is estimated to occur in 6% of married women ages 15–44 years.[10]

Available nonprescription products for ovulation prediction (Table 48–3) include ovulation detection devices, basal thermometers, and urine tests.[11–14] Each detection method has a different mechanism of action and method of use. Women should pick their preferred method.

PATIENT EDUCATION FOR

Pregnancy Tests

Avoidance of Incorrect Results

- The most accurate results will be obtained by waiting at least 1 week after the date of the expected period. Performing the test earlier may produce false-negative results.
- Try to test the urine sample immediately after collection.
- If the sample must be tested later, store it in the refrigerator, but allow the sample to warm to room temperature for 20–30 minutes before testing. Chilled urine may produce false-negative results. Be careful not to redisperse or shake up any sediment present in the sample.

Usage Guidelines

- Unless package instructions specify otherwise, use the first morning urine, because the levels of hCG, if present, will be concentrated at that time.
- If testing occurs at other times of the day, restrict fluid intake 4–6 hours before urine collection.
- Check the expiration date of the packaging. Remove test stick from packaging just before use. Remove cap from absorbent tip.
- Apply urine to testing device using whichever of the following methods is specified in package instructions: Hold test stick in the urine stream for designated time, or collect urine in a clean collection cup and dip the stick in the urine.
- After the urine is applied to the stick, lay the testing device on a flat surface. Wait the recommended time (1–5 minutes) before reading the results. Waiting the maximum allowed time may improve the sensitivity of the test.
- After reading the results, discard the testing device. If the test result is negative, test again in 1 week if menstruation has not started.

When to Seek Medical Attention

- If the second test is negative and menstruation has not begun, consult a health care provider.

Source: References 8 and 9.

Saliva microscopy and home saliva monitors are also available. These two products are not discussed here, because the results obtained are not reliable or the data on accuracy are conflicting.

Basal Thermometry

For many years, women have measured basal body temperature (BBT) to predict the time of ovulation. Resting BBT is usually between 96.0°F (35.6°C) and 97.5°F (36.4°C) during the first part of the female reproductive cycle. Approximately 24–48 hours after ovulation, it rises to a level closer to normal (i.e., 98.6°F [37.0°C]).[13]

Usage Considerations

Mechanism of Action

When using basal thermometry, women take their temperature (orally, rectally, or vaginally) with a basal thermometer each morning before arising. These temperature measurements are then

TABLE 48-3 **Selected Nonprescription Ovulation Prediction Tests and Devices**

Trade Name	Reaction Time	Product Features
Clearblue EasyDigital Ovulation Test	3 minutes	7-day kit or 1-month kit. Urine test sticks; clear and easy to read with no lines to interpret; digital smiley face technology; highly sensitive and easy to read with 97% of study volunteers correctly reading result and considered most preferred test.[10]
Clearblue Easy Fertility Monitor	5 minutes	Reusable monitor. Urine test sticks; typically predicts 2-day window for peak or high fertility level; stores daily fertility information; easy to read; tests for LH and E3G, an estrogen metabolite. More expensive touchscreen version with alarm reminders also available.
Clearblue Advanced Digital Ovulation Test	5 minutes	1- or 2-month supply available. Urine test sticks + holder, tests for LH and E3G, an estrogen metabolite; typically identifies 4 fertile days.
Answer 1-Step Ovulation	5 minutes	7-day kit. Urine test sticks; predicts ovulation within 24–36 hours.
Accu-Clear Early Ovulation Predictor Test	3 minutes	5-day kit. Urine test sticks; predicts ovulation within 24–48 hours.
First Response 1-Step Ovulation Predictor Test	5 minutes	7-day kit or 1-month supply kit. Urine test sticks; predicts ovulation within 24–36 hours; Some versions include 1 pregnancy test stick; digital ovulation test also available.
Nexcare Basal Thermometer	1 minute	Digital thermometer. Auto memory for last reading; continuous beep to indicate it is working; signals when done; large lighted display.
OV-Watch	Measures chloride ions every 30 minutes up to 12 readings	Lightweight watch that is worn during sleep; detects LH surge up to 4 days prior to ovulation; easy to use and read.

Key: E3G = Estrone-3-glucuronide; LH = luteinizing hormone.
Source: References 11–14.

plotted graphically. A rise in temperature signals that ovulation has occurred. When the increase occurs, women who want to become pregnant should have intercourse as soon as possible to maximize their chances of conception.

Accuracy Rate

The only equipment necessary for monitoring BBT is a basal thermometer, which has smaller gradations than a regular thermometer (i.e., 0.1 degree vs. 0.2). Although basal thermometry is a relatively simple method of ovulation prediction, interpreting temperature data can be confusing. The temperature increase that follows ovulation is small (0.4°F–1.0°F [0.2°C–0.6°C]). Women who have trouble reading a thermometer may miss the rise altogether; in this case, a digital model should be used.

Interferences

Several factors, such as emotions, movements, and infections, can influence the basal temperature. Eating, drinking, talking, and smoking should be postponed until after each measurement is obtained.

Usage Guidelines

See the box "Patient Education for Ovulation Prediction Tests and Devices."

Product Selection Guidelines

Digital thermometers that track multiple temperature readings for the user are available, although they are more expensive than digital thermometers that lack this feature.

Urinary Hormone Tests

Ovulation prediction tests that use urine samples to estimate the time of ovulation are marketed to women who are having difficulty conceiving and need to pinpoint ovulation.

Usage Considerations

Mechanism of Action

Urine-based ovulation prediction tests use antibodies specific to luteinizing hormone (LH) to detect the surge in the level of LH. An enzyme-linked immunosorbent assay (ELISA) elicits a color change that indicates the amount of LH in the urine. The LH surge is revealed by a difference in color or color intensity from that noted on the previous day of testing. The intensity of color on the test stick is directly proportional to the amount of LH in the urine sample. The standard digital test has a similar mechanism of action; when LH is detected in urine, the test stick shows a blue surge line that is read by the digital device. The digital device will display a smiley face, which means that LH has been detected and a woman's chances for conceiving are increased over the next 48 hours. This device also sets an individualized threshold for measuring the user's LH readings and compares them from baseline. The digital device helps to decrease human error. Generally, early morning collection of urine is recommended, because the LH surge usually begins early in the day, and the urine concentration is relatively consistent at this time. Some products do not specify a time of day but require only that a consistent time of day be used.

Testing should begin 2–4 days before the estimated day of ovulation. The kit contains directions to determine when to begin testing; the starting date is based on the average length of the past three menstrual cycles. If the cycle varies by more than 3–4 days each month, the woman should use the shortest menstrual cycle to determine the starting date.

The Clearblue Advanced Digital Ovulation Test and Clearblue Fertility Monitor both increase the window for ovulation detection by measuring two hormones, LH and estrone-3-glucuronide (E3G), a component of estrogen. E3G levels rise and fall in a pattern similar to that of LH but peak before LH, thus expanding the window of detection. The advanced digital product uses a test holder with disposable test sticks that are inserted into the holder for reading. The test holder contains special software that tracks changes in a woman's hormones from baseline in order to display peak and high fertility trends. The Clearblue Fertility Monitor is a small, palm-size device with a light-emitting diode screen that allows the woman to use urine test sticks that she then inserts into the monitor for results. To accurately predict ovulation, the patient must establish a baseline using data about fluctuations in her hormone levels. For the first month, the test monitor will instruct the woman to test daily for 10–20 consecutive days, starting on approximately the sixth day after the beginning of menstruation. Using these data, the monitor calculates the time window during which the woman is most likely to conceive. After establishing her baseline, the woman tests for 10–20 days each month, depending on her cycle length. Each day's results are displayed as low, high, or peak fertility. A low result indicates a small chance of conception; a high result indicates an increased chance of conception. This reading is typically displayed for 1–5 days, leading up to the peak fertility period for each cycle. A peak fertility reading indicates the highest chance of conception and is usually observed 2 days before ovulation.

Interferences

Medications used to promote ovulation (e.g., menotropins) artificially elevate LH and may cause false-positive results in ovulation prediction tests that measure only LH. The true LH surge can be detected in patients receiving clomiphene as long as testing does not begin until the second day after the drug therapy ends. Medical conditions associated with high levels of LH, such as menopause and polycystic ovarian syndrome (PCOS), may cause false-positive results for ovulation. Pregnancy can also cause a false-positive result for ovulation. If the patient has recently discontinued using oral contraceptives, the start of ovulation may be delayed for one to two cycles. Therefore, it would not be appropriate to use a home ovulation prediction test until fertilization has been attempted unsuccessfully for 1–2 months after discontinuation of the oral contraceptives.

PCOS, medications that affect the cycle (e.g., oral contraceptives, certain fertility treatments, estrogen-containing medications), impaired liver or kidney function (which alters levels of E3G), breastfeeding, tetracycline, and perimenopause may produce false-positive results with the Clearblue Fertility Monitor. Women who have recently been pregnant, stopped breastfeeding, or stopped using hormonal contraception should consider waiting until they have at least two consecutive natural menstrual cycles (lasting 21–42 days) before using the Clearblue Fertility Monitor.

Usage Guidelines

See the box "Patient Education for Ovulation Prediction Tests and Devices."

Product Selection Guidelines

The available ovulation prediction tests vary in the length of time needed to complete the test, method of applying urine to the test stick, number of individual tests provided, and method for reading results. Patients with longer cycles may benefit from purchasing kits that contain more testing sticks.

The Clearblue Fertility Monitor and Clearblue Advanced Digital Ovulation Test have some possible advantages over the traditional ovulation prediction kits, which detect only LH. The traditional kits identify the 24- to 48-hour window around ovulation. Both Clearblue products identify a larger window of several days and do not require that patients interpret color changes. In addition, they measure both LH and E3G, increasing the specificity of ovulation prediction. However, no studies have proved that these advantages increase a woman's chance of accurately identifying ovulation and, ultimately, conceiving. The initial cost of the Clearblue Fertility Monitor is higher than that of the traditional ovulation prediction kits, which detect only LH, but it is reusable for an indefinite period, with only the additional expense of more test sticks.

In an evaluation of four ovulation prediction kits, one study found that the Clearblue Digital Ovulation Test was the most preferred by study participants and easiest to read.[11]

Wristwatch Ovulation Prediction Device

OV-Watch, which is worn on the wrist, uses a specialized biosensor to detect and measure the fluctuation of chloride ions to predict ovulation.

Usage Considerations

Mechanism of Action

During a woman's cycle, numerous electrolytes in perspiration fluctuate. One of the electrolytes, chloride, peaks at various times throughout the monthly cycle.[14] Approximately 5 days before ovulation, a surge in chloride ions occurs. The OV-Watch has a biosensor that detects the chloride ion surge transdermally. The woman should begin wearing the watch at least 6 hours during sleep, starting on the first, second, or third day of the menstrual cycle. Chloride ion data are recorded every 30 minutes.

Accuracy Rate

The OV-Watch underwent clinical testing to be cleared as an acceptable device by FDA. Research concluded that the watch was equivalent to the other products that measured LH. However, compared with these products, the watch detected fertility up to 4 days prior to ovulation. Finally, the data suggest that approximately two-thirds of patients who used the watch were more likely to become pregnant within 6 months.[14]

Interferences

Factors such as excessive moisture, hormonal contraceptives, menopause, liver and kidney disease, breastfeeding, and PCOS can affect the accuracy of the watch.

Usage Guidelines

See the box "Patient Education for Ovulation Prediction Tests and Devices."

Product Selection Guidelines

The OV-Watch uses advanced technology to help predict a woman's fertile window. In addition, the more fertile days that a woman can identify, the greater are her chances of becoming pregnant.

Assessment of Female Fertility Test Use

The patient should be asked privately about her reasons for using an ovulation prediction test. If the reason is difficulty in conceiving, the patient should be asked whether she has consulted a health care specialist about a possible fertility problem and whether she has previously used ovulation prediction tests or devices. Questions about other possible pathology and medication use are appropriate to determine possible interferences with test results or temperature measurements. Case 48–1 illustrates assessment of a patient who wishes to become pregnant.

Patient Counseling for Female Fertility Tests

To use ovulation prediction products effectively, a woman must know approximately when ovulation occurs or be willing to track three menstrual cycles to determine when it occurs. The HCP should explain hormonal fluctuations during the cycle and how they relate to the use of ovulation prediction tests and devices. The provider should also explain the reason for the number of tests or measurements that must be performed with each type of product. Finally, counseling should emphasize consistent use of the products for at least 3 months to achieve accurate results. The box "Patient Education for Ovulation Prediction Tests and Devices" lists specific information to provide patients.

Evaluation of Patient Outcomes With Female Fertility Tests

Ovulation prediction products should not be used for more than 3 months. If conception does not occur within this period, the woman should see an HCP.

MALE FERTILITY TESTS

Sperm concentration is one of the many factors used to determine male fertility. Because many additional factors play a role in male infertility, a positive test for sperm count is not a guarantee of fertility. A decreased sperm concentration can result from epididymitis, orchitis, hormone imbalances, anabolic steroid use, and many other reasons.

CASE 48-1

Relevant Evaluation Criteria	Scenario/Model Outcome
Collect	
1. Gather essential information about the patient's symptoms and medical history, including	
a. Description of symptom(s) (i.e., nature, onset, duration, severity, associated symptoms)	Patient has been trying to become pregnant for 2 months. She asks if the ovulation kits can help.
b. Medical history, including family history	Menstrual cycle: 29 days; regular cycle in the past. She has regular intercourse with her husband of 1 year.
c. Patient's identity	Blair Jones
d. Patient's age, gender, height, and weight	27 years old, female, 5 ft 5 in., 155 lb
e. Patient's occupation	Electrical engineer
f. Concurrent medical conditions, prescription and nonprescription medications, and dietary supplements	No current medical conditions; multivitamin daily
g. Prior use of diagnostic/monitoring test	Has never used any home diagnostic tests.
h. Potential problems with performing/interpreting test	Lauren does not know how to use an ovulation prediction test.
Assess	
2. Determine whether self-testing is appropriate.	Self-testing is appropriate.
3. Identify exclusions for self-treatment.	None
4. Formulate a comprehensive list of therapeutic alternatives for the primary problem to determine whether triage to a medical provider is required, and share this information with the patient or caregiver.	Options include (1) Recommend an ovulation test today. Educate the patient to follow all manufacturer's instructions when performing the self-test. (2) Advise the patient to make an appointment with her HCP if she does not become pregnant within 1 year. (3) Take no action.
Plan	
5. Select an optimal therapeutic alternative to address the patient's problem, taking into account patient preferences.	Because the patient likes technology, she is interested in trying a fertility monitor.
Implement	
6. Describe the testing procedure to the patient.	
a. Specific instructions	"When you perform the test, follow the instructions carefully."
b. How to avoid incorrect results	See the box "Patient Education for Pregnancy Tests."
Solicit follow-up questions from the patient or caregiver.	"How long should I do the tests before seeing a doctor?"
Answer the patient's or caregiver's questions.	"It can take up to a year for couples to conceive without the help of ovulation prediction. If you are consistently able to predict ovulation with the monitor for 3 months and have not become pregnant, you should make an appointment with your health care provider."
Follow-up: Monitor and Evaluate	
7. Assess patient outcome.	"You can call if you have any questions while doing the test or are concerned about the results."

Key: HCP = Health care provider.

PATIENT EDUCATION FOR Ovulation Prediction Tests and Devices

Basal Thermometers

Avoidance of Incorrect Results

- Do not move while taking temperature measurements.
- Note that emotions can affect temperature measurements.
- If fever is present, discontinue the measurements until the fever is resolved. Resume measurements on the first day of the menstrual cycle that occurs after the fever is gone.
- Do not eat, drink, talk, or smoke within 30 minutes of taking temperature measurements.

Usage Guidelines

- Read the instructions thoroughly before using the thermometer.
- Choose one method of taking temperatures (orally, vaginally, rectally), and use that method consistently.
- Take temperature readings at approximately the same time each morning. Take temperature just before rising each morning after at least 5 hours of sleep. If using a regular basal thermometer, plot the temperatures on a graph. A rise in temperature indicates that ovulation has occurred.

Ovulation Prediction Tests

Avoidance of Incorrect Results

- Fertility medications, PCOS, menopause, and pregnancy can cause false-positive results for ovulation.
- With the Clearblue Easy Fertility Monitor, estrogen-containing medications, impaired liver or kidney function, breastfeeding, tetracycline, and perimenopause can cause false-positive results.
- Recent pregnancy or discontinuation of oral contraceptives or breastfeeding will delay ovulation for one or two cycles. Start testing after two natural menstrual cycles have occurred.

Usage Guidelines (Except Clearblue Easy Fertility Monitor)

- Start using the test 2–3 days before ovulation is expected.
- Follow the manufacturer's specific directions for the timing of urine collection. If the first morning urine is not tested, restrict fluid intake for at least 4 hours before testing, and avoid urinating until you are ready to test the urine so that the urine will not be diluted.
- Test the urine sample immediately after collection.
- If immediate testing is not feasible, refrigerate urine for the length of time specified in the product's directions. Allow refrigerated sample to stand at room temperature for 20–30 minutes before beginning the test.
- Do not shake up any sediment that may be present in the sample.
- Either hold a test stick in the urine stream for the specified time, or collect urine in a collection cup and dip the stick in the urine.
- After the urine is placed on the testing device, read the results in 3–5 minutes, depending on the manufacturer's instructions.
- Watch for the test's first significant increase in color intensity or, if using a digital test, the display of the "smiley face." Either result indicates that the surge of LH has occurred and that ovulation will occur within 1 or 2 days.
- Once the LH surge is detected, discontinue testing. Remaining tests can be used later, if necessary.
- If the LH surge is not detected, carefully review the testing instructions to ensure that they were performed properly.
- If the testing procedure was accurate, ovulation may not have occurred or testing may have occurred too late in the cycle. Consider testing for a longer period and earlier in the next cycle to increase the chances of detecting the LH surge.

Usage Guidelines for Clearblue Easy Fertility Monitor Test

- For the first month, begin testing on the sixth day after menstruation starts; the monitor will indicate how many total days you should test.
- For subsequent months, test the number of days indicated by the monitor.
- Remove test stick from packaging just before use.
- Hold the test stick in the urine stream; insert stick in monitor.
- Discard test stick after use.

OV-Watch Fertility Predictor Device

Avoidance of Incorrect Results

- Fertility medications, hormonal contraceptives, menopause, impaired liver and kidney function, breastfeeding, and PCOS may interfere with results.
- Do not expose the watch to water or excessive moisture. Wait 1 hour after exercising or showering before wearing the watch.

Usage Guidelines

- Before using the watch, read thoroughly the manufacturer's instructions for attaching the sensor and programming the device.
- Use the watch on the first, second, or third day of the menstrual period.

Key: LH = Luteinizing hormone; PCOS = polycystic ovarian syndrome.
Source: References 11–14.

Usage Considerations

The male fertility test measures sperm concentration as either above or below the cutoff of 20 million sperm cells per milliliter, which is the World Health Organization criterion for determining low sperm count.[15] Two test results of fewer than 20 million sperm cells per milliliter obtained at least 3 days apart, but not more than 7 days apart, may indicate male infertility.[16]

Mechanism of Action

The test works by detecting the concentration of a sperm-specific protein (antigen SP-10) in the semen, which is then used to determine the sperm count.[17] The semen is mixed with a buffer to help release the specific protein from the sperm. The mixture then binds to a colloidal gold compound in the test well and flows through the test. If the sample contains more than 20 million cells per milliliter, a reddish line appears, indicating a positive result. The test kit contains all the necessary supplies for the test: a testing device, testing solution, transfer device, and sperm collection cup.

Accuracy Rate

Testing performed by the manufacturer found the overall accuracy of the test to be 98%.[17]

Interferences

No interferences that can cause false-positive or negative results are known.

Usage Guidelines

See the box "Patient Education for Male Fertility Tests."

Product Selection Guidelines

SpermCheck is the only male fertility test currently on the market. Because this test requires the user to determine visually whether a line is present, patients with visual difficulties should seek assistance in interpreting the test results.

Assessment of Male Fertility Test Use

The patient should be asked privately whether he has consulted an HCP about a possible fertility problem and whether he has previously used male fertility tests.

Patient Counseling for Male Fertility Tests

The patient should be advised that a positive test does not account for sperm motility, morphology, and other factors that contribute to male fertility. The box "Patient Education for Male Fertility Tests" lists specific information to provide patients.

Evaluation of Patient Outcomes With Male Fertility Tests

If a negative result is obtained, the patient should contact his HCP or a fertility specialist. If a negative result is obtained but the patient is trying to increase his sperm count, he can test his fertility every 3 months.

FECAL OCCULT BLOOD TESTS

Colorectal cancer is the third leading cause of cancer death in the United States.[18] One early and common symptom of colorectal cancer is bleeding. Checking for hidden (occult) blood in the stool is an easy way to screen for a potential colon problem. Fecal occult blood tests (FOBTs) can be used as an adjunct to more invasive tests to detect colorectal cancer and other causes of gastrointestinal (GI) bleeding.

Colorectal cancer occurs most commonly in patients with a history of colorectal cancer in a first-degree relative, adenomatous intestinal polyps, certain inherited genes, or inflammatory bowel disease.[19] The incidence of colorectal cancer has been associated with advancing age, consumption of high amounts of red and processed meat, overweight/obesity, physical inactivity, smoking, and heavy alcohol use.[19]

Usage Considerations

Two types of nonprescription FOBTs are available: pseudoperoxidase–based toilet test (referred to as FOBT in the following discussion) and immunochemical-based FOBT (iFOBT), also known as fecal immunochemical test. Both kinds of tests are noninvasive and easy to use in the privacy of the home.

Accuracy Rate

The sensitivity and specificity of FOBT using guaiac testing (Hemocult cards) for colorectal cancer detection varies from 0.13 to 1 and 0.69 to 0.99, respectively.[20] The figures for the iFOBT are from 0.42 to 0.94 and 0.4 to 1, respectively. FOBT has better diagnostic performance for detecting distal colon cancer than proximal disease.

PATIENT EDUCATION FOR Male Fertility Tests

Avoidance of Incorrect Results

- Collect a semen sample between 2 and 7 days after the last ejaculation.
- Test within 3 hours of sample collection.

Usage Guidelines

- The semen sample is collected by masturbation, with semen directed into the liquefaction cup.
- Because freshly ejaculated semen is gel-like, the sample must be allowed to sit for 20 minutes, during which it will thin to a liquid consistency for testing.
- Gently stir the cup with the semen transfer device at least 10 times.
- Insert the semen transfer device into the sample cup, and withdraw semen to the level of the black line, while trying to avoid creating any air bubbles.
- Gently add the semen to the upright SpermCheck solution bottle. Gently mix the solution by turning the bottle upside down at least 5–10 times. Let the solution bottle stand for 2 minutes before completing the next step.
- Add 6 drops of the solution to the sample well on the SpermCheck device that is labeled "S."
- Read results exactly 7 minutes after adding the solution.
- To read the test, make sure there is a reddish line beside the "C" (Control) position on the device. If a control line is not present, the test did not work accurately. If a reddish line appears next to the "T" (test) position on the device, the result is positive (sperm ≥20 million/mL). If no line is present at the test position, the sample is negative (sperm ≤20 million/mL). Do not compare the faintness or darkness of the lines between the control and test positions. The presence of a line is a positive test result.

When to Seek Medical Attention

- If a negative test is obtained, see a health care provider for evaluation and further testing.

Source: Reference 16.

Mechanism of Action

Blood may be present on the surface or contained within the stool matrix. In general, matrix blood originates in the upper GI tract, whereas surface blood comes from the lower tract. FOBT kits are more likely to detect blood from lower GI abnormalities. The FOBT toilet test detects blood in feces with a pseudo-peroxidase reaction utilizing a chromogen that, when oxidized by hemoglobin, produces a blue-green color. The appearance of this color indicates a positive test.[21–22] This type of kit is based on the premise that a significant amount of fecal blood from stool will remain on the surface of the toilet bowl water after a bowel movement.

The iFOBT uses antibodies to detect human hemoglobin protein in stool. This test reacts to part of the human hemoglobin protein (heme), which is found in red blood cells, and it is also less likely to react to bleeding from parts of the upper digestive tract, such as the stomach. With this test, stool is sampled from toilet tissue after a bowel movement.

Interferences

Blood in the stool can signify a number of conditions in addition to cancer of the colon and rectum, including ulcers, Crohn's disease, colitis, anal fissures, diverticulitis, and hemorrhoids. Any of these conditions can give a positive result for an FOBT.

Women who are menstruating should delay testing until menses has ceased. Menstrual blood that is present in the toilet bowl water or contaminates the stool sample can produce a positive result.

Aspirin, nonsteroidal anti-inflammatory drugs (NSAIDs), and steroids may cause sufficient gastric bleeding to produce positive results. These medications should ideally be avoided for at least 2–3 days before testing and during the test period. However, studies do not suggest a benefit in withholding these agents and have not directly assessed the impact on sensitivity or specificity.[23] Rectally administered medications should also be avoided.

The FOBT toilet tests are not specific for human blood and may theoretically produce false-positive results if red meat is consumed. However, a meta-analysis of dietary restriction studies found no difference in response rates between restricting and not restricting meat consumption before physician-based testing.[24] The manufacturer's instructions say no dietary restrictions are necessary.[21] Toilet bowl cleaners may also produce false-positive results in the toilet tests. The box "Patient Education for Fecal Occult Blood Tests" lists measures for avoiding inaccurate test results.

Usage Guidelines

See the box "Patient Education for Fecal Occult Blood Tests."

Product Selection Guidelines

All tests are similar in cost. Patients who do not want to use sample stool from toilet paper may wish to use the toilet test kits.

Assessment of Fecal Occult Blood Test Use

For most patients, colon cancer screening should start at 50 years of age and be conducted every 5–10 years; in those at high risk, screening should begin at age 40 or 45.[25–27] The US Preventive Services Task Force recommends the use of FOBT, sigmoidoscopy, or colonoscopy for screening, but these recommendations are currently under revision.[26] Because of better sensitivity, the American College of Gastroenterology recommends that colonoscopy rather than FOBT be used to screen for colon cancer.[25] The American Cancer Society recommends FOBT yearly, colonoscopy every 10 years, or other screening tests such as a virtual colonoscopy every 5 years as options for people 50 years of age and older who are at average risk of colon cancer.[27] For those at increased risk, FOBT is not recommended. Patients seeking FOBT information should be assessed for risk factors for colon cancer. Those with risk factors should be encouraged to have a screening test other than FOBT. Determining the potential for false test results is an important consideration. False-negative tests could delay necessary treatment, whereas false-positive tests could cause unwarranted anxiety and expensive follow-up testing.

Patient Counseling for Fecal Occult Blood Tests

When counseling a patient on the use of FOBTs, the HCP should emphasize the importance of following package instructions carefully. The box "Patient Education for Fecal Occult Blood Tests" lists specific information to provide patients.

Evaluation of Patient Outcomes With Fecal Occult Blood Tests

A patient evaluating the results of an FOBT must remember that the test is a screening method and is not specific to a particular disease. A positive test result may indicate any medical condition that causes a loss of blood through the GI system. The primary value of FOBT is to alert patients and HCPs that a thorough workup may be needed. The kits are not intended to replace other diagnostic procedures. Patients should be advised to contact their HCP if a positive test result is obtained.

CHOLESTEROL TESTS

Elevated levels of low-density lipoprotein cholesterol (LDL-C) and triglycerides and low levels of high-density lipoprotein cholesterol (HDL-C) are major contributors to the development of atherosclerotic heart disease, which can result in heart attack and stroke. Thirteen percent of American adults have high cholesterol.[28] The American College of Cardiology/American Heart Association Cardiovascular risk assessment guidelines recommend that all adults without known cardiovascular disease have a lipid profile measured every 4–6 years, starting at age 20.[29] A home cholesterol test is one means of achieving this critical step to minimize the risk for cardiovascular disease. However, this test should not replace a complete lipid panel conducted by an HCP.

Because elevated cholesterol is a chronic condition that requires lifestyle modification and, frequently, medication for treatment, adhering to a treatment plan can be difficult for patients. Home cholesterol tests can help them monitor the efficacy of and adherence to diet, exercise, and medication plans.

PATIENT EDUCATION FOR Fecal Occult Blood Tests

Avoidance of Incorrect Results

- Do not perform test during times of known bleeding, such as hemorrhoidal or menstrual bleeding.
- Increase dietary fiber intake for several days before testing. Roughage increases the accuracy of the test by stimulating bleeding from lesions that might not otherwise bleed.
- Because bleeding from cancerous lesions may be intermittent, perform the test on three consecutive bowel movements to increase the chance of detecting a possible lesion.
- Complete all three stool tests, even if the first two produce negative results.
- Do not take nonprescription medications such as aspirin and NSAIDs for 2–3 days before testing and during testing.
- Some prescription medications can cause bleeding and may need to be discontinued before testing. Consult a health care provider about which medications to stop before performing the test.

Toilet Test Products (EZ-Detect)

- Remove toilet tank cleansers or deodorizers, and flush toilet twice before testing.
- Keep test pads in original foil pouch until time of testing.
- Before testing, use one test pad to perform a water quality check. Hold the pad by its corners and drop it into the toilet bowl. If any trace of blue appears in the cross-shaped area when the pad is placed in the toilet water, use another toilet to complete the testing. Perform this water quality check on the second toilet as well.
- Immediately after a bowel movement, place a pad in the toilet bowl, printed side up. After 2 minutes, check for the appearance of a blue cross on the test pad (positive result).
- If color changes differ from the blue cross, discard the pad and repeat the test after the next bowel movement.
- Repeat the test on the next two bowel movements.
- If results are negative for all three tests, use remaining pad to perform a quality check of the test pads using the positive control chemical package that is provided. Flush the toilet and empty the contents of the package into the bowl as it refills. Float the remaining test pad in the water, printed side up. After 2 minutes, check for a blue cross, which indicates the test pads are working properly. If the blue cross does not appear, call the product manufacturer's assistance line provided with the product.

Stool Application Product (Second-generation FIT)

- After a bowel movement, wipe the anal area as you normally do, and retain a small amount of stool on toilet paper.
- Unscrew cap/wand from buffer tube.
- Collect a small sample of stool onto the grooves of the buffer tube cap/wand.
- Return cap to tube and screw tightly. Shake tube for 3 seconds. Unscrew smaller clear cap at top of tube.
- Apply 3 drops from tube to sample well.
- Read results after 5 minutes. There should be a red line at "C," which indicates the test is working. A positive test will also have a line at "T." Do not read results if 10 minutes has elapsed.

When to Seek Medical Attention

- Notify a health care provider if any of the tests are positive.

Source: References 21 and 22.

Usage Considerations

Some nonprescription cholesterol tests (Table 48–4) measure only total cholesterol, whereas others also measure LDL-C, HDL-C, and triglycerides.[30–35] Individuals with diabetes might want to consider a device such as the CardioChek, which measures glucose levels in addition to cholesterol and triglyceride levels. The CholesTrak and First Check kits allow patients to measure their total blood cholesterol levels at home. Check Up America offers a self-collected, laboratory-performed test for a complete lipid profile.

Mechanism of Action

With the total cholesterol test cassettes, cholesterol present in a blood sample is converted into hydrogen peroxide through a chemical reaction involving cholesterol esterase and cholesterol oxidase.[30,31] The peroxide then reacts with horseradish peroxidase and a dye to produce the color that rises along the cholesterol test's measurement scale. The test cassette has two separate indicator spots that change color to show that the test is functioning properly. One of the indicator spots also indicates completion of the test, signaling that it is time to read the scale.

CardioChek, Accutrend Plus, and Q. Steps Cholesterol Biometer all use a reflectance photometer that reads the color intensity of the chemical test reaction.[32–34] Similar to a glucose meter, the results of the test are displayed on a screen. Check Up America's lipid profile is performed by a Clinical Laboratory Improvement Act (CLIA)–certified laboratory.[35]

TABLE 48-4 Selected Nonprescription Cholesterol Tests

Trade Name	Product Features
CholesTrak Home Cholesterol Test; First Check Home Cholesterol Test	Measures total cholesterol; not reusable; includes test cassette, lancet, and chart for interpreting test results from a drop of blood; chart is specific for test cassette and should not be reused.
CardioChek	Measures total cholesterol, HDL-C, and triglycerides; can also measure glucose and ketones; stores results; reusable; separate test strip and corresponding color-coded memory chip required for each type of test.
Accutrend Plus and Cholesterol Biometer	Measures total cholesterol; can also measure glucose; stores results; reusable; separate test strip required for each type of test; Accutrend Plus has low and high control solutions.
Check Up America Cholesterol Panel	Lipid profile (total cholesterol, triglycerides, HDL-C, LDL-C) results are obtained after mailing sample to laboratory; not reusable; contains lancet and sample collection cassette.

Key: HDL-C = High-density lipoprotein cholesterol; LDL-C = low-density lipoprotein cholesterol.
Source: References 30–35.

Accuracy Rate

The accuracy rate of home cholesterol tests is debated. Except for Check Up America, which is mailed to a laboratory, all products are FDA-approved for home use, are CLIA-waived devices, and are rated substantially equivalent to a laboratory-based cholesterol test. A published study of the CholesTrak device found that untrained patients obtained results that correlated well with a laboratory-based cholesterol reference method.[36] Several years ago, *Consumer Reports* tested the CholesTrak, First Check, and CardioChek kits. The first two, which are essentially the same device, gave results that varied no more than 15% from laboratory values. The CardioChek yielded results that were "often wide of the mark."[37] The report provided no more specifics. The professional version of the CardioChek (CardioChek PA) has been tested against another point-of-care device (Cholestech LDX) and laboratory measurements and did not meet the National Cholesterol Education Program (NCEP) accuracy goal.[38]

Interferences

Good fingerstick technique is necessary to avoid erroneous results with cholesterol tests. Two or three hanging drops of blood are needed, but excessive squeezing and milking of the finger will negatively affect the quality of the blood sample. If sufficient blood cannot be obtained from the first fingerstick, the patient should use a different finger. A low cholesterol value may result if the blood sample is too small or if it takes longer than 5 minutes to collect the necessary amount of blood.

The patient should avoid doses of 500 mg or more of vitamin C before the test to avoid obtaining an artificially low result. Vitamin C slows the development of the color reaction by slowing the rate at which peroxide is produced and has been shown to interfere with all home-based tests.

Usage Guidelines

See the box "Patient Education for Cholesterol Tests."

Product Selection Guidelines

Although significantly more expensive than individual total cholesterol test cassette kits, the cholesterol meters are reusable with the purchase of additional testing materials and will store test results. Some of the meters have the ability to test for HDL-C and triglycerides, whereas the other home tests measure only total cholesterol. Check Up America provides a lipid profile done in a certified laboratory, but results are not immediately available.

Assessment of Cholesterol Test Use

Whether the patient has been diagnosed with or has some reason to be concerned about hypercholesterolemia should be determined before a cholesterol test is recommended. Any factors that could affect the test results should also be determined.

Patient Counseling for Cholesterol Tests

Counseling about cholesterol tests should emphasize the importance of properly collecting blood samples. Patients should also be advised to seek assistance with the fingerstick, if needed. As further assurance of accurate test results, patients should be advised of factors that can cause inaccurate test results. The box "Patient Education for Cholesterol Tests" lists specific information to provide patients.

PATIENT EDUCATION FOR Cholesterol Tests

Avoidance of Incorrect Results

- If two or three hanging drops of blood cannot be obtained, or if it takes longer than 5 minutes to collect this amount of blood, do not perform the test.
- Do not excessively squeeze or milk the finger.
- If taking vitamin C in doses of 500 mg or more, do not take the dose within 4 hours of testing.
- The lancet is a biohazard; dispose of it in a puncture-resistant container.

Usage Guidelines

- Before starting the test, wash your hands thoroughly with soap and warm water, and then dry them.
- To stabilize the cholesterol level, sit and relax for 5 minutes before performing the test.
- CardioChek Test: Insert the memory chip corresponding to the desired test into the meter; then turn on the meter.
- Lance the outside of one fingertip, and wipe away the first sign of blood with the gauze pad. Then apply blood to the testing device as quickly as possible. For test cassettes (CholesTrak/First Check), fill the well of the test cassette. For cholesterol meters, apply enough blood to cover the testing area of a strip. For the Check Up America Test, place enough blood to fill the well on the test device and to turn the indicator window red.
- Test cassettes: Wait at least 2 minutes, but no more than 4 minutes, before pulling the clear plastic tab on the right side of the cassette. Pull the tab until it clicks into place and a red line appears. Use a timepiece with a second hand for accurate timing. Wait another 10–12 minutes. When the "END" indicator turns green, measure the height of the purple column against the scale printed on the cassette. Use the result chart included in the kit to interpret the reading.
- Cholesterol meter: A test strip may need to be inserted before applying blood for the meter to read the bar code. The test strip can be removed to apply the blood sample. The meter displays the test results in approximately 1–3 minutes.
- Check Up America Test: Allow blood to dry on the test cassette. Seal the device in the provided mailing pouch along with the completed paperwork. Mail to the laboratory. Results will be available online in approximately 1 week.
- Dispose of the lancet in a puncture-resistant container.

When to Seek Medical Attention

- If the total cholesterol reading is 200 mg/dL or greater, HDL-C is 40 mg/dL or less, or triglycerides are 150 mg/dL or greater, see a health care provider for evaluation and further testing.

Key: HDL-C = High-density lipoprotein cholesterol.
Source: References 30–35.

Evaluation of Patient Outcomes With Cholesterol Tests

Any patient who obtains a total cholesterol result of 200 mg/dL or greater, an HDL-C of 40 mg/dL or less, or triglycerides of 150 mg/dL or greater should see an HCP for a full lipid profile and appropriate medical workup. Patients should not adjust their cholesterol-lowering medications based on results of a home test without consulting their HCP.

URINARY TRACT INFECTION TESTS

Urinary tract infections (UTIs) are the cause of 8–10 million visits to HCPs every year.[39] Women have a shorter urethra compared with men and are therefore more likely to contract UTIs because of retrograde migration of bacteria from the skin. Conditions that increase risk of UTIs include pregnancy, diabetes, urinary stones, urinary obstructions such as those caused by an enlarged prostate, presence of urinary catheters, and a history of UTIs.[40]

The gram-negative bacterium *Escherichia coli* is responsible for 90% of UTIs.[39] Other gram-positive and gram-negative bacteria account for the other 20% of causative organisms. Symptoms of a UTI include pain on urination, the sensation of an urgent need to urinate, frequent urination, blood in the urine, and lower abdominal pain or discomfort.

Two primary uses for UTI tests are (1) early detection of an infection in patients with a history of recurrent UTIs or risk factors associated with UTIs and (2) confirmation that an infection has been cured by antibiotic therapy.

Usage Considerations

Only one type of UTI test is currently available.

Mechanism of Action

The UTI test (AZO Test Strips, store brands) detects both nitrite and leukocyte esterase (LE), an enzyme unique to *leukocytes* (white blood cells).[41] White blood cells may be found in the urine when a UTI is present. Gram-negative bacteria reduce nitrate in the urine to nitrite. In the test strip, arsanilic acid reacts with urinary nitrite to form a diazonium compound, which in turn reacts with another chemical on the strip to produce a pink color. A positive test requires a bacterial concentration of 10^5 per milliliter of urine. LE detection helps identify infections with gram-positive organisms that would be missed with testing for only nitrites.

Accuracy Rate

Combining nitrite and LE in one test increases overall sensitivity compared with either alone. Sensitivity has been reported to be 68%–90% when used by an HCP.[42]

Interferences

A strict vegetarian diet that provides insufficient urinary nitrates can cause false-negative nitrite results with a UTI test. Tetracycline, along with doses of vitamin C in excess of 250 mg, may also produce a false-negative reading for nitrites, because ascorbic acid blocks the nitrite test reaction. Doses of vitamin C in excess of 500 mg within 24 hours of testing may result in a false-negative result for the LE test by blocking the development of the color reaction.[41] The patient should allow 10 hours between the last dose of vitamin C and the test procedure. Dyes or medications such as phenazopyridine, occasionally used by patients with UTIs, may cause a false-positive result by changing the sensor pad to pink.

Usage Guidelines

See the box "Patient Education for Urinary Tract Infection Tests."

Product Selection Guidelines

UTI tests are small test strips. The AZO test strips have a small, attached handle that may make them easy to hold in the urine stream.

Assessment of Urinary Tract Infection Tests

The patient's reason for using a UTI test should be determined before a test is recommended. If the patient is testing for a suspected UTI, the patient's symptoms and risk factors for UTIs should be evaluated. If symptoms of a UTI are present, the patient should be referred to his or her HCP immediately for evaluation and treatment. If the patient is testing to find out whether a treated UTI has been cured, the patient's adherence to the therapy should be assessed. The patient's diet and medication use are important factors to evaluate for possible interference with test results.

Patient Counseling for Urinary Tract Infection Tests

If the sensor pad is to be immersed in a cup of urine, counseling on the use of UTI tests should emphasize the importance of collecting a clean sample of midstream urine in a clean, unwaxed container. A patient with visual difficulties should be advised to seek assistance in interpreting test results. As further assurance of accurate test results, patients should be advised of medical and dietary factors that can cause inaccurate test results. The box "Patient Education for Urinary Tract Infection Tests" lists specific information to provide patients.

Evaluation of Patient Outcomes With Urinary Tract Infection Tests

Because UTI tests will detect only about 90% of infections, the patient should contact an HCP if a negative result is obtained but UTI symptoms persist. If a positive result is obtained, the patient should contact an HCP immediately for evaluation and treatment.

PATIENT EDUCATION FOR Urinary Tract Infection Tests

Avoidance of Incorrect Results

- Persons on a strict vegetarian diet or tetracycline may not obtain accurate results.
- Certain dyes or medications, such as phenazopyridine, may cause a false-positive result by changing the sensor pad to pink.
- Do not take 250 mg or more of vitamin C within 24 hours of testing.
- Women should not use the test during menses, because menstrual blood will cause a false-positive result.

Usage Guidelines

- Clean the genital area thoroughly before collecting a urine sample.
- Test the first urine of the morning or, for later testing, use urine held in the bladder for at least 4 hours.
- To improve sensitivity, test on 3 consecutive days if the test on the previous day was negative.
- Pass the test strip through the urine stream, or immerse sensor pad for 1 second in urine collected in a clean cup.
- Do not touch the sensor pad with your fingers, because skin oils can interfere with the test reaction.
- Make sure urine completely covers the pad.
- Wait the indicated time (30–60 seconds); then compare the color on the sensor pad with the color chart provided.
- Wait no longer than 3 minutes to read the test strip, and ignore any color changes that occur after that time.

When to Seek Medical Attention

- Contact a health care provider immediately for evaluation and treatment of any positive test.
- If the test is negative but symptoms persist, see a health care provider immediately for evaluation and treatment.

Source: Reference 41.

HUMAN IMMUNODEFICIENCY VIRUS TESTS

In 2014, new cases of human immunodeficiency virus (HIV) infections in the United States were estimated at 37,600 compared with 45,700 in 2008. At the end of 2014, an estimated 1.1 million people in the United States were living with HIV, and an estimated 15% of these cases were undiagnosed.[43] Home HIV tests allow a person to test for HIV in privacy.

Acquired immunodeficiency syndrome (AIDS), an incurable disease caused by HIV infection, destroys the body's immune system. HIV infection can be contracted by contact with infected body fluids such as blood or semen. People at risk for contracting the virus include those who (1) share needles or syringes for the purpose of injecting drugs, including steroids; (2) have sexual intercourse with a person infected with HIV, with someone who injects drugs, or with multiple partners; (3) had a blood transfusion anytime between 1978 and May 1985; and (4) were born to a mother infected with HIV.

Usage Considerations

Home test kits that require saliva or blood samples for HIV detection are currently available. Home Access HIV Test and Home Access Express HIV Test Systems require a blood sample and are mailed off for testing. OraQuick is a saliva-based kit that provides an immediate result.

Mechanism of Action

The HIV tests detect antibodies to the virus. Because 3 weeks to 6 months may be required for an exposed individual to develop sufficient antibodies for detection, the time of possible exposure to the virus must be considered in determining when to perform the test.

The saliva test uses technology similar to that used in home pregnancy tests to detect antibodies to both HIV-1 and HIV-2.[44] Using a lateral flow process, the saliva specimen is wicked up by the device; HIV antibodies, if present, bind to the colloidal gold particles. The bound HIV antibodies then bind to an HIV antigen "T" line forming a visible red band. After collection, the home HIV test blood samples are mailed to a certified laboratory for processing. Positive samples are rescreened twice. Repeated positive samples are confirmed with an immunofluorescent assay.[45]

Interferences

Providing an inadequate blood sample (i.e., incompletely filling the circle on the blood sample card) or inadequately swabbing the gums to provide an adequate saliva sample may cause inaccurate results.

Usage Guidelines

See the box "Patient Education for HIV Tests."

Product Selection Guidelines

Many people will prefer to use the saliva test, because it gives faster results, does not require a fingerstick, and has a price similar to that of the Home Access test. For the blood tests, the two available HIV tests differ in price and turnaround time to obtain results. The first test, Home Access, takes approximately 7 business days to obtain the results. The second, Home Access Express, takes approximately 3 business days. The Home Access sample is sent to the testing laboratory by regular mail, whereas the Home Access Express sample is shipped through Federal Express. Consequently, the Home Access Express version costs more.

Assessment of HIV Test Use

The elapsed time since possible exposure to the HIV virus should be determined before an HIV test is recommended. The patient may not know all the risk factors for HIV infection; therefore, whether the patient has engaged in any activities that increase risk for contracting HIV should be tactfully determined. The patient should be asked about medical disorders that might rule out the use of a fingerstick-based test, such as an anticoagulation or bleeding disorder, or physical limitations that might interfere with performing the test.

Patient Counseling for HIV Tests

Counseling on the use of HIV blood tests should emphasize the importance of applying enough blood on the specimen card to ensure an accurate reading. Patients should also be advised of the fragility of blood samples and not to delay mailing the specimen card. Counseling for the saliva test should emphasize the importance of adequately swabbing the gums with the test stick. The box "Patient Education for HIV Tests" lists specific information to provide patients.

Evaluation of Patient Outcomes With HIV Tests

A patient with a positive result should see an HCP to be retested for confirmation of HIV infection. Infected patients should be counseled on precautions to avoid infecting others. Patients with negative results should confirm that sufficient time has passed since the potential exposure.

HEPATITIS C TESTS

Hepatitis C (HCV) is one of six identified hepatitis viruses. With an estimated 2.7–3.9 million chronically infected individuals, HCV infection is the most common blood-borne infection in the United States.[46] Risk factors for hepatitis C infection include use of injectable drugs; receipt of clotting factor concentrate produced before 1987; blood transfusion, long-term hemodialysis, or organ transplant before 1992; sexual intercourse with multiple partners; birth by a mother infected with hepatitis C; and occupational exposure to blood.[46]

Hepatitis C induces liver damage by causing hepatic cell necrosis and inflammation, which over time may progress to fibrosis, cirrhosis, and hepatocellular carcinoma. Of people infected with hepatitis C, 75%–85% are likely to progress to the chronic disease state.[46] Clinically, hepatitis C may go undetected for many years; liver disease may be advanced by the time symptoms arise. Because of very high rates of infection, CDC recommends that all adults born between 1945 and 1965 (Baby Boomers) be screened for hepatitis C.[46]

Usage Considerations

Home Access Hepatitis C Check is a single-use test kit containing two lancets, a blood sample card, a gauze pad, an adhesive bandage, and a postage-paid envelope. After collection, the blood

PATIENT EDUCATION FOR HIV Tests

Precautions—Blood Tests

- Do not share the test lancet with other individuals. Do not allow the blood being tested to contact other individuals.
- The lancet is a biohazard; dispose of it in a puncture-resistant container.

Avoidance of Incorrect Results—Saliva Test

- Do not open any of the packets until you are ready to begin the test.
- Do not eat, drink, or use oral care products (such as mouthwash, toothpaste, or whitening strips) for 30 minutes before starting the test.
- Remove dental products such as dentures or retainers that cover gums.
- To prevent a false-positive result, swab each gum only once.

Usage Guidelines—Blood Tests

- Call the product manufacturer's toll-free number to register and receive pretest counseling. The manufacturer's customer representative will ask for the confidential code included in the kit.
- Using alcohol, clean the fingertip chosen for puncture. Allow alcohol to dry.
- Prick the cleaned fingertip using the lancet provided, and place a few drops of blood on the blood specimen card. Fill the circle on the card completely to ensure a readable test. Examine the back of the card to ensure that the blood soaked through. If it did not, place more blood on the front of the card. If a second fingerstick is needed, use the second lancet provided in the kit.
- Allow the card to air dry for 30 minutes; place the sample in the specimen return pouch, and seal the pouch in the prepaid and addressed shipping package. Be sure that the processing laboratory receives the specimen within 10 days of sampling.
- To obtain the results, call the manufacturer's toll-free number 3–7 business days after mailing the specimen, depending on which test kit was used.
- Note that counseling is available 24 hours a day, for both negative and positive results, and counseling is included in the cost of the testing unit.

Usage Guidelines—Saliva Tests

- A timer or watch is needed.
- Remove the test tube from packaging, pop it open, and insert it into the holder. Hold the test tube upright to avoid spilling the liquid that is inside.
- Remove the test stick from packaging. Do not touch the test pad.
- Swipe the test pad along upper and lower gums. Swipe each gum only once.
- Insert the test stick into the test tube with the test window facing forward. Start timing.
- Read the test result in the test window at 20 minutes. After 40 minutes, the results may be invalid.
- The test kit provides guidelines for how to read the results and what the results mean. One line at C is negative. A line at C and T is positive.
- Note that counseling on performing the test is available 24 hours a day from the company.

When to Seek Medical Attention

- If the test is positive, see a health care provider immediately for evaluation and treatment. Avoid activities that can result in transfer of blood or other body fluids to other individuals.

Source: References 44 and 45.

sample is mailed to a certified laboratory for processing. Each kit also includes a unique personal identification number, which the purchaser uses to register the kit and access test results.

Mechanism of Action

The kit tests for presence of antibodies to the hepatitis C virus, not the virus itself. The Hepatitis C Check uses an ELISA to test for antibodies and then confirms the results with a recombinant immunoblot assay.[47] Because 6 months may be required to develop sufficient antibodies for detection, the time since possible exposure to the virus must be considered in determining when to perform the test.

Interferences

Providing an inadequate blood sample (i.e., incompletely filling the circle on the blood sample card) may cause inaccurate results.

Usage Guidelines

See the box "Patient Education for Hepatitis C Tests."

Product Selection Guidelines

Hepatitis C Check is the only test kit currently available for hepatitis C detection.

Assessment of Hepatitis C Test Use: A Case-Based Approach

A patient who recently has been infected may receive a false-negative result, because antibodies to the virus have not had sufficient time to form. Clinical studies on file with the manufacturer report no false-positive results.[47] The patient may not know all the risk factors for hepatitis C; therefore, whether the patient has engaged in any activities that can cause the disease should be tactfully determined. The patient should be asked about medical disorders that might rule out use of a fingerstick-based test or physical limitations that could interfere with performing the test. Case 48–2 is an example of assessment of a patient who wishes to test for hepatitis C infection.

Patient Counseling for Hepatitis C Tests

Patients should be advised of the fragility of blood samples and not to delay mailing the specimen card. The box "Patient Education for Hepatitis C Tests" lists specific information to provide patients.

Evaluation of Patient Outcomes With Hepatitis C Tests

Patients who test positive should be referred to an HCP, given that treatment options are available only by prescription. Infected patients should be counseled on precautions to avoid infection of others. These patients should also be advised to avoid alcohol and other drugs that may advance the progression of liver disease. They should also be tested for and vaccinated against other forms of hepatitis, such as the hepatitis A and B viruses.

DRUG ABUSE TESTS

An estimated 9.4% of Americans abuse drugs, whether legal or illegal.[28] The symptoms of drug use are varied but may include withdrawal from normal activities, fatigue, red eyes, drowsiness, slurred speech, and chronic cough. The National Institute of Drug Abuse (www.nida.nih.gov) is a good resource for specific symptoms for the various drugs of abuse. Drug abuse tests may allow parents and caregivers to detect drug use early enough to affect the course of addiction.

Usage Considerations

Numerous products for detecting use of drugs are available in retail stores and pharmacies and through the internet. Table 48–5 lists examples of tests and the substances that each test identifies.

Home drug tests are marketed primarily to parents as an aid for determining drug use in their children. These tests are a means of obtaining results anonymously when drug use is suspected. Home drug testing, however, is not a substitute for open communication between parents and children regarding drug use.

Users of these tests may have questions about how soon drugs can be detected after consumption and how long they can be detected after being used. Clearance rates for common drugs of abuse are given in Table 48–6.[48] These data are only guidelines, however, and the times can vary significantly from these estimates based on how long the person has been taking the drug, the amount used, or the person's metabolism.

Samples of urine or hair are collected at home. The hair tests and some of the urine tests are mailed to a clinical laboratory, with results obtained by telephone or over the internet. For some of the urine tests, the user conducts a preliminary screening test in the home and then mails positive samples to a laboratory for confirmation. Other urine tests are performed only at home. Saliva tests are available, but they are currently marketed only to drug testing programs and employers.

Some of the test kits include telephone counseling (1) to help parents recognize the signs of drug use, (2) to assist in creating a family drug policy, and (3) to emphasize that parents should use the test to develop trust and open communication within their families, rather than to intimidate with the threat of random testing. Some telephone counseling programs provide referrals to rehabilitation and counseling services in the family's community.

Mechanism of Action

For the home urine tests, an immunochromatographic assay similar to the home pregnancy and ovulation tests is used for initial screening of a sample. Available testing devices include (1) a test cassette to which urine is applied and (2) a test device that is placed in the urine sample. In each test, a positive result for a particular drug is the absence of a line next to the drug name in the testing area. For a negative test, a line appears by the drug name and in the control area.

CASE 48-2

Relevant Evaluation Criteria	Scenario/Model Outcome
Collect	
1. Gather essential information about the patient's symptoms and medical history, including	
a. Description of symptom(s) (i.e., nature, onset, duration, severity, associated symptoms)	Patient recently read an article about the high rate of hepatitis C infections in Baby Boomers.
b. Medical history, including family history	He has heart disease, high cholesterol, atrial fibrillation, and hypertension. He did have a blood transfusion years ago but is evasive when asked about other risk factors.
c. Patient's identity	Jeff Martin
d. Patient's age, gender, height, and weight	68 years old, male, 5 ft 7 in., 180 lb
e. Patient's dietary habits	n/a
f. Concurrent medical conditions, prescription and nonprescription medications, and dietary supplements	Simvastatin 20 mg, ezetimibe 10 mg, losartan 50 mg, warfarin 5 mg daily (adherence verified by refill records)
g. Prior use of diagnostic/monitoring test	Jeff has never used any home tests.
h. Potential problems with performing/interpreting test	He wears reading glasses to read fine print. His wife could help him read the instructions and complete the test.
Assess	
2. Determine whether self-testing is appropriate.	Although he should be screened for hepatitis C because of his age group, self-testing is not appropriate.
3. Identify exclusions for self-treatment.	Use of warfarin
4. Formulate a comprehensive list of therapeutic alternatives for the primary problem to determine whether triage to a medical provider is required, and share this information with the patient or caregiver.	Options include (1) Refer patient for hepatitis C testing. (2) Take no action.
Plan	
5. Select an optimal therapeutic alternative to address the patient's problem, taking into account patient preferences.	The patient understands why self-testing is not appropriate. He has an appointment with his HCP in 4 months and will ask for the test at that time.
Follow-up: Monitor and Evaluate	
6. Assess patient outcome.	Pharmacist will check with the patient at his next pharmacy visit to see if the test was performed or is scheduled.

Key: HCP = Health care provider; n/a = not applicable.

PATIENT EDUCATION FOR Hepatitis C Tests

Precautions

- Do not share the test lancet with other individuals.
- Do not allow the blood being tested to contact other individuals.
- The lancet is considered a biohazard; dispose of it in a puncture-resistant container.

Usage Guidelines

- Register the PIN (personal identification number) with the manufacturer by calling the provided toll-free telephone number and following the automated directions.
- Remain seated during the testing process to prevent falling if dizziness occurs.
- Before starting the test, wash your hands thoroughly with soap and warm water, and then dry them.
- Date the blood sample card.
- Lance the side of one of your middle fingers.
- Apply a sufficient number of blood drops until both the front and back of the circular area on the testing card are saturated.
- Allow the sample to dry at least 30 minutes before sealing it in the pouch and mailing it.
- Within 4–10 business days after mailing the sample, call the toll-free number provided, using the PIN to access the test results. Test results are available for up to 1 year.
- Note that counseling is included in the cost of the testing unit and is available 24 hours a day, for both negative and positive results.

When to Seek Medical Attention

- If the test is positive, see a health care provider immediately for evaluation and treatment. Avoid activities that can result in transfer of blood or other body fluids to other individuals.

Source: Reference 47.

TABLE 48-5 Selected Nonprescription Home Drug Abuse Tests

Product (website)	Time to Result	Body Site	Testing Location	Substances Detected
At Home Drug Test (www.phamatech.com)	10 minutes for initial screen; 5–7 days for laboratory confirmation	Urine	Home; send away for confirmation	Multiple-substances kits: 6 panel kit: Amphetamine, cocaine, ecstasy, marijuana, methamphetamine, opiates 12 panel kit: Amphetamine, barbiturates, benzodiazepines, cocaine, ecstasy, marijuana, methadone, methamphetamine, MDA (3,4-Methylenedioxyamphetamine), opiates, oxycodone, phencyclidine Single-substance kits: marijuana or cocaine
Dr. Brown's Home Drug Testing System (www.drbrowns.com)	5–7 days	Urine	Send away	Amphetamines, cocaine, codeine, heroin, marijuana, morphine, phencyclidine
PDT-90 Personal Drug Testing Service (www.psychemedics.com)	5–7 days	Hair	Send away	Amphetamines, cocaine, marijuana, methamphetamines opiates, phencyclidine
HairConfirm Regular, Express, and Prescription (www.hairconfirm.com)	5–7 days	Hair	Send away	HairConfirm Regular: 7 illicit drugs: amphetamines, cocaine, ecstasy, marijuana, methamphetamines, opiates, phencyclidine HairConfirm Express: 7 illicit drugs listed above plus overnight shipping HairConfirm Prescription: 7 illicit drugs listed above plus 5 prescription drugs: Dilaudid (hydromorphone); Lorcet/Lortab, Vicodin (hydrocodone); Oxycontin, Percocet/Percodan (oxycodone)

Source: References 49–52.

TABLE 48-6 Examples of Estimated Times for Positive Drug Test

Drug	How soon after taking drug will a positive drug test occur?	How long after taking drug will a drug test continue to be positive?
Amphetamine, methamphetamine	4-6 hours	2-3 days
Barbiturates	2-4 hours	1-3 weeks
Benzodiazepine	2-7 hours	1-4 days
Cocaine	2-6 hours	2-3 days
Ecstasy	2-7 hours	2-4 days
Marijuana	1-3 hours	1-7 days
Methadone	3-8 hours	1-3 days
Opiates	2-6 hours	1-3 days
Oxycodone	1-3 hours	1-2 days
Phencyclidine	4-6 hours	7-14 days

Source: Reference 48.

The laboratories use an enzyme-multiplied immunoassay technique to detect drugs in the urine samples. Gas chromatography–mass spectrometry is then used to identify the specific drug. Positive home urine samples sent to clinical laboratories for confirmation are checked for evidence of adulteration.[49–51] Substances such as water or household chemicals can be added to urine samples in an attempt to mask drug use.

Home urine tests detect drug use that occurred from several hours before testing to within 2–3 days of testing. The amount of drug found in the urine is affected by the time since consumption, the amount taken, and the amount of water consumed before sampling. Test results are reported as only positive or negative for a drug. Quantity or route of ingestion is not determined.

Hair testing detects trace amounts of ingested drugs that become trapped in the core of the hair shaft as it grows at an average rate of ½ inch per month. Drug use over a 90-day period can be determined from a hair sample of 1½ inches.[52] The presence of drugs is determined by radioimmunoassay techniques, and then gas chromatography–mass spectrometry analysis identifies the specific substance. Hair tests report positive or negative results for a drug. Positive results are reported as a number indicating low, medium, or high levels of use for all drugs except marijuana, which is reported only as positive or negative.

Usage Guidelines

See the box "Patient Education for Drug Abuse Tests."

Interferences

Ingestion of decongestants, dextromethorphan, antidiarrheals, or cough medicines containing codeine may cause false-positive results for home drug abuse tests. These items contain substances structurally related to certain drugs of abuse. Consumption of large quantities of poppy seeds or poppy seed paste may or may not cause a false-positive result for opiates, depending on the test's sensitivity. Sensitivity standards for opiates have been raised to reduce the possibility of false-positive results.

Product Selection Guidelines

The criteria for selecting one drug abuse test over another include the drugs that are suspected of being used, the type of suspected use (i.e., casual vs. chronic), the length of time since last use, and the possibility that the suspected drug user tampered with the sample. The list of drugs that may be identified varies with each kit. These tests can test for a single drug or up to 12 drugs.

In general, urine tests are better for detecting low-level, casual drug use. Hair testing detects longer-term use. It takes at least 5–7 days for hair to grow far enough from the scalp for testing purposes.

Urine samples are subject to tampering by adding chemicals, diluting with water, or substituting someone else's urine sample. Some of the test kits include a temperature strip on the urine collection cup to ensure the sample is at body temperature. Parents may accompany their child to the bathroom to collect the urine sample. Hair samples, if taken directly from the person being tested, are not subject to tampering. Parents should weigh the possibility of tampering when deciding which type of test to choose.

Assessment of Drug Abuse Test Use

The length of time of suspected drug use and the types of drugs that are suspected will determine which type of drug abuse test to recommend. Whether the suspected user is likely to tamper with urine samples should also be determined. Finally, whether the suspected user takes legal prescription or nonprescription medications that may interfere with the test should be determined.

Patient Counseling for Drug Abuse Tests

When parents or caregivers ask for assistance in selecting a drug abuse test, HCPs should offer clinical advice and information about family counseling agencies. Counseling should emphasize the limitations of the tests for confirming drug use and, in the case of urine tests, for identifying anything more than the type of drug that is being abused. The box "Patient Education for Drug Abuse Tests" lists specific information to provide patients.

Evaluation of Patient Outcomes With Drug Abuse Tests

If a positive result is obtained with a drug abuse test, parents or caregivers need to consider potential problems with the test itself before concluding that drug use is confirmed. In addition, they must not assume that a negative result is accurate. Parents should also consider the testing window when evaluating results.

PATIENT EDUCATION FOR Drug Abuse Tests

Avoidance of Incorrect Results

- Drug tests on urine samples report only a positive or negative outcome. Neither the quantity of drug taken nor the method in which it was taken is determined.
- Drug tests on hair samples can report a low-, medium-, or high-level of drug use, but the use could have occurred as long as 90 days before testing.
- Cough medications that contain codeine or dextromethorphan, decongestants, antidiarrheals, narcotic analgesics, and possibly poppy seeds may cause false-positive test results.

Usage Guidelines for Urine Drug Abuse Tests

- Collect urine using the collection device included with the test. Do not take urine from the toilet.
- Check the temperature of the urine sample immediately after collection using the temperature strip, if included. If the sample is not between 90°F (32°C) and 100°F (38°C), adulteration may have occurred.
- Immerse the test card in the urine sample for 10 seconds or until visible migration across the test panels has occurred. Place the device on a flat surface or leave it immersed in the sample. Do not allow urine to exceed the "max line."
- Read the results when the "results ready" indicator changes to a pinkish red. Do not read the results 15 minutes or more after this indicator changes color or after the "results expired" indicator changes color.
- If no line appears in the control region, the test is invalid and should be repeated with a new card.

Usage Guidelines for Hair Drug Abuse Tests

- Collect a hair sample, ½-inch wide and one strand deep, from the crown of the head, as close to the scalp as possible.
- Align the cut ends of the hair sample and place the sample in the collection package as directed. Do not collect hair from a hairbrush, comb, or clothing; there is no guarantee that the hair is actually from the person to be tested.
- Results are available approximately 5 days after receipt by the laboratory. To access results, call the manufacturer's toll-free number and provide the code number accompanying the kit.

When to Seek Medical Attention

- If the test is positive, seek the services of a drug rehabilitation organization.

Source: References 49–52.

BLOOD PRESSURE MONITORS

Hypertension is often an asymptomatic disease. The eighth report of the Joint National Committee on Prevention, Detection, Evaluation and Treatment of High Blood Pressure (JNC 8) no longer defines a specific blood pressure value for being hypertensive, but the report does recommend goal blood pressures of less than 140/90 for persons younger than 60 years of age and 150/90 for those older than 60.[53]

Thirty-two percent of Americans 20 years of age and older have hypertension.[54] Approximately 17% of people with hypertension are unaware of their condition; almost 23.5% are not receiving treatment; and 45.9% have not achieved blood pressure control.[54] The reasons for the lack of adequate control are multiple, but a significant factor is lack of patient motivation to take steps to control blood pressure, especially if the patient is asymptomatic, which leads to nonadherence with treatment strategies.

The consequences of untreated hypertension are well documented. Long-standing elevations in blood pressure can lead to damage to the heart, kidneys, lungs, eyes, and blood vessels, and to an increase in morbidity and mortality.

Treatment of high blood pressure often involves significant lifestyle changes (diet, exercise). Medications may cause adverse effects that impact adherence. Patient education and empowerment play a large role in improving patient adherence with efforts to control hypertension. Adherence, in turn, helps reduce morbidity and mortality, maintains or improves the patient's quality of life, and improves the patient's use of health care resources.

Teaching patients to take their own blood pressure at home is an excellent means of achieving blood pressure control: home blood pressure monitoring gives patients a sense of control over their health and allows them to measure their progress toward a target blood pressure. Three general advantages of measuring blood pressure at home are the ability (1) to distinguish sustained hypertension from "white-coat hypertension" (i.e., measurements affected by being in the HCP's office); (2) to assess response to antihypertensive medication; and (3) to improve patient adherence to treatment.

Usage Considerations

Of the three categories of blood pressure monitors (mercury column, aneroid, digital), the most popular choices for home use are aneroid and digital monitors. Monitors that measure pressure at the wrist and fingers have become popular, but the systolic and diastolic pressures vary substantially in different parts of the arterial tree. Finger monitors have so far been found to be inaccurate and are not recommended.[55] Wrist monitors are typically smaller than the arm devices and can be used in obese people, because wrist diameter is little affected by obesity.[55]

Mechanism of Action

Blood pressure readings include two types of pressures: *systolic,* which indicates pressure at the time of contraction of the heart cavities, and *diastolic,* which indicates pressure at the time of dilation of the heart cavities. Blood pressure is measured indirectly by two methods: *auscultatory* (measurement of sound) and *oscillometric* (measurement of vibration). Mercury column and aneroid meters involve auscultation with the use of a stethoscope to detect *Korotkoff's sounds,* which are produced by the motion of the arterial wall in response to changes in arterial pressure. *Oscillometric sensors,* which are often used with digital meters, measure blood pressure by detecting blood surges underneath the cuff as it is deflated. The detection device, which is usually indicated on the cuff with a tab or other marking, is placed directly over the brachial artery. The brachial artery can be found by palpating 1–2 inches above and just to the inside of the antecubital space. As cuff pressure increases during the measurement procedure, the brachial artery is compressed and blood flow is obstructed. As cuff pressure is gradually released, blood flow is reestablished and Korotkoff's sounds can be heard in different phases. Phase I, which corresponds to systolic pressure, can be identified when at least two consecutive "beats" are heard as cuff pressure is decreased. The nature of the sounds changes over the next three phases. Diastolic pressure is identified at the point the sounds disappear (Phase V).

Interferences

Stress, tobacco smoking, and ingestion of caffeine-containing beverages can increase blood pressure. Some medications (e.g., pseudoephedrine) may also increase blood pressure.

Usage Guidelines

The actual measurement of blood pressure is a relatively simple procedure; however, many people consistently do it incorrectly. Blood pressure is naturally variable. Therefore, proper technique is essential to reduce measurement variability and improve the quality of results. The normal range for blood pressure is established in patients seated in the resting state; any variation from this setting can produce inaccurate results.

Using the appropriate size cuff is essential to accurately measure a patient's blood pressure (Table 48–7). If the cuff is too small, blood pressure readings can be overestimated significantly by as much as 20–30 mm Hg. Several monitors are supplied with a large cuff; many others allow a large cuff to be purchased separately. For patients with arms too large for the largest size cuff,

TABLE 48–7 Arm Circumferences to Determine Appropriate Blood Pressure Cuff Size

Arm Circumference (adult)[a]	Cuff Size
22–26 cm	Small adult cuff
27–34 cm	Regular adult cuff
35–44 cm	Large adult cuff
≥45 cm	Thigh cuff[b]

[a] Determine arm circumference by measuring around the midpoint of the upper arm. Remeasure the patient's arm periodically, especially if he or she has recently gained or lost significant weight.

[b] Consider a wrist monitor for patients whose arm circumference is >45 cm.

Source: Reference 55.

a wrist monitor may be a useful alternative. To obtain accurate readings with wrist cuffs, the patient must hold the wrist at heart level during the reading. Because these devices are also highly sensitive to changes in the wrist level, it is best to support the arm on a table with a pillow that will raise the wrist to the appropriate level. For the person who is doing the actual monitoring, following the steps outlined in the box "Patient Education for Self-Monitoring of Blood Pressure" will help improve the accuracy of blood pressure readings, regardless of whether they are taken in the HCP's office, the pharmacy, or the home.

Product Selection Guidelines

Of the three types of blood pressure–measuring devices, no single type is best for every patient. The choice of device is individualized according to characteristics such as the patient's ability and willingness to learn, physical disabilities, patient preference, and the cost of the device. Mercury column devices are expensive and, as discussed in the next section, have other disadvantages for home use. In general, aneroid devices are the least expensive. Depending on its features, a digital device can cost as much as a mercury column device. A discussion of the pros and cons of all three types of devices follows.

Mercury Column Devices

The mercury column blood pressure monitor is still the reference standard in blood pressure measurement. This monitor typically comes with a cuff and an inflation bulb. The tubing from the cuff is attached to a column of mercury encased in a calibrated vertical glass tube.

Although mercury monitors are the most accurate and reliable of the devices, their routine use for home measurement is discouraged, because they are cumbersome and pose the risk of mercury toxicity should the glass tubing break. They also require good eyesight and hearing for effective use. If the mercury does not rest at zero when the cuff is lying flat and completely deflated, the device needs recalibration.

Aneroid Devices

Next to mercury column monitors, aneroid devices are the most accurate and reliable. They are light, portable, and very affordable, and they pose no risk from mercury toxicity. They include several features that make patient instruction much easier. First, most devices come with a stethoscope attached to the cuff, which frees the patient from having to hold the bell of the stethoscope in place. Second, a D-ring on the cuff allows a single user to place the cuff on the arm easily. Third, a few manufacturers offer a gauge attached to the inflation bulb, making it easier to manipulate the equipment, because there are fewer pieces to control. These monitors are considered the option of choice for home use, but they do require careful patient instruction and follow-up. Good eyesight and hearing are necessary for accurate readings with standard models. For patients with reduced visual capacity, however, devices with large-type print on the face of the gauge are available.

At the bottom of the face of each aneroid device is a small box. When the cuff is completely deflated and lying on the table, the needle of the gauge should rest in the box. If the needle is outside the box, the gauge needs recalibration. Many manufacturers sell recalibration tools to allow HCPs to adjust the devices.

Digital Devices

With advancing technology, digital devices have become more accurate, reliable, and easy to use; as a result, they have skyrocketed in popularity. These devices include *semiautomatic* (manually inflating), *fully automatic* (autoinflating), wrist, and finger blood pressure monitors. Features such as printouts, pulse monitor, digital clock, automated inflation and deflation, memory, large display, and D-ring for the cuff differentiate many of the devices. These features significantly affect the price.

A major drawback to digital monitors is the user's inability to determine whether the device is out of calibration. Patients should be advised to have their monitors checked at least yearly by an HCP for accuracy.

If recommending a digital device, the provider should check the manufacturer's specifications to ensure that the monitor meets at least the accuracy standards set by the American National Standards Institute (ANSI). The ANSI standards for digital sphygmomanometers state that blood pressure readings between 20 and 250 mm Hg must not differ by more than 3 mm Hg or 2%, whichever is greater.[56]

Assessment of Blood Pressure Self-Monitoring

Assessment should include determination of (1) why a patient wants to use a blood pressure monitor, (2) whether the patient has physical impairments that can interfere with proper use of the monitor, and (3) the patient's ability to comprehend and follow instructions.

Patient Counseling for Blood Pressure Self-Monitoring

The HCP should emphasize the importance of tracking blood pressure values to monitor control of hypertension. Regular self-monitoring of blood pressure will illustrate positive effects of lifestyle changes and medication use in controlling the disorder. This reinforcement can improve patient adherence with prescribed therapies. The patient should be shown the proper technique for blood pressure monitoring and be encouraged to return for a follow-up evaluation of his or her technique. Because of white coat hypertension, patients who measure blood pressure at home usually obtain lower results than those taken at the provider's office. In the home setting, a blood pressure greater than 135/85 mm Hg should be considered elevated.[55] The box "Patient Education for Self-Monitoring of Blood Pressure" lists specific information to provide patients.

Evaluation of Patient Outcomes for Self-Monitoring of Blood Pressure

Patients measuring blood pressure for diagnostic and monitoring purposes should be instructed on how to track values and how to discuss the values with an HCP. Patients monitoring their blood pressure should be cautioned not to adjust their medications unless

PATIENT EDUCATION FOR Self-Monitoring of Blood Pressure

Precautions and Avoidance of Incorrect Results

- Keep a log of blood pressure readings and any circumstances that might have affected the reading (e.g., feeling nervous or being late for work).
- If home readings are being performed for diagnostic purposes, take readings at different times throughout the day and under different circumstances.
- If readings are being done to determine adequacy of antihypertensive therapy, take the reading at the same time of day, preferably in the early morning soon after arising from bed.
- Allow plenty of time to relax before taking a blood pressure reading. Feelings of stress or pressure can elevate the blood pressure.
- Do not use tobacco products or drink caffeine-containing beverages for at least 30 minutes before taking a measurement. These activities can increase blood pressure.
- Wait 10–15 minutes after a bath and 30 minutes after eating to take a measurement. These activities can lower blood pressure.
- Some medications may increase blood pressure. Be alert for possible changes in blood pressure readings when starting or stopping medications.

Usage Guidelines

- Make sure the room is at a comfortable temperature.
- Sit in a comfortable chair, with your back supported and your feet facing straight ahead and placed flat on the floor.
- If using an arm cuff, place the arm to be measured on a table, making sure your upper arm is at heart level. Remove restrictive clothing from the arm.
- If using a wrist cuff, place pillows under the arm to be measured to bring the wrist up to heart level.
- Place the cuff on the arm to be measured. The cuff should be snug but not tight enough to restrict blood flow. Use the guidelines in Table 48–7 for selecting cuff size.
- Rest for at least 5 minutes in this position.
- Measure the blood pressure as directed by the product instructions. If using a stethoscope, listen for the Korotkoff's sounds as described here:
  - Phase 1: Sound begins as a soft tapping. Record the systolic pressure when two taps are heard in sequence.
  - Phase 2: Tapping sound becomes louder and is accompanied by a swishing sound or murmur.
  - Phase 3: Tapping sounds persist, but the swishing or murmur sound stops.
  - Phase 4: There is muffling or softening of tapping sounds.
  - Phase 5: Sound stops. Record the diastolic pressure when the sound stops.
- Using the same arm, take two to three measurements separated by at least 2 minutes.
- Record the results, arm used, time and date of measurement, and name and time of last dose of any medications, including antihypertensive medications.
- Do not adjust blood pressure medications based on home measurements unless specifically instructed to do so by a health care provider.

When to Seek Medical Attention

- See a health care provider immediately for evaluation and treatment if readings are above limits set by your health care provider or above the limits stated in national guidelines, and if you are having symptoms such as headache or blurred vision.

Source: References 55.

instructed otherwise. Patients should be instructed to immediately contact their HCP if they obtain elevated values and have any symptoms of high blood pressure, such as headache or blurred vision. Patient counseling and follow-up can improve outcomes in hypertensive patients by (1) motivating them to perform home monitoring of blood pressure; (2) guiding them in product selection; (3) training them to use devices appropriately; and (4) facilitating communication between the patient, the patient's family, and the patient's HCP regarding any antihypertensive therapy.

MISCELLANEOUS HOME TESTS

As the market for home test products and shopping over the internet have exploded, new tests are becoming available with increasing frequency. Selected miscellaneous home tests are described in Table 48–8. Instructions for use are generally available from the manufacturer's website or a site that sells the product. Following the general guidelines given in this chapter will also help patients obtain accurate results.

Key Points for Home Testing and Monitoring Devices

- To advise patients properly on selecting and using home testing or monitoring products, HCPs must be familiar with the procedures for each available product.
- Manufacturers continually introduce new products and modify current ones to provide more user-friendly versions. To keep up to date, providers should request product information from manufacturers by calling their toll-free numbers, visiting their websites, or contacting their sales representatives.
- FDA's website should also be checked frequently for problem reports, updates, and news on home tests.
- Patients who are using home tests or devices should be encouraged to follow instructions carefully and to contact either their HCP or the manufacturer's toll-free number for assistance, if needed.
- HCPs should stress that the patient is self-testing, not self-diagnosing. Positive test results should be reported immediately for definitive diagnosis and management. Negative test results should be questioned when the patient is experiencing symptoms of a suspected condition.
- If there is any question about the results, the patient should seek the advice of an HCP.

TABLE 48–8 Selected Miscellaneous Nonprescription Home Tests

Test	Purpose	Important Points	Additional Information
Alcohol screening tests (breath, saliva)	Prevent inappropriate alcohol consumption	Put nothing in mouth 15 minutes before or during the test. Follow timing directions carefully and use a timing device.	Semiquantitative BAC; saliva test strips can be used to detect alcohol in drinks.
Visiderm	Monitor moles for changes over time	Use a transparent overlay to trace outline of individual moles; record color and other details. Do subsequent examinations of each mole on same overlay.	Test includes transparent overlays, pen, color chart, instructions, and storage box.
Breast Self-Examination Aid	Make breast self-examination easier and more comfortable	Examine breasts monthly. Self-examination does not take place of mammogram and professional examination.	Two-layer polyurethane breast shield or glove contains a small amount of silicone lubricant to reduce friction. Some kits come with instructional video (Aware, Sensa Touch).
Monistat Complete Care Vaginal Health Test	Detect pH of vaginal secretions	pH 4.5 + symptoms suggest yeast. pH ≥ 5 + symptoms suggest bacterial vaginosis or trichomoniasis.	Those with first-time yeast infection and those with pH ≥5 should see HCP for diagnosis. See Chapter 8 for additional information
TobacAlert/NicAlert (www.tobacalert.com, nymox.com)	Detect tobacco use or exposure	Test detects cotine, a metabolite of nicotine; test detects nicotine use or exposure in previous 48–72 hours. Dip strip in urine (TobacAlert, NicAlert) or saliva (NicAlert) sample, and read results in specified time.	Use of nicotine patch or gum can affect results. Secondhand smoke exposure may cause a positive result.
IDENTIGENE DNA Paternity Test Collection Kit	Check paternity of a child	Collect cheek cell samples from each participant: alleged father, child, and biological mother. Swabs are mailed to laboratory.	Kit is not available in all states. Results are available 3–5 days after sample is received by laboratory. Results are not valid for legal purposes (requires verified collection procedure and additional costs).
Menopause Test	Detect FSH in urine	Positive test = FSH level > 25 IU/L, which may indicate a woman is menopausal. FSH levels change during the menstrual cycle, so the test should be done twice 1–2 weeks apart to confirm results.	Not a definitive diagnostic test for menopause. The diagnosis would need to be confirmed by the woman's HCP.
Strep A Test	Detect strep throat infections	Same rapid test kit as that used in medical settings. Includes positive and negative control. Results provided in 10 minutes.	Diagnosis would need to be confirmed by HCP.
Home Electrocardiogram Monitor (www.theheartcheck.com)	Detect and record heart rhythm	Consumer and prescription versions. Device electrodes are placed on thumbs or on one thumb and skin of chest near heart.	Device should be used in conjunction with HCP monitoring.

Key: BAC = Blood alcohol concentration; FSH = follicle-stimulating hormone; HCP = health care provider.

REFERENCES

1. Top 10 OTC brand for diagnostics by revenue in the U.S. in 2013. Available at: http://www.statistia.com. Accessed June 24, 2017.
2. Cole LA. The utility of six over-the-counter (home) pregnancy tests. *Clin Lab Med.* 2011;49(8):1317–22.
3. Cole L, Sutton-Riley J, Khanlian S, et al. Sensitivity of over-the-counter pregnancy tests: comparison of utility and marketing messages. *J Am Pharm Assoc.* 2005;45(5):608–15.
4. Johnson S, Cushion M, Bond S, et al. Comparison of analytical sensitivity and women's interpretation of home pregnancy tests. *Clin Chem Lab Med.* 2015;53(3):391–402.
5. Cole L, Khanlian S, Sutton J, et al. Accuracy of home pregnancy tests at the time of a missed menses. *Am J Obstet Gynecol.* 2004;190(1):100–5.
6. Wilcox AJ, Baird DD, Dunson D, et al. Natural limits of pregnancy testing in relation to the expected menstrual period. *JAMA.* 2001;286(14):1759–61.
7. Wallace L, Zite N, Homewood V. Making sense of home pregnancy test instructions. *J Womens Health.* 2009;18(3):323–68.
8. Clearblue [product information]. Cincinnati, OH: Proctor and Gamble; 2011.
9. Fact Plus [product information]. Cincinnati, OH: Proctor and Gamble; 2008.
10. Martinez G, Daniels K, Chandra A. Fertility of men and women aged 15–44 years in the United States: National Survey of Family Growth, 2006–2010. *National Health Statistics Reports.* 2012;51. Hyattsville, MD: National Center for Health Statistics.
11. Johnson S, Ellis J, Godbert S, et al. Comparison of a digital ovulation test with three popular line ovulation tests to investigate user accuracy and certainty. *Expert Opin Med Diagn.* 2011;5(6):467–73.
12. Accu-Clear [product information]. Geneva, Switzerland: Swiss Precision Diagnostics GmbH; 2008–2012.
13. Nexcare Basal Digital Thermometer [product information]. Franklin Lakes, NJ: 2007.
14. OV Watch [product information]. Watersound, FL: Health Watch Systems, Inc; 2011.
15. Cooper T, Noonan E, Eckardstein S, et al. WHO reference values for human semen characteristics. *Human Reproductive Update* 2010;16(3):231–45.
16. SpermCheck [product information]. Bellingham, WA: Fairhaven Health; 2012–2013.
17. Coppola MA, Klotz KL, Kim KA, et al. SpermCheck Fertility, an immunodiagnostic home test that detects normozoospermia and severe oligozoospermia. *Hum Reprod.* 2010;25(4):853–61.
18. American Cancer Society. Cancer facts and figures 2017. Available at: https://www.cancer.org/research/cancer-facts-statistics/all-cancer-facts-figures/cancer-facts-figures-2017.html. Accessed June 24 2017.
19. American Cancer Society. Colorectal cancer risk factors. Available at: https://www.cancer.org/cancer/colon-rectal-cancer/causes-risks-prevention/risk-factors.html. Accessed June 24, 2017.
20. Khakimov N, Khasanova G, Ershova K, et al. Screening for colon cancer: a test for occult blood. *Int J Risk Saf Med.* 2015;27(Suppl 1):S110–1.
21. EZ-Detect [product information]. Newport Beach, CA: Biomerica; 2000–2001.
22. Second generation FIT Quick Guide [product information]. Madison, TN: Pinnacle BioLabs; 2015.
23. Konrad G, Katz A. Are medication restrictions before FOBT necessary? Practical advice based on a systematic review of the literature. *Can Fam Physician.* 2012;58(9):939–48.
24. Konrad G. Dietary interventions for fecal occult blood test screening. Systematic review of the literature. *Can Fam Physician.* 2010;56(3):229–38.
25. Rex DK, Johnson DA, Anderson JC, et al. American College of Gastroenterology guidelines for colorectal cancer screening 2008. *Am J Gastroenterol.* 2009;104(3):739–50.
26. U.S. Preventive Services Task Force. Final recommendation statement. Colorectal cancer: screening. June 2016. Available at: https://www.uspreventiveservicestaskforce.org/Page/Document/RecommendationStatementFinal/colorectal-cancer-screening2. Accessed June 24, 2017.
27. American Cancer Society. Recommendations for Colorectal Cancer Early Detection. March 2017. Available at: https://www.cancer.org/content/cancer/en/cancer/colon-rectal-cancer/detection-diagnosis-staging/acs-recommendations.html. Accessed June 24, 2017.
28. National Center for Health Statistics. *Health, United States, 2014: With Special Feature on Adults Aged 55–64.* Hyattsville, MD: National Center for Health Statistics; 2015.
29. Goff D, Lloyd-Jones D, Bennett G, et al. 2013 ACC/AHA Guideline on the Assessment of Cardiovascular Risk in Adults. *Circulation* 2014;129:S49–73.
30. CholesTrak [product information]. Vista, CA: Accutech; 2008.
31. First Check Home Cholesterol Test [product information]. Waltham, MA: First Check Diagnostics; 2013.
32. CardioChek [product information]. Indianapolis, IN: Polymer Technology Systems; 2010.
33. Accutrend Plus [product information]. Indianapolis, IN: Roche Diagnostics; 2012.
34. Q. Steps Cholesterol Biometer [product information]. Fremont, CA: Biomedix Inc.; 2004.
35. Check Up America Cholesterol Panel [product information]. Hoffman Estates, IL: Home Access Health.
36. McNamara JR, Warnick GR, Leary ET, et al. Multicenter evaluation of a patient-administered test for blood cholesterol measurement. *Prev Med.* 1996;25(5):583–92.
37. Do home cholesterol tests work? *Consum Rep.* August 2003:9.
38. Whitehead S, Ford C, Gama R. A combined laboratory and field evaluation of the Cholestech LDX and CardioChek PA point-of-care testing lipid and glucose analysers. *Ann Clin Biochem* 2014:51(Pt 1):54–7.
39. Centers for Disease Control and Prevention. *Urinary Tract Infections.* Available at: http://www.cdc.gov. Accessed February 17, 2016.
40. Gupta K, Trautner BW. Urinary tract infections, pyelonephritis, and prostatitis. In: Longo DL, Fauci AS, Kasper DL, et al., eds. *Harrison's Principles of Internal Medicine.* 19th ed. New York, NY: McGraw-Hill; 2015.
41. AZO Test Strips [product information]. Cromwell, CT: I-Health, Inc.; 2016.
42. St John A, Boyd JC, Lowes AJ, Price CP. The use of urinary dipstick tests to exclude urinary tract infection: a systematic review of the literature. *Am J Clin Pathol* 2006;125(3):428–36.
43. Centers for Disease Control and Prevention. HIV basics: basic statistics. Available at: https://www.cdc.gov/hiv/basics/statistics.html. Accessed June 24, 2016.
44. OraQuick In Home HIV Test. [product information]. Bethlehem, PA: OraSure Technologies, Inc.; 2012.
45. Home Access Express HIV Test System [product information]. Hoffman Estates, IL: Home Access Health.
46. Centers for Disease Control and Prevention. Hepatitis C FAQ for health professionals: Overview and statistics. Available at: https://www.cdc.gov/hepatitis/hcv/hcvfaq.htm#section2. Accessed June 24, 2017.
47. Home Access Hepatitis C Check [product information]. Hoffman Estates, IL: Home Access Health.
48. U.S. Food and Drug Administration. Drugs of abuse home use test. Available at: http://www.fda.gov/MedicalDevices/ProductsandMedicalProcedures/InVitroDiagnostics/HomeUseTests/ucm125722.htm. Accessed June 24, 2017.
49. At Home Drug Test [product information]. San Diego, CA: Pharmatech; 2010.
50. Dr. Brown's Home Drug Testing System [product information]. Telecare. Available at: http://www.drbrowns.com. Accessed June 24, 2017.
51. PDT-90 Personal Drug Testing Service [product information]. Acton, MA: Psychemedics; 2012.
52. HairConfirm [product information]. San Diego, CA: Confirm Biosciences.
53. James PA, Oparil S, Carter BL, et al. 2014 evidence based guideline for the management of high blood pressure in adults: report from the panel members appointed to the Eighth Joint National Committee (JNC 8). *JAMA.* 2014:311(5):507–20. Available at: http://jama.jamanetwork.com/article.aspx?articleid=1791497. Accessed June 24, 2017.
54. Mozaffarian D, Benjamin EJ, Go AS, et al; American Heart Association Statistics Committee and Stroke Statistics Subcommittee. Heart disease and stroke statistics—2016 update: a report from the American Heart Association. *Circulation.* 2016;133(4):e38–360. doi: 10.1161/CIR.0000000000000350.
55. American Heart Association. AHA scientific statement. Recommendations for blood pressure measurement in humans and experimental animals, part 1: blood pressure measurement in humans: a statement for professionals from the Subcommittee of Professional and Public Education of the American Heart Association Council on High Blood Pressure Research. *Circulation.* 2005;111:697–716.
56. Association for the Advancement of Medical Instrumentation. Manual, Electronic, or Automated Sphygmomanometers. Arlington, VA: American National Standards Institute; 2008:1–84.

CHAPTER 49

ADULT URINARY INCONTINENCE AND SUPPLIES

CHRISTINE K. O'NEIL

Urinary incontinence (UI) is defined as the symptom of any involuntary leakage of urine.[1] Although often mistakenly thought of as a problem of aging, UI affects people of all ages, socioeconomic backgrounds, and ethnicities.[2] An estimated 17 million people in the United States are affected by UI,[3] whereas 42.2 million may suffer from *overactive bladder* (OAB), a strong desire to void.[4]

UI is an underdiagnosed and underreported condition that has major psychosocial and economic effects. Feelings of embarrassment, denial, and misinformation prevent many people from seeking help, which may lead to anxiety, depression, and, possibly, social isolation. Severe UI usually results in a loss of self-esteem and the ability to maintain an independent lifestyle. In addition, it is generally recognized as a strong predictor of nursing home admission of older people.[3]

Direct costs associated with UI include the expenses for diagnosis, specific treatment, routine care, rehabilitation, and hospital and nursing home admissions. The direct costs of treating OAB with UI in adults older than 25 years were estimated at $65.9 billion in 2007.[5]

Despite the high prevalence of UI, less than half of community-dwelling adults with UI consult their health care provider.[6] Many accept the symptoms as a natural part of aging and use self-care strategies with little or no health professional guidance. Although they are reluctant to talk about UI, Americans spend $1.1 billion annually on disposable incontinence products (e.g., pads, shields, guards, undergarments, briefs).[7]

Pathophysiology of Urinary Incontinence

Urination is a complex process, involving a coordinated effort by the bladder, urethra, and muscular components of the lower urinary tract, brain, and spinal cord.[8] Urine produced by the kidneys is propelled through the ureters to the bladder. The *detrusor muscle*, the smooth muscle layer of the bladder, gives tone to the bladder, relaxing as the bladder fills with urine and contracting during urination. The *bladder neck,* which joins the bladder and the urethra, is surrounded by smooth muscle, referred to as the internal sphincter, which either constricts to hold urine in the bladder or relaxes, permitting urine to flow through the urethra. Voluntary control of urination, or *micturition,* is maintained by contraction of the *external sphincter,* a striated muscle located at mid-urethral length. When relaxed, the urethra, which is surrounded by both smooth and striated muscle, allows urine to leave the body.

The bladder and the internal sphincter are innervated by the autonomic nervous system, and the external sphincter is innervated by the somatic or voluntary nervous system. Parasympathetic and sympathetic nerves innervate the smooth muscle of the bladder and urethra. Both α-adrenergic and β-adrenergic receptors are present in the urinary structures. The alpha receptors are located in the base of the bladder and the proximal urethra, and the beta receptors are found primarily in the body of the bladder detrusor. Stimulation of the alpha receptors causes contraction of the smooth muscles in the bladder neck and urethra, thus closing the bladder outlet. Stimulation of the beta receptors results in smooth muscle relaxation and allows the bladder to fill. Thus, sympathetic stimulation causes the bladder to retain urine. Parasympathetic cholinergic receptors are located throughout the bladder. Stimulation of these receptors causes the detrusor to contract, emptying the bladder. The *sacral center,* lying between vertebrae S2 and S4, acts as the relay center for information to and from the bladder, pelvic floor, and brain.

The capacity of the bladder is approximately 400–500 mL. When the bladder fills, stretch receptors in the detrusor wall transmit signals to the brain through the spinal cord, initiating the urge to urinate when the bladder is approximately half full. Under normal circumstances, adults can delay voiding for 30–60 minutes as a result of the short sacral reflex, which diminishes the urge to urinate by increasing contraction of the external sphincter and relaxing the detrusor muscle of the bladder. Bladder emptying is initiated voluntarily, causing relaxation of the external sphincter and contraction of the detrusor. Normal urination results in complete emptying of the bladder, with little or no residual urine (≤50 mL). Any disruption in the integration of musculoskeletal and neurologic function can lead to loss of control of normal bladder function and UI.[9]

Clinical Presentation of Urinary Incontinence

UI is a symptom that can be caused by external factors and by anatomic, physiologic, and pathologic factors that affect the urinary tract.[2,10–12] In many cases, multiple and interacting factors contribute to UI. The risk of UI is strongly associated with aging. Additional risk factors for UI, some at least partially reversible, have been identified (Table 49–1).[2,10–12] Identification of the cause(s) of UI is essential for the assessment and successful management of UI.

Age-related changes in the bladder and urinary tract may contribute to an older person's vulnerability to UI. With age, the

TABLE 49–1 Risk Factors for Urinary Incontinence

Medical Disorders or Procedures	
Benign prostatic hyperplasia (BPH)/transurethral resection of the prostate (TURP)/prostatectomy	
Childhood nocturnal enuresis	
Diabetes	
Fecal impaction	
Immobility/chronic degenerative disease	
Impaired cognition, acute or chronic	
Metabolic disorders (hyperglycemia, hypercalcemia)	
Neurologic disorders (spinal cord injury, neuropathy)	
Obesity (moderate-morbid)	
Pregnancy/vaginal delivery/episiotomy	
Stroke	
Physiologic Factors	
Estrogen depletion	
High fluid intake (leading to polyuria and bladder capacity overload)	
Low fluid intake (leading to concentrated urine and bladder irritation that worsens symptoms)	
Pelvic floor muscle weakness	
Lifestyle Factors	
High-impact physical activities	
Smoking	
Other Factors	
Caucasian race	
Environmental barriers	
Medications (Table 49–2)	

Source: Adapted from references 2 and 10–12.

kidney's ability to concentrate urine diminishes, resulting in larger urine volumes. In addition, age-related hypotrophic changes in bladder tissue lead to frequent urination and nocturia, whereas decreased muscle tone of the bladder, as well as the bladder sphincters and pelvic muscles, contributes to the potential for reduced urine control. This loss of control, combined with diminished mobility and reaction time, predisposes older people to UI.[13]

In women, the loss of estrogen causes a decrease in bladder outlet and urethral resistance, as well as a decline in pelvic musculature—all of which increase the likelihood of UI. In addition, estrogen loss results in atrophic changes in the vaginal and urethral mucosa, disrupting the vaginal flora and leading to atrophic vaginitis and chronic urethritis. These conditions, in turn, may cause urinary frequency and urgency, dysuria, urinary tract infections, and UI. The short female urethra exerts less resistance to intravesicular pressure compared with the longer male urethra. Consequently, obesity, chronic cough, and jarring exercise, which all increase intra-abdominal pressure, result in an extra load on the bladder. As such, these factors can overwhelm the relatively low resistance offered by the short female urethra. Childbirth, gynecologic procedures, and muscle atrophy from aging also weaken the female pelvic floor muscles, thereby decreasing support for the bladder. Without adequate support, positioning of the bladder becomes distorted (known as *cystocele* or *anterior wall prolapse*) and can result in urethral kinking, with subsequent poor bladder emptying. These conditions may result in chronic obstruction of the bladder, again leading to UI from urine volume overload.

Men often develop prostatic enlargement beginning in their middle to late 40s, which results in urethral obstruction, leading to decreased urinary flow rates, increased residual volumes, detrusor instability, and possibly overflow incontinence. Paradoxically, prostatectomy to relieve bothersome symptoms related to benign prostatic hyperplasia (BPH) can result in stress incontinence caused by incidental injury to the internal sphincter.

UI can be described broadly as transient or chronic. *Transient UI* usually is of sudden onset and secondary to acute illness (e.g., urinary tract infections) or to any disease that causes acute confusion (e.g., respiratory disease, myocardial infarction, septicemia) or immobility, preventing the person from reaching a toilet independently or in time. Many other conditions and medications can cause or contribute to transient UI (Table 49–2).[2,9] Managing these conditions may resolve UI in some patients but only reduce the severity of symptoms in others. Chronic UI often is related to neurologic or other chronic conditions, such as intrinsic sphincter deficiency, BPH, or cystocele.[14] UI can be classified as OAB, stress incontinence, mixed incontinence (OAB plus stress incontinence), overflow incontinence, or functional incontinence, depending on the underlying etiologies.

Recognition of signs and symptoms of UI is an essential first step in providing treatment advice. Patients often delay discussion or do not seek medical evaluation of UI with their health care providers. Therefore, it is important for providers to inquire about

TABLE 49–2 Reversible Conditions That Cause or Contribute to Urinary Incontinence

Conditions Affecting the Lower Urinary Tract	
Urinary tract infections, atrophic vaginitis/urethritis, fecal impaction, pelvic floor prolapse, hyperglycemia, hypercalcemia	
Drug Adverse effects	
Polyuria, frequency, urgency: caffeine, diuretics, alcohol, acetylcholinesterase inhibitors	
Urinary retention: anticholinergics, antidepressants, hypnotics/sedatives, antipsychotics, narcotics, muscle relaxants, antihypertensives (calcium channel blockers), β-adrenergic agonists, α-adrenergic agonists	
Urethral relaxation: α-adrenergic blockers	
Urethral pressure imbalance (stress incontinence): cough from ACE inhibitors	
Increased Urine Production	
Metabolic disorders (e.g., hyperglycemia, hypercalcemia), excessive fluid intake, volume overload, venous insufficiency with edema leading to nocturia	
Inability or Unwillingness to Reach a Toilet	
Dementia, delirium, illness/injury that interferes with mobility, psychological conditions	

Key: ACE = Angiotensin-converting enzyme.
Source: References 2 and 9.

potential UI symptoms when such conditions are suspected based on clinical evidence or patient inquiries. Open-ended questions such as "What problems are you having, if any, with your bladder?" and "How often do you experience urine leakage?" can be used to begin this dialog. An awareness of signs such as the odor of urine or appearance of wetness is also necessary to identify potential patients suffering from UI. Table 49–3 lists observed and reported symptoms commonly associated with particular types of UI. Encouraging the use of a 24-hour voiding diary, paper or electronic, is a helpful tool in diagnosing and managing UI.[15,16] Voiding dairies permit the patient to document fluid intake, amount of urine voided, episodes of urine leakage, urge to urinate, and activity at the time of leakage or sense of urgency.

OAB occurs in both men and women, and its incidence increases with age. OAB is characterized by sudden and profound urinary urgency, frequency (urinating more than 8 times daily), nocturia (two or more awakenings at night to pass urine), or UI; the condition often, but not always, is accompanied by *urge incontinence* (involuntary urine leakage with urgency).[2,9,13] OAB usually, but not always, is attributable to uninhibited contractions of the detrusor muscle, referred to as *detrusor instability.* Other terms describing detrusor instability are *detrusor hyperreflexia, detrusor hyperactivity with impaired bladder contractility,* and *bladder instability.*

Neurogenic causes of detrusor instability include dementia, stroke, parkinsonism, suprasacral spinal cord injury, multiple sclerosis, and medullary lesions. Detrusor instability of neurologic origin is referred to as *hyperreflexia.* Nonneurogenic causes of detrusor instability include bladder irritation caused by infection or interstitial cystitis (*bladder pain syndrome*), obstruction (e.g., BPH, cystocele), bladder stones, and tumors. Excessive beverage intake and some therapeutic agents (e.g., diuretics, alcohol) can exacerbate symptoms of urge incontinence as a result of increased filling of the bladder. Bethanechol can also lead to urge incontinence through cholinergically mediated contraction of bladder smooth muscle.

Stress incontinence is characterized by involuntary leakage of urine with sudden increases in abdominal pressure associated with sneezing, laughing, coughing, exercising, and lifting. Stress incontinence is the most frequently encountered type of UI in women, except in the very old (>75 years), in whom OAB is most common. Symptoms of stress incontinence may occur in some men after transurethral resection of the prostate and radical prostatectomy.[13] Symptoms in women are exacerbated by pregnancy and obesity, which also increase intra-abdominal pressure. This involuntary leakage is believed to be caused by hypermobility of the bladder neck or weakness of the urethral sphincter and pelvic floor muscles. Hypermobility refers to displacement of the bladder neck and urethra during physical exertion; it occurs when the supporting pelvic muscles have been weakened as a result of vaginal childbirth and aging. The weakening of the urethral sphincter can be secondary to vaginal or urologic surgery, trauma, aging, or inadequate estrogen, or it may be neurologic in etiology.[17] Drug-related causes of stress incontinence include α-adrenergic antagonists such as prazosin, terazosin, doxazosin, tamsulosin, and alfuzosin, which cause urethral relaxation (Table 49–2).

Overflow incontinence, an involuntary urine loss associated with overdistention of the bladder, is observed in 7%–11% of incontinent older patients.[2] Symptoms include dribbling, reduced force and caliber of urinary stream, urgency, and a sensation of incomplete voiding. The two main causes are outlet obstruction and/or an underactive bladder (detrusor) muscle. Outlet obstruction can be caused by BPH, urogenital tumors, pelvic organ prolapse, or previous anti-incontinence surgery. Dysfunctional bladder contractility can result from diabetic or alcoholic neuropathy, lower spinal cord injury, radical pelvic surgery, or medications with anticholinergic properties, such as antihistamines, antipsychotics, narcotics, tricyclic antidepressants, muscle relaxants, and medications used to treat urge incontinence. These medications can cause overflow incontinence by blocking cholinergically mediated bladder contractions, thereby inhibiting normal bladder function.

Mixed incontinence, most common in women, consists of the combination of OAB and stress incontinence.[2] Although the term *mixed UI* generally is applied to women, men with outlet obstruction resulting from BPH may exhibit mixed symptoms of OAB and overflow incontinence. Men may also exhibit mixed symptoms as a result of stress UI attributable to radical prostatectomy or transurethral resection of the prostate combined with OAB.

Functional incontinence is described as urine loss caused by factors such as physical or cognitive impairment, which interfere with a person's ability to reach toilet facilities in time or to perform toileting tasks.[2] Causes of this type of UI are many and include stroke, diminished mobility, impaired cognitive function or perception, environmental barriers, use of sedative and hypotensive agents, poorly controlled severe pain, and psychological unwillingness to release urine in the proper place. Because many functionally impaired people may have other types of UI, functional incontinence should be a diagnosis of exclusion.

The consequences of UI are considerable. Many people are embarrassed by such a condition and refrain from discussing their urinary problems with their primary care providers (PCPs). Some

TABLE 49–3 Common Signs and Symptoms of Urinary Incontinence (UI) by Type

Type of UI	Urgency	Frequency	Volume of Loss	Nocturia	Other
Urge	Frequent	>8 times per day	Large amount of urine loss: >100 mL and may empty completely	>1 time per night	Inability to reach toilet following urge to void
Stress	Occasional	Urine leakage during physical activity, lifting, coughing, sneezing; if severe, urine loss on ambulating	Small–moderate urine loss, depending on level of activity	Rare	Ability to reach toilet in time to complete void
Overflow	Hesitancy	Straining to void	Decreased or incomplete urine stream; dribbling	Frequent	Sensation of bladder or abdominal fullness, and incomplete bladder emptying

people with UI believe it is a normal consequence of aging, rather than a symptom of underlying disease or anatomic change. Social isolation occurs because the incontinent patient avoids social interaction to prevent the embarrassment and rejection that often accompany UI. In turn, social isolation leads to depression. Intimate contact and sexual activity with the patient's partner can also decrease. Attempts to limit episodes of involuntary urine loss by restricting fluid intake can cause dehydration and hypotension, whereas skin irritation and ulceration caused by long exposure to urine result in "diaper rash" and possibly pressure injuries.[2]

The caregivers of incontinent older patients are under stress because of the tedious and time-consuming care needed to deal with the problems of UI at home. Often, the loss of urine control leads to a drastic reduction in quality of life, and in some cases, placement in a long-term care facility.[2,18] Falls and fractures may be potential risks associated with repeated trips to the bathroom caused by UI and urgency symptoms in the absence of incontinence.

Treatment of Adult Urinary Incontinence

Treatment Goals

The goals of treatment of UI are to cure incontinence or to reduce the severity of symptoms, avoid complications, and improve the patient's quality of life. When incontinence aids are used as part of self-management in UI treatment, additional goals are to control or treat skin breakdown (diaper rash), control the odor of leaked urine, and contain urine in the undergarment.

General Treatment Approach

Treatment is individualized for the type of UI. The four major categories of intervention are behavioral modification, use of devices, pharmacologic treatment, and surgical treatment. A recent publication provides a systematic review of nonsurgical treatments for UI in women.[19] Figure 49–1 outlines the self-management of adult UI.

Nonpharmacologic Therapy

Behavioral techniques decrease the frequency of UI in most patients, have no reported adverse effects, and do not limit future therapies.[2] These techniques generally require patient and caregiver involvement and continued practice to be most successful. Three types of behavioral techniques, listed in order of increasing need for patient involvement, are toileting assistance, bladder training, and pelvic floor muscle training. Behavioral techniques now are the accepted first-line therapy in treating all forms of UI except overflow incontinence.[20] A behavioral modification program involving pelvic floor muscle training and behavioral techniques was found to prevent the development of UI in continent older women.[21] Providers should educate patients about the role of behavioral therapy in the prevention and management of UI.

Toileting assistance includes routine or scheduled voiding performed at fixed, regular intervals (every 2–4 hours); habit training, which is voiding scheduled to match patterns in those who have natural voiding patterns; and prompted voiding. In prompted voiding, patients are trained to void only if the need is voiced on direct questioning. They are checked for wetness and praised for maintaining continence and trying to void.

Bladder training consists of education, scheduled voiding with systematic delay, and positive reinforcement. Patients are taught to delay voiding when the urge occurs and to use tactics to increase urine volume and the interval between voids. Bladder training is recommended for urge or mixed incontinence but often is difficult to achieve in cognitively impaired or frail older people.

Pelvic floor muscle training aims to improve urethral closure pressure by activating the striated muscles of the urethra and the underlying pelvic floor muscles. Two components of training have been established. Early improvement (reduction of urine leakage within 1 week of beginning pelvic floor muscle exercises) may be achieved by some women who learn "the knack maneuver," or volitional precontraction. The *knack maneuver* describes learning to contract pelvic floor muscles in anticipation of and during increases in intra-abdominal pressure (e.g., coughing). This maneuver alone has demonstrated the capacity to reduce stress incontinence.[22] In addition, pelvic floor muscle training, also known as Kegel exercises or pelvic floor exercises, is designed to strengthen the voluntary periurethral and perivaginal muscles, giving the patient more control of micturition and reducing UI.[2] Kegel exercises, which have been used successfully for stress and OAB, are performed by squeezing the pelvic muscles as if to stop the flow of urine. The contractions should be held for about 10 seconds and then released for 10 seconds; 3–4 sets of 10 contractions per day are generally recommended.[2,23] It is important to advise patients that the response to pelvic muscle exercises is delayed.

The exercises may be augmented by the use of vaginal weights or biofeedback techniques. Biofeedback can facilitate learning pelvic muscle exercises. Direct electrical stimulation of the pelvic floor muscles with vaginal or anal probes or surface electrodes has been used with limited success in stress, urge, and mixed UI. Radiofrequency energy treatment (Lyrette, formerly Renessa) is available in a urologist's office and is a nonsurgical approach to stress UI.[24] The treatment, which uses low temperature to cause natural collagen to become firmer, produces improvements in 3 of 4 women and nearly 60% can eliminate the use of pads.[25]

Another option available only through a PCP's office is the NeoControl pelvic floor therapy system.[26] This is a pulsating magnetic chair that uses directed magnetic fields to induce pelvic muscle contractions. Patients generally require treatments twice a week for about 20–30 minutes for a total of 8 weeks or more. This option is approved by the Food and Drug Administration (FDA) for the treatment of stress, OAB, and mixed UI.

Application of mechanical pressure to support the urethra is evident in the age-old advice to women with stress incontinence to cross their legs before coughing or sneezing to prevent urine leakage.[27] Similarly, various devices have been used for UI, including elevating devices to support the bladder neck (pessary, tampon, prosthesis); urethral occlusive devices (urethral plug or insert, caps, expandable urethral devices, urethral shields); external collection systems (condom catheters, female urinals); penile compression devices; and catheterization (intermittent, indwelling, suprapubic).[2] Poise Impressa Bladder Supports are the first nonprescription internal product in the United States cleared by FDA for the temporary management of stress urinary incontinence (SUI).[28] The core of this bladder support is made from flexible, medical-grade silicone, surrounded by a soft, non-absorbent polypropylene covering with a polyester and rayon string to help make insertion and removal easy. Each bladder support comes in a smooth plastic applicator (like a tampon) and is inserted into the

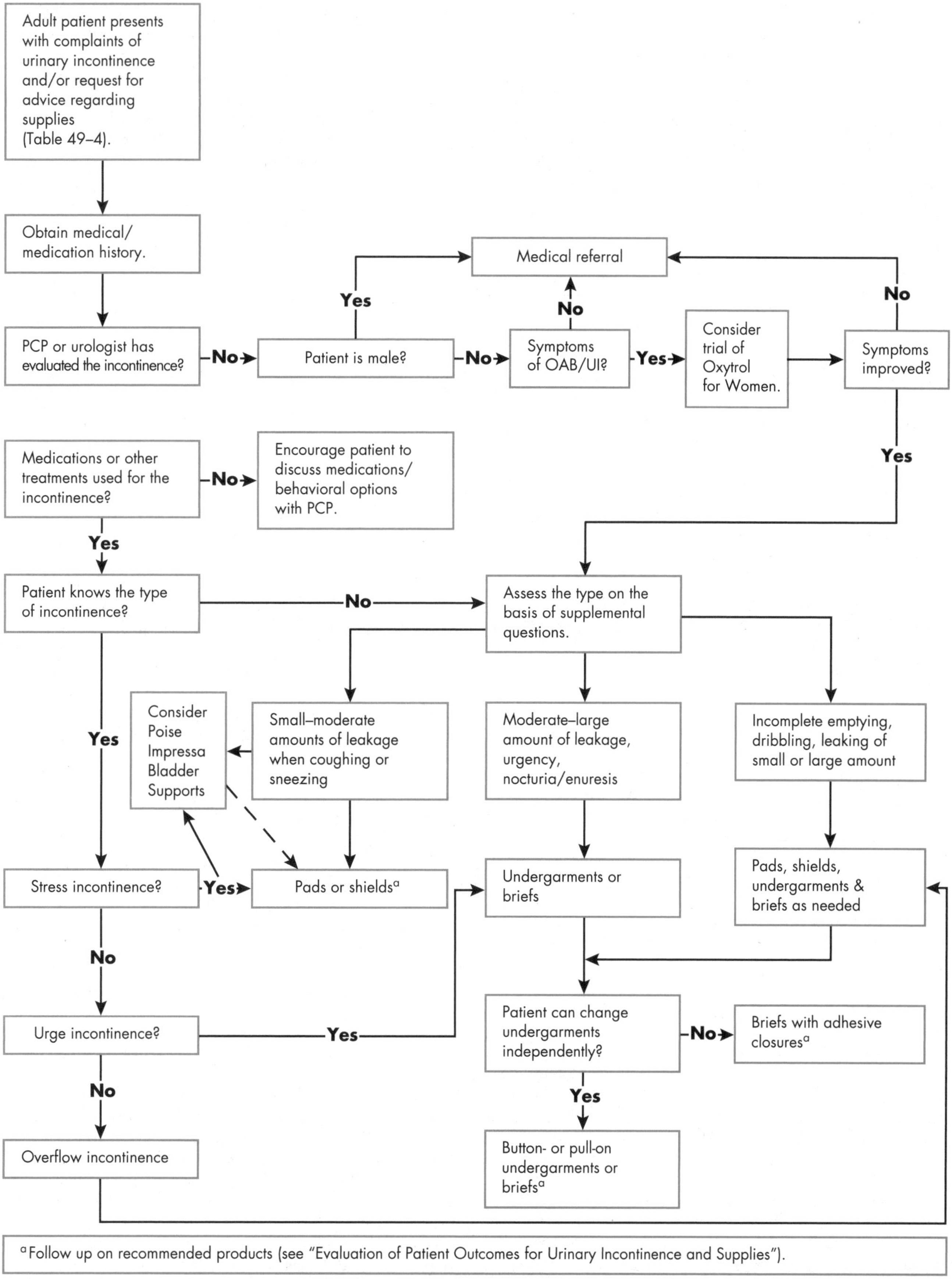

FIGURE 49–1 Self-care for adult urinary incontinence. Key: OAB = Overactive bladder; PCP = primary care provider; UI = urinary incontinence.

vagina the same way to gently lift and give support to the urethra. Designed to reduce or stop urine leakage in women with SUI, Impressa is available in three different sizes to adapt to a woman's unique internal shape. A recent review of mechanical devices found inconsistent results, insufficient evidence to compare one device with another, and no evidence to compare mechanical devices with other forms of treatment.[29]

Although surgery is uncommon in the treatment of OAB, both stress and overflow incontinence can be treated successfully by surgery. Surgery is an option when nonpharmacologic and pharmacologic therapies have failed or the patient wants definitive treatment. The aims of continence surgery are to elevate the bladder neck, support the urethra, and increase urethral resistance.[2,30] Some surgical options include urethral bulking agents (collagen), sling operation, tension-free vaginal tape, artificial sphincter insertion, needle bladder-neck suspension, retropubic suspension, urinary diversion, and bladder denervation. It should be noted that surgical treatment for stress incontinence can instigate or exacerbate symptoms of urgency.

Pharmacologic Therapy

The type of UI influences the choice of treatments. For that reason, an overview of the pharmacologic measures for specific types of UI is presented here. Most medications used to treat these disorders are prescription products; however, a nonprescription form of oxybutynin, Oxytrol for Women, was approved in 2013. Inappropriate use of systemic nonprescription products and incorrect use of absorbent undergarments and pads before a proper evaluation may result in unnecessary expense, inappropriate treatment, and possibly unnecessary changes in the patient's lifestyle and psychological well-being.

OAB or urge incontinence may be treated with anticholinergic medications, which facilitate urine storage by decreasing uninhibited detrusor contractions. Oxybutynin (Oxytrol for Women) provides a nonprescription option for women ages 18 years and older with urinary symptoms consistent with OAB. The transdermal patch is applied every 4 days to a clean, dry, and smooth area of the skin on the abdomen, hips, or buttocks. Application sites need to be rotated with each patch. Common adverse effects include skin irritation at the patch application site, constipation, and dry mouth. Sleepiness, dizziness, and blurry vision may also occur. Thus, driving or operating machinery is not advised until patients know how they will react to the patch. If symptoms do not improve, women should seek a medical referral.[31]

Prescription anticholinergic medications such as darifenacin, oxybutynin chloride, solifenacin, tolterodine, fesoterodine, or trospium are used frequently for OAB and urge UI. Mirabegron, a beta-3 adrenergic agonist approved for the treatment of OAB and urge UI, is an alternative to anticholinergic medications. For patients who do not respond or who cannot take anticholinergic medication, onabotulinumtoxinA offers significant relief from symptoms of OAB and urge UI.[32]

Other prescription medications that have less evidence of clinical efficacy and raise concerns about risks of adverse effects include propantheline, imipramine, hyoscyamine, and nifedipine. Flavoxate, FDA approved for urinary tract symptoms, is not effective according to the results of four placebo-controlled trials.[30] Diphenhydramine (see Chapter 11) and dicyclomine are used occasionally. Providers should counsel patients about the potential adverse effects that occur more frequently with diphenhydramine than with the prescription products. Sedation, dry mouth (a problem for denture users and patients with gastroesophageal reflux disease, dysphagia, or stroke), dizziness, constipation, and confusion can be significant problems in older patients. Contraindications to the use of diphenhydramine and other anticholinergic medications include many conditions (e.g., narrow-angle glaucoma, peptic ulcer, urinary tract obstruction, gastroesophageal reflux disease, uncontrolled hyperthyroidism) that occur more often in older patients than in other patients. Because of these concerns, diphenhydramine and other anticholinergic medications are considered potentially inappropriate medications in older patients and are included in the most recent release of the Beers list.[33]

Stress incontinence often is treated with agents that increase outflow resistance through alpha-receptor stimulation that enhances contraction of the bladder-neck muscles.[2] A commonly recommended nonprescription drug is pseudoephedrine (see Chapter 11).[2,17] The dose of pseudoephedrine is 15–30 mg 3 times daily, starting with the lowest dose, especially in older people. Use of nonprescription medications for UI is an off-label indication and must be approved by a PCP. Caution should be used, however, when initiating such therapy in patients with hypertension and/or cardiac arrhythmias. Providers should advise patients to monitor their blood pressure and pulse, and to report any new occurrences of heart palpitations or fainting. Common adverse effects of pseudoephedrine include insomnia, headache, tachycardia, elevated blood pressure, dizziness, nervousness, agitation, and tremor.

In women, only topical estrogen should be advised, because placebo-controlled studies have shown that oral estrogen therapy is not effective and that systemic therapy is associated with potentially serious adverse effects, including venous thromboembolism, heart attack, stroke, and breast cancer. Topical vaginal estrogen therapy is most useful in stress UI with underlying vaginitis and urethritis caused by estrogen deficiency; several randomized controlled trials of vaginal estrogen have shown a decrease in urgency and incontinence.[34,35] Therapy with estrogen vaginal cream is usually initiated with daily application and tapered to several times weekly applications; benefits are usually seen in 4–6 weeks. Other vaginal estrogen options include the vaginal ring and vaginal tablets. Estrogen can be used in combination with α-adrenergic agonists; however, the combination is only slightly more effective and can be associated with more adverse effects and increased therapy cost. The antidepressant imipramine, which also acts as an adrenergic agonist, has been suggested when α-adrenergic agonists and estrogens have failed. Duloxetine, a selective serotonin and norepinephrine reuptake inhibitor currently approved for the treatment of depression, postherpetic neuropathy, and diabetic neuropathy, is moderately effective in managing stress UI.[36] If medical treatment fails, surgical correction may be possible.

The treatment of overflow incontinence is directed by the underlying cause. In BPH, α-adrenergic antagonists (terazosin, doxazosin, tamsulosin, alfuzosin, silodosin, prazosin) or 5-alpha-reductase inhibitors (finasteride, dutasteride) can be used to reduce the degree of outlet obstruction. Compared with 5-alpha-reductase inhibitors, α-adrenergic antagonists have a much faster onset of effect (several days). Because of a relatively high rate of orthostatic hypotension, prazosin is not recommended for therapy of UI. Prescription agents, such as bethanechol chloride, may be initiated if the bladder has insufficient contractile strength, such as after general anesthesia. Its efficacy is not well established in long-standing hypotonic bladder, however, and it is associated with potentially serious adverse effects. In neurogenic bladder, bethanechol appears to be most effective when starting therapy as soon as possible after the occurrence of incontinence following the neurologic event. Surgery for BPH is often necessary. Catheterization, usually intermittent, is combined with frequent attempts to void as a last resort when medical and surgical corrections have failed.

Treatment of functional and iatrogenic incontinence requires evaluating the patient's entire medical status, medication history, and environment. UI resulting from medications can be resolved by initiating alternative treatments. Underlying dysfunctions, such as pain related to rheumatoid arthritis and decreased mobility, can be remedied by medical and environmental changes that make using the toilet possible or easier within the limitations of the patient's functional status. Often an assessment by physical or occupational therapists can be useful in enhancing physical function.

Use of Urinary Incontinence Supplies

Absorbent undergarments and pads are used to protect clothing, bedding, and furniture while allowing the patient to have independence and mobility. Although absorbent products are beneficial, they should be used only after a thorough and complete physical examination. Medicare, Medicaid, and other private insurers typically cover catheters and related supplies, but Medicare does not cover absorbent undergarments or pads, except during hospital and skilled long-term care visits. Medicaid will cover such bladder control supplies, but coverage varies by state. Prematurely initiating the use of absorbent protective products relieves the discomfort and obscures the cause of UI. Because correction of the cause may be possible, the premature acceptance of UI may have significant financial, social, and psychological consequences.

Product Selection Guidelines

The type of absorbent product selected depends on several factors[2]:

- Type and severity of UI
- Functional status
- Gender
- Availability of caregivers
- Patient preference
- Cost
- Convenience

Health care providers need to discuss these factors with patients and their caregivers when helping them select absorbent garments and pads, which are available as reusable or disposable products (Table 49–4). This discussion is particularly important for low-income patients, who often do not have the economic flexibility to purchase absorbent products; they may be forced to resort to toilet paper or tissue products, an ineffective substitute. Many people attempt to extend the life of disposable products by layering flushable tissue over the pad. The tissue is also easier to dispose of in public places. However, its reduced wicking capacity can expose the skin to more moisture and thus create the potential for breakdown. Some patients may be inclined to use low-cost menstrual pads that may be effective in some cases; however, these products contain materials that are specific to absorbing blood, not urine. Given the wide variety of available products, a resource guide published by the National Association for Continence (NAFC) may be invaluable in helping patients to select a product.[37]

In 2012, NAFC recommended the following eight national quality performance standards for disposable adult absorbent products[38]:

1. *Rewet rate:* a measure of a product's ability to withstand incontinent episodes between changes
2. *Rate of acquisition:* a measure of the speed at which urine is drawn away from the skin
3. *Retention capacity:* a measure of a product's capacity to hold fluid

TABLE 49–4 Selected Adult Incontinence Product Features[a]

Trade Name	Absorbency	Size	Characteristics
Undergarments			
Assurance Slip-On Protective Undergarment[b]	Moderate–heavy leakage	One size	One-piece design; no buttons or tapes
Attends Undergarments Super Absorbency	Moderate leakage		Reusable elastic belts
Depend Undergarments Easy Fit Elastic Leg/Adjustable Straps Regular & Extra Absorbency	Moderate leakage	One size; fits hip sizes up to 65 in.	Soft, cloth-like outer cover; reusable hook and loop strap tabs
Depend Undergarments Elastic Leg/ Button Straps Regular & Extra Absorbency	Moderate leakage	One size; fits hip sizes up to 65 in.	Soft, cloth-like outer cover; reusable button strap tabs
Depend Undergarments Elastic Leg Extra Absorbency	Moderate leakage	One size	Soft, cloth-like outer cover; reusable button strap tabs
Depend Underwear Extra & Super Plus Absorbency	Heavy leakage	S/M, L	Feels and wears like underwear
Depend Refastenable Underwear Extra & Super Plus Absorbency	Heavy leakage	S/M, L/XL	Feels and wears like underwear; 4 refastenable tabs
Prevail Underwear	Heavy leakage	S, M, L	For men and women; look and feel like underwear; pull-on

(continued)

TABLE 49-4 **Selected Adult Incontinence Product Features[a]** *(continued)*

Trade Name	Absorbency	Size	Characteristics
Briefs			
Attends Briefs	Heavy leakage	Y, S, M, L	Refastenable tapes
Attends Briefs with Waistband	Heavy leakage	M, L	Waistband
Depend Fitted Briefs Regular & Overnight Absorbency	Heavy leakage; overnight absorbency absorbs 30% more urine than regular absorbency	M, L	Six refastenable tapes plus elastic leg and waist; wetness indicator
TENA Briefs	Heavy leakage	Y, S, M, L	Refastenable tabs
Pads			
Attends Pads	Light leakage; medium-, extra-, super absorbency	8.5, 10.5, 12.5 14.5, 18 in. long	
Poise Liners	Very light absorbency	6.5 in. long	
Poise Extra Coverage Liners	Very light absorbency	7.5 in. long	
Poise Thin Pads Light Absorbency	Light leakage	8.5 in. long	Elasticized sides
Poise Pads Regular Absorbency	Light leakage	8.5 in. long	Elasticized sides
Poise Pads Extra Absorbency	Light leakage	9.5 in. long	Elasticized sides; one end wider
Poise Pads Extra Plus Absorbency	Light–moderate leakage	11 in. long	Elasticized sides; one end wider
Poise Pads with Side Shields Ultra Absorbency	Light–moderate leakage	11 in. long	
Poise Pads with Side Shields Ultra Plus Absorbency	Moderate leakage	13 in. long	Pad-like comfort with guard-like absorbency; one end wider
Serenity/TENA Dry Active Liners	Light leakage	Regular and long	
Serenity/TENA Active Ultra Thin Pads	Light–moderate leakage	Regular and long	
Serenity/TENA Stylish Ultra Thin Pads with Wings	Light leakage	One size	Form fitting, sleek, and super absorbent
Serenity/TENA Anywhere Ultra Thin Pads	Heavy leakage	Long	
Serenity/TENA Anywhere Ultra Thin Pads	Moderate leakage	Regular	
Serenity/TENA Pads Moderate	Moderate leakage	Regular and long	
Serenity/TENA Pads Heavy	Heavy leakage	Regular and long	
Serenity/TENA Ultimate Pads	Heavy leakage	One size	
Serenity/TENA Overnight Pads	Heavy leakage; overnight	One size	Longest pad
Serenity/TENA InstaDRY Heavy Pads	Heavy leakage	One size	Fast-absorbing pad
Guards			
Attends Guards Super Absorbency	Light–moderate leakage	One size	Curved fit
Conveen Drip Collector	Dribbling or light leakage; adheres to underwear; designed for men	3- and 4-oz capacity	
Depend Guards for Men	Light–moderate leakage	One size	Anatomic design with elasticized pouch and cup-like fit
Serenity/TENA Guards Super Absorbency	Moderate–heavy leakage	One size	
Serenity Guards Super Plus Absorbency	Heavy leakage	One size	

Key: Y = Youth; S = small; M = medium; L = large.

[a] Products change often; for current product availability, refer to websites (i.e., www.depend.com, www.poise.com, www.serenity.com).

[b] Manufacturer markets other products similar to the Depend line but offers a lower price point.

4. Sizing options: sizes ranging from youth and small adult to extra-large and double-extra-large adult
5. Safety: no components, including additives, that are listed in any federal regulatory agency as being considered "unsafe"
6. Presence of a *closure system:* mechanism that allows the product to be opened and refastened
7. *Breathable zones:* an acceptable minimum air flow in side "wings" of the product sufficient to release trapped body heat and gaseous body perspiration in the pelvic region
8. Performance of elastics: provision of evidence of fit and functionality of containment of body waste, without sacrificing comfort

The disposable product market has been a multimillion-dollar industry since the 1990s. These products work in the same manner as children's disposable diapers. They are designed to absorb urine; provide a moisture barrier to protect clothes, bedding, and furniture; and minimize skin contact with urine. For maximum absorbency, products containing an absorptive gel of superabsorbent polymers may be preferable. Urine is jelled in the matrix of the absorbent layer, minimizing its contact with skin. Reusable incontinence undergarments may offer a more affordable option. These products resemble underpants with a waterproof crotch and are designed to hold a reusable panty liner. The newest option is reusable incontinence undergarments that resemble standard underwear but have the absorbency of disposable briefs. These undergarments have a unique crotch design made of several layers of wicking fabric that quickly pulls moisture away from the skin. They are available for men and women in a variety of leakage control levels. Reusable incontinence underwear is constructed of waterproof outer fabrics ranging from lace to nylon floral prints, making them an attractive and affordable option for patients with an active lifestyle. A comparative evaluation of the performance and cost-effectiveness of four key absorbent product designs demonstrated significant and substantial differences between products and considerable individual variability in preference. Cost-effective management with absorbent products may best be achieved by allowing users to choose combinations of designs for different circumstances.[39]

The capacity of each disposable product corresponds to the needs of the patient:

- Guards/shields: 2–12 oz. (60–360 mL), light–heavy capacity
- Undergarments: 12–18 oz. (360–540 mL), moderate–heavy capacity
- Briefs: 28–36 oz. (840–1100 mL), moderate–heavy capacity

Patients with small amounts of leakage (e.g., dribbling), as occurs in stress or overflow incontinence and after urologic surgical procedures, may require only a pad or shield.[40,41] A recent systematic review of absorbent products suggested that disposable insert pads are best for leak-through prevention; they are also the most acceptable and preferred design for women with light UI.[42] In a similar study, guards were a preferred product for light UI in men.[43] If larger amounts of urine are lost with UI, as often occurs with detrusor instability, products with a larger capacity would be more appropriate. Many products designed for overnight (heavy) use tend to have the largest capacities.[37] Booster or doubler pads or inserts are also available to prevent leaks and increase the absorbency of current absorbent products.

Another important issue is the functional capacity of the patient. If the patient needs assistance with absorbent garments, the caregiver may find that briefs or diapers with "roll-on" bed application and adhesive closures are useful. Securing the product may be an important issue. Close-fitting underwear is recommended. Some garments or shields have adhesive strips or belts to hold them in place. The use of belts may require assistance from a caregiver. Of course, comfort and leg security from urine leakage are important. Many product lines offer elastic legs or contoured shapes. Caregivers and patients should consider products designed for the differences between male and female anatomy when selecting large-capacity products.[40,41]

Protective underpads often are used in conjunction with briefs and undergarments for extended duration activities, such as sleeping and sitting. Both bed and chair pads are available, and the provider should inquire about the need for additional protection. The underpad should have a known capacity, a waterproof duration of several hours, and an ability to remain intact when wet. Bed pads are available in sizes from 16 by 24 in. to 30 by 36 in. For chairs, a 16- by 18-in. pad should be used.[41]

Complications From Absorbent Products

Because the use of absorbent products increases the risk of skin irritation and maceration, these products should be checked every 2 hours. With continual urine loss, it is recommended that the absorbent material be changed every 2–4 hours. The use of skin protectants (barrier creams, ointments), as in diaper rash, is appropriate. If a rash occurs, the same treatment as that described for infants is indicated (see Chapter 36).

Urine odor is an embarrassing problem. Nonprescription products containing chlorophyll (e.g., Derifil, Pals, Nullo) or vitamin C can be recommended to help decrease urine odor. However, frequent checks for wetness and prompt changes of soiled pads and garments are preferable to efforts to mask the odor.

The healing of skin wounds may be delayed in the patient with skin wetted by urine. Any skin breakdown needs to be reported to the PCP. This serious complication should not be treated with nonprescription products without medical supervision.

UI products that are not available from the pharmacy or specialty supply store may be obtained by contacting the National Association for Continence (NAFC), PO Box 1019, Charleston, SC 29402-1019; 1-843-377-0900, 1-800-BLADDER; fax: 1-843-377-0905; or www.nafc.org.

Complementary Therapies

Nutritional deficiencies of protein, calcium, vitamin C, zinc, magnesium, and vitamin B_{12} have been proposed as possibly contributing to the development of UI.[44] Of these, the relationship between vitamin B_{12} deficiency and UI has been established.[45] A B_{12} deficiency may lead to diminished neurosensory input regarding bladder fullness or to inappropriate neurologic stimulation of the bladder, causing detrusor instability. Many factors, such as spicy and acidic foods (e.g., caffeine, alcohol, citrus fruits), tobacco, dyes (e.g., Federal Food, Drug, and Cosmetic Yellow No. 5), food preservatives, and sugar substitutes (i.e., aspartame), may cause urinary frequency and urgency with the potential for UI.

Several herbal treatments have been suggested for UI, including phytoestrogens (e.g., soybean, flaxseed), saw palmetto and pygeum (African plum), St. John's wort, and bearberry (uva-ursi) teas. Good clinical evidence from recent rigorous studies showed that saw palmetto is not effective in improving lower urinary tract symptoms related to BPH.[46,47] In addition, there is no evidence from controlled studies that other herbal products significantly improve lower urinary tract symptoms.[48] Patients should be advised to consult with their PCPs before using any of these products for UI. An in-depth discussion of saw palmetto and pygeum is presented in Chapter 51.

Assessment of Adult Urinary Incontinence and Supplies: A Case-Based Approach

Because of the public's general lack of sufficient medical knowledge about the different types of UI, some patients (or their caregivers) may attempt self-diagnosis and treatment without consulting their PCPs. Self-diagnosis obviously could lead to inappropriate treatment. Therefore, it is imperative that providers inquire about a proper medical evaluation before recommending nonprescription products, including absorbent products. A PCP must recommend use of nonprescription medications for off-label indications.

Armed with the patient's history and proper diagnosis, the provider can answer questions appropriately and help in the selection and proper use of devices and medications for treating this disorder.

Cases 49–1 and 49–2 illustrate the assessment of adult patients with UI.

Patient Counseling for Adult Urinary Incontinence and Supplies

The PCP's role in self-treatment of UI includes educating patients about UI; recommending medical evaluation, as appropriate, that is based on an initial evaluation of signs and symptoms; assisting patients and caregivers in selecting products to reduce the risk of urine leaking to outer garments; and avoiding aggravating factors. Patients should be provided with information to help them understand UI. The box Patient Education for Adult Urinary Incontinence and Supplies lists specific information to provide patients regarding the use of incontinence supplies. An excellent resource for patient education is the Simon Foundation for Continence, PO Box 815, Wilmette, IL 60091; 1-800-23Simon; or www.simonfoundation.org.

CASE 49–1

Relevant Evaluation Criteria	Scenario/Model Outcome
Information Gathering	
1. Gather essential information about the patient's symptoms and medical history, including	
a. Description of symptom(s) (i.e., nature, onset, duration, severity, associated symptoms)	Patient complains of episodes of a weak bladder and light urine leakage. The first incident occurred after the birth of her third child. As a result, she refrains from many activities that she once enjoyed, particularly sports and dancing. She has consulted her gynecologist but is not interested in any surgery for stress incontinence at this time.
b. Description of any factors that seem to precipitate, exacerbate, and/or relieve the patient's symptom(s)	The "leakage" occurs when she lifts her children, coughs, sneezes, or laughs. No leakage occurs at any other times.
c. Description of the patient's efforts to relieve the symptoms	"I have been using panty liners, but they don't seem to protect my clothes. I am so embarrassed."
d. Patient's identity	Amelia Watt
e. Patient's age, gender, height, and weight	54 years old, female, 5 ft 5 in., 171 lb
f. Patient's occupation	Interior designer
g. Patient's dietary habits	Vegetarian diet, 3 cups of coffee/tea per day; 1 glass of wine daily
h. Patient's sleep habits	Occasional nighttime awakenings caused by hot flushes.
i. Concurrent medical conditions, prescription and nonprescription medications, and dietary supplements	Occasional use of acetaminophen for morning stiffness; vitamin D 2000 IU daily
j. Allergies	NKA
k. History of other adverse reactions to medications	None
l. Other (describe) ______	Lives with husband and children.
Assessment and Triage	
2. Differentiate patient's signs/symptoms and correctly identify the patient's primary problem(s).	Characteristics of Mrs. Watt's urine leakage are consistent with stress incontinence.
3. Identify exclusions for self-treatment.	None. However, Mrs. Watt should be encouraged to seek a diagnosis for her UI before relying on incontinence products.

CASE 49-1 *continued*

Relevant Evaluation Criteria	Scenario/Model Outcome
4. Formulate a comprehensive list of therapeutic alternatives for the primary problem to determine whether triage to a medical provider is required, and share this information with the patient or caregiver.	Options include (1) Refer Mrs. Watt to her PCP/gynecologist for evaluation of stress incontinence. (2) Use nondrug measures and products to manage the symptoms. (3) Use nondrug measures and products until Mrs. Watt sees her PCP. (4) Take no action.
Plan	
5. Select an optimal therapeutic alternative to address the patient's problem, taking into account patient preferences.	See Figure 49–1. Mrs. Watt should be encouraged to try Poise Impressa Bladder Supports before activities. She should be encouraged to learn pelvic floor muscle exercises and to use pads, shields, or reusable incontinence underwear, as needed, for light urine leakage. These products would offer more protection than panty liners. She should be counseled on the benefits of caffeine reduction, weight reduction, and pelvic exercises.
6. Describe the recommended therapeutic approach to the patient or caregiver.	"Once you have tried Impressa, consult your primary care provider if symptoms persist. An incontinence pad or shield may be appropriate for additional protection."
7. Explain to the patient or caregiver the rationale for selecting the recommended therapeutic approach from the considered therapeutic alternatives.	"If Impressa does not control your limited bladder leakage, medical evaluation is necessary to determine the type of incontinence and the need for a prescription medication or device."
Patient Education	
8. When recommending self-care with nonprescription medications and/or nondrug therapy, convey accurate information to the patient or caregiver:	See the box "Patient Education for Adult Urinary Incontinence and Supplies." Poise Impressa Bladder Supports are recommended for the self-care of symptoms of stress incontinence. Advise the patient not to use the product if she ■ Is younger than 21 years ■ Is pregnant, may become pregnant, or has given birth in the past 3 months ■ Has experienced unusual or unexpected vaginal bleeding within the last 6 months ■ Has pain or a burning sensation when she urinates (symptoms indicative of a *urinary tract infection*) ■ Is experiencing malodorous vaginal discharge, or irritation, soreness, or itching in the vaginal area (symptoms indicative of a *vaginal infection*) ■ Had vaginal surgery within the past 3 months ■ Has already been diagnosed by her PCP with a severely dry (*atrophic*) vagina
a. Appropriate dose and frequency of administration	Poise Impressa Bladder Supports are available in three sizes. Advise Mrs. Watt that selecting the right size is important in providing the most comfortable solution. a. "Start with the sizing kit." b. "Use size 1 first. If it feels comfortable and you have little or no urine leakage, then size 1 is the correct size for you." c. "If the product does not feel comfortable or if you still experience leakage, continue to try the next larger size until you find the size that is right for you." "Use only one support at a time, and do not use the same support more than once." See the box "Patient Education for Adult Urinary Incontinence and Supplies."

CASE 49-1 *continued*

Relevant Evaluation Criteria	Scenario/Model Outcome
b. Maximum number of days the therapy should be employed	The patient should not use Poise Impressa bladder supports for more than 8 hours in a 24-hour period. Advise Mrs. Watt to see her PCP if use of the bladder supports for 14 days does not reduce her bladder leakage. "You may have a type of incontinence other than stress urinary incontinence that requires different treatment." See the box Patient Education for Adult Urinary Incontinence and Supplies.
c. Product administration procedures	"If the Poise Impressa Bladder Supports are effective, you still should not ■ Use a support during your period or if you have any vaginal bleeding ■ Use a support with a tampon ■ Use the same support more than once ■ Use more than one support at a time ■ Use a support during sexual intercourse ■ Use the product if the package is damaged" See the box Patient Education for Adult Urinary Incontinence and Supplies.
d. Expected time to onset of relief	"Symptoms may improve within 2 weeks. See your primary care provider if using Poise Impressa Bladder Supports does not reduce your bladder leakage after 14 days of use. You may have a type of incontinence other than stress urinary incontinence that requires different treatment."
e. Degree of relief that can be reasonably expected	"Results will be different for every woman, because Poise Impressa Bladder Supports can reduce leakage in some women, stop leakage in others, and may not work for some." See the box Patient Education for Adult Urinary Incontinence and Supplies.
f. Most common adverse effects	"Mild and temporary adverse effects when using Poise Impressa Bladder Supports for the first few times include ■ Small blood spots on the product ■ Mild discomfort ■ Vaginal soreness These symptoms typically do not last more than 14 days."
g. Adverse effects that warrant medical intervention should they occur	"If you experience any of the following adverse effects, remove the bladder support device and call your primary care provider: ■ Pain or burning when urinating ■ Vaginal discharge that smells bad ■ Irritation or itching in your vagina ■ Vaginal bleeding between your monthly periods ■ Pain in your vagina ■ Increased bladder leakage" See the box Patient Education for Adult Urinary Incontinence and Supplies.
h. Patient options in the event that condition worsens or persists	"Remove the Poise Bladder Support immediately if you have a fever of 102.0°F (38.9°C) AND one or more of the following symptoms: ■ Aching muscles or joints ■ Redness of your eyes ■ Sore throat ■ Weakness, fainting, or dizziness ■ A rash that looks like sunburn ■ Vomiting ■ Diarrhea"

CASE 49-1 *continued*

Relevant Evaluation Criteria	Scenario/Model Outcome
	"Call your primary care provider immediately, because you may have toxic shock syndrome (TSS). TSS is a rare but serious disease that can cause death if your primary care provider does not treat it right away. Increased risk of TSS is associated with products worn in the vagina. However, an association with use of this product and TSS has not been established."
	"If urinary symptoms persist, see your primary care provider or urologist for further follow-up. If urine loss is continual, change absorbent undergarments every 2–4 hours."
i. product storage requirements	n/a
j. specific nondrug measures	See the box Patient Education for Adult Urinary Incontinence and Supplies for behavioral measures to reduce and improve incontinence symptoms.
Solicit follow-up questions from patient or caregiver.	(1) "What if the symptoms don't improve?"
	(2) "What if the incontinence product does not provide enough protection?"
Answer patient's or caregiver's questions.	(1) "If symptoms do not improve, see your primary care provider."
	(2) "You may select a product with higher absorbency according to the amount of urine leakage." (See Table 49–4.)
Evaluation of Patient Outcome	
9. Assess patient outcome.	"If symptoms do not improve within 2 weeks of using Impressa, consult your primary care provider for further evaluation and treatment."

Key: n/a = Not applicable; NKA = no known allergies; PCP = primary care provider; UI = urinary incontinence.

CASE 49-2

Relevant Evaluation Criteria	Scenario/Model Outcome
Information Gathering	
1. Gather essential information about the patient's symptoms and medical history, including	
a. Description of symptom(s) (i.e., nature, onset, duration, severity, associated symptoms)	Patient wants to use an herbal product for a recent problem of "dribbling and inability to empty my bladder." He heard about a product for urinary heath during a recent radio broadcast. He has been quite healthy, and this new problem is affecting his social life.
b. Description of any factors that seem to precipitate, exacerbate, and/or relieve the patient's symptom(s)	The dribbling occurs throughout the day. He often wakes up 2–3 times per night to urinate.
c. Description of the patient's efforts to relieve the symptoms	Frequent trips to the bathroom
d. Patient's identity	Joe Walker
e. Patient's age, gender, height, and weight	70 years old, male, 5 ft 11 in., 220 lb
f. Patient's occupation	Retired
g. Patient's dietary habits	Whiskey, 2–3 drinks on weekends
h. Patient's sleep habits	Frequent nighttime awakenings to urinate
i. Concurrent medical conditions, prescription and nonprescription medications, and dietary supplements	Benign prostatic hyperplasia: tamsulosin (Flomax) 0.4 mg HS; hypertension: currently takes lisinopril 10 mg daily.
j. Allergies	NKA
k. History of other adverse reactions to medications	None
l. Other (describe) ______	

CASE 49-2 *continued*

Relevant Evaluation Criteria	Scenario/Model Outcome
Assessment and Triage	
2. Differentiate patient's signs/symptoms, and correctly identify the patient's primary problem(s).	Mr. Walker's urine leakage is consistent with symptoms of BPH. He is currently on tamsulosin (Flomax) and has not had symptoms; he should see his PCP or urologist for reevaluation of the therapy prior to starting any dietary supplement or other nonprescription treatment.
3. Identify exclusions for self-treatment.	Mr. Walker has been evaluated by a PCP or urologist and is currently receiving therapy for BPH.
4. Formulate a comprehensive list of therapeutic alternatives for the primary problem to determine whether triage to a medical provider is required, and share this information with the patient or caregiver.	Options include (1) Refer Mr. Walker for further evaluation for BPH therapy. (2) Recommend nondrug measures and products to control his symptoms. (3) Recommend nondrug measures and products until he can see his PCP. (4) Take no action.
Plan	
5. Select an optimal therapeutic alternative to address the patient's problem, taking into account patient preferences.	Mr. Walker should consult a PCP or other health care provider for further evaluation prior to using any nonprescription medication, prescription medication, or incontinence product.
6. Describe the recommended therapeutic approach to the patient or caregiver.	"Once current therapy has been evaluated and other causes eliminated, alternative prescription drug therapy may be suggested for reducing the symptoms of BPH. An absorbent guard may be appropriate for persistent symptoms."
7. Explain to the patient or caregiver the rationale for selecting the recommended therapeutic approach from the considered therapeutic alternatives.	"Medical evaluation is necessary to assess the effectiveness of your current regimen and determine the need for another drug therapy option."
Patient Education	
8. When recommending self-care with nonprescription medications and/or nondrug therapy, convey accurate information to the patient or caregiver:	See the box "Patient Education for Adult Urinary Incontinence and Supplies."
a. Appropriate dose and frequency of administration	See the box "Patient Education for Adult Urinary Incontinence and Supplies."
b. Maximum number of days the therapy should be employed	See the box "Patient Education for Adult Urinary Incontinence and Supplies."
c. Product administration procedures	See the box "Patient Education for Adult Urinary Incontinence and Supplies."
d. Expected time to onset of relief	n/a
e. Degree of relief that can be reasonably expected	See the box "Patient Education for Adult Urinary Incontinence and Supplies."
f. Most common adverse effects	"You may experience irritation, rash, maceration, and breakdown of the affected skin."
g. Adverse effects that warrant medical intervention should they occur	"You should check for skin irritation every 2 hours." See the box "Patient Education for Adult Urinary Incontinence and Supplies."
h. Patient options in the event that condition worsens or persists	"If urine loss is continual, change absorbent undergarments every 2–4 hours. See your primary care provider or urologist for further follow-up."
i. Product storage requirements	n/a

CASE 49-2 *continued*

Relevant Evaluation Criteria	Scenario/Model Outcome
j. Specific nondrug measures	See the box "Patient Education for Adult Urinary Incontinence and Supplies."
Solicit follow-up questions from patient or caregiver.	"What if the incontinence product does not provide enough protection?"
Answer patient's or caregiver's questions.	"You may select a different product with higher absorbency based on the amount of urine leakage." (See Table 49–4.)
Evaluation of Patient Outcome	
9. Assess patient outcome.	Contact the patient in a couple of days to ensure that he made an appointment and sought medical care

Key: BPH = Benign prostatic hyperplasia; n/a = not applicable; NKA = no known allergies; PCP = primary care provider.

Evaluation of Patient Outcomes for Adult Urinary Incontinence and Supplies

At follow-up, the provider should find out whether the pharmacologic therapy is effective, whether the recommended incontinence product is comfortable and easy to use, and whether leakage from the undergarment or odor is a problem. If leakage is occurring, the absorbency and/or type of product should be reassessed. Patients who have problems with odor may need to use deodorizers. The patient or caregiver should also be asked whether the skin, especially in the perivaginal and perianal areas, is being checked for breakdown. Redness or skin irritation call for the use of skin protectants. Questioning about occurrence of urinary tract or vaginal infections is also appropriate. Such infections may indicate a need to change undergarments more often or to use another type of incontinence product. These measures will prevent prolonged skin contact with urine. In addition, the provider should monitor the effectiveness of other prescription medications and behavioral therapies for UI. The patient should be asked about adverse effects associated with the specific medication he or she may be prescribed.

Providers should also evaluate whether the use of incontinence products and other treatments has allowed patients to resume their normal lifestyles and social interactions. If these objectives

PATIENT EDUCATION FOR Adult Urinary Incontinence and Supplies

The objectives of self-treatment are (1) to reduce or eliminate symptoms of urinary incontinence (UI), (2) to control or treat skin irritation caused by contact with urine, (3) to control the odor of urine leaked from the bladder, (4) to control leakage of urine to outer garments, and (5) to prevent other complications such as falls and social isolation. For most patients, carefully following product instructions and the self-care measures listed here will help to ensure optimal therapeutic outcomes.

- Consult a primary care provider or urologist for a thorough examination before resorting to permanent use of absorbent undergarments or shields. Many cases of UI are reversible with treatment.
- Absorbent products are designed to absorb urine; to provide a moisture barrier to protect clothes, bedding, and furniture; and to minimize skin contact with urine.
- Base selection of absorbent products on the amount of leaked urine:
  - Guards/shields: 2–12 ounces (60–360 mL), light–heavy capacity
  - Undergarments: 12–18 ounces (360–540 mL), moderate–heavy capacity
  - Briefs: 28–36 ounces (840–1000 mL), moderate–heavy capacity
- Choose briefs or diapers with roll-on bed application and adhesive closures (for patients who are unable to change themselves).
- If additional protection is needed during sleeping and sitting, select absorbent bed or chair pads to use with absorbent undergarments.
- Check skin for irritation or maceration every 2 hours, even when absorbent garments are used.
- If urine loss is continual, change absorbent undergarments every 2–4 hours, and consult your primary care provider or urologist if UI symptoms worsen.
- If desired, use skin protectants labeled for diaper rash to protect the skin.
- If desired, use products containing chlorophyll, such as Derifil, Pals, and Nullo, to help decrease odor. However, continue frequent skin checks and frequent changes of absorbent undergarments.
- If pressure injuries (open sores) occur in an immobile patient, the caregiver should not attempt to treat the ulcers with nonprescription products and should instead consult a primary care provider.
- Identify and eliminate foods, liquids, or other substances that can irritate the bladder (e.g., coffee, tea, soda, alcohol, chocolate, acidic juices, tomato-based sauces, spicy food, artificial sweeteners, nicotine).
- Avoid excessive intake of liquid. Drink enough to produce about a cup of urine every 3–4 waking hours on average. Do not drink large amounts of liquid after 5 PM.
- Avoid products that irritate the urethra and bladder. Use cotton underwear, avoid scented powders or bath products, and use white toilet paper.
- Follow instructions for behavioral therapy and medications for incontinence if prescribed by your primary care provider or urologist.

are not being met after an adequate duration of any pharmacotherapy, the medication dose and type should be reviewed. Alternative absorbent products should also be considered. The patient should be encouraged to seek further advice from his or her PCP on treatment options.

Key Points for Adult Urinary Incontinence and Supplies

- UI is a common treatable condition that is often cured or improved with therapy.
- Because the cause of UI may be multifactorial, the patient should receive a comprehensive medical evaluation before a therapy plan is developed.
- A variety of treatment options, including drug therapy, behavioral therapies, devices, incontinence aids, and surgery, are available.
- Incontinence aids are designed to absorb urine; to provide a moisture barrier to protect clothes, bedding, and furniture; and to minimize skin contact with urine.
- The selection of absorbent products is based on the amount of urine leakage.
- Providers can play an important role in educating patients about UI; performing assessment and triage and referring for medical evaluation, if needed; counseling on the selection and appropriate use of prescription and nonprescription incontinence products and the avoidance of aggravating factors; and monitoring patient response.

REFERENCES

1. Abrams P, Cardozo L, Fall M et al. The standardisation of terminology of lower urinary tract dysfunction: report from the standardisation subcommittee of the international continence society. *Neurourol Urodynam.* 2002;21(2):167–78. doi:10.1002/nau.10052.
2. Shaban A, Drake MJ, Hashim H. The medical management of urinary incontinence. *Auton Neurosci.* 2010;152(1–2):4–10. doi:10.1016/j.autneu.2009.09.022.
3. Gaugler JE, Duval S, Anderson KA, et al. Predicting nursing home admission in the US: a meta-analysis. *BMC Geriatr.* 2007;7:13. doi:10.1186/1471-2318-7-13.
4. Onukwugha E, Zuckerman IH, McNally D, et al. The total economic burden of overactive bladder in the United States: a disease-specific approach. *Am J Manag Care.* 2009;15(4 Suppl):S90–7. PMID: 19355803.Available at: http://www.ajmc.com/journals/supplement/2009/A220_09mar_OAB/A220_09mar_OnukS90toS97/. Accessed May 18, 2017.
5. Coyne KS, Wein A, Nicholson S, et al. Economic burden of urgency urinary incontinence in the United States: a systematic review. *J Manag Care Pharm.* 2014;20(2):130–40. doi: 10.18553/jmcp.2014.20.2.130.
6. Koch LH. Help-seeking behaviors of women with urinary incontinence: an integrative literature review. *J Midwifery Womens Health.* 2006;51(6): e39–e44. doi: 10.1016/j.jmwh.2006.06.004.
7. Lee SY, Phanumus D, Fields SD. Urinary incontinence: a primary care guide to managing acute and chronic symptoms in older adults. *Geriatrics.* 2000;55(11):65–72. PMID: 11086473.
8. de Groat WC, Yoshimura N. Pharmacology of the lower urinary tract. *Annu Rev Pharmacol Toxicol.* 2001;41:691–721. doi: 10.1146/annurev.pharmtox.41.1.691.
9. Couture JA, Valiquette L. Urinary incontinence. *Ann Pharmacother.* 2000;34(5):646–55. doi: 10.1345/aph.19176.
10. Holroyd-Leduc JM, Strauss SE. Management of urinary incontinence in women. *JAMA.* 2004;291(8):986–95. doi:10.1001/jama.291.8.986
11. Grodstein F, Fretts R, Lifford K, et al. Association of age, race, and obstetric history with urinary symptoms among women in the Nurses' Health Study. *Am J Obstet Gynecol.* 2003;189(2):428–34. doi: http://dx.doi.org/10.1067/S0002-9378(03)00361-2.
12. Sampselle CM, Harlow SD, Skurnick J, et al. Urinary incontinence predictors and life impact in ethnically diverse perimenopausal women. *Obstet Gynecol.* 2002;100(6):1230–8. PMID: 12468167.
13. Staskin DR. Overactive bladder in the elderly: a guide to pharmacological management. *Drugs Aging.* 2005;22(12):1013–28. PMID: 16363885.
14. DeLancey JO, Miller JM, Kearney R, et al. Vaginal birth and de novo stress incontinence: relative contributions of urethral dysfunction and mobility. *Obstet Gynecol.* 2007;110(2 pt 1):354–62. doi: 10.1097/01.AOG.0000270120.60522.55.
15. American Urogynecological Society. Intake and voiding diary. Available at: http://www.oabcentral.org/resources/AUGS_Voiding_Diary.pdf. Accessed June 24, 2017.
16. iP voidingdiary. Synappz Medical Apps. Available at: http://www.ip-voiding-diary.com. Accessed June 24, 2017.
17. Culligan PJ, Heit M. Urinary incontinence in women: evaluation and management. *Am Fam Physician.* 2000;62(11):2433–44. PMID: 11130230. Available at: http://www.aafp.org/afp/2000/1201/p2433.html. Accessed May 18, 2017.
18. Palmer MH. Urinary incontinence: quality improvement in nursing homes: where have we been? Where are we going? *Urol Nurs.* 2008;28(6):439–44, 453. PMID: 19241782.
19. Shamilyan TA, Kane, RL, Wyman J, et al. Systematic review: randomized, controlled trials of nonsurgical treatments for urinary incontinence in women. *Ann Intern Med.* 2008;148(6):459–73. PMID: 18268288.
20. Syan R, Brucker BM. Guideline of guidelines: urinary incontinence. *BJU Int.* 2016;117(1):20–33. doi: 10.1111/bju.13187.
21. Diokno AC, Samselle CM, Herzog AR, et al. Prevention of urinary incontinence by behavioral modification program: a randomized, controlled trial among older women in the community. *J Urol.* 2004;171(3):1165–71. doi:10.1097/01.ju.0000111503.73803.c2.
22. Miller J, Sampselle C, Ashton-Miller J, et al. Clarification and confirmation of the knack maneuver: the effect of volitional pelvic floor muscle contraction to preempt urine expected stress incontinence. *Int Urogynecol J.* 2008;19(6):773–82. doi:10.1007/s00192-007-0525-3.
23. Information from your family doctor: exercising your pelvic muscles. *Am Fam Physician.* 2000;62(11):2447. Available at: http://www.aafp.org/afp/2000/1201/p2447.html. Accessed May 18, 2017.
24. *Lyrette*™: Minimally invasive treatment for stress urinary incontinence. Los Alamitos, California: Pacific Coast Urology Medical Center. Available at: http://www.pacificcoasturology.com/lyrette/. Accessed May 18, 2017.
25. Elser D, Mitchell G, Miklos J, et al. Nonsurgical transurethral radiofrequency collagen denaturation: results at three years after treatment. *Adv Urol.* 2011; 2011:872057. doi: 10.1155/2011/872057.
26. NeoControl pelvic floor rehabilitation therapy (extracorporeal magnetic innervation). Munchen, Germany: Kitalpha Med. Available at: http://www.neocontrol.de/neocontrol.php. Accessed June 24, 2017.
27. Norton PA, Baker JE. Postural changes reduce leakage in women with stress urinary incontinence. *Obstet Gynecol.* 1994;84(5):770–4. PMID: 7936510.
28. Poise Impressa bladder supports. Neenah, WI: Kimberly-Clark. Available at: http://www.poise.com/products/impressa. Accessed June 24, 2017.
29. Shaikh S, Ong EK, Glavind K, et al. Mechanical devices for urinary incontinence in women. *Cochrane Database Syst Rev.* 2006;3:CD001756. doi:10.1002/14651858.CD001576.
30. Smith PP, McCrery RJ, Appell RA. Current trends in the evaluation and management of female urinary incontinence. *CMAJ.* 2006;175(10): 1233–40. doi: 10.1503/cmaj.060034.
31. Oxytrol for Women. Dublin, Ireland: Allergan. Available at: http://www.oxytrolforwomen.com. Accessed June 24, 2017.
32. Nitti V, Dmochowski R, Herschorn S, et al. OnabotulinumtoxinA for the treatment of patients with overactive bladder and urinary incontinence: results of a phase 3, randomized, placebo controlled trial. EMBARK Study Group. *J Urology.* 2013;189(6):2186–93. doi: 10.1016/j.juro.2013.05.062
33. American Geriatrics Society 2015 Beers Criteria Update Expert Panel. American Geriatrics Society 2015 updated criteria for potentially inappropriate medication use in older adults. *J Am Geriatr Soc.* 2015:63(11): 2227–46. doi: 10.1111/jgs.13702.
34. Moehrer B, Hextall A, Jackson S. Oestrogens for urinary incontinence in women. *Cochrane Database Syst Rev.* 2003;2:CD001405. doi:10.1002/14651858.CD001405.

35. The North American Menopause Society. The role of local vaginal estrogen for treatment of vaginal atrophy: 2007 position statement of the North American Menopause Society. *Menopause.* 2007;14(3 pt 1):357–69. doi: 10.1097/gme.0b013e31805170eb.
36. McCormick PL, Keating GM. Duloxetine: in stress urinary incontinence. *Drugs.* 2004;64(22):2567–73. PMID: 15516154.
37. National Association for Continence. *Resource Guide: Products and Services for Incontinence.* Charleston, SC: National Association for Continence. Available at: http://www.nafc.org/online-store/consumer-publications-and-products/nafc-educational-booklets/resource-guide-products-and-services-for-incontinence. Accessed June 24, 2017.
38. Muller N, McInnis E. The development of national quality performance standards for disposable absorbent products for adult incontinence. *Ostomy Wound Manage.* 2013;59(9):40–55. PMID: 24018391. Available at: http://www.o-wm.com/article/development-national-quality-performance-standards-disposable-absorbent-products-adult-incon. Accessed May 18, 2017.
39. Fader M, Cottenden A, Getliffe K, et al. Absorbent products for urinary/faecal incontinence: a comparative evaluation of key product designs. *Health Technol Assess.* 2008;12(29):1–208. doi: 10.1002/nau.20918.
40. Newman DK. Bladder dysfunction in women. Products and devices play important role. *Adv Nurse Pract.* 2006;14(5):55–6, 58, 60–2. PMID: 16972428.
41. Fader M, Bliss D, Cottenden A, et al. Continence products: research priorities to improve the lives of people with urinary and/or fecal leakage. *Neurourol Urodynam.* 2010;29:640–44. doi: 10.1002/nau.20918.
42. Fader M, Cottenden AM, Getliffe K. Absorbent products for light urinary incontinence in women. *Cochrane Database Syst Rev.* 2007;2:CD001406. doi:10.1002/14651858.CD001406.
43. Fader M, Macaulay M, Pettersson L, et al. A multi-centre evaluation of absorbent products for men with light urinary incontinence. *Neurourol Urodyn.* 2006;25(7):689–95. doi: 10.1002/nau.20259.
44. Bottomley JM. Complementary nutrition in treating urinary incontinence. *Top Geriatr Rehab.* 2000;16:61–77.
45. Kesiktas N, Karan A, Erkan H, et al. Is there a relationship between vitamin B12 and stress urinary incontinence? *Low Urin Tract Symptoms.* 2012;4(2):55–8. doi: 10.1111/j.1757-5672.2011.00116.x.
46. Barry MJ, Meleth S, Lee JY et al. Effect of increasing doses of saw palmetto extract on lower urinary tract symptoms: a randomized trial. *JAMA.* 2011;306(12):1344–51. doi: 10.1001/jama.2011.1364.
47. Tacklind J, MacDonald R, Rutks I, et al. Serenoa repens for benign prostatic hyperplasia. *Cochrane Database Syst Rev.* 2009;2:CD001423. doi:10.1002/14651858.CD001423.pub2.
48. Kane CJ, Raheem OA, Bent S, et al. What do I tell patients about saw palmetto for benign prostatic hyperplasia? *Urol Clin North Am.* 2011; 38(3):261–77. doi: 10.1016/j.ucl.2011.04.005.

section

XI

COMPLEMENTARY THERAPIES

CHAPTER 50

INTRODUCTION TO DIETARY SUPPLEMENTS

CANDY TSOUROUNIS AND CATHI DENNEHY

The Food and Drug Administration (FDA) defines *dietary supplements* (DS) as vitamins, minerals, herbs or other botanicals, and amino acids; dietary substances used to supplement the diet by increasing dietary intake or concentrates, metabolites, constituents, and extracts; or any combination of these stated ingredients.[1] Many terms have been used to describe DS, including *nutraceuticals, natural products, supplements, herbs, botanicals,* and *phytochemicals.* DS are most often grouped into the natural products category of complementary and alternative medicine (CAM) or integrative health (IH), according to the National Institutes of Health (NIH).[2] The term *complementary* refers to the use of natural products in addition to conventional medicine; *alternative* is the use of natural products in place of conventional medicine; *integrative* combines both natural and conventional approaches in a coordinated and purposeful way.[2] For the purposes of this chapter, herbs, vitamins, and similar products will be referred to as DS. This designation is also used by FDA as it relates to the intended use, namely for oral use only and for supplementing the diet. Indeed, DS are used by consumers not only to supplement the diet but also to maintain health and wellness. Some consumers also use DS to treat symptoms of medical conditions, despite FDA legislation that prohibits DS manufacturers from marketing products for this purpose unless the specific DS have undergone extensive review and been preapproved by FDA for a specified health claim.

Use of Dietary Supplements

Prevalence and Indications for Use

The National Health Interview Survey (NHIS), which is administered every 5 years to approximately 34,000–40,000 U.S. citizens, includes questions on complementary health approaches. In the 2012 survey, the use of non-vitamin and non-mineral natural products was 17.7% in adults older than 18 years and 4.9% in children ages 4–17 years.[3,4] Importantly, this survey omitted vitamins and minerals, which are the most common form of DS used by consumers. A 2014 consumer survey of approximately 2000 adults conducted by the Council for Responsible Nutrition estimated that DS use in adults is closer to 68%, with 75% of supplement users taking a multivitamin product.[5] In children ages 2–8 years, about 40% are given DS containing vitamins or minerals, despite generally having adequate nutrient intake.[6]

The 2007–2010 National Health and Nutrition Examination Survey assessed motivations for adults to use DS.[7] The primary reasons cited were to improve overall health (45%), maintain health (33%), and promote bone health (25%). Among adults ages 60 years and older, DS were used for site-specific conditions involving the bones, heart, and joints, whereas younger adults, ages 20–39 years, used DS for energy and immunity. Women were frequent users of calcium for bone health, whereas men used DS for heart health and lowering of cholesterol levels.

The 2012 NHIS cited the following indications for CAM use in children in order of prevalence: back or neck pain, other musculoskeletal disorders, head or chest cold, anxiety or stress, attention-deficit/hyperactivity disorder, and insomnia.[4] When DS were considered as a separate CAM modality, indications for use in children were less specific and involved diverse health conditions.[4]

Commonly Used Dietary Supplements

In 2014, the DS industry was estimated at $36.7 billion, with sales of $14.3 billion for individual vitamin and mineral products, $5.7 billion for combination vitamin–mineral products with or without other ingredients, and $6.4 billion for herbs and/or botanical supplements.[8] This represents a continued increase in growth of the DS industry for the past decade, but an overall slowing of growth in more recent years to 5.9% in 2015 and 5.1% in 2014.[8] Reports of top DS sales differ according to the purchase location.[8] Sales data, however, may differ from actual consumer-use data. The most commonly used non-vitamin, non-mineral supplements in adults include fish oil, glucosamine, and chondroitin or a combination of these; pre- or probiotics; melatonin; and coenzyme Q10.[3] In children, the most commonly used non-vitamin, non-mineral products are fish oil, melatonin, pre- and probiotics, echinacea, and garlic.[4] Popular single-ingredient vitamins and minerals include vitamin D, calcium, and vitamin C.

Among all DS, vitamins and minerals remain the top-selling supplements, primarily because they are used across all life stages. Many Americans do not consume sufficient nutrient-dense foods, such as fruits and vegetables, resulting in inadequate intake of several vitamins and minerals relative to their estimated average requirements or adequate intake levels set by the Institute of Medicine.[9] Specifically, the 2015 report on dietary guidelines for Americans characterized a shortfall of the following nutrients in the American diet: vitamins A, D, E, and C; folate; calcium; magnesium; fiber; and potassium.[9] Recognition of these commonly used DS in adults and children will benefit pharmacists who are likely to be asked to assist with product selection, directions for proper use, and safety considerations.

Attitudes and Predictors of Use

Many studies have measured predictors of CAM use and, more specifically, use of natural products such as DS.[3,7] For most U.S. adults, common predictors for DS use include being female; being 45–64 years of age; having a college or higher degree; being of White, Asian, Pacific Islander, American Indian, or Alaskan Native descent; living in the western United States (i.e., West North Central, Mountain, and Pacific states); and having a current self-rated health status of very good to excellent.[3,7] Having a higher socioeconomic status, defined as not poor or near poor, and having private health insurance are also predictors of high DS use.[7] Users of DS are also more likely to be physically active and are less likely to smoke.[7]

Among children, use of non-vitamin, non-mineral natural products was twice as likely to be reported if the parent also used a CAM modality (9% vs. 4%).[4] When vitamins and minerals were included, predictors of use in children included being from a family with a higher level of parental education and family income, being from a family with private health insurance, living in the western United States, and being non-Hispanic White.[4] DS use was more common in children who have a higher disease burden, more health conditions, and more frequent primary care provider visits in the last 12 months.[4]

Older adults, ages 61–69 years, are frequent DS users and are more likely to have chronic conditions and to use concomitant prescription medications.[10] As such, this population is at an increased risk for drug and disease state interactions with DS. Individuals who cited general wellness as their rationale for use were 16 times more likely to consume DS. Other factors that appear to be highly predictive of DS use include having an attitude that the DS will work and having a history of receiving health care from CAM providers.[10] The findings suggest that the most important predictor of use is preservation of health, regardless of an individual's assessment of his or her own health status, medical history, or use of concomitant medications.[9,10]

Television was the most commonly reported source of DS information (73%), followed by magazines and radio (both 30%), newspapers (13%), friends (8%), and store displays (5%).[10] Users of DS may not report this use to their health care providers (HCPs); nondisclosure to HCPs is estimated to be 24.9% for DS, with the most common reasons for nondisclosure being a lack of provider inquiry and feeling that the provider did not need to know.[11] These data confirm the importance of obtaining a complete medication history that includes use of DS and prescription and nonprescription drugs. The nondisclosure rate is reported to increase if the provider seems disinterested, appears judgmental of IH use, or lacks sufficient knowledge about these therapies.[11]

Legislation and Regulatory Issues

FDA regulates both finished (ready to be sold) DS products and individual dietary ingredients that are used to make DS products. Importantly, FDA regulates DS under a different set of regulations than those covering conventional foods and medications.

Dietary Supplement Health and Education Act

In 1994, the Dietary Supplement Health and Education Act (DSHEA) was approved by Congress and signed into law.[1] This act allowed FDA to regulate DS under the purview of the Center for Food Safety and Applied Nutrition. As a result, DS were excluded from the strict purity and potency standards that are applied to prescription and nonprescription drugs by the Center for Drug Evaluation and Research. DS had to meet only the standards that applied to food preparation. Any additional standards regarding purity and potency were the sole responsibility of the manufacturer. The lack of strict good manufacturing practice standards created problems with DS content, purity, potency, consistency, and actual identity, as well as contamination, herb misidentification, and sub- and supratherapeutic effects. The lack of strict standards and limited oversight of the manufacturing process created a buyer-beware market, placing the consumer at risk and often alienating conventional HCPs to the use of IH therapies, and also led to the misconception that DS are not regulated by FDA.

Another major difference between DS and prescription and nonprescription drugs is the level of evidence required to demonstrate safety and efficacy. For prescription and nonprescription drugs, clinical trials are required to demonstrate evidence of a drug's safety and efficacy prior to its marketing. Although DS manufacturers are prohibited from marketing unsafe or ineffective products, clinical trials are not generally required to prove the safety and efficacy of DS products prior to their marketing. Some exceptions do exist such as new DS ingredients or DS with health and nutrient content claims. The DS manufacturer is responsible for the product's safety and efficacy; FDA assumes a postmarketing surveillance role and must prove that a particular DS is not safe in order to restrict its use or remove it from the market.

New Dietary Supplement Ingredients

DS ingredients that were sold in the United States prior to October 15, 1994, are not required to be reviewed for safety by FDA before being marketed; they are assumed to be safe based on a history of use in humans. For any new DS ingredient that was not on the market prior to October 15, 1994, a manufacturer must notify FDA 75 days in advance of its intent to market the product.[1] The manufacturer must also provide FDA with evidence that the DS is safe in humans when used as directed.[1] Unfortunately, a comprehensive list of DS ingredients that were sold prior to this date is not available. As a result, the decision whether a product contains a new ingredient is left up to the manufacturer. Since the approval of DSHEA, more than 85,000 DS have come on the market, yet up until 2011, FDA had received only 700 premarket notifications during this period.[12] This stark disparity between newly marketed DS and premarket notifications led to the creation of a guidance document for industry regarding new dietary ingredients. In 2011, FDA issued comprehensive guidance that outlines specific recommendations that must be submitted in new dietary ingredient notifications. The guidance document outlines the specific materials that should be submitted to FDA and makes recommendations for the types of safety evidence that should be submitted for new DS ingredients taken short term, long term, or intermittently. Submission of available information on genotoxicity, teratogenicity, mutagenicity, and toxicology for a dietary ingredient is also recommended.[12]

Current Good Manufacturing Practice

DSHEA enactment required the establishment of current good manufacturing practice (cGMP) standards for the DS industry. In 2007, FDA issued a final rule on proposed changes to cGMP standards for DS.[13] Among the changes, DS must be manufactured in a quality manner without adulterants or impurities; they must be labeled accurately; and raw materials need to be evaluated by the manufacturer. These changes have helped to better regulate manufacturing practices, especially with regard to setting limits on the presence of bacteria, pesticides, and heavy metals. In 2013, researchers tested 44 DS products marketed in both the United States and Canada using DNA barcoding technology; in many products containing herbs, they found content discrepancies, herb substitution, and contaminants or use of fillers in place of active ingredients.[14] These findings were concerning as DS products marketed in the United States are required to meet cGMP standards as outlined in DSHEA. Most manufacturers achieve this requirement through their manufacturing and production processes. To combat cGMP concerns, some manufacturers take extra steps to have their DS products tested by external quality assurance programs so their product can carry a seal of approval verifying compliance with cGMP standards. These programs are discussed in the section "Quality Assurance Programs."

Labeling

FDA has primary responsibility for regulating claims found on packaging, package labeling, inserts, and other promotional materials that are distributed at the point of sale. The Federal Trade Commission (FTC) has primary responsibility for advertising claims made through print and broadcast advertisements, infomercials, catalogs, and other direct marketing materials.[15] FTC requires DS claims of safety and efficacy to be supported by "competent and reliable scientific evidence." This evidence is defined as "tests, analyses, research, studies or other evidence based on the expertise of professionals in the relevant area that have been conducted and evaluated in an objective manner by qualified individuals, using procedures generally accepted to yield accurate and reliable results."[15] Complaints against DS advertising may be filed with FTC online.

All DS marketed in the United States must meet supplement labeling requirements.[1] The labels must list (1) the name of the product as well as the word *dietary supplement;* (2) the net quantity of contents; (3) the manufacturer's, packer's, or distributor's name and place of business; and (4) directions for use. In addition, each label must also contain a supplement facts panel that describes the serving size, the list of dietary ingredients, amount per serving size, and the percent daily value, if one is established (Figure 50–1).

Plant-based DS should indicate the plant's scientific name, or Latin binomial (i.e., genus and species), and the specific plant part used. Manufacturers may market a combination of DS ingredients as a proprietary blend. Although the individual ingredients in the proprietary blend are listed, the actual quantity of each ingredient is not disclosed. Under DSHEA, the total weight of the blend and the components of the blend, in order of predominance by weight, are required. Fillers, artificial colors, sweeteners, flavors, or binders should also be listed in descending order of predominance. Consistent with the trend in formulating proprietary blends, many multivitamin products are being combined with DS.

When a DS does not follow labeling requirements, the product is considered misbranded.[1] DS manufacturers are not allowed to make claims that their product will diagnose, cure, mitigate, treat, or prevent disease.[1] These claims would require the product to adhere to the regulations related to a drug, and the product would be subject to all the regulatory processes necessary to demonstrate safety and efficacy. Other examples of misbranding include DS that do not conform to labeling requirements; fail to contain the name or place of business of the manufacturer, packer, or distributor; or fail to include accurate statements regarding the quantity of the contents.

The claims for all DS products fall under one of three types: (1) health claim, (2) nutrient content claim, or (3) structure–function claim.[16] Health claims and nutrient content claims require FDA approval, whereas structure–function claims do not. A manufacturer must notify FDA of the exact wording of any structure–function claim within 30 days after the product is marketed. Product labels that contain these claims must also carry a disclaimer: "This statement has not been evaluated by the FDA. This product is not intended to diagnose, treat, cure or prevent disease."

Health claims describe the relationship between a food, food component, or DS ingredient and the resulting reduction in risk of a disease or health-related condition. Claiming that a diet low in saturated fat and cholesterol that includes 25 g of soy protein daily may reduce the risk of heart disease is an example of an approved health claim. Nutrient content claims describe the relative amount of a nutrient or dietary substance in a product. For example, "very low sodium" means the product is required to have 35 mg or less of sodium per reference amount. Finally, a structure–function claim describes how a product may maintain the normal healthy structure or function of the body without discussing a specific disease state. A supplement manufacturer may claim that the product "supports healthy cholesterol levels" but is prohibited from indicating that the supplement may "reduce high cholesterol levels."

Dietary Supplement and Nonprescription Drug Consumer Protection Act

One of the most important changes to the supplement industry involves the Dietary Supplement and Nonprescription Drug Consumer Protection Act (Public Law 109-462), which was signed into law on December 22, 2006.[17] This law requires manufacturers, packers, or distributors of DS to submit to FDA reports of serious adverse events that are based on specific information received from the public. Serious adverse events are defined as death, a life-threatening situation, a hospitalization, a persistent or significant disability or incapacity, a congenital anomaly or birth defect, or an adverse event that, based on reasonable medical judgment, requires medical or surgical intervention to prevent such serious outcomes. Increased reporting of adverse events may better characterize the frequency and type of serious adverse events associated with DS. FDA actively evaluates trends in serious adverse events so that appropriate corrective action may be taken. Consumers and HCPs are also encouraged to report DS-related adverse events through FDA's MedWatch adverse event reporting program (www.fda.gov/medwatch).[18]

Production Issues

Plant Species and Parts

A HCP should explain that herbal products typically carry two names, the common name and the Latin binomial. An example would be a product such as St. John's wort (common name), which is also known as *Hypericum perforatum* (Latin genus and species name). Some product labels may list only the Latin name, which can be confusing to a consumer who is unfamiliar with this terminology. When consumers enter a pharmacy and search for an echinacea product, they may encounter single-ingredient

How do you read a supplement label?

Serving size is the manufacturer's suggested serving expressed in the appropriate unit (tablet, capsule, softgel, packet, teaspoonful).

Amount Per Serving heads the listing of nutrients contained in the supplement, followed by the quantity present in each serving.

International Unit (IU) is a standard unit of measure for fat soluble vitamins (A, D and E).

Milligram (mg) and microgram (mcg) are units of measurement for water soluble vitamins (C and B complex) and minerals. A milligram is equal to .001 grams. A microgram is equal to .001 milligrams.

Percent Daily Value (DV) tells what percentage of the recommended daily intake for each nutrient for adults and children ages 4 and up is provided by the supplement.

An asterisk under the "Percent Daily Value" heading indicates that a Daily Value is not established for that nutrient.

Supplement Facts

Serving Size 1 tablet

Suggested Use: Adults, take one tablet per day with meal

Amount Per Serving	% Daily Value
Vitamin A 5000 I.U.	
50% as Beta Carotene	100%
Vitamin C 250 mg	417%
Vitamin D 400 I.U.	100%
Vitamin E 200 I.U.	667%
Vitamin K 80 mcg	100%
Thiamin 5 mg	333%
Riboflavin 5 mg	294%
Niacin 20 mg	100%
Vitamin B_6 5 mg	250%
Folic acid 400 mcg	100%
Vitamin B_{12} 6 mcg	100%
Biotin 150 mcg	50%
Pantothenic Acid 10 mg	100%
Calcium 200 mg	20%
Iron 18 mg	100%
Phosphorus 200 mg	20%
Iodine 150 mcg	100%
Selenium 35 mcg	50%
Magnesium 200 mg	50%
Zinc 15 mg	100%
Copper 2 mg	100%
Boron 150 mcg	*

* Daily Value not established

Ingredients: vitamin A acetate, beta carotene, vitamin D, dl-alpha tocopherol acetate, ascorbic acid, thiamin mononitrate, riboflavin, niacinamide, pyridoxine hydrochloride, vitamin B12, biotin, d-calcium pantothenate, potassium chloride, dicalcium phosphate, potassium iodine, ferrous fumarate, magnesisum oxide, copper sulfate, zinc oxide, manganese sulfate, sodium selenate, chromium chloride, sodium molybdate, microcrystalline cellulose, calcium carbonate, sodium carboxymethyl cellulose

Storage: Keep tightly closed in dry place; do not expose to excessive heat

KEEP OUT OF REACH OF CHILDREN

Expiration date: JUN 2016

Company V, Cityville, New York 01010

The list of all ingredients includes nutrients and other ingredients used to formulate the supplement, in decreasing order by weight.

All supplements should be stored in a cool, dry place in their original containers, out of the reach of children and should be used before the expiration date to assure full potency.

The manufacturer's or distributor's name and place of business or phone number are required to appear on the label.

FIGURE **50–1** Statutory labeling format for certain dietary supplements. (Source: Food and Drug Administration. Dietary supplement labeling guide. Available at: http://www.fda.gov/Food/GuidanceRegulation/GuidanceDocumentsRegulatoryInformation/DietarySupplements/ucm2006823.htm. Accessed June 24, 2017.)

products that contain *Echinacea pallida, Echinacea purpurea,* or *Echinacea angustifolia;* products that contain a mixture of two or all of these species; and products that contain echinacea as one of many listed supplement ingredients. In the case of echinacea, single-ingredient products involving the above-ground parts of *E. purpurea,* formulated as an alcohol extract of the fresh pressed juice, have been the most widely studied. According to one meta-analysis, the above-ground parts of *E. purpurea* demonstrate some evidence of efficacy, albeit weak, in reducing cold symptoms in adults when administered at the first sign of symptoms.[19] The other two species of echinacea and combinations involving these species, with or without *E. purpurea,* have not demonstrated consistent benefits in clinical trials for treating colds.[19]

Common Product Formulations

The content of any DS is based on the raw starting material and how the material is subsequently processed or formulated. Plant-based DS such as echinacea and ginseng have greater variability in their composition than single-ingredient nonbotanical products such as creatine or melatonin. This variability is caused by the chemical composition of botanical DS, which is influenced by the plant's growing conditions, the plant species, the specific plant part used, and the time of harvest.

Knowing which plant species is preferred or which part of the plant to use can be based on historical precedent when clinical trial data are lacking. In developing countries, plant-based medicine is common, and information regarding preferred plant species, preferred plant part, and proper use is handed down from generation to generation, setting a historical precedent for use. An estimated 25% of modern drugs are plant derived, and 50% are derived from natural products (e.g., plants, animals, microbes, and their derivatives).[20] In developing countries, such as those in Africa, the use of plants as drugs is as high as 80%.[20] Use of herbs based on historical precedent is also common in the practice of midwifery. Few clinical trials exist on the use of DS in pregnant and lactating women and in children. The decision to use DS based on historical precedent is something providers must discuss with their patients.

Method of Preparation

The method in which a DS is manufactured will ultimately affect its final chemical composition and potential efficacy. Some formulations may be well studied, whereas others may not have been studied at all. The most common herbal formulations that a consumer will encounter are made either directly from the fresh plant (e.g., expressed juice, tincture, tea) or from the dried plant (e.g., fluid extract or tincture, evaporated extract [capsules, tablets], tea).[21] Tinctures are most commonly prepared by combining chopped herbs with alcohol. This type of formulation should be avoided in persons taking sedating medications or medications that carry disulfiram reaction warnings. Tinctures should also be used cautiously in special populations such as infants, children, and older people. Most of the common non–plant-based DS, such as vitamins, minerals, glucosamine, creatine, coenzyme Q10, and melatonin, are manufactured as tablets or capsules; these DS represent compounds that are structurally similar to or identical to compounds naturally found in the human body.

Freshly pressed juice formulations are prepared by pressing the herb and collecting the liquid that is removed.[21] This type of preparation often takes a large amount of the herb to create a substantial portion of juice. In the case of *E. purpurea,* the best-studied formulation is an alcohol extract of the freshly pressed juice.[19] A potential advantage of the alcohol extract is that the presence of alcohol increases the product's shelf life.

Tea formulations can be prepared from the root, leaf, bark, and/or fruit of a plant. Most often they are prepared as an *infusion* by pouring boiling water over the fresh or dried leaf portions of one or more plant species and then letting the herb steep for a small amount of time.[21] This process releases the water-soluble constituents into the tea. The potency is determined by the steeping time and the amount of herb used. The term *decoction* may be used when the plant parts are placed in cold water, brought to a boil, and then simmered for a period of time.[21] Common single-herb tea formulations include chamomile, ginger, peppermint, green tea, or black tea. Multi-ingredient blends that are customized to a specific person's ailment are commonly used in traditional Chinese medicine and may also be administered as teas.

Extracts are intended to concentrate the effects of an herb and can be prepared by soaking fresh or dried plant parts in alcohol, water, alcohol/water mixtures, or oil.[21] The extraction liquid is then reserved and the plant material discarded. Tinctures are fluid extracts in which alcohol is typically used as the extraction medium.[21] Chemicals that seep into the extraction liquid are specific to the solution used. If the extracted liquid is evaporated and dried, it can be formulated into tablets or capsules.[21] Extracts and tinctures may list the extraction ratio on the package label. For example, a 5:1 ratio would indicate that 5 parts of herb were used to prepare 1 part of the extract. *Ginkgo biloba* is prepared as a dried extract in tablet form. Ginkgo is typically standardized to a 50:1 extract ratio, meaning that 50 parts of the ginkgo leaf were used to prepare 1 part of the extract.[21] Garlic is available in multiple formulations, the most popular being a dried powdered extract in tablet or capsule form and an aged garlic extract. The chemical composition of the powdered extract will differ from that of the aged extract because of the differences in method of preparation. This variance in composition, in turn, may influence the efficacy of each product.

Standardization

The process of standardization is reserved primarily for plant-based DS, because herbs contain many active and inactive constituents.[21] For specific DS, standardization involves identifying specific chemicals or "markers" that may possess therapeutic activity, isolating them, and then formulating them into a final and consistent product. Standardization can occur only if the chemical markers that contribute to the pharmacologic effect have been identified. For example, a *G. biloba* product may be standardized to contain 6% terpene lactones and 24% flavonoid glycosides, whereas a chastetree berry product may not list any standardized markers at all. The identified active chemical markers may change over time as new research is performed. For example, the active antidepressant marker for St. John's wort was initially thought to be hypericin but is now considered to be hyperforin. Bottles of St. John's wort may list one or both of these standardizations on the package label. Interestingly, no legal or regulatory definition is accepted as it relates to standardization of DS. Claiming that a product is standardized does not necessarily mean a uniform manufacturing process was used. DS verification programs, however, may be helpful in determining compliance with package labeling and actual product composition.

Common Quality Control Issue: Adulteration

According to DSHEA, adulteration of a DS occurs when (1) the DS presents a significant or unreasonable risk of illness or injury when used in accordance with the suggested labeling, (2) the DS is a new entity and lacks adequate evidence to ensure its safety of use, (3) the DS has been declared an imminent hazard by the Department of Health and Human Services Secretary, or (4) the DS contains a dietary ingredient that is present in sufficient quantity to render the product poisonous or deleterious to human health, as described for adulterated foods in the Federal Food, Drug, and Cosmetic Act.[1] Adulteration of DS has occurred both intentionally and unintentionally. Examples of unintentional adulterants include heavy metals introduced at the time of cultivation or during the manufacturing process.[22] Heavy metals from environmental pollution can leach from contaminated soil into a plant as the plant grows.[23] In an analysis of 230 Ayurvedic medicines purchased over the Internet, 21% of the Indian-manufactured medicines and 22% of the U.S.-manufactured medicines contained lead, mercury, or arsenic.[22] Heavy metals may also be added to traditional medicine products with the intent of promoting good health. In traditional *rasa shastra* Ayurvedic medicine, addition of heavy metals is standard practice.[23] In this instance, the presence of heavy metals would not be considered adulteration, because they were added intentionally and with the intent of promoting good health. However, this practice could still lead to heavy metal contamination of the product user if the content exceeds recommended levels for heavy metal exposure set by state or national health standards.[23]

Intentional adulteration can occur when a manufacturer substitutes a different DS for an ingredient that is in short supply or is too expensive (e.g., economic adulteration). It can also occur when a prescription drug is added to the product to enhance its efficacy. Traditional Chinese medicines have frequently been found to contain heavy metals and undeclared drugs.[24] A survey of FDA Class I drug recalls performed between 2004 and 2012 found that 50% of all drug recalls involved DS products.[25] A Class I drug recall involves products containing a drug compound that is likely to result in serious health consequences or death.[25] These recalls most commonly involved products manufactured in the United States and marketed for sexual enhancement, bodybuilding, and weight loss. DS used for weight loss and energy are problematic, causing 71.8% of emergency department visits related to DS and resulting in palpitations, chest pain, or tachycardia in predominantly young patients, ages 20–34 years.[24] Violations of cGMP standards have been documented for nearly half of the DS manufacturing firms inspected by FDA.[25] The agency is addressing this issue by issuing targeted marketing about adulterated supplements to both consumers and HCPs and by creating multinational enforcement groups who target suppliers of commonly adulterated supplements.[25]

Quality Assurance Programs

Several organizations have developed quality assurance programs to assess analytical reference standards and to certify DS composition. These programs indicate whether the DS product contents match the label contents; unfortunately DS safety or efficacy cannot be ensured. These programs also do not address product quality between different batches or lots, because only a single batch is tested at any one time. Most quality assurance programs offer a "voluntary third party verification program" to manufacturers who pay to have their products tested. Products that pass are then allowed to carry a verification seal on the product label.

U.S. Pharmacopeia Dietary Supplement Verification Program

In 2002, the U.S. Pharmacopeia (USP) initiated a voluntary Dietary Supplements Verification Program.[26] The purpose of the program is to provide consumers with a method for identifying DS that have passed rigorous standards for purity, accuracy of ingredient labeling, and cGMP. Products earning USP certification carry a distinctive seal of approval on the product label. These products are certified to contain the listed ingredients in the indicated amounts, to be bioavailable and free of contaminants, and to have been manufactured under appropriate conditions. As of 2016, a total of 16 DS manufacturers are regular program participants. The USP will periodically conduct audits of certified products to ensure continuing adherence to quality standards. Approved products can be found at the USP website (www.usp.org/USPVerified/dietarySupplements).

ConsumerLab.com

ConsumerLab.com (CL) is an independent company that tests products related to health, wellness, and nutrition, such as DS.[27] Products are tested on the basis of identity, purity, and consistency with the labeled ingredients. The test results are posted on their website, www.consumerlab.com/aboutcl.asp, with new results available every 4–6 weeks. Manufacturers are allowed to license the CL seal of approval for a product that passes the review. To continue to carry the approval seal, a product must pass random sample testing every 12 months. The site provides free access to some names of a few products in each category that have passed testing, whereas names of products that fail testing are available only to subscribers. The company is not affiliated with manufacturers of any DS, health, or nutrition products.

NSF International

NSF was established more than 66 years ago to standardize sanitation and food safety requirements. Today, NSF International (www.nsf.org) is an independent, nonprofit organization that provides certifications of DS and food and water quality.[28] This organization verifies that the DS product contains the labeled ingredients and that contaminants and unlisted ingredients are not present. Any DS product that meets certification standards is allowed to carry the NSF certification seal of approval on the label. NSF works with professional sports teams to test athletic enhancement supplements.

Hazards From Dietary Supplements

False Advertising and Quackery

Manufacturers who make DS health claims sometimes ignore the regulations established by FDA and FTC and market products using false or misleading claims. FTC requires all advertising to be truthful, not misleading, and based on sound scientific evidence. The weight-loss DS market is one example in which false or misleading health claims are commonly identified.[29] Historically, this type of practice might be considered *quackery*, which implies that the person promoting use of the product knows it to be ineffective and is still promoting its use. In the case of some DS, manufacturers may believe, with or without strong clinical support, that their products are effective for a wide variety of ailments.

Consumers and providers should be wary of information found on online sites that market DS products. Some retail sites have been shown to be unreliable and may list disease claims, may fail to cite the standard disclaimer, and may lack referenced information.[30] Consumers should be wary of products that contain any of the characteristics listed in Table 50–1.[29,31] In addition, consumers should consult a reliable drug information resource, as well as their HCP, to confirm whether the health claims have a scientific basis. Consumers and providers can go to the NIH Office of Dietary Supplements site and sign up to receive FDA and FTC press releases for products that have been identified as containing adulterants, such as prescription drugs, or for manufacturers that have been issued warnings or recalls for product quality.[29] This online site also provides tips on how to evaluate health information on the Internet.[29] FDA has also created supplement categories that should be viewed with scrutiny because of a history of prior violations or problems.[31] These supplement categories are listed in Table 50–2. A consumer or provider who wishes to file a complaint related to false advertising should contact FTC.[15]

Hazards Introduced by the Consumer

Exceeding the recommended dietary allowance for a vitamin or mineral supplement or taking more of a supplement than is directed on the label can occur intentionally or accidentally. Accidental over-supplementation is more likely to occur when a consumer is taking more than one multi-ingredient product containing similar ingredients. Regardless of how it occurs, over-supplementation should be discouraged, because an adverse event may result. Overuse of some DS has serious consequences. For example, overuse of colloidal silver has led to irreversible blue-gray skin discoloration.[32] Overuse of calcium or vitamin D supplements over short periods may cause hypercalcemia. In addition, concern exists that excessive calcium supplementation over long periods of time may contribute to coronary artery calcification.[33] As mentioned previously, adverse events should be reported by consumers and health care professionals to MedWatch.[18] For most DS, individual case reports and postmarketing surveillance provide the best means of identifying adverse events and drug interactions. Consumers should be advised to monitor for acute adverse events for up to 2 weeks after initiating a new DS and to continue monitoring while using the product.

TABLE 50–1 Characteristics of Supplements Making Fraudulent or Misleading Claims

- List specific disease states or allude to the product's use for a disease usually treated with prescription drug therapy.
- State that supplement's efficacy is similar to, or supplement can be used as an alternative to, a prescription or nonprescription drug.
- List a wide variety of unrelated clinical conditions for use.
- State only benefits and no harmful effects.
- Neglect to provide expiration date, lot number, and contact information for the manufacturer on the package label.
- Use pseudo-medical terminology such as *detoxify, purify*, or *improves body chemistry*.
- Use terms such as *miraculous discovery, revolutionary therapy*, or *breakthrough treatment*, which suggest that the product has superior efficacy to standard care.
- Suggest that the product is more expensive because it works so well.
- Use personal testimonials in place of sound scientific evidence to support product claims.
- Promise quick relief of a health condition.
- Promote natural content as being superior to conventional medicine.
- Provide a money-back guarantee or satisfaction guarantee, but marketers of fraudulent products often change their business location.
- Make accusations that pharmaceutical drug manufacturers and health care providers are working together to defraud consumers and steer consumers away from healthier dietary supplement options.

TABLE 50–2 Categories of Supplements That FDA Considers "Clearly Problematic"

- Treatments for life-threatening diseases (e.g., HIV, cancer) or serious medical conditions such as Alzheimer disease
- Weight-loss products
- Chelation products
- Treatments for behavioral disorders such as attention-deficit/hyperactivity disorder or autism
- Treatments for intellectual disability or Down syndrome
- Colloidal minerals and silver products
- Supplements for addiction (e.g., smoking, drinking)
- Supplements for body builders
- Supplements for sexual enhancement (e.g., impotence)

Key: FDA = Food and Drug Administration; HIV = human immunodeficiency virus.

Product Hazards: Adverse Effects and Drug Interactions

The fact that herbal DS are derived from a natural source does not guarantee safety. Adverse effects are often linked to the pharmacology of the supplement, as was noted when products containing ephedra were removed from the market because of their association with stroke and myocardial infarction.[34] Other DS may be harmful in that they contain chemicals that are toxic when ingested. Pyrrolizidine alkaloids present in *Symphytum officinale* (comfrey), *Borago officinalis* (borage), *Tussilago farfara* (coltsfoot), and *Senecio aureus* (golden ragwort or life root) have been associated with case reports of hepatotoxicity.[35] If an adverse event is suspected, product testing is essential to rule out possible plant misidentification; adulteration with prescription or nonprescription drugs; or contamination with heavy metals, microbial contaminants, and pesticides that can occur during production.[36]

Interactions between DS and conventional medications may have a pharmacodynamic or pharmacokinetic basis. Pharmacodynamic interactions can occur when a supplement's pharmacology is similar to or opposite that of a drug the consumer is taking. For example, both St. John's wort and L-tryptophan have been linked to case reports of serotonin syndrome in persons taking these products with prescription psychotropic drugs.[37,38] Additive effects have occurred, or could theoretically occur, in persons combining central nervous system depressants with DS that have sedative properties, such as melatonin or valerian, or in persons combining drugs that have antiplatelet or anticoagulant activity with DS that have antiplatelet properties (e.g., fish oil, flaxseed oil, garlic, ginseng, ginkgo, ginger).[39] Case reports of a DS opposing the effect of a drug or adversely influencing an existing disease state have been reported infrequently in the literature. Theoretical concerns are cited as a reason to avoid DS that enhance immune system activity such as echinacea in persons who have autoimmune disorders or require immunosuppressants.[40] Finally, DS may have pharmacokinetic interactions. St. John's wort induces multiple cytochrome P450 isoenzymes, as well as the P-glycoprotein drug transporter system.[39]

Communication Issues

Counseling on Dietary Supplements

The primary consideration in counseling consumers on DS is to recognize the importance of respecting the person's beliefs and values so that a trusting, nonjudgmental relationship can develop. The person must feel comfortable telling the provider about any use of DS. Providers should ask about all therapies being used, including DS, because consumers may not routinely disclose this information. Providers must also be able to provide recommendations regarding DS, when information is available. The risk of adverse effects versus the potential for positive effects must be considered and clearly explained. As an example, if a consumer wishes to take a DS that has *demonstrated both positive and negative outcomes in clinical trials, but lacks* documented adverse effects or drug interactions, a provider may support DS use with the caveat that it may or may not be of benefit. The consumer should be advised to monitor for perceived benefit and adverse effects. If no benefits are observed within the expected time frame, the DS should be discontinued. Providers should be less inclined to support use of a DS whose efficacy is not supported by evidence and should discourage the use of unsafe products and practices. Importantly, providers do not control access to DS, and consumers may choose to use any available DS. In many instances, providers may be in the position of educating a consumer about DS even though they believe that the product should not be used. In these situations, counseling on expectations and adverse effects is essential. For example, educating consumers on the early signs of a serious adverse effect will enable them to recognize a problem and discontinue the DS to minimize harm. Consumers should always be advised to seek medical care for serious conditions.

Consumers should read labels carefully and ask questions. Providers should be aware of the potential for confusion related to DS labels and claims, and counsel consumers in a way that lessens confusion. *Thymus* is an example of a term that might be dangerous if misunderstood. *Thymus vulgaris* is the Latin name for garden thyme. On a supplement label, "*Thymus extract*" may refer to an extract of the herbs thyme, Spanish thyme, or wild thyme, products with relatively few adverse effect when used in small doses. However, "thymus extract" may refer to a preparation made from animal thymus gland that is marketed to enhance immune function, a product with considerable quality and safety concerns.

In addition to these broad counseling issues, the following points should be emphasized. First, providers should emphasize that most self-care with DS should be for a limited period. If a problem persists, the consumer should seek medical care. Second, consumers should inform their provider before taking DS for a condition that is also being treated with a prescription drug. Third, consumers should be informed that FDA does not require DS manufacturers to submit data demonstrating efficacy or safety before the product is marketed, unless the product contains a new dietary ingredient that was not on the market prior to October 15, 1994. Quality and consistency of DS products remain a concern but may improve with the new cGMP standards. The following points should be used in counseling consumers who wish to use a DS:

- Purchase products that have either a seal of quality on the label, acquired through a program such as the USP's Dietary Supplements Verification Program or NSF International's certification program, or that meet their content claim as assessed by ConsumerLab.com.
- Purchase from large, reputable companies. These companies have the resources to meet strict manufacturing standards, have a reputation to uphold, and are more likely to follow quality assurance procedures. Companies that also manufacture prescription or nonprescription drugs (e.g., drugstore chain brands) are more likely to have cGMP standards in place and to follow these procedures when producing DS.
- Once a quality DS has been selected, continue to use the same brand and formulation. Although this approach does not guarantee a lack of potential quality issues, given that variability between batches can occur, it does increase the likelihood of a consistent product and dose. Providers working with consumers who have not had positive results with use of a DS might consider a trial of a different brand that is appropriate for the specific symptom before determining that the supplement is ineffective for that consumer.
- Know the DS products that you are using and tell your health care provider about them.
- Report any adverse effects related to DS use to your health care provider.

Additional recommendations for counseling can be found in Table 50–3. Cases 50–1 and 50–2 provide examples of how to counsel consumers who wish to use DS

Considerations for Special Population Groups

This section provides a brief overview of issues regarding the use of DS by different consumers. The lack of data on safety and efficacy in these groups, as well as the current regulatory issues, underscores the need for comprehensive assessment of the consumer's health status and knowledgeable counseling.

Older Adults

Although many older adults are healthy and living independently, some may have a significant burden of disease. The latter may have age- and disease-related physiologic declines such as impaired kidney function. Older individuals may be chronically taking multiple prescription and nonprescription drugs, making a thorough medical history essential. The potential for drug–food and drug–DS interactions, age-related functional declines, and concomitant diseases should be considered in counseling older adults about DS.

Children

Use of DS by children presents unique challenges. The central nervous system of a child may be sensitive to many drugs and chemicals. Little research is available regarding the safe and effective use of DS in children, making evidence-based recommendations difficult. In addition, from a practical perspective, an appropriate pediatric dosage of a DS product cannot be determined

TABLE 50-3 General Recommendations for Consumers

Appropriate Use

- Read all labels carefully; never take more than the recommended amount.
- Never share DS with others.
- Do not select a product that lacks dosing recommendations on the label.
- Avoid products that do not carry a lot number or expiration date.
- Discard products 1 year from date of purchase if no other expiration date is present.
- Select products that list the manufacturer's name, address, and telephone number.
- Store products in a dry environment out of direct sunlight and away from young children and pets.

Special Groups

- Always seek the advice of a pediatrician before using a DS in children.
- Avoid DS if you are pregnant or breastfeeding or are trying to become pregnant.
- Speak to your health care provider if you are trying to treat a life-threatening condition, such as cancer or HIV.

Adverse Effects

- The term *natural* does not mean safe; be diligent and report any unusual experiences to your health care provider.
- If you are allergic to plants, weeds, and/or pollen, ask your provider before using a DS.

Interactions

- If you are taking a prescription medicine, do not take a DS for the same condition.
- When possible, avoid taking multi-ingredient preparations; select single-ingredient products that list the strength per dose.
- Do not take these products with alcohol.
- Check with your health care provider if you are taking "blood-thinning" drugs; some DS may interact with these drugs.
- Always inform your primary care provider of the products you are taking; keep a list if necessary or bring them with you to your appointment.

Expectations

- Never use these products in place of proper rest and nutrition; eat a balanced diet.
- Do not expect a cure or unrealistic results; these agents are not cure-alls.
- If it sounds too good to be true, it probably is; use discretion when evaluating claims.
- Keep a diary to track the effectiveness and adverse effects of DS.

Key: DS = Dietary supplements; HIV = human immunodeficiency virus.

if the content of the product is in question. Finally, DS should have childproof safety closures because accidental ingestions may occur in young children.

Pregnant and Lactating Women

Use of DS by a woman who is planning to become pregnant or is already pregnant presents several dilemmas. Throughout the world, herbal DS have been used to maintain health during pregnancy, prevent miscarriages, and induce labor. In the United States, concern has focused on minimizing fetal exposures to prescription and nonprescription drugs, as well as DS. Although many natural products have been used in pregnancy, little published data exist on their safety with regard to the developing embryo and fetus. As part of standard preconception care, a woman should be asked about her use of DS, especially if her nutritional status might be affected at the time of conception (e.g., folic acid intake) or her ability to become pregnant might be affected (e.g., DS effects on ovulation). The most important issue concerning DS use during pregnancy and lactation is the uncertainty about the exact content in any given product batch or brand. Currently, providers should advise women to limit their use of DS to products that have reasonable proof of safety and efficacy for use during pregnancy and lactation.

Kidney Disease

Many Americans have chronic kidney disease (CKD) caused by diseases such as diabetes. CKD presents many challenges to the safe use of many prescription and nonprescription drugs. Most commonly, the individual may be unable to eliminate the drug appropriately, potentially resulting in supratherapeutic concentrations. This effect is also true for hepatically metabolized drugs with active, renally eliminated metabolites. When a patient with CKD requires dialysis, the absorption, distribution, and hepatic metabolism of drugs may also be altered. In addition, many herbs possess antiplatelet properties that might increase the risk of bleeding in CKD.[39]

Liver Disease

The effects of liver disease on DS pharmacokinetics have not been adequately studied. Many DS products contain combination ingredients; studying and evaluating the effects of liver disease on the pharmacokinetics of combination DS present unique challenges. For this reason, DS should be avoided or used cautiously in patients with compromised liver function. Some DS products can affect the ability of the liver to metabolize other medications, which can lead to drug interactions. DS products containing known hepatotoxic ingredients should be avoided. No DS have been found to be clinically effective in reversing liver disease or in preventing liver damage.

Surgery

A detailed preoperative history that includes questions related to DS use should be obtained from all patients undergoing surgery. Supplements that are known to affect sedation or platelet function or that may possibly affect the metabolism of anesthetic agents should be discontinued 2 weeks prior to the procedure. Other DS that the patient is taking should be reviewed by the provider to avoid potential harm.

Reliable Information Resources

The following resources may be used for general information, ongoing research, regulatory updates and alerts, and information on DS composition. Among these, Micromedex (Alternative Medicine), Natural Medicines, and ConsumerLab.com require a paid subscription.

CASE 50-1

Patient Symptoms and History

Ms. Smith is a 29-year-old woman who would like to select a melatonin product for her insomnia. Her health care provider recommended that she try melatonin. For the past 2 weeks she has had difficulty falling asleep. Her usual bedtime is 11 PM, yet she eventually falls asleep around 3 AM and has to wake up by 5 AM in order to get ready for work. This sleep schedule has left her feeling extremely exhausted and unable to focus, and she is very drowsy by 4 PM when she has to drive home. She has not tried anything for her insomnia but has tried to read in bed to help her fall asleep. She has been reading her work e-mail and reviewing work-related documents, because this helps her catch up for the next day. She has no known drug allergies. Ms. Smith states that she does not use products that contain nicotine, alcohol, or caffeine. She takes drospirenone/ethinyl estradiol (Yaz) once daily and is in excellent health. She does not exercise as she is very tired from the lack of sleep. Ms. Smith notes that several melatonin products are on the shelf and would like assistance in selecting the best product.

Clinical Considerations

Ms. Smith appears to be suffering from episodic sleep-onset insomnia. She has not taken anything for the insomnia, and her symptoms have continued for the past 2 weeks. The insomnia is impacting her quality of life as she does not feel rested in the morning, she is not functional during the day, and the insomnia is placing her health at risk while driving. Ms. Smith also reports reading work e-mail and work materials in bed to help her sleep, which may be increasing her stress level and not helping her relax.

Ms. Smith should begin by following the principles of good sleep hygiene before initiating melatonin. She should use her bed for sleeping and intimacy only, not for reading her work-related e-mail or other work-related materials. She should also establish a regular sleep pattern by going to bed and arising at the same time daily, even on the weekends. Ms. Smith should maintain a comfortable room environment and engage only in relaxing activities before bed. She may wish to read a book that helps her relax before bed. She should avoid reading anything on an electronic device (e.g., computer screens, tablets, smartphones), because electronic devices emit bright light, which can delay sleep onset. Ms. Smith should talk with her health care provider about starting an exercise program. Exercise has been shown to relieve stress and may help her fall asleep. She should avoid exercising within 2–4 hours of bedtime. Ms. Smith does not use alcohol, caffeine, or nicotine, which can contribute to insomnia. If she is unable to sleep within the first 2 hours, she should avoid watching the clock. Rather, she should get out of bed and perform a relaxing activity until she feels tired.

If, after implementing the principles of good sleep hygiene, Ms. Smith continues to suffer from sleep-onset insomnia, she may consider melatonin. Ms. Smith should select a melatonin product that has been approved by one of the three DS quality assurance programs: U.S. Pharmacopeia Dietary Supplement Verification Process, ConsumerLab.com, or NSF International. Some melatonin products may carry the seal of approval on the label. When a seal of approval is not present, a good way to verity the quality of the product is to visit the website of each quality assurance program to verify whether the product is approved. Ms. Smith should review the label of the melatonin DS carefully. It should list the active ingredient and the strength of each ingredient provided in each tablet. The manufacturer's name and address and the daily recommended dose should be listed. In some instances, the packer's or distributor's information may be listed instead.

Melatonin may help with sleep-onset insomnia when taken 30 minutes before bedtime. It should be taken with bedroom lights off, because room light can affect the activity of melatonin. If Ms. Smith does not feel somnolent within 1 hour, she can repeat the dose one time. If she does not become somnolent, she should avoid taking any more melatonin.

Because melatonin is short acting, it tends to cause less early morning drowsiness the following day. Rarely, melatonin may lead to adverse effects, including headache, dizziness, nausea, and drowsiness. Ms. Smith should avoid driving for 4–5 hours after taking a dose of melatonin. This means that she should avoid taking melatonin after 1 AM if she will be driving at 6 AM. Ms. Smith should maintain a diary to track the dose taken, the time given, the quality of sleep, and whether she experienced any adverse effects the next day. Melatonin should be used for 2–3 nights consecutively, and then Ms. Smith should skip a night to evaluate sleep quality. If melatonin helps her sleep quality, she may continue taking it for 10 days. Long-term use of melatonin for sleep-onset insomnia in adults has not been studied and is not recommended. There are no interactions between melatonin and her oral contraceptive; however, Ms. Smith should inform her health care providers that she will be taking melatonin, because it may affect the activity of some medications.

If Ms. Smith continues to have insomnia despite following the principles of good sleep hygiene and taking melatonin, she should talk with her health care provider.

Micromedex, Alternative Medicines

Micromedex (Truven Health Analytics, Inc., Ann Arbor, MI) provides drug information on all types of DS, including herbs, vitamins, minerals, Chinese medicine, and acupuncture. This resource provides information about DS dosing, pharmacokinetics, interactions, and clinical use, along with primary literature citations. The content undergoes extensive review and is updated quarterly. The database is searchable by DS ingredient(s) and trade name.[41]

CARDS, NIH Office of Dietary Supplements

The Computer Access to Research on Dietary Supplements (CARDS) database contains federally funded research specific to DS. Information found in CARDS is provided from many government agencies that sponsor DS research, including but not limited to the NIH Office of Dietary Supplements. The database is searchable by DS ingredient, health outcome, study type, or names of research investigators. A record of completed and published research studies on DS is maintained within the database.[42]

CASE 50-2

Patient Complaint and History

Mr. Hartman is a 74-year-old man who just came from visiting his primary care provider (PCP) where he was told that he has early-onset dementia from Alzheimer disease. He and his PCP are in favor of using an integrative health approach and have decided to start *Ginkgo biloba,* standardized extract, 240 mg daily, instead of an acetylcholinesterase inhibitor. He brings two products to the counter, one is called MindOptimum and the other is labeled ginkgo biloba. You are aware that he routinely picks up refills of his prescription medications for blood pressure (benazepril), cholesterol reduction (simvastatin), and type 2 diabetes (metformin) on time. He would like your help in selecting the best product that meets his PCP's recommendations and is seeking reassurance that the new supplement is safe to use with his other prescription drugs.

You evaluate the label on the MindOptimum product and find that it is a proprietary blend with *Hypericum perforatum* listed as the first ingredient, but also includes *G. biloba* as the second ingredient. The other product is a single-ingredient gingko biloba product from a large nutraceutical manufacturing company that is known to you.

Clinical Considerations

The ingredient listed first in a proprietary blend is present in the greatest quantity. In general, the actual amount of each ingredient in a proprietary blend is not listed, but the total weight of the blend is listed. In addition, the contents are listed in the order of the most prevalent to the least prevalent ingredient. Evaluating the first three ingredients in a blend is a good place to start. If the ingredients listed are unfamiliar, one of the drug information resources listed in this chapter can be used to evaluate the ingredients. *Hypericum perforatum* is the Latin binomial name (genus and species) for St. John's wort. Compared with placebo, this DS has been shown to be efficacious in relieving symptoms of mild–moderate depression in some clinical trials. St. John's wort may enhance the metabolism of several drugs through cytochrome P450 induction and could lead to reduced efficacy of some of his prescription medicines. Because the proprietary blend does not list the actual amount of ginkgo per serving and lists only the amount of the blend per serving, it is best not to select this product. This product also has ingredients that are not needed in this patient and could lead to supplement–drug interactions.

In reviewing the Supplement Facts panel of the other product, you are seeking evidence of standardization, correct formulation, and the presence of any third-party verification quality assurance program, such as U.S. Pharmacopeia Dietary Supplement Verification Process, ConsumerLab.com, or NSF International. Using the Lexicomp natural products database, you see that a standardized extract of ginkgo biloba should be prepared from the leaf of the tree and standardized to contain 24% flavone glycosides and 6% terpene lactones. The product that Mr. Hartman selected bears this standardization, a USP stamp, and is a leaf formulation with 240 mg of extract per capsule. Lexicomp also describes evidence of a small placebo-controlled trial in healthy volunteers that found no significant alteration in lipid-lowering efficacy with 14 days administration of *G. biloba* extract and simvastatin. Because of the short duration of this small trial, you advise Mr. Hartman to work with his PCP to monitor his cholesterol levels over the next 3 months to ensure that that his levels are still well controlled. Sending a message to his PCP is also advisable. The database does not list any other drug interactions that would be significant with Mr. Hartman's medication profile. Because this herb has antiplatelet properties, if Mr. Hartman were to be started on a prescription drug in the future such as warfarin, this would be a significant consideration with the use of *G. biloba.*

Cochrane Database of Systematic Reviews

The Cochrane Database of Systematic Reviews is accessible through Medline and offers evidence-based analyses of DS. These reports provide detailed information on trials that were included and excluded from the analysis and on the methodology used.[43] One advantage of this database is that statements that support or refute the use of a specific DS are clearly expressed. This database requires a subscription for access and many providers may have difficulty understanding the style and arrangement of the information that supports the analyses.

ConsumerLab.com

ConsumerLab.com provides access to an encyclopedia of *Natural and Alternative Treatments.* The information in this encyclopedia is evidence based and well referenced. It is a useful resource for both consumers and HCPs.[27]

Dietary Supplement Ingredient Database

The Dietary Supplement Ingredient Database (DSID) was created by a group of federal agencies and research organizations to estimate the levels of ingredients found in DS products. DSID provides information on analyzed levels of nutrients found in adult multivitamins and minerals used in the United States. The database is intended for use in research applications that are appropriate for conducting population-based studies on nutrient intake as opposed to assessing individual products. The data are grouped by nutrient levels rather than by product name.[44]

Dietary Supplement Label Database

The Dietary Supplement Label Database (DSLD) was created by the National Library of Medicine and includes information from the labels of more than 50,000 DS products. DSLD is intended to help consumers and health care professionals identify ingredients found in brand-name DS. Information in this database is based on the ingredients declared by the DS manufacturer and includes both active and inactive ingredients. DS ingredients are linked to MedlinePlus and PubMed to allow users to investigate the dietary ingredients and evaluate the primary literature pertaining to them. For each DS product listed, the database provides the manufacturer's name and contact information. The DSLD also provides links to fact sheets published by FDA, the NIH Office of Dietary Supplements, National Center for Complementary and Integrative Health (NCCIH), and the National Cancer Institute.[45]

Lexicomp, Natural Products

This database can be searched for more than 400 commonly used DS and is intended for use by HCPs. It is peer reviewed by an expert panel and is fully referenced to the primary literature. It includes a natural products database and printable patient education information. The database is searchable by ingredient (both vitamin and mineral and non-vitamin and mineral ingredients), brand name, and even specific extract formulations. This resource may be used to locate a wide variety of information on efficacy, safety, interactions, formulations, and dosing.[46]

MedlinePlus

MedlinePlus, published by NIH, is designed for consumers and contains information regarding diseases, conditions, and wellness. The medication and DS information is provided in consumer-friendly language, includes both plant-based and other DS, and contains a summary of the science behind each ingredient. Directories, a medical encyclopedia, and a medical dictionary are available in several languages.[47]

Natural Medicines

Natural Medicines, formerly Natural Medicines Comprehensive Database and Natural Standard (Somerville, MA), is published by the Therapeutic Research Center (Stockton, CA).[40] Prior to 2015, the two leading information resources on DS were the Natural Medicines Comprehensive Database and the Natural Standard. In 2015, these two databases were combined into one electronic format and renamed Natural Medicines. This resource is an international research collaboration of providers from many disciplines, including those trained in Western- and Asian-based forms of care. The database provides a comprehensive listing of single-ingredient and combination DS products and their associated adverse effects, drug–supplement interactions, and more. Commercially available DS products are listed for both the United States and Canada. Recommendations for DS efficacy are graded to reflect the type and quality of the clinical evidence on which they are based. In addition to reviews of DS, the database also includes monographs on other IH modalities and a dictionary of terms. Each monograph has an accompanying consumer handout that is available in Spanish, French, and English languages.

National Center for Complementary and Integrative Health

NCCIH is part of NIH and is one of the federal government's leading agencies in promoting evidence-based research on IH therapies. This online site provides information on clinical trials, opportunities for research and funding, training opportunities for IH providers, and health information on IH modalities. DS monographs that contain evidence-based summaries are available in the health information section linked from MedlinePlus.[48]

Office of Dietary Supplements, National Institutes of Health

The NIH Office of Dietary Supplements is a comprehensive site for general information on DS. The online site contains information regarding health and nutrition and decision-making approaches for DS treatment options and nutrient recommendations. Importantly, the site provides evidence-based fact sheets on many DS, including vitamins and botanicals. In addition, the site provides resources for researchers of DS and information on DS training and career development opportunities.[49]

PubMed Subset for Dietary Supplements

The NIH Office of Dietary Supplements instituted a joint project with the National Library of Medicine to create the PubMed subset for DS. This subset succeeds the International Bibliographic Information on Dietary Supplements database, which was a collaboration between the Office of Dietary Supplements and the U.S. Department of Agriculture National Agricultural Library. The subset was created to improve access to DS-related literature and incorporates journals indexed in Medline that contain this content.[50]

Key Points for Dietary Supplements

- DS use is common among consumers, making it essential for all providers to be knowledgeable about the most frequently used products. This education should include information about evidenced-based resources and where to report adverse effects, drug interactions, or suspected fraudulent health claims.
- Regulation under DSHEA has created a marketplace in which product safety, efficacy, and quality can vary or be unknown.
- HCPs are in a unique position to counsel consumers on DS and should take an open, nonjudgmental, evidence-based approach.
- Obtaining a DS history should be part of the overall drug history.
- Counseling recommendations should include consideration of overall scientific support, historical use, specific patient groups, potential for adverse effects, and potential for interactions with other medications or medical illnesses.

REFERENCES

1. U.S. Food and Drug Administration. Dietary Supplement Health and Education Act of 1994 (Pub. L. No. 103-417, 103rd Congress). Available at: http://www.fda.gov/regulatoryinformation/legislation/significant amendmentstothefdcact/ucm148003.htm. Accessed April 6, 2016.
2. National Center for Complementary and Integrative Health. Complementary, alternative, or integrative health: what's in a name? Available at: https://nccih.nih.gov/health/integrative-health/. Updated June 28, 2016. Accessed June 24, 2017.
3. Clarke TC, Black LI, Stussman BJ, et al. Trends in the use of complementary health approaches among adults: United States, 2002–2012. *Natl Health Stat Report.* 2015 Feb 10;(79):1–16. PMCID: PMC4573565. Available at: https://www.ncbi.nlm.nih.gov/pmc/articles/PMC4573565/. Accessed June 24, 2017.
4. Black LI, Clarke TC, Barnes PM, et al. Use of complementary health approaches among children aged 4–17 years in the United States: National Health Interview Survey, 2007–2012. *Natl Health Stat Report.* 2015 Feb 10;(78):1–19.
5. Council for Responsible Nutrition (CRN). The CRN consumer survey on dietary supplements: 2014. Available at: http://www.crnusa.org/CRN consumersurvey/2014. Accessed June 24, 2017.
6. Bailey RL, Fulgoni VL 3rd, Keast DR, et al. Do dietary supplements improve micronutrient sufficiency in children and adolescents? *J Pediatr.* 2012;161(5):837–2. doi: 10.1016/j.jpeds.2012.05.009.

7. Bailey RL, Gahche JJ, Miller PE, et al. Why US adults use dietary supplements. *JAMA Intern Med.* 2013;173(5):355–1. doi: 10.1001/jamainternmed.2013.2299.
8. Supplement business report 2015. *Nutrit Business J.* 2015;1–320.
9. Dietary Guidelines Advisory Committee. Scientific report of the 2015 dietary guidelines advisory committee: executive summary. Available at: http://health.gov/dietaryguidelines/2015-scientific-report/02-executive-summary.asp. Accessed June 24, 2017.
10. Marinac JS, Buchinger CL, Godfrey LA, et al. Herbal products and dietary supplements: a survey of use, attitudes and knowledge among older adults. *J Am Osteopath Assoc.* 2007;107(1):13–3. PMID: 17299031.
11. Jou J, Johnson P. Nondisclosure of complementary and alternative medicine use to primary care physicians: findings from the 2012 National Health Interview Survey. *JAMA Intern Med.* 2016;176(4):545–6. doi: 10.1001/jamainternmed.2015.8593.
12. U.S. Food and Drug Administration. Draft guidance for industry: dietary supplements: new dietary ingredient notifications and related issues. Available at: http://www.fda.gov/Food/GuidanceRegulation/GuidanceDocumentsRegulatoryInformation/DietarySupplements/ucm257563.htm#iii-scope. Updated August 2016. Accessed June 24, 2017.
13. U.S. Food and Drug Administration. Current good manufacturing practice in manufacturing, packaging, labeling, or holding operations for dietary supplements: final rule. *Fed Reg.* 2007;72(121):34752–8. Available at: http://www.fda.gov/Food/GuidanceRegulation/CGMP/ucm079496.htm. Accessed June 24, 2017.
14. Newmaster SG, Grguric M, Shanmughanandhan D, et al. DNA barcoding detects contamination and substitution in North American herbal products. *BMC Med.* 2013;11:222. doi: 10.1186/1741-7015-11-222.
15. Federal Trade Commission. Dietary supplements: an advertising guide for industry. Available at: http://business.ftc.gov/documents/bus09-dietary-supplements-advertising-guide-industry. Updated April 2001. Accessed June 24, 2017.
16. U.S. Food and Drug Administration. Label claims for conventional foods and dietary supplements. Available at: http://www.fda.gov/Food/IngredientsPackagingLabeling/LabelingNutrition/ucm111447.htm. Updated April 11, 2016. Accessed June 24, 2017.
17. U.S. Food and Drug Administration. Dietary Supplement and Non-Prescription Drug Consumer Protection Act (Pub. L. No. 109-462, 109th Congress). Available at: http://www.fda.gov/downloads/AboutFDA/CentersOffices/CDER/ucm102797.pdf. December 22, 2006. Accessed June 24, 2017.
18. U.S. Food and Drug Administration. MedWatch: The FDA safety information and adverse event reporting program. Available at: http://www.fda.gov/medwatch. Accessed June 24, 2017.
19. Karsch-Völk M, Barrett B, Linde K. Echinacea for preventing and treating the common cold. *JAMA.* 2015;313(6):618–9. doi: 10.1001/jama.2014.17145.
20. Gurib-Fakim A. Medicinal plants: traditions of yesterday and drugs of tomorrow. *Mol Aspects Med.* 2006;27(1):1–3. doi: 10.1016/j.mam.2005.07.008.
21. Schulz V, Hansel R, Blumenthal M, eds. *Rational Phytotherapy: A Reference Guide for Physicians and Pharmacists.* 2nd ed. Berlin Heidelberg, Germany: Springer-Verlag; 2004.
22. Saper RB, Phillips RS, Sehgal A, et al. Lead, mercury, and arsenic in U.S. and Indian manufactured Ayurvedic medicines sold via the Internet. *JAMA.* 2008;300(8):915–23. doi: 10.1001/jama.300.8.915.
23. Genius SJ, Schwalfenberg G, Siy AK, et al. Toxic element contamination of natural health products and pharmaceutical preparations. *PLoS One.* 2012;7(11):e49676. doi: 10.1371/journal.pone.0049676.
24. Geller A, Shehab N, Weidle N et al. Emergency department visits for adverse events related to dietary supplements. *N Engl J Med.* 2015;373(16):1531–0. doi: 10.1056/NEJMsa1504267.
25. Harel Z, Harel S, Wald R, et al. The frequency and characteristics of dietary supplement recalls in the United States. *JAMA Intern Med.* 2013;173(10):926–8. doi: 10.1001/jamainternmed.2013.379.
26. U.S. Pharmacopeia Convention. USP verification services. Available at: http://www.usp.org/usp-verification-services. Accessed June 24, 2017.
27. Consumer.Lab.com. About Consumer.Lab.com. Available at: http://www.consumerlab.com/aboutcl.asp. Accessed June 24, 2017.
28. NSF International. Dietary supplement safety, certification process. Available at: http://www.nsf.org/services/by-industry/dietary-supplements/supplement-safety. Accessed June 24, 2017.
29. National Institutes of Health (NIH) Office of Dietary Supplements. Consumer protection. Available at: http://ods.od.nih.gov/HealthInformation/consumerprotection.sec.aspx. Accessed June 24, 2017.
30. Morris CA, Avorn J. Internet marketing of herbal products. *JAMA.* 2003;290(11):1505–9. doi: 10.1001/jama.290.11.1505.
31. U.S. Food and Drug Administration. Health fraud consumer updates. Available at: http://www.fda.gov/ForConsumers/ProtectYourself/HealthFraud/ucm267375.htm#3-tab. Accessed June 24, 2017.
32. Chung IS, Lee MY, Jung HR. Three systemic argyria cases after ingestion of colloidal silver solution. *Int J Dermatol.* 2010;49(10):1175–7. doi: 10.1111/j.1365-4632.2009.04380.x.
33. Wang L, Manson JE, Sesso HD. Calcium intake and risk of cardiovascular disease: a review of prospective studies and randomized clinical trials. *Am J Cardiovasc Drugs.* 2012;12(12):105–6. doi: 10.2165/11595400-000000000-00000.
34. Siegner AW Jr. The Food and Drug Administration's actions on ephedra and androstenedione: understanding their potential impacts on the protections of the Dietary Supplement Health and Education Act. *Food Drug Law J.* 2004;59(4):617–8. PMID: 15880877.
35. Chitturi S, Farrell G. Hepatotoxic slimming aids and other herbal hepatotoxins. *J Gastroenterol Hepatol.* 2008;23(3):366–3. doi: 10.1111/j.1440-1746.2008.05310.x.
36. van Breemen RB, Fong HHS, Farnsworth NR. Ensuring the safety of botanical dietary supplements. *Am J Clin Nutr.* 2008;87(2):509S–3S. PMID: 18258648.
37. Schulz V. Safety of St. John's wort extract compared to synthetic antidepressants. *Phytomedicine.* 2006;13(3):199–4. doi: 10.1016/j.phymed.2005.07.005.
38. Fernstrom JD. Effects and side effects associated with the non-nutritional use of tryptophan by humans. *J Nutr.* 2012;142(12):2236S–4S. doi: 10.3945/jn.111.157065.
39. Haller CA. Clinical approach to adverse events and interactions related to herbal and dietary supplements. *Clin Toxicol (Phila).* 2006;44(5):605–0. doi: 10.1080/15563650600795545.
40. Natural Medicines. Database search engine. Available at: https://naturalmedicines.therapeuticresearch.com. Accessed April 6, 2016.
41. Micromedex, Alternative Medicine. Database search engine. Available at: http://www.micromedexsolutions.com. Accessed April 6, 2016.
42. NIH Office of Dietary Supplements. Computer access to research on dietary supplements (CARDS) database. Available at: http://ods.od.nih.gov/Research/CARDS_Database.aspx. Accessed April 6, 2016.
43. Cochrane Library. Cochrane database of systematic reviews. Available at: http://www.cochranelibrary.com/cochrane-database-of-systematic-reviews/. Accessed June 24, 2017.
44. NIH Office of Dietary Supplements. Dietary supplement ingredient database. Available at: https://dietarysupplementdatabase.usda.nih.gov/. Accessed June 24, 2017.
45. NIH Office of Dietary Supplements. Dietary Supplement Label Database (DSLD). Available at: https://ods.od.nih.gov/Research/Dietary_Supplement_Label_Database.aspx. Accessed March 2, 2017.
46. Lexicomp Online. Wolters Kluwer clinical drug information: natural products. Available at: http://www.wolterskluwercdi.com. Accessed July 21, 2016.
47. U.S. National Library of Medicine. Medline Plus database search engine. Available at: http://medlineplus.gov. Accessed June 24, 2017.
48. National Center for Complementary and Integrative Health. Complementary, alternative, or integrative health: what's in a name? Available at: https://nccih.nih.gov/health/integrative-health/. Accessed June 24, 2017.
49. NIH Office of Dietary Supplements. Dietary supplement fact sheets. Available at: http://ods.od.nih.gov. Accessed June 24, 2017.
50. NIH Office of Dietary Supplements. A new PubMed subset for dietary supplements. Available at: http://ods.od.nih.gov/health_information/ibids.aspx. Accessed June 24, 2017.

CHAPTER 51

NATURAL PRODUCTS

CYDNEY E. McQUEEN AND KATHERINE KELLY ORR

This chapter uses the organ system approach outlined in Table 51–1. This approach is based on a review of natural products of importance in pharmacy practice. The products discussed were chosen because they have evidence to support their use, are widely promoted either with or without evidence supporting use, or present known or theoretical safety concerns.

CARDIOVASCULAR SYSTEM

Coenzyme Q10

Therapeutic Uses

Consumers primarily use coenzyme Q10 (CoQ10) for cardiovascular conditions, as a general antioxidant, and for reduction of statin-associated adverse effects. Additionally, it has been investigated for use in migraine prevention, Parkinson disease, and breast cancer, and in reduction of chemotherapy-associated adverse effects.

Physiologic Activity

CoQ10 (also called ubiquinone) is converted to ubiquinol in the body and is found in every cell, primarily in mitochondria, with greatest concentrations in heart, kidney, liver, and muscle.[1] The rate-limiting cofactor in mitochondrial adenosine triphosphate (ATP) formation, CoQ10 is involved in many energy production functions and regeneration of antioxidants such as vitamin E. Low plasma CoQ10 levels are common in people with migraines and may be predictive of mortality in patients with chronic heart failure (HF).[2] Statins decrease CoQ10 biosynthesis and lower serum concentrations, but not always in muscle tissue; decreases may differ in extent among statins.[3] CoQ10 stabilizes membranes and may have vasodilatory and inotropic effects.[4]

Dosage and Product Considerations

For HF, cardiomyopathy, or hypertension, the dosage is generally 100 mg taken 2–3 times daily with meals to aid absorption, but dosages up to 1200 mg/day have been used safely for some neurologic conditions.[5] To counteract depletion by statins, the dosage is 50–100 mg/day, and for migraine prevention, 100 mg/day for children and 300 mg/day for adults. Products meeting United States Pharmacopeia (USP) standards should be recommended.

Safety Considerations

Gastrointestinal (GI) effects from CoQ10 use may be minimized by splitting large (>100 mg) doses. Adverse effects are mild, including nausea, GI distress, anorexia, headache, irritability, and dizziness in less than 1% of patients. Mild liver enzyme increases have been reported. CoQ10 use should be avoided in pregnancy and lactation because safety information is lacking. Potential drug interactions with CoQ10 are listed in Table 51–2.[5–7]

Summary of Clinical Evidence

Evidence for CoQ10 in HF is contradictory. Studies have shown excellent results as indicated by decreased levels of cardiovascular health markers, such as endothelial function and C-reactive protein levels, whereas trials examining symptoms or ejection fraction have demonstrated both positive and negative results when CoQ10 was added to standard therapies.[8,9]

One large, well-designed, 2-year study examined short- and long-term effects in patients with HF taking 300 mg/day CoQ10 or placebo.[10] The groups had similar improvements in symptoms or function at 16 weeks, although at 106 weeks, 58% of CoQ10 patients had improved at least one New York Heart Association (NYHA) class compared with 45% of patients receiving placebo. At 106 weeks, the risk of cardiovascular events was reduced by 43% in the CoQ10 group compared with placebo, as was the risk of cardiovascular death, 9% versus 16%.

Whether supplemental CoQ10 can reduce adverse effects associated with statins remains controversial. Some studies support CoQ10's effects to reverse statin-associated adverse effects, with or without statin discontinuation.[11,12] A 2015 meta-analysis of 6 trials concluded that myalgia or other adverse effects were not significantly reduced, and an additional trial in patients with confirmed statin myopathy caused by simvastatin found no differences between CoQ10 600 mg/day and placebo after 8 weeks.[13] Genetic differences may contribute to the variable responses to CoQ10 treatment.[14]

Although the true efficacy is unknown, CoQ10's favorable adverse effect profile does support a trial of adjunctive use in HF or for reduction of statin-associated adverse effects. These uses, as well as a dose and duration for the trial period, should be discussed with the health care provider (HCP) before beginning treatment.[5]

TABLE 51-1 Chapter Supplements Grouped by Organ Systems

System/Systemic Effect or Action	Supplement
Cardiovascular system	Coenzyme Q10
	Fish oil
	Garlic
	Green coffee bean extract
	Red yeast rice
Central nervous system	Butterbur
	Feverfew
	Ginkgo
	Melatonin
	St. John's wort
	Valerian
Digestive system	Ginger
	Milk thistle
	Peppermint
Endocrine system	Alpha lipoic acid
	Cinnamon
Immune modulators	Echinacea
	Elderberry
Physical and mental performance enhancers	Eleuthero
	Asian ginseng
	Green tea
Kidney, urinary tract, and prostate	African plum
	Cranberry
	DHEA
	Saw palmetto
Musculoskeletal system	Glucosamine and chondroitin
	MSM
	SAMe
	Turmeric/curcumin
Skin conditions	Aloe vera
	Tea tree oil
Weight-loss supplements	*Garcinia cambogia*/hydroxycitric acid
	Raspberry ketone
Women's health	Black cohosh
	Chaste tree berry
	Evening primrose oil
	Fenugreek
	Phytoestrogens

Key: DHEA, Dehydroepiandrosterone; MSM, methylsulfonylmethane; SAMe, *S*-adenosyl-L-methionine.

Fish Oil

Fish oil is a source of omega-3 fatty acids, primarily docosahexaenoic acid (DHA) and eicosapentaenoic acid (EPA).

Therapeutic Uses

Fish oil is used to lower triglyceride (TG) levels, improve cardiac health, aid in the treatment of depression, and relieve inflammatory conditions such as rheumatoid arthritis and psoriasis. American diets tend to be low in omega-3 fatty acids and high in omega-6 fatty acids. The American Heart Association recommends a minimum intake of fatty fish twice weekly for heart health.[15] Consumers who do not eat fatty fish can take supplements to improve the omega-3:omega-6 ratio.

Physiologic Activity

Omega-3 fatty acids may decrease intestinal cholesterol absorption and inhibit enzymes involved in synthesis, excretion, and degradation of very-low-density lipoproteins (VLDLs), thereby decreasing other lipoproteins including low-density lipoproteins (LDLs).[16] The mechanism of hypotriglyceridemic action through peroxisome proliferator–activated receptors may be responsible also for improvements in glucose concentrations and insulin resistance.[17]

Intake of EPA and DHA in fish oil influences the production and concentrations of inflammatory response cytokines. Competitive inhibition of arachidonic acid decreases production of thromboxane A_2 and leukotriene B_4, while effects at another part of the production cascade increase thromboxane A_3 and prostaglandin E_3. Overall, actions can be summarized as increasing noninflammatory and decreasing proinflammatory cytokines. Plaque inflammation is decreased through the mediators, resolvins and protectins, which are solely derived from omega-3 fatty acids.[18]

Dosage and Product Considerations

The usual recommendation for fish oil is 1–2 g/day; for hyperlipidemia, dosages of 2–4 g/day in divided doses are used. Most studies have used products with an EPA:DHA ratio of 1.2:1 or 1.5:1. The EPA and DHA amounts may not equal the stated total dose per capsule because of excipients and additional components; however, high-quality products will be close to the total. For example, a "1 gram fish oil" product labeled to contain "480 mg EPA and 370 mg DHA" per capsule would be within the acceptable ratios, while a "1 gram fish oil" product with "250 mg EPA and 180 mg DHA" per capsule would not contain adequate amounts. For vegetarian and vegan patients, DHA and DHA/EPA products made from algae are available; DHA/EPA amounts may be lower, so total dosages of the algal oil may need to be higher.

Enteric-coated capsules taken with meals or at bedtime are recommended to minimize the common "fish burp" effect. Anecdotally, some patients have success with freezing the capsules. Data on mercury and other toxins in fish have increased concerns about quality of these supplements. Because mercury is insoluble in oil, it collects primarily in flesh, while most fish oil is extracted from the skin. Supplements tested have had no or barely detectable concentrations of mercury.[19] Dioxin and pesticides can accumulate in the oil, so a high-quality product meeting USP standards may limit exposure to these toxins.[20]

Supplements made from krill oil, which may be better absorbed, are often promoted as superior to fish oil. Although

TABLE 51–2 **Selected Dietary Supplement–Drug Interactions**

Dietary Supplement	Known Interactions/Results[a]	Theoretical Interactions/Results[b]
African plum (pygeum)	n/d	Potential risk for increased adverse effects when combined with finasteride or dutasteride
Alpha lipoic acid	Increased bioavailability of valproate	SMBG recommended in patients taking antihyperglycemic drugs
		Potential chelating activity with minerals and antacids
		Possible interference with conversion of thyroxine to triiodothyronine
		Possible reduction of effectiveness of some chemotherapy agents
Black cohosh		Possible potentiation of antihypertensive agents
		May increase toxicity of doxorubicin and docetaxel
		May decrease effectiveness of cisplatin
		Avoid with hepatotoxic drugs
Butterbur		Possible interaction with anticholinergic drugs or antimigraine medications
		Avoid with known inducers of CYP3A4; possible pyrrolizidine increases
Chasteberry		Possible interference with HT or OCPs
		Possible interaction with antipsychotics, dopamine agonists and antagonists, and metoclopramide because of dopaminergic activity
Cinnamon		Additive effects with antihyperglycemic agents
Chondroitin		Possible increased risk of bleeding if taken with antithrombotic agents
Coenzyme Q10		Possible vitamin K–like procoagulant effects if taken with warfarin; monitor INR initially
Cranberry		Possible increased INR and risk of bleeding in people taking warfarin
		Possible CYP2C9 inhibition
		May alter excretion of weakly alkaline drugs or neutralize effects of antacids
DHEA	Triazolam: increased blood levels	Interference with hormonal or antihormonal therapies
	Antidepressants; increased risk of mania	May increase risk of thromboembolism with OCPs
		Possible increased levels of CYP3A4 substrates
Echinacea		Possible interaction with immunomodulating therapies
		CYP3A4 substrates with low oral bioavailability: verapamil, cyclosporine, tacrolimus. Effects on CYP1A2, CYP2C9, or CYP3A4 are likely to be clinically insignificant.
Elderberry		Possible additive effects with antihypertensive and antihyperglycemic agents; increase monitoring
Eleuthero ("Siberian ginseng")	Digoxin: possible false elevation in plasma levels (assay dependent)	SMBG recommended in patients taking antihyperglycemic agents
	Caffeine: increased CNS stimulation	Possible inhibition of CYP1A2, CYP2C9, CYP3A4, and CYP2D6
		Possible inhibition of P-glycoprotein
		Possible additive effects with antithrombotic agents
Evening primrose oil		Possible additive effects if taken with other antithrombotic agents or herbs
		Possible increased risk of seizure possible with phenothiazines
		Potential additive effects to antihypertensives

(continued)

TABLE 51-2 **Selected Dietary Supplement–Drug Interactions** *(continued)*

Dietary Supplement	Known Interactions/Results[a]	Theoretical Interactions/Results[b]
Fenugreek		Possible additive effects if taken with other antithrombotic agents or herbs Avoid with antihyperglycemic drugs because of additive effects
Feverfew		Possible additive effects if taken with other antithrombotic agents or herbs Possible inhibition of CYP1A2, CYP2C8, CYP2C9, CYP2C19, CYP2D6, and CYP3A4
Fish oil		Possible additive effects primarily at dosages >4 g/day if taken with antithrombotic agents
Garcinia cambogia/HCA	SSRIs: case report of serotonin syndrome I	Possible additive effects when used with antihyperglycemic agents
Garlic	Warfarin: increased INR in case reports Saquinavir: 50% decrease in levels OCPs: decreased effectiveness	Contradictory evidence regarding induction of drugs metabolized through CYP3A4 and CYP2D6 May inhibit isoniazid absorption
Ginger	Antithrombotic agents: possible additive effect Nifedipine: decreased platelet aggregation	Avoid with antihyperglycemic drugs because of additive effects
Ginkgo	Antithrombotic agents: possible additive effect (contradictory evidence) Atorvastatin: decreased clearance, though efficacy does not seem to be decreased Efavirenz: decreased levels Omeprazole: decreased levels Trazodone: case report of coma in patient taking low-dose trazodone	Excessive ingestion associated with seizures; avoid in patients with a history of seizures or on drugs that may lower seizure threshold Potential additive effects with antihypertensive drugs, although paradoxical hypertension has been reported with HCTZ, possible increase in levels of nifedipine Possible reduction concentrations of ritonavir, lansoprazole, and tolbutamide
Ginseng (*Panax ginseng*)	Glucose-lowering drugs: possible lowered BG levels in type 2 diabetes mellitus; SMBG levels required Phenelzine: possible headache, tremor, and mania in case report Imatinib: increased toxicity	Unpredictable effects on concurrent antithrombotic agents Possible interference with antipsychotics and immunosuppressants Possible inhibition of CYP1A1, CYP2D6, and CYP3A4
Glucosamine	Warfarin: increased bleeding risk in individuals with variant CYP2C9 alleles	SMBG recommended for first few days of use in patients taking antihyperglycemic drugs
Green coffee bean extract		Antihypertensive agents: possible additive effects Possible decreased absorption of alendronate
Green tea	Decongestants: additive stimulant effects	Possible antagonism of warfarin's effect Possible antagonism of concurrent sedatives related to caffeine content Possible reduction in serum folate levels
Melatonin	Nifedipine: reduced delivery via the GITS Fluvoxamine, MAOIs, and tricyclic antidepressants: increase melatonin BZDPs, sodium valproate, and beta blockers: decrease nighttime levels	Caffeine or OCP use: various effects on melatonin levels Verapamil may decrease melatonin Possible interaction with immunosuppressant drugs related to immunostimulating properties
Milk thistle		Inhibition of CYP2C9, CYP2D6, and CYP3A4 is unlikely; evidence is contradictory
Peppermint	Decreased absorption of iron salts Drugs that increase gastric pH: premature dissolution of enteric-coated peppermint oil capsules	Possible inhibition of CYP3A4

TABLE 51–2 **Selected Dietary Supplement–Drug Interactions** *(continued)*

Dietary Supplement	Known Interactions/Results[a]	Theoretical Interactions/Results[b]
Phytoestrogens (red clover, others)		Possible increased risk of bleeding in patients taking antithrombotic agents with red clover–based products
Raspberry ketone		Possible additive effects with antiglycemic agents
Red yeast rice	Additive activity when used with statins	CYP3A4 inhibitors: possible increased levels and adverse effects Gemfibrozil: possible increased adverse effects
SAMe	Antidepressants and 5-HT_1 agonists: increased risk of serotonin syndrome	Risk of additive adverse effects with monoamine oxidase inhibitors Avoid concomitant use with corticosteroids due to possible effects on glucocorticoid concentrations
Saw palmetto		Potential interaction with hormonal or antihormonal therapies in men and women Possible additive effects when used with antithrombotic agents
St. John's wort	CYP3A4 substrates: significantly decreased drug levels and effects (e.g., alprazolam, amitriptyline, atorvastatin, erythromycin, finasteride, imatinib, irinotecan, methadone, nifedipine, simvastatin, tacrolimus, verapamil, voriconazole, warfarin, zolpidem) Antidepressants: increased risk of serotonin syndromes Cyclosporine: decreased blood levels of immunosuppressant leading to transplant graft rejection OCPs and HT: decreased activity Protease inhibitors, nonnucleoside reverse transcriptase inhibitors, and nonstructural protein 5A or 5B inhibitors: decreased serum levels	Possible increased risk of serotonin syndrome if taken with 5-HT_1 agonists, dextromethorphan, meperidine, and tramadol Digoxin: decreased intestinal absorption, decreased levels Possible decreased levels and effect of amiodarone, theophylline, and proton pump inhibitors Monitoring for fexofenadine toxicity recommended if taken concomitantly Morphine: increased narcotic-induced sleep time in animal studies Use with other photosensitizing agents contraindicated
Turmeric	Sulfasalazine: significantly increased blood levels	Possible increased effects with antithrombotic agents Possible P-glycoprotein inhibition
Valerian		Possible increased sedative effect if taken with alcohol or other CNS depressants (BZDPs) Possible inhibition of CYP3A4

Key: BG = Blood glucose; BZDP = benzodiazepine; CNS = central nervous system; CYP = cytochrome P450; DHEA = dehydroepiandrosterone; GITS = gastrointestinal therapeutic system; HCA = hydroxycitric acid; HCTZ = hydrochlorothiazide; HT = hormone therapy; 5-HT_1 = 5-hydroxytryptamine$_1$; INR = international normalized ratio; MAOI = monoamine oxidase inhibitor; OCP = oral contraceptive pill; SAMe = S-adenosyl-L-methionine; SMBG = self-monitoring of blood glucose; SSRI = selective serotonin reuptake inhibitor.

[a] Based on human studies and/or validated case reports.

[b] Extrapolated from animal or in vitro studies.

these have demonstrated similar effects in animal studies and some human studies, human clinical trials are needed before any recommendations can be made.[21] Krill oil is more expensive than fish oil.

Safety Considerations

Fish oil products are generally safe; the most common adverse effects are belching with fishy halitosis and GI distress. With more than 4 g/day, an increased risk of bleeding could be present, so patients taking antithrombotic agents are recommended to use no more than 3 g/day and to be monitored closely. However, some trial evidence suggests that 4 or 6.9 g/day in combination with aspirin and heparin or with warfarin does not result in increased bleeding events.[18]

Summary of Clinical Evidence

Fish oil's greatest effect is on TG levels. A recent meta-analysis examining 38 trials found that dietary ingestion of 4 g or greater of fish oil daily resulted in reductions of 9%–26% in TG levels, while 1–5 g/day of fish oil supplements were associated with decreases of 4%–51%.[22] Earlier meta-analyses reported decreases of 14%–29%, with greater lowering of VLDL levels.[23,24] Total cholesterol (TC) reductions range from 0% to 11% with high-density lipoprotein (HDL) levels either unchanged or increased modestly (<10%).[25] Effects on LDL levels are variable, with most studies noting small decreases.

After significant cardiovascular risk reduction was noted in the Italian GISSI-Prevenzione trial, many studies evaluated cardiovascular outcomes with fish oil. Disease management has changed considerably since that time, which may explain the conflicting results reported in subsequent clinical trials. Over the past decade, meta-analyses of fish oil trials have had conflicting conclusions regarding its cardiovascular risk reduction.[26] Several trials demonstrated increased lipid lowering when fish oil was added to statin therapy and one large (N = 18,645) study demonstrated a 53% reduction in heart disease in patients with elevated TG and low HDL levels.[27] Other studies found no additional benefit either for lipid lowering or for reduction of cardiovascular risk.[28] One analysis suggested that fish oil may only reduce cardiovascular risk in patients who are low in omega-3 fatty acids, and that no additional protective effects occur in patients already taking statins, possibly through a competitive interference because of increased arachidonic acid.[28]

Patients on hemodialysis experience heightened risk of thrombosis in arteriovenous (AV) grafts for vascular access. A meta-analysis of 13 controlled trials using dosages of 1.3–6 g/day of fish oil reported a decreased risk of AV graft thrombosis (risk ratio [RR] = 0.71 [CI 0.52–0.97], $P = 0.03$) and a decreased risk of cardiovascular events in this high risk population (RR = 0.41 [CI 0.26–0.66], $P = 0.0002$).[29]

Overall, fish oil may safely be recommended to aid in TG reduction and to increase omega-3 dietary intake. Patients who are interested in fish oil specifically for reduction of general cardiovascular risk should be counseled that the potential benefit may be low and may be affected by many factors, including concomitant statin therapy.

Garlic

Therapeutic Uses

Garlic products derived from dried or fresh bulbs of *Allium sativum* are promoted for hyperlipidemia, hypertension, and type 2 diabetes mellitus, as well as for immune function and prevention of various cancers.

Physiologic Activity

Garlic bulbs contain an odorless sulfur-containing amino acid derivative alliin (*S*-allyl-L-cysteine sulfoxide). When a garlic clove is crushed, the enzyme alliinase is released, converting alliin to pungent allicin, the main component of garlic's volatile oil. Allicin is used as a product quality marker and is not the only active compound; other substances such as S-allycysteine (SAC) also exert pharmacologic effects. In animal and in vitro models, garlic possesses antiplatelet and anti-infective properties. Garlic's prevention of lipid oxidation may be as important to cardiovascular health as its hypolipidemic and antihypertensive activity.[30] Garlic increases hydrogen sulfide, a vasodilator, enhances nitric oxide production, and may inhibit angiotensin-converting enzyme.[31]

Dosage and Product Considerations

Differences in dosage forms may be responsible for the varied outcomes from clinical trials. Only products similar to those used in clinical trials should be used: either powdered garlic standardized to allicin content of 1%–1.6%, providing 3–5 mg of allicin per day, or aged garlic extracts (AGE) containing at least 1.2 mg SAC should be recommended.[32] Enteric-coated products may help to decrease "garlic breath" and may possibly provide more benefit for lipid reduction.

Safety Considerations

Although well tolerated, garlic may cause GI effects including nausea, reflux, vomiting, and heartburn, especially with higher dosages or in the first week of therapy. Garlic breath and body odor may also occur. Allergic reactions have been reported rarely.

Garlic should be stopped 10–14 days prior to surgical procedures to avoid excess bleeding. Patients taking antithrombotic agents should use garlic supplements with caution because of potential bleeding risk, but dietary amounts do not affect platelet function.[33,34]

Effects on cytochrome P450 (CYP) isoenzymes are unclear, but enzyme induction is possible; drug profiles should be reviewed for potentially severe interactions before garlic is initiated. Table 51–2 lists potential drug interactions.

Summary of Clinical Evidence

Multiple trials have examined effects of garlic supplements on lipid levels. A 2013 meta-analysis of 37 trials concluded that garlic reduces TC levels by 15 mg/dL. Studies of 13–52 weeks in duration reported reductions up to 19.63 mg/dL; the decreases in LDL levels were more modest at 7–9 mg/dL.[32] Trials of 2–8 weeks in duration demonstrated no difference from placebo. A subgroup analysis suggested that aged garlic extracts may be more beneficial than garlic powder products, with little to no effect for garlic oil and raw garlic.[32] Overall, patients with TC levels higher than 200 mg/dL experienced greater reductions.

With respect to hypertension, a 2016 meta-analysis of nine trials concluded that garlic reduces systolic blood pressure (SBP) and diastolic blood pressure (DBP) by a mean of 8.7 and 6.1 mm Hg, respectively, in hypertensive patients compared with placebo, while normotensive individuals had SBP and DBP reductions of 5.1 and 2.5 mm Hg, respectively.[35] A 2015 meta-analysis concluded SBP and DBP mean reductions with garlic were 9.36 and 3.82 mm Hg, respectively; the authors stated reductions were similar to those in a meta-analysis of 354 short-term studies of prescription antihypertensive agents.[36,37]

A 2016 trial evaluated blood pressure responses in 88 individuals receiving 1.2 g/day of AGE for 12 weeks. Responders were classified as those with reductions of more than 3% in SBP and DBP.[38] The mean SBP reduction was 5 mm Hg ($P = 0.016$ compared with placebo). In the responder group, mean SBP lowering was 11.5 mm Hg, with a 6.3 mm Hg decline in DBP ($P < 0.001$). Overall, the evidence does support that garlic may be a suitable option for individuals with mild hypertension, mild hypercholesterolemia, or both although long-term outcome studies are not available.

Green Coffee Bean Extract

Therapeutic Uses

Green coffee bean extract has been promoted primarily for weight loss. Although some animal studies provide some support, no recommendations for weight loss can be made. Because early animal studies revealed effects on blood pressure, research has begun into green coffee bean extract for hypertension.

Physiologic Activity

The active components in green coffee bean extract are chlorogenic acids (CGAs). One third undergoes intestinal absorption and is metabolized to quinic, caffeic, and ferulic acids. Ferulic acid increases vasoreactivity and has hypotensive effects, likely through endothelial nitric oxide mechanisms. Although regular roasted coffee contains some CGA, it does not have antihypertensive effects, because hydroxyhydroquinone, which counteracts the antihypertensive effects of CGA, is created during the roasting process.[39]

CGA also inhibits the glucose-6-phosphatase system and may have some lipolytic activity although blood glucose or insulin response is unchanged.[40,41]

Dosage and Product Considerations

The optimal dosage has not been determined and trials in hypertension have used green coffee bean extract containing 140 mg of CGA.[42–44] A dosage of 5 mg/kg of CGA was used safely in a trial of a combination product, but this amount is not recommended.[41]

Safety Considerations

No adverse events have been reported in the hypertension studies, although data on safety is limited. The potential for drug interactions has not been investigated.

Summary of Clinical Evidence

A human trial tested green coffee bean extract containing 140 mg/day of CGA in 20 healthy, normotensive men for 4 months.[41] Although blood pressure decreased slightly at each study visit, changes were not significant. Lipid and blood chemistry parameters did not change in the green coffee bean extract group, except for a decrease in homocysteine, a potential cardiovascular disease risk factor which fell from 1.3 mg/L to 1.07 mg/L ($P < 0.01$).

Green coffee bean extract has exhibited a dose-response effect in mild hypertension.[44] Subjects (N = 117) were randomized to placebo or 25, 50, or 100 mg of CGA. All green coffee bean extract doses resulted in significant decreases in SBP of 3.2, 4.7, and 5.6 mm Hg, respectively, and in DBP of 2.9, 3.2, and 3.9 mm Hg.

A 480-mg dose of green coffee bean extract containing 140 mg/day of CGA was tested in 28 adult men with mild hypertension in a placebo-controlled clinical trial.[45] Blood pressure did not change in the placebo group, but the mean blood pressure in the CGA group decreased from 195/91 mm Hg at baseline to 137/84 mm Hg at 4 weeks and 135/84 mm Hg at 12 weeks (SBP $P < 0.001$, DBP $P < 0.05$). No changes occurred in pulse rate, body mass index (BMI), lipid levels, or blood chemistry.

A 2015 meta-analysis of seven trials, including the three just discussed as well as two others using CGA-enriched coffee drinks, concluded that CGA lowers SBP and DBP with a moderate effect size in Asian populations.[46] At this time, the human research in hypertension is promising, but the optimal dosage and long-term safety have not been determined. As a result, the use of green coffee bean extract cannot be recommended, and patients who choose to use it or CGA products should be monitored for adverse effects.

Red Yeast Rice

Monascus purpureus, a yeast that grows on fermented rice and gives Peking duck its red hue, is used in traditional Chinese medicine.

Therapeutic Uses

Red yeast rice is used to lower lipid concentrations.

Physiologic Activity

Red yeast rice contains multiple components; monacolin K, a naturally occurring lovastatin analogue is the most important. The standard dosing for most products would normally contain less than 5 mg/day of monacolin K. As a result, this cannot be solely responsible for the extent of lipid-lowering effects reported in clinical trials. Multiple other mechanisms are possible, including increased bile acid excretion.

Dosage and Product Considerations

For hyperlipidemia, the dosage is 1.2–2.4 g/day in 2 doses. In the United States, certain red yeast rice products have been declared illegal, because they contained an "unauthorized drug."[47] As a result, many manufacturers no longer ensure their products contain a standardized amount of monacolin K, making the choice of a high-quality, effective product more difficult.[47]

Safety Considerations

Adverse effects associated with red yeast rice include allergic reactions, headache, and mild GI symptoms including bloating, flatulence, and heartburn. Increased liver function enzymes have been reported, so monitoring liver function 1–2 months after starting red yeast rice, and annually thereafter, is recommended.[47] Patients with heavy daily alcohol intake (more than two drinks) should not use red yeast rice because of potential increased hepatotoxicity risk. Any use of red yeast rice is contraindicated in pregnancy.[48]

The *M. purpureus* yeast can also generate the nephrotoxin, citrinin, during fermentation.[49] Only red yeast rice brands that have been tested to be free of citrinin should be used; patients with kidney disease should not use red yeast rice.

At least three studies have found that red yeast rice can be safely used in patients unable to take statins. Rare reports of rhabdomyolysis with red yeast rice exist, which may be associated with products with higher monacolin K content.[50–52] Initial increased monitoring is appropriate if used in a patient with previous statin-induced myalgia.

Summary of Clinical Evidence

Multiple studies have demonstrated that red yeast rice lowers lipid concentrations. A 2015 meta-analysis reported a mean

A WORD ABOUT Resveratrol

Interest in this polyphenol from grapes and berries began with research into the hypothetical cardioprotective effects of red wines. Higher dietary intake has been associated with lower levels of lipids, blood pressure, and glucose, as well as a lower heart rate.[a] Resveratrol, known to be an antioxidant, affects dilation of blood vessels, has anti-inflammatory activity, and may increase insulin sensitivity.[b,c] Clinical data do not yet include long-term outcomes such as cardiac morbidity or mortality. In small studies, cardiovascular risk markers, such as lipid levels, apolipoprotein A-1, tumor necrosis factor α, C-reactive protein, and interleukin-10, were all improved with use of resveratrol.[b,d] Although trials have used dosages ranging from 8 to 1000 mg, the optimum dosage has not been determined. Resveratrol does seem to be very safe, with headache being the only reported adverse effect in trials.

[a] Zamora-Ros R, Urpi-Sarda M, Lamuela-Raventós RM, et al. High urinary levels of resveratrol metabolites are associated with a reduction in the prevalence of cardiovascular risk factors in high-risk patients. *Pharmacol Res.* 2012;65(6):315–20. doi: 10.1016/j.phrs.2012.03.009.

[b] Magyar K, Halmosi R, Palfi A, et al. Cardioprotection by resveratrol: a human clinical trial in patients with stable coronary artery disease. *Clin Hemorheol Microcirc.* 2012;50(3):179–87. doi: 10.3233/CH-2011-1424.

[c] Brasnyó P, Molnár GA, Mohás M, et al. Resveratrol improves insulin sensitivity, reduces oxidative stress and activates the Akt pathway in type 2 diabetic patients. *Br J Nutr.* 2011;106(3):383–9. doi: 10.1017/S0007114511000316.

[d] Tomé-Carneiro J, Gonzálvez M, Larrosa M, et al. One-year consumption of a grape nutraceutical containing resveratrol improves the inflammatory and fibrinolytic status of patients in primary prevention of cardiovascular disease. *Am J Cardiol.* 2012;110(3):356–63. doi: 10.1016/j.amjcard.2012.03.030.

reduction of 39.44 mg/dL in LDL-cholesterol levels compared with placebo and noted LDL lowering was not different from statin use.[53] In a 2016 systematic review of 10 trials of red yeast rice versus simvastatin, examining effects on TC, LDL, HDL, and TG, both simvastatin and red yeast rice identified similar effects on all lipid measures.[54]

Because the increases in HDL cholesterol (HDL-C) levels have not been as large as the decreases in other lipids, patients who are at greater cardiac risk because of low HDL-C levels are not good candidates for red yeast rice. Whether red yeast rice alone possesses the long-term benefits for cardiovascular risk reduction similar to statins is yet to be determined.

CENTRAL NERVOUS SYSTEM

Butterbur

Petasites hybridus, also known as butterbur, is native to marshy areas in northern Asia, Europe, and parts of North America. It is a member of the Asteraceae/Compositae family.

Therapeutic Uses

Butterbur is used to prevent migraines and treat allergic rhinitis and asthma.

Physiologic Activity

Petasin and isopetasin are isolated from butterbur's rhizomes, roots, and leaves. Extracts also contain volatile oils, tannins, flavonoids, and pyrrolizidine alkaloids (PAs). Petasin may reduce spasms in smooth muscle and vascular walls and also inhibit leukotriene synthesis. Isopetasin decreases prostaglandin synthesis, thereby reducing inflammation. Both compounds have an affinity for cerebral blood vessels.[55]

Dosage and Product Considerations

For migraine prevention, studies have used standardized extracts of butterbur containing a minimum of petasin 7.5 mg and isopetasin 7.5 mg per 50 mg tablet or capsule. Dosages of standardized butterbur ranging from 50–75 mg twice daily are used for 4–6 months, and then tapered until the migraine incidence increases. The maximum study duration has been 12–16 weeks.[55] Standardized petasin (Ze 339) 8–16 mg has been administered 3–4 times daily for allergic rhinitis.[56,57]

Safety Considerations

Butterbur is well tolerated with minor GI symptoms most commonly reported, followed by skin changes and dizziness.[55] PAs and their N-oxides are toxic compounds in butterbur extracts that can cause serious hepatotoxicity and carcinogenesis. Products labeled as PA-free should be recommended.[58] Patients with an allergy to ragweed and related plants in the Asteraceae/Compositae family should avoid butterbur. Its use should also be avoided during pregnancy and lactation because of the potential for hepatotoxicity.

Summary of Clinical Evidence

The American Academy of Neurology and the American Headache Society consider butterbur effective for the prevention of migraine, with the highest evidence level of A based on two randomized controlled trials.[59] Studies including children and adolescents have also shown positive results with lower quality studies.[60] In patients with seasonal allergic rhinitis, short-term studies of butterbur suggest similar efficacy as to cetirizine and fexofenadine.[56,57]

Feverfew

Tanacetum parthenium, also known as feverfew, is a member of the Asteraceae/Compositae family. The plant is native to the Balkans and is now found throughout the world.

Therapeutic Uses

Feverfew is used to prevent migraines and treat dysmenorrhea, arthritis, and psoriasis.

Physiologic Activity

The activity of feverfew for migraine prevention involves multiple many mechanisms. Parthenolide, a sesquiterpene lactone, is the most abundant and biologically active component and likely contributes anti-inflammatory benefits. Other active components include flavonoids, volatile oils, and additional sesquiterpene lactones. Feverfew may have effects on prostaglandin synthesis, platelet aggregation, serotonin release, histamine release, and vascular smooth muscle contraction.[61]

Dosage and Product Considerations

Studies have used feverfew leaf 50–100 mg/day in divided doses or 6.25 mg CO_2-standardized extract (MIG-99) of 0.2%–0.35% of parthenolide 2–3 times daily.[62] Standardization of a product to its parthenolide content has not appeared to be necessary, as content has varied throughout studies. Feverfew must be taken continuously for migraine prophylaxis and is not effective for treatment of acute migraine attacks.

Safety Considerations

GI adverse effects may result from ingestion of feverfew. Oral ulcers can occur from chewing fresh leaves. Post-feverfew syndrome has been reported after abrupt withdrawal from chronic use, resulting in anxiety, headaches, insomnia, and muscle stiffness. Patients who are allergic to plants in the Asteraceae/Compositae family should avoid use of feverfew, as should women who are pregnant or breastfeeding.[61] Possible antiplatelet effects have been identified, so patients taking antithrombotic agents should use feverfew with caution.[63,61]

Summary of Clinical Evidence

A previous Cochrane review found insufficient evidence to support feverfew for the prevention of migraines, although an update included a well-designed study of MIG-99 resulting in an overall decrease of 0.6 migraines per month compared with placebo.[62] The long-term safety and efficacy has not been established and the American Academy of Neurology and the American Headache Society consider MIG-99 probably effective for prevention of migraine, with an evidence level of B.[59]

Ginkgo

Ginkgo biloba is a tree and the only living member of the family Ginkgoaceae.

Therapeutic Uses

Ginkgo has been used for Alzheimer's disease (AD), vascular dementia, attention-deficit/hyperactivity disorder (ADHD), tardive dyskinesia, intermittent claudication, tinnitus, acute mountain sickness, and age-related macular degeneration.

Physiologic Activity

The standardized *G. biloba* (EGb 761) concentrated (50:1) leaf extract contains ginkgolides (A, B, C, and M) and bilobalide. These constituents may be responsible for neuroprotective properties reported with the leaf extract. Ginkgolide B is a potent platelet-activating factor antagonist. The extract also contains bioflavonoids and flavone glycosides, such as quercetin, 3-methyl quercetin, and kaempferol. The flavonoid fractions may possess antioxidant and free radical scavenger effects.[64]

Dosage and Product Considerations

Recommended dosages for dementias, intermittent claudication, and ADHD range between 120 and 240 mg/day of ginkgo leaf extract in 2–3 divided doses. EGb 761, used in many clinical trials, is available containing 24% ginkgo flavone glycosides and 6% terpenoids.[61]

Safety Considerations

Mild GI adverse effects, headache, dizziness, and allergic skin reactions have been reported with ginkgo.[65] Ginkgo should be avoided during pregnancy and lactation because of the lack of safety information. Several potential drug interactions with ginkgo are listed in Table 51–2.[65,66]

Increased bleeding risk has been associated with use of ginkgo. A large retrospective analysis found bleeding risk increased about 40% when concurrently taken with antithrombotic agents.[67] Patients taking antithrombotic agents should use ginkgo with caution and its use should be stopped at least 7–10 days before any surgical procedure.[63]

Summary of Clinical Evidence

A meta-analysis and systematic review evaluated studies comparing the efficacy and safety of ginkgo in patients with dementia or cognitive decline. Nine trials were included with EGb 761 as an intervention demonstrating improvement in cognition, activities of daily living, and Clinicians' Global Impression of Change (CGIC) scale with 240 mg/day after 6 months of treatment. The AD subgroup did not reach significance in these outcomes.[68] The Ginkgo Evaluation of Memory (GEM) study evaluated 120 mg of standardized ginkgo extract twice daily versus placebo in more than 3000 community-dwelling adults ages 72–96 years. Rates of change were similar in the two groups.[69] Older adults with normal cognition are unlikely to benefit from the use of ginkgo.

Melatonin

Therapeutic Uses

Melatonin, a hormone produced by the pineal gland, is synthesized from tryptophan via a serotonin pathway. Melatonin has Food and Drug Administration (FDA) orphan drug status for sleep disorders in blind patients. The dietary supplement (DS) melatonin is primarily used for insomnia, prevention of "jet lag," and sleep issues related to shift work.

Physiologic Activity

Melatonin regulates sleep and circadian rhythms. Its release is induced by darkness and suppressed by light, especially blue light emitted by phone and computer screens. Exogenous administration stimulates sleep regulation mechanisms. Melatonin does not generally cause feelings of drowsiness, rather sleep attempts are more successful. A potent antioxidant, melatonin has regulatory effects on sexual development and ovulation, and may have effects on bone regulation.[70,71]

Dosage and Product Considerations

For insomnia, 0.3–5 mg is taken orally 30–60 minutes prior to bedtime. For jet lag, dosage is 2–5 mg the evening (between 5:00 and 10:00 PM) of arrival day at the destination and at bedtime for the following 2–5 days. The dosage for occasional insomnia is unclear as supraphysiologic concentrations are produced by 0.3 mg and higher doses may not be more effective.[72]

Most supplements are synthetically produced, but melatonin extracted from bovine pineal glands should be avoided because of added risk of bacterial contamination and bovine spongiform encephalitis (mad cow disease). Some wine varieties contain small amounts of melatonin naturally produced during fermentation.

Safety Considerations

Rare adverse effects include nausea and vomiting, headache, tachycardia, irritability, dysthymia and worsening of depressive symptoms, and morning grogginess. Long-term use is only recommended under supervision of a primary care provider.

Melatonin use in adolescents is controversial because of hormonal effects, and use should be discussed first with an HCP. Pregnant and breastfeeding women should avoid melatonin.

Melatonin may increase effectiveness of some chemo- or radiotherapies for cancer and help reduce toxicities of agents such as doxorubicin and cisplatin.[73,74] Information regarding chemotherapy changes rapidly, so patients should first discuss melatonin with their oncologists.

Summary of Clinical Evidence

Melatonin's evidence for occasional insomnia in generally healthy people is variable. One meta-analysis concluded melatonin produced small, clinically significant improvements in sleep quality.[72] More consistent beneficial responses have been demonstrated in chronic sleep disorders, or in children and adults with developmental disabilities, neurologic disorders, or autism, including improved sleep and daytime behaviors.[75,76] Depressed patients with sleep disorders may experience additional benefits for mood.[77] One study of 791 older patients, ages 55–80 years, reported responses to melatonin regardless of their endogenous levels.[78] Additionally, prolonged-release melatonin has improved sleep quality, daytime alertness, and psychomotor performance in older adults.[79] In patients treated with beta blockers, 2.5 mg of melatonin for 3 weeks improved sleep time and efficiency.[80] Because of the minor adverse effect profile, melatonin may be an option on a trial basis for many individuals, with appropriate counseling that effects may be small.

Melatonin can decrease jet lag when crossing five or more time zones, effects are greater for eastward travel than westward, and individual responses vary. The amount and timing of daylight exposure after arrival can decrease the benefits.[81] Melatonin may not be as effective as zolpidem for sleep improvement or daytime tiredness.[82]

Despite some positive results in trials, the overall clinical evidence does not support melatonin's use for insomnia caused by shift work.

St. John's Wort

Hypericum perforatum, also known as St. John's wort, is a perennial with more than 400 species that grow wild throughout Europe, Asia, North America, and South America. The yellow flowers and the leaves contain the highest levels of medicinally useful compounds. St. John's wort (SJW) is classified in the Clusiaceae family but may also be listed under the Hypericaceae family.

Therapeutic Uses

SJW is used to treat depression, pain, anxiety, obsessive-compulsive disorder, menopause symptoms, and premenstrual syndrome.

Physiologic Activity

Although hypericin was previously considered to have antidepressant activity, evidence now indicates that hyperforin and related compounds are primarily responsible. Other potential biologically active constituents include flavonoids and its derivatives, as well as procyanidins tannins, volatile oils, amino acids, phenylpropanes, and xanthones. SJW may modulate serotonin, dopamine, and norepinephrine. Additional data suggest SJW may also activate gamma aminobutyric acid (GABA) and glutamate receptors and potentially inhibit monoamine oxidase inhibitor (MAO).[83]

Dosage and Product Considerations

The dosage of SJW for adults with mild to moderate depression is 900–1800 mg/day of standardized extract of 0.3% hypericin or 2%–5% hyperforin. It should be taken in three divided doses with meals. Extracts commonly used in clinical studies include LI 160, ZE 117, WS 5570, STW3, and STW3-VI. The content of hypericin and hyperforin varies in commercial preparations, and products may not be interchangeable.[84] As with prescription antidepressants, the therapeutic effects of SJW are not evident for several weeks. Depression should never be self-diagnosed or self-treated. Patients should seek appropriate medical care before using SJW.

Safety Considerations

An analysis of randomized trials found rates of adverse effects in patients taking SJW that were similar to those for placebo. In addition, rates for SJW were lower compared with selective serotonin reuptake inhibitors (SSRIs).[85] The most commonly reported adverse effects include nausea, fatigue, and skin reactions.[86] Photosensitivity reactions have been reported, although evidence is contradictory, patients should limit their exposure to sun and apply sunscreen.[87] SJW should be avoided in patients with bipolar disorder and schizophrenia. As with SSRIs, SJW may cause sexual dysfunction. Abrupt discontinuation after chronic use may result in withdrawal symptoms similar to those of conventional antidepressants. Limited evidence is available to assess the safety of SJW during pregnancy and lactation.

Interactions with SJW are well documented and clinically significant (Table 51–2). SJW is a potent inducer of CYP3A4, resulting in significantly lower concentrations of drugs metabolized through this pathway.[86] The extent of CYP3A4 induction may correlate to hyperforin dose and varies among products. SJW may also induce P-glycoprotein transport proteins, resulting in lower serum concentrations of drugs. Additional evidence suggests induction of CYP2C19. If taken with other serotonergic agents, SJW may increase the risk of developing serotonin syndrome.[86]

Summary of Clinical Evidence

SJW may be as effective as many antidepressants with fewer adverse effects for mild to moderate depression. A Cochrane review evaluating *Hypericum* extracts for major depression included 18 placebo-controlled trials and 17 studies with an active control. SJW had a significant benefit compared with placebo and similar efficacy to standard antidepressants for mild to moderate depression. The rates for adverse effects and trial discontinuation were also lower with SJW than with older antidepressants, indicating *Hypericum* extract may be more tolerable. In addition, the results vary depending on the country of origin, with German-speaking countries showing more positive outcomes. Conclusions cannot be made regarding severe depression.[88] Similar results have been noted with WS 5572, LI 160, WS 5570, and ZE 117 *Hypericum* extracts when compared with placebo and antidepressants. Evidence supports efficacy for mild to moderate depression, with efficacy comparable to that of fluoxetine, sertraline, and citalopram, but with better tolerability.[89] Because of its drug interactions and the potential seriousness of depression, SJW is not an appropriate choice for many patients.

Valerian

Native to Europe and Asia, valerian grows in most parts of the world. More than 200 plant species belong to the genus *Valeriana*. The most common plant used for medicinal purposes is *Valeriana officinalis* from the Valerianaceae family.

Therapeutic Uses

Valerian is used for alleviating insomnia and anxiety.

Physiologic Activity

The central nervous system (CNS) activity of valerian may be the result of valepotriates and sesquiterpene constituents of the volatile oils. Other active components include alkaloids, furofuran ligans, and free amino acids, including GABA. Valeric acid and other components likely interact with GABA receptors in the brain, with valproates and valeric acid producing sedation.[90] Valerian may also have barbiturate-like CNS depressant effects.

Dosage and Product Considerations

Most clinical trials for insomnia use valerian root extract 400–900 mg, administered 30–120 minutes before bedtime. Teas can be prepared from dried roots, although they often have an unpleasant taste and smell. Combination products with hops or lemon balm are commonly marketed.

Safety Considerations

Valerian is generally well-tolerated with headache, excitability, and paradoxical insomnia occurring infrequently. Benzodiazepine-like withdrawal symptoms have been reported after discontinuation of valerian and residual daytime sedation has been associated with higher dosages. *Valeriana officinalis* preparations are safe despite the known in vitro cytotoxic activity of valepotriates, which are generally not found in products. Chronic administration has been linked to hepatotoxicity, although reports include combination products and the role of valerian is unclear. Valerian can potentiate the effects of other CNS depressants and should not be taken concomitantly. Pregnant women should avoid the use of valerian because of potential induction of uterine contractions.[65]

A WORD ABOUT

Kava

Kava is derived from the rhizome and roots of *Piper methysticum* and is widely used by Pacific Islanders as a social and ceremonial tranquilizing beverage; it has been used to treat mild anxiety and sleep disturbances.[a] A meta-analysis comparison of kava extract WS 1490 with a placebo reported efficacy (odds ratio 3.3 [95% CI 2.09–5.22]); however, the differences in the Hamilton Anxiety (HAM-A) scores overall were not significant. Women and younger patients showed the most improvement.[b] In 2002, the Center for Food Safety and Nutrition issued a warning advising consumers and professionals of the risk of severe liver injury associated with kava-containing supplements. Germany, Switzerland, Canada, Australia, and France have restricted the sale of kava products in response to case reports of liver failure associated with use.[c] Several factors as to the origin of liver injury are in question. These factors include aqueous versus acetone or ethanol extracts, continuous high doses, inappropriate raw products, and potential contaminants. No updates to the consumer advisory have been made.[d] Until further data that identify the cause of liver injuries are available, patients should avoid taking kava.

[a] Sarris J, LaPorte E, Schweitzer I. Kava: a comprehensive review of efficacy, safety, and psychopharmacology. *Aust N Z J Psychiatry.* 2011;45(1): 27–35. doi: 10.3109/00048674.2010.522554.

[b] Witte S, Loew D, Gaus W. Meta-analysis of the efficacy of the acetonic kava-kava extract WS1490 in patients with non-psychotic anxiety disorders. *Phytother Res.* 2005;19(3):183–8. doi: 10.1002/ptr.1609.

[c] Centers for Disease Control and Prevention. Hepatic toxicity possibly associated with kava-containing products—United States, Germany, and Switzerland, 1999–2002. *MMWR Morb Mortal Wkly Rep.* 2002;51(47):1065–7. Available at: https://www.cdc.gov/mmwr/preview/mmwrhtml/mm5147a1.htm. Accessed June 25, 2017.

[d] Teschke R, Lebot V. Proposal for a kava quality standardization code. *Food Chem Toxicol.* 2011;49(10):2503–16. doi: 10.1016/j.fct.2011.06.075.

Summary of Clinical Evidence

A meta-analysis of 18 randomized, placebo-controlled trials evaluated the effect of valerian on insomnia. Eight trials were of high quality. Subjective improvements were reported for insomnia, although the overall effectiveness of valerian could not be assessed.[91] A study of older adults found *V. officinalis* to be inferior to temazepam or diphenhydramine.[92]

DIGESTIVE SYSTEM

Ginger

Ginger (*Zingiber officinale*) is a perennial from the Zingiberaceae family whose rhizomes and roots are used medicinally.

Therapeutic Uses

The primary use of ginger has been to relieve nausea and vomiting associated with pregnancy, motion sickness, chemotherapy, and surgery. Ginger has also been used for indigestion, colic, and arthritis.

Physiologic Activity

Ginger rhizomes possess a volatile oil that contains sesquiterpene hydrocarbons, including zingiberene and alpha curcumene with lesser amounts of farnesene, beta sesquiphellandrene, and beta bisabolene. Ginger also contains an oleoresin with nonvolatile pungent components, including gingerol, shogaols, and zingerone. Galanolactone, a diterpenoid isolated from ginger, and 6-shogaol have anti-5-hydroxytriptamine activity in the GI tract, which possibly contributes to ginger's antiemetic activity. Ginger does not affect GI motility or increase gastric emptying. The 6-shogaol and 6-gingerol components inhibit cyclooxygenase (COX) and lipoxygenase pathways, resulting in anti-inflammatory actions and potential inhibition of platelet thromboxane.[93]

Dosage and Product Considerations

Dried ginger 250 mg taken 4 times daily has been used for nausea and vomiting in pregnancy. For motion sickness, a typical dosage is 500 mg of dried powdered ginger root taken 30 minutes before travel, followed by 1–2 additional 500 mg capsules as needed every 4 hours. Daily dosages greater than 4 g should be avoided.

Safety Considerations

Mild heartburn and belching have been reported with ginger. Ginger may increase the risk of hypoglycemia.[65] Ginger may alter platelet function at dosages greater than 1 g/day.[63] Although findings are mixed, ginger should be used with caution by individuals also taking antithrombotic agents.

Randomized controlled trials have not identified significant adverse effects on pregnancy outcomes between ginger and placebo or pyridoxine.[94,95] A large Norwegian population-based cohort study found no increase in malformations, fetal death, premature birth, low birth weight, or Apgar scores below 7. About 45% ingested ginger during the first trimester, although timing of exposure and dosing was lacking. A small, but significant, increase in vaginal bleeding was noted after week 17 (7.8% vs. 5.8%) compared with controls.[96]

Summary of Clinical Evidence

Mixed results have been found for ginger's efficacy in the management of postoperative and chemotherapy-induced nausea and vomiting. A meta-analysis evaluated a fixed dose of ginger in the management of postoperative nausea and vomiting providing evidence that at least 1 g of ginger was effective.[97] A systematic review of five randomized, controlled trials encompassing more than 800 subjects compared ginger with metoclopramide or placebo for treatment of chemotherapy-induced nausea and vomiting. Ginger did not control the severity or incidence of acute nausea.[98] Other studies support its value as an adjunct in patients receiving highly emetogenic chemotherapy demonstrating a significant delay and reduction in severity of symptoms when ginger powder or oil capsules were used in addition to ondansetron and dexamethasone.[99,100]

A systematic review and meta-analysis of pregnancy-induced nausea and vomiting evaluated 12 randomized controlled clinical trials. Studies varied in size, dosage of ginger, duration, and comparative treatments (placebo, pyridoxine, dimenhydrinate, or metoclopramide). Use of ginger in early pregnancy improved symptoms of nausea, but not overall vomiting episodes compared with placebo. In comparison to pyridoxine, no differences were noted from two studies included in the meta-analysis. Daily dosages of less than 1500 mg were most effective.[95] A Cochrane review concluded that ginger may have a role in early pregnancy for nausea and vomiting.[101] The American College of Obstetricians and Gynecologists (ACOG) practice guidelines includes ginger as an option with beneficial effects as level evidence B, suggesting limited or inconsistent evidence, in treating nausea and vomiting in pregnancy.[102] As the effectiveness of ginger for hyperemesis gravidarum is limited, ginger should not be recommended for this condition.

Milk Thistle

Silybum marianum, or milk thistle, is a member of the Asteraceae/Compositae family.

Therapeutic Uses

Milk thistle has been used to treat liver disease, including hepatitis and cirrhosis. In Europe, it is used to treat poisoning by the mushroom *Amanita phalloides* (death cap). Milk thistle has been used as a liver protective agent for exposure to alcohol, acetaminophen, and carbon tetrachloride.

Physiologic Activity

Milk thistle's seeds and fruit, and to a lesser extent, the leaves and stems contain several compounds, collectively referred to as silymarin. Three major flavonolignans include silybin, silydianin, and silychristin.[103] These biologically active compounds may have antioxidant, antifibrotic, and anti-inflammatory activity, in addition to other beneficial effects such as regulation of cell permeability and inhibition of mitochondrial injury. Stimulation of nucleolar polymerase A, resulting in increased ribosomal protein synthesis, stimulates liver regeneration and the formation of new hepatocytes. The antioxidant properties of silymarin may be the primary beneficial effect.

Dosage and Product Considerations

The average dosage is silymarin 150 mg taken 3 times daily for cirrhosis and silybin (silibinin) 240 mg twice daily for hepatitis. Milk thistle preparations contain varying amounts of a concentrated seed extract, standardized to flavonolignans 70%–80% calculated as silymarin; approximately 70% is silybin. Multiple products of silymarin and silybin have been used in clinical studies, but they may not be available in the United States, even with identical standardization. Liver disease resulting from alcohol, acetaminophen, and other drugs or chemicals is potentially fatal, and patients should be cautioned against self-treatment with milk thistle.

Safety Considerations

Milk thistle is generally well tolerated. Pregnant women and patients with an allergy to ragweed and other members of the Asteraceae/Compositae family should avoid the use of milk thistle. The product may stimulate lactation, although evidence is limited.[104] Most, but not all, studies indicate that milk thistle does not inhibit several CYP isoenzymes and P-glycoprotein, thereby reducing the likelihood of drug interactions.[66]

Summary of Clinical Evidence

Evidence to support the use of milk thistle in liver disease is limited. A Cochrane review of 18 randomized controlled studies investigated its effect on liver disease caused by alcohol or hepatitis B or C viral infection. Reductions in mortality or complications of liver disease or changes in liver histology were not identified. Liver-related mortality was significantly reduced with inclusion of all trials but not in the 5 high-quality trials.[105] In a randomized, placebo-controlled trial of patients with chronic hepatitis C virus who did not respond to interferon therapy, treatment consisted of either 420 mg or 700 mg of silymarin daily for 6 months; the results did not demonstrate reduction in serum alanine aminotransferase levels, hepatitis C virus RNA levels, or changes in quality of life.[106] Milk thistle has not been compared with the new treatments for hepatitis C and should never be used in place of antiviral therapy.

Peppermint

Mentha piperita, or peppermint, is a member of the mint family Lamiaceae. It has been cultivated for its fragrant volatile oil, which is extracted primarily from leaves of the plant.

Therapeutic Uses

Both peppermint leaf and oil have been used for treatment of irritable bowel syndrome (IBS), nonulcerative dyspepsia, colonic spasm, and tension headache.

Physiologic Activity

The activity of peppermint may be a result of its 0.5%–4% essential oil. The oil or leaf preparations should be standardized to contain not less than 44% menthol. Menthol stereoisomers are also present, including 3% *d*-neomenthol and menthone, menthofuran, eucalyptol, and limonene. The mechanism of action of peppermint involves direct relaxation of GI smooth muscle.

Dosage and Product Considerations

The usual dosage of peppermint oil enteric-coated capsules for IBS is 0.2–0.4 mL (187–374 mg) taken 3 times daily 15–30 minutes before meals. Enteric-coated preparations reduce risk of heartburn. Clinical trials have studied 8–16 mL of peppermint oil solution as an antispasmodic.[107]

Safety Considerations

Heartburn may be attributed to relaxation of the lower esophageal sphincter. Patients who have severe preexisting gastroesophageal conditions should avoid use of peppermint oil. Peppermint leaf tea or topical products should be used with caution in infants and small children because of possible laryngeal and bronchial spasms from volatilized menthol. The oil may also irritate mucous membranes. Data suggest that peppermint may decrease activity of CYP3A4 for drugs such as felodipine.[66] The ingestion of peppermint may decrease absorption of iron.[33] Antacids or other medications that increase stomach pH may affect dissolution of enteric-coated capsules.

Summary of Clinical Evidence

A systematic review and meta-analysis of nine studies with enteric-coated peppermint oil capsule demonstrated short-term safety and efficacy in patients with IBS. Significant differences were found in global improvement of IBS symptoms (RR 2.23 [95% CI 1.78–2.81], 392 patients) and another abdominal pain (RR 2.14 [95% CI 1.64–2.79], 357 patients) compared with placebo.[108] A higher rate of adverse events were reported in the peppermint oil groups, with heartburn the most common symptom.

ENDOCRINE SYSTEM

Alpha Lipoic Acid

Therapeutic Uses

Alpha lipoic acid, or thioctic acid, is an endogenous antioxidant promoted for diabetes. Both intravenous (I.V.) and oral dosage forms have been studied for diabetic peripheral neuropathy.

Physiologic Activity

Alpha lipoic acid, synthesized from linoleic acid, is a cofactor for glucose metabolism enzymes. Small amounts exist in plant and animal sources with the greatest amounts occurring attached to lysine in spinach and broccoli.[109] Alpha lipoic acid has both hydrophilic and lipophilic properties. These allow it to serve as an antioxidant within both lipid membranes and aqueous environments, in constant regenerative balance with its reduced form, dihydrolipoic acid. Alpha lipoic acid acts on glucose transporters and stimulates glucose uptake by various mechanisms, including effects on glucose transporter-1 (GLUT-1) and GLUT-4 receptors. In addition to improved nerve conduction and blood flow, human studies have shown improvement in insulin sensitivity and oral glucose tolerance tests.[109,110]

Dosage and Product Considerations

With oral bioavailability of 30%, 600 mg taken 3 times daily is comparable to the 600 mg I.V. dosage used in many European trials for diabetic neuropathy.[109,110] Food decreases absorption, so alpha lipoic acid should be taken on an empty stomach.[111] It must be separated 2–3 hours from antacids or other mineral-containing supplements because of its chelating activity.[111]

Safety Considerations

Adverse effects are mild and include headache, nausea, diarrhea, and rash. Patients who wish to add alpha lipoic acid to antidiabetic treatments should first discuss its use with their HCP. More frequent monitoring of glucose concentrations is advised during initial weeks of therapy as additive hypoglycemic effects may occur. Alpha lipoic acid can inhibit conversion of thyroxine to triiodothyronine and may displace thyroxine from serum-binding protein; patients with thyroid conditions should avoid this supplement.

Summary of Clinical Evidence

Evidence for oral alpha lipoic acid for diabetic neuropathy is somewhat contradictory. Three meta-analyses concluded that I.V. and oral supplementation is beneficial, with improvement in total symptom scores, neuropathy impairment scores, and short-term symptoms of pain and parathesia.[112–114] A 2-year study found improvements in nerve conduction but not neuropathic symptoms. [112–114] The largest (N= 460), most rigorous study of 4 years suggested alpha lipoic acid may be more useful in preventing progression of neuropathy rather than acute pain treatment.[115] A study comparing alpha lipoic acid to carbamazepine and pregabalin noted pain severity on a visual analog scale (VAS) score was significantly improved from baseline for alpha lipoic acid and pregabalin.[116] A 4-month trial found patients who significantly responded to 4 weeks of 600 mg alpha lipoic acid taken 3 times daily were able to maintain benefits when taking 600 mg once daily.[117] At the lower dosage, burning pain and paresthesias continued to improve; week 20 scores were significantly improved over week 4, while numbness and lancinating pain scores were similar to week 4. Alpha lipoic acid may be considered a treatment option for diabetic neuropathy.

In several neuropathy trials, the reductions in glucose and hemoglobin have not been significant.[112–114] Two recent small trials documented clinically significant lowering of fasting blood glucose (~29 mg/mL) and hemoglobin A1C (–0.6%) when alpha lipoic acid was added to standard antidiabetic medications.[118,119] A dose-response was present, with 1200 mg/day providing the most benefit. Although a recommendation for glucose control cannot be made, alpha lipoic acid's good safety profile supports its use in individual patients.

Cinnamon (*Cinnamomum cassia* or *C. aromaticum*)

Therapeutic Uses

Cinnamon, specifically *Cinnamomum cassia,* the type most commonly found in grocery spice aisles, is used to help lower blood glucose.

Physiologic Activity

Both *C. cassia* and true cinnamon (also known as Ceylon cinnamon, *Cinnamomum verum,* or *Cinnamomum zeylanicum*), have components with differing mechanisms of action to affect glucose and have had similar results in preclinical studies.[120,121] A proanthocyanidin, cinnamtannin B1, is involved in triggering autophosphorylation of the insulin receptor to increase insulin sensitivity.[121] Cinnamaldehyde increases cellular glucose uptake by stimulating GLUT-1 and GLUT-4 receptors.[121] Water-soluble extracts of both *C. cassia* and *C. verum* activate peroxisome proliferator-activated receptor alpha (PPAR-alpha) and PPAR-gamma in a manner similar to that of pioglitazone and display inhibition of amylase and sucrose.[121] Whole cinnamon may delay gastric emptying. Cinnamon inhibits inactivation of insulin receptors by tyrosine phosphatase, and anti-inflammatory actions occur through changes in multiple cytokines involved in the inflammatory process.[120]

Dosage and Product Considerations

The dosage of aqueous extract, the form that may be most effective, is 0.5–1 g/day of *C. cassia* or *C. verum.* The dosage of ground cinnamon (*C. cassia*) is 2–6 g given in divided doses, either in capsules or in food. A half-teaspoonful is approximately 1 g.[122]

Safety Considerations

Patients should not confuse cinnamon supplements with cinnamon oil, as hypersensitivity reactions to the oil can occur, as well as pediatric poisoning from ingestion.[122] Other than an allergic reaction of rash, no adverse events have been reported in trials lasting up to 4 months. One case report exists of probable medication-induced hepatitis; cinnamon is known to contain coumarins (much greater amounts in *C. cassia* than in *C. verum*) that can be hepatotoxic.[123] Potentiation of hypoglycemic reactions in patients on antihyperglycemic medications is theoretically possible.

Summary of Clinical Evidence

Cinnamomum verum has not received the same evaluations as *C. cassia* and its use is more controversial. One clinical trial of *C. verum* found no effect on glucose or insulin levels, while a human laboratory study did note reductions in the postprandial glycemia AUC.[124,125]

Clinical trials of *C. cassia* have had contradictory results for glucose control. Some results may be associated with differences in the dosage or dosage form with negative trials using 1–1.5 g/day, and positive trials using 3–6 g/day or equivalent aqueous extract.[126–128] A well-designed trial of 2 g/day of ground cinnamon added to standard antidiabetic medications reduced mean hemoglobin A1C from 8.22% to 7.86% after 12 weeks, significantly greater than placebo.[129] A 3-month trial of low doses of cinnamon aqueous extract (120 and 360 mg/day) added to sulfonylurea therapy significantly reduced fasting glucose and hemoglobin A1C levels compared with placebo.[130]

Overall, the evidence indicates that the effect size of cinnamon on fasting plasma glucose or hemoglobin A1C is small.[127] The favorable safety profile suggests that cinnamon could be considered for adjunctive therapy in some patients, especially those attempting to control blood glucose through lifestyle changes.

IMMUNE MODULATORS

Echinacea

Echinacea species include *Echinacea purpurea, Echinacea angustifolia,* and *Echinacea pallida.* Roots, leaves, and flowers are all used medicinally. Depending on the species, the above-ground parts may have more activity.

Therapeutic Uses

Echinacea is used to prevent and treat colds and other respiratory infections.

Physiologic Activity

Echinacea has multiple components targeting the nonspecific cellular immune system, including alkylamides, caffeic acid derivatives such as chicoric acid, flavonoids, glycoproteins, and polysaccharides. Multiple mechanisms of action are involved, including increased cytokine secretion, lymphocyte activity, and phagocytosis. Direct inactivation of viruses, bacteria, and fungi has been observed.[131] Anti-inflammatory activities and decreases in mucin production are likely responsible for decreased symptoms of upper respiratory infections.[131] Some of the immunostimulatory activity of echinacea is caused by the lipopolysaccharides and xanthienopyran from the endophytic bacteria that live within the plant.[132] The activity is lost when extracts from plants grown from sterilized seed are used. The bacterial load may vary between plants, and the extraction processes may affect the content of these components, which may explain the varied results from clinical trials.

Dosage and Product Considerations

Products labeled "echinacea" may be chemically different plants or plant parts, making comparisons difficult. The optimal standardization and dosage of echinacea is unknown. Standardized concentrates, such as Echinaforce, generally perform better in trials. Echinacea is available in single- and multi-ingredient formulations such as teas, extracts, juices, throat sprays, capsules, and tablets; each formulation has its own dosing regimen. Many echinacea products in the United States are less concentrated or are labeled for use at lower dosages than used in trials and may be ineffective if used as directed. For the greatest efficacy, all formulations must be taken at the first sign of illness.

Safety Considerations

Allergic reactions may occur. Patients with a history of asthma or atopy should avoid echinacea; a severe allergy to the Asteraceae/Compositae family, which includes ragweed and chrysanthemums, is a contraindication. Adverse effects include mild GI discomfort, tingling sensation of the tongue with liquid preparations, and headache. More serious reactions are possible; one patient developed acute cholestatic hepatitis after taking an echinacea root product for 5 days while ill with a flu-like syndrome.[133] The hepatitis resolved quickly after echinacea was stopped. Use of echinacea should be avoided in patients with severe systemic illnesses such as human immunodeficiency virus (HIV) infection or acquired immunodeficiency syndrome (AIDS), multiple sclerosis, tuberculosis, and autoimmune disorders, and in patients taking immunosuppressants, although this concern is based on case reports and theory.[134] Echinacea exhibits some effects on P-glycoprotein transport and several intestinal and hepatic CYP450 systems and except for drugs with a narrow therapeutic range, these effects are not likely to be significant.[135] A systematic review of echinacea use during pregnancy found no increase in the rates of major malformations.[136]

Summary of Clinical Evidence

Individual trials for either treatment or prevention of colds or upper respiratory infections have had widely variable results, making conclusions difficult. In part, this may be a result of disparate dosages, concentrations, plant species and parts, or extraction methods used for the study products. For prevention, a 2015 meta-analysis examining the effect of echinacea on the risk of recurrent infections when used continuously for 2–4 months or in repetitive 10-day treatments over 4 months concluded that treatment resulted in a 35% decrease in the risk of recurrent infections compared with placebo ($P < 0.0001$).[137]

For treatment, the evidence is also mixed. A 2007 meta-analysis of 14 randomized placebo-controlled studies found a significant reduction in duration of 1.4 days, and the risk of cold development was reduced by 58%.[138] The most recent Cochrane review determined that treatment data was so heterogeneous that pooling could not be performed and concluded effects were of questionable clinical relevance.[139] Further study will have to determine the true effectiveness of treatment, but current treatment data does indicate that best results occur when echinacea is administered at the first sign of symptoms.

Echinacea's immunostimulatory effects were tested in a pilot study in adults with respiratory disease that compared rates of influenza- and parainfluenza-like symptoms and respiratory complications. Groups were prophylactically given flu vaccine, a hydroalcoholic root extract of *E. angustifolia* roots, or both. Rates of symptoms were decreased for echinacea-only and echinacea+vaccine groups compared with the vaccine-alone group.[140] Parainfluenza-like symptoms occurred in 5 patients in the vaccine-only group and in only 1 patient in each of the echinacea-only and echinacea+vaccine groups.

Elderberry

Therapeutic Uses

Juice or extracts of the *Sambucus nigra* berry are used primarily for prevention or treatment of influenza and other upper respiratory illnesses.

Physiologic Activity

Elderberries contain vitamins C, B_2, B_6, folic acid, and beta carotene, among others, as well as multiple flavonoids and anthocyanins.[141] The activities of elderberry include inhibition of replication of viruses, increased production of anti-inflammatory and inflammatory cytokines, strong antioxidant capacity, increased viral antibodies, and inhibition of hemagglutination of the influenza virus, which prevents entry into cells.[141] Liquid extracts have inhibited growth of several gram-positive and gram-negative bacteria.[142]

Dosage and Product Considerations

Clinical trials have been performed with at least 4 elderberry dosage forms: a spray-dried elderberry juice (400 mg given 3 times daily, 10% anthocyanins), a syrup standardized to flavonoid content (Sambucol), an encapsulated extract (125 mg anthocyanin), and an infusion prepared daily from dried elderberries.[143–145] The optimal standardization and dosage form has not been determined.

Safety Considerations

Commercially available elderberry extracts are well tolerated, with few adverse effects reported.[144,145] Insufficiently cooked or unripe berries, stems, or leaves contain cyanogenic glycosides, which are metabolized in the GI tract to cyanide; reports exist of not only nausea and vomiting, but dizziness, weakness, and stupor with home-prepared juices and extracts.[146] See Table 51–2 for possible drug interactions.

Summary of Clinical Evidence

The first study of elderberry extract (Sambucol) used 30 mL (15 mL for children) daily for 3 days in patients reporting symptoms during an outbreak of influenza B. The duration of fever was 4 days versus 6 days in the treatment and placebo groups, respectively. After 3 days, a complete cure was noted in 46.7% of elderberry-treated patients and 16.7% in the placebo group.[143] The second study (N = 60), during an influenza A epidemic, used a VAS to assess symptom improvement and found that elderberry-treated patients reached scores closer to pronounced improvement (10 on the 0–10 scale) within 3–4 days, whereas placebo-treated patients reached similar scores after 7–8 days.[147] Rescue medications including a nasal spray and analgesic were used by 21 and 26 patients, respectively, in the placebo group and by 5 and 7 patients in the elderberry group.

A combination elderberry and echinacea hot drink product was tested against oseltamivir in a randomized, double-dummy noninferiority trial of 473 patients with clinically diagnosed influenza.[148] Alleviation of symptoms was similar at 5 or 10 days: 50.2% versus 48.8%, and 90.1% versus 84.8% in the hot drink and oseltamivir groups, respectively. A subanalysis of patients with laboratory-confirmed influenza noted noninferiority at days 5 and 10, and the hot drink group experienced significantly greater recovery at day 10 than the oseltamivir group, 95% versus 76.2%, respectively. Complication rates were 2.5% and 6.5% in the hot drink and oseltamivir groups. With its mild adverse effect profile, elderberry extracts may be an appropriate option for individual patients.

PHYSICAL AND MENTAL PERFORMANCE ENHANCERS

Eleuthero (Siberian Ginseng)

Eleutherococcus senticosus from the Araliaceae family is often referred to as *Acanthopanax senticosus* or Siberian ginseng. The plant is not a genus of *Panax*, as are Asian and American ginseng species. *Eleutherococcus* is found in eastern Siberia, northeastern China, Korea, and Hokkaido Island in Japan.

Therapeutic Uses

Eleuthero's traditional use is as an adaptogen for improvement of athletic performance, chronic stress, upper respiratory conditions, and immune deficiency. Other uses include treatment of herpes simplex type 2 infections, blood pressure, prevention of atherosclerosis, and diabetes mellitus.

Physiologic Activity

The active compounds of eleuthero, derived primarily from the root and leaf, are referred to as eleutherosides (subtypes A to M). Flavonoids, hydroxycinnamates, and other constituents such as sesamin, B-sitosterol, hederasaponin B, and isofraxidin may also have biological activity. Animal studies and in vitro analysis suggest these compounds have antiplatelet, immunostimulant, and antioxidant properties.[149]

Dosage and Product Considerations

Commercial products are often standardized to eleutheroside B and/or E content at a dosage of 300–400 mg/day. A 33% ethanolic extract 10 mL taken 3 times daily has also been used. After 2 months of daily use, patients should discontinue the product for a minimum of 2 weeks.[149]

Safety Considerations

Both drowsiness and stimulant effects have been reported with eleuthero. Because of its variable effects on blood pressure, eleuthero should be avoided in patients with hypertension.

Theoretically, patients with diabetes mellitus should be monitored for hypoglycemia.[149] Safety data are lacking for use during pregnancy and lactation. In patients taking digoxin, eleuthero may interfere with digoxin assays because of structural likeness of its glycosides.[66]

Summary of Clinical Evidence

Well-designed, randomized clinical trials documenting the safety and efficacy of eleuthero are lacking. In one study, 144 subjects were assigned 120 mg/day *E. senticosus* root extract, professional stress management training, or combination of both. Participants suffered from chronic stress and fatigue resulting in impaired work capacity. All treatment groups improved similarly from baseline at weeks 2 and 8 in most parameters related to performance and stress; mental fatigue and alertness were significantly better in the combination therapy compared with eleuthero alone.[150]

In a small 6-month study, *Eleutherococcus* extract taken once daily demonstrated a beneficial effect on frequency, severity, and duration of herpes simplex type 2 infections.[151] Other double-blind, placebo-controlled studies have evaluated eleuthero in fixed combination with andrographis for upper respiratory tract infections.[152] Improvements have been demonstrated on most symptoms; cough only improved in the study with a combination product including echinacea purpurea.[149,152,153]

Asian Ginseng (*Panax ginseng*)

The root and rhizome of Asian ginseng (*P. ginseng* C. A. Meyer) is from the family Araliaceae and is exported primarily from Korea, China, and Japan.

Therapeutic Uses

Asian ginseng has been used to improve mental and physical stress, anemia, diabetes mellitus, immune response, insomnia, and impotence, and for cancer prevention.

Physiologic Activity

The constituents likely responsible for ginseng's adaptogen activity are triterpenoid saponins, including ginsenosides. At least 30 ginsenosides, also referred to as panaxosides, have been identified. Additional constituents include carbohydrates, B vitamins, and flavonoids.[154]

Dosage and Product Considerations

Ginseng extracts are standardized to 4% ginsenosides administered at 200 mg/day in divided doses. Crude powdered root has been used in dosages of 2–3 g/day. Decoctions and tea preparations are also commonly used.[154]

Safety Considerations

Adverse effects include insomnia, headache, blood pressure changes, anorexia, rash, mastalgia, and menstrual abnormalities. Large dosages can result in gastric upset and CNS stimulation. Ginseng should be used with caution in patients with cardiovascular disease, diabetes mellitus, or acute illness. Ginseng abuse and misuse has been described in ginseng users and prolonged use is not recommended.[155] Ginseng should not be used during pregnancy or lactation because of a lack of data and concern about its potential estrogenic effects.[156] Several potential drug interactions are listed in Table 51–2.[65,66,154]

Summary of Clinical Evidence

A systematic review of four randomized controlled trials of ginseng in patients with type 2 diabetes mellitus found an overall lack of an effect on fasting blood glucose, hemoglobin A1C, or 2-hour postprandial glucose.[157] A second systematic review and meta-analysis of 16 trials, involving both diabetic and healthy subjects, evaluated various measures of glucose control. Significant improvements were noted in fasting glucose, but not in hemoglobin A1C values or insulin resistance.[158]

For erectile dysfunction, a systematic review of seven randomized controlled trials found significant benefit with Asian ginseng, although the review noted limitations of a small sample size and trial quality.[159]

Five trials were included in a Cochrane review of the role of *P. ginseng* for cognition; the majority of subjects were healthy with cognitive impairment or dementia. The data could not be pooled because of varied dosing regimens, outcomes, and study durations. Although ginseng improved some end points related to cognitive function, quality of life, and behavior, the overall evidence does not support its use.[160] A systematic review and meta-analysis of 4 randomized, controlled trials of ginseng in patients with AD in addition to standard treatments did not identify a benefit.[161]

Green Tea

Native to southeastern Asia, the tea shrub *Camellia sinensis* belongs to the family Theaceae. Tea leaves are heated immediately after harvesting and then mechanically rolled and crushed before drying to produce green tea. Black tea is produced by allowing the leaves to wilt before they are rolled and left in a humid environment for several hours. This process promotes fermentation and a gradual change in color to reddish-brown. Oolong, another commonly available tea, is a partially fermented tea.

Therapeutic Uses

Green tea is considered a performance enhancer because of the stimulant effect from caffeine. Green tea has also been used to prevent cardiovascular disease, cancer, and liver disorders.

Physiologic Activity

In addition to caffeine, green tea contains polyphenolic compounds including flavonols, also known as catechins, flavonoids, and phenolic acids. The most prevalent flavonols include epicatechin, epicatechin-3-gallate, epigallocatechin, and epigallocatechin-3-gallate (or EGCG). These components have antioxidant and antitumor effects.[162] Catechins and caffeine may each contribute to weight loss.[163]

Dosage and Product Considerations

Dosages of green tea in epidemiologic studies vary between 1 and 10 cups daily. The preferred dosage is 3–5 cups daily, or up to 1200 mL/day, including a minimum of 250 mg/day of catechins.[164] Green tea extract supplements are standardized to polyphenol content and retain effects similar to those of green tea while reducing exposure to caffeine.[162]

Safety Considerations

Ingestion of large quantities of green tea can cause adverse GI symptoms as well as CNS and cardiac stimulation because of the caffeine content. One 8-ounce cup of green tea contains 24–40 mg of caffeine. In comparison, an 8-ounce cup of black tea has 14–61 mg of caffeine and an 8-ounce cup of coffee can range from 95–200 mg on average.[165] Green tea should be avoided if other stimulating drugs are ingested. Green tea extracts have been associated with liver toxicity.[166] Serum folate levels have been reduced by green tea.[66] As a result, green tea should be used cautiously during pregnancy and lactation because of caffeine consumption and potential folic acid concerns. Green tea in large dosages may antagonize the effects of warfarin because of small amounts of vitamin K.[65]

Summary of Clinical Evidence

Epidemiologic data suggest that daily consumption of green tea may protect against cardiovascular and metabolic diseases.[167]

A WORD ABOUT

Kratom

The leaves of kratom (*Mitragyna speciosa*), a Southeast Asian tree, were historically used for pain treatment, but current use is primarily recreational. The major alkaloid mitragynine is psychoactive and has opioid-like properties; heroin addicts in Malaysia will sometimes use kratom as a substitute although it is also highly addictive.[a] Despite being illegal in a number of countries, kratom has become a recreational drug option, easily obtainable over the Internet or locally as an "herbal incense." Reported adverse effects of kratom include cases of cholestatic hepatitis and acute cholecystitis, as well as incidences of increased blood pressure, kidney toxicity, impaired cognition, cardiotoxicity, primary hypothyroidism, liver failure, seizures, and coma.[b–d] When combined with O-desmethyltramadol in the drug called "krypton," death has resulted. A number of drug metabolic and pharmacodynamic drug interactions are possible. Potentially beneficial activities of mitragynine are being investigated in animal studies, but currently its use cannot be recommended.

[a] Singh D, Müller CP, Vicknasingam BK, et al. Social functioning of kratom (*Mitragyna speciosa*) users in Malaysia. *J Psychoactive Drugs.* 2015; 47(2):125–31. doi: 10.1080/02791072.2015.1012610.

[b] Arens A, Gerona R, Meier K, Smollin C. Acute cholecystitis associated with kratom abuse. *Clin Toxicol.* 2015;53(7):661.

[c] Cinosi E, Martinotti G, Simonato P, et al. Following "the roots" of kratom (*Mitragyna speciosa*): the evolution of an enhancer from a traditional use to increase work and productivity in Southeast Asia to a recreational psychoactive drug in Western countries. *Biomed Res Int.* 2015:968786. doi: 10.1155/2015/968786.

[d] Ulbricht C, Costa D, Dao J, et al. An evidence-based systematic review of kratom (*Mitragyna speciosa*) by the Natural Standard Research Collaboration. *J Diet Suppl.* 2013;10(2):152–70. doi: 10.3109/19390211.2013.793541.

Green and black teas were evaluated for primary prevention of cardiovascular disease by the Cochrane Heart Group.[168] Seven randomized, controlled trials were included with green tea or green tea extract as intervention for at least 3 months. A significant reduction in TC and LDL-cholesterol levels was noted, as well as small reduction in mean SBP (–3.18 mm Hg [95% CI –5.25, –1.11]) and DBP (–2.81 mm Hg [95% CI –3.77, –1.86]). Cardiovascular events were not reported, presumably because of the short durations of the studies. Another systematic review and meta-analysis of randomized, controlled trials evaluating green tea's effect on blood pressure and cholesterol reported similar findings.[169] A Cochrane review found that green tea products had no significant effects for weight loss and weight maintenance in obese patients.[163]

The consumption of green tea has been studied with regard to reducing the incidence of breast, prostate, lung, bladder, ovarian, digestive, and oral cancers. A Cochrane review of 51 studies that included 1.6 million subjects found conflicting evidence that green tea consumption affects overall cancer prevention.[164] Although some evidence has suggested a positive effect on prostate, lung, pancreatic, and colorectal cancers, many studies were observational in nature and performed in Asia where green tea consumption is high.

KIDNEY, URINARY TRACT, AND PROSTATE

African Plum

African plum is derived from the bark of *Prunus africana*, a member of the Rosaceae family.

Therapeutic Uses

Pygeum (African plum tree) bark has been used to treat benign prostatic hyperplasia (BPH).

Physiologic Activity

Pygeum bark contains phytosterols; pentacyclic triterpenes, including ursolic and oleanic acids; and ferulic acid esters, including docosanol and tetracosanol. Phytosterols may compete with androgen precursors and inhibit prostaglandin synthesis in the prostate. Triterpenes may have anti-inflammatory properties. Ferulic acid esters reduce concentrations of prolactin and prostate cholesterol, a precursor to testosterone synthesis.[170,171]

Dosage and Product Considerations

Products are standardized to contain 14% triterpenes and 0.5% *n*-docosanol; the average dosage is 50–100 mg twice daily.[170]

Safety Considerations

Adverse effects include diarrhea, constipation, and gastric pain. Men presenting with prostate symptoms should contact their HCP before starting pygeum to rule out prostate cancer. It is unclear if pygeum affects prostate-specific antigen concentrations.

Summary of Clinical Evidence

Pygeum has improved urinary flow, void volumes, residual volumes, nocturia, daytime frequency, and subjective symptom assessments of BPH. Larger studies that include standardized dosages, active comparisons, and adequate durations are needed to fully assess its efficacy.[172]

Cranberry

Cranberry (*Vaccinium macrocarpon*) is an evergreen bush native to North America and belongs to the family Ericaceae.

Therapeutic Uses

Cranberry has been used to prevent and treat urinary tract infections (UTIs).

Physiologic Activity

Cranberry contains proanthocyanidins, and epicatechin is the primary proanthocyanidin found in cranberry extracts. Evidence suggests that cranberry blocks bacteria, *Escherichia coli*, in particular, from adhering to bladder, kidneys, and urethra. Fructose found in cranberry juice may also alter bacterial adhesion.[173]

Dosage and Product Considerations

Many studies have used unsweetened cranberry juice. Cranberry juice cocktail is about 30% pure cranberry juice and contains sugar; it is unknown if this product will demonstrate the same effects. Efficacy may be based on the proanthocyanidin content. For prevention of UTI, the dosage of cranberry juice is 300–900 mL/day. Encapsulated cranberry formulations at a dosage of about 400 mg twice daily may be preferred to avoid the sugar content of juices.

Safety Considerations

Evidence suggests that regular use of cranberry concentrate tablets might increase risk of kidney stones. Patients may experience diarrhea with large daily doses.[65] Theoretically, cranberry juice may alter excretion of weakly alkaline drugs or neutralize effects of antacids. Case reports have suggested cranberry may cause bleeding in patients taking antithrombotic agents; pharmacokinetic and pharmacodynamic evidence has not supported this finding.[66,174]

Summary of Clinical Evidence

A Cochrane review of 24 studies, with 13 included in a meta-analysis, concluded preventive use of cranberry products does not significantly reduce the overall risk of UTIs or in subgroups of women or children with recurrent UTIs, older adults, pregnant women, cancer patients, and catheterized patients. The long-term use of cranberry, specifically juice, is not well tolerated, potentially resulting in high dropout rates in studies.[175] An additional consideration with negative studies is whether the tablet or capsule products contained adequate proanthocyanidins to be effective. Randomized, controlled studies published since the Cochrane review have reported usefulness in preventing UTIs in women with recurrent infections, high-risk of UTIs in long-term care settings, and after gynecological surgery requiring catheterization.[176–178] Cranberry products should not be used to treat UTIs, and instead patients should be referred to their HCP.[179]

Dehydroepiandrosterone

Therapeutic Uses

Dehydroepiandrosterone (DHEA) is a steroid hormone secreted by the adrenal cortex that declines with advancing age. Transformation to androgens and estrogens occurs in peripheral tissues and is regulated both systemically and locally.[180] The DS form of DHEA is marketed to treat sexual dysfunction or improve sexual performance, to combat physical and mental symptoms of aging, and to enhance athletic performance or increase muscle mass.

Physiologic Activity

In general, exogenous use of DHEA in women increases testosterone concentrations more than those of estrogen, whereas in men the reverse is true. The extent to which androgen and estrogen transformation occurs depends largely on a patient's baseline hormone concentrations. In women, route of administration and menopausal status affect transformation; more androgens than estrogens are formed in postmenopausal women.[181]

Dosage and Product Considerations

For most uses, the dosage is 25–100 mg once daily. Because of greater risk of serious adverse effects with dosages greater than 25 mg, patients should use larger dosages only under the guidance of an HCP.[182]

Most DHEA is synthetic, but some animal-extracted products exist and should be avoided because of the risk of contamination. Wild yam products are falsely promoted as DHEA or hormone precursors because wild yam contains diosgenin. This was once used by pharmaceutical manufacturers to produce estrogens and androgens, but the necessary chemical reactions do not occur in vivo. To further complicate patient education, some wild yam plants do contain very small amounts of naturally occurring DHEA.

Safety Considerations

The adverse effects of DHEA are sex hormone–related. Women may experience hirsutism, voice deepening (generally irreversible), increased acne, and menstrual changes, while men report gynecomastia and testicular changes. If hormone-associated adverse effects appear, DHEA should be discontinued. Other adverse effects include increases in liver function enzymes, prostate growth, and possibly HDL-C, and headache, nasal congestion, and insomnia.[183] At least four reports of mania requiring hospitalization exist, so DHEA is contraindicated in bipolar disorder and should be avoided in any mood disorder.[182] DHEA should be avoided by patients with a history of hormone-sensitive cancer, taking hormonal or hormone-blocking medications, or in pregnant or lactating women.

Summary of Clinical Evidence

Low levels of DHEA have been associated with a greater risk for erectile dysfunction (ED); however, evidence for the effectiveness of DHEA supplementation for ED is contradictory. In 2 trials, improvement was noted when the ED was caused by hypertension or unknown causes, but not when it was caused by diabetes mellitus or a neurologic disease.[184] Studies measuring outcomes such as arousal, desire, sexual activity, and ability to climax have had both positive and negative results.[180]

In healthy premenopausal women, oral DHEA does not improve sexual arousal or function.[185] In postmenopausal women, a small 1-year study of 10 mg/day DHEA found improvement on the McCoy Female Sexuality Questionnaire total scores, with increases in intercourse frequency.[186] Other studies in postmenopausal women have noted improvement in arousal, desire, sexual activity, and ability to climax with oral DHEA.[180]

In addition to sexual effects, low DHEA levels may be associated with decreased bone mineral density (BMD), higher fasting glucose levels, ischemic heart disease, and all-cause mortality in older men and women.[180] Treatment with DHEA generally increases hip and spine BMD (by 1.14% and 1.09%, respectively) in both men and women.[187] Strength and body composition may be improved in older men and women when DHEA supplementation is combined with exercise.[188,189] In addition, some study participants have observed improved skin health, such as increased epidermal thickness and sebum production with oral DHEA; topical use may also improve aging skin.[190]

Saw Palmetto

Saw palmetto (*Serenoa repens*), a dwarf palm tree from the Arecaceae family, is native to the southeast coastal region of the United States.

Therapeutic Uses

Saw palmetto has been used to treat BPH.

Physiologic Activity

The lipophilic extracts from the ripened fruit contain saturated and unsaturated fatty acids and plant sterols. Although the active compounds have not been identified, they are likely present in the lipophilic extract. Saw palmetto does not reduce prostate-specific antigen concentrations. Saw palmetto inhibits 5-alpha-reductase and cytosolic androgen receptor binding; it also has local antiestrogenic and anti-inflammatory effects on the prostate.[191]

Dosage and Product Considerations

The usual dosage is 160 mg twice daily or 320 mg once daily. Saw palmetto products should contain 80%–95% standardized fatty acids.

Safety Considerations

In comparative studies, saw palmetto was better tolerated than finasteride and tamsulosin. Mild GI complaints are most commonly reported, also fatigue and headache.[192] Although an 18-month study with 3 times the usual dosages of saw palmetto showed little toxicity, case reports of pancreatitis, hepatotoxicity, and coagulopathy have been reported.[193] Significant bleeding has been reported with saw palmetto, so its use in individuals taking antithrombotic agents should be avoided.[65] Patients taking androgenic drugs should also avoid its use. Men with prostate symptoms should contact their provider to rule out prostate cancer before starting saw palmetto. Saw palmetto is occasionally used in multi-ingredient products intended for women. Because of the inhibition of 5-alpha-reductase, it should be considered absolutely contraindicated in pregnancy and also should not be used in lactation.

Summary of Clinical Evidence

In a Cochrane review of 32 randomized controlled trials ranging from 4 to 72 weeks with more than 5000 men, saw palmetto was not effective for treating urinary symptoms, increasing peak urine flow, or reducing prostate size.[194] The meta-analysis included 2 high-quality trials of 582 men and based on the American Urological Association Symptom Score Index, demonstrated no difference in lower urinary tract symptoms for those taking saw palmetto compared with placebo. A 72-week study at 2–3 times the usual dose of 320 mg/day found insignificant differences in lower urinary tract symptoms, including nocturnal symptoms. Three high-quality trials assessing peak urine flow in 667 men also found no change compared with placebo. No difference was noted in prostate size after a 12-month trial. Overall, the evidence does not support use of saw palmetto for BPH symptoms.

MUSCULOSKELETAL SYSTEM

Glucosamine and Chondroitin

Therapeutic Uses

Glucosamine and chondroitin are commonly used together in supplements for osteoarthritis (OA) and joint health.

Physiologic Activity

Both glucosamine, an endogenous mucopolysaccharide, and chondroitin sulfate, a glycosaminoglycan, can serve as "building material" for cartilage production, in addition to other mechanisms of action. Glucosamine stimulates chondrocytes to produce cartilage and synoviocytes to produce synovial fluid and hyaluronic acid, inhibits matrix metalloproteinase, and modulates activities of inflammatory cytokines.[195] Glucosamine sulfate, as well as glucosamine sulfate/chondroitin sulfate, increases the receptor activator of nuclear factor kappa B ligand (NF-kappa B) to reduce bone resorption by osteoclasts more than glucosamine hydrochloride.[196]

Chondroitin sulfate inhibits leukocyte elastase, an enzyme involved in cartilage degradation, and bone resorption by osteoclasts, stimulates chondrocytes, reduces inflammation via inhibition of the translocation of NF-kappa B involved in activating B cells, and donates sulfur, essential for creation of the sulfur bonds used in cartilage synthesis.[197,198]

An in vivo pharmacoproteomics study determined that glucosamine and chondroitin used together have synergistic benefits on cartilage metabolism.[199] A meta-analysis of clinical studies has concluded that both long-term glucosamine sulfate and chondroitin use can slow progression of cartilage degradation in knee OA.[200]

Dosage and Product Considerations

For OA, the most common dosage is 1500 mg of glucosamine and 1200 mg of chondroitin sulfate daily, either once or in divided doses. This may be increased to 2000 mg of glucosamine and 1600 mg of chondroitin for larger individuals; greater amounts provide no additional benefit. If glucosamine monotherapy is desired, the sulfate salt should be used, rather than the hydrochloride, as the evidence is greater for efficacy. The daily dosages for glucosamine sulfate, glucosamine hydrochloride, or chondroitin monotherapy are the same as when used in combination. Products should be taken with food if nausea or GI upset occurs.

Neither glucosamine sulfate nor chondroitin sulfate, nor their combination, will provide pain relief as quickly as nonsteroidal anti-inflammatory drugs (NSAIDs) or acetaminophen, so concurrent analgesic therapy should be continued as needed. Effects may not be experienced for 6–8 weeks, with full benefits not evident for 4–6 months. If benefits are not noted after 6 months of therapy, discontinue therapy.

Both glucosamine sulfate and chondroitin sulfate are available in prescription-grade forms in Europe and these types have demonstrated greater success in clinical trials.[201] These forms are usually available in the United States only through Internet purchase; the products available on store shelves are of lower quality and the effect from treatment should be correspondingly lower. Patients using glucosamine and/or chondroitin should be encouraged to purchase only products displaying the USP Verified seal, tested by a third-party laboratory, or brands used in successful clinical trials.

Safety Considerations

Adverse effects include mild GI upset, nausea, diarrhea, and constipation for both components, which can often be alleviated by taking in divided doses with meals. Drowsiness, headache, and skin reactions have been infrequently reported with glucosamine, while allergic reactions, edema, nausea, heartburn, and hair loss have been reported with chondroitin sulfate. Chondroitin is often produced from bovine trachea, so there is a slight microbial contamination risk. Because trachea contains little neural tissue, risk of bovine spongiform encephalitis is minimal.

Glucosamine is manufactured from shellfish chitin or produced synthetically. Some products claim to be allergen-free, because processing removes allergenic material. Two studies tested this claim using shellfish-derived products and found no reactions in individuals with documented shellfish allergies.[202] Because source materials may change even for a particular manufacturer, patients with severe shellfish allergies should avoid glucosamine and use chondroitin monotherapy.

Pregnant or lactating women should avoid both glucosamine and chondroitin because of a lack of safety data. There are no known interactions.

Summary of Clinical Evidence

Glucosamine sulfate, glucosamine hydrochloride, and chondroitin sulfate have been examined separately with varying results. Currently, OA treatment guidelines from the Osteoarthritis Research Society International and the European League Against Rheumatism include pharmaceutical-grade crystalline glucosamine sulfate as an initial option, while the American College of Rheumatology does not differentiate between forms and considers glucosamine recommendations as premature.[196,203] The benefits of glucosamine sulfate treatment may extend beyond symptom reduction. When patients who had participated in two 3-year studies of a pharmaceutical-grade crystalline glucosamine sulfate product were followed for 5 years, there was a 57% reduction in the number of patients needing knee joint replacement compared with placebo.[203]

The overall evidence, including from the 2-year Glucosamine/Chondroitin Arthritis Intervention Trial (GAIT) funded by the National Institutes of Health and meta-analyses of other trials, does not support use of glucosamine hydrochloride monotherapy.[204,205] Chondroitin monotherapy decreases the rate of degradation of knee cartilage and reduces pain and stiffness in hand OA.[206,207]

The greatest benefits may be seen in combination treatment with either salt of glucosamine plus chondroitin. One trial of 606 patients with knee OA with moderate to severe pain compared glucosamine hydrochloride/chondroitin, 500/400 mg taken 3 times daily, to celecoxib 200 mg/day for 6 months.[208] The Western Ontario and McMaster Universities Arthritis Index (WOMAC) scores for pain, stiffness, and function were all decreased similarly at 6 months in the glucosamine hydrochloride/chondroitin and celecoxib groups respectively, 51.1% versus 50.2%, 46.9% versus 49.2%, and 45.5% versus 46.4%. The patient or physician global assessments were similar in the groups. In the first month, rescue medications were used more often by patients in the glucosamine hydrochloride/chondroitin group. After that period, use of rescue medications was similar between the groups.

The question of whether glucosamine sulfate/chondroitin is more efficacious than glucosamine hydrochloride/chondroitin was addressed in an open-label, noninferiority study involving 909 participants. The interventions were glucosamine sulfate/chondroitin sulfate given once daily (Artrolive 1500/1200 mg sachet) or 3 times daily (Artrolive 500/400 mg capsules) compared with glucosamine hydrochloride/chondroitin sulfate (Cosamin DS 500/400 mg capsules) given 3 times daily for 16 weeks.[209] At study end, all treatment groups had achieved significant reductions from baseline in pain VAS ($P = 0.001$), Lequesne Index scores ($P = 0.001$), and patient and physician global assessment VAS (both $P < 0.05$), with no differences between groups.

Glucosamine sulfate/chondroitin and glucosamine hydrochloride/chondroitin, products, chondroitin sulfate monotherapy, and crystalline glucosamine sulfate monotherapy should be considered as potential treatment options for patients with mild to moderate OA symptoms.

Methylsulfonylmethane

Therapeutic Uses

Methylsulfonylmethane (MSM) occurs naturally in foods and is a major metabolite of dimethylsulfoxide (DMSO), an industrial solvent. Arthritic workers began using DMSO topically, and MSM was developed in an attempt to avoid DMSO's toxicity and unpleasant adverse effects.[210] MSM is included in arthritis supplements despite little clinical evidence.

Physiologic Activity

Intestinal bacteria break down MSM to release sulfur, which is then incorporated into amino acids such as cysteine. Sulfur is essential for cartilage bonding and animal studies have found lower sulfur levels in arthritic cartilage. Preclinical studies have demonstrated anti-inflammatory effects such as reduced production of interleukin-6 (IL-6) and tumor necrosis factor alpha (TNFα), decreased cyclooxygenase-2 (COX-2) expression, and inhibition of NF-kappa B. MSM decreases apoptosis in macrophages, but with a biphasic response; higher doses may have detrimental effects.[211,212]

Dosage and Product Considerations

Dosages of MSM used in OA studies have varied from 1500 to 3000 mg/day in one or divided doses.[213] A patient choosing to use MSM should not exceed 3000 mg/day. MSM can be destroyed by water or excessive heat in the manufacturing process or during storage, so purchasing from a reliable manufacturer and proper storage are essential. Smaller amounts of MSM are common in combination products for OA.

Safety Considerations

Adverse effects include headache, pruritus, nausea, and diarrhea. Use in pregnancy and lactation should be avoided because of a lack of safety information. No drug interactions are known.

Summary of Clinical Evidence

One 12-week trial of 118 participants compared MSM with glucosamine sulfate, placebo, and the combination of MSM and glucosamine and reported significant improvement in pain and functioning in all groups but placebo. Improvement was greater in the combination group than with MSM or glucosamine alone.[213] A placebo-controlled pilot trial of 50 patients noted greater improvement with MSM.[213] A trial in 120 patients examined a combination of 5 g of MSM and 7.2 mg of boswellic acids daily compared with glucosamine sulfate 1500 mg/day.[214] Decreases in pain severity measured by VAS were significant for both groups, but not significantly different from each other. Other outcome results, such as Lequesne Index scores or maximum distance walked, followed a similar pattern. Overall, the evidence is insufficient to recommend MSM alone or in combination with other therapies.

S-Adenosyl-L-Methionine

Therapeutic Uses

S-Adenosyl-L-methionine (SAMe) is an endogenous substance formed from L-methionine and ATP. SAMe is marketed for OA and depression.

Physiologic Activity

SAMe is produced primarily in the liver. Liver disease and low vitamin B_{12} or folate levels may decrease concentrations.[215] For OA, SAMe stimulates chondrocytes to produce proteoglycans; reduces cartilage degradation enzymes, such as matrix metalloproteinase-3 in serum and synovial fluid; and has anti-inflammatory effects, such as decreased TNFα, and IL-1β.[215,216]

SAMe donates methyl groups to neurotransmitters and catecholamines. Neurotransmitter levels in the brain, including norepinephrine, dopamine, and serotonin, increase, which may contribute to its antidepressant effects.

Dosage and Product Considerations

Most OA trials used dosages of 400–800 mg/day in divided doses, whereas dosages for depression are 1200–1600 mg/day.[217]

Safety Considerations

Adverse effects include nausea, diarrhea, and heartburn. Less frequently, dry mouth, headache, dizziness, nervousness, insomnia, cognitive impairment, and a switch to mania in patients with bipolar disorder have been reported.[218] SAMe is also associated with hypomania or severe mania in subjects with no personal or family history of mania or bipolar disorder; one report of mixed mania with suicidal ideation occurred within 2 weeks.[219,220] These effects may be dose-related because mania and hypomania has not been reported with the lower dosages used in OA trials, but instead with higher dosages for depression. Patients who use SAMe for OA should take the lowest dosage providing relief and no more than 800 mg/day.

Use in pregnancy or lactation should be avoided. Potential drug interactions are listed in Table 51–2.

Summary of Clinical Evidence

Many early OA trials with positive results were of short duration and poor design and used injectable dosage forms or combinations of I.V. and oral therapies.[221] When oral SAMe was compared with NSAIDs or a COX-2 inhibitor, restoration of functionality and decreased pain were similar, although with slower onset.[222] A more rigorous trial compared SAMe 1200 mg/day to nabumetone.[223] Pain measured on a 40-mm VAS was significantly decreased to a similar extent in the SAMe (−13 mm) and nabumetone (−15.7 mm) groups at 8 weeks. The WOMAC score also decreased similarly in the SAMe and nabumetone groups (–6.9 mm and −9.3 mm, respectively; $P = 0.459$). Changes occurred more slowly in the SAMe group; the WOMAC change was only −3 mm at 4 weeks compared with –6.4 mm for nabumetone. A meta-analysis concluded that SAMe's clinical effects may be small.[221] Until additional information on adverse effects is available, SAMe should not be recommended.

Turmeric and Curcumin

The names curcumin and turmeric are often used interchangeably, especially for the spice used in cooking. Curcumin is the primary curcuminoid present in the turmeric plant, *Curcuma longa*.[224]

Therapeutic Uses

Turmeric extracts and curcumin are primarily used for arthritis and inflammatory conditions.

Physiologic Activity

Curcumin has anti-inflammatory activity via inhibition of arachidonic acid, lipoxygenase, COX, NF-kappa B, TNFα, and interleukins.[224] In a study of patients with knee OA, curcumin extract 30 mg taken 3 times daily decreased the COX-2 secretion into synovial fluid to the same extent as diclofenac 25 mg taken 3 times daily.[225] Antioxidant activity is strong, and extracts have antihyperlipidemic, antitumor, antibacterial, and antidiabetic effects. Distribution in the body after ingestion is fairly low, although higher when administered with oils; researchers have developed a nanoparticle formulation with increased bioavailability.[224]

Dosage and Product Considerations

An optimal dosage has not been determined. Clinical trials demonstrating benefit have used 1000–1500 mg/day in divided doses.

Safety Considerations

The most common adverse effects are GI discomfort and nausea. Human studies have shown good tolerance with dosages as high as 12,000 mg/day.[224] The World Health Organization lists daily intake 0–3 mg/kg per day as acceptable. Curcumin inhibits platelet aggregation in vitro and in vivo, so patients on antithrombotic agents should use curcumin cautiously.[226]

Summary of Clinical Evidence

A noninferiority trial (N = 367) compared 1500 mg of curcumin extract daily to 1200 mg of ibuprofen daily for 4 weeks.[227] The WOMAC total, pain, stiffness, and function scores were all similar between the curcumin and ibuprofen groups; 64.3% and 63.8% of curcumin and ibuprofen-treated patients, respectively, rated themselves as "improved" on the global assessment. Adverse events were similar except the curcumin-treated patients reported less abdominal pain and distention (10.8% vs. 18.1%, $P = 0.046$).

A polysaccharide-rich curcumin extract was examined in an OA trial in 120 patients.[228] Patients were randomized into 3 groups to receive 500 mg curcumin extract, 750 mg glucosamine sulfate, curcumin extract/glucosamine sulfate, or placebo, each twice daily for 42 days. The VAS pain scores were significantly reduced from baseline in all treatment groups, with the greatest reduction in the curcumin extract group, 66.5 – 19.48 ($P < 0.01$). The WOMAC scores were also significantly improved in the curcumin extract group, 54.97 – 17.14. The pain and WOMAC score reductions for glucosamine were also significantly better than baseline, but less so than curcumin extract; the combination treatment was less effective than either treatment alone, so a synergistic or additive effect was not demonstrated.

The evidence for curcumin and turmeric is promising, especially given its safety record. It may be considered an appropriate option for some patients with mild OA symptoms.

SKIN CONDITIONS

Aloe Vera

Aloe vera or *Aloe barbadensis,* commonly called aloe vera, is a succulent perennial, endemic to desert regions. Found in the leaf mucilage is a viscous, clear gel that has been historically used since ancient Egypt times for dermatologic conditions. It is a member of the Liliaceae family, also known as the desert lily.[229]

Therapeutic Uses

Aloe vera gel has been used topically for wound healing, including cuts, scrapes, and minor burns. Oral aloe products had been approved as a nonprescription stimulant laxative ingredient, but this dosage form was removed in 2002 from the nonprescription drug monographs because of a lack of safety and efficacy data.[230]

Physiological Activity

Aloe vera gel is derived from the mucilage of the plant and contains immunostimulating polysaccharides, called glucomannan, which contribute to collagen production, stimulate fibroblast growth factor, and improve transversal connections promoting skin healing. It is also rich in vitamins E, C, amino acids, and other antioxidants. Aloe vera may have anti-inflammatory and antimicrobial effects.[229] The outer skin of the plant, the latex, contains anthraquinone glycosides including aloin, aloe-emodin, and barbaloin responsible for laxative actions. Whole leaf extract contains both the mucilage and latex.[231]

Dosage and Product Concerns

Aloe vera gel is applied topically 2–3 times per day for the treatment of minor cuts, scrapes, and burns. Aloe vera is a component in many beauty and nonprescription products as an inactive ingredient. The International Aloe Science Council will certify products based on labeling, aloe content, aloe source, and quality standards defined by the Council. It sets criteria of less than 10 ppm of aloin for oral products and 50 ppm for topical formulations.[232]

Safety Considerations

Topical aloe vera is generally well tolerated, with occasional adverse effects of rashes and skin irritations, especially if the person has an allergy to members of the Liliaceae family such as lilies, garlic, or onions. Oral administration may cause laxative effects, GI upset, hypoglycemia, or hypokalemia related to the presence of anthraquinones. Case reports of hepatotoxicity have been attributed to oral aloe use.[231] Drug interactions have been reported with hypoglycemic, antiretroviral, and antithrombotic agents.[65] The consumption of oral aloe should be avoided because safety data are lacking.

Summary of Clinical Evidence

A Cochrane systematic review of randomized, controlled studies evaluated 7 trials involving 347 subjects using aloe or aloe-derived products, either as topical gels or wound dressing, for wound healing. Five trials included patients with burns, hemorrhoidectomy, and skin biopsies. In a comparison of aloe with silver sulfadiazine, no difference in the duration of burn healing was noted. Healing time was significantly decreased after hemorrhoidectomy in aloe group (RR 16.33 days [95% CI 3.46–77.15]). No difference in the completion of healing of skin biopsy sites was found. Two trials evaluating chronic wounds found no difference or significant delay in time to healing.[233]

An analysis of four trials comprising 371 subjects identified benefits in healing of first- and second-degree burns. Studies were combined and data analyzed using weighted mean differences (WMDs) on healing time. The WMD on the healing time was significantly decreased by 8.79 days in the aloe vera group versus the control group (95% CI 2.51, 15.07). Using active comparison control subjects, aloe demonstrated benefit over silver sulfadiazine and petrolatum (Vaseline) gauze. The trials were small and of variable quality.[234]

Overall, topical aloe vera is well tolerated, but evidence to support its efficacy in acute wound healing is mixed. It may be a useful adjunct to treatment in selected patients who are appropriate for self-care.

Tea Tree Oil

Tea tree oil (TTO) is derived from leaves of the tree *Melaleuca alternifolia* from the family Myrtaceae. The tea tree is not related to the plant used to make black and green teas.

Therapeutic Uses

TTO has been used as a topical anti-infective agent.

Physiologic Activity

TTO's major active component is terpinen-4-ol, which has displayed broad-spectrum antimicrobial activity against bacteria, fungus, viruses, and protozoa. Terpinen-4-ol has also demonstrated anti-inflammatory properties in decreasing TNF, IL-1, IL-8, IL-10, and prostaglandin E2. TTO constituents such as alpha-terpinene, alpha-terpinolene, and gamma-terpinene may have antioxidant properties.[235]

Dosage and Product Concerns

The oil is applied topically once or twice daily in concentrations of 0.4%–100%, depending on the condition and area of treatment. For acne, a 5% concentration is applied daily. For athlete's foot, TTO solution 25%–50% is applied twice daily for 4 weeks. For fungal toenail infections, TTO 100% has been used twice daily for 6 months.

Safety Considerations

Skin irritation may occur in sensitive patients, especially at higher concentrations. Although the oil can be used safely on oral mucosa, it should not be swallowed because ingesting small amounts may cause confusion, ataxia, and a systemic contact dermatitis that resolves slowly.[235] Prepubertal gynecomastia occurred in 3 boys using topical tea tree and lavender oils and resolved on discontinuation.[236]

Summary of Clinical Evidence

TTO may be effective for athlete's foot and other fungal infections of the skin, hair (dandruff), and nails.[237–239] For onychomycosis, TTO was compared with clotrimazole 1% solution and after 6 months had similar culture and clinical resolutions.[239] Evidence supporting TTO use for fungal conditions is older and has not been compared with current treatment options; it may be an option for individuals who are not tolerating current therapies for the treatment of athlete's foot or onychomycosis. In the treatment of mild to moderate acne, daily application of a TTO gel 5% for 45 days significantly reduced the total acne lesion count and acne severity index compared with placebo.[240]

WEIGHT LOSS

Garcinia cambogia/ Hydroxycitric Acid

Therapeutic Uses

Garcinia cambogia extracts, a source of hydroxycitric acid, are marketed for weight loss and are often included in supplements promoted for weight and glycemic control in patients with diabetes mellitus.

Physiologic Activity

Preclinical studies have shown that the (–)-hydroxycitric acid isomer decreases lipogenesis by competitively inhibiting ATP citrate lyase, essential for transformation of carbohydrates to fatty acids.[241] Hydroxycitric acid or *G. cambogia* extracts may decrease appetite through serotonin reuptake inhibition, delayed glucose absorption, and decreased postprandial plasma glucose levels. Human trials have not reported increased satiety from hydroxycitric acid alone.[241] Effects on glucose metabolism and levels have been variable in weight-loss studies.[242]

Dosage and Product Considerations

The optimal dose of *G. cambogia* extracts or hydroxycitric acid is unknown. Clinical trials have used dosages from 285 mg hydroxycitric acid alone to *G. cambogia* extracts containing 2800 mg hydroxycitric acid. *G. cambogia* extracts and hydroxycitric acid are often combined with other herbal or mineral ingredients.

Safety Considerations

Few adverse effects have been reported in clinical trials and a comprehensive review of toxicity studies concluded that *G. cambogia* extract/hydroxycitric acid is safe to use short term and is classified as "no observed adverse effect level."[243] However, one patient taking a *G. cambogia* extract–containing supplement experienced acute liver failure requiring transplant that was assessed to be "probably" related to the supplement.[244] A *G. cambogia* supplement was also linked to development of catecholamine-induced cardiomyopathy in a previously healthy adult.[246] Potential drug interactions are listed in Table 51–2.

Summary of Clinical Evidence

Many trials examining *G. cambogia* extracts or hydroxycitric acid have been small and of short duration. In one placebo-controlled trial on the effects on appetite in 89 mildly overweight women, subjects received 2.4 g/day of *G. cambogia* extract containing 1.3 g/day of hydroxycitric acid in 3 doses taken 30–60 minutes before meals.[246] At 12 weeks, weight loss for the treatment and placebo groups was 3.7 kg and 2.4 kg ($P = 0.026$). Another placebo-controlled study used 3 g/day *G. cambogia* extract containing 50% hydroxycitric acid in 3 doses taken 30 minutes before meals in men and women following a high-fiber low-calorie diet.[247] At 12 weeks, both groups had lost a similar amount of weight, 4.1 kg with placebo and 3.2 kg in the *G. cambogia* extract group.

Summarizing the evidence is difficult, as studies have used different extracts, doses, or supplement combinations. Some trials with lower (750 mg) hydroxycitric acid dosages are associated with greater weight loss, and that the effect may be smaller in men and more obese subjects.[247] As a result of the uncertain efficacy and safety of *G. cambogia* extracts and hydroxycitric acid, these products should not be recommended for weight loss.

Raspberry Ketone

Therapeutic Uses

Raspberry ketone is a flavoring agent with structural similarity to both synephrine and capsaicin that is promoted for weight loss.

Physiologic Activity

Preclinical studies have identified increased norepinephrine-stimulated adiponectin secretion, increased lipolysis in adipocytes, and decreased pancreatic lipase, potentially resulting in decreased fat absorption.[248] Antioxidant activity is also present and may play a role in weight management, as obesity is associated with increased oxidative stress.[249]

Dosage and Product Considerations

The optimal dosage of raspberry ketone is unknown.

Safety Considerations

Little is known about raspberry ketone's safety for DS use in humans. One case report exists of a healthy adult man who developed insomnia, jitteriness, and palpitations about 1 week after starting a raspberry ketone supplement.[250] Sinus tachycardia with QT and QRS normal intervals was documented 3 weeks later; symptoms resolved after discontinuation of the supplement. A review of the UK's National Poisons Information Service revealed increasing numbers of raspberry ketone reports, with symptoms of nausea or vomiting, diarrhea, abdominal pain, dizziness, fever, shortness of breath, and palpitations.[251] Potential drug interactions are listed in Table 51–2.

Summary of Clinical Evidence

One human study has assessed effects of raspberry ketones as a single agent. The study included 60 Iraqi women and compared placebo, L-carnitine 1000 mg/day, and 500 mg raspberry ketone.[249] All patients followed a similar low-calorie diet. At 12 weeks, all groups had significant weight reductions compared with baseline; the placebo group lost 3.2 kg (3.79%) while the raspberry ketone group lost 4.26 kg (5.1%), and the L-carnitine group 5.94 kg (7.38%). Weight lost in the raspberry ketone group was similar to placebo, although the difference in waist circumference was –4.31% and –2.57%, respectively, (P <0.05). L-carnitine demonstrated a greater effect, with a 7.73% reduction in circumference.

At this time, questions about its safety and efficacy remain, so patients should be discouraged from using raspberry ketone products.

WOMEN'S HEALTH

Black Cohosh

Black cohosh is made from the dried rhizome and roots of *Cimicifuga racemosa*, formerly *Actaea racemosa*. It is a member of the Ranunculaceae (buttercup) family.

Therapeutic Uses

Black cohosh has been used to treat the symptoms of premenstrual syndrome, dysmenorrhea, menopause, and rheumatoid arthritis.

Physiologic Activity

The active components of black cohosh rhizomes are triterpene glycosides, including acetein, cimicifugoside, and 27-deoxyacetin. Isoflavones such as formononetin are often present, but they may be absent from commercial products. Other constituents include isoferulic and salicylic acids, tannins, resin, starch, and sugars.[252] Black cohosh extract may also act as a partial serotonin agonist.[253] Black cohosh probably does not exhibit estrogenic activity and has no effect on vaginal epithelium, endometrium, or hormone concentrations.[254]

Dosage and Product Considerations

Black cohosh, as a standardized extract, is usually taken as 40 mg/day in 1–2 doses. One proprietary preparation is Remifemin. The extract is standardized to 1 mg of triterpene glycosides, calculated as 27-deoxyactein, per 20-mg extract tablet.[255]

Safety Considerations

Adverse effects are mild and include GI complaints, headache, rash, and weight gain. Hepatitis, seizures, and cardiovascular disease have been reported in patients taking combination products including black cohosh, although causal relationship has not been established.[256] Because of case reports of acute hepatitis with black cohosh, the USP Botanical Dietary Supplements and Herbal Medicines Expert Committee recommended a cautionary statement regarding potential hepatotoxicity be placed on product labels.[257] Further evaluations have suggested lack of product quality may have contributed, with the wrong plant being used.[258] The use of black cohosh for longer than 6 months is not recommended because of the lack of long-term safety studies. Data on drug interactions with black cohosh are limited, with the exception of possible additive effects with tamoxifen.[256] Unprocessed black cohosh plants contain small amounts of salicylic acid, but it is unknown if it is present in commercial products. Data on concurrent use with estrogens or progestins are not available. The use of black cohosh should be avoided during pregnancy and lactation because of its potential hormonal effects.[255]

Summary of Clinical Evidence

Several clinical trials have evaluated black cohosh alone and in combination products for menopausal symptoms, with mixed results. A systematic review of black cohosh included 16 randomized controlled trials with 2027 perimenopausal or postmenopausal women.[259] Efficacy was compared against placebo, hormone therapy, red clover, and fluoxetine. Analysis found the median dose of 40 mg/day of black cohosh for a 23-week average. For hot flushes and menopausal scores, no significant difference was noted between black cohosh and placebo while hormone therapy significantly reduced these outcomes. Other data provided inconclusive results as to the efficacy of black cohosh.[259]

Multi-ingredient product comparisons with placebo, hormonal therapy, and fluoxetine lack standardized dosing and have poor methodologic quality or small differences compared with placebo, making it difficult to establish efficacy. Benefits from other constituents in multi-ingredient products and SJW may be responsible for improvement in symptoms.[253] Combination with SJW has demonstrated an improvement in climacteric symptoms.[260] The ACOG practice guideline for managing menopausal symptoms stated insufficient evidence exists to support use of natural products.[261]

The safety and efficacy of black cohosh in women who have had breast cancer remains controversial. A systematic review in women with a history of breast cancer found inconclusive evidence to support safety and efficacy, although the product did not exert estrogenic effects.[262] A second systematic review of women with or without greater risk of breast cancer found the use of black cohosh did not increase risk of developing cancer.[263] The long-term effects on cardiovascular disease, osteoporosis, and breast cancer are unknown.

Chasteberry

Chaste tree (*Vitex agnus-castus*), commonly referred to as vitex, is a member of the Verbenaceae family. The dried ripe fruits, or berries, and the leaves are the medicinally useful parts of the plant.

Therapeutic Uses

Chasteberry has been used to treat symptoms of premenstrual syndrome (PMS), premenstrual dysphoric disorder (PMDD), dysmenorrhea, mastalgia, and menopausal symptoms.

Physiologic Activity

The fruits contain essential oils, diterpenes, iridoid glycosides, and flavonoids. Effects on menstrual regulation are likely caused by the dopaminergic compounds diterpenes, which are responsible for suppressing prolactin release by binding to the dopamine-2 receptor. Chasteberry may have weak estrogenic activity.[264]

Dosage and Product Considerations

Clinical trials have used 20–40 mg of the extract daily. The standardization of chasteberry has not been well established. It is available alone or in combination products.

Safety Considerations

GI complaints occur occasionally with use of chasteberry. Other symptoms include dry mouth, headache, rashes, itching, acne, menstrual disorders, and agitation. The use of chasteberry should be avoided during pregnancy and lactation because of insufficient data supporting safety. Chasteberry may theoretically interact with medications impacting dopamine and hormone replacement therapies or oral contraceptives.[265]

Summary of Clinical Evidence

Evidence for chasteberry, in combination with other herbals, for menopausal symptoms is mixed. A randomized, double-blind, placebo-controlled parallel trial studied combination SJW (*H. perforatum*) and chasteberry administered twice daily over 16 weeks in 100 perimenopausal and postmenopausal women. Symptoms did not differ between the groups regarding the primary end point of hot flushes.[266] Phyto-Female Complex, standardized extracts of black cohosh, dong quai, milk thistle, red clover, American ginseng, and chasteberry, has been studied in 50 premenopausal and postmenopausal women in a randomized, placebo-controlled trial. Improvements in hot flushes, night sweats, and sleep quality were reported, with no changes on vaginal ultrasonography, estradiol, follicle-stimulating hormone, liver enzymes, or thyroid-stimulating hormone.[267]

Chasteberry extract may be effective in PMS, PMDD, and latent hyperprolactinemia. A systematic review of seven trials of PMS found chasteberry to be more effective than placebo, pyridoxine, or magnesium. In PMDD, data were conflicting in two trials with comparison to fluoxetine, one being as effective. Chasteberry was more effective than placebo in one trial, and as effective as bromocriptine in another, for the treatment of hyperprolactinemia and associated clinical markers. Methodologic quality has been limited by study sizes and variable treatment measures.[268]

Evening Primrose Oil

Evening primrose (*Oenothera biennis*) is a member of the primrose family Onagraceae and is used for its high content of essential fatty acids. The seed oils of black currant (*Ribes nigrum*) and borage (*Borago officinalis*) are also used for similar purposes.

Therapeutic Uses

Evening primrose oil (EPO) has been used for mastalgia, PMS, menopause, preeclampsia, diabetic neuropathy, chronic fatigue syndrome, and atopic dermatitis.

Physiologic Activity

The oil from evening primrose seeds consists of omega-6 essential fatty acids, primarily 65%–75% linoleic acid and 7%–10% gamma linolenic acid. These components are thought to be responsible for anti-inflammatory activity.[269,270] The seed oil contains smaller amounts of palmitic, oleic, and stearic acids, as well as campesterol and beta sitosterol.[270]

Dosage and Product Considerations

In clinical trials, daily dosages of EPO 2–4 g have been used as a liquid or capsule. A standardized product, Efamol, a 1 g capsule, contains 0.62 g linoleic acid, 0.05 g gamma linolenic acid, and 0.062 g oleic acid.[269]

Safety Considerations

Adverse effects include headache, nausea, diarrhea, and occasional abdominal pain. EPO products may possess antiplatelet effects and should be used with caution in patients taking antithrombotic agents. Seizures have been reported in people taking EPO, so individuals taking anticonvulsants should avoid its use.[65,66] Use of EPO for cervical ripening during labor may be associated with adverse pregnancy outcomes including prolonged rupture of membranes and vacuum extraction.[270]

Summary of Clinical Evidence

Few studies exist of EPO's benefit on mastalgia. A randomized pilot placebo-controlled study found improvement in cyclic mastalgia with EPO 3 g, taken alone or in combination with vitamin E 1200 IU over 6 months.[271] A large double-blind, randomized, placebo-controlled trial comparing a branded British product containing gamma linolenic acid with or without antioxidant vitamins found no significant changes in reported pain in patients with moderate–severe mastalgia. A large placebo effect was noted, with 40% of subjects reporting improvement without therapy.[272]

A Cochrane review of 19 studies using oral EPO and borage oil concluded neither was effective for the treatment of atopic eczema. Studies of EPO found no improvement in global eczema symptoms recorded by visual analogue scales.[273]

Fenugreek

Fenugreek (*Trigonella foenum-graecum*) has a long history of use as a spice and a medicine in India, China, and Northern Africa. Both leaves and seeds may have medicinal properties.[274]

Therapeutic Uses

Fenugreek has been used for diabetes mellitus, hyperlipidemia, GI conditions, and stimulation of breast milk production.[275]

Physiologic Activity

An active constituent of fenugreek, 4-hydroxyisoleucine, may contribute to the hypoglycemic effects by stimulating glucose-induced insulin release and reducing insulin resistance.[274] Saponins converted to sapogenins in the GI tract may decrease cholesterol levels through activation of biliary cholesterol secretion. Fenugreek seeds are high in fiber, possibly delaying glucose absorption or binding cholesterol.[275] Lactation effects may be the result of increased sweat production impacting the milk duct or by phytoestrogens and diosgenin found in fenugreek.[104]

Dosage and Product Considerations

Dosages have varied, with fenugreek seed powder capsules 2.5 g twice daily or seed powder 25 g/day in 2 divided doses used in studies. Defatted seeds have also been used at 100 g/day in 2 equally divided doses. Fenugreek can also be administered in a tea.[275] For increasing milk supply, 2–3 capsules (580–610 mg per capsule) can be administered 3–4 times per day.[104]

Safety Considerations

Fenugreek is generally safe when used in meal preparation. When fenugreek is consumed, urine, sweat, and breast milk have been noted to smell like maple syrup, which is caused by sotolone excretion. This effect also occurs in breastfeeding infants, which has led to mistaken cases of maple syrup urine disease. Patients with an allergy to chickpeas should avoid fenugreek because of possible cross-reactivity; inhalation of the powder has resulted in bronchospasm. Fenugreek should be avoided during pregnancy because of potential oxytocic and uterine stimulant effects. Hypoglycemia or hypokalemia may result from use. The high-fiber content can bind with drugs and decrease absorption.[275] Fenugreek may increase risk of bleeding in patients taking antithrombotic agents.[66]

Summary of Clinical Evidence

Although fenugreek is promoted to stimulate production of breast milk, evidence is limited.[104] A small trial of immediate postpartum mothers and nursing newborns compared a treatment group receiving a tea containing fenugreek with placebo and control groups. Infants in the fenugreek group had significantly less weight loss and regained birth weight earlier, and mothers had higher breast milk volume at 3 days compared with placebo and control groups.[276] Other components present in the tea may have contributed to findings as well. Small studies with varying dosages have noted potential benefit in type 2 diabetes mellitus.[277]

Phytoestrogens

Phytoestrogens are found in many different plants; supplements have been derived primarily from soy (*Glycine max*) and red clover (*Trifolium pratense*).

Therapeutic Uses

Phytoestrogens have been used mainly for symptoms associated with menopause and related bone health. Phytoestrogens may also have a role in preventing prostate cancer. Soy is also used for its potential cardiovascular benefits.

Physiologic Activity

Soy-based phytoestrogens are composed of isoflavones such as genistein, daidzein, and glycitein. Red clover–based products have greater content of the isoflavones biochanin A and formononetin.[278] These compounds have effects including estrogenic, antiestrogenic, antioxidant, and anticancer activity.

Dosage and Product Considerations

A recommended dosage of phytoestrogen has not been established. Phytoestrogen products contain varying amounts and types of isoflavones. Products derived from soy and red clover sources may have different effects. The benefits from soy are primarily from dietary sources, not from supplements.

Safety Considerations

Phytoestrogen products derived from soy or red clover are well tolerated. GI complaints and allergic reactions may occur. The long-term safety of phytoestrogens is not established, especially with respect to the risk of estrogen-dependent cancers and thromboembolic disease. The safety of phytoestrogen supplements in women with hormone-sensitive cancers is unknown, and their use should be avoided.[65] Red clover may increase the risk of bleeding, especially if antithrombotic agents are taken concomitantly, although evidence of this interaction is lacking.[66]

Summary of Clinical Evidence

Purported benefits of phytoestrogens, especially soy-based products, are derived from population-based observational studies of dietary patterns. The lifetime risk of any disease is unlikely to be related solely to the presence or absence of one dietary component such as isoflavones. The phytoestrogen content in foods, especially of the biologically active isoflavones, varies significantly even in soy foods.

The most common use of phytoestrogens is for managing menopausal symptoms. A large meta-analysis and systematic review of 63 randomized, controlled studies and more than 6000 women evaluated the effectiveness of plant-based agents. Daily hot flash frequency and vaginal dryness scores using pooled mean differences both improved significantly in the phytoestrogen groups, although night sweats did not.[279]

The effect of soy isoflavones on the risk of osteoporosis has yielded mixed findings. A double-blind, placebo-controlled study randomized 389 postmenopausal women with osteopenia to receive placebo or genistein 54 mg/day. Significant changes were observed in the anteroposterior lumbar spine, the femoral neck, and urinary markers, with no documented changes in endometrial thickness.[280] A follow-up study at 3 years continued to show benefit on bone loss, with no significant changes in breast health.[281] Soy isoflavones 120 mg/day did not demonstrate a benefit on lumbar spine, total proximal femur, and total body BMD in 432 postmenopausal women without osteoporosis in a double-blind, placebo-controlled trial. Improvement was found only at the femoral neck.[282] A fixed combination of genistein and daidzein compared with placebo did not show a benefit on the BMD of the lumbar spine or femur after 2 years of use in Taiwanese postmenopausal women.[283]

The ingestion of at least 25 g of soy protein daily as part of a diet low in saturated fat and cholesterol may reduce the risk of

A WORD ABOUT Piperine and Its Effects on Drug Therapy

Piperine, the main alkaloid in black pepper (*Piper nigrum*), demonstrates nonspecific inhibition of cytochrome P450 enzymes and strongly inhibits P-glycoprotein, leading to increased absorption of many oral drugs and increased drug concentrations.[a] Piperine also inhibits bacterial efflux pumps, which could increase the effectiveness of antibiotic therapy.[b] DS manufacturers are including *Piper nigrum* extracts, piperine, or BioPerine, a patented extract, in many DS products to increase absorption of the supplements or prolong their effects. Patients taking DS products containing piperine must also consider their impact on any prescription medications. When taken with piperine, phenytoin concentrations were doubled in one study, whereas the area under the curve (AUC) of nevirapine increased by 170%.[a,c]

[a] Bhardwaj RK, Glaeser H, Becquemont L, et al. Piperine, a major constituent of black pepper, inhibits human P-glycoprotein and CYP3A4. *J Pharmacol Exp Ther.* 2002;302(2):645–50. doi: 10.1124/jpet.102.034728.

[b] Khamenah B, Iranshahy M, Ghandadi M, et al. Investigation of the antibacterial activity and efflux pump inhibitory effect of co-loaded piperine and gentamicin nanoliposomes in methicillin-resistant Staphylococcus aureus. *Drug Dev Ind Pharm.* 2015;41(6):989–94. doi: 10.3109/03639045.2014.920025.

[c] Kasibhatta R, Naidu MUR. Influence of piperine on the pharmacokinetics of nevirapine under fasting conditions: a randomised, crossover, placebo-controlled study. *Drugs R D.* 2007;8(6):383–91. doi: 10.2165/00126839-200708060-00006.

coronary heart disease. The effect of phytoestrogen DS on the risk of myocardial infarction is unclear.[284]

Epidemiologic research has indicated consumption of soy products has a role in decreasing breast cancer risk although concerns exist that estrogenic activity will increase recurrence. The potential effect likely will depend on the specific isoflavone, timing of exposure, genetic factors, and whether estrogen receptors are positive or negative for cancer. Dietary consumption of soy similar to that in Asian populations does not appear to increase cancer recurrence, nor does it interact with tamoxifen or anastrozole.[285] Another review concluded overall safety is promising because endometrial, uterine, and breast cancer risk do not appear to be increased. Dietary soy intake may even be associated with a decrease in endometrial or uterine cancers, however, it should be used with caution at the present time.[286] Observational data in a meta-analysis suggested that soy food consumption may reduce prostate cancer risk.[287]

Assessment of Natural Product Use: A Case-Based Approach

As stated in Chapter 50, the HCP should determine the patient's reasons for purchasing a natural product. The appropriateness of supplements must be determined especially for a child, a pregnant woman, or an older adult. If a medical condition is being treated and use of a supplement is appropriate, the patient should be encouraged to involve the HCP in the use of the supplement. Information about possible allergies to plant materials, current drug therapy, and comorbid conditions will identify possible contraindications. If self-treatment is appropriate, the provider should review the length of therapy and recommended dosages with the patient. Cases 51–1 and 51–2 provide examples of assessment of patients who are considering use of a natural product.

CASE 51-1

Relevant Evaluation Criteria	Scenario/Model Outcome
Collect	
1. Gather essential information about the patient's symptoms and medical history, including	A patient reports that his cholesterol level has not decreased as much as his PCP wants. His PCP has given him a new prescription for an increased dosage of simvastatin.
a. Description of symptom(s) (i.e., nature, onset, duration, severity, associated symptoms)	"I just need to come down 7 or 8 more points."
b. Description of any factors that seem to precipitate, exacerbate, and/or relieve the patient's symptom(s)	None
c. Description of the patient's efforts to relieve the symptoms	The patient follows a low-fat, low-cholesterol diet and exercises regularly. He also takes fish oil 1 g/day.
d. Patient's identity	R. Jakob Bjornsen
e. Patient's age, gender, height, and weight	66 years old, male, 5 ft 11 in., 176 lb
f. Patient's occupation	Retired plumber
g. Patient's dietary habits	Low-fat, low-cholesterol diet
h. Patient's sleep habits	Usually gets 7.5–8 hours of sleep per night; has insomnia 4–5 times per year.
i. Concurrent medical conditions, prescription and nonprescription medications, and dietary supplements	HTN, well controlled on lisinopril 10 mg/day; osteoarthritis in hands, treated with PRN ibuprofen, naproxen, or APAP; Centrum Silver 1 tab daily; enteric-coated fish oil 1 g at bedtime; simvastatin 20 mg/day
j. Allergies	NKDA; no known food or plant allergies

Relevant Evaluation Criteria	Scenario/Model Outcome
k. History of other adverse reactions to medications	Intolerant of erythromycin (severe nausea and vomiting requiring change in antibiotic)
l. Other (describe) _______	Patient comes to your pharmacy counter with two products, red yeast rice and garlic. He states that he does not want to increase his simvastatin dose, because at first diagnosis several years ago, he was prescribed a 40 mg dose and felt quite fatigued and "brain dead" much of the time. He has felt fine on the 20 mg dose and says, "I *really* don't want to increase that again!" He wants to know which of the two natural medicines would be better for him to take to get his cholesterol down a little lower.
Assess	
2. Differentiate patient's signs and symptoms, and correctly identify the patient's primary problem(s).	Hyperlipidemia, uncontrolled; osteoarthritis, mild and adequately treated with PRN medications; HTN, controlled; lack of education regarding dietary supplements
3. Identify exclusions for self-treatment.	The patient has a contraindication to a therapy in which he is interested.
4. Formulate a comprehensive list of therapeutic alternatives for the primary problem to determine whether triage to a health care provider is required, and share this information with the patient or caregiver.	Options include (1) Have patient continue current antihyperlipidemic prescription, diet, and exercise, and add a supplement therapy for a trial period. Have patient discuss plan with PCP before proceeding. (2) Fill new antihyperlipidemic prescription, have patient continue current diet and exercise therapy, and suggest adding coenzyme Q10 to the patient's regimen. (3) Fill new antihyperlipidemic prescription, and have patient continue current diet and exercise therapy. (4) Take no action.
Plan	
5. Select an optimal therapeutic alternative to address the patient's problem, taking into account patient preferences.	Suggest patient add a garlic supplement to his regimen.
6. Describe the recommended therapeutic approach to the patient or caregiver.	"Begin taking a garlic supplement, either a powdered garlic that will provide 3–5 mg/day of allicin or 1.2 g/day of an aged garlic extract containing a minimum of 1.2 mg S-allylcysteine." "You should continue the low-fat diet and regular exercise to control your hyperlipidemia and HTN."
7. Explain to the patient or caregiver the rationale for selecting the recommended therapeutic approach from the considered therapeutic alternatives.	"The red yeast rice product contains a statin similar to the simvastatin that you are currently taking, so it would not be appropriate to take them at the same time."
Implement	
8. When recommending self-care with nonprescription medications and/or nondrug therapy, convey accurate information to the patient or caregiver.	
Solicit follow-up questions from the patient or caregiver.	"What if this doesn't get my cholesterol down enough?"
Answer the patient's or caregiver's questions.	"If your cholesterol doesn't reach the goal set by your PCP, then we will stop the garlic, fill the new simvastatin prescription at the higher dose, and have you start taking coenzyme Q10. Simvastatin is known to decrease cholesterol levels and that may be associated with adverse effects, such as the fatigue you experienced with the previous 40 mg dose. Some patients are better able to tolerate statins when they take them with coenzyme Q10."
Follow-up: Monitor and Evaluate	
9. Assess patient outcome.	Patient should have his lipid levels checked in 6–8 weeks to determine whether the addition of garlic is providing sufficient benefit. If not, he may need to take the higher simvastatin dose and coenzyme Q10.

Key: APAP = Acetaminophen; HTN = hypertension; NKDA = no known drug allergies; PCP = primary care provider; PRN = as needed.

CASE 51-2

Relevant Evaluation Criteria	Scenario/Model Outcome
Collect	
1. Gather essential information about the patient's symptoms and medical history, including	
a. Description of symptom(s) (i.e., nature, onset, duration, severity, associated symptoms)	Patient believes she has another UTI. She describes feeling the urge to use the bathroom frequently, with only a small amount of urine output. She also noticed a burning sensation when she urinated last night.
b. Description of any factors that seem to precipitate, exacerbate, and/or relieve the patient's symptom(s)	She cannot identify anything that specifically precipitated the infection. She thinks the orange juice that she drank earlier may have aggravated her symptoms. Nothing has relieved her discomfort or urgency.
c. Description of the patient's efforts to relieve the symptoms	The patient has done nothing to relieve the symptoms. She says she does not want to go back to her provider. She is holding a cranberry product labeled "urinary tract health."
d. Patient's identity	Vivian Bailey
e. Patient's age, gender, height, and weight	22 years old, female, 5 ft 2 in., 120 lb
f. Patient's occupation	College student
g. Patient's dietary habits	Generally healthy diet; occasional alcohol
h. Patient's sleep habits	Approximately 6 hours of sleep per night
i. Concurrent medical conditions, prescription and nonprescription medications, and dietary supplements	No concurrent medical conditions; history of previous UTI a few months ago that was treated with a prescription antibiotic (she does not remember the name). She is taking Ortho Tri-Cyclen Lo daily for birth control.
j. Allergies	NKA
k. History of other adverse reactions to medications	Phenazopyridine caused gastrointestinal upset.
l. Other (describe) ______	Patient is sexually active.
Assess	
2. Differentiate patient's signs and symptoms, and correctly identify the patient's primary problem(s).	Vivian is likely experiencing a UTI, which is more likely to occur in females and those who are sexually active.
3. Identify exclusions for self-treatment.	Self-treatment is not appropriate for a UTI. She wants to use a cranberry product to avoid going back to her provider.
4. Formulate a comprehensive list of therapeutic alternatives for the primary problem to determine whether triage to a health care provider is required, and share this information with the patient or caregiver.	Options include (1) Refer Vivian to an appropriate HCP. (2) Recommend self-care with a dietary supplement and nondrug measures. (3) Recommend self-care until Vivian can see an appropriate provider. (4) Take no action.
Plan	
5. Select an optimal therapeutic alternative to address the patient's problem, taking into account patient preferences.	Patient should consult an HCP.
6. Describe the recommended therapeutic approach to the patient or caregiver.	"You should consult your primary care provider for treatment of your urinary tract infection."
7. Explain to the patient or caregiver the rationale for selecting the recommended therapeutic approach from the considered therapeutic alternatives.	"This option is best because your problem cannot be treated with dietary supplements. You likely have a bacterial infection that requires a prescription antibiotic. Cranberry products, including juice or concentrated tablets, will not cure the infection."
Implement	
8. When recommending self-care with nonprescription medications and/or nondrug therapy, convey accurate information to the patient or caregiver.	"Increasing water intake and using a warm heating pad on your abdomen may help symptoms until you see your primary care provider."

CASE 51-2 continued

Relevant Evaluation Criteria	Scenario/Model Outcome
Solicit follow-up questions from the patient or caregiver.	"Is there anything I can do to prevent this from happening? This is the second time in the past few months."
Answer the patient's or caregiver's questions.	"Evidence has been mixed, but some studies have found cranberry may be a useful preventive measure in patients with recurrent urinary tract infections. However, these products may cause gastrointestinal upset. If you like cranberry juice and want to incorporate it into your diet, select a product with a low sugar content. Tablets are also an option; however, different brands may contain different levels of proanthocyanidins, an active component that appears to be beneficial."
Follow-up: Monitor and Evaluate	
9. Assess patient outcome.	Contact the patient in a day or two to ensure that she made an appointment with her PCP.

Key: HCP = Health care provider; NKA = no known allergies; PCP = primary care provider; UTI = urinary tract infection.

REFERENCES

1. Ayer A, Macdonald P, Stocker R. CoQ_{10} function and role in heart failure and ischemic heart disease. *Ann Rev Nutr.* 2015;35:175–213. doi: 10.1146/annurev-nutr-071714-034258.
2. Molyneux SL, Florkowski CM, George PM, et al. Coenzyme Q10: an independent predictor of mortality in chronic heart failure. *J Am Coll Cardiol.* 2008;52(18):1435–41. doi: 10.1016/j.jacc.2008.07.044.
3. Banach M, Serban C, Ursoniu S, et al. Statin therapy and plasma coenzyme Q10 concentrations: a systematic review and meta-analysis of placebo-controlled trials. *Pharmacologic Res.* 2015;99:329–36. doi: 10.1016/j.phrs.2015.07.008.
4. Turunen M, Olsson J, Dallner G. Metabolism and function of coenzyme Q. *Biochim Biophys Acta.* 2004;1660(1-2):171–90. PMID: 14757233.
5. Saha SP, Whayne TF. Coenzyme Q-10 in human health: supporting evidence? *South Med J.* 2016;109(1):17–21. doi: 10.14423/SMJ.0000000000000393.
6. Engelsen J. Effect of coenzyme Q10 and *Ginkgo biloba* on warfarin dosage in stable, long-term warfarin treated outpatients. A randomized, double-blind, placebo-crossover trial. *Thromb Haemost.* 2002;87(6):1075–6. PMID: 12083489.
7. Young JM, Florkowski CM, Molyneux SL, et al. A randomized, double-blind, placebo-controlled crossover study of coenzyme Q10 therapy in hypertensive patients with the metabolic syndrome. *Am J Hypertens.* 2012;25(2):261–70. doi: 10.1038/ajh.2011.209.
8. Belardinelli R, Mucaj A, Lacalaprice F, et al. Coenzyme Q10 and exercise training in chronic heart failure. *Eur Heart J.* 2006;27(22):2675–81. doi: 10.1093/eurheartj/ehl158.
9. Gao L, Mao Q, Cao J, et al. Effects of coenzyme Q10 on vascular endothelial function in humans: a meta-analysis of randomized controlled trials. *Atherosclerosis.* 2012;221(2):311–6. doi: 10.1016/j.atherosclerosis.2011.10.027.
10. Mortensen SA, Rosenfeldt F, Kumar A, et al. The effect of coenzyme Q_{10} on morbidity and mortality in chronic heart failure. *JACC Heart Fail.* 2014;2(6):641–9. doi: 10.1016/j.jchf.2014.06.008.
11. Langsjoen PH, Langsjoen JO, Langsjoen AM, et al. Treatment of statin adverse effects with supplemental coenzyme Q10 and statin drug discontinuation. *Biofactors.* 2005;25(1-4):147–52. doi: 10.1002/biof.5520250116.
12. Kelly P, Vasu S, Getato M. et al. Coenzyme Q10 improves myopathic pain in statin treated patients. *J Am Coll Cardiol.* 2005;45:3A.
13. Taylor BA, Lorson L, White CM, et al. A randomized trial of coenzyme Q10 in patients with confirmed statin myopathy. *Atherosclerosis.* 2015;238(2):329–35. doi: 10.1016/j.atherosclerosis.2014.
14. Ruaño G, Windemuth A, Wu, AH, et al. Mechanisms of stain-induced myalgia assessed by physiogenomic associations. *Atherosclerosis.* 2011;218(2):451–6. doi: 10.1016/j.atherosclerosis.2011.07.007.
15. Lichtenstein AH, Appel LJ, Brands M, et al. Diet and lifestyle recommendations revision 2006: a scientific statement from the American Heart Association Nutrition Committee. *Circulation.* 2006;114(1):82–96. doi: 10.1161/CIRCULATIONAHA.106.176158.
16. Adkins Y, Kelley DS. Mechanisms underlying the cardioprotective effects of omega-3 polyunsaturated fatty acids. *J Nutr Biochem.* 2010;21(9):781–92. doi: 10.1016/j.jnutbio.2009.12.004.
17. Siriwardhana N, Kalupahana NS, Moustaid-Moussa N. Health benefits of n-3 polyunsaturated fatty acids: eicosapentaenoic acid and docosahexaenoic acid. *Adv Food Nutr Res.* 2012;65:211–22. doi: 10.1016/B978-0-12-416003-3.00013-5.
18. Weitz D, Weintraub H, Fisher E, et al. Fish oil for the treatment of cardiovascular disease. *Cardiol Rev.* 2010;18(5):258–63. doi: 10.1097/CRD.0b013e3181ea0de0.
19. Smutna M, Kruzikova K, Marsalek P, et al. Fish oil and cod liver as safe and healthy food supplements. *Neuro Endocrinol Lett.* 2009;30(Suppl 1):156–62. PMID: 20027164.
20. Melanson SF, Lewandrowski EL, Flood JG, et al. Measurement of organochlorines in commercial over-the-counter fish oil preparations: implications for dietary and therapeutic recommendations for omega-3 fatty acids and a review of the literature. *Arch Pathol Lab Med.* 2005;129(1):74–7. doi: 10.1043/1543-2165(2005)129<74:MOOICO>2.0.CO;2.
21. Ulven SM, Holven KB. Comparison of bioavailability of krill oil versus fish oil and health effect. *Vasc Health Risk Manag.* 2015;11:511–24. doi: 10.2147/VHRM.S85165. eCollection 2015.
22. Leslie MA, Cohen CJA, Liddle DM, et al. A review of the effect of omega-3 polyunsaturated fatty acids on blood triacylglycerol levels in normolipidemic and borderline hyperlipidemic individuals. *Lipids Health Dis.* 2015;14:53. doi: 10.1186/s12944-015-0049-7.
23. Hartweg J, Farmer AJ, Perera R, et al. Meta-analysis of the effects of n-3 polyunsaturated fatty acids on lipoproteins and other emerging lipid cardiovascular risk markers in patients with type 2 diabetes. *Diabetologia.* 2007;50(8):1593–602. doi: 10.1007/s00125-007-0695-z.
24. Eslick GD, Howe PRC, Smith C, et al. Benefits of fish oil supplementation in hyperlipidemia: a systematic review and meta-analysis. *Int J Cardiol.* 2009;136(1):4–16. doi: 10.1016/j.ijcard.2008.03.092.
25. Lewis A, Lookinland S, Beckstrand RL, et al. Treatment of hypertriglyceridemia with omega-3 fatty acids: a systematic review. *J Am Acad Nurse Pract.* 2004;16(9):384–95. doi: 10.1111/j.1745-7599.2004.tb00388.x.

26. Khawaja OA, Gaziano JM, Djoussé L. N-3 fatty acids for prevention of cardiovascular disease. *Curr Atherslero Rep.* 2014;16(11):450. doi: 10.1007/s11883-014-0450-0.
27. Minihane AM. Fish oil omega-3 fatty acids and cardio-metabolic health, alone or with statins. *Eur J Clin Nutr.* 2013;67(5):536–40. doi: 10.1038/ejcn.2013.19.
28. de Lorgeril M, Salen P, Defaye P, et al. Recent findings on the health effects of omega-3 fatty acids and statins, and their interactions: do statins inhibit omega-3? *BMC Med.* 2013;11:15. doi: 10.1186/1741-7015-11-5.
29. He L, Li M, Lin, M, et al. Effect of fish oil supplement in maintenance hemodialysis patients: a systematic review and meta-analysis of published randomized controlled trials. *Eur J Clin Pharmacol.* 2016;72(2): 129–39. doi: 10.1007/s00228-015-1976-y.
30. Hosseini A, Hosseinzadeh H. A review on the effects of *Allium sativum* (Garlic) in metabolic syndrome. *J Endocrinol Invest.* 2015;38(11): 1147–57. doi: 10.1007/s40618-015-0313-8.
31. Shouk R, Abdou A, Shetty K, et al. Mechanisms underlying the anti-hypertensive effects of garlic bioactives. *Nutr Res.* 2014;34(2):106–15. doi: 10.1016/j.nutres.2013.12.005.
32. Ried K, Toben C, Fakler P. Effect of garlic on serum lipids: an updated meta-analysis. *Nutr Rev.* 2013;71(5):282–99. doi: 10.1111/nure.12012.
33. Boullata J. Natural health product interactions with medication. *Nutr Clin Pract.* 2005;20(1):33–51. doi: 10.1177/011542650502000133.
34. Scharbert G, Kalb ML, Duris M, et al. Garlic at dietary doses does not impair platelet function. *Anesth Analg.* 2007;105(5):1214–8. doi: 10.1213/01.ane.0000287253.92211.06.
35. Ried K. Garlic lowers blood pressure in hypertensive individuals, regulates serum cholesterol, and stimulates immunity: an updated meta-analysis and review. *J Nutr.* 2016;146(2):389S–396S. doi: 10.3945/jn.114.202192.
36. Rohner A, Ried K, Sobenin IA, et al. A systematic review and meta-analysis on the effects of garlic preparations on blood pressure in individuals with hypertension. *Am J Hyperten.* 2015;28(3):414–23. doi: 10.1093/ajh/hpu165.
37. Law MR, Wald NJ, Morris JK, et al. Value of low dose combination treatment with blood pressure lowering drugs: analysis of 354 randomised trials. *BMJ.* 2003;326(7404):1427. doi: 10.1136/bmj.326.7404.1427.
38. Ried K, Travica N, Sali A. The effect of aged garlic extract on blood pressure and other cardiovascular risk factors in uncontrolled hypertensives: the AGE at Heart trial. *Integr Blood Press Control.* 2016;9:9–21. doi: 10.2147/IBPC.S93335.
39. Zhao Y, Wang J, Ballevre O, et al. Antihypertensive effects and mechanisms of chlorogenic acids. *Hypertens Res.* 2012;35(4):370–4.
40. Flanagan J, Bily A, Rolland Y, et al. Lipolytic activity of Svetol, a decaffeinated green coffee bean extract. *Phytother Res.* 2014;28(6):946–8. doi: 10.1002/ptr.5085.
41. Beam JR, Gibson AL, Kerksick CM, et al. Effect of post-exercise caffeine and green coffee bean extract consumption on blood glucose and insulin concentrations. *Nutrition.* 2015;31(2):292–7. doi: 10.1016/j.nut.2014.07.012.
42. Ochiai R, Jokura H, Suzuki A, et al. Green coffee bean extract improves human vasoreactivity. *Hypertens Res.* 2004;27(10):731–7. doi: 10.1291/hypres.27.731.
43. Loader TB, Taylor CG, Zahradka P, et al. Chlorogenic acid from coffee beans: evaluating the evidence for a blood pressure-regulating health claim. *Nutr Rev.* 2017;75(1):114–33. doi: 10.1093/nutrit/nuw057.
44. Kozuma K, Tsuchiya S, Kohuri J, et al. Antihypertensive effect of green coffee bean extract on mildly hypertensive subjects. *Hypertens Res.* 2005;28(9):711–8. doi: 10.1291/hypres.28.711.
45. Watanabe T, Arai Y, Mitsui Y, et al. The blood pressure-lowering effect and safety of chlorogenic acid from green coffee bean extract in essential hypertension. *Clin Exp Hypertens.* 2006;28(5):439–49. doi: 10.1080/10641960600798655.
46. Onakpoya I, Spencer EA, Thompson MJ, et al. The effect of chlorogenic acid on blood pressure: a systematic review and meta-analysis of randomized clinical trials. *J Hum Hypertens.* 2015;29(2):77–81. doi: 10.1038/jhh.2014.46.
47. Gordon RY, Cooperman T, Obermeyer W, et al. Marked variability of monacolin levels in commercial red yeast rice products. *Arch Intern Med.*2010;170(19):1722–7. doi: 10.1001/archinternmed.2010.382.
48. Kazmin A, Garcia-Bournissen F, Koren G. Risks of statin use during pregnancy: a systematic review. *J Obstet Gynaecol Can.* 2007;29(11): 906–8. doi: 10.1016/S1701-2163(16)32656-1.
49. Patakova P. Monascus secondary metabolites: production and biological activity. *J Ind Microbiol Biotechnol.* 2013;40(2):169–81. doi: 10.1007/s10295-012-1216-8.
50. Venero CV, Venero JV, Wortham DC, et al. Lipid-lowering efficacy of red yeast rice in a population intolerant to statins. *Am J Cardiol.* 2010;105(5):664–6. doi: 10.1016/j.amjcard.2009.10.045.
51. Halbert SC, French B, Gordon RY, et al. Tolerability of red yeast rice (2,400 mg twice daily) versus pravastatin (20 mg twice daily) in patients with previous statin intolerance. *Am J Cardiol.* 2010;105(2):198–204. doi: 10.1016/j.amjcard.2009.08.672.
52. Becker DJ, Gordon RY, Halbert SC, et al. Red yeast rice for dyslipidemia in statin-intolerant patients: a randomized trial. *Ann Intern Med.* 2009;150(12):830–9. doi: 10.7326/0003-4819-150-12-200906160-00006.
53. Gerards MC, Terlou RJ, Yu H, et al. Traditional Chinese lipid-lowering agent red yeast rice results in significant LDL reduction but safety is uncertain—a systematic review and meta-analysis. *Atherosclerosis.* 2015;240(2):415–23. doi: 10.1016/j.atherosclerosis.2015.04.004.
54. Ong YC, Aziz Z. Systematic review of red yeast rice compared with simvastatin in dyslipidaemia. *J Clin Pharm Ther.* 2016;41(2):170–9. doi:10.111/jcpt.12374.
55. Sutherland A, Sweet BV. Butterbur: an alternative therapy for migraine prevention. *Am J Health Syst Pharm.* 2010;67(9):705–11. doi: 10.2146/ajhp090136.
56. Schapowal A. Randomised controlled trial of butterbur and cetirizine for treating seasonal allergic rhinitis. *BMJ.* 2002;324(7330):114–6. doi: 10.1136/bmj.324.7330.144.
57. Schapowal A. Treating intermittent allergic rhinitis: a prospective, randomized, placebo and antihistamine-controlled study of butterbur extract Ze 339. *Phytother Res.* 2005;19(6):530–7. doi: 10.1002/ptr.1705.
58. Avula B, Wang YH, Wang M, et al. Simultaneous determination of sesquiterpenes and pyrrolizidine alkaloids from the rhizomes of Petasites hybridus (L.) G.M. et Sch. and dietary supplements using UPLC-UV and HPLCTOF-MS methods. *J Pharm Biomed Anal.* 2012;70:53–63. doi: 10.1016/j.jpba.2012.05.021.
59. Holland S, Silberstein SD, Freitag F, et al. Evidence-based guideline update: NSAIDs and other complementary treatments for episodic migraine prevention in adults: report of the Quality Standards Subcommittee of the American Academy of Neurology and the American Headache Society. *Neurology.* 2012;78(17):1346–53. doi: 10.1212/WNL.0b013e3182535d0c.
60. Orr SL, Venkateswaren S. Nutraceuticals in prophylaxis of pediatric migraine: Evidence-based review and recommendations. *Cephalalgia.* 2014;34(8):568–83. doi: 10.1177/0333102413519512.
61. Pareek A, Suthar M, Rathore GS, et al. Feverfew (Tanacetum parthenium L.): a systematic review. *Pharmacogn Rev.* 2011;5(9):103–10. doi: 10.4103/0973-7847.79105.
62. Wider B, Pittler M, Ernst E. Feverfew for preventing migraine. *Cochrane Database Syst Rev.* 2015;4:CD002286. doi: 10.1002/14651858.CD002286.pub3.
63. Ciocon JO, Ciocon DG, Galindo DJ. Dietary supplements in primary care. Botanicals can affect surgical outcomes and follow-up. *Geriatrics.* 2004;59(9):20–4. PMID: 15461234.
64. Chan PC, Xia Q, Fu PP. Ginkgo biloba leave extract: biological, medicinal, and toxicological effects. *J Environ Sci Health C Environ Carcinog Ecotoxicol Rev.* 2007;25(3):211–44. doi: 10.1080/10590500701569414.
65. Ulbricht C, Chao W, Costa D, et al. Clinical evidence of herb-drug interactions: a systematic review by the Natural Standard Research Collaboration. *Curr Drug Metab.* 2008;9(10):1063–120. doi: 10.2174/138920008786927785.
66. Izzo AA. Interactions between herbs and conventional drugs: overview of the clinical data. *Med Princ Pract.* 2012;21(5):404–28. doi: 10.1159/000334488.

67. Stoddard GJ, Archer M, Shane-McWhorter L, et al. Ginkgo and warfarin interaction in a large veterans administration population. *AMIA Annu Symp Proc.* 2015;2015:1174–83
68. Tan MS, Yu JT, Tan CC, et al. Efficacy and adverse effects of gingko biloba for cognitive impairment and dementia: A systematic review and meta-analysis. *J Alzheimers Dis.* 2015;43(2):589–603. doi: 10.3233/JAD-140837.
69. DeKosky ST, Williamson JD, Fitzpatrick AL, et al. *Ginkgo biloba* for prevention of dementia: a randomized controlled trial. *JAMA.* 2008; 300(19):2253–2262. doi: 10.1001/jama.2008.683.
70. Luboshitzky R, Lavie P. Melatonin and sex hormone interrelationships—a review. *J Ped Endocrinol.* 1999;12:355–62.
71. Diaz Lopez B, Diaz Rodriguez E, Urquijo C, et al. Melatonin influences on the neuroendocrine-reproductive axis. *Ann N Y Acad Sci.* 2005;1057:337–64. doi: 10.1196/annals.1356.026.
72. Kotlarczyk MP, Lassila HC, O'Neil CK, et al. Melatonin osteoporosis prevention study (MOPS): a randomized, double-blind, placebo-controlled study examining the effects of melatonin on bone health and quality of life in perimenopausal women. *J Pineal Res.* 2012;52(4):414–26. doi: 10.1111/j.1600-079X.2011.00956.x.
73. Brzezinski A, Vangel MG, Wurtman RJ, et al. Effect of exogenous melatonin on sleep: a meta-analysis. *Sleep Med Rev.* 2005;9(1):41–50. doi: 10.1016/j.smrv.2004.06.004.
74. Wang Y, Jin B, Ai F, et al. The efficacy and safety of melatonin in concurrent chemotherapy or radiotherapy for solid tumors: a meta-analysis of randomized controlled trials. *Cancer Chemother Pharmacol.* 2012;69(5):1213–20. doi: 10.1007/s00280-012-1828-8.
75. Sanchez-Barcelo EJ, Mediavilla MD, Alonso-Gonzalez C, et al. Melatonin uses in oncology: breast cancer prevention and reduction of the side effects of chemotherapy and radiation. *Expert Opin Investig Drugs.* 2012;21(6):819–31. doi: 10.1517/13543784.2012.681045.
76. Braam W, Didden R, Maas AP, et al. Melatonin decreases daytime challenging behavior in persons with intellectual disability and chronic insomnia. *J Intellect Disabil Res.* 2010;54(1):52–9. doi: 10.1111/j.1365-2788.2009.01223.x.
77. Malow B, Adkins KW, McGrew SG, et al. Melatonin for sleep in children with autism: a controlled trial examining dose, tolerability, and outcomes. *J Autism Dev Disord.* 2012;42(8):1729–37. doi: 10.1007/s10803-011-1418-3.
78. Serfaty MA, Osborne D, Buszewicz MJ, et al. A randomized double-blind placebo controlled trial of treatment as usual plus exogenous slow-release melatonin (6 mg) or placebo for sleep disturbance and depressed mood. *Int Clin Psychopharmacol.* 2010;25(3):132–42. doi: 10.1097/YIC.0b013e32832c260b.
79. Wade AG, Crawford G, Ford I, et al. Prolonged release melatonin in the treatment of primary insomnia: evaluation of the age cut-off for short- and long-term response. *Curr Med Res Opin.* 2011;27(1):87–98. doi: 10.1185/03007995.2010.537317.
80. Luthringer R, Muzet M, Zisapel N, et al. The effect of prolonged-release melatonin on sleep measures and psychomotor performance in elderly patients with insomnia. *Int Clin Psychopharmacol.* 2009;24(5):239–49. doi: 10.1097/YIC.0b013e32832e9b08.
81. Scheer FA, Morris CJ, Garcia JI, et al. Repeated melatonin supplementation improves sleep in hypertensive patients treated with beta-blockers: a randomized controlled trial. *Sleep.* 2012;35(10):1395–1402. doi: 10.5665/sleep.2122.
82. Herxheimer A, Petrie K. Melatonin for the prevention and treatment of jet lag. *Cochrane Database Syst Rev.* 2002;2:CD001520. doi: 10.1002/14651858.CD001520.
83. Linde K. St. John's wort—an overview. *Forsch Komplementmed.* 2009; 16(3):146–55. doi: 10.1159/000209290.
84. Wurglics M, Westerhoff K, Kaunzinger A, et al. Batch-to-batch reproducibility of St. John's wort preparations. *Pharmacopsychiatry.* 2001;34(Suppl 1):S152–6.doi: 10.1055/s-2001-15453.
85. Knuppel L, Linde K. Adverse effects of St. John's wort: a systematic review. *J Clin Psychiatry.* 2004;65(11):1470–9. doi: 10.4088/JCP.v65n1105.
86. Russo E, Scicchitano F, Whalley BJ, et al. Hypericum perforatum: pharmacokinetic, mechanism of action, tolerability, and clinical drug-drug interactions. *Phytother Res.* 2014;28(5):643–55. doi: 10.1002/ptr.5050.
87. Schulz HU, Schürer M, Bässler D, et al. Investigation of the effect on photosensitivity following multiple oral dosing of two different hypericum extracts in healthy men. *Arzneimittelforschung.* 2006;56(3):212–21. doi:10.1055/s-0031-1296713.
88. Linde K, Berner M, Kriston L. St. John's wort for major depression. *Cochrane Database Syst Rev.* 2008;4:CD000448. doi: 10.1002/14651858.CD000448.pub3.
89. Kasper S, Caraci F, Forti B, et al. Efficacy and tolerability of Hypericum extract for the treatment of mild to moderate depression. *Eur Neuropsychopharmacol.* 2010;20(11):747–65. doi: 10.1016/j.euroneuro.2010.07.005.
90. Hadley S, Petry JJ. Valerian. *Am Fam Physician.* 2003;67(8):1755–8. PMID: 12725454.
91. Fernández-San-Martín MI, Masa-Font R, Palacios-Soler L, et al. Effectiveness of valerian on insomnia: a meta-analysis of randomized placebo-controlled trials. *Sleep Med.* 2010;11(6):505–11. doi: 10.1016/j.sleep.2009.12.009.
92. Glass J, Sproule B, Herrmann N, et al. Acute pharmacological effects of temazepam, diphenhydramine, and valerian in healthy elderly subjects. *J Clin Psychoparmacol.* 2003;23(3):260–8. doi: 10.1097/01.jcp.0000084033.22282.b6.
93. Chrubasik S, Pittler MH, Roufogalis BD. *Zingiberis rhizoma:* a comprehensive review on the ginger effect and efficacy profiles. *Phytomedicine.* 2005;12(9):684–701. doi: 10.1016/j.phymed.2004.07.009.
94. Ding M, Leach M, Bradley H. The effectiveness and safety of ginger for pregnancy-induced nausea and vomiting: A systematic review. *Women Birth.* 2013;26(1):e26–30. doi: 10.1016/j.wombi.2012.08.001.
95. Viljoen E, Visser J, Koen N, et al. A systematic review and meta-analysis of the effect and safety of ginger in the treatment of pregnancy-associated nausea and vomiting. *Nutr J.* 2014;13:20. doi: 10.1186/1475-2891-13-20.
96. Heitmann K, Nordeng H, Holst L. Safety of ginger use in pregnancy: results from a large population-based cohort study. *Eur J Clin Pharmacol.* 2013;69(2):269–77. doi: 10.1007/s00228-012-1331-5.
97. Caiyakunapruk N, Kitikannakorn N, Nathisuwan S, et al. The efficacy of ginger for the prevention of postoperative nausea and vomiting: a meta-analysis. *Am J Obstet Gynecol.* 2006;194(1):95–9. doi: 10.1016/j.ajog.2005.06.046.
98. Lee J, Oh H. Ginger as an antiemetic modality for chemotherapy-induced nausea and vomiting: a systematic review and meta-analysis. *Oncol Nurs Forum.* 2013;40(2):163–70. doi: 10.1188/13.ONF.163-170.
99. Pillai AK, Sharma KK, Gupta YK, et al. Anti-emetic effect of ginger powder versus placebo as an add-on therapy in children and young adults receiving high emetogenic chemotherapy. *Pediatr Blood Cancer.* 2010;56(2):234–8. doi: 10.1002/pbc.22778.
100. Ryan JL, Heckler CE, Roscoe JA, et al. Ginger (Zingiber officinale) reduces acute chemotherapy-induced nausea: a URCC CCOP study of 576 patients. *Support Care Cancer.* 2012;20(7):1479–89. doi: 10.1007/s00520-011-1236-3.
101. Matthews A, Haas DM, O'Mathúna DP, et al. Interventions for nausea and vomiting in early pregnancy. *Cochrane Database Syst Rev.* 2014;3:CD007575. doi: 10.1002/14651858.CD007575.pub3.
102. American College of Obstetricians and Gynecologists. Practice bulletin no. 153: nausea and vomiting of pregnancy. *Obstet Gynecol.* 2015; 126(3):687–8. doi: 10.1097/01.AOG.0000471177.80067.19.
103. Abenavoli L, Capasso R, Milic N, et al. Milk thistle in liver diseases: past, present, future. *Phytother Res.* 2010;24(10):1423–32. doi: 10.1002/ptr.3207.
104. Forinash AB, Yancey AM, Barnes KN, et al. The use of galactogogues in the breastfeeding mother. *Ann Pharmacother.* 2012;46(10):1392–404. doi: 10.1345/aph.1R167.
105. Rambaldi A, Jacobs BP, Gluud C. Milk thistle for alcoholic and/or hepatitis B or C virus liver diseases. *Cochrane Database Syst Rev.* 2007; 4:CD003620. doi: 10.1002/14651858.CD003620.pub3.
106. Fried MW, Navarro VJ, Afdhal N, et al. Effect of silymarin (milk thistle) on liver disease in patients with chronic hepatitis C unsuccessfully treated with interferon therapy: a randomized controlled trial. *JAMA.* 2012;308(3):274–82. doi: 10.1001/jama.2012.8265.
107. Keifer D, Ulbricht C, Abrams TR, et al. Peppermint (Mentha piperita): an evidence-based systematic review by the Natural Standard Research Collaboration. *J Herb Pharmacother.* 2007;7(2):91–143. doi: 10.1080/J157v07n02_07.

108. Khanna R, MacDonald JK, Levesque BG. Peppermint oil for the treatment of irritable bowel syndrome: a systematic review and meta-analysis. *J Clin Gastroenterol.* 2014;48(6):505–12. doi: 10.1097/MCG.0b013e3182a88357.
109. Rochette L, Ghibu S, Muresan A, et al. Alpha-lipoic acid: molecular mechanisms and therapeutic potential in diabetes. *Can J Physiol Pharmacol.* 2015;93(12):1021–7. doi: 10.1139/cjpp-2014-0353.
110. Papanas N, Ziegler D. Efficacy of α-lipoic acid in diabetic neuropathy. *Expert Opin Pharmacother.* 2014;15(18):2721–31. doi: 10.1517/14656566.2014.972935.
111. Gleiter CH, Schug BS, Hermann R, et al. Influence of food intake on the bioavailability of thioctic acid enantiomers. *Eur J Clin Pharmacol.* 1996;50(6):513–4. doi: 10.1007/s002280050151.
112. McIlduff CE, Rutkove SB. Critical appraisal of the use of alpha lipoic acid (thioctic acid) in the treatment of symptomatic diabetic polyneuropathy. *Ther Clin Risk Manag.* 2011;7:377–85. doi: 10.2147/TCRM.S11325.
113. Han T, Bai J, Liu W, et al. A systematic review and meta-analysis of alpha-lipoic acid in the treatment of diabetic peripheral neuropathy. *Eur J Endocrinol.* 2012;167(4):465–71. doi: 10.1530/EJE-12-0555.
114. Mijnhout GS, Kollen BJ, Alkhalaf A, et al. Alpha lipoic acid for symptomatic peripheral neuropathy in patients with diabetes: a meta-analysis of randomized controlled trials. *Intl J Endocrinol.* 2012:456279. doi: 10.1155/2012/456279.
115. Ziegler D, Low PA, Litchy WJ, et al. Efficacy and safety of antioxidant treatment with alpha-lipoic acid over 4 years in diabetic polyneuropathy: the NATHAN 1 trial. *Diabetes Care.* 2011;34(9):2054–60. doi: 10.2337/dc11-0503.
116. Patel N, Mishra V, Patel P, et al. A study of the use of carbamazepine, pregabalin and alpha lipoic acid in patients of diabetic neuropathy. *J Diabetes Metab Disord.* 2014;13:62. doi: 10.1186/2251-6581-13-62.
117. Garcia-Alcala H, Santos Vichido CI, Macedo SI, et al. Treatment of α-lipoic acid over 16 weeks in type 2 diabetic patients with symptomatic polyneuropathy who responded to initial 4-week high-dose loading. *J Diabetes Res.* 2015:189857. doi: 10.1155/2015/189857.
118. Ansar H, Mazloom Z, Kazemi F, et al. Effect of alpha-lipoic acid on blood glucose, insulin resistance, and glutathione peroxidase of type 2 diabetic patients. *Saudi Med J.* 2011;32(6):584–8. PMID: 21666939.
119. Porasuphatana S, Suddee S, Nartnampong A, et al. Glycemic and oxidative status of patients with type 2 diabetes mellitus following oral administration of alpha-lipoic acid: a randomized double-blinded placebo-controlled study. *Asia Pac J Clin Nutr.* 2012;21(1):12–21. PMID: 22374556.
120. Rafehi H, Ververis K, Karagiannis TC. Controversies surrounding the clinical potential of cinnamon for the management of diabetes. *Diabetes Obes Metab.* 2012;14(6):493–9. doi: 10.1111/j.1463-1326.2011.01538.x.
121. Medagama AB. The glycaemic outcomes of cinnamon, a review of the experimental evidence and clinical trials. *Nutr. J.* 2015;14:108. doi: 10.1186/s12937-015-0098-9.
122. Chase CK, McQueen CE. The use of cinnamon in diabetes. *Am J Health Syst Pharm.* 2007;64(10):1033–35. doi: 10.2146/ajhp060538.
123. Brancheau D, Patel B, Zughaib M. Do cinnamon supplements cause acute hepatitis? *Am J Case Rep.* 2015;16:250–4. doi: 10.12659/AJCR.892804.
124. Wickenberg J, Lindstedt S, Berntorp K, et al. Ceylon cinnamon does not affect postprandial plasma glucose or insulin in subjects with impaired glucose tolerance. *Br J Nutr.* 2012;107(12):1845–9. doi: 10.1017/S0007114511005113.
125. Beejmohum V, Peytavy-Izard M, Mignon C, et al. Acute effect of Ceylon cinnamon extract on postprandial glycemia: alpha-amylase inhibition, starch tolerance test in rats, and randomized crossover clinical trial in healthy volunteers. *BMC Complement Altern Med.* 2014;14:351. doi: 10.1186/1472-6882-14-351.
126. Leach MJ, Kumar S. Cinnamon for diabetes mellitus. *Cochrane Database Syst Rev.* 2012;9:CD007170. doi: 10.1002/14651858.CD007170.pub2.
127. Allen RW, Schwartzman E, Baker WL, et al. Cinnamon use in type 2 diabetes: an updated systematic review and meta-analysis. *Ann Fam Med.* 2013;11(5):452–9. doi: 10.1370/afm.1517.
128. Davis PA, Yokoyama W. Cinnamon intake lowers fasting blood glucose: meta-analysis. *J Med Food.* 2011;14(9):884–9. doi: 10.1089/jmf.2010.0180.
129. Akilen R, Tsiami A, Devendra D, et al. Glycated haemoglobin and blood pressure-lowering effect of cinnamon in multi-ethnic type 2 diabetic patients in the UK: a randomized, placebo-controlled, double-blind clinical trial. *Diabetic Med.* 2010;27(10):1159–67. doi: 10.1111/j.1464-5491.2010.03079.x.
130. Lu T, Sheng H, Wu J, et al. Cinnamon extract improves fasting blood glucose and glycosylated hemoglobin level in Chinese patients with type 2 diabetes. *Nutr Res.* 2012;32(6):408–12. doi: 10.1016/j.nutres.2012.05.003.
131. Hudson JB. Applications of the phytomedicine Echinacea purpurea (purple coneflower) in infectious diseases. *J Biomed Biotech.* 2012:769896. doi: 10.1155/2012/769896.
132. Todd DA, Gulledge TV, Britton ER, et al. Ethanolic *Echinacea purpurea* extract contain a mixture of cytokine suppressive and cytokine-inducing compounds, including some that originate from endophytic bacteria. *PLoS ONE.* 2015;10(5):e0124276. doi: 10.1371/journal.pone.0124276.
133. Gabranis I, Koufakis T, Papakrivos I, et al. Echinacea-associated acute cholestatic hepatitis. *J Postgrad Med.* 2015;61(3):211–2. doi: 10.4103/0022-3859.159430.
134. Lee A, Werth V. Activation of autoimmunity following use of immunostimulatory herbal supplements. *Arch Dermatol.* 2004;140(6):723–7. doi: 10.1001/archderm.140.6.723.
135. Hermann R, von Richter O. Clinical evidence of herbal drugs as perpetrators of pharmacokinetic drug interactions. *Planta Med.* 2012;78(13):1458–77. doi: 10.1055/s-0032-1315117.
136. Perri D, Dugoua JJ, Mills E, et al. Safety and efficacy of echinacea (*Echinacea angustafolia, E. purpurea* and *E. pallida*) during pregnancy and lactation. *Can J Clin Pharmacol.* 2006;13(3):e262–7. PMID: 17085774.
137. Schapowal A, Klein P, Johnston SL. Echinacea reduces the risk of recurrent respiratory tract infections and complications: a meta-analysis of randomized controlled trials. *Adv Ther.* 2015;32(3):187–200. doi: 10.1007/s12325-015-0194-4.
138. Shah SA, Sander S, White CM, et al. Evaluation of echinacea for the prevention and treatment of the common cold: a meta-analysis. *Lancet Infect Dis.* 2007;7(7):473–80. doi: 10.1016/S1473-3099(07)70160-3.
139. Karsch-Völk M, Barrett B, Kiefer D, et al. Echinacea for preventing and treating the common cold. *Cochrane Database Syst Rev.* 2014;2:CD000530. doi: 10.1002/14651858.CD000530.pub3.
140. Di Pierro F, Rapacioli G, Ferrara T, et al. Use of a standardized extract from *Echinacea angustifolia* (Polinacea) for the prevention of respiratory tract infections. *Altern Med Rev.* 2012;17(1):36–41. PMID: 22502621.
141. Ulbricht C, Basch E, Cheung L, et al. An evidence-based systematic review of elderberry and elderflower (*Sambucus nigra*) by the Natural Standard Research Collaboration. *J Diet Suppl.* 2014;11(1):80–120. doi: 10.3109/19390211.2013.859852.
142. Krawitz C, Abu Mraheil M, Stein M, et al. Inhibitory activity of a standardized elderberry liquid extract against clinically-relevant human respiratory bacterial pathogens and influenza A and B viruses. *BMC Complement Altern Med.* 2011;11:16. doi: 10.1186/1472-6882-11-16.
143. Zakay-Rones Z, Varsano N, Zlotnik M, et al. Inhibition of several strains of influenza virus in vitro and reduction of symptoms by an elderberry extract (*Sambucus nigra* L.) during an outbreak of influenza B Panama. *J Altern Complement Med.* 1995;1(4):361–9. doi: 10.1089/acm.1995.1.361.
144. Curtis PJ, Kroon PA, Hollands WJ, et al. Cardiovascular disease risk biomarkers and liver and kidney function are not altered in postmenopausal women after ingesting an elderberry extract rich in anthocyanins for 12 weeks. *J Nutr.* 2009;139(12):2266–71. doi: 10.3945/jn.109.113126.
145. Ivanova D, Tasinov O, Kiselova-Kaneva Y. Improved lipid profile and increased serum antioxidant capacity in healthy volunteers after *Sambucus ebulus* L. fruit infusion consumption. *Int J Food Sci Nutr.* 2014;65(6):740–4. doi: 10.3109/09637486.2014.898256.
146. Vlachojannis JE, Cameron M, Chrubasik S. A systematic review on the *Sambuci fructus* effect and efficacy profiles. *Phytother Res.* 2010;24(1):1–8. doi: 10.1002/ptr.2729.
147. Zakay-Rones Z, Thom E, Wollan T, et al. Randomized study of the efficacy and safety of oral elderberry extract in the treatment of influenza A and B virus infections. *J Int Med Res.* 2004;32(2):132–40. doi: 10.1177/147323000403200205.

148. Rauš K, Pleschka S, Klein P, et al. Effect of an echinacea-based hot drink versus oseltamivir in influenza treatment: a randomized, double-blind, double-dummy, multicenter, noninferiority clinical trial. *Curr Ther Res Clin Exp.* 2015;77:66–72. doi: 10.1016/j.curtheres.2015.04.001.
149. *Eleutherococcus senticosus* [monograph]. *Altern Med Rev.* 2006;11(2): 151–5. PMID: 16813463.
150. Schaffler K, Wolf OT, Burkart M. No benefit adding *Eleutherococcus senticosus* to stress management training in stress-related fatigue/weakness, impaired work or concentration, a randomized controlled study. *Pharmacopsychiatry.* 2013;46(5):181–90. doi: 10.1055/s-0033–1347178.
151. Williams M. Immunoprotection against herpes simplex type II infection by eleutherococcus root extract. *Int J Altern Complement Med.* 2001;13:9–12.
152. Gabrielian ES, Shukarian AK, Goukasova GI, et al. A double blind, placebo-controlled study of Andrographis paniculata fixed combination Kan Jang in the treatment of acute upper respiratory tract infections including sinusitis. *Phytomedicine.* 2002;9(7):589–97. doi: 10.1078/094471102321616391.
153. Barth A, Hovhannisyan A, Jamalyan K, et al. Antitussive effect of a fixed combination of *Justicia adhatoda, Echinacea purpurea* and *Eleutherococcus senticosus* extracts in patients with acute upper respiratory tract infection: a comparative, randomized, double-blind, placebo-controlled study. *Phytomedicine.* 2015;22(13):1195–200. doi: 10.1016/j.phymed.2015.10.001.
154. *Panax ginseng* [monograph]. *Altern Med Rev.* 2009;14(2):172–6. PMID: 19594226.
155. Paik DJ, Lee CH. Review of cases of patient risk associated with ginseng abuse and misuse. *J Ginseng Res.* 2015;39(2):89–93. doi: 10.1016/j.jgr.2014.11.005.
156. Seely D, Dugoua JJ, Perri D, et al. Safety and efficacy of panax ginseng during pregnancy and lactation. *Can J Clin Pharmacol.* 2008;15(1): e87–94. PMID: 18204104.
157. Kim S, Shin BC, et al. Red ginseng for type 2 diabetes mellitus: a systematic review of randomized controlled trials. *Chin J Integr Med.* 2011;17(12):937–44. doi: 10.1007/s11655-011-0937-2.
158. Shishtar E, Sievenpiper JL, Djedovic V, et al. The effect of ginseng (the genus panax) on glycemic control: a systematic review and meta-analysis of randomized controlled clinical trials. *PLoS One.* 2014;9(9):e107391. doi: 10.1371/journal.pone.0107391.
159. Jang DJ, Lee MS, Shin BC, et al. Red ginseng for treating erectile dysfunction: a systematic review. *Br J Clin Pharmacol.* 2008;66(4): 444–50. doi: 10.1111/j.1365-2125.2008.03236.x.
160. Geng J, Dong J, Ni H, et al. Ginseng for cognition. *Cochrane Database Syst Rev.* 2010;(12):CD007769. doi: 10.1002/14651858.CD007769.pub2.
161. Wang Y, Yang G, Gong J, et al. Ginseng for Alzheimer's disease: a systematic review and meta-analysis of randomized controlled trials. *Curr Top Med Chem* 2016;16(5):529–36. doi: 10.2174/15680266156661508 13143753.
162. Henning S, Niu Y, Lee N, et al. Bioavailability and antioxidant activity of tea flavanols after consumption of green tea, black tea, or a green tea extract supplement. *Am J Clin Nutr.* 2004;80(6):1558–64.
163. Jurgens TM, Whelan AM, Killian L, et al. Green tea for weight loss and weight maintenance in overweight or obese adults. *Cochrane Database Syst Rev.* 2012;12:CD008650. doi: 10.1002/14651858.CD008650.pub2.
164. Boehm K, Borrelli F, Ernst E, et al. Green tea (*Camellia sinensis*) for the prevention of cancer. *Cochrane Database Syst Rev.* 2009;3:CD005004. doi: 10.1002/14651858.CD005004.pub2.
165. Mayo Clinic. Caffeine content for coffee, tea, soda and more. Available at: http://www.mayoclinic.org/healthy-lifestyle/nutrition-and-healthy-eating/in-depth/caffeine/art-20049372. Accessed March 22, 2016.
166. Sarma DN, Barrett ML, Chavez ML, et al. Safety of green tea extracts: a systematic review by the US Pharmacopeia. *Drug Saf.* 2008;31(6): 469–84. doi: 10.2165/00002018-200831060-00003.
167. Wolfram S. Effects of green tea and EGCG on cardiovascular and metabolic health. *J Am Coll Nutr.* 2007;26(4):373S–88S. doi: 10.1080/07315724.2007.10719626.
168. Hartley L, Flowers N, Holmes J, et al. Green tea and black tea for the primary prevention of cardiovascular disease. *Cochrane Database Syst Rev.* 2013;6:CD009934. doi: 10.1002/14651858.CD009934.pub2.
169. Onakpoya I, Spencer E, Heneghan C, et al. The effect of green tea on blood pressure and lipid profile: a systematic review and meta-analysis of randomized clinical trials. *Nutr Metab Cardiovasc Dis.* 2014;24(8): 823–36. doi: 10.1016/j.numecd.2014.01.016.
170. Strong KM. African plum and benign prostatic hypertrophy. *J Herb Pharmacother.* 2004;4(1):41–6. doi: 10.1080/J157v04n01_05.
171. *Pygeum africanum* (*Prunus africana*) (African plum tree) [monograph]. *Altern Med Rev.* 2002;7(1):71–4. PMID: 11896748.
172. Wilt T, Ishani A, MacDonald R, et al. *Pygeum africanum* for benign prostatic hyperplasia. *Cochrane Database Syst Rev.* 2002;1:CD001044. doi: 10.1002/14651858.CD001044.
173. Howell AB. Bioactive compounds in cranberries and their role in prevention of urinary tract infections. *Mol Nutr Food Res.* 2007;51(6):732–7. doi: 10.1002/mnfr.200700038.
174. Haber SL, Cauthon KA, Raney EC. Cranberry and warfarin interaction: a case report and review of the literature. *Consult Pharm.* 2012;27(1): 58–65. doi: 10.4140/TCP.n.2012.58.
175. Jepson R, Williams G, Craig J. Cranberries for preventing urinary tract infections. *Cochrane Database Syst Rev.* 2012;10:CD001321. doi: 10.1002/14651858.CD001321.
176. Takahashi S, Hamasuna R, Yasuda M, et al. A randomized clinical trial to evaluate the preventive effect of cranberry juice (UR65) for patients with recurrent urinary tract infection. *J Infect Chemother.* 2013;19(1): 112–7. doi: 10.1007/s10156-012-0467-7.
177. Caljouw MA, van den Hout WB, Putter H, et al. Effectiveness of cranberry capsules to prevent urinary tract infections in vulnerable older persons: a double-blind randomized placebo-controlled trial in long-term care facilities. *J Am Geriatr Soc.* 2014;62(1):103–10. doi: 10.1111/jgs.12593.
178. Foxman B, Cronenwett AE, Spino C, et al. Cranberry juice capsules and urinary tract infection after surgery: results of a randomized trial. *Am J Obstet Gynecol.* 2015;213(2):194.e1–8. doi: 10.1016/j.ajog.2015.04.003.
179. Jepson RG, Mihaljevic L, Craig J. Cranberries for treating urinary tract infections. *Cochrane Database Syst Rev.* 2010;2:CD001322. doi: 10.1002/14651858.CD001322.
180. Samaras N, Samaras D, Frangos E, et al. A review of age-related dehydroepiandrosterone decline and its association with well-known geriatric syndromes: is treatment beneficial? *Rejuvenation Res.* 2013;16(4):285–94. doi: 10.1089/rej.2013.1425.
181. Pluchino N, Drakopoulos P, Petignat P, et al. DHEA supplementation in menopause. *Curr Obstet Gynecol Rep.* 2014;3(4):232–7. doi: 10.1007/s13669-014-0095-6.
182. Dean CE. Prasterone (DHEA) and mania. *Ann Pharmacother.* 2000; 34(12):1419–22. doi: 10.1345/aph.10115.
183. Acacio BD, Stanczyk FZ, Mullin P, et al. Pharmacokinetics of dehydroepiandrosterone and its metabolites after long-term daily oral administration to healthy young men. *Fertil Steril.* 2004;81(3):595–604. doi: 10.1016/j.fertnstert.2003.07.035.
184. Reiter WJ, Scheatzl G, Mark I, et al. Dehydroepiandrosterone in the treatment of erectile dysfunction in patients with different organic etiologies. *Urol Res.* 2001;29(4):278–81. doi: 10.1007/s002400100189.
185. Panjari M, Davis SR. DHEA for postmenopausal women: a review of the evidence. *Maturitas.* 2010;66(2):172–9. doi: 10.1016/j.maturitas.2009.12.017.
186. Genazzani AR, Stomati M, Valentino V, et al. Effect of 1-year, low-dose DHEA therapy on climacteric symptoms and female sexuality. *Climacteric.* 2011;14(6):661–8. doi: 10.3109/13697137.2011.579649.
187. Jankowski CM, Gozansky WS, Kittelson JM, et al. Increases in bone mineral density in response to oral dehydroepiandrosterone replacement in older adults appear to be mediated by serum estrogens. *J Clin Endocrinol Metab.* 2008;93(12):4767–73. doi: 10.1210/jc.2007-2614.
188. Kenny AM, Boxer RX, Kleppinger A, et al. Dehydroepiandrosterone combined with exercise improves muscle strength and physical function in frail older women. *J Am Geriatr Soc.* 2010;58(9):1707–14. doi: 10.1111/j.1532-5415.2010.03019.x.
189. von Mühlen D, Laughlin GA, Kritz-Silverstein D, et al. Effect of dehydroepiandrosterone supplementation on bone mineral density, bone markers, and body composition in older adults: the DAWN trial. *Osteoporosis Int.* 2008;19(5):699–707. doi: 10.1007/s00198-007-0520-z.

190. El-Alfy M, Deloche C, Azzi L, et al. Skin responses to topical dehydroepiandrosterone: implications in antiaging treatment? *Brit J Dermatol.* 2010;163(5):968–76. doi: 10.1111/j.1365-2133.2010.09972.x.
191. Fong YK, Milani S, Djavan B. Role of phytotherapy in men with lower urinary tract symptoms. *Curr Opin Urol.* 2005;15(1):45–8. doi: 10.1097/00042307-200501000-00011.
192. Agbabiaka TB, Pittler MH, Wider B, et al. *Serenoa repens* (saw palmetto): A systematic review of adverse events. *Drug Saf.* 2009;32(8):637–47. doi: 10.2165/00002018-200932080-00003.
193. Avins AL, Lee JY, Meyers CM, et al. Safety and toxicity in the CAMUS trial. *J Urol.* 2013;189(4):1415–20. doi: 10.1016/j.juro.2012.10.002.
194. Tacklind J, Macdonald R, Rutks I, et al. *Serenoa repens* for benign prostatic hyperplasia. *Cochrane Database Syst Rev.* 2012;12:CD001423. doi: 10.1002/14651858.CD001423.pub3.
195. Nagaoka I, Igarashi M, Sakamoto K. Biological activities of glucosamine and its related substances. *Adv Food Nutr Res.* 2012;65:337–52. doi: 10.1016/B978-0-12-416003-3.00022-6.
196. Henrotin Y, Mobasheri A, Marty M. Is there any scientific evidence for the use of glucosamine in the management of human osteoarthritis? *Arthritis Res Ther.* 2012;14(1):201. doi: 10.1186/ar3657.
197. Volpi N. Anti-inflammatory activity of chondroitin sulphate: new functions from an old natural molecule. *Inflammopharmacology.* 2011;19(6): 299–306. doi: 10.1007/s10787-011-0098-0.
198. Martel-Pelletier J, Farran A, Montell E, et al. Discrepancies in composition and biological effects of different formulations of chondroitin sulfate. *Molecules.* 2015;20(3):4277–89. doi: 10.3390/molecules20034277.
199. Calamia V, Mateos J, Fernández-Puente P, et al. A pharmacoproteomic study confirms the synergistic effect of chondroitin sulfate and glucosamine. *Sci Rep.* 2014;4:5069. doi: 10.1038/srep05069.
200. Lee YH, Woo JH, Choi SJ, et al. Effect of glucosamine or chondroitin sulfate on the osteoarthritis progression: a meta-analysis. *Rheumatol Int.* 2010;30(3):357–63. doi: 10.1007/s00296-009-0969-5.
201. Eriksen P, Bartels EM, Altman RD, et al. Risk of bias and brand explain the observed inconsistency in trials on glucosamine for symptomatic relief of osteoarthritis: a meta-analysis of placebo-controlled trials. *Arthritis Care Res (Hoboken).* 2014;66(12):1844–55. doi: 10.1002/acr.22376.
202. Villacis J, Rice TR, Bucci LR, et al. Do shrimp-allergic individuals tolerate shrimp-derived glucosamine? *Clin Exper Allergy.* 2006;36(11): 1457–61. doi: 10.1111/j.1365-2222.2006.02590.x.
203. Bruyére O, Altman RD, Reginster JY. Efficacy and safety of glucosamine sulfate in the management of osteoarthritis: evidence from real-life setting trials and surveys. *Semin Arthritis Rheum.* 2016;45(4 Suppl):S12–7. doi: 10.1016/j.semarthrit.2015.11.011.
204. Wandel S, Jüni P, Tendal B, et al. Effects of glucosamine, chondroitin, or placebo in patients with osteoarthritis of hip or knee: network meta-analysis. *BMJ.* 2010;34:c4675. doi: 10.1136/bmj.c4675.
205. Sawitzke AD, Shi H, Finco MF, et al. Clinical efficacy and safety of glucosamine, chondroitin sulfate, their combination, celecoxib or placebo taken to treat osteoarthritis of the knee: 2-year results from GAIT. *Ann Rheum Dis.* 2010;69(8):1459–64. doi: 10.1136/ard.2009.120469.
206. Hochberg Mc. Structure-modifying effects of chondroitin sulfate in knee osteoarthritis: an updated meta-analysis of randomized placebo-controlled trials of 2-year duration. *Osteoarthritis Cartilage.* 2010;18(Suppl 1): S28–31. doi: 10.1016/j.joca.2010.02.016.
207. Gabay C, Medinger-Sadowski C, Gascon D, et al. Symptomatic effects of chondroitin 4 and chondroitin 6 sulfate on hand osteoarthritis: a randomized, double-blind, placebo-controlled clinical trial at a single center. *Arthritis Rheum.* 2011;63(11):3383–91. doi: 10.1002/art.30574.
208. Hochberg MC, Martel-Pelletier J, Monfort J, et al. Combined chondroitin sulfate and glucosamine for painful knee osteoarthritis: a multicentre, randomized, double-blind, non-inferiority trial versus celecoxib. *Ann Rheum Dis.* 2016;75(1):37–44. doi: 10.1136/annrheumdis-2014-206792.
209. Provenza JR, Shinjo SM, Silva JM, et al. Combined glucosamine and chondroitin sulfate, once or three times daily, provides clinically relevant analgesia in knee osteoarthritis. *Clin Rheumatol,* 2015;34(8):1455–62. doi: 10.1007/s10067-014-2757-1.
210. Ely A, Lockwood B. What is the evidence for the safety and efficacy of dimethylsulfoxide and methylsulfonylmethane in pain relief? *Pharm J.* 2002;269(7223):685–7.
211. Karabay AZ, Aktan F, Sunguroğlu A, et al. Methylsulfonylmethane modulates apoptosis of LPS/IFN-γ-activated RAW 264.7 macrophage-like cells by targeting p53, Bax, Bcl-2, cytochrome c and PARP proteins. *Immunopharmacol Immunotoxicol.* 2014;36(6):379–389. doi: 10.3109/08923973.2014.956752.
212. Kim YH, Kim DH, Lim H, et al. The anti-inflammatory effects of methylsulfonylmethane on lipopolysaccharide-induced responses in murine macrophages. *Biol Pharm Bull.* 2009;32(4):651–6. doi: 10.1248/bpb.32.651.
213. Brien S, Prescott P, Bashir N, et al. Systematic review of the nutritional supplements dimethylsulfoxide (DMSO) and methylsulfonylmethane (MSM) in the treatment of osteoarthritis. *Osteoarthritis Cartilage.* 2008; 16(11):1277–88. doi: 10.1016/j.joca.2008.03.002.
214. Notarnicola A, Maccagnano G, Moretti L, et al. Methylsulfonylmethane and boswellic acids versus glucosamine sulfate in the treatment of knee arthritis: randomized trial. *Int J Immunopathol Pharmacol.* 2015;29(1):140–6. doi: 10.1177/0394632015622215.
215. Hosea Blewett HJ. Exploring the mechanisms behind S-adenosylmethionine (SAMe) in the treatment of osteoarthritis. *Crit Rev Food Sci Nutr.* 2008;48(5):458–63. doi: 10.1080/10408390701429526.
216. Zhang M, Li L, Huang J-Y, et al. Protective effect of S-adenosyl-L-methionine combined with meloxicam on knee osteoarthritis in rats. *Chin J New Drugs.* 2015;24(18):2142–6 and 2152.
217. Williams A, Girard C, Jui D, et al. S-Adenosylmethionine (SAMe) as treatment for depression: a systematic review. *Med Clin Exp.*2005;28(3): 132–9. PMID: 16021987.
218. Brown RP, Gerbarg P, Bottiglieri T. S-Adenosylmethionine (SAMe) for depression. *Psychiatr Ann.* 2002;32(1):29–44.doi: 10.3928/0048-5713-20020101-07.
219. Kagan BL, Sultzer DL, Rosenlicht N, et al. Oral *S*-adenosylmethionine in depression: a randomized, double-blind, placebo-controlled trial. *Am J Psychiatry.* 1990;147(5):591–5. doi: 10.1176/ajp.147.5.591.
220. Gorën JL, Stoll AL, Damico KE, et al. Bioavailability and lack of toxicity of S-adenosyl-L-methionine (SAMe) in humans. *Pharmacotherapy.* 2004;24(11):1501–7. doi: 10.1592/phco.24.16.1501.50943.
221. Rutjes AW, Nüesch E, Reichenbach S, et al. S-adenosylmethionine for osteoarthritis of the knee or hip. *Cochrane Database Syst Rev.* 2009;4:CD007321. doi: 10.1002/14651858.CD007321.pub2.
222. Najm WI, Reinsch S, Hoehler F, et al. S-Adenosyl methionine (SAMe) versus celecoxib for the treatment of osteoarthritis symptoms: a double-blind cross-over trial. *BMC Musculoskelet Disord.* 2004;5:6. doi: 10.1186/1471-2474-5-6.
223. Kim J, Lee EY, Koh EM, et al. Comparative clinical trial of S-adenosylmethionine versus nabumetone for the treatment of knee osteoarthritis: an 8-week, multicenter, randomized, double-blind, double-dummy, phase IV study in Korean patients. *Clin Ther.* 2009;31(12):2860–72. doi: 10.1016/j.clinthera.2009.12.016.
224. Agrawal S, Goel RK. Curcumin and its protective and therapeutic uses. *Nat J Physiol Pharm Pharmacol.* 2016;6(1):1–8. doi: 10.5455/njppp.2016.6.3005201596.
225. Kertia N, Asdie AH, Rochmah W, et al. Ability of curcuminoid compared to diclofenac sodium in reducing the secretion of cyclooxygenase-2 enzyme by synovial fluids' monocytes of patients with osteoarthritis. *Acta Med Indones.* 2012;44(2):105–113. PMID: 22745140.
226. Lopez HL. Nutritional interventions to prevent and treat osteoarthritis. Part II: focus on micronutrients and supportive nutraceuticals. *PM R.* 2012;4(5 Suppl):S155–68. doi: 10.1016/j.pmrj.2012.02.023.
227. Kuptniratsaikul V, Dajpratham P, Taechaarpornkul W, et al. Efficacy and safety of Curcuma domestica extracts compared with ibuprofen in patients with knee osteoarthritis: a multicenter study. *Clin Interv Aging.* 2014; 9:451–8. doi: 10.2147/CIA.S58535.
228. Madhu K, Chanda K, Saji MJ. Safety and efficacy of Curcuma long extract in the treatment of painful knee osteoarthritis: a randomized, placebo-controlled trial. *Inflammopharmacology.* 2013;21(2):129–36. doi: 10.1007/s10787-012-0163-3.
229. Hashemi SA, Madani SA, Abediankenari S. The review of properties of aloe vera in healing cutaneous wounds. *Biomed Res Int.* 2015:714216. doi: 10.1155/2015/714216.
230. U.S. Food and Drug Administration. Status of certain additional over-the-counter drug category II and III active ingredients. Final rule. *Fed*

Reg. 2002;67(90):31125–7. Available at: https://www.gpo.gov/fdsys/pkg/FR-2002-05-09/pdf/02-11510.pdf. Accessed June 25, 2017.

231. Guo X, Mei N. Aloe vera: a review of toxicity and adverse clinical effects. *J Environ Sci Health C Environ Carcinog Ecotoxicol Rev.* 2016;34(2):77–96. doi: 10.1080/10590501.2016.1166826.
232. International Aloe Science Council. Certification program. Available at: http://www.iasc.org/Certification.aspx. Accessed June 25, 2017.
233. Dat AD, Poon F, Pham KB, et al. Aloe vera for treating acute and chronic wounds. *Cochrane Database Syst Rev.* 2012;2:CD008762. doi: 10.1002/14651858.CD008762.pub2.
234. Maenthaisong R, Chaiyakunapruk N, Niruntraporn S, et al. The efficacy of aloe vera used for burn wound healing: a systematic review. *Burns.* 2007;33(6):713–8. doi: 10.1016/j.burns.2006.10.384.
235. Pazyar N, Yaghoobi R, Bagherani N, et al. A review of applications of tea tree oil in dermatology. *Int J Dermatol.* 2013;52(7):784–90. doi: 10.1111/j.1365-4632.2012.05654.x.
236. Henley DV, Lipson N, Korach KS, et al. Prepubertal gynecomastia linked to lavender and tea tree oils. *N Engl J Med.* 2007;356(5):479–85. doi: 10.1056/NEJMoa064725.
237. Satchell AC, Saurajen A, Bell C, et al. Treatment of interdigital tinea pedis with 25% and 50% tea tree oil solution: a randomized, placebo-controlled, blinded study. *Australas J Dermatol.* 2002;43(3):175–8. doi: 10.1046/j.1440-0960.2002.00590.x.
238. Satchell AC, Saurajen A, Bell C, et al. Treatment of dandruff with 5% tea tree oil shampoo. *J Am Acad Dermatol.* 2002;47(6):852–5. doi: 10.1067/mjd.2002.122734.
239. Buck DS, Nidorf DM, Addino JG. Comparison of two topical preparations for the treatment of onychomycosis: *Melaleuca alternifolia* (tea tree) oil and clotrimazole. *J Fam Pract.* 1994;38(6):601–5. PMID: 8195735
240. Enshaieh S, Jooya A, Siadat AH, et al. The efficacy of 5% topical tea tree oil gel in mild to moderate acne vulgaris: a randomized, double-blind placebo-controlled study. *Indian J Dermatol Venereol Leprol.* 2007;73(1):22–5. doi: 10.4103/0378-6323.30646.
241. Semwal RB, Semwal KL, Vermaak I, et al. A comprehensive scientific overview of *Garcinia cambogia*. *Fitoterapia.* 2015;102:134–48. doi: 10.1016/j.fitote.2015.02.012.
242. Chuah LO, Ho WY, Beh BK, et al. Updates on antiobesity effect of *Garcinia* origin (-)-HCA. *Evid Based Complement Altern Med.* 2013:751658. doi: 10.1155/2013/751658.
243. Chuah LO, Yeap SK, Ho WY, et al. In vitro and in vivo toxicity of *Garcinia* or hydroxycitric acid: a review. *Evid Based Complement Altern Med.* 2012:197920. doi: 10.1155/2012/197920.
244. Corey R, Werner KT, Singer A, et al. Acute liver failure associated with Garcinia cambogia use. *Ann Hepatol.* 2016;15(1):123–6. doi: 10.5604/16652681.1184287
245. Joseph D, Joseph M, Levine M. Stress induced cardiomyopathy after ingestion of garcinia cambogia. *Clin Toxicol.* 2014;52(7):739–40.
246. Mattes RD, Bormann L. Effects of (-)-hydroxycitric acid on appetitive variables. *Physiol Behav.* 2000;71(1-2):87–94. doi: 10.1016/S0031-9384(00)00321-8.
247. Heymsfield SB, Allison DB, Vasselli JR, et al. *Garcinia cambogia* (hydroxycitric acid) as a potential antiobesity agent. *JAMA.* 1998;280(18):1596–1600. doi: 10.1001/jama.280.18.1596.
248. Park KS. Raspberry ketone increases both lipolysis and fatty acid oxidation in 3T3-L1 adipocytes. *Planta Med.* 2010;76(15):1654–8. doi: 10.1055/s-0030-1249860.
249. Khazaal FAK, Mosah HA, Sahib HB, et al. Effect of raspberry ketones and L-carnitine on oxidative stress and body weight in Iraqi obese patients. *Int J Pharm Sci Rev Res.* 2015;31(2):69–75.
250. Takematsu M, Smith SW, Hoffman RS, et al. Berries that weren't that sweet after all: a case of raspberry ketone intoxication. *Clin Toxicol.* 2013;51(4):284.
251. Jones S, Thomas AM, Vale JA, et al. Analysis of telephone enquiries to the UK National Poisons Information Service (NPIS) concerning raspberry ketone weight loss supplements (2011–2014). *Clin Toxicol.* 2015;53(4):244.
252. Li JX, Yu ZY. Cimicifugae rhizoma: from origins, bioactive constituents to clinical outcomes. *Curr Med Chem.* 2006;13(24):2927–51. doi: 10.2174/092986706778521869.
253. Palacio C, Masri G, Mooradian AD. Black cohosh for the management of menopausal symptoms: a systematic review of clinical trials. *Drugs Aging.* 2009;26(1):23–36. doi: 10.2165/0002512-200926010-00002.
254. Roberts H. Safety of herbal medicinal products in women with breast cancer. *Maturitas.* 2010;66(4):363–9. doi: 10.1016/j.maturitas.2010.02.010.
255. Ulbricht C, Windsor RC. An evidence-based systematic review of black cohosh (Cimicifuga racemosa, Actaea racemosa) by the Natural Standard Research Collaboration. *J Diet Suppl.* 2015;12(3):265–358. doi: 10.3109/19390211.2014.946731.
256. Borrelli F, Ernst E. Black cohosh (*Cimicifuga racemosa*): a systematic review of adverse events. *Am J Obstet Gynecol.* 2008;199(5):455–66. doi: 10.1016/j.ajog.2008.05.007.
257. Mahady GB, Low Dog T, Barrett ML, et al. United States Pharmacopeia review of the black cohosh case reports of hepatotoxicity. *Menopause.* 2008;15(4 Pt 1):628–38. doi: 10.1097/gme.0b013e31816054bf.
258. Teschke R, Schwarzenboeck A, Schmidt-Taenzer W, et al. Herb induced liver injury presumably caused by black cohosh: a survey of initially purported cases and herbal quality specifications. *Ann Hepatol.* 2011;10(3):249–59. PMID: 21677326.
259. Leach MJ, Moore V. Black cohosh (Cimicifuga spp.) for menopausal symptoms. *Cochrane Database Syst Rev.* 2012;9:CD007244. doi: 10.1002/14651858.CD007244.pub2.
260. Laakmann E, Grajecki D, Doege K, et al. Efficacy of Cimicifuga racemosa, Hypericum perforatum and Agnus castus in the treatment of climacteric complaints: a systematic review. *Gynecol Endocrinol.* 2012;28(9):703–9. doi: 10.3109/09513590.2011.650772.
261. American College of Obstetricians and Gynecologists. ACOG Practice Bulletin No. 141: management of menopausal symptoms. *Obstet Gynecol.* 2014;123(1):202–16. doi: 10.1097/01.AOG.0000441353.20693.78.
262. Walji R, Boon H, Guns E, et al. Black cohosh (*Cimicifuga racemosa* [L.] Nutt.): safety and efficacy for cancer patients. *Support Care Cancer.* 2007;15(8):913–21. doi: 10.1007/s00520-007-0286-z.
263. Fritz H, Seely D, McGowan J, et al. Black cohosh and breast cancer: a systematic review. *Integr Cancer Ther.* 2014;13(1):12–29. doi: 10.1177/1534735413477191.
264. van Die MD, Burger HG, Teede HJ, et al. Vitex agnus-castus (Chaste-Tree/Berry) in the treatment of menopause-related complaints. *J Altern Complement Med.* 2009;15(8):853–62. doi: 10.1089/acm.2008.0447.
265. Daniele C, Thompson Coon J, Pittler MH, et al. Vitex agnus castus: a systematic review of adverse events. *Drug Saf.* 2005;28(4):319–32. doi: 10.2165/00002018-200528040-00004.
266. van Die MD, Burger HG, Bone KM, et al. Hypericum perforatum with Vitex agnus-castus in menopausal symptoms: a randomized, controlled trial. *Menopause.* 2009;16(1):156–63. doi: 10.1097/gme.0b013e31817fa9e0.
267. Rotem C, Kaplan B. Phyto-Female Complex for the relief of hot flushes, night sweats and quality of sleep: randomized, controlled, double-blind pilot study. *Gynecol Endocrinol.* 2007;23(2):117–22. doi: 10.1080/09513590701200900.
268. van Die MD, Burger HG, Teede HJ, Bone KM. Vitex agnus-castus extracts for female reproductive disorders: a systematic review of clinical trials. *Planta Med.* 2013;79(7):562–75. doi: 10.1055/s-0032-1327831.
269. Bayles B, Usatine R. Evening primrose oil. *Am Fam Physician.* 2009;80(12):1405–8. PMID: 20000302.
270. Stonemetz D. A review of the clinical efficacy of evening primrose. *Holist Nurs Pract.* 2008;22(3):171–4. doi: 10.1097/01.HNP.0000318026.45527.07.
271. Pruthi S, Wahner-Roedler DL, Torkelson CJ, et al. Vitamin E and evening primrose oil for management of cyclical mastalgia: a randomized pilot study. *Altern Med Rev.* 2010;15(1):59–67. PMID: 20359269.
272. Goyal A, Mansel RE; Efamast Study Group. A randomized multicenter study of gamolenic acid (Efamast) with and without antioxidant vitamins and minerals in the management of mastalgia. *Breast J.* 2005;11(1):41–7. doi: 10.1111/j.1075-122X.2005.21492.x.
273. Bamford JT, Ray S, Musekiwa A, et al. Oral evening primrose oil and borage oil for eczema. *Cochrane Database Syst Rev.* 2013;4:CD004416. doi: 10.1002/14651858.CD004416.pub2.

274. Yadav UC, Baquer NZ. Pharmacological effects of Trigonella foenum-graecum L. in health and disease. *Pharm Biol.* 2014;52(2):243–54. doi: 10.3109/13880209.2013.826247.
275. Ulbricht C, Basch E, Burke D, et al. Fenugreek (*Trigonella foenum-graecum* L. Leguminosae): an evidence-based systematic review by the natural standard research collaboration. *J Herb Pharmacother.* 2007;7(3-4):143–77. doi: 10.1080/15228940802142852.
276. Turkyilmaz C, Onal E, Hirfanoglu IM, et al. The effect of galactagogue herbal tea on breast milk production and short-term catch-up of birth weight in the first week of life. *J Altern Complement Med.* 2011;17(2): 139–42. doi: 10.1089/acm.2010.0090.
277. Haber SL, Keonavong J. Fenugreek use in patients with diabetes mellitus. *Am J Health Syst Pharm.* 2013; 70(14):1196, 1198, 1200, 1202-3. doi: 10.2146/ajhp120523.
278. Panay N. Taking an integrated approach: managing women with phytoestrogens. *Climacteric.* 2011;14(Suppl 2):2–7. doi: 10.3109/13697137.2011.626367.
279. Franco OH, Chowdhury R, Troup J, et al. Use of plant-based therapies and menopausal symptoms: a systematic review and meta-analysis. *JAMA.* 2016;315(23):2554–63. doi: 10.1001/jama.2016.8012.
280. Marini H, Minutoli L, Polito F, et al. Effects of the phytoestrogen genistein on bone metabolism in osteopenic postmenopausal women: a randomized trial. *Ann Intern Med.* 2007;146(12):839–47. doi: 10.7326/0003-4819-146-12-200706190-00005.
281. Marini H, Bitto A, Altavilla D, et al. Breast safety and efficacy of genistein aglycone for postmenopausal bone loss: a follow-up study. *J Clin Endocrinol Metab.* 2008;93(12):4787–96. doi: 10.1210/jc.2008-1087.
282. Alekel DL, Van Loan MD, Koehler KJ, et al. The soy isoflavones for reducing bone loss (SIRBL) study: a 3-y randomized controlled trial in postmenopausal women. *Am J Clin Nutr.* 2010;91(1):218–30. doi: 10.3945/ajcn.2009.28306.
283. Tai TY, Tsai KS, Tu ST, et al. The effect of soy isoflavone on bone mineral density in postmenopausal Taiwanese women with bone loss: a 2-year randomized double-blind placebo-controlled study. *Osteoporos Int.* 2012;23(5):1571–80. doi: 10.1007/s00198-011-1750-7.
284. Sacks FM, Lichtenstein A, Van Horn L, et al. Soy protein, isoflavones, and cardiovascular health: an American Heart Association Science Advisory for professionals from the Nutrition Committee. *Circulation.* 2006;113(7):1034–44. doi: 10.1161/CIRCULATIONAHA.106.171052.
285. Magee PJ, Rowland I. Soy products in the management of breast cancer. *Curr Opin Clin Nutr Metab Care.* 2012;15(6):586–91. doi: 10.1097/MCO.0b013e328359156f.
286. Eden JA. Phytoestrogens for menopausal symptoms: a review. *Mauritas.* 2012;72(2):157–9. doi: 10.1016/j.maturitas.2012.03.006.
287. Yan L, Spitznagel EL. Soy consumption and prostate cancer risk in men: a revisit of a meta-analysis. *Am J Clin Nutr.* 2009;89(4):1155–63. doi: 10.3945/ajcn.2008.27029.

CHAPTER 52

COMMON COMPLEMENTARY AND INTEGRATIVE MEDICINE HEALTH SYSTEMS

CATHERINE ULBRICHT AND EUNJI MICHELLE KO

The term *complementary and integrative medicine* (CIM) refers to a broad domain of healing practices that include diverse health systems, modalities, and practices, and their accompanying theories and beliefs.[1–3] CIM includes many modalities beyond simply the use of dietary supplements. *Complementary medicine* refers to using a non-mainstream approach together with conventional medicine. *Integrative medicine* is defined as integrating nontraditional approaches into conventional medicine.[2] Other terms used to describe CIM include *folkloric, holistic, irregular, nonconventional, non-Western, traditional, unorthodox,* and *unproven medicine.* Common CIM therapies and health systems include homeopathy, naturopathy, traditional Chinese medicine, acupuncture, chiropractic care, Ayurveda, and massage. This chapter presents a brief overview of common types of CIM other than dietary supplements, which are discussed in Chapter 51.

Overview of Common CIM Health Systems

Major Categories

In the United States, the National Center for Complementary and Integrative Health (NCCIH) classifies CIM therapies into three broad categories.[2] These include natural products, mind–body practices, and other complementary health approaches. Natural products include herbal medicines, or botanicals; nonbotanicals; minerals; vitamins; and other products such as probiotics. The mind–body practices are diverse and feature procedures or techniques that are taught or conducted by a trained practitioner or teacher. Examples of mind–body medicine include chiropractic manipulation, acupuncture, guided imagery, hypnotherapy, *qi gong, tai chi,* yoga, and massage therapy, among many others. The third category is especially broad; it includes traditional healers, energy therapies such as Reiki, and whole medical systems such as Ayurveda, TCM, homeopathy, and naturopathy.[2] The NCCIH website (https://nccih.nih.gov) contains extensive information on many forms of CIM.

Healing systems encompass complete sets of theories and practices. A system focuses on a philosophy or lifestyle, such as the power of nature or the presence of energy in the body. Some CIM therapies have been integrated into conventional medicine. Many prescription drugs originally came from natural products; examples include digoxin from the foxglove plant, paclitaxel from the bark of the yew tree, yohimbine from yohimbe bark, oseltamivir from Chinese star anise, etoposide and teniposide derived from *Podophyllum peltatum,* and vincristine and vinblastine derived from *Catharanthus roseus.*[4]

Potential Risks and Benefits

CIM is often considered a form of preventive medicine and is widely used to maintain health and reduce disease risk.[2] The attraction of CIM includes the potential to treat diseases for which conventional therapies have been ineffective. CIM may also provide an increased sense of patient empowerment and participation, and a widespread belief exists that CIM represents safe and natural therapeutic approaches. Cancer patients have cited the media as influencing their decisions to try CIM therapies. In addition, some patients use CIM techniques, such as meditation and prayer, to cope with chronic or untreatable illnesses.[3]

Although some CIM therapies are supported by basic science and clinical evidence, many CIM therapies have not been subjected to rigorous testing. For example, natural products may potentially cause adverse effects or have clinically significant interactions with drugs, foods, or other supplements. Therefore, CIM therapies should not be used concurrently with drugs and should not be used in place of proven conventional therapies without medical supervision.

Research Issues

Many CIM approaches have not been fully evaluated. In 1992, the U.S. Congress established the Office of Alternative Medicine within the National Institutes of Health (NIH) and provided a budget of $2 million to rigorously evaluate CIM practices. In 1998, with the creation of NCCIH, Congress elevated the status of the Office of Alternative Medicine to an NIH center with a budget of $50 million for fiscal year 1999. The federal appropriations for NCCIH reached $124.1 million for fiscal year 2015. The mission of NCCIH is to "define, through rigorous scientific investigation, the usefulness and safety of complementary and integrative health interventions and their roles in improving health and health care."[5]

In addition, the National Cancer Institute (NCI) established the Office of Cancer Complementary and Alternative Medicine (OCCAM) in October 1998 to coordinate and enhance the activities of NCI and to increase the amount of high-quality cancer research and information on the use of CIM. According to OCCAM, in fiscal year 2010, NCI supported $105,341,737 in CIM-related research. This represents more than 382 projects in the form of grants, cooperative agreements, supplements, or contracts. Other NIH institutes also contribute funds to CIM research, with estimates of almost $25 billion for all institutes and centers combined.[1]

Despite this investment, evidence of the safety and efficacy of CIM may be difficult to obtain. This challenge may be partly related to the fact that many CIM studies are reported in foreign languages and in journals that are not peer reviewed. To conduct evidence-based assessments on CIM, authors of systematic reviews and meta-analyses often broaden literature searches to include languages other than English. Several databases may be searched in addition to PubMed or MEDLINE. Researchers may also use guides and validated scales, such as the Jadad scale, which has been used to rate the quality of the available studies concerning CIM therapies.[6]

Another issue in evaluating CIM research is the lack of standardization. Many individual therapies involve a variety of techniques or dosages, making comparisons difficult. Some types of CIM, such as Ayurveda, do not require providers to be licensed or formally trained, which may contribute to the variable research results.

Experimental design is the most problematic issue in CIM research. The metaphysical aspects of some CIM therapies, such as the harmony between the body and the universe in Ayurveda, are difficult to test with scientific methods.[7] Integral elements of clinical research, such as placebo control and double blinding, are difficult to conduct in many CIM studies. For example, the participatory nature of meditation prevents blinding of the subject to the active treatment.[8] Double blinding is a central problem with modalities such as acupuncture, because this therapy cannot be easily delivered by a provider blinded to the intervention. The Jadad score is sometimes modified for application to acupuncture studies because of the difficulty in blinding the acupuncturist.[9] In such cases, modified Jadad scoring may include awarding one point if the trial is single blinded or if outcomes are assessed by a blinded investigator rather than the acupuncturist.

With respect to the challenge of a placebo-controlled study for CIM therapies such as acupuncture, researchers have developed sham treatments to approximate subject blinding. For acupuncture, sham treatment typically involves placement of needles at non-active sites or at a specific distance, usually about 1 inch, from the active sites in the study, whereas depth and stimulation remain the same. Other sham acupuncture techniques involve treatment at actual acupuncture points but without needle penetration. Critics of this approach argue that even pressure at acupuncture points may elicit effects. Although some studies have demonstrated that sham procedures achieved blinding of subjects, methods used to create sham acupuncture vary widely. Sham acupuncture often is not regarded as a true placebo, because the patient is subjected to physical stimulation, and studies have shown that this technique also elicits effects.[10] *Acupressure* is an alternative therapy technique based on energy flow through the body, similar to acupuncture. In place of needle penetration, acupressure uses massage stimulation at acupuncture points.[11]

Working With CIM Providers

Ideally, conventional and CIM providers should work collaboratively for the benefit of the patient. Pharmacists and other health care providers (HCPs) should have an objective attitude toward CIM providers, especially given that some techniques are now provided in conventional medical centers. An example of an integrative approach is a clinic that includes both conventional and CIM providers. To meet patient demand, conventional providers may refer patients to CIM therapies, such as therapeutic massage or acupuncture.

Individuals who use CIM may also lack a clear understanding about the therapies. A survey among users of homeopathy in England showed that nearly 10% of users were confused about what constitutes a homeopathic product.[12] Patients should feel comfortable discussing potential CIM therapies with their conventional HCPs, and an increasing number of these providers now integrate certain evidence-based CIM techniques into their own practices. Unfortunately, many HCPs lack the resources and training to respond to patients' CIM inquiries.

Homeopathy

Homeopathy is a distinct system of medicine with its own pharmacopoeia and principles of practice. The term *homeopathy* comes from the two Greek words *homoios* (similar) and *pathos* (suffering or disease). Dr. Samuel Hahnemann developed homeopathy in the early 1800s and also coined the term *allopathy* as a synonym for conventional medicine. Homeopathy is based on the principle of "like cures like" or the "law of similars." This principle maintains that if a substance produces the symptoms of an illness in large doses, that same substance can cure it in very small doses. The more dilute a homeopathic medicine is, the greater is its potency. The efficacy of homeopathic medicines is believed to depend not only on the dilution factor but also on vigorous shaking, or *succussion*, which is performed with each dilution.

The homeopathic principle of "like cures like" is often compared with *vaccination*, which involves administration of antigenic material to induce immunity to infectious agents. However, this comparison is not entirely accurate. Vaccines typically contain measurable levels of attenuated or killed pathogens (or their purified antigens) and are used for prophylaxis. In contrast, homeopathic preparations are often so dilute that they contain statistically negligible amounts of the purported active ingredients. In addition, homeopathic remedies are generally used to treat an existing illness rather than for prophylaxis. One exception is Oscillococcinum, a homeopathic preparation derived from duck heart and liver, which is used to both prevent and treat influenza, although evidence of its efficacy is lacking.[13]

Although homeopathic medicines are generally intended to be ingested, they are not classified as dietary supplements. The Food and Drug Administration (FDA) regulates homeopathic medicines under sections 201(g) and 201(j) of the Federal Food, Drug, and Cosmetic Act as drugs recognized in the official *United States Pharmacopoeia* (USP), *Homoeopathic Pharmacopoeia of the United States* (HPUS), or *National Formulary* (NF). For homeopathic drugs, the premarket approval process is distinct from the approval process for conventional drugs. Homeopathic drugs are approved with the publication of a monograph by the Homeopathic Pharmacopoeia Convention of the United States (HPCUS) in HPUS. For a homeopathic drug to be included in HPUS, it must be manufactured according to approved methods of preparation and determined by HPCUS to be safe and effective. The safety and the efficacy of a homeopathic drug are determined by procedures called provings (or research procedures in the HPUS), which determine dosages necessary to induce symptoms in healthy individuals. Evidence from homeopathic provings is subject to verification by foundations for the clinical practice of homeopathy; however, according to FDA, "compliance with requirements of the HPUS, USP, or NF does not establish that it has been shown by appropriate means to be safe, effective, and not misbranded for its intended use."[14]

As with conventional drugs, homeopathic remedies may be sold without a prescription if they are intended to treat self-limiting conditions such as headaches and colds. Most homeopathic remedies are available without a prescription, whereas about 5% require prescriptions from medical care providers.[14] Homeopathic medicines are commonly found in integrative pharmacies that stock dietary supplements and alternative remedies along with standard drugs. Chain pharmacies and health food markets may also carry homeopathic medicines, including pediatric and veterinary formulations.[14]

Homeopathic product sales steadily increased by 16% between 2008 and 2013, with Americans spending $6.4 billion on these products in 2012.[15] Despite the widespread use of homeopathic products, particularly in children, surveys have demonstrated that confusion exists about what constitutes a homeopathic product, which suggests better patient education is needed.[12]

Practice

Medicines used in homeopathy are derived from many substances, including botanical, mineral, pharmaceutical, and zoological sources. These substances are serially diluted and successed (or *triturated*), which is thought to increase the strength or potency of the medication. This process is called attenuation or potentization. After each attenuation step, the preparation is given a higher number, so a substance that was attenuated 4 times would be designated as 4X, 4C, or LM4 depending on the dilution factor.[14] The decimal (1:10 dilutions) and centesimal (1:100 dilutions) scales of attenuation are used to make X and C potencies, respectively (Figure 52–1). The letter M means 1000C, not the use of 1:1000 dilutions in the attenuation process. A 1:50,000 dilution is represented by the potency LM, which is derived by combining Roman numerals L and M for 50 and 1000, respectively (although the actual Roman numeral LM means 1000 minus 50, or 950). The method for preparing LM potencies is illustrated in Figure 52–2. Although many homeopathic medicines are derived from highly toxic materials such as aconite and arnica, the final preparations are often so dilute that they are well below toxic dosages.

Training

More than 30 schools in North America offer training in homeopathy, and the Accreditation Commission for Homeopathic Education in North America (ACHENA, formerly Council on Homeopathy Education [CHE]) continually develops professional standards for homeopathic education. Currently, the site lists four accredited homeopathic schools and five schools that are seeking accreditation. The Council for Homeopathic Certification offers a Certificate in Classical Homeopathy (CCH) and provides listings of certified homeopathic practitioners on their website for use by other HCPs to identify qualified homeopaths.

Certification with CCH is not recognized by any state as a license to practice homeopathy. Arizona, Connecticut, and Nevada require that homeopaths also be licensed allopathic or osteopathic HCPs. Health freedom acts in some states, such as State of California Senate Bill 577, protect the rights of professionals without medical licenses to practice homeopathy and other modalities that the state deems harmless. Most other states lack specific regulatory language for homeopathy; therefore, homeopathy falls under the statutes regulating the practice of medicine.

Theory and Evidence

Because homeopathic preparations contain little-to-no active ingredient, critics argue that any demonstrated efficacy is simply a placebo effect. Proponents of homeopathy state that trials have demonstrated effectiveness in infants or animals, and that these subjects are unlikely to have preconceived expectations that may influence their perceptions. Overall, the effectiveness of homeopathy has not been demonstrated consistently in randomized controlled trials. A 2010 analysis of six reviews in the Cochrane

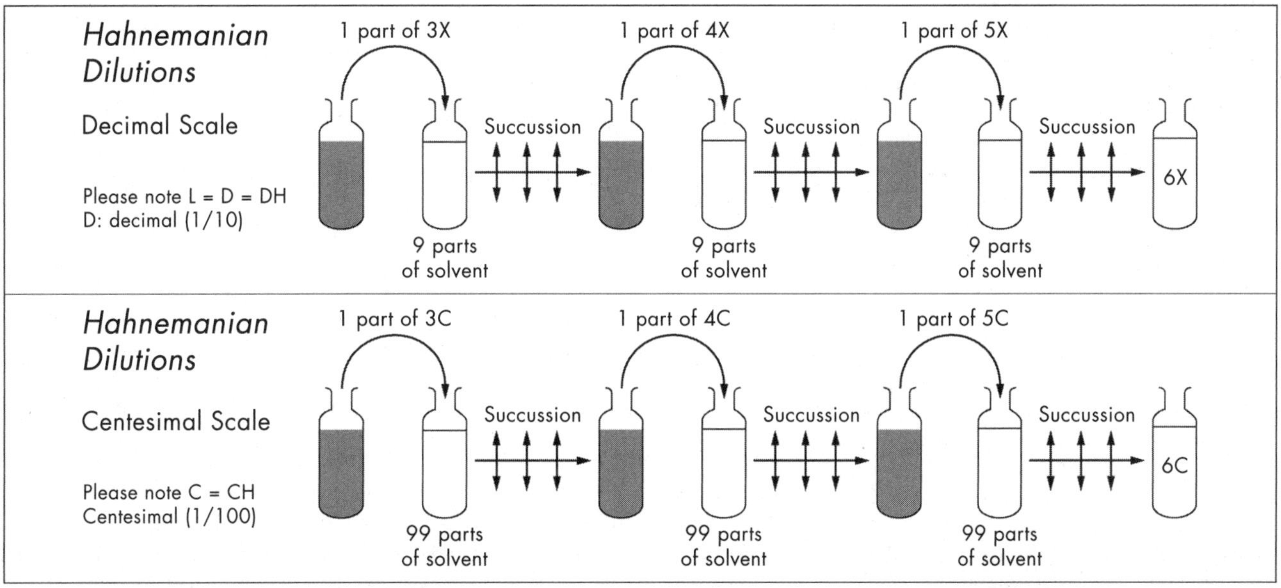

FIGURE 52–1 Method for making homeopathic X and C potencies. Decimal scale, designated by an *X* or *D*, involves dilutions of 1:10 for each attenuation (dilution with succussion) step taken to make the desired X potency. Centesimal scale, designated by *C*, involves dilutions of 1:100 for each attenuation step taken to make the desired C potency. (Source: Reprinted with permission from *Introduction to Homeopathic Medicines for Pharmacists*. Newtown Square, PA: Boiron Institute; 2001:9.)

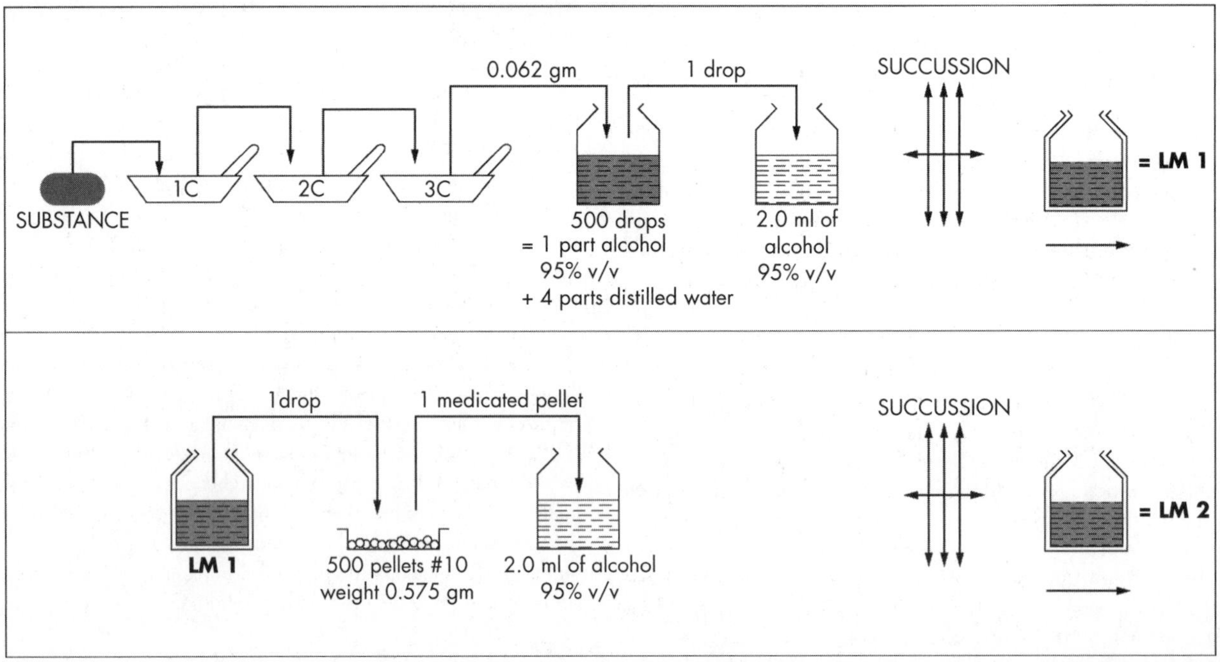

FIGURE 52-2 Method for making homeopathic LM potencies. The 50-Millesimal scale, designated by LM or Q, involves a complex attenuation process using incremental dilutions of 1:50,000 with succussion. (Source: Reprinted with permission from *The Homeopathic Pharmacopoeia of the United States.* Southeastern, PA: The Homeopathic Pharmacopoeia Convention of the United States Revision Service; December 2004:40.)

Database of Systematic Reviews concluded that the evidence suggests the effects of homeopathic therapies are similar to those of placebo.[16] A 2014 systematic review and meta-analysis of placebo-controlled randomized controlled trials of individualized homeopathic therapies concluded that the overall quality of the scientific evidence that support homeopathic therapies as being distinguishable from placebo effect are low or unclear, preventing firm conclusions.[17] Citing the contradictory results of clinical trials and the overall lack of evidence determined by systematic reviews and meta-analyses, NCCIH has stated that homeopathy has not been definitively proven to treat any clinical condition. Similarly, the American Medical Association and the American Academy of Pediatrics have neither accepted nor rejected homeopathy in the treatment of any medical condition.[18]

Safety

For most homeopathic medicines, the risk of toxicity is low because of the extremely dilute nature of the homeopathic remedies. Studies have suggested that adverse effects are less frequent in patients receiving homeopathic treatments than in those receiving conventional care.[19] The popular cold remedy Zicam has been labeled homeopathic, but some formulations contain significant levels of zinc. The nasal spray formulation containing zinc gluconate is known to cause irreversible damage to human nasal tissue.[20] According to FDA, more than 100 reports of loss of sense of smell have been associated with the use of this product, and this dosage form has since been withdrawn from the U.S. market. Homeopathic remedies are regulated as drugs under the Federal Food, Drug and Cosmetic Act (FDCA). However, under its current policy, FDA does not evaluate the remedies for safety or effectiveness. FDA enforcement policies for homeopathic drugs are described in the agency's compliance policy guide *Conditions Under Which Homeopathic Drugs May be Marketed* (CPG 7132.15).[21] According to a National Health and Medical Research Council study, patients who use only homeopathic products may put their health at risk if they reject, exclude, or delay treatments that have scientifically proven safety and efficacy.[15]

Naturopathy

The term *naturopathy* was coined in the late 1890s by German priest Sebastian Kneipp, who practiced herbal medicine and water therapies. Dr. Benedict Lust, who studied under Kneipp, purportedly purchased the rights to naturopathic medicine from another of Kneipp's students. In 1902, Dr. Lust opened the American School of Naturopathy in New York City. Because he was instrumental in promoting this field of medicine, Dr. Lust is generally credited as the founder of naturopathy.

Traditional naturopathy is a philosophy of life and an approach to living that encourages lifestyles and therapies as close to nature as possible. A system of naturopathic therapy employs natural forces such as light, heat, air, water, and massage. Naturopathy focuses primarily on building health rather than on treating disease.

The practice of naturopathic medicine emerges from six underlying principles of healing that distinguish the profession from other medical approaches. These principles are based on the observation of the nature of health and disease and are continually reexamined in light of scientific analysis. The first principle is that the body has the inherent ability to maintain and restore health.

Second, the naturopathic HCP aims to identify and treat the cause rather than the symptoms of a disease. The third principle states that methods designed to treat only the symptoms may be harmful and should be avoided or minimized. Fourth, the HCP treats the whole person, taking into account the physical, spiritual, mental, and social aspects of the individual. The fifth principle is that the naturopath educates and encourages patients to take responsibility for their own health. Finally, the naturopath assesses risk factors and hereditary susceptibility to disease and makes appropriate interventions to prevent further harm or risk to patients.

Practice

In most cases of disease or wellness, nutritional counseling and support are major components of naturopathic treatments. Naturopathic HCPs use dietetics, fasting, and nutritional supplementation in practice. Botanical medicine and homeopathy may also be used.

Naturopathic medicine has its own methods of therapeutic manipulation of the muscles, bones, and spine. HCPs use ultrasound, acupuncture, *diathermy* (electrically induced heat), exercise, massage, water, heat, cold, air, and gentle electrical pulses. Naturopathic HCPs also provide natural childbirth care. They offer prenatal and postnatal care using modern diagnostic techniques. In some states, naturopaths may perform minor outpatient surgeries, such as repair of superficial wounds or removal of foreign bodies or cysts.

Because naturopaths believe that mental attitudes and emotional states may influence or cause physical illnesses, they may incorporate counseling, nutritional balancing, stress management, hypnotherapy, biofeedback, and other therapies to help patients heal on the psychological level.

Naturopaths may prescribe substances that are deemed appropriate by the Naturopathic Formulary Advisory Peer Committee. Listed substances depend on state law and vary among states. Some state-specific regulations, such as the Naturopathic Physician Practice Act Rule of Utah,[22] allow naturopaths to prescribe only medicines listed in the *Naturopathic Physician Formulary.*

Training

In North America, seven schools offer training for the Doctor of Naturopathic Medicine (ND) degree. These include Bastyr University (Seattle, Washington); Boucher Institute of Naturopathic Medicine (Vancouver, British Columbia); the Canadian College of Naturopathic Medicine (Toronto, Ontario); National University of Natural Medicine (Portland, Oregon); National University of Health Sciences (Chicago, Illinois); Southwest College of Naturopathic Medicine (Phoenix, Arizona); and University of Bridgeport College of Naturopathic Medicine (Bridgeport, Connecticut).

Similar to allopathic medical schools, admission into a naturopathic training program requires four years of undergraduate study that includes premedical coursework. The ND degree consists of 4 years of postgraduate training, which includes about 4500 hours of academic and clinical training. Academic training includes courses such as anatomy, biochemistry, microbiology, and pathology. Clinical training encompasses various alternative modalities, including herbal therapy and homeopathy, in addition to mainstream clinical training such as that in cardiology and nutrition. Naturopathic HCPs are educated in modern methods of diagnostic testing and imaging, including radiology, ultrasound, and other imaging techniques. Some naturopaths may participate in residency programs, including integrative programs that train NDs in conventional medical settings.

In addition to a standard medical curriculum, a naturopath must study holistic therapies that have a strong emphasis on preventing disease and optimizing wellness. The ND is required to complete training in clinical nutrition, acupuncture, homeopathic medicine, botanical medicine, psychology, and counseling. Before they can practice, naturopathic HCPs must pass board examinations set by the North American Board of Naturopathic Examiners, and most states require NDs to complete continuing education hours to renew their licenses.

The licensing of naturopathic HCPs varies among states. According to the Association of Accredited Naturopathic Medical Colleges (https://aanmc.org/careers/licensure) and the Council on Naturopathic Medical Education (http://www.cnme.org/faq.html), the practice of naturopathic medicine is allowed in 16 states (Alaska, Arizona, California, Connecticut, Hawaii, Idaho, Kansas, Maine, Minnesota, Montana, New Hampshire, North Dakota, Oregon, Utah, Vermont, Washington) and 4 provinces (British Columbia, Manitoba, Ontario, Saskatchewan).

Because of its popularity, more HCPs trained in conventional medicine or other CIM fields are incorporating naturopathic treatments into their practices. HCPs who hold degrees in osteopathy, chiropractic, acupuncture, dentistry, and veterinary medicine may seek additional training in naturopathy; they sometimes use terms such as *holistic, natural,* or *integrative* to promote their practices.

Theory and Evidence

The individual methods used in naturopathic medicine vary in their effectiveness. A proper diet may help prevent heart disease; this measure is recommended in both conventional and naturopathic medicine. However, other forms of naturopathic treatment may not be more effective than conventional medicine. For example, acupuncture may help to reduce pain in some instances, but it is not widely recommended for use in place of standard analgesics for extreme pain or in surgery.[23] Some naturopathic treatments may be more effective than conventional therapies, as shown with a combination naturopathic treatment for anxiety that includes nutrition counseling, relaxation techniques, and vitamin and herbal supplementation.[24]

Safety

The safety of naturopathic remedies depends on the treatment and the condition. Naturopathic methods are generally considered safer alternatives for some conventional drugs or treatments. The safety of other approaches such as fasting or other dietary restrictions depends on the individual. As with all CIM therapies, naturopathic treatments should not be used in place of proven therapies for serious medical conditions.

Traditional Chinese Medicine

Chinese medicine is a broad term encompassing many different modalities and traditions of healing, including herbal medicine and acupuncture.[4,25] These therapies share a common root in Chinese philosophy, including Taoism, Confucianism, and Buddhism, and may date back more than 5000 years.

In the 1940s and 1950s, the Chinese government undertook an effort to coalesce diverse forms of Chinese medicine into a unified system to be officially defined as traditional Chinese medicine (TCM). The intent was to integrate traditional providers into an organized health system and to provide care for a large population by using familiar and inexpensive methods.

Although TCM is considered to be a complementary or alternative medicine in most of the Western world, in China the term for TCM literally means "central medicine." TCM and Western medicine are commonly used side by side in modern China. As a result, compared with Western countries, China is relatively advanced in using alternative medicine. The most prominent focus of TCM is the treatment of major illnesses, including cancer and heart disease. According to the World Health Organization, TCM is fully integrated into the Chinese health system and is practiced in 95% of Chinese hospitals.[26]

Technique

TCM emphasizes herbal medicine. Herbs are usually given as pills, extracts, capsules, tinctures, or powders, which may be used directly or combined with food or other treatments. More than 2000 different types of herbs are used in Chinese medicine, with 400 frequently used and 50 considered "fundamental" herbs.[27] Some Chinese herbs have received attention in Western medicine for treating serious disorders. For example, the *Monascus purpureus* fungus, found in red yeast rice, is a natural source of lovastatin. Bevirimat, derived from the Chinese herb *Syzygium claviflorum,* is in a new class of drugs called maturation inhibitors and is being investigated in ongoing clinical trials in human immunodeficiency virus (HIV).[28]

TCM incorporates not only herbs but also minerals, metals, and animal products into therapeutic preparations. The use of animal products has become more infrequent in recent years, in part because of restrictions on certain species, particularly endangered species.

Acupuncture is also considered a form of TCM, although it is regarded as more of a supportive treatment to herbal therapy. Many varieties of acupuncture exist both in Chinese and Western medicine. Classic acupuncture, also known as five-element acupuncture, uses a different needling technique and relies on acupuncture without the use of herbs. Needles used in Japanese acupuncture are smaller than those of other forms of acupuncture. Medical acupuncture refers to an acupuncture therapy that uses knowledge of pathology, anatomy, and physiology, while removing certain components of TCM. Auricular acupuncture treats the entire body through acupuncture points in the ears only, and electroacupuncture uses electrical currents attached to acupuncture needles. As with many forms of TCM, acupuncture may require multiple treatments and long-term follow-up for symptom improvement and health maintenance.

Cupping and moxibustion are commonly used to complement acupuncture, but these techniques may also be used independently in TCM. They share the principle of using heat to stimulate circulation to break up congestion or stagnation of blood and *chi* (or *qi*), which is the life force central to health and well-being in TCM. Cupping has some relation to the massage technique *tuina,* which uses rapid skin pinching at points on the back to break up congestion and stimulate circulation. Cupping may also be used over acupuncture points or elsewhere. Popular in the United States, moxibustion involves the burning of dried moxa (mugwort), either on or near the skin, and sometimes in conjunction with cupping or acupuncture on specific points.[29]

TCM providers may use other modalities such as meditation and martial arts. *Tai chi chuan* (or *tai chi*) is a meditative form of martial arts that incorporates the theories of *yin* and *yang* from both Taoism and Confucianism. *Tai chi* is practiced to improve balance, coordination, and relaxation, and overall well-being. TCM may also incorporate *feng shui,* which is the art of arranging furniture and objects to increase health and prosperity.

Training

The Accreditation Commission of Acupuncture and Oriental Medicine (ACAOM) accredits professional acupuncture programs and is recognized by the U.S. Department of Education. According to the ACAOM, acupuncture and Oriental medicine is a 3- or 4-year master's degree program, offered by over 70 accredited or candidate colleges in the United States (http://www.naturalhealers.com/natural-health-careers/article/acupuncture-licensure). The National Certification Commission for Acupuncture and Oriental Medicine (NCCAOM) offers four independent certification programs, including Acupuncture, Chinese Herbology, Oriental Medicine, and Asian Bodywork Therapy (http://www.nccaom.org; select Certification Brochure). Acupuncturists who pass national examinations administered by NCCAOM are entitled to identify themselves as board certified in their discipline and as diplomates of the NCCAOM.

Licenses to practice acupuncture are granted by individual states. Although requirements vary, many states require acupuncturists to pass the NCCAOM examinations and obtain continuing education.

Theory and Evidence

Taoism, Confucianism, and Buddhism provided the basis for the development of Chinese medical theory. According to these philosophies, nature and the laws that govern the ongoing, harmonious flow of life energy through the natural world also govern the body and health. The person is viewed as an ecosystem that is embedded in the larger ecosystem of nature and is therefore subject to the same laws. The life force called *chi* (*qi*) circulates through the body and enlivens it. Health is a function of a balanced, harmonious flow of *chi,* and illness results when there is a blockage or an imbalance in the flow of *chi. Yin* and *yang* are opposite and complementary qualities of life energy (*chi*). *Yin* is regarded as the feminine principle and *yang,* the masculine principle. The human being has a system of pathways called meridians, sometimes referred to as channels, through which *chi* flows. Meridians correspond with specific organs or organ systems (organ networks). Health is believed to be an ongoing process of maintaining balance and harmony of the circulation of *chi* through all the organs and systems of the body. In TCM theory, the body has five organ networks, each corresponding with a particular element.

Despite the growing popularity of TCM in the West, its effectiveness remains debatable. Scientific evidence supports the use of acupuncture for several indications including osteoarthritis and various types of pain and nausea. The American Cancer Society states "clinical studies have found that acupuncture may help treat nausea caused by chemotherapy drugs and surgical anesthesia." Moxibustion, which is traditionally used to turn breech babies, has been used with some success, although systematic reviews and meta-analyses have yielded insufficient evidence to support its efficacy.[29] In general, few well-designed trials of TCM herbal formulas have been conducted and the need for improving the methodological quality of TCM research has been identified.[30] A 2013 assessment of the research found that 41 of 70 systematic reviews of the scientific evidence (including 19 of 26 reviews on acupuncture for a variety of conditions and 22 of 42 reviews on Chinese herbal medicine) were unable to reach conclusions about whether the technique worked for the condition under investigation because of insufficient good-quality evidence.[31] The other 29 systematic reviews (including 7 of 26 reviews on acupuncture and 20 of 42 reviews on TCM herbal medicine) suggested possible benefits but could not reach definite conclusions because of the small quantity or poor quality of the studies.[31]

Safety

Adverse events with acupuncture, including with cupping and moxibustion, are rare. Needles must be sterile and disposable needles are often used to reduce the risk of disease transmission. Acupuncture should be avoided or used cautiously in individuals with heart disease, seizures, infections, bleeding disorders, or neurologic disorders, or among individuals using antithrombotic drugs because of theoretical or reported adverse effects. Acupuncture should not be performed on areas that have received radiation therapy and for conditions of unknown medical origin. Caution is advised during pregnancy. Frail older adults or otherwise medically complex patients should use acupuncture with caution. Electroacupuncture should be avoided in patients with an arrhythmia or seizure disorder and in patients with pacemakers.

Cupping commonly leaves a temporary bruising of the skin. Moxibustion may also leave a temporary discoloration on the skin, which may be washed off or will disappear on its own. Historically, some traditional providers of moxibustion have intentionally employed more aggressive use of the technique to an extent that might leave minor scarring, but this aggressive form of practice is not regularly used in the West.

Chinese herbs have been associated with adverse effects. In April 2004, FDA banned the sale of products containing ephedra or ma huang (*Ephedra sinica*) in response to more than 18,000 adverse event reports.[32] The U.S. Poison Control Centers has reported that ephedra-related adverse events resulting in major adverse effects or death declined 98% from 10,326 poisonings in 2002 to 180 in 2013.[32] Some Chinese herbal products have contained toxins or heavy metals.[31] In addition, prescription drugs, such as corticosteroids, have been included in the preparations but not listed as ingredients.[33] Patients should purchase Chinese herbs from trustworthy sources and should be aware that Chinese herbs can interact with other herbs, foods, and drugs.

Chiropractic Care

Chiropractic focuses on the relationship between spinal structure and body function mediated by the nervous system. It originated in 1895 with D. D. Palmer, a popular hands-on healer practicing in Davenport, Iowa. The formulation of *chiropractic* combined the Greek *cheir* (hand) and *praxis* (practice). Palmer's original philosophy described the approach as connecting "man the spiritual" to "man the physical" by eliminating interference to the flow of "Innate Intelligence" through each individual. This innate intelligence, an almost metaphysical phenomenon, was thought to flow through the nervous system. The clearer the nervous system is, the more the innate intelligence can express itself and fully enliven the person's body and organs.[34]

Important distinctions exist between the profession of chiropractic, chiropractic care, and spinal manipulation. A chiropractor delivers chiropractic care that is a full range of treatment delivered in one or more therapeutic encounters. Treatment includes procedures and techniques of assessment and a tailored mix of therapeutic interventions to improve a patient's health status. The term *spinal manipulation* or *spinal adjustment* does not operationally define the profession or chiropractic care, although it is a well-known procedure. Chiropractic care also includes other procedures, such as exercise, dietary advice, ergonomic and lifestyle advice, supplements, all forms of physical therapy and rehabilitation intervention, and referral to other providers as necessary.[34]

Techniques

Patients usually lie face down on a Cox table, which is similar to a massage table with an open space in which to place the face. Depending on the technique used, chiropractic visits may last 15 minutes to 1 hour or more. Chiropractors may see patients up to 3 times a week initially and then less frequently over time.

Patients can be diagnosed by different procedures including X-ray, computed tomography, magnetic resonance imaging, electrical current, and ultrasound therapy. Thermography may also be used, followed by treatment with ice packs and heat packs.

More than 100 chiropractic and spinal manipulative adjusting techniques may be employed. Spinal manipulative therapy uses many techniques to apply force to an area of the spine joint. Massage or mobilization of soft tissue is used in techniques such as myofascial trigger point therapy, cross-friction massage, active release therapy, muscle stripping, Rolfing, or other forms of structural integration. Mechanical traction or the use of external resistance on the spine may also be used. The cracking sound has typically been associated with cavitation in the spinal zygapophyseal (the neural arch between the joint processes) joints. The cracking or popping of a joint has not been proven to be essential to a clinically effective manipulation.[35]

Training

Chiropractic is one of the largest CIM professions in the United States. According to the U.S. Department of Labor, an estimated 32,960 chiropractors were practicing in 2016.[36] The Council on Chiropractic Education (CCE) accredits programs and institutions offering the Doctor of Chiropractic degree, which currently includes 15 schools in the United States (CCEUS) and two in Canada (CCEC) (http://www.cce-usa.org/DCP_Representatives.html; http://www.chirofed.ca/english/accreditation.html). According to the Federation of Chiropractic Licensing Boards, all 50 states have formal statutes that recognize and regulate the practice of chiropractic (http://directory.fclb.org/Statistics.aspx).

The Doctor of Chiropractic degree requires the completion of didactic coursework and clinical training totaling a minimum of 4200 instructional hours. Clinical training with actual patients typically lasts a minimum of 1 year. Specialty training is available through residency programs, which may require an additional 2–3 years of clinical training. Before they are allowed to practice, doctors of chiropractic must pass national board examinations and become licensed. Chiropractors generally do not prescribe drugs, but those who are also licensed naturopaths or other health care professionals may prescribe remedies according to their respective state regulations (https://www.acatoday.org/Patients/Why-Choose-Chiropractic/Chiropractic-Qualifications).

Theory and Evidence

Designing clinical trials to evaluate the efficacy of chiropractic is difficult, primarily because of the issues in developing an appropriate control. Other major issues include a potentially strong placebo effect and the high rate of spontaneous recovery. In addition, patients often seek chiropractic treatment for conditions with poorly understood pathologies such as fibromyalgia; available evidence is insufficient to support the use of chiropractic for this condition.[37] For low back pain, sufficient evidence from both blinded and nonblinded trials supports the use of spinal manipulation, although the benefits are modest and of uncertain clinical significance.[38] Chiropractic has been used to treat asthma, colic, ear infection, headache, whiplash, and hypertension, although evidence is insufficient to support efficacy for these conditions.

Safety

The safety of chiropractic is controversial. Some systematic reviews show that spinal manipulation is associated with mild–moderate adverse effects. The most common serious adverse effects with spinal manipulation are vertebral artery dissection and stroke (VADS).[39] A 2010 review revealed 26 deaths associated with chiropractic spinal manipulation, and more fatalities may be unpublished.[40] However, despite the increasing popularity of chiropractic and its association with potentially fatal adverse events such as VADS, myelopathy, vertebral disc extrusion, and epidural hematoma, few studies have properly evaluated the safety of chiropractic.[41] Whether the adverse effects are directly related to spinal manipulation or to sampling bias of patients is unclear. Case-control studies suggested a causal role[40]: patients predisposed to VADS may be more likely to seek chiropractic treatment, which suggests a potential sampling bias.[42] A 2009 systematic review showed that adverse events occurred with a frequency of 33%–60.9%, but serious adverse events were rare, as few as 1.46 serious adverse events and 2.68 deaths for every 10 million manipulations.[41] Although this study did not support a strong causal relationship between chiropractic manipulation and the adverse events, the authors stated further high-quality studies are needed to assess its safety.

Patients with osteoporosis or any type of acute arthritis should either avoid chiropractic adjustment or use it cautiously because of the risk of fracture. Caution is also warranted in patients with bleeding disorders, migraines, and tumors or metastases to the spine. Patients with symptoms of vertebrobasilar vascular insufficiency, aneurysms, arteritis, or unstable spondylolisthesis should avoid chiropractic care. Patients receiving anticoagulant therapy should also be advised to avoid chiropractic care.

A final consideration with this health system is that chiropractors have traditionally discouraged the use of routine vaccinations. In a 2011 study of 12,164 adults identified as chiropractic users, only 41% received vaccinations within the previous year.[43] Although this attitude may be less likely now, Western HCPs, including pharmacists, should be aware of this aspect of chiropractic care.

Ayurveda

Ayurveda originated in India more than 5000 years ago and is probably the world's oldest system of natural medicine.[44] When translated, *Ayurveda* means science of life, which stems from the spiritual teachings known as the Vedas. Ayurveda may be the original basis for Chinese medicine and is an integrated system of specific theories and techniques that employ diet, herbs, exercise, meditation, yoga, and massage or bodywork. The goal of Ayurveda is to achieve optimal health on physical, psychological, and spiritual levels.

In India, Ayurveda involves the eight principal branches of medicine: pediatrics, gynecology, obstetrics, ophthalmology, geriatrics, otolaryngology, general medicine, and surgery. In Western countries, the practice of Ayurveda is less focused on its spiritual roots than on its use as a form of CIM. Ayurveda relies on the individual's willingness to participate in lifestyle and behavior changes.

Technique

Ayurveda teaches that vital energy (*prana*) is the basis of all life and healing.[44] As *prana* circulates throughout the human body, it is governed by the five elements of earth, air, fire, water, and ether. The five elements combine with one another into pairs called *doshas* that include *vata* (ether and air), *pitta* (fire and water), and *kapha* (earth and water). Health is thought to be a state of balance and harmony among the five elements, and illness occurs when there is an imbalance or lack of harmony among them.

The regulation of diet as a form of therapy is a central idea in Ayurveda. An individual's temperament and mental and spiritual development can be influenced by the quality and quantity of food consumed. An important principle in Ayurveda is that "there is nothing in the world that is not a medicine or food." Foods and herbs are described in terms of their energetic qualities rather than chemical properties. Sweet foods (called *madhura*) provide nourishment and coolness and also aid in increasing body weight. Sour foods (called *amla*) provide warmth and aid weight gain. Salty foods (*lavana*) provide warmth, stimulate the senses, and aid weight gain. In contrast, bitter foods (*katu*) provide coolness and help weight loss. Pungent foods (*tikta*) also aid weight loss but provide warmth and stimulation. Numerous herbs and spices including turmeric and cumin are used in Ayurveda.[44]

Ayurveda holds that each 24-hour cycle is divided into 4-hour segments governed by the *doshas*. These time periods are believed to correspond with nature. Ayurvedic providers guide patients to plan their activities to be in harmony with these natural principles of timing.[44]

A provider usually interviews the patient about his or her medical history. The provider then palpates the patient's wrist to determine subtle qualities of the pulse. Providers may also evaluate the appearance of the tongue, face, lips, nails, or eyes. Laboratory tests of blood, urine, and stools may be used to help with diagnosis. The initial consultation is usually the longest and lasts from 45 to 90 minutes or longer. Follow-up consultations may be spaced by several weeks or months to monitor the individual's progress. Follow-up will usually be brief office visits involving a diagnostic review and an adjustment of the regimen.[44]

Training

In India, more than 150 undergraduate and 30 postgraduate institutions for Ayurvedic medicine exist, and the standard length of training is at least 5 years. Despite the abundance of institutions, the standard of Ayurvedic education in India is poorly structured and largely unregulated, which has resulted in a global negative perception of the practice.[45]

According to NCCIH, no national standard for Ayurvedic training or certification exists in the United States. Ayurveda is practiced in Western medicine by HCPs who are licensed in a variety of disciplines.[44] Allopathic and osteopathic HCPs, naturopaths, acupuncturists, primary care providers, massage therapists, and chiropractors may all practice Ayurveda. Health counselors, educators, or consultants may also incorporate Ayurveda into their practices without specific licensing. In Western countries, two major approaches to training and practice exist. The first is offered by diverse teachers and providers, many of whom are either from India or were trained there. The second consists of devotees of Maharishi Mahesh Yogi, the Indian spiritual teacher who introduced Transcendental Meditation (TM) to the West. In 1980, this group coined the term *Maharishi Ayur-Ved,* a practice that incorporates TM as part of an Ayurvedic approach.

Theory and Evidence

Some of the more metaphysical aspects of Ayurveda, such as harmony between the body and the universe, are difficult to assess with modern scientific methods.[7] Several herbal formulations have been studied in Western-style clinical trials and, currently, evidence is inadequate to recommend Ayurveda for any indication.

Safety

Many different Ayurvedic herbs exist, and they are frequently taken in combination with other herbs and/or minerals. Safety and toxicity will vary depending on the herb and its preparation. In general, Ayurvedic herbal medicines should be used cautiously, because their potencies may not be tested or standardized. Therapeutic levels of sildenafil have been detected in Ayurvedic herbal preparations used for aphrodisiac purposes.[46] Patients should purchase Ayurvedic herbs from trustworthy sources and should be aware that Ayurvedic herbs can interact with other herbs, foods, and drugs. For example, ginger, which is commonly used in Ayurveda, may increase the risk of bleeding when used with antithrombotic drugs.

Heavy metal contamination continues to be a concern in Ayurvedic medicines. In addition to herbs, Ayurvedic formulas known as *rasa shastra* may also contain metals such as arsenic, mercury, or zinc. Providers claim that these medicines are safe when properly prepared and administered. According to the U.S. Centers for Disease Control and Prevention, 12 cases of lead poisoning in five states were associated with Ayurvedic medicines from 2000 to 2003.[47] Even herbal Ayurvedic formulas may contain heavy metals; one study found that 20% of purported herb-only formulas contained detectable metals compared with 40% of *rasa shastra* medicines.[47] Consequently, patients are advised to use Ayurvedic herbs cautiously. Products that have USP seals of quality approval have been tested and should not contain unacceptable levels of harmful metals. Product testing information is also available from sites such as ConsumerLab.com (see Chapter 50).

Massage

Soft tissue manipulation has been practiced for thousands of years in diverse cultures. Chinese use of massage dates to 1600 BC, and Hippocrates referred to the importance of primary care providers being experienced with "rubbing" as early as 400 BC.

Massage spread throughout Europe during the Renaissance and was introduced in the United States in the 1850s. By the early 1930s, massage became a less prominent part of Western medicine. Renewed interest in therapeutic massage emerged in the 1970s, particularly among athletes to promote well-being, relaxation, analgesia, stress relief, healing of musculoskeletal injuries, sleep enhancement, and quality of life. Massage is one of the most common forms of CIM therapy used in the United States.

A common goal of massage therapy is to help the body heal itself. Touch is fundamental to massage therapy and is used by therapists to locate painful or tense areas, to determine how much pressure to apply, and to establish a therapeutic relationship with patients.

Technique

Different therapeutic techniques can be classified as massage therapy. Most involve the application of fixed or moving pressure or manipulation of the patients' muscles and connective tissues. Providers may use their hands or other areas such as forearms, elbows, or feet. Lubricants may be used to aid the smoothness of massage strokes. Examples of massage therapy include Swedish massage, sports massage, deep tissue massage, and trigger point massage.

Training

Training requirements for massage therapy vary in the United States, but they generally involve 500–1000 hours for certification by the National Certification Board for Therapeutic Massage and Bodywork. More than 1000 massage training programs exist, and some have received accreditation by the Commission on Massage Therapy Accreditation, which is recognized by the U.S. Department of Education. Upon fulfilling the necessary requirements, massage therapists receive the designation of Nationally Certified in Therapeutic Massage and Bodywork. A national examination is available from the National Certification Board for Therapeutic Massage and Bodywork. Most states require massage therapists to be certified before practicing.

Theory and Evidence

Research on massage therapy is limited, and published studies frequently use a variety of techniques and trial designs. The effectiveness of massage has not been established for any health condition, although it remains popular for improving relaxation, mood, and overall well-being, particularly in palliative care.[48]

Safety

Adverse effects have been reported with massage. For example, fractures, discomfort, bruising, swelling of massaged tissues, and liver hematoma have been reported. Vigorous massage should be avoided in patients with bleeding disorders, peripheral vascular disease, or thrombocytopenia, or in those receiving antithrombotic therapy. According to preliminary data, blood pressure may increase in healthy patients following vigorous massage (e.g., trigger point therapy, which focuses on painful muscle knots); however, in patients with hypertension, massage may lower blood pressure. Areas that should not be massaged include those with osteoporotic and other fractures, open or healing skin wounds, skin infections, recent surgery, or blood clots. Massage and other touch-based therapies should be used cautiously in patients with a history of physical abuse. Women who are pregnant should consult their obstetrician before beginning massage therapy. Allergies or skin irritation can occur with the oils used in massages, such as olive and mineral oil.

Massage has not been evaluated as a method to diagnose medical conditions. Massage should not be used as a substitute for more proven therapies for medical conditions.

Conclusion

Patients increasingly seek care from CIM providers and health systems. Although some historical and scientific evidence supports the effectiveness of some approaches, general statements are difficult to make on the safety and efficacy of CIM. Important components of

TABLE 52-1 Common Health Issues with Evidence of Benefit from CIM

Condition	CIM Treatment
Osteoarthritis	Acupuncture
Chronic pain, fibromyalgia, postoperative pain	Acupuncture
Nausea	Acupressure
Low back pain	Chiropractic
Quality of life in cancer patients	Massage
Anxiety and stress	Therapeutic touch

Key: CIM, Complementary and integrative medicine.
Source: Reference 4.

clinical trials such as placebo controls and blinding are difficult to achieve for some forms of CIM therapy and, as a result, evidence is limited. Because the use of CIM continues to increase, both patients and providers should be informed about the potential risks and benefits of CIM techniques. Table 52–1 lists common evidence-based uses of CIM health systems. Cases 52–1 and 52–2 are examples of disorders that are amenable to CIM therapies.

More patients are using the internet for health information before consulting HCPs. As information has become increasingly available, patients have increased their responsibility for their health decisions and should be encouraged to tell their HCP whether they are also using any CIM approaches to their health. Similarly, all Western HCPs, including pharmacists, must be knowledgeable about CIM health systems and the evidence that supports or refutes their use.

Key Points for CIM Health Systems

- The term *complementary and integrative medicine* (CIM) is a broad group of healing philosophies, diagnostic approaches, and therapeutic interventions that are not generally considered part of the conventional Western health system. Common CIM approaches include homeopathy, naturopathy, TCM and acupuncture, chiropractic care, Ayurveda, and massage.
- Homeopathy is based on the principle of "like cures like," which states that if a substance produces the symptoms of an illness in large doses, that same substance can cure it in very minute dosages. The efficacy of homeopathy has not been determined for any clinical condition, although the risk of toxicity is low.
- Naturopathy employs natural forces such as light, heat, air, and water through nutrition, botanical medicine, psychotherapy, acupuncture, homeopathy, massage, and spinal manipulation; this therapy focuses on building health rather than on treating

CASE 52-1

Relevant Evaluation Criteria	Scenario/Model Outcome
Collect	
1. Gather essential information about the patient's symptoms and medical history, including	
a. Description of symptom(s) (i.e., nature, onset, duration, severity, associated symptoms)	The patient comes to the pharmacy seeking advice to help treat his symptoms of insomnia. He states that he works the evening shift as security officer and is unable to fall asleep after returning home. He also mentions that his job has been very stressful. He comes to the pharmacy seeking advice on ways to ease his stress.
b. Description of any factors that seem to precipitate, exacerbate, and/or relieve the patient's symptom(s)	The insomnia and stress is consistent with his type of work and schedule. He explains that he feels sleep deprived and tired during his shift, yet once he returns home he is no longer able to fall asleep. He does not want to take drugs or supplements.
c. Description of the patient's efforts to relieve the symptoms	He states that he has tried taking diphenhydramine without relief.
d. Patient's identity	Steve Russell
e. Patient's age, gender, height, and weight	36 years old, male, 5 ft 9 in., 181 lb
f. Patient's occupation	Security officer
g. Patient's dietary habits	Mostly fast food or frozen foods; he does not do much cooking. He is a frequent soda drinker.
h. Patient's sleep habits	Unable to fall asleep after working evening shift, feeling stressed
i. Concurrent medical conditions, prescription and nonprescription medications, and dietary supplements	None
j. Allergies	None
k. History of other adverse reactions to medications	None
l. Other (describe) ______	n/a

CASE 52-1 *continued*

Relevant Evaluation Criteria	Scenario/Model Outcome
Assess	
2. Differentiate patient's signs/symptoms, and correctly identify the patient's primary problem(s).	Insomnia, work-related stress
3. Identify exclusions for self-treatment.	None
4. Formulate a comprehensive list of therapeutic alternatives for the primary problem to determine whether triage to a health care provider is required, and share this information with the patient or caregiver.	Options include (1) Refer the patient to his HCP or to an integrative medicine provider such as a naturopath. (2) Recommend sleep hygiene practices, including exercising regularly, limiting alcohol and caffeine consumption, and establishing a consistent sleep–wake pattern. (3) Advise the patient to consider relaxation therapy, massage, or meditation. (4) Recommend self-care until the patient can see an appropriate provider. (5) Take no action.
Plan	
5. Select an optimal therapeutic alternative to address the patient's problem, taking into account patient preferences.	Recommend sleep hygiene best practices. Suggest meditation, relaxation therapy, massage therapy.
6. Describe the recommended therapeutic approach to the patient or caregiver.	■ "Proper sleep hygiene should help your insomnia: avoid stimulants such as caffeine. ■ Limit alcohol intake. ■ Regular exercise can promote good sleep. ■ Associate bed with sleep; do not read in bed. ■ Avoid using any electronic devices close to bedtime. ■ Meditation: many programs are available." "A naturopath may be able to help you manage the stress as well as improve your sleep through diet and lifestyle changes."
7. Explain to the patient or caregiver the rationale for selecting the recommended therapeutic approach from the considered therapeutic alternatives.	"Previously you were taking diphenhydramine. This is okay for occasional use." "Meditation may help to reduce some of your stress-related symptoms and help regulate sleep." [Give the patient a pamphlet on meditation programs available in the area.]
Implement	
8. When recommending self-care with nonprescription medications and/or nondrug therapy, convey accurate information to the patient or caregiver.	"The good sleep hygiene practices may help with your symptoms and just require consistency to see an effect." "Meditation practices may require training, but they will likely help with your stress and other concerns."
Solicit follow-up questions from the patient or caregiver.	"How long will it take to see the effect?"
Answer the patient's or caregiver's questions.	"Responses are variable and it is important to be consistent in following the sleep hygiene practices."
Follow-up: Monitor and Evaluate	
9. Assess patient outcome.	Ask the patient to call to update you on his response to your recommendations. Or you could call him in a week to evaluate the outcome.

Key: HCP = Health care provider; n/a = not applicable.

CASE 52-2

Relevant Evaluation Criteria	Scenario/Model Outcome
Collect	
1. Gather essential information about the patient's symptoms and medical history, including	
a. Description of symptom(s) (i.e., nature, onset, duration, severity, associated symptoms)	Patient presents to pharmacy with a persistent pain in his lower back. The pain tends to be achy and dull, and it comes and goes. At times the pain is 8 out of 10, preventing him from wanting to get up and do his daily activities. Sometimes it radiates down his legs and feels as though a nerve is pinched somewhere. He thinks he remembers the pain starting after he strained his back shoveling out his driveway, and it became worse after he slipped on some ice this past winter. The pain is so much of a problem that he does not feel as though he gets a full night's sleep.
b. Description of any factors that seem to precipitate, exacerbate, and/or relieve the patient's symptom(s)	The pain tends to be bad in the morning, and is alleviated a bit as he moves around and loosens up throughout the day. But it gets worse at the end of the day if he pushes it too much.
c. Description of the patient's efforts to relieve the symptoms	The patient has tried taking naproxen and only gets some relief. He states that his wife also told him to try an analgesic topical cream, which did not give him any relief.
d. Patient's identity	Adam Smith
e. Patient's age, gender, height, and weight	57 years old, male, 5 ft 8 in., 215 lb
f. Patient's occupation	Sales executive
g. Patient's dietary habits	Eats mostly red meat, some vegetables, and a few baked goods daily.
h. Patient's sleep habits	5–7 hours nightly
i. Concurrent medical conditions, prescription and nonprescription medications, and dietary supplements	Hyperlipidemia diagnosed at age 45: atorvastatin 40 mg/day; back pain, self-diagnosed: naproxen 220 mg/day PRN; 1 multivitamin daily
j. Allergies	Shellfish
k. History of other adverse reactions to medications	None
l. Other (describe) ______	n/a
Assess	
2. Differentiate patient's signs and symptoms, and correctly identify the patient's primary problem(s).	Patient is suffering from back pain in the lower lumbar region, which may be caused by a pinched nerve due to a compressed disc or some residual inflammation from his fall.
3. Identify exclusions for self-treatment.	Symptoms are persistent. Patient tried OTC pain management and did not get resolution of all symptoms. The pain is now disrupting his sleep cycle.
4. Formulate a comprehensive list of therapeutic alternatives for the primary problem to determine whether triage to a health care provider is required, and share this information with the patient or caregiver.	Options include (1) Refer the patient to his HCP and, as appropriate, to a chiropractor or acupuncturist. (2) Recommend self-care with a nondrug measure. (3) Recommend self-care until the patient can see an appropriate HCP. (4) Recommend other pain relievers and hot packs.
Plan	
5. Select an optimal therapeutic alternative to address the patient's problem, taking into account patient preferences.	Patient should consult his HCP, as well as try chiropractic treatment or acupuncture for his pain.
6. Describe the recommended therapeutic approach to the patient or caregiver.	"You should consult your regular health care provider for possible referral to a massage, acupuncture, or chiropractic practitioner. Acupuncture may be a good option. In the meantime, try alternating hot packs to seek some relief from pain caused by the injury. Prevent further back strain."
7. Explain to the patient or caregiver the rationale for selecting the recommended therapeutic approach from the considered therapeutic alternatives.	"This option is best because your problem is becoming more severe and debilitating. You do not want to have to lose sleep because of pain, which can further contribute to increased pain during the day and is not conducive to a balanced lifestyle."

CASE 52-2 *continued*

Relevant Evaluation Criteria	Scenario/Model Outcome
Implement	
8. When recommending self-care with nonprescription medications and/or nondrug therapy, convey accurate information to the patient or caregiver.	Provide an evidence-based patient education handout on chiropractic, acupuncture, physical therapy, and orthopedic care so the patient may explore multiple options with his regular HCP.
Solicit follow-up questions from the patient or caregiver.	"Is there anything I can do to keep this condition from getting worse?"
Answer the patient's or caregiver's questions.	"Avoid heavy lifting or other daily activities that you have noticed exacerbate the condition. Explore multiple integrative therapies to try to help your back pain before relying on nonprescription or prescription drugs. This approach will help to prevent adverse effects."
Follow-up: Monitor and Evaluate	
9. Assess patient outcome.	Contact the patient in a day or two to ensure that he made an appointment and sought medical care.

Key: HCP = Health care provider; n/a = not applicable; OTC = over-the-counter; PRN = as needed.

disease. Naturopathy is based on six principles: (1) the healing power of nature, (2) identifying and treating the cause, (3) doing no harm, (4) treating the whole person, (5) the primary care provider as teacher, and (6) preventing disease.

- TCM includes herbal medicine as well as techniques such as acupuncture, exercise, massage, moxibustion, and cupping. TCM focuses on the life force (*chi*), which is thought to circulate through the body through meridians (channels) connecting all major organs. *Chi* consists of *yin* and *yang*, which are opposite and complementary qualities. Illness is believed to result when these forces are unbalanced. An acupuncturist inserts sterilized needles into channels of energy to try to restore balance to the patient's *chi*.
- Chiropractic focuses on the relationship between spinal structure and body function mediated by the nervous system. Spinal manipulation is a well-known procedure, but chiropractic care also includes other procedures, including all forms of physical therapy and rehabilitation intervention. Spinal manipulation may be helpful for back pain.
- Ayurveda is an integrated system employing diet, herbs, exercise, meditation, yoga, and massage or bodywork. Ayurveda teaches that vital energy (*prana*) is the basis of all life and healing. As *prana* circulates throughout the body, it is governed by the five elements of earth, air, fire, water, and ether. The five elements combine with one another into pairs called *doshas*, which include *vata* (ether and air), *pitta* (fire and water), and *kapha* (earth and water).
- Touch is fundamental to massage therapy and is used by massage therapists to locate painful or tense areas, to determine how much pressure to apply, and to establish a therapeutic relationship with patients.

REFERENCES

1. Ulbricht CE, Cohen L, Lee R. Complementary, alternative, and integrative therapies in cancer care. In: Devita VT, ed. *Devita, Hellman, and Rosenberg's Cancer: Principles & Practice of Oncology.* 8th ed. Philadelphia, PA: Wolters Kluwer/Lippincott Williams & Wilkins; 2008.
2. National Center for Complementary and Integrative Health. Complementary, alternative, or integrative health: what's in a name? Available at: https://nccih.nih.gov/health/integrative-health/. Accessed June 24, 2017.
3. Cassileth BR. 'Complementary' or 'alternative'? It makes a difference in cancer care. *Complement Ther Med.* 1999;7(1):35–7. doi: 10.1016/S0965-2299(99)80056-9.
4. Ulbricht C, Seamon E. *Natural Standard Herbal Pharmacotherapy: An Evidence-Based Approach.* St. Louis, MO: Mosby/Elsevier; 2009.
5. National Center for Complementary and Integrative Health. NCCIH funding: appropriations history. Available at: https://nccih.nih.gov/about/budget/appropriations.htm. Accessed January 7, 2017.
6. Jadad AR, Moore RA, Carroll D, et al. Assessing the quality of reports of randomized clinical trials: is blinding necessary? *Control Clin Trials.* 1996;17(1):1–12. doi: 10.1016/0197-2456(95)00134-4.
7. Valiathan MS, Thatte U. Ayurveda: the time to experiment. *Int J Ayurveda Res.* 2010;1(1):3. doi: 10.4103/0974-7788.59935.
8. Mehling WE, DiBlasi Z, Hecht F. Bias control in trials of bodywork: a review of methodological issues. *J Altern Complement Med.* 2005;11(2):333–42. doi: 10.1089/acm.2005.11.333.
9. Schnyer RN, Allen JJ. Bridging the gap in complementary and alternative medicine research: manualization as a means of promoting standardization and flexibility of treatment in clinical trials of acupuncture. *J Altern Complement Med.* 2002;8(5):623–34. doi: 10.1089/107555302320825147.
10. Birch S. A review and analysis of placebo treatments, placebo effects, and placebo controls in trials of medical procedures when sham is not inert. *J Altern Complement Med.* 2006;12(3):303–10. doi: 10.1089/act.2006.12.303.
11. Lee EJ, Frazier SK. The efficacy of acupressure for symptom management: a systematic review. *J Pain Symptom Manage.* 2011;42(4): 589–603. doi: 10.1016/j.jpainsymman.2011.01.007.
12. Thompson EA, Bishop JL, Northstone K. The use of homeopathic products in childhood: data generated over 8.5 years from the Avon Longitudinal Study of Parents and Children (ALSPAC). *J Altern Complement Med.* 2010;16(1):69–79. doi: 10.1089/acm.2009.0007.
13. Ulbricht C, Chao W, Clark A, et al. Oscillococcinum: an evidence-based systematic review by the Natural Standard Research Collaboration. *Altern Complement Ther.* 2011;17(1):41–9. doi: 10.1089/act.2011.17107.
14. Borneman JP, Field RI. Regulation of homeopathic drug products. *Am J Health Syst Pharm.* 2006;63(1):86–91. doi: 10.2146/ajhp050105.
15. Lindsay RA, De Dora M, Blumner R; Center for Inquiry. Examining advertising for over-the-counter homeopathic products. September 21, 2015. Available at: https://www.ftc.gov/system/files/documents/public_comments/2015/11/00517-99779.pdf. Accessed Jun 24, 2017.
16. Ernst E. Homeopathy: what does the "best" evidence tell us? *Med J Aust.* 2010;192(8):458–60. PMID: 20402610.

17. Mathie RT, Lloyd SM, Legg LA, et al. Randomised placebo-controlled trials of individualised homeopathic treatment: systematic review and meta-analysis. *Syst Rev.* 2014;3(142):1-16. doi: 10.1186/2046-4053-3-142.
18. Stehlin I. Homeopathy: real medicine or empty promises? *FDA Consum.* 1996;30:15–9.
19. Marian F, Joost K, Saini KD, et al. Patient satisfaction and side effects in primary care: an observational study comparing homeopathy and conventional medicine. *BMC Complement Altern Med.* 2008;8:52. doi: 10.1186/1472-6882-8-52.
20. Lim JH, Davis GE, Wang Z, et al. Zicam-induced damage to mouse and human nasal tissue. *PLoS One.* 2009;4(10):e7647. doi: 10.1371/journal.pone.0007647.
21. National Center for Complementary and Integrative Health. Homeopathy. Available at: https://nccih.nih.gov/health/homeopathy#hed3. Accessed August 25, 2017.
22. Utah Department of Administrative Services, Office of Administrative Rules. R156-71-101: Naturopathic Physician Practice Act Rule. Available at: https://rules.utah.gov/publicat/code/r156/r156-71.htm. Accessed June 24, 2017.
23. Wang SM, Kain ZN, White P. Acupuncture analgesia, I: the scientific basis. *Anesth Analg.* 2008;106(2):602–10. doi: 10.1213/01.ane.0000277493.42335.7b.
24. Cooley K, Szczurko O, Perri D, et al. Naturopathic care for anxiety: a randomized controlled trial ISRCTN78958974. *PLoS One.* 2009;4(8):e6628. doi: 10.1371/journal.pone.0006628.
25. Shea JL. Applying evidence-based medicine to traditional Chinese medicine: debate and strategy. *J Altern Complement Med.* 2006;12(3):255–63. doi: 10.1089/act.2006.12.255.
26. Xutian S, Zhang J, Louise W. New exploration and understanding of traditional Chinese medicine. *Am J Chin Med.* 2009;37(3):411–26. doi: 10.1142/S0192415X09006941.
27. Hucker CO. *China's Imperial Past: An Introduction to Chinese History and Culture.* Stanford, CA: Stanford University Press; 1997.
28. Yu D, Morris-Natschke SL, Lee KH. New developments in natural products-based anti-AIDS research. *Med Res Rev.* 2007;27(1):108–32. doi: 10.1002/med.20075.
29. Coyle ME, Smith CA, Peat B. Cephalic version by moxibustion for breech presentation. *Cochrane Database Syst Rev.* 2005;2:CD003928. doi: 10.1002/14651858.CD3928.
30. Xue CC, Zhang AL, Greenwood KM, et al. Traditional Chinese medicine: an update on clinical evidence. *J Altern Complement Med.* 2010;16(3):301–12. doi: 10.1089/acm.2009.0293.
31. National Center for Complementary and Integrative Health. Traditional Chinese medicine: in depth. Bethesda, MD: U.S. Department of Health and Human Services, National Institutes of Health; 2013. Publication No: D248. Available at: https://nccih.nih.gov/health/whatiscam/chinesemed.htm. Accessed June 24, 2017.
32. Zell-Kanter M, Quigley MA, Leikin JB. Reduction in ephedra poisonings after FDA ban. *N Engl J Med.* 2015;372(22):2172–4. doi: 10.1056/NEJMc1502505.
33. Keane FM, Munn SE, du Vivier AW, et al. Analysis of Chinese herbal creams prescribed for dermatological conditions. *BMJ.* 1999;318(7183):563–4. doi: 10.1136/bmj.318.7183.563.
34. Holisticonline. Chiropractic, history. Available at: holisticonline.com/chiropractic/chiro_history.htm. Accessed June 24, 2017.
35. Ventola CL. Current issues regarding complementary and alternative medicine (CAM) in the United States: part 1: the widespread use of CAM and the need for better-informed health care professionals to provide patient counseling. *PT.* 2010;35(8):461–8. PMCID: PMC2957758.
36. U.S. Department of Labor, Bureau of Labor Statistics. Occupational Employment and Wages, May 2016. Available at: https://www.bls.gov/oes/current/oes291011.htm. Accessed August 25, 2017.
37. Ernst E. Chiropractic treatment for fibromyalgia: a systematic review. *Clin Rheumatol.* 2009;28(10):1175–8. doi: 10.1007/s10067-009-1217-9.
38. Walker BF, French SD, Grant W, et al. Combined chiropractic interventions for low-back pain. *Cochrane Database Syst Rev.* 2010;4:CD005427. doi: 10.1002/14651858.CD005427.pub2.
39. Paciaroni M, Bogousslavsky J. Cerebrovascular complications of neck manipulation. *Eur Neurol.* 2009;61(2):112–8. doi: 10.1159/000180314.
40. Ernst E. Deaths after chiropractic: a review of published cases. *Int J Clin Pract.* 2010;64(8):1162–5. doi: 10.1111/j.1742-1241.2010.02352.x.
41. Gouveia LO, Castanho P, Ferreira JJ. Safety of chiropractic interventions: a systematic review. *Spine (Phila PA 1976).* 2009;34(11):E405–13. doi: 10.1097/BRS.0b013e3181a16d63.
42. Murphy DR. Current understanding of the relationship between cervical manipulation and stroke: what does it mean for the chiropractic profession? *Chiropr Osteopat.* 2010;18:22. doi: 10.1186/1746-1340-18-22.
43. Davis M, Smith M, Weeks W. Influenza vaccination among chiropractic patients and other users of complementary and alternative medicine: are chiropractic patients really different? *Prev Med.* 2012;54(1):5–8. doi: 10.1016/j.ypmed.2011.01.007.
44. Sharma H, Chandola HM, Singh G, et al. Utilization of Ayurveda in health care: an approach for prevention, health promotion, and treatment of disease, part 1: Ayurveda, the science of life. *J Altern Complement Med.* 2007;13(9):1011–9. doi: 10.1089/acm.2007.7017-A.
45. Patwardhan K, Gehlot S, Singh G, et al. Global challenges of graduate level Ayurvedic education: a survey. *Int J Ayurveda Res.* 2010;1(1):49–54. doi: 10.4103/0974-7788.59945.
46. Savaliya AA, Shah RP, Prasad B, et al. Screening of Indian aphrodisiac ayurvedic/herbal healthcare products for adulteration with sildenafil, tadalafil and/or vardenafil using LC/PDA and extracted ion LC-MS/TOF. *J Pharm Biomed Anal.* 2010;52(3):406–9. doi: 10.1016/j.jpba.2009.05.021.
47. Saper RB, Phillips RS, Sehgal A, et al. Lead, mercury, and arsenic in US- and Indian-manufactured Ayurvedic medicines sold via the Internet. *JAMA.* 2008;300(8):915–23. doi: 10.1001/jama.300.8.915.
48. Gray RA. The use of massage therapy in palliative care. *Complement Ther Nurs Midwifery.* 2000;6(2):77–82. doi: 10.1054/ctnm.2000.0483.

INDEX

Page numbers followed by *t* and *f* indicate tables and figures, respectively. Numbers preceded by "CP" refer to color photographs found in the Color Plates.

D

O

X

Y

Z

NOTES

NOTES

NOTES

NOTES